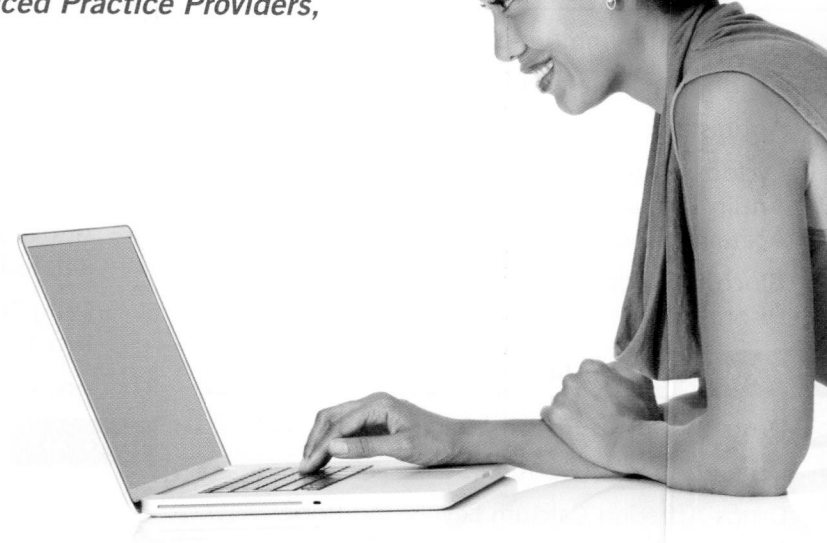

Lehne's Pharmacotherapeutics *for* Advanced Practice Providers

Laura D. Rosenthal, DNP, ACNP, FAANP
Assistant Professor, College of Nursing
University of Colorado, Anschutz Medical Campus
Denver, Colorado

Jacqueline Rosenjack Burchum, DNSc, FNP-BC, CNE
Associate Professor, College of Nursing
Department of Advanced Practice and Doctoral Studies
University of Tennessee Health Science Center
Memphis, Tennessee

ELSEVIER

ELSEVIER

3251 Riverport Lane
St. Louis, Missouri 63043

Lehne's Pharmacotherapeutics for Advanced Practice Providers ISBN: 978-0-323-44783-6

Notices

Knowledge and best practice in this field are constantly changing. As new research and experience broaden our understanding, changes in research methods, professional practices, or medical treatment may become necessary.

Practitioners and researchers must always rely on their own experience and knowledge in evaluating and using any information, methods, compounds, or experiments described herein. In using such information or methods they should be mindful of their own safety and the safety of others, including parties for whom they have a professional responsibility.

With respect to any drug or pharmaceutical products identified, readers are advised to check the most current information provided (i) on procedures featured or (ii) by the manufacturer of each product to be administered, to verify the recommended dose or formula, the method and duration of administration, and contraindications. It is the responsibility of practitioners, relying on their own experience and knowledge of their patients, to make diagnoses, to determine dosages and the best treatment for each individual patient, and to take all appropriate safety precautions.

To the fullest extent of the law, neither the Publisher nor the authors, contributors, or editors, assume any liability for any injury and/or damage to persons or property as a matter of products liability, negligence or otherwise, or from any use or operation of any methods, products, instructions, or ideas contained in the material herein.

Library of Congress Cataloging-in-Publication Data

International Standard Book Number: 978-0-323-44783-6

Executive Content Strategist: Lee Henderson
Senior Content Development Manager: Laurie Gower
Content Development Specialist: Jennifer Wade
Publishing Services Manager: Jeff Patterson
Senior Project Manager: Anne Konopka
Design Direction: Ashley Miner

Printed in China

Last digit is the print number: 9 8 7 6 5 4 3 2 1

For Alli and Sky, who bring sunshine into my life.

LDR

To my remarkable students. It excites me to know that the future of nursing is in your most capable hands.

JRB

Acknowledgments

We would like to acknowledge the support of our colleagues at Elsevier, including Executive Content Strategist Lee Henderson; Content Development Specialist Jennifer Wade; and Senior Project Manager Anne Konopka. We would also like to thank Cassie Carey for all of her production assistance. Finally, we would like to express our gratitude to Richard A. Lehne for his dedication to the Lehne Pharmacology series. Without his work, this text would not be possible.

About the Authors

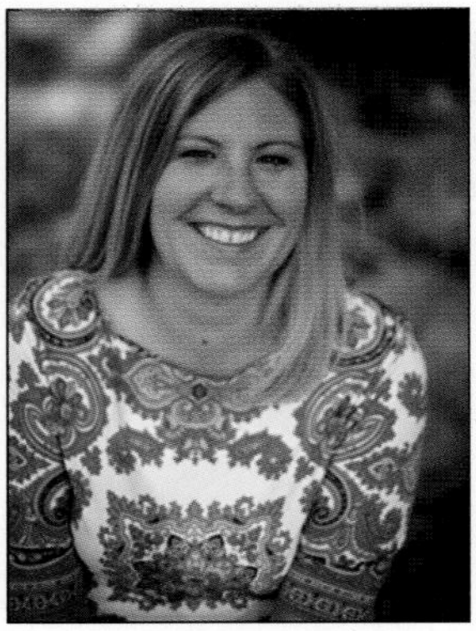

Laura Rosenthal, DNP, ACNP, FAANP, has been a registered nurse since graduating with her Bachelor of Science degree in Nursing from the University of Michigan in 2000. She completed her Master of Science degree in Nursing in 2006 at Case Western Reserve University in Cleveland, Ohio. She finished her nursing education at the University of Colorado, College of Nursing, graduating with her Doctor of Nursing Practice degree in 2011. Her background includes practice in acute care and inpatient medicine. While working as a nurse practitioner at the University of Colorado Hospital, she assisted in developing one of the first fellowships for advanced practice clinicians in hospital medicine. Dr. Rosenthal serves as an assistant professor at the University of Colorado, College of Nursing, where she teaches within the undergraduate and graduate programs. She received the Dean's Award for Excellence in Teaching in 2013. She is the co-chair of the Allied Health Committee at the University of Colorado Hospital. In her spare time, Dr. Rosenthal enjoys running, skiing, and fostering retired greyhounds for Colorado Greyhound Adoption.

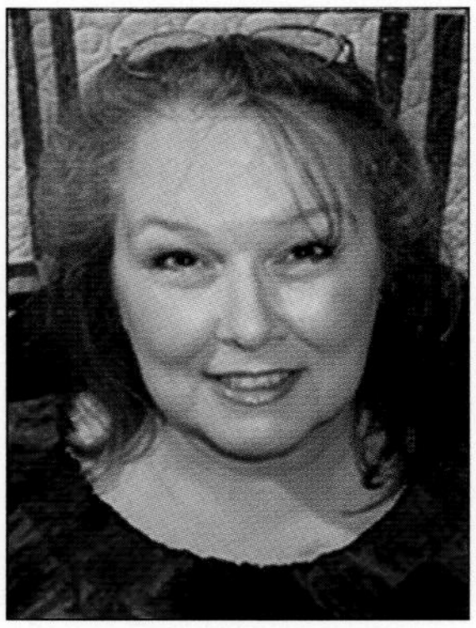

Jacqueline Lee Rosenjack Burchum, DNSc, FNP-BC, CNE, earned the Bachelor of Science in Nursing degree from Union University in Jackson, Tennessee, and both the Masters of Science in Nursing and the Doctor of Nursing Science degree from the University of Tennessee Health Science Center (UTHSC) in Memphis, Tennessee. Dr. Burchum holds certification as a Family Nurse Practitioner (FNP-BC) and Certified Nurse Educator (CNE). She is a faculty member in the Department of Advanced Practice and Doctoral Studies of the College of Nursing at UTHSC.

As a nurse practitioner and researcher, Dr. Burchum's work has centered on addressing the needs of vulnerable populations with a special focus on immigrant and refugee populations. As an educator, Dr. Burchum has a special interest in online teaching and nursing program quality. She has received awards for excellence in teaching from both student and professional organizations. She has served as a National Council Licensure Examination-RN (NCLEX-RN®) Item Writer and Expert Network Panel Consultant. She currently serves as an On-Site Evaluator for the Commission on Collegiate Nursing Education (CCNE), a national accreditation agency that accredits nursing education programs. Her favorite activities center on spending time with her husband, son, and other family members. She also enjoys designing and making quilts in her spare time.

Contributor and Reviewers

CONTRIBUTOR

Courtney Quiring, BSP, BCGP
College of Pharmacy and Nutrition
University of Saskatchewan
Saskatoon, Saskatchewan
Canada
Appendix: Canadian Drug Information

REVIEWERS

Sameeya Ahmed-Winston, MSN, CPNP, CPHON, BMTCN
Pediatric Nurse Practitioner
Blood Marrow and Transplant Department
Children's National Health System
Washington, DC

Diane Daddario, MSN, ANP-C, ACNS-BC, RN-BC, CMSRN
Hospitalist CRNP in Behavioral Health
Holy Spirit Hospital,
Camp Hill, Pennsylvania;
Adjunct Nursing Faculty
College of Nursing
Pennsylvania State University
University Park, Pennsylvania

Abimbola Farinde, PhD
Professor
College of Business
Columbia Southern University
Orange Beach, Alabama

Margaret M. Gingrich, RN, MSN, CRNP
Professor of Nursing
Nursing Department
Harrisburg Area Community College
Harrisburg, Pennsylvania

James Anthony Graves, PharmD
Staff/Clinical Pharmacist
Inpatient Pharmacy
St. Mary Health Center
Jefferson City, Missouri

Bradley R. Harrell, DNP, APRN, ACNP-BC
Clinical Associate Professor
Loewenberg College of Nursing
University of Memphis
Memphis, Tennessee

Kathleen Sanders Jordan, DNP, MS, FNP-BC, ENP-BC, SANE-P
Clinical Assistant Professor
Graduate School of Nursing
The University of North Carolina at Charlotte
Charlotte, North Carolina;
Nurse Practitioner
Emergency Department
Mid-Atlantic Emergency Medicine Associates
Charlotte, North Carolina

Terry A. Kania, MSN, CRNA, RN
Associate Professor of Nursing
Nursing Department
Joliet Junior College
Joliet, Illinois

Pamela L. King, PhD, RN, MSN, APRN
Family Nurse Practitioner, Pediatric Nurse Practitioner
Nursing Department
Spalding University
Louisville, Kentucky

Rosemary K. Lee, DNP, ARNP-BC, CCNS, CCRN
Clinical Nurse Specialist
Critical Care Department
Homestead Hospital
Homestead, Florida

Katie L. Mysen, DNP, FNP-BC
Adjunct Instructor
Oakland University
School of Nursing
Rochester, Michigan

Patricia Rouen, PhD, FNP-BC
Associate Professor
College of Health Professions, McAuley School of Nursing
University of Detroit Mercy
Detroit, Michigan

Meera K. Shah, PharmD
Pharmacist
School of Pharmacy
University of Missouri–Kansas City
Kansas City, Missouri

Cory G. Sheeler, MSN, RN, FNP-BC, CNE
Lecturer
School of Nursing
University of North Carolina at Charlotte
Charlotte, North Carolina

Crystal Sherman, DNP, RN
Associate Professor
Department of Nursing
Shawnee State University
Portsmouth, Ohio

Paula D. Silver, BS Biology, PharmD
Medical Instructor
Medical Assisting/LPN and RN Departments
Medical Careers School of Health Sciences and Technology
ECPI University
Newport News, Virginia

Allison White, PharmD
Pharmacist
Kansas City, Missouri

Preface

Pharmacology and pharmacotherapeutics pervade all phases of advanced practice and relate directly to patient care and education. Despite their importance, many students—and even some teachers—are often uncomfortable with these subjects because traditional texts have stressed *memorizing* rather than *understanding*. In this text, the guiding principle is to establish further understanding of drugs and their use in patient care.

This text has two major objectives: to help you, the advanced practice student, establish a continued knowledge base in the basic science of drugs, and to show you how that knowledge can be applied in clinical practice. The methods by which these goals are achieved are described here.

LAYING FOUNDATIONS IN BASIC PRINCIPLES

To understand drugs, you need a solid foundation in basic pharmacologic principles. To help you establish that foundation, the book has major chapters on the following topics: basic principles that apply to all drugs (Chapters 4 through 6), basic principles of drug therapy across the life span (Chapters 7 through 9), basic principles of neuropharmacology (Chapter 10), and basic principles of antimicrobial therapy (Chapter 68).

REVIEWING PHYSIOLOGY AND PATHOPHYSIOLOGY

To understand the actions of a drug, it is useful to understand the biologic systems that the drug influences. Accordingly, for all major drug families, relevant physiology and pathophysiology are reviewed. In almost all cases, these reviews are presented at the beginning of each chapter rather than in a systems review at the beginning of a unit. This juxtaposition of pharmacology, physiology, and pathophysiology is designed to help you understand how these topics interrelate.

TEACHING THROUGH PROTOTYPES

Within each drug family, we can usually identify a prototype—that is, a drug that embodies characteristics shared by all members of the group. Because other family members are similar to the prototype, to know the prototype is to know the basic properties of all family members.

The benefits of teaching through prototypes can be appreciated with an example. Let's consider the nonsteroidal anti-inflammatory drugs (NSAIDs), a family that includes aspirin, ibuprofen [Motrin], naproxen [Aleve], celecoxib [Celebrex], and more than 20 other drugs. Traditionally, information on these drugs is presented in a series of paragraphs describing each drug in turn. When attempting to study from such a list, you are likely to learn many drug names and little else; the important concept of similarity among family members is easily lost. In this text, the family prototype—aspirin—is discussed first and in depth. After this, the small ways in which individual NSAIDs differ from aspirin are pointed out. Not only is this approach more efficient than the traditional approach, it is also more effective, in that similarities among family members are emphasized.

LARGE PRINT AND SMALL PRINT: A WAY TO FOCUS ON ESSENTIALS

Pharmacology is exceptionally rich in detail. There are many drug families, each with multiple members and each member with its own catalog of indications, contraindications, adverse effects, and drug interactions. This abundance of detail confronts teachers with the difficult question of what to teach and students with the equally difficult question of what to study. Attempting to answer these questions can frustrate teachers and students alike. Even worse, in the presence of myriad details, basic concepts can be obscured.

To help you focus on essentials, there are two sizes of type. Large type is intended to say, "On your first exposure to this topic, this is the core of information you should learn." Small type is intended to say, "Here is additional information that you may want to learn after mastering the material in large type." As a rule, we reserve large print for prototypes, basic principles of pharmacology, and reviews of physiology and pathophysiology. We use small print for secondary information about the prototypes and for discussion of drugs that are not prototypes. This technique allows the book to contain a large body of detail without having that detail cloud the big picture. Furthermore, because the technique highlights essentials, it minimizes questions about what to teach and what to study.

The use of large and small print is especially valuable for discussing adverse effects and drug interactions. Most drugs are associated with many adverse effects and interactions. As a rule, however, only a few of these are noteworthy. In traditional texts, practically all adverse effects and interactions are presented, creating long and tedious lists. In this text, we use large print to highlight the few adverse effects and interactions that are especially characteristic; the rest are noted briefly in small print. Rather than overwhelming you with long and forbidding lists, this text delineates a moderate body of information that's truly important, and thereby facilitates comprehension.

USING CLINICAL REALITY TO PRIORITIZE CONTENT

This book contains two broad categories of information: pharmacology (i.e., basic science about drugs) and therapeutics (i.e., clinical use of drugs). To ensure that content is clinically relevant, we use evidence-based treatment guidelines as a basis for deciding what to stress and what to play down. Unfortunately, clinical practice is a moving target: when effective new drugs are introduced, and when clinical trials reveal new benefits or new risks of older drugs, the guidelines change—and so we have to work hard to keep this book current. Despite our best efforts, the book and clinical reality may not always agree. Some treatments discussed here will be considered inappropriate before the second edition comes out. Furthermore, in areas where controversy exists, the treatments discussed here may be considered inappropriate by some clinicians right now.

SPECIAL FEATURES

- **Prototype Drugs:** Denoted in green boxes; these key drugs are easy to locate.
- **Black Box Warnings:** This feature draws the reader's attention to important safety concerns related to contraindications and adverse effects.
- **Patient Education:** These boxes offer important information to provide to patients regarding their therapy.
- **Patient-Centered Care Across the Life Span:** Tables in many chapters highlight care concerns for patients throughout their lives, from infancy to older adulthood.
- **Canadian trade names** are identified by a **maple-leaf icon.**

TEACHING SUPPLEMENTS FOR INSTRUCTORS

- The Instructor Resources for the first edition are available online and include **a Test Bank**, **a PowerPoint Collection**, and **an Image Collection.**

WAYS TO USE THIS TEXTBOOK

Thanks to its focus on essentials, this text is especially well suited to serve as the primary text for a course dedicated specifically to pharmacology and pharmacotherapeutics. In addition, the book's focused approach makes it a valuable resource for pharmacologic instruction within an integrated curriculum and for self-directed learning by students, teachers, and practitioners.

How is this focus achieved? Four primary techniques are employed: (1) teaching through prototypes, (2) using standard print for essential information and small print for secondary information, (3) limiting discussion of adverse effects and drug interactions to information that matters most, and (4) using evidence-based clinical guidelines to determine what content to stress.

Students often feel that pharmacology is one of the most difficult classes to master. Pharmacotherapeutics can be an unpopular subject because of the vast and rapidly changing area of content. We hope that this book makes the subjects of pharmacology and pharmacotherapeutics easier for you to master and more enjoyable for you to understand by allowing you to focus on the most important, umbrella concepts of pharmacology and pharmacotherapeutics as they relate to the care and safety of patients and the management of their health problems.

Laura D. Rosenthal
Jacqueline Rosenjack Burchum

Contents

UNIT IV Peripheral Nervous System Drugs

UNIT I

Introduction

CHAPTER 1

Prescriptive Authority

Jacqueline Rosenjack Burchum, DNSc, FNP-BC, CNE

Our purpose in writing this book is to prepare advanced practice providers to provide safe and competent medication therapy to patients. This role requires the ability to select, prescribe, and manage medications. In this chapter we examine issues surrounding prescriptive authority and how those issues affect this fundamental aspect of comprehensive patient care.

WHAT IS PRESCRIPTIVE AUTHORITY?

Prescriptive authority is the legal right to prescribe drugs. Full prescriptive authority affords the legal right to prescribe independently and without limitation. Physicians have full prescriptive authority. For nonphysician providers, the degree of prescriptive authority varies. Some have full prescriptive authority; however, for many, prescriptive authority is restricted. Limitations are generally tied to oversight by a doctor of medicine (MD) or doctor of osteopathy (DO) as part of the provider's scope of practice.

Recall that there are two components of prescriptive authority: (1) the right to prescribe independently and (2) the right to prescribe without limitation. The provider who prescribes independently is not subject to rules requiring physician supervision or collaboration. The provider who prescribes without limitation may prescribe any drugs, including controlled drugs, with the exception of Schedule I drugs which have no current medical use.

Full practice authority is sometimes interpreted differently for advanced practice registered nurses (APRNs) and physician assistants (PAs) because supervisory requirements vary for the two professions. (See Box 1.1 for information on other professions seeking and obtaining prescriptive authority). PAs are required to practice and prescribe under the supervision of a physician. All PAs, including those in a solo practice, must have a supervising physician who can be reached by telephone or other means of telecommunication. (See *Guidelines for State Regulation of Physician Assistants* available at https://www.aapa.org/Workarea/DownloadAsset.aspx?id=795 for additional information.) If the PA-physician arrangement does not limit drugs that may be prescribed and if the law allows the PA to prescribe Schedule II to V drugs, the PA may enjoy a type of quasi-full prescriptive authority. Indeed, some have referred to this as full prescriptive authority; however, the issue of supervision still applies. Hence, PAs do not have the legal right to prescribe independently of a supervisory arrangement. Even for those in solo practice, there is always the possibility of dissolution of the PA-physician arrangement. In the event this occurs, the PA must affiliate with another physician or physician group in order to continue prescribing.

Whether APRNs possess full prescriptive authority depends on their legal right to prescribe without a supervisory or collaborative requirement. APRNs are *educated* to practice and prescribe independently without supervision; however, some state laws require that they practice in collaboration with or under the supervision of a physician. In these situations, some physicians limit the types of drugs that the APRN can prescribe. State laws may place additional restrictions with regard to controlled drugs.

Table 1.1 provides prescriptive authority status for PAs and the four categories of APRNs—clinical nurse specialist, certified registered nurse anesthetist, certified nurse midwife, and certified nurse practitioner. Information regarding the right to prescribe controlled drugs is available at http://www.deadiversion.usdoj.gov/drugreg/practioners.

PRESCRIPTIVE AUTHORITY REGULATIONS

Prescriptive authority is determined by state law. As a result of differences from state to state, advanced practice providers may have full prescriptive authority in some states yet face significant restrictions in other states. The stark differences particularly affect providers who serve in *locum tenens* staffing positions or who have practices in two contiguous states.

The regulation of prescriptive authority is under the jurisdiction of a health professional board. This may be the State Board of Nursing, the State Board of Medicine, or the State Board of Pharmacy, as determined by each state.

Although the federal government controls drug regulation, it has no control over prescriptive authority. However, several organizations have appealed for changes that would place scope of practice and prescriptive authority under federal regulation in an effort to expand prescriptive authority and the scope of practice of advanced practice providers. The Institute

BOX 1.1 ■ SELECTED PROFESSIONS SEEKING AND OBTAINING PRESCRIPTIVE AUTHORITY

APRNs and PAs are not the only professions concerned with prescriptive authority. The number of professions seeking to obtain or expand prescriptive authority has increased dramatically in the past decade. Here is the current status of a few of those:

- *Chiropractors:* New Mexico approved the new title of "certified advanced practice chiropractic physician" to identify chiropractors with prescriptive authority. For additional information see New Mexico State Law Title 16, Chapter 4, Part 15 (16.4.15.7B) at http://164.64.110.239/nmac/parts/title16/16.004.0015.htm.
- *Naturopathic doctors (NDs):* Several states, including California, Hawaii, Oregon, and Maine, have given prescriptive authority to NDs. Pending legislative action is available at http://www.naturopathic.org/lac.
- *Pharmacists:* California, Montana, New Mexico, North Carolina, North Dakota, and Oregon give pharmacists varying degrees of prescriptive authority. For additional information see https://www.nabp.net/news/tagged/prescribing-authority.
- *Psychologists*: Illinois, New Mexico, and Louisiana have given psychologists limited prescriptive authority. See http://www.apapracticecentral.org/advocacy/authority.

of Medicine (IOM), for example, advocated for federal regulation in their report, *The Future of Nursing: Focus on Scope of Practice.* After noting problems with the "patchwork of state regulations," they wrote:

The federal government has a compelling interest in the regulatory environment for health care professions because of its responsibility to patients covered by federal programs. ... Equally important is the responsibility to all American taxpayers who fund the care provided under these programs to ensure that their tax dollars are spent efficiently. ... Scope-of-practice regulations in all states should reflect the full extent not only of nurses but of each profession's education and training.

THE CASE FOR FULL PRESCRIPTIVE AUTHORITY

Advanced practice providers complete rigorous programs of study, largely in accredited programs that meet stringent national standards. Although there are differences in each program, all include common components. For example, they require extensive education focused on assessment, diagnosis, and management of health problems. Diagnostic reasoning, critical thinking, and procedural skills are evaluated in both didactic and clinical courses. National examinations validate the ability to provide safe and competent care. Licensure ensures that providers comply with standards of practice that promote the public health and safety. In short, advanced practice providers are prepared to fully implement the advanced practice role in their profession.

Limited prescriptive authority creates numerous barriers to quality, affordable, and accessible patient care. For example, restrictions on the distance of the APRN or PA from the physician providing supervision or collaboration may prevent outreach to areas of greatest need. A requirement to obtain the physician's cosignature on prescriptions can increase patient waits. Despite the use of terms such as *collaborative* arrangement, these relationships create a situation in which one partner holds the power. In the event of dissolution of the arrangement, the ultimate loss is commonly assumed by the advanced practice provider rather than the physician.

In 2010, the Association of American Medical Colleges commissioned a report projecting the future of the physician workforce. The report, *The Complexities of Physician Supply and Demand: Projections from 2013 to 2025,* was released in 2015. Several of the key findings have important implications for nonphysician providers.

- By 2025, the shortage of physicians will range between 46,100 and 90,400. In primary care alone, a 12,500 to 31,100 physician shortage is anticipated. *(The lower numbers on these ranges reflect an increase in APRNs and PAs used to help offset physician shortages.)*
- As the Affordable Care Act is fully implemented, the demand for provider coverage will increase.

These findings echo the dire circumstances reported in the 2013 Department of Health and Human Services report, *Projecting the Supply and Demand for Primary Care Practitioners through 2020,* which concluded that full utilization of nurse practitioners and PAs can reduce the physician shortage.

In this scenario in which physician demands are excessive, requiring oversight for other providers may be untenable. To adequately meet the demands for future health care needs, APRNs and PAs will need broader practice privileges than some states currently allow. This includes an imperative to afford full prescriptive authority.

PRESCRIPTIVE AUTHORITY AND RESPONSIBILITY

The possession of full prescriptive authority requires a somber responsibility. Whether you are reading this book as a student or as a practicing provider, it is essential to recognize the full obligation this requires. The safe and competent practice of prescribing and managing medications requires a sound understanding of drugs and the conditions that they are used to manage. It is our goal to help you lay that foundation. In the coming chapters, you will read about rational drug selection, writing prescriptions, and promoting positive outcomes. Then we will delve into the heart of pharmacology through a study of pharmacokinetics and pharmacodynamics as we prepare you for the study of individual drug categories.

TABLE 1.1 ▪ Advanced Practice Provider Prescriptive Authority by State

State	Clinical Nurse Specialists (CNS)	Certified Registered Nurse Anesthetists (CRNA)	Certified Nurse Midwives (CNM)	Certified Nurse Practitioners (CNP)	Physician Assistants (PAs)
AL	FA	NA	LA	LA	PL
AK	FA	FA	FA	FA	PL
AZ	FA	LA	FA	FA	PL
AR	FA	LA	LA	LA	SR
CA	ND	NA	LA	LA	PL
CO	FA	FA	FA	FA	PL
CT	FA	FA	FA	FA	PL
DE	LA	LA	LA	FA	PL
FL	NA	LA	LA	LA	SR
GA	LA	LA	LA	LA	SR
HI	FA	FA	FA	FA	PL
ID	FA	FA	FA	FA	PL
IL	LA	LA	LA	LA	PL
IN	LA	LA	LA	LA	PL
IA	FA	FA	FA	FA	SR
KS	LA	NA	LA	LA	PL
KY	FA	LA	LA	LA	SR
LA	LA	LA	LA	LA	PL
ME	FA	NA	FA	FA	SR
MD	FA	NA	FA	LA	PL
MA	LA	LA	FA	LA	PL
MI	ND	NA	LA	LA	PL
MN	FA	FA	FA	FA	PL
MS	ND	NA	LA	LA	PL
MO	LA	LA	LA	LA	SR
MT	FA	FA	FA	FA	PL
NE	FA	FA	LA	FA	PL
NV	FA	FA	FA	FA	PL
NH	ND	FA	FA	FA	PL
NJ	LA	NA	LA	LA	PL
NM	FA	FA	FA	FA	PL
NY	ND	ND	LA	LA	PL
NC	FA	NA	LA	LA	PL
ND	FA	FA	FA	FA	PL
OH	LA	LA	LA	LA	PL
OK	FA	LA	LA	LA	SR
OR	FA	FA	FA	FA	PL
PA	NA	ND	LA	LA	PL
RI	FA	FA	FA	FA	PL
SC	LA	LA	LA	LA	PL
SD	LA	NA	LA	LA	PL
TN	LA	LA	LA	LA	PL
TX	LA	LA	LA	LA	PL
UT	FA	FA	FA	FA	PL
VT	FA	FA	FA	FA	PL
VA	NA	NA	LA	LA	PL
WA	ND	FA	FA	FA	PL
WV	FA	LA	LA	LA	SR
WI	FA	LA	LA	LA	PL
WY	FA	FA	FA	FA	PL

FA, full authority; LA, limited authority (due to supervisory requirements or state restrictions); NA, no authority; ND, no data or state does not recognize as an advanced practice registered nurse; NSR, no state restrictions; PL, any restrictions are determined at the practice level with the supervising physician; SR, state restrictions.

Sources: https://www.ncsbn.org/5410.htm; https://www.ncsbn.org/5408.htm; https://ncsbn.org/5409.htm; https://ncsbn.org/5411.htm; http://kff.org/other/state-indicator/physician-assistant-scope-of-practice-laws

CHAPTER

2 Rational Drug Selection and Prescription Writing

Laura D. Rosenthal, DNP, ACNP, FAANP

THE RESPONSIBILITY OF PRESCRIBING

As a practitioner, you will assume great responsibility when caring for patients. The ability to prescribe medications is both a privilege and a burden. Although you may be familiar with many drugs through your previous practice as a registered nurse or other member of the health care field, giving medications and prescribing medications are two very different things. There are many different issues to consider when writing a prescription, many of which we discuss in this chapter or in the previous chapter regarding prescriptive authority.

The best way to keep your patients (and yourself) safe is to be prudent and deliberate in your decision-making process. Have a documented provider-patient relationship with the person for whom you are prescribing. Do not prescribe medications for family or friends, or for yourself. Document a thorough history and physical examination in your records. Include any discussions you have with the patient regarding risk factors, side effects, or therapy options. Have a documented plan regarding drug monitoring or titration, if applicable. If you consult additional providers, note that you did so. Finally, use the considerations provided in the following box to assist in safely and rationally choosing one medication over another.

DRUG SELECTION

Cost

The cost of medications in the United States has risen steeply within the past 10 years. Increasing cost is related to multiple factors, including corporate competition and proactive increases in anticipation of the Affordable Care Act (ACA). It is also noted that one of the reasons people do not adhere to their prescribed medication regimen is its excessive cost. Often we are so concerned with obtaining the right diagnosis and making our patient well that we overlook key pieces of information, including patient financial status. When patients cannot afford the drug you prescribe, they may not get well, even though they want to be compliant. It is of critical importance that providers ask patients if they have difficulty obtaining their medication because it is cost prohibitive.

If you find that your patient is having difficulty purchasing the prescribed medications, consider changing pharmacies or drug regimens. The cost of a drug can vary widely between pharmacies, even within the same city. In addition, many corporations have created generic $4 lists or special prescription programs that allow patients to fill their medications for a reasonable cost. In addition, all health plans through the ACA are required to include prescription drug coverage, although these vary greatly. As a prescriber, you need to be familiar with the local resources for medication assistance and low-cost medications.

Guidelines

When in doubt, follow current guidelines for the treatment of a particular disease or symptom. Almost all medical and nursing societies have published guidelines, including the American Heart Association, the American College of Cardiology, the Infectious Diseases Society of America, and the American Diabetes Association. It is the provider's responsibility to keep abreast of new recommendations or changes in guidelines and to incorporate these into their prescribing practices. Although closely following the guidelines is desirable, we must always take into account that our patients may not fit well into these guidelines and that individualized care is always best. In these cases, it is important to document the rationale for deviating from standard of care.

Availability

Every facility and pharmacy provides drugs according to a selected formulary. This formulary is selected by a panel of pharmacists and providers and may be subject to following guidelines created by regulatory agencies, such as the Centers for Medicare and Medicaid Services (CMS). The formulary may also depend on regional and national drug supplies, drug costs and available rebates, and the presence of generic medications on the market.

In short, the drug you want may not be available in your facility or at a specific pharmacy. This can affect your choice in medications. Become familiar with the formulary where you are employed, and know that it can change over time. Often there are substitutes or similar medications you can order in place of what you originally intended. For example, omeprazole may be indicated for the treatment of erosive esophagitis, but the formulary contains esomeprazole instead.

Interactions

As noted throughout this text, there are very few medications that do not interact with either another medication or a food.

Helpful Applications and Websites for Safe Prescribing

Websites

Epocrates: http://www.epocrates.com/
LexiComp: http://online.lexi.com/action/home
Pepid: http://www.pepid.com/
Physicians' Desk Reference (PDR): http://www.pdr.net/
UptoDate: http://www.uptodate.com/contents/search

Applications for Tablets, Phones

Centers for Disease Control and Prevention Antibiotic Guidelines
Elsevier Clinical Pharmacology
Epocrates
Pepid
Prescriber's Letter

Polypharmacy greatly increases the risk for interactions. Some of these interactions are negligible, but some can have life-threatening consequences. It is of crucial importance to ask the patient about *all* current drugs, including over-the-counter (OTC) medications and other herbal preparations. Many patients do not consider OTC or alternative pharmaceuticals as "medications" and may not mention them unless you ask specifically.

When adding a new medication to a patient regimen, check for significant interactions. There are many resources that allow checks for interactions between multiple medications or foods at one time. If there is a low-risk interaction identified, you may find it acceptable to discuss this with your patient, document the conversation, and then prescribe the medication. If there is a relative or absolute contraindication to the proposed drug combination, it is best to choose an alternative if at all possible.

Side Effects

All drugs have side effects. Some are adverse, and some may be beneficial. In addition, one patient may experience adverse effects to a medication, whereas another patient may not. It is important to note the pertinent side effects for each medication and to ask your patients about presence of symptoms after initiating, stopping, or changing a medication dose. When assessing the risk-to-benefit ratio of a medication, one must consider the severity of the side effects. If a patient started on a new antihypertensive medication has a decreased blood pressure, and therefore improvement in hypertension, but experiences fainting, a decrease in dose or a different medication should be considered.

Allergies

At times, guidelines may suggest a particular drug for a specific ailment. Unfortunately, your patient may have an allergy to that medication or class of drug. It is of critical importance to determine the type of reaction and to document in the patient's chart. Then, selection of an appropriate drug may begin.

In the case of severe allergy, such as anaphylaxis or swelling of the face, these drugs are absolutely contraindicated. But in the case of the patient who experienced vomiting or other similar reactions, the drug may be used again if necessary. The desired choice would be to use an alternate medication that is just as effective. For example, a patient with pyelonephritis who is allergic to penicillin can benefit from a fluoroquinolone instead.

Liver and Renal Function

Many drugs are metabolized and eliminated by the liver and kidneys. If these systems are impaired, this can lead to increased adverse effects and possible medication overdose. Frequently, drugs have special decreased doses or different dosing schedules for patients with hepatic or renal impairment. This is known as *hepatic dosing* or *renal dosing*. Despite the known safety of decreasing doses in some drugs, if there is a different option available, it is prudent to choose a different medication. For example, morphine sulfate is highly metabolized by the kidneys. For patients with renal impairment, morphine can be used to treat pain, but the better choice would be fentanyl because fentanyl does not require a dose reduction in patients with renal impairment. Although some drugs are safe to give or can be used with caution in patients with hepatic or renal dysfunction, other drugs are contraindicated in these patients and must be avoided at all costs.

Need for Monitoring

Some drugs require frequent monitoring at initiation, or throughout the duration of treatment. Some examples of these medications include warfarin, lithium, opioids, and immunosuppressive therapies (tacrolimus, sirolimus). When levels of these drugs are not within therapeutic range, serious patient harm can occur. If a patient does not have the ability to attend frequent laboratory appointments, cannot take their medications reliably, or is not easily reachable by phone or electronically, it may be best to try and avoid these medications if possible.

Special Populations

Populations that deserve special mention when thinking about medications include pregnant or nursing mothers, pediatrics, and older adults. These populations are addressed in depth in Unit III, Drug Therapy Across the Life Span. In addition, Life Span Tables are present in many of the chapters throughout the text to alert you to special considerations.

PRESCRIPTIONS

Necessities

When writing any prescription, there are key elements that must be present to compose a complete prescription. An example of a common template for a written prescription is provided in Fig. 2.1. These elements include the following:

- Prescriber name, license number, and contact information
- Prescriber U.S. Drug Enforcement Administration (DEA) number, if applicable
- Patient name and date of birth

UNIVERSITY CLINIC
Robert Smith, FNP-BC
1777 E. 17th Avenue
Las Vegas, CO 87777
Phone: 777-777-7777 Fax: 777-777-7778

Patient Name:____________________ Date:__________
Allergies:____________________
Medical Record#: Date of Birth:__________
Medication:____________________ Strength:______ Quantity:
Directions for Use: 0 DAW

Indication for use: Refills:________
Prescriber Signature:____________________ DEA#
License#____________ NPI #____________
Contact #/Pager #____________

Figure 2.1 ■ **Common example of a written prescription.**

- Patient allergies
- Name of medication
- Indication of medication (*example:* atenolol for hypertension)
- Medication strength (*example:* 25 mg, 500 mg/mL)
- Dose of medication and frequency (*example:* 12.5 mg once daily)
- Number of tablets or capsules to dispense
- Number of refills

If using an electronic medical record (EMR) to complete prescriptions, many of these elements will be mandatory for the provider, although many will already be completed by the EMR, including prescriber name and contact information. It is important to note the indication for the medication because many drugs are used for more than one purpose. This allows for the patient as well as other providers to understand your intent for prescribing this particular drug.

Types of Prescriptions

Telephone

A common and convenient way to create a new prescription or prescription refill is by telephone. A prescription can be called in to a pharmacy by you or a specified designee. This is often done by leaving a message with the correct information. Although this is a different way of prescribing, the necessities remain the same (see earlier section "Necessities"). Certain medications cannot be prescribed or refilled by telephone. These include medications within the Schedule II category. Patients must have a written prescription for these medications. The only exception to this rule is during an emergency. In this case a telephone order can be used for a limited amount of medication, but a written prescription must be presented to the pharmacy within 7 days.

Written

Providers have been writing prescriptions in the United States since the 1700s. Patients even received scripts during Prohibition in the 1920s to purchase alcohol for medicinal use (Fig. 2.2). Interestingly enough, these paper scripts did not look much different than they do today. This is because the required elements for a complete prescription have not changed over the years. Although health care is making the transition to electronic prescriptions, many providers still use written scripts to prescribe medication. Written prescriptions, like telephone calls or electronic scripts, contain all the necessary elements as described earlier in this chapter. Although all the correct prompts for information may be prepopulated on your script, there are still some important points to consider. If you use a script with a different provider name or a generic script, make sure your name and contact information are printed legibly on the paper. Write all prescriptions in ink or indelible pencil. Avoid abbreviations such as U (units), MSO_4 (morphine), or QD (daily) because these can increase errors and are therefore no longer acceptable. For a list of abbreviations to avoid, see Table 2.1.

In addition, never write prescriptions on presigned scripts or presign blank scripts for other providers or staff. Although this may seem like a convenient way to ensure availability to patients at all times, it is ultimately an unsafe practice. Finally, many facilities provide tamper-resistant scripts, and some states require their use, especially in the prevention of substance misuse and abuse. A few tamper-resistant security features include Hidden Message Technology, which appears when the script is copied on a copy machine; Anti-Copy Coin Rub, which appears when rubbed with a coin; and distinctive security backgrounds. To learn more about these features, visit http://rxsecurityfeatures.com/.

E-Prescribing

With the advent of the EMR, many pharmacies now have capabilities to accept electronic prescriptions. In fact CMS provides incentives for using an EMR to prescribe medications. This program, called *Meaningful Use,* is thought to contribute to increased patient safety and improved patient outcomes.

Using an EMR allows the provider to select a specific, patient-selected pharmacy. After the correct medication information is entered, the prescription is automatically sent to the selected pharmacy. This is beneficial because there is direct

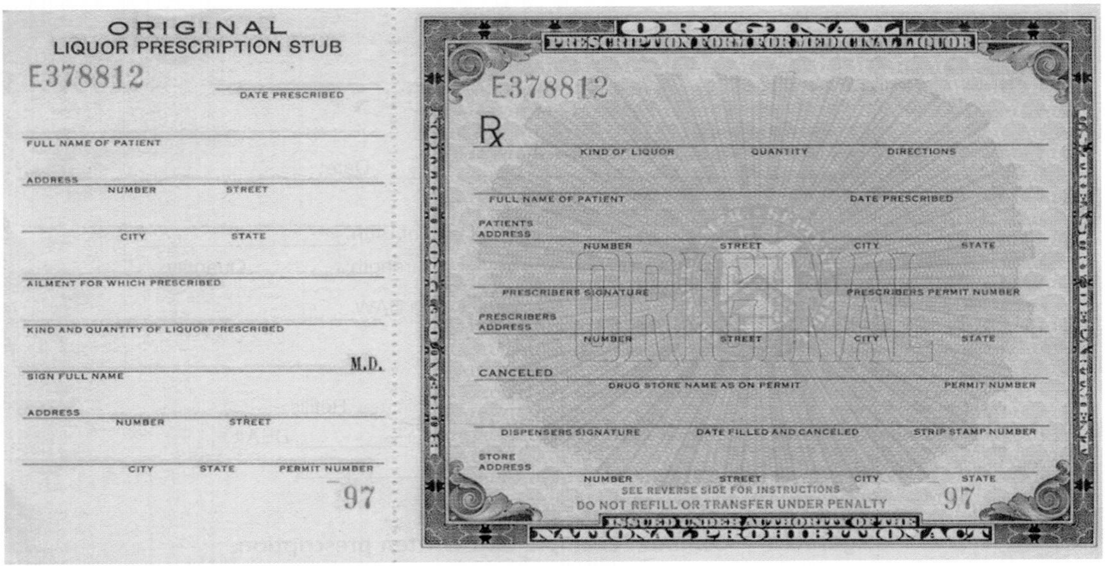

Figure 2.2 ■ Prescription for alcohol during the 1920s Prohibition era.
(From http://www.smithsonianmag.com/history/during-prohibition-your-doctor-could-write-you-prescription-booze-180947940/?no-ist.)

TABLE 2.1 ■ Abbreviations and Figures to Avoid

Do *Not* Use	Preferred
U	Units
IU	International units
QD	Daily
QOD	Every other day
Trailing zero (X.0 mg)	Never trail (X mg)
Lack of leading zero (.X mg)	Always lead with a zero before a decimal point (0.X mg)
MS, MSO_4, $MgSO_4$	Morphine sulfate, magnesium sulfate
AS, AD, AU	Left ear, right ear, both ears
OS, OD, OU	Left eye, right eye, both eyes

transmission of information, making error less likely. Also, the prescription can be ready for the patient when the patient leaves the facility—the patient does not need to drop off the paper script and then wait for a medication fill. Limitations to e-prescribing include scheduled medications, which still require a prescription on tamper-resistant paper. In addition, many health care organizations still do not have a functional EMR, and many pharmacies still do not have the software capabilities to process these requests. In these cases, paper prescriptions are still necessary.

Refills

There are a few things to consider when refilling a prescription. Questions you should ask yourself include the following:

- Is this a newer medication for this patient?
- Am I changing dose or frequency of the medication?
- Am I adding new medications to their regimen?
- Is the patient having undesired side effects?
- When do I expect to follow up with this patient?
- If the patient is requesting a refill by telephone, when was the last time I saw this patient? Do I need to see the patient again before refill?
- Is this a Schedule II medication?

If the answer to any of these questions is "yes," consider a shorter time between refills (1 to 3 months). The exception to this question is with Schedule II medications. These are not eligible for refills and must have a new prescription each renewal period. When changing or adding to current medication regimens, it is prudent to follow up with the patient by phone or in person to assess changes. This time can be used to discuss new or increased side effects, check vital signs, obtain laboratory work, or make further adjustments. When a medication, such as warfarin, requires frequent monitoring with drug levels, an even shorter refill allotment is reasonable. If the patient has been maintained on the current dose of a medication for some time and remains stable, it is likely acceptable to continue to refill that medication for a longer time period (e.g., 12 months).

ASSISTANCE

Applications for Tablets and Phones

This textbook will be paramount in your learning, but it may not be convenient to carry around in the clinical setting. Although we encourage you to use this text to the fullest extent, there are many new applications and websites available to assist providers with safe prescribing (see Table 2.1). It must be noted, however, that all these tools still require common sense and good judgment on the part of the prescriber. As stated previously, one must take into account the individual patient as well as multiple other factors, including cost, side effects, and medication formularies. An application can assist you with the basic suggestions in dosing and duration, but ultimately there is no substitute for sound practice.

Collaboration

As reflected in this chapter, writing a prescription safely can be complicated. It is strongly encouraged that you use all available resources, including your colleagues. Developing a relationship with your pharmacist can be one of the most helpful and fruitful relationships you cultivate. Because this is their specialty, pharmacists will likely have additional information on formulary and drug interactions as well as suggestions for adequate medication dosing. In some practices, pharmacists are responsible for medication initiation and titration based on standardized protocols.

Infectious disease (ID) specialists can also be a helpful resource. Choosing an appropriate antimicrobial agent for a specific infectious process is often difficult for a new practitioner. A local ID specialist can provide guidance on resistance patterns, common local microbial flora, and correct doses, as well as on duration of treatment for specific infections.

CHAPTER

3 Promoting Positive Outcomes of Drug Therapy

Jacqueline Rosenjack Burchum, DNSc, FNP-BC, CNE

Selecting and prescribing the most appropriate drug (see Chapter 2) is just the first step in providing safe and competent medication therapy. Ensuring positive outcomes requires establishing a medication education plan, monitoring positive and negative patient responses, identifying and addressing issues of nonadherence, and managing the patient's complete medication regimen.

MEDICATION EDUCATION

Probably no other provider action influences the patient's commitment to carry out a medication plan more than medication education. This not only provides an opportunity to explain the importance of the medication but also allows the provider to dispel rumors about medications that often lead to therapy failures. Moreover, education reduces medication errors by empowering patients with accurate information and clear guidelines.

Medication Education Components

There are basic components that should be included when teaching about any new medication. These are (1) medication name, (2) purpose, (3) dosing regimen, (4) administration, (5) adverse effects, (6) any special storage needs, (7) associated laboratory testing, (8) food or drug interactions, and (9) duration of therapy. Each of these is discussed in the following sections.

Medication Name

Patients need to know the name of the medication they are taking. Unfortunately, when taking a medication history, we still have patients who refer to medications by their understood purpose (e.g., "blood pressure pill") rather than by their name. This creates a challenge for the provider who needs to select appropriate therapy. It also increases the risk for medication errors. If we teach patients the medication names, we can avoid this concern.

Both the generic name and the brand (trade) name should be given, or at least included in written handouts. This knowledge can be especially important for the patient who travels and may be treated by providers unfamiliar with the patient's history. Knowing both empowers the patient to catch medication errors in the event that two different providers prescribe the same generic drug under different brand names.

Purpose

Patients are more likely to participate in activities when they know those activities produce positive outcomes. The same is true of taking medications. Knowing the reason the medication is prescribed propels the patient to follow through with the medication plan because the patient is aware that this action helps to achieve the therapeutic goal.

Dosing

The dosing regimen needs to be reviewed with the patient even though it is written on the prescription label. Doing this ensures that the patient understands how to take the medication and provides an opportunity for the patient to ask questions.

It is important to be specific when explaining the dosing regimen. For example, "four times a day" may be interpreted in various ways by different people. Can the medication be taken every 4 hours for four doses, or does it need to be spaced out evenly to every 6 hours? Does "once a day" mean that it can be taken at any time, or it is better to take the medication in the morning or evening hours? Patients need to know what to do if a dose is accidentally skipped. This is also a good time to explain why drugs should be taken exactly as prescribed.

Administration

A common patient concern is whether medication should be taken with or without food. This routine information should be provided for all drugs.

Patients also need to be informed of common administration needs that many of us take for granted. For example, suspensions should be shaken (or rolled, if shaking causes foaming) to equally disperse ingredients before administration.

Finally, some drugs require a special apparatus for administration. Inhaled drugs are a common example. Patients need to see how these are administered and should be able to repeat a demonstration before leaving with a prescription. Many manufacturers provide a "dummy" device for teaching purposes.

Adverse Effects

Some providers and other health care workers hesitate to discuss a drug's potential adverse effects. Some fear that doing so will lead to a patient's refusal to take the medications. Although that concern is understandable, and the consequences may well be true, patients have a right to know of potential harms that may result from therapy. Therefore providers are ethically obligated to divulge adverse effects and other risks. That said, often the approach used in discussing these can make a difference in how patients view them.

You probably know patients who worry about taking drugs when the product labeling (i.e., package insert) lists dozens of adverse effects. Patients may not know that, for most drugs, most adverse effects occur in less than 1% to 2% of those taking the drug. Most patients are unaware that the long list of adverse effects represents all effects reported during clinical trials, regardless of whether a direct association to the drug is known. Furthermore, labeling doesn't mention that sometimes the incidence of adverse effects in the placebo group is similarly high. For example, in clinical trials of lovastatin, 1.8% of subjects taking 40 mg reported myalgias; however, 1.7% of subjects taking a placebo also reported myalgias.

When discussing adverse effects, focus on the adverse effects that are common and avoid undue attention on rare and unanticipated effects. If complex effects such as liver injury or pancytopenia may occur, teach patients the signs and symptoms to report. Let patients know that many adverse effects – most commonly nausea and sedation – are usually temporary and go away with continued medication use. In these discussions, it is also beneficial to emphasize benefits over risks. Patients are often willing to endure short term adverse effects for long term health improvement.

Storage

Storage is an important concern for some drugs. For example, some antibiotic suspensions, insulins, and rectal suppositories need to be refrigerated. Medications such as sublingual nitroglycerin and dabigatran [Pradaxa] need to be stored in their original container to prevent drug breakdown and loss of potency.

Laboratory Testing

Laboratory testing is sometimes necessary to determine whether a medication remains safe and effective. For example, liver enzymes may need to be checked periodically for drugs that can cause liver damage. Serum drug levels may need to be checked when maintaining therapeutic levels is challenging.

Patients need to know if special testing will be needed. They also need to know why the monitoring is necessary because those who understand the purpose are more likely to adhere to testing schedules. We recommend teaching what, when, where, why, and how when giving instructions. (See Box 3.1.)

Food or Drug Interactions

Many medications interact with certain foods or other drugs (including alcohol and other recreational drugs). Patients need to know of any potential interactions and the consequence of those interactions. They also need to know if the problem with interactions can be solved by taking substances further apart or whether they need to avoid an interacting food or drug for the duration of therapy. For example, antacids may be taken with most drugs as long as administration is separated by 2 hours; however, patients taking metronidazole must avoid alcohol for the duration of therapy.

BOX 3.1 ▪ PATIENT TEACHING FOR DRUG MONITORING

When testing is needed for monitoring, include the following when providing patient teaching.

What: What test is needed?

Patients like to know what test is needed. Rather than telling them that a blood test is needed, let them know the type of blood test, e.g. a test of thyroid function or cholesterol levels.

When: When is testing required?

Testing can disrupt normal routines. Patients need to know, in advance, how often testing is needed so they can make plans.

Where: Where will testing take place?

In some practices, testing takes place at locations other than the primary clinic. Patients who are unfamiliar with the area need directions to the testing site and where to go after arrival.

Why: Why is testing necessary?

Testing is often expensive and disruptive to daily lives. These barriers are common reasons that patients miss appointments. If they understand the need for testing, they are more likely to adhere to testing schedules.

How: How does the patient prepare for testing?

Some tests require special preparation. For example, many blood tests require fasting. If exercise testing is needed, patients should be told to bring comfortable shoes. It is important to let patients know of anything they need to do prior to arrival.

Duration of Therapy

It is important to let the patient know if medication therapy is being prescribed for a short time (e.g., antibiotics for an acute infection) or whether ongoing long-term medication therapy is anticipated (e.g., thyroid hormone therapy for hypothyroidism). Failure to recognize the need for prolonged therapy is a common reason patients stop medications prematurely when a prescription runs out.

Written Instructions

Medication information is notoriously easy to forget, especially for patients taking numerous medications. We recommend accompanying all verbal education with written instructions. For those who are unable to read due to literacy or vision problems, video or audio instructions can be used.

Best practices in developing written patient education materials abound in the literature. Table 3.1 provides a list of those for which there is greatest consensus. An excellent resource for writing patient education materials is available at http://www.cdc.gov/healthliteracy/pdf/Simply_Put.pdf.

MONITORING

As mentioned in Chapter 2, monitoring is an important consideration in medication therapy. Ongoing monitoring of positive and negative patient responses—and acting on those

TABLE 3.1 ■ Best Practices in Developing Written Patient Education Materials

Practice	Rationale
Limit content	Focus on main points. Include only the most important-to-know content.
Place important information first	People tend to remember the first things they read and may become distracted toward the end.
Write in active voice	Active voice is more direct. Passive voice is less dynamic and may be confusing.
Include adequate white space	White space does not contain text or images. White space makes the page feel less cluttered and less overwhelming.
Use meaningful illustrations	Illustrations are a useful way to break up text. Select images or drawings that have a purpose or that reinforce a point in the handout.
Avoid professional terminology	Use common terms in short, simple sentences that patients can easily understand.
Check for readability	Materials should be written at a lower education level that can be understood by most patients. Information for increasing readability is available at http://www.cdc.gov/healthliteracy/pdf/Simply_Put.pdf

responses in ways that increase benefit or decrease risk—is essential to ensure optimal outcomes.

There are three primary reasons for drug monitoring: (1) determining therapeutic dosage, (2) evaluating medication adequacy, and (3) identifying adverse effects. Each of these purposes is discussed in the following sections. Table 3.2 provides some common examples of drugs that require periodic laboratory monitoring.

Determining Therapeutic Dosage

Many drugs have a narrow therapeutic index (NTI) (see Chapter 4). Examples include carbamazepine, digoxin, lithium, phenytoin, and theophylline. For these drugs, the difference between an effective dose and a lethal dose is small.

To ensure safety, periodic measurement of serum drug levels is needed when drugs with a NTI are prescribed. This not only determines whether the drug is in a therapeutic range but also provides an opportunity for fine-tuning of dosage. If a drug is nearing a toxic level or a subtherapeutic level, the provider will make a dosage adjustment accordingly. How often monitoring is needed varies for each drug. Additionally, patient factors such as poor liver or renal function may determine the frequency of drug level monitoring.

For some drugs with a NTI, a therapeutic dosage is determined by means other than the serum drug level. Warfarin is a drug that illustrates this method. Instead of ordering a serum warfarin level, optimal dosing is determined by measures of prothrombin time with international normalized ratio (PT/INR).

Evaluating Medication Adequacy

For some drugs, evaluation of effectiveness can be determined easily. For example, if an analgesic is given, effectiveness is determined by asking the patient to rate the pain on a scale of 0 to 10. Similarly, the adequacy of an antihypertensive medication can be evaluated by checking the patient's blood pressure. Evaluating medication adequacy is not so simple for some conditions, however.

Some conditions do not cause obvious signs or symptoms. Hyperlipidemia is a common example; signs and symptoms often do not appear until after decades of accumulated damage have occurred. Other conditions may be manifested by signs and symptoms that are not easily quantifiable. A common example of this condition is hyperglycemia associated with diabetes. Some people display obvious signs and symptoms when hyperglycemic, whereas for others, the evidence is much more subtle. For conditions such as hyperlipidemia and hyperglycemia, laboratory testing offers a precisely quantifiable measure that can be used to gauge the effectiveness of medication therapy. A hemoglobin A_{1c} level can be used to evaluate glucose control, for example, and lipid panels can used to determine the effectiveness of hyperlipidemia management.

Identifying Adverse Effects

One of the most common uses of drug monitoring is that of monitoring for harm. This is a proactive undertaking to identify problems early, before they progress to the point of harm.

Many drugs are potentially dangerous. For these, monitoring depends on the type of potential injury. For example, if a drug can cause liver injury, periodic monitoring of liver enzymes (and possibly other tests of liver function) is needed. If a drug can cause bone marrow suppression, periodic monitoring of a complete blood count to assess for anemia, leukopenia, or thrombocytopenia is warranted. In addition, baseline laboratory studies are done before initiating therapy.

ADHERENCE

Medication nonadherence costs the U.S. health care system approximately $290 billion each year. It is often directly responsible for disease exacerbations, avoidable hospitalizations, transitioning to long-term (i.e., "nursing home") care, and premature deaths.

Medication adherence can be defined as the extent to which patients take their medications as prescribed by the provider and agreed to by the patient.[1] The patient who adheres to the agreed-on medication regimen takes the medication in the prescribed dose at the prescribed frequency for the length of time indicated.

In 2013, the National Community Pharmacists Association (NCPA) released *Medication Adherence in America: A National Report Card* (available at http://www.ncpa.co/adherence/AdherenceReportCard_Full.pdf with yearly progress reports at http://www.ncpanet.org/solutions/adherence-simplify-my-meds). The NCPA report identifies six

[1]The addition of "agreed to by the patient" distinguishes the definition of medication adherence from medication compliance. The concept of medication compliance has fallen out of favor because it views the provider from the perspective of an authoritarian who dictates treatment rather than a provider who makes decisions that consider the patient's preferences and values.

TABLE 3.2 ▪ Selected Medications That Require Periodic Laboratory Monitoring

Drug or Drug Category	Laboratory Testing	Reason for Monitoring
ACEIs and ARBs	Potassium	These drugs can cause hyperkalemia.
	Serum creatinine	Renal perfusion is dependent on angiotensin in some patients; increased creatinine may require change in medication.
Amiodarone	Liver function	Hepatotoxicity is an adverse effect.
	Thyroid function	Either hypothyroidism or hyperthyroidism may occur.
	Pulmonary function and chest radiographs	Pulmonary toxicity is not uncommon; effects may be permanent.
Antidiabetic drugs	Serum glucose Hemoglobin A_{1c}	Determination of glucose control is needed.
Anticonvulsants	Serum drug levels	Determination of therapeutic dosage is needed. Some have narrow therapeutic index.
Digoxin	Digoxin level	The drugs have a narrow therapeutic index.
	Serum electrolytes if at risk	Hypokalemia, hypomagnesemia, and hypocalcemia can increase toxicity risk.
Diuretics, potassium-sparing	Serum electrolytes	Hyperkalemia can reach dangerous levels. Hypocalcemia and hypomagnesemia may occur.
Diuretics, thiazide and loop	Serum electrolytes	Hypokalemia, hypomagnesemia, and hyponatremia are common. Thiazide diuretics can cause hypercalcemia; loop diuretics can cause hypocalcemia.
Lithium	CBC	Lithium can cause leukocyte elevation.
	Lithium level	The drug has a narrow therapeutic index.
	Thyroid function	Both hypothyroidism and hyperthyroidism may occur.
	Renal function	Renal damage is a serious adverse effect.
	Serum electrolytes	Nephrogenic diabetes insipidus may occur; hyponatremia can create complications.
Methotrexate	CBC	Pancytopenia, or a decrease of any of the blood cell types, may occur.
	Liver function	Hepatotoxicity is an adverse effect.
	Renal function	Renal toxicity is an adverse effect.
NSAIDS (long-term use)	CBC	Anemia may occur, especially if there is bleeding, which may be occult.
	Serum creatinine	Prostaglandin inhibition may decrease renal perfusion, causing injury.
	Liver function	Rare but serious liver injury has occurred.
Statins	Liver function	Elevations in liver enzymes may be associated with injury.
	Creatine kinase	Creatine kinase can determine whether muscle pain is caused by injury secondary to drug use.
	Lipid panel	Lipids are checked to determine effect.
Thiazolidinediones	Liver function	These drugs are associated with a risk for hepatotoxicity.
Thyroid hormone	TSH, T_4	Monitoring is needed to optimize therapy.
Warfarin	PT/INR	Monitoring is needed to maintain therapeutic range.

ACEI, angiotensin-converting enzyme inhibitor; ARB, angiotensin receptor blocker; CBC, complete blood count; PT/INR, prothrombin time/international normalized ratio; TSH, thyroid-stimulating hormone; T_4, thyroxine.

nonadherent behaviors. They are, in the percentage of frequency, as follows:

- Missed a dose (57%)
- Forgot to take a dose (30%)
- Did not refill the medication in time (28%)
- Took a lower than prescribed dose (22%)
- Did not refill the medication (20%)
- Stopped taking the medication (14%)

The reasons given by patients to explain their nonadherence provide additional insight. Again, in the frequency of occurrence, they are as follows:

- Forgot to take it (42%)
- Ran out (34%)
- Was away from home (27%)
- Was trying to save money (22%)
- Didn't like the side effects (21%)
- Was too busy (17%)
- The medicine wasn't working (17%)
- Didn't believe the medicine was necessary (16%)
- Didn't like taking the medicine (12%)

These documents can offer valuable insight for the health care provider. Moreover, they beg the question, "What could the provider have done differently to address issues of nonadherence proactively?"

In examining these, five primary patterns emerge. These are: (1) forgetfulness, (2) lack of planning, (3) cost, (4) dissatisfaction, and (5) altered dosing. An honest and open discussion that respects both the patient and provider perspectives can be an important facilitator to promoting positive outcomes. Individualized solutions that address the specific patient's concerns are those most likely to be successful.

Forgetfulness

The most common reason cited for nonadherence was that the patient simply forgot to take the medication. Studies have demonstrated that medications are easier to remember if they are aligned with common daily activities. For example, morning medications may be taken on first arising (if they should be taken on an empty stomach) or with breakfast (if they should be taken with food). Doing this establishes habits, which are more difficult to forget.

Several memory aids are available to help patients remember to take their medications. Drug organizers are probably the most common tool used. If these are filled at the beginning of each week, the patient can tell at a glance if medications have been taken on any given day.

Numerous apps are also available for various electronic devices. These can be programmed to alarm or deliver a verbal message when it is time to take a drug.

Some patients have found that medication administration records (MARs), similar to MARs used by nurses in hospitals, can be helpful. One company (https://www.medactionplan.com) offers a free online service that patients can use to set up personalized MARs that include the option to receive reminders by email or text messaging.

Lack of Planning

Aligned closely with forgetfulness is the lack of planning. In this category, we include those statements aligned with failure to refill medications whether because the patient was too busy, away from home, or ran out for other reasons.

Most pharmacies offer reminder notices, either by email or automated phone calls, as part of their regular services. If being "too busy" is a concern, a pharmacy that offers a home delivery service or a mail delivery service is a viable solution.

Cost

As mentioned in Chapter 2, costs should be considered initially when selecting an appropriate drug. Sometimes, however, there are no adequate substitutions for a necessary but expensive drug. Fortunately, prescription assistance programs (PAPs), also called *patient assistance programs* and *pharmaceutical assistance programs*, are widely available. These offer steeply discounted drugs for those who meet eligibility requirements.

There are three sources for PAPs: pharmaceutical companies, government-run programs, and nonprofit organizations. Table 3.3 offers a program sampling. If you do not find what you need here, your likely best resource for reliable information is a local pharmacist. Warn patients to beware of discount cards that are not affiliated with known reputable organizations. Unfortunately, some criminals use applications for fake cards for illegal purposes.

Dissatisfaction

The issue of dissatisfaction as a reason for nonadherence highlights the need to identify what medications are taken and to discuss any concerns with the patient at each encounter. It is essential to uncover the reason for dissatisfaction (e.g., adverse effects, inconvenient dosing, or a perception that a drug is ineffective). Often the problem can be easily addressed by simple interventions. For example, taking medications with food can reduce adverse effects of nausea and gastrointestinal distress in many instances. Changing to a sustained-release drug may be all that is necessary to address problems with inconvenient dosing.

If the patient believes a drug is ineffective, it becomes important to discuss patient expectations of drug therapy and what can be realistically achieved. For some conditions (e.g., obesity), change may come slowly. For others (e.g., hypertension), the medication may cause the patient to feel worse without a perceived benefit. If the drug is truly an important one, this may be a good time to explore with the patient any consequences of not taking the drug and whether the patient is willing to assume those risks. In some instances, the patient may decide to assume those risks rather than to take the medication. It is within the patient's right to do so.

Altered Dosing

We were concerned to see that more than 20% of patients took lower than the prescribed dose. The reasons were not made clear; however, the consequence is this: A subtherapeutic dose

TABLE 3.3 ■ Patient Assistance Programs

PHARMACEUTICAL PROGRAMS	
Allergan	http://www.allergan.com/responsibility/patient-resources/patient-assistance-programs
AstraZeneca	http://www.astrazeneca-us.com/medicines/help-affording-your-medicines
Boehringer Ingelheim	us.boehringer-ingelheim.com/our_responsibility/patients-families.html
Johnson & Johnson	http://www.jjpaf.org
Merck	http://www.merckhelps.com
Novartis	http://www.patientassistancenow.com/index.jsp
Pfizer	http://www.pfizer.com/health/financial_assistance_programs/patient_assistance_programs
Takeda	http://www.takeda.us/responsibility/patient_assistance_program.aspx
GOVERNMENT PROGRAMS	
Medicare	https://www.medicare.gov/pharmaceutical-assistance-program
State-run programs	http://www.ncsl.org/research/health/state-pharmaceutical-assistance-programs.aspx
NONPROFIT ORGANIZATIONS	
American Association of Retired Persons (AARP)	http://advantages.aarp.org/en/brand.aarp-prescription-discounts-provided-by-catamaran-an-optumrx-company.html
NeedyMeds	http://www.needymeds.org
Partnership for Prescription Assistance	https://www.pparx.org
RxAssist	http://www.rxassist.org

is no better than no dose at all! Most drugs must reach a level sufficient to cause a therapeutic effect. If the drug does not reach that level, it is not helping. In the case of certain antimicrobial drugs, subtherapeutic levels may cause harm if the bacteria develop resistance as a result.

This finding emphasizes the necessity of not only reviewing which medications are taken at each encounter but also asking whether the medications are taken as prescribed. If dosing is altered, it is imperative to determine how and why, and then to educate the patient regarding how alterations in dosing affect outcomes.

MANAGING MEDICATION THERAPY

In addition to the medication review undertaken at each patient encounter, a more comprehensive and deliberate review is needed periodically (at least annually). This review should be approached with the intent purpose of determining whether there are better options for medication therapy. Inherent questions that must be asked about each drug include the following:

- Is each medication accomplishing its intended purpose?
- Is each medication still necessary?
  - Has the patient's condition changed?
  - Do adverse effects or risks outweigh the benefits that some drugs provide?
  - What would happen if some medications were no longer prescribed?
- What problems does each medication create for the patient?
  - Is a medication problem amplified by other drugs the patient is taking?
  - If a medication is necessary but problematic, are drugs with fewer adverse effects available?
- If polypharmacy is an issue, are there ways to decrease the number of medications?
  - Will a combination drug simplify management?
  - Is a single drug available (and desirable) for management of two different conditions?

Ideally, these reviews should be carried out in collaboration with the patient or patient's family so that nothing is overlooked. Medication regimens can then be optimized to eliminate unnecessary drugs, add new drugs, if necessary, and ultimately improve patient satisfaction with care.

SUMMARY

We have examined four opportunities to promote positive outcomes in drug therapy. Patients need adequate drug education in order to take drugs correctly and to avoid complications associated with therapy. Monitoring provides a method of ensuring safe and effective therapy. Promoting adherence, by addressing common causes of nonadherence proactively, can ensure ongoing therapy without interruption. Finally, scheduled medication reviews with the intent to optimize medication regimens, based on patient experiences and needs, can help to promote positive outcomes.

UNIT II

Basic Principles of Pharmacology

CHAPTER 4

Pharmacokinetics, Pharmacodynamics, and Drug Interactions

Jacqueline Rosenjack Burchum, DNSc, FNP-BC, CNE

PHARMACOKINETICS

Pharmacokinetics is the study of drug movement throughout the body.[1] There are four basic pharmacokinetic processes: absorption, distribution, metabolism, and excretion (Fig. 4.1). *Absorption* is defined as the movement of a drug from its site of administration into the blood. *Distribution* is defined as drug movement from the blood to the interstitial space of tissues and from there into cells. *Metabolism* (biotransformation) is defined as enzymatically mediated alteration of drug structure. *Excretion* is the movement of drugs and their metabolites out of the body. The combination of metabolism and excretion is called *elimination.* The four pharmacokinetic processes, acting in concert, determine the concentration of a drug at its sites of action.

APPLICATION OF PHARMACOKINETICS IN PHARMACOTHERAPEUTICS

By applying knowledge of pharmacokinetics to drug therapy, we can help maximize beneficial effects and minimize harm. Recall that the intensity of the response to a drug is directly related to the concentration of the drug at its site of action. To maximize beneficial effects, a drug must achieve concentrations that are high enough to elicit desired responses; to minimize harm, we must avoid concentrations that are too high. This balance is achieved by selecting the most appropriate route, dosage, and dosing schedule.

[1]Fundamental pharmacologic concepts are typically covered in undergraduate courses; however, experience has demonstrated that a refresher in the basic principles of pharmacokinetics, pharmacodynamics, and drug interactions is usually helpful. Because it is a refresher, the information in this chapter is relatively brief. A more expansive discussion of this content is found in *Lehne's Pharmacology for Nursing Care,* 9th edition.

PASSAGE OF DRUGS ACROSS MEMBRANES

All four phases of pharmacokinetics—absorption, distribution, metabolism, and excretion—involve drug movement. To move throughout the body, drugs must cross membranes. Drugs must cross membranes to enter the blood from their site of administration. When in the blood, drugs must cross membranes to leave the vascular system and reach their sites of action. In addition, drugs must cross membranes to undergo metabolism and excretion. Accordingly, the factors that determine the passage of drugs across biologic membranes have a profound influence on all aspects of pharmacokinetics.

Biologic membranes are composed of layers of individual cells. The cells composing most membranes are very close to one another—so close, in fact, that drugs must usually pass *through* cells, rather than between them, to cross the membrane. Hence the ability of a drug to cross a biologic membrane is determined primarily by its ability to pass through single cells.

Three Ways to Cross a Cell Membrane

The three most important ways by which drugs cross cell membranes are (1) passage through channels or pores, (2) passage with the aid of a transport system, and (3) direct penetration of the membrane. Of the three, direct penetration of the membrane is most common.

Channels and Pores

Very few drugs cross membranes through channels or pores. The channels in membranes are extremely small and are specific for certain molecules. Consequently, only the smallest of compounds, such as potassium and sodium, can pass through these channels, and then only if the channel is the right one.

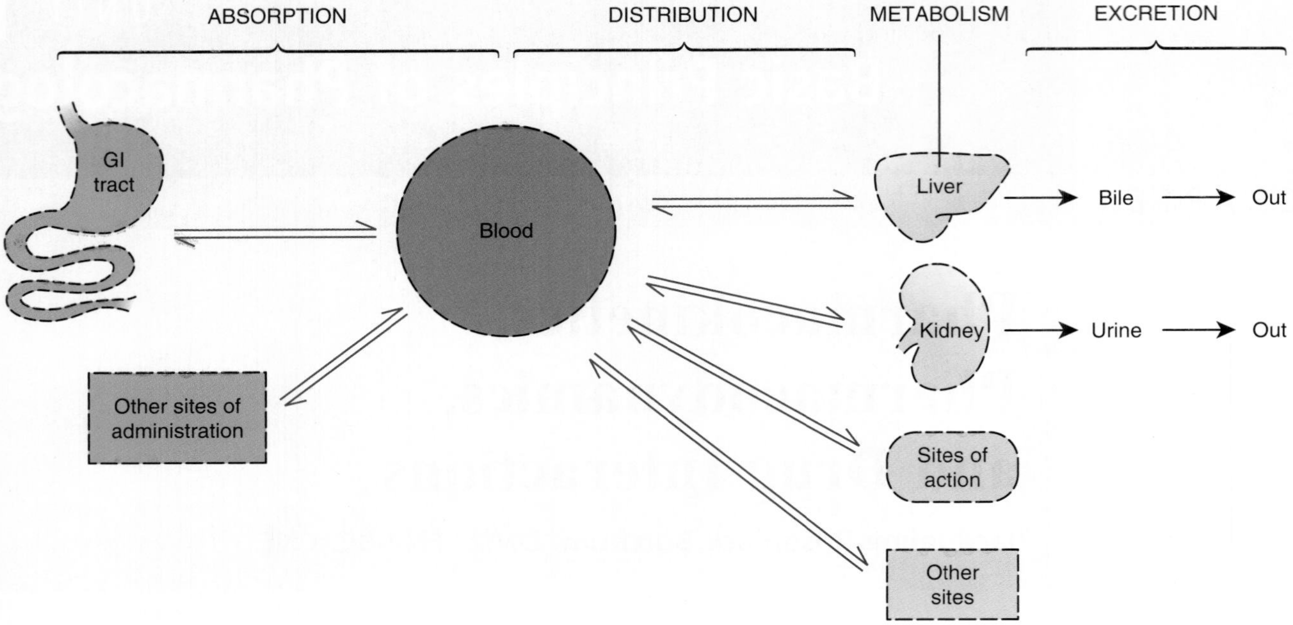

Figure 4.1 ■ The four basic pharmacokinetic processes. *Dotted lines* represent membranes that must be crossed as drugs move throughout the body.

Transport Systems

Transport systems are carriers that can move drugs from one side of the cell membrane to the other side. All transport systems are selective. Whether a transporter will carry a particular drug depends on the drug's structure.

Transport systems are an important means of drug transit. For example, certain orally administered drugs could not be absorbed unless there were transport systems to move them across the membranes that separate the lumen of the intestine from the blood. A number of drugs could not reach intracellular sites of action without a transport system to move them across the cell membrane. One transporter, known as *P-glycoprotein* (PGP) or *multidrug transporter protein,* deserves special mention. PGP is a transmembrane protein that transports a wide variety of drugs *out* of cells.

Direct Penetration of the Membrane

For most drugs, movement throughout the body is dependent on the ability to penetrate membranes directly because (1) most drugs are too large to pass through channels or pores, and (2) most drugs lack transport systems to help them cross all of the membranes that separate them from their sites of action, metabolism, and excretion.

A general rule in chemistry states that "like dissolves like." Membranes are composed primarily of lipids; therefore, to directly penetrate membranes, a drug must be *lipid soluble* (lipophilic).

Certain kinds of molecules are *not* lipid soluble and therefore cannot penetrate membranes. This group consists of *polar molecules* and *ions.*

Polar Molecules

Polar molecules are molecules that have no *net* charge; however, they have an uneven *distribution* of electrical charge. That is, positive and negative charges within the molecule tend to congregate separately from one another. Water is the classic example. As depicted in Fig. 4.1, the electrons (negative charges) in the water molecule spend more time in the vicinity of the oxygen atom than in the vicinity of the two hydrogen atoms. As a result, the area around the oxygen atom tends to be negatively charged, whereas the area around the hydrogen atoms tends to be positively charged. In accord with the "like dissolves like" rule, polar molecules will dissolve in *polar* solvents (such as water) but not in *nonpolar* solvents (such as lipids).

Ions

Ions are defined as molecules that have a *net electrical charge* (either positive or negative). Except for very small molecules, *ions are unable to cross membranes;* therefore, they must become nonionized in order to cross from one side to the other. Many drugs are either weak organic acids or weak organic bases, which can exist in charged and uncharged forms. Whether a weak acid or base carries an electrical charge is determined by the pH of the surrounding medium. Acids tend to ionize in basic (alkaline) media, whereas bases tend to ionize in acidic media. Therefore drugs that are weak acids are best absorbed in an acidic environment such as gastric acid because they remain in a nonionized form. When aspirin molecules pass from the stomach into the small intestine, where the environment is relatively alkaline, more of the molecules change to their ionized form. As a result, absorption of aspirin from the intestine is impeded.

Ion Trapping (pH Partitioning)

Because the ionization of drugs is pH dependent, when the pH of the fluid on one side of a membrane differs from the pH of the fluid on the other side, drug molecules tend to accumulate on the side where the pH most favors their ionization. Accordingly, because acidic drugs tend to ionize in basic media, and because basic drugs tend to ionize in acidic media, *when there is a pH gradient between two sides of a membrane,* the following occur:

- Acidic drugs accumulate on the alkaline side.
- Basic drugs accumulate on the acidic side.

The process whereby a drug accumulates on the side of a membrane where the pH most favors its ionization is referred to as *ion trapping* or *pH partitioning.*

ABSORPTION

Absorption is defined as *the movement of a drug from its site of administration into the systemic circulation.* The *rate* of absorption determines how *soon* effects will begin. The *amount* of absorption helps determine how *intense* effects will be. Two other terms associated with absorption are *chemical equivalence* and *bioavailability.* Drug preparations are considered *chemically equivalent* if they contain the same amount of the identical chemical compound (drug). Preparations are considered equal in *bioavailability* if the drug they contain is absorbed at the same rate and to the same extent. It is possible for two formulations of the same drug to be chemically equivalent while differing in bioavailability. The concept of bioavailability is discussed further in Chapter 6.

Factors Affecting Drug Absorption

The rate at which a drug undergoes absorption is influenced by the physical and chemical properties of the drug and by physiologic and anatomic factors at the absorption site.

Rate of Dissolution

Before a drug can be absorbed, it must first dissolve. Hence, the rate of dissolution helps determine the rate of absorption. Drugs in formulations that allow rapid dissolution have a faster onset than drugs formulated for slow dissolution.

Surface Area

The surface area available for absorption is a major determinant of the rate of absorption. When the surface area is larger, absorption is faster. For this reason, absorption of orally administered drugs is usually greater from the small intestine rather than from the stomach. (Recall that the small intestine, because of its lining of microvilli, has an extremely large surface area, whereas the surface area of the stomach is relatively small.)

Blood Flow

Drugs are absorbed most rapidly from sites where blood flow is high because blood containing a newly absorbed drug will be replaced rapidly by drug-free blood, thereby maintaining a large gradient between the concentration of drug outside the blood and the concentration of drug in the blood. The greater the concentration gradient, the more rapid absorption will be.

Lipid Solubility

As a rule, highly lipid-soluble drugs are absorbed more rapidly than drugs whose lipid solubility is low. This occurs because lipid-soluble drugs can readily cross the membranes that separate them from the blood, whereas drugs of low lipid solubility cannot.

pH Partitioning

pH partitioning can influence drug absorption. Absorption will be enhanced when the difference between the pH of plasma and the pH at the site of administration is such that drug molecules will have a greater tendency to be ionized in the plasma.

Characteristics of Commonly Used Routes of Administration

For each of the major routes of administration—oral (PO), intravenous (IV), intramuscular (IM), and subcutaneous (subQ)—the pattern of drug absorption (i.e., the rate and extent of absorption) is unique. Consequently, the route by which a drug is administered significantly affects both the onset and the intensity of effects. The distinguishing characteristics of the four major routes are summarized in Table 4.1. Additional routes of administration (e.g., topical, transdermal, inhaled) each have unique characteristics that are addressed throughout the book as we discuss specific drugs that employ them.

DISTRIBUTION

Distribution is defined as *the movement of drugs from the systemic circulation to the site of drug action.* Drug distribution is determined by three major factors: blood flow to tissues, the ability of a drug to exit the vascular system, and, to a lesser extent, the ability of a drug to enter cells.

Blood Flow to Tissues

In the first phase of distribution, drugs are carried by the blood to the tissues and organs of the body. The rate at which drugs are delivered to a particular tissue is determined by blood flow to that tissue. Because most tissues are well perfused, regional blood flow is rarely a limiting factor in drug distribution.

There are two pathologic conditions—abscesses and tumors—in which low regional blood flow can affect drug therapy. An abscess has no internal blood vessels; therefore, because abscesses lack a blood supply, antibiotics cannot reach the bacteria within. Accordingly, if drug therapy is to be effective, the abscess must usually be surgically drained.

Solid tumors have a limited blood supply. Although blood flow to the outer regions of tumors is relatively high, blood flow becomes progressively lower toward the core. As a result, it may not be possible to achieve high drug levels deep inside tumors. Limited blood flow is a major reason that solid tumors are resistant to drug therapy.

TABLE 4.1 ▪ Properties of Major Routes of Drug Administration

Route	Barriers to Absorption	Absorption Pattern	Advantages	Disadvantages
PARENTERAL				
Intravenous (IV)	None (absorption is bypassed)	Instantaneous	Rapid onset, and hence ideal for emergencies Precise control over drug levels Permits use of large fluid volumes Permits use of irritant drugs	Irreversible Expensive Inconvenient Difficult to do, and hence poorly suited for self-administration Risk for fluid overload, infection, and embolism Drug must be water soluble
Intramuscular (IM)	Capillary wall (easy to pass)	Rapid with water-soluble drugs Slow with poorly soluble drugs	Permits use of poorly soluble drugs Permits use of depot preparations	Possible discomfort Inconvenient Potential for injury
Subcutaneous (subQ)	Same as IM	Same as IM	Same as IM	Same as IM
ENTERAL				
Oral (PO)	Epithelial lining of gastrointestinal tract; capillary wall	Slow and variable	Easy Convenient Inexpensive Ideal for self-medication Potentially reversible, and hence safer than parenteral routes	Variability Inactivation of some drugs by gastric acid and digestive enzymes Possible nausea and vomiting from local irritation Patient must be conscious and cooperative.

Exiting the Vascular System

After a drug has been delivered to an organ or tissue by blood circulation, the next step is to exit the vasculature. Because most drugs do not produce their effects within the blood, the ability to leave the vascular system is an important determinant of drug actions. Drugs in the vascular system leave the blood at capillary beds.

Typical Capillary Beds

Most capillary beds offer no resistance to the departure of drugs because, in most tissues, drugs can leave the vasculature simply by passing through pores in the capillary wall. Because drugs pass *between* capillary cells rather than *through* them, movement into the interstitial space is not impeded. The exit of drugs from a typical capillary bed is depicted in Fig. 4.2.

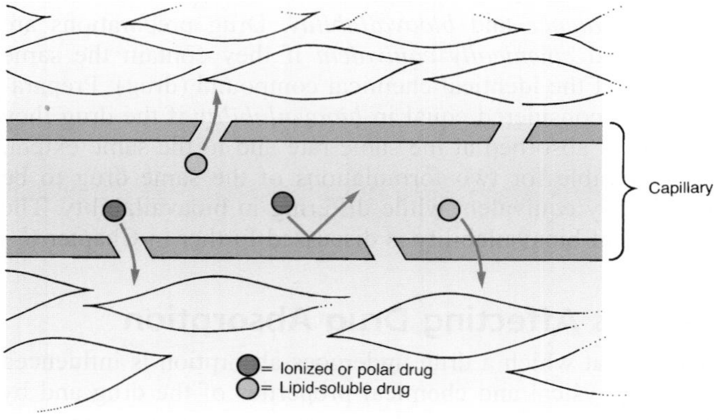

Figure 4.2 ▪ Drug movement at typical capillary beds. In most capillary beds, "large" gaps exist between the cells that compose the capillary wall. Drugs and other molecules can pass freely into and out of the bloodstream through these gaps. As illustrated, lipid-soluble compounds can also pass directly through the cells of the capillary wall.

The Blood-Brain Barrier

The term *blood-brain barrier* (BBB) refers to the unique anatomy of capillaries in the central nervous system (CNS). As shown in Fig. 4.3, there are *tight junctions* between the cells that compose the walls of most capillaries in the CNS. These junctions are so tight that they prevent drug passage. Consequently, to leave the blood and reach sites of action within the brain, a drug must be able to pass *through* cells of the capillary wall. Only drugs that are *lipid soluble* or have a *transport system* can cross the BBB to a significant degree.

Recent evidence indicates that, in addition to tight junctions, the BBB has another protective component: *PGP.* As noted earlier, PGP is a transporter that pumps a variety of drugs out of cells. In capillaries of the CNS, PGP pumps drugs back into the blood and thereby limits their access to the brain.

The BBB is not fully developed at birth. As a result, newborns have heightened sensitivity to medicines that act on the brain. Likewise, neonates are especially vulnerable to CNS toxicity.

Placental Drug Transfer

The membranes of the placenta separate the maternal circulation from the fetal circulation (Fig. 4.4). *However, the membranes of the placenta do NOT constitute an absolute barrier to the passage of drugs.* The same factors that determine the movement of drugs across other membranes determine the movement of drugs across the placenta. Accordingly, lipid-soluble, nonionized compounds readily pass from the maternal bloodstream into the blood of the fetus. In contrast, compounds that are ionized, highly polar, or protein bound are largely excluded—as are drugs that are substrates for the PGP transporter that can pump a variety of drugs out of placental cells into the maternal blood.

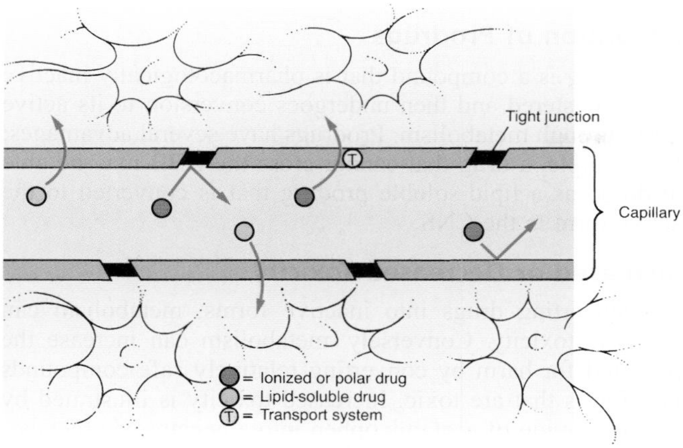

Figure 4.3 ▪ Drug movement across the blood-brain barrier.
Tight junctions between cells that compose the walls of capillaries in the central nervous system prevent drugs from passing between cells to exit the vascular system. Consequently, to reach sites of action within the brain, a drug must pass directly through cells of the capillary wall. To do this, the drug must be lipid soluble or be able to use an existing transport system.

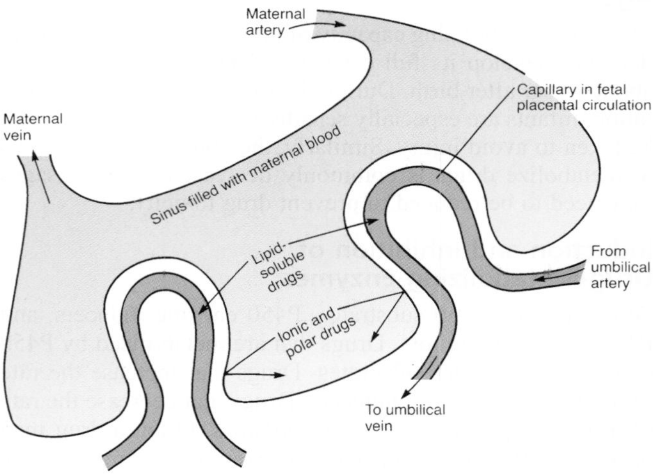

Figure 4.4 ▪ Placental drug transfer.
To enter the fetal circulation, drugs must cross membranes of the maternal and fetal vascular systems. Lipid-soluble drugs can readily cross these membranes and enter the fetal blood, whereas ions and polar molecules are prevented from reaching the fetal blood.

Protein Binding

Drugs can form reversible bonds with various proteins in the body. Of all the proteins with which drugs can bind, *plasma albumin* is the most important. Like other proteins, albumin is a large molecule. Because of its size, albumin is too large to leave the bloodstream.

Fig. 4.5 depicts the binding of drug molecules to albumin. Note that the drug molecules are much smaller than albumin. As indicated by the two-way arrows, binding between albumin and drugs is *reversible.* Hence, drugs may be *bound* or *unbound* (free).

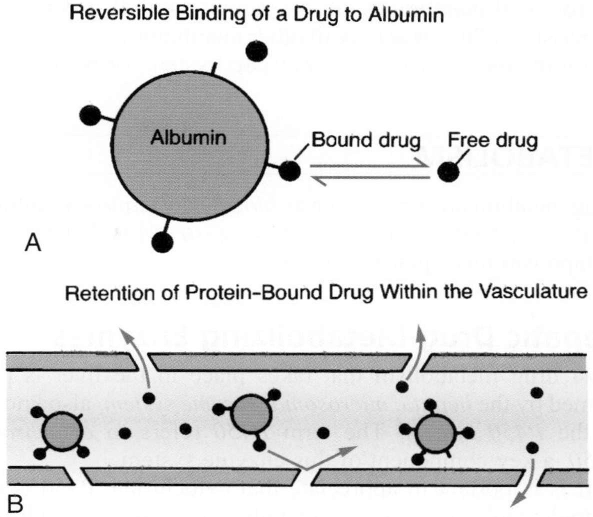

Figure 4.5 ▪ Protein binding of drugs.
A, Albumin is the most prevalent protein in plasma and the most important of the proteins to which drugs bind. **B,** Only unbound (free) drug molecules can leave the vascular system. Bound molecules are too large to fit through the pores in the capillary wall.

Even though a drug can bind albumin, only some molecules will be bound at any moment. The percentage of drug molecules that are bound is determined by the strength of the attraction between albumin and the drug. For example, the attraction between albumin and the anticoagulant warfarin is strong, causing nearly all (99%) of the warfarin molecules in plasma to be bound, leaving only 1% free. On the other hand, the attraction between the antibiotic gentamicin and albumin is relatively weak; less than 10% of the gentamicin molecules in plasma are bound, leaving more than 90% free.

An important consequence of protein binding is restriction of drug distribution. Because albumin is too large to leave the bloodstream, drug molecules that are bound to albumin cannot leave either (see Fig. 4.5B). As a result, bound molecules cannot reach their sites of action or undergo metabolism or excretion until the drug-protein bond is broken so that the drug is free to leave the circulation.

In addition to restricting drug distribution, protein binding can be a source of drug interactions. As suggested by Fig. 4.5A, each molecule of albumin has only a few sites to which drug molecules can bind. Because the number of binding sites is limited, drugs with the ability to bind albumin will compete with one another for those sites. As a result, one drug can displace another from albumin, causing the free concentration of the displaced drug to rise, thus increasing the intensity of drug responses. If plasma drug levels rise sufficiently, toxicity can result.

Entering Cells

Many drugs produce their effects by binding with receptors located on the external surface of the cell membrane; however, some drugs must enter cells to reach their sites of action, and practically all drugs must enter cells to undergo metabolism and excretion. The factors that determine the ability of a drug to cross cell membranes are the same factors that determine the passage of drugs across all other membranes, namely, lipid solubility, the presence of a transport system, or both.

METABOLISM

Drug metabolism, also known as *biotransformation,* is defined as *the enzymatic alteration of drug structure.* Most drug metabolism takes place in the liver.

Hepatic Drug-Metabolizing Enzymes

Most drug metabolism that takes place in the liver is performed by the *hepatic microsomal enzyme system,* also known as the *P450 system.* The term *P450* refers to *cytochrome P450,* a key component of this enzyme system.

It is important to appreciate that cytochrome P450 is not a single molecular entity, but rather a group of 12 closely related enzyme families. Three of the cytochrome P450 (CYP) families—designated CYP1, CYP2, and CYP3—metabolize drugs. The other nine families metabolize endogenous compounds (e.g., steroids, fatty acids). Each of the three P450 families that metabolize drugs is composed of multiple forms, each of which metabolizes only certain drugs. To identify the individual forms of cytochrome P450, designations such as CYP1A2, CYP2D6, and CYP3A4 are used to indicate specific members of the CYP1, CYP2, and CYP3 families, respectively.

Therapeutic Consequences of Drug Metabolism

Drug metabolism has six possible consequences of therapeutic significance:

- Accelerated renal excretion of drugs
- Drug inactivation
- Increased therapeutic action
- Activation of prodrugs
- Increased toxicity
- Decreased toxicity

Accelerated Renal Drug Excretion

The most important consequence of drug metabolism is promotion of renal drug excretion. The kidneys, which are the major organs of drug excretion, are unable to excrete drugs that are highly lipid soluble. Hence, by converting lipid-soluble drugs into more hydrophilic (water-soluble) forms, metabolic conversion can accelerate renal excretion of many agents.

Drug Inactivation

Drug metabolism can convert pharmacologically active compounds to inactive forms. This is the most common end result of drug metabolism.

Increased Therapeutic Action

Metabolism can increase the effectiveness of some drugs. For example, metabolism converts codeine into morphine. The analgesic activity of morphine is so much greater than that of codeine that formation of morphine may account for virtually all the pain relief that occurs after codeine administration.

Activation of Prodrugs

A *prodrug* is a compound that is pharmacologically inactive as administered and then undergoes conversion to its active form through metabolism. Prodrugs have several advantages; for example, a drug that cannot cross the BBB may be able to do so as a lipid-soluble prodrug that is converted to the active form in the CNS.

Increased or Decreased Toxicity

By converting drugs into inactive forms, metabolism can decrease toxicity. Conversely, metabolism can increase the potential for harm by converting relatively safe compounds into forms that are toxic. Increased toxicity is illustrated by the conversion of acetaminophen into a hepatotoxic metabolite. It is this product of metabolism, and not acetaminophen itself, that causes injury when acetaminophen is taken in overdose.

Special Considerations in Drug Metabolism

Several factors can influence the rate at which drugs are metabolized. These must be accounted for in drug therapy.

Age

The drug-metabolizing capacity of infants is limited. The liver does not develop its full capacity to metabolize drugs until about 1 year after birth. During the time before hepatic maturation, infants are especially sensitive to drugs, and care must be taken to avoid injury. Similarly, the ability of older adults to metabolize drugs is commonly decreased. Drug dosages may need to be reduced to prevent drug toxicity.

Induction and Inhibition of Drug-Metabolizing Enzymes

Drugs may be P450 substrates, P450 enzyme inducers, and P450 enzyme inhibitors. Drugs that are metabolized by P450 hepatic enzymes are substrates. Drugs that increase the rate of drug metabolism are inducers. Drugs that decrease the rate of drug metabolism are called *inhibitors.* Often a drug may have more than one property. For example, a drug may be both a substrate and an inducer.

Inducers act on the liver to stimulate enzyme synthesis. This process is known as *induction.* By increasing the rate of drug metabolism, the amount of active drug is decreased and plasma drug levels fall. If dosage adjustments are not made to accommodate for this, a drug may not achieve therapeutic levels.

Inhibitors act on the liver through a process known as *inhibition.* By slowing the rate of metabolism, inhibition can cause an increase in active drug accumulation. This can lead to an increase in adverse effects and toxicity.

First-Pass Effect

The term *first-pass effect* refers to the rapid hepatic inactivation of certain oral drugs. When drugs are absorbed from the gastrointestinal tract, they are carried directly to the liver through the hepatic portal vein before they enter the systemic circulation. If the capacity of the liver to metabolize a drug is extremely high, that drug can be completely inactivated on its first pass through the liver. As a result, no therapeutic effects can occur. To circumvent the first-pass effect, a drug that undergoes rapid hepatic metabolism is often administered parenterally. This permits the drug to temporarily bypass the liver, thereby allowing it to reach therapeutic levels in the systemic circulation before being metabolized.

Nutritional Status

Hepatic drug-metabolizing enzymes require a number of cofactors to function. In the malnourished patient, these cofactors may be deficient, causing drug metabolism to be compromised.

Competition Between Drugs

When two drugs are metabolized by the same metabolic pathway, they may compete with each other for metabolism and may thereby decrease the rate at which one or both agents are metabolized. If metabolism is depressed enough, a drug can accumulate to dangerous levels.

Enterohepatic Recirculation

As noted earlier and depicted in Fig. 4.6, enterohepatic recirculation is a repeating cycle in which a drug is transported from the liver into the duodenum (through the bile duct) and then back to the liver (through the portal blood). It is important to note, however, that only certain drugs are affected. Specifically, the process is limited to drugs that have undergone *glucuronidation,* a process that converts lipid-soluble drugs to water-soluble drugs by binding them to glucuronic acid. After glucuronidation, these drugs can enter the bile and then pass to the duodenum. In the intestine, some drugs can be hydrolyzed by intestinal beta-glucuronidase, an enzyme that breaks the bond between the original drug and the glucuronide moiety, thereby releasing the free drug. Because the free drug is more lipid soluble than the glucuronidated form, the free drug can undergo reabsorption across the intestinal wall, followed by transport back to the liver, where the cycle can start again. Because of enterohepatic recycling, drugs can remain in the body much longer than they otherwise would.

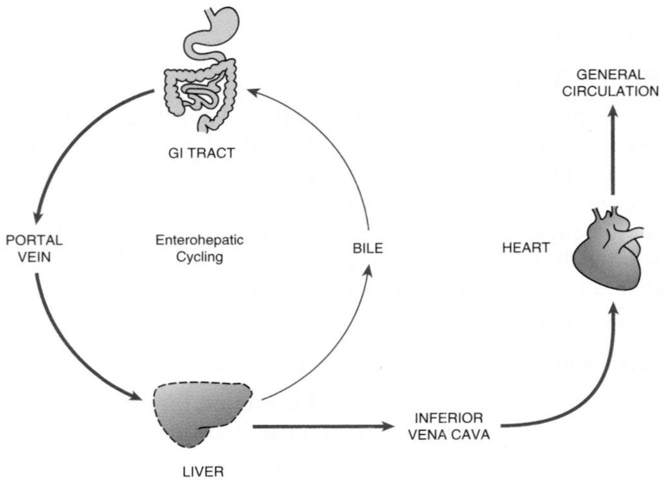

Figure 4.6 ▪ Movement of drugs after gastrointestinal (GI) absorption.

All drugs absorbed from sites along the GI tract—stomach, small intestine, and large intestine (but not the oral mucosa or distal rectum)—must go through the liver, through the portal vein, on their way to the heart and then the general circulation. For some drugs, passage is uneventful. Others undergo extensive hepatic metabolism. And still others undergo *enterohepatic recirculation,* a repeating cycle in which a drug moves from the liver into the duodenum (through the bile duct) and then back to the liver (through the portal blood). As discussed in the text under *Enterohepatic Recirculation,* the process is limited to drugs that have first undergone hepatic glucuronidation.

EXCRETION

Drug excretion is defined as *the removal of drugs from the body.* Drugs and their metabolites can exit the body in urine, bile, sweat, saliva, breast milk, and expired air. The most important organ for drug excretion is the kidney.

Renal Drug Excretion

The kidneys account for the majority of drug excretion. When the kidneys are healthy, they serve to limit the duration of action of many drugs. Conversely, if renal failure occurs, both the duration and intensity of drug responses may increase.

Steps in Renal Drug Excretion

Urinary excretion is the net result of three processes: (1) glomerular filtration, (2) passive tubular reabsorption, and (3) active tubular secretion.

Glomerular Filtration

Renal excretion begins at the glomerulus of the kidney tubule. As blood flows through the glomerular capillaries, fluids and small molecules—including drugs—are forced through the pores of the capillary wall. This process, called *glomerular filtration,* moves drugs from the blood into the tubular urine. Blood cells and large molecules (e.g., proteins) are too big to pass through the capillary pores and therefore do not undergo filtration. Because large molecules are not filtered, drugs bound to albumin remain in the blood.

Passive Tubular Reabsorption

As depicted in Fig. 4.7, the vessels that deliver blood to the glomerulus return to proximity with the renal tubule at a point distal to the glomerulus. At this distal site, drug concentrations in the blood are lower than drug concentrations in the tubule. This concentration gradient acts as a driving force to move drugs from the lumen of the tubule back into the blood. Because lipid-soluble drugs can readily cross the membranes that compose the tubular and vascular walls, *drugs that are lipid soluble undergo passive reabsorption from the tubule back into the blood.* In contrast, drugs that are not lipid soluble (ions and polar compounds) remain in the urine to be excreted.

Active Tubular Secretion

There are active transport systems in the kidney tubules that pump drugs from the blood to the tubular urine. These pumps have a relatively high capacity and play a significant role in excreting certain compounds.

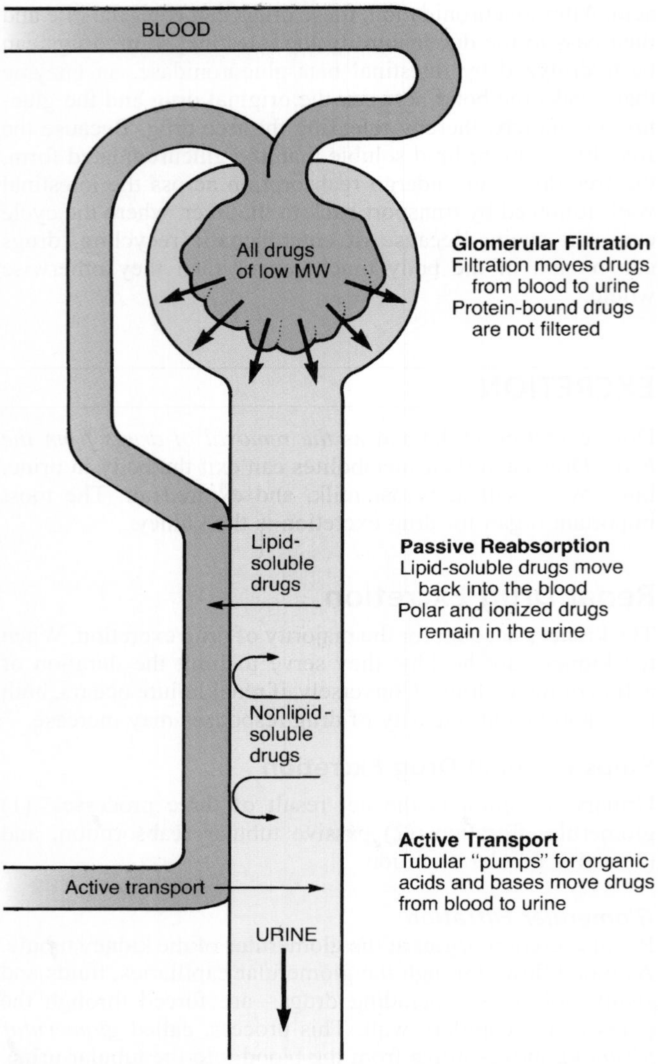

Figure 4.7 ▪ Renal drug excretion. MW, molecular weight.

Factors That Modify Renal Drug Excretion

Renal drug excretion varies from patient to patient. Conditions such as chronic renal disease may cause profound alterations. Three other important factors to consider are pH-dependent ionization, competition for active tubular transport, and patient age.

pH-Dependent Ionization

The phenomenon of pH-dependent ionization can be used to accelerate renal excretion of drugs. Recall that passive tubular reabsorption is limited to lipid-soluble compounds. Because ions are not lipid soluble, drugs that are ionized at the pH of tubular urine will remain in the tubule and be excreted. Consequently, by manipulating urinary pH in such a way as to promote the ionization of a drug, we can decrease passive reabsorption back into the blood and can thereby hasten the drug's elimination. This principle has been employed to promote the excretion of poisons as well as medications that have been taken in toxic doses.

Competition for Active Tubular Transport

Competition between drugs for active tubular transport can delay renal excretion, thereby prolonging effects. The active transport systems of the renal tubules can be envisioned as motor-driven revolving doors that carry drugs from the plasma into the renal tubules. These "revolving doors" can carry only a limited number of drug molecules per unit of time. Accordingly, if there are too many molecules present, some must wait their turn. Because of competition, if we administer two drugs at the same time, and if both drugs use the same transport system, excretion of each will be delayed by the presence of the other.

Age

The kidneys of newborns are not fully developed. Until their kidneys reach full capacity (a few months after birth), infants have a limited capacity to excrete drugs. This must be accounted for when medicating an infant.

In old age, renal function often declines. Older adults have smaller kidneys and fewer nephrons. The loss of nephrons results in decreased blood filtration. Additionally, vessel changes such as atherosclerosis reduce renal blood flow. As a result, renal excretion of drugs is decreased.

Nonrenal Routes of Drug Excretion

In most cases, excretion of drugs by nonrenal routes has minimal clinical significance. However, in certain situations, nonrenal excretion can have important therapeutic and toxicologic consequences.

Breast Milk

Some drugs taken by breast-feeding women can undergo excretion into milk. As a result, breastfeeding can expose the nursing infant to drugs. The factors that influence the appearance of drugs in breast milk are the same factors that determine the passage of drugs across membranes. Accordingly, lipid-soluble drugs have ready access to breast milk, whereas drugs that are polar, ionized, or protein bound cannot enter in significant amounts.

Other Nonrenal Routes of Excretion

The *bile* is an important route of excretion for certain drugs. Because bile is secreted into the small intestine, drugs that do not undergo enterohepatic recirculation leave the body in the feces.

The *lungs* are the major route by which volatile anesthetics are excreted. Alcohol is partially eliminated by this route.

Small amounts of drugs can appear in *sweat* and *saliva.* These routes have little therapeutic or toxicologic significance.

TIME COURSE OF DRUG RESPONSES

It is possible to regulate the time at which drug responses start, the time they are most intense, and the time they cease. Because the four pharmacokinetic processes—absorption, distribution, metabolism, and excretion—determine how much drug will be at its sites of action at any given time, these processes are the major determinants of the time course over which drug responses take place.

Plasma Drug Levels

In most cases, the time course of drug action bears a direct relationship to the concentration of a drug in the blood. Hence, before discussing the time course per se, we need to review several important concepts related to plasma drug levels.

Clinical Significance of Plasma Drug Levels

Providers frequently monitor plasma drug levels in efforts to regulate drug responses. When measurements indicate that drug levels are inappropriate, these levels can be adjusted up or down by changing dosage size, dosage timing, or both.

The practice of regulating plasma drug levels to control drug responses should seem a bit odd, given that (1) drug responses are related to drug concentrations at sites of action and (2) the site of action of most drugs is not in the blood. More often than not, it is a practical impossibility to measure drug concentrations at sites of action. Experience has shown that, for most drugs, *there is a direct correlation between therapeutic and toxic responses and the amount of drug present in plasma.* Therefore, although we cannot usually measure drug concentrations at sites of action, we *can* determine plasma drug concentrations that, in turn, are highly predictive of therapeutic and toxic responses. Accordingly, the dosing objective is commonly spoken of in terms of achieving a specific plasma level of a drug.

Two Plasma Drug Levels Defined

Two plasma drug levels are of special importance: (1) the minimum effective concentration, and (2) the toxic concentration. These levels are depicted in Fig. 4.8.

Minimum Effective Concentration

The minimum effective concentration (MEC) is defined as *the plasma drug level below which therapeutic effects will not occur.* Hence, to be of benefit, a drug must be present in concentrations at or above the MEC.

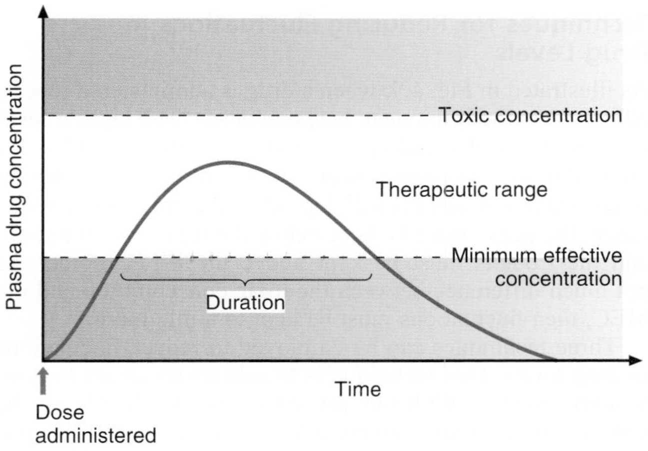

Figure 4.8 ■ Single-dose time course.

Toxic Concentration

Toxicity occurs when plasma drug levels climb too high. The plasma level at which toxic effects begin is termed the *toxic concentration.* Doses must be kept small enough so that the toxic concentration is not reached.

Therapeutic Range

As indicated in Fig. 4.8, there is a range of plasma drug levels, falling between the MEC and the toxic concentration, which is termed the *therapeutic range.* When plasma levels are within the therapeutic range, there is enough drug present to produce therapeutic responses but not so much that toxicity results. *The objective of drug dosing is to maintain plasma drug levels within the therapeutic range.*

The width of the therapeutic range is a major determinant of the ease with which a drug can be used safely. Drugs that have a narrow therapeutic range are difficult to administer safely. Conversely, drugs that have a wide therapeutic range can be administered safely with relative ease. The principle is the same as that of the therapeutic index discussed in Chapter 3. The therapeutic range is quantified, or measured, by the therapeutic index.

Understanding the concept of therapeutic range can facilitate patient care. Because drugs with a narrow therapeutic range are more dangerous than drugs with a wide therapeutic range, patients taking drugs with a narrow therapeutic range are the most likely to require intervention for drug-related complications. The provider who is aware of this fact can focus additional attention on monitoring these patients for signs and symptoms of toxicity.

Single-Dose Time Course

Fig. 4.8 shows how plasma drug levels change over time after a single dose of an oral medication. Drug levels rise as the medicine undergoes absorption. Drug levels then decline as metabolism and excretion eliminate the drug from the body.

Because responses cannot occur until plasma drug levels have reached the MEC, there is a latent period between drug administration and onset of effects. The extent of this delay is determined by the rate of absorption.

The duration of effects is determined largely by the combination of metabolism and excretion. As long as drug levels remain above the MEC, therapeutic responses will be maintained; when levels fall below the MEC, benefits will cease. Because metabolism and excretion are the processes most responsible for causing plasma drug levels to fall, these processes are the primary determinants of how long drug effects will persist.

Drug Half-Life

Before proceeding to the topic of multiple dosing, we need to discuss the concept of half-life. When a patient ceases drug use, the combination of metabolism and excretion will cause the amount of drug in the body to decline. The half-life of a drug is an index of just how rapidly that decline occurs for most drugs. (The concept of half-life does not apply to the elimination of all drugs. A few agents, most notably ethanol (alcohol), leave the body at a *constant rate,* regardless of how much is present. The implications of this kind of decline for ethanol are discussed in Chapter 31.

Drug half-life is defined as *the time required for the amount of drug in the body to decrease by 50%.* A few drugs have half-lives that are extremely short—on the order of minutes or less. In contrast, the half-lives of some drugs exceed 1 week.

Note that, in our definition of half-life, a *percentage*—not a specific *amount*—of drug is lost during one half-life. That is, the half-life does not specify, for example, that 2 g or 18 mg will leave the body in a given time. Rather, the half-life tells us that, no matter what the amount of drug in the body may be, half (50%) will leave during a specified period of time (the half-life). The actual amount of drug that is lost during one half-life depends on just how much drug is present: the more drug in the body, the larger the amount lost during one half-life.

The concept of half-life is best understood through an example. Morphine provides a good illustration. The half-life of morphine is approximately 3 hours. By definition, this means that body stores of morphine will decrease by 50% every 3 hours—regardless of how much morphine is in the body. If there are 50 mg of morphine in the body, 25 mg (50% of 50 mg) will be lost in 3 hours; if there are only 2 mg of morphine in the body, only 1 mg (50% of 2 mg) will be lost in 3 hours. Note that, in both cases, morphine levels drop by 50% during an interval of one half-life. However, the actual *amount* lost is larger when total body stores of the drug are higher.

The half-life of a drug determines the dosing interval (i.e., how much time separates each dose). For drugs with a short half-life, the dosing interval must be correspondingly short. If a long dosing interval is used, drug levels will fall below the MEC between doses, and therapeutic effects will be lost. Conversely, if a drug has a long half-life, a long time can separate doses without loss of benefits.

Drug Levels Produced With Repeated Doses

Multiple dosing leads to drug accumulation. When a patient takes a single dose of a drug, plasma levels simply go up and then come back down. In contrast, when a patient takes repeated doses of a drug, the process is more complex and results in drug accumulation. The factors that determine the rate and extent of accumulation are considered next.

The Process by Which Plateau Drug Levels Are Achieved

Administering repeated doses will cause a drug to build up in the body until a *plateau* (steady level) has been achieved. What causes drug levels to reach plateau? If a second dose of a drug is administered before all of the prior dose has been eliminated, total body stores of that drug will be higher after the second dose than after the initial dose. As succeeding doses are administered, drug levels will climb even higher. The drug will continue to accumulate until a state has been achieved in which the amount of drug eliminated between doses equals the amount administered. *When the amount of drug eliminated between doses equals the dose administered, average drug levels will remain constant and plateau will have been reached* (Fig. 4.9).

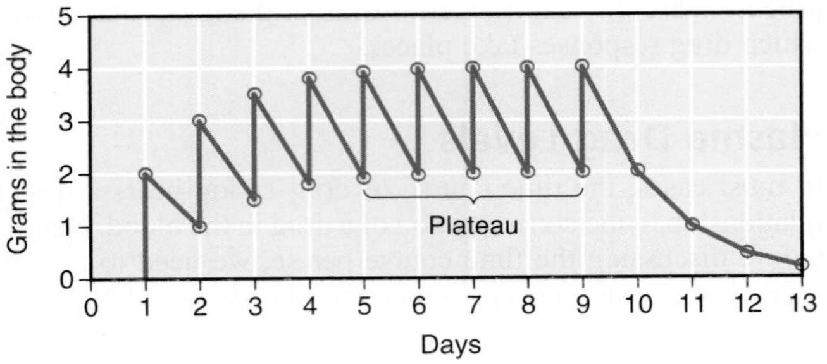

Figure 4.9 ■ Drug accumulation with repeated administration.
The drug has a half-life of 1 day. The dosing schedule is 2 g given once a day on days 1 through 9. Note that plateau is reached at about the beginning of day 5 (i.e., after four half-lives). Note also that, when administration is discontinued, it takes about 4 days (four half-lives) for most (94%) of the drug to leave the body.

Time to Plateau

When a drug is administered repeatedly in the same dose, *plateau will be reached in approximately four half-lives.* For the hypothetical agent illustrated in Fig. 4.9, total body stores approached their peak near the beginning of day 5, or approximately 4 full days after treatment began. Because the half-life of this drug is 1 day, reaching plateau in 4 days is equivalent to reaching plateau in four half-lives.

As long as dosage remains constant, the time required to reach plateau is independent of dosage size. Put another way, the time required to reach plateau when giving repeated large doses of a particular drug is identical to the time required to reach plateau when giving repeated small doses of that drug. Referring to the drug in Fig. 4.9, just as it took four half-lives (4 days) to reach plateau when a dose of 2 g was administered daily, it would also take four half-lives to reach plateau if a dose of 4 g were administered daily. It is true that the *height* of the plateau would be greater if a 4-g dose were given, but the time required to reach plateau would not be altered by the increase in dosage. To confirm this statement, substitute a dose of 4 g in the previous exercise and see when plateau is reached.

Techniques for Reducing Fluctuations in Drug Levels

As illustrated in Fig. 4.9, when a drug is administered repeatedly, its level will fluctuate between doses. The highest level is referred to as the *peak concentration,* and the lowest level is referred to as the *trough concentration.* The acceptable height of the peaks and troughs will depend on the drug's therapeutic range: the peaks must be kept below the toxic concentration, and the troughs must be kept above the MEC. If there is not much difference between the toxic concentration and the MEC, then fluctuations must be kept to a minimum.

Three techniques can be employed to reduce fluctuations in drug levels. One technique is to *administer drugs by continuous infusion.* With this procedure, plasma levels can be kept nearly constant. Another is to *administer a depot preparation,* which releases the drug slowly and steadily. The third is to *reduce both the size of each dose and the dosing interval* (keeping the total daily dose constant). For example, rather than giving the drug from Fig. 4.9 in 2-g doses once every 24 hours, we could give this drug in 1-g doses every 12 hours. With this altered dosing schedule, the total daily dose would remain unchanged, as would total body stores at plateau. However, instead of fluctuating over a range of 2 g between doses, levels would fluctuate over a range of 1 g.

Loading Doses Versus Maintenance Doses

As discussed previously, if we administer a drug in repeated doses of *equal size,* an interval equivalent to about four half-lives is required to achieve plateau. When plateau must be achieved more quickly, a large initial dose can be administered. This large initial dose is called a *loading dose.* After high drug levels have been established with a loading dose, plateau can be maintained by giving smaller doses. These smaller doses are referred to as *maintenance doses.*

The claim that use of a loading dose will shorten the time to plateau may appear to contradict an earlier statement, which said that the time to plateau is not affected by dosage size. However, there is no contradiction. For any *specified dosage,* it will always take about four half-lives to reach plateau. When a loading dose is administered followed by maintenance doses, the plateau is not reached *for the loading dose.* Rather, we have simply used the loading dose to rapidly produce a drug level equivalent to the plateau level for a smaller dose. To achieve plateau level for the loading dose, it would be necessary to either administer repeated doses equivalent to the loading dose for a period of four half-lives or administer a dose even larger than the original loading dose.

Decline From Plateau

When drug administration is discontinued, most (94%) of the drug in the body will be eliminated over an interval equal to about four half-lives. The time required for drugs to leave the body is important when toxicity develops. If a drug has a short half-life, body stores will decline rapidly, thereby making management of overdose less difficult. When an overdose of a drug with a long half-life occurs, however, toxic levels of the drug will remain in the body for a long time. Additional management may be needed in these instances.

PHARMACODYNAMICS

Pharmacodynamics is the study of the biochemical and physiologic effects of drugs on the body and the molecular mechanisms by which those effects are produced. To participate rationally in achieving the therapeutic objective, an understanding of pharmacodynamics is essential.

DOSE-RESPONSE RELATIONSHIPS

The dose-response relationship (i.e., the relationship between the size of an administered dose and the intensity of the response produced) is a fundamental concern in therapeutics. Dose-response relationships determine the minimal amount of drug needed to elicit a response, the maximal response a drug can elicit, and how much to increase the dosage to produce the desired increase in response.

Basic Features of the Dose-Response Relationship

The basic characteristics of dose-response relationships are illustrated in Fig. 4.10. Part A shows dose-response data plotted on *linear* coordinates. Part B shows the same data plotted on *semilogarithmic* coordinates (i.e., the scale on which dosage is plotted is logarithmic rather than linear). The most obvious and important characteristic revealed by these curves is that the dose-response relationship is *graded.* That is, as the dosage increases, the response becomes progressively larger. Because drug responses are graded, therapeutic effects can be adjusted to fit the needs of each patient by raising or lowering the dosage until a response of the desired intensity is achieved.

As indicated in Fig. 4.10, the dose-response relationship can be viewed as having three phases. Phase 1 (see Fig. 4.10B) occurs at low doses. The curve is flat during this phase because doses are too low to elicit a measurable response. During phase 2, an increase in dose elicits a corresponding increase in the response. This is the phase during which the dose-response relationship is graded. As the dose goes higher, eventually a point is reached where an increase in dose is unable to elicit a further increase in response. At this point, the curve flattens out into phase 3.

Maximal Efficacy and Relative Potency

Dose-response curves reveal two characteristic properties of drugs: *maximal efficacy* and *relative potency.* Curves that reflect these properties are shown in Fig. 4.11.

Maximal Efficacy

Maximal efficacy is defined as *the largest effect that a drug can produce.* Maximal efficacy is indicated by the *height* of the dose-response curve.

The concept of maximal efficacy is illustrated by the dose-response curves for meperidine [Demerol] and pentazocine [Talwin], two morphine-like pain relievers (see Fig. 4.11A). As you can see, the curve for pentazocine levels off at a maximal height below that of the curve for meperidine. This tells us that the maximal degree of pain relief we can achieve with pentazocine is smaller than the maximal degree of pain relief we can achieve with meperidine. Put another way, no matter how much pentazocine we administer, we can never produce the degree of pain relief that we can with meperidine. Accordingly, we would say that meperidine has greater maximal efficacy than pentazocine.

Despite what intuition might tell us, a drug with very high maximal efficacy is not always more desirable than a drug with lower efficacy. Recall that we want to match the intensity of the response to the patient's needs. This may be difficult to do with a drug that produces extremely intense responses. For example, certain diuretics (e.g., furosemide) have such high maximal efficacy that they can cause dehydration. If we only want to mobilize a modest volume of water, a diuretic with lower maximal efficacy (e.g., hydrochlorothiazide) would be preferred. Similarly, in a patient with a mild headache, we

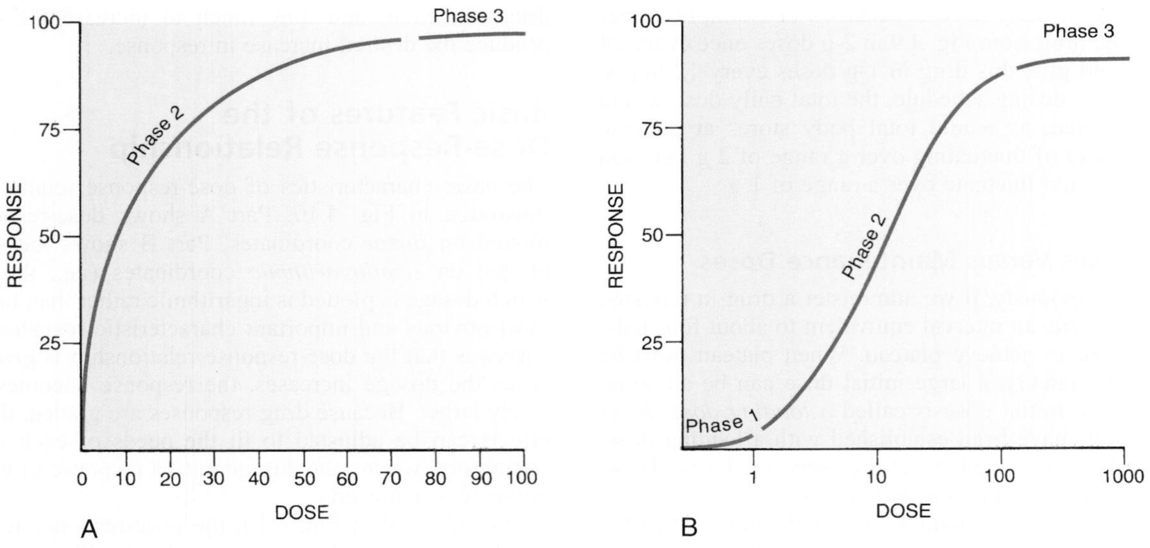

Figure 4.10 ▪ Basic components of the dose-response curve.
A, A dose-response curve with dose plotted on a linear scale. **B,** The same dose-response relationship shown in **A** but with the dose plotted on a logarithmic scale. Note the three phases of the dose-response curve: ***Phase 1,*** The curve is relatively flat; doses are too low to elicit a significant response. ***Phase 2,*** The curve climbs upward as bigger doses elicit correspondingly bigger responses. ***Phase 3,*** The curve levels off; bigger doses are unable to elicit a further increase in response. (Phase 1 is not indicated in **A** because very low doses cannot be shown on a linear scale.)

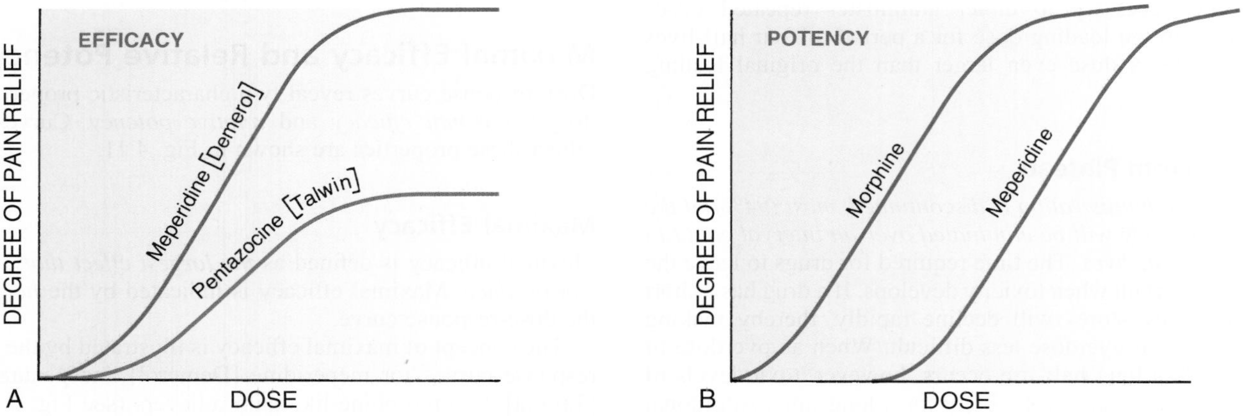

Figure 4.11 ▪ Dose-response curves demonstrating efficacy and potency.
A, Efficacy, or maximal efficacy, is an index of the maximal response a drug can produce. The efficacy of a drug is indicated by the height of its dose-response curve. In this example, meperidine has greater efficacy than pentazocine. Efficacy is an important quality in a drug. **B,** Potency is an index of how much drug must be administered to elicit a desired response. In this example, achieving pain relief with meperidine requires higher doses than with morphine. We would say that morphine is more potent than meperidine. Note that, if administered in sufficiently high doses, meperidine can produce just as much pain relief as morphine. Potency is usually not an important quality in a drug.

would not select a powerful analgesic (e.g., morphine) for relief. Rather, we would select an analgesic with lower maximal efficacy, such as aspirin.

Relative Potency

The term *potency* refers to the amount of drug we must give to elicit an effect. Potency is indicated by the relative position of the dose-response curve along the *x* (dose) axis.

The concept of potency is illustrated by the curves in Fig. 4.11B. These curves plot doses for two analgesics—morphine and meperidine—versus the degree of pain relief achieved. As you can see, for any particular degree of pain relief, the required dose of meperidine is larger than the required dose of morphine. Because morphine produces pain relief at lower doses than meperidine, we would say that morphine is more potent than meperidine. That is, a potent drug is one that produces its effects at low doses.

Potency is rarely an important characteristic of a drug. The only consequence of having greater potency is that a drug with greater potency can be given in smaller doses.

It is important to note that the potency of a drug implies nothing about its maximal efficacy! Potency and efficacy are completely independent qualities. Drug A can be more effective than drug B even though drug B may be more potent. Also, drugs A and B can be equally effective even though one may be more potent. As we saw in Fig. 4.11B, although meperidine happens to be less potent than morphine, the maximal degree of pain relief that we can achieve with these drugs is identical.

A final comment on the word *potency* is in order. In everyday parlance, people tend to use the word *potent* to express the pharmacologic concept of effectiveness. That is, when most people say, "This drug is very potent," what they mean is, "This drug produces powerful effects." They do not mean, "This drug produces its effects at low doses." In pharmacology, we use the words *potent* and *potency* with the specific and appropriate terminology.

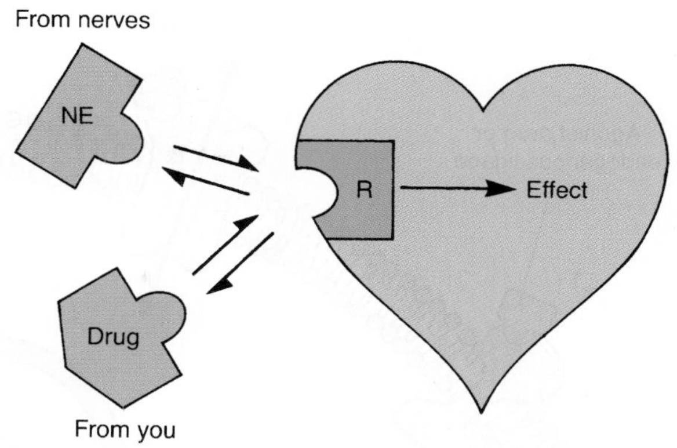

Figure 4.12 ▪ Interaction of drugs with receptors for norepinephrine.
Under physiologic conditions, cardiac output can be increased by the binding of norepinephrine (NE) to receptors (R) on the heart. Norepinephrine is supplied to these receptors by nerves. These same receptors can be acted on by drugs, which can either mimic the actions of endogenous NE (and thereby increase cardiac output) or block the actions of endogenous NE (and thereby reduce cardiac output).

DRUG-RECEPTOR INTERACTIONS

Introduction to Drug Receptors

Drugs produce their effects by interacting with other chemicals. Receptors are the special chemical sites in the body that most drugs interact with to produce effects.

We can define a receptor as *any functional macromolecule in a cell to which a drug binds to produce its effects.* However, although the formal definition of a receptor encompasses all functional macromolecules, the term *receptor* is generally reserved for the body's own receptors for hormones, neurotransmitters, and other regulatory molecules. The other macromolecules to which drugs bind, such as enzymes and ribosomes, can be thought of simply as target molecules, rather than as true receptors.

Binding of a drug to its receptor is usually *reversible.* Receptors are activated by interaction with other molecules (Fig. 4.12). Under physiologic conditions, endogenous compounds (neurotransmitters, hormones, other regulatory molecules) are the molecules that bind to receptors to produce a response. When a drug is the molecule that binds to a receptor, all that it can do is mimic or block the actions of endogenous regulatory molecules. By doing so, the drug will either increase or decrease the rate of the physiologic activity normally controlled by that receptor. Because drug action is limited to mimicking or blocking the body's own regulatory molecules, drugs cannot give cells new functions. In other words, drugs cannot make the body do anything that it is not already capable of doing.[2]

Receptors and Selectivity of Drug Action

Selectivity, the ability to elicit only the response for which a drug is given, is a highly desirable characteristic of a drug, in that the more selective a drug is, the fewer side effects it will produce. Selective drug action is possible in large part because drugs act through specific receptors. There are receptors for each neurotransmitter (e.g., norepinephrine [NE], acetylcholine, dopamine); there are receptors for each hormone (e.g., progesterone, insulin, thyrotropin); and there are receptors for all of the other molecules the body uses to regulate physiologic processes (e.g., histamine, prostaglandins, leukotrienes). As a rule, each type of receptor participates in the regulation of just a few processes (Fig. 4.13). If a drug interacts with only one type of receptor, and if that receptor type regulates just a few processes, then the effects of the drug will be limited. Conversely, if a drug interacts with several different receptor types, then that drug is likely to elicit a wide variety of responses.

How can a drug interact with one receptor type and not with others? In some important ways, a receptor is analogous to a lock and a drug is analogous to a key for that lock: just as only keys with the proper profile can fit a particular lock, only those drugs with the proper size, shape, and physical properties can bind to a particular receptor (Fig. 4.14).

Theories of Drug-Receptor Interaction

In the discussion that follows, we consider two theories of drug-receptor interaction: (1) the simple occupancy theory and (2) the modified occupancy theory. These theories help explain dose-response relationships and the ability of drugs to mimic or block the actions of endogenous regulatory molecules.

Simple Occupancy Theory

The simple occupancy theory of drug-receptor interaction states that (1) the intensity of the response to a drug is proportional to the number of receptors occupied by that drug and (2) a maximal response will occur when *all* available receptors have been occupied. This relationship between

[2]The only exception to this rule is gene therapy. By inserting genes into cells, we actually can make them do something they were previously incapable of doing.

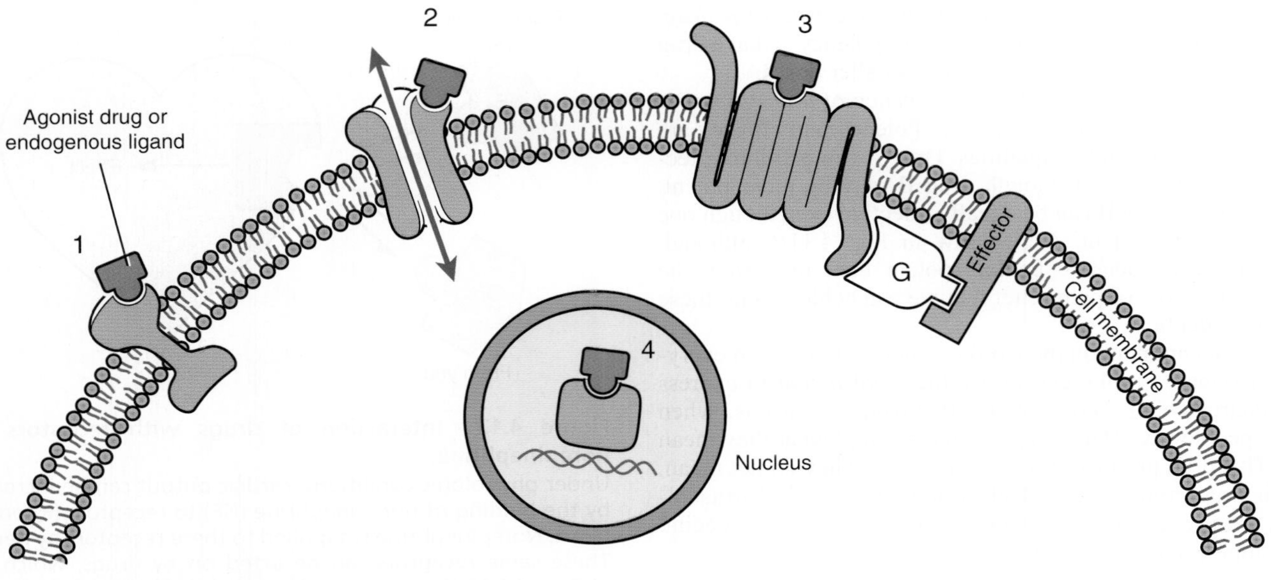

Figure 4.13 ■ The four primary receptor families.
1, Cell membrane–embedded enzyme. **2,** Ligand-gated ion channel. **3,** G protein–coupled receptor system (G, G protein). **4,** Transcription factor. (See text for details.)

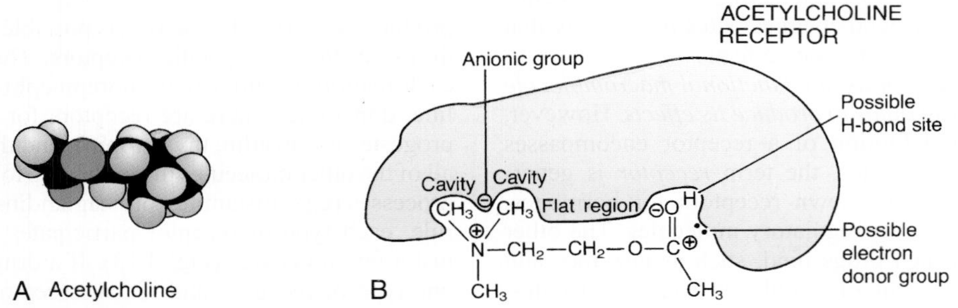

Figure 4.14 ■ Interaction of acetylcholine with its receptor.
A, Three-dimensional model of the acetylcholine molecule. **B,** Binding of acetylcholine to its receptor. Note how the shape of acetylcholine closely matches the shape of the receptor. Note also how the positive charges on acetylcholine align with the negative sites on the receptor.

receptor occupancy and the intensity of the response is depicted in Fig. 4.15.

Although certain aspects of dose-response relationships can be explained by the simple occupancy theory, other important phenomena cannot. Specifically, there is nothing in this theory to explain why one drug should be more potent than another. In addition, this theory cannot explain how one drug can have higher maximal efficacy than another. That is, according to this theory, two drugs acting at the same receptor should produce the same maximal effect, provided that their dosages were high enough to produce 100% receptor occupancy. However, we have already seen this is not true. As illustrated in Fig. 4.11A, there is a dose of pentazocine above which no further increase in response can be elicited. Presumably, all receptors are occupied when the dose-response curve levels off. However, at 100% receptor occupancy, the response elicited by pentazocine is less than that elicited by meperidine. Simple occupancy theory cannot account for this difference.

Modified Occupancy Theory

The modified occupancy theory of drug-receptor interaction explains certain observations that cannot be accounted for with the simple occupancy theory. The modified theory ascribes two qualities to drugs: *affinity* and *intrinsic activity.* The term *affinity* refers to the strength of the attraction between a drug and its receptor. *Intrinsic activity* refers to the ability of a drug to activate the receptor after binding. *Affinity and intrinsic activity are independent properties.*

Affinity

As noted, the term *affinity* refers to the strength of the attraction between a drug and its receptor. Drugs with high affinity are strongly attracted to their receptors. Conversely, drugs with low affinity are weakly attracted.

The affinity of a drug for its receptor is reflected in its *potency.* Because they are strongly attracted to their receptors, drugs with high affinity can bind to their receptors when

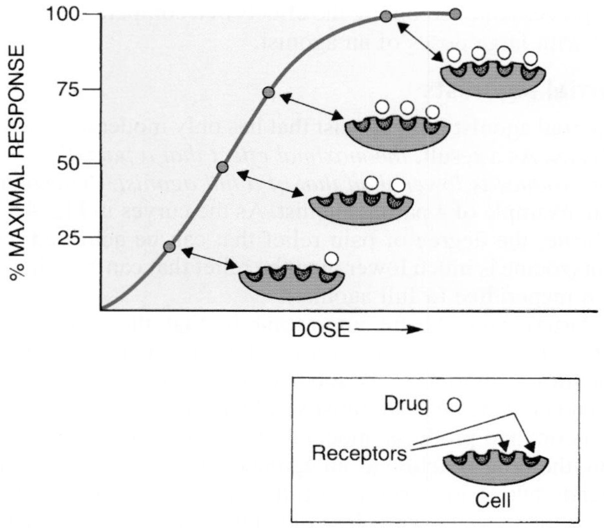

Figure 4.15 ■ Model of simple occupancy theory.
The simple occupancy theory states that the intensity of response to a drug is proportional to the number of receptors occupied; maximal response is reached with 100% receptor occupancy. Because the hypothetical cell in this figure has only four receptors, maximal response is achieved when all four receptors are occupied. (*Note:* Real cells have thousands of receptors.)

present in low concentrations. Because they bind to receptors at low concentrations, drugs with high affinity are effective in low doses. That is, *drugs with high affinity are very potent.* Conversely, drugs with low affinity must be present in high concentrations to bind to their receptors. Accordingly, these drugs are less potent.

Intrinsic Activity

The term *intrinsic activity* refers to the ability of a drug to activate a receptor upon binding. Drugs with high intrinsic activity cause intense receptor activation. Conversely, drugs with low intrinsic activity cause only slight activation.

The intrinsic activity of a drug is reflected in its *maximal efficacy.* Drugs with high intrinsic activity have high maximal efficacy. That is, by causing intense receptor activation, they are able to cause intense responses. Conversely, if intrinsic activity is low, maximal efficacy will be low as well.

It should be noted that, under the modified occupancy theory, the intensity of the response to a drug is still related to the number of receptors occupied. The wrinkle added by the modified theory is that intensity is also related to the ability of the drug to activate receptors after binding has occurred. Under the modified theory, two drugs can occupy the same number of receptors but produce effects of different intensity; the drug with greater intrinsic activity will produce the more intense response.

Agonists, Antagonists, and Partial Agonists

As previously noted, when drugs bind to receptors they can do one of two things: they can either *mimic* the action of endogenous regulatory molecules or they can *block* the action of endogenous regulatory molecules. Drugs that mimic the body's own regulatory molecules are called *agonists.* Drugs that block the actions of endogenous regulators are called *antagonists.* Like agonists, *partial agonists* also mimic the actions of endogenous regulatory molecules, but they produce responses of intermediate intensity.

Agonists

Agonists are molecules that activate receptors. Because neurotransmitters, hormones, and other endogenous regulators activate the receptors to which they bind, all of these compounds are considered agonists. When drugs act as agonists, they simply bind to receptors and mimic the actions of the body's own regulatory molecules. Dobutamine, for example, is a drug that mimics the action of NE at receptors on the heart, thereby causing heart rate and force of contraction to increase.

In terms of the modified occupancy theory, an agonist is a drug that has both *affinity* and *high intrinsic activity.* Affinity allows the agonist to bind to receptors, whereas intrinsic activity allows the bound agonist to activate or turn on receptor function.

Antagonists

Antagonists produce their effects by preventing receptor activation by endogenous regulatory molecules and drugs. Antagonists have virtually no effects of their own on receptor function.

In terms of the modified occupancy theory, an antagonist is a drug with affinity for a receptor but with no intrinsic activity. Affinity allows the antagonist to bind to receptors, but lack of intrinsic activity prevents the bound antagonist from causing receptor activation.

Although antagonists do not cause receptor activation, they most certainly *do* produce pharmacologic effects. Antagonists produce their effects by *preventing the activation of receptors* by endogenous regulatory molecules. Antihistamines, for example, are histamine receptor antagonists that suppress allergy symptoms by binding to receptors for histamine, thereby preventing activation of these receptors by histamine released in response to allergens.

It is important to note that the response to an antagonist is determined by how much *agonist* is present. Because antagonists act by preventing receptor activation, *if there is no agonist present, administration of an antagonist will have no observable effect;* the drug will bind to its receptors, but nothing will happen. On the other hand, if receptors are undergoing activation by agonists, administration of an antagonist will shut the process down, resulting in an observable response. An example is the use of the opioid antagonist naloxone, which is used to block opioid receptors in the event of an opioid overdose.

Antagonists can be subdivided into two major classes: (1) noncompetitive antagonists and (2) competitive antagonists. Most antagonists are competitive.

Noncompetitive (Insurmountable) Antagonists

Noncompetitive antagonists bind *irreversibly* to receptors. The effect of irreversible binding is equivalent to reducing the total number of receptors available for activation by an agonist. Because the intensity of the response to an agonist is proportional to the total number of receptors occupied, and because noncompetitive antagonists decrease the number of receptors available for activation, noncompetitive antagonists *reduce the maximal response* that an agonist can elicit. If sufficient antagonist is present, agonist effects will be blocked completely. Dose-response curves illustrating inhibition by a noncompetitive antagonist are shown in Fig. 4.16A.

Because the binding of noncompetitive antagonists is irreversible, inhibition by these agents cannot be overcome, no matter how much agonist may be available.

Although noncompetitive antagonists bind irreversibly, this does not mean that their effects last forever. Cells are constantly breaking down old receptors and synthesizing new ones. Consequently, the effects of noncompetitive antagonists wear off as the receptors to which they are bound are replaced. Because the life cycle of a receptor can be relatively short, the effects of noncompetitive antagonists m ay subside in a few days. Still, this can be a long time for some functions; therefore, these agents are rarely used therapeutically.

Competitive (Surmountable) Antagonists

Competitive antagonists bind *reversibly* to receptors. As their name implies, competitive antagonists produce receptor blockade by competing with agonists for receptor binding. If an agonist and a competitive antagonist have equal affinity for a particular receptor, then the receptor will be occupied by whichever agent—agonist or antagonist—is present in the highest concentration. If there are more antagonist molecules present than agonist molecules, antagonist molecules will occupy the receptors and receptor activation will be blocked. Conversely, if agonist molecules outnumber the antagonists, receptors will be occupied mainly by the agonist and little inhibition will occur.

Because competitive antagonists bind reversibly to receptors, the inhibition they cause is *surmountable.* In the presence of sufficiently high amounts of agonist, agonist molecules will occupy all receptors and inhibition will be completely overcome. The dose-response curves shown in Fig. 4.16B illustrate the process of overcoming the effects of a competitive antagonist with large doses of an agonist.

Partial Agonists

A partial agonist is an agonist that has only moderate intrinsic activity. As a result, *the maximal effect that a partial agonist can produce is lower than that of a full agonist.* Pentazocine is an example of a partial agonist. As the curves in Fig. 4.11A indicate, the degree of pain relief that can be achieved with pentazocine is much lower than the relief that can be achieved with meperidine (a full agonist).

Partial agonists are interesting in that they can act as *antagonists* as well as *agonists.* For this reason, they are sometimes referred to as agonists-antagonists. For example, when pentazocine is administered by itself, it occupies opioid receptors and produces moderate relief of pain. In this situation, the drug is acting as an agonist. However, if a patient is already taking meperidine (a full agonist at opioid receptors) and is then given a large dose of pentazocine, pentazocine will occupy the opioid receptors and prevent their activation by meperidine. As a result, rather than experiencing the high degree of pain relief that meperidine can produce, the patient will experience only the limited relief that pentazocine can produce. In this situation, pentazocine is acting as both an agonist (producing moderate pain relief) and an antagonist (blocking the higher degree of relief that could have been achieved with meperidine by itself).

Regulation of Receptor Sensitivity

Receptors are dynamic components of the cell. In response to continuous activation or continuous inhibition, the number of receptors on the cell surface can change, as can their sensitivity to agonist molecules. For example, when the receptors of a cell are continually exposed to an *agonist,* the cell usually becomes less responsive. When this occurs, the cell is said to be *desensitized* or *refractory,* or to have

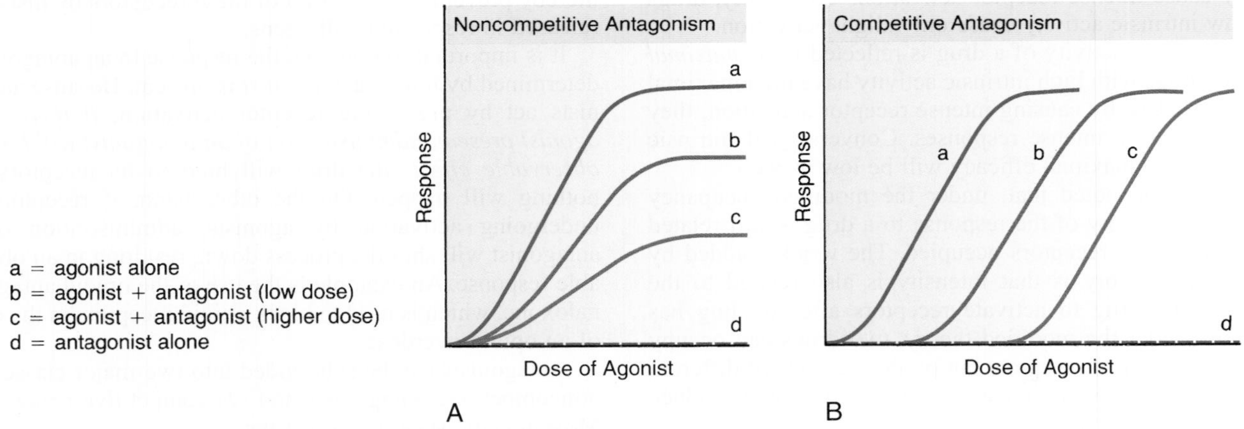

Figure 4.16 ■ Dose-response curves in the presence of competitive and noncompetitive antagonists.
A, Effect of a noncompetitive antagonist on the dose-response curve of an agonist. Note that noncompetitive antagonists decrease the maximal response achievable with an agonist. **B,** Effect of a competitive antagonist on the dose-response curve of an agonist. Note that the maximal response achievable with the agonist is not reduced. Competitive antagonists simply increase the amount of agonist required to produce any given intensity of response.

undergone *downregulation.* Several mechanisms may be responsible, including destruction of receptors by the cell and modification of receptors such that they respond less fully. Continuous exposure to antagonists has the opposite effect, causing the cell to become *hypersensitive* (also referred to as *supersensitive*). One mechanism that can cause hypersensitivity is synthesis of more receptors.

DRUG RESPONSES THAT DO NOT INVOLVE RECEPTORS

Although the effects of most drugs result from drug-receptor interactions, some drugs do not act through receptors. Rather, they act through simple physical or chemical interactions with other small molecules.

Common examples of these drugs include antacids, antiseptics, saline laxatives, and chelating agents. Antacids neutralize gastric acidity by direct chemical interaction with stomach acid. The antiseptic action of ethyl alcohol results from precipitating bacterial proteins. Magnesium sulfate, a powerful laxative, acts by retaining water in the intestinal lumen through an osmotic effect. Dimercaprol, a chelating agent, prevents toxicity from heavy metals (e.g., arsenic, mercury) by forming complexes with these compounds. All of these pharmacologic effects are the result of simple physical or chemical interactions, and not interactions with cellular receptors.

INTERPATIENT VARIABILITY IN DRUG RESPONSES

The dose required to produce a therapeutic response can vary substantially from patient to patient because people differ from one another. In this section we consider interpatient variation as a general issue. The specific kinds of differences that underlie variability in drug responses are discussed in Chapter 6.

To promote the therapeutic objective, you must be alert to interpatient variation in drug responses. Because of interpatient variation, it is not possible to predict exactly how an individual patient will respond to medication. The provider who appreciates the reality of interpatient variability will be better prepared to anticipate, evaluate, and respond appropriately to each patient's therapeutic needs.

Fig. 4.17 illustrates an example of interpatient variability in response to a drug. Fig. 4.17A represents incremental increases in the milligram dose of drug to elevated gastric pH coupled with the number of patients who had a therapeutic response (pH of 5) at each dose. In Fig. 4.17B, these results are plotted on a *frequency distribution curve.* We can see from the curve that a wide range of doses is required to produce the desired response in all subjects. For some subjects, a dose of only 100 mg was sufficient to produce the target response. For other subjects, the therapeutic end point was not achieved until the dose totaled 240 mg.

The ED_{50}

The dose at the middle of the frequency distribution curve is termed the *ED_{50}* (see Fig. 4.17B). (ED_{50} is an abbreviation for *average effective dose.*) The ED_{50} is defined as *the dose that is required to produce a defined therapeutic response in 50% of the population.* In the case of the drug in our example, the ED_{50} was 170 mg—the dose needed to elevate gastric pH to a value of 5 in 50% of the 100 people tested.

The ED_{50} can be considered a standard dose and, as such, is frequently the dose selected for initial treatment. After evaluating a patient's response to this standard dose, we can then adjust subsequent doses up or down to meet the patient's needs.

Dose of Drug (mg)	Number of Subjects Responding at Each Dose
100	2
120	6
140	17
160	25
180	25
200	17
220	6
240	2

A

B

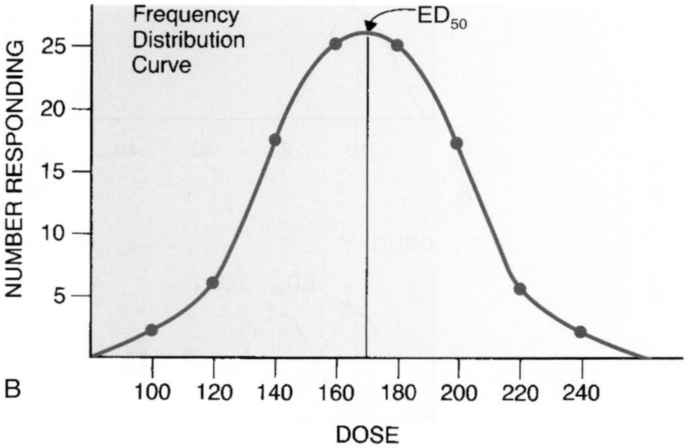

Figure 4.17 ▪ Interpatient variation in drug responses.
A, Data from tests of a hypothetical acid suppressant in 100 patients. The goal of the study is to determine the dosage required by each patient to elevate gastric pH to 5. Note the wide variability in doses needed to produce the target response for the 100 subjects. **B,** Frequency distribution curve for the data in **A.** The dose at the middle of the curve is termed the ED_{50}—the dose that will produce a predefined intensity of response in 50% of the population.

Clinical Implications of Interpatient Variability

Interpatient variation has four important clinical consequences. As a provider you should be aware of these implications:

- The initial dose of a drug is necessarily an approximation. Subsequent doses may need to be fine-tuned based on the patient's response.
- When given an average effective dose (ED_{50}), some patients will be undertreated, whereas others will have received more drug than they need. Accordingly, when therapy is initiated with a dose equivalent to the ED_{50}, it is especially important to evaluate the response. Patients who fail to respond may need an increase in dosage. Conversely, patients who show signs of toxicity will need a dosage reduction.
- Because drug responses are not completely predictable, you must monitor the patient's response for both positive effects and adverse effects to determine whether too much or too little medication has been administered. In other words, dosage should be adjusted on the basis of the patient's response and not just on the basis of clinical guidelines.

THE THERAPEUTIC INDEX

The therapeutic index is a measure of a drug's safety. The therapeutic index is defined as *the ratio of a drug's LD_{50} to its ED_{50}*. (The LD_{50}, or average lethal dose, is the dose that is lethal to 50% of the subjects treated.) A large (or high or wide) therapeutic index indicates that a drug is relatively safe. Conversely, a small (or low or narrow) therapeutic index indicates that a drug is relatively unsafe.

The concept of therapeutic index is illustrated by the frequency distribution curves in Fig. 4.18. Part A of the figure shows curves for therapeutic and lethal responses to drug X. Part B shows equivalent curves for drug Y. As you can see in Fig. 4.18A, the average lethal dose (100 mg) for drug X is much larger than the average therapeutic dose (10 mg). Because this drug's lethal dose is much larger than its therapeutic dose, common sense tells us that the drug should be relatively safe. The safety of this drug is reflected in its high therapeutic index, which is 10. In contrast, drug Y is unsafe. As shown in Fig. 4.18B, the average lethal dose for drug Y (20 mg) is only twice the average therapeutic dose (10 mg). Hence, for drug Y, a dose only twice the ED_{50} could be lethal to 50% of those treated. Clearly, drug Y is not safe. This lack of safety is reflected in its low therapeutic index.

The curves for drug Y illustrate a phenomenon that is even more important than the therapeutic index. As you can see, there is *overlap* between the curve for therapeutic effects and the curve for lethal effects. This overlap tells us that the high doses needed to produce therapeutic effects in some people may be large enough to cause death in others. The message here is that, if a drug is to be truly safe, the highest dose required to produce therapeutic effects must be substantially lower than the lowest dose required to produce death.

DRUG INTERACTION

DRUG-DRUG INTERACTIONS

Drug-drug interactions can occur whenever a patient takes two or more drugs. Some interactions are both intended and desired, as when we combine drugs to treat hypertension. In contrast, some interactions are both unintended and undesired.

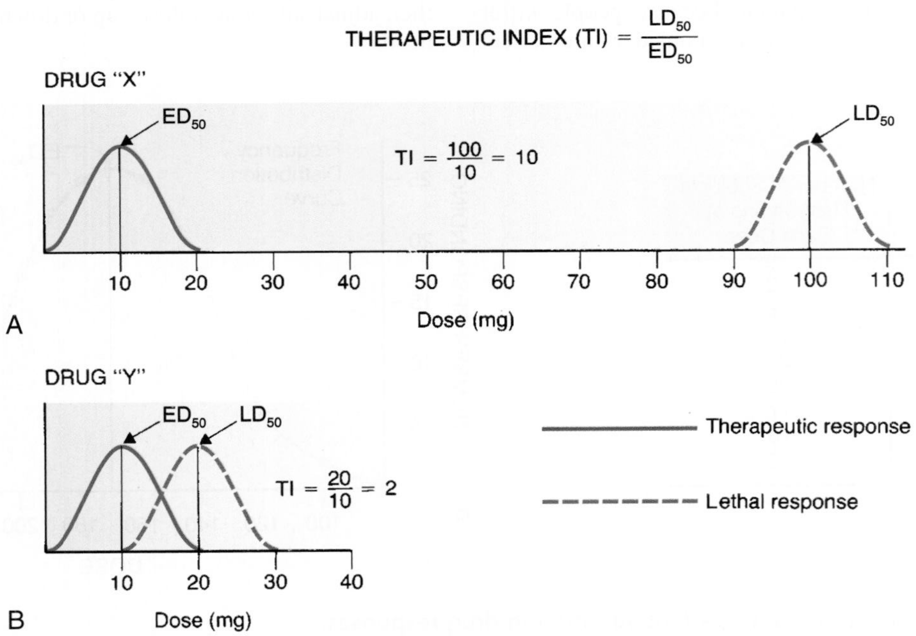

Figure 4.18 ■ The therapeutic index.
A, Frequency distribution curves indicating the ED_{50} and LD_{50} for drug X. Because its LD_{50} is much greater than its ED_{50}, drug X is relatively safe. **B,** Frequency distribution curves indicating the ED_{50} and LD_{50} for drug Y. Because its LD_{50} is very close to its ED_{50}, drug Y is not very safe. Also note the overlap between the effective-dose curve and the lethal-dose curve.

Consequences of Drug-Drug Interactions

When two drugs interact, there are three possible outcomes: (1) one drug may intensify the effects of the other, (2) one drug may reduce the effects of the other, or (3) the combination may produce a new response not seen with either drug alone.

Intensification of Effects

When one drug intensifies, or potentiates, the effects of the other, this type of interaction is often termed *potentiative.* Potentiative interactions may be beneficial or detrimental.

Increased Therapeutic Effects

The interaction between sulbactam and ampicillin represents a beneficial potentiative interaction. When administered alone, ampicillin undergoes rapid inactivation by bacterial enzymes. Sulbactam inhibits those enzymes and thereby prolongs and intensifies ampicillin's therapeutic effects.

Increased Adverse Effects

The interaction between aspirin and warfarin represents a potentially detrimental potentiative interaction. Both aspirin and warfarin suppress formation of blood clots; aspirin does this through antiplatelet activity, and warfarin does this through anticoagulant activity. As a result, if aspirin and warfarin are taken concurrently, the risk for bleeding is significantly increased.

Reduction of Effects

Interactions that result in reduced drug effects are often termed *inhibitory.* As with potentiative interactions, inhibitory interactions can be beneficial or detrimental. Inhibitory interactions that reduce toxicity are beneficial. Conversely, inhibitory interactions that reduce therapeutic effects are detrimental.

Reduced Therapeutic Effects

The interaction between propranolol and albuterol represents a detrimental inhibitory interaction. Albuterol is taken by people with asthma to dilate the bronchi. Propranolol, a drug for cardiovascular disorders, can act in the lung to block the effects of albuterol. Hence, if propranolol and albuterol are taken together, propranolol can reduce albuterol's therapeutic effects.

Reduced Adverse Effects

The use of naloxone to treat morphine overdose is an excellent example of a beneficial inhibitory interaction. When administered in excessive dosage, morphine can produce coma, profound respiratory depression, and eventual death. Naloxone blocks morphine's actions and can completely reverse all symptoms of toxicity.

Creation of a Unique Response

Rarely, the combination of two drugs produces a new response not seen with either agent alone. To illustrate, let's consider the combination of alcohol with disulfiram [Antabuse], a drug used to treat alcoholism. When alcohol and disulfiram are combined, a host of unpleasant and dangerous responses can result; however, these effects do not occur when disulfiram or alcohol is used alone.

Basic Mechanisms of Drug-Drug Interactions

Drugs can interact through four basic mechanisms: (1) direct chemical or physical interaction, (2) pharmacokinetic interaction, (3) pharmacodynamic interaction, and (4) combined toxicity.

Direct Chemical or Physical Interactions

Some drugs, because of their physical or chemical properties, can undergo direct interaction with other drugs. Direct physical and chemical interactions usually render both drugs inactive.

Direct interactions occur most commonly when drugs are combined in IV solutions. Frequently, the interaction produces a precipitate; however, direct drug interactions may not always leave visible evidence. Hence you cannot rely on simple inspection to reveal all direct interactions. Because drugs can interact in solution, *it is essential to consider and verify drug incompatibilities when ordering medications.*

The same kinds of interactions that can take place when drugs are mixed together in an IV solution can also occur when incompatible drugs are taken by other routes. However, because drugs are diluted in body water after administration, and because dilution decreases chemical interactions, significant interactions within the patient are much less likely than in IV solutions.

Pharmacokinetic Interactions

Drug interactions can affect all four of the basic pharmacokinetic processes. That is, when two drugs are taken together, one may alter the absorption, distribution, metabolism, or excretion of the other.

Altered Absorption

Drug absorption may be enhanced or reduced by drug interactions. There are several mechanisms by which one drug can alter the absorption of another.

- By elevating gastric pH, antacids can decrease the ionization of basic drugs in the stomach, increasing the ability of basic drugs to cross membranes and be absorbed. Antacids have the opposite effect on acidic drugs.
- Laxatives can reduce absorption of other oral drugs by accelerating their passage through the intestine.
- Drugs that depress peristalsis (e.g., morphine, atropine) prolong drug transit time in the intestine, thereby increasing the time for absorption.
- Drugs that induce vomiting can decrease absorption of oral drugs.
- Orally administered adsorbent drugs that do not undergo absorption (e.g., cholestyramine) can adsorb other drugs onto themselves, thereby preventing absorption of the other drugs into the blood.
- Drugs that reduce regional blood flow can reduce absorption of other drugs from that region. For example, when epinephrine is injected together with a local anesthetic, the epinephrine causes local vasoconstriction, thereby reducing regional blood flow and delaying absorption of the anesthetic.

Altered Distribution

There are two principal mechanisms by which one drug can alter the distribution of another: (1) competition for protein binding and (2) alteration of extracellular pH.

Competition for Protein Binding. When two drugs bind to the same site on plasma albumin, coadministration of those drugs produces competition for binding. As a result, binding of one or both agents is reduced, causing plasma levels of free drug to rise. In theory, the increase in free drug can intensify effects. However, because the newly freed drug usually undergoes rapid elimination, the increase in plasma levels of free drug is rarely sustained or significant unless the patient has liver problems that interfere with drug metabolism or has renal problems that interfere with drug excretion.

Alteration of Extracellular pH. A drug with the ability to change extracellular pH can alter the distribution of other drugs. For example, if a drug were to increase extracellular pH, that drug would increase the ionization of acidic drugs in extracellular fluids (i.e., plasma and interstitial fluid). As a result, acidic drugs would be drawn from within cells (where the pH was below that of the extracellular fluid) into the extracellular space. Hence, the alteration in pH would change drug distribution.

The ability of drugs to alter pH and thereby alter the distribution of other drugs can be put to practical use in the management of poisoning. For example, symptoms of aspirin toxicity can be reduced with sodium bicarbonate, a drug that elevates extracellular pH. By increasing the pH outside cells, bicarbonate causes aspirin to move from intracellular sites into the interstitial fluid and plasma, thereby minimizing injury to cells.

Altered Metabolism

Altered metabolism is one of the most important—and most complex—mechanisms by which drugs interact. Some drugs *increase* the metabolism of other drugs, and some drugs *decrease* the metabolism of other drugs. Drugs that increase the metabolism of other drugs do so by inducing synthesis of hepatic drug-metabolizing enzymes. Drugs that decrease the metabolism of other drugs do so by inhibiting those enzymes.

As discussed earlier in this chapter, the majority of drug metabolism is catalyzed by the cytochrome P450 enzymes, which are composed of a large number of isoenzyme families (CYP1, CYP2, and CYP3) that are further divided into specific forms. Five isoenzyme forms are responsible for the metabolism of most drugs: CYP1A2, CYP2C9, CYP2C19, CYP2D6, and CYP3A4. Table 4.2 lists major drugs that are metabolized by each isoenzyme and indicates drugs that can inhibit or induce those isoenzymes.

Induction of CYP Enzymes

In our discussion of metabolism earlier in the chapter, you learned about induction of CYP enzymes.

When it is essential that an inducing agent is taken with another medicine, dosage of the other medicine may need adjustment. For example, if a woman taking oral contraceptives were to begin taking phenobarbital, induction of drug metabolism by phenobarbital would accelerate metabolism of the contraceptive, thereby lowering its level. If drug metabolism were increased enough, protection against pregnancy would be lost. To maintain contraceptive efficacy, dosage of the contraceptive should be increased. Conversely, when a patient *discontinues* an inducing agent, dosages of other drugs may need to be *lowered.* If dosage is not reduced, drug levels may climb dangerously high as rates of hepatic metabolism decline to their baseline (noninduced) values.

Inhibition of CYP Enzymes

If drug A inhibits the metabolism of drug B, then levels of drug B will rise. The result may be beneficial or harmful. The interactions of ketoconazole (an antifungal drug) and cyclosporine (an expensive immunosuppressant) provide an interesting case in point. Ketoconazole inhibits CYP3A4, the CYP isoenzyme that metabolizes cyclosporine. If ketoconazole is combined with cyclosporine, the serum drug level of cyclosporine will rise. In this instance inhibition of CYP3A4 allows us to achieve therapeutic drug levels at lower doses, thereby greatly reducing the cost of treatment.

Although inhibition of drug metabolism can be beneficial, as a rule inhibition has undesirable results. That is, in most cases, when an inhibitor increases the level of another drug, the outcome is toxicity. Accordingly, when a patient is taking an inhibitor along with his or her other medicines, you should be alert for possible adverse effects. Unfortunately, because the number of possible interactions of this type is large, keeping track is a challenge. The safest practice is to check for drug interactions in one of the reliable software applications that are widely available.

Altered Renal Excretion

Drugs can alter all three phases of renal excretion: filtration, reabsorption, and active secretion. By doing so, one drug can alter the renal excretion of another. Glomerular filtration can be decreased by drugs that reduce cardiac output: a reduction in cardiac output decreases renal perfusion, which decreases drug filtration at the glomerulus, which in turn decreases the rate of drug excretion. By altering urinary pH, one drug can alter the ionization of another and thereby increase or decrease the extent to which that drug undergoes passive tubular reabsorption. Finally, competition between two drugs for active tubular secretion can decrease the renal excretion of both agents.

Interactions That Involve P-Glycoprotein

As discussed previously in this chapter, PGP is a transmembrane protein that transports a wide variety of drugs *out* of cells, including cells of the intestinal epithelium, placenta, BBB, liver, and kidney tubules. Like P450 isoenzymes, PGP is subject to induction and inhibition by drugs. In fact (and curiously), most of the drugs that induce or inhibit P450 have the same effect on PGP. Drugs that *induce* PGP can have the following effects on other drugs:

- *Reduced absorption*—by increasing drug export from cells of the intestinal epithelium into the intestinal lumen
- *Reduced fetal drug exposure*—by increasing drug export from placental cells into the maternal blood
- *Reduced brain drug exposure*—by increasing drug export from cells of brain capillaries into the blood
- *Increased drug elimination*—by increasing drug export from liver into the bile and from renal tubular cells into the urine

Drugs that inhibit PGP will have opposite effects.

Pharmacodynamic Interactions

By influencing pharmacodynamic processes, one drug can alter the effects of another. Pharmacodynamic interactions are of two basic types: (1) interactions in which the interacting drugs act at the *same* site and (2) interactions in which the interacting drugs act at *separate* sites. Pharmacodynamic interactions may be potentiative or inhibitory and can be of great clinical significance.

TABLE 4.2 ▪ Drugs That Are Important Substrates, Inhibitors, or Inducers of Specific CYP Isoenzymes

CYP	Substrates	Inhibitors	Inducers
CYP1A2	***CNS Drugs:*** amitriptyline, clomipramine, clozapine, desipramine, duloxetine, fluvoxamine, haloperidol, imipramine, methadone, ramelteon, rasagiline, ropinirole, tacrine ***Others:*** theophylline, tizanidine, warfarin	Acyclovir Ciprofloxacin Ethinyl estradiol Fluvoxamine Isoniazid Norfloxacin Oral contraceptives Zafirlukast Zileuton	Carbamazepine Phenobarbital Phenytoin Primidone Rifampin Ritonavir Tobacco St. John's wort
CYP2C9	Diazepam, phenytoin, ramelteon, voriconazole, warfarin	Amiodarone Azole antifungals Efavirenz Fenofibrate Fluorouracil Fluoxetine Fluvastatin Fluvoxamine Gemfibrozil Isoniazid Leflunomide Zafirlukast	Aprepitant Carbamazepine Phenobarbital Phenytoin Primidone Rifampin Rifapentine Ritonavir St. John's wort
CYP2C19	Citalopram, clopidogrel, methadone, phenytoin, thioridazine, voriconazole	Chloramphenicol Cimetidine Esomeprazole Etravirine Felbamate Fluconazole Fluoxetine Fluvoxamine Isoniazid Ketoconazole Lansoprazole Modafinil Omeprazole Ticlopidine Voriconazole	Carbamazepine Phenobarbital Phenytoin St. John's wort Tipranavir/ritonavir
CYP2D6	***CNS Drugs:*** amitriptyline, atomoxetine, clozapine, desipramine, donepezil, doxepin, duloxetine, fentanyl, haloperidol, iloperidone, imipramine, meperidine, nortriptyline, tetrabenazine, thioridazine, tramadol, trazodone ***Antidysrhythmic Drugs:*** flecainide, mexiletine, propafenone ***Beta Blocker:*** metoprolol *Opioids:* codeine, dextromethorphan, hydrocodone	Amiodarone Cimetidine Darifenacin Darunavir/ritonavir Duloxetine Fluoxetine Methadone Paroxetine Propranolol Quinidine Ritonavir Sertraline Tipranavir/ritonavir	Not an inducible enzyme
CYP3A4	***Antibacterials/Antifungals:*** clarithromycin, erythromycin, ketoconazole, itraconazole, rifabutin, telithromycin, voriconazole ***Anticancer Drugs:*** busulfan, dasatinib, doxorubicin, erlotinib, etoposide, ixabepilone, lapatinib, paclitaxel, pazopanib, romidepsin, sunitinib, tamoxifen, vinblastine, vincristine ***Calcium Channel Blockers:*** amlodipine, felodipine, isradipine, nifedipine, nimodipine, nisoldipine, verapamil ***Drugs for HIV Infection:*** amprenavir, darunavir, etravirine, indinavir, maraviroc, nelfinavir, ritonavir, saquinavir, tipranavir ***Drugs for Erectile Dysfunction:*** sildenafil, tadalafil, vardenafil ***Drugs for Urge Incontinence:*** darifenacin, fesoterodine, solifenacin, tolterodine ***Immunosuppressants:*** cyclosporine, everolimus, sirolimus, tacrolimus ***Opioids:*** alfentanil, alfuzosin, fentanyl, methadone, oxycodone ***Sedative-Hypnotics:*** alprazolam, eszopiclone, midazolam, ramelteon, triazolam ***Statins:*** atorvastatin, lovastatin, simvastatin ***Antidysrhythmics Drugs:*** disopyramide, dronedarone, lidocaine, quinidine ***Others:*** aprepitant, bosentan, cinacalcet, cisapride, colchicine, conivaptan, dihydroergotamine, dronabinol, eplerenone, ergotamine, estrogens, ethosuximide, fluticasone, guanfacine, iloperidone, ondansetron, oral contraceptives, pimozide, ranolazine, saxagliptin, sertraline, silodosin, tiagabine, tolvaptan, trazodone, warfarin	Amiodarone Amprenavir Aprepitant Atazanavir Azole antifungals Chloramphenicol Cimetidine Clarithromycin Conivaptan Cyclosporine Darunavir/ritonavir Delavirdine Diltiazem Dronedarone Erythromycin Fluvoxamine Fosamprenavir Grapefruit juice Indinavir Isoniazid Methylprednisolone Nefazodone Nelfinavir Nicardipine Nifedipine Norfloxacin Pazopanib Prednisone Quinine Quinupristin/dalfopristin Ritonavir Saquinavir Telithromycin Tipranavir/ritonavir Verapamil	Amprenavir Aprepitant Bosentan Carbamazepine Dexamethasone Efavirenz Ethosuximide Etravirine Garlic supplements Nevirapine Oxcarbazepine Phenobarbital Phenytoin Primidone Rifabutin Rifampin Rifapentine Ritonavir St. John's wort

CNS, central nervous system; HIV, human immunodeficiency virus.

Interactions at the Same Receptor

Interactions that occur at the same receptor are almost always *inhibitory*. Inhibition occurs when an antagonist drug blocks access of an agonist drug to its receptor. There are many agonist-antagonist interactions of clinical importance. Some reduce therapeutic effects and are therefore undesirable. Others reduce toxicity and are of obvious benefit. The interaction between naloxone and morphine noted previously is an example of a beneficial inhibitory interaction: by blocking access of morphine to its receptors, naloxone can reverse all symptoms of morphine overdose.

Interactions Resulting From Actions at Separate Sites

Even though two drugs have different mechanisms of action and act at separate sites, if both drugs influence the same physiologic process, then one drug can alter responses produced by the other. Interactions resulting from effects produced at different sites may be potentiative or inhibitory.

The interaction between morphine and diazepam [Valium] illustrates a potentiative interaction resulting from concurrent use of drugs that act at separate sites. Morphine and diazepam are CNS depressants, but these drugs do not share the same mechanism of action. Hence, when these agents are administered together, the ability of each to depress CNS function reinforces the depressant effects of the other. This potentiative interaction can result in profound CNS depression.

The interaction between two diuretics—hydrochlorothiazide and spironolactone—illustrates how the effects of a drug acting at one site can counteract the effects of a second drug acting at a different site. Hydrochlorothiazide acts on the distal convoluted tubule of the nephron to increase excretion of potassium. Acting at a different site in the kidney, spironolactone works to decrease renal excretion of potassium. Consequently, when these two drugs are administered together, the potassium-sparing effects of spironolactone tend to balance the potassium-wasting effects of hydrochlorothiazide, leaving renal excretion of potassium at about the same level it would have been had no drugs been given at all.

Combined Toxicity

If drug A and drug B are both toxic to the same organ, then taking them together will cause more injury than if they were not combined. For example, when we treat tuberculosis with isoniazid and rifampin, both of which are hepatotoxic, the potential to cause liver injury is greater than it would be if we used just one of the drugs. As a rule, drugs with overlapping toxicity are not used together. Unfortunately, when treating tuberculosis, the combination is essential.

Clinical Significance of Drug-Drug Interactions

Clearly, drug interactions have the potential to affect the outcome of therapy. As a result of drug-drug interactions, the intensity of responses may be increased or reduced. Interactions that increase therapeutic effects or reduce toxicity are desirable. Conversely, interactions that reduce therapeutic effects or increase toxicity are detrimental.

Interactions are especially important for drugs that have a narrow therapeutic range. For these agents, an interaction that produces a modest increase in drug levels can cause toxicity. Conversely, an interaction that produces a modest decrease in drug levels can cause therapeutic failure.

Although a large number of important interactions have been documented, many more are yet to be identified. Therefore, if a patient develops unusual symptoms, it is wise to suspect that a drug interaction may be the cause—especially because yet another drug might be given to control the new symptoms.

Minimizing Adverse Drug-Drug Interactions

We can minimize adverse interactions in several ways. The most obvious is to minimize the number of drugs a patient receives. A second and equally important way to avoid detrimental interactions is to take a thorough drug history. A history that identifies all drugs the patient is taking, including illicit and over-the-counter preparations, allows the provider to adjust the regimen accordingly. Additional measures for reducing adverse interactions include adjusting the dosage when an inducer of metabolism is added to or deleted from the regimen, adjusting the timing of administration to minimize interference with absorption, monitoring for early signs of toxicity when combinations of toxic agents cannot be avoided, and being especially vigilant when the patient is taking a drug with a narrow therapeutic range.

DRUG-FOOD INTERACTIONS

Drug-food interactions are both important and poorly understood. They are important because they can result in toxicity or therapeutic failure. They are poorly understood because research has been largely lacking.

Effects of Food on Drug Absorption

Decreased Absorption

Food frequently decreases the *rate* of drug absorption and occasionally decreases the *extent* of absorption. Reducing the rate of absorption merely delays the onset of effects; peak effects are not lowered. In contrast, reducing the extent of absorption reduces the intensity of peak responses.

The interaction between calcium-containing foods and tetracycline antibiotics is a classic example of food reducing drug absorption. Tetracyclines bind with calcium to form an insoluble and nonabsorbable complex. Hence, if tetracyclines are administered with milk products or calcium supplements, absorption is reduced and antibacterial effects may be lost.

High-fiber foods can reduce absorption of some drugs. For example, absorption of digoxin [Lanoxin], used for cardiac disorders, is reduced significantly by wheat bran, rolled oats, and sunflower seeds. This reduced absorption can result in therapeutic failure.

Increased Absorption

With some drugs, food increases the extent of absorption. When this occurs, peak effects are heightened. For example, a high-calorie meal more than doubles the absorption of saquinavir [Invirase], a drug for HIV infection. If saquinavir is taken without food, absorption may be insufficient for antiviral activity.

Effects of Food on Drug Metabolism: The Grapefruit Juice Effect

Grapefruit juice can inhibit the metabolism of certain drugs, thereby raising their blood levels. Four compounds have been identified as the responsible agents: two furanocoumarins (*bergapten* and *6′,7′-dihydroxybergamottin)* and two flavonoids (*naringin* and *naringenin*). This effect is *not* seen with other citrus juices, including orange juice.

Grapefruit juice raises drug levels mainly by inhibiting CYP3A4 metabolism. CYP3A4 is an isoenzyme of cytochrome P450 found in the liver and the intestinal wall. Inhibition of the *intestinal* isoenzyme is much greater than inhibition of the liver isoenzyme. By inhibiting CYP3A4, grapefruit juice decreases the intestinal metabolism of many drugs (Table 4.3) and thereby increases the amount available for absorption. As a result, blood levels of these drugs rise, causing peak effects to be more intense. Because inhibition of CYP3A4 in the liver is minimal, grapefruit juice does not usually affect metabolism of drugs after they have been absorbed. Importantly, grapefruit juice has little or no effect on drugs administered intravenously. Why? Because, with IV administration, intestinal metabolism is not involved. Inhibition of CYP3A4 is dose dependent; the more grapefruit juice the patient drinks, the greater the inhibition.

Inhibition of CYP3A4 persists after grapefruit juice is consumed, so the problem cannot be easily resolved by scheduling medication hours after drinking the juice. In fact, when grapefruit juice is consumed on a regular basis, inhibition can persist up to 3 days after the last drink.

The effects of grapefruit juice vary considerably among patients because levels of CYP3A4 show great individual variation. In patients with very little CYP3A4, inhibition by grapefruit juice may be sufficient to stop metabolism completely. As a result, large increases in drug levels may occur. Conversely, in patients with an abundance of CYP3A4, metabolism may continue more or less normally, despite inhibition by grapefruit juice.

The effects of grapefruit juice also vary considerably among CYP3A4 substrates. In one study, coadministration of grapefruit juice produced a 406% increase in blood levels of the calcium channel blocker felodipine [Plendil]. For some other drugs metabolized by these isoenzymes, the effects are negligible.

The clinical consequences of inhibition may be good or bad. As indicated in Table 4.3, by elevating levels of certain drugs, grapefruit juice can increase the risk for serious toxicity. On the other hand, by increasing levels of two drugs—saquinavir and cyclosporine—grapefruit juice can intensify therapeutic effects to promote positive outcomes.

What should providers do if the drugs they are prescribing can be affected by grapefruit juice? Unless a predictable effect is known or desirable, prudence dictates advising patients to avoid grapefruit juice entirely.

Effects of Food on Drug Toxicity

Drug-food interactions sometimes increase toxicity. The most dramatic example is the interaction between monoamine oxidase (MAO) inhibitors and foods rich in tyramine (e.g.,

TABLE 4.3 ▪ Some Drugs Whose Levels Can Be Increased by Grapefruit Juice

Drug	Indications	Potential Consequences of Increased Drug Levels
Dihydropyridine CCBs: amlodipine, felodipine, nicardipine, nifedipine, nimodipine, nisoldipine	Hypertension; angina pectoris	Toxicity: flushing, headache, tachycardia, hypotension
Nondihydropyridine CCBs: diltiazem, verapamil	Hypertension; angina pectoris	Toxicity: bradycardia, AV heart block, hypotension, constipation
Statins: lovastatin, simvastatin (minimal effect on atorvastatin, fluvastatin, pravastatin, or rosuvastatin)	Cholesterol reduction	Toxicity: headache, GI disturbances, liver and muscle toxicity
Amiodarone	Cardiac dysrhythmias	Toxicity
Caffeine	Prevents sleepiness	Toxicity: restlessness, insomnia, convulsions, tachycardia
Carbamazepine	Seizures; bipolar disorder	Toxicity: ataxia, drowsiness, nausea, vomiting, tremor
Buspirone	Anxiety	Drowsiness, dysphoria
Triazolam	Anxiety; insomnia	Increased sedation
Midazolam	Induction of anesthesia; conscious sedation	Increased sedation
Saquinavir	HIV infection	Increased therapeutic effect
Cyclosporine	Prevents rejection of organ transplants	Increased therapeutic effects; if levels rise too high, renal and hepatic toxicity will occur
Sirolimus and tacrolimus	Prevent rejection of organ transplants	Toxicity
SSRIs: fluoxetine, fluvoxamine, sertraline	Depression	Toxicity: serotonin syndrome
Pimozide	Tourette syndrome	Toxicity: QT prolongation resulting in a life-threatening ventricular dysrhythmia
Praziquantel	Schistosomiasis	Toxicity
Dextromethorphan	Cough	Toxicity
Sildenafil	Erectile dysfunction	Toxicity

AV, atrioventricular; CCBs, calcium channel blockers; GI, gastrointestinal; HIV, human immunodeficiency virus; SSRIs, selective serotonin reuptake inhibitors.

aged cheeses, yeast extracts, Chianti wine). If an MAO inhibitor is combined with these foods, blood pressure can rise to a life-threatening level. To avoid disaster, patients taking MAO inhibitors must be warned about the consequences of consuming tyramine-rich foods and must be given a list of foods to strictly avoid (see Chapter 25). Other drug-food combinations that can increase toxicity include the following:

- Theophylline (an asthma medicine) plus caffeine, which can result in excessive CNS excitation
- Potassium-sparing diuretics (e.g., spironolactone) plus salt substitutes, which can result in dangerously high potassium levels
- Aluminum-containing antacids (e.g., Maalox) plus citrus beverages (e.g., orange juice), which can result in excessive absorption of aluminum

Effects of Food on Drug Action

Although most drug-food interactions concern drug absorption or drug metabolism, food may also (rarely) have a direct effect on drug action. For example, foods rich in vitamin K (e.g., broccoli, Brussels sprouts, cabbage) can reduce the effects of warfarin, an anticoagulant. This occurs because warfarin inhibits vitamin K–dependent clotting factors. Accordingly, when vitamin K is more abundant, warfarin is less able to inhibit the clotting factors, and therapeutic effects decline.

Timing of Drug Administration With Respect to Meals

Administration of drugs at the appropriate time with respect to meals is an important part of drug therapy. As discussed, the absorption of some drugs can be significantly decreased by food, and hence these drugs should be administered on an empty stomach (i.e., at least 1 hour before or 2 hours after a meal). Conversely, the absorption of other drugs can be increased by food, and hence these drugs should be administered with meals.

Many drugs cause stomach upset when taken without food. If food does not significantly reduce their absorption, then these drugs should be administered with meals. However, if food does reduce their absorption, then we have a difficult choice: we can administer them with food and thereby reduce stomach upset, but also reduce absorption—or, we can administer them without food and thereby improve absorption, but also increase stomach upset. Unfortunately, the correct choice is not obvious. The best solution, when possible, may be to select an alternative drug that doesn't upset the stomach.

DRUG-SUPPLEMENT INTERACTIONS

Dietary supplements (herbal medicines and other nonconventional remedies) create the potential for frequent and significant interactions with conventional drugs. Of greatest concern are interactions that reduce beneficial responses to conventional drugs and interactions that increase toxicity. These interactions occur through the same pharmacokinetic and pharmacodynamic mechanisms by which conventional drugs interact with each other. Unfortunately, reliable information about dietary supplements is largely lacking, including information on interactions with conventional agents. Interactions that *have* been well documented are discussed as appropriate throughout this text.

CHAPTER

5

Adverse Drug Reactions and Medication Errors

Jacqueline Rosenjack Burchum, DNSc, FNP-BC, CNE

In this chapter we discuss two related issues of drug safety: (1) adverse drug reactions (ADRs), also known as *adverse drug events*, and (2) medication errors, a major cause of ADRs. We begin with ADRs and then discuss medication errors.

ADVERSE DRUG REACTIONS

An ADR, as defined by the World Health Organization, is any noxious, unintended, and undesired effect that occurs at normal drug doses. Adverse reactions can range in intensity from mildly annoying to life threatening. Among the more mild reactions are drowsiness, nausea, itching, and rash. Severe reactions include potentially fatal conditions such as neutropenia, hepatocellular injury, cardiac dysrhythmias, anaphylaxis, and hemorrhage.

Scope of the Problem

A 2011 statistical brief by the Agency for Healthcare Research and Quality highlighted a dramatic rise in ADRs despite interventions to decrease their incidence. More than 800,000 outpatients sought emergency treatment because of ADRs. Among hospitalized inpatients, 1,735,500 experienced adverse outcomes due to drug reactions and medication errors, and of these, more than 53,800 patients died. Many of these incidences were preventable, but fortunately, when drugs are carefully prescribed and patients are well educated on proper use, many ADRs can be avoided or minimized.

Definitions

Side Effect

A side effect is formally defined as *a nearly unavoidable secondary drug effect produced at therapeutic doses.* Common examples include drowsiness caused by traditional antihistamines and gastric irritation caused by aspirin. Side effects are generally predictable, and their intensity is dose dependent. Some side effects develop soon after drug use starts, whereas others may not appear until a drug has been taken for weeks or months.

Toxicity

The formal definition of toxicity is *the degree of detrimental physiologic effects caused by excessive drug dosing.* Examples include profound respiratory depression from an overdose of morphine and severe hypoglycemia from an overdose of insulin. Although the formal definition of toxicity includes only those severe reactions that occur when dosage is excessive, in everyday language the term *toxicity* has come to mean any severe ADR, regardless of the dose that caused it. For example, when administered in therapeutic doses, many anticancer drugs cause neutropenia, thereby putting the patient at high risk for infection. This neutropenia may be called "toxicity" even though it was produced when dosage was therapeutic.

Allergic Reaction

An allergic reaction is an immune response. For an allergic reaction to occur, there must be prior sensitization of the immune system. After the immune system has been sensitized to a drug, reexposure to that drug can trigger an allergic response. The intensity of allergic reactions can range from mild itching to severe rash to anaphylaxis. Estimates suggest that less than 10% of ADRs are of the allergic type.

The intensity of an allergic reaction is determined primarily by the degree of sensitization of the immune system, not by drug dosage. Put another way, *the intensity of allergic reactions is largely independent of dosage.* As a result, a dose that elicits a very strong reaction in one allergic patient may elicit a very mild reaction in another. Furthermore, because a patient's sensitivity to a drug can change over time, a dose that elicits a mild reaction early in treatment may produce an intense reaction later on.

Very few medications cause severe allergic reactions. In fact, most serious reactions are caused by just one drug family—the *penicillins.* Other drugs noted for causing allergic reactions include the nonsteroidal antiinflammatory drugs (e.g., aspirin) and the sulfonamide group of compounds, which includes certain diuretics, antibiotics, and oral hypoglycemic agents.

Idiosyncratic Effect

An idiosyncratic effect is defined as *an uncommon drug response resulting from a genetic predisposition.* An example of an idiosyncratic effect occurs in people with glucose-6-phosphate dehydrogenase (G6PD) deficiency. G6PD deficiency is an X-linked inherited condition that occurs primarily in people with African and Mediterranean ancestry. When people with G6PD deficiency take drugs such as sulfonamides or aspirin, they develop varying degrees of red blood cell hemolysis, which may become life threatening.

Paradoxical Effect

A paradoxical effect is the opposite of the intended drug response. A common example is the insomnia and excitement that may occur when some children and older adults are given benzodiazepines for sedation.

Iatrogenic Disease

An iatrogenic disease is a disease that occurs as the result of medical care or treatment. The term *iatrogenic disease* is also used to denote *a disease produced by drugs.*

Iatrogenic diseases are nearly identical to naturally occurring diseases. For example, patients taking certain antipsychotic drugs may develop a syndrome whose symptoms closely resemble those of Parkinson disease.

Physical Dependence

Physical dependence is a state in which the body has adapted to drug exposure in such a way that an abstinence syndrome will result if drug use is discontinued. Physical dependence develops during long-term use of certain drugs, such as opioids, alcohol, barbiturates, and amphetamines. The precise nature of the abstinence syndrome is determined by the drug involved.

Although physical dependence is usually associated with opioids, these are not the only dependence-inducing drugs. A variety of other centrally acting drugs (e.g., ethanol, barbiturates, amphetamines) can promote dependence. Furthermore, some drugs that work outside the central nervous system can cause physical dependence of a sort. Because a variety of drugs can cause physical dependence of one type or another, and because withdrawal reactions have the potential for harm, *patients should be warned against abrupt discontinuation of any medication without first consulting a health professional.*

Carcinogenic Effect

The term *carcinogenic effect* refers to the ability of certain medications and environmental chemicals to cause cancers. Fortunately, only a few therapeutic agents are carcinogenic. Ironically, several of the drugs used to *treat* cancer are among those with the greatest carcinogenic potential.

Evaluating drugs for the ability to cause cancer is extremely difficult. Evidence of neoplastic disease may not appear until 20 or more years after initial exposure to a cancer-causing compound.

Teratogenic Effect

A *teratogenic effect* is a drug-induced birth defect. Medicines and other chemicals capable of causing birth defects are called teratogens. Teratogenesis is discussed in Chapter 7.

Organ-Specific Toxicity

Many drugs are toxic to specific organs. Common examples include injury to the kidneys caused by amphotericin B (an antifungal drug), injury to the heart caused by doxorubicin (an anticancer drug), injury to the lungs caused by amiodarone (an antidysrhythmic drug), and injury to the inner ear caused by aminoglycoside antibiotics (e.g., gentamicin). Patients using these drugs should be monitored for signs of developing injury. In addition, patients should be educated about these signs and advised to seek medical attention if they appear.

Two types of organ-specific toxicity deserve special comment. These are (1) injury to the liver and (2) altered cardiac function, as evidenced by a prolonged QT interval on the electrocardiogram. Both are discussed next.

Hepatotoxic Drugs

As some drugs undergo metabolism by the liver, they are converted to toxic products that can injure liver cells. These drugs are called *hepatotoxic drugs*.

In the United States, drugs are the leading cause of acute liver failure, a rare condition that can rapidly prove fatal. Fortunately, liver failure from using known hepatotoxic drugs is rare, with an incidence of less than 1 in 50,000. (Drugs that cause liver failure more often than this are removed from the market—unless they are indicated for a life-threatening illness.) More than 50 drugs are known to be hepatotoxic. Some examples are listed in Table 5.1.

Combining a hepatotoxic drug with certain other drugs may increase the risk of liver damage. Acetaminophen [Tylenol] is a hepatotoxic drug that can damage the liver when taken in excessive doses. When taken in therapeutic doses, acetaminophen does not usually create a risk for liver injury; however, if the drug is taken with just two or three alcoholic beverages, severe liver injury can result.

QT Interval Drugs

The term *QT interval drugs*—or simply *QT drugs*—refers to the ability of some medications to prolong the QT interval on the electrocardiogram, thereby creating a risk for serious dysrhythmias. The QT interval is a measure of the time required for the ventricles to repolarize after each contraction. When the QT interval is prolonged (more than 470 msec for postpubertal males or more than 480 msec for postpubertal females), patients can develop a dysrhythmia known as *torsades de pointes,* which can progress to potentially fatal ventricular fibrillation.

More than 100 drugs are known to cause QT prolongation, torsades de pointes, or both. As shown in Table 5.2, QT drugs are found in many drug families. Several QT drugs have been withdrawn from the market because of deaths linked to their use, and use of another QT drug—cisapride [Propulsid]—is now restricted. To reduce the risks from QT drugs, the U.S. Food and Drug Administration (FDA) now requires that all new drugs be tested for the ability to cause QT prolongation.

Identifying Adverse Drug Reactions

It can be very difficult to determine whether a specific drug is responsible for an observed adverse event because other factors—especially the underlying illness and other drugs being taken—could be the actual cause. To help determine whether a particular drug is responsible, the following questions should be considered:

- Did symptoms appear shortly after the drug was first used?
- Did symptoms abate when the drug was discontinued?
- Did symptoms reappear when the drug was reinstituted?
- Is the illness itself sufficient to explain the event?
- Are other drugs in the regimen sufficient to explain the event?

If the answers reveal a temporal relationship between the presence of the drug and the adverse event, and if the event cannot be explained by the illness itself or by other drugs in

TABLE 5.1 ▪ Some Hepatotoxic Drugs

STATINS AND OTHER LIPID-LOWERING DRUGS	**ANTIMICROBIAL DRUGS**
Atorvastatin [Lipitor]	Amoxicillin–clavulanic acid [Augmentin]
Fenofibrate [TriCor, Trilipix, Lipidil EZ]	Erythromycin
Fluvastatin [Lescol]	Minocycline [Minocin]
Gemfibrozil [Lopid]	Nitrofurantoin [Macrodantin, Macrobid]
Lovastatin [Mevacor]	Penicillin
Niacin [Niaspan, others]	Trimethoprim-sulfamethoxazole [Septra, Bactrim]
Pitavastatin [Livalo]	**DRUGS FOR TUBERCULOSIS**
Pravastatin [Pravachol]	Isoniazid
Simvastatin [Zocor]	Pyrazinamide
ORAL ANTIDIABETIC DRUGS	Rifampin [Rifadin]
Acarbose [Precose, Glucobay]	**IMMUNOSUPPRESSANTS**
Pioglitazone [Actos]	Azathioprine [Imuran]
Rosiglitazone [Avandia]	Leflunomide [Arava]
ANTISEIZURE DRUGS	Methotrexate [Rheumatrex]
Carbamazepine [Tegretol]	**ANTIRETROVIRAL DRUGS**
Felbamate [Felbatol]	Nevirapine [Viramune]
Phenytoin [Dilantin]	Ritonavir [Norvir]
Valproic acid [Depakene, others]	**OTHER DRUGS**
ANTIFUNGAL DRUGS	Acetaminophen [Tylenol], but only when combined with alcohol or taken in excessive dose
Fluconazole [Diflucan]	Amiodarone [Cordarone]
Griseofulvin [Grifulvin V, Gris-PEG]	Baclofen [Lioresal, Gablofen]
Itraconazole [Sporanox]	Celecoxib [Celebrex]
Ketoconazole [Nizoral]	Diclofenac [Voltaren]
Terbinafine [Lamisil]	Labetalol [Trandate]
ANTIGOUT DRUGS	Lisinopril [Prinivil, Zestril]
Allopurinol [Zyloprim]	Losartan [Cozaar]
Febuxostat [Uloric]	Methyldopa [Aldomet]
ANTIDEPRESSANT/ANTIPSYCHOTIC DRUGS	Omeprazole [Prilosec]
Buproprion [Wellbutrin, Zyban]	Procainamide
Duloxetine [Cymbalta]	Tamoxifen [Nolvadex]
Nefazodone	Testosterone
Trazodone	Zileuton [Zyflo]
Tricyclic antidepressants	

the regimen, then there is a high probability that the drug under suspicion is indeed the culprit. Unfortunately, this process is limited. It can only identify adverse effects that occur while the drug is being used; it cannot identify adverse events that develop years after drug withdrawal. Nor can it identify effects that develop slowly over the course of prolonged drug use.

Adverse Reactions to New Drugs

Preclinical and clinical trials of new drugs cannot detect all of the ADRs that a drug may be able to cause. In fact, about 50% of all new drugs have serious ADRs that are not revealed during phase 1 and phase 3 trials.

Because newly released drugs may have as-yet unreported adverse effects, you should be alert for unusual responses when prescribing new drugs. If the patient develops new symptoms, it is wise to suspect that the drug may be responsible—even if the symptoms are not described in the literature. It is a good practice to initially check postmarket drug evaluations at www.fda.gov/Drugs/GuidanceCompliance RegulatoryInformation/Surveillance/ucm204091.htm to determine whether serious problems have been reported. If the drug is especially new, however, you may be the first provider to have observed the effect. If you suspect a drug of causing a previously unknown adverse effect, you should report the effect to MedWatch, the FDA Medical Products Reporting Program. You can file your report online at www.fda.gov/medwatch. Because voluntary reporting by health care professionals is an important mechanism for bringing ADRs to light, you should report all suspected ADRs, even if absolute proof of the drug's complicity has not been established.

Ways to Minimize Adverse Drug Reactions

The responsibility for reducing ADRs lies with everyone associated with drug production and use. The pharmaceutical industry must strive to produce the safest medicines possible; the provider must select the least harmful medicine for a particular patient and provide clear instructions for its use; the nurse must evaluate patients for ADRs and educate patients in ways to avoid or minimize harm; and patients and their families must take medication only as directed, watch for signs that an ADR may be developing, and seek medical attention if one appears.

When patients are using drugs that are toxic to specific organs, function of the target organ should be monitored.

TABLE 5.2 ▪ Drugs That Prolong the QT Interval, Induce Torsades De Pointes, or Both

CARDIOVASCULAR: ANTIDYSRHYTHMICS
Amiodarone [Cordarone]
Disopyramide [Norpace]
Dofetilide [Tikosyn]
Dronedarone [Multaq]
Flecainide [Tambocor]
Ibutilide [Corvert]
Mexiletine [Mexitil]
Procainamide [Procan, Pronestyl]
Quinidine
Sotalol [Betapace]

CARDIOVASCULAR: ACE INHIBITORS/CCBS
Bepridil [Vascor]
Isradipine [DynaCirc]
Moexipril
Nicardipine [Cardene]

ANTIBIOTICS
Azithromycin [Zithromax]
Clarithromycin [Biaxin]
Erythromycin
Gemifloxacin [Factive]
Levofloxacin [Levaquin]
Moxifloxacin [Avelox]
Ofloxacin [Floxin]
Telithromycin [Ketek]

ANTIFUNGAL DRUGS
Fluconazole [Diflucan]
Voriconazole [Vfend]

ANTIDEPRESSANTS
Amitriptyline [Elavil]
Citalopram [Celexa]
Desipramine [Norpramin]
Doxepin [Sinequan]
Escitalopram [Lexapro]
Fluoxetine [Prozac]
Imipramine [Tofranil]
Mirtazepine [Remeron]
Protriptyline [Pamelor, Aventyl]
Sertraline [Zoloft]
Trimipramine [Surmontil]
Venlafaxine [Effexor]

ANTIPSYCHOTICS
Chlorpromazine [Thorazine]
Clozapine [Clozaril]
Haloperidol [Haldol]
Iloperidone [Fanapt]
Paliperidone [Invega]
Pimozide [Orap]
Quetiapine [Seroquel]
Risperidone [Risperdal]
Thioridazine [Mellaril]
Ziprasidone [Geodon]

ANTIEMETICS/ANTINAUSEA DRUGS
Dolasetron [Anzemet]
Domperidone [Motilium] 🍁
Droperidol [Inapsine]
Granisetron [Kytril]
Ondansetron [Zofran]

ANTICANCER DRUGS
Arsenic trioxide [Trisenox]
Eribulin [Halaven]
Lapatinib [Tykerb]
Nilotinib [Tasigna]
Sunitinib [Sutent]
Tamoxifen [Nolvadex]
Vandetanib [Caprelsa]
Vorinostat [Zolinza]

DRUGS FOR ADHD
Amphetamine/dextroamphetamine [Adderall]
Atomoxetine [Strattera]
Dexmethylphenidate [Focalin]
Dextroamphetamine [Dexedrine]
Methylphenidate [Ritalin, Concerta]

NASAL DECONGESTANTS
Phenylephrine [Neo-Synephrine, Sudafed PE]
Pseudoephedrine [Sudafed]

OTHER DRUGS
Alfuzosin [Uroxatral]
Amantadine [Symmetrel]
Chloroquine [Aralen]
Cisapride [Propulsid]*
Cocaine
Felbamate [Felbatol]
Fingolimod [Gilenya]
Foscarnet [Foscavir]
Fosphenytoin [Cerebyx]
Galantamine [Razadyne]
Halofantrine [Halfan]
Indapamide [Lozol]
Lithium [Lithobid, Eskalith]
Methadone [Dolophine]
Midodrine [ProAmatine]
Octreotide [Sandostatin]
Pasireotide [Signifor]
Pentamidine [Pentam, Nebupent]
Phentermine [Fastin]
Ranolazine [Ranexa]
Ritodrine [Yutopar]
Salmeterol [Serevent]
Saquinavir [Invirase]
Solifenacin [Vesicare]
Tacrolimus [Prograf]
Terbutaline
Tizanidine [Zanaflex]
Tolterodine [Detrol]
Vardenafil [Levitra]

*Restricted availability.
ACE, angiotensin-converting enzyme; ADHD, attention-deficit/hyperactivity disorder; CCB, calcium channel blocker.

The liver, kidneys, and bone marrow are important sites of drug toxicity. For drugs that are toxic to the liver, the patient should be monitored for signs and symptoms of liver damage (jaundice, dark urine, light-colored stools, nausea, vomiting, malaise, abdominal discomfort, loss of appetite), and periodic tests of liver function (e.g., *aspartate aminotransferase* [AST] and *alanine aminotransferase* [ALT]) should be performed. For drugs that are toxic to the kidneys, the patient should undergo routine urinalysis and measurement of serum creatinine or creatinine clearance. For drugs that are toxic to bone marrow, periodic complete blood cell counts are required.

Adverse effects can be reduced by individualizing therapy. When choosing a drug for a particular patient, the provider must balance the drug's risks and benefits. Drugs that are likely to harm a specific patient should be avoided unless the benefit of the drug exceeds the risk for injury.

Special Alerts and Management Guidelines

In an effort to decrease harm associated with drugs that cause serious adverse effects, the FDA requires special alerts and management guidelines. These may take the form of a *Medication Guide* for patients, a *boxed warning* to alert providers, or a *Risk Evaluation and Mitigation Strategy* (REMS), which can involve patients, providers, and pharmacists.

Medication Guides

Medication Guides, commonly called MedGuides, are FDA-approved documents created to educate patients about how to minimize harm from potentially dangerous drugs. In addition, a MedGuide is required when the FDA has determined that (1) patient adherence to directions for drug use is essential for efficacy or (2) patients need to know about potentially serious effects when deciding to use a drug.

All MedGuides use a standard format that provides information under the following main headings:

- What is the most important information I should know about (*name of drug*)?
- What is (*name of drug*)? Include a description of the drug and its indications.
- Who should not take (*name of drug*)?
- How should I take (*name of drug*)? Include importance of adherence to dosing instructions, special instructions about administration, what to do in case of overdose, and what to do if a dose is missed.
- What should I avoid while taking (*name of drug*)? Include activities (e.g., driving, sunbathing), other drugs, foods, pregnancy, and breastfeeding.
- What are the possible or reasonably likely side effects of (*name of drug*)?
- General information about the safe and effective use of prescription drugs.

Additional headings may be added by the manufacturer as appropriate, with the approval of the FDA. MedGuides for all drug products that require one are available online at *www.fda.gov/Drugs/DrugSafety/UCM085729.*The MedGuide should be provided whenever a prescription is filled, and even when drug samples are handed out.

Boxed Warnings

The *boxed warning,* also known as a *black box warning,* is the strongest safety warning a drug can carry and still remain on the market. Text for the warning is presented inside a box with a heavy black border. The FDA requires a boxed warning on drugs with serious or life-threatening risks. The purpose of the warning is to alert providers to (1) potentially severe side effects (e.g., life-threatening dysrhythmias, suicidality, major fetal harm) as well as (2) ways to prevent or reduce harm (e.g., avoiding a teratogenic drug during pregnancy). The boxed warning provides a *concise summary* of the adverse effects of concern. A boxed warning must appear prominently on the package insert, on the product label, and even in magazine advertising. Drugs that have a boxed warning must also have a MedGuide.

Risk Evaluation and Mitigation Strategies

A REMS is simply a plan to minimize drug-induced harm. For most drugs that have a REMS, a MedGuide is all that is needed. For a few drugs, however, the REMS may have additional components. For example, the REMS for the antiacne drug isotretinoin has provisions that pertain to the patient, provider, and pharmacist. This program, known as iPledge, is needed because isotretinoin can cause serious birth defects. The iPledge program was designed to ensure that patients who are pregnant, or may become pregnant, will not have access to the drug. Details of the iPledge program are presented in Chapter 85. All REMS that have received FDA approval can be found online at www.fda.gov/Drugs/DrugSafety/PostmarketDrugSafetyInformationforPatientsandProviders/ucm111350.htm.

MEDICATION ERRORS

Medication errors are a major cause of morbidity and mortality. According to the Institute of Medicine (IOM), every year medication errors injure at least 1.5 million Americans and kill an estimated 7000. The financial costs are staggering: among hospitalized patients alone, treatment of drug-related injuries costs at least $3.5 billion a year.

What Is a Medication Error?

The National Coordinating Council for Medication Error Reporting and Prevention (NCC MERP) defines a medication error as "any preventable event that may cause or lead to inappropriate medication use or patient harm, while the medication is in the control of the healthcare professional, patient, or consumer. Such events may be related to professional practice, healthcare products, procedures, and systems, including prescribing; order communication; product labeling, packaging and nomenclature; compounding; dispensing; distribution; administration; education; monitoring; and use." Note that, by this definition, medication errors can be made by many people—beginning with workers in the pharmaceutical industry, followed by people in the health care delivery system, and ending with patients and their family members. In this chapter, we focus on medication errors attributed to health care providers. These typically fall into one of the following categories:

Prescribing Practices

- Inappropriate drug selection
- Error in drug dosage
- Lack of clear instructions
- Illegible writing

Oversight

- Failure to keep an up-to-date medication list
- Failure to continue or discontinue medications
- Absence of medication reconciliation

Communication
- Inadequate or unclear instructions
- Failure to verify drugs that sound alike
- Inadequate patient education

Ways to Reduce Medication Errors

Organizations throughout many countries are working to design and implement measures to reduce medication errors. Changes having the most dramatic effect have been those that focused on the IOM recommendations to (1) help and encourage patients and their families to be active, informed members of the healthcare team, and (2) give health care providers the tools and information needed to prescribe, dispense, and administer drugs as safely as possible.

Implementation of technology to reduce errors has had remarkable success, as well. For example, replacing handwritten medication orders with a computerized order entry system has reduced medication errors by 50%. Using bar-code systems that match the patient's armband bar code to a drug bar code has decreased medication errors in some institutions by as much as 85%.

Targeted interventions to address provider-related errors can be employed to decrease medication errors by health care providers. These are provided in Table 5.4.

Incorporating *medication reconciliation* (Box 5.1) has resulted in decreasing medication errors by 70% and reducing ADRs by 15%.

TABLE 5.3 ▪ Examples of Drugs With Names That Sound Alike or Look Alike*

Amicar	*Omacar*
Anaspaz	*Antispas*
Celebrex	*Cerebyx*
Clinoril	*Clozaril*
Cycloserine	Cyclosporine
Depo-Estradiol	*Depo-Testadiol*
Dioval	*Diovan*
Estratab	*Estratest*
Etidronate	Etretinate
Flomax	*Volmax*
Lamisil	*Lamictal*
Levoxine	*Levoxyl*
Lithobid	*Lithostat*
Lodine	Iodine
Naprelan	*Naprosyn*
Nasarel	*Nizoral*
Neoral	*Neosar*
Nicoderm	*Nitroderm*
Sarafem	*Serophene*
Serentil	*Seroquel*
Tamiflu	*Theraflu*
Tramadol	*Toradol*

*Trade names are italicized; generic names are not.

TABLE 5.4 ▪ Provider-Related Medication Errors and Interventions

Errors	Interventions
PRESCRIBING PRACTICES	
Inappropriate drug selection	Verify that the drug selected is the drug intended. (See Table 5.3 for a list of drugs that look or sound like other drugs.)
	Drug information changes frequently; make sure that drug references are authoritative and up to date.
	Verify allergies when ordering new medications. Display allergies prominently in the patient record.
	Check for interactions of new medications against all currently prescribed medications, over-the-counter medications, herbal remedies, nutritional supplements, and recreational drugs that the patient is taking. Authoritative drug interaction application software is recommended.
	Verify that patients can afford the medication; otherwise, this increases the likelihood of errors due to taking subtherapeutic doses, if filled at all.
	Consider individualized patient factors (e.g., age, pregnancy, comorbidities) when selecting the most appropriate drug.
Error in drug dosage	Verify unit of measure (e.g., milligram versus microgram).
	Verify height and weight and verify unit of measure (e.g., kilograms versus pounds) for dosage calculations.
	Verify decimal placement; follow the ISMP recommendations in Table 5.5.
Lack of clear labeling instructions	Incorporate ISMP-recommended substitutions for any error-prone abbreviations. (See Table 5.5.)
	Write precise and detailed instructions. Avoid "Take as directed" and similar nonspecific labeling.
	Request large font labeling for patients who have difficulty reading small print.
Illegible writing	Use print instead of cursive writing.
	Check spelling, placement of decimals, and clarity of numerals.
	Convert to computerized provider order entry at earliest possibility.
OVERSIGHT	
Failure to keep an up-to-date medication list	When taking a medication history, assess not only how a medication is prescribed to be taken but also how the patient actually takes it in order to identify discrepancies and why they occur.
	Include dates when drugs are stopped, started, or altered, as well as the reasons for these changes.
Failure to continue/ discontinue medications	Update patient medications at every visit and compare this list with prior lists to identify drugs that should have been continued or that should be discontinued or weaned.
	Avoid polypharmacy when possible; determine whether all drugs prescribed are necessary and if new drugs are truly needed.
Absence of medication reconciliation	Medication reconciliation should occur any time there is a transfer of patients to another provider or to another facility. (See Box 5.1.)
	Develop interprofessional relationships to facilitate communication regarding reconciliation needs.

TABLE 5.4 ▪ Provider-Related Medication Errors and Interventions—cont'd

Errors	Interventions
COMMUNICATION	
Inadequate or unclear instructions	Reserve verbal orders for emergency situations. When verbal orders are required, have the nurse repeat them to ensure that they are understood and are what you intended.
Inadequate patient education	Develop strong collaborative partnerships with patients (or their caretakers) and consider their perspectives and preferences when making treatment decisions. Verify patient understanding of teaching by repeating instructions or demonstrating procedures. Provide handouts to reinforce teaching. These should be written at the 5th grade level or, at most, the 8th grade level.

BOX 5.1 ▪ MEDICATION RECONCILIATION

What Is Medication Reconciliation and When Is It Done?

Medication reconciliation is the process of comparing a list of all medications that a patient is currently taking with a list of new medications that are about to be provided. Reconciliation is conducted whenever a patient undergoes a *transition in care* in which new medications may be ordered or existing orders may be changed. Transitions in care include hospital admission, hospital discharge, moving to a different level of care within a hospital, transfer to another facility, or discharge home.

How Is Medication Reconciliation Conducted?

There are five steps:

Step 1. Create a list of current medications. For each drug, include the name, indication, route, dosage size, and dosing interval. For patients entering a hospital, the list would consist of all medications being taken at home, including vitamins, herbal products, and prescription and nonprescription drugs.

Step 2. Create a list of all medications to be prescribed in the new setting.

Step 3. Compare the medications on both lists.

Step 4. Adjust medications based on the comparison. For example, the provider would discontinue drugs that are duplicates or inappropriate and would avoid drugs that can interact adversely.

Step 5. When the next transition in care occurs, provide the updated, reconciled list to the patient and the new provider. By consulting the list, the new provider will be less likely to omit a prescribed medication or commit a dosing error and will be less likely to prescribe a new medication that might duplicate or negate the effects of a current medication or interact with a current medication to cause a serious adverse event.

Every time a new transition in care occurs, reconciliation should be conducted again.

Does Medication Reconciliation Reduce Medication Errors?

Definitely. Roughly 60% of medication errors occur when patients undergo a transition in care. Medication reconciliation can eliminate most of these errors.

Should Medication Reconciliation Be Conducted at Discharge?

When patients leave a facility, they should receive a single, clear, comprehensive list of *all* medications they will be taking after discharge. The list should include any medications ordered at the time of discharge, as well as any other medications the patient will be taking, including over-the-counter drugs, vitamins, and herbal products and other nutritional supplements. In addition, the list should include all prescription medications that the patient had been taking at home but had been temporarily discontinued during the episode of care. The discharge list should *not* include drugs that had been used during the episode of care but are no longer needed. The patient and, with the patient's permission, the next provider of care, should receive the discharge list so that the new provider will be able to continue the reconciliation process.

Many medication errors result from using error-prone abbreviations, symbols, and dose designations. To address this concern, the Institute for Safe Medical Practices (ISMP) and the FDA together compiled a list of error-prone abbreviations, symbols, and dose designations (Table 5.5) and have recommended against their use. This list includes eight entries (at the top of Table 5.5) that have been *banned* by The Joint Commission (TJC). These banned abbreviations can no longer be used by hospitals and other organizations that require TJC accreditation. The full list is available online at www.ismp.org/tools/errorproneabbreviations.pdf.

A wealth of information is available on reducing medication errors. See Table 5.6 for some good places to start.

How to Report a Medication Error

You can report a medication error through the MER Program, a nationwide system run by the ISMP. All reporting is confidential and can be done by phone or through the Internet. Details on submitting a report are available at www.ismp.org/orderForms/reporterrortoISMP.asp. The MER Program encourages participation by all health care providers, including pharmacists, nurses, physicians, and students. The objective is not to establish blame, but instead to improve patient safety by increasing our knowledge of medication errors. All information gathered by the MER Program is forwarded to the FDA, the ISMP, and the product manufacturer.

TABLE 5.5 ▪ Abbreviations, Symbols, and Dose Designations That Can Promote Medication Errors

Abbreviations, Symbols, or Dose Designations	Intended Meaning	Potential Misinterpretation	Preferred Alternative
ABBREVIATIONS AND NOTATIONS FOR WHICH THE ALTERNATIVE *MUST* BE USED (TJC MANDATED)			
U or u	Unit	Misread as 0 or 4 (e.g., 4U seen as 40; 4u seen as 44); mistaken to mean "cc" so dose given in volume instead of units (e.g., 4u mistaken to mean 4 cc)	Write "unit"
IU	International unit	Misread as IV (intravenous) or "10"	Write "international unit"
q.d./Q.D.	Every day	Misread as q.i.d. (four times a day)	Write "daily"
q.o.d./Q.O.D.	Every other day	Misread as q.d. (daily) or q.i.d. (four times a day)	Write "every other day"
MS or MSO_4	Morphine sulfate	Mistaken as magnesium sulfate	Write "morphine sulfate"
$MgSO_4$	Magnesium sulfate	Mistaken as morphine sulfate	Write "magnesium sulfate"
Trailing zero after final decimal point (e.g., 1.0 mg)	1 mg	Mistaken as 10 mg if the decimal point is missed	Never write a zero by itself after a decimal point
Leading decimal point not preceded by a zero (e.g., .5 mg)	0.5 mg	Mistaken as 5 mg if the decimal point is missed	Write "0" before a leading decimal point
SOME ABBREVIATIONS AND NOTATIONS FOR WHICH THE ALTERNATIVE IS *RECOMMENDED* (BUT NOT YET TJC MANDATED)			
µg	Microgram	Mistaken as "mg"	Write "mcg"
cc	Cubic centimeters	Mistaken as "u" (units)	Write "mL"
IN	Intranasal	Mistaken as "IM" or "IV"	Write "intranasal" or "NAS"
H.S.; hs	Half-strength; at bedtime	Mistaken as opposite of what was intended	Write "half-strength" or "at bedtime"
qhs	At bedtime	Mistaken as qhr (every hour)	Write "at bedtime"
q1d	Daily	Mistaken as q.i.d. (four times daily)	Write "daily"
q6PM, etc.	Nightly at 6 PM	Mistaken as every 6 hours	Write "nightly at 6 PM"
T.I.W.	Three times a week	Mistaken as three times a day or twice weekly	Write "three times weekly"
SC, SQ, sub q	Subcutaneous	SC mistaken as "SL" (sublingual); SQ mistaken as "5 every"; the "q" in "sub q" mistaken as "every" (e.g., a heparin dose ordered "sub q 2 hours before surgery" mistaken as "every 2 hours before surgery")	Write "subQ," "sub-Q," "subcut," or "subcutaneously"; write "every"
D/C	Discharge or discontinue	Premature discontinuation of medications if D/C (intended to mean "discharge") has been interpreted as "discontinued" when followed by a list of discharge medications	Write "discharge" or "discontinue"
AD, AS, AU	Right ear, left ear, each ear	Mistaken as OD, OS, OU (right eye, left eye, each eye)	Write "right ear," "left ear," or "each ear"
OD, OS, OU	Right eye, left eye, each eye	Mistaken as AD, AS, AU (right ear, left ear, each ear)	Write "right eye," "left eye," or "each eye"
Per os	By mouth, orally	The "os" can be mistaken as "left eye" (OS = oculus sinister)	Write "PO," "by mouth," or "orally"
> or <	Greater than or less than	Mistaken for the opposite	Write "greater than" or "less than"
AZT	Zidovudine [Retrovir]	Mistaken as azathioprine or aztreonam	Write complete drug name
CPZ	Prochlorperazine [Compazine]	Mistaken as chlorpromazine	Write complete drug name
ARA A	Vidarabine	Mistaken as cytarabine (ARAC)	Write complete drug name
HCT	Hydrocortisone	Mistaken as hydrochlorothiazide	Write complete drug name
HCTZ	Hydrochlorothiazide	Mistaken as hydrocortisone	Write complete drug name

TJC, The Joint Commission.
Adapted from a list compiled by the Institute for Safe Medication Practices. The official TJC list is available at http://www.jointcommission.org/assets/1/18/dnu_list.pdf. The complete ISMP list is available at www.ismp.org/tools/errorproneabbreviations.pdf.

TABLE 5.6 ▪ Resources on Decreasing Medication Errors

Resource	Location
Agency for Healthcare Research and Quality's Patient Safety Network	www.psnet.ahrq.gov
Institute for Safe Medication Practices	www.ismp.org
Institute for Healthcare Improvement *Medication Reconciliation Information and Tools*	http://www.ihi.org/topics/adesmedicationreconciliation/Pages/default.aspx
National Coordinating Council for Medication Error Reporting and Prevention	www.nccmerp.org
Institute of Medicine: *Reducing Medication Errors* ("The IOM Report")	www.nap.edu/catalog.php?record_id511623
The Joint Commission: *Resources Related to Medication Errors*	www.jointcommission.org/topics/default.aspx?k=660
U.S. Food and Drug Administration: *Medication Errors Related to Drugs*	www.fda.gov/Drugs/DrugSafety/MedicationErrors/default.htm

CHAPTER

6 Individual Variation in Drug Responses

Jacqueline Rosenjack Burchum, DNSc, FNP-BC, CNE

In this chapter, we discuss the major factors that can cause one patient to respond to drugs differently than another. With this information, you will be better prepared to reduce individual variation in drug responses, thereby maximizing the benefits of treatment and reducing the potential for harm.

BODY WEIGHT AND COMPOSITION

The intensity of the response to a drug is determined in large part by the concentration of the drug at its sites of action—the higher the concentration, the more intense the response; therefore, body size can be a significant determinant of drug effects. If we give the same dose to a small person and a large person, the drug will achieve a higher concentration in the small person and therefore will produce more intense effects. The potential consequences are that we will produce toxicity in the smaller person and undertreat the larger person. To compensate for this potential source of individual variation, the size of the patient should be considered when prescribing drug dosage.

Adjustments in dosage are typically based on body surface area because surface area determinations account not only for the patient's weight but also for the patient's relative amount of body adiposity. Because percentage of body fat can change drug distribution, and because altered distribution can change the concentration of a drug at its sites of action, dosage adjustments based on body surface area provide a more precise means of controlling drug responses than do adjustments based on weight alone.

AGE

Drug sensitivity varies with age. Infants and older adults are especially sensitive to drugs. In the very young patient, heightened drug sensitivity is the result of organ immaturity. In older adults, heightened sensitivity results largely from decline in organ function. Other factors that affect sensitivity in older adults are the presence of multiple comorbidities and treatment with multiple drugs. The clinical challenge created by heightened drug sensitivity in very young or in older adult patients is the subject of Chapters 8 and 9.

PATHOPHYSIOLOGY

Physiologic alterations can modify drug responses. Four pathologic conditions, in particular, may have a profound effect: (1) kidney disease, (2) liver disease, (3) acid-base imbalance, and (4) altered electrolyte status.

Kidney Disease

Kidney disease can reduce drug excretion, causing drugs to accumulate in the body. If dosage is not lowered, drugs may accumulate to toxic levels. Accordingly, if a patient is taking a drug that is eliminated by the kidneys, and if renal function declines, dosage must be decreased.

Liver Disease

Like kidney disease, liver disease can cause drugs to accumulate. This occurs because the liver is the major site of drug metabolism. Therefore, if liver function declines, the rate of metabolism will decline, causing drug levels to climb. Accordingly, to prevent accumulation to toxic levels, dosage of drugs eliminated through hepatic metabolism must be reduced or discontinued if liver disease develops.

Acid-Base Imbalance

By altering pH partitioning (see Chapter 4), changes in acid-base status can alter the absorption, distribution, metabolism, and excretion of drugs. Because of pH partitioning, if there is a difference in pH on two sides of a membrane, a drug will accumulate on the side where the pH most favors its ionization. Because acidic drugs ionize in alkaline media, acidic drugs will accumulate on the alkaline side of the membrane. Conversely, basic drugs will accumulate on the acidic side.

Altered Electrolyte Status

Electrolytes (e.g., potassium, sodium, calcium, magnesium, phosphorus) have important roles in cell physiology. Consequently, when electrolyte levels become disturbed, multiple cellular processes can be disrupted. Excitable tissues (nerves and muscles) are especially sensitive to alterations in electrolyte status. Given that disturbances in electrolyte balance can have widespread effects on cell physiology, we might expect that electrolyte imbalances would cause profound and widespread effects on responses to drugs. However, this does not seem to be the case; examples in which electrolyte changes have a significant effect on drug responses are rare. An exception is digoxin in the presence of hypokalemia. When potassium levels are low, the ability of digoxin to induce dysrhythmias is greatly increased. Accordingly, all patients receiving digoxin must undergo regular measurement of serum potassium to ensure that levels remain within a safe range.

TOLERANCE

Tolerance is a *decreased responsiveness to a drug as a result of repeated drug administration.* Patients who are tolerant to a drug require higher doses to produce effects equivalent to those that could be achieved with lower doses before tolerance developed. There are three categories of drug tolerance: (1) pharmacodynamic tolerance, (2) metabolic tolerance, and (3) tachyphylaxis.

Pharmacodynamic Tolerance

The term *pharmacodynamic tolerance* refers to the familiar type of tolerance associated with long-term administration of drugs such as morphine and heroin. Pharmacodynamic tolerance is the result of adaptive processes that occur in response to chronic receptor occupation. Because increased drug levels are required to produce an effective response, the minimum effective concentration (MEC) of a drug becomes abnormally high.

Metabolic Tolerance

Metabolic tolerance is defined as tolerance resulting from accelerated drug metabolism. This form of tolerance is brought about by the ability of certain drugs (e.g., barbiturates) to induce synthesis of hepatic drug-metabolizing enzymes, thereby causing rates of drug metabolism to increase. Because of increased metabolism, dosage must be increased to maintain therapeutic drug levels. Unlike pharmacodynamic tolerance, which causes the MEC to increase, metabolic tolerance does not affect the MEC.

Tachyphylaxis

Tachyphylaxis is a reduction in drug responsiveness brought on by repeated dosing over a short time. This is unlike pharmacodynamic tolerance and metabolic tolerance, which take days or longer to develop. Transdermal nitroglycerin provides a good example of tachyphylaxis. When nitroglycerin is administered using a transdermal patch, effects are lost in less than 24 hours if the patch is left in place around the clock. As discussed in Chapter 43 the loss of effect results from depletion of a cofactor required for nitroglycerin to act. When nitroglycerin is administered on an intermittent schedule, rather than continuously, the cofactor can be replenished between doses, and no loss of effect occurs.

PLACEBO EFFECT

A *placebo* is devoid of intrinsic pharmacologic activity; therefore any response that a patient may have to a placebo is based solely on the patient's psychological reaction to the idea of taking a medication and not to any direct physiologic or biochemical action of the placebo itself. The primary use of the placebo is as a control preparation during clinical trials.

In pharmacology, the *placebo effect* is defined as that component of a drug response that is caused by psychological factors and not by the biochemical or physiologic properties of the drug. It is widely believed that, with practically all medications, some fraction of the total response results from a placebo effect. Although placebo effects are determined by psychological factors and not physiologic responses to the inactive placebo, the presence of a placebo response does not imply that a patient's original pathology was imaginary.

Not all placebo responses are beneficial. If a patient believes that a medication is going to be effective, then placebo responses are likely to help promote recovery. Conversely, if a patient is convinced that a particular medication is ineffective or perhaps even harmful, then placebo effects are likely to detract from his or her progress.

Because the placebo effect depends on the patient's attitude toward medicine, fostering a positive attitude may help promote beneficial effects. In this regard, it is desirable that all members of the health care team present the patient with an optimistic (but realistic) assessment of the effects that therapy is likely to produce.

VARIABILITY IN ABSORPTION

Both the rate and extent of drug absorption can vary among patients. As a result, both the timing and intensity of responses can be changed.

Bioavailability

The term *bioavailability* refers to the amount of active drug that reaches the systemic circulation from its site of administration. Different formulations of the same drug can vary in bioavailability. Factors such as tablet disintegration time, enteric coatings, and sustained-release formulations can alter bioavailability and can thereby make drug responses variable.

Differences in bioavailability occur primarily with oral preparations rather than parenteral preparations. Fortunately, even with oral agents, when differences in bioavailability do exist between preparations, those differences are usually so small that they lack clinical significance.

Differences in bioavailability are of greatest concern for drugs with a narrow therapeutic range because with these agents, a relatively small change in drug level can produce a significant change in response: a small decline in drug level may cause therapeutic failure, whereas a small increase in drug level may cause toxicity. Under these conditions, differences in bioavailability could have a significant effect.

Individual Causes of Variable Absorption

Individual variations that affect the speed and degree of drug absorption affect bioavailability and can thereby lead to variations in drug responses. Alterations in gastric pH can affect absorption through the pH partitioning effect. For drugs that undergo absorption in the intestine, absorption will be delayed when gastric emptying time is prolonged. Diarrhea can reduce absorption by accelerating transport of drugs through the intestine. Conversely, constipation may enhance absorption of some drugs by prolonging the time available for absorption.

GENETICS AND PHARMACOGENOMICS

A patient's unique genetic makeup can lead to drug responses that are qualitatively and quantitatively different from those of the population at large. Adverse effects and therapeutic effects may be increased or reduced. Idiosyncratic responses to drugs may also occur.

Pharmacogenomics is the study of how genetic variations can affect individual responses to drugs. Although pharmacogenomics is a relatively young science, it has already produced clinically relevant information—information that can be used to enhance therapeutic effects and reduce harm. As a result, genetic testing is now done routinely for some drugs. In fact, for a few drugs, such as maraviroc [Selzentry] and trastuzumab [Herceptin], the U.S. Food and Drug Administration (FDA) now *requires* genetic testing before use, and for a few other drugs, including warfarin [Coumadin] and carbamazepine [Tegretol], genetic testing is recommended but not required.

In the discussion that follows, we look at ways in which genetic variations can influence an individual's responses to drugs, and then indicate how pharmacogenomic tests may be used to guide treatment (Table 6.1).

Genetic Variants That Alter Drug Metabolism

The most common mechanism by which genetic variants modify drug responses is by altering drug metabolism. These gene-based changes can either accelerate or slow the metabolism of many drugs. The usual consequence is either a reduction in benefits or an increase in toxicity.

For drugs that have a high therapeutic index (TI), altered rates of metabolism may have little effect on the clinical outcome. However, if the TI is low or narrow, then relatively small increases in drug levels can lead to toxicity, and relatively small decreases in drug levels can lead to therapeutic

TABLE 6.1 ■ Examples of How Genetic Variations Can Affect Drugs Responses

Genetic Variation	Drug Affected	Effect of the Genetic Variation	Explanation	FDA Stand on Genetic Testing
VARIANTS THAT ALTER DRUG METABOLISM				
CYP2D6 variants	Tamoxifen [Nolvadex]	Reduced therapeutic effect	Women with inadequate CYP2D6 activity cannot convert tamoxifen to its active form; therefore the drug cannot adequately protect them from breast cancer.	No recommendation
CYP2C19 variants	Clopidogrel [Plavix]	Reduced therapeutic effect	Patients with inadequate CYP2C19 activity cannot convert clopidogrel to its active form; therefore the drug cannot protect them against cardiovascular events.	Recommended
CYP2C9 variants	Warfarin [Coumadin]	Increased toxicity	In patients with abnormal CYP2C9, warfarin may accumulate to a level that causes bleeding.	Recommended
TMPT variants	Thiopurines (e.g., thioguanine, mercaptopurine)	Increased toxicity	In patients with reduced TPMT activity, thiopurines can accumulate to levels that cause severe bone marrow toxicity.	Recommended
VARIANTS THAT ALTER DRUG TARGETS ON NORMAL CELLS				
ADRB1 variants	Metoprolol and other beta blockers	Increased therapeutic effect	$Beta_1$ receptors produced by ADRB1 variant genes respond more intensely to beta agonists, causing enhanced effects of blockade by beta antagonists.	No recommendation
VKORC1 variants	Warfarin [Coumadin]	Increased drug sensitivity	Variant VKORC1 is readily inhibited by warfarin, allowing anticoagulation with a reduced warfarin dosage.	Recommended
VARIANTS THAT ALTER DRUG TARGETS ON CANCER CELLS OR VIRUSES				
HER2 overexpression	Trastuzumab [Herceptin]	Increased therapeutic effect	Trastuzumab only acts against breast cancers that overexpress HER2.	Required
EGFR expression	Cetuximab [Erbitux]	Increased therapeutic effect	Cetuximab only works against colorectal cancers that express EGFR.	Required
CCR5 tropism	Maraviroc [Selzentry]	Increased therapeutic effect	Maraviroc only acts against HIV strains that express CCR5.	Required
VARIANTS THAT ALTER IMMUNE RESPONSES TO DRUGS				
HLA-B*1502	Carbamazepine [Tegretol, Carbatrol]	Increased toxicity	The HLA-B*1502 variant increases the risk for life-threatening skin reactions in patients taking carbamazepine.	Recommended for patients of Asian descent
HLA-B*5701	Abacavir [Ziagen]	Increased toxicity	The HLA-B*5701 variant increases the risk for fatal hypersensitivity reactions in patients taking abacavir.	Recommended

ADRB1, $beta_1$-adrenergic receptor; CCR5, chemokine receptor 5; CYP2C9, 2C9 isozyme of cytochrome P450 (CYP); CYP2C19, 2C19 isozyme of CYP; CYP2D6, 2D6 isozyme of CYP; EGFR, epidermal growth factor receptor; FDA, U.S. Food and Drug Administration; HER2, human epidermal growth factor receptor type 2; HLA-B*1502, human leukocyte antigen B*1502; HLA-B*5701, human leukocyte antigen B*5701; TPMT, thiopurine methyltransferase; VKORC1, vitamin K epoxide reductase complex 1.

failure. In these cases, altered rates of metabolism can be significant.

The following examples show how a genetically determined variation in drug metabolism can *reduce the benefits* of therapy.

- Variants in the gene that codes for cytochrome P450-2D6 (CYP2D6) can greatly reduce the benefits of tamoxifen [Soltamox, Nolvadex-D ♣], a drug used to prevent breast cancer recurrence. Here's how. To work, tamoxifen must first be converted to its active form—endoxifen—by CYP2D6. Women with an inherited deficiency in the CYP2D6 gene cannot activate the drug well, so they get minimal benefit from treatment. In one study, the cancer recurrence rate in these poor metabolizers was 9.5 times higher than in good metabolizers. Who are the poor metabolizers? Between 8% and 10% of women of European ancestry have gene variants that prevent them from metabolizing tamoxifen to endoxifen. At this time, the FDA neither requires nor recommends testing for variants in the CYP2D6 gene. However, a test kit is available.
- Variants of the gene that codes for CYP2C19 can greatly reduce the benefits of clopidogrel [Plavix], a drug that prevents platelet aggregation. Like tamoxifen, clopidogrel is a prodrug that must undergo conversion to an active form. With clopidogrel, the conversion is catalyzed by CYP2C19. Unfortunately, about 25% of patients produce a variant form of the enzyme—CYP2C19*2. As a result, these people experience a weak antiplatelet response, which places them at increased risk for stroke, myocardial infarction, and other events. People with this genetic variation should use a different antiplatelet drug.
- Among Americans of European heritage, about 52% metabolize isoniazid (a drug for tuberculosis) slowly and 48% metabolize it rapidly. Why? Because, owing to genetic differences, these people produce two different forms of *N*-acetyltransferase-2, the enzyme that metabolizes isoniazid. If dosage is not adjusted for these differences, the rapid metabolizers may experience treatment failure and the slow metabolizers may experience toxicity.
- About 1 in 14 people of European heritage have a form of CYP2D6 that is unable to convert codeine into morphine, the active form of codeine. As a result, codeine cannot relieve pain in these people.

The following examples show how a genetically determined variation in drug metabolism can *increase drug toxicity*.

- Variants in the gene that codes for CYP2C9 can increase the risk for toxicity (bleeding) from *warfarin* [Coumadin], an anticoagulant with a narrow TI. Bleeding occurs because (1) warfarin is inactivated by CYP2D9 and (2) patients with altered CYP2D9 genes produce a form of the enzyme that metabolizes warfarin slowly, allowing it to accumulate to dangerous levels. To reduce bleeding risk, the FDA now recommends that patients be tested for variants of the CYP2C9 gene. It should be noted, however, that in this case outcomes using expensive genetic tests are no better than outcomes using cheaper traditional tests, which directly measure the effect of warfarin on coagulation.
- Variants in the gene that codes for *thiopurine methyltransferase* (TPMT) can reduce TPMT activity and can thereby delay the metabolic inactivation of two thiopurine anticancer drugs: *thioguanine* [generic only] and *mercaptopurine* [Purinethol]. As a result, in patients with inherited TPMT deficiency, standard doses of thiopurine or mercaptopurine can accumulate to high levels, posing a risk for potentially fatal bone marrow damage. To reduce risk, the FDA recommends testing for TPMT variants before using either drug. Patients who are found to be TPMT deficient should be given these drugs in reduced dosage.
- In the United States, about 1% of the population produces a form of *dihydropyrimidine dehydrogenase* that does a poor job of metabolizing *fluorouracil,* a drug used to treat cancer. Several people with this inherited difference, while receiving standard doses of fluorouracil, have died from central nervous system injury owing to accumulation of the drug to toxic levels.

Genetic Variants That Alter Drug Targets

Genetic variations can alter the structure of drug receptors and other target molecules and can thereby influence drug responses. These variants have been documented in normal cells and in cancer cells and viruses.

Genetic variants that affect drug targets on *normal cells* are illustrated by these two examples.

- Variants in the genes that code for the *beta$_1$-adrenergic receptor* (ADRB1) produce receptors that are hyperresponsive to activation, which can be a mixed blessing. The bad news is that, in people with hypertension, activation of these receptors may produce an exaggerated *increase* in blood pressure. The good news is that, in people with hypertension, blockade of these receptors will therefore produce an exaggerated *decrease* in blood pressure. Population studies indicate that variant ADRB1 receptors occur more often in people of European ancestry than in people of African ancestry, which may explain why *beta blockers* work better, on average, against hypertension in people with light skin than in people with dark skin.
- The anticoagulant *warfarin* works by inhibiting *vitamin K epoxide reductase complex 1* (VKORC1). Variant genes that code for VKORC1 produce a form of the enzyme that can be easily inhibited, and hence anticoagulation can be achieved with low warfarin doses. If normal doses are given, anticoagulation will be excessive, and bleeding could result. To reduce risk, the FDA recommends testing for variants in the VKORC1 gene before warfarin is used.

Genetic variants that affect drug targets on *cancer cells* and *viruses* are illustrated by these three examples.

- *Trastuzumab* [Herceptin], used for breast cancer, only works against tumors that overexpress *human epidermal growth factor receptor type 2* (HER2). The HER2 protein, which serves as a receptor for hormones that stimulate tumor growth, is overexpressed in about 25% of breast cancer patients. Overexpression of HER2 is associated with a poor prognosis but also predicts a better response to trastuzumab. Accordingly, the FDA requires a positive test result for HER2 overexpression before trastuzumab is used.
- *Cetuximab* [Erbitux], used mainly for metastatic colorectal cancer, only works against tumors that express the *epidermal growth factor receptor* (EGFR). All other tumors are unresponsive. Accordingly, the FDA requires evidence of EGFR expression if the drug is to be used.
- *Maraviroc* [Selzentry], a drug for HIV infection, works by binding with a viral surface protein known as *chemokine*

receptor 5 (CCR5), which certain strains of HIV require for entry into immune cells. HIV strains that use CCR5 are known as being *CCR5 tropic.* If maraviroc is to be of benefit, patients must be infected with one of these strains. Accordingly, before maraviroc is used, the FDA requires that testing be done to confirm that the infecting strain is indeed CCR5 tropic.

Genetic Variants That Alter Immune Responses to Drugs

Genetic variants that affect the immune system can increase the risk for severe hypersensitivity reactions to certain drugs. Two examples follow.

- *Carbamazepine* [Tegretol, Carbatrol], used for epilepsy and bipolar disorder, can cause life-threatening skin reactions in some patients—specifically, patients of Asian ancestry who carry genes that code for an unusual *human leukocyte antigen* (HLA) known as *HLA-B*1502.* (HLA molecules are essential elements of the immune system.) Although the mechanism underlying toxicity is unclear, a good guess is that interaction between HLA-B*1502 molecules and carbamazepine (or a metabolite) may trigger a cellular immune response. To reduce risk, the FDA recommends that patients of Asian descent be screened for the HLA-B*1502 gene before carbamazepine is used. If the test is positive, carbamazepine should be avoided.
- *Abacavir* [Ziagen], used for HIV infection, can cause potentially fatal hypersensitivity reactions in patients who have a variant gene that codes for HLA-B*5701. Accordingly, the FDA recommends screening for the variant gene before using this drug. If the test is positive, abacavir should be avoided.

In the future, pharmacogenomic analysis of each patient may allow us to engage in revolutionary personalized medicine that addresses the individual patient's genotype. For the present, however, although many advances have been made in pharmacogenomic knowledge, the science is still relatively new (as science goes). Nevertheless, the rapid expanse of knowledge in this area is astonishing. See Table 6.2 for resources to help you keep abreast of changes in this field.

GENDER- AND RACE-RELATED VARIATIONS

Gender- and race-related differences in drug responses are, ultimately, genetically based. Our discussion of pharmacogenomics continues with a focus on these important topics.

Gender

Men and women can respond differently to the same drug. A drug may be more effective in men than in women, or vice versa. Likewise, adverse effects may be more intense in men than in women, or vice versa. Unfortunately, for most drugs, we do not have adequate knowledge about gender-related differences because, before 1997 when the FDA pressured drug companies to include women in trials of new drugs, essentially all drug research was done in men. Since that time, research has demonstrated that significant gender-related differences really do exist. Here are four examples.

- When used to treat heart failure, digoxin may *increase* mortality in women while having no effect on mortality in men.
- Alcohol is metabolized more slowly by women than by men. As a result, a woman who drinks the same amount as a man (on a weight-adjusted basis) will become more intoxicated.
- Certain opioid analgesics (e.g., pentazocine, nalbuphine) are much more effective in women than in men. As a result, pain relief can be achieved at lower doses in women.
- Quinidine causes greater QT interval prolongation in women than in men. As a result, women given the drug are more likely to develop torsades de pointes, a potentially fatal cardiac dysrhythmia.

Although there is still a lack of adequate data related to drug effects in women, information generated by these drug trials, coupled with current and future trials, will permit drug therapy in women to be more rational than is possible today. In the meantime, clinicians must keep in mind that the information currently available may fail to accurately predict responses in female patients. Accordingly, clinicians should

TABLE 6.2 ■ Pharmacogenomic Resources for Health Care Providers

Organization	Resource	Website
Clinical Pharmacogenetics Implementation Consortium (CPIC)	Guidelines to assist providers in using genetic testing to optimize drug therapy	https://www.pharmgkb.org/page/cpic https://www.pharmgkb.org/view/dosing-guidelines.do?source=CPIC#
U.S. Food and Drug Administration (FDA)	*Table of Pharmacogenomic Biomarkers in Drug Labeling*	http://www.fda.gov/drugs/scienceresearch/researchareas/pharmacogenetics/ucm083378.htm
Genetics/Genomics Competency Center (G2C2)	Genetics and genomics resource-specific search engine	http://g-2-c-2.org
Genetics in Primary Care Institute (GPCI)	Multiple resources for application into primary practice	https://geneticsinprimarycare.aap.org
Personalized Medicine Coalition	Variety of resources including a table that links drugs, biomarkers, and indications	http://www.personalizedmedicinecoalition.org http://www.personalizedmedicinecoalition.org/Userfiles/PMC-Corporate/file/pmc_personalized_medicine_drugs_genes.pdf
Pharmacogenomics Knowledgebase (PharmGKB)	A wealth of information including a listing of drugs having labels with genetic information approved by the FDA and Health Canada (Santé Canada)	https://www.pharmgkb.org https://www.pharmgkb.org/view/drug-labels.do

remain alert for treatment failures and unexpected adverse effects.

Race

In general, race is not very helpful as a basis for predicting individual variation in drug responses. To start with, race is nearly impossible to define. Do we define it by skin color and other superficial characteristics? Or do we define it by group genetics? If we define race by skin color, how dark must skin be, for example, to define a patient as "black?" On the other hand, if we define race by group genetics, how many ancestors of African heritage must a patient have to be considered genetically "black?" And what about most people, whose ancestry is ethnically heterogeneous? Latinos, for example, represent a mix of ethnic backgrounds from three continents.

What we really care about is not race per se, but rather the specific genetic and psychosocial factors—shared by many members of an ethnic group—that influence drug responses. Armed with this knowledge, we can identify group members who share those genetic or psychosocial factors and tailor drug therapy accordingly. Perhaps more importantly, application of this knowledge is not limited to members of the ethnic group from which the knowledge arose: we can use it in the management of *all* patients, regardless of ethnic background. How can this be? Owing to ethnic heterogeneity, these factors are not limited to members of any one race. Hence, when we know about a factor (e.g., a specific genetic variation), we can screen all patients for it, and, if it's present, adjust drug therapy as indicated.

This discussion of race-based therapy would be incomplete without mentioning BiDil, a fixed-dose combination of two vasodilators: isosorbide dinitrate (ISDN) and hydralazine, both of which have been available separately for years. In 2005 BiDil became the first drug product approved by the FDA for treating members of just one race, specifically, African Americans. Approval was based on results of the African-American Heart Failure Trial (A-HeFT), which showed that, in self-described black patients, adding ISDN plus hydralazine to standard therapy of heart failure reduced 1-year mortality by 43%—a very impressive and welcome result. Does BiDil benefit African Americans more than other Americans? We do not know; only patients of African ancestry were enrolled in A-HeFT, so the comparison cannot be made. The bottom line? Even though BiDil is approved for treating a specific racial group, there is no proof that it would not work just as well (or even better) in some other group.

COMORBIDITIES AND DRUG INTERACTIONS

Individuals often have two or more medical conditions or disease processes. When this occurs, drugs taken to manage one condition may complicate management of the other condition. As an example, if a person who has both asthma and hypertension is prescribed a nonselective beta-adrenergic antagonist (beta blocker) to control blood pressure, this may worsen the patient's asthma symptoms if the dose is sufficient to cause airway constriction. This illustrates the necessity for the provider to consider the whole patient, not only the disease being treated, when selecting drug therapy.

Because patients with comorbidities often take multiple medications, there is the increased likelihood of drug interactions. Drug interactions can be an important source of variability. The mechanisms by which one drug can alter the effects of another and the clinical consequences of drug interactions are discussed at length in Chapter 4.

UNIT III

Drug Therapy Across the Life Span

CHAPTER 7

Drug Therapy During Pregnancy and Breastfeeding

Jacqueline Rosenjack Burchum, DNSc, FNP-BC, CNE

This chapter addresses drug therapy in women who are pregnant or breastfeeding. The clinical challenge is to provide effective treatment for the patient while avoiding harm to the fetus or nursing infant. Unfortunately, meeting this challenge is confounded by a shortage of reliable data on drug toxicity during pregnancy or breastfeeding.

DRUG THERAPY DURING PREGNANCY: BASIC CONSIDERATIONS

Drug use during pregnancy is common: about two thirds of pregnant patients take at least one medication, and the majority take more. Some drugs are used to treat pregnancy-related conditions, such as nausea, constipation, and preeclampsia. Some are used to treat chronic disorders, such as hypertension, diabetes, and epilepsy. Still others are used for management of invasive conditions such as infectious diseases or cancer. In addition to taking these therapeutic agents, pregnant patients may use drugs of abuse, such as alcohol, cocaine, and heroin.

Drug therapy in pregnancy presents a vexing dilemma. In pregnant patients, as in all other patients, the benefits of treatment must balance the risks. Of course, when drugs are used during pregnancy, risks apply to the fetus as well. Unfortunately, most drugs have not been tested during pregnancy. As a result, the risks for most drugs are unknown—hence the dilemma: the provider is obliged to balance risks versus benefits, without always knowing what the risks really are.

Despite the imposing challenge of balancing risks versus benefits, drug therapy during pregnancy cannot and should not be avoided. Because the health of the fetus depends on the health of the mother, conditions that threaten the mother's health must be addressed. Chronic asthma is a good example. Uncontrolled maternal asthma is far more dangerous to the fetus than the drugs used to treat it. The incidence of stillbirth is doubled among pregnant patients who do not take medications for asthma control.

One of the greatest challenges in identifying drug effects on a developing fetus has been the lack of clinical trials, which, by their nature, would put the developing fetus at risk. Current research often focuses on comparing histories of women who have had children with and without birth defects. An example is the National Birth Defects Prevention Study (http://www.nbdps.org) which is examining births from 1997 to 2011. Another is the Birth Defects Study to Evaluate Pregnancy Exposures (http://www.cdc.gov/ncbddd/birthdefects/bd-steps.html), which began collecting data on children born January 2014 and beyond. Additionally, there are a number of pregnancy registries in which a woman who needs to take a drug while pregnant can enroll. This allows researchers to monitor pregnancy outcomes associated with a drug. The U.S. Food and Drug Administration (FDA) provides a list of pregnancy exposure registries at http://www.fda.gov/ScienceResearch/SpecialTopics/WomensHealthResearch/ucm134848.htm. Although some are devoted to a single drug and its effect on pregnancy and the fetus, many of these study multiple drugs.

Physiologic Changes During Pregnancy and Their Effects on Drug Disposition and Dosing

Pregnancy brings on physiologic changes that can alter drug disposition. Changes in the kidney, liver, and gastrointestinal (GI) tract are of particular interest. Because of these changes, a compensatory change in dosage may be needed.

By the third trimester, renal blood flow is doubled, causing a large increase in glomerular filtration rate. As a result, there is accelerated clearance of drugs that are eliminated by glomerular filtration. Elimination of lithium, for example, is increased by 100%. To compensate for accelerated excretion, dosage must be increased.

For some drugs, hepatic metabolism increases during pregnancy. Three antiseizure drugs—phenytoin, carbamazepine, and valproic acid—provide examples.

Tone and motility of the bowel decrease in pregnancy, causing intestinal transit time to increase. Because of prolonged transit, there is more time for drugs to be absorbed. In theory, this could increase levels of drugs whose absorption is normally poor. Similarly, there is more time for reabsorption of drugs that undergo enterohepatic recirculation, possibly resulting in a prolongation of drug effects. In both cases, a reduction in dosage might be needed.

Placental Drug Transfer

The factors that determine drug passage across the membranes of the placenta are the same factors that determine drug passage across all other membranes. Accordingly, drugs that are lipid soluble cross the placenta easily, whereas drugs that are ionized, highly polar, or protein bound cross with difficulty. Nonetheless, for practical purposes, the provider should assume that *any drug taken during pregnancy will reach the fetus.*

Adverse Reactions During Pregnancy

Not only are pregnant patients subject to the same adverse effects as nonpregnant patients, but they may also suffer effects unique to pregnancy. For example, when heparin (an anticoagulant) is taken by pregnant patients, it can cause osteoporosis, which in turn can cause compression fractures of the spine. Use of prostaglandins (e.g., misoprostol), which stimulate uterine contraction, can cause abortion. Conversely, use of aspirin near term can suppress contractions in labor. In addition, aspirin increases the risk for serious bleeding.

Drugs taken during pregnancy can adversely affect the patient as well as the fetus. Regular use of dependence-producing drugs (e.g., heroin, barbiturates, alcohol) during pregnancy can result in the birth of a drug-dependent infant. If the newborn's dependence is not supported with drugs, a withdrawal syndrome will ensue. Symptoms include shrill crying, vomiting, and extreme irritability. The neonate should be weaned from dependence by giving progressively smaller doses of the drug on which he or she is dependent. Additionally, certain pain relievers used during delivery can depress respiration in the neonate. The infant must be closely monitored until respiration is normal.

The drug effect of greatest concern is teratogenesis. This is the production of birth defects in the fetus.

DRUG THERAPY DURING PREGNANCY: TERATOGENESIS

The term *teratogenesis* is derived from *teras,* the Greek word for monster. Translated literally, teratogenesis means *to produce a monster.* Consistent with this derivation, we usually think of birth defects in terms of gross malformations, such as cleft palate, clubfoot, and hydrocephalus.

Incidence and Causes of Congenital Anomalies

The incidence of *major* structural abnormalities (e.g., abnormalities that are life threatening or require surgical correction) is between 1% and 3%. Half of these are obvious and are reported at birth. The other half involve internal organs (e.g., heart, liver, GI tract) and are not discovered until later in life or at autopsy. The incidence of minor structural abnormalities is unknown, as is the incidence of functional abnormalities (e.g., growth delay, intellectual disabilities).

Congenital anomalies have multiple causes, including genetic predisposition, environmental chemicals, and drugs. Genetic factors account for about 25% of all birth defects. Of the genetically based anomalies, Down syndrome is the most common. Less than 1% of all birth defects are caused by drugs. For most congenital anomalies, the cause is unknown.

Teratogenesis and Stage of Development

Fetal sensitivity to teratogens changes during development; thus the effect of a teratogen is highly dependent on when the drug is given. As shown in Fig. 7.1, development occurs in three major stages: the *preimplantation/presomite period* (conception through week 2), the *embryonic period* (weeks 3 through 8), and the *fetal period* (week 9 through term). During the preimplantation/presomite period, teratogens act in an all-or-nothing fashion. That is, if the dose is sufficiently high, the result is death of the conceptus. Conversely, if the dose is sublethal, the conceptus is likely to recover fully.

Gross malformations are produced by exposure to teratogens during the *embryonic period* (roughly the first trimester). This is the time when the basic shape of internal organs and other structures is being established. Because the fetus is especially vulnerable during the embryonic period, pregnant patients must take special care to avoid teratogen exposure during this time.

Teratogen exposure during the *fetal period* (i.e., the second and third trimesters) usually disrupts *function* rather than gross anatomy. Of the developmental processes that occur in the fetal period, growth and development of the brain are especially important. Disruption of brain development can result in learning deficits and behavioral abnormalities.

Identification of Teratogens

For the following reasons, human teratogens are extremely difficult to identify:

- The incidence of congenital anomalies is generally low.
- Animal tests may not be applicable to humans.
- Prolonged drug exposure may be required.
- Teratogenic effects may be delayed.
- Behavioral effects are difficult to document.
- Controlled experiments cannot be done in humans.

As a result, only a few drugs are considered *proven* teratogens. Drugs whose teratogenicity has been documented (or at least is highly suspected) are listed in Table 7.1. It is important to note, however, that *lack of proof of teratogenicity does not mean that a drug is safe*—it only means that the available data are insufficient to make a definitive judgment. Conversely, *proof of teratogenicity does not mean that every exposure will result in a birth defect.* In fact, with most teratogens, the risk for malformation after exposure is only about 10%.

To prove that a drug is a teratogen, three criteria must be met:

- The drug must cause a characteristic set of malformations.
- The drug must act only during a specific window of vulnerability (e.g., weeks 4 through 7 of gestation).
- The incidence of malformations should increase with increasing dosage and duration of exposure.

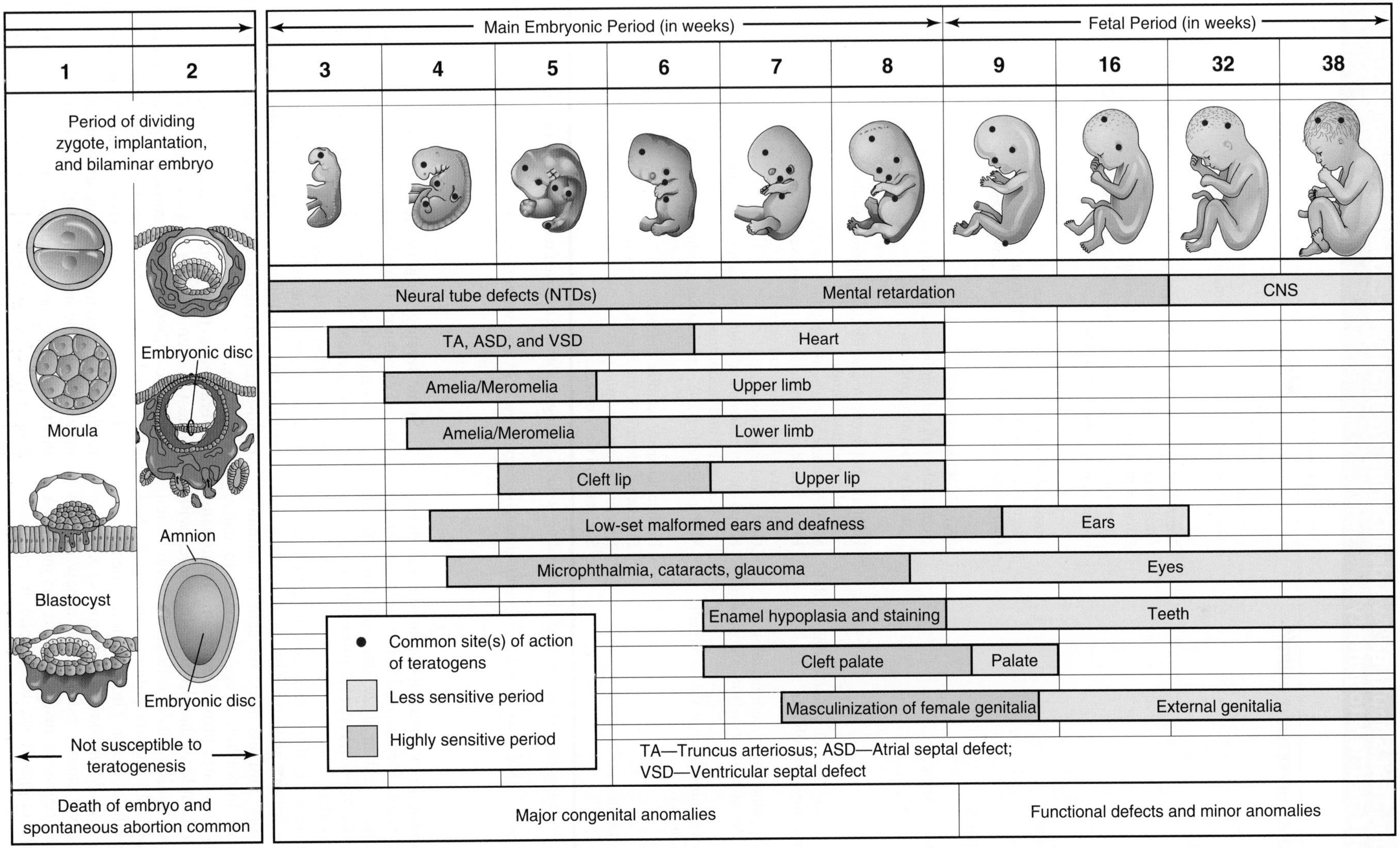

Figure 7.1 ▪ Effects of teratogens at various stages of development of the fetus. (From Moore K, Persaud TVN, Torchia M. The Developing Human: Clinically Oriented Embryology, 9th ed. Philadelphia: Elsevier, 2012, with permission.)

TABLE 7.1 ■ Drugs That Should Be Avoided During Pregnancy Because of Proven or Strongly Suspected Teratogenicity*

Drug	Teratogenic Effect
ANTICANCER/IMMUNOSUPPRESSANT DRUGS	
Cyclophosphamide	CNS malformation, secondary cancer
Methotrexate	CNS and limb malformations
Thalidomide	Shortened limbs, internal organ defects
ANTISEIZURE DRUGS	
Carbamazepine	Neural tube defects, craniofacial defects, malformations of the heart, hypospadias
Phenytoin	Growth delay, CNS defects
Topiramate	Growth delay, cleft lip with cleft palate
Valproic acid	Neural tube defects, craniofacial defects, malformations of the heart and extremities, and hypospadias
SEX HORMONES	
Androgens (e.g., danazol)	Masculinization of the female fetus
Diethylstilbestrol	Vaginal carcinoma in female offspring
Estrogens	Congenital defects of female reproductive organs
ANTIMICROBIAL DRUGS	
Tetracycline	Tooth and bone anomalies
Trimethoprim-sulfamethoxazole	Neural tube defects, cardiovascular malformations, cleft palate, clubfoot, and urinary tract abnormalities
OTHER DRUGS	
Alcohol	Fetal alcohol syndrome, stillbirth, spontaneous abortion, low birth weight, intellectual disabilities
5-Alpha-reductase inhibitors (e.g., dutasteride, finasteride)	Malformations of external genitalia in males
Angiotensin-converting enzyme inhibitors	Renal failure, renal tubular dysgenesis, skull hypoplasia (from exposure during the second and third trimesters)
Antithyroid drugs (propylthiouracil, methimazole)	Goiter and hypothyroidism
HMG CoA reductase inhibitors (atorvastatin, simvastatin)	Facial malformations and CNS anomalies, including holoprosencephaly (single-lobed brain) and neural tube defects
Isotretinoin and other vitamin A derivatives (etretinate, megadoses of vitamin A)	Multiple defects (CNS, craniofacial, cardiovascular, others)
Lithium	Epstein anomaly (cardiac defects)
NSAIDs	Premature closure of the ductus arteriosus
Oral hypoglycemic drugs (e.g., tolbutamide)	Neonatal hypoglycemia
Warfarin	Skeletal and CNS defects

*The absence of a drug from this table does not mean that the drug is not a teratogen. For most proven teratogens, the risk for a congenital anomaly is only 10%.

CNS, central nervous system; HMG CoA, 3-hydroxy-3methylglutaryl coenzyme A; NSAIDs, nonsteroidal antiinflammatory drugs.

Obviously, we cannot do experiments on humans to determine whether a drug meets these criteria. The best we can do is systematically collect and analyze data on drugs taken during pregnancy in the hope that useful information on teratogenicity will be revealed.

Studies in animals may be of limited value, in part because teratogenicity may be species specific. That is, drugs that are teratogens in laboratory animals may be safe in humans. Conversely, and more important, drugs that fail to cause anomalies in animals may later prove teratogenic in humans. The most notorious example is thalidomide. In studies with pregnant animals, thalidomide was harmless; however, when thalidomide was taken by pregnant patients, about 30% had babies with severe malformations. The take-home message is this: *lack of teratogenicity in animals is not proof of safety in humans.* Accordingly, we cannot assume that a new drug is safe for use in human pregnancy just because it has met FDA requirements, which are based on tests done in pregnant animals.

Some teratogens act quickly, whereas others require prolonged exposure. Thalidomide represents a fast-acting teratogen: a single dose can cause malformation. In contrast, alcohol (ethanol) must be taken repeatedly in high doses if gross malformation is to result. (Lower doses of alcohol may produce subtle anomalies.) Because a single exposure to a rapid-acting teratogen can produce obvious malformation, rapid-acting teratogens are easier to identify than slow-acting teratogens.

Teratogens that produce delayed effects are among the hardest to identify. The best example is diethylstilbestrol, an estrogenic substance that causes vaginal cancer in female offspring 18 years or so after they were born.

Teratogens that affect behavior may be nearly impossible to identify. Behavioral changes are often delayed and therefore may not become apparent until the child goes to school. By this time, it may be difficult to establish a correlation between drug use during pregnancy and the behavioral deficit. Furthermore, if the deficit is subtle, it may not even be recognized.

Although we have been discussing the effect of teratogens, it is important to note that drug-related effects are not limited to the distortions of gross anatomy caused by teratogens. Drugs may also include neurobehavioral and metabolic anomalies. For example, benzodiazepines taken late in pregnancy may cause hypoglycemia and respiratory complications along with a hypotonic state that is commonly called *floppy infant syndrome*. The aminoglycoside streptomycin provides another example. Although the teratogen risk of aminoglycosides is low, children born to women taking streptomycin have been born with congenital deafness. Some drugs taken by pregnant women may be dangerous (e.g., the anticoagulant warfarin has been associated with fetal hemorrhage) or life threatening (e.g., misoprostol, a drug taken to protect the stomach of people taking nonsteroidal antiinflammatory drugs [NSAIDs]) can cause a spontaneous abortion.

FDA Pregnancy Risk Categories

In 1979, the FDA established a system for classifying drugs according to their probable risks to the fetus. According to this system, *drugs can be put into one of five risk categories: A, B, C, D,* and *X* (Table 7.2). Drugs in Risk Category A are the least dangerous; controlled studies have been done in pregnant patients and have failed to demonstrate a risk for fetal harm. In contrast, drugs in Category X are the most dangerous; these drugs are known to cause human fetal harm, and their risk to the fetus outweighs any possible therapeutic benefit. Drugs in Categories B, C, and D are progressively more dangerous than drugs in Category A and less dangerous than drugs in Category X. The law does not require classification of drugs that were in use before 1983, so many drugs are not classified. Although this rating system is helpful, it is far from ideal.

TABLE 7.2 ■ FDA Pregnancy Risk Categories

Category	Category Description
A	*Remote risk for fetal harm:* Controlled studies in women have been done and have failed to demonstrate a risk for fetal harm during the first trimester, and there is no evidence of risk in later trimesters.
B	*Slightly more risk than A:* Animal studies show no fetal risk, but controlled studies have not been done in women. *or* Animal studies do show a risk for fetal harm, but controlled studies in women have failed to demonstrate a risk during the first trimester, and there is no evidence of risk in later trimesters.
C	*Greater risk than B:* Animal studies show a risk for fetal harm, but no controlled studies have been done in women. *or* No studies have been done in women or animals.
D	*Proven risk for fetal harm:* Studies in women show proof of fetal damage, but the potential benefits of use during pregnancy may be acceptable despite the risks (e.g., treatment of life-threatening disease for which safer drugs are ineffective). A statement on risk will appear in the WARNINGS section of drug labeling.
X	*Proven risk for fetal harm:* Studies in women or animals show definite risk for fetal abnormality. *or* Adverse reaction reports indicate evidence of fetal risk. The risks clearly outweigh any possible benefit. A statement on risk will appear in the CONTRAINDICATIONS section of drug labeling.

FDA Pregnancy and Lactation Labeling Rule

In December 2014, the FDA issued the Pregnancy and Lactation Labeling Rule (PLLR) providing new guidance for labeling. This rule phased out the Pregnancy Risk Categories beginning June 30, 2015. All newly approved drugs must follow the PLLR guidance for labeling. Manufacturers of previously used drugs are allowed a transition period during which they may continue to use Pregnancy Risk Categories. By 2020, all drugs will cease using Pregnancy Risk Category labeling. Those drugs approved on or after June 30, 2001 must be converted to the new PLLR format. Drugs approved before June 30, 2001 must remove the Pregnancy Risk Category letter while keeping other pregnancy labeling information.

The PLLR requires three sections for labeling: (1) pregnancy, (2) lactation, and (3) females and males of reproductive potential. These are further divided into subsections containing specified content (Table 7.3). The full report is available at http://www.fda.gov/downloads/drugs/guidancecomplianceregulatoryinformation/guidances/ucm450636.pdf.

Minimizing the Drug Risk During Pregnancy

A first step in decreasing drug risk during pregnancy is to develop a comprehensive list of current drugs used. It is crucial to include not only prescription drugs but also over-the-counter and nutritional supplements, as well as recreational drug use, at every visit. A drug as common as vitamin A is dangerous when taken in excess. Vitamin A, which is designated Pregnancy Risk Factor X, can cause craniofacial defects and central nervous system, cardiac, and thymus abnormalities.

If pregnancy status is unknown and a high-risk drug is recommended for management of a condition, a pregnancy test should be performed before prescribing. As noted, some disease states (e.g., epilepsy, asthma, diabetes) pose a greater risk to fetal health than the drugs used for treatment. However, even with these disorders, in which drug therapy reduces the risk for disease-induced fetal harm, we must still take steps to minimize harm from drugs. Accordingly, drugs that pose a high risk for danger to the developing embryo or fetus should be discontinued and safer alternatives substituted.

Sometimes the use of a high-risk drug is unavoidable. Some anticancer drugs, for example, are highly toxic to the developing fetus, yet cannot be ethically withheld from the pregnant patient. If a patient elects to use such drugs, termination of pregnancy should be considered. Reducing the risk for dangerous drug effects also applies to female patients who are *not* pregnant because about 50% of pregnancies are unintended. Accordingly, if a patient of reproductive age is taking a teratogenic medication, she should be educated about the

TABLE 7.3 ▪ FDA Pregnancy and Lactation Labeling Rule Requirements

Sections	Subsections	Headings and/or Content
Pregnancy	Pregnancy Exposure Registry *(This subsection is omitted if there are no known pregnancy exposure registries for the drug.)*	*If a pregnancy exposure registry exists, the following sentence will be included.* "There is a pregnancy exposure registry that monitors pregnancy outcomes in women exposed to (name of drug) during pregnancy." *The statement is followed by registry enrollment information.*
	Risk Summary *(This subsection is required.)*	*Risk summaries are statements that summarize outcomes for the following content relative to drug dosage, length of time drug was taken, and weeks of gestation when drug was taken as well as known pharmacologic mechanisms of action.* Human data Animal data Pharmacology
	Clinical Considerations *(This subsection is omitted if none of the headings is applicable.)*	*Information is provided for the following five headings.* Disease-associated maternal and/or embryo/fetal risk Dose adjustments during pregnancy and the postpartum period Maternal adverse reactions Fetal/neonatal adverse reactions Labor or delivery *(Any heading that is not applicable is omitted.)*
	Data *(This subsection is omitted if none of the headings is applicable.)*	*This section describes research that served as a source of data for Risk Summaries. The following categories are included.* a. Human data b. Animal data *(Any heading that is not applicable is omitted.)*
Lactation	Risk Summary *(This subsection is required.)*	*Risk summaries are statements that summarize outcomes for the following content.* Presence of drug in human milk Effects of drug on the breastfed child Effects of drug on milk production/excretion Risk and benefit statement
	Clinical Considerations *(This subsection is omitted if none of the headings is applicable.)*	*Information is provided for the following headings.* Minimizing exposure Monitoring for adverse reactions *(Any heading that is not applicable is omitted.)*
	Data *(This subsection is omitted if none of the headings is applicable.)*	*This section expands on the Risk Summary and Clinical Considerations subsections. There are no defined headings.*
Females and males of reproductive potential	*(There is no defined subsection for this section.)*	*The following headings are included to address the need for pregnancy testing or contraception and adverse effects associated with preimplantation loss or adverse effects on fertility.* a. Pregnancy testing b. Contraception c. Infertility *(Any heading that is not applicable is omitted.)*

Adapted from U.S. Department of Health and Human Services, Food and Drug Administration. (2015, June). Appendix A: Organization and Format for Pregnancy, Lactation, and Females and Males of Reproductive Potential Subsections. *Pregnancy, Lactation, and Reproductive Potential: Labeling for Human Prescription Drug and Biological Products—Content and Format.* Available at http://www.fda.gov/downloads/drugs/guidancecomplianceregulatoryinformation/guidances/ucm450636.pdf.

teratogenic risk as well as the necessity of using at least one reliable form of birth control.

Responding to Teratogen Exposure

When a pregnant patient has been exposed to a known teratogen, the first step is to determine exactly when the drug was taken and exactly when the pregnancy began. If drug exposure was not during the period of organogenesis (i.e., weeks 3 through 8), the patient should be reassured that the risk of drug-induced malformation is minimal.

What should be done if the exposure *did* occur during organogenesis? First, a reference (such as FDA-approved prescribing information for the drug) should be consulted to determine the type of malformation expected. Next, at least two ultrasound scans should be done to assess the extent of injury. If the malformation is severe, termination of pregnancy should be considered. If the malformation is minor (e.g., cleft palate), it may be correctable by surgery, either shortly after birth or later in childhood.

DRUG THERAPY DURING BREASTFEEDING

Drugs taken by lactating patients can be excreted in breast milk. Although nearly all drugs can enter breast milk, the extent of entry varies greatly. The factors that determine entry into breast milk are the same factors that determine passage of drugs across membranes. Accordingly, drugs that are lipid soluble enter breast milk readily, whereas drugs that are ionized, highly polar, or protein bound tend to be excluded. If drug concentrations in milk are high enough, a pharmacologic effect can occur in the infant, raising the possibility of harm. Unfortunately, relatively little systematic research has been done on this issue. As a result, although a few drugs are known to be hazardous (Table 7.4), the possible danger posed by many others remains undetermined.

Fortunately, most drugs detected in milk are in concentrations that are too low to cause harm. Still, prudence is in order: if the nursing patient can avoid drugs, she should. Moreover, when drugs *must* be used, steps should be taken to minimize risk. These include the following:

- Dosing immediately *after* breastfeeding (to minimize drug concentrations in milk at the next feeding)
- Avoiding drugs that have a long half-life
- Avoiding sustained-release formulations
- Choosing drugs that tend to be excluded from milk
- Choosing drugs that are least likely to affect the infant (Table 7.5)
- Avoiding drugs that are known to be hazardous (see Table 7.4)
- Using the lowest effective dosage for the shortest possible time
- Abandoning plans to breastfeed if a necessary drug is known to be harmful to the child

TABLE 7.4 ■ Drugs That Are Contraindicated During Breastfeeding

CONTROLLED SUBSTANCES
Amphetamine
Cocaine
Heroin
Marijuana
Phencyclidine

ANTICANCER AGENTS/IMMUNOSUPPRESSANTS
Cyclophosphamide
Cyclosporine
Doxorubicin
Methotrexate

OTHERS
Atenolol
Bromocriptine
Ergotamine
Lithium
Nicotine
Radioactive compounds (temporary cessation)

TABLE 7.5 ■ Drugs of Choice for Breastfeeding Patients*

Drug Category	Drugs and Drug Groups of Choice	Comments
Analgesic drugs	Acetaminophen, ibuprofen, flurbiprofen, ketorolac, mefenamic acid, sumatriptan, morphine	Sumatriptan may be given for migraine. Morphine may be given for severe pain.
Anticoagulant drugs	Warfarin, acenocoumarol ♣, heparin (unfractionated)	Among breastfed infants whose mothers were taking warfarin, the drug was undetectable in plasma and bleeding time was not affected. The large molecular size of unfractionated heparin decreases the amount excreted in breast milk. Furthermore, it is not bioavailable from the GI tract, so heparin in breast milk is not systemically absorbed.
Antidepressant drugs	Sertraline, paroxetine, TCAs	Fluoxetine [Prozac] may be given if other SSRIs are ineffective; however, caution is needed because levels are higher in breast milk than levels of other SSRIs. Infant risk with TCAs cannot be ruled out; however, no significant adverse effects have been reported.
Antiepileptic drugs	Carbamazepine, phenytoin, valproic acid	The estimated level of exposure to these drugs in infants is less than 10% of the therapeutic dose standardized by weight.
Antihistamines (histamine-1 blockers)	Loratadine, fexofenadine	First-generation antihistamines are associated with irritability or sedation and may decrease milk supply.
Antimicrobial drugs	Penicillins, cephalosporins, aminoglycosides, macrolides	Avoid chloramphenicol and tetracycline.
Beta-adrenergic antagonists	Labetalol, metoprolol, propranolol	Angiotensin-converting enzyme inhibitors and calcium channel–blocking agents are also considered safe.
Endocrine drugs	Propylthiouracil, insulin, levothyroxine	The estimated level of exposure to propylthiouracil in breastfeeding infants is less than 1% of the therapeutic dose standardized by weight; thyroid function of the infant is not affected.
Glucocorticoids	Prednisolone and prednisone	The amount of prednisolone the infant would ingest in breast milk is less than 0.1% of the therapeutic dose standardized by weight.

*This list is not exhaustive. Cases of overdoses of these drugs must be assessed on an individual basis.
GI, gastrointestinal; SSRI, selective serotonin reuptake inhibitor; TCA, tricyclic antidepressant.

CHAPTER

8 Drug Therapy in Pediatric Patients

Jacqueline Rosenjack Burchum, DNSc, FNP-BC, CNE

Patients who are very young respond differently to drugs than do the rest of the population. Most differences are *quantitative.* Specifically, younger patients are more sensitive to drugs than adult patients, and they show greater individual variation. Drug sensitivity in the very young results largely from *organ system immaturity.* Because of heightened drug sensitivity, they are at increased risk for adverse drug reactions. In this chapter we discuss the physiologic factors that underlie heightened drug sensitivity in pediatric patients and ways to promote safe and effective drug use.

Pediatrics covers all patients up to age 16 years. Because of ongoing growth and development, pediatric patients in different age groups present different therapeutic challenges. Traditionally, the pediatric population is subdivided into six groups:

- Premature infants (less than 36 weeks' gestational age)
- Full-term infants (36 to 40 weeks' gestational age)
- Neonates (first 4 postnatal weeks)
- Infants (postnatal weeks 5 to 52)
- Children (1 to 12 years)
- Adolescents (12 to 16 years)

Not surprisingly, as young patients grow older, they become more like adults physiologically, and hence more like adults with regard to drug therapy. Conversely, the very young—those younger than 1 year, and especially those younger than 1 month—are very different from adults. If drug therapy in these patients is to be safe and effective, we must account for these differences.

Managing pediatric drug therapy is made even more difficult by insufficient drug information. To address this deficit, the U.S. Food and Drug Administration (FDA) Safety and Innovation Act of 2012 permanently reauthorized two laws previously enacted by Congress to promote drug research in children: the Best Pharmaceuticals for Children Act (BPCA) and the Pediatric Research Equity Act (PREA). Additionally, in 2012, the Institutes of Medicine (IOM) published a synopsis of findings from previous research conducted under the BPCA and PREA. This report is available at www.iom.edu/Reports/2012/Safe-and-Effective-Medicines-for-Children.aspx.

As more studies are done, the gaps in our knowledge will shrink. In the meantime, we must still treat children with drugs—even though we lack the information needed to prescribe rationally. Similar to drug therapy during pregnancy, providers must try to balance benefits and risks, without precisely knowing what the benefits and risks really are.

PHARMACOKINETICS: NEONATES AND INFANTS

Pharmacokinetic factors determine the concentration of a drug at its sites of action and hence determine the intensity and duration of responses. If drug levels are elevated, responses will be more intense. If drug elimination is delayed, responses will be prolonged. Because the organ systems that regulate drug levels are not fully developed in the very young, these patients are at risk for both possibilities: drug effects that are unusually intense *and* prolonged. By accounting for pharmacokinetic differences in the very young, we can increase the chances that drug therapy will be both effective and safe.

Fig. 8.1 illustrates how drug levels differ between infants and adults after administration of doses adjusted for body weight. When a drug is administered *intravenously,* levels decline more slowly in the infant than in the adult. As a result, drug levels in the infant remain above the minimum effective concentration (MEC) longer than in the adult, thereby causing effects to be prolonged. When a drug is administered *subcutaneously,* not only do levels in the infant remain above the MEC *longer* than in the adult, but these levels also rise *higher,* causing effects to be more intense as well as prolonged. From these illustrations, it is clear that adjustment of dosage for infants on the basis of body size alone is not sufficient to achieve safe results.

If small body size is not the major reason for heightened drug sensitivity in infants, what is? The increased sensitivity of infants is due largely to the immature state of five pharmacokinetic processes: (1) drug absorption, (2) protein binding of drugs, (3) exclusion of drugs from the central nervous system (CNS) by the blood-brain barrier, (4) hepatic drug metabolism, and (5) renal drug excretion.

Absorption

Oral Administration

Gastrointestinal physiology in the infant is very different from that in the adult. As a result, drug absorption may be enhanced or impeded, depending on the physicochemical properties of the drug involved.

Gastric emptying time is both prolonged and irregular in early infancy, and then gradually reaches adult values by 6 to 8 months. For drugs that are absorbed primarily from the stomach, delayed gastric emptying enhances absorption. On the other hand, for drugs that are absorbed primarily from the intestine, absorption is delayed. Because gastric emptying time is irregular, the precise effect on absorption is not predictable.

Gastric acidity is very low 24 hours after birth and does not reach adult values for 2 years. Because of low acidity, absorption of acid-labile drugs is increased.

Intramuscular Administration

Drug absorption after intramuscular injection in the *neonate* is *slow* and *erratic.* Delayed absorption is due in part to low

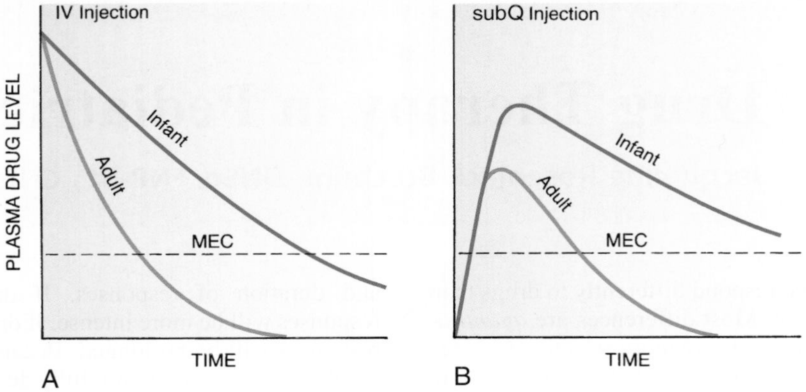

Figure 8.1 ■ Comparison of plasma drug levels in adults and infants. **A,** Plasma drug levels after intravenous injection. Dosage was adjusted for body weight. Note that plasma levels remain above the minimum effective concentration (MEC) much longer in the infant. **B,** Plasma drug levels after subcutaneous injection. Dosage was adjusted for body weight. Note that both the maximal drug level and the duration of action are greater in the infant.

blood flow through muscle during the first days of postnatal life. By early *infancy,* absorption of intramuscular drugs becomes more *rapid* than in neonates and adults.

Transdermal Absorption

Drug absorption through the skin is more rapid and complete in infants than in older children and adults. The stratum corneum of the infant's skin is very thin, and blood flow to the skin is greater in infants than in older patients. Because of this enhanced absorption, infants are at increased risk for toxicity from topical drugs.

Distribution

Protein Binding

Binding of drugs to albumin and other plasma proteins is limited in the infant because (1) the amount of serum albumin is relatively low and (2) endogenous compounds (e.g., fatty acids, bilirubin) compete with drugs for available binding sites. Consequently, drugs that ordinarily undergo extensive protein binding in adults undergo much less binding in infants. As a result, the concentration of *free* levels of such drugs is relatively high in the infant, thereby intensifying effects. To ensure that effects are not too intense, dosages in infants should be reduced. Protein-binding capacity reaches adult values within 10 to 12 months.

Blood-Brain Barrier

The blood-brain barrier is not fully developed at birth. As a result, drugs and other chemicals have relatively easy access to the CNS, making the infant especially sensitive to drugs that affect CNS function. Accordingly, all medicines employed for their CNS effects (e.g., morphine, phenobarbital) should be given in reduced dosage. Dosage should also be reduced for drugs used for actions *outside* the CNS if those drugs are capable of producing CNS toxicity as a side effect.

Hepatic Metabolism

The drug-metabolizing capacity of newborns is low. As a result, neonates are especially sensitive to drugs that are eliminated primarily by hepatic metabolism. When these drugs are used, dosages must be reduced. The capacity of the liver to metabolize many drugs increases rapidly about 1 month after birth and approaches adult levels a few months later. Complete maturation of the liver develops by 1 year.

Renal Excretion

Renal drug excretion is significantly reduced at birth. Renal blood flow, glomerular filtration, and active tubular secretion are all low during infancy. Because the drug-excreting capacity of infants is limited, drugs that are eliminated primarily by renal excretion must be given in reduced dosage or at longer dosing intervals, or both. Adult levels of renal function are achieved by 1 year.

PHARMACOKINETICS: CHILDREN 1 YEAR AND OLDER

By age 1 year, most pharmacokinetic parameters in children are similar to those in adults. Therefore drug sensitivity in children older than 1 year is more like that of adults than that of the very young. Although pharmacokinetically similar to adults, children do differ in one important way: they metabolize drugs *faster* than adults. Drug-metabolizing capacity is markedly elevated until age 2 years and then gradually declines. A further sharp decline takes place at puberty, when adult values are reached. Because of enhanced drug metabolism in children, an increase in dosage or a reduction in dosing interval may be needed for drugs that are eliminated by hepatic metabolism.

ADVERSE DRUG REACTIONS

Like adults, pediatric patients are subject to adverse reactions when drug levels rise too high. In addition, pediatric patients are vulnerable to unique adverse effects related to organ system immaturity and to ongoing growth and development. Among these age-related effects are growth suppression

TABLE 8.1 ■ Adverse Drug Reactions Unique to Pediatric Patients

Drug	Adverse Effect
Androgens	Premature puberty in males; reduced adult height from premature epiphyseal closure
Aspirin and other salicylates	Severe intoxication from acute overdose (acidosis, hyperthermia, respiratory depression); Reye syndrome in children with chickenpox or influenza
Chloramphenicol	Gray syndrome (neonates and infants)
Fluoroquinolones	Tendon rupture
Glucocorticoids	Growth suppression with prolonged use
Hexachlorophene	Central nervous system toxicity (infants)
Nalidixic acid	Cartilage erosion
Phenothiazines	Sudden infant death syndrome
Promethazine	Pronounced respiratory depression in children younger than 2 years
Sulfonamides	Kernicterus (neonates)
Tetracyclines	Staining of developing teeth

(caused by glucocorticoids), discoloration of developing teeth (caused by tetracyclines), and kernicterus (caused by sulfonamides). Table 8.1 presents a list of drugs that can cause unique adverse effects in pediatric patients of various ages. These drugs should be avoided in patients whose age puts them at risk.

DOSAGE DETERMINATION

Because of the pharmacokinetic factors discussed previously, dosage selection for pediatric patients can be challenging. Selecting a dosage is especially difficult in the very young because pharmacokinetic factors are undergoing rapid change.

Pediatric doses have been established for a few drugs, but not for most. For drugs that do not have an established pediatric dose, dosage can be extrapolated from adult doses. The method of conversion employed most commonly is based on body surface area (BSA):

$$\text{Child's BSA} \times \text{Adult dosage} \div 1.73\ \text{m}^2 = \text{Pediatric dosage}$$

Please note that initial pediatric doses—whether based on established pediatric doses or extrapolated from adult doses—are at best an *approximation.* Subsequent doses must be adjusted on the basis of clinical outcome and plasma drug concentrations. These adjustments are especially important in neonates and younger infants. If dosage adjustments are to be optimal, it is essential that we monitor the patient for therapeutic and adverse responses as a component of optimizing dosage.

PROMOTING ADHERENCE

Achieving accurate and timely dosing requires informed participation of the child's caregiver and, to the extent possible, active involvement of the child as well. Effective education is critical. The following issues should be addressed:

- Dosage size and timing
- Route and technique of administration
- Duration of treatment
- Drug storage
- The nature and time course of desired responses
- The nature and time course of adverse responses

Written instructions should be provided to reinforce verbal instructions. For techniques of administration that are difficult, a demonstration should be made, after which the child's caregivers should repeat the procedure to ensure they understand. With young children, spills and spitting out are common causes of inaccurate dosing; parents should be taught to estimate the amount of drug lost and to readminister that amount, being careful not to overcompensate. When more than one person is helping medicate a child, all participants should be warned against multiple dosing. Multiple dosing can be avoided by maintaining a drug administration chart. With some disorders—especially infections—symptoms may resolve before the prescribed course of treatment has been completed. Parents should be instructed to complete the full course nonetheless. Additional strategies to promote adherence are presented in Table 8.2.

TABLE 8.2 ▪ Strategies to Promote Medication Adherence in Children

STRATEGIES FOR PROVIDERS

Prescribe drugs that can be taken once daily or less often, when possible.
Consider drug costs and insurance coverage when choosing medications; discuss options with the caregiver.
Use drug information sheets to reinforce verbal instructions.
Give caregivers age-appropriate and condition-specific reading or coloring books to teach children.

STRATEGIES FOR CAREGIVERS

Suggest medication reminders to avoid missed doses, such as pillboxes, calendars, computer alert systems.
Recommend a reward system to prompt the child to take medication, such as stickers.
Provide pleasant-tasting medication when possible. If the medication is unpalatable, consider the following:

- Suggest keeping it refrigerated, even if not required for storage.
- Administer with food to mask taste, unless contraindicated.
- Have the child suck on a frozen treat to decrease taste sensation before administration.
- Offer a treat to "get the taste out" immediately after taking the medication.
- Praise the child for taking the medication well.

STRATEGIES FOR OLDER CHILDREN AND ADOLESCENTS

Simplify medication regimens, when possible.
Treat the patient with respect and develop trust.
Teach and reinforce necessary skills (e.g., inhaler administration, insulin injection) to improve confidence.
Provide developmentally appropriate information, games, software, and videos to reinforce teaching.
Proactively address adverse effects when possible and collaborate with the patient on preferred methods to manage them when they occur.
Set up networks to connect the child or adolescent with others managing similar illnesses and medication regimens.
Employ an interprofessional team approach for support and encouragement.

CHAPTER

9 Drug Therapy in Geriatric Patients

Jacqueline Rosenjack Burchum, DNSc, FNP-BC, CNE

Drug use among older adults (those 65 years and older) is disproportionately high. Whereas older adults constitute only 12.8% of the U.S. population, they consume 33% of the nation's prescribed drugs. Reasons for this intensive use of drugs include increased severity of illness, multiple pathologies, and excessive prescribing.

Drug therapy in older adults represents a special therapeutic challenge. As a rule, older patients are more sensitive to drugs than are younger adults, and they show wider individual variation. In addition, older adults experience more adverse drug reactions and drug-drug interactions. The principal factors underlying these complications are (1) altered pharmacokinetics (secondary to organ system degeneration), (2) multiple and severe illnesses, (3) multidrug therapy, and (4) poor adherence. To help ensure that drug therapy is as safe and effective as possible, *individualization of treatment is essential: each patient must be monitored for desired and adverse responses, and the regimen must be adjusted accordingly.* Because older adults often suffer from incurable chronic illnesses, the usual objective is to reduce symptoms and improve quality of life.

PHARMACOKINETIC CHANGES IN OLDER ADULTS

The aging process can affect all phases of pharmacokinetics. From early adulthood on, there is a gradual, progressive decline in organ function. This decline can alter the absorption, distribution, metabolism, and excretion of drugs. As a rule, these pharmacokinetic changes increase drug sensitivity (largely from reduced hepatic and renal drug elimination). It should be noted, however, that the extent of change varies greatly among patients: pharmacokinetic changes may be minimal in patients who have remained physically fit, whereas they may be dramatic in patients who have aged less fortunately. Accordingly, you should keep in mind that age-related changes in pharmacokinetics are not only a potential source of increased sensitivity to drugs but also a potential source of increased variability. The physiologic changes that underlie alterations in pharmacokinetics are summarized in Table 9.1.

Absorption

Altered gastrointestinal absorption is not a major factor in drug sensitivity in older adults. As a rule, the *percentage* of an oral dose that becomes absorbed does not usually change with age. However, the *rate* of absorption may be slowed (because of delayed gastric emptying and reduced splanchnic blood flow). As a result, drug responses may be somewhat delayed. Gastric acidity is reduced in older adults and may alter the absorption of certain drugs. For example, some drug formulations require high acidity to dissolve, and hence their absorption may be reduced.

Distribution

Four major factors can alter drug distribution in older adults: (1) increased percent body fat, (2) decreased percent lean body mass, (3) decreased total body water, and (4) reduced concentration of serum albumin. The increase in body fat seen in older adults provides a storage depot for *lipid-soluble* drugs (e.g., propranolol). As a result, plasma levels of these drugs are reduced, causing a reduction in responses. Because of the decline in lean body mass and total body water, *water-soluble* drugs (e.g., ethanol) become distributed in a smaller volume than in younger adults. As a result, the concentration of these drugs is increased, causing effects to be more intense. Although albumin levels are only slightly reduced in healthy older adults, these levels can be significantly reduced in older adults who are malnourished. Because of reduced albumin levels, sites for protein binding of drugs decrease, causing levels of free drug to rise. As a result, drug effects may be more intense.

Metabolism

Rates of hepatic drug metabolism tend to decline with age. Principal reasons are reduced hepatic blood flow, reduced liver mass, and decreased activity of some hepatic enzymes. Because liver function is diminished, the half-lives of certain drugs may be increased, thereby prolonging responses. Responses to oral drugs that ordinarily undergo extensive first-pass metabolism may be enhanced because fewer drugs are inactivated before entering the systemic circulation. Please note, however, that the degree of decline in drug metabolism varies greatly among individuals. As a result, we cannot predict whether drug responses will be significantly reduced in any particular patient.

Excretion

Renal function, and hence renal drug excretion, undergoes progressive decline beginning in early adulthood. *Drug accumulation secondary to reduced renal excretion is the most important cause of adverse drug reactions in older adults.* The decline in renal function is the result of reductions in renal blood flow, glomerular filtration rate, active tubular secretion, and number of nephrons. Renal pathology can further compromise kidney function. The degree of decline in renal function varies greatly among individuals. Accordingly, when patients are taking drugs that are eliminated primarily

TABLE 9.1 ▪ Physiologic Changes That Can Affect Pharmacokinetics in Older Adults

ABSORPTION OF DRUGS
Increased gastric pH
Decreased absorptive surface area
Decreased splanchnic blood flow
Decreased gastrointestinal motility
Delayed gastric emptying
DISTRIBUTION OF DRUGS
Increased body fat
Decreased lean body mass
Decreased total body water
Decreased serum albumin
Decreased cardiac output
METABOLISM OF DRUGS
Decreased hepatic blood flow
Decreased hepatic mass
Decreased activity of hepatic enzymes
EXCRETION OF DRUGS
Decreased renal blood flow
Decreased glomerular filtration rate
Decreased tubular secretion
Decreased number of nephrons

by the kidneys, renal function should be assessed. In older adults, the proper index of renal function is *creatinine clearance,* not *serum creatinine levels.* Creatinine levels do not adequately reflect kidney function in older adults because the source of serum creatinine—lean muscle mass—declines in parallel with the decline in kidney function. Accordingly, creatinine levels may be normal even though renal function is greatly reduced.

PHARMACODYNAMIC CHANGES IN OLDER ADULTS

Alterations in receptor properties may underlie altered sensitivity to some drugs. However, information on such pharmacodynamic changes is limited. In support of the possibility of altered pharmacodynamics is the observation that beta-adrenergic blocking agents (drugs used primarily for cardiac disorders) are *less* effective in older adults than in younger adults, even when present in the same concentrations. Possible explanations for this observation include (1) a reduction in the number of beta receptors and (2) a reduction in the affinity of beta receptors for beta-receptor blocking agents. Other drugs (warfarin, certain central nervous system depressants) produce effects that are more intense in older adults, suggesting a possible increase in receptor number, receptor affinity, or both. Unfortunately, our knowledge of pharmacodynamic changes in older adults is restricted to a few families of drugs.

ADVERSE DRUG REACTIONS AND DRUG INTERACTIONS

Adverse drug reactions (ADRs) are 7 times more common in older adults than in younger adults, accounting for about 16% of hospital admissions among older individuals and 50% of all medication-related deaths. Most of these reactions are dose related, not idiosyncratic. Symptoms in older adults are often nonspecific (e.g., dizziness, cognitive impairment), making identification of ADRs difficult.

Perhaps surprisingly, the increase in ADRs seen in older adults is not the direct result of aging. Rather, multiple factors predispose older patients to ADRs, the most important of which follow:

- Drug accumulation secondary to reduced renal function
- Polypharmacy (treatment with multiple drugs)
- Greater severity of illness
- The presence of comorbidities
- Greater use of drugs that have a low therapeutic index (e.g., digoxin, a drug for heart failure)
- Increased individual variation secondary to altered pharmacokinetics
- Inadequate supervision of long-term therapy
- Poor patient adherence

Most ADRs in older adults are avoidable. Measures that can reduce their incidence include the following:

- Taking a thorough drug history, including over-the-counter medications, herbal remedies, and dietary supplements
- Accounting for the pharmacokinetic and pharmacodynamic changes that occur with aging
- Initiating therapy with low doses and titrating upward gradually ("start low and go slow")
- Monitoring clinical responses and plasma drug levels to provide a rational basis for dosage adjustment
- Employing the simplest medication regimen possible
- Monitoring for drug-drug interactions and iatrogenic illness
- Periodically reviewing the need for continued drug therapy, and discontinuing medications as appropriate
- Encouraging the patient to dispose of old medications
- Taking steps to promote adherence (discussed later)
- Avoiding drugs included in *Beers Criteria for Potentially Inappropriate Medication Use in Older Adults* (the Beers list)

The *Beers list* identifies drugs with a high likelihood of causing adverse effects in older adults. Accordingly, drugs on this list should generally be avoided in adults older than 65 years except when the benefits are significantly greater than the risks. A partial listing of these drugs appears in Table 9.2. The full list, updated in 2015, is available online at http://onlinelibrary.wiley.com/doi/10.1111/jgs.13702/pdf.

PROMOTING ADHERENCE

Between 26% and 59% of older adult patients fail to take their medicines as prescribed. Some patients never fill their prescriptions, some fail to refill their prescriptions, and some don't follow the prescribed dosing schedule. Nonadherence can result in therapeutic failure (from underdosing or erratic dosing) or toxicity (from overdosing). Of the two possibilities, underdosing with resulting therapeutic failure is by far (90%) the more common. Problems arising from nonadherence account for up to 10% of all hospital admissions, and their management may cost more than $100 billion a year.

Multiple factors underlie nonadherence to the prescribed regimen (Table 9.3). Among these are forgetfulness; failure to comprehend instructions (because of intellectual, visual, or

TABLE 9.2 ■ Some Drugs to Generally Avoid in Older Adults

Drugs	Reason for Concern	Alternative Treatments
ANALGESICS		
Indomethacin [Indocin] Ketorolac [Toradol] Non–COX-2 selective NSAIDs (e.g., ibuprofen, aspirin >325 mg/day)	Risk of GI bleeding, especially with long-term use; some may contribute to heart failure	Mild pain: acetaminophen, codeine, COX-2–selective inhibitors if no heart failure risk, *short-term* use of *low-dose* NSAIDs
Meperidine [Demerol]	Not effective at usual doses, risk for neurotoxicity, confusion, delirium	Moderate to severe pain: morphine, oxycodone, hydrocodone
TRICYCLIC ANTIDEPRESSANTS, FIRST GENERATION		
Amitriptyline Clomipramine [Anafranil] Doxepin (>6 mg/day) Imipramine [Tofranil]	Anticholinergic effects (constipation, urinary retention, blurred vision), risk for cognitive impairment, delirium, syncope	SSRIs with shorter half-life, SNRIs, or other antidepressants
ANTIHISTAMINES, FIRST GENERATION		
Chlorpheniramine [Chlor-Trimeton (Chlor-Tripolon ♣), Teldrin] Diphenhydramine [Benadryl] Hydroxyzine [Vistaril, Atarax ♣] Promethazine [Phenergan]	Anticholinergic effects: constipation, urinary retention, blurred vision	Second-generation antihistamines, such as cetirizine [Zyrtec], fexofenadine [Allegra], or loratadine [Claritin]
ANTIHYPERTENSIVES, ALPHA-ADRENERGIC BLOCKING AGENTS		
Alpha$_1$ blockers (e.g., doxazosin [Cardura], prazosin [Minipress], terazosin [Hytrin])	High risk for orthostatic hypotension and falls; less dangerous drugs are available	Thiazide diuretic, ACE inhibitor, beta-adrenergic blocker, calcium channel blocker
Centrally acting alpha$_2$ agonists (e.g., clonidine [Catapres], methyldopa)	Risk for bradycardia, orthostatic hypotension, adverse CNS effects, depression, sedation	
SEDATIVE-HYPNOTICS		
Barbiturates	Physical dependence; compared with other hypnotics, higher risk for falls, confusion, cognitive impairment	Short-term zolpidem [Ambien], zaleplon [Sonata], or eszopiclone [Lunesta] Low-dose ramelteon [Rozerem] or doxepin Nonpharmacologic interventions (e.g., cognitive behavioral therapy)
Benzodiazepines, both short acting (e.g., alprazolam [Xanax], lorazepam [Ativan]) and long acting (e.g., chlordiazepoxide [Librium], diazepam [Valium])	Sedation, cognitive impairment, risk for falls, delirium risk	Low-dose ramelteon [Rozerem] or doxepin Nonpharmacologic interventions (e.g., cognitive behavioral therapy)
DRUGS FOR URGE INCONTINENCE		
Oxybutynin [Ditropan] Tolterodine [Detrol]	Anticholinergic effects, urinary retention, confusion, hallucinations, sedation	Behavioral therapy (e.g., bladder retraining, urge suppression)
MUSCLE RELAXANTS		
Carisoprodol [Soma] Cyclobenzaprine Metaxalone [Skelaxin] Methocarbamol [Robaxin]	Anticholinergic effects, sedation, cognitive impairment; may not be effective at tolerable dosage	Antispasmodics, such as baclofen [Lioresal] Nonpharmacologic interventions (e.g., exercises, proper body mechanics)
PROTON PUMP INHIBITORS		
Esomeprazole [Nexium] Lansoprazole [Prevacid] Omeprazole [Prilosec]	Increased risk for *Clostridium difficile* infection, decreased bone integrity, and fractures	Histamine-2 receptor antagonists (e.g., famotidine [Pepcid], ranitidine [Zantac]) Nonpharmacologic interventions (e.g., deleting foods that increase gastric acidity such as high-fat foods and deleting substances that lower esophageal sphincter pressure such as alcohol)

ACE, angiotensin-converting enzyme; CNS, central nervous system; COX-2, cyclooxygenase-2; GI, gastrointestinal; NSAIDs, nonsteroidal antiinflammatory drugs; SNRI, serotonin/norepinephrine reuptake inhibitor; SSRI, selective serotonin reuptake inhibitor.
Adapted from American Geriatrics Society 2015 updated Beers criteria for potentially inappropriate medication use in older adults. J Am Geriatr Soc 2015;63:62227-62246. (*Note:* The original document lists many drugs in addition to those in this table.)

TABLE 9.3 ■ Factors That Contribute to Poor Adherence in Older Adults

- Multiple chronic disorders
- Multiple prescription medications
- Multiple doses per day for each medication
- Drug packaging that is difficult to open
- Multiple prescribers
- Changes in the regimen (addition of drugs, changes in dosage size or timing)
- Cognitive or physical impairment (reduction in memory, hearing, visual acuity, color discrimination, or manual dexterity)
- Living alone
- Recent discharge from hospital
- Low literacy
- Inability to pay for drugs
- Personal conviction that a drug is unnecessary or the dosage too high
- Presence of side effects

auditory impairment); inability to pay for medications; and use of complex regimens (several drugs taken several times a day). All of these factors can contribute to *unintentional* nonadherence. However, in most cases (about 75%), nonadherence among older adults is *intentional.* The principal reason given for intentional nonadherence is the patient's conviction that the drug was simply not needed in the dosage prescribed. Unpleasant side effects and expense also contribute to intentional nonadherence.

Several measures can promote adherence, including the following:

- Simplifying the regimen so that the number of drugs and doses per day is as small as possible
- Explaining the treatment plan using clear, concise verbal and written instructions
- Choosing an appropriate dosage form (e.g., a liquid formulation if the patient has difficulty swallowing)
- Requesting that the pharmacist label drug containers using a large print size and provide containers that are easy to open by patients with impaired dexterity (e.g., those with arthritis)
- Suggesting the use of a calendar, diary, or pill counter to record drug administration
- Asking the patient if he or she has access to a pharmacy and can afford the medication
- Enlisting the aid of a friend, relative, or visiting health care professional
- Monitoring for therapeutic responses, adverse reactions, and plasma drug levels

It must be noted, however, that the benefits of these measures will be restricted primarily to patients whose nonadherence is *unintentional.* Unfortunately, these measures are generally inapplicable to the patient whose nonadherence is *intentional.* For these patients, intensive education may help.

UNIT IV

Peripheral Nervous System Drugs

CHAPTER 10

Basic Principles of Neuropharmacology

Jacqueline Rosenjack Burchum, DNSc, FNP-BC, CNE

Neuropharmacology can be defined as *the study of drugs that alter processes controlled by the nervous system.* Neuropharmacologic drugs produce effects equivalent to those produced by excitation or suppression of neuronal activity. Neuropharmacologic agents can be divided into two broad categories: (1) peripheral nervous system (PNS) drugs and (2) central nervous system (CNS) drugs.

The neuropharmacologic drugs constitute a large and important family of therapeutic agents. These drugs are used to treat conditions ranging from depression to epilepsy to hypertension to asthma. The clinical significance of these agents is reflected in the fact that more than 25% of this text is dedicated to them.

Why do we have so many neuropharmacologic drugs? Because the nervous system participates in the regulation of practically all bodily processes, practically all bodily processes can be influenced by drugs that alter neuronal regulation. By mimicking or blocking neuronal regulation, neuropharmacologic drugs can modify such diverse processes as skeletal muscle contraction, cardiac output, vascular tone, respiration, gastrointestinal function, uterine motility, glandular secretion, and functions unique to the CNS, such as ideation, mood, and perception of pain. Given the broad spectrum of processes that neuropharmacologic drugs can alter, and given the potential benefits to be gained by manipulating those processes, it is no surprise that neuropharmacologic drugs have widespread clinical applications.

We begin our study of neuropharmacology by discussing PNS drugs (Chapters 11 through 15), after which we discuss CNS drugs (Chapters 16 through 33). The principal rationale for this order of presentation is that our understanding of PNS pharmacology is much clearer than our understanding of CNS pharmacology. Why? Because the PNS is less complex than the CNS, and more accessible to experimentation. By placing our initial focus on the PNS, we can establish a firm knowledge base in neuropharmacology before proceeding to the less definitive and vastly more complex realm of CNS pharmacology.

HOW NEURONS REGULATE PHYSIOLOGIC PROCESSES

As a rule, if we want to understand the effects of a drug on a particular physiologic process, we must first understand the process itself. Accordingly, if we wish to understand the effects of drugs on neuronal regulation of bodily function, we must first understand how neurons regulate bodily function when drugs are absent.

Fig. 10.1 illustrates the basic process by which neurons elicit responses from other cells. The figure depicts two cells: a neuron and a postsynaptic cell. The postsynaptic cell might be another neuron, a muscle cell, or a cell within a secretory gland. As indicated, there are two basic steps—*axonal conduction* and *synaptic transmission*—in the process by which the neuron influences the behavior of the postsynaptic cell. Axonal conduction is simply the process of conducting an action potential down the axon of the neuron. Synaptic transmission is the process by which information is carried across the gap between the neuron and the postsynaptic cell. As shown in the figure, synaptic transmission requires the release of neurotransmitter molecules from the axon terminal followed by binding of these molecules to receptors on the postsynaptic cell. As a result of transmitter-receptor binding, a series of events is initiated in the postsynaptic cell, leading to a change in its behavior. The precise nature of the change depends on the identity of the neurotransmitter and the type of cell involved. If the postsynaptic cell is another neuron, it may increase or decrease its firing rate; if the cell is part of a muscle, it may contract or relax; and if the cell is glandular, it may increase or decrease secretion.

BASIC MECHANISMS BY WHICH NEUROPHARMACOLOGIC AGENTS ACT

Sites of Action: Axons Versus Synapses

To influence a process under neuronal control, a drug can alter one of two basic neuronal activities: axonal conduction or

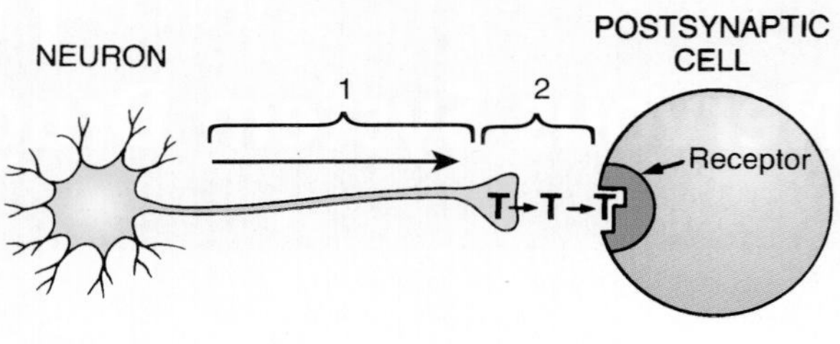

Figure 10.1 ■ How neurons regulate other cells. There are two basic steps in the process by which neurons elicit responses from other cells: (1) axonal conduction and (2) synaptic transmission. (T, neurotransmitter.)

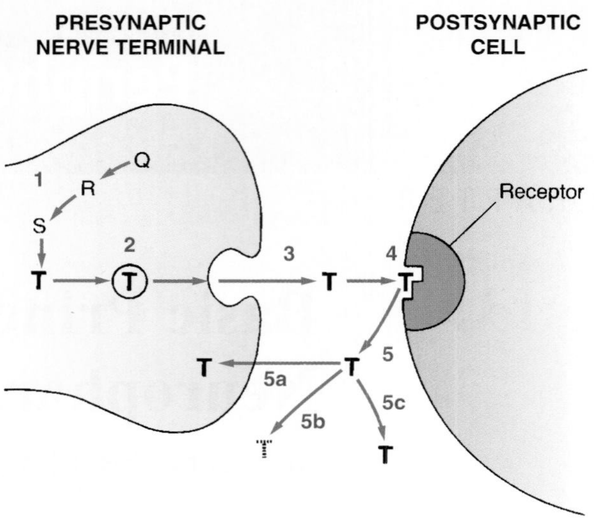

Figure 10.2 ■ Steps in synaptic transmission. *Step 1,* Synthesis of transmitter (T) from precursor molecules (Q, R, and S). *Step 2,* Storage of transmitter in vesicles. *Step 3,* Release of transmitter: in response to an action potential, vesicles fuse with the terminal membrane and discharge their contents into the synaptic gap. *Step 4,* Action at receptor: transmitter binds (reversibly) to its receptor on the postsynaptic cell, causing a response in that cell. *Step 5,* Termination of transmission: transmitter dissociates from its receptor and is then removed from the synaptic gap by (*a*) reuptake into the nerve terminal, (*b*) enzymatic degradation, or (*c*) diffusion away from the gap.

synaptic transmission. *Most neuropharmacologic agents act by altering synaptic transmission.* Only a few alter axonal conduction. This is to our advantage because drugs that alter synaptic transmission can produce effects that are much more *selective* than those produced by drugs that alter axonal conduction.

Axonal Conduction

Drugs that act by altering axonal conduction are not very selective. Recall that the process of conducting an impulse along an axon is essentially the same in all neurons. As a consequence, a drug that alters axonal conduction will affect conduction in all nerves to which it has access. Such a drug cannot produce selective effects.

Local anesthetics are drugs that work by altering (decreasing) axonal conduction. Because these agents produce nonselective inhibition of axonal conduction, they suppress transmission in any nerve they reach. Hence, although local anesthetics are certainly valuable, their indications are limited.

Synaptic Transmission

In contrast to drugs that alter axonal conduction, drugs that alter synaptic transmission can produce effects that are highly selective. Why? Because synapses, unlike axons, differ from one another. Synapses at different sites employ different transmitters. In addition, for most transmitters, the body employs more than one type of receptor. Hence, by using a drug that selectively influences a specific type of neurotransmitter or receptor, we can alter one neuronally regulated process while leaving most others unchanged. Because of their relative selectivity, drugs that alter synaptic transmission have many uses.

Receptors

The ability of a neuron to influence the behavior of another cell depends, ultimately, on the ability of that neuron to alter receptor activity on the target cell. As discussed, neurons alter receptor activity by releasing transmitter molecules, which diffuse across the synaptic gap and bind to receptors on the postsynaptic cell. If the target cell lacked receptors for the transmitter that a neuron released, that neuron would be unable to affect the target cell.

The effects of neuropharmacologic drugs, like those of neurons, depend on altering receptor activity. That is, no matter what its precise mechanism of action, a neuropharmacologic drug ultimately works by influencing receptor activity on target cells. This concept is central to understanding the actions of neuropharmacologic drugs. In fact, this concept is so critical to our understanding of neuropharmacologic agents that I will repeat it: *the effect of a drug on a neuronally regulated process is dependent on the ability of that drug to directly or indirectly influence receptor activity on target cells.*

Steps in Synaptic Transmission

To understand how drugs alter receptor activity, we must first understand the steps by which synaptic transmission takes place because it is by modifying these steps that neuropharmacologic drugs influence receptor function. The steps in synaptic transmission are shown in Fig. 10.2.

Step 1: Transmitter Synthesis

For synaptic transmission to take place, molecules of transmitter must be present in the nerve terminal. Hence we can look on transmitter synthesis as the first step in transmission. In the figure, the letters Q, R, and S represent the precursor molecules from which the transmitter (T) is made.

Step 2: Transmitter Storage

After transmitter is synthesized, it must be stored until the time of its release. Transmitter storage takes place within vesicles—tiny packets present in the axon terminal. Each nerve terminal contains a large number of transmitter-filled vesicles.

Step 3: Transmitter Release

Release of transmitter is triggered by the arrival of an action potential at the axon terminal. The action potential initiates a process in which vesicles undergo fusion with the terminal membrane, causing release of their contents into the synaptic gap. Each action potential causes only a small fraction of all vesicles present in the axon terminal to discharge their contents.

Step 4: Receptor Binding

After release, transmitter molecules diffuse across the synaptic gap and then undergo *reversible* binding to receptors on the postsynaptic cell. This binding initiates a cascade of events that result in altered behavior of the postsynaptic cell.

Step 5: Termination of Transmission

Transmission is terminated by dissociation of transmitter from its receptors, followed by removal of free transmitter from the synaptic gap. Transmitter can be removed from the synaptic gap by three processes: (1) reuptake, (2) enzymatic degradation, and (3) diffusion. In those synapses where transmission is terminated by reuptake, axon terminals contain "pumps" that transport transmitter molecules back into the neuron from which they were released (Step 5a in Fig. 10.2). After reuptake, molecules of transmitter may be degraded, or they may be packaged in vesicles for reuse. In synapses where transmitter is cleared by enzymatic degradation (Step 5b), the synapse contains large quantities of transmitter-inactivating enzymes. Although simple diffusion away from the synaptic gap (Step 5c) is a potential means of terminating transmitter action, this process is very slow and generally of little significance.

TABLE 10.1 ▪ Effects of Drugs on Synaptic Transmission and the Resulting Effect on Receptor Activation

Step of Synaptic Transmission	Drug Action	Effect on Receptor Activation*
1. Synthesis of transmitter	Increased synthesis of T	Increase
	Decreased synthesis of T	Decrease
	Synthesis of "super" T	Increase
2. Storage of transmitter	Reduced storage of T	Decrease
3. Release of transmitter	Promotion of T release	Increase
	Inhibition of T release	Decrease
4. Binding to receptor	Direct receptor activation	Increase
	Enhanced response to T	Increase
	Blockade of T binding	Decrease
5. Termination of transmission	Blockade of T reuptake	Increase
	Inhibition of T breakdown	Increase

*Receptor activation is defined as producing an effect equivalent to that produced by the natural transmitter that acts on a particular receptor.
T, transmitter.

Effects of Drugs on the Steps of Synaptic Transmission

As emphatically noted, all neuropharmacologic agents (except local anesthetics) produce their effects by directly or indirectly altering receptor activity. We also noted that the way in which drugs alter receptor activity is by interfering with synaptic transmission. Because synaptic transmission has multiple steps, the process offers a number of potential targets for drugs. In this section, we examine the specific ways in which drugs can alter the steps of synaptic transmission.

Before discussing specific mechanisms by which drugs can alter receptor activity, we need to understand what drugs are capable of doing to receptors in general terms. From the broadest perspective, when a drug influences receptor function, that drug can do just one of two things: it can enhance receptor activation, or it can reduce receptor activation. What do we mean by receptor activation? For our purposes, we can define *activation* as *an effect on receptor function equivalent to that produced by the natural neurotransmitter at a particular synapse.* Hence a drug whose effects mimic the effects of a natural transmitter would be said to *increase* receptor activation. Conversely, a drug whose effects were equivalent to reducing the amount of natural transmitter available for receptor binding would be said to *decrease* receptor activation.

Please note that activation of a receptor does not necessarily mean that a physiologic process will go faster; receptor activation can also make a process go slower. For example, when the neurotransmitter acetylcholine activates cholinergic receptors on the heart, the heart rate will decline. Similarly, a drug that mimics acetylcholine at receptors on the heart will cause the heart to beat more slowly.

Having defined receptor activation, we are ready to discuss the mechanisms by which drugs, acting on specific steps of synaptic transmission, can increase or decrease receptor activity (Table 10.1). As we consider these mechanisms one by one, their commonsense nature should become apparent.

Transmitter Synthesis

There are three different effects that drugs are known to have on transmitter synthesis. They can (1) increase transmitter synthesis, (2) decrease transmitter synthesis, or (3) cause the synthesis of transmitter molecules that are more effective than the natural transmitter itself.

A drug that increases transmitter synthesis will cause receptor activation to increase. The process is this: As a result of increased transmitter synthesis, storage vesicles will contain transmitter in abnormally high amounts. Hence, when an action potential reaches the axon terminal, more transmitter will be released, and therefore more transmitter will be available to receptors on the postsynaptic cell, causing activation of those receptors to increase. Conversely, a drug that decreases transmitter synthesis will cause the transmitter content of vesicles to decline, resulting in reduced transmitter release and decreased receptor activation.

Some drugs can cause neurons to synthesize transmitter molecules whose structure is different from that of normal transmitter molecules. For example, by acting as substrates for enzymes in the axon terminal, drugs can be converted into "super" transmitters (molecules whose ability to activate receptors is greater than that of the naturally occurring transmitter at a particular site). Release of these supertransmitters will cause receptor activation to increase.

Transmitter Storage

Drugs that interfere with transmitter storage will cause receptor activation to decrease. This occurs because disruption of storage depletes vesicles of their transmitter content, thereby decreasing the amount of transmitter available for release.

Transmitter Release

Drugs can either *promote* or *inhibit* transmitter release. Drugs that promote release will increase receptor activation. Conversely, drugs that inhibit release will reduce receptor activation. The amphetamines represent drugs that act by promoting transmitter release. Botulinum toxin, in contrast, acts by inhibiting transmitter release.

Receptor Binding

Many drugs act directly at receptors. These agents can either (1) bind to receptors and cause activation, (2) bind to receptors and thereby block receptor activation by other agents, or (3) bind to receptor components and thereby enhance receptor activation by the natural transmitter at the site.

In the terminology introduced in Chapter 4, drugs that directly activate receptors are called *agonists,* whereas drugs that prevent receptor activation are called *antagonists.* The direct-acting receptor agonists and antagonists constitute the largest and most important groups of neuropharmacologic drugs. There is no single name or category for drugs that bind to receptors to enhance natural transmitter effects.

Examples of drugs that act directly at receptors are numerous. Drugs that bind to receptors and cause *activation* include morphine (used for its effects on the CNS), epinephrine (used mainly for its effects on the cardiovascular system), and insulin (used for its effects in diabetes). Drugs that bind to and block receptors to *prevent* their activation include naloxone (used to treat overdose with opioid drugs), antihistamines (used to treat allergic disorders), and metoprolol (used to treat hypertension, angina pectoris, and cardiac dysrhythmias). Benzodiazepines are excellent examples of drugs that bind to receptors and thereby enhance the actions of a natural transmitter. Drugs in this family, which includes diazepam [Valium] and related agents, are used to treat anxiety, seizure disorders, and muscle spasm.

Termination of Transmitter Action

Drugs can interfere with the termination of transmitter action by two mechanisms: (1) blockade of transmitter reuptake and (2) inhibition of transmitter degradation. Drugs that act by either mechanism will increase transmitter availability, thereby causing receptor activation to increase.

MULTIPLE RECEPTOR TYPES AND SELECTIVITY OF DRUG ACTION

As we discussed in Chapter 4, selectivity is one of the most desirable qualities a drug can have. A selective drug is able to alter a specific disease process while leaving other physiologic processes largely unaffected.

Many neuropharmacologic agents display a high degree of selectivity. This selectivity is possible because the nervous system works through multiple types of receptors to regulate processes under its control. The relationship between multiple receptor types and selective drug action is illustrated by Mort and Merv, whose unique physiologies are depicted in Fig. 10.3. Let's begin with Mort. Mort can perform four functions: he can pump blood, digest food, shake hands, and empty his

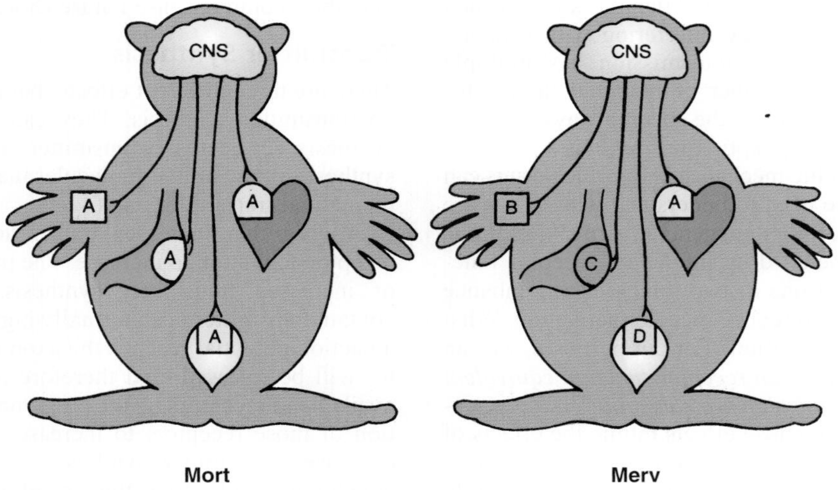

Figure 10.3 ■ Multiple drug receptors and selective drug action.
All of the **Mort** organs are regulated through activation of type A receptors. Drugs that affect type A receptors on one organ will affect type A receptors on all other organs. Hence, selective drug action is impossible. **Merv** has four types of receptors (A, B, C, and D) to regulate his four organs. A drug that acts at one type of receptor will not affect the others. Hence, selective drug action is possible.

bladder. All four functions are under neuronal control, and, in all cases, that control is exerted by activation of the same type of receptor (designated A).

As long as Mort remains healthy, having only one type of receptor to regulate his various functions is no problem. Selective *physiologic* regulation can be achieved simply by sending impulses down the appropriate nerves. When there is a need to increase cardiac output, impulses are sent down the nerve to his heart; when digestion is needed, impulses are sent down the nerve to his stomach; and so forth.

Although having only one receptor type is no disadvantage when all is well, if Mort gets sick, having only one receptor type creates a therapeutic challenge. Let's assume he develops heart disease and we need to give a drug that will help increase cardiac output. To stimulate cardiac function, we need to administer a drug that will activate receptors on his heart. Unfortunately, because the receptors on his heart are the same as the receptors on his other organs, a drug that stimulates cardiac function will stimulate his other organs, too. Consequently, any attempt to improve cardiac output with drugs will necessarily be accompanied by side effects. These will range from silly (compulsive handshaking) to embarrassing (enuresis) to hazardous (gastric ulcers). Please note that all of these undesirable effects are the direct result of Mort having a nervous system that works through just one type of receptor to regulate all organs. That is, the presence of only one receptor type has made selective drug action impossible.

Now let's consider Merv. Although Merv appears to be Mort's twin, Merv differs in one important way: whereas all functions in Mort are regulated through just one type of receptor, Merv employs different receptors to control each of his four functions. Because of this simple but important difference, the selective drug action that was impossible with Mort can be achieved easily with Merv. We can, for example, selectively enhance cardiac function in Merv without risking the side effects to which Mort was predisposed. This can be done simply by administering an agonist agent that binds selectively to receptors on the heart (type A receptors). If this medication is sufficiently selective for type A receptors, it will not interact with receptor types B, C, or D. Hence, function in structures regulated by those receptors will be unaffected. Note that our ability to produce selective drug action in Merv is made possible because his nervous system works through different types of receptors to regulate function in his various organs. The message from this example is clear: *the more types of receptors we have to work with, the greater our chances of producing selective drug effects.*

AN APPROACH TO LEARNING ABOUT PERIPHERAL NERVOUS SYSTEM DRUGS

As discussed, to understand the ways in which drugs can alter a process under neuronal control, we must first understand how the nervous system itself regulates that process. Accordingly, when preparing to study PNS pharmacology, you must first establish a working knowledge of the PNS itself. In particular, you need to know two basic types of information about PNS function. First, you need to know the types of receptors through which the PNS works when influencing the function of a specific organ. Second, you need to know what the normal response to activation of those receptors is. All of the information you need about PNS function is reviewed in Chapter 11.

To understand any particular PNS drug, you need three types of information: (1) the type (or types) of receptor through which the drug acts; (2) the normal response to activation of those receptors; and (3) what the drug in question does to receptor function (i.e., does it increase or decrease receptor activation?). Armed with these three types of information, you can predict the major effects of any PNS drug.

An example will illustrate this process. Let's consider the drug named *isoproterenol.* The first information we need is the identity of the receptors at which isoproterenol acts. Isoproterenol acts at two types of receptors, named beta_1- and beta_2-adrenergic receptors. Next, we need to know the normal responses to activation of these receptors. The most prominent responses to activation of beta_1 receptors are *increased heart rate* and *increased force of cardiac contraction.* The primary responses to activation of beta_2 receptors are *bronchial dilation* and *elevation of blood glucose levels.* Lastly, we need to know whether isoproterenol increases or decreases the activation of beta_1 and beta_2 receptors. At both types of receptor, isoproterenol causes *activation.* Armed with these three primary pieces of information about isoproterenol, we can now predict the principal effects of this drug. By *activating* beta_1 and beta_2 receptors, isoproterenol can elicit three major responses: (1) increased cardiac output (by increasing heart rate and force of contraction); (2) dilation of the bronchi; and (3) elevation of blood glucose.

From this example, you can see how easy it is to predict the effects of a PNS drug. Accordingly, I strongly encourage you to take the approach suggested when studying these agents. That is, for each PNS drug, you should learn (1) the identity of the receptors at which that drug acts, (2) the normal responses to activation of those receptors, and (3) whether the drug increases or decreases receptor activation.

CHAPTER

11 Physiology of the Peripheral Nervous System

Jacqueline Rosenjack Burchum, DNSc, FNP-BC, CNE

To understand peripheral nervous system (PNS) drugs, we must first understand the PNS itself. The purpose of this chapter is to help you develop that understanding.

It's not uncommon for students to be at least slightly apprehensive about studying the PNS—especially the autonomic component. This book's approach to teaching the information is untraditional. Hopefully, it will make your work easier.

Because our ultimate goal concerns pharmacology—and not physiology—we do not address everything there is to know about the PNS. Rather, we limit the discussion to those aspects of PNS physiology that have a direct bearing on your ability to understand drugs.

DIVISIONS OF THE NERVOUS SYSTEM

The nervous system has two main divisions, the *central nervous system* (CNS) and the *peripheral nervous system.* The PNS has two major subdivisions: (1) the *somatic motor system* and (2) the *autonomic nervous system.* The autonomic nervous system is further subdivided into the *parasympathetic nervous system* and the *sympathetic nervous system.* The somatic motor system controls voluntary movement of muscles. The two subdivisions of the autonomic nervous system regulate many involuntary processes.

The autonomic nervous system is the principal focus of this chapter. The somatic motor system is also considered, but discussion is brief.

OVERVIEW OF AUTONOMIC NERVOUS SYSTEM FUNCTIONS

The autonomic nervous system has three principal functions: (1) regulation of the *heart;* (2) regulation of *secretory glands* (salivary, gastric, sweat, and bronchial glands); and (3) regulation of *smooth muscles* (muscles of the bronchi, blood vessels, urogenital system, and gastrointestinal [GI] tract). These regulatory activities are shared between the sympathetic and parasympathetic divisions of the autonomic nervous system.

Functions of the Parasympathetic Nervous System

The parasympathetic nervous system performs seven regulatory functions that have particular relevance to drugs. Specifically, stimulation of appropriate parasympathetic nerves causes the following:

- Slowing of heart rate
- Increased gastric secretion
- Emptying of the bladder
- Emptying of the bowel
- Focusing the eye for near vision
- Constricting the pupil
- Contracting bronchial smooth muscle

Just how the parasympathetic nervous system elicits these responses is discussed later in the section "Functions of Cholinergic Receptor Subtypes."

From the previous discussion we can see that the parasympathetic nervous system is concerned primarily with what might be called the "housekeeping" chores of the body (digestion of food and excretion of wastes). In addition, the system helps control vision and conserve energy (by reducing cardiac work).

Therapeutic agents that alter parasympathetic nervous system function are used primarily for their effects on the GI tract, bladder, and eye. Occasionally, these drugs are also used for effects on the heart and lungs.

A variety of poisons act by mimicking or blocking effects of parasympathetic stimulation. Among these are insecticides, nerve gases, and toxic compounds found in certain mushrooms and plants.

Functions of the Sympathetic Nervous System

The sympathetic nervous system has three main functions:

- Regulating the cardiovascular system
- Regulating body temperature
- Implementing the acute stress response (commonly called a "fight-or-flight" reaction)

The sympathetic nervous system exerts multiple influences on the heart and blood vessels. Stimulation of sympathetic nerves to the heart increases cardiac output. Stimulation of sympathetic nerves to arterioles and veins causes vasoconstriction. Release of epinephrine from the adrenal medulla results in vasoconstriction in most vascular beds and vasodilation in certain others. By influencing the heart and blood vessels, the sympathetic nervous system can achieve three homeostatic objectives:

- Maintenance of blood flow to the brain
- Redistribution of blood flow during exercise
- Compensation for loss of blood, primarily by causing vasoconstriction

The sympathetic nervous system helps regulate body temperature in three ways: (1) By regulating blood flow to the skin, sympathetic nerves can increase or decrease heat loss. By *dilating* surface vessels, sympathetic nerves increase blood flow to the skin and thereby accelerate heat loss. Conversely, *constricting* cutaneous vessels conserves heat. (2) Sympathetic nerves to sweat glands promote secretion of sweat, thereby helping the body cool. (3) By inducing piloerection (erection of hair), sympathetic nerves can promote heat conservation.

When we are faced with an acute stress-inducing situation, the sympathetic nervous system orchestrates the fight-or-flight response, which consists of the following:

- Increasing heart rate and blood pressure
- Shunting blood away from the skin and viscera and into skeletal muscles
- Dilating the bronchi to improve oxygenation
- Dilating the pupils (perhaps to enhance visual acuity)
- Mobilizing stored energy, thereby providing glucose for the brain and fatty acids for muscles

The sensation of being "cold with fear" is brought on by shunting of blood away from the skin. The phrase "wide-eyed with fear" may be based on pupillary dilation.

Many therapeutic agents produce their effects by altering functions under sympathetic control. These drugs are used primarily for effects on the heart, blood vessels, and lungs. Agents that alter cardiovascular function are used to treat hypertension, heart failure, angina pectoris, and other disorders. Drugs affecting the lungs are used primarily for asthma.

BASIC MECHANISMS BY WHICH THE AUTONOMIC NERVOUS SYSTEM REGULATES PHYSIOLOGIC PROCESSES

To understand how drugs influence processes under autonomic control, we must first understand how the autonomic nervous system itself regulates those activities. The basic mechanisms by which the autonomic nervous system regulates physiologic processes are discussed next.

Patterns of Innervation and Control

Most structures under autonomic control are innervated by sympathetic nerves *and* parasympathetic nerves. The relative influence of sympathetic and parasympathetic nerves depends on the organ under consideration.

In many organs that receive dual innervation, the influence of sympathetic nerves *opposes* that of parasympathetic nerves. For example, in the heart, *sympathetic* nerves *increase* heart rate, whereas *parasympathetic* nerves *slow* heart rate (Fig. 11.1).

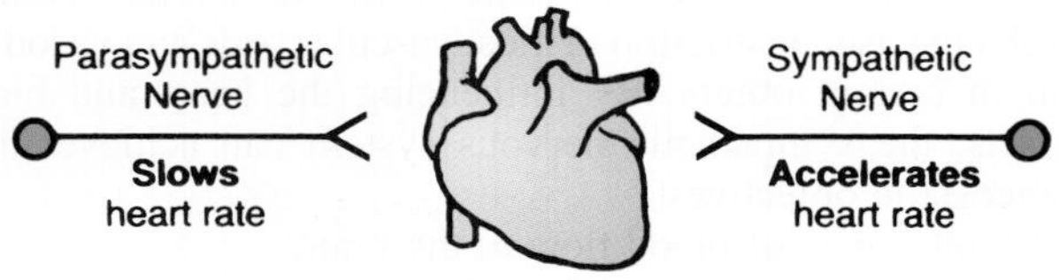

Figure 11.1 ■ Opposing effects of parasympathetic and sympathetic nerves.

In some organs that receive nerves from both divisions of the autonomic nervous system, the effects of sympathetic and parasympathetic nerves are *complementary*, rather than opposite. For example, in the male reproductive system, erection is regulated by parasympathetic nerves, whereas ejaculation is controlled by sympathetic nerves. If attempts at reproduction are to succeed, cooperative interaction of both systems is needed.

A few structures under autonomic control receive innervation from only one division. The principal example is blood vessels, which are innervated exclusively by sympathetic nerves.

In summary, there are three basic patterns of autonomic innervation and regulation:

- Innervation by *both* divisions of the autonomic nervous system in which the effects of the two divisions are *opposed*
- Innervation by *both* divisions of the autonomic nervous system in which the effects of the two divisions are *complementary*
- Innervation and regulation by *only one* division of the autonomic nervous system

Feedback Regulation

Feedback regulation is a process that allows a system to adjust itself by responding to incoming information. Practically all physiologic processes are regulated at least in part by feedback control.

Fig. 11.2 depicts a feedback loop typical of those used by the autonomic nervous system. The main elements of this loop are (1) a *sensor*, (2) an *effector*, and (3) *neurons* connecting the sensor to the effector. The purpose of the sensor is to monitor the status of a physiologic process. Information picked up by the sensor is sent to the CNS (spinal cord and brain), where it is integrated with other relevant information. Signals (instructions for change) are then sent from the CNS along nerves of the autonomic system to the effector. In response to these instructions, the effector makes appropriate adjustments in the process. The entire procedure is called a *reflex*.

Baroreceptor Reflex

From a pharmacologic perspective, the most important feedback loop of the autonomic nervous system is one that helps regulate blood pressure. This system is referred to as the *baroreceptor reflex*. (Baroreceptors are receptors that sense

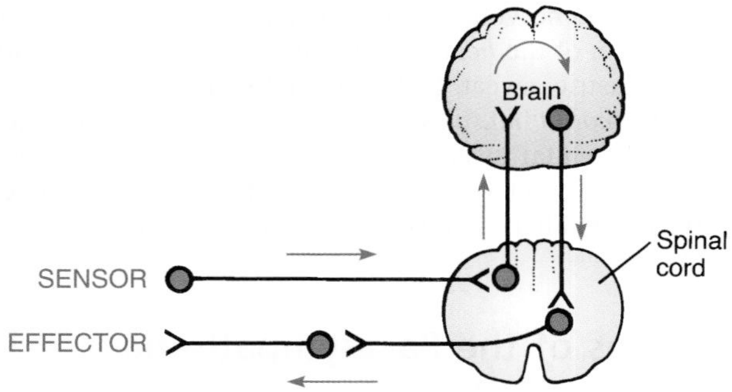

Figure 11.2 ■ Feedback loop of the autonomic nervous system.

blood pressure.) This reflex is important to us because it frequently opposes our attempts to modify blood pressure with drugs.

Feedback (reflex) control of blood pressure is achieved as follows: (1) Baroreceptors located in the carotid sinus and aortic arch monitor changes in blood pressure and send this information to the brain. (2) In response, the brain sends impulses along nerves of the autonomic nervous system, instructing the heart and blood vessels to behave in a way that restores blood pressure to normal. Accordingly, when blood pressure *falls,* the baroreceptor reflex causes vasoconstriction and increases cardiac output. Both actions help bring blood pressure back up. Conversely, when blood pressure *rises* too high, the baroreceptor reflex causes vasodilation and reduces cardiac output, thereby causing blood pressure to drop. The baroreceptor reflex is discussed in greater detail in Chapter 34.

Autonomic Tone

Autonomic tone is the steady, day-to-day influence exerted by the autonomic nervous system on a particular organ or organ system. Autonomic tone provides a basal level of control over which reflex regulation is superimposed.

When an organ is innervated by both divisions of the autonomic nervous system, one division—either sympathetic or parasympathetic—provides most of the basal control, thereby obviating conflicting instruction. Recall that, when an organ receives nerves from both divisions of the autonomic nervous system, those nerves frequently exert opposing influences. If both divisions were to send impulses simultaneously, the resultant conflicting instructions would be counterproductive (like running heating and air conditioning simultaneously). By having only one division of the autonomic nervous system provide the basal control to an organ, conflicting signals are avoided.

The branch of the autonomic nervous system that controls organ function most of the time is said to provide the *predominant tone* to that organ. *In most organs, the parasympathetic nervous system provides the predominant tone.* The vascular system, which is regulated almost exclusively by the *sympathetic* nervous system, is the principal exception.

ANATOMIC CONSIDERATIONS

Although we know a great deal about the anatomy of the PNS, very little of this information helps us understand PNS drugs. The few details that *do* pertain to pharmacology are shown in Fig. 11.3.

Parasympathetic Nervous System

Pharmacologically relevant aspects of parasympathetic anatomy are shown in Fig. 11.3. Note that there are *two* neurons in the pathway leading from the spinal cord to organs innervated by parasympathetic nerves. The junction (synapse) between these two neurons occurs within a structure called a *ganglion.* (A ganglion is simply a mass of nerve cell bodies.) The neurons that go from the spinal cord to the parasympathetic ganglia are called *preganglionic neurons,* whereas the neurons that go from the ganglia to effector organs are called *postganglionic neurons.* The anatomy of the parasympathetic nervous system offers two general sites at which drugs can act: (1) the synapses between preganglionic neurons and postganglionic neurons and (2) the junctions between postganglionic neurons and their effector organs.

Sympathetic Nervous System

Pharmacologically relevant aspects of sympathetic nervous system anatomy are illustrated in Fig. 11.3. As you can see, these features are nearly identical to those of the parasympathetic nervous system. Like the parasympathetic nervous system, the sympathetic nervous system employs two neurons

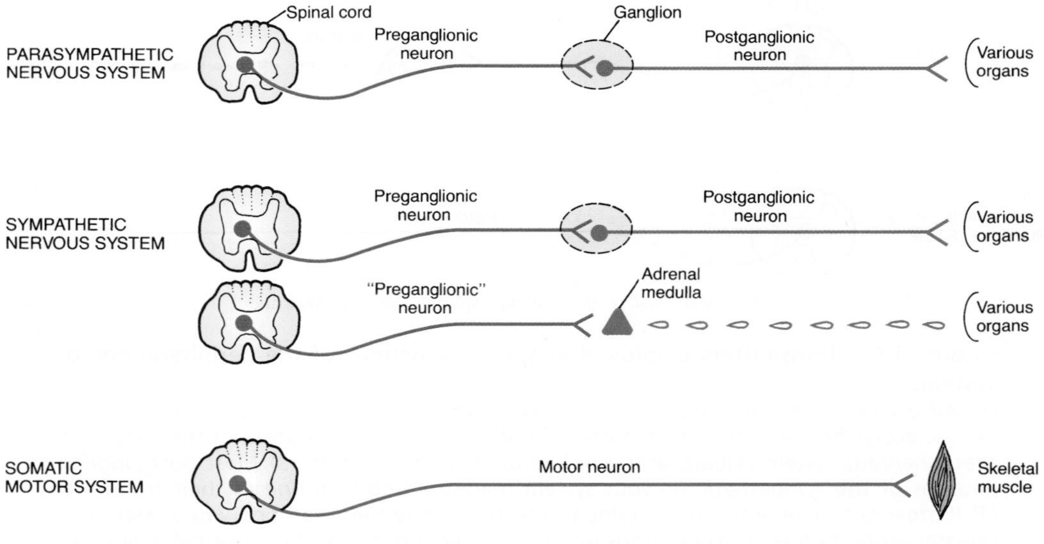

Figure 11.3 ■ The basic anatomy of the parasympathetic and sympathetic nervous systems and the somatic motor system.

in the pathways leading from the spinal cord to organs under its control. As with the parasympathetic nervous system, the junctions between those neurons are located in *ganglia.* Neurons leading from the spinal cord to the sympathetic ganglia are termed *preganglionic neurons,* and neurons leading from ganglia to effector organs are termed *postganglionic neurons.*

The *medulla of the adrenal gland* is a feature of the sympathetic nervous system that requires comment. Although not a neuron per se, the adrenal medulla can be looked on as the functional equivalent of a postganglionic neuron of the sympathetic nervous system. (The adrenal medulla influences the body by releasing epinephrine into the bloodstream, which then produces effects much like those that occur in response to stimulation of postganglionic sympathetic nerves.) Because the adrenal medulla is similar in function to a postganglionic neuron, the nerve leading from the spinal cord to the adrenal gland is commonly referred to as a preganglionic neuron, even though there is no ganglion in this pathway.

As with the parasympathetic nervous system, drugs that affect the sympathetic nervous system have two general sites of action: (1) the synapses between preganglionic and postganglionic neurons (including the adrenal medulla), and (2) the junctions between postganglionic neurons and their effector organs.

Somatic Motor System

Pharmacologically relevant anatomy of the somatic motor system is depicted in Fig. 11.3. Note that there is *only one* neuron in the pathway from the spinal cord to the muscles innervated by somatic motor nerves. Because this pathway contains only one neuron, peripherally acting drugs that affect somatic motor system function have only one site of action: the *neuromuscular junction* (i.e., the junction between the somatic motor nerve and the muscle).

INTRODUCTION TO TRANSMITTERS OF THE PERIPHERAL NERVOUS SYSTEM

The PNS employs three neurotransmitters: *acetylcholine, norepinephrine,* and *epinephrine.* Any given junction in the PNS uses only one of these transmitter substances. A fourth compound—*dopamine*—may also serve as a PNS transmitter, but this role has not been demonstrated conclusively.

To understand PNS pharmacology, it is necessary to know the identity of the transmitter employed at each of the junctions of the PNS. This information is shown in Fig. 11.4. As indicated, acetylcholine is the transmitter employed at most junctions of the PNS. Acetylcholine is the transmitter released

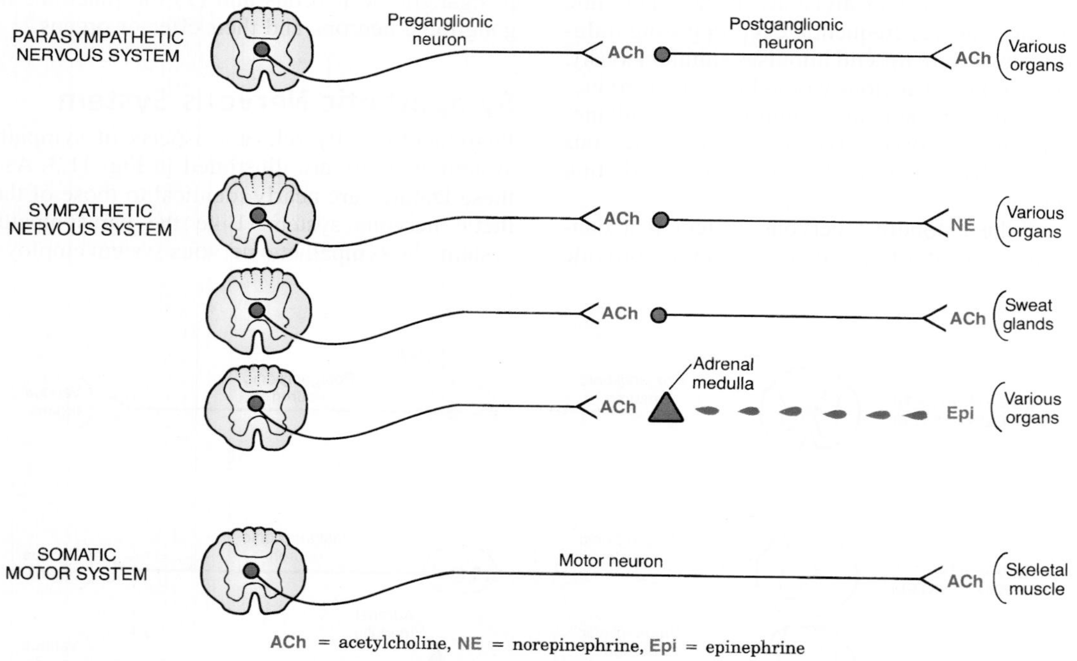

Figure 11.4 ■ Transmitters employed at specific junctions of the peripheral nervous system.

(1) *All preganglionic* neurons of the *parasympathetic* and *sympathetic* nervous systems release *acetylcholine* as their transmitter. (2) *All postganglionic* neurons of the *parasympathetic* nervous system release *acetylcholine* as their transmitter. (3) *Most postganglionic* neurons of the *sympathetic* nervous system release *norepinephrine* as their transmitter. (4) *Postganglionic* neurons of the sympathetic nervous system that innervate *sweat glands* release *acetylcholine* as their transmitter. (5) *Epinephrine* is the principal transmitter released by the *adrenal medulla.* (6) *All motor neurons* to *skeletal muscles* release *acetylcholine* as their transmitter.

by (1) all preganglionic neurons of the parasympathetic nervous system, (2) all preganglionic neurons of the sympathetic nervous system, (3) all postganglionic neurons of the parasympathetic nervous system, (4) all motor neurons to skeletal muscles, and (5) most postganglionic neurons of the sympathetic nervous system that go to sweat glands.

Norepinephrine is the transmitter released by practically all postganglionic neurons of the sympathetic nervous system. The only exceptions are the postganglionic sympathetic neurons that go to sweat glands, which employ acetylcholine as their transmitter.

Epinephrine is the major transmitter released by the adrenal medulla. (The adrenal medulla also releases some norepinephrine.)

INTRODUCTION TO RECEPTORS OF THE PERIPHERAL NERVOUS SYSTEM

The PNS works through several different types of receptors. Understanding these receptors is central to understanding PNS pharmacology. All effort that you invest in learning about these receptors now will be rewarded as we discuss PNS drugs in later chapters. Much of what follows is based on the information in Fig. 11.4.

Primary Receptor Types: Cholinergic Receptors and Adrenergic Receptors

There are two basic categories of receptors associated with the PNS: *cholinergic receptors* and *adrenergic receptors.* Cholinergic receptors are defined as receptors that mediate responses to acetylcholine. These receptors mediate responses at all junctions where acetylcholine is the transmitter. Adrenergic receptors are defined as receptors that mediate responses to epinephrine (adrenaline) and norepinephrine. These receptors mediate responses at all junctions where norepinephrine or epinephrine is the transmitter.

Subtypes of Cholinergic and Adrenergic Receptors

Not all cholinergic receptors are the same; likewise, not all adrenergic receptors are the same. For each of these two major receptor classes there are receptor subtypes. There are three major subtypes of cholinergic receptors, referred to as nicotinic_N, nicotinic_M, and muscarinic.[1] There are four major subtypes of adrenergic receptors, referred to as alpha_1, alpha_2, beta_1, and beta_2.

In addition to the four major subtypes of adrenergic receptors, there is another adrenergic receptor type, referred to as the *dopamine* receptor. Although dopamine receptors are classified as adrenergic, these receptors do not respond to epinephrine or norepinephrine. Rather, they respond only to dopamine, a neurotransmitter found primarily in the CNS.

[1]Evidence indicates that muscarinic receptors, like nicotinic receptors, come in subtypes. Five have been identified. Of these, only three—designated M_1, M_2, and M_3—have clearly identified functions. At this time, practically all drugs that affect muscarinic receptors are nonselective. Accordingly, because our understanding of these receptors is limited, and because drugs that can selectively alter their function are few, we will not discuss muscarinic receptor subtypes further in this chapter. However, we will discuss them in Chapter 12, in the context of drugs for overactive bladder.

EXPLORING THE CONCEPT OF RECEPTOR SUBTYPES

The concept of receptor subtypes is important and potentially confusing. In this section we discuss what a receptor subtype is and why receptor subtypes matter.

What Do We Mean by "Receptor Subtype"?

Receptors that respond to the same transmitter but nonetheless are different from one another would be called *receptor subtypes*. For example, peripheral receptors that respond to acetylcholine can be found (1) in ganglia of the autonomic nervous system, (2) at neuromuscular junctions, and (3) on organs regulated by the parasympathetic nervous system. However, even though all of these receptors can be activated by acetylcholine, there is clear evidence that the receptors at these three sites are, in fact, different from one another. Hence, although all of these receptors belong to the same major receptor category (cholinergic), they are sufficiently different as to constitute distinct receptor subtypes.

How Do We Know That Receptor Subtypes Exist?

Historically, our knowledge of receptor subtypes came from observing responses to drugs. In fact, were it not for drugs, receptor subtypes might never have been discovered.

Table 11.1 illustrates the types of drug responses that led to the realization that receptor subtypes exist. These data summarize the results of an experiment designed to study the effects of a natural transmitter (acetylcholine) and a series of drugs (nicotine, muscarine, *d*-tubocurarine, and atropine) on two tissues: skeletal muscle and ciliary muscle. (The ciliary muscle is the muscle responsible for focusing the eye for near vision.) Although skeletal muscle and ciliary muscle both contract in response to acetylcholine, these tissues differ in their responses to drugs. In the discussion that follows, we examine the selective responses of these tissues to drugs and see how those responses reveal the existence of receptor subtypes.

At synapses on skeletal muscle and ciliary muscle, acetylcholine is the transmitter employed by neurons to

TABLE 11.1 ▪ Responses of Skeletal Muscle and Ciliary Muscle to a Series of Drugs

	Response	
Drug	**Skeletal Muscle**	**Ciliary Muscle**
Acetylcholine	Contraction	Contraction
Nicotine	Contraction	No response
Muscarine	No response	Contraction
Acetylcholine		
After *d*-tubocurarine	No response	Contraction
After atropine	Contraction	No response

elicit contraction. Because both types of muscle respond to acetylcholine, it is safe to conclude that both muscles have receptors for this substance. Because acetylcholine is the natural transmitter for these receptors, we would classify these receptors as *cholinergic.*

What do the effects of nicotine on skeletal muscle and ciliary muscle suggest? The effects of nicotine on these muscles suggest four possible conclusions: (1) Because skeletal muscle contracts in response to nicotine, we can conclude that skeletal muscle has receptors at which nicotine can act. (2) Because ciliary muscle does *not* respond to nicotine, we can tentatively conclude that ciliary muscle does not have receptors for nicotine. (3) Because nicotine mimics the effects of acetylcholine on skeletal muscle, we can conclude that nicotine may act at the same skeletal muscle receptors where acetylcholine acts. (4) Because both skeletal and ciliary muscle have receptors for acetylcholine, and because nicotine appears to act only at the acetylcholine receptors on skeletal muscle, we can tentatively conclude that the acetylcholine receptors on skeletal muscle are different from the acetylcholine receptors on ciliary muscle.

What do the responses to muscarine suggest? The conclusions that can be drawn regarding responses to muscarine are exactly parallel to those drawn for nicotine. These conclusions are that (1) ciliary muscle has receptors that respond to muscarine, (2) skeletal muscle may not have receptors for muscarine, (3) muscarine may be acting at the same receptors on ciliary muscle where acetylcholine acts, and (4) the receptors for acetylcholine on ciliary muscle may be different from the receptors for acetylcholine on skeletal muscle.

The responses of skeletal muscle and ciliary muscle to nicotine and muscarine suggest, but do not prove, that the cholinergic receptors on these two tissues are different. However, the responses of these two tissues to d-*tubocurarine* and *atropine,* both of which are receptor *blocking agents,* eliminate any doubts as to the presence of cholinergic receptor subtypes. When both types of muscle are pretreated with *d*-tubocurarine and then exposed to acetylcholine, the response to acetylcholine is blocked in skeletal muscle but not in ciliary muscle. Tubocurarine pretreatment does not reduce the ability of acetylcholine to stimulate ciliary muscle. Conversely, pretreatment with atropine selectively blocks the response to acetylcholine in ciliary muscle—but atropine does nothing to prevent acetylcholine from stimulating receptors on skeletal muscle. Because tubocurarine can selectively block cholinergic receptors in skeletal muscle, whereas atropine can selectively block cholinergic receptors in ciliary muscle, we can conclude with certainty that the receptors for acetylcholine in these two types of muscle must be different.

The data just discussed illustrate the essential role of drugs in revealing the presence of receptor subtypes. If acetylcholine were the only probe that we had, all that we would have been able to observe is that both skeletal muscle and ciliary muscle can respond to this agent. This simple observation would provide no basis for suspecting that the receptors for acetylcholine in these two tissues were different. It is only through the use of selectively acting drugs that the presence of receptor subtypes was initially revealed.

Today, the technology for identifying receptors and their subtypes is extremely sophisticated—not that studies like the one just discussed are no longer of value. In addition to performing traditional drug-based studies, scientists are now cloning receptors using DNA hybridization technology. As you can imagine, this allows us to understand receptors in ways that were unthinkable in the past.

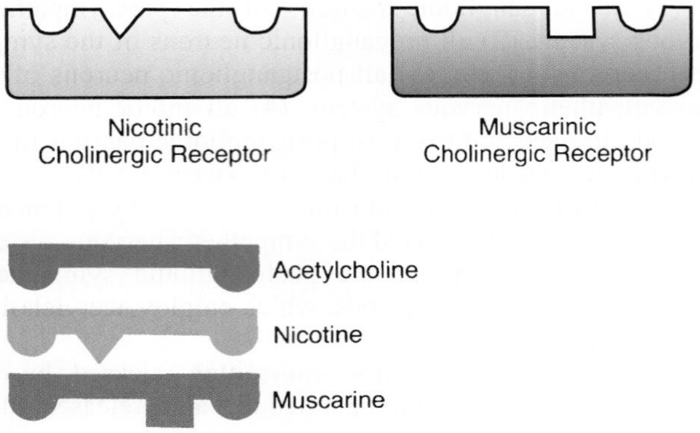

Figure 11.5 ■ Drug structure and receptor selectivity. The relationship between structure and receptor selectivity is shown. The structure of acetylcholine allows this transmitter to interact with both receptor subtypes. In contrast, because of their unique structures, nicotine and muscarine are selective for the cholinergic receptor subtypes whose structure complements their own.

How Can Drugs Be More Selective Than Natural Transmitters at Receptor Subtypes?

Drugs achieve their selectivity for receptor subtypes by having structures that are different from those of natural transmitters. The relationship between structure and receptor selectivity is illustrated in Fig. 11.5. Drawings are used to represent drugs (nicotine and muscarine), receptor subtypes (nicotinic and muscarinic), and acetylcholine (the natural transmitter at nicotinic and muscarinic receptors). From the structures shown, we can easily imagine how acetylcholine is able to interact with both kinds of receptor subtypes, whereas nicotine and muscarine can interact only with the receptor subtypes whose structure is complementary to their own. By synthesizing chemicals that are structurally related to natural transmitters, pharmaceutical chemists have been able to produce drugs that are more selective for specific receptor subtypes than are the natural transmitters that act at those sites.

Why Do Receptor Subtypes Exist, and Why Do They Matter?

The physiologic benefits of having multiple receptor subtypes for the same transmitter are not immediately obvious. In fact, as noted previously, were it not for drugs, we probably wouldn't know that receptor subtypes existed at all. Although receptor subtypes are of uncertain physiologic relevance, from the viewpoint of therapeutics, receptor subtypes are invaluable.

The presence of receptor subtypes makes possible a dramatic increase in drug selectivity. For example, thanks to the existence of subtypes of cholinergic receptors (and the development of drugs selective for those receptor subtypes),

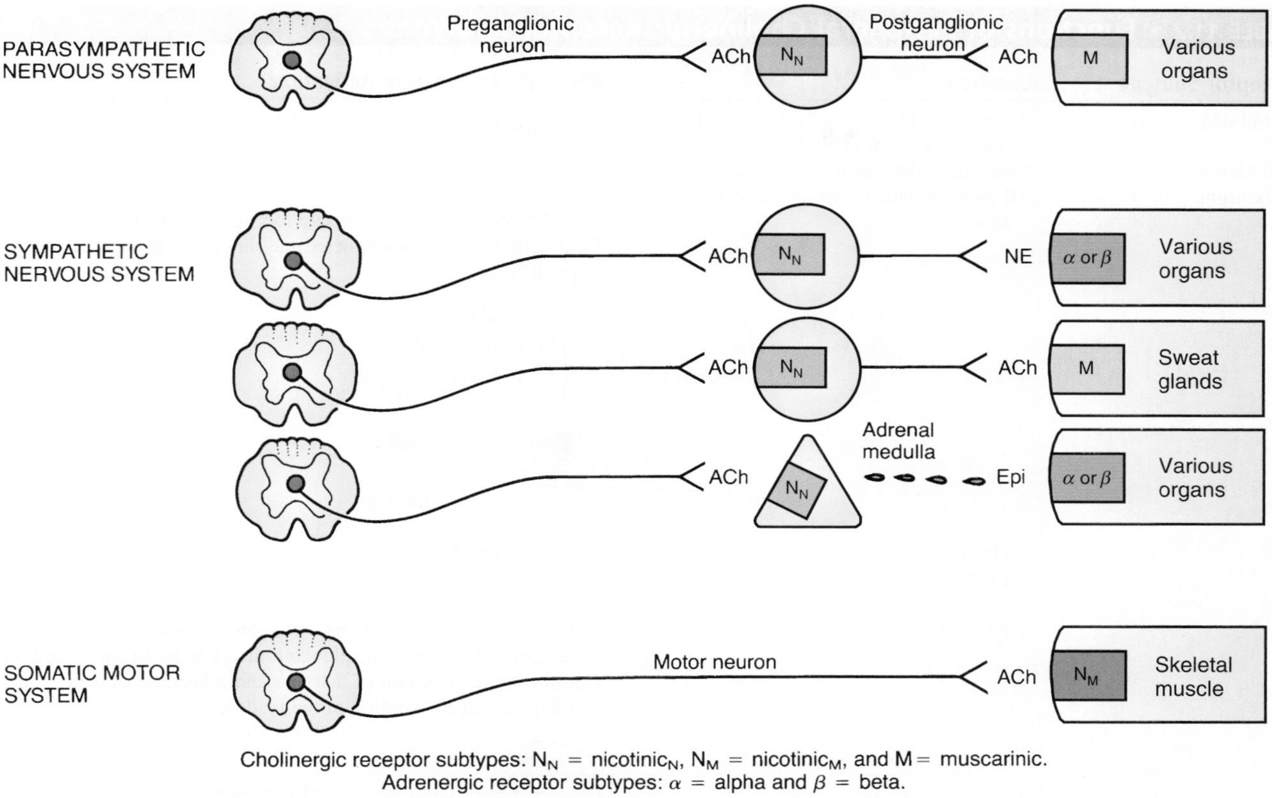

Figure 11.6 ■ Locations of cholinergic and adrenergic receptor subtypes. (1) *Nicotinic$_N$* receptors are located on the *cell bodies of all postganglionic neurons* of the *parasympathetic* and *sympathetic* nervous systems. *Nicotinic$_N$* receptors are also located on cells of the *adrenal medulla.* (2) *Nicotinic$_M$* receptors are located on *skeletal muscle.* (3) *Muscarinic* receptors are located on *all organs* regulated by the *parasympathetic* nervous system (i.e., organs innervated by postganglionic parasympathetic nerves). *Muscarinic* receptors are also located on *sweat glands.* (4) *Adrenergic* receptors—*alpha, beta,* or both—are located on *all organs* (except sweat glands) regulated by the *sympathetic* nervous system (i.e., organs innervated by postganglionic sympathetic nerves). *Adrenergic* receptors are also located on organs regulated by epinephrine released from the *adrenal medulla.*

it is possible to influence the activity of certain cholinergic receptors (e.g., receptors of the neuromuscular junction) without altering the activity of all other cholinergic receptors (e.g., the cholinergic receptors found in all autonomic ganglia and all target organs of the parasympathetic nervous system). Were it not for the existence of receptor subtypes, a drug that acted on cholinergic receptors at one site would alter the activity of cholinergic receptors at all other sites. Clearly, the existence of receptor subtypes for a particular transmitter makes possible drug actions that are much more selective than could be achieved if all of the receptors for that transmitter were the same. (Recall our discussion of Mort and Merv in Chapter 10.)

LOCATIONS OF RECEPTOR SUBTYPES

Because many of the drugs discussed in later chapters are selective for specific receptor subtypes, knowledge of the sites at which specific receptor subtypes are located will help us predict which organs a drug will affect. Accordingly, in laying our foundation for studying PNS drugs, it is important to learn the sites at which the subtypes of adrenergic and cholinergic receptors are located. This information is shown in Fig. 11.6. You will find it helpful to master the content of this figure before proceeding. (In the interest of minimizing confusion, subtypes of adrenergic receptors in Fig. 11.6 are listed simply as alpha and beta rather than as alpha$_1$, alpha$_2$, beta$_1$, and beta$_2$. The locations of all four subtypes of adrenergic receptors are discussed in the section that follows.)

FUNCTIONS OF CHOLINERGIC AND ADRENERGIC RECEPTOR SUBTYPES

Knowledge of receptor function is essential for understanding PNS drugs. By knowing the receptors at which a drug acts, and by knowing what those receptors do, we can predict the major effects of any PNS drug.

Tables 11.2 and 11.3 show the pharmacologically relevant functions of PNS receptors. Table 11.2 summarizes responses elicited by activation of *cholinergic* receptor subtypes.

TABLE 11.2 ▪ Functions of Peripheral Cholinergic Receptor Subtypes

Receptor Subtype	Location	Response to Receptor Activation
$Nicotinic_N$	All autonomic nervous system ganglia and the adrenal medulla	Stimulation of parasympathetic and sympathetic postganglionic nerves and release of epinephrine from the adrenal medulla
$Nicotinic_M$	Neuromuscular junction	Contraction of skeletal muscle
Muscarinic	All parasympathetic target organs:	
	Eye	Contraction of the ciliary muscle focuses the lens for near vision Contraction of the iris sphincter muscle causes miosis (decreased pupil diameter)

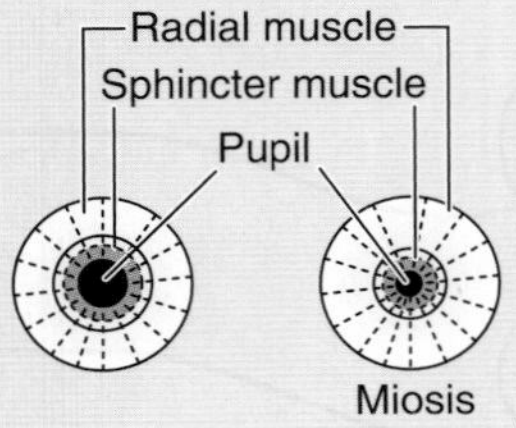

	Heart	Decreased rate
	Lung	Constriction of bronchi Promotion of secretions
	Bladder	Contraction of detrusor increases bladder pressure Relaxation of trigone and sphincter allows urine to leave the bladder Coordinated contraction of detrusor and relaxation of trigone and sphincter causes voiding of the bladder

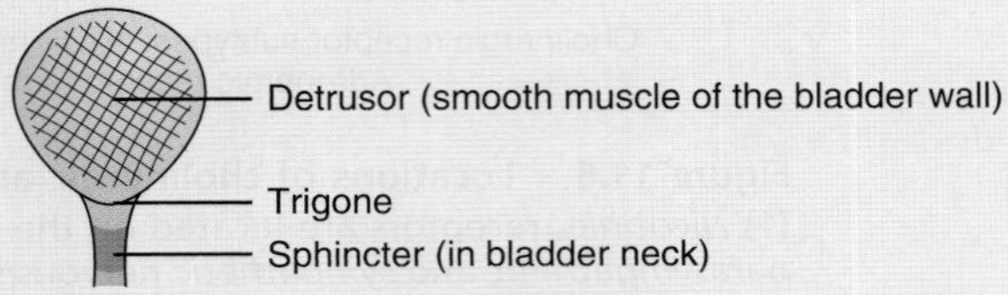

	Gastrointestinal tract	Salivation Increased gastric secretions Increased intestinal tone and motility Defecation
	Sweat glands*	Generalized sweating
	Sex organs	Erection
	Blood vessels†	Vasodilation

*Although sweating is due primarily to stimulation of muscarinic receptors by acetylcholine, the nerves that supply acetylcholine to sweat glands belong to the sympathetic nervous system rather than the parasympathetic nervous system.
†Cholinergic receptors on blood vessels are not associated with the nervous system.

Table 11.3 summarizes responses to activation of *adrenergic* receptor subtypes. You should master Table 11.2 before studying cholinergic drugs (Chapter 12). And you should master Table 11.3 before studying adrenergic drugs (Chapters 13, 14, and 15). If you master these tables in preparation for learning about PNS drugs, you will find the process of learning the pharmacology relatively simple. Conversely, if you attempt to study the pharmacology without first mastering the appropriate table, you are likely to meet with frustration.

Functions of Cholinergic Receptor Subtypes

Table 11.2 shows the pharmacologically relevant responses to activation of the three major subtypes of cholinergic receptors: $nicotinic_N$, $nicotinic_M$, and muscarinic.

We can group responses to cholinergic receptor activation into three major categories based on the subtype of receptor involved:

- Activation of *nicotinic*$_N$ (neuronal) receptors promotes *ganglionic transmission* at all ganglia of the sympathetic and parasympathetic nervous systems. In addition, activation of $nicotinic_N$ receptors promotes *release of epinephrine from the adrenal medulla.*
- Activation of *nicotinic*$_M$ (muscle) receptors causes *contraction of skeletal muscle.*
- Activation of *muscarinic* receptors, which are located on target organs of the parasympathetic nervous system, elicits an appropriate response from the organ involved. Specifically, muscarinic activation causes (1) increased glandular secretions (from pulmonary, gastric, intestinal, and sweat glands); (2) contraction of smooth muscle in the

TABLE 11.3 ■ Functions of Peripheral Adrenergic Receptor Subtypes

Receptor Subtype	Location	Response to Receptor Activation
Alpha$_1$	Eye	Contraction of the radial muscle of the iris causes mydriasis (increased pupil size)
	Arterioles Skin Viscera Mucous membranes	Constriction
	Veins	Constriction
	Sex organs, male	Ejaculation
	Prostatic capsule	Contraction
	Bladder	Contraction of trigone and sphincter
Alpha$_2$	Presynaptic nerve terminals*	Inhibition of transmitter release
Beta$_1$	Heart	Increased rate Increased force of contraction Increased AV conduction velocity
	Kidney	Release of renin
Beta$_2$	Arterioles Heart Lung Skeletal muscle	Dilation
	Bronchi	Dilation
	Uterus	Relaxation
	Liver	Glycogenolysis
	Skeletal muscle	Enhanced contraction, glycogenolysis
Dopamine	Kidney	Dilation of kidney vasculature

*Alpha$_2$ receptors in the central nervous system are postsynaptic.
AV, atrioventricular; NE, norepinephrine; R, receptor.

bronchi and GI tract; (3) slowing of heart rate; (4) contraction of the sphincter muscle of the iris, resulting in miosis (reduction in pupillary diameter); (5) contraction of the ciliary muscle of the eye, causing the lens to focus for near vision; (6) dilation of blood vessels; and (7) voiding of the urinary bladder (by causing contraction of the detrusor muscle [which forms the bladder wall] and relaxation of the trigone and sphincter muscles [which block the bladder neck when contracted]).

Muscarinic cholinergic receptors on blood vessels require additional comment. These receptors are not associated with the nervous system in any way. That is, no autonomic nerves terminate at vascular muscarinic receptors. It is not at all clear as to how, or even if, these receptors are activated physiologically. However, regardless of their physiologic relevance, the cholinergic receptors on blood vessels do have *pharmacologic* significance because drugs that are able to activate these receptors cause vasodilation, which in turn causes blood pressure to fall.

Functions of Adrenergic Receptor Subtypes

Adrenergic receptor subtypes and their functions are shown in Table 11.3.

Alpha$_1$ Receptors

Alpha$_1$ receptors are located in the eyes, blood vessels, male sex organs, prostatic capsule, and bladder (trigone and sphincter).

Ocular alpha$_1$ receptors are present on the radial muscle of the iris. Activation of these receptors leads to *mydriasis* (dilation of the pupil). As depicted in Table 11.3, the fibers of the radial muscle are arranged like the spokes of a wheel. Because of this configuration, contraction of the radial muscle causes the pupil to enlarge. (If you have difficulty remembering that *mydriasis* means pupillary enlargement, whereas *miosis* means pupillary constriction, just remember that mydriasis [dilation] is a bigger word than miosis and that mydriasis contains a "d" for dilation.)

Alpha$_1$ receptors are present on veins and on arterioles in many capillary beds. Activation of alpha$_1$ receptors in blood vessels produces *vasoconstriction.*

Activation of alpha$_1$ receptors in the sexual apparatus of males causes *ejaculation.* Activation of alpha$_1$ receptors in smooth muscle of the bladder (trigone and sphincter) and prostatic capsule causes *contraction.*

Alpha$_2$ Receptors

Alpha$_2$ receptors of the PNS are located on nerve terminals (see Table 11.3) and not on the organs innervated by the autonomic nervous system. Because alpha$_2$ receptors are located on nerve terminals, these receptors are referred to as *presynaptic* or *prejunctional.* The function of these receptors is to *regulate transmitter release.* As depicted in Table 11.3, norepinephrine can bind to alpha$_2$ receptors located on the same neuron from which the norepinephrine was released. The consequence of this norepinephrine-receptor interaction is suppression of further norepinephrine release. Hence, presynaptic alpha$_2$ receptors can help reduce transmitter release when too much transmitter has accumulated in the synaptic gap. Drug effects resulting from activation of *peripheral* alpha$_2$ receptors are of minimal clinical significance.

Alpha$_2$ receptors are also present in the CNS. In contrast to peripheral alpha$_2$ receptors, central alpha$_2$ receptors are therapeutically relevant. We will consider these receptors in later chapters.

Beta$_1$ Receptors

Beta$_1$ receptors are located in the heart and the kidney. Cardiac beta$_1$ receptors have great therapeutic significance. Activation of these receptors *increases heart rate, force of contraction,* and *velocity of impulse conduction through the atrioventricular node.*

Activation of beta$_1$ receptors in the kidney causes *release of renin* into the blood. Because renin promotes synthesis of angiotensin, a powerful vasoconstrictor, activation of renal beta$_1$ receptors is a means by which the nervous system helps elevate blood pressure. (The role of renin in the regulation of blood pressure is discussed in depth in Chapter 36.)

Beta$_2$ Receptors

Beta$_2$ receptors mediate several important processes. Activation of beta$_2$ receptors in the lung leads to *bronchial dilation.* Activation of beta$_2$ receptors in the uterus causes *relaxation uterine smooth muscle.* Activation of beta$_2$ receptors in of arterioles of the heart, lungs, and skeletal muscles causes *vasodilation* (an effect opposite to that of alpha$_1$ activation). Activation of beta$_2$ receptors in the liver and skeletal muscle promotes *glycogenolysis* (breakdown of glycogen into glucose), thereby increasing blood levels of glucose. In addition, activation of beta$_2$ receptors in skeletal muscle enhances *contraction.*

Dopamine Receptors

In the periphery, the only dopamine receptors of clinical significance are located in the vasculature of the kidney. Activation of these receptors *dilates renal blood vessels,* enhancing renal perfusion.

In the CNS, receptors for dopamine are of great therapeutic significance. The functions of these receptors are discussed in Chapters 17 and 24.

RECEPTOR SPECIFICITY OF THE ADRENERGIC TRANSMITTERS

The receptor specificity of adrenergic transmitters is more complex than the receptor specificity of acetylcholine. Whereas acetylcholine can activate all three subtypes of cholinergic receptors, not every adrenergic transmitter (epinephrine, norepinephrine, dopamine) can interact with each of the five subtypes of adrenergic receptors.

Receptor specificity of adrenergic transmitters is as follows: (1) *epinephrine* can activate all alpha and beta receptors, but not dopamine receptors; (2) *norepinephrine* can activate alpha$_1$, alpha$_2$, and beta$_1$ receptors, but not beta$_2$ or dopamine receptors; and (3) *dopamine* can activate alpha$_1$, beta$_1$, and dopamine receptors. (Note that dopamine itself is the only transmitter capable of activating dopamine receptors.) Receptor specificity of the adrenergic transmitters is shown in Table 11.4.

Knowing that epinephrine is the only transmitter that acts at beta$_2$ receptors can serve as an aid to remembering the functions of this receptor subtype. Recall that epinephrine is released from the adrenal medulla—not from neurons—and that the function of epinephrine is to prepare the body for fight or flight. Accordingly, because epinephrine is the only transmitter that activates beta$_2$ receptors, and because epinephrine is released only in preparation for fight or flight, times of fight or flight will be the only occasions on which beta$_2$ receptors will undergo significant physiologic activation. As it turns out, the physiologic changes elicited by beta$_2$ activation are precisely those needed for success in the fight-or-flight response. Specifically, activation of beta$_2$ receptors will (1) dilate blood vessels in the heart, lungs, and skeletal muscles, thereby increasing blood flow to these organs; (2) dilate the bronchi, thereby increasing oxygenation; (3) increase glycogenolysis, thereby increasing available energy; and (4) relax uterine smooth muscle, thereby preventing delivery (a process that would be inconvenient for a pregnant woman preparing to fight or flee). Accordingly, if you think of the physiologic requirements for success during fight or flight, you will have a good picture of the responses that beta$_2$ activation can cause.

TRANSMITTER LIFE CYCLES

In this section we consider the life cycles of acetylcholine, norepinephrine, and epinephrine. Because a number of drugs produce their effects by interfering with specific phases of the transmitters' life cycles, knowledge of these cycles helps us understand drug actions.

Life Cycle of Acetylcholine

The life cycle of acetylcholine (ACh) is depicted in Fig. 11.7. The cycle begins with synthesis of ACh from two precursors: choline and acetylcoenzyme A. After synthesis, ACh is stored in vesicles and later released in response to an action potential. After release, ACh binds to receptors (nicotinic$_N$, nicotinic$_M$, or muscarinic) located on the postjunctional cell.

TABLE 11.4 ■ Receptor Specificity of Adrenergic Transmitters*

Transmitter	Alpha$_1$	Alpha$_2$	Beta$_1$	Beta$_2$	Dopamine
Epinephrine	←———	———	———	———→	
Norepinephrine	←———	———	———→		
Dopamine	←→		←→		←→

**Arrows* indicate the range of receptors that the transmitters can activate.

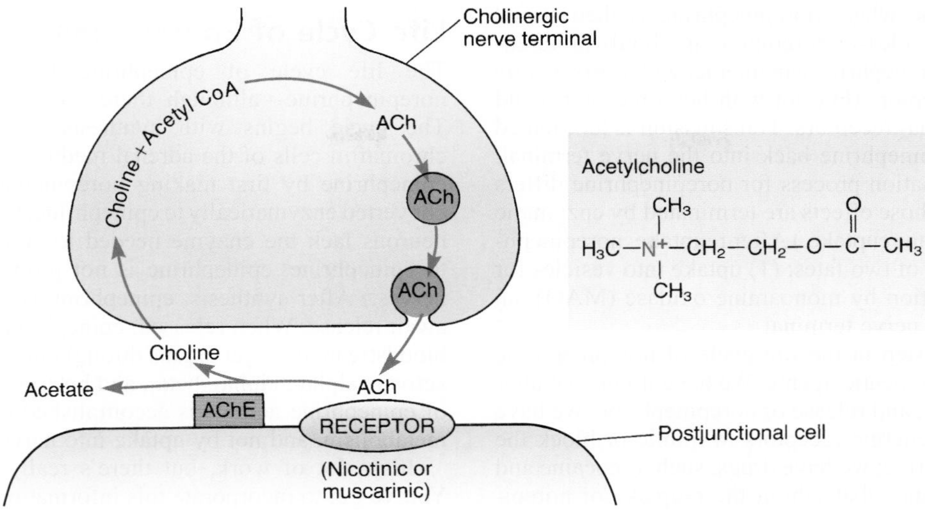

Figure 11.7 ▪ Life cycle of acetylcholine.
Transmission is terminated by enzymatic degradation of acetylcholine (Ach) and not by uptake of intact ACh back into the nerve terminal. (Acetyl CoA, acetylcoenzyme A; AChE, acetylcholinesterase.)

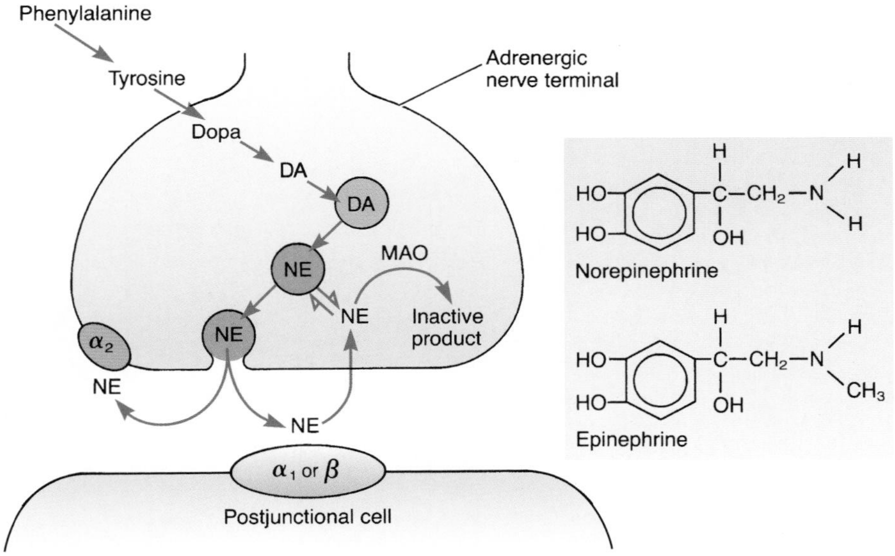

Figure 11.8 ▪ Life cycle of norepinephrine.
Note that transmission mediated by norepinephrine (NE) is terminated by reuptake of NE into the nerve terminal, and not by enzymatic degradation. Be aware that, although postsynaptic cells may have alpha$_1$, beta$_1$, and beta$_2$ receptors, NE can only activate postsynaptic alpha$_1$ and beta$_1$ receptors; physiologic activation of beta$_2$ receptors is done by epinephrine. (DA, dopamine; MAO, monoamine oxidase.)

Upon dissociating from its receptors, ACh is destroyed almost instantaneously by *acetylcholinesterase* (AChE), an enzyme present in abundance on the surface of the postjunctional cell. AChE degrades ACh into two inactive products: acetate and choline. Uptake of choline into the cholinergic nerve terminal completes the life cycle of ACh. Note that an inactive substance (choline), and not the active transmitter (ACh), is taken back up for reuse.

Therapeutic and toxic agents can interfere with the ACh life cycle at several points. Botulinum toxin inhibits ACh release. A number of medicines and poisons act at cholinergic receptors to mimic or block the actions of ACh. Several therapeutic and toxic agents act by inhibiting AChE, thereby causing ACh to accumulate in the junctional gap.

Life Cycle of Norepinephrine

The life cycle of norepinephrine is depicted in Fig. 11.8. As indicated, the cycle begins with synthesis of norepinephrine from a series of precursors. The final step of synthesis takes place within vesicles, where norepinephrine is then stored before release. After release, norepinephrine binds to adrenergic receptors. Norepinephrine can interact with *postsynaptic* alpha$_1$ and beta$_1$ receptors (but not with beta$_2$ receptors) and with *presynaptic* alpha$_2$ receptors. Transmission is terminated by *reuptake* of norepinephrine back into the nerve terminal. (Note that the termination process for norepinephrine differs from that for ACh, whose effects are terminated by enzymatic degradation rather than reuptake.) After reuptake, norepinephrine can undergo one of two fates: (1) uptake into vesicles for reuse or (2) inactivation by monoamine oxidase (MAO), an enzyme found in the nerve terminal.

Practically every step in the life cycle of norepinephrine can be altered by therapeutic agents. We have drugs that alter the synthesis, storage, and release of norepinephrine; we have drugs that act at adrenergic receptors to mimic or block the effects of norepinephrine; we have drugs, such as cocaine and tricyclic antidepressants, that inhibit the reuptake of norepinephrine (and thereby intensify transmission); and we have drugs that inhibit the breakdown of norepinephrine by MAO, causing an increase in the amount of transmitter available for release.

Life Cycle of Epinephrine

The life cycle of epinephrine is much like that of norepinephrine—although there are significant differences. The cycle begins with synthesis of epinephrine within chromaffin cells of the adrenal medulla. These cells produce epinephrine by first making norepinephrine, which is then converted enzymatically to epinephrine. (Because sympathetic neurons lack the enzyme needed to convert norepinephrine to epinephrine, epinephrine is not produced in sympathetic nerves.) After synthesis, epinephrine is stored in vesicles to await release. When released, epinephrine travels through the bloodstream to target organs throughout the body, where it can activate alpha$_1$, alpha$_2$, beta$_1$, and beta$_2$ receptors. Termination of epinephrine actions is accomplished primarily by hepatic metabolism, and not by uptake into nerves.

It's a lot of work, but there's really no way around it: You've got to incorporate this information into your personal database (i.e., memorize it).

CHAPTER

12 Muscarinic Agonists and Antagonists

Jacqueline Rosenjack Burchum, DNSc, FNP-BC, CNE

INTRODUCTION TO CHOLINERGIC DRUGS

Cholinergic drugs are agents that influence the activity of cholinergic receptors. Most of these drugs act directly at cholinergic receptors, where they either mimic or block the actions of acetylcholine. The remainder—the cholinesterase inhibitors—activate cholinergic receptors indirectly by preventing the breakdown of acetylcholine.

The cholinergic drugs have both therapeutic and toxicologic significance. Therapeutic applications are limited but valuable. The toxicology of cholinergic drugs is extensive, encompassing such agents as nicotine, insecticides, and compounds designed for chemical warfare.

There are six categories of cholinergic drugs. These categories are muscarinic agonists, muscarinic antagonists, cholinesterase inhibitors, ganglionic stimulating agents, ganglionic blocking agents, and neuromuscular blocking agents.

The *muscarinic agonists,* represented by bethanechol, selectively mimic the effects of acetylcholine at muscarinic receptors. The *muscarinic antagonists,* represented by atropine, selectively block the effects of acetylcholine (and other muscarinic agonists) at muscarinic receptors. The *cholinesterase inhibitors,* represented by neostigmine and physostigmine, prevent the breakdown of acetylcholine by acetylcholinesterase. As a result, more acetylcholine remains available to activate cholinergic receptors.

Ganglionic stimulating agents, represented by nicotine, selectively mimic the effects of acetylcholine at $nicotinic_N$ (neuronal) receptors of autonomic ganglia. These drugs have little therapeutic value beyond the use of nicotine in smoking cessation programs (see Chapter 32). *Ganglionic blocking agents,* represented by mecamylamine, selectively block ganglionic $nicotinic_N$ receptors. *Neuromuscular blocking agents,* represented by *d*-tubocurarine and succinylcholine, selectively block the effects of acetylcholine at $nicotinic_M$ (muscle) receptors at the neuromuscular junction. Ganglionic and neuromuscular blocking agents are used in specialty settings and are beyond the scope of this text.

Table 12.1 is your key to understanding the cholinergic drugs. It lists the three major subtypes of cholinergic receptors (muscarinic, $nicotinic_N$, and $nicotinic_M$) and indicates the following for each receptor type: (1) location, (2) responses to activation, (3) drugs that produce activation (agonists), and (4) drugs that prevent activation (antagonists). This information, along with the detailed information on cholinergic receptor function summarized in Table 11.2 in Chapter 11, is just about all you need to predict the actions of cholinergic drugs.

An example will demonstrate the combined value of Tables 12.1 and 11.2. Let's consider bethanechol. As shown in Table 12.1, bethanechol is a selective *agonist* at *muscarinic* cholinergic receptors. Referring to Table 11.2, we see that activation of muscarinic receptors can produce the following: ocular effects (miosis and ciliary muscle contraction), slowing of heart rate, bronchial constriction, urination, glandular secretion, stimulation of the gastrointestinal (GI) tract, and vasodilation. Because bethanechol *activates* muscarinic receptors, the drug is capable of eliciting all of these responses. Therefore, by knowing which receptors bethanechol activates (from Table 12.1), and by knowing what those receptors do (from Table 11.2), you can predict the kinds of responses you might expect bethanechol to produce.

In the chapters that follow, we will employ the approach just described. That is, for each cholinergic drug discussed, you will want to know (1) the receptors that the drug affects, (2) the normal responses to activation of those receptors, and (3) whether the drug in question increases or decreases receptor activation. All of this information is contained in Tables 12.1 and 11.2. If you learn this information now, you will be prepared to follow discussions in succeeding chapters with relative ease.

MUSCARINIC AGONISTS, CHOLINESTERASE INHIBITORS, AND MUSCARINIC ANTAGONISTS

The muscarinic agonists and antagonists produce their effects through *direct* interaction with muscarinic receptors. The muscarinic agonists cause receptor activation; the antagonists produce receptor blockade. Like the muscarinic agonists, another group of drugs—the cholinesterase inhibitors—can also cause receptor activation, but they do so by an *indirect* mechanism.

Muscarinic Agonists

The muscarinic agonists bind to muscarinic receptors and thereby cause receptor activation. Because nearly all muscarinic receptors are associated with the parasympathetic nervous system, responses to muscarinic agonists closely resemble those produced by stimulation of parasympathetic

PATIENT-CENTERED CARE ACROSS THE LIFE SPAN

Anticholinergic Drugs

Life Stage	Patient Care Concerns
Pregnant women	The U.S. Food and Drug Administration Pregnancy Risk Category for cholinergic and anticholinergic drugs ranges from B to C.
Breastfeeding women	Anticholinergics may inhibit lactation in some women, resulting in decreased production of breast milk.
Older adults	Anticholinergic drugs have been designated as potentially inappropriate for use in geriatric patients. They can cause confusion, blurred vision, tachycardia, urinary retention, and constipation. Many of these complicate preexisting conditions (e.g., urinary retention secondary to benign prostatic hyperplasia) and increase the risk for other conditions (e.g., narrow-angle glaucoma risk secondary to pupil dilation and heat-related illness secondary to hyperthermia and impaired sweating mechanisms).

TABLE 12.1 ▪ Cholinergic Drugs and Their Receptors

	Receptor Subtype		
	Muscarinic	**Nicotinic$_N$**	**Nicotinic$_M$**
Receptor Location	Sweat glands Blood vessels All organs regulated by the parasympathetic nervous system	All ganglia of the autonomic nervous system	Neuromuscular junctions (NMJs)
Effects of Receptor Activation	Many, including: ↓ Heart rate ↑ Gland secretion Smooth muscle contraction	Promotes ganglionic transmission	Skeletal muscle contraction
Receptor Agonists	Bethanechol	Nicotine	(Nicotine*)
Receptor Antagonists	Atropine	Mecamylamine	*d*-Tubocurarine, succinylcholine
Indirect-Acting Cholinomimetics	Cholinesterase inhibitors: physostigmine, neostigmine, and other cholinesterase inhibitors can activate *all* cholinergic receptors (by causing accumulation of acetylcholine at cholinergic junctions)		

*The doses of nicotine needed to activate nicotinic$_M$ receptors of the NMJs are much higher than the doses needed to activate nicotinic$_N$ receptors in autonomic ganglia.

nerves. Accordingly, muscarinic agonists are also known as *parasympathomimetic agents.*

Bethanechol

Bethanechol [Urecholine, Duvoid ♣] embodies the properties that typify all muscarinic agonists and will serve as our prototype for the group.

Mechanism of Action

Bethanechol is a direct-acting muscarinic agonist. The drug binds reversibly to muscarinic cholinergic receptors to cause activation. At therapeutic doses, bethanechol acts selectively at muscarinic receptors, having little or no effect on nicotinic receptors, either in ganglia or in skeletal muscle.

Pharmacologic Effects

Bethanechol can elicit all of the responses typical of muscarinic receptor activation. Accordingly, we can readily predict the effects of bethanechol by knowing the information on muscarinic responses summarized in Table 11.2.

The principal structures affected by muscarinic activation are the *heart, exocrine glands, smooth muscles,* and *eyes.* Muscarinic agonists act on the heart to cause bradycardia (decreased heart rate) and on exocrine glands to increase sweating, salivation, bronchial secretions, and secretion of gastric acid. In smooth muscles of the lungs and GI tract, muscarinic agonists promote contraction. The result is constriction of the bronchi and increased tone and motility of GI smooth muscle. In the bladder, muscarinic activation causes *contraction* of the detrusor muscle and *relaxation* of the trigone and sphincter; the result is bladder emptying. In vascular smooth muscle, these drugs cause relaxation; the resultant vasodilation can produce hypotension. Activation of muscarinic receptors in the eyes has two effects: (1) miosis (pupillary constriction), and (2) contraction of the ciliary muscle, resulting in accommodation for near vision. (The ciliary muscle, which is attached to the lens, focuses the eyes for near vision by altering lens curvature.)

Pharmacokinetics

Bethanechol is available for oral administration. Effects begin in 30 to 60 minutes and persist for about 1 hour. Because bethanechol is a quaternary ammonium compound (Fig. 12.1), the drug crosses membranes poorly. As a result, only a small fraction of each dose is absorbed.

Preparations, Dosage, and Administration

Preparation and dosing of bethanechol and other cholinesterase inhibitors is provided in Table 12.2. Administration guidelines are also provided.

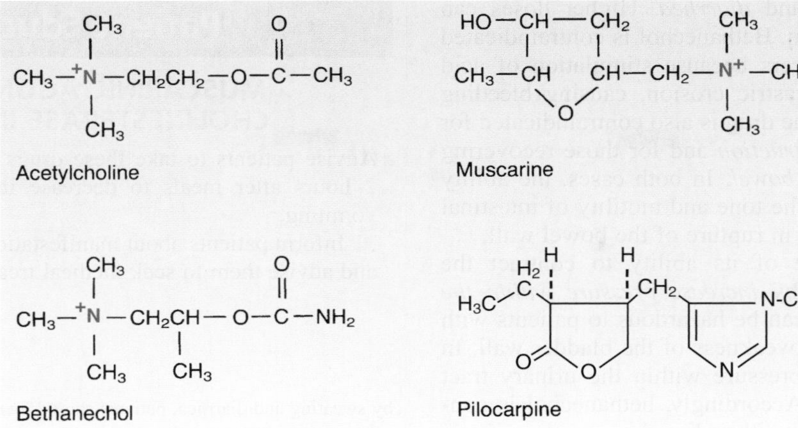

Figure 12.1 ▪ Structures of muscarinic agonists.
Note that, with the exception of pilocarpine, all of these agents are quaternary ammonium compounds and always carry a positive charge. Because of this charge, these compounds cross membranes poorly.

TABLE 12.2 ▪ Preparation, Dosage, and Administration of Muscarinic Agonists

Drug Class or Drug	Preparation	Dosage	Administration
MUSCARINIC AGONISTS			
Bethanechol [Urecholine, Duvoid ♣]	Tablets: 5, 10, 25, and 50 mg	10–50 mg 3–4 times a day	1 hour before meals or 2 hours after to prevent nausea and vomiting
Cevimeline [Evoxac]	Capsules: 30 mg	30 mg 3 times a day	May be given without regard to food. Food decreases the rate of absorption but not the amount absorbed.
Pilocarpine ophthalmic [Isopto Carpine, Diocarpine ♣, Pilopine HS]	Solution: 1% in 15 mL, 2% in 15 mL, & 4% in 15 mL Gel: 4%	Solution: 1–2 drops to affected eye up to 6 times a day Gel: apply a 0.5-inch ribbon onto the lower conjunctival sac at bedtime	Apply pressure to lacrimal area for 1–2 minutes after administration. If both solution and gel are needed, patient should apply the solution first and wait 5 minutes before applying the gel.
Pilocarpine systemic [Salagen]	Tablets: 5 mg, 7.5 mg	Sjögren syndrome: 5 mg 4 times a day Postradiotherapy for cancer: 5 mg 3 times a day initially; may be titrated upward to 10 mg 3 times a day	Avoid administration with high-fat meals due to decreased rate of absorption.

Therapeutic Uses

Although bethanechol can produce a broad spectrum of pharmacologic effects, the drug is approved only for urinary retention.

Urinary Retention. Bethanechol relieves urinary retention by activating muscarinic receptors of the urinary tract. Muscarinic activation relaxes the trigone and sphincter muscles and increases voiding pressure by contracting the detrusor muscle, which composes the bladder wall. It is approved to treat urinary retention in postoperative and postpartum patients and to treat retention secondary to neurogenic atony of the bladder. The drug should not be used to treat urinary retention caused by physical obstruction of the urinary tract because increased pressure in the tract in the presence of blockage could cause injury.

GI Uses. Bethanechol has been used off-label to treat *gastroesophageal reflux.* Benefits may result from increased esophageal motility and increased pressure in the lower esophageal sphincter.

Bethanechol can help treat disorders associated with GI paralysis. Benefits derive from increased tone and motility of GI smooth muscle. Specific applications are *adynamic ileus, gastric atony,* and *postoperative abdominal distention.* Bethanechol should not be given if physical obstruction of the GI tract is present because, in the presence of blockage, increased propulsive contractions might result in damage to the intestinal wall.

Adverse Effects

In theory, bethanechol can produce the full range of muscarinic responses as side effects. However, with oral dosing, side effects are relatively rare.

Cardiovascular System. Bethanechol can cause *hypotension* (secondary to vasodilation) and *bradycardia.* Accordingly, the drug is contraindicated for patients with low blood pressure or low cardiac output.

GI System. At usual therapeutic doses, bethanechol can cause *excessive salivation, increased secretion of gastric acid, abdominal cramps,* and *diarrhea.* Higher doses can cause involuntary defecation. Bethanechol is contraindicated in patients with gastric ulcers because stimulation of acid secretion could intensify gastric erosion, causing bleeding and possibly perforation. The drug is also contraindicated for patients with *intestinal obstruction* and for those recovering from recent *surgery of the bowel.* In both cases, the ability of bethanechol to increase the tone and motility of intestinal smooth muscle could result in rupture of the bowel wall.

Urinary Tract. Because of its ability to contract the bladder detrusor and thereby *increase pressure within the urinary tract,* bethanechol can be hazardous to patients with urinary tract obstruction or weakness of the bladder wall. In both groups, elevation of pressure within the urinary tract could rupture the bladder. Accordingly, bethanechol is contraindicated for patients with either disorder.

Exacerbation of Asthma. By activating muscarinic receptors in the lungs, bethanechol can cause bronchoconstriction. Accordingly, the drug is contraindicated for patients with latent or active asthma. Of course, it stands to reason that muscarinic agonists may also complicate other respiratory disorders.

Dysrhythmias in Hyperthyroid Patients. Bethanechol is contraindicated for people with hyperthyroidism. *If given to patients with this condition, bethanechol may increase heart rate to the point of initiating a dysrhythmia. (Note that increased heart rate is opposite to the effect that muscarinic agonists have in most patients.)* The mechanism of dysrhythmia induction is explained here.

When hyperthyroid patients are given bethanechol, their initial cardiovascular responses are like those of anyone else: bradycardia and hypotension. In reaction to hypotension, the baroreceptor reflex attempts to return blood pressure to normal. Part of this reflex involves the release of norepinephrine from sympathetic nerves that regulate heart rate. In patients who are not hyperthyroid, norepinephrine release serves to increase cardiac output and thus helps restore blood pressure. However, in hyperthyroid patients, norepinephrine can induce cardiac dysrhythmias. The reason for this unusual response is that, in hyperthyroid patients, the heart is exquisitely sensitive to the effects of norepinephrine, and hence relatively small amounts can cause stimulation sufficient to elicit a dysrhythmia.

Other Muscarinic Agonists

Cevimeline

Actions and Uses

Cevimeline [Evoxac] is a derivative of acetylcholine with actions much like those of bethanechol. The drug is indicated for relief of xerostomia (dry mouth) in patients with Sjögren syndrome, an autoimmune disorder characterized by xerostomia. It has also been used to manage keratoconjunctivitis sicca (inflammation of the cornea and conjunctiva) and dry eye. Dry mouth, left untreated, can lead to multiple complications, including periodontal disease, dental caries, altered taste, oral ulcers and candidiasis, and difficulty eating and speaking. Cevimeline relieves dry mouth by activating muscarinic receptors on residual healthy tissue in salivary glands, thereby promoting salivation. Because it stimulates salivation, cevimeline may also benefit patients with xerostomia induced by radiation therapy for head and neck cancer, although the drug is not approved for this use. The drug also increases tear production, which can help relieve keratoconjunctivitis and dry eye.

Adverse Effects

Adverse effects result from activating muscarinic receptors and hence are similar to those of bethanechol. The most common effects are excessive sweating, nausea, rhinitis, and diarrhea. To compensate for fluid loss caused by sweating and diarrhea, patients should increase fluid intake. Like bethanechol, cevimeline promotes miosis (constriction of the pupil) and may also cause blurred vision. Both actions can make driving dangerous, especially at night.

Activation of cardiac muscarinic receptors can reduce heart rate and slow cardiac conduction. Accordingly, cevimeline should be used with caution in patients with a history of heart disease.

Because muscarinic activation increases airway resistance, cevimeline is contraindicated for patients with uncontrolled asthma and should be used with caution in patients with controlled asthma, chronic bronchitis, or chronic obstructive pulmonary disease (COPD). Cevimeline is also contraindicated for people with both narrow-angle glaucoma and iritis.

Drug Interactions

Cevimeline can intensify cardiac depression caused by beta blockers because both drugs decrease heart rate and cardiac conduction.

Beneficial effects of cevimeline can be antagonized by drugs that block muscarinic receptors. Among these are atropine, tricyclic antidepressants (e.g., imipramine), antihistamines (e.g., diphenhydramine), and phenothiazine antipsychotics (e.g., chlorpromazine).

Pilocarpine

Pilocarpine is a muscarinic agonist used mainly for topical therapy of glaucoma, an ophthalmic disorder characterized by elevated intraocular pressure (IOP) with subsequent injury to the optic nerve. The basic pharmacology of pilocarpine and its use in glaucoma are discussed in Chapter 84.

In addition to its use in glaucoma, oral pilocarpine is approved for treatment of dry mouth resulting from Sjögren syndrome or from salivary gland damage caused by radiation therapy of head and neck cancer. For these applications, pilocarpine is available under the trade name Salagen. It may also be given to manage dry mouth secondary to head and neck cancer. At lower doses, the principal adverse effect is sweating. However, if dosage is excessive, pilocarpine can produce the full spectrum of muscarinic effects.

> **Patient Education**
>
> **MUSCARINIC AGONISTS AND CHOLINESTERASE INHIBITORS**
>
> Advise patients to take these drugs 1 hour before meals or 2 hours after meals to decrease incidence of nausea and vomiting.
>
> Inform patients about manifestations of muscarinic excess and advise them to seek medical treatment if they occur.

Cholinesterase Inhibitors

Cholinesterase inhibitors are drugs that prevent the degradation of acetylcholine by acetylcholinesterase (also known simply as cholinesterase). Cholinesterase inhibitors are also known as *anticholinesterase* drugs. By preventing the breakdown of acetylcholine, cholinesterase inhibitors increase the amount of acetylcholine available to activate receptors, thus enhancing cholinergic action. Because cholinesterase inhibitors do not bind directly with cholinergic receptors, they are viewed as indirect-acting cholinergic agonists. Use of cholinesterase inhibitors results in transmission at all cholinergic junctions (muscarinic, ganglionic, and neuromuscular), so these drugs can elicit a broad spectrum of responses. Because they lack selectivity, cholinesterase inhibitors have limited therapeutic applications.

There are two basic categories of cholinesterase inhibitors: (1) *reversible inhibitors* and (2) *irreversible inhibitors.* The reversible inhibitors produce effects of moderate duration, and the irreversible inhibitors produce effects of long duration.

Reversible Cholinesterase Inhibitors

Neostigmine

Neostigmine [Bloxiverz, Prostigmin] typifies the reversible cholinesterase inhibitors and will serve as our prototype for the group. The principal indication of Prostigmin is management of *myasthenia gravis* (MG). Bloxiverz is used to reverse the actions of nondepolarizing neuromuscular blockade after surgery; however, this use is beyond the scope of this book.

Chemistry. As shown in Fig. 12.2, neostigmine contains a quaternary nitrogen atom and hence always carries a positive charge. Because of this charge, neostigmine cannot readily cross membranes, including those of the GI tract, blood-brain barrier, and placenta. Consequently, neostigmine is absorbed poorly after oral administration and has minimal effects on the brain and fetus.

Mechanism of Action. Neostigmine and the other reversible cholinesterase inhibitors act as substrates for cholinesterase. As indicated in Fig. 12.2, the normal function of cholinesterase is to break down acetylcholine into choline and acetic acid. (This process is called a *hydrolysis reaction* because of the water molecule involved.) The overall reaction between acetylcholine and cholinesterase is extremely fast. As a result, one molecule of cholinesterase can break down a huge amount of acetylcholine in a very short time.

The reaction between neostigmine and cholinesterase is much like the reaction between acetylcholine and cholinesterase. The only difference is that cholinesterase splits neostigmine more slowly than it splits acetylcholine. Hence, after neostigmine becomes bound to cholinesterase, the drug remains in place for a relatively long time. Because cholinesterase remains bound until it finally succeeds in degrading neostigmine, less cholinesterase is available to catalyze the breakdown of acetylcholine. As a result, more acetylcholine is available to activate cholinergic receptors.

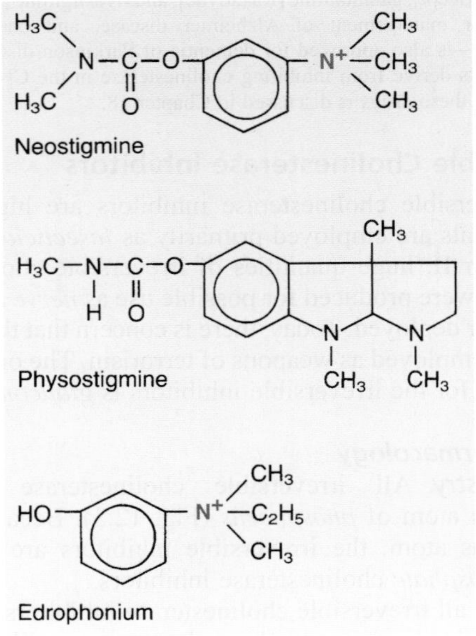

Figure 12.2 ■ Structural formulas of reversible cholinesterase inhibitors.
Note that neostigmine and edrophonium are quaternary ammonium compounds, but physostigmine is not. What does this difference imply about the relative abilities of these drugs to cross membranes, including the blood-brain barrier?

Pharmacologic Effects. By decreasing breakdown of acetylcholine, neostigmine and the other cholinesterase inhibitors make more acetylcholine available, and this can intensify transmission at virtually all junctions where acetylcholine is the transmitter. In sufficient doses, cholinesterase inhibitors can produce skeletal muscle stimulation, ganglionic stimulation, activation of peripheral muscarinic receptors, and activation of cholinergic receptors in the central nervous system (CNS). However, when used *therapeutically,* cholinesterase inhibitors usually affect only muscarinic receptors on organs and nicotinic receptors of the neuromuscular junction (NMJ). Ganglionic transmission and CNS function are usually unaltered.

MUSCARINIC RESPONSES. Muscarinic effects of the cholinesterase inhibitors are identical to those of the direct-acting muscarinic agonists. By preventing breakdown of acetylcholine, cholinesterase inhibitors can cause bradycardia, bronchial constriction, urinary urgency, increased glandular secretions, increased tone and motility of GI smooth muscle, miosis, and focusing of the lens for near vision.

NEUROMUSCULAR EFFECTS. The effects of cholinesterase inhibitors on skeletal muscle are dose dependent. At *therapeutic* doses, these drugs *increase* force of contraction. In contrast, *toxic* doses *reduce* force of contraction. Contractile force is reduced because excessive amounts of acetylcholine at the NMJ keep the motor end plate in a state of constant depolarization, causing depolarizing neuromuscular blockade.

CENTRAL NERVOUS SYSTEM. Effects on the CNS vary with drug concentration. *Therapeutic* levels can produce mild *stimulation,* whereas *toxic* levels *depress* the CNS, including the areas that regulate respiration. However, keep in mind that, for CNS effects to occur, the inhibitor must first penetrate the blood-brain barrier, which some cholinesterase inhibitors can do only when present in very high concentrations.

Pharmacokinetics. Neostigmine may be administered by intramuscular (IM), intravenous (IV), or subcutaneous (subQ) injection. Because neostigmine carries a positive charge, the drug is poorly absorbed after oral administration; hence oral formulations have been discontinued in the United States, although they remain available in some other countries. After it is absorbed, neostigmine can reach sites of action at the NMJ and peripheral muscarinic receptors, but cannot cross the blood-brain barrier to affect the CNS. Duration of action is 2 to 4 hours. Neostigmine is eliminated by enzymatic degradation by cholinesterase.

Preparation, Dosage, and Administration. Preparation and dosage of neostigmine and other cholinesterase inhibitors are provided in Table 12.3. Administration guidelines are also provided.

Therapeutic Uses

MYASTHENIA GRAVIS. MG is a major indication for neostigmine and several other reversible cholinesterase inhibitors. Treatment of MG is discussed separately.

Adverse Effects

EXCESSIVE MUSCARINIC STIMULATION. Accumulation of acetylcholine at muscarinic receptors can result in excessive salivation, increased gastric secretions, increased tone and motility of the GI tract, urinary urgency, bradycardia, sweating, miosis, and spasm of accommodation (focusing of the lens for near vision). If necessary, these responses can be suppressed with atropine.

TABLE 12.3 ▪ Preparation, Dosage, and Administration of Cholinesterase Inhibitors

Drug Class or Drug	Preparation	Dosage	Administration
CHOLINESTERASE INHIBITORS			
Neostigmine [Prostigmin]	Prostigmin: 0.5-mg/mL solution available in 1-mL and 10-mL vials Generic: 0.5 mg/mL and 1 mg/mL, both in 10-mL vials	Myasthenia gravis treatment (highly individualized): 0.5 mg IM or subQ initially with additional dosing based on patient response. Typical dosing is 15–375 mg/day in divided doses	Timing administration so that peak effects occur at meal time may help with eating and swallowing
Physostigmine	1 mg/mL in 2-mL vials	Reversal of anticholinergic toxicity: adults—0.5–2 mg IM or IV Children: 0.02 mg/kg Dose may be repeated every 10–30 minutes as needed	Rapid IV administration can cause respiratory distress, bradycardia, and seizures. Limit rate to 1 mg/min in adults or 0.5 mg/min in children.
Pyridostigmine [Mestinon Regonol, Mestinon-SR ♣]	Syrup: 60 mg/5 mL Tablet IR: 60 mg Tablet ER: 180 mg	Myasthenia gravis treatment (highly individualized) IR: 60–1,500 mg/day Typical dosing 600 mg/day divided into 5 doses ER: 180–540 mg once or twice a day (It may be necessary to use both IR and ER dosing to sustain effects)	Take the ER tablets whole.

ER, extended release; IM, intramuscular; IR, immediate release; IV, intravenous; subQ, subcutaneous.

NEUROMUSCULAR BLOCKADE. If administered in toxic doses, cholinesterase inhibitors can cause accumulation of acetylcholine in amounts sufficient to produce depolarizing neuromuscular blockade. Paralysis of the respiratory muscles can be fatal.

Precautions and Contraindications. Most of the precautions and contraindications regarding the cholinesterase inhibitors are the same as those for the direct-acting muscarinic agonists. These include obstruction of the GI tract, obstruction of the urinary tract, peptic ulcer disease, asthma, coronary insufficiency, and hyperthyroidism.

Drug Interactions

MUSCARINIC ANTAGONISTS. The effects of cholinesterase inhibitors at muscarinic receptors are opposite to those of atropine (and all other muscarinic antagonists). Consequently, cholinesterase inhibitors can be used to overcome excessive muscarinic blockade caused by atropine. Conversely, atropine can be used to reduce excessive muscarinic stimulation caused by cholinesterase inhibitors.

Other Reversible Cholinesterase Inhibitors

Physostigmine. The basic pharmacology of physostigmine is identical to that of neostigmine. In contrast to neostigmine, physostigmine is *not* a quaternary ammonium compound and hence does *not* carry a charge. Because physostigmine is uncharged, physostigmine readily crosses membranes, whereas neostigmine does not.

Physostigmine is the drug of choice for treating *poisoning by atropine and other drugs that cause muscarinic blockade,* including antihistamines and phenothiazine antipsychotics—but *not* tricyclic antidepressants, owing to a risk for causing seizures and cardiotoxicity. Physostigmine counteracts antimuscarinic poisoning by causing acetylcholine to build up at muscarinic junctions. The accumulated acetylcholine competes with the muscarinic blocker for receptor binding and thereby reverses receptor blockade. Physostigmine is preferred to neostigmine because, lacking a charge, physostigmine is able to cross the blood-brain barrier to reverse muscarinic blockade in the CNS.

Edrophonium and Pyridostigmine. Edrophonium [Enlon, Tensilon ♣] and pyridostigmine [Mestinon] have pharmacologic effects much like those of neostigmine. One of these drugs—edrophonium—is noteworthy for its very brief duration of action. Edrophonium is also unique in that it is indicated for diagnosis, but not treatment, of MG. In current practice, though, edrophonium is not commonly used for this purpose because better and more accurate testing is now available.

Drugs for Alzheimer Disease. Three cholinesterase inhibitors—donepezil [Aricept], galantamine [Razadyne], and rivastigmine [Exelon]—are approved for management of Alzheimer disease, and one of them—rivastigmine—is also approved for dementia of Parkinson disease. With all three, benefits derive from inhibiting cholinesterase in the CNS. The pharmacology of these drugs is discussed in Chapter 18.

Irreversible Cholinesterase Inhibitors

The irreversible cholinesterase inhibitors are highly toxic. These agents are employed primarily as *insecticides.* During World War II, huge quantities of irreversible cholinesterase inhibitors were produced for possible use as *nerve agents,* but were never deployed. Today, there is concern that these agents might be employed as weapons of terrorism. The only clinical indication for the irreversible inhibitors is *glaucoma.*

Basic Pharmacology

Chemistry. All irreversible cholinesterase inhibitors contain an atom of *phosphorus* (Fig. 12.3). Because of this phosphorus atom, the irreversible inhibitors are known as *organophosphate* cholinesterase inhibitors.

Almost all irreversible cholinesterase inhibitors are *highly lipid soluble.* As a result, these drugs are readily absorbed from all routes of administration. They can even be absorbed directly through the skin. Easy absorption, coupled with high toxicity, is what makes these drugs good insecticides—and gives them potential as agents of chemical warfare. After they are absorbed, the organophosphate inhibitors have ready access to all tissues and organs, including the CNS.

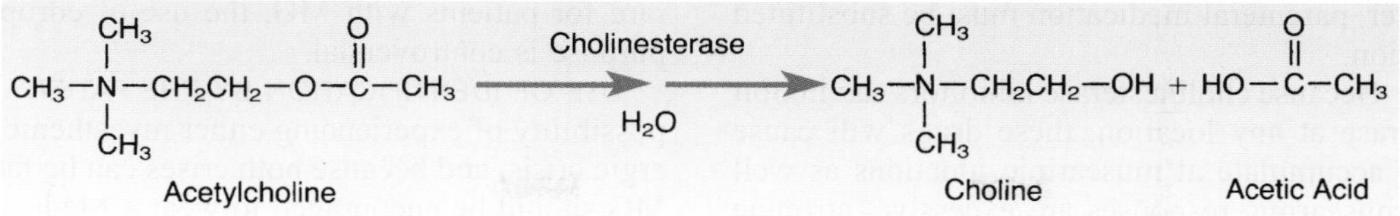

Figure 12.3 ■ Hydrolysis of acetylcholine by cholinesterase.

Mechanism of Action. The irreversible cholinesterase inhibitors bind to the active center of cholinesterase, preventing the enzyme from hydrolyzing acetylcholine. Although these drugs can be split from cholinesterase, the splitting reaction takes place *extremely* slowly. Hence, under normal conditions, their binding to cholinesterase can be considered irreversible. Because binding is irreversible, effects persist until new molecules of cholinesterase can be synthesized.

Although we normally consider the bond between irreversible inhibitors and cholinesterase permanent, this bond can, in fact, be broken. To break the bond and reverse the inhibition of cholinesterase, we must administer *pralidoxime,* a cholinesterase reactivator.

Pharmacologic Effects. The irreversible cholinesterase inhibitors produce essentially the same spectrum of effects as the reversible inhibitors. The principal difference is that responses to irreversible inhibitors last a long time, whereas responses to reversible inhibitors are brief.

Therapeutic Uses. As mentioned previously, the irreversible cholinesterase inhibitors have only one indication: treatment of *glaucoma.* And for that indication, only one drug—echothiophate—is available. The limited indications for irreversible cholinesterase inhibitors should be no surprise given their potential for harm. The use of echothiophate for glaucoma is discussed in Chapter 84.

Toxicology of Cholinesterase Inhibitors

Sources of Poisoning

Poisoning by organophosphate cholinesterase inhibitors is a common occurrence. Agricultural workers have been poisoned by accidental ingestion of organophosphate insecticides and by absorption of these lipid-soluble compounds through the skin. In addition, because organophosphate insecticides are readily available to the general public, poisoning may occur accidentally or from attempted homicide or suicide. Exposure could also occur if these drugs were used as instruments of warfare or terrorism.

Symptoms

Toxic doses of irreversible cholinesterase inhibitors produce excessive muscarinic, nicotinic, and CNS effects. This condition, known as a *cholinergic crisis,* is characterized by *excessive muscarinic stimulation* and *depolarizing neuromuscular blockade.* Overstimulation of muscarinic receptors results in profuse secretions from salivary and bronchial glands, involuntary urination and defecation, laryngospasm, and bronchoconstriction. Prominent nicotinic effects reflect nicotinic activity at neuromuscular junctions resulting in muscle weakness, fasciculations, cramps, and twitching. Neuromuscular blockade can result in paralysis, followed by death from apnea. CNS effects may range from anxiety and confusion to delirium. Convulsions of CNS origin precede paralysis and apnea.

Treatment

Pharmacologic treatment involves giving *atropine* to reduce muscarinic stimulation, giving *pralidoxime* to reverse inhibition of cholinesterase (primarily at the NMJ), and giving a benzodiazepine such as *diazepam* to suppress convulsions. Respiratory depression from cholinesterase inhibitors cannot be managed with drugs. Rather, treatment consists of mechanical ventilation with oxygen.

Pralidoxime. Pralidoxime is a specific antidote to poisoning by the irreversible (organophosphate) cholinesterase inhibitors; the drug is *not* effective against poisoning by reversible cholinesterase inhibitors. In poisoning by irreversible inhibitors, benefits derive from causing the inhibitor to dissociate from the active center of cholinesterase. Reversal is most effective at the NMJ. Pralidoxime is much less effective at reversing cholinesterase inhibition at muscarinic and ganglionic sites. Furthermore, because pralidoxime is a quaternary ammonium compound, it cannot cross the blood-brain barrier and therefore cannot reverse cholinesterase inhibition in the CNS. To be effective, pralidoxime must be administered soon after organophosphate poisoning has occurred.

Myasthenia Gravis

Pathophysiology

MG is a neuromuscular disorder characterized by fluctuating muscle weakness and a predisposition to rapid fatigue. Common symptoms include ptosis (drooping eyelids), difficulty swallowing, and weakness of skeletal muscles. Patients with severe MG may have difficulty breathing owing to weakness of the muscles of respiration.

Symptoms of MG result from an autoimmune process in which the patient's immune system produces antibodies that attack nicotinic$_M$ receptors on skeletal muscle. As a result, the number of functional receptors at the NMJ is reduced by 70% to 90%, causing muscle weakness.

Treatment With Cholinesterase Inhibitors

Beneficial Effects. Reversible cholinesterase inhibitors (e.g., neostigmine) are the mainstay of therapy. By preventing acetylcholine inactivation, anticholinesterase agents can intensify the effects of acetylcholine released from motor neurons, increasing muscle strength. Cholinesterase inhibitors do not cure MG. Rather, they only produce symptomatic relief, so patients usually need therapy lifelong.

When working with patients with MG, keep in mind that muscle strength may be insufficient to permit swallowing. Accordingly, you should assess the ability to swallow before prescribing oral medications. If the patient is unable to swallow the water, parenteral medication must be substituted for oral medication.

Side Effects. Because cholinesterase inhibitors can inhibit acetylcholinesterase at any location, these drugs will cause acetylcholine to accumulate at muscarinic junctions as well as at NMJs. If muscarinic responses are excessive, atropine may be given to suppress them. However, atropine should not be employed *routinely* because the drug can mask the early signs (e.g., excessive salivation) of overdose with anticholinesterase agents.

Dosage Adjustment. In the treatment of MG, establishing an optimal dosage for cholinesterase inhibitors can be a challenge. Dosage determination is accomplished by administering a small initial dose followed by additional small doses until an optimal level of muscle function has been achieved. Important signs of improvement include increased ease of swallowing and increased ability to raise the eyelids. You can help establish a correct dosage by having the patient or family keep records of (1) times of drug administration, (2) times at which fatigue occurs, (3) the state of muscle strength before and after drug administration, and (4) signs of excessive muscarinic stimulation.

To maintain optimal responses, patients must occasionally modify dosage themselves. To do this, they must be taught to recognize signs of undermedication (ptosis, difficulty in swallowing) and signs of overmedication (excessive salivation and other muscarinic responses). Patients may also need to modify dosage in anticipation of exertion. For example, they may find it necessary to take supplementary medication 30 to 60 minutes before activities such as eating or shopping.

Myasthenic Crisis and Cholinergic Crisis

MYASTHENIC CRISIS. Patients who are inadequately medicated may experience myasthenic crisis, a state characterized by extreme muscle weakness caused by insufficient acetylcholine at the NMJ. Left untreated, myasthenic crisis can result in death from paralysis of the muscles of respiration. A cholinesterase inhibitor (e.g., neostigmine) is used to relieve the crisis.

CHOLINERGIC CRISIS. As noted previously, overdose with a cholinesterase inhibitor can produce cholinergic crisis. Like myasthenic crisis, cholinergic crisis is characterized by extreme muscle weakness or frank paralysis. In addition, cholinergic crisis is accompanied by signs of excessive muscarinic stimulation. Treatment consists of respiratory support plus atropine. The offending cholinesterase inhibitor should be withheld until muscle strength has returned.

DISTINGUISHING MYASTHENIC CRISIS FROM CHOLINERGIC CRISIS. Because myasthenic crisis and cholinergic crisis share similar symptoms (muscle weakness or paralysis), but are treated very differently, it is essential to distinguish between them. A history of medication use or signs of excessive muscarinic stimulation are usually sufficient to permit a differential diagnosis. If these clues are inadequate, the provider may elect to administer a challenging dose of *edrophonium,* an ultrashort-acting cholinesterase inhibitor. If edrophonium-induced elevation of acetylcholine levels alleviates symptoms, the crisis is myasthenic. Conversely, if edrophonium intensifies symptoms, the crisis is cholinergic. Because the symptoms of cholinergic crisis will be made even worse by edrophonium and could be life-threatening, atropine and oxygen should be immediately available whenever edrophonium is used for this test. For this reason, and because cholinergic crisis is relatively rare for patients with MG, the use of edrophonium for this purpose is controversial.

USE OF IDENTIFICATION BY THE PATIENT. Because of the possibility of experiencing either myasthenic crisis or cholinergic crisis, and because both crises can be fatal, patients with MG should be encouraged to wear a Medic Alert bracelet or some other form of identification to inform emergency medical personnel of their condition.

Toxicology of Muscarinic Agonists

Sources of Muscarinic Poisoning

Muscarinic poisoning can result from ingestion of certain mushrooms (e.g., *Inocybe* and *Clitocybe* spp.) and from overdose with two kinds of medications: (1) direct-acting muscarinic agonists (e.g., bethanechol, pilocarpine), and (2) cholinesterase inhibitors (indirect-acting cholinomimetics).

Symptoms

Manifestations of muscarinic poisoning result from excessive activation of muscarinic receptors. Prominent symptoms are (1) respiratory (bronchospasm and excessive bronchial secretions); (2) cardiovascular (bradycardia and hypotension); (3) gastrointestinal (profuse salivation, nausea and vomiting, abdominal pain, diarrhea, and fecal incontinence); (4) genitourinary (excessive urination and urinary incontinence); integumentary (diaphoresis); and visual (lacrimation and miosis). Severe poisoning can produce cardiovascular collapse. (Mnemonics for muscarinic poisoning are presented in Box 12.1.)

Treatment

Management is direct and specific: administer *atropine* (a selective muscarinic blocking agent) and provide supportive

BOX 12.1 ▪ MUSCARINIC (CHOLINERGIC) TOXICITY

Muscarinic (cholinergic) toxicity can be caused by either muscarinic agonists or cholinesterase inhibitors. Some common mnemonics can help you to identify this potentially dangerous condition.

Mnemonic 1: Dumbels

Diaphoresis/**D**iarrhea
Urination
Miosis
Bradycardia/**B**ronchospasm/**B**ronchorrhea
Emesis
Lacrimation
Salivation

Mnemonic 2: Sludge and the Killer Bs

Salivation
Lacrimation
Urination
Diaphoresis/**D**iarrhea
Gastrointestinal cramping
Emesis
Bradycardia
Bronchospasm
Bronchorrhea

therapy. By blocking access of muscarinic agonists to their receptors, atropine can reverse most signs of toxicity.

Muscarinic Antagonists (Anticholinergic Drugs)

Muscarinic antagonists competitively block the actions of acetylcholine at muscarinic receptors. Because most muscarinic receptors are located on structures innervated by parasympathetic nerves, the muscarinic antagonists are also known as *parasympatholytic drugs*. Additional names for these agents are *antimuscarinic drugs, muscarinic blockers,* and *anticholinergic drugs.*

The term *anticholinergic* can be a source of confusion and requires comment. This term is unfortunate in that it implies blockade at *all* cholinergic receptors. However, as normally used, the term *anticholinergic* only denotes blockade of *muscarinic* receptors. Therefore, when a drug is characterized as being anticholinergic, you can take this to mean that it produces selective *muscarinic* blockade—and not blockade of all cholinergic receptors. In this chapter, the terms *muscarinic antagonist* and *anticholinergic agent* are used interchangeably.

Atropine

Atropine [AtroPen, others] is the best-known muscarinic antagonist and will serve as our prototype for the group. The actions of all other muscarinic blockers are much like those of this drug.

Atropine is found naturally in a variety of plants, including *Atropa belladonna* (deadly nightshade) and *Datura stramonium* (also known as Jimson weed, stinkweed, and devil's apple). Because of its presence in *A. belladonna,* atropine is referred to as a *belladonna alkaloid.*

Mechanism of Action

Atropine produces its effects through competitive blockade at muscarinic receptors. Like all other receptor antagonists, atropine has no direct effects of its own. Rather, all responses to atropine result from *preventing receptor activation* by endogenous acetylcholine (or by drugs that act as muscarinic agonists).

At therapeutic doses, atropine produces selective blockade of muscarinic cholinergic receptors. However, if the dosage is sufficiently high, the drug will produce some blockade of nicotinic receptors, too.

Pharmacologic Effects

Because atropine acts by causing muscarinic receptor blockade, its effects are opposite to those caused by muscarinic activation. Accordingly, we can readily predict the effects of atropine by knowing the normal responses to muscarinic receptor activation (see Table 11.2) and by knowing that atropine will reverse those responses. Like the muscarinic agonists, the muscarinic antagonists exert their influence primarily on the *heart, exocrine glands, smooth muscles,* and *eyes.*

Heart. Atropine *increases heart rate.* Because activation of cardiac muscarinic receptors decreases heart rate, blockade of these receptors will cause heart rate to increase.

Exocrine Glands. Atropine *decreases secretion* from salivary glands, bronchial glands, sweat glands, and the acid-secreting cells of the stomach. Note that these effects are opposite to those of muscarinic agonists, which increase secretion from exocrine glands.

Smooth Muscle. By preventing activation of muscarinic receptors on smooth muscle, atropine causes *relaxation of the bronchi, decreased tone of the urinary bladder detrusor,* and *decreased tone and motility of the GI tract.* In the absence of an exogenous muscarinic agonist (e.g., bethanechol), muscarinic blockade has no effect on vascular smooth muscle tone because there is no parasympathetic innervation to muscarinic receptors in blood vessels.

Eyes. Blockade of muscarinic receptors on the iris sphincter causes *mydriasis* (dilation of the pupil). Blockade of muscarinic receptors on the ciliary muscle produces *cycloplegia* (relaxation of the ciliary muscle), thereby focusing the lens for far vision.

Central Nervous System. At therapeutic doses, atropine can cause mild *CNS excitation.* Toxic doses can cause *hallucinations* and *delirium,* which can resemble psychosis. Extremely high doses can result in coma, respiratory arrest, and death.

Dose Dependency of Muscarinic Blockade. It is important to note that not all muscarinic receptors are equally sensitive to blockade by atropine and most other anticholinergic drugs: at some sites, muscarinic receptors can be blocked with relatively low doses; whereas at other sites, much higher doses are needed. Table 12.4 indicates the sequence in which specific muscarinic receptors are blocked as the dose of atropine is increased.

Differences in receptor sensitivity to muscarinic blockers are of clinical significance. As indicated in Table 12.4, the doses needed to block muscarinic receptors in the stomach and bronchial smooth muscle are higher than the doses needed to block muscarinic receptors at all other locations. Accordingly, if we want to use atropine to treat peptic ulcer disease (by suppressing gastric acid secretion) or asthma (by dilating the bronchi), we cannot do so without also affecting the heart, exocrine glands, many smooth muscles, and the eyes. Because of these obligatory side effects, atropine and most other muscarinic antagonists are not preferred drugs for treating peptic ulcers or asthma.

TABLE 12.4 ▪ Relationship Between Dosage and Responses to Atropine

Dosage of Atropine	Response Produced
Low dose	Salivary glands—decreased secretion
↓	Sweat glands—decreased secretion
High dose	Bronchial glands—decreased secretion
	Heart—increased rate
	Eyes—mydriasis, blurred vision
	Urinary tract—interference with voiding
	Intestines—decreased tone and motility
	Lungs—dilation of bronchi*
	Stomach—decreased acid secretion*

*Doses of atropine that are high enough to dilate the bronchi or decrease gastric acid secretion will also affect all other structures under muscarinic control. As a result, atropine and most other muscarinic antagonists are not very desirable for treating peptic ulcer disease or asthma.

Pharmacokinetics

Atropine may be administered topically (to the eye), and parenterally (IM, IV, and subQ routes). The drug is rapidly absorbed after administration and distributes to all tissues, including the CNS. Elimination is by a combination of hepatic metabolism and urinary excretion. Atropine has a half-life of approximately 3 hours.

Therapeutic Uses

Preanesthetic Medication. The cardiac effects of atropine can help during surgery. Procedures that stimulate baroreceptors of the carotid body can initiate reflex slowing of the heart, resulting in profound bradycardia. Because this reflex is mediated by muscarinic receptors on the heart, pretreatment with atropine can prevent a dangerous reduction in heart rate.

Certain anesthetics irritate the respiratory tract and thereby stimulate secretion from salivary, nasal, pharyngeal, and bronchial glands. If these secretions are sufficiently profuse, they can interfere with respiration. By blocking muscarinic receptors on secretory glands, atropine can help prevent excessive secretions. Fortunately, modern anesthetics are much less irritating. The availability of these new anesthetics has greatly reduced the use of atropine for this purpose during anesthesia.

Disorders of the Eyes. By blocking muscarinic receptors in the eyes, atropine can cause mydriasis and paralysis of the ciliary muscle. Both actions can be of help during eye examinations and ocular surgery. The ophthalmic uses of atropine and other muscarinic antagonists are discussed in Chapter 84.

Bradycardia. Atropine can accelerate heart rate in certain patients with bradycardia. Heart rate is increased because blockade of cardiac muscarinic receptors reverses parasympathetic slowing of the heart.

Intestinal Hypertonicity and Hypermotility. By blocking muscarinic receptors in the intestine, atropine can decrease both the tone and motility of intestinal smooth muscle. This can be beneficial in conditions characterized by excessive intestinal motility, such as mild dysentery and diverticulitis. When taken for these disorders, atropine can reduce both the frequency of bowel movements and associated abdominal cramps.

Muscarinic Agonist Poisoning. Atropine is a specific antidote to poisoning by agents that activate muscarinic receptors. By blocking muscarinic receptors, atropine can reverse all signs of muscarinic poisoning. An atropine autoinjector (Atropen) is approved for use in people exposed to the irreversible cholinesterase inhibitor nerve agents or insecticides discussed previously. (See Box 12.2.)

Peptic Ulcer Disease. Because it can suppress secretion of gastric acid, atropine has been used to treat peptic ulcer disease. Unfortunately, when administered in doses that are strong enough to block the muscarinic receptors that regulate secretion of gastric acid, atropine also blocks most other muscarinic receptors. Therefore use of atropine in treatment of ulcers is associated with a broad range of antimuscarinic side effects (dry mouth, blurred vision, urinary retention, constipation, and so on). Because of these side effects, atropine is not a first-choice drug for ulcer therapy. Rather, atropine is reserved for rare cases in which symptoms cannot be relieved with preferred medications (e.g., antibiotics, histamine-2 receptor antagonists, proton pump inhibitors).

Asthma. By blocking bronchial muscarinic receptors, atropine can promote bronchial dilation, thereby improving respiration in patients with asthma. Unfortunately, in addition to dilating the bronchi, atropine also causes drying and thickening of bronchial secretions, effects that can be harmful to patients with asthma. Furthermore, when given in the doses needed to dilate the bronchi, atropine causes a variety of antimuscarinic side effects. Because of the potential for harm, and because superior medicines are available, atropine is rarely used for asthma.

BOX 12.2 ■ ATROPEN FOR CHOLINESTERASE INHIBITOR POISONING

The AtroPen is a prefilled autoinjector indicated for intramuscular treatment of poisoning with an organophosphate cholinesterase inhibitor (nerve agent or insecticide). Four strengths are available: 0.25 and 0.5 mg (for children weighing <40 pounds), 1 mg (for children 40–90 pounds), and 2 mg (for adults and children >90 pounds). The AtroPen should be used immediately on exposure or if exposure is strongly suspected. Injections are administered into the lateral thigh, directly through clothing if necessary.

Dosing is determined by symptom severity and weight. Dosage by weight is as follows:

- <6.8 kg (<15 lb): administer 0.25 mg/dose
- 6.8 to 18 kg (15–40 lb): administer 0.5 mg/dose
- 18 to 41 kg (40–90 lb): administer 1 mg/dose
- >41 kg (>90 lb): administer 2 mg/dose

Multiple doses are often required. If symptoms are severe, three weight-based doses should be administered rapidly. If symptoms are mild, one dose should be given; if severe symptoms develop afterward, additional doses can be given up to a maximum of three doses.

Biliary Colic. Biliary colic is characterized by intense abdominal pain brought on by passage of a gallstone through the bile duct. In some cases, atropine may be combined with analgesics such as morphine to relax biliary tract smooth muscle, thereby helping alleviate discomfort.

Adverse Effects

Most adverse effects of atropine and other anticholinergic drugs are the direct result of muscarinic receptor blockade. Accordingly, these effects can be predicted from your knowledge of muscarinic receptor function.

Xerostomia (Dry Mouth). Blockade of muscarinic receptors on salivary glands can inhibit salivation, thereby causing dry mouth. Not only is this uncomfortable, it also can impede swallowing and can promote tooth decay, gum problems, and oral infections. Patients should be informed that dryness can be alleviated by sipping fluids, chewing specially formulated sugar-free gum (e.g., Altoids Chewing Gum, Biotene Dry Mouth Gum), treating the mouth with a saliva substitute (e.g., Salivart, Biotene Gel), and using an alcohol-free mouthwash (Biotene mouthwash). Owing to increased risk for tooth decay, patients should avoid sugary gum and hard candy.

Blurred Vision and Photophobia. Blockade of muscarinic receptors on the ciliary muscle and the sphincter of the iris can paralyze these muscles. Paralysis of the ciliary muscle focuses the eye for far vision, causing nearby objects to appear blurred. Patients should be forewarned about this effect and advised to avoid hazardous activities if vision is impaired.

Additionally, paralysis of the iris sphincter prevents constriction of the pupil, thereby rendering the eye unable to adapt to bright light. Patients should be advised to wear dark glasses if photophobia is a problem. Room lighting for hospitalized patients should be kept low.

Elevation of Intraocular Pressure. Paralysis of the iris sphincter can raise IOP by a mechanism discussed in Chapter 84. Because they can increase IOP, anticholinergic drugs are contraindicated for patients with glaucoma, a disease characterized by abnormally high IOP. In addition, these drugs should be used with caution in patients who may not have glaucoma per se but for whom a predisposition to glaucoma may be present.

Urinary Retention. Blockade of muscarinic receptors in the urinary tract reduces pressure within the bladder and increases the tone of the urinary sphincter and trigone. These effects can produce urinary hesitancy or urinary retention. In the event of severe urinary retention, catheterization or treatment with a muscarinic agonist (e.g., bethanechol) may be required. Patients should be advised that urinary retention can be minimized by voiding just before taking their medication.

Constipation. Muscarinic blockade decreases the tone and motility of intestinal smooth muscle. The resultant delay in transit through the intestine can produce constipation. Patients should be informed that constipation can be minimized by increasing dietary fiber, fluids, and physical activity. A laxative may be needed if constipation is severe. Because of their ability to decrease smooth muscle tone, muscarinic antagonists are contraindicated for patients with intestinal atony, a condition in which intestinal tone is already low.

Anhidrosis. Blockade of muscarinic receptors on sweat glands can produce anhidrosis (a deficiency or absence of sweat). Because sweating is necessary for cooling, people who cannot sweat are at risk for hyperthermia. Patients should be warned of this possibility and advised to avoid activities that might lead to overheating (e.g., exercising on a hot day).

Tachycardia. Blockade of cardiac muscarinic receptors eliminates parasympathetic influence on the heart. By removing the "braking" influence of parasympathetic nerves, anticholinergic agents can cause tachycardia. Exercise caution in patients with preexisting tachycardia.

Asthma. In patients with asthma, antimuscarinic drugs can cause thickening and drying of bronchial secretions and can thereby cause bronchial plugging. Consequently, although muscarinic antagonists can be used to treat asthma, they can also do harm.

Drug Interactions. A number of drugs that are not classified as muscarinic antagonists can nonetheless produce significant muscarinic blockade. Among these are antihistamines, phenothiazine antipsychotics, and tricyclic antidepressants. Because of their prominent anticholinergic actions, these drugs can greatly enhance the antimuscarinic effects of atropine and related agents. Accordingly, it is wise to avoid combined use of atropine with other drugs that can cause muscarinic blockade.

Preparations, Dosage, and Administration

General Systemic Therapy. Atropine sulfate is available in solution (0.05–1 mg/mL) for IM, IV, and subQ administration.

Muscarinic Antagonists for Overactive Bladder

Overactive Bladder: Characteristics and Overview of Treatment

Overactive bladder (OAB)—also known as urgency incontinence—is a disorder with four major symptoms: urinary urgency (a sudden, compelling desire to urinate), urinary frequency (voiding 8 or more times in 24 hours), nocturia (waking 2 or more times to void), and urge incontinence (involuntary urine leakage associated with a strong urge to void). In most cases, urge incontinence results from *involuntary contractions of the bladder detrusor* (the smooth muscle component of the bladder wall). These contractions are often referred to as detrusor instability or detrusor overactivity. Urge incontinence should not be confused with *stress incontinence,* defined as involuntary urine leakage caused by activities (e.g., exertion, sneezing, coughing, laughter) that increase pressure within the abdominal cavity, or *overflow incontinence,* which is the involuntary leakage of urine from an overly distended bladder.

OAB is a common disorder, affecting up to one third of Americans. The condition can develop at any age but is most prevalent in older populations. Among people ages 40 to 44 years, symptoms are reported by 3% of men and 9% of women. In comparison, among those 75 years and older, symptoms are reported by 42% of men and 31% of women. Because urine leakage, the most disturbing symptom, is both unpredictable and potentially embarrassing, many people with OAB curtail travel, social activities, and even work.

OAB has two primary modes of treatment: *behavioral therapy* and *drug therapy* (Fig. 12.4). Behavioral therapy, which is at least as effective as drug therapy and lacks side effects, should be tried first. Behavioral interventions include scheduled voiding, timing fluid intake, doing Kegel exercises (to strengthen pelvic floor muscles), and avoiding caffeine, a diuretic that may also increase detrusor activity. As a rule, drugs should be reserved for patients who don't respond adequately to behavioral measures. If behavioral therapy and drugs are inadequate, a provider may offer specialized treatments (e.g., sacral neuromodulation, peripheral tibial nerve stimulation).

Introduction to Anticholinergic Therapy of OAB

When drug therapy *is* indicated, *anticholinergic agents* (e.g., oxybutynin, tolterodine) are indicated. These drugs block muscarinic receptors on the bladder detrusor and thereby inhibit bladder contractions and the urge to void.

Unfortunately, drugs that block muscarinic receptors in the bladder can also block muscarinic receptors elsewhere and cause the typical anticholinergic side effects previously described. Anticholinergic side effects can be reduced in at least three ways: (1) using long-acting formulations, (2) using drugs that don't cross the blood-brain barrier, and (3) using drugs that are selective for muscarinic receptors in the bladder. Long-acting formulations (e.g., extended-release capsules, transdermal patches) reduce side effects by providing a steady but relatively low level of drug, thereby avoiding the high peak levels that can cause intense side effects. Drugs that can't cross the blood-brain barrier are unable to cause CNS effects.

What about drugs that are selective for muscarinic receptors in the bladder? To answer this question, we must first discuss muscarinic receptor subtypes. As noted in Chapter 11, there are five known muscarinic receptor subtypes. However, only three—designated M_1, M_2, and M_3—have clearly identified functions. Locations of these receptor subtypes, and responses to their activation and blockade, are shown in

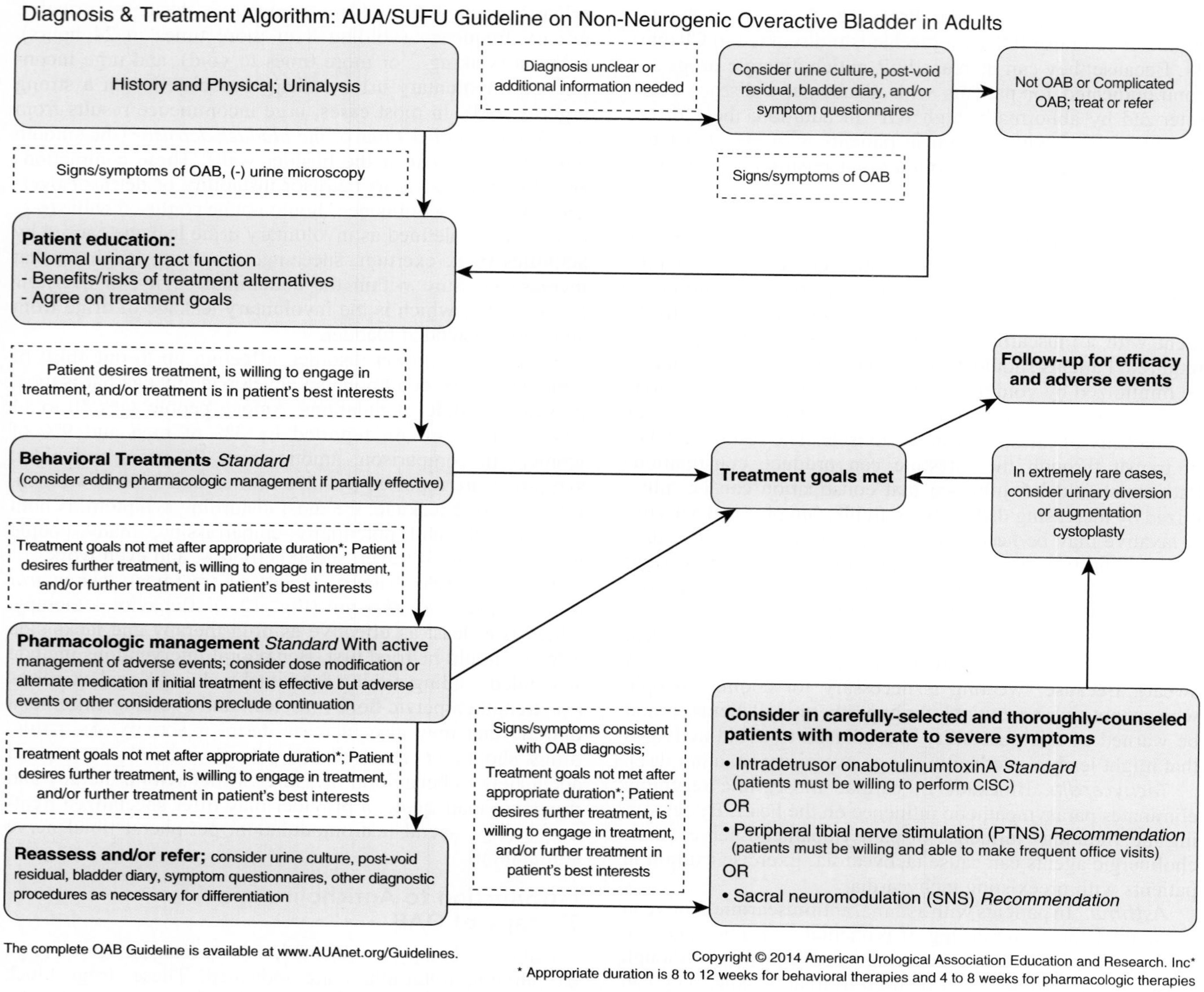

Figure 12.4 ■ **Algorithm for management of overactive bladder.**
(From the American Urologic Association. https://www.auanet.org/common/pdf/education/clinical-guidance/Overactive-Bladder-Algorithm.pdf.)

Table 12.5. As indicated, M_3 receptors are the most widely distributed, being found in salivary glands, the bladder detrusor, GI smooth muscle, and the eyes. M_2 receptors are found only in the heart, and M_1 receptors are found in salivary glands and the CNS. At each location, responses to receptor activation are the same as we discussed in Chapter 11—although, in that chapter, we didn't identify the receptors by subtype; rather, we called all of them *muscarinic.*

With this background, we can consider how receptor selectivity might decrease anticholinergic side effects of drugs for OAB. To be beneficial, an anticholinergic agent must block muscarinic receptors in the bladder detrusor. That is, it must block the M_3 receptor subtype. Because M_3 receptors are also found in GI smooth muscle, the eyes, and salivary glands, an M_3-selective blocker will still have some unwanted anticholinergic effects, namely, constipation (from reducing bowel motility), blurred vision and photophobia (from preventing contraction of the ciliary muscle and iris sphincter), dry eyes (from blocking tear production), and *some* degree of dry mouth (from blocking salivary gland M_3 receptors, while sparing salivary M_1 receptors). What an M_3-selective blocker will *not* do is cause tachycardia (because muscarinic receptors in the heart are the M_2 type) or impairment of CNS function (because muscarinic receptors in the brain are primarily the M_1 type).

Specific Anticholinergic Drugs for Overactive Bladder

In the United States six anticholinergic drugs are approved specifically for OAB (Table 12.6). All six work by M_3-muscarinic receptor blockade, although most block M_1 and M_2 receptors as well. With all of these drugs, we want sufficient M_3 blockade to reduce symptoms of OAB, but not so much as to cause urinary retention. You should be aware that

TABLE 12.5 ▪ Muscarinic Receptor Subtypes

Muscarinic Subtype	Location	Response to Activation	Impact of Blockade
M_1	Salivary glands	Salivation	Dry mouth
	CNS	Enhanced cognition	Confusion, hallucinations
M_2	Heart	Bradycardia	Tachycardia
M_3	Salivary glands	Salivation	Dry mouth
	Bladder: detrusor	Contraction (increased pressure)	Relaxation (decreased pressure)
	GI smooth muscle	Increased tone and motility	Decreased tone and motility (constipation)
	Eyes: iris sphincter	Contraction (miosis)	Relaxation (mydriasis)
	Eyes: ciliary muscle	Contraction (accommodation)	Relaxation (blurred vision)
	Eyes: lacrimal gland	Tearing	Dry eyes

CNS, central nervous system; GI, gastrointestinal.

TABLE 12.6 ▪ Anticholinergic Drugs for Overactive Bladder

Generic and Trade Names	Formulation	Dosage: Initial	Dosage: Maximum	Administration
HIGHLY M_3 SELECTIVE				
Darifenacin				
Enablex	ER tablets	7.5 mg once daily	15 mg once daily	Swallow whole. May be taken with or without food.
PRIMARILY M_3 SELECTIVE				
Oxybutynin				
(generic only)	Syrup	5 mg 2–3 times/day	5 mg 4 times/day	May be taken with or without food.
(generic only)	IR tablets	5 mg 2–3 times/day	5 mg 4 times/day	May be taken with or without food.
Ditropan XL	ER tablets	5 mg once daily	30 mg once daily*	Swallow whole. May be taken with or without food.
Oxytrol	Transdermal patch	1 patch twice weekly (delivers 3 mg/day)	1 patch twice weekly	*Apply to dry, intact skin of the abdomen, hip, or buttock. Rotate sites.*
Gelnique	Topical gel	3%: 3 pumps once daily 10%: one 100-mg/1-g gel packet once daily	100 mg once daily	Discard any gel dispensed when priming the pump. Apply to dry, intact, unshaven skin of the abdomen, upper arm, shoulder, or thigh. Rotate sites. Cover site to avoid drug transfer to others.
Solifenacin				
VESIcare	Tablets	5 mg once daily	10 mg once daily	Swallow whole. May be taken with or without food.
NONSELECTIVE				
Fesoterodine				
Toviaz	ER tablets	4 mg once daily	8 mg once daily	Swallow whole. May be taken with or without food.
Tolterodine				
Detrol	IR tablets	1–2 mg twice daily	2 mg twice daily	May be taken with or without food.
Detrol LA	ER capsules	2–4 mg once daily	4 mg once daily	Swallow whole. May be taken with or without food.
Trospium				
(generic only in U.S.) Trosec ♣	Tablets	20 mg twice daily†	20 mg twice daily	Take 1 hour before meals on an empty stomach.
Sanctura XR ♣	ER capsules	60 mg once daily	60 mg once daily†	Take in the morning with a full glass of water. Do not take within 2 hours of consuming alcohol.

*Titrate dose upward as needed and tolerated.
†For patients with severe renal impairment, decrease dosage to 20 mg once daily at bedtime.
ER, extended release; IR, immediate release.

responses to these agents are relatively modest and, for many patients, only slightly better than a placebo. None of the anticholinergics used for OAB is clearly superior to the others. However, if one anticholinergic fails to reduce symptoms, success may occur with a different anticholinergic approved for OAB.

Oxybutynin

Oxybutynin [Ditropan XL, Gelnique, Oxytrol] is an anticholinergic agent that acts primarily at M_3 muscarinic receptors. The drug is approved only for OAB. Benefits derive from blocking M_3 receptors on the bladder detrusor.

Oxybutynin is rapidly absorbed from the GI tract, achieving peak plasma levels about 1 hour after dosing. However, despite rapid absorption, absolute bioavailability is low (about 6%) because oxybutynin undergoes extensive first-pass metabolism—both in the gut wall and liver—primarily by CYP3A4, the 3A4 isoenzyme of cytochrome P450. One metabolite—*N*-desethyloxybutynin—is highly active, especially against muscarinic receptors in the salivary glands. Oxybutynin is very lipid soluble; therefore it can penetrate the blood-brain barrier. The drug has a short half-life (2–3 hours), and hence multiple daily doses are required.

Anticholinergic side effects are common. The incidence of dry mouth is very high, in part because of muscarinic blockade by oxybutynin itself, and in part because of blockade by *N*-desethyloxybutynin. Other common side effects include constipation, tachycardia, urinary hesitancy, urinary retention, mydriasis, blurred vision, and dry eyes. In the CNS, cholinergic blockade can result in confusion, hallucinations, insomnia, and nervousness. In postmarketing reports of CNS effects, hallucinations and agitation were prominent among reports involving pediatric patients, whereas hallucinations, confusion, and sedation were prominent among reports involving older-adult patients. Combined use of oxybutynin with other anticholinergic agents (e.g., antihistamines, tricyclic antidepressants, phenothiazine antipsychotics) can intensify all anticholinergic side effects.

Drugs that inhibit or induce CYP3A4 may alter oxybutynin blood levels and may thereby either increase toxicity (inhibitors of CYP3A4) or reduce effectiveness (inducers of CYP3A4).

Oxybutynin is available in five formulations. Two are short acting (syrup and immediate-release [IR] tablets), and three are long acting (transdermal patch, topical gel, and extended-release [ER] tablets). Dosing of oxybutynin and other drugs for OAB is provided in Table 12.6.

Anticholinergic side effects are less intense with the long-acting products. These long-acting formulations of oxybutynin have special characteristics worth noting.

Extended-Release Tablets. Oxybutynin ER tablets [Ditropan XL] are as effective as the IR tablets and somewhat better tolerated. The ER tablets have an insoluble shell that is eliminated intact in the feces. Patients should be informed of this fact.

Transdermal Patch. The oxybutynin transdermal system [Oxytrol] contains 39 mg of oxybutynin and delivers 3.9 mg/day. Owing to its high lipid solubility, oxybutynin from the patch is readily absorbed directly through the skin. A new patch is applied twice weekly to dry, intact skin of the abdomen, hip, or buttock, rotating the site with each change. Reduction of OAB symptoms is about the same as with the ER tablets.

Pharmacokinetically, the patch is unique in two ways. First, absorption is both slow and steady, and hence the patch produces low but stable blood levels of the drug. Second, transdermal absorption bypasses metabolism in the intestinal wall and delays metabolism in the liver. As a result, levels of *N*-desethyloxybutynin, the active metabolite, are less than 20% of those achieved with oral therapy.

Transdermal oxybutynin is generally well tolerated. The most common side effect is application-site pruritus. The incidence of dry mouth is much lower than with the oral formulations, presumably because (1) formation of *N*-desethyloxybutynin is low and (2) high peak levels of oxybutynin itself are avoided. Rates of constipation, blurred vision, and CNS effects are also low.

Topical Gel. Topical oxybutynin gel [Gelnique] is much like the transdermal patch. As with the patch, oxybutynin is absorbed directly through the skin. Stable blood levels are achieved after 10 days of daily application. The most common side effects are application-site reactions and dry mouth. Other reactions include dizziness, headache, and constipation.

Gelnique should be applied to dry, intact skin of the abdomen, upper arm or shoulder, or thigh—but not to recently shaved skin—using a different site each day. Advise patients to wash their hands immediately after application and to avoid showering for at least 1 hour. Applying a sunscreen before or after dosing does not alter efficacy. Topical oxybutynin can be transferred to another person through direct contact. To avoid transfer, patients should cover the application site with clothing.

Darifenacin

Of the anticholinergic agents used for OAB, darifenacin [Enablex] displays the greatest degree of M_3 selectivity. As a result, the drug can reduce OAB symptoms while having no effect on M_1 receptors in the brain or M_2 receptors in the heart. However, darifenacin does block M_3 receptors outside the bladder, so it can still cause dry mouth, constipation, and other M_3-related effects.

Clinical benefits are similar to those of oxybutynin and tolterodine. On average, treatment reduces episodes of urge incontinence from 15/week down to 7/week (using 7.5 mg/day) and from 17/week down to 6/week (using 15 mg/day).

Darifenacin is administered orally in ER tablets. Absorption is adequate (15%–19%) and not affected by food. In the blood, darifenacin is 98% protein bound. The drug undergoes extensive hepatic metabolism, primarily by CYP3A4. The resulting inactive metabolites are excreted in the urine (60%) and feces (40%). The drug's half-life is approximately 12 hours.

Darifenacin is relatively well tolerated. The most common side effect is dry mouth. Constipation is also common. Other adverse effects include dyspepsia, gastritis, and headache. Darifenacin has little or no effect on memory, reaction time, word recognition, or cognition. The drug does not increase heart rate.

Levels of darifenacin can be raised significantly by strong inhibitors of CYP3A4. Among these are azole antifungal drugs (e.g., ketoconazole, itraconazole), certain protease inhibitors used for HIV/AIDS (e.g., ritonavir, nelfinavir), and clarithromycin (a macrolide antibiotic). If darifenacin is combined with any of these, its dosage must be kept low.

In patients with moderate liver impairment and in those taking powerful inhibitors of CYP3A4, dosage should be kept low. In patients with severe liver impairment, darifenacin should be avoided.

Solifenacin

Solifenacin [VESIcare] is very similar to darifenacin, although it's not quite as M_3 selective. In clinical trials, the drug reduced episodes of urge incontinence from 18/week down to 8/week (using 5 mg/day) and from 20/week down to 8/week (using 10 mg/day).

Solifenacin undergoes nearly complete absorption after oral dosing, achieving peak plasma levels in 3 to 6 hours. In the blood, the drug is highly (98%) protein bound. Like darifenacin, solifenacin undergoes extensive metabolism by hepatic CYP3A4. The resulting inactive metabolites are excreted in the urine (62%) and feces (23%). Solifenacin has a long half-life (about 50 hours) and hence can be administered just once a day.

The most common adverse effects are dry mouth, constipation, and blurred vision. Dyspepsia, urinary retention, headache, and nasal dryness occur infrequently. Rarely, solifenacin has caused potentially fatal angioedema of the face, lips, tongue, and larynx. At high doses (10–30 mg/day), solifenacin can prolong the QT interval, thereby posing a risk for a fatal dysrhythmia. Accordingly, caution is needed in patients with a history of QT prolongation and in those taking other QT-prolonging drugs. As with darifenacin, levels of solifenacin can be increased by strong inhibitors of CYP3A4 (e.g., ketoconazole, ritonavir, clarithromycin).

Solifenacin should be swallowed intact with liquid. Dosing may be done with or without food. For patients with moderate hepatic impairment or severe renal impairment and for those taking a powerful CYP3A4 inhibitor, dosage should not exceed 5 mg/day. For patients with severe hepatic impairment, solifenacin should be not be used.

Tolterodine

Tolterodine [Detrol, Detrol LA] is a nonselective muscarinic antagonist approved only for OAB. Like oxybutynin, tolterodine is available in short- and long-acting formulations. Anticholinergic side effects are less intense with the long-acting form.

Immediate-Release Tablets. In patients with OAB, tolterodine IR tablets [Detrol] can reduce the incidence of urge incontinence, urinary frequency, and urinary urgency. However, benefits are modest.

Tolterodine is rapidly but variably absorbed from the GI tract. Plasma levels peak 1 to 2 hours after dosing. After absorption, the drug undergoes conversion to 5-hydroxymethyl tolterodine, its active form. The active metabolite is later inactivated by CYP3A4 and CYP2D6 (the 2D6 isoenzyme of cytochrome P450). Parent drug and metabolites are eliminated in the urine (77%) and feces (17%). Tolterodine has a relatively short half-life.

Anticholinergic side effects with tolterodine affect fewer patients compared with other anticholinergics prescribed for OAB. For example, dry mouth occurs in 35% of patients taking IR tolterodine versus 70% with IR oxybutynin. At a dosage of 2 mg twice daily, the most common side effects are dry mouth, constipation, and dry eyes. Effects on the CNS—somnolence, vertigo, dizziness—occur infrequently. The incidence of both tachycardia and urinary retention is less than 1%. Anticholinergic effects can be intensified by concurrent use of other drugs with anticholinergic actions (e.g., antihistamines, tricyclic antidepressants, phenothiazine antipsychotics). Drugs that inhibit CYP3A4 (e.g., erythromycin, ketoconazole) can raise levels of tolterodine and can thereby intensify beneficial and adverse effects.

In addition to its anticholinergic effects, tolterodine can prolong the QT interval and can thereby promote serious cardiac dysrhythmias. Because of this risk, dosage should not exceed 4 mg/day.

Tolterodine is available as both IR tablets [Detrol] and ER capsules [Detrol LA]. Standard dosing is in Table 12.6; however, dosage should be decreased for patients with significant hepatic or renal impairment and for those taking a strong inhibitor of CYP3A4.

Fesoterodine

Fesoterodine [Toviaz] is a nonselective muscarinic antagonist very similar to tolterodine. Both fesoterodine and tolterodine are used only for OAB, and, at a dosage of 4 mg/day, both are equally effective. Furthermore, both agents undergo conversion to the same active metabolite—5-hydroxymethyl tolterodine—which is later inactivated by CYP3A4 and CYP2D6. In patients taking a strong inhibitor of CYP3A4 (e.g., ketoconazole, clarithromycin), beneficial and adverse effects are increased. Conversely, in patients taking a strong inducer of CYP3A4 (e.g., rifampin, carbamazepine), beneficial and adverse effects are reduced. As with tolterodine, the most common side effect is dry mouth. Another common side effect is constipation. Less common side effects include dizziness, fatigue, and blurred vision. Unlike tolterodine, fesoterodine has not been associated with QT prolongation and hence probably does not pose a risk for dysrhythmia.

Trospium

Trospium [Sanctura XR, Trosec ♣] is a nonselective muscarinic blocker indicated only for OAB. Like oxybutynin and tolterodine, trospium is available in short- and long-acting formulations. Anticholinergic side effects are less intense with the long-acting form. Compared with other drugs for OAB, trospium is notable for its low bioavailability, lack of CNS effects, and lack of metabolism-related interactions with other drugs.

Immediate-Release Tablets. Trospium IR tablets [Trosec] reduce episodes of urge incontinence from 27/week down to 12/week (compared with 30/week down to 16/week with placebo). Reductions in urinary frequency are minimal.

Trospium is a quaternary ammonium compound (always carries a positive charge), so it crosses membranes poorly. After oral dosing, absorption is poor (only 10%) on an empty stomach and is greatly reduced (70%–80%) by food. Plasma levels peak 3.5 to 6 hours after dosing and decline with a half-life of 18 hours. Trospium does not undergo hepatic metabolism and is eliminated unchanged in the urine.

Trospium IR tablets are generally well tolerated. The most common side effects are dry mouth and constipation. Rarely, the drug causes dry eyes and urinary retention. Owing to its positive charge, trospium cannot cross the blood-brain barrier and hence is devoid of CNS effects.

Few studies of drug interactions have been done. However, because trospium is eliminated by the kidneys, we can assume it may compete with other drugs that undergo renal tubular excretion. Among these are vancomycin (an antibiotic), metformin (used for diabetes), and digoxin and procainamide (both used for cardiac disorders). Because trospium is not metabolized, the drug is unlikely to influence hepatic metabolism of other agents.

Extended-Release Capsules. Trospium ER capsules [Sanctura XR ♣] are as effective as the IR tablets, and cause less dry mouth. The incidence of constipation and other side effects is about the same. Ethanol can increase the peak serum levels; therefore trospium ER should not be taken within 2 hours of consuming alcohol.

Other Muscarinic Antagonists

Scopolamine

Scopolamine is an anticholinergic drug with actions much like those of atropine, but with two exceptions. First, whereas therapeutic doses of atropine produce mild CNS excitation, therapeutic doses of scopolamine produce sedation. And second, scopolamine suppresses emesis and motion sickness, whereas atropine does not. Principal uses for scopolamine are motion sickness (see Chapter 64), production of cycloplegia and mydriasis for ophthalmic procedures (see Chapter 84), and production of preanesthetic sedation and obstetric amnesia.

Ipratropium Bromide

Ipratropium [Atrovent] is an anticholinergic drug used to treat asthma, COPD, and rhinitis caused by allergies or the common cold. The drug is administered by inhalation for asthma and COPD and by nasal spray for rhinitis. Systemic absorption is minimal for both formulations. As a result, therapy is not associated with typical antimuscarinic side effects (dry mouth, blurred vision, urinary hesitancy, constipation, and so forth). Ipratropium is discussed fully in Chapter 60.

Antisecretory Anticholinergics

Muscarinic blockers can be used to suppress gastric acid secretion in patients with peptic ulcer disease. However, because superior antiulcer drugs are available, and because anticholinergic agents produce significant side effects, most of these drugs have been withdrawn. Today, only four agents—glycopyrrolate [Robinul, Cuvposa], mepenzolate [Cantil], methscopolamine [Pamine], and propantheline [generic]—remain on the market. All four are administered orally, and one—glycopyrrolate—may also be given by IM or IV route. Glycopyrrolate oral solution [Cuvposa] is also approved for reducing severe drooling in children with chronic severe neurologic disorders. The drug is also approved for reducing salivation caused by anesthesia. Although it was originally approved as an adjunct in treatment of peptic ulcer disease, it is no longer indicated for this purpose.

Dicyclomine

Dicyclomine [Bentyl, Bentylol] is indicated for irritable bowel syndrome (spastic colon, mucous colitis) and functional bowel disorders (diarrhea, hypermotility). Administration may be oral (20–40 mg 4 times a day) or by IM injection (10–20 mg 4 times a day for 1–2 days followed by conversion to oral therapy).

Mydriatic Cycloplegics

Five muscarinic antagonists—atropine, homatropine, scopolamine, cyclopentolate, and tropicamide—are employed to produce mydriasis and cycloplegia in ophthalmic procedures. These applications are discussed in Chapter 84.

Centrally Acting Anticholinergics

Several anticholinergic drugs, including benztropine [Cogentin] and trihexyphenidyl, are used to treat Parkinson disease and drug-induced parkinsonism. Benefits derive from blockade of muscarinic receptors in the CNS. The centrally acting anticholinergics and their use in Parkinson disease are discussed in Chapter 17.

Patient Education

MUSCARINIC ANTAGONISTS (ANTICHOLINERGICS)

- Teach patients that dry mouth can be relieved by sipping fluids, chewing sugar-free gum, treating the mouth with a saliva substitute, and using an alcohol-free mouthwash. Owing to increased risk for tooth decay, advise patients to avoid sugared gum, hard candy, and cough drops.
- Because these drugs can cause blurred vision, advise patients to avoid hazardous activities if vision is impaired. Recommend wearing sunglasses to decrease discomfort due to glare and excessive light related to pupil dilation. Indoors, lights may need to be turned down.
- Advise patients that urinary retention can be minimized by voiding just before taking anticholinergic medication.
- Counsel patients that constipation can be reduced by increasing dietary fiber and fluids and can be treated with a laxative if severe. Reinforce the need for adequate fluids if fiber supplements are taken to avoid worsening constipation.
- Caution patients to avoid vigorous exercise in warm environments to prevent hyperthermia. Health related illness is a particular concern amount older patients taking anticholinergic drugs.

Toxicology of Muscarinic Antagonists

Sources of Antimuscarinic Poisoning

Sources of poisoning include natural products (e.g., *A. belladonna, D. stramonium*), selective antimuscarinic drugs (e.g., atropine, scopolamine), and other drugs with pronounced antimuscarinic properties (e.g., antihistamines, phenothiazines, tricyclic antidepressants).

Symptoms

Symptoms of antimuscarinic poisoning, which are the direct result of excessive muscarinic blockade, include dry mouth, blurred vision, photophobia secondary to mydriasis, hyperthermia, CNS effects (hallucinations, delirium), and skin that is hot, dry, and flushed. Death results from respiratory depression secondary to blockade of cholinergic receptors in the brain. (See Box 12.3 for a mnemonic to help you remember antimuscarinic poisoning.)

Treatment

Treatment consists of (1) minimizing intestinal absorption of the antimuscarinic agent and (2) administering an antidote. Minimizing absorption is accomplished by administering activated charcoal, which will adsorb the poison within the intestine, thereby preventing its absorption into the blood.

The most effective antidote to antimuscarinic poisoning is *physostigmine,* an inhibitor of acetylcholinesterase. By inhibiting cholinesterase, physostigmine causes acetylcholine to accumulate at all cholinergic junctions. As acetylcholine builds up, it competes with the antimuscarinic agent for receptor binding, thereby reversing excessive muscarinic blockade.

Warning

It is important to differentiate between antimuscarinic poisoning, which often resembles psychosis (hallucinations, delirium), and an actual psychotic episode. We need to make the differential diagnosis because some antipsychotic drugs have antimuscarinic properties of their own and hence will intensify symptoms if given to a victim of antimuscarinic poisoning. Fortunately, because a true psychotic episode is not ordinarily associated with signs of excessive muscarinic blockade (dry mouth, hyperthermia, dry skin, and so forth), differentiation is not usually difficult.

BOX 12.3 ▪ ANTIMUSCARINIC (ANTICHOLINERGIC) TOXICITY

A mnemonic is commonly used to remember the signs and symptoms of antimuscarinic (anticholinergic) toxicity.

Hot as a hare (hyperthermia)
Dry as a bone (dry eyes, dry mouth, dry skin)
Red as a beet (flushed face)
Blind as a bat (mydriasis)
Mad as a hatter (delirium)

Prescribing and Monitoring Considerations

Bethanechol

Assessment

Therapeutic Goal. Treatment of nonobstructive urinary retention.

Identifying High-Risk Patients

Bethanechol is *contraindicated* for patients with peptic ulcer disease, urinary tract obstruction, intestinal obstruction, coronary insufficiency, hypotension, asthma, and hyperthyroidism.

Administration Considerations

Nausea and vomiting may occur if taken with meals. Taking on an empty stomach is advised.

Ongoing Monitoring and Interventions

Minimizing Adverse Effects. Excessive muscarinic activation can cause salivation, sweating, urinary urgency, bradycardia, and hypotension. Monitor blood pressure and pulse rate. Observe for signs of muscarinic excess and treat or decrease dosage as indicated.

Management of Acute Toxicity. Overdose produces manifestations of excessive muscarinic stimulation (salivation, sweating, involuntary urination and defecation, bradycardia, severe hypotension). Treat with parenteral atropine and supportive measures.

Reversible Cholinesterase Inhibitors

Assessment

Therapeutic Goal. Cholinesterase inhibitors are used to treat myasthenia gravis, glaucoma, Alzheimer disease, Parkinson disease dementia, and poisoning by muscarinic antagonists and, in specialty areas, to reverse competitive (nondepolarizing) neuromuscular blockade. Applications of individual agents are shown in Table 12.7.

Baseline Data

MYASTHENIA GRAVIS. Determine the extent of neuromuscular dysfunction by assessing muscle strength, fatigue, ptosis, and ability to swallow.

TABLE 12.7 ▪ Clinical Applications of Cholinesterase Inhibitors

Generic Name [Trade Name]	Routes	Myasthenia Gravis: Diagnosis	Myasthenia Gravis: Treatment	Glaucoma	Reversal of Competitive Neuromuscular Blockade	Antidote to Poisoning by Muscarinic Antagonists	Alzheimer Disease
REVERSIBLE INHIBITORS							
Neostigmine [Prostigmin]	PO, IM, IV, subQ		✓		✓		
Pyridostigmine [Mestinon]	PO		✓				
Edrophonium [Enlon]	IM, IV	✓			✓		
Physostigmine [generic]	IM, IV					✓	
Donepezil [Aricept]*	PO						✓
Galantamine [Razadyne]	PO						✓
Rivastigmine [Exelon]*	PO, Transdermal						✓
IRREVERSIBLE INHIBITOR							
Echothiophate [Phospholine Iodide]	Topical			✓			

*Also used for Parkinson disease dementia.
IM, intramuscular; IV, intravenous; PO, oral; subQ, subcutaneous.

Identifying High-Risk Patients. Cholinesterase inhibitors are *contraindicated* for patients with mechanical obstruction of the intestine or urinary tract. Exercise *caution* in patients with peptic ulcer disease, bradycardia, asthma, or hyperthyroidism.

Administration and Dosage Considerations in Myasthenia Gravis. If swallowing is impaired, substitute a parenteral medication. Monitor for therapeutic responses and adjust the dosage accordingly.

Treating Muscarinic Antagonist Poisoning. Physostigmine is the drug of choice for this indication. The usual dose is 2 mg administered by IM or slow IV injection.

Measures to Enhance Therapeutic Effects

Myasthenia Gravis

PROMOTING COMPLIANCE. Inform patients that MG is not usually curable, so treatment is lifelong. Encourage patients to take their medication as prescribed and to play an active role in dosage adjustment.

USING IDENTIFICATION. Because patients with MG are at risk for fatal complications (cholinergic crisis, myasthenic crisis), encourage them to wear a Medic Alert bracelet or similar identification to inform emergency medical personnel of their condition.

Ongoing Monitoring and Interventions

Evaluating Therapeutic Effects

MYASTHENIA GRAVIS. Monitor and record (1) times of drug administration; (2) times at which fatigue occurs; (3) state of muscle strength, ptosis, and ability to swallow; and (4) signs of excessive muscarinic stimulation. Dosage is increased or decreased based on these observations.

Monitor for *myasthenic crisis* (extreme muscle weakness, paralysis of respiratory muscles), which can occur when cholinesterase inhibitor dosage is insufficient. Manage with respiratory support and increased dosage.

Be certain to distinguish myasthenic crisis from cholinergic crisis. This is done by observing for signs of excessive muscarinic stimulation, which will accompany cholinergic crisis but not myasthenic crisis.

Minimizing Adverse Effects

EXCESSIVE MUSCARINIC STIMULATION. Accumulation of acetylcholine at muscarinic receptors can cause profuse salivation, increased tone and motility of the gut, urinary urgency, sweating, miosis, spasm of accommodation, bronchoconstriction, and bradycardia. Excessive muscarinic responses can be managed with *atropine.*

CHOLINERGIC CRISIS. This condition results from cholinesterase inhibitor overdose. Manifestations are skeletal muscle paralysis (from depolarizing neuromuscular blockade) and signs of excessive muscarinic stimulation (e.g., salivation, sweating, miosis, bradycardia).

Manage with mechanical ventilation and atropine. Cholinergic crisis must be distinguished from myasthenic crisis.

Atropine and Other Muscarinic Antagonists (Anticholinergic Drugs)

Assessment

Therapeutic Goal. Atropine has many applications, including treatment of bradycardia, biliary colic, intestinal hypertonicity and hypermotility, and muscarinic agonist poisoning.

Identifying High-Risk Patients

Atropine and other muscarinic antagonists are *contraindicated* for patients with glaucoma, intestinal atony, urinary tract obstruction, and tachycardia. Use with *caution* in patients with asthma.

Administration Considerations

Dry mouth from muscarinic blockade may interfere with swallowing. Advise patients to moisten the mouth by sipping water before oral administration.

Ongoing Monitoring and Interventions

Minimizing Adverse Effects

XEROSTOMIA (DRY MOUTH). Decreased salivation can dry the mouth. Common interventions such as sipping fluids frequently, chewing gum, and sucking on hard candies will usually alleviate symptoms. Saliva substitutes are available for severe cases.

BLURRED VISION. Paralysis of the ciliary muscle may reduce visual acuity. Patients should not participate in activities such as driving where good vision is necessary.

PHOTOPHOBIA. Muscarinic blockade prevents the pupil from constricting in response to bright light. Keep room lighting low to reduce visual discomfort. Sunglasses are often required.

URINARY RETENTION. Muscarinic blockade in the urinary tract can cause urinary hesitancy or retention If urinary retention is severe, catheterization or treatment with bethanechol (a muscarinic agonist) may be required. Keep in mind, however, that a muscarinic agonist will also counteract positive effects of anticholinergics.

CONSTIPATION. Reduced tone and motility of the gut may cause constipation. Increasing fluids, fiber, and activity will be helpful.

HYPERTHERMIA. Suppression of sweating may result in hyperthermia.

TACHYCARDIA. Blockade of cardiac muscarinic receptors can accelerate heart rate. Monitor pulse and report significant increases.

Minimizing Adverse Interactions. Antihistamines, tricyclic antidepressants, and *phenothiazines* have prominent antimuscarinic actions. Combining these agents with atropine and other anticholinergic drugs can cause excessive muscarinic blockade.

Management of Acute Toxicity

Symptoms. Overdose produces dry mouth, blurred vision, photophobia, hyperthermia, hallucinations, and delirium; the skin becomes hot, dry, and flushed. Differentiate muscarinic antagonist poisoning from psychosis!

Treatment. Treatment centers on limiting absorption of ingested poison (e.g., by giving activated charcoal to adsorb the drug) and administering physostigmine, an inhibitor of acetylcholinesterase.

CHAPTER

13 Adrenergic Agonists

Jacqueline Rosenjack Burchum, DNSc, FNP-BC, CNE

Adrenergic agonists produce their effects by activating adrenergic receptors. Because the sympathetic nervous system acts through these same receptors, responses to adrenergic agonists and responses to stimulation of the sympathetic nervous system are very similar. Because of this similarity, adrenergic agonists are often referred to as *sympathomimetics.* Adrenergic agonists have a broad spectrum of indications, ranging from heart failure to asthma to preterm labor.

Learning about adrenergic agonists can be a challenge. To facilitate the process, our approach to these drugs has four stages. We begin with the general mechanisms by which drugs can activate adrenergic receptors. Next we establish an overview of the major adrenergic agonists, focusing on their receptor specificity and chemical classification. After that, we address the adrenergic receptors themselves; for each receptor type—$alpha_1$, $alpha_2$, $beta_1$, $beta_2$, and dopamine—we discuss the beneficial and harmful effects that can result from receptor activation. Finally, we integrate all of this information by discussing the characteristic properties of representative sympathomimetic drugs.

This chapter is intended only as an *introduction* to the adrenergic agonists. Our objective is to discuss the basic properties of the sympathomimetic drugs and establish an overview of their applications and adverse effects. In later chapters, we will discuss the clinical applications of these agents in greater depth.

MECHANISMS OF ADRENERGIC RECEPTOR ACTIVATION

Drugs can activate adrenergic receptors by four basic mechanisms: (1) direct receptor binding, (2) promotion of norepinephrine (NE) release, (3) blockade of NE reuptake, and (4) inhibition of NE inactivation. Note that only the first mechanism is *direct.* With the other three mechanisms, receptor activation occurs by an *indirect* process. Examples of drugs that act by these four mechanisms are presented in Table 13.1.

Direct Receptor Binding

Direct interaction with receptors is the most common mechanism by which drugs activate peripheral adrenergic receptors. The direct-acting receptor stimulants produce their effects by binding to adrenergic receptors and mimicking the actions of natural transmitters (NE, epinephrine, dopamine). All of the drugs discussed in this chapter activate receptors directly.

Promotion of Norepinephrine Release

By acting on terminals of sympathetic nerves to cause NE release, drugs can bring about indirect activation of adrenergic receptors. Agents that act by this mechanism include amphetamines and ephedrine. (Ephedrine can also activate adrenergic receptors directly.)

Inhibition of Norepinephrine Reuptake

Recall that reuptake of NE into terminals of sympathetic nerves is the major mechanism for terminating adrenergic transmission. By blocking NE reuptake, drugs can cause NE to accumulate within the synaptic gap and can thereby increase receptor activation. Agents that act by this mechanism include cocaine and the tricyclic antidepressants.

Inhibition of Norepinephrine Inactivation

As discussed in Chapter 11, some of the NE in terminals of adrenergic neurons is subject to inactivation by monoamine oxidase (MAO). Hence drugs that inhibit MAO can increase the amount of NE available for release and enhance receptor activation. (In addition to being present in sympathetic nerves, MAO is present in the liver and the intestinal wall. The significance of MAO at these other sites is considered later.)

In this chapter, which focuses on *peripherally* acting sympathomimetics, nearly all of the drugs discussed act exclusively by *direct* receptor activation. The only exception is *ephedrine,* a drug that works by a combination of direct receptor activation and promotion of NE release.

Most of the indirect-acting adrenergic agonists are used for their ability to activate adrenergic receptors in the central nervous system (CNS)—not for their effects in the periphery. The indirect-acting sympathomimetics (e.g., amphetamine, cocaine) are mentioned here to emphasize that, although these agents are employed for effects on the brain, they can and will cause activation of adrenergic receptors in the periphery. Peripheral activation is responsible for certain toxicities of these drugs (e.g., cardiac dysrhythmias, hypertension).

OVERVIEW OF THE ADRENERGIC AGONISTS

Chemical Classification: Catecholamines Versus Noncatecholamines

The adrenergic agonists fall into two major chemical classes: catecholamines and noncatecholamines. The catecholamines and noncatecholamines differ in three important respects: (1) availability for oral use, (2) duration of action, and (3) ability to act in the CNS. Accordingly, if we know to which category a particular adrenergic agonist belongs, we will know three of its prominent features.

TABLE 13.1 ▪ Mechanisms of Adrenergic Receptor Activation

Mechanism of Stimulation	Examples
DIRECT MECHANISM	
Receptor activation through direct binding	Dopamine Epinephrine Isoproterenol Ephedrine*
INDIRECT MECHANISMS	
Promotion of NE release	Amphetamine Ephedrine*
Inhibition of NE reuptake	Cocaine Tricyclic antidepressants
Inhibition of MAO	MAO inhibitors

*Ephedrine is a mixed-acting drug that activates receptors directly and by promoting release of norephinephrine.
MAO, monoamine oxidase; NE, norepinephrine.

Catecholamines

The catecholamines are so named because they contain a *catechol* group and an *amine* group. A catechol group is simply a benzene ring that has hydroxyl groups on two adjacent carbons. The amine component of the catecholamines is *ethylamine.* Structural formulas for each of the major catecholamines—epinephrine, NE, isoproterenol, dopamine, and dobutamine—are shown in Fig. 13.1. Because of their chemistry, all catecholamines have three properties in common: (1) they cannot be used orally, (2) they have a brief duration of action, and (3) they cannot cross the blood-brain barrier.

The actions of two enzymes—*monoamine oxidase* and *catechol-*O*-methyltransferase* (COMT)—explain why the catecholamines have short half-lives and cannot be used orally. MAO and COMT are located in the liver and in the intestinal wall. Both enzymes are very active and quickly destroy catecholamines administered by any route. Because these enzymes are located in the liver and intestinal wall, catecholamines that are administered orally become inactivated before they can reach the systemic circulation. Hence catecholamines are ineffective if given by mouth. Because of rapid inactivation by MAO and COMT, three catecholamines—NE, dopamine, and dobutamine—are effective only if administered by continuous infusion. Administration by other parenteral routes (e.g., subcutaneously, intramuscularly) will not yield adequate blood levels, owing to rapid hepatic inactivation.

Catecholamines are polar molecules, so they cannot cross the blood-brain barrier. (Recall from Chapter 4 that polar compounds penetrate membranes poorly.) The polar nature of the catecholamines is due to the hydroxyl groups on the catechol portion of the molecule. Because they cannot cross the blood-brain barrier, catecholamines have minimal effects on the CNS.

Be aware that catecholamine-containing solutions, which are colorless when first prepared, turn pink or brown over time. This pigmentation is caused by oxidation of the catecholamine molecule. *Catecholamine solutions should be discarded as soon as discoloration develops.* The only exception is dobutamine, which can be used up to 24 hours after the solution was made, even if discoloration appears.

Noncatecholamines

The noncatecholamines have ethylamine in their structure (see Fig. 13.1), but do not contain the catechol moiety that characterizes the catecholamines. Here we discuss three noncatecholamines: ephedrine, albuterol, and phenylephrine.

The noncatecholamines differ from the catecholamines in three important respects. First, because they lack a catechol group, noncatecholamines are not substrates for COMT and are metabolized slowly by MAO. As a result, the half-lives of noncatecholamines are much longer than those of catecholamines. Second, because they do not undergo rapid degradation by MAO and COMT, noncatecholamines can be given orally, whereas catecholamines cannot. Third, noncatecholamines are considerably less polar than catecholamines and hence are more able to cross the blood-brain barrier.

Receptor Specificity

To understand the actions of individual adrenergic agonists, we need to know their receptor specificity. Variability in receptor specificity among the adrenergic agonists can be illustrated with three drugs: albuterol, isoproterenol, and epinephrine. Albuterol is highly selective, acting at $beta_2$ receptors only. Isoproterenol is less selective, acting at $beta_1$ receptors and $beta_2$ receptors. Epinephrine is even less selective, acting at all four adrenergic receptor subtypes: $alpha_1$, $alpha_2$, $beta_1$, and $beta_2$.

The receptor specificities of the major adrenergic agonists are shown in Table 13.2. In the upper part of the table, receptor specificity is presented in tabular form. In the lower part, the same information is presented schematically. By learning this content, you will be well on your way to understanding the pharmacology of the sympathomimetic drugs.

Note that the concept of receptor specificity is relative, not absolute. The ability of a drug to selectively activate certain receptors to the exclusion of others depends on the dosage: at low doses, selectivity is maximal; as dosage increases, selectivity declines. For example, when albuterol is administered in low to moderate doses, the drug is highly selective for $beta_2$-adrenergic receptors. However, if the dosage is high, albuterol will activate $beta_1$ receptors as well. The information on receptor specificity in Table 13.2 refers to usual therapeutic doses. So-called selective agents will activate additional adrenergic receptors if the dosage is abnormally high.

THERAPEUTIC APPLICATIONS AND ADVERSE EFFECTS OF ADRENERGIC RECEPTOR ACTIVATION

In this section we discuss the responses—both therapeutic and adverse—that can be elicited with sympathomimetic drugs. Because many adrenergic agonists activate more than one type of receptor (see Table 13.2), it could be quite confusing if we were to talk about the effects of the sympathomimetics while employing specific drugs as examples. Consequently, rather than attempting to structure this presentation around representative drugs, we discuss the actions of the adrenergic agonists one receptor at a time. Our discussion begins with

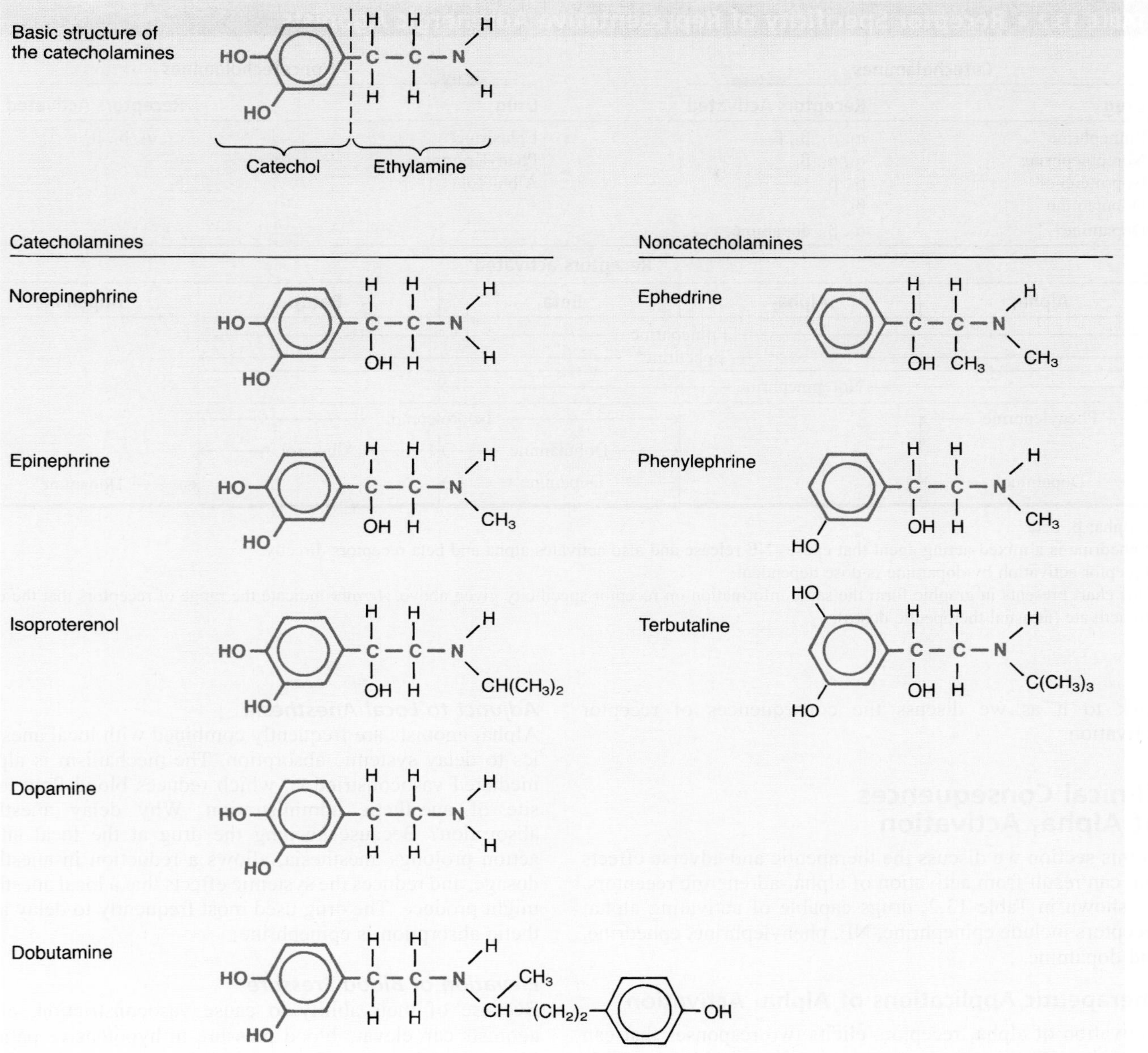

Figure 13.1 ■ Structures of representative catecholamines and noncatecholamines. *Catecholamines:* All of the catecholamines share the same basic chemical formula. Because of their biochemical properties, the catecholamines cannot be used orally, cannot cross the blood-brain barrier, and have short half-lives (owing to rapid inactivation by monoamine oxidase [MAO] and catechol-*O*-methyltransferase [COMT]). *Noncatecholamines:* Although structurally similar to catecholamines, noncatecholamines differ from catecholamines in three important ways: they can be used orally; they can cross the blood-brain barrier; and, because they are not rapidly metabolized by MAO or COMT, they have much longer half-lives.

alpha$_1$ receptors, and then moves to alpha$_2$ receptors, beta$_1$ receptors, beta$_2$ receptors, and finally dopamine receptors. For each receptor type, we discuss both the therapeutic and adverse responses that can result from receptor activation.

To understand the effects of any specific adrenergic agonist, all you need are two types of information: (1) the identity of the receptors at which the drug acts and (2) the effects produced by activating those receptors. Combining these two types of information will reveal a profile of drug action. This is the same approach to understanding neuropharmacologic agents that we discussed in Chapter 10.

Before you continue, I encourage you to review Table 11.3 in Chapter 11. We are about to discuss the clinical consequences of adrenergic receptor activation, and Table 11.3 shows the responses to activation of those receptors. If you choose not to memorize Table 11.3 now, be prepared to refer

TABLE 13.2 ▪ Receptor Specificity of Representative Adrenergic Agonists

Catecholamines		Noncatecholamines	
Drug	**Receptors Activated**	**Drug**	**Receptors Activated**
Epinephrine	α_1, α_2, β_1, β_2	Ephedrine*	α_1, α_2, β_1, β_2
Norepinephrine	α_1, α_2, β_1	Phenylephrine	α_1
Isoproterenol	β_1, β_2	Albuterol	β_2
Dobutamine	β_1		
Dopamine†	α_1, β_1, dopamine		

Receptors activated‡

Alpha$_1$	Alpha$_2$	Beta$_1$	Beta$_2$	Dopamine
←	Epinephrine		→	
←	Ephedrine*		→	
←	Norepinephrine	→		
← Phenylephrine →		←	Isoproterenol →	
		← Dobutamine →	← Albuterol →	
← Dopamine† →		← Dopamine† →		← Dopamine† →

α, alpha; β, beta.

*Ephedrine is a mixed-acting agent that causes NE release and also activates alpha and beta receptors directly.

†Receptor activation by dopamine is dose dependent.

‡This chart presents in graphic form the same information on receptor specificity given above. *Arrows* indicate the range of receptors that the drugs can activate (at usual therapeutic doses).

back to it as we discuss the consequences of receptor activation.

Clinical Consequences of Alpha$_1$ Activation

In this section we discuss the therapeutic and adverse effects that can result from activation of alpha$_1$-adrenergic receptors. As shown in Table 13.2, drugs capable of activating alpha$_1$ receptors include epinephrine, NE, phenylephrine, ephedrine, and dopamine.

Therapeutic Applications of Alpha$_1$ Activation

Activation of alpha$_1$ receptors elicits two responses that can be of therapeutic use: (1) *vasoconstriction* (in blood vessels of the skin, viscera, and mucous membranes); and (2) *mydriasis.* Of the two, vasoconstriction is the one for which alpha$_1$ agonists are used most often. Using these drugs for mydriasis is rare.

Hemostasis

Hemostasis is defined as the arrest of bleeding, which alpha$_1$ agonists support through vasoconstriction. Alpha$_1$ agonists are given to stop bleeding primarily in the skin and mucous membranes. Epinephrine, applied topically, is the alpha$_1$ agonist used most for this purpose.

Nasal Decongestion

Nasal congestion results from dilation and engorgement of blood vessels in the nasal mucosa. Drugs can relieve congestion by causing alpha$_1$-mediated vasoconstriction. Specific alpha$_1$-activating agents employed as nasal decongestants include phenylephrine (administered topically) and pseudoephedrine (administered orally).

Adjunct to Local Anesthesia

Alpha$_1$ agonists are frequently combined with local anesthetics to delay systemic absorption. The mechanism is alpha$_1$-mediated vasoconstriction, which reduces blood flow to the site of anesthetic administration. Why delay anesthetic absorption? Because keeping the drug at the local site of action prolongs anesthesia, allows a reduction in anesthetic dosage, and reduces the systemic effects that a local anesthetic might produce. The drug used most frequently to delay anesthetic absorption is epinephrine.

Elevation of Blood Pressure

Because of their ability to cause vasoconstriction, alpha$_1$ agonists can elevate blood pressure in hypotensive patients. Please note, however, that alpha$_1$ agonists are not the primary therapy for hypotension. Rather, they are reserved for situations in which fluid replacement and other measures either are contraindicated or have failed to restore blood pressure to a satisfactory level.

Mydriasis

Activation of alpha$_1$ receptors on the radial muscle of the iris causes mydriasis (dilation of the pupil), which can facilitate eye examinations and ocular surgery. Note that producing mydriasis is the only clinical use of alpha$_1$ activation that is not based on vasoconstriction.

Adverse Effects of Alpha$_1$ Activation

All of the adverse effects caused by alpha$_1$ activation result directly or indirectly from vasoconstriction.

Hypertension

Alpha$_1$ agonists can produce hypertension by causing widespread vasoconstriction. Severe hypertension is most likely with parenteral dosing. Accordingly, when alpha$_1$ agonists are given intravenously, the patient's cardiac rhythm must be monitored continuously, and other indicators of cardiovascular status and perfusion (e.g., blood pressure, peripheral pulses, urine output) should be assessed frequently.

Necrosis

If the IV line used to administer an alpha$_1$ agonist becomes extravasated, seepage of the drug into the surrounding tissues may result in necrosis (tissue death). The cause is lack of blood flow to the affected area secondary to intense local vasoconstriction. If extravasation occurs, the area should be infiltrated with an alpha$_1$-blocking agent (e.g., phentolamine), which will counteract alpha$_1$-mediated vasoconstriction and thereby help minimize injury.

Bradycardia

Alpha$_1$ agonists can cause reflex slowing of the heart. The mechanism is this: alpha$_1$-mediated vasoconstriction elevates blood pressure, which triggers the baroreceptor reflex, causing heart rate to decline. In patients with marginal cardiac reserve, the decrease in cardiac output may compromise tissue perfusion.

Clinical Consequences of Alpha$_2$ Activation

Alpha$_2$ receptors in the periphery are located *presynaptically,* and their activation inhibits NE release. Several adrenergic agonists (e.g., epinephrine, NE) are capable of causing alpha$_2$ activation. However, their ability to activate alpha$_2$ receptors in the periphery has little clinical significance because there are no therapeutic applications related to activation of peripheral alpha$_2$ receptors. Furthermore, activation of these receptors rarely causes significant adverse effects.

In contrast to alpha$_2$ receptors in the *periphery,* alpha$_2$ receptors in the *CNS* are of great clinical significance. By activating central alpha$_2$ receptors, we can produce two useful effects: (1) *reduction* of sympathetic outflow to the heart and blood vessels and (2) relief of severe pain. The central alpha$_2$ agonists used for effects on the heart and blood vessels, and the agents used to relieve pain, are discussed in Chapters 15 and 22, respectively.

Clinical Consequences of Beta$_1$ Activation

All of the clinically relevant responses to activation of beta$_1$ receptors result from activating beta$_1$ receptors in the *heart;* activation of renal beta$_1$ receptors is not associated with either beneficial or adverse effects. As indicated in Table 13.2, beta$_1$ receptors can be activated by epinephrine, NE, isoproterenol, dopamine, dobutamine, and ephedrine.

Therapeutic Applications of Beta$_1$ Activation

Heart Failure

Heart failure is characterized by a reduction in the force of myocardial contraction, resulting in insufficient cardiac output. Because activation of beta$_1$ receptors in the heart has a positive inotropic effect (i.e., increases the force of contraction), drugs that activate these receptors can improve cardiac performance.

Shock

This condition is characterized by profound hypotension and greatly reduced tissue perfusion. The primary goal of treatment is to maintain blood flow to vital organs. By increasing heart rate and force of contraction, beta$_1$ stimulants can increase cardiac output and can thereby improve tissue perfusion.

Atrioventricular Heart Block

Atrioventricular (AV) heart block is a condition in which impulse conduction from the atria to the ventricles is either impeded or blocked entirely. As a consequence, the ventricles are no longer driven at an appropriate rate. Because activation of cardiac beta$_1$ receptors can enhance impulse conduction through the AV node, beta$_1$ stimulants can help overcome AV block. It should be noted, however, that drugs are only a temporary form of treatment. For long-term management, a pacemaker is implanted.

Cardiac Arrest

By activating cardiac beta$_1$ receptors, drugs have a role in initiating contraction in asystole or pulseless ventricular rhythms. It should be noted, however, that drugs are not the preferred treatment. Initial management focuses on cardiopulmonary resuscitation, external pacing, or defibrillation (whichever is applicable), and identification and treatment of the underlying cause (e.g., hypoxia, severe acidosis, drug overdose). When a beta$_1$ agonist *is* indicated, epinephrine, administered intravenously, is the preferred drug. If IV access is not possible, epinephrine can be injected directly into the heart or endotracheally.

Adverse Effects of Beta$_1$ Activation

All of the adverse effects of beta$_1$ activation result from activating beta$_1$ receptors in the heart. Activating renal beta$_1$ receptors is not associated with untoward effects.

Altered Heart Rate or Rhythm

Overstimulation of cardiac beta$_1$ receptors can produce *tachycardia* (excessive heart rate) and *dysrhythmias* (irregular heartbeat).

Angina Pectoris

In some patients, drugs that activate beta$_1$ receptors can precipitate an attack of angina pectoris, a condition characterized by substernal pain in the region of the heart. Anginal pain occurs when cardiac oxygen supply (blood flow) is insufficient to meet cardiac oxygen needs. The most common cause of angina is coronary atherosclerosis (accumulation of lipids and other substances in coronary arteries). Because beta$_1$ agonists increase cardiac oxygen demand (by increasing heart rate and force of contraction), patients with compromised coronary circulation are at risk for an anginal attack.

Clinical Consequences of Beta$_2$ Activation

Applications of beta$_2$ activation are limited to the *lungs* and the *uterus.* Drugs used for their beta$_2$-activating ability include epinephrine, isoproterenol, and albuterol.

Therapeutic Applications of Beta$_2$ Activation

Asthma

Asthma is a chronic condition characterized by inflammation and bronchoconstriction occurring in response to a variety of stimuli. During a severe attack, the airflow reduction can be life threatening. Because drugs that activate $beta_2$ receptors in the lungs promote bronchodilation, these drugs can help relieve or prevent asthma attacks.

For therapy of asthma, adrenergic agonists that are *selective for $beta_2$ receptors* (e.g., albuterol) are preferred to less selective agents (e.g., isoproterenol). This is especially true for patients who also suffer from *angina pectoris* or *tachycardia* because drugs that can activate $beta_1$ receptors would aggravate these cardiac disorders.

Most $beta_2$ agonists used to treat asthma are administered by *inhalation.* This route is desirable in that it helps minimize adverse systemic effects. It should be noted, however, that inhalation does not guarantee safety: Serious systemic toxicity can result from overdosing with inhaled sympathomimetics, so patients must be warned against inhaling too much drug.

Delay of Preterm Labor

Activation of $beta_2$ receptors in the uterus relaxes uterine smooth muscle. This action can be employed to delay preterm labor.

Adverse Effects of $Beta_2$ Activation

Hyperglycemia

The most important adverse response to $beta_2$ activation is hyperglycemia (elevation of blood glucose). The mechanism is activation of $beta_2$ receptors in the liver and skeletal muscles, which promotes breakdown of glycogen into glucose. As a rule, $beta_2$ agonists cause hyperglycemia only in patients with *diabetes;* in patients with normal pancreatic function, insulin release will maintain blood glucose at an appropriate level. If hyperglycemia develops in the patient with diabetes, medications used for glucose control will need to be adjusted.

Tremor

Tremor is the most common side effect of $beta_2$ agonists. It occurs because activation of $beta_2$ receptors in skeletal muscle enhances contraction. This effect can be confounding for patients with diabetes because tremor is a common symptom of hypoglycemia; however, when due to $beta_2$ activation, it may be accompanied by hyperglycemia. Fortunately, the tremor generally fades over time and can be minimized by initiating therapy at low doses.

Clinical Consequences of Dopamine Receptor Activation

Activation of peripheral dopamine receptors causes dilation of the renal vasculature. This effect is employed in the treatment of *shock:* by dilating renal blood vessels, we can improve renal perfusion and can thereby reduce the risk for renal failure. *Dopamine* is the only drug available that can activate dopamine receptors. It should be noted that, when dopamine is given to treat shock, the drug also enhances cardiac performance because it activates $beta_1$ receptors in the heart.

Multiple Receptor Activation: Treatment of Anaphylactic Shock

Pathophysiology of Anaphylaxis

Anaphylactic shock is a manifestation of severe allergy. The reaction is characterized by *hypotension* (from widespread vasodilation), *bronchoconstriction,* and *edema of the glottis.* Although histamine contributes to these responses, symptoms are due largely to release of other mediators (e.g., leukotrienes). Anaphylaxis can be triggered by a variety of substances, including bee venom, wasp venom, latex rubber, certain foods (e.g., peanuts, shellfish), and certain drugs (e.g., penicillins).

Treatment

Epinephrine, injected intramuscularly or intravenously, is the treatment of choice for anaphylactic shock. Benefits derive from activating three types of adrenergic receptors: $alpha_1$, $beta_1$, and $beta_2$. By activating these receptors, epinephrine can reverse the most severe manifestations of the anaphylactic reaction. Activation of $beta_1$ receptors increases cardiac output, helping elevate blood pressure. Blood pressure is also increased because epinephrine promotes $alpha_1$-mediated vasoconstriction. In addition to increasing blood pressure, vasoconstriction helps suppress glottal edema. By activating $beta_2$ receptors, epinephrine can counteract bronchoconstriction. Individuals who are prone to severe allergic responses should carry an epinephrine autoinjector (e.g., EpiPen) at all times. Antihistamines are not especially useful against anaphylaxis because histamine is only one of several contributors to the reaction.

PROPERTIES OF REPRESENTATIVE ADRENERGIC AGONISTS

Our aim in this section is to establish an overview of the adrenergic agonists. The information is presented in the form of "drug digests" that highlight characteristic features of representative sympathomimetic agents. Some of these drugs are used in specialty areas; however, the choices of representative drugs will increase understanding of adrenergic receptor activation. This knowledge will be helpful for later chapters.

As noted, there are two keys to understanding individual adrenergic agonists: (1) knowledge of the receptors that the drug can activate and (2) knowledge of the therapeutic and adverse effects that receptor activation can elicit. By integrating these two types of information, you can easily predict the spectrum of effects that a particular drug can produce.

Unfortunately, knowing the effects that a drug is *capable* of producing does not always indicate how that drug is *actually used* in a clinical setting. Safer alternatives are often available. For example, NE can activate $alpha_1$ receptors and can therefore produce mydriasis, but safer drugs are available for this purpose. Similarly, although isoproterenol is capable of producing uterine relaxation through $beta_2$ activation, it is no longer used for this purpose because safer drugs are available. Because receptor specificity is not always a predictor of the therapeutic applications of a particular adrenergic agonist, for each of the drugs discussed next, approved clinical applications are indicated.

Epinephrine

- *Receptor specificity:* $alpha_1$, $alpha_2$, $beta_1$, $beta_2$
- *Chemical classification:* catecholamine

Epinephrine [Adrenalin, others] was among the first adrenergic agonists employed clinically and can be considered the prototype of the sympathomimetic drugs. Because of its prototypic status, epinephrine is discussed in detail.

Therapeutic Uses

Epinephrine can activate all four subtypes of adrenergic receptors. As a consequence, the drug can produce a broad spectrum of beneficial sympathomimetic effects:

- Because it can cause $alpha_1$-mediated vasoconstriction, epinephrine is used to (1) delay absorption of local anesthetics, (2) control superficial bleeding, and (3) elevate blood pressure.
- Because it can activate $beta_1$ receptors, epinephrine may be used to (1) overcome AV heart block and (2) restore cardiac function in patients in cardiac arrest experiencing ventricular fibrillation, pulseless ventricular tachycardia, pulseless electrical activity, or asystole.
- Activation of $beta_2$ receptors in the lung promotes bronchodilation, which can be useful in patients with asthma (although epinephrine is not the drug of choice for this purpose).
- Because it can activate a combination of alpha and beta receptors, epinephrine is the treatment of choice for anaphylactic shock.

Pharmacokinetics

Absorption

Epinephrine may be administered topically or by injection. The drug cannot be given orally because epinephrine and other catecholamines undergo destruction by MAO and COMT before reaching the systemic circulation. After subcutaneous injection, absorption is slow owing to epinephrine-induced local vasoconstriction. Absorption is more rapid after intramuscular injection and is immediate with IV administration.

Inactivation

Epinephrine has a short half-life because of two processes: enzymatic inactivation and uptake into adrenergic nerves. The enzymes that inactivate epinephrine and other catecholamines are MAO and COMT.

Adverse Effects

Because it can activate the four major adrenergic receptor subtypes, epinephrine can produce multiple adverse effects.

Hypertensive Crisis

Vasoconstriction secondary to excessive $alpha_1$ activation can produce a dramatic increase in blood pressure. Cerebral hemorrhage can occur. Because of the potential for severe hypertension, patients receiving *parenteral* epinephrine must undergo continuous cardiovascular monitoring with frequent assessment of vital signs.

Dysrhythmias

Excessive activation of $beta_1$ receptors in the heart can produce dysrhythmias. Because of their sensitivity to catecholamines, hyperthyroid patients are at high risk for epinephrine-induced dysrhythmias.

Angina Pectoris

By activating $beta_1$ receptors in the heart, epinephrine can increase cardiac work and oxygen demand. If the increase in oxygen demand is significant, an anginal attack may ensue. Provocation of angina is especially likely in patients with coronary atherosclerosis.

Post-Extravasation Necrosis

If an IV line containing epinephrine becomes extravasated, the ensuing localized vasoconstriction may result in necrosis. Because of this possibility, the IV site should be monitored closely. If extravasation occurs, injury can be minimized by local injection of phentolamine, an alpha-adrenergic antagonist.

Hyperglycemia

In patients with diabetes, epinephrine can cause hyperglycemia. How? By causing breakdown of glycogen secondary to activation of $beta_2$ receptors in liver and skeletal muscle. If hyperglycemia develops, dosage adjustments will need to be made for medications used to manage diabetes.

Drug Interactions

MAO Inhibitors

As their name implies, MAO inhibitors suppress the activity of MAO. These drugs are used primarily to treat depression (see Chapter 25). Because MAO is one of the enzymes that inactivate epinephrine and other catecholamines, inhibition of MAO will prolong and intensify epinephrine's effects. In most situations, patients receiving an MAO inhibitor should not receive epinephrine.

Tricyclic Antidepressants

Tricyclic antidepressants block the uptake of catecholamines into adrenergic neurons. Because neuronal uptake is one mechanism by which the actions of NE and other catecholamines are terminated, blocking uptake can intensify and prolong epinephrine's effects. Accordingly, patients receiving a tricyclic antidepressant may require a reduction in epinephrine dosage.

General Anesthetics

Several inhalation anesthetics render the myocardium hypersensitive to activation by $beta_1$ agonists. When the heart is in this hypersensitive state, exposure to epinephrine and other $beta_1$ agonists can cause tachydysrhythmias.

Alpha-Adrenergic Blocking Agents

Drugs that block alpha-adrenergic receptors can prevent alpha-adrenergic receptor activation by epinephrine. Alpha blockers (e.g., phentolamine) can be used to treat toxicity (e.g., hypertension, local vasoconstriction) caused by excessive epinephrine-induced alpha activation.

Beta-Adrenergic Blocking Agents

Drugs that block beta-adrenergic receptors can prevent beta-adrenergic receptor activation by epinephrine. Beta-blocking agents (e.g., metoprolol) can reduce adverse effects (e.g., dysrhythmias, anginal pain) caused by epinephrine and other $beta_1$ agonists.

Treatment of anaphylaxis using an epinephrine autoinjector is discussed in Box 13.1.

Norepinephrine

- *Receptor specificity:* $alpha_1$, $alpha_2$, $beta_1$
- *Chemical classification:* catecholamine

BOX 13.1 ▪ THE EPIPEN: DON'T LEAVE HOME WITHOUT IT!

The EpiPen is an epinephrine autoinjector, one of three brands available in the United States.* It is indicated for emergency treatment of anaphylaxis, a life-threatening allergic reaction caused by severe hypersensitivity to insect venoms (e.g., from bees), certain foods (e.g., peanuts, shellfish), and certain drugs (especially penicillins). Every year, anaphylaxis kills about 6000 Americans: 125 who have food allergies, between 40 and 400 who have venom allergies, and more than 5400 who have penicillin allergy. Could most of these deaths be avoided? Yes—through immediate injection of epinephrine. Unfortunately, many of the people at risk don't carry an epinephrine injector, and many of those who do aren't sure how to use it. By encouraging highly allergic patients to carry an EpiPen, and by teaching them when and how to use it, you could well save someone's life.

EpiPen Description and Dosage

The EpiPen autoinjector is a single-use delivery device, featuring a spring-activated needle, designed for intramuscular injection of epinephrine. Two strengths are available. The larger one, sold as EpiPen, delivers a 0.3-mg dose (for individuals weighing 66 pounds or more). The smaller one, sold as EpiPen Jr, delivers a 0.15-mg dose (for individuals between 33 and 66 pounds). If one injection fails to completely reverse symptoms, a second injection (using a second EpiPen) may be given. The EpiPen is available only by prescription.

EpiPen Storage and Replacement

Epinephrine is sensitive to extreme heat and light, so the EpiPen should be stored at room temperature in a dark place. This is not to infer that the device should be left in this environment until needed; when the patient will be in an area where an encounter with an antigen is possible, it is essential to take the EpiPen along. The factory-issue storage tube provides additional protection from ultraviolet light. Refrigeration can compromise the injection mechanism and should be avoided. If the epinephrine solution turns brown, if a precipitate forms, or if the expiration date has passed, the unit should be replaced. (The distributor offers a free service to remind patients when their EpiPen is about to expire.)

Who Should Carry an EpiPen and When Should They Use It?

Anyone who has experienced a severe, systemic allergic reaction should *always* carry at least one epinephrine autoinjector. Anaphylaxis can develop within minutes of allergen exposure. To prevent a full-blown reaction, epinephrine should be injected as soon as early symptoms appear (e.g., swelling, shortness of breath). People who do not carry an EpiPen, and hence must wait for an emergency response team, greatly increase their risk for death.

What's the Self-Injection Procedure?

The EpiPen autoinjector is a tubular device with three prominent external features: a black tip (the needle comes out through this end), a clear window (for examining the epinephrine solution), and a gray cap (which prevents activation until being removed).

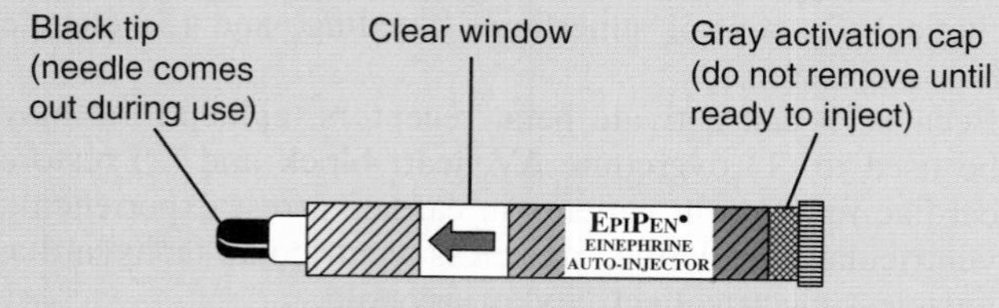

Injections are made into the outer thigh as follows:

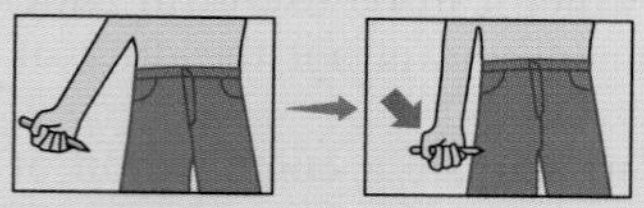

1. Form a fist around the unit with the black tip pointing down.
2. With the free hand, pull off the gray activation cap.
3. Jab the device firmly into the outer thigh, at an angle perpendicular to the thigh, and hold it there for 10 seconds. (The injection may be made directly through clothing.)
4. Remove the unit and massage the area for 10 seconds to facilitate absorption.

To ensure the injection was made, examine the used EpiPen: if the needle is projecting through the black tip, the procedure was a success; if the needle is not projecting, jab the device in again. *Note:* The EpiPen contains 2 mL of epinephrine solution, but only 0.3 mL is actually injected. Hence, even after a successful injection, the device will not be empty.

What Should Be Done After the Injection?

After epinephrine injection, it is important to get immediate medical attention. The effects of epinephrine begin to fade in 10 to 20 minutes, and anaphylactic reactions can be biphasic and prolonged. To ensure a good outcome, hospitalization (up to 6 hours) is recommended. Hospital staff should be informed that epinephrine has been injected and should be shown the used EpiPen (to confirm the dosage). A systemic glucocorticoid may be given to manage delayed or persistent symptoms.

Does Intramuscular Epinephrine Have Side Effects?

Yes. The injection itself may cause discomfort, and the epinephrine may cause tachycardia, palpitations, and a feeling of nervousness. It may also cause sweating, dizziness, headache, nausea, and vomiting.

*In addition to the EpiPen, two other epinephrine auto-injectors—*Adrenaclick* and *Twinject*—are available. The Adrenaclick injector is nearly identical to the EpiPen. Twinject differs from the other two products in that it can deliver two separate doses. The first dose is injected automatically, just as with EpiPen and Adrenaclick. The second dose, if needed, is injected manually.

Norepinephrine [Levophed] is similar to epinephrine in several respects. With regard to receptor specificity, NE differs from epinephrine only in that NE does not activate beta$_2$ receptors. Accordingly, NE can elicit all of the responses that epinephrine can, except those that are beta$_2$ mediated. Because NE is a catecholamine, the drug is subject to rapid inactivation by MAO and COMT and hence cannot be given orally. Adverse effects are nearly identical to those of epinephrine: tachydysrhythmias, angina, hypertension, and local necrosis on extravasation. In contrast to epinephrine, NE does not promote hyperglycemia, a response that is beta$_2$ mediated. As with epinephrine, responses to NE can be modified by MAO inhibitors, tricyclic antidepressants, general anesthetics, and adrenergic blocking agents.

Despite its similarity to epinephrine, NE has limited clinical applications. The only recognized indications are hypotensive states and cardiac arrest.

Isoproterenol

- *Receptor specificity:* beta$_1$ and beta$_2$
- *Chemical classification:* catecholamine

Isoproterenol [Isuprel] differs significantly from NE and epinephrine in that isoproterenol acts only at beta-adrenergic receptors. Isoproterenol was the first beta-selective agent employed clinically and will serve as our prototype of the beta-selective adrenergic agonists.

Therapeutic Uses

Cardiovascular

By activating beta$_1$ receptors in the heart, isoproterenol can benefit patients with cardiovascular disorders. Specifically, it is used to manage AV heart block, to improve outcomes in cardiac arrest, and to increase cardiac output during shock.

Adverse Effects

Because isoproterenol does not activate alpha-adrenergic receptors, it produces fewer adverse effects than NE or epinephrine. The major undesired responses, caused by activating beta$_1$ receptors in the heart, are *tachydysrhythmias* and *angina pectoris.* In patients with diabetes, isoproterenol can cause *hyperglycemia* by promoting beta$_2$-mediated glycogenolysis.

Drug Interactions

The major drug interactions of isoproterenol are nearly identical to those of epinephrine. Effects are enhanced by MAO inhibitors and tricyclic antidepressants and reduced by beta-adrenergic blocking agents. Like epinephrine, isoproterenol can cause dysrhythmias in patients receiving certain inhalation anesthetics.

Dopamine

- *Receptor specificity:* dopamine, beta$_1$, and, at high doses, alpha$_1$
- *Chemical classification:* catecholamine

Receptor Specificity

Dopamine has *dose-dependent* receptor specificity. When administered in low therapeutic doses, dopamine acts on dopamine receptors only. At moderate therapeutic doses, dopamine activates beta$_1$ receptors in addition to dopamine receptors. And at very high doses, dopamine activates alpha$_1$ receptors along with beta$_1$ and dopamine receptors.

Therapeutic Uses

Shock

The major indication for dopamine is shock. Benefits derive from effects on the heart and renal blood vessels. By activating beta$_1$ receptors in the heart, dopamine can increase cardiac output, improving tissue perfusion. By activating dopamine receptors in the kidney, dopamine can dilate renal blood vessels, improving renal perfusion; however, studies indicate that it is not effective in preventing acute renal failure. Moreover, at very high doses that activate alpha$_1$ receptors, vasoconstriction may decrease renal perfusion, overriding the effects of dopamine activation. Therefore monitoring urine output is an essential component of care for patients on this drug.

Heart Failure

Heart failure is characterized by reduced tissue perfusion secondary to reduced cardiac output. Dopamine can help alleviate symptoms by activating beta$_1$ receptors on the heart, which increases myocardial contractility and thereby increases cardiac output.

Adverse Effects

The most common adverse effects of dopamine—*tachycardia, dysrhythmias,* and *anginal pain*—result from activation of beta$_1$ receptors in the heart. Because of its cardiac actions, dopamine is contraindicated for patients with tachydysrhythmias or ventricular fibrillation. Because high concentrations of dopamine cause alpha$_1$ activation, extravasation may result in *necrosis* from localized vasoconstriction. Tissue injury can be minimized by local infiltration of phentolamine, an alpha-adrenergic antagonist.

Drug Interactions

MAO inhibitors can intensify the effects of dopamine on the heart and blood vessels. If a patient is receiving an MAO inhibitor, the dosage of dopamine must be reduced by at least 90%. Tricyclic antidepressants can also intensify dopamine's actions, but not to the extent seen with MAO inhibitors. Certain general anesthetics can sensitize the myocardium to stimulation by dopamine and other catecholamines, thereby increasing the risk for dysrhythmias. Diuretics can complement the beneficial effects of dopamine on the kidney.

Dobutamine

- *Receptor specificity:* beta$_1$
- *Chemical classification:* catecholamine

Actions and Uses

At therapeutic doses, dobutamine causes selective activation of beta$_1$-adrenergic receptors. The only indication for the drug is heart failure.

Adverse Effects

The major adverse effect is tachycardia. Blood pressure and the electrocardiogram (ECG) should be monitored closely.

Drug Interactions

Effects of dobutamine on the heart and blood vessels are intensified greatly by MAO inhibitors. Accordingly, in patients receiving an MAO inhibitor, dobutamine dosage must be reduced at least 90%. Concurrent use of tricyclic antidepressants may cause a moderate increase in the cardiovascular effects. Certain general anesthetics can sensitize the myocardium to stimulation by dobutamine, thereby increasing the risk for dysrhythmias.

Phenylephrine

- *Receptor specificity:* alpha$_1$
- *Chemical classification:* noncatecholamine

Phenylephrine [Neo-Synephrine, others] is a selective alpha$_1$ agonist. The drug can be administered locally to reduce nasal congestion and parenterally to elevate blood pressure. In addition, phenylephrine eye drops can be used to dilate the pupil. Also, phenylephrine can be coadministered with local anesthetics to delay anesthetic absorption.

Albuterol

- *Receptor specificity:* $beta_2$
- *Chemical classification:* noncatecholamine

Therapeutic Uses

Asthma

Albuterol [Proventil, Ventolin, VoSpire, others] can reduce airway resistance in asthma by causing $beta_2$-mediated bronchodilation. Because albuterol is relatively selective for $beta_2$ receptors, it produces much less activation of cardiac $beta_1$ receptors than does isoproterenol. As a result, albuterol and other $beta_2$-selective agents have replaced isoproterenol for therapy of asthma. Remember, however, that receptor selectivity is only relative: if administered in large doses, albuterol will lose selectivity and activate $beta_1$ receptors as well as $beta_2$ receptors. Accordingly, patients should be warned not to exceed recommended doses because doing so may cause undesired cardiac stimulation. Preparations and dosages for asthma are presented in Chapter 60.

Adverse Effects

Adverse effects are minimal at therapeutic doses. *Tremor* is most common. If dosage is excessive, albuterol can cause *tachycardia* by activating $beta_1$ receptors in the heart.

Ephedrine

- *Receptor specificity:* $alpha_1$, $alpha_2$, $beta_1$, $beta_2$
- *Chemical classification:* noncatecholamine

Ephedrine is referred to as a mixed-acting drug because it activates adrenergic receptors by direct and indirect mechanisms. Direct activation results from binding of the drug to alpha and beta receptors. Indirect activation results from release of NE from adrenergic neurons.

Owing to the development of more selective adrenergic agonists, uses for ephedrine are limited. By promoting beta2-mediated bronchodilation, ephedrine can benefit patients with asthma. By activating a combination of alpha and beta receptors, ephedrine can improve hemodynamic status in patients with shock. It may also be used to manage anesthesia-induced hypotension.

Because ephedrine activates the same receptors as epinephrine, both drugs share the same adverse effects: hypertension, dysrhythmias, angina, and hyperglycemia. In addition, because ephedrine can cross the blood-brain barrier, it can act in the CNS to cause insomnia.

All of the drugs presented here are also discussed in chapters that address specific applications (Table 13.3).

TABLE 13.3 ▪ Discussion of Adrenergic Agonists in Other Chapters

Drug Class	Discussion Topic	Chapter
$Alpha_1$ agonists	Nasal congestion	61
	Ophthalmology	84
$Alpha_2$ agonists	Cardiovascular effects	34
	Hypertension	39
	Ophthalmology	84
$Beta_1$ agonists	Heart failure	40
$Beta_2$ agonists	Asthma	60
Amphetamines	Basic pharmacology	16
	Attention-deficit/hyperactivity disorder	29
	Drug abuse	33
	Appetite suppression	66

PRESCRIBING AND MONITORING CONSIDERATIONS

Epinephrine

Therapeutic Goal

Epinephrine has multiple indications. The major use is treatment of *anaphylaxis*. Other uses include *control of superficial bleeding, delay of local anesthetic absorption,* and *management of cardiac arrest.*

Identifying High-Risk Patients

Epinephrine must be used with *great caution* in patients with hyperthyroidism, cardiac dysrhythmias, organic heart disease, or hypertension. *Caution* is also needed in patients with angina pectoris or diabetes and in those receiving MAO inhibitors, tricyclic antidepressants, or general anesthetics.

Administration Considerations

The concentration of epinephrine solutions varies according to the route of administration (see Table 13.3). To avoid serious injury, check solution strength to ensure that the concentration is appropriate for the intended route.

Epinephrine solutions oxidize over time, causing them to turn pink or brown. Discard discolored solutions.

Ongoing Monitoring and Interventions

Evaluating Therapeutic Effects

Monitor heart rate, blood pressure, and, if appropriate, ECG monitor. In hospital settings, for patients receiving IV epinephrine, monitor cardiovascular status continuously.

Minimizing Adverse Effects

Cardiovascular Effects. By stimulating the heart, epinephrine can cause *anginal pain, tachycardia,* and *dysrhythmias.* These responses can be reduced with a beta-adrenergic blocking agent (e.g., metoprolol).

By activating $alpha_1$ receptors on blood vessels, epinephrine can cause intense vasoconstriction, which can result in *severe hypertension.* Blood pressure can be lowered with an alpha-adrenergic blocking agent.

Necrosis. If an IV line delivering epinephrine becomes extravasated, necrosis may result. Exercise care to avoid extravasation. If extravasation occurs, infiltrate the region with phentolamine to minimize injury.

Hyperglycemia. Epinephrine may cause hyperglycemia in patients with diabetes. If hyperglycemia develops, adjustment of antidiabetic medications may be needed.

Minimizing Adverse Interactions

MAO Inhibitors and Tricyclic Antidepressants. These drugs prolong and intensify the actions of epinephrine. Patients taking these antidepressants require a reduction in epinephrine dosage.

General Anesthetics. When combined with certain general anesthetics, epinephrine can induce cardiac dysrhythmias. Dysrhythmias may respond to a $beta_1$-adrenergic blocker.

Dopamine

Therapeutic Goal

Dopamine is used to improve hemodynamic status in patients with *shock* or *heart failure*. Benefits derive from enhanced cardiac performance and increased renal perfusion.

Baseline Data

Full assessment of cardiac, hemodynamic, and renal status is needed.

Identifying High-Risk Patients

Dopamine is *contraindicated* for patients with tachydysrhythmias or ventricular fibrillation. Use with *extreme caution* in patients with organic heart disease, hyperthyroidism, or hypertension and in patients receiving MAO inhibitors. *Caution* is also needed in patients with angina pectoris and in those receiving tricyclic antidepressants or general anesthetics.

Administration Considerations

Administer by continuous infusion, employing an infusion pump to control flow rate.

If extravasation occurs, stop the infusion immediately and infiltrate the region with an alpha-adrenergic antagonist (e.g., phentolamine).

Ongoing Monitoring and Interventions

Evaluating Therapeutic Effects

Monitor cardiovascular status continuously. Increased urine output is one index of success. Diuretics may complement the beneficial effects of dopamine on the kidney.

Minimizing Adverse Effects

Cardiovascular Effects. By stimulating the heart, dopamine may cause *anginal pain, tachycardia,* or *dysrhythmias*. These reactions can be decreased with a beta-adrenergic blocking agent.

Necrosis. If the IV line delivering dopamine becomes extravasated, necrosis may result. Exercise care to avoid extravasation. If extravasation occurs, infiltrate the region with phentolamine.

Minimizing Adverse Interactions

MAO Inhibitors. Concurrent use of MAO inhibitors and dopamine can result in severe cardiovascular toxicity. If a patient is taking an MAO inhibitor, dopamine dosage must be reduced by at least 90%.

Tricyclic Antidepressants. These drugs prolong and intensify the actions of dopamine. Patients receiving them may require a reduction in dopamine dosage.

General Anesthetics. When combined with certain general anesthetics, dopamine can induce dysrhythmias. These may respond to a $beta_1$-adrenergic blocker.

Dobutamine

Therapeutic Goal

Improvement of hemodynamic status in patients with heart failure.

Baseline Data

Full assessment of cardiac, renal, and hemodynamic status is needed.

Identifying High-Risk Patients

Use with *great caution* in patients with organic heart disease, hyperthyroidism, tachydysrhythmias, or hypertension and in those taking an MAO inhibitor. *Caution* is also needed in patients with angina pectoris and in those receiving tricyclic antidepressants or general anesthetics.

Administration Considerations

Administer by continuous IV infusion. Dilute concentrated solutions before use. Adjust the infusion rate on the basis of the cardiovascular response.

Ongoing Monitoring and Interventions

Evaluating Therapeutic Effects

Monitor cardiac function (heart rate, ECG), blood pressure, and urine output. When possible, monitor central venous pressure and pulmonary wedge pressure.

Minimizing Adverse Effects

Major adverse effects are *tachycardia* and *dysrhythmias*. Monitor the ECG and blood pressure closely. Adverse cardiac effects can be reduced with a beta-adrenergic antagonist.

Minimizing Adverse Interactions

MAO Inhibitors. Concurrent use of an MAO inhibitor with dobutamine can cause severe cardiovascular toxicity. If a patient is taking an MAO inhibitor, dobutamine dosage must be reduced by at least 90%.

Tricyclic Antidepressants. These drugs can prolong and intensify the actions of dobutamine. Patients receiving them may require a reduction in dobutamine dosage.

General Anesthetics. When combined with certain general anesthetics, dobutamine can cause cardiac dysrhythmias. These may respond to a $beta_1$-adrenergic antagonist.

CHAPTER

14 Adrenergic Antagonists

Jacqueline Rosenjack Burchum, DNSc, FNP-BC, CNE

The adrenergic antagonists cause direct blockade of adrenergic receptors. With one exception, all of the adrenergic antagonists produce *reversible* (competitive) blockade.

Unlike many adrenergic agonists, which act at alpha- *and* beta-adrenergic receptors, most adrenergic antagonists are more selective. As a result, the adrenergic antagonists can be neatly divided into two major groups (Table 14.1): (1) *alpha-adrenergic blocking agents* (drugs that produce selective blockade of alpha-adrenergic receptors); and (2) *beta-adrenergic blocking agents* (drugs that produce selective blockade of beta receptors).[a]

Our approach to the adrenergic antagonists mirrors the approach we took with the adrenergic agonists. We begin by discussing the therapeutic and adverse effects that can result from alpha- and beta-adrenergic blockade, after which we discuss the individual drugs that produce receptor blockade.

It is much easier to understand responses to the adrenergic drugs if you first understand the responses to activation of adrenergic receptors. Accordingly, if you have not yet mastered Table 11.3 in Chapter 11, you should do so now (or be prepared to consult the table as we proceed).

ALPHA-ADRENERGIC ANTAGONISTS

Therapeutic and Adverse Responses to Alpha Blockade

In this section we discuss the beneficial and adverse responses that can result from blockade of alpha-adrenergic receptors. Then, properties of individual alpha-blocking agents are discussed.

Therapeutic Applications of Alpha Blockade

Most clinically useful responses to alpha-adrenergic antagonists result from blockade of $alpha_1$ receptors on blood vessels. Blockade of $alpha_1$ receptors in the bladder and prostate can help those with benign prostatic hyperplasia (BPH). Blockade of $alpha_1$ receptors in the eyes and blockade of $alpha_2$ receptors have no recognized therapeutic applications.

Essential Hypertension

Hypertension (high blood pressure) can be treated with a variety of drugs, including the alpha-adrenergic antagonists. Alpha antagonists lower blood pressure by causing vasodilation by blocking $alpha_1$ receptors on arterioles and veins. Dilation of arterioles reduces arterial pressure directly. Dilation of veins lowers arterial pressure by an indirect process: in response to venous dilation, return of blood to the heart decreases, thereby decreasing cardiac output, which in turn reduces arterial pressure. The role of alpha-adrenergic blockers in essential hypertension is discussed further in Chapter 39.

Reversal of Toxicity From Alpha$_1$ Agonists

Overdose with an alpha-adrenergic agonist (e.g., epinephrine) can produce *hypertension* secondary to excessive activation of $alpha_1$ receptors on blood vessels. When this occurs, blood pressure can be lowered by reversing the vasoconstriction with an alpha-blocking agent.

If an intravenous (IV) line containing an alpha agonist becomes extravasated, necrosis can occur secondary to intense local vasoconstriction. By infiltrating the region with phentolamine (an alpha-adrenergic antagonist), we can block the vasoconstriction and thereby prevent injury.

BPH

BPH results from proliferation of cells in the prostate gland. Symptoms include dysuria, increased frequency of daytime urination, nocturia, urinary hesitancy, urinary urgency, a sensation of incomplete voiding, and a reduction in the size and force of the urinary stream. All of these symptoms can be improved with drugs that block $alpha_1$ receptors. Benefits derive from reduced contraction of smooth muscle in the prostatic capsule and the bladder neck (trigone and sphincter). Please note that BPH and its treatment are discussed in Chapter 51.

Pheochromocytoma

A pheochromocytoma is a catecholamine-secreting tumor derived from cells of the sympathetic nervous system. These tumors are usually located in the adrenal medulla. If secretion of catecholamines (epinephrine, norepinephrine) is sufficiently great, persistent hypertension can result. The principal cause of hypertension is activation of $alpha_1$ receptors on blood vessels, although activation of $beta_1$ receptors on the heart can also contribute. The preferred treatment is surgical removal of the tumor, but alpha-adrenergic blockers may also be employed.

Alpha-blocking agents have two roles in managing pheochromocytoma. First, in patients with inoperable tumors, alpha blockers are given long term to suppress hypertension. Second, when surgery is indicated, alpha blockers are administered preoperatively to reduce the risk for acute hypertension during the procedure. This is necessary because the surgical patient is at risk because manipulation of the tumor can cause massive catecholamine release.

[a]Only two adrenergic antagonists—carvedilol and labetalol—act as alpha *and* beta receptors.

TABLE 14.1 ▪ Receptor Specificity of Adrenergic Antagonists

Category	Drugs	Receptors Blocked
ALPHA-ADRENERGIC BLOCKING AGENTS		
Nonselective agents	Phenoxybenzamine	$alpha_1$, $alpha_2$
	Phentolamine	$alpha_1$, $alpha_2$
$Alpha_1$-selective agents	Alfuzosin	$alpha_1$
	Doxazosin	$alpha_1$
	Prazosin	$alpha_1$
	Silodosin	$alpha_1$
	Tamsulosin	$alpha_1$
	Terazosin	$alpha_1$
BETA-ADRENERGIC BLOCKING AGENTS		
Nonselective agents	Carteolol	$beta_1$, $beta_2$
	Nadolol	$beta_1$, $beta_2$
	Pindolol	$beta_1$, $beta_2$
	Propranolol	$beta_1$, $beta_2$
	Sotalol	$beta_1$, $beta_2$
	Timolol	$beta_1$, $beta_2$
	Carvedilol	$beta_1$, $beta_2$, $alpha_1$
	Labetalol	$beta_1$, $beta_2$, $alpha_1$
$Beta_1$-selective agents	Acebutolol	$beta_1$
	Atenolol	$beta_1$
	Betaxolol	$beta_1$
	Bisoprolol	$beta_1$
	Esmolol	$beta_1$
	Metoprolol	$beta_1$
	Nebivolol	$beta_1$

Raynaud Disease

Raynaud disease is a peripheral vascular disorder characterized by vasospasm in the toes and fingers. Prominent symptoms are local sensations of pain and cold. Alpha blockers can suppress symptoms by preventing alpha-mediated vasoconstriction. It should be noted, however, that although alpha blockers can relieve symptoms of Raynaud disease, they are generally ineffective against other peripheral vascular disorders that involve inappropriate vasoconstriction.

Adverse Effects of Alpha Blockade

The most significant adverse effects of the alpha-adrenergic antagonists result from blockade of $alpha_1$ receptors. Detrimental effects associated with $alpha_2$ blockade are minor.

Adverse Effects of $Alpha_1$ Blockade

Orthostatic Hypotension. Orthostatic (postural) hypotension is the most serious adverse response to alpha-adrenergic blockade. This hypotension can reduce blood flow to the brain, causing dizziness, lightheadedness, and even syncope (fainting).

The cause of orthostatic hypotension is blockade of alpha receptors on *veins,* which reduces muscle tone in the venous wall. Because of reduced venous tone, blood tends to pool (accumulate) in veins when the patient assumes an erect posture. As a result, return of blood to the heart is reduced, which decreases cardiac output, which in turn causes blood pressure to fall.

Patients should be informed about symptoms of orthostatic hypotension (lightheadedness or dizziness on standing) and be advised to sit or lie down if these occur. In addition, patients should be informed that orthostatic hypotension can be minimized by avoiding abrupt transitions from a supine or sitting position to an erect posture.

Reflex Tachycardia. Alpha-adrenergic antagonists can increase heart rate by triggering the baroreceptor reflex. The mechanism is this: (1) blockade of vascular $alpha_1$ receptors causes vasodilation; (2) vasodilation reduces blood pressure; and (3) baroreceptors sense the reduction in blood pressure and, in an attempt to restore normal pressure, initiate a reflex increase in heart rate via the autonomic nervous system. If necessary, reflex tachycardia can be suppressed with a beta-adrenergic blocking agent.

Nasal Congestion. Alpha blockade can dilate the blood vessels of the nasal mucosa, producing nasal congestion.

Inhibition of Ejaculation. Because activation of $alpha_1$ receptors is required for ejaculation (see Table 11.3), blockade of these receptors can cause sexual dysfunction. This form of dysfunction is reversible and resolves when the alpha blocker is withdrawn. If a patient deems the adverse sexual effects of alpha blockade unacceptable, a change in medication will be required. Because males may be reluctant to discuss such concerns, a tactful interview may be needed to discern whether drug-induced sexual dysfunction is discouraging drug use.

Sodium Retention and Increased Blood Volume. By reducing blood pressure, alpha blockers can promote renal retention of sodium and water, thereby causing blood volume to increase. The steps in this process are as follows: (1) by reducing blood pressure, $alpha_1$ blockers decrease renal blood flow; (2) in response to reduced renal perfusion, the kidney excretes less sodium and water; and (3) the resultant retention of sodium and water increases blood volume. As a result, blood pressure is elevated, blood flow to the kidney is increased, and, as far as the kidney is concerned, all is well. Unfortunately, when alpha blockers are used to treat hypertension (which they often are), this compensatory elevation in blood pressure can negate beneficial effects. To prevent the kidney from "neutralizing" hypotensive actions, alpha-blocking agents are usually combined with a diuretic when used in patients with hypertension.

Adverse Effects of $Alpha_2$ Blockade

The most significant adverse effect associated with $alpha_2$ blockade is potentiation of the reflex tachycardia that can occur in response to blockade of $alpha_1$ receptors. Why does $alpha_2$ blockade intensify reflex tachycardia? Recall that peripheral $alpha_2$ receptors are located presynaptically and that activation of these receptors inhibits norepinephrine release. Hence, if $alpha_2$ receptors are blocked, release of norepinephrine will increase. Because the reflex tachycardia caused by $alpha_1$ blockade is ultimately the result of increased firing of the sympathetic nerves to the heart, and because $alpha_2$ blockade will cause each nerve impulse to release a greater amount of norepinephrine, $alpha_2$ blockade will potentiate reflex tachycardia initiated by blockade of $alpha_1$ receptors. Accordingly, drugs such as phentolamine, which block $alpha_2$ as well as $alpha_1$ receptors, cause greater reflex tachycardia than do drugs that block $alpha_1$ receptors only.

Properties of Individual Alpha Blockers

Eight alpha-adrenergic antagonists are employed clinically. Because the alpha blockers often cause postural hypotension, therapeutic uses are limited.

As indicated in Table 14.1, the alpha-adrenergic blocking agents can be subdivided into two major groups. One group, represented by *prazosin,* contains drugs that produce *selective $alpha_1$ blockade.* The second group, represented by *phentolamine,* consists of *nonselective alpha blockers,* which block $alpha_1$ *and* $alpha_2$ receptors.

Prazosin

Actions and Uses

Prazosin [Minipress], our prototype, is a competitive antagonist that produces selective blockade of $alpha_1$-adrenergic receptors. The results are dilation of arterioles and veins and relaxation of smooth muscle in the bladder neck (trigone and sphincter) and prostatic capsule. Prazosin is approved only for hypertension, but it can also benefit men with BPH.

Pharmacokinetics

Prazosin is administered orally. Antihypertensive effects peak in 1 to 3 hours and persist for 10 hours. The drug undergoes extensive hepatic metabolism followed by excretion in the bile. Only 10% is eliminated in the urine. The half-life is 2 to 3 hours.

Adverse Effects

Blockade of $alpha_1$ receptors can cause *orthostatic hypotension, reflex tachycardia,* and *nasal congestion.* The most serious of these is hypotension. Patients should be educated about the symptoms of orthostatic hypotension and be advised to sit or lie down if they occur. Also, patients should be informed that orthostatic hypotension can be minimized by moving slowly when changing from a supine or sitting position to an upright position.

About 1% of patients lose consciousness 30 to 60 minutes after receiving their initial prazosin dose. This "first-dose" effect is the result of severe postural hypotension. To minimize the first-dose effect, the initial dose should be small (no more than 1 mg). Subsequent doses can be gradually increased with little risk for fainting. Patients who are starting treatment should be forewarned about the first-dose effect and advised to avoid driving and other hazardous activities for 12 to 24 hours. Administering the initial dose immediately before going to bed eliminates the risk for a first-dose effect.

Terazosin

Actions and Uses

Like prazosin, terazosin is a selective, competitive antagonist at $alpha_1$-adrenergic receptors. The drug is approved for hypertension and BPH.

Pharmacokinetics

Peak effects develop 1 to 2 hours after oral dosing. The drug's half-life is prolonged (9 to 12 hours), allowing benefits to be maintained with just one dose a day. Terazosin undergoes hepatic metabolism followed by excretion in the bile and urine.

Adverse Effects

Like other alpha-blocking agents, terazosin can cause orthostatic hypotension, reflex tachycardia, and nasal congestion. In addition, terazosin is associated with a high incidence (16%) of headache. As with prazosin, the first dose can cause profound hypotension. To minimize this first-dose effect, the initial dose should be administered at bedtime.

Doxazosin

Actions and Uses

Doxazosin [Cardura, Cardura XL] is a selective, competitive inhibitor of $alpha_1$-adrenergic receptors. The drug is indicated for hypertension and BPH.

Pharmacokinetics

Doxazosin is administered orally, and peak effects develop in 2 to 3 hours. Its half-life is prolonged (22 hours), so once-a-day dosing is adequate. In the blood, most (98%) of the drug is protein bound. Doxazosin undergoes extensive hepatic metabolism followed by biliary excretion.

Adverse Effects

Like prazosin and terazosin, doxazosin can cause orthostatic hypotension, reflex tachycardia, and nasal congestion. As with prazosin and terazosin, the first dose can cause profound hypotension, which can be minimized by giving the initial dose at bedtime.

Tamsulosin

Actions and Uses

Tamsulosin [Flomax] is an $alpha_1$-adrenergic antagonist that causes "selective" blockade of $alpha_1$ receptors on smooth muscle of the bladder neck (trigone and sphincter), prostatic capsule, and prostatic urethra; blockade of vascular $alpha_1$ receptors is weak. The drug is approved only for BPH. It is not useful for hypertension. In men with BPH, tamsulosin increases urine flow rate and decreases residual urine volume. Maximum benefits develop within 2 weeks.

Pharmacokinetics

Tamsulosin is administered orally, and absorption is slow. Food further decreases the rate and extent of absorption. The drug is metabolized in the liver and excreted in the urine.

Adverse Effects

The most common adverse effects are headache and dizziness. Between 8% and 18% of patients experience abnormal ejaculation (ejaculation failure, ejaculation decrease, retrograde ejaculation). In addition, the drug is associated with increased incidence of rhinitis.

Drug Interactions

Combined use with cimetidine increases tamsulosin serum levels, which may cause toxicity. Combined use with hypotensive drugs—including phosphodiesterase type 5 (PDE-5) inhibitors such as sildenafil [Viagra]—may cause a significant reduction in blood pressure.

Alfuzosin

Actions and Uses

Like tamsulosin, alfuzosin [Uroxatral, Xatral ♣] is an $alpha_1$ blocker with selectivity for $alpha_1$ receptors in the prostate and urinary tract. At recommended doses, blockade of $alpha_1$ receptors on blood vessels is weak. Therefore, alfuzosin is indicated only for BPH.

Pharmacokinetics

Alfuzosin is formulated in extended-release tablets, and hence absorption is slow. Plasma levels peak 8 hours after dosing. Bioavailability is 49%. Alfuzosin undergoes extensive hepatic metabolism, primarily by CYP3A4, an isoenzyme of cytochrome P450. Most (70%) of each dose is eliminated in the feces as inactive metabolites. A small fraction leaves unchanged in the urine. The half-life is 10 hours.

In patients with moderate to severe hepatic impairment, alfuzosin levels increase threefold to fourfold. The drug is contraindicated for these patients.

Adverse Effects

Alfuzosin is generally well tolerated. The most common adverse effect is dizziness. Syncope and clinically significant hypotension are rare. Unlike tamsulosin, alfuzosin does not interfere with ejaculation. Doses 4 times greater than recommended can prolong the QT interval and might thereby pose a risk for ventricular dysrhythmias.

Drug Interactions

Levels of alfuzosin are markedly raised by powerful inhibitors of CYP3A4. Among these are erythromycin, clarithromycin, itraconazole, ketoconazole, nefazodone, and the HIV protease inhibitors, such as ritonavir. Concurrent use of alfuzosin with these drugs is contraindicated.

Although alfuzosin does not lower blood pressure much, combining it with other hypotensive agents could produce a more dramatic reduction. Accordingly, such combinations should be used with caution. Drugs of concern include organic nitrates, antihypertensive agents, and the PDE-5 inhibitors used for sexual dysfunction (e.g., sildenafil [Viagra]).

Silodosin

Actions and Uses

Silodosin [Rapaflo] is an alpha-adrenergic antagonist that selectively blocks $alpha_1$ receptors in the prostate, bladder, and urethra. Blockade of vascular alpha receptors is weak. The drug is indicated only for BPH.

Adverse Effects
Silodosin is generally well tolerated. However, like tamsulosin, silodosin can greatly reduce or eliminate release of semen during orgasm. This effect reverses when the drug is discontinued. Although blockade of vascular alpha receptors is usually minimal, silodosin can produce dizziness, lightheadedness, and nasal congestion.

Phentolamine
Actions and Uses
Like prazosin, phentolamine [OraVerse, Rogitine ♣] is a competitive adrenergic antagonist. However, in contrast to prazosin, phentolamine blocks $alpha_2$ receptors as well as $alpha_1$ receptors. Phentolamine has three approved applications: (1) diagnosis and treatment of pheochromocytoma; (2) prevention of tissue necrosis after extravasation of drugs that produce $alpha_1$-mediated vasoconstriction (e.g., norepinephrine); and (3) reversal of soft tissue anesthesia. (Local anesthetics are often combined with epinephrine, which prolongs anesthetic action by causing $alpha_1$-mediated vasoconstriction. Phentolamine blocks epinephrine-mediated vasoconstriction and thereby increases local blood flow, which increases the rate of anesthetic removal.)

Adverse Effects
Like prazosin, phentolamine can produce the typical adverse effects associated with alpha-adrenergic blockade: orthostatic hypotension, reflex tachycardia, nasal congestion, and inhibition of ejaculation. Because it blocks $alpha_2$ receptors, phentolamine produces greater reflex tachycardia than prazosin. If reflex tachycardia is especially severe, heart rate can be reduced with a beta blocker. Because tachycardia can aggravate angina pectoris and myocardial infarction (MI), phentolamine is contraindicated for patients with either disorder.

Overdose can produce profound hypotension. If necessary, blood pressure can be elevated with norepinephrine. Epinephrine should not be used because the drug can cause blood pressure to drop even further. In the presence of $alpha_1$ blockade, the ability of epinephrine to promote vasodilation (through activation of vascular $beta_2$ receptors) may outweigh the ability of epinephrine to cause vasoconstriction (through activation of vascular $alpha_1$ receptors). Further lowering of blood pressure is not a significant problem with norepinephrine because norepinephrine does not activate $beta_2$ receptors.

Phenoxybenzamine
Actions and Uses
Phenoxybenzamine [Dibenzyline] is an old drug that, like phentolamine, blocks $alpha_1$ and $alpha_2$ receptors. However, unlike all of the other alpha-adrenergic antagonists, phenoxybenzamine is a noncompetitive receptor antagonist. Hence receptor blockade is not reversible. As a result, the effects of phenoxybenzamine are long lasting. (Responses to a single dose can persist for several days.) Effects subside as newly synthesized receptors replace the ones that have been irreversibly blocked. Phenoxybenzamine is approved only for pheochromocytoma.

Adverse Effects
Like the other alpha-adrenergic antagonists, phenoxybenzamine can produce orthostatic hypotension, reflex tachycardia, nasal congestion, and inhibition of ejaculation. Reflex tachycardia is greater than that caused by prazosin and about equal to that caused by phentolamine.

> **Patient Education**
>
> **$ALPHA_1$-ADRENERGIC ANTAGONISTS**
>
> Forewarn patients about first-dose hypotension. Advise them to sit or lie down if dizziness or lightheadedness occurs on standing. Teach patients to move slowly when changing from a supine or sitting position to an upright posture. Urge them to avoid driving and other hazardous activities for 12 to 24 hours after the initial dose. Reinforce the importance of taking the initial dose at bedtime to minimize the first-dose effect.
>
> Outpatients need to be taught how to monitor heart rate and blood pressure. Instruct them to hold the drug and notify the provider if sustained bradycardia or hypotension develop.

If dosage is excessive, phenoxybenzamine, like phentolamine, will cause profound hypotension. Furthermore, because hypotension is the result of irreversible $alpha_1$ blockade, it cannot be corrected with an $alpha_1$ agonist. To restore blood pressure, patients must be given intravenous fluids, which elevate blood pressure by increasing blood volume.

BETA-ADRENERGIC ANTAGONISTS

Therapeutic and Adverse Responses to Beta Blockade

In this section we consider the beneficial and adverse responses that can result from blockade of beta-adrenergic receptors. Then we examine the properties of individual beta blockers.

Therapeutic Applications of Beta Blockade

Practically all of the therapeutic effects of the beta-adrenergic antagonists result from blockade of $beta_1$ receptors in the heart. The major consequences of blocking these receptors are (1) reduced heart rate, (2) reduced force of contraction, and (3) reduced velocity of impulse conduction through the atrioventricular (AV) node. Because of these effects, beta blockers are useful in a variety of cardiovascular disorders.

Angina Pectoris
Angina pectoris (cardiac pain due to ischemia) occurs when oxygen supplied to the heart through coronary circulation is insufficient to meet cardiac oxygen demand. Anginal attacks can be precipitated by exertion, intense emotion, and other factors. Beta-adrenergic blockers are a mainstay of antianginal therapy. By blocking $beta_1$ receptors in the heart, these drugs decrease cardiac workload. This reduces oxygen demand, bringing it back into balance with oxygen supply and thereby preventing ischemia and pain.

Hypertension
For years, beta blockers were considered drugs of choice for hypertension. However, more recent data indicate they are less beneficial than previously believed.

The exact mechanism by which beta blockers reduce blood pressure is not known. Older proposed mechanisms include reduction of cardiac output through blockade of $beta_1$ receptors in the heart and suppression of renin release through blockade of $beta_1$ receptors in the kidney (see Chapter 36 for a discussion of the role of renin in blood pressure control). More recently, we have learned that, with long-term use, beta blockers reduce peripheral vascular resistance, which could account for much of their antihypertensive effects.

Cardiac Dysrhythmias
Beta-adrenergic blocking agents are especially useful for treating dysrhythmias that involve excessive electrical activity in the sinus node and atria. By blocking cardiac $beta_1$ receptors, these drugs can (1) decrease the rate of sinus nodal discharge and (2) suppress conduction of atrial impulses through the AV node, thereby preventing the ventricles from being driven at an excessive rate.

Myocardial Infarction
An MI is a region of myocardial necrosis caused by localized interruption of blood flow to the heart wall. Treatment with a beta blocker can reduce pain, infarct size, mortality, and the risk for reinfarction. To be effective, therapy with a beta

blocker must begin soon after an MI has occurred and should be continued for several years.

Reduction of Perioperative Mortality

Beta blockers may decrease the risk for mortality associated with noncardiac surgery in high-risk patients. In the DECREASE-IV trial, pretreatment with bisoprolol reduced the incidence of perioperative MI and death. However, for treatment to be both safe and effective, dosing should begin *early* (several days to weeks before surgery) and *doses should be low initially and then titrated up* (to achieve a resting heart rate of 60 to 80 beats/minute). In addition, treatment should continue for 1 month after surgery. As shown in an earlier trial, known as POISE, if the beta blocker is started *late* (just before surgery), and if the doses are *large,* such treatment can actually *increase* the risk for perioperative mortality.

Heart Failure

Beta blockers are now considered standard therapy for heart failure. This application is relatively new and may come as a surprise to some readers because, until recently, heart failure was considered an absolute *contraindication* to beta blockers. At this time, only three beta blockers—carvedilol, bisoprolol, and metoprolol—have been shown effective for heart failure.

Hyperthyroidism

Hyperthyroidism (excessive production of thyroid hormone) is associated with an increase in the sensitivity of the heart to catecholamines (e.g., norepinephrine, epinephrine). As a result, normal levels of sympathetic activity to the heart can generate tachydysrhythmias and angina pectoris. Blockade of cardiac beta$_1$ receptors suppresses these responses.

Migraine Prophylaxis

When taken prophylactically, beta-adrenergic blocking agents can reduce the frequency and intensity of migraine attacks. However, although beta blockers are effective as prophylaxis, these drugs are not able to abort a migraine headache after it has begun. The mechanism by which beta blockers prevent migraine is not known.

Performance Anxiety

Public speakers and other performers sometimes experience performance anxiety ("stage fright"). Prominent symptoms are tachycardia, tremors, and sweating brought on by generalized discharge of the sympathetic nervous system. Some of you may experience similar symptoms when taking tests. Beta blockers help prevent performance anxiety—including test anxiety—by preventing beta$_1$-mediated tachycardia.

Pheochromocytoma

As discussed earlier, a pheochromocytoma secretes large amounts of catecholamines, which can cause excessive stimulation of the heart. Cardiac stimulation can be prevented by beta$_1$ blockade.

Glaucoma

Beta blockers are important drugs for treating glaucoma, a condition characterized by elevated intraocular pressure with subsequent injury to the optic nerve. The group of beta blockers used in glaucoma (see Table 14.2) is different from the group of beta blockers discussed here.

TABLE 14.2 ▪ Clinical Pharmacology of the Beta-Adrenergic Blocking Agents

Generic Name	Trade Name	Receptors Blocked	ISA	Lipid Solubility	Half-Life (hr)	Route*	Maintenance Dosage in Hypertension†
FIRST-GENERATION: NONSELECTIVE BETA BLOCKERS							
Carteolol	Cartrol	beta$_1$, beta$_2$	++	Low	6	PO	2.5 mg/day
Nadolol	Corgard	beta$_1$, beta$_2$	0	Low	20–24	PO	40 mg/day
Pindolol	Visken	beta$_1$, beta$_2$	+++	Moderate	3–4	PO	10 mg twice/day
Propranolol (IR)	generic only	beta$_1$, beta$_2$	0	High	3–5	PO, IV	60 mg twice/day
Propranolol (ER)	Inderal LA, InnoPran XL					PO	80 mg/day
Sotalol	Betapace, Betapace AF	beta$_1$, beta$_2$	0	High	12	PO	Not for hypertension
Timolol	Blocadren	beta$_1$, beta$_2$	0	Low	4	PO	20 mg twice/day
SECOND-GENERATION: CARDIOSELECTIVE BETA BLOCKERS							
Acebutolol	Sectral	beta$_1$	+	Moderate	3–4	PO	400 mg/day
Atenolol	Tenormin	beta$_1$	0	Low	6–9	PO, IV	50 mg/day
Betaxolol	Kerlone	beta$_1$	0	Low	14–22	PO	10 mg/day
Bisoprolol	Zebeta	beta$_1$	0	Moderate	9–12	PO	5 mg/day
Esmolol	Brevibloc	beta$_1$	0	Low	0.15	IV	Not for hypertension
Metoprolol (IR)	Lopressor, Betaloc 🍁	beta$_1$	0	High	3–7	PO, IV	100 mg/day
Metoprolol (SR)	Toprol XL					PO	100 mg/day
THIRD-GENERATION: BETA BLOCKERS WITH VASODILATING ACTIONS							
Carvedilol (IR)	Coreg	beta$_1$, beta$_2$, alpha$_1$	0	Moderate	5–11	PO	12.5 mg twice/day
Carvedilol (SR)	Coreg CR					PO	40 mg/day
Labetalol	Normodyne, Trandate	beta$_1$, beta$_2$, alpha$_1$	0	Low	6–8	PO, IV	300 mg twice/day
Nebivolol	Bystolic	beta$_1$	0	High	12–19	PO	20 mg/day

*Oral administration is used for essential hypertension. Intravenous administration is reserved for acute myocardial infarction (atenolol, metoprolol), cardiac dysrhythmias (esmolol, propranolol), and severe hypertension (labetalol).

†These are the lowest doses normally used for maintenance in hypertension.

ER, extended release; IR, immediate release; ISA, intrinsic sympathomimetic activity (partial agonist activity); PO, orally; SR, sustained release.

Adverse Effects of Beta Blockade

Although therapeutic responses to beta blockers are due almost entirely to blockade of $beta_1$ receptors, adverse effects involve both $beta_1$ and $beta_2$ blockade. Consequently, the nonselective beta-adrenergic blocking agents (drugs that block $beta_1$ *and* $beta_2$ receptors) produce a broader spectrum of adverse effects than do the "cardioselective" beta-adrenergic antagonists (drugs that block only $beta_1$ receptors at therapeutic doses).

Adverse Effects of $Beta_1$ Blockade

All of the adverse effects of $beta_1$ blockade are the result of blocking $beta_1$ receptors in the heart. Blockade of renal $beta_1$ receptors is not a concern.

Bradycardia. Blockade of cardiac $beta_1$ receptors can produce bradycardia (excessively slow heart rate). If necessary, heart rate can be increased using a beta-adrenergic agonist, such as isoproterenol, and atropine (a muscarinic antagonist). Isoproterenol competes with the beta blocker for cardiac $beta_1$ receptors, thereby promoting cardiac stimulation. By blocking muscarinic receptors on the heart, atropine prevents slowing of the heart by the parasympathetic nervous system.

Reduced Cardiac Output. $Beta_1$ blockade can reduce cardiac output by decreasing heart rate and the force of myocardial contraction. Because they can decrease cardiac output, *beta blockers must be used with great caution in patients with heart failure or reduced cardiac reserve.* In both cases, any further decrease in cardiac output could result in insufficient tissue perfusion.

Precipitation of Heart Failure. In some patients, suppression of cardiac function with a beta blocker can be so great as to cause heart failure. Patients should be informed about the early signs of heart failure (shortness of breath, night coughs, swelling of the extremities) and instructed to notify the prescriber if these occur. It is important to appreciate that, although beta blockers can precipitate heart failure, they are also used to *treat* heart failure.

AV Heart Block. AV heart block is defined as a delay in the conduction of electrical impulses through the AV node. In its most severe form, AV block prevents *all* atrial impulses from reaching the ventricles. Because blockade of cardiac $beta_1$ receptors can suppress AV conduction, production of AV block is a potential complication of beta-blocker therapy. These drugs are contraindicated for patients with preexisting AV block.

Rebound Cardiac Excitation. Long-term use of beta blockers can sensitize the heart to catecholamines. As a result, if a beta blocker is withdrawn *abruptly,* anginal pain or ventricular dysrhythmias may develop. This phenomenon of increased cardiac activity in response to abrupt cessation of beta-blocker therapy is referred to as *rebound excitation.* The risk for rebound excitation can be minimized by withdrawing these drugs gradually (e.g., by tapering the dosage over a period of 1 to 2 weeks). If rebound excitation occurs, dosing should be temporarily resumed. Patients should be warned against abrupt cessation of treatment. Also, they should be advised to carry an adequate supply of their beta blocker when traveling.

Adverse Effects of $Beta_2$ Blockade

Bronchoconstriction. Blockade of $beta_2$ receptors in the lungs can cause constriction of the bronchi. (Recall that activation of these receptors promotes bronchodilation.) For most people, the degree of bronchoconstriction is insignificant. However, when bronchial $beta_2$ receptors are blocked in patients with asthma, the resulting increase in airway resistance can be life threatening. Accordingly, *drugs that block $beta_2$ receptors* are contraindicated for people with asthma. If these individuals must use a beta blocker, they should use an agent that is $beta_1$ selective (e.g., metoprolol).

Hypoglycemia From Inhibition of Glycogenolysis. Epinephrine, acting at $beta_2$ receptors in skeletal muscle and the liver, can stimulate glycogenolysis (breakdown of glycogen into glucose). $Beta_2$ blockade will inhibit this process, posing a risk for hypoglycemia in susceptible individuals. Although suppression of $beta_2$-mediated glycogenolysis is inconsequential for most people, interference with this process can be detrimental to patients with *diabetes.* These people are especially dependent on $beta_2$-mediated glycogenolysis as a way to overcome insulin-induced hypoglycemia. If the patient with diabetes requires a beta blocker, a $beta_1$-selective agent should be chosen.

Adverse Effects in Neonates From $Beta_1$ and $Beta_2$ Blockade

Use of beta blockers during pregnancy can have residual effects on the newborn infant. Specifically, because beta blockers can remain in the circulation for several days after birth, neonates may be at risk for bradycardia (from $beta_1$ blockade), respiratory distress (from $beta_2$ blockade), and hypoglycemia (from $beta_2$ blockade). Accordingly, for 3 to 5 days after birth, newborns should be closely monitored for these effects. Adverse neonatal effects have been observed with at least one beta blocker (betaxolol) and may be a risk with others as well.

Properties of Individual Beta Blockers

The beta-adrenergic antagonists can be subdivided into three groups:

- *First-generation (nonselective) beta blockers* (e.g., propranolol), which block $beta_1$ and $beta_2$ receptors
- *Second-generation (cardioselective) beta blockers* (e.g., metoprolol), which produce selective blockade of $beta_1$ receptors (at usual doses)
- *Third-generation (vasodilating) beta blockers* (e.g., carvedilol), which act on blood vessels to cause dilation, but may produce nonselective or cardioselective beta blockade

Our discussion of the individual beta blockers focuses on two prototypes: propranolol and metoprolol. Properties of these and other beta blockers are shown in Tables 14.2 and 14.3.

Propranolol

Propranolol [Inderal LA, InnoPran XL], our prototype of the first-generation beta blockers, produces *nonselective* beta blockade. That is, this drug blocks both $beta_1$- *and* $beta_2$-adrenergic receptors. Propranolol was the first beta blocker to receive widespread clinical use and remains one of our most important beta-blocking agents.

Pharmacologic Effects

By blocking *cardiac* $beta_1$ receptors, propranolol can *reduce heart rate, decrease the force of ventricular contraction,* and

TABLE 14.3 ▪ Beta-Adrenergic Blocking Agents: Summary of Therapeutic Uses

	Hypertension	Angina Pectoris	Myocardial Infarction or Prophylaxis	Cardiac Dysrhythmia/ Rate Control	Heart Failure	Glaucoma	Migraine Prophylaxis	Hyperthyroidism/ Thyrotoxicosis	Performance Anxiety	Tremor or Movement Disorder
FIRST-GENERATION: NONSELECTIVE BETA BLOCKERS										
Carteolol						A				
Nadolol	A	A		O			O	O		
Pindolol	A	O*		O						
Propranolol	A	A	A	A			A	O	O	O
Sotalol				A						
Timolol	A	A	A	O		A	A			
SECOND-GENERATION: CARDIOSELECTIVE BETA BLOCKERS										
Acebutolol	A	O		A				O		
Atenolol	A	A	A	O						
Betaxolol	A	O		O		A				
Bisoprolol	A	O		O	O					
Esmolol				A				O		
Metoprolol	A	A	A	O	A		O	O		O
THIRD-GENERATION: BETA BLOCKERS WITH VASODILATING ACTIONS										
Carvedilol	A	O		O						
Labetalol	A									
Nebivolol	A									

*Approved for use in Canada but not in the United States.
A, U.S. Food and Drug Administration–approved use; O, Off-label use.

suppress impulse conduction through the AV node. The net effect is a reduction in cardiac output.

By blocking *renal* $beta_1$ receptors, propranolol can *suppress secretion of renin*.

By blocking $beta_2$ receptors, propranolol can produce three major effects: (1) *bronchoconstriction* (through $beta_2$ blockade in the lungs), (2) *vasoconstriction* (through $beta_2$ blockade on certain blood vessels), and (3) *reduced glycogenolysis* (through $beta_2$ blockade in skeletal muscle and liver).

Pharmacokinetics

Propranolol is *highly lipid soluble* and therefore can readily cross membranes. The drug is well absorbed after oral administration, but, because of extensive metabolism on its first pass through the liver, less than 30% of each dose reaches the systemic circulation. Because of its ability to cross membranes, propranolol is widely distributed to all tissues and organs, including the central nervous system (CNS). Propranolol undergoes hepatic metabolism followed by excretion in the urine.

Therapeutic Uses

Practically all of the applications of propranolol are based on blockade of $beta_1$ receptors in the heart. The most important indications are *hypertension, angina pectoris, cardiac dysrhythmias,* and *myocardial infarction*. The role of propranolol and other beta blockers in these disorders is discussed in Chapters 23, 39, 41, 43, and 88. Additional indications include prevention of migraine headache and performance anxiety.

Adverse Effects

The most serious adverse effects result from blockade of $beta_1$ receptors in the heart and blockade of $beta_2$ receptors in the lungs.

Bradycardia. $Beta_1$ blockade in the heart can cause bradycardia. Heart rate should be assessed before each dose. If the heart rate is below normal, the drug should be held and the prescriber should be notified. If necessary, heart rate can be increased by administering atropine and isoproterenol.

AV Heart Block. By slowing conduction of impulses through the AV node, propranolol can cause AV heart block. The drug is contraindicated for patients with preexisting AV block (if the block is greater than first degree).

Heart Failure. In patients with heart disease, suppression of myocardial contractility by propranolol can result in heart failure. Patients should be informed about the early signs of heart failure (shortness of breath on mild exertion or when lying supine, night coughs, swelling of the extremities, weight gain from fluid retention) and instructed to notify the prescriber if these occur. Propranolol is generally contraindicated for patients with preexisting heart failure (although other beta blockers are used to *treat* heart failure).

Rebound Cardiac Excitation. Abrupt withdrawal of propranolol can cause rebound excitation of the heart, resulting in tachycardia and ventricular dysrhythmias. This problem is especially dangerous for patients with preexisting cardiac ischemia. To avoid rebound excitation, propranolol should be withdrawn slowly by giving progressively smaller doses over 1 to 2 weeks. Patients should be warned against abrupt cessation of treatment. In addition, they should be advised to carry an adequate supply of propranolol when traveling.

Bronchoconstriction. Blockade of $beta_2$ receptors in the lungs can cause bronchoconstriction. As a rule, increased airway resistance is hazardous only to patients with asthma and other obstructive pulmonary disorders.

Inhibition of Glycogenolysis. Blockade of $beta_2$ receptors in skeletal muscle and the liver can inhibit glycogenolysis. This effect can be dangerous for people with diabetes (see later).

CNS Effects. Because of its lipid solubility, propranolol can readily cross the blood-brain barrier and hence has ready access sites in the CNS. However, although propranolol is reputed to cause a variety of CNS reactions—depression, insomnia, nightmares, and hallucinations—these reactions are, in fact, very rare. Because of the possible risk for depression, prudence dictates avoiding propranolol in patients who already have this disorder.

Effects in Neonates. Propranolol crosses the placental barrier. Using propranolol and other beta blockers during pregnancy may put the neonate at risk for bradycardia, respiratory distress, and hypoglycemia. Neonates should be closely monitored for these effects.

Precautions, Warnings, and Contraindications

Severe Allergy. Propranolol should be avoided in patients with a history of severe allergic reactions (anaphylaxis). Recall that epinephrine, the drug of choice for anaphylaxis, relieves symptoms in large part by activating $beta_1$ receptors in the heart and $beta_2$ receptors in the lungs. If these receptors are blocked by propranolol, the ability of epinephrine to help will be impaired.

Diabetes. Propranolol can be detrimental to diabetic patients in two ways. First, by blocking $beta_2$ receptors in muscle and liver, propranolol can suppress glycogenolysis, thereby eliminating an important mechanism for correcting insulin-induced hypoglycemia. Second, by blocking $beta_1$ receptors, propranolol can suppress tachycardia, tremors, and perspiration, which normally serve as an early warning signal that blood glucose levels are falling too low. (When glucose drops below a safe level, the sympathetic nervous system is activated, causing these symptoms.) By "masking" symptoms of hypoglycemia, propranolol can delay awareness of hypoglycemia, thereby compromising the patient's ability to correct the problem in a timely fashion. Patients with diabetes who take propranolol should be warned that these common symptoms may no longer be a reliable indicator of hypoglycemia. In addition, they should be taught to recognize alternative symptoms (hunger, fatigue, poor concentration) that blood glucose is falling perilously low.

Cardiac, Respiratory, and Psychiatric Disorders. Propranolol can exacerbate *heart failure, AV heart block, sinus bradycardia, asthma,* and *bronchospasm*. Accordingly, the drug is contraindicated for patients with these disorders. In addition, propranolol should be used with caution in patients with a history of *depression*.

Drug Interactions

Calcium Channel Blockers. The cardiac effects of two calcium channel blockers—verapamil and diltiazem—are identical to those of propranolol: reduction of heart rate, suppression of AV conduction, and suppression of myocardial contractility. When propranolol is combined with either of these drugs, excessive cardiosuppression may result.

Insulin. As discussed previously, propranolol can impede early recognition of insulin-induced hypoglycemia. In addition, propranolol can block glycogenolysis, the body's mechanism for correcting hypoglycemia.

General Dosing Considerations

Establishing an effective propranolol dosage is difficult for two reasons: (1) patients vary widely in their requirements for propranolol and (2) there is a poor correlation between blood levels of propranolol and therapeutic responses. The explanation for these observations is that responses to propranolol are dependent on the activity of the sympathetic nervous system. If sympathetic activity is high, then the dose needed to reduce receptor activation will be high. Conversely, if sympathetic activity is low, then low doses will usually be sufficient to produce receptor blockade. Because sympathetic activity varies among patients, propranolol requirements vary also. Accordingly, the dosage must be adjusted by monitoring the patient's response, and not by relying on dosing information in a drug reference.

Metoprolol

Metoprolol [Lopressor, Toprol XL], our prototype of the second-generation beta blockers, produces selective blockade of $beta_1$ receptors in the heart. At usual therapeutic doses, the drug does not cause $beta_2$ blockade. Please note, however, that selectivity for $beta_1$ receptors is not absolute: at higher doses, metoprolol and the other cardioselective agents will block $beta_2$ receptors as well. Because their effects on $beta_2$ receptors are normally minimal, cardioselective agents are not likely to cause bronchoconstriction or hypoglycemia. Accordingly, these drugs are preferred to the nonselective beta blockers for patients with asthma or diabetes.

Pharmacologic Effects

By blocking cardiac $beta_1$ receptors, metoprolol has the same impact on the heart as propranolol: it reduces heart rate, force of contraction, and conduction velocity through the AV node. Also like propranolol, metoprolol reduces secretion of renin by the kidney. In contrast to propranolol, metoprolol does not block bronchial $beta_2$ receptors at usual doses and therefore does not increase airway resistance.

Pharmacokinetics

Metoprolol is very lipid soluble and well absorbed after oral administration. Like propranolol, metoprolol undergoes extensive metabolism on its first pass through the liver. As a result, only 40% of an oral dose reaches the systemic circulation. Elimination is by hepatic metabolism and renal excretion.

Therapeutic Uses

The primary indication for metoprolol is *hypertension.* The drug is also approved for *angina pectoris, heart failure,* and *myocardial infarction.*

Adverse Effects

Major adverse effects involve the heart. Like propranolol, metoprolol can cause *bradycardia, reduced cardiac output, AV heart block,* and *rebound cardiac excitation after abrupt withdrawal.* Also, even though metoprolol is approved for *treating* heart failure, it can *cause* heart failure if used incautiously. In contrast to propranolol, metoprolol causes minimal bronchoconstriction and does not interfere with $beta_2$-mediated glycogenolysis.

Precautions, Warnings, and Contraindications

Like propranolol, metoprolol is contraindicated for patients with *sinus bradycardia* and *AV block greater than first degree.* In addition, it should be used with great care in patients with *heart failure.* Because metoprolol produces only minimal blockade of $beta_2$ receptors, the drug is safer than propranolol for patients with asthma or a history of severe allergic reactions. In addition, because metoprolol does not suppress $beta_2$-mediated glycogenolysis, it can be used more safely than propranolol by patients with diabetes. Please note, however, that metoprolol, like propranolol, will mask common signs and symptoms of hypoglycemia, thereby depriving the diabetic patient of an early indication that hypoglycemia is developing.

Other Beta-Adrenergic Blockers

In the United States, 16 beta blockers are approved for cardiovascular disorders (hypertension, angina pectoris, cardiac dysrhythmias, MI). Principal differences among these drugs concern receptor specificity, pharmacokinetics, indications, side effects, intrinsic sympathomimetic activity, and the ability to cause vasodilation.

In addition to the agents used for cardiovascular disorders, there is a group of beta blockers used for glaucoma (see Chapter 84).

Properties of the beta blockers employed for cardiovascular disorders are discussed later.

Receptor Specificity

With regard to receptor specificity, beta blockers fall into two groups: nonselective agents and cardioselective agents. The nonselective agents block $beta_1$ *and* $beta_2$ receptors, whereas the cardioselective agents block $beta_1$ receptors only when prescribed at usual doses. Because of their limited side effects, the cardioselective agents are preferred for patients with asthma or diabetes. Two beta blockers—*labetalol* and *carvedilol*—differ from all the others in that they block *alpha*-adrenergic receptors in addition to beta receptors. The receptor specificity of individual beta blockers is indicated in Tables 14.1 and 14.2.

Pharmacokinetics

Pharmacokinetic properties of the beta blockers are shown in Table 14.2. The relative lipid solubility of these agents is of particular importance. The drugs with high solubility (e.g., propranolol, metoprolol) have two prominent features: (1) they penetrate the blood-brain barrier with ease and (2) they are eliminated primarily by hepatic metabolism. Conversely, the drugs with low lipid solubility (e.g., nadolol, atenolol) penetrate the blood-brain barrier poorly and are eliminated primarily by renal excretion.

BLACK BOX WARNING: SOTALOL [BETAPACE, BETAPACE AF]

When starting or restarting sotalol, patients should be in a facility that can provide continuous electrocardiogram monitoring and cardiopulmonary resuscitation for a minimum of 3 days to minimize problems associated with induced arrhythmia.

Creatinine clearance should be established before initiating this drug.

Betapace cannot be substituted for Betapace AF when treating atrial fibrillation.

PATIENT-CENTERED CARE ACROSS THE LIFE SPAN

Adrenergic Antagonists

Life Stage	Patient Care Concerns
Pregnant women	Atenolol is classified as Pregnancy Risk Category D. It crosses the placenta and has been associated with a number of fetal and neonatal risks, including intrauterine growth restriction, bradycardia, hypoglycemia, and respiratory depression.
Breastfeeding women	Betaxolol is more extensively excreted into breast milk than other beta blockers. When a beta blocker is necessary, it may be better to prescribe an alternate beta-blocking agent when prescribing to breastfeeding mothers.
Older adults	The following drugs have been identified as potentially inappropriate for use in geriatric patients: the alpha$_1$ blockers doxazosin, prazosin, and terazosin; and the beta blocker sotalol.

Therapeutic Uses

Principal indications for the beta-adrenergic blockers are *hypertension, angina pectoris,* and *cardiac dysrhythmias.* Other uses include prophylaxis of *migraine headache,* treatment of *myocardial infarction,* symptom suppression in individuals with *situational anxiety* (e.g., stage fright), and treatment of *heart failure* (see Chapter 40). Approved and investigational uses of the beta blockers are shown in Table 14.3.

Esmolol and *sotalol* differ from the other beta blockers in that they are not used for hypertension. Because of its very short half-life (15 minutes), *esmolol* is clearly unsuited for treating hypertension, which requires maintenance of blood levels throughout the day, every day, for an indefinite time. The only approved indication for esmolol is emergency intravenous therapy of *supraventricular tachycardia. Sotalol* is approved for *ventricular dysrhythmias* and for maintenance of normal sinus rhythm in patients who previously experienced symptomatic atrial fibrillation or atrial flutter. Esmolol and sotalol are discussed in Chapter 41.

Adverse Effects

By blocking beta$_1$ receptors in the heart, all of the beta blockers can cause *bradycardia, AV heart block,* and, rarely, *heart failure.* By blocking beta$_2$ receptors in the lung, the nonselective agents can cause significant *bronchoconstriction* in patients with asthma or chronic obstructive pulmonary disease. In addition, by blocking beta$_2$ receptors in the liver and skeletal muscle, the *nonselective* agents can *inhibit glycogenolysis,* compromising the ability of diabetic patients to compensate for insulin-induced hypoglycemia. Because of their ability to block alpha-adrenergic receptors, *carvedilol* and *labetalol* can cause *postural hypotension.*

Although *CNS effects* (insomnia, depression) can occur with all beta blockers, these effects are rare and are most likely with the more lipid-soluble agents. Abrupt discontinuation of any beta blocker can produce *rebound cardiac excitation.* Accordingly, all beta blockers should be withdrawn slowly (by tapering the dosage over 1 to 2 weeks).

Intrinsic Sympathomimetic Activity (Partial Agonist Activity)

The term *intrinsic sympathomimetic activity* (ISA) refers to the ability of certain beta blockers—especially *pindolol*—to act as *partial agonists* at beta-adrenergic receptors. (A partial agonist is a drug that, when bound to a receptor, produces a limited degree of receptor activation while preventing strong agonists from binding to that receptor to cause full activation.)

In contrast to other beta blockers, agents with ISA have very little effect on resting heart rate and cardiac output. When patients are at rest, stimulation of the heart by the sympathetic nervous system is low. If an ordinary beta blocker is given, it will block sympathetic stimulation, causing heart rate and cardiac output to decline. However, if a beta blocker has ISA, its own ability to cause limited receptor activation will compensate for blocking receptor activation by the sympathetic nervous system, and, consequently, resting heart rate and cardiac output are not reduced.

Because of their ability to provide a low level of cardiac stimulation, beta blockers with ISA are preferred to other beta blockers for use in patients with bradycardia. Conversely, these agents should not be given to patients with MI because their ability to cause even limited cardiac stimulation can be detrimental.

Vasodilation

The third-generation beta blockers—*carvedilol, labetalol,* and *nebivolol*—can dilate blood vessels. Two mechanisms are employed: carvedilol and labetalol block vascular alpha$_1$ receptors; nebivolol promotes synthesis and release of nitric oxide from the vascular epithelium. The exact clinical benefit of vasodilation by these drugs has not been clarified.

All of the drugs presented in this chapter are also discussed in chapters that address specific applications (Table 14.4).

TABLE 14.4 ▪ Discussion of Adrenergic Antagonists in Other Chapters

Drug Class	Discussion Topic	Chapter
ALPHA-ADRENERGIC BLOCKING AGENTS		
Nonselective agents	Vasodilators	38
Alpha$_1$-selective agents	Vasodilators	38
	Hypertension	39
	Benign prostatic hypertrophy	51
BETA-ADRENERGIC BLOCKING AGENTS		
Nonselective agents	Migraine headache	23
	Hypertension	39
	Dysrhythmias	41
	Angina	43
	Glaucoma	84
Beta$_1$-selective agents	Migraine headache	23
	Hypertension	39
	Heart failure	40
	Dysrhythmias	41
	Angina	43
	Myocardial infarction	88

BLACK BOX WARNING: ATENOLOL, METOPROLOL, NADOLOL, TIMOLOL

Abrupt discontinuation may cause exacerbation of angina and increases the risk for myocardial infarction.

Patient Education

BETA BLOCKERS

$Beta_1$ blockade can mask early signs and symptoms of hypoglycemia by preventing common tachycardia, tremors, and perspiration. Warn patients with diabetes that tachycardia, tremors, and perspiration cannot be relied on as an indicator of impending hypoglycemia, and teach them to recognize other indicators (e.g. hunger, fatigue, poor concentration) that blood glucose is falling dangerously low.

Inform patients about early signs of heart failure (shortness of breath, night coughs, swelling of the extremities), and instruct them to notify the provider if these occur.

Warn patients against abruptly discontinuing beta blockers because this may cause tachycardia and other dysrhythmias. Advise patients, when traveling, to carry an adequate supply of medication plus a copy of their prescription.

PRESCRIBING AND MONITORING CONSIDERATIONS

$Alpha_1$-Adrenergic Antagonists

Alfuzosin
Doxazosin
Prazosin
Silodosin
Tamsulosin
Terazosin

Therapeutic Goal

Doxazosin, Prazosin, Terazosin

These drugs reduce blood pressure in patients with *essential hypertension.*

Doxazosin, Terazosin, Alfuzosin, Silodosin, Tamsulosin

These drugs reduce symptoms in patients with BPH.

Baseline Data

Essential Hypertension

Determine blood pressure and heart rate.

BPH

Determine the degree of nocturia, daytime frequency, hesitance, intermittency, terminal dribbling (at the end of voiding), urgency, impairment of size and force of urinary stream, dysuria, and sensation of incomplete voiding.

Identifying High-Risk Patients

The only contraindication is hypersensitivity to these drugs.

Ongoing Monitoring and Interventions

Evaluating Therapeutic Effects

Essential Hypertension. Evaluate by monitoring blood pressure.

BPH. Evaluate for improvement in the symptoms listed later under "Baseline Data."

Minimizing Adverse Effects

Orthostatic Hypotension. $Alpha_1$ blockade can cause postural hypotension. Effects may be minimized by having patients sit or lie down if these occur. Patients need to move slowly when changing from a supine or sitting position to an upright posture.

First-Dose Effect. The first dose may cause fainting from severe orthostatic hypotension. This can be minimized by prescribing the first dose to be taken at bedtime.

Beta-Adrenergic Antagonists

Acebutolol
Atenolol
Betaxolol
Bisoprolol
Carteolol
Carvedilol
Esmolol
Labetalol
Metoprolol
Nadolol
Nebivolol
Pindolol
Propranolol
Sotalol
Timolol

Except where noted, the implications here apply to all beta-adrenergic blocking agents.

Therapeutic Goal

Principal indications are *hypertension, angina pectoris, heart failure,* and *cardiac dysrhythmias.* Indications for individual agents are shown in Table 14.3.

Baseline Data

All Patients

Determine heart rate.

Hypertension

Determine standing and supine blood pressure and heart rate.

Angina Pectoris

Determine the incidence, severity, and circumstances of anginal attacks.

Cardiac Dysrhythmias

Obtain a baseline electrocardiogram (ECG).

Identifying High-Risk Patients

All beta blockers are *contraindicated* for patients with sinus bradycardia or AV heart block greater than first degree and must be used with *great caution* in patients with heart failure.

Use with *caution* (especially the nonselective agents) in patients with asthma, bronchospasm, diabetes, or a history of severe allergic reactions. Use all beta blockers with *caution* in patients with a history of depression and in those taking calcium channel blockers.

Ongoing Monitoring and Interventions

Evaluating Therapeutic Effects

Hypertension. Monitor blood pressure and heart rate before each dose. Advise outpatients to monitor and record blood pressure and heart rate daily.

Angina Pectoris. Advise patients to record the incidence, circumstances, and severity of any anginal attacks. Inadequate control of angina may indicate a need to increase dosage. Other medications may need to be adjusted or added.

Cardiac Dysrhythmias. Monitor for improvement in the ECG.

Minimizing Adverse Effects

Bradycardia. $Beta_1$ blockade can reduce heart rate. Decrease dosage if bradycardia is sustained. If bradycardia is severe, withhold medication. If necessary, administer atropine and isoproterenol to restore heart rate.

AV Heart Block. $Beta_1$ blockade can decrease AV conduction. Carefully weigh benefits versus risks if first degree AV block develops. Discontinue beta blockers for patients who develop AV block greater than first degree.

Heart Failure. Suppression of myocardial contractility can cause heart failure. Development of signs or symptoms of heart failure (e.g. shortness of breath, orthopnea, and peripheral edema) may require medication adjustment or discontinuation.

Rebound Cardiac Excitation. Abrupt withdrawal of beta blockers can cause tachycardia and ventricular dysrhythmias. Taper off gradually when discontinuing this drug.

Postural Hypotension. By blocking alpha-adrenergic receptors, *carvedilol* and *labetalol* can cause postural hypotension. As mentioned previously, these alpha-adrenergic effects may be minimized by having patients sit or lie down if these occur. Patients need to move slowly when changing from a supine or sitting position to an upright posture.

Bronchoconstriction. $Beta_2$ blockade can cause substantial airway constriction in patients with asthma. The risk for bronchoconstriction is much lower with the cardioselective agents than with the nonselective agents, so cardioselective drugs should be preferentially prescribed for patients with asthma and other respiratory problems.

Effects in Diabetic Patients. $Beta_1$ blockade can mask early signs and symptoms of hypoglycemia by preventing common tachycardia, tremors, and perspiration. Patients will need to rely on indicators such as hunger and poor concentration to identify hypoglycemia. It may be necessary to monitor fingerstick glucose more closely until recognition is well-established. $Beta_2$ blockade can prevent glycogenolysis, an emergency means of increasing blood glucose. Patients may need to reduce their insulin dosage. Cardioselective beta blockers are preferred to nonselective agents in patients with diabetes.

Effects in Neonates. Maternal use of *betaxolol* during pregnancy may cause bradycardia, respiratory distress, and hypoglycemia in the infant. Accordingly, for 3 to 5 days after birth, newborns should be closely monitored for these effects. Beta blockers other than betaxolol may pose a similar risk.

CNS Effects. Rarely, beta blockers cause depression, insomnia, and nightmares. If these occur, switching to a beta blocker with low lipid solubility may help (see Table 14.2).

Minimizing Adverse Interactions

Calcium Channel Blockers. Two calcium channel blockers—verapamil and diltiazem—can intensify the cardiosuppressant effects of the beta blockers. Use these combinations with caution.

Insulin. Beta blockers can prevent the compensatory glycogenolysis that normally occurs in response to insulin-induced hypoglycemia. Patients with diabetes may need reductions in insulin dosage.

CHAPTER

15

Indirect-Acting Antiadrenergic Agents

Jacqueline Rosenjack Burchum, DNSc, FNP-BC, CNE

The indirect-acting antiadrenergic agents are drugs that prevent the activation of peripheral adrenergic receptors, but by mechanisms that do not involve direct interaction with peripheral receptors. There are two categories of indirect-acting antiadrenergic drugs. The first group—*centrally acting alpha₂ agonists*—consists of drugs that act within the central nervous system (CNS) to reduce the outflow of impulses along sympathetic neurons. The second group—*adrenergic neuron-blocking agents*—consists of drugs that act within the terminals of sympathetic neurons to decrease norepinephrine (NE) release. With both groups, the net result is reduced activation of peripheral adrenergic receptors. Hence the pharmacologic effects of the indirect-acting adrenergic blocking agents are very similar to those of drugs that block adrenergic receptors directly.

CENTRALLY ACTING ALPHA$_2$ AGONISTS

The drugs discussed in this section act within the CNS to reduce the firing of sympathetic neurons. Their primary use is for hypertension.

How can an adrenergic agonist act as an antiadrenergic agent? Alpha$_2$ receptors in the CNS are located on *presynaptic* nerve terminals. As NE accumulates in the synapse, it activates alpha$_2$ receptors. This activation signals that adequate NE is available. As a result, synthesis of NE is decreased. The decrease of available NE results in vasodilation, which in turn decreases blood pressure.

Why are we discussing centrally acting drugs in a unit on peripheral nervous system pharmacology? Because the effects of these drugs are ultimately the result of decreased activation of alpha- and beta-adrenergic receptors in the periphery. That is, by inhibiting the firing of sympathetic neurons, the centrally acting agents decrease the release of NE from sympathetic nerves and thereby decrease activation of peripheral adrenergic receptors. Therefore, although these drugs act within the CNS, their effects are like those of the direct-acting adrenergic receptor blockers. Accordingly, it seems appropriate to discuss these agents in the context of peripheral nervous system pharmacology, rather than presenting them in the context of CNS drugs.

Clonidine

Clonidine [Catapres, Catapres-TTS, Duraclon, Kapvay, Dixarit ♣] is a centrally acting alpha$_2$ agonist with three approved indications: *hypertension, severe pain,* and *attention-deficit/hyperactivity disorder (ADHD).* For treatment of hypertension, the drug is sold as *Catapres.* For treatment of pain, it is sold as *Duraclon* for epidural administration. For management of ADHD, *Kapvay* is used. Use for hypertension is discussed here. Use against pain is discussed in Chapter 22. Use in ADHD management is discussed in Chapter 29.

Clonidine is not used as often as many antihypertensive drugs; however, it has important indications in the management of severe hypertension. Except for rare instances of rebound hypertension, the drug is generally free of serious adverse effects. Dosing is done orally or by transdermal patch.

Mechanism of Antihypertensive Action

Clonidine is an alpha$_2$-adrenergic agonist that causes selective activation of alpha$_2$ receptors in the CNS—specifically, in brainstem areas associated with autonomic regulation of the cardiovascular system. By activating central alpha$_2$ receptors, clonidine reduces sympathetic outflow to blood vessels and to the heart.

Pharmacologic Effects

The most significant effects of clonidine concern the heart and vascular system. By suppressing the firing of sympathetic nerves to the heart, clonidine can cause *bradycardia* and *a decrease in cardiac output.* By suppressing sympathetic regulation of blood vessels, the drug promotes *vasodilation.* The net result of cardiac suppression and vasodilation is *decreased blood pressure.* Blood pressure is reduced in both supine and standing subjects. Because the hypotensive effects of clonidine are not posture dependent, orthostatic hypotension is minimal.

Pharmacokinetics

Clonidine is very lipid soluble. As a result, the drug is readily absorbed after oral dosing and is widely distributed throughout the body, including the CNS. Hypotensive responses begin 30 to 60 minutes after administration and peak in 4 hours. Effects of a single dose may persist as long as 1 day. Clonidine is eliminated by a combination of hepatic metabolism and renal excretion.

Therapeutic Uses

Clonidine has three *approved* applications: treatment of hypertension (its main use), relief of severe pain, and management of ADHD. It has been used off-label for managing opioid and methadone withdrawal, facilitating smoking cessation, treating conduct disorder and oppositional defiant disorder in children, and treating Tourette syndrome, a CNS

Patient Education

CLONIDINE

Advise the patient to take the major portion of the daily dose at bedtime to minimize daytime sedation. For transdermal clonidine, instruct the patient to apply transdermal patches to hairless, intact skin on the upper arm or torso, and to apply a new patch every 7 days.

Have patient record blood pressure daily and call the clinic if hypotension develops. Warn patients against abruptly discontinuing beta blockers because this may cause tachycardia and other dysrhythmias. Advise patients, when traveling, to carry an adequate supply of medication plus a copy of their prescription.

Inform patients about possible CNS depression. Warn them to avoid hazardous activities if alertness is reduced.

Dry mouth can be significant. Inform patients that discomfort can be reduced by chewing sugarless chewing gum, sucking hard candy, and taking frequent sips of fluids.

disease characterized by uncontrollable tics and verbal outbursts that are frequently obscene.

Adverse Effects

Drowsiness

CNS depression is common. About 35% of patients experience drowsiness; an additional 8% experience outright sedation. These responses become less intense with continued drug use. Patients in their early weeks of treatment should be advised to avoid hazardous activities if alertness is impaired.

Xerostomia

Xerostomia is common, occurring in about 40% of patients. The reaction usually diminishes over the first 2 to 4 weeks of therapy. Although not dangerous, xerostomia can be annoying enough to discourage drug use. Patients should be advised that discomfort can be reduced by chewing gum, sucking hard candy, and taking frequent sips of fluids.

Rebound Hypertension

Rebound hypertension is characterized by a large increase in blood pressure occurring in response to abrupt clonidine withdrawal. This rare but serious reaction is caused by overactivity of the sympathetic nervous system and can be accompanied by nervousness, tachycardia, and sweating. Left untreated, the reaction may persist for a week or more. If blood pressure climbs dangerously high, it should be lowered with a combination of alpha- and beta-adrenergic blocking agents. Rebound effects can be avoided by withdrawing clonidine slowly (over 2 to 4 days). Patients should be informed about rebound hypertension and warned not to discontinue clonidine without consulting the prescriber.

Use in Pregnancy

Clonidine is embryotoxic in animals. Because of the possibility of fetal harm, clonidine is not recommended for pregnant women. Pregnancy should be ruled out before clonidine is given.

Abuse

People who abuse cocaine, opioids (e.g., morphine, heroin), and other drugs frequently abuse clonidine as well. At high doses, clonidine can cause subjective effects—euphoria, sedation, hallucinations—that some individuals find desirable. In addition, clonidine can intensify the subjective effects of some abused drugs, including benzodiazepines, cocaine, and opioids. Because clonidine costs less than these drugs, the combination allows abusers to get high for less money.

Other Adverse Effects

Clonidine can cause a variety of adverse effects, including constipation, impotence, gynecomastia, and adverse CNS effects (e.g., vivid dreams, nightmares, anxiety, depression). Localized skin reactions are common with transdermal clonidine patches.

Preparations, Dosage, and Administration

Preparations

Clonidine hydrochloride is available in oral and transdermal formulations and as a solution for epidural administration (see Table 15.1). Oral clonidine is marketed as Catapres. Transdermal clonidine [Catapres-TTS] is available as patches that deliver 0.1, 0.2, and 0.3 mg/24 hours, respectively. Duraclon is supplied as 100-mcg/mL and 500-mcg/mL solutions for epidural administration. Kapvay is an extended-release preparation.

Guanfacine

The pharmacology of guanfacine [Intuniv, Tenex] is very similar to that of clonidine. Like clonidine, guanfacine is indicated for hypertension. In addition, guanfacine, marketed as Intuniv, is used for ADHD. Benefits in hypertension derive from activating brainstem alpha$_2$-adrenergic receptors, an action that reduces sympathetic outflow to the heart and blood vessels. The result is a reduction in cardiac output and blood pressure. Both drugs have the same major adverse effects as clonidine: sedation and dry mouth. In addition, both can cause rebound hypertension after abrupt withdrawal.

Methyldopa and Methyldopate

Methyldopa is an oral antihypertensive agent that lowers blood pressure by acting at sites within the CNS. Two side effects—hemolytic anemia and hepatic necrosis—can be severe. Methyldopate, an intravenous agent, is nearly identical to methyldopa in structure and pharmacologic effects. In the discussion below, the term *methyldopa* is used in reference to both methyldopate and methyldopa.

Mechanism of Action

Methyldopa works much like clonidine. Like clonidine, methyldopa inhibits sympathetic outflow from the CNS by causing alpha$_2$ activation in the brain. However, methyldopa differs from clonidine in that methyldopa itself is not an alpha$_2$ agonist. Thus, before it can act, methyldopa must first be taken up into brainstem neurons, where it is converted to methylnorepinephrine, a compound that *is* an effective alpha$_2$ agonist. Release of methylnorepinephrine results in alpha$_2$ activation.

Pharmacologic Effects

The most prominent response to methyldopa is a drop in blood pressure. The principal mechanism is vasodilation, not cardiosuppression. Vasodilation occurs because of reduced sympathetic stimulation of blood vessels. At usual therapeutic doses, methyldopa does not decrease heart rate or cardiac output. The hemodynamic effects of methyldopa are very much like those of clonidine: both drugs lower blood pressure in supine and standing subjects, and both produce relatively little orthostatic hypotension.

TABLE 15.1 ▪ Preparation, Dosage, and Administration of Indirect-Acting Antiadrenergic Agents

Drug Class or Drug	Preparation	Dosage	Administration
CENTRALLY ACTING ALPHA$_2$ AGONISTS			
Clonidine [Catapres, Catapres-TTS-1, Catapres-TTS-2, Catapres-TTS-3, Kapvay, Dixarit ✦]	Tablets IR: 0.1 mg, 0.2 mg, 0.3 mg Tablets ER: 0.1 mg, 0.2 mg Transdermal patch: 2.5-mg patch delivers 0.1 mg/24 hours 5-mg patch delivers 0.2 mg/24 hours 7.5-mg patch delivers 0.3 mg/24 hours	IR: 0.1 mg twice a day; typical maintenance dose 0.1-0.8 mg/day in divided doses ER: 0.1-0.4 mg/day Patches: 1 every 7 days	May be taken with or without food. When immediate-release (twice-daily) dosing is used, taking most of the daily dose at bedtime can minimize daytime sedation. Patches should be applied to hairless, intact skin on the upper arm or torso.
Guanfacine	Tablets: 1 mg, 2 mg	Usual dose: 1 mg/day	Take IR tablets at bedtime to minimize daytime sedation. Do not administer with grapefruit juice.
Methyldopa	Tablets: 250 mg, 500 mg	Initial dose: 250 mg 2-3 times a day Maintenance does: 0.5-2 g in 2-4 divided doses	May be taken without regard to meals. If dosage is increased, scheduling the increase at bedtime can decrease daytime drowsiness.
ADRENERGIC NEURON-BLOCKING AGENT			
Reserpine	Tablets: 0.1 mg, 0.25 mg	0.5 mg/day for 1-2 weeks, then increase as needed Maintenance dose: 0.1-0.25 mg daily	May be administered with food if gastrointestinal upset occurs.

Therapeutic Use

The only indication for methyldopa is *hypertension.* Studies regarding methyldopa use in pregnant patients have shown improved outcomes without fetal harm, so the American Congress of Obstetricians and Gynecologists has designated methyldopa as a preferred drug in management of hypertension during pregnancy.

Adverse Effects

Positive Coombs Test and Hemolytic Anemia

A positive Coombs test[a] develops in 10% to 20% of patients who take methyldopa chronically. A Coombs test should be performed before treatment and 6 to 12 months later. Blood counts (hematocrit, hemoglobin, or red cell count) should also be obtained before treatment and periodically thereafter. If the test turns positive, it usually occurs between 6 and 12 months of treatment. Of the patients who have a positive Coombs test, about 5% develop hemolytic anemia. Coombs-positive patients who do not develop hemolytic anemia may continue methyldopa treatment. However, if hemolytic anemia does develop, methyldopa should be withdrawn immediately. For most patients, hemolytic anemia quickly resolves after withdrawal, although the Coombs test may remain positive for months.

Hepatotoxicity

Methyldopa has been associated with hepatitis, jaundice, and, rarely, fatal hepatic necrosis. All patients should undergo periodic assessment of liver function. If signs of hepatotoxicity appear, methyldopa should be discontinued immediately. Liver function usually normalizes after drug withdrawal.

[a]The Coombs test detects the presence of antibodies directed against the patient's own red blood cells. These antibodies can cause hemolysis (i.e., red blood cell lysis).

Other Adverse Effects

Methyldopa can cause xerostomia, sexual dysfunction, orthostatic hypotension, and a variety of CNS effects, including drowsiness, reduced mental acuity, nightmares, and depression. These responses are not usually dangerous, but they can detract from adherence.

ADRENERGIC NEURON-BLOCKING AGENTS

The adrenergic neuron-blocking agents act presynaptically to reduce the release of NE from sympathetic neurons. These drugs have little or no effect on the release of epinephrine from the adrenal medulla. Reserpine is the only adrenergic neuron blocker available.

Reserpine

Manufacture of reserpine was discontinued in the U.S. in 2016. We cover it here because it remains available until stock is depleted or expired. Reserpine is a naturally occurring compound prepared from the root of Rauwolfia serpentina, a shrub indigenous to India. Because of its source, reserpine is classified as a Rauwolfia alkaloid. The primary indication for reserpine is hypertension. The side effect of greatest concern is severe depression.

Mechanism of Action

Reserpine causes depletion of NE from postganglionic sympathetic neurons. By doing so, the drug can decrease activation of practically all adrenergic receptors. Hence, the effects of reserpine closely resemble those produced by a combination of alpha- and beta-adrenergic blockade.

Reserpine depletes NE in two ways. First, the drug acts on vesicles within the nerve terminal to cause displacement of stored NE, thereby exposing the transmitter to destruction by monoamine oxidase. Second, reserpine suppresses NE synthesis by blocking the uptake of dopamine (the immediate precursor of NE) into presynaptic vesicles, which contain the enzymes needed to convert dopamine into NE (Fig. 15.1). A week or two may be required to produce maximal transmitter depletion.

In addition to its peripheral effects, reserpine can cause depletion of serotonin and catecholamines from neurons in the CNS. Depletion of these CNS transmitters underlies the most serious side effect of reserpine—deep emotional depression—and also explains the occasional use of reserpine in psychiatry.

Pharmacologic Effects

Peripheral Effects

By depleting sympathetic neurons of NE, reserpine decreases the activation of alpha- and beta-adrenergic receptors. Decreased activation of beta receptors slows heart rate and reduces cardiac output. Decreased alpha activation promotes vasodilation. All three effects cause a decrease in blood pressure.

Effects on the CNS

Reserpine produces sedation and a state of indifference to the environment. In addition, the drug can cause severe depression. These effects are thought to result from depletion of catecholamines and serotonin from neurons in the brain.

Therapeutic Uses

Hypertension

The principal indication for reserpine is hypertension. Benefits result from vasodilation and reduced cardiac workload. Because these effects occur secondary to depletion of NE, and because transmitter depletion occurs slowly, full antihypertensive responses can take a week or more to develop. Conversely, when reserpine is discontinued, effects may persist for several weeks as the NE content of sympathetic neurons becomes replenished. Because its side effects can be severe, and because more desirable drugs are available (see Chapter 39), reserpine is not a preferred drug for hypertension.

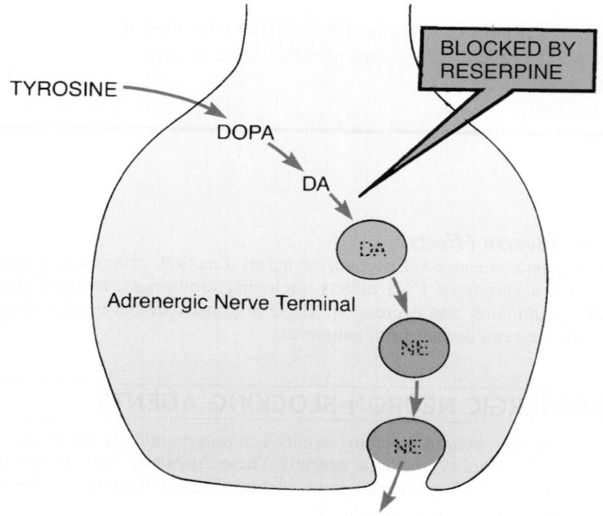

Figure 15.1 ■ Mechanism of reserpine action. Reserpine depletes neurons of norepinephrine (NE) by two mechanisms: (1) Reserpine blocks the uptake of dopamine (DA) into vesicles, preventing NE synthesis. (2) Reserpine also displaces NE from vesicles, thereby allowing degradation of NE by monoamine oxidase present in the nerve terminal (not shown).

Psychotic States

Reserpine can be used to treat agitated psychotic patients, such as those suffering from certain forms of schizophrenia. However, because more effective drugs are available, reserpine is rarely employed in psychotherapy.

Adverse Effects

Depression

Reserpine can produce severe depression that may persist for months after the drug is withdrawn. Suicide has occurred. All patients should be informed about the risk for depression. Also, they should be educated about signs of depression (e.g., early morning insomnia, loss of appetite, change in mood) and instructed to notify the prescriber immediately if these develop. Because of the risk for suicide, patients who develop depression may require hospitalization. Reserpine is contraindicated for patients with a history of depressive disorders. The risk for depression can be minimized by keeping the dosage low (0.25 mg/day or less).

Cardiovascular Effects

Depletion of NE from sympathetic neurons can result in bradycardia, orthostatic hypotension, and nasal congestion. Bradycardia is caused by decreased activation of $beta_1$ receptors in the heart. Hypotension and nasal congestion result from vasodilation secondary to decreased activation of alpha receptors on blood vessels. Patients should be informed that orthostatic hypotension, the most serious cardiovascular effect, can be minimized by moving slowly when changing from a seated or supine position to an upright position. In addition, patients should be advised to sit or lie down if lightheadedness or dizziness occurs.

Gastrointestinal Effects

By mechanisms that are not understood, reserpine can stimulate several aspects of gastrointestinal function. The drug can increase secretion of gastric acid, which may result in ulcer formation. In addition, reserpine can increase the tone and motility of intestinal smooth muscle, causing cramps and diarrhea.

PRESCRIBING AND MONITORING CONSIDERATIONS

Clonidine

Therapeutic Goal

Clonidine is used to reduce blood pressure in hypertensive patients.[b]

Baseline Data

Determine blood pressure and heart rate.

[b]Clonidine is also used to relieve severe pain and to manage ADHD.

PATIENT-CENTERED CARE ACROSS THE LIFE SPAN

Considerations for Indirect-Acting Antiadrenergic Agents

Life Stage	Considerations or Concerns
Children	Centrally acting agonists are approved for use in children 6 years and older, although clonidine has been used in children as young as 5 years (for conduct/oppositional defiance disorders). Although reserpine is sometimes given to children, it is not recommended unless other drugs fail.
Pregnant women	Guanfacine and methyldopa (noninjectable) are Pregnancy Risk Category B drugs. Clonidine is a Pregnancy Risk Category C drug; however, embryotoxicity in some animals raises concerns. Other drugs are preferable.
Breastfeeding women	Clonidine is excreted in relatively large amounts in breast milk. Breastfeeding is not recommended for women taking clonidine, especially if large doses are required, and should be avoided altogether in women breastfeeding premature infants.
Older adults	The Beers Criteria recommend avoidance of centrally acting alpha blockers in patients 65 years and older. When reserpine, an adrenergic neuron-blocking drug, is required, the Beers Criteria recommend maximal dosing at 0.1 mg/day.

Identifying High-Risk Patients

Clonidine is embryotoxic to animals and should not be used during pregnancy. Rule out pregnancy before initiating treatment.

Ongoing Monitoring and Interventions

Evaluating Therapeutic Effects

Monitor blood pressure and heart rate before each dose. Advise outpatients to monitor and record blood pressure and heart rate daily.

Minimizing Adverse Effects

Drowsiness and Sedation. CNS depression increases the risk of accidents. Safety precautions should be initiated for patients at risk of falls. Outpatients should refrain from hazardous activities if alertness is reduced.

Xerostomia. Dry mouth is common. This can be relieved by taking frequent sips of fluids, chewing sugarless gum, and sucking on hard candy.

Rebound Hypertension. Severe hypertension occurs rarely after abrupt clonidine withdrawal. Treat with a combination of alpha- and beta-adrenergic blockers. To avoid rebound hypertension, withdraw clonidine slowly (over 2 to 4 days).

Abuse. People who abuse cocaine, opioids, and other drugs frequently abuse clonidine as well. Be alert for signs of clonidine abuse (e.g., questionable or frequent requests for a prescription).

Methyldopa

Therapeutic Goal

Reduction of blood pressure in hypertensive patients.

Baseline Data

Obtain baseline values for blood pressure, heart rate, blood counts (hematocrit, hemoglobin, or red cell count), Coombs test, and liver function tests.

Identifying High-Risk Patients

Methyldopa is *contraindicated* for patients with active liver disease or a history of methyldopa-induced liver dysfunction.

Administration Considerations

Routes

Oral. Methyldopa is used for routine management of hypertension.

Intravenous. Methyldopa is used for hypertensive emergencies.

Administration. Most patients receiving oral therapy require divided (two to four) daily doses. For some patients, blood pressure can be controlled with a single daily dose at bedtime.

Ongoing Evaluation and Interventions

Evaluating Therapeutic Effects

Monitor blood pressure.

Minimizing Adverse Effects

Hemolytic Anemia. If hemolysis occurs, withdraw methyldopa immediately; hemolytic anemia usually resolves quickly. Obtain a Coombs test before treatment and 6 to 12 months later. Obtain blood counts (hematocrit, hemoglobin, or red cell count) before treatment and periodically thereafter.

Hepatotoxicity. Methyldopa can cause hepatitis, jaundice, and fatal hepatic necrosis. Assess liver function before treatment and periodically thereafter. If liver dysfunction develops, discontinue methyldopa immediately. In most cases, liver function returns to normal soon.

UNIT V

Central Nervous System Drugs

CHAPTER 16

Introduction to Central Nervous System Pharmacology

Jacqueline Rosenjack Burchum, DNSc, FNP-BC, CNE

Central nervous system (CNS) drugs—agents that act on the brain and spinal cord—are used for medical and nonmedical purposes. Medical applications include relief of pain, suppression of seizures, production of anesthesia, and treatment of psychiatric disorders. CNS drugs are used nonmedically for their stimulant, depressant, euphoriant, and other "mind-altering" abilities.

Despite the widespread use of CNS drugs, knowledge of these agents is limited. Much of our ignorance stems from the anatomic and neurochemical complexity of the brain and spinal cord. (There are more than 50 billion neurons in the cerebral hemispheres alone.) We are a long way from fully understanding both the CNS and the drugs used to affect it.

TRANSMITTERS OF THE CENTRAL NERVOUS SYSTEM

In contrast to the peripheral nervous system, in which only 3 compounds—acetylcholine, norepinephrine, and epinephrine—serve as neurotransmitters, the CNS contains at least 21 compounds that serve as neurotransmitters (Box 16.1). Furthermore, there are numerous sites within the CNS for which no transmitter has been identified, so it is clear that additional compounds, yet to be discovered, also mediate central neurotransmission.

None of the compounds believed to be CNS neurotransmitters has actually been *proved* to serve this function. The reason for uncertainty lies with the technical difficulties involved in CNS research. However, although absolute proof may be lacking, the evidence supporting a neurotransmitter role for several compounds (e.g., dopamine, norepinephrine, enkephalins) is completely convincing.

Although much is known about the actions of CNS transmitters at various sites in the brain and spinal cord, it is not usually possible to precisely relate these known actions to behavioral or psychological processes. For example, we know the locations of specific CNS sites at which norepinephrine appears to act as a transmitter, and we know the effect of norepinephrine at most of these sites (suppression of neuronal excitability), but we do not know the precise relationship between suppression of neuronal excitability at each of these sites and the effect of that suppression on the overt function of the organism. This example shows the state of our knowledge of CNS transmitter function: we have a great deal of detailed information about the biochemistry and electrophysiology of CNS transmitters, but we are as yet unable to assemble those details into a completely meaningful picture.

THE BLOOD-BRAIN BARRIER

The blood-brain barrier impedes the entry of drugs into the brain. Passage across the barrier is limited to lipid-soluble agents and to drugs that cross by way of specific transport systems. Protein-bound drugs and highly ionized drugs cannot cross.

From a therapeutic perspective, the blood-brain barrier is a mixed blessing. The barrier protects the brain from injury by potentially toxic substances, but it can also be a significant obstacle to entry of therapeutic agents.

The blood-brain barrier is not fully developed at birth. Accordingly, infants are much more sensitive to CNS drugs than are older children and adults.

HOW DO CENTRAL NERVOUS SYSTEM DRUGS PRODUCE THERAPEUTIC EFFECTS?

Although much is known about the biochemical and electrophysiologic effects of CNS drugs, in most cases we cannot state with certainty the relationship between these effects and production of beneficial responses. Why? To fully understand how a drug alters symptoms, we need to understand, at a biochemical and physiologic level, the pathophysiology of the disorder being treated. In the case of most CNS disorders, our knowledge is limited: we do not fully understand the brain in either health or disease. Therefore we must exercise caution

BOX 16.1 ■ NEUROTRANSMITTERS OF THE CENTRAL NERVOUS SYSTEM

Monoamines
Dopamine
Epinephrine
Norepinephrine
Serotonin

Amino Acids
Aspartate
GABA
Glutamate
Glycine

Purines
Adenosine
Adenosine monophosphate
Adenosine triphosphate

Opioid Peptides
Dynorphins
Endorphins
Enkephalins

Nonopioid Peptides
Neurotensin
Oxytocin
Somatostatin
Substance P
Vasopressin

Others
Acetylcholine
Histamine

GABA, gamma-aminobutyric acid.

when attempting to assign a precise mechanism for a drug's therapeutic effects.

Although we can't state with certainty how CNS drugs act, we do have sufficient data to permit formulation of plausible hypotheses. Consequently, as we study CNS drugs, proposed mechanisms of action are presented. Keep in mind, however, that these mechanisms are tentative, representing our best guess based on available data. As we learn more, it is almost certain that these concepts will be modified, if not discarded.

ADAPTATION OF THE CENTRAL NERVOUS SYSTEM TO PROLONGED DRUG EXPOSURE

When CNS drugs are taken chronically, their effects may differ from those produced during initial use. These altered effects are the result of adaptive changes that occur in the brain in response to prolonged drug exposure. The brain's ability to adapt to drugs can produce alterations in therapeutic effects and side effects. Adaptive changes are often beneficial, although they can also be detrimental.

Increased Therapeutic Effects

Certain drugs used in psychiatry—antipsychotics and antidepressants—must be taken for several weeks before full therapeutic effects develop. Beneficial responses may be delayed because they result from adaptive changes, not from direct effects of drugs on synaptic function. Hence full therapeutic effects are not seen until the CNS has had time to modify in response to prolonged drug exposure.

Decreased Side Effects

When CNS drugs are taken chronically, the intensity of side effects may decrease (while therapeutic effects remain undiminished). For example, phenobarbital (an antiseizure drug) produces sedation during the initial phase of therapy; however, with continued treatment, sedation declines while full protection from seizures is retained. Adaptations within the brain are believed to underlie this phenomenon.

Tolerance and Physical Dependence

Tolerance and physical dependence are special manifestations of CNS adaptation. *Tolerance* is a decreased response occurring in the course of prolonged drug use. *Physical dependence* is a state in which abrupt discontinuation of drug use will precipitate a withdrawal syndrome. The kinds of adaptive changes that underlie tolerance and dependence are such that, after they have taken place, continued drug use is required for the brain to function "normally." If drug use is stopped, the drug-adapted brain can no longer function properly, and withdrawal syndrome ensues. The withdrawal reaction continues until the adaptive changes have had time to revert, restoring the CNS to its pretreatment state.

DEVELOPMENT OF NEW PSYCHOTHERAPEUTIC DRUGS

Because of deficiencies in our knowledge of the neurochemical and physiologic changes that underlie mental disease, it is impossible to take a rational approach to the development of truly new (nonderivative) psychotherapeutic agents. History bears this out: virtually all of the major advances in psychopharmacology have been serendipitous.

In addition to our relative ignorance about the neurochemical and physiologic correlates of mental illness, two other factors contribute to the difficulty in generating truly new psychotherapeutic agents. First, in contrast to many other diseases, we lack adequate animal models of mental illness. Accordingly, animal research is not likely to reveal new types of psychotherapeutic agents. Second, mentally healthy individuals cannot be used as subjects to assess potential psychotherapeutic agents because most psychotherapeutic drugs either have no effect on healthy individuals or produce paradoxical effects.

After a new drug has been found, variations on that agent can be developed systematically: (1) structural analogs of the new agent are synthesized; (2) these analogs are run through biochemical and physiologic screening tests to determine whether they possess activity similar to that of the parent compound; and (3) after serious toxicity has been ruled out, promising agents are tested in humans for possible psychotherapeutic activity. Using this procedure, it is possible to develop drugs that have fewer side effects than the original drug and perhaps even superior therapeutic effects. However, although this procedure may produce small advances, it is not likely to yield a major therapeutic breakthrough.

APPROACHING THE STUDY OF CENTRAL NERVOUS SYSTEM DRUGS

Because our understanding of the CNS is less complete than our understanding of the peripheral nervous system, our approach to studying CNS drugs differs from the approach we took with peripheral nervous system agents. When we studied the pharmacology of the peripheral nervous system, we emphasized the importance of understanding transmitters and their receptors before embarking on a study of drugs. Because our knowledge of CNS transmitters is insufficient to allow this approach, rather than making a detailed examination of CNS transmitters before we study CNS drugs, we will discuss drugs and transmitters concurrently. Hence, for now, all that you need to know about CNS transmitters is that (1) there are a lot of them, (2) their precise functional roles are not clear, and (3) their complexity makes it difficult for us to know with certainty just how CNS drugs produce their beneficial effects.

CHAPTER

17

Drugs for Parkinson Disease

Jacqueline Rosenjack Burchum, DNSc, FNP-BC, CNE

Parkinson disease (PD) is a slowly progressive neurodegenerative disorder that afflicts more than 1 million Americans, making it second only to Alzheimer disease as the most common degenerative disease of neurons. Cardinal symptoms are tremor, rigidity, postural instability, and slowed movement. In addition to these motor symptoms, most patients also experience nonmotor symptoms, especially autonomic disturbances, sleep disturbances, depression, psychosis, and dementia. Years before functional impairment develops, patients may experience early symptoms of PD, including loss of smell, excessive salivation, clumsiness of the hands, worsening of handwriting, bothersome tremor, slower gait, and reduced voice volume. Symptoms first appear in middle age and progress relentlessly. The underlying cause of motor symptoms is loss of dopaminergic neurons in the substantia nigra. Although there is no cure for motor symptoms, drug therapy can maintain functional mobility for years and can thereby substantially prolong quality of life and life expectancy.

PATHOPHYSIOLOGY THAT UNDERLIES MOTOR SYMPTOMS

Motor symptoms result from damage to the *extrapyramidal system,* a complex neuronal network that helps regulate movement. When extrapyramidal function is disrupted, *dyskinesias* (disorders of movement) result. The dyskinesias that characterize PD are tremor at rest, rigidity, postural instability, and bradykinesia (slowed movement). In severe PD, bradykinesia may progress to *akinesia*—complete absence of movement.

In people with PD, neurotransmission is disrupted primarily in the brain's *striatum.* A simplified model of striatal neurotransmission is depicted in Fig. 17.1A. As indicated, proper function of the striatum requires a balance between two neurotransmitters: *dopamine* and *acetylcholine.* Dopamine is an *inhibitory* transmitter; acetylcholine is *excitatory.* The neurons that release dopamine inhibit neurons that release gamma-aminobutyric acid (GABA), another inhibitory transmitter. In contrast, the neurons that release acetylcholine excite the neurons that release GABA. Movement is normal when the inhibitory influence of dopamine and the excitatory influence of acetylcholine are in balance. In PD, there is an imbalance between dopamine and acetylcholine in the striatum (Fig. 17.1B). As noted, the imbalance results from *degeneration of the neurons in the substantia nigra that supply dopamine to the striatum.* In the absence of dopamine, the excitatory influence of acetylcholine goes unopposed, causing excessive stimulation of the neurons that release GABA. Overactivity of these GABAergic neurons contributes to the motor symptoms that characterize PD. That said, between 70% and 80% of these neurons must be lost before PD becomes clinically recognizable. Because this loss takes place over 5 to 20 years, neuronal degeneration begins long before overt motor symptoms appear.

What causes degeneration of dopaminergic neurons? No one knows for sure. However, some evidence strongly implicates *alpha-synuclein*—a potentially toxic protein synthesized by dopaminergic neurons. Under normal conditions, alpha-synuclein is rapidly degraded. As a result, it doesn't accumulate, and no harm occurs. Degradation of alpha-synuclein requires two other proteins: *parkin* and *ubiquitin.* (Parkin is an enzyme that catalyzes the binding of alpha-synuclein to ubiquitin. When bound to ubiquitin, alpha-synuclein can be degraded.) If any of these proteins—alpha-synuclein, parkin, or ubiquitin—is defective, degradation of alpha-synuclein cannot take place. When this occurs, alpha-synuclein accumulates inside the cell, forming neurotoxic fibrils. At autopsy, these fibrils are visible as *Lewy bodies,* which are characteristic of PD pathology. Failure to degrade alpha-synuclein appears to result from two causes: genetic vulnerability and toxins in the environment. Defective genes coding for all three proteins have been found in families with inherited forms of PD. In people with PD that is not inherited, environmental toxins may explain the inability to degrade alpha-synuclein.

As discussed in Chapter 24, movement disorders similar to those of PD can occur as side effects of antipsychotic drugs. These dyskinesias, which are referred to as *extrapyramidal side effects,* result from blockade of dopamine receptors in the striatum. This drug-induced parkinsonism can be managed with some of the drugs used to treat PD.

OVERVIEW OF MOTOR SYMPTOM MANAGEMENT

Therapeutic Goal

Ideally, treatment would reverse neuronal degeneration, or at least prevent further degeneration, and control symptoms. Unfortunately, the ideal treatment doesn't exist: we have no drugs that can prevent neuronal damage or reverse damage that has already occurred. Drugs can only provide symptomatic relief; they do not cure PD. Furthermore, there is no convincing proof that any current drug can delay disease progression. Hence the goal of pharmacologic therapy is simply to improve the patient's ability to carry out activities of daily living. Drug selection and dosage are determined by the extent to which PD interferes with work, walking, dressing, eating, bathing, and other activities. Drugs benefit the

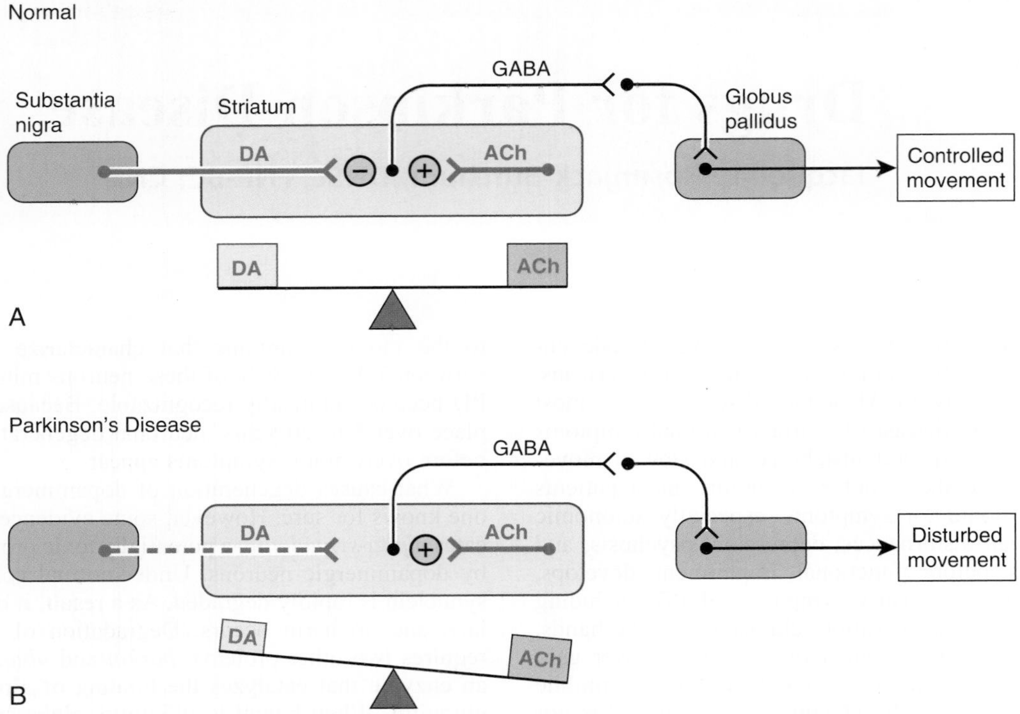

Figure 17.1 ▪ A model of neurotransmission in the healthy striatum and parkinsonian striatum.
A, In the healthy striatum, dopamine (DA) released from neurons originating in the substantia nigra *inhibits* the firing of neurons in the striatum that release gamma-aminobutyric acid (GABA). Conversely, neurons located within the striatum, which release acetylcholine (ACh), *excite* the GABAergic neurons. Therefore, under normal conditions, the inhibitory actions of DA are balanced by the excitatory actions of ACh, and controlled movement results. **B,** In Parkinson disease, the neurons that supply DA to the striatum degenerate. In the absence of sufficient DA, the excitatory effects of ACh go unopposed, and disturbed movement results.

patient primarily by improving bradykinesia, gait disturbance, and postural instability. Tremor and rigidity, although disturbing, are less disabling.

Drugs Employed

Given the neurochemical basis of parkinsonism—too little striatal dopamine and too much acetylcholine—the approach to treatment is obvious: give drugs that can restore the functional balance between dopamine and acetylcholine. To accomplish this, two types of drugs are used: (1) *dopaminergic agents* (i.e., drugs that directly or indirectly activate dopamine receptors) and (2) *anticholinergic agents* (i.e., drugs that block receptors for acetylcholine). Of the two groups, dopaminergic agents are by far the more widely employed.

As shown in Table 17.1, dopaminergic drugs act by several mechanisms: levodopa is converted to dopamine, which activates dopamine receptors directly; inhibitors of monoamine oxidase-B (MAO-B) prevent dopamine breakdown; amantadine promotes dopamine release (and may also block dopamine reuptake); and the inhibitors of catechol-*O*-methyltransferase (COMT) enhance the effects of levodopa by blocking its degradation.

In contrast to the dopaminergic drugs, which act by multiple mechanisms, all of the anticholinergic agents share the same mechanism: blockade of muscarinic receptors in the striatum.

Clinical Guidelines

Management of PD is generally under the guidance of a neurologist who oversees pharmacologic management. Other providers are responsible for differing aspects of care, including management of primary care needs and monitoring of patient status. Thus it is important for all providers involved in care to have a familiarity of drugs used to manage PD. The American Academy of Neurology (AAN) has developed a set of evidence-based guidelines for the treatment of PD and management of individual manifestations of the disease (see https://www.aan.com/Guidelines). The recommendations that follow are based on these guidelines. Lifespan considerations are summarized in the Patient-Centered Care Across the Lifespan box for Parkinson's Disease.

Drug Selection

Initial Treatment

For patients with mild symptoms, treatment can begin with an MAO-B inhibitor. MAO-B inhibitors confer mild, symptomatic benefit.

TABLE 17.1 ■ Dopaminergic Agents for Parkinson Disease

Drug	Mechanism of Action	Therapeutic Role
DOPAMINE REPLACEMENT		
Levodopa/carbidopa	Levodopa undergoes conversion to DA in the brain and then activates DA receptors (carbidopa blocks destruction of levodopa in the periphery)	First-line drug, or supplement to a dopamine agonist
DOPAMINE AGONISTS		
Nonergot Derivatives Apomorphine Pramipexole Ropinirole Rotigotine	Directly activate DA receptors	Pramipexole and ropinirole are first-line drugs, or supplements to levodopa. Apomorphine—a subQ nonergot agent—is reserved for rescue therapy during "off" times. Ergot derivatives are generally avoided.
Ergot Derivatives Bromocriptine Cabergoline		
COMT INHIBITORS		
Entacapone Tolcapone	Inhibit breakdown of levodopa by COMT	Adjunct to levodopa to decrease "wearing off"; entacapone is more effective and safer than tolcapone
MAO-B INHIBITORS		
Rasagiline Selegiline	Inhibit breakdown of DA by MAO-B	Used in newly diagnosed patients and for managing "off" times during levodopa therapy
DOPAMINE RELEASER		
Amantadine	Promotes release of DA from remaining DA neurons; may also block DA reuptake	May help reduce levodopa-induced dyskinesias

COMT, catechol-*O*-methyltransferase; DA, dopamine; MAO-B, type B monoamine oxidase.

PATIENT-CENTERED CARE ACROSS THE LIFE SPAN

Drugs for Parkinson Disease

Life Stage	Considerations or Concerns
Children	Juvenile PD in patients younger than 18 years is extremely rare; therefore, many drugs for PD have not been tested in children. Only amantadine, benztropine, and bromocriptine have approval for pediatric populations. Selegiline is contraindicated in children younger than 12 years.
Pregnant women	Bromocriptine and cabergoline are FDA Pregnancy Risk Category B (although the manufacturer recommends stopping them after pregnancy is determined). All other drugs in this chapter are FDA Pregnancy Risk Category C owing to adverse events in animal studies. Of note, it is rare for a woman of childbearing age to develop PD.
Breastfeeding women	Bromocriptine and cabergoline interfere with lactation. Anticholinergics such as benztropine can suppress lactation. Breastfeeding is not recommended for women taking other drugs in this chapter.
Older adults	The average age of PD diagnosis is 62 years; therefore, most prescriptions are written for older adults. Adverse effects tend to be more common and more serious in these patients. Beers criteria designate anticholinergic drugs (e.g., benztropine and trihexyphenidyl) as potentially inappropriate for use in geriatric patients.

For patients with more severe symptoms, treatment should begin with either levodopa (combined with carbidopa) or a dopamine agonist. Levodopa is more effective than the dopamine agonists, but long-term use carries a higher risk for disabling dyskinesias. Hence the choice must be tailored to the patient: if improving motor function is the primary objective, then levodopa is preferred. However, if drug-induced dyskinesias are a primary concern, then a dopamine agonist would be preferred.

Management of Motor Fluctuations

Long-term treatment with levodopa or dopamine agonists is associated with two types of motor fluctuations: *"off" times* (loss of symptom relief) and *drug-induced dyskinesias* (involuntary movements). "Off" times can be reduced with three types of drugs: dopamine agonists, COMT inhibitors, and MAO-B inhibitors. Evidence of efficacy is strongest for entacapone (a COMT inhibitor) and rasagiline (an MAO-B inhibitor). The only drug recommended for dyskinesias is amantadine.

Neuroprotection

To date, there is no definitive proof that any drug can protect dopaminergic neurons from progressive degeneration. However, although no drug has yet been proved to provide neuroprotective effects for people with PD, studies suggest that some drugs are promising. For example, MAO-B inhibitors have provided neuroprotective effects in animal studies. Similarly, dopamine agonists have demonstrated neuroprotective effects in laboratory studies. For both drug categories, however, clinical studies in humans have been inconclusive. A growing body of research with levodopa supports a likely role for neuroprotection; however, because some studies demonstrate toxic effects in patients with PD, the risks may outweigh the benefits when given for this purpose.

PHARMACOLOGY OF THE DRUGS USED FOR MOTOR SYMPTOMS

Levodopa

Levodopa was introduced in the 1960s and has been a cornerstone of PD treatment ever since. Unfortunately, although the drug is highly effective, beneficial effects diminish over time.

Use in Parkinson Disease

Beneficial Effects

Levodopa is the most effective drug for PD. At the beginning of treatment, about 75% of patients experience a 50% reduction in symptom severity. Levodopa is so effective, in fact, that a diagnosis of PD should be questioned if the patient fails to respond.

Full therapeutic responses may take several months to develop. Consequently, although the effects of levodopa can be significant, patients should not expect immediate improvement. Rather, they should be informed that beneficial effects are likely to increase steadily over the first few months.

In contrast to the dramatic improvements seen during initial therapy, long-term therapy with levodopa has been disappointing. Although symptoms may be well controlled during the first 2 years of treatment, by the end of year 5, ability to function may deteriorate to pretreatment levels. This probably reflects disease progression and not development of tolerance to levodopa.

Acute Loss of Effect

Acute loss of effect occurs in two patterns: gradual loss and abrupt loss. Gradual loss—"wearing off"—develops near the end of the dosing interval and simply indicates that drug levels have declined to a subtherapeutic value. Wearing off can be minimized in three ways: (1) shortening the dosing interval, (2) giving a drug that prolongs levodopa's plasma half-life (e.g., entacapone), and (3) giving a direct-acting dopamine agonist.

Abrupt loss of effect, often referred to as the "on-off" phenomenon, can occur at any time during the dosing interval—even while drug levels are high. "Off" times may last from minutes to hours. Over the course of treatment, "off" periods are likely to increase in both intensity and frequency. Drugs that can help reduce "off" times are listed in Table 17.2. As discussed later, avoiding high-protein meals may also help.

TABLE 17.2 ▪ Drugs for Motor Complications of Levodopa Therapy

Drug	Drug Class
DRUGS FOR "OFF" TIMES	
Definitely Effective	
Entacapone	COMT inhibitor
Rasagiline	MAO-B inhibitor
Probably Effective	
Rotigotine	DA agonist
Pramipexole	DA agonist
Ropinirole	DA agonist
Tolcapone	COMT inhibitor
Possibly Effective	
Apomorphine	DA agonist
Cabergoline	DA agonist
Selegiline	MAO-B inhibitor
DRUG FOR LEVODOPA-INDUCED DYSKINESIAS	
Amantadine	DA-releasing agent

COMT, catechol-*O*-methyltransferase; DA, dopamine; MAO-B, type B monoamine oxidase.

Mechanism of Action

Levodopa reduces symptoms by increasing dopamine synthesis in the striatum (Fig. 17.2). Levodopa enters the brain through an active transport system that carries it across the blood-brain barrier. When in the brain, the drug undergoes uptake into the remaining dopaminergic nerve terminals that remain in the striatum. After uptake, levodopa, which has no direct effects of its own, is converted to dopamine, its active form. As dopamine, levodopa helps restore a proper balance between dopamine and acetylcholine.

Conversion of levodopa to dopamine is depicted in Fig. 17.3. As indicated, the enzyme that catalyzes the reaction is called a *decarboxylase* (because it removes a carboxyl group from levodopa). The activity of decarboxylases is enhanced by *pyridoxine* (vitamin B_6).

Why is PD treated with levodopa and not with dopamine itself? There are two reasons. First, dopamine cannot cross the blood-brain barrier (see Fig. 17.2). As noted, levodopa crosses the barrier by means of an active transport system, a system that does not transport dopamine. Second, dopamine has such a short half-life in the blood that it would be impractical to use even if it could cross the blood-brain barrier.

Pharmacokinetics

Levodopa is administered orally and undergoes rapid absorption from the small intestine. Food delays absorption by slowing gastric emptying. Furthermore, because neutral amino acids compete with levodopa for intestinal absorption (and for transport across the blood-brain barrier as well), high-protein foods will reduce therapeutic effects.

Only a small fraction of each dose reaches the brain. Most is metabolized in the periphery, primarily by *decarboxylase enzymes* and to a lesser extent by COMT. Peripheral decarboxylases convert levodopa into dopamine, an active metabolite. In contrast, COMT converts levodopa into an inactive metabolite. Like the enzymes that decarboxylate levodopa within the brain, peripheral decarboxylases work faster in the presence of pyridoxine. Because of peripheral metabolism, less than 2% of each dose enters the brain if levodopa is given alone. Fortunately, levodopa is now available only in combination preparations with either carbidopa or carbidopa and entacapone. These additional agents decrease the amount of

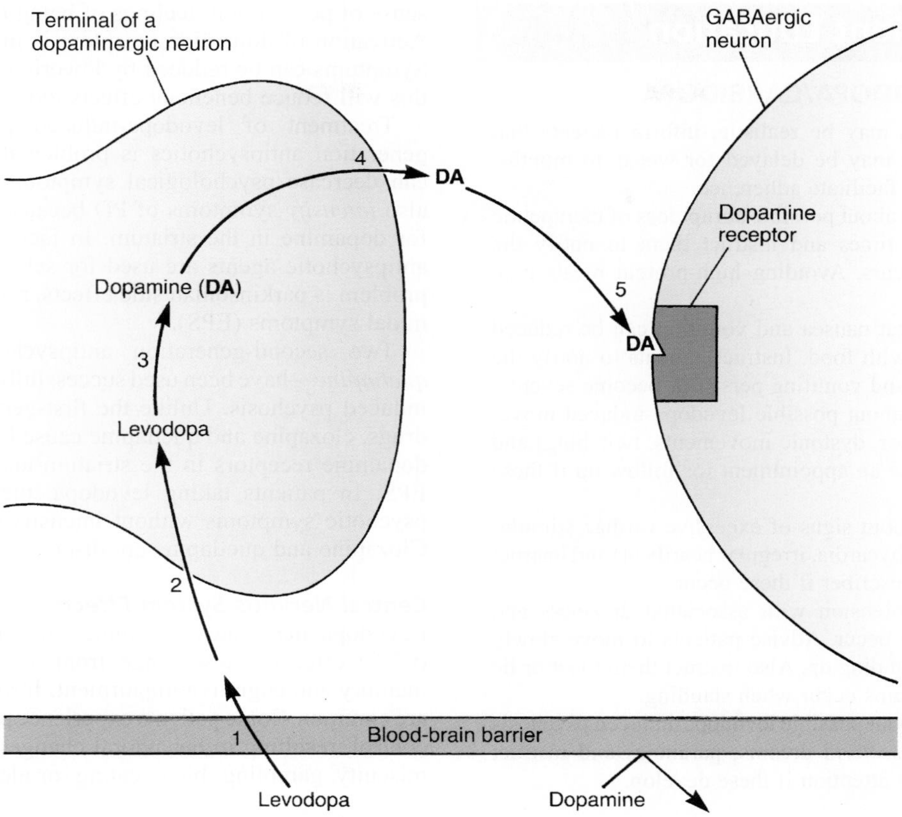

Figure 17.2 ■ Steps leading to alteration of CNS function by levodopa. To produce its beneficial effects in PD, levodopa must be (1) transported across the blood-brain barrier; (2) taken up by dopaminergic nerve terminals in the striatum; (3) converted into dopamine; (4) released into the synaptic space; and (5) bound to dopamine receptors on striatal GABAergic neurons, causing them to fire at a slower rate. Note that dopamine itself is unable to cross the blood-brain barrier, and hence cannot be used to treat PD.

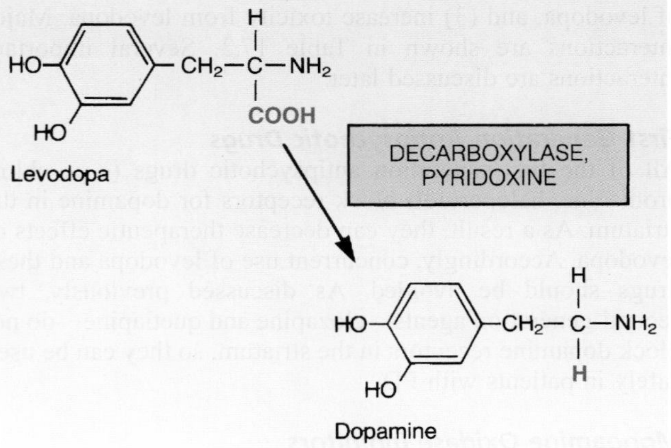

Figure 17.3 ■ Conversion of levodopa to dopamine. Decarboxylases present in the brain, liver, and intestine convert levodopa into dopamine. Pyridoxine (vitamin B6) accelerates the reaction.

decarboxylation in the periphery so that more of the drug can enter the CNS. This is discussed in greater detail later in the chapter.

Adverse Effects

Most side effects of levodopa are dose dependent. Older-adult patients, who are the primary users of levodopa, are especially sensitive to adverse effects.

Nausea and Vomiting

Most patients experience nausea and vomiting early in treatment. The cause is activation of dopamine receptors in the chemoreceptor trigger zone (CTZ) of the medulla. Nausea and vomiting can be reduced by administering levodopa in low initial doses and with meals. (Food delays levodopa absorption, causing a decrease in peak plasma drug levels and a corresponding decrease in stimulation of the CTZ.) However, because administration with food can reduce therapeutic effects by decreasing levodopa absorption, administration with meals should be avoided if possible. Giving additional carbidopa (without levodopa) can help reduce nausea and vomiting. Why carbidopa helps is unknown.

Patient Education

LEVODOPA/CARBIDOPA

So that expectations may be realistic, inform patients that benefits of levodopa may be delayed for weeks to months. This knowledge will facilitate adherence.

Forewarn patients about possible abrupt loss of therapeutic effects during "off" times and instruct them to notify the prescriber if this occurs. Avoiding high-protein meals may help.

Inform patients that nausea and vomiting can be reduced by taking levodopa with food. Instruct patients to notify the prescriber if nausea and vomiting persist or become severe.

Counsel patients about possible levodopa-induced movement disorders (tremor, dystonic movements, twitching) and instruct them to make an appointment for follow up if these develop.

Inform patients about signs of excessive cardiac stimulation (palpitations, tachycardia, irregular heartbeat) and instruct them to notify the prescriber if these occur.

Explain that hypotension with associated dizziness and lightheadedness may occur. Advise patients to move slowly when sitting up or standing up. Also instruct them to sit or lie down if these symptoms occur when standing.

Inform patients about possible levodopa-induced psychosis (visual hallucinations, vivid dreams, paranoia) and instruct them to seek medical attention if these develop.

Dyskinesias

Ironically, levodopa, which is given to *alleviate* movement disorders, actually *causes* movement disorders in many patients. About 80% develop involuntary movements within the first year. Some dyskinesias are just annoying (e.g., head bobbing, tics, grimacing), whereas others can be disabling (e.g., ballismus, a rapid involuntary jerking or flinging of proximal muscle groups, or choreoathetosis, a slow involuntary writhing movement). These dyskinesias develop just before or soon after optimal levodopa dosage has been achieved. Dyskinesias can be managed in three ways. First, the dosage of levodopa can be reduced. However, dosage reduction may allow PD symptoms to reemerge. Second, we can give amantadine (see later), which can reduce dyskinesias in some patients. If these measures fail, the remaining options are usually surgery and electrical stimulation.

Cardiovascular Effects

Postural hypotension is common early in treatment. The underlying mechanism is unknown. Hypotension can be reduced by increasing intake of salt and water. An alpha-adrenergic agonist can help, too.

Conversion of levodopa to dopamine in the periphery can produce excessive activation of $beta_1$ receptors in the heart. *Dysrhythmias* can result, especially in patients with heart disease.

Psychosis

Psychosis develops in about 20% of patients. Prominent symptoms are visual hallucinations, vivid dreams or nightmares, and paranoid ideation (fears of personal endangerment, sense of persecution, feelings of being followed or spied on). Activation of dopamine receptors is in some way involved. Symptoms can be reduced by lowering levodopa dosage, but this will reduce beneficial effects too.

Treatment of levodopa-induced psychosis with first-generation antipsychotics is problematic. Yes, these agents can decrease psychological symptoms. However, they will also *intensify* symptoms of PD because they block receptors for dopamine in the striatum. In fact, when first-generation antipsychotic agents are used for schizophrenia, the biggest problem is parkinsonian side effects, referred to as extrapyramidal symptoms (EPS).

Two second-generation antipsychotics—*clozapine* and *quetiapine*—have been used successfully to manage levodopa-induced psychosis. Unlike the first-generation antipsychotic drugs, clozapine and quetiapine cause little or no blockade of dopamine receptors in the striatum and hence do not cause EPS. In patients taking levodopa, these drugs can reduce psychotic symptoms without intensifying symptoms of PD. Clozapine and quetiapine are discussed in Chapter 24.

Central Nervous System Effects

Levodopa may cause a number of central nervous system (CNS) effects. These range from anxiety and agitation to memory and cognitive impairment. Insomnia and nightmares are common. Some patients experience problems with impulse control, resulting in behavioral changes associated with promiscuity, gambling, binge eating, or alcohol abuse.

Other Adverse Effects

Levodopa may *darken sweat and urine;* patients should be informed about this harmless effect. Some studies suggest that levodopa can *activate malignant melanoma;* however, others have failed to support this finding. Until more is known, it is important to perform a careful skin assessment of patients who are prescribed levodopa.

Drug Interactions

Interactions between levodopa and other drugs can (1) increase beneficial effects of levodopa, (2) decrease beneficial effects of levodopa, and (3) increase toxicity from levodopa. Major interactions are shown in Table 17.3. Several important interactions are discussed later.

First-Generation Antipsychotic Drugs

All of the first-generation antipsychotic drugs (e.g., chlorpromazine, haloperidol) block receptors for dopamine in the striatum. As a result, they can decrease therapeutic effects of levodopa. Accordingly, concurrent use of levodopa and these drugs should be avoided. As discussed previously, two second-generation agents—clozapine and quetiapine—do not block dopamine receptors in the striatum, so they can be used safely in patients with PD.

Monoamine Oxidase Inhibitors

Levodopa can cause a hypertensive crisis if administered to an individual taking a *nonselective* inhibitor of monoamine oxidase (MAO). The mechanism is as follows: (1) levodopa elevates neuronal stores of dopamine and norepinephrine (NE) by promoting synthesis of both transmitters. (2) Because intraneuronal MAO serves to inactivate dopamine and NE, inhibition of MAO allows elevated neuronal stores of these

TABLE 17.3 ▪ Major Drug Interactions of Levodopa

Drug Category	Drug	Mechanism of Interaction
Drugs that *increase* beneficial effects of levodopa	Carbidopa	Inhibits peripheral decarboxylation of levodopa
	Entacapone, tolcapone	Inhibit destruction of levodopa by COMT in the intestine and peripheral tissues
	Rotigotine, apomorphine, bromocriptine, cabergoline, pramipexole, ropinirole	Stimulate dopamine receptors directly and thereby add to the effects of dopamine derived from levodopa
	Amantadine	Promotes release of dopamine
	Anticholinergic drugs	Block cholinergic receptors in the CNS and thereby help restore the balance between dopamine and ACh
Drugs that *decrease* beneficial effects of levodopa	Antipsychotic drugs*	Block dopamine receptors in the striatum
Drugs that *increase* levodopa toxicity	MAO inhibitors (especially *nonselective* MAO inhibitors)	Inhibition of MAO increases the risk for severe levodopa-induced hypertension

ACh, acetylcholine; CNS, central nervous system; COMT, catechol-*O*-methyltransferase; MAO, monoamine oxidase.
*First-generation antipsychotic agents block dopamine receptors in the striatum and can thereby nullify the therapeutic effects of levodopa. Two second-generation antipsychotics—clozapine [Clozaril] and quetiapine [Seroquel]—do not block dopamine receptors in the striatum and thus do not nullify the therapeutic effects of levodopa.

transmitters to grow even larger. (3) Because both dopamine and NE promote vasoconstriction, release of these agents in supranormal amounts can lead to massive vasoconstriction, thereby causing blood pressure to rise dangerously high. To avoid hypertensive crisis, nonselective MAO inhibitors should be withdrawn at least 2 weeks before giving levodopa.

Anticholinergic Drugs

As discussed previously, excessive stimulation of cholinergic receptors contributes to the dyskinesias of PD. Therefore, by blocking these receptors, anticholinergic agents can enhance responses to levodopa.

Pyridoxine

You may read advice to limit pyridoxine (vitamin B_6). It is true that pyridoxine can decrease the amount of levodopa available to reach the CNS by accelerating decarboxylation of levodopa in the periphery. However, because levodopa is now always combined with carbidopa, a drug that suppresses decarboxylase activity, this potential interaction is no longer a clinical concern.

Food Interactions

High-protein meals can reduce therapeutic responses to levodopa. Neutral amino acids compete with levodopa for absorption from the intestine and for transport across the blood-brain barrier. Therefore a high-protein meal can significantly reduce both the amount of levodopa absorbed and the amount transported into the brain. It has been suggested that a high-protein meal could trigger an abrupt loss of effect (i.e., an "off" episode). Accordingly, patients should be advised to spread their protein consumption evenly throughout the day.

Preparations

At one time levodopa was available as a single drug. However, these single-drug preparations have been withdrawn from the market. Levodopa is now available only in combination preparations, either levodopa/carbidopa or levodopa/carbidopa/entacapone.

Levodopa/Carbidopa

The combination of levodopa plus carbidopa is our most effective therapy for PD. Levodopa plus carbidopa is available under three trade names: *Rytary, Sinemet,* and *Duopa.*

Mechanism of Action

Carbidopa has no therapeutic effects of its own; however, carbidopa inhibits decarboxylation of levodopa in the intestine and peripheral tissues, making more levodopa available to the CNS. Carbidopa does not prevent the conversion of levodopa to dopamine by decarboxylases in the brain because carbidopa is unable to cross the blood-brain barrier.

The effect of carbidopa is shown schematically in Fig. 17.4, which compares the fate of levodopa in the presence and absence of carbidopa. As mentioned previously, in the absence of carbidopa, about 98% of levodopa is lost in the periphery, leaving only 2% available to the brain. Why is levodopa lost? Primarily because decarboxylases in the gastrointestinal (GI) tract and peripheral tissues convert it to dopamine, which cannot cross the blood-brain barrier. When these decarboxylases are inhibited by carbidopa, only 90% of levodopa is lost in the periphery, leaving 10% for actions in the brain.

Advantages of Carbidopa

The combination of carbidopa plus levodopa is superior to levodopa alone in three ways:

- By increasing the fraction of levodopa available for actions in the CNS, carbidopa allows the dosage of levodopa to be reduced by about 75%. In the example in Fig. 17.4, to provide 10 mg of dopamine to the brain, we must administer 500 mg of levodopa if carbidopa is absent, but only 100 mg if carbidopa is present.
- By reducing production of dopamine in the periphery, carbidopa reduces cardiovascular responses to levodopa as well as nausea and vomiting.
- By causing direct inhibition of decarboxylase, carbidopa eliminates concerns about decreasing the effects of levodopa by taking a vitamin preparation that contains pyridoxine.

Disadvantages of Carbidopa

Carbidopa has no adverse effects of its own. Accordingly, any adverse responses from carbidopa/levodopa are the result of potentiating the effects of levodopa. When levodopa is combined with carbidopa, abnormal movements and psychiatric disturbances can occur sooner and can be more intense than with levodopa alone.

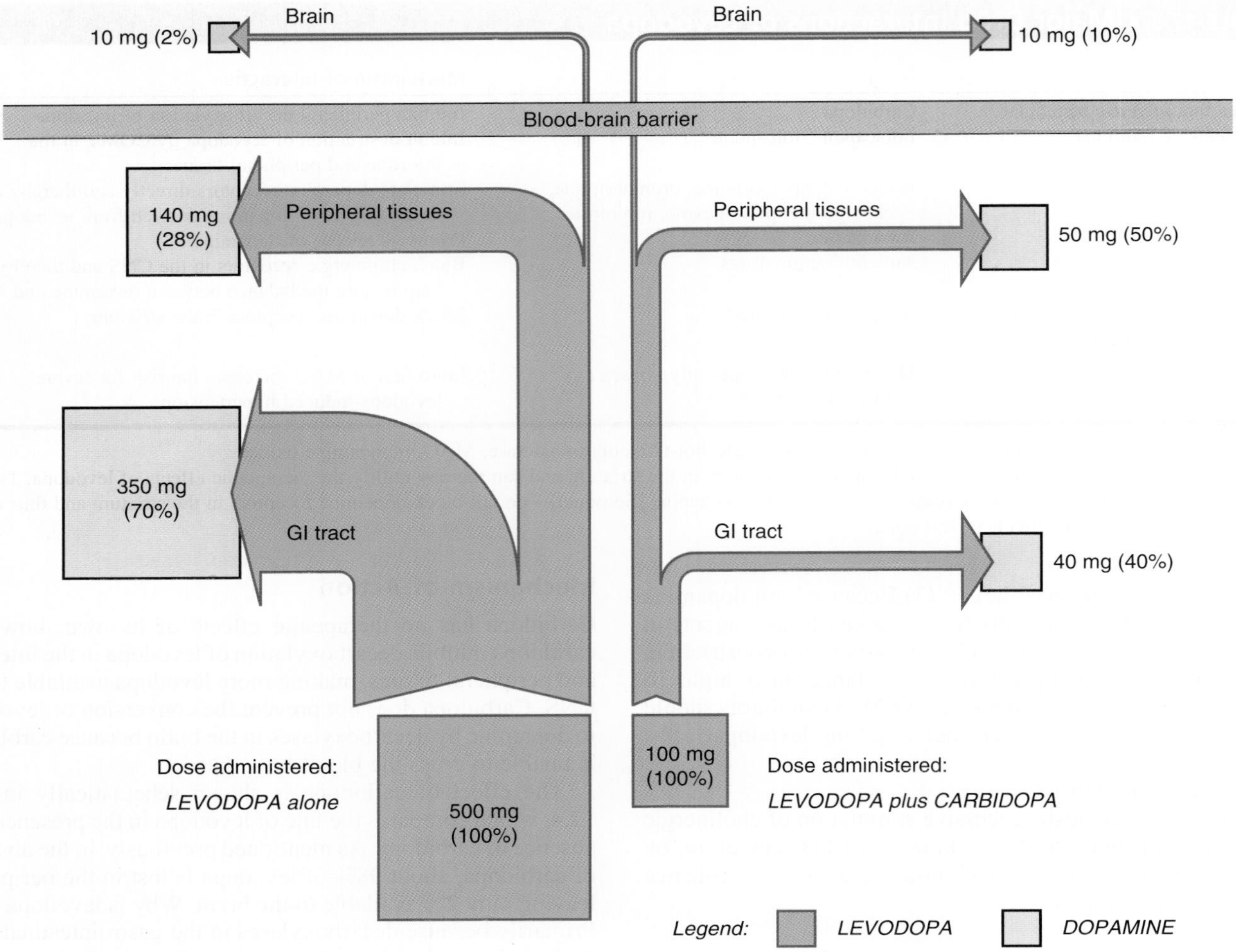

Figure 17.4 ■ Fate of levodopa in the presence and absence of carbidopa. In the absence of carbidopa, 98% of an administered dose of levodopa is metabolized in intestinal and peripheral tissues—either by decarboxylases or COMT—leaving only 2% for actions in the brain. Therefore, to deliver 10 mg of levodopa to the brain, the dose of levodopa must be large (500 mg). By inhibiting intestinal and peripheral decarboxylases, carbidopa increases the percentage of levodopa available to the brain. Thus, the dose needed to deliver 10 mg is greatly reduced (to 100 mg in this example). Since carbidopa cannot cross the blood-brain barrier, it does not suppress conversion of levodopa to dopamine in the brain. Furthermore, since carbidopa reduces peripheral production of dopamine (from 140 mg to 50 mg in this example), peripheral toxicity (nausea, cardiovascular effects) is greatly reduced.

Preparations, Dosage, and Administration

Preparations, dosage, and administration of levodopa/carbidopa, and other drugs used in management of PD are provided in Table 17.4.

Carbidopa Alone

Carbidopa without levodopa, sold as Lodosyn, is available by special request. When carbidopa is added to levodopa/carbidopa, carbidopa can reduce levodopa-induced nausea and vomiting. It also allows smaller doses of levodopa to be used while promoting a more prompt response.

Dopamine Agonists

Dopamine agonists are first-line drugs for PD. Beneficial effects result from direct activation of dopamine receptors in the striatum. For patients with mild or moderate symptoms, dopamine agonists are drugs of first choice. Although dopamine agonists are less effective than levodopa, they still have advantages. Specifically, in contrast to levodopa, they aren't dependent on enzymatic conversion to become active, aren't converted to potentially toxic metabolites, and don't compete with dietary proteins for uptake from the intestine or transport across the blood-brain barrier. In addition, when used long term, dopamine agonists have a lower incidence of response failures and are less likely to cause disabling dyskinesias. However, dopamine agonists do cause serious side effects—especially hallucinations, daytime sleepiness, and postural hypotension. As a result, these drugs are usually reserved for younger patients, who tolerate their side effects better than do the older patients.

The dopamine agonists fall into two groups: derivatives of ergot (an alkaloid found in plants) and nonergot derivatives. The nonergot derivatives—*pramipexole, ropinirole, rotigotine,*

TABLE 17.4 ▪ Preparation, Dosage, and Administration of Drugs for Parkinson Disease

Drug Name	Preparation	Daily Dosage	Administration
LEVODOPA COMBINATIONS			
Levodopa/carbidopa [Sinemet, Rytary, Duopa, Duodopa ♣]	Sinemet (IR): 10 mg carbidopa/100 mg levodopa; 25 mg carbidopa/100 mg levodopa; 25 mg carbidopa/250 mg levodopa Sinemet CR: 25 mg carbidopa/100 mg levodopa; 50 mg carbidopa/200 mg levodopa Rytary: carbidopa 23.75 mg/levodopa 95 mg; carbidopa 36.25 mg/levodopa 145 mg; carbidopa 48.75 mg/levodopa 195 mg; carbidopa 61.25 mg/levodopa 245 mg Duopa enteral suspension: carbidopa 4.63 mg/levodopa 20 mg/mL Duodopa ♣ intestinal gel: carbidopa 5 mg/levodopa 20 mg/1 mL	Dosage is highly individualized. Typical dosage is 1 tablet daily or every other day initially and then gradually increased up to a maximum of 8 tablets a day, regardless of strength, administered in divided doses. Duopa and Duodopa are both highly individualized to the patient with dosage adjustments sometimes made on a daily basis.	Food reduces absorption; give on an empty stomach. Duopa enteral suspension and Duodopa intestinal gel are administered via PEG-J tube infusion.
Levodopa/carbidopa/entacapone [Stalevo]	Stalevo 50: carbidopa 12.5 mg/levodopa 50 mg/ entacapone 200 mg Stalevo 75: carbidopa 18.75 mg/levodopa 75 mg/entacapone 200 mg Stalevo 100: carbidopa 25 mg/levodopa 100 mg/ entacapone 200 mg Stalevo 125: carbidopa 31.25 mg/ levodopa 125 mg/entacapone 200 mg Stalevo 150: carbidopa 37.5 mg/ levodopa 150 mg/entacapone 200 Stalevo 200: carbidopa 50 mg/levodopa 200 mg/entacapone 200 mg	Dosage is highly individualized. Typical dosage is 1 tablet of any strength at each dosing interval up to a maximum daily limit of 8 tablets of Stalevo 50 to Stalevo 150 or 6 tablets of Stalevo 200. Dosing intervals are determined by patient response.	May be given with or without food; however, foods that are high in fat may delay absorption. Tablets should be swallowed whole.
DOPAMINE AGONISTS: ERGOT DERIVATIVES			
Bromocriptine [Cycloset, Parlodel]	Cycloset: 0.8-mg tablet Parlodel: 5-mg capsule	Initial: 1.25 mg twice daily. Gradually increase dosage to achieve desired response or until side effects become intolerable. Maintenance: 30 mg–100 mg/day.	Administer with food or meals to decrease GI symptoms. Cycloset should be administered within 2 hours of awakening.
Cabergoline [Dostinex ♣, generic in U.S.]	0.5-mg tablet	Initial: 1 mg daily. Increase using 0.5–1 mg at 1–2 week intervals. Maintenance: 2–3 mg/day.	Administer with food or meals to decrease GI symptoms.
DOPAMINE AGONISTS: NONERGOT DERIVATIVES			
Pramipexole [Mirapex, Mirapex ER]	IR tablets: 0.125 mg, 0.25 mg, 0.5 mg, 0.75 mg, 1 mg, and 1.5 mg ER tablets: 0.375 mg, 0.75 mg, 1.5 mg, 2.25 mg, 3 mg, and 4.5 mg	IR tablets: 0.125 mg 3 times/day initially, and then increased over 7 weeks to a maximum of 1.5 mg 3 times/day. ER tablets: 0.375 mg once daily initially, and then gradually increased to a maximum of 4.5 mg once daily. Reduced dosage for significant renal impairment.	May be taken with or without food; however, food decreases GI upset. ER formulation should be swallowed whole.
Ropinirole [Requip, Requip XL]	IR tablets: 0.25 mg, 0.5 mg, 1 mg, 2 mg, 3 mg, 4 mg, and 5 mg ER tablets: 2 mg, 4 mg, 6 mg, 8 mg, and 12 mg	IR tablets: 0.25 mg 3 times a day initially. Can increase over several months to a maximum of 8 mg 3 times a day. ER tablets: 2 mg once a day initially. Can increase over several months to a maximum of 24 mg once a day.	May be taken with or without food; however, food decreases GI upset. ER formulation should be swallowed whole.
Rotigotine [Neupro]	24-hour transdermal patch: 1 mg, 2 mg, 3 mg, 4 mg, 6 mg, or 8 mg	Early-stage PD: Usual starting dose is one 2-mg patch every 24 hours. Increase by 2 mg weekly until lowest effective dose is attained or until maximal dose of 6 mg/24 hr. Advanced-stage PD: Usual starting dose is one 4-mg patch every 24 hours. Increased by 2 mg weekly up to a maximum of 8 mg/24 hr. If it becomes necessary to discontinue treatment, withdrawal should be done at the same rate of 2 mg/wk.	Apply to skin that is clean, dry, hairless, and free of abrasions or cuts. To decrease skin reactions, rotate site with each application. Allow at least a 2-week lapse before applying the patch to a site used previously.

Continued

TABLE 17.4 ■ Preparation, Dosage, and Administration of Drugs for Parkinson Disease—cont'd

Drug Name	Preparation	Daily Dosage	Administration
Apomorphine [Apokyn]	10 mg/mL in 3-mL cartridges to be used with a multidose injector pen (provided)	2–6 mg (0.2–0.6 mL) subQ for each "off" episode. Maximum: 5 doses a day	Package labeling states that all patients should take an antiemetic (e.g., trimethobenzamide, 300 mg 3 times a day), starting 3 days before the first apomorphine dose.
COMT INHIBITORS			
Entacapone [Comtan]	200 mg tablets	Initial: 200 mg Can increase to a maximum of 8 doses (1600 mg) a day.	May be taken with or without food. Should be taken with each dose of levodopa/carbidopa.
Tolcapone [Tasmar]	100-mg tablets	100 mg 3 times a day. Increase to 200 mg 3 times a day, if needed.	May be taken with or without food. The first dose should be administered in the morning along with levodopa/carbidopa. The next two doses are taken 6 and 12 hours later.
MAO-B INHIBITORS			
Selegiline [Eldepryl, Zelapar]	Capsule: (Eldepryl, generic): 5 mg Tablet (generic): 5 mg Dispersible tablet (Zelapar): 1.25 mg (A 24-hour patch marketed as Emsam is available, but this is not approved for management of PD.)	5 mg taken with breakfast and lunch, for a total of 10 mg a day. This dosage produces complete inhibition of MAO-B, and hence larger doses are unnecessary. Orally disintegrating tablets: 1.25 mg once a day for 6 weeks. Can increase to a maximal dose of 2.5 mg daily, if needed.	Dispersible tablet should be place on top of tongue and allowed to dissolve. Take dispersible tablet before breakfast and allow at least 5 minutes before drinking or eating after administration.
Rasagiline [Azilect]	0.5- and 1-mg tablets	Monotherapy: usual dosage is 1 mg once a day or 0.5 mg daily for mild hepatic impairment. Adjunctive therapy with levodopa: 0.5 mg daily initially. Increase to 1 mg daily, if needed.	May be taken with or without food.
ANTIVIRAL AGENT			
Amantadine [generic]	Tablet: 100 mg Capsules: 100 mg Syrup: 10 mg/mL	100 mg twice daily initially. May increase to 400 mg/day in divided doses. Dosage for patients taking high doses of other drugs for PD: 100 mg/day initially. May increase to 200 mg/day in divided doses.	May be taken with or without food; however, food decreases GI upset.
CENTRALLY ACTING ANTICHOLINERGIC DRUGS			
Benztropine [Cogentin]	Tablet: 0.5 mg, 1 mg, 2 mg Solution for injection: 1 mg/mL in 2-mL vials	Initial: 0.5–1 mg at bedtime. May increase by 0.5 mg every 5–6 days to a maximal dose of 6 mg/day.	May be taken with or without food. IM injection is preferable because, for PD, IV injection doesn't provide an advantage.
Trihexyphenidyl [generic]	Tablet: 2 mg, 5 mg Elixir: 0.4/mL	Initial: 1 mg once a day. May increase by 2 mg every 3–5 days to a maximal dose of 15 mg/day.	May be taken with or without food.

CR, controlled release; ER, extended release; GI, gastrointestinal; IR, immediate release; PEG, percutaneous endoscopic gastrostomy; PD, Parkinson disease, subQ, subcutaneous.

and *apomorphine*—are highly selective for dopamine receptors. In contrast, the ergot derivatives—*bromocriptine* and *cabergoline*—are less selective: in addition to activating dopamine receptors, these drugs cause mild *blockage* of serotonergic and alpha-adrenergic receptors. Because of their selectivity, the nonergot derivatives cause fewer side effects than the ergot derivatives and hence are preferred.

Prototype Drugs

Dopaminergic Drugs
Levodopa (increases dopamine [DA] synthesis)
Carbidopa (blocks levodopa destruction)
Pramipexole (DA receptor agonist)
Entacapone (inhibits catechol-*O*-methyltransferase)
Selegiline (inhibits monoamine oxidase-B)
Amantadine (promotes DA release)

Centrally Acting Anticholinergic Drugs
Benztropine

Nonergot Derivatives: Pramipexole, Ropinirole, Rotigotine, and Apomorphine

Pramipexole

Actions and Uses. Pramipexole [Mirapex] is a nonergot dopamine receptor agonist. The drug is used alone in early-stage PD and is combined with levodopa in advanced-stage PD. Pramipexole binds selectively to dopamine-2 (D_2) and dopamine-3 (D_3) receptors. Binding to D_2 receptors underlies therapeutic effects. The significance of D_3 binding is unknown. When used as monotherapy in early PD, pramipexole can produce significant improvement in motor performance. When combined with levodopa in advanced PD, the drug can reduce fluctuations in motor control and may permit a reduction in levodopa dosage. In both cases, maximal benefits take several weeks to develop. Compared with levodopa, pramipexole is less effective at controlling motor symptoms of PD, but is also less likely to cause motor fluctuations.

In addition to its use in PD, pramipexole is approved for patients with moderate to severe *restless legs syndrome* (RLS), a sensorimotor disorder characterized by unpleasant leg sensations that create an urge to move the legs in an effort to ease discomfort. Symptoms are usually more intense in the evening and often disrupt sleep. People with severe RLS experience sleep loss, daytime exhaustion, and diminished quality of life.

Pharmacokinetics. Pramipexole is rapidly absorbed, and plasma levels peak in 1 to 2 hours. Food reduces the speed of absorption but not the extent. Pramipexole undergoes wide distribution and achieves a high concentration in red blood cells. The drug is eliminated unchanged in the urine.

Adverse Effects and Interactions. Pramipexole can produce a variety of adverse effects, primarily by activating dopamine receptors. The most common effects seen when pramipexole is used *alone* are nausea, dizziness, daytime somnolence, insomnia, constipation, weakness, and hallucinations. When the drug is *combined with levodopa,* about half of patients experience orthostatic hypotension and dyskinesias, which are not seen when the drug is used by itself. In addition, the incidence of hallucinations nearly doubles.

A few patients have reported *sleep attacks* (overwhelming and irresistible sleepiness that comes on without warning). Sleep attacks can be a real danger for people who are driving. Sleep attacks should not be equated with the normal sleepiness that occurs with dopaminergic agents. Patients who experience a sleep attack should inform their prescriber.

Pramipexole has been associated with *impulse control disorders,* including compulsive gambling, shopping, binge eating, and hypersexuality. These behaviors are dose related, begin about 9 months after starting pramipexole, and reverse when the drug is discontinued. Risk factors include younger adulthood, a family or personal history of alcohol abuse, and a personality trait called novelty seeking, characterized by impulsivity, a quick temper, and a low threshold for boredom. Before prescribing pramipexole, clinicians should screen patients for compulsive behaviors.

Cimetidine (a drug for peptic ulcer disease) can inhibit renal excretion of pramipexole, thereby increasing its blood level.

Ropinirole

Actions, Uses, and Adverse Effects. Ropinirole [Requip], a nonergot dopamine agonist, is similar to pramipexole with respect to receptor specificity, mechanism of action, indications, and adverse effects. Like pramipexole, ropinirole is highly selective for D_2 and D_3 receptors, and both drugs share the same indications: PD and RLS. In patients with PD, ropinirole can be used as monotherapy (in early PD) and as an adjunct to levodopa (in advanced PD). In contrast to pramipexole, which is eliminated entirely by renal excretion, ropinirole is eliminated by hepatic metabolism. Some adverse effects are more common than with pramipexole. When ropinirole is used alone, the most common effects are nausea, dizziness, somnolence, and hallucinations. Rarely, sleep attacks occur. When ropinirole is combined with levodopa, the most important side effects are dyskinesias, hallucinations, and postural hypotension. Note that these occur less frequently than when pramipexole is combined with levodopa. Like pramipexole, ropinirole can promote compulsive gambling, shopping, eating, and hypersexuality. Animal tests indicate that ropinirole can harm the developing fetus. Accordingly, the drug should not be used during pregnancy.

Rotigotine

Actions and Uses. Rotigotine [Neupro] is a nonergot dopamine agonist that is specific for selected dopamine receptors. Although the exact mechanism of action is unknown, it is believed that rotigotine improves dopamine transmission by activating postsynaptic dopamine receptors in the substantia nigra. Rotigotine is approved for management of PD from early to advanced stages. It is also approved for management of moderate to severe primary RLS.

Pharmacokinetics. Because first-pass metabolism of rotigotine is extensive, oral formulations are not manufactured. Rotigotine is currently available as a transdermal patch. The time from application to peak is typically 15 to 18 hours but may range from 4 to 27 hours. Approximately 90% of the drug is protein bound. Rotigotine has a half-life of approximately 5 to 7 hours after patch removal. Excretion occurs in both urine (>70%) and feces.

Adverse Effects. The most common adverse effects are associated with the CNS and neuromuscular systems. These include a variety of sleep disorders, dizziness, headache, dose-related hallucinations, and dose-related dyskinesia. Orthostatic hypotension and peripheral edema may occur. Nausea and vomiting are common, especially when beginning the drug. Some patients develop skin reactions at the site of application, and hyperhidrosis (excessive perspiration) may occur.

Apomorphine

Actions and Therapeutic Use. Apomorphine [Apokyn] is a nonergot dopamine agonist approved for acute treatment of hypomobility during "off" episodes in patients with advanced PD. Unlike other dopamine agonists, the drug is not given by mouth (PO) and is not indicated for routine PD management. When tested in patients experiencing at least 2 hours of "off" time a day, apomorphine produced a 62% improvement in PD rating scores, compared with no improvement in patients receiving placebo. Benefits were sustained during 4 weeks of use. Apomorphine is a derivative of morphine but is devoid of typical opioid effects (e.g., analgesia, euphoria, respiratory depression).

Pharmacokinetics. Apomorphine is highly lipophilic but undergoes extensive first-pass metabolism and hence is ineffective when taken orally. After subcutaneous (subQ) injection, the drug undergoes rapid, complete absorption. Effects begin in 10 to 20 minutes and persist about 1 hour. The drug's half-life is about 40 minutes.

Adverse Effects. The most common adverse effects are injection-site reactions, hallucinations, yawning, drowsiness, dyskinesias, rhinorrhea, and nausea and vomiting. During clinical trials, there was a 4% incidence of serious cardiovascular events: angina, myocardial infarction, cardiac arrest, or sudden death. Postural hypotension and fainting occurred in 2% of patients. Like other dopamine agonists, apomorphine poses a risk for daytime sleep attacks. In addition, apomorphine can promote hypersexuality and enhanced erections (the drug is used in Europe to treat erectile dysfunction). Rarely, apomorphine causes priapism (sustained, painful erection), possibly requiring surgical intervention.

Combined Use With an Antiemetic. To prevent nausea and vomiting during clinical trials, nearly all patients were treated with an antiemetic, starting 3 days before the first dose of apomorphine. The antiemetic chosen was trimethobenzamide [Tigan, others]. Two classes of antiemetics cannot be used: serotonin receptor antagonists (e.g., ondansetron [Zofran]) and dopamine receptor antagonists (e.g., prochlorperazine [Compazine]). Serotonin receptor antagonists will increase the risk for postural hypotension while having no effect on the nausea, and dopamine receptor antagonists will decrease the effectiveness of apomorphine and most other drugs for PD. About half the trial participants discontinued the antiemetic at some point but continued taking apomorphine.

Ergot Derivatives: Bromocriptine and Cabergoline

Two ergot derivatives—bromocriptine and cabergoline—are used to manage PD. Bromocriptine is approved for PD; cabergoline is not. These drugs are poorly tolerated, so their use is limited. The side-effect profile of the ergot derivatives differs from that of the nonergot agents because, in addition to activating dopamine receptors, the ergot drugs cause mild blockade of serotonergic and alpha-adrenergic receptors.

Bromocriptine. Bromocriptine [Cycloset, Parlodel], a derivative of ergot, is a direct-acting dopamine agonist. Beneficial effects derive from activating dopamine receptors in the striatum. Responses are equivalent to those seen with pramipexole and ropinirole. Bromocriptine is used alone in early PD and in combination with levodopa in advanced PD. When combined with levodopa, bromocriptine can prolong therapeutic responses and reduce motor fluctuations. In addition, because bromocriptine allows the dosage of levodopa to be reduced, the incidence of levodopa-induced dyskinesias may be reduced too.

Adverse effects are dose dependent and are seen in 30% to 50% of patients. Nausea is most common. The most common dose-limiting effects are psychological reactions (confusion, nightmares, agitation, hallucinations, paranoid delusions). These occur in about 30% of patients and are most likely when the dosage is high. Like levodopa, bromocriptine can cause dyskinesias and postural hypotension. Rarely, bromocriptine causes retroperitoneal fibrosis, pulmonary infiltrates, a Raynaud-like phenomenon, and erythromelalgia (vasodilation in the feet, and sometimes hands, resulting in swelling, redness, warmth, and burning pain). In addition, the ergot derivatives have been associated with valvular heart disease. The probable cause is activation of serotonin receptors on heart valves.

Cabergoline. Cabergoline, a drug approved for treatment of hyperprolactinemic disorders, is used occasionally in PD, although it is not approved by the U.S. Food and Drug Administration (FDA) for this disorder. According to the AAN guidelines, the drug is "possibly effective" for improving "off" times during levodopa therapy; however, the supporting evidence is weak. Consequently, cabergoline is rarely used unless other management attempts have failed. Common side effects are headaches, dizziness, nausea, and weakness. A more concerning adverse effect is the development of cardiac valve regurgitation and subsequent development of heart failure. Pulmonary and pericardial fibrosis have also occurred.

Catechol-*O*-Methyltransferase Inhibitors

Two COMT inhibitors are available: entacapone and tolcapone. With both drugs, benefits derive from inhibiting metabolism of levodopa in the periphery; these drugs have no direct therapeutic effects of their own. Entacapone is safer and more effective than tolcapone and hence is preferred.

Entacapone

Actions and Therapeutic Use

Entacapone [Comtan] is a selective, reversible inhibitor of COMT indicated only for use with levodopa. Like carbidopa, entacapone inhibits metabolism of levodopa in the intestine and peripheral tissues. However, the drugs inhibit different enzymes: carbidopa inhibits decarboxylases, whereas entacapone inhibits COMT. By inhibiting COMT, entacapone prolongs the plasma half-life of levodopa and thereby prolongs the time that levodopa is available to the brain. In addition, entacapone increases levodopa availability by a second mechanism: By inhibiting COMT, entacapone decreases production of levodopa metabolites that compete with levodopa for transport across the blood-brain barrier. In clinical trials, entacapone increased the half-life of levodopa by 50% to 75% and thereby caused levodopa blood levels to be more stable and sustained. As a result, "wearing off" was delayed and "on" times were extended. Entacapone may also permit a reduction in levodopa dosage.

Pharmacokinetics

Entacapone is rapidly absorbed and reaches peak levels in 2 hours. Elimination is by hepatic metabolism followed by excretion in the feces and urine. The plasma half-life is 1.5 to 3.5 hours.

Adverse Effects

Most adverse effects result from increasing levodopa levels, although some are caused by entacapone itself. By increasing levodopa levels, entacapone can cause dyskinesias, orthostatic hypotension, nausea, hallucinations, sleep disturbances, and impulse control disorders (see "Pramipexole"). These can be managed by decreasing levodopa dosage. Entacopone should not be stopped abruptly, though. Doing so can result in a significant worsening of symptoms.

Entacapone itself has fewer adverse effects. The most common are vomiting, diarrhea, constipation, and yellow-orange discoloration of the urine.

Drug Interactions

Because it inhibits COMT, entacapone can, in theory, increase levels of drugs metabolized by COMT. In addition to levodopa, these include methyldopa (an antihypertensive agent), dobutamine (an adrenergic agonist), and isoproterenol (a beta-adrenergic agonist). If entacapone is combined with these drugs, a reduction in their dosages may be needed.

Tolcapone

Actions and Therapeutic Use

Tolcapone [Tasmar] is a COMT inhibitor used only in conjunction with levodopa—and only if safer agents are ineffective or inappropriate. As with entacapone, benefits derive from inhibiting levodopa metabolism in the periphery, which prolongs levodopa availability. When given to patients taking levodopa, tolcapone improves motor function and may allow a reduction in levodopa dosage. For many patients, the drug reduces the "wearing-off" effect that can occur with levodopa, thereby extending levodopa "on" times by as much as 2.9 hours a day. Unfortunately, although tolcapone is effective, it is also potentially dangerous: deaths from liver failure have occurred. Because it carries a serious risk, tolcapone should be reserved for patients who cannot be treated, or treated adequately, with safer drugs. When tolcapone is used, treatment should be limited to 3 weeks in the absence of a beneficial response.

Pharmacokinetics

Tolcapone is well absorbed after oral dosing. Plasma levels peak in 2 hours. In the blood, tolcapone is highly bound (>99.9%) to plasma proteins. The drug undergoes extensive hepatic metabolism followed by renal excretion. The plasma half-life is 2 to 3 hours.

Adverse Effects

Liver Failure. Tolcapone can cause severe hepatocellular injury, which is sometimes fatal. Because of this risk, a black box warning is mandated by the FDA. Before treatment, patients should be fully apprised of the risks. They also should be informed about signs of emergent liver dysfunction (persistent nausea, fatigue, lethargy, anorexia, jaundice, dark urine) and instructed to report these immediately. Patients with preexisting liver dysfunction should not take the drug. If liver injury is diagnosed, tolcapone should be discontinued and never used again.

BLACK BOX WARNING: TOLCAPONE [TASMAR]

Tolcapone increase the risk for hepatotoxicity. Liver injury and failure may be fatal. Close monitoring is required. Tolcapone should be discontinued if clinical signs or symptoms of liver injury occur or if AST or ALT elevation is twice the upper range of normal.

Laboratory monitoring of liver enzymes is required. Tests for serum alanine aminotransferase (ALT) and aspartate aminotransferase (AST) should be conducted before treatment and then throughout treatment as follows: every 2 weeks for the first year, every 4 weeks for the next 6 months, and every 8 weeks thereafter. If ALT or AST levels exceed the upper limit of normal, tolcapone should be discontinued. Monitoring may not prevent liver injury, but early detection and immediate drug withdrawal can minimize harm.

Other Adverse Effects. By increasing the availability of levodopa, tolcapone can intensify levodopa-related effects, especially dyskinesias, orthostatic hypotension, nausea, hallucinations, sleep disturbances, and impulse control disorders (see "Pramipexole"); a reduction in levodopa dosage may be required. Tolcapone itself can cause diarrhea, hematuria, and yellow-orange discoloration of the urine. Abrupt withdrawal of tolcapone can produce symptoms that resemble neuroleptic malignant syndrome (fever, muscular rigidity, altered consciousness). In rats, large doses have caused renal tubular necrosis and tumors of the kidneys and uterus.

Levodopa/Carbidopa/Entacapone

Levodopa, carbidopa, and entacapone are now available in fixed-dose combinations sold as Stalevo. As discussed earlier, both carbidopa and entacapone inhibit the enzymatic degradation of levodopa and thereby enhance therapeutic effects. The triple combination is more convenient than taking levodopa/carbidopa and entacapone separately, and it costs a little less, too. Unfortunately, Stalevo is available only in immediate-release tablets and only in specific strengths (see Table 17.4).

Patients who need more flexibility in their regimen cannot be treated with Stalevo, nor can patients who require a sustained-release formulation.

Monoamine Oxidase-B Inhibitors

The MAO-B inhibitors—selegiline and rasagiline—are considered first-line drugs for PD even though benefits are modest. When combined with levodopa, they can reduce the wearing-off effect.

Selegiline

Selegiline [Eldepryl, Zelapar], also known as *deprenyl,* was the first MAO inhibitor approved for PD. The drug may be used alone or in combination with levodopa. In both cases, improvement of motor function is modest. There is some evidence suggesting that selegiline may delay neurodegeneration and hence may delay disease progression. However, conclusive proof of neuroprotection is lacking. Nonetheless, current guidelines suggest trying selegiline in newly diagnosed patients, just in case the drug *does* confer some protection.

Actions and Use

Selegiline causes *selective, irreversible* inhibition of MAO-B, the enzyme that inactivates dopamine in the striatum. Another form of MAO, known as monoamine oxidase-A (MAO-A), inactivates NE and serotonin. As discussed in Chapter 25, nonselective inhibitors of MAO (i.e., drugs that inhibit MAO-A *and* MAO-B) are used to treat depression—and pose a risk for hypertensive crisis as a side effect. Because selegiline is a selective inhibitor of MAO-B, the drug is not an antidepressant and, *at recommended doses,* poses little or no risk for hypertensive crisis.

Selegiline appears to benefit patients with PD in two ways. First, when used as an adjunct to levodopa, selegiline can suppress destruction of dopamine derived from levodopa. The mechanism is inhibition of MAO-B. By helping preserve dopamine, selegiline can prolong the effects of levodopa and can thereby decrease fluctuations in motor control. Unfortunately, these benefits decline dramatically within 12 to 24 months.

In addition to preserving dopamine, there is some hope that selegiline may delay the progression of PD. When used early in the disease, selegiline can delay the need for levodopa. This may reflect a delay in the progression of the disease, or it may simply reflect direct symptomatic relief from selegiline itself.

If selegiline does slow the progression of PD, what might be the mechanism? In experimental animals, selegiline can prevent development of parkinsonism after exposure to 1-methyl-4-phenyl-1,2,3,6-tetrahydropyridine (MPTP), a neurotoxin that causes selective degeneration of dopaminergic neurons. (Humans accidentally exposed to MPTP develop severe parkinsonism.) Neuronal degeneration is not caused by MPTP itself, but rather by a toxic metabolite. Formation of this metabolite is catalyzed by MAO-B. By inhibiting MAO-B, selegiline prevents formation of the toxic metabolite and thereby protects against neuronal injury. If selegiline delays progression of PD, this mechanism could explain the effect. That is, just as selegiline protects animals by suppressing formation of a neurotoxic metabolite of MPTP, the drug may delay progression of PD by suppressing formation of a neurotoxic metabolite of an as-yet unidentified compound.

Pharmacokinetics

For treatment of PD, selegiline is available in two oral formulations (tablets and capsules) and in orally disintegrating tablets (ODTs).

Tablets and Capsules. Selegiline in tablets [generic only] and capsules [Eldepryl] undergoes rapid GI absorption, travels to the brain, and quickly penetrates the blood-brain barrier. Irreversible inhibition of MAO-B follows. Selegiline undergoes hepatic metabolism followed by renal excretion. Two metabolites—l-amphetamine and l-methamphetamine—are CNS stimulants. These metabolites, which do not appear to have therapeutic effects, can be harmful. Because selegiline causes irreversible inhibition of MAO-B, effects persist until more MAO-B can be synthesized.

Orally Disintegrating Tablets. Unlike selegiline in tablets and capsules, which is absorbed from the GI tract, selegiline in ODTs [Zelapar] is absorbed through the oral mucosa. As a result, bioavailability is higher than with tablets and capsules, and hence doses can be lower. Otherwise, the pharmacokinetics of selegiline in ODTs, tablets, and capsules are identical.

Adverse Effects

When selegiline is used alone, the principal adverse effect is insomnia, presumably because of CNS excitation by amphetamine and methamphetamine. Insomnia can be minimized by administering the last daily dose no later than noon. Other adverse effects include orthostatic hypotension, dizziness, and GI symptoms. Patients taking selegiline ODTs may experience irritation of the buccal mucosa.

Hypertensive Crisis. Although selegiline is selective for MAO-B, high doses can inhibit MAO-A, which creates a risk for hypertensive crisis, especially in younger patients. As discussed in Chapter 25, when a patient is taking an MAO inhibitor, hypertensive crisis can be triggered by ingesting foods that contain tyramine and by taking certain drugs, including sympathomimetics. Accordingly, patients should be instructed to avoid these foods and drugs, both while taking selegiline and for 2 weeks after stopping it.

BLACK BOX WARNING: SELEGILINE [ELDEPRYL, EMSAM, ZELAPAR]

Antidepressants are associated with an increased risk for suicide in patients younger than 24 years. Selegiline, an antidepressant as well as a drug for PD, is included in this warning.

Selegiline carries an increased risk for hypertensive crisis in younger patients and is contraindicated for children younger than 12 years.

Drug Interactions

Levodopa. When used with levodopa, selegiline can intensify adverse responses to levodopa-derived dopamine. These reactions—orthostatic hypotension, dyskinesias, and psychological disturbances (hallucinations, confusion)—can be reduced by decreasing the dosage of levodopa.

Meperidine. Like the nonselective MAO inhibitors, selegiline can cause a dangerous interaction with meperidine [Demerol]. Symptoms include stupor, rigidity, agitation, and hyperthermia. The combination should be avoided.

Selective Serotonin Reuptake Inhibitors (SSRIs). Selegiline should not be combined with SSRIs such as fluoxetine [Prozac]. The combination of an MAO-B inhibitor plus an SSRI can cause fatal serotonin syndrome. Accordingly, SSRIs should be withdrawn at least 5 weeks before giving selegiline.

Rasagiline

Actions and Therapeutic Use

Rasagiline [Azilect] is another MAO-B inhibitor for PD. Like selegiline, rasagiline is a selective, irreversible inhibitor of MAO-B. Benefits derive from preserving dopamine in the brain. The drug is approved for initial monotherapy of PD and for combined use with levodopa. Rasagiline is similar to selegiline in most regards. As with selegiline, benefits are modest. The drugs differ primarily in that rasagiline is not converted to amphetamine or methamphetamine.

Pharmacokinetics

Rasagiline is rapidly absorbed, with a bioavailability of 36%. In the liver, the drug undergoes nearly complete metabolism by CYP1A2 (the 1A2 isozyme of cytochrome P450). Hepatic impairment and drugs that inhibit CYP1A2 will delay metabolism of rasagiline, causing blood levels of the drug to rise. The drug should be decreased by half in mild hepatic impairment. *Patients with moderate to severe hepatic impairment should not use this drug.*

In contrast to selegiline, rasagiline is not metabolized to amphetamine derivatives. Excretion is primarily through the urine (62%) and feces (7%). The plasma half-life is 3 hours. However, because rasagiline causes irreversible inhibition of MAO-B, clinical effects persist until new MAO-B is synthesized.

Adverse Effects

When used as monotherapy, rasagiline is generally well tolerated. The most common side effects are headache, arthralgia, dyspepsia, depression, and flu-like symptoms. Unlike selegiline, rasagiline does not cause insomnia.

When rasagiline is combined with levodopa, side effects increase. The most common additional reactions are dyskinesias, accidental injury, nausea, orthostatic hypotension, constipation, weight loss, and hallucinations. Like selegiline, rasagiline may pose a risk for hypertensive crisis (owing to inhibition of MAO-A, especially at higher doses), and hence patients should be instructed to avoid tyramine-containing foods and certain drugs, including sympathomimetic agents.

Rasagiline may increase the risk for malignant melanoma, a potentially deadly cancer of the skin. Periodic monitoring of the skin is recommended.

Drug and Food Interactions

Rasagiline has the potential to interact adversely with multiple drugs. Drugs that should be used with caution include the following:

- *Levodopa.* Like selegiline, rasagiline can intensify adverse responses to levodopa-derived dopamine. If the patient develops dopaminergic side effects, including dyskinesias or hallucinations, reducing the dosage of levodopa, not rasagiline, should be considered.
- *CYP1A2 inhibitors,* Blood levels of rasagiline can be raised by ciprofloxacin and other drugs that inhibit CYP1A2, the hepatic enzyme that inactivates rasagiline. For patients taking these drugs, the daily dosage should be reduced.

Drugs and foods that are contraindicated include the following:

- *MAO inhibitors.* Combining rasagiline with another MAO inhibitor increases the risk for hypertensive crisis. At least 2 weeks should separate use of these drugs.
- *Sympathomimetics.* These drugs (e.g., amphetamines, ephedrine, phenylephrine, pseudoephedrine) increase the risk for hypertensive crisis and must be avoided.
- *Tyramine-containing foods.* These agents increase the risk for hypertensive crisis and must be avoided.
- *Antidepressants.* Combining rasagiline with mirtazapine, SSRIs, serotonin-norepinephrine reuptake inhibitors, and tricyclic antidepressants may pose a risk for hyperpyrexia and death. These drugs should be discontinued at least 2 weeks before starting rasagiline. Fluoxetine (an SSRI) should be discontinued at least 5 weeks before starting rasagiline.
- *Analgesics.* Combining rasagiline with meperidine, methadone, or tramadol may pose a risk for serious reactions, including coma, respiratory depression, convulsions, hypertension, hypotension, and even death. At least 2 weeks should separate use of these drugs.
- *Dextromethorphan.* Combining rasagiline with dextromethorphan may pose a risk for brief episodes of psychosis and bizarre behavior.
- *Cyclobenzaprine.* This drug is structurally related to the tricyclic antidepressants, so it should be avoided.

Amantadine

Actions and Uses

Amantadine [generic], formerly available as Symmetrel, was developed as an antiviral agent and was later found effective in PD. Possible mechanisms include inhibition of dopamine uptake, stimulation of dopamine release, blockade of cholinergic receptors, antagonism of *N*-methyl-D-aspartate (NMDA) receptors, and blockade of glutamate receptors. Responses develop rapidly—often within 2 to 3 days—but are much less profound than with levodopa or the dopamine agonists. Furthermore, responses may begin to diminish within 3 to 6 months. Accordingly, amantadine is not considered a first-line agent. However, the drug may be helpful for managing dyskinesias caused by levodopa.

Adverse Effects

Amantadine can cause adverse CNS effects (confusion, lightheadedness, anxiety) and peripheral effects that are thought to result from muscarinic blockade (blurred vision, urinary retention, dry mouth, constipation). All of these are generally mild when amantadine is used alone. However, if amantadine is combined with an anticholinergic agent, both the CNS and peripheral responses will be intensified.

Patients taking amantadine for 1 month or longer often develop livedo reticularis, a condition characterized by mottled discoloration of the skin. Livedo reticularis is benign and gradually subsides after amantadine withdrawal.

Amantadine often loses effectiveness after several months. If effects diminish, they can be restored by increasing the dosage or by interrupting treatment for several weeks.

Centrally Acting Anticholinergic Drugs

Anticholinergic drugs have been used in PD since 1867, making them the oldest medicines for this disease. These drugs alleviate symptoms by blocking muscarinic receptors in the striatum, thereby improving the balance between dopamine and acetylcholine. Anticholinergic drugs can reduce tremor and possibly rigidity, but not bradykinesia. These drugs are less effective than levodopa or the dopamine agonists but are better tolerated. Today, anticholinergics are used as second-line therapy for tremor. They are most appropriate for younger patients with mild symptoms. Anticholinergics are generally avoided in older patients, who are intolerant of CNS side effects (sedation, confusion, delusions, and hallucinations).

Although the anticholinergic drugs used today are somewhat selective for cholinergic receptors in the CNS, they can also block cholinergic receptors in the periphery. As a result, they can cause dry mouth, blurred vision, photophobia, urinary retention, constipation, and tachycardia. These effects are usually dose limiting. Blockade of cholinergic receptors in the eye may precipitate or aggravate glaucoma. Accordingly, intraocular pressure should be measured periodically. Peripheral anticholinergic effects are discussed in Chapter 12.

The anticholinergic agents used most often are benztropine [Cogentin] and trihexyphenidyl, formerly available as Artane. Providers need to be aware that if anticholinergic drugs are discontinued abruptly, symptoms of parkinsonism may be intensified.

NONMOTOR SYMPTOMS AND THEIR MANAGEMENT

In addition to experiencing characteristic motor symptoms, about 90% of patients with PD develop nonmotor symptoms, notably autonomic disturbances, sleep disturbances, depression, dementia, and psychosis. Management is addressed in two evidence-based AAN guidelines: *Practice Parameter: Evaluation and Treatment of Depression, Psychosis, and Dementia in Parkinson Disease* and *Practice Parameter: Treatment of Nonmotor Symptoms of Parkinson Disease.*

Autonomic Symptoms

Disruption of autonomic function can produce a variety of symptoms, including constipation, urinary incontinence, drooling, orthostatic hypotension, cold intolerance, and erectile dysfunction. The intensity of these symptoms increases in parallel with the intensity of motor symptoms. Erectile function can be managed with sildenafil [Viagra] and other inhibitors of type 5 phosphodiesterase (see Chapter 51). Orthostatic hypotension can be improved by increasing intake of salt and fluid, and possibly by taking fludrocortisone, a mineralocorticoid. Urinary incontinence may improve with oxybutynin and other peripherally acting anticholinergic drugs (see Chapter 12). Constipation can be managed by getting regular exercise and maintaining adequate intake of fluid and fiber. Polyethylene glycol (an osmotic laxative) or a stool softener (e.g., docusate) may also be tried (see Chapter 63).

Sleep Disturbances

PD is associated with excessive daytime sleepiness (EDS), periodic limb movements of sleep (PLMS), and insomnia (difficulty falling asleep and staying asleep). EDS may respond to modafinil [Provigil, Alertec ♣], a nonamphetamine CNS stimulant (see Chapter 29). For PLMS, levodopa/carbidopa should be considered; the nonergot dopamine agonists—pramipexole and ropinirole—may also help. Insomnia may be improved by levodopa/carbidopa and melatonin (see Chapter 27). Levodopa/carbidopa helps by reducing motor symptoms that can impair sleep. Melatonin helps by making people feel they are sleeping better, even though objective measures of sleep quality may not improve.

Depression

About 50% of PD patients develop depression, partly in reaction to having a debilitating disease and partly due to the disease process itself. According to the AAN guidelines, only one drug—amitriptyline—has been proved effective in these patients. Unfortunately, amitriptyline, a tricyclic antidepressant, has anticholinergic effects that can exacerbate dementia and antiadrenergic effects that can exacerbate orthostatic hypotension. Data for other antidepressants, including SSRIs and bupropion, are insufficient to prove or disprove efficacy in PD.

Dementia

Dementia occurs in 40% of PD patients. The AAN guidelines recommend considering treatment with two drugs: donepezil and rivastigmine. Both drugs are cholinesterase inhibitors developed for Alzheimer disease (see Chapter 18). In patients with PD, these drugs can produce a modest improvement in cognitive function, without causing significant worsening of motor symptoms, even though these drugs increase availability of acetylcholine at central synapses.

Psychosis

In patients with PD, psychosis is usually caused by the drugs taken to control motor symptoms. Most of these drugs—levodopa, dopamine agonists, amantadine, and anticholinergic drugs—can cause hallucinations. Therefore, if psychosis develops, dopamine agonists, amantadine, and anticholinergic drugs should be withdrawn, and the dosage of levodopa should be reduced to the lowest effective amount. If antipsychotic medication is needed, first-generation antipsychotics should be avoided because all of these drugs block receptors for dopamine and hence can intensify motor symptoms. Accordingly, the AAN guidelines recommend considering two second-generation antipsychotics: clozapine and quetiapine. Because clozapine can cause agranulocytosis, many clinicians prefer quetiapine. The guidelines recommend against routine use of olanzapine, another second-generation agent. The antipsychotic drugs are discussed in Chapter 24.

PRESCRIBING AND MONITORING CONSIDERATIONS

Levodopa/Carbidopa [Sinemet, Parcopa]

Therapeutic Goal

The goal of treatment is to improve the patient's ability to carry out activities of daily living. Levodopa does not cure PD or delay its progression.

Baseline Data

Assess motor symptoms—bradykinesia, akinesia, postural instability, tremor, rigidity—and the extent to which they interfere with activities of daily living (e.g., ability to work, dress, bathe, walk).

Identifying High-Risk Patients

Because some studies suggest that levodopa and MAO inhibitors can activate malignant melanoma, for patients taking these drugs it is important to perform a careful skin assessment and to monitor the skin for changes.

Exercise *caution* in patients with cardiac disease and psychiatric disorders and in patients taking selective MAO-B inhibitors.

Administration Concerns

Motor symptoms may make self-medication challenging. The patient may require assistive devices for opening medication containers. Request pharmacist to avoid using childproof containers. If appropriate, involve family members in medicating outpatients.

Ongoing Monitoring and Interventions

Evaluating Therapeutic Effects

Evaluate for improvements in activities of daily living and for reductions in bradykinesia, postural instability, tremor, and rigidity.

Managing Acute Loss of Effect

"Off" times can be reduced by combining levodopa/carbidopa with a dopamine agonist (e.g., pramipexole), a COMT inhibitor (e.g., entacapone), or an MAO-B inhibitor (e.g., rasagiline). Notify the prescribing specialist of increasing problems.

Minimizing Adverse Effects

Nausea and Vomiting. Recommend that medications be taken with food if nausea and vomiting are a problem.

Dyskinesias. Giving amantadine may help with dyskinesias. Consult the prescribing specialist about a possible reduction in dosage.

Orthostatic Hypotension and Dysrhythmias. Monitor orthostatic vital signs at each clinic visit. If the patient reports palpitations or if dysrhythmias are suspected, an ECG or monitoring may be indicated. Notify the prescriber of the development of new dysrhythmias.

Psychosis. Notify the prescriber of psychosis or other mental status changes. The prescriber may recommend treatment with clozapine or quetiapine.

Minimizing Adverse Interactions

First-Generation Antipsychotic Drugs. These can block responses to levodopa and should be avoided. Two second-generation antipsychotics—clozapine and quetiapine—can be used safely.

MAO Inhibitors. Concurrent use of levodopa and a nonselective MAO inhibitor can produce severe hypertension. Withdraw nonselective MAO inhibitors at least 2 weeks before initiating levodopa.

Anticholinergic Drugs. These can enhance therapeutic responses to levodopa, but they also increase the risk for adverse psychiatric effects.

High-Protein Meals. Amino acids compete with levodopa for absorption from the intestine and for transport across the blood-brain barrier.

Dopamine Agonists

Therapeutic Goal

The goal of treatment is to improve the patient's ability to carry out activities of daily living. Dopamine agonists do not cure PD or delay its progression.

Apomorphine is reserved for rescue treatment of hypomobility during "off" episodes in patients with advanced PD.

Baseline Data

Assess motor symptoms—bradykinesia, akinesia, postural instability, tremor, rigidity—and the extent to which these interfere with activities of daily living (e.g., ability to work, dress, bathe, walk).

Identifying High-Risk Patients

Use *all dopamine agonists* with *caution* in older-adult patients and in those with psychiatric disorders. Use *pramipexole* with *caution* in patients with kidney dysfunction. Avoid *ropinirole* during pregnancy. Use *pramipexole* and *ropinirole* with *caution* in patients prone to compulsive behavior.

Administration Concerns

Parkinsonism may make self-medication difficult. Assistive devices may be needed. If appropriate, involve family members in medicating outpatients.

To minimize adverse effects, dosage should be low initially and then gradually increased.

Reduce dosage of pramipexole in patients with significant renal dysfunction.

Ongoing Evaluation and Interventions

Evaluating Therapeutic Effects

Evaluate for improvements in activities of daily living and for reductions in bradykinesia, postural instability, tremor, and rigidity.

Minimizing Adverse Effects

Nausea and Vomiting. Nausea and vomiting and orthostatic hypotension are addressed through teaching. (See Patient Education: Dopamine Agonists). If symptoms persist or if other complications occur (e.g., dyskinesias, hallucinations, or sleep attacks), the prescriber should be notified. Medication adjustments may be necessary.

Patient Education

DOPAMINE AGONISTS

Inform patients that nausea and vomiting can be reduced by taking oral dopamine agonists with food. Instruct them to notify the prescriber if nausea and vomiting persist or become severe. Patients taking apomorphine may pretreat with trimethobenzamide [Tigan], an antiemetic.

Inform patients about symptoms of orthostatic hypotension (dizziness, lightheadedness on standing) and advise them to sit or lie down if these occur. Advise patients to move slowly when sitting up or standing up.

Explain about the potential for movement disorders (tremor, dystonic movements, twitching) and instruct patients to notify the prescriber if these develop.

Forewarn patients that dopamine agonists can cause hallucinations, especially in older adults, and instruct them to notify the prescriber if these develop.

Warn patients that pramipexole, ropinirole, rotigotine, and apomorphine may cause sleep attacks. If a sleep attack occurs, patients should inform the prescriber and avoid potentially hazardous activities (e.g., driving).

Inform patients of childbearing age that ropinirole may harm the developing fetus, and advise them to use effective birth control.

Fetal Injury. If pregnancy occurs and will be continued, switching to a dopamine agonist other than ropinirole is advised.

Impulse Control Disorders. *Pramipexole* and *ropinirole* may induce *compulsive, self-rewarding behaviors,* including compulsive gambling, eating, shopping, and hypersexuality. Risk factors include relative youth, a family or personal history of alcohol abuse, and a novelty-seeking personality. Before prescribing these drugs, clinicians should screen patient for compulsive behaviors.

CHAPTER

18 Drugs for Alzheimer Disease

Jacqueline Rosenjack Burchum, DNSc, FNP-BC, CNE

Alzheimer disease (AD) is a devastating illness characterized by progressive memory loss, impaired thinking, neuropsychiatric symptoms (e.g., hallucinations, delusions), and inability to perform routine tasks of daily living. More than 5 million older Americans have AD. It is the sixth leading cause of death, with an annual cost of about $226 billion. Major pathologic findings are cerebral atrophy, degeneration of cholinergic neurons, and the presence of neuritic plaques and neurofibrillary tangles—all of which begin to develop years before clinical symptoms appear. This neuronal damage is irreversible, so AD cannot be cured. Drugs in current use do little to relieve symptoms or prevent neuronal loss. Furthermore, for many patients there is no significant delay in the progression of AD or cognitive decline.

PATHOPHYSIOLOGY

The underlying cause of AD is still unknown. Scientists have discovered important pieces of the AD puzzle, but still don't know how they fit together. It may well be that AD results from a combination of factors, rather than from a single cause.

Degeneration of Neurons

Neuronal degeneration occurs in the hippocampus early in AD, followed later by degeneration of neurons in the cerebral cortex and subsequent decline in cerebral volume. The hippocampus serves an important role in memory. The cerebral cortex is central to speech, perception, reasoning, and other higher functions. As hippocampal neurons degenerate, short-term memory begins to fail. As cortical neurons degenerate, patients begin having difficulty with language. With advancing cortical degeneration, more severe symptoms appear. These include complete loss of speech, loss of bladder and bowel control, and complete inability for self-care. AD eventually destroys enough brain function to cause death.

Reduced Cholinergic Transmission

In patients with advanced AD, levels of acetylcholine are 90% below normal. Loss of acetylcholine is significant for two reasons. First, acetylcholine is an important transmitter in the hippocampus and cerebral cortex, regions where neuronal degeneration occurs. Second, acetylcholine is critical to forming memories, and its decline has been linked to memory loss. However, cholinergic transmission is essentially normal in patients with mild AD. Hence, loss of cholinergic function cannot explain the cognitive deficits that occur early in the disease process.

Beta-Amyloid and Neuritic Plaques

Neuritic plaques, which form outside of neurons, are a hallmark of AD. These spherical bodies are composed of a central core of *beta-amyloid* (a protein fragment) surrounded by neuron remnants. Neuritic plaques are seen mainly in the hippocampus and cerebral cortex.

In patients with AD, beta-amyloid is present in high levels and may contribute to neuronal injury. Accumulation of beta-amyloid begins early in the disease process, perhaps 10 to 20 years before the first symptoms of AD appear. Because of the central role that beta-amyloid appears to play in AD, treatments directed against beta-amyloid are in development.

Neurofibrillary Tangles and Tau

Like neuritic plaques, neurofibrillary tangles are a prominent feature of AD. These tangles, which form inside of neurons, result when the orderly arrangement of microtubules becomes disrupted (Fig. 18.1). The underlying cause is production of an abnormal form of tau, a protein that, in healthy neurons, forms cross-bridges between microtubules and thereby keeps their configuration stable. In patients with AD, tau twists into paired helical filaments that form tangles.

Apolipoprotein E4

Apolipoprotein E (apoE), long known for its role in cholesterol transport, may also contribute to AD. ApoE has three forms, named apoE2, apoE3, and apoE4. Only one form—apoE4—is associated with AD. Genetic research has shown that individuals with one or two copies of the gene that codes for apoE4 are at increased risk for AD; however, many people with AD do not have the gene for apoE4.

Endoplasmic Reticulum–Associated Binding Protein

The discovery of endoplasmic reticulum–associated binding protein (ERAB) adds another piece to the AD puzzle. ERAB is present in high concentration in the brains of patients with AD. These high concentrations of ERAB enhance the neurotoxic effects of beta-amyloid.

Homocysteine

Elevated plasma levels of homocysteine are associated with an increased risk for AD. Fortunately, the risk can be easily reduced: levels of homocysteine can be lowered by eating foods rich in folic acid and vitamins B_6 and B_{12}, or by taking dietary supplements that contain these compounds.

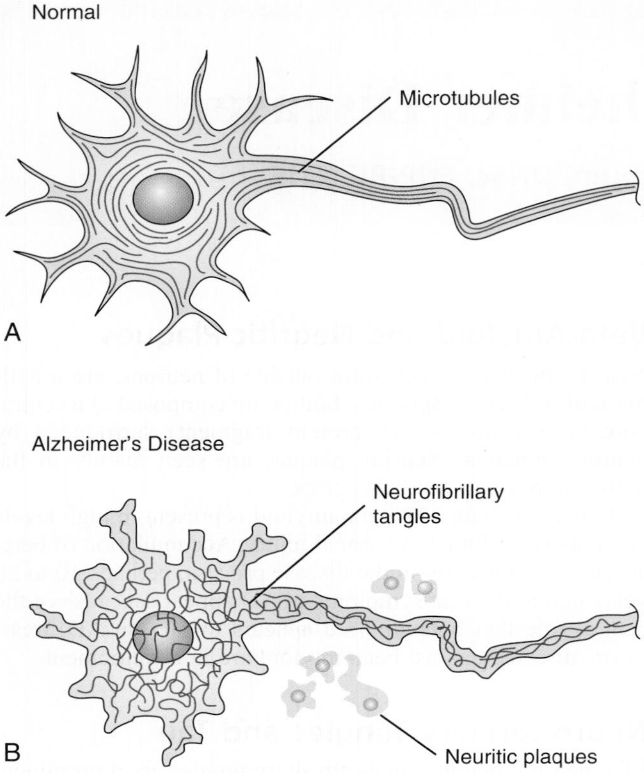

Figure 18.1 ▪ Histologic changes in Alzheimer disease. **A,** Healthy neuron. **B,** Neuron affected by Alzheimer disease, showing characteristic intracellular neurofibrillary tangles. Note also extracellular neuritic plaques.

RISK FACTORS AND SYMPTOMS

Risk Factors

The major known risk factor for AD is advancing age. In 90% of patients, the age of onset is 65 years or older. After age 65 years, the risk for AD increases exponentially, doubling every 10 years until age 85 to 90 years, after which the risk for getting AD levels off or declines. The only other known risk factor is a family history of AD. Being female *may* be a risk factor. However, the higher incidence of AD in women may occur simply because women generally live longer than men. Other possible risk factors include head injury, low educational level, production of apoE4, high levels of homocysteine, low levels of folic acid, estrogen/progestin therapy, sedentary lifestyle, and nicotine in cigarette smoke.

Symptoms

AD is a disease in which symptoms progress relentlessly from mild to moderate to severe (Table 18.1). Symptoms typically begin after age 65 years but may appear in people as young as 40 years. Early in the disease, patients begin to experience memory loss and confusion. They may be disoriented and get lost in familiar surroundings. Judgment becomes impaired, and personality may change. As the disease progresses, patients have increasing difficulty with self-care. Between 70% and 90% eventually develop behavior problems (wandering, pacing, agitation, screaming). Symptoms may intensify in the evening, a phenomenon known as *sundowning*. In the final stages of AD, the patient is unable to recognize close family members or communicate in any way. All sense of identity is lost, and the individual is completely dependent on others for survival. The time from onset of symptoms to death may be 20 years or longer, but it is usually 4 to 8 years. Although there is no clearly effective therapy for *core symptoms,* other symptoms (e.g., incontinence, depression) can be treated.

TABLE 18.1 ▪ Symptoms of Alzheimer Disease

MILD SYMPTOMS	Confusion and memory loss Disorientation; getting lost in familiar surroundings Problems with routine tasks Changes in personality and judgment
MODERATE SYMPTOMS	Difficulty with activities of daily living, such as feeding and bathing Anxiety, suspiciousness, agitation Sleep disturbances Wandering, pacing Difficulty recognizing family and friends
SEVERE SYMPTOMS	Loss of speech Loss of appetite; weight loss Loss of bladder and bowel control Total dependence on caregiver

DRUGS FOR COGNITIVE IMPAIRMENT

Ideally, the goal of AD treatment is to improve symptoms and reverse cognitive decline (See Fig. 18.2). Unfortunately, available drugs cannot do this. At best, drugs currently in use may slow loss of memory and cognition and prolong independent function. However, for many patients, even these modest goals are elusive.

Four drugs are approved for treating AD dementia. Three of the drugs—donepezil, galantamine, and rivastigmine—are cholinesterase inhibitors. The fourth drug—memantine—blocks neuronal receptors for *N*-methyl-D-aspartate (NMDA). Treatment of dementia with these drugs can yield improvement that is statistically significant but clinically marginal. As one expert put it, benefits of these drugs are equivalent to losing half a pound after taking a weight loss drug for 6 months. Given the modest benefits of these drugs, evidence-based clinical guidelines do not recommend that all patients receive drug therapy; this decision is left to the patient, family, and prescriber. No single drug is more effective than the others, so selection should be based on tolerability, ease of use, and cost. Research has not established an optimal treatment duration. Properties of the cholinesterase inhibitors and memantine are shown in Table 18.2.

Cholinesterase Inhibitors

The cholinesterase inhibitors were the first drugs approved by the U.S. Food and Drug Administration (FDA) to treat AD. Three cholinesterase inhibitors are available.

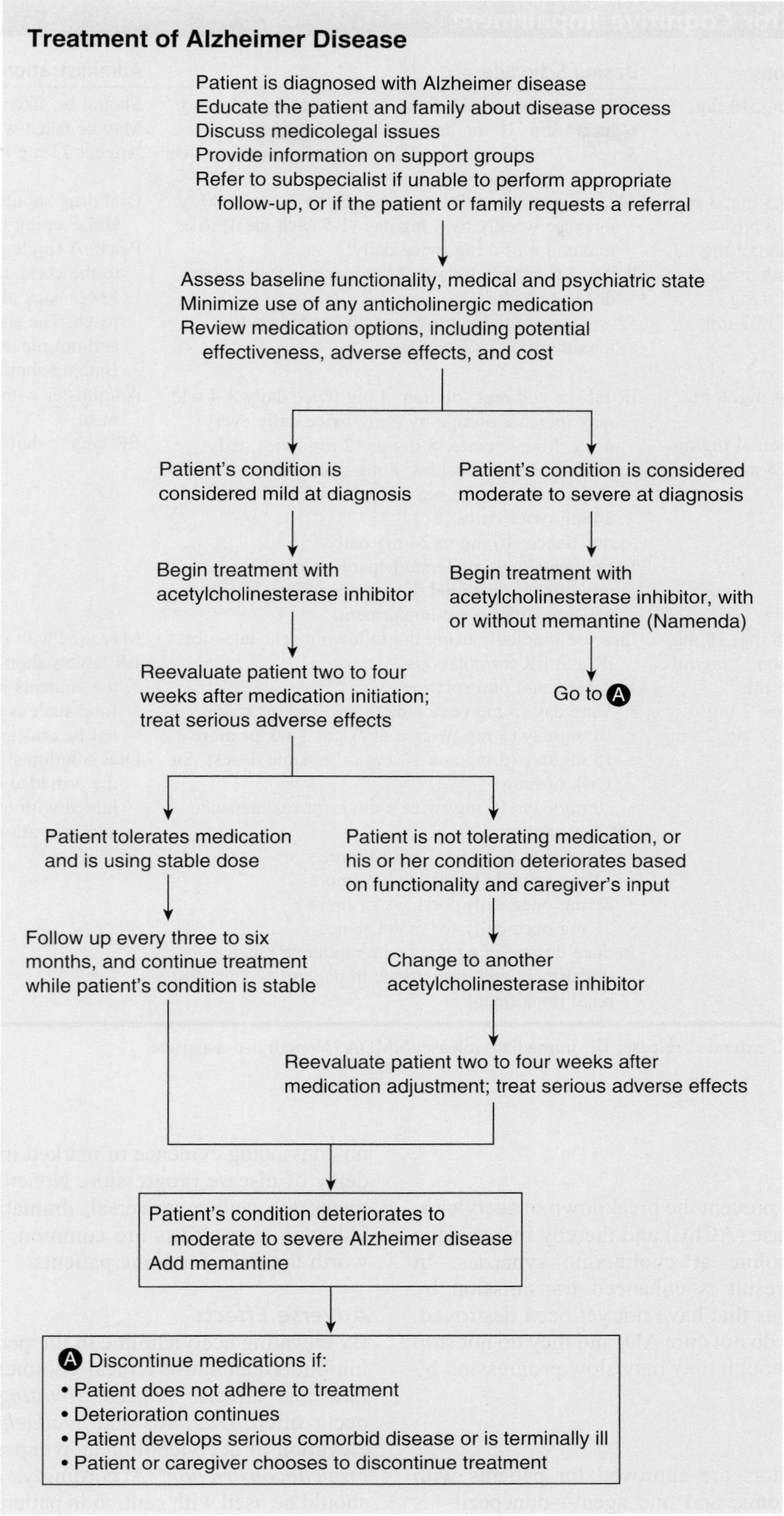
Treatment of Alzheimer Disease
Patient is diagnosed with Alzheimer disease
Educate the patient and family about disease process
Discuss medicolegal issues
Provide information on support groups
Refer to subspecialist if unable to perform appropriate follow-up, or if the patient or family requests a referral
Assess baseline functionality, medical and psychiatric state
Minimize use of any anticholinergic medication
Review medication options, including potential effectiveness, adverse effects, and cost
Patient's condition is considered mild at diagnosis
Patient's condition is considered moderate to severe at diagnosis
Begin treatment with acetylcholinesterase inhibitor
Begin treatment with acetylcholinesterase inhibitor, with or without memantine (Namenda)
Reevaluate patient two to four weeks after medication initiation; treat serious adverse effects
Go to A
Patient tolerates medication and is using stable dose
Patient is not tolerating medication, or his or her condition deteriorates based on functionality and caregiver's input
Follow up every three to six months, and continue treatment while patient's condition is stable
Change to another acetylcholinesterase inhibitor
Reevaluate patient two to four weeks after medication adjustment; treat serious adverse effects
Patient's condition deteriorates to moderate to severe Alzheimer disease
Add memantine
A Discontinue medications if:
• Patient does not adhere to treatment
• Deterioration continues
• Patient develops serious comorbid disease or is terminally ill
• Patient or caregiver chooses to discontinue treatment

Figure 18.2 ■ Source: American Family Physician available online at http://www.aafp.org/afp/2011/0615/p1403.pdf.

TABLE 18.2 ▪ Drugs for Cognitive Impairment

Drug	Preparations	Dosing Schedule	Administration
Donepezil [Aricept]	Tablet: 5 mg, 10 mg, 23 mg	*Mild to moderate AD:* 5 mg daily. After 4-6 wk, may increase to 10 mg daily *Severe AD:* 10 mg daily. After 3 months, may increase to 23 mg daily	Should be taken at bedtime. May be taken with or without food. Aricept 23 mg must be swallowed whole.
Rivastigmine [Exelon]	Capsule: 1.5 mg, 3 mg, 4.5 mg, 6 mg Oral solution: 2 mg/mL 24-hr transdermal patch: 4.6 mg, 9.5 mg, 13.3 mg	*Mild to moderate AD:* Oral: 1.5 mg twice daily. May increase weekly by 3 mg/day (1.5 each meal) to a maximum of 6 mg twice daily Patch: 4.6-mg patch daily. May increase to a higher dose, if needed *Severe AD:* Initially 4.6-mg patch titrated up to a maximum of 13.3 mg daily	Oral drug should be taken with morning and evening meal. Patch: A single patch is applied once daily to the chest, upper arm, upper back, or lower back after removing the previous patch. The site should be changed daily, and not repeated for at least 14 days. Bathing should not affect treatment.
Galantamine [Razadyne, Razadyne ER]	IR tablet: 4 mg, 8 mg, 12 mg Oral solution: 4 mg/mL ER tablet: 8 mg, 16 mg, 24 mg	IR tablets and oral solution: 4 mg twice daily × 4 wk; may increase dosage by 4 mg twice daily every 4 wk. Maintenance: 8 mg to 12 mg twice daily Extended-release capsules: 8 mg once daily × 4 wk; may increase to 16 mg daily × 4 wk and then to 24 mg twice daily Maintenance: 16 mg to 24 mg daily For patients with moderate hepatic or renal impairment, maximal dose is 16 mg/day. Avoid in patients with severe impairment.	Administer with morning and evening meal. ER tablets should be swallowed whole.
Memantine [Namenda, Namenda XR]	IR tablet: 5 mg, 10 mg Oral solution: 2 mg/mL, 10 mg/5 mL ER capsules: 7 mg, 14 mg, 21 mg, 28 mg	Increase gradually using the following schedules for IR and ER formulations. IR tablets and oral solution: • 5 mg/day (5 mg once a day), for 1 wk or more • 10 mg/day (5 mg twice a day), for 1 wk or more • 15 mg/day (5 mg and 10 mg in separate doses), for 1 wk or more • 20 mg/day (10 mg twice a day), for maintenance ER capsules: • 7 mg once daily for 1 wk or more • 14 mg once daily for 1 wk or more • 21 mg once daily for 1 wk or more • 21 mg once daily for maintenance Reduce dosage in patients with moderate renal impairment and discontinue in patients with severe renal impairment.	May take with or without food. ER tablets should be swallowed whole *or* the contents may be emptied into a soft food such as applesauce. Contents must not be crushed or chewed. Oral solution should be administered using the provided device. It should not be mixed with other solutions for administration.

AD, Alzheimer's disease; ER, extended release; IR, immediate release; NMDA, *N*-methyl-D-aspartate.

Group Properties

Mechanism of Action

Cholinesterase inhibitors prevent the breakdown of acetylcholine by acetylcholinesterase (AChE) and thereby increase the availability of acetylcholine at cholinergic synapses. In patients with AD, the result is enhanced transmission by central cholinergic neurons that have not yet been destroyed. Cholinesterase inhibitors do not cure AD, and they do not stop disease progression—although they may slow progression by a few months.

Therapeutic Effect

All cholinesterase inhibitors are approved for patients with *mild to moderate* symptoms, and one agent—donepezil—is also approved for those with *severe* symptoms. Unfortunately, treatment only benefits 1 in 12 patients. Among those who do benefit, improvements are seen in quality of life and cognitive functions (e.g., memory, thought, reasoning). However, these improvements are modest and short lasting. There is no convincing evidence of marked improvement or significant delay of disease progression. Nonetheless, although improvements are neither universal, dramatic, nor long lasting, and although side effects are common, the benefits may still be worth the risks for some patients.

Adverse Effects

By elevating acetylcholine in the periphery, all cholinesterase inhibitors can cause typical cholinergic side effects. Gastrointestinal effects—*nausea, vomiting, dyspepsia, diarrhea*—occur often. *Dizziness* and *headache* are also common. The elevation of acetylcholine at synapses in the lungs can cause *bronchoconstriction.* Accordingly, cholinesterase inhibitors should be used with caution in patients with asthma or chronic obstructive pulmonary disease (COPD).

Cardiovascular effects, although uncommon, are a serious concern. Increased activation of cholinergic receptors in the heart can cause symptomatic bradycardia, leading to fainting, falls, fall-related fractures, and pacemaker placement. If a patient is experiencing bradycardia, fainting, or falls, drug withdrawal may be indicated, especially if cognitive benefits are lacking.

Drug Interactions

Drugs that block cholinergic receptors (e.g., anticholinergic agents, first-generation antihistamines, tricyclic antidepressants, conventional antipsychotics) can reduce therapeutic effects and should be avoided.

Dosage and Duration of Treatment

Dosage should be carefully titrated, and treatment should continue as long as clinically indicated. The highest doses produce the greatest benefits—but also the most intense side effects. Accordingly, dosage should be low initially and then gradually increased to the highest tolerable amount. Treatment can continue indefinitely or until side effects become intolerable or benefits are lost.

Properties of Individual Cholinesterase Inhibitors

These drugs have not been directly compared with one another for efficacy. However, they appear to offer equivalent benefits. Accordingly, selection among them is based on side effects, ease of dosing, and cost.

Donepezil

Donepezil [Aricept] is indicated for mild, moderate, or severe AD. The drug causes reversible inhibition of AChE—but is more selective for the form of AChE found in the brain than that found in the periphery. Like other cholinesterase inhibitors, donepezil does not affect the underlying disease process.

Donepezil is well absorbed after oral administration and undergoes metabolism by hepatic cytochrome P450 enzymes as a CYP2D6 and CYP3A4 substrate. Elimination is mainly in the urine and partly in the bile. Donepezil has a prolonged plasma half-life (about 60 hours) and hence can be administered just once a day.

Although donepezil is somewhat selective for brain cholinesterase, it can still cause peripheral cholinergic effects; nausea and diarrhea are most common. Like other drugs in this class, donepezil can cause bradycardia, fainting, falls, and fall-related fractures. To minimize side effects, patients are stabilized on the initial dosage for 1 to 3 months before an increase in dosage.

Rivastigmine

Rivastigmine [Exelon] is approved for AD and for dementia of Parkinson disease. Unlike donepezil, which causes reversible inhibition of AChE, rivastigmine causes irreversible inhibition. As with other cholinesterase inhibitors, benefits in AD are modest.

Rivastigmine is available in tablets and solution for oral dosing and a patch for transdermal dosing. Oral rivastigmine is well absorbed from the gastrointestinal tract, especially in the presence of food. With the patch, blood levels are lower and steadier than with oral therapy, which improves tolerance. The patch is also beneficial for patients with difficulty swallowing. Because 50% of the starting dose remains in the patch after 24 hours, it is essential to remove an old patch before a new one is applied to avoid toxicity.

In contrast to other cholinesterase inhibitors, rivastigmine is converted to inactive metabolites by AChE, and not by cytochrome P450 enzymes in the liver. The half-life is short—about 1.5 hours. Elimination is in the urine.

Like other cholinesterase inhibitors, rivastigmine can cause peripheral cholinergic side effects. These occur with more frequency compared with the other two drugs. With oral dosing, the most common cholinergic effects are nausea, vomiting, diarrhea, abdominal pain, and anorexia. Weight loss (7% of initial weight) occurs in 18% to 26% of patients. By enhancing cholinergic transmission, rivastigmine can intensify symptoms in patients with peptic ulcer disease, bradycardia, sick sinus syndrome, urinary obstruction, and lung disease; caution is advised. Like other drugs in this class, rivastigmine can cause bradycardia, fainting, falls, and fall-related fractures. Blood levels are lower with transdermal dosing than with oral dosing, and hence the intensity of side effects is lower as well. Rivastigmine has no significant drug interactions, probably because it does not interact with hepatic drug-metabolizing enzymes.

Galantamine

Galantamine [Razadyne, Razadyne ER] is a reversible cholinesterase inhibitor indicated for mild to moderate AD. The drug is prepared by extraction from daffodil bulbs. In clinical trials, galantamine improved cognitive function, behavioral symptoms, quality of life, and ability to perform activities of daily living. However, as with other cholinesterase inhibitors, benefits were modest and short lasting.

Galantamine is rapidly and completely absorbed after oral administration. Protein binding in plasma is low. Elimination is by CYP2D6 and CYP3A4 hepatic enzymes. Excretion is renal. Moderate to severe hepatic or renal impairment delays elimination and increases blood levels. Therefore dosage should be decreased for patients with moderate hepatic or renal impairment and avoided with severe impairment. In healthy adults, the half-life is about 7 hours.

The most common adverse effects are nausea, vomiting, diarrhea, anorexia, and weight loss. Nausea and other gastrointestinal complaints are greater than with donepezil, but less than with oral rivastigmine. By increasing cholinergic stimulation in the heart, galantamine can cause bradycardia, fainting, falls, and fall-related fractures. Like other cholinesterase inhibitors, galantamine can cause bronchoconstriction and hence must be used with caution in patients with asthma or COPD. Drugs that block cholinergic receptors (e.g., anticholinergics, first-generation antihistamines, tricyclic antidepressants, conventional antipsychotics) can reduce therapeutic effects and should be avoided.

Memantine

Memantine [Namenda, Namenda XR] is a first-in-class NMDA receptor antagonist. Unlike the cholinesterase inhibitors, which can be used for mild AD, memantine is indicated only for *moderate or severe* AD. We don't yet know if memantine is more effective than the cholinesterase inhibitors, but we do know it's better tolerated. Although memantine helps treat symptoms of AD, there is no evidence that it modifies the underlying disease process.

Therapeutic Effects

In patients with moderate to severe AD, memantine appears to confer modest benefits. For many patients, the drug can slow the decline in function, and, in some cases, it may actually cause symptoms to improve. In one study, patients taking memantine for 28 weeks scored higher on tests of cognitive function and day-to-day function than did those taking placebo, suggesting that memantine slowed functional decline. In another study, treatment with memantine plus donepezil (a cholinesterase inhibitor) was compared with donepezil alone. The result? After 24 weeks, those taking the combination showed less decline in cognitive and day-to-day function than those taking donepezil alone, suggesting that either (1) the two agents confer independent benefits or (2) they act synergistically to enhance each other's effects. Of note, although memantine can benefit patients with moderate to severe AD, it does not benefit patients with mild AD.

Mechanism of Action

Memantine modulates the effects of glutamate (the major excitatory transmitter in the central nervous system) at NMDA receptors, which are believed to play a critical role in learning and memory. The NMDA receptor—a transmembrane protein with a central channel—regulates calcium entry into neurons. Binding of glutamate to the receptor promotes calcium influx.

Under healthy conditions, an action potential releases a burst of glutamate into the synaptic space. Glutamate then binds with the NMDA receptor and displaces magnesium from the receptor channel, permitting calcium entry (Fig. 18.3A). Glutamate then quickly dissociates from the receptor, permitting magnesium to reblock the channel, and thereby prevents further calcium influx. The brief period of calcium entry constitutes a "signal" in the learning and memory process.

Under pathologic conditions, there is slow but steady leakage of glutamate from the presynaptic neuron and from surrounding glia. As a result, the channel in the NMDA

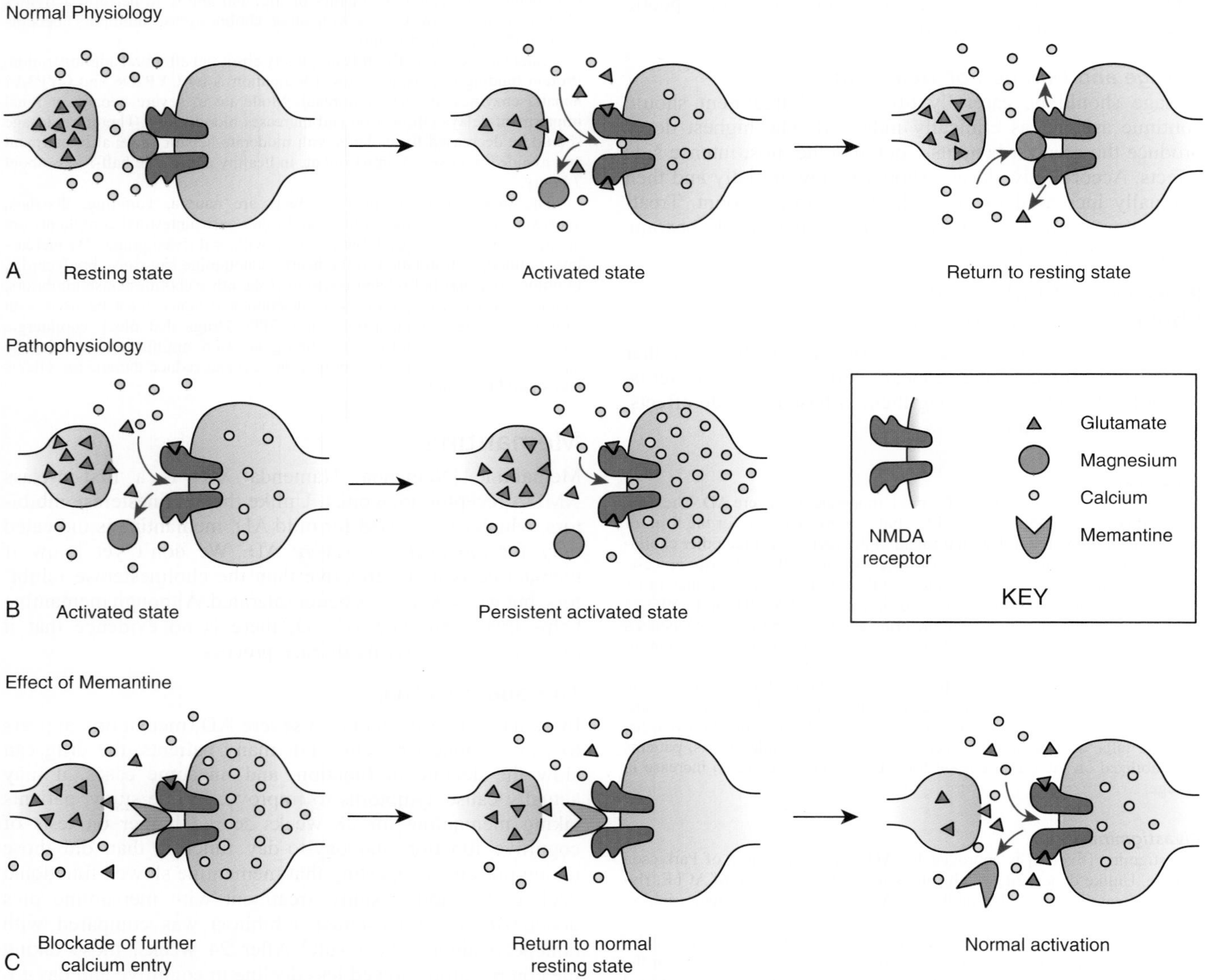

Figure 18.3 ■ Memantine mechanism of action.
A, *Normal physiology.* In the resting postsynaptic neuron, magnesium occupies the *N*-methyl-D-aspartate (NMDA) receptor channel, blocking calcium entry. Binding of glutamate to the receptor displaces magnesium, allowing calcium to enter. When glutamate dissociates from the receptor, magnesium returns to the channel and blocks further calcium inflow. The brief period of calcium entry constitutes a "signal" in the learning and memory process. **B,** *Pathophysiology.* Slow but steady leakage of glutamate from the presynaptic neuron keeps the NMDA receptor in a constantly activated state, thereby allowing excessive calcium influx, which can impair memory and learning and can eventually cause neuronal death. **C,** *Effect of memantine.* Memantine blocks calcium entry when extracellular glutamate is low and thereby stops further calcium entry, which allows intracellular calcium levels to normalize. When a burst of glutamate is released in response to an action potential, the resulting high level of glutamate is able to displace memantine, causing a brief period of calcium entry. Not shown: When glutamate diffuses away, memantine reblocks the channel and thereby stops further calcium entry, despite continuing low levels of glutamate in the synapse.

receptor is kept open, allowing excessive influx of calcium (see Fig. 18.3B). High intracellular calcium has two effects: (1) impaired learning and memory (because the "noise" created by excessive calcium overpowers the "signal" created when calcium enters in response to glutamate released by a nerve impulse); and (2) neurodegeneration (because too much intracellular calcium is toxic).

How does memantine help? It blocks calcium influx when extracellular glutamate is low, but permits calcium influx when extracellular glutamate is high. As shown in Figure 18.3C, when the glutamate level is low, memantine is able to occupy the NMDA receptor channel and thereby block the steady entry of calcium. As a result, the level of intracellular calcium is able to normalize. Then, when a burst of glutamate is released in response to an action potential, the resulting high level of extracellular glutamate is able to displace memantine, causing a brief period of calcium entry. Because intracellular calcium is now low, normal signaling can occur. When glutamate diffuses away from the receptor, memantine reblocks the channel and thereby stops further calcium entry, despite continuing low levels of glutamate in the synapse.

Pharmacokinetics

Memantine is well absorbed after oral dosing, both in the presence and absence of food. Plasma levels peak in 3 to 7 hours. The drug undergoes little metabolism and is excreted largely unchanged in the urine. The half-life is long—60 to 80 hours. Clearance is reduced in patients with renal impairment.

Adverse Effects

Memantine is well tolerated. The most common side effects are dizziness, headache, confusion, and constipation. In clinical trials, the incidence of these effects was about the same as in patients taking placebo.

Drug Interactions

In theory, combining memantine with another NMDA antagonist, such as amantadine or ketamine, could have an undesirable additive effect. Accordingly, such combinations should be used with caution.

Sodium bicarbonate and other drugs that alkalinize the urine can greatly decrease the renal excretion of memantine. Accumulation of the drug to toxic levels might result.

DRUGS FOR NEUROPSYCHIATRIC SYMPTOMS

Neuropsychiatric symptoms (e.g., agitation, aggression, delusions, hallucinations) occur in more than 80% of people with AD. Although multiple drug classes—antipsychotics, cholinesterase inhibitors, mood stabilizers, antidepressants, anxiolytics, NMDA receptor antagonists—have been tried as treatment, very few are effective, and even then benefits are limited. There *is* convincing evidence that neuropsychiatric symptoms can be reduced with two atypical antipsychotics: *risperidone* [Risperdal] and *olanzapine* [Zyprexa]. However, benefits are modest, and these drugs slightly *increase* mortality, mainly from cardiovascular events and infection. Cholinesterase inhibitors may offer modest help. There is little or no evidence for a benefit from conventional antipsychotics (e.g., haloperidol, chlorpromazine), mood stabilizers (valproate, carbamazepine, lithium), antidepressants, or memantine.

CAN WE PREVENT ALZHEIMER DISEASE OR DELAY COGNITIVE DECLINE?

In 2010, an expert panel released a report (*Preventing Alzheimer's Disease and Cognitive Decline*) stating that we have no good evidence supporting the association of any *modifiable* factor—diet, exercise, social interaction, economic status, nutritional supplements, medications, environmental toxins—with reduced risk for AD. However, this discouraging conclusion does not mean that all available interventions have been proved not to work. Rather, it means that the evidence is too meager to prove that some interventions *might* work. Table 18.3 shows the panel's conclusions regarding certain interventions, indicating the effect of the intervention and the quality of the research involved.

TABLE 18.3 ▪ Interventions to Delay the Onset of Alzheimer's Disease or Slow Cognitive Decline

Intervention	Effect	Quality of Evidence
POTENTIAL INTERVENTIONS TO DELAY ONSET OF ALZHEIMER DISEASE		
Nutrition		
Mediterranean diet	Possible benefit	Low
Light to moderate alcohol intake	Possible benefit	Low
Folic acid	Possible benefit	Low
Ginkgo biloba	No benefit	High
Vitamin E	No benefit	Moderate
Homocysteine	No benefit	Low
Vitamin B_{12}	No benefit	Low
Vitamin C	No benefit	Low
Omega-3 fatty acids	No benefit	Low
Beta-carotene	No benefit	Low
Medications		
Statins	Possible benefit	Low
Cholinesterase inhibitors	No benefit	Moderate
Antihypertensives	No benefit	Low
Celecoxib, naproxen	Increased risk	Low
Estrogen alone	No benefit	Low
Estrogen plus progestin	Increased risk	Moderate
Social and Behavioral Factors		
Cognitive training	Small protective effect	Low
Physical activity	Small protective effect	Low
POTENTIAL INTERVENTIONS TO IMPROVE OR MAINTAIN COGNITIVE FUNCTION		
Nutrition		
Vitamin E	No effect or no consistent effect across trials	High
Vitamin B_6	No effect or no consistent effect across trials	Moderate
Vitamin B_{12}	No effect or no consistent effect across trials	Moderate
Folic acid	No effect or no consistent effect across trials	Moderate
Medications		
Cholinesterase inhibitors	No benefit	Moderate
Statins	No benefit	High
Estrogen	No benefit	High
Antihypertensives	No benefit	Low
NSAIDs	No benefit or increased risk	Low
Social and Behavioral Factors		
Cognitive training	Small protective effect	High
Physical activity	Small protective effect	Low
Noncognitive, nonphysical leisure activity	Small protective effect	Low

NSAIDs, nonsteroidal antiinflammatory drugs.
Modified from Williams JW, Plassman BL, Burke J, et al. Preventing Alzheimer's Disease and Cognitive Decline: Evidence Report/Technology Assessment No. 193. (Prepared by the Duke Evidence-based Practice Center under Contract No. HHSA 290-2007-10066-I.) AHRQ Publication No. 10-E005. Rockville, MD: Agency for Healthcare Research and Quality, 2010.

CHAPTER

19 Drugs for Epilepsy

Jacqueline Rosenjack Burchum, DNSc, FNP-BC, CNE

The term *epilepsy* refers to a group of chronic neurologic disorders characterized by recurrent seizures, brought on by excessive excitability of neurons in the brain. Symptoms can range from brief periods of unconsciousness to violent convulsions. Patients may also experience problems with learning, memory, and mood, which can be just as troubling as their seizures.

In the United States about 2.9 million people have epilepsy, according to the Centers for Disease Control and Prevention. The incidence is highest in the very young and in older adults. Between 60% and 70% of patients can be rendered free of seizures with drugs. Unfortunately, this means that 30% to 40% cannot. The total direct and indirect costs of epilepsy are estimated at $15.5 billion a year.

The terms *seizure* and *convulsion* are not synonymous. *Seizure* is a general term that applies to all types of epileptic events. In contrast, *convulsion* has a more limited meaning, applying only to abnormal motor phenomena, for example, the jerking movements that occur during a tonic-clonic attack. Accordingly, although all convulsions may be called seizures, it is not correct to call all seizures convulsions. Absence seizures, for example, manifest as brief periods of unconsciousness, which may or may not be accompanied by involuntary movements. Because not all epileptic seizures involve convulsions, we will refer to the agents used to treat epilepsy as *antiepileptic drugs* (AEDs), rather than anticonvulsants.

SEIZURE GENERATION

Seizures are initiated by synchronous, high-frequency discharge from a group of hyperexcitable neurons, called a *focus.* A focus may result from several causes, including congenital defects, hypoxia at birth, head trauma, brain infection, stroke, cancer, and genetic disorders. Seizures occur when discharge from a focus spreads to other brain areas, thereby recruiting normal neurons to discharge abnormally. The overt manifestations of any particular seizure disorder depend on the location of the seizure focus and the neuronal connections to that focus. The connections to the focus determine the brain areas to which seizure activity can spread.

TYPES OF SEIZURES

Seizure can be divided into two broad categories: *partial (focal) seizures* and *generalized seizures.* In partial seizures, seizure activity undergoes a very limited spread to adjacent cortical areas beyond the focus. In generalized seizures, focal seizure activity is conducted widely throughout both hemispheres. As a rule, partial seizures and generalized seizures are treated with different drugs (Table 19.1).

Partial Seizures

Partial seizures fall into three groups: simple partial seizures, complex partial seizures, and partial seizures that evolve into secondarily generalized seizures.

Simple Partial Seizures

These seizures manifest with discrete symptoms that are determined by the brain region involved. Hence the patient may experience discrete motor symptoms (e.g., twitching thumb), sensory symptoms (e.g., local numbness; auditory, visual, or olfactory hallucinations), autonomic symptoms (e.g., nausea, flushing, salivation, urinary incontinence), or psychoillusory symptoms (e.g., feelings of unreality, fear, or depression). Simple partial seizures are distinguished from complex partial seizures in that there is *no loss of consciousness.* These seizures persist for 20 to 60 seconds.

Complex Partial Seizures

These seizures are characterized by *impaired consciousness* and lack of responsiveness. At seizure onset, the patient becomes motionless and stares with a fixed gaze. This state is followed by a period of *automatism,* in which the patient performs repetitive, purposeless movements, such as lip smacking or hand wringing. Seizures last 45 to 90 seconds.

Secondarily Generalized Seizures

These seizures begin as simple or complex partial seizures and then evolve into generalized tonic-clonic seizures. Consciousness is lost. These seizures last 1 to 2 minutes.

Generalized Seizures

Generalized seizures may be convulsive or nonconvulsive. As a rule, they produce immediate loss of consciousness. The major generalized seizures are discussed briefly later.

Tonic-Clonic Seizures

In tonic-clonic seizures (formerly known as grand mal seizures), neuronal discharge spreads throughout both hemispheres of the cerebral cortex. These seizures manifest as major convulsions, characterized by a period of muscle rigidity (tonic phase) followed by synchronous muscle jerks (clonic phase). Tonic-clonic seizures often cause urination, but not defecation. Convulsions may be preceded by a loud

TABLE 19.1 ■ Drugs for Specific Types of Seizures

Seizure Type	Drugs Used for Treatment: Traditional AEDs	Newer AEDs
PARTIAL		
Simple partial, complex partial, and secondarily generalized	Carbamazepine Fosphenytoin Phenobarbital Phenytoin Primidone Valproic acid	Ezogabine Felbamate Gabapentin Lacosamide Lamotrigine Levetiracetam Oxcarbazepine Pregabalin Tiagabine Topiramate Vigabatrin Zonisamide
PRIMARY GENERALIZED		
Tonic-clonic	Carbamazepine Fosphenytoin Phenobarbital Phenytoin Primidone Valproic acid	Lamotrigine Levetiracetam Topiramate
Absence	Ethosuximide Valproic acid	Lamotrigine
Myoclonic	Valproic acid	Lamotrigine Levetiracetam Topiramate

AEDs, antiepileptic drugs.

cry, caused by forceful expiration of air across the vocal cords. Tonic-clonic seizures are accompanied by marked impairment of consciousness and are followed by a period of central nervous system (CNS) depression, referred to as the *postictal state.* The seizure itself typically lasts 90 seconds or less.

Absence Seizures (Petit Mal)

Absence seizures are characterized by loss of consciousness for a brief time (10–30 seconds). Seizures usually involve mild, symmetrical motor activity (e.g., eye blinking) but may occur with no motor activity at all. The patient may experience hundreds of absence attacks a day. Absence seizures occur primarily in children and usually cease during the early teen years.

Atonic Seizures

These seizures are characterized by sudden loss of muscle tone. If seizure activity is limited to the muscles of the neck, "head drop" occurs. However, if the muscles of the limbs and trunk are involved, a "drop attack" can occur, causing the patient to suddenly collapse. Atonic seizures occur mainly in children.

Myoclonic Seizures

These seizures consist of sudden muscle contraction that lasts for just 1 second. Seizure activity may be limited to one limb (focal myoclonus), or it may involve the entire body (massive myoclonus).

Status Epilepticus

Status epilepticus (SE) is defined as a seizure that persists for 15 to 30 minutes or longer or a series of recurrent seizures during which the patient does not regain consciousness. There are several types of SE, including generalized convulsive SE, absence SE, and myoclonic SE.

Febrile Seizures

Fever-associated seizures are common among children aged 6 months to 5 years. Febrile seizures typically manifest as generalized tonic-clonic convulsions of short duration. Children who experience these seizures are *not* at high risk for developing epilepsy later in life.

Mixed Seizures: Lennox-Gastaut Syndrome

Lennox-Gastaut syndrome is a severe form of epilepsy that usually develops during the preschool years. The syndrome is characterized by developmental delay and a mixture of partial and generalized seizures. Seizure types include partial, atonic, tonic, generalized tonic-clonic, and atypical absence. In children with Lennox-Gastaut syndrome, seizures can be very difficult to manage.

HOW ANTIEPILEPTIC DRUGS WORK

We have long known that AEDs can (1) suppress discharge of neurons within a seizure focus and (2) suppress propagation of seizure activity from the focus to other areas of the brain. However, until recently we didn't know how these effects were achieved. It now appears that nearly all AEDs act through five basic mechanisms: suppression of sodium influx, suppression of calcium influx, promotion of potassium efflux, blockade of receptors for glutamate, and potentiation or increase of gamma-aminobutyric acid (GABA). Categorization of AEDs by mechanism of action, when known, is displayed in Box 19.1.

Suppression of Sodium Influx

Before discussing AED actions, we need to review sodium channel physiology. Neuronal action potentials are propagated by influx of sodium through sodium channels, which are gated pores in the cell membrane that control sodium entry. For sodium influx to occur, the channel must be in an *activated state.* Immediately after sodium entry, the channel goes into an *inactivated state,* during which further sodium entry is prevented. Under normal circumstances, the inactive channel very quickly returns to the activated state, thereby permitting more sodium entry and propagation of another action potential.

Several AEDs, including phenytoin, carbamazepine, and lamotrigine, reversibly bind to sodium channels while they are in the inactivated state and thereby prolong channel inactivation. By delaying return to the active state, these drugs decrease the ability of neurons to fire at high frequency. As a result, seizures that depend on high-frequency discharge are suppressed.

BOX 19.1 ▪ CATEGORIZATION OF ANTIEPILEPTIC DRUGS BY MECHANISM OF ACTION

Drugs That Affect Sodium Influx

Phenytoin
Lamotrigine
Carbamazepine
Eslicarbazepine
Oxcarbazepine
Lacosamide
Rufinamide
Zonisamide
Topiramate*

Drugs That Affect Calcium Influx

Ethosuximide

Drugs That Affect Potassium Efflux

Ezogabine

Drugs That Affect GABA Activity

Benzodiazepines (e.g. diazepam)
Barbiturates (e.g. phenobarbital)
Gabapentin
Tiagabine
Vigabatrin
Valproic acid

Drugs That Affect Glutamate Receptors

Perampanel
Felbamate
Topiramate*

Drugs With Uncertain Mechanisms of Action

Pregabalin
Levetiracetam

*Drug possesses more than one mechanism of action

Suppression of Calcium Influx

In axon terminals, influx of calcium through voltage-gated calcium channels promotes transmitter release. Hence drugs that block these calcium channels can suppress transmission. Ethosuximide acts by this mechanism.

Promotion of Potassium Efflux

During an action potential, influx of sodium causes neurons to depolarize, and then efflux of potassium causes neurons to repolarize. One AED—ezogabine (retigabine)—acts on voltage-gated potassium channels to facilitate potassium efflux. This action is believed to underlie the drug's ability to slow repetitive neuronal firing and thereby provide seizure control.

Antagonism of Glutamate

Glutamic acid (glutamate) is the primary excitatory transmitter in the CNS. The compound works through two receptors: (1) *N*-methyl-D-aspartate (NMDA) receptors and (2) alpha-amino-3-hydroxy-5-methyl-4-isoxazole propionic acid (AMPA) receptors. Perampanel is an AMPA glutamate receptor antagonist. Two other drugs—felbamate and topiramate—block the actions of glutamate at NMDA receptors and thereby suppress neuronal excitation.

Potentiation of Gamma-Aminobutyric Acid

Several AEDs potentiate the actions of GABA, an inhibitory neurotransmitter that is widely distributed throughout the brain. By augmenting the inhibitory influence of GABA, these drugs decrease neuronal excitability and thereby suppress seizure activity. Drugs increase the influence of GABA by several mechanisms. Benzodiazepines and barbiturates enhance the effects of GABA by mechanisms that involve direct binding to GABA receptors. Gabapentin promotes GABA release. Tiagabine inhibits GABA reuptake, and vigabatrin inhibits the enzyme that degrades GABA and thereby increases GABA availability.

BASIC THERAPEUTIC CONSIDERATIONS

Therapeutic Goal and Treatment Options

The goal in treating epilepsy is to reduce seizures to an extent that enables the patient to live a normal or nearly normal life. Ideally, treatment should eliminate seizures entirely. However, this may not be possible without causing intolerable side effects. Therefore we must balance the desire for complete seizure control against the acceptability of side effects.

Epilepsy may be treated with drugs or with nondrug therapies. As noted, drugs can benefit 60% to 70% of patients. This means that, of the 2.9 million Americans with epilepsy, between 870,000 and 1,160,000 *cannot* be treated successfully with drugs. For these people, nondrug therapy may well help. Three options exist: neurosurgery, vagus nerve stimulation, and the ketogenic diet. Of the three, neurosurgery has the best success rate, but vagus nerve stimulation is used most widely.

Diagnosis and Drug Selection

Control of seizures requires proper drug selection. As indicated in Table 19.1, many AEDs are selective for specific seizure disorders. Phenytoin, for example, is useful for treating tonic-clonic and partial seizures but not absence seizures. Conversely, ethosuximide is active against absence seizures but not against tonic-clonic or partial seizures. Only one drug—valproic acid—appears effective against practically all forms of epilepsy. Because most AEDs are selective for certain seizure disorders, effective treatment requires a proper match between the drug and the seizure. To make this match, the seizure type must be accurately diagnosed.

Making a diagnosis requires physical, neurologic, and laboratory evaluations along with a thorough history. The history should determine the age at which seizures began, the frequency and duration of seizure events, precipitating factors, and times when seizures occur. Physical and neurologic evaluations may reveal signs of head injury or other disorders that could underlie seizure activity, although in many patients the physical and neurologic evaluations may be normal. An electroencephalogram is essential for diagnosis. Other diagnostic tests that may be employed include computed tomography, positron emission tomography, and magnetic resonance imaging.

Pharmacologic management with AEDs is highly individualized. Very often, patients must try several AEDs before a regimen that is both effective and well tolerated can be established. Initial treatment should be done with just one AED. If this drug fails, it should be discontinued and a different AED should be tried. If this second drug fails, two options are open: (1) treatment with a third AED alone or (2) treatment with a combination of AEDs.

Drug Evaluation

After an AED has been selected, a trial period is needed to determine its effectiveness. During this time there is no guarantee that seizures will be controlled. Until seizure control is certain, the patient should be warned not to participate in driving and other activities that could be hazardous should a seizure occur.

Maintenance of a seizure frequency chart is important. The chart should be kept by the patient or a family member and should contain a complete record of all seizure events. This record can be used to help guide the provider in optimizing pharmacologic management.

During the process of drug evaluation, adjustments in dosage are often needed. No drug should be considered ineffective until it has been tested in sufficiently high dosages and for a reasonable time. Knowledge of plasma drug levels can be a valuable tool for establishing dosage and evaluating the effectiveness of a specific drug.

Monitoring Plasma Drug Levels

Safe and effective levels have been firmly established for most AEDs (see Table 19.2). Monitoring these levels can help guide dosage adjustments.

TABLE 19.2 ■ Clinical Pharmacology of the Oral Antiepileptic Drugs

Drug	Preparations	Product Name	Daily Dosing[a]	Daily Maintenance Dosage[a] Adults (mg)	Daily Maintenance Dosage[a] Children (mg/kg)	Target Serum Level (mcg/mL)	Induces Hepatic Drug Metabolism
TRADITIONAL AEDS							
Carbamazepine	IR tablets: 200 mg Chewable tablets: 100 mg ER tablets: 100, 200, 400 mg ER capsules: 100, 200, 300 mg Oral suspension: 20 mg/mL	Tegretol Epitol Tegretol XR, Tegretol CR 🍁 Carbatrol Equetro	3 times 3 times 2 times 2 times 2 times	800–1200	10–35	4–12	Yes
Ethosuximide	Capsules: 250 mg Syrup: 250 mg/5 mL	Zarontin	1 or 2 times	750	20	40–100	No
Phenobarbital	Tablets: 15 mg, 16.2 mg, 30 mg, 32.4 mg, 60 mg, 64.8 mg, 97.2 mg, 100 mg Elixir: 20 mg/5 mL Oral solution: 20 mg/5 mL Solution for injection: 65 mg/mL, 130 mg/mL	Generic only	1 or 2 times	50–120	3–8	15–45	Yes
Phenytoin	Chewable tablets: 50 mg Capsules: 30, 100, 200, 300 mg Oral suspension: 125 mg/5 mL Solution for injection: 50 mg/mL	Dilantin-125 Dilantin Infatab Phenytek (ER capsules) Dilantin (ER capsules)	2 or 3 times 2 or 3 times 1 time 1 time	300–600	4–8	10–20	Yes
Fosphenytoin	Solution for injection: 100 mg PE/2 mL, 500 mg						
Primidone	Tablets: 50 mg, 250 mg	Mysoline	3 or 4 times	500–750	10–25	5–12[b]	Yes
Valproic acid	See Table 19–4	Depakene Depakote, Epival 🍁 Depakote ER Stavzor	3 or 4 times 3 or 4 times 2 times 2 or 3 times	500–3000	15–60	50–100	No
NEWER AEDS							
Ezogabine	Tablets: 50 mg, 200 mg, 300 mg, 400 mg	Potiga	3 times	600–1200	ND	ND	No
Felbamate	Tablets: 400 mg, 600 mg Oral suspension: 600 mg/5 mL	Felbatol	3 or 4 times	1200–3600	15–45	ND	Yes

TABLE 19.2 ■ Clinical Pharmacology of the Oral Antiepileptic Drugs—cont'd

Drug	Preparations	Product Name	Daily Dosing[a]	Daily Maintenance Dosage[a]: Adults (mg)	Daily Maintenance Dosage[a]: Children (mg/kg)	Target Serum Level (mcg/mL)	Induces Hepatic Drug Metabolism
Gabapentin	Tablets: 600 mg, 800 mg Capsule: 100 mg, 300 mg, 400 mg, 600 mg, 800 mg Oral solution: 250 mg/5 mL	Neurontin	3 times	1200–3600	25–50	12–20	No
Lacosamide	Tablets: 50 mg, 100 mg, 150 mg, 200 mg Oral solution: 10 mg/mL IV solution: 200 mg/20 mL	Vimpat	2 times	200–400	ND	ND	No
Lamotrigine	Tablets: 25 mg, 100 mg, 150 mg, 200 mg Chewable tablets: 5 mg, 25 mg ODT: 25 mg, 50 mg, 100 mg, 200 mg ER tablet: 25 mg, 50 mg, 100 mg, 200 mg, 250 mg, 300 mg	Lamictal, Lamictal ODT Lamictal XR	2 times 1 time	400–600[c,d]	5[c,d]	3–14	No
Levetiracetam	IR tablet: 250 mg, 500 mg, 750 mg, 1000 mg ER tablets: 500 mg, 750 mg ODT: 250 mg, 500 mg, 750 mg, 1000 mg Oral solution: 100 mg/mL IV solution: 500 mg/5 mL, 500 mg/100 mL, 1 g/100 mL, 1.5 g/100 mL	Keppra Keppra XR	2 times 1 time	2000–3000	40–100	10–40	No
Oxcarbazepine	IR tablets: 150 mg, 300 mg, 600 mg ER tablets: 150 mg, 300 mg, 600 mg Oral suspension: 300 mg/5 mL	Trileptal Oxtellar XR	2 times 1 time	900–2400 1200–2400	30–46 20–29 kg: 900 mg/day; 29.1–39 kg: 1200 mg/day; >39 kg: 1800 mg/day	3–40	Yes[e]
Pregabalin	Capsule: 25 mg, 50 mg, 75 mg, 100 mg, 150 mg, 200 mg, 225 mg, 300 mg Oral solution: 20 mg/mL	Lyrica	2 or 3 times	150–600	ND	ND	No
Rufinamide	Tablets: 200 mg, 400 mg Oral suspension: 40 mg/mL	Banzel	2 times	3200	45	ND	Yes[f]
Tiagabine	Tablets: 2 mg, 4 mg, 12 mg, 16 mg	Gabitril	2–4 times	16–32	0.4[d]	ND	No
Topiramate	Tablets: 25 mg, 50 mg, 100 mg, 200 mg Sprinkle capsule: 15 mg, 25 mg ER sprinkle capsule: 25 mg, 50 mg, 100 mg, 150 mg, 200 mg ER capsule: 25 mg, 50 mg, 100 mg, 200 mg	Topamax, Trokendi XR, Qudexy XR	2 times	100–400	3–9	5–25	No
Vigabatrin	Tablets: 500 mg Solution: 500 mg	Sabril	2 times	3000–6000	50–150	ND	Yes
Zonisamide	Capsules: 25 mg, 50 mg, 100 mg	Zonegran	1 or 2 times	200–400	4–12	10–40	No
Eslicarbazepine	Tablets: 400 mg, 600 mg, 800 mg	Aptiom	1 time	800–1600	N/A	ND	Yes
Perampanel	Tablets: 2 mg, 4 mg, 6 mg, 8 mg, 10 mg, 12 mg	Fycompa	1 time	8–12	N/A	N/D	No

[a]Dosing for AEDs is highly individualized. These represent averages, which may be subtherapeutic for some patients but toxic for others.
[b]Target serum level is 5 to 12 mcg/mL for primidone itself, and 15 to 40 mcg/mL for phenobarbital derived from primidone.
[c]Dosage must be decreased in patients taking valproic acid.
[d]Dosage must be increased in patients taking drugs that induce hepatic drug-metabolizing enzymes.
[e]Oxcarbazepine does not induce enzymes that metabolize AEDs but does induce enzymes that metabolize other drugs.
[f]Rufinamide produces mild induction of CYP3A4.
AED, antiepileptic drug; CR, controlled release; ER, extended release; IR, immediate release; IV, intravenous; ND, not determined; ODT, orally disintegrating tablet; XR, extended release; PE, phenytoin equivalent.

Monitoring plasma drug levels is especially helpful when treating major convulsive disorders (e.g., tonic-clonic seizures). Because these seizures can be dangerous, and because delay of therapy may allow the condition to worsen, rapid control of seizures is desirable. However, because these seizures occur infrequently, a long time may be needed to establish control if clinical outcome is relied on as the only means of determining an effective dosage. By adjusting initial doses on the basis of plasma drug levels (rather than on the basis of seizure control), we can readily achieve drug levels that are likely to be effective, thereby increasing our chances of establishing control quickly.

Measurements of plasma drug levels are less important for determining effective dosages for absence seizures. Because absence seizures occur very frequently (up to several hundred a day), observation of the patient is the best means for establishing an effective dosage: if seizures stop, dosage is sufficient; if seizures continue, it is likely that more drug is needed.

In addition to serving as a guide for dosage adjustment, knowledge of plasma drug levels can serve as an aid to (1) monitoring patient adherence, (2) determining the cause of lost seizure control, and (3) identifying causes of toxicity, especially in patients taking more than one drug.

Promoting Patient Adherence

Epilepsy is a chronic condition that requires regular and continuous therapy. As a result, seizure control is highly dependent on patient adherence. In fact, it is estimated that nonadherence accounts for about 50% of all treatment failures. Accordingly, promoting adherence should be a priority for all members of the health care team. Measures that can help include the following:

- Educating patients and families about the chronic nature of epilepsy and the importance of adhering to the prescribed regimen
- Monitoring plasma drug levels to encourage and evaluate adherence
- Deepening patient and family involvement by having them maintain a seizure frequency chart

Withdrawing Antiepileptic Drugs

Some forms of epilepsy undergo spontaneous remission, and hence discontinuing treatment may eventually be appropriate. Unfortunately, there are no firm guidelines to indicate the most appropriate time to withdraw AEDs. However, after the decision to discontinue treatment has been made, agreement does exist on how drug withdrawal should be accomplished. The most important rule is that *AEDs be withdrawn slowly* (over a period of 6 weeks to several months). Failure to gradually reduce dosage is a frequent cause of SE. If the patient is taking two drugs to control seizures, they should be withdrawn sequentially, not simultaneously.

Suicide Risk With Antiepileptic Drugs

In 2008, the U.S. Food and Drug Administration (FDA) warned that all AEDs can increase suicidal thoughts and behavior. However, data gathered since 2008 suggest that the risk may be lower than previously believed and may apply only to certain AEDs.

Since the FDA issued its warning, other large studies have been conducted to clarify the relationship between AEDs and suicidality. Unfortunately, these studies have yielded conflicting results. Nonetheless, they do suggest three things. First, only some AEDs—especially topiramate and lamotrigine—are likely to increase suicidality, not all AEDs as warned by the FDA. Second, the risk for suicidal behavior may be related more to the illness than the medication: by analyzing data on 5,130,795 patients, researchers in the United Kingdom found that AEDs produced a small increase in suicidal behavior in patients with *depression,* but did *not* increase suicidal behavior in patients with *epilepsy* or *bipolar disorder.* And third, even if AEDs do promote suicidality, AED-related suicide attempts and completed suicides are very rare.

Given the uncertainty regarding AEDs and suicidality, what should the clinician do? Because epilepsy itself carries a risk for suicide, and because patients with epilepsy often have depression or anxiety (which increases the risk for suicide), prudence dictates screening all patients for suicide risk, whether or not AEDs increase that risk. In addition, after treatment begins, all patients should be monitored for increased anxiety, agitation, mania, and hostility—signs that may indicate the emergence or worsening of depression—and an increased risk for suicidal thoughts or behavior. Patients, families, and caregivers should be alerted to these signs and advised to report them immediately. Finally, two AEDs—topiramate and lamotrigine—should be used with special caution, given their significant association with suicidality.

CLASSIFICATION OF ANTIEPILEPTIC DRUGS

The AEDs can be grouped into two major categories: *traditional AEDs* and *newer AEDs.* The traditional group has seven major members. The group of newer AEDs has 13 members. As shown in Table 19.3, both groups have their advantages and disadvantages. For example, clinical experience with the older AEDs is more extensive than with the newer ones, and the older drugs cost less. Both facts make the older drugs attractive. However, the older AEDs also have drawbacks, including troublesome side effects and complex drug interactions. Of importance, drugs in both groups appear equally effective—although few direct comparisons have been made. The bottom line? Neither group is clearly superior. Hence, when selecting an AED, drugs in both groups should be considered.

TRADITIONAL ANTIEPILEPTIC DRUGS

The traditional AEDs have been in use for decades. Because of this extensive clinical experience, the efficacy and therapeutic niche of the traditional AEDs are well established. As a result, these drugs are prescribed more widely than the newer AEDs.

Although familiarity makes the traditional AEDs appealing, these drugs do have drawbacks. In general, they are less well tolerated than the newer AEDs, and they pose a greater risk to the developing fetus. Furthermore, owing to effects on drug-metabolizing enzymes (either induction or inhibition), they have complex interactions with other drugs, including other AEDs.

TABLE 19.3 ▪ Comparison of Traditional and Newer Antiepileptic Drugs

Area of Comparison	AED Group	
	Traditional AEDs*	Newer AEDs†
Efficacy	Well established	Equally good (probably), but less well established
Clinical experience	Extensive	Less extensive
Therapeutic niche	Well established	Evolving
Tolerability	Less well tolerated	Better tolerated (usually)
Pharmacokinetics	Often complex	Less complex
Drug interactions	Extensive, owing to induction of drug-metabolizing enzymes	Limited, owing to little or no induction of drug-metabolizing enzymes
Safety in pregnancy	Less safe	Safer
Cost	Less expensive	More expensive

*Carbamazepine, ethosuximide, phenobarbital, fosphenytoin, phenytoin, primidone, and valproic acid.

†Ezogabine, felbamate, gabapentin, lacosamide, lamotrigine, levetiracetam, oxcarbazepine, pregabalin, rufinamide, tiagabine, topiramate, vigabatrin, and zonisamide.

In the discussion that follows, we focus on the major traditional AEDs. They are phenytoin, fosphenytoin, carbamazepine, valproic acid, ethosuximide, phenobarbital, and primidone.

Prototype Drugs

DRUGS FOR EPILEPSY

Traditional Agents

Phenytoin
Carbamazepine
Valproic acid
Ethosuximide
Phenobarbital
Diazepam (intravenous)

Newer Agents

Oxcarbazepine
Lamotrigine

Phenytoin

Phenytoin [Dilantin, Phenytek] is our most widely used AED, despite having tricky kinetics and troublesome side effects. The drug is active against partial seizures as well as primary generalized tonic-clonic seizures. Phenytoin is of historical importance in that it was the first drug to suppress seizures without depressing the entire CNS. Consequently, phenytoin heralded the development of selective medications that could treat epilepsy while leaving most CNS functions undiminished.

Mechanism of Action

At the concentrations achieved clinically, phenytoin causes selective inhibition of sodium channels. Specifically, the drug slows recovery of sodium channels from the inactive state back to the active state. As a result, entry of sodium into neurons is inhibited, and hence action potentials are suppressed. Blockade of sodium entry is limited to neurons that are hyperactive. As a result, the drug suppresses activity of seizure-generating neurons while leaving healthy neurons unaffected.

Pharmacokinetics

Phenytoin has unusual pharmacokinetics that must be accounted for in therapy. Absorption varies substantially among patients. In addition, because of saturation kinetics, small changes in dosage can produce disproportionately large changes in serum drug levels. As a result, a dosage that is both effective and safe is difficult to establish.

Absorption

Absorption varies between the different oral formulations of phenytoin. With the oral suspension and chewable tablets absorption is relatively fast, whereas with the extended-release capsules absorption is delayed and prolonged.

In the past, there was concern that absorption also varied between preparations of phenytoin made by different manufacturers. However, it is now clear that all FDA-approved equivalent products have equivalent bioavailability. As a result, switching from one brand of phenytoin to another produces no more variability than switching between different lots of phenytoin produced by the same manufacturer.

Metabolism

The capacity of the liver to metabolize phenytoin is very limited. Doses of phenytoin needed to produce therapeutic effects are only slightly smaller than the doses needed to saturate the hepatic enzymes that metabolize phenytoin. Consequently, if phenytoin is administered in doses only slightly greater than those needed for therapeutic effects, the liver's capacity to metabolize the drug will be overwhelmed, causing plasma levels of phenytoin to rise dramatically. This unusual relationship between dosage and plasma levels is illustrated in Fig. 19.1A. As you can see, after plasma levels have reached the therapeutic range, small changes in dosage produce large changes in plasma levels. As a result, small increases in dosage can cause toxicity, and small decreases can cause therapeutic failure. This relationship makes it difficult to establish and maintain a dosage that is both safe and effective.

The relationship between dosage and plasma levels that exists for most drugs is detailed in Fig. 19.1B. As indicated, this relationship is *linear,* in contrast to the nonlinear relationship that exists for phenytoin. Accordingly, for most drugs, if the patient is taking doses that produce plasma levels that are within the therapeutic range, small deviations from that dosage produce only small deviations in plasma drug levels. Because of this relationship, with most drugs it is relatively easy to maintain plasma levels that are safe and effective.

Because of saturation kinetics, the half-life of phenytoin varies with dosage. At low doses, the half-life is relatively short—about 8 hours. However, at higher doses, the half-life becomes prolonged—in some cases up to 60 hours. At higher doses, there is more drug present than the liver can process. As a result, metabolism is delayed, causing the half-life to increase.

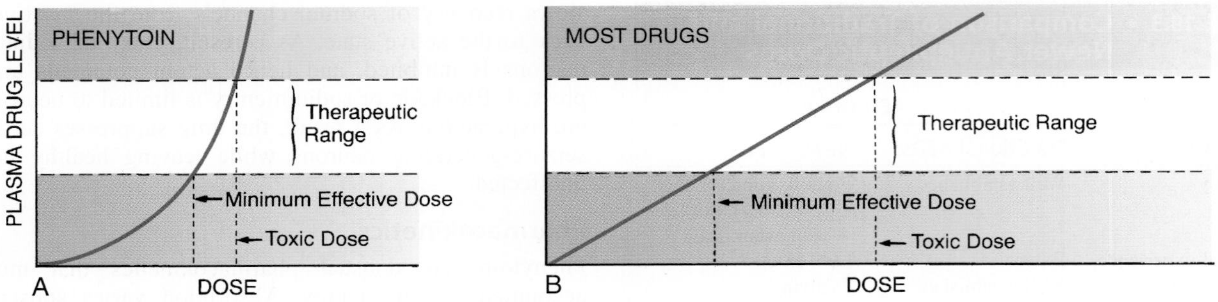

Figure 19.1 ■ Relationship between dose and plasma level for phenytoin compared with most other drugs.
A, Within the therapeutic range, small increments in phenytoin dosage produce sharp increases in plasma drug levels. This relationship makes it difficult to maintain plasma phenytoin levels within the therapeutic range. **B,** Within the therapeutic range, small increments in dosage of most drugs produce small increases in drug levels. With this relationship, moderate fluctuations in dosage are unlikely to result in either toxicity or therapeutic failure.

Therapeutic Uses

Epilepsy

Phenytoin can be used to treat all major forms of epilepsy except absence seizures. The drug is especially effective against tonic-clonic seizures, and phenytoin is a drug of choice for treating these seizures in adults and older children. (Carbamazepine is preferred to phenytoin for treating tonic-clonic seizures in young children.) Although phenytoin can be used to treat simple and complex partial seizures, the drug is less effective against these seizures than against tonic-clonic seizures. Phenytoin can be administered by intravenous (IV) injection to treat generalized convulsive SE, but other drugs are preferred.

Cardiac Dysrhythmias

Phenytoin is active against certain types of dysrhythmias. Antidysrhythmic applications are discussed in Chapter 41.

Adverse Effects

Effects on the CNS

Although phenytoin acts on the CNS in a relatively selective fashion to suppress seizures, the drug can still cause CNS side effects—especially when dosage is excessive. At therapeutic levels (10–20 mcg/mL), sedation and other CNS effects are mild. At plasma levels above 20 mcg/mL, toxicity can occur. Nystagmus (continuous back-and-forth movements of the eyes) is relatively common. Other manifestations of excessive dosage include sedation, ataxia (staggering gait), diplopia (double vision), and cognitive impairment.

Gingival Hyperplasia

Gingival hyperplasia (excessive growth of gum tissue) is characterized by swelling, tenderness, and bleeding of the gums. In extreme cases, patients require gingivectomy (surgical removal of excess gum tissue). Gingival hyperplasia is seen in about 20% of patients who take phenytoin. Can risk be reduced? Possibly. Risk may be minimized by good oral hygiene, including dental flossing and gum massage. Patients should be taught these techniques and encouraged to practice them. Supplemental folic acid is often recommended for this adverse effect based on studies that demonstrated that supplemental folic acid (0.5 mg/day) reduces gingival overgrowth. However, other research did not demonstrate this benefit. A subsequent Cochrane review established that only 15 of the studies met inclusion criteria and even those had issues with methodological quality. Their conclusion: Current evidence is insufficient to support the use of folic acid to prevent gingival hyperplasia so additional randomized control trial are needed.

Dermatologic Effects

Between 2% and 5% of patients develop a morbilliform (measles-like) rash. Rarely, morbilliform rash progresses to much more severe reactions: *Stevens-Johnson syndrome* (SJS) or *toxic epidermal necrolysis* (TEN). FDA labeling warns that the risk for developing SJS or TEN is strongly associated with a genetic mutation known as *human leukocyte antigen (HLA)-B*1502,* which occurs almost exclusively in people of Asian descent. For this reason, phenytoin should not be prescribed for patients known to have this mutation.

Effects in Pregnancy

Phenytoin is a teratogen. It can cause cleft palate, heart malformations, and *fetal hydantoin syndrome,* characterized by growth deficiency, motor or mental deficiency, microcephaly, craniofacial distortion, positional deformities of the limbs, hypoplasia of the nails and fingers, and impaired neurodevelopment. Because of these effects, phenytoin is classified in FDA Pregnancy Risk Category D and hence should be used during pregnancy only if safer alternatives are not effective and if the benefits of seizure control are deemed to outweigh the risk to the fetus.

Phenytoin can decrease synthesis of vitamin K–dependent clotting factors and can thereby cause *bleeding tendencies in newborns.* The risk for neonatal bleeding can be decreased by giving prophylactic vitamin K to the mother for 1 month before and during delivery and to the infant immediately after delivery.

Cardiovascular Effects

When phenytoin is administered by IV injection (to treat SE), cardiac dysrhythmias and hypotension may result. These dangerous responses can be minimized by injecting phenytoin no faster than 50 mg/min.

BLACK BOX WARNING: PHENYTOIN [DILANTIN, PHENYTEK] AND FOSPHENYTOIN [CEREBYX]

When administered intravenously at rates exceeding 50 mg/min in adults, or at the slower rate of either 1 to 3 mg/kg/min *or* 50 mg/min in children, phenytoin can cause severe hypotension and cardiac dysrhythmias. Cardiac monitoring should be in place before administration.

Other Adverse Effects

Hirsutism (overgrowth of hair in unusual places) can be a disturbing response, especially in young women. Interference with vitamin D metabolism may cause rickets and osteomalacia (softening of the bones). Interference with vitamin K metabolism can lower prothrombin levels, thereby causing bleeding tendencies in newborns. Very rarely, liver damage may occur, probably because of drug allergy.

Drug Interactions

Phenytoin interacts with a large number of drugs. The more important interactions are discussed here.

Interactions Resulting From Induction of Hepatic Drug-Metabolizing Enzymes

Phenytoin stimulates synthesis of hepatic drug-metabolizing enzymes. As a result, phenytoin can decrease the effects of other drugs, including *oral contraceptives, warfarin* (an anticoagulant), and *glucocorticoids* (antiinflammatory and immunosuppressive drugs). Because avoiding pregnancy is desirable while taking antiseizure medications, and because phenytoin can decrease the effectiveness of oral contraceptives, the provider may need to increase the contraceptive dosage, or a switch to an alternative form of contraception may need to be made.

Drugs That Increase Plasma Levels of Phenytoin

Because the therapeutic range of phenytoin is narrow, slight increases in phenytoin levels can cause toxicity. Consequently, caution must be exercised when phenytoin is used with drugs that can increase its level. Drugs known to elevate phenytoin levels include *diazepam* (an antianxiety agent and AED), *isoniazid* (a drug for tuberculosis), *cimetidine* (a drug for gastric ulcers), and *alcohol* (when taken acutely). These agents increase phenytoin levels by reducing the rate at which phenytoin is metabolized. *Valproic acid* (an AED) elevates levels of free phenytoin by displacing phenytoin from binding sites on plasma proteins.

Drugs That Decrease Plasma Levels of Phenytoin

Carbamazepine, phenobarbital, and *alcohol* (when used chronically) can accelerate the metabolism of phenytoin, thereby decreasing its level. Breakthrough seizures can result.

CNS Depressants

The depressant effects of *alcohol, barbiturates,* and *other CNS depressants* will add with those of phenytoin. Advise patients to avoid alcohol and all other drugs with CNS-depressant actions.

Preparations, Dosage, and Administration

Preparations

There are a large number of phenytoin products on the market. Phenytoin products made by different manufacturers have equivalent bioavailability. Therefore, although switching between products from different manufacturers was a concern in the past, it is not a concern today.

Dosage

Dosing is highly individualized. Plasma drug levels are often monitored as an aid to establishing dosage. *The dosing objective is to produce levels between 10 and 20 mcg/mL.* Levels below 10 mcg/mL are too low to control seizures; levels above 20 mcg/mL produce toxicity. Because phenytoin has a relatively narrow therapeutic range (between 10 and 20 mcg/mL), and because of the nonlinear relationship between phenytoin dosage and phenytoin plasma levels, after a safe and effective dosage has been established, the patient should adhere to it rigidly.

When treatment is discontinued, dosage should be reduced gradually. Abrupt withdrawal may precipitate seizures.

Administration

Oral preparations may cause gastric discomfort. Patients should be informed that gastric upset can be reduced by administering phenytoin with or immediately after a meal. Patients using the oral suspension should shake it well before dispensing because failure to do so can result in uneven dosing.

Fosphenytoin

Fosphenytoin [Cerebyx] is a prodrug that is converted to phenytoin when metabolized. It is recommended as a substitute for oral phenytoin when the oral route is contraindicated. Because it is converted to phenytoin, the mechanism of action, therapeutic and adverse effects, and drug interactions are the same as those of phenytoin.

Pharmacokinetics

Pharmacokinetic properties are essentially the same as phenytoin after conversion. There are a few differences that are attributable to the prodrug in its nonhydrolyzed state.

Absorption

Fosphenytoin is available for parenteral administration only. Unlike phenytoin, fosphenytoin may be administered by the intramuscular (IM) route. This provides an advantage in that, if IV access is unattainable, the drug is rapidly absorbed after IM administration. Bioavailability is 100% using either the IM or the IV route.

Metabolism

Fosphenytoin is rapidly hydrolyzed to phenytoin. Its conversion half-life is 15 minutes.

Distribution

Fosphenytoin is 95% to 99% protein bound. Because it is more highly protein bound than phenytoin, protein binding with fosphenytoin may displace phenytoin from protein binding sites, resulting in a transient increase in free (unbound, active) phenytoin.

Adverse Effects

Adverse effects of fosphenytoin are the same as those of phenytoin, with one notable exception. During IV infusion, temporary paresthesias and itching, especially in the groin area, may occur. This infusion-related reaction will resolve when the infusion rate is decreased or within 10 minutes after completion of the infusion.

Dosage and Administration

Fosphenytoin has a unique dosing system. Although 150 mg of fosphenytoin will hydrolyze to 100 mg of phenytoin, rather than use standard milligram dosing, fosphenytoin is dosed in phenytoin equivalents (PE). Using this alternative, fosphenytoin 1 mg PE equals phenytoin 1 mg.

Unlike phenytoin, the IV formulation of fosphenytoin is compatible with standard IV solutions. When the drug is administered IM, the full dose may need to be divided into 2 to 4 separate injections.

Carbamazepine

Carbamazepine [Tegretol, Tegretol-XR, Tegretol CR ♣, Carbatrol, Epitol, Equetro] is a cornerstone of epilepsy therapy. The drug is active against partial seizures and tonic-clonic seizures but not absence seizures.

Mechanism of Action

Carbamazepine suppresses high-frequency neuronal discharge in and around seizure foci. The mechanism appears to be the same as that of phenytoin: delayed recovery of sodium channels from their inactivated state.

Pharmacokinetics

Absorption of carbamazepine is delayed and variable. Levels peak 4 to 12 hours after dosing. Overall bioavailability is about 80%. The drug distributes well to tissues.

Elimination is by hepatic metabolism. Carbamazepine is unusual in that its half-life decreases as therapy progresses. During the initial phase of treatment, the half-life is about 40 hours. With continued treatment, the half-life decreases to about 15 hours because carbamazepine, like phenytoin and phenobarbital, induces hepatic drug-metabolizing enzymes. By increasing its own metabolism, carbamazepine causes its own half-life to decline.

Therapeutic Uses

Epilepsy

Carbamazepine is effective against tonic-clonic, simple partial, and complex partial seizures. Because the drug causes fewer adverse effects than phenytoin and phenobarbital, it is often preferred to these agents. Many prescribers consider carbamazepine the drug of first choice for partial seizures. Carbamazepine is not effective against absence, myoclonic, or atonic seizures.

Bipolar Disorder

Carbamazepine can provide symptomatic control in patients with bipolar disorder (manic-depressive illness) and is often effective in patients who are refractory to lithium. The role of carbamazepine in bipolar disorder is discussed in Chapter 26.

Trigeminal and Glossopharyngeal Neuralgias

A neuralgia is a severe, stabbing pain that occurs along the course of a nerve. Carbamazepine can reduce neuralgia associated with the trigeminal and glossopharyngeal nerves. The mechanism is unknown. It should be noted that, although carbamazepine can reduce pain in these specific neuralgias, it is not generally effective as an analgesic and is not indicated for other kinds of pain.

Adverse Effects

CNS Effects

In contrast to phenytoin and phenobarbital, carbamazepine has minimal effects on cognitive function. This is a primary reason for selecting carbamazepine over other antiseizure drugs.

Carbamazepine can cause a variety of *neurologic effects,* including visual disturbances (nystagmus, blurred vision, diplopia), ataxia, vertigo, unsteadiness, and headache. These reactions are common during the first weeks of treatment, affecting 35% to 50% of patients. Fortunately, tolerance usually develops with continued use. These effects can be minimized by initiating therapy at low doses and giving the largest portion of the daily dose at bedtime.

Hematologic Effects

Carbamazepine-induced bone marrow suppression can cause *leukopenia, anemia,* and *thrombocytopenia.* However, serious reactions are rare. Thrombocytopenia and anemia, which have an incidence of 5%, respond to drug discontinuation. Leukopenia, which has an incidence of 10%, is usually transient and subsides even with continued drug use. Accordingly, carbamazepine should not be withdrawn unless the white blood cell count drops below $3000/mm^3$.

Fatal *aplastic anemia* has occurred during carbamazepine therapy. This reaction is extremely rare, having an incidence of 1 in 200,000.

To monitor for serious hematologic effects, complete blood counts should be performed before treatment and periodically thereafter. Patients with preexisting hematologic abnormalities should not use this drug. Patients should be informed about manifestations of hematologic abnormalities (fever, sore throat, pallor, weakness, infection, easy bruising, petechiae) and instructed to notify the prescriber if these occur.

Birth Defects

Carbamazepine is teratogenic. In humans, the drug is associated with a 2.6-fold increase in the risk for spina bifida, a neural tube defect. Because it can harm the fetus, carbamazepine is classified in FDA Pregnancy Risk Category D and hence should be used only if the benefits of seizure control are deemed to outweigh risks to the fetus.

Hypoosmolarity

Carbamazepine can inhibit renal excretion of water, apparently by promoting secretion of antidiuretic hormone. Water retention can reduce the osmolarity of blood and other body fluids, thereby posing a threat to patients with heart failure. Periodic monitoring of serum sodium levels is recommended.

Dermatologic Effects

Carbamazepine has been associated with several dermatologic effects, including morbilliform rash (10% incidence), photosensitivity reactions, SJS, and TEN. Mild reactions can often be treated with prednisone (an antiinflammatory agent) or an antihistamine. Severe reactions—SJS and TEN—necessitate drug withdrawal.

BLACK BOX WARNING: CARBAMAZEPINE [CARBATROL, EPITOL, EQUETRO, TEGRETOL]

Carbamazepine may cause serious skin reactions such as SJS and TEN. Fatalities may occur. The risk for a reaction is strongly associated with the HLA-B*1502 variant of the HLA-B gene that is found predominantly in people of Asian ancestry.

Aplastic anemia and agranulocytosis occurred in patients taking carbamazepine. Incidence is rare (±2–6 patients for each 1 million taking the drug.)

A major risk factor for SJS and TEN is HLA-B*1502, a genetic variation seen primarily in people of Asian descent. Among people with the variant gene, about 5% develop SJS or TEN with carbamazepine. Accordingly, to reduce the risk for severe reactions, the FDA recommends that, before receiving carbamazepine, patients of Asian descent be tested for HLA-B*1502. Of note, this was the first time that the FDA recommended genetic screening for a major drug. As discussed previously, the presence of HLA-B*1502 *may* also increase the risk for SJS and TEN in patients taking phenytoin. Accordingly, phenytoin should not be used as an alternative to carbamazepine in patients with the mutation.

Drug-Drug and Drug-Food Interactions

Induction of Drug-Metabolizing Enzymes

Carbamazepine induces hepatic drug-metabolizing enzymes and hence can increase the rate at which it and other drugs are inactivated. Accelerated inactivation of *oral contraceptives* and *warfarin* is of particular concern.

Phenytoin and Phenobarbital

Both phenytoin and phenobarbital induce hepatic drug metabolism. Thus, if either drug is taken with carbamazepine, induction of metabolism is likely to be greater than with carbamazepine alone. Accordingly, phenytoin and phenobarbital can further accelerate the metabolism of carbamazepine, thereby decreasing its effects.

Grapefruit Juice

As discussed in Chapter 4, grapefruit juice can inhibit the metabolism of many drugs, thereby causing their plasma levels to rise. Grapefruit juice can increase peak and trough levels of carbamazepine by 40%. Advise patients to avoid grapefruit juice.

Dosage and Administration

Carbamazepine should be administered with meals to reduce gastric upset. Administering the largest portion of the daily dose at bedtime can help reduce adverse CNS effects. Carbamazepine suspension should not be administered with other liquid-formulation medicines.

To minimize side effects, dosage is low initially and then increased gradually (every 1–3 weeks) until seizure control is achieved.

Valproic Acid

Valproic acid [Depakene, Depakote, Depakote ER, Depacon, Stavzor, Epival ♣] is an important AED used widely to treat all major seizure types. In addition to its use in epilepsy, valproic acid is used for bipolar disorder and migraine headache.

Nomenclature

Valproic acid is available in three closely related chemical forms (Table 19.4): (1) valproic acid; (2) the sodium salt of valproic acid, known as *valproate;* and (3) *divalproex sodium,* a combination of valproic acid plus its sodium salt. All three forms have identical antiseizure actions. In this chapter, the term *valproic acid* is used in reference to all three.

Mechanism of Action

The exact mechanism of valproic acid is unknown. Though several mechanisms have been suggested, most experts now believe it may augment the inhibitory influence of GABA or increase GABA concentration in the brain.

Pharmacokinetics

Valproic acid is readily absorbed from the gastrointestinal (GI) tract and is widely distributed throughout the body. The drug undergoes extensive hepatic metabolism followed by renal excretion.

Therapeutic responses are often seen at plasma levels of 50 to 100 mcg/mL. However, the correlation between plasma levels and therapeutic effects is not very narrow.

TABLE 19.4 ■ Oral Preparations of Valproic Acid and Its Derivatives

Chemical Form	Trade Name	Product Description	Comments
Valproic acid	Depakene	Capsules (250 mg)	Immediate release; GI upset is common.
	Stavzor	Capsules, delayed release, enteric coated (125, 250, 500 mg)	Capsule is smaller and easier to swallow than Depakote and Depakote ER tablets. Enteric coating may reduce GI upset, but there are no clinical data to show that Stavzor is better tolerated than Depakene.
Valproate	Depakene	Syrup (250 mg/5 mL)	Immediate release; GI upset is common.
Divalproex sodium	Depakote, Epival ♣	Tablets, delayed release, enteric coated (125, 250, 500 mg)	Released over 8–12 hr, so *not* for once-daily administration. *Not interchangeable with Depakote ER* (extended-release tablets) because rate of drug release is different. Less GI upset than Depakene.
	Depakote ER	Tablets, extended release, enteric coated (250 and 500 mg)	Released over 18–24 hr, so *can* be administered once daily. *Not interchangeable with regular Depakote* (delayed-release tablets) because rate of drug release is different. Not approved for epilepsy (but used anyway). Less GI upset than Depakene.
	Depakote	"Sprinkle" capsules containing enteric-coated granules (125 mg)	Immediate release. Less GI upset than Depakene. May swallow capsule whole or open and sprinkle granules on a small amount (1 tsp) of soft food.

GI, gastrointestinal.

Therapeutic Uses

Seizure Disorders

Valproic acid is considered a first-line drug for all partial and generalized seizures.

Bipolar Disorder

Like carbamazepine, valproic acid can provide symptomatic control in patients with bipolar disorder (manic-depressive illness). This application is discussed in Chapter 26.

Migraine

Valproic acid is approved for prophylaxis of migraine (see Chapter 23).

Adverse Effects

Valproic acid is generally well tolerated and causes minimal sedation and cognitive impairment. Gastrointestinal effects are most common. Hepatotoxicity and pancreatitis are rare but serious.

BLACK BOX WARNING: VALPROATE AND VALPROIC ACID [DEPACON, DEPAKENE, DEPAKOTE, STAVZOR]

Fatal hepatic failure has occurred; young children and patients with mitochondrial disease are at increased risk.

Fatal and rapidly progressing pancreatitis has occurred. Common symptoms include nausea, vomiting, anorexia, and abdominal pain.

Valproate is highly teratogenic. Neonates who survive may have major congenital malformations and decreased mental capacity.

Gastrointestinal Effects

Nausea, vomiting, and indigestion are common but transient. These effects are most intense with formulations that are not enteric coated. Gastrointestinal reactions can be minimized by administering valproic acid with food and by using an enteric-coated product (see Table 19.4).

Hepatotoxicity

Rarely, valproic acid has been associated with fatal liver failure. Most deaths have occurred within the first few months of therapy. The overall incidence of fatal hepatotoxicity is about 1 in 40,000. However, in high-risk patients—children younger than 2 years receiving multidrug therapy—the incidence is much higher: 1 in 500. To minimize the risk for fatal liver injury, the following guidelines have been established:

- Don't use valproic acid in conjunction with other drugs in children younger than 2 years.
- Don't use valproic acid in patients with preexisting liver dysfunction.
- Evaluate liver function at baseline and periodically thereafter. (Unfortunately, monitoring liver function may fail to provide advance warning of severe hepatotoxicity. Fatal liver failure can develop so rapidly that it is not preceded by an abnormal test result.)
- Inform patients about signs and symptoms of liver injury (reduced appetite, malaise, nausea, abdominal pain, jaundice) and instruct them to notify the prescriber if these develop.
- Use valproic acid in the lowest effective dosage.

Pancreatitis

Life-threatening pancreatitis may develop in children and adults. Some cases have been hemorrhagic, progressing rapidly from initial symptoms to death. Pancreatitis can develop soon after starting therapy or after years of drug use. Patients should be informed about signs of pancreatitis (abdominal pain, nausea, vomiting, anorexia) and instructed to obtain immediate evaluation if these develop. If pancreatitis is diagnosed, valproic acid should be withdrawn, and alternative medication should be substituted as indicated.

Pregnancy-Related Harm

Valproic acid is *highly teratogenic,* especially when taken during the first trimester. The risk for a major congenital malformation is 4 times higher than with other AEDs. Neural tube defects (e.g., spina bifida) are the greatest concern. The risk is 1 in 20 among women taking valproic acid, versus 1 in 1000 among women in the general population. In addition to neural tube defects, valproic acid can cause five other major congenital malformations: atrial septal defect, cleft palate, hypospadias, polydactyly, and craniosynostosis.

Exposure to valproic acid in utero can *impair cognitive function.* Children exposed to valproic acid had IQ scores that were significantly lower than those of children exposed to other AEDs (carbamazepine, phenytoin, or lamotrigine). These deficits persist for at least 4.5 years, and perhaps longer.

Valproic acid is classified in FDA Pregnancy Risk Category D and should be avoided by women of childbearing potential—unless it is the only AED that will work. Women who *must* use the drug should use an effective form of contraception and should take folic acid supplements to help protect against neural tube damage in case pregnancy occurs. (See Patient Care across the Lifespan.)

Hyperammonemia

Combining valproic acid with topiramate poses a risk for hyperammonemia (excessive ammonia in the blood), which may occur with or without encephalopathy. Symptoms include vomiting, lethargy, altered level of consciousness, and altered cognitive function. If these symptoms develop, hyperammonemic encephalopathy should be suspected, and blood ammonia should be measured. As a rule, symptoms abate after removal of either drug.

Other Adverse Effects

Valproic acid may cause rash, weight gain, hair loss, tremor, and blood dyscrasias (leukopenia, thrombocytopenia, red blood cell aplasia). Significant CNS effects are uncommon.

Drug Interactions

Phenobarbital

Valproic acid decreases the rate at which phenobarbital is metabolized. Blood levels of phenobarbital may rise by 40%, resulting in significant CNS depression. When the combination is used, levels of phenobarbital should be monitored, and, if they rise too high, phenobarbital dosage should be reduced.

Phenytoin

Valproic acid can displace phenytoin from binding sites on plasma proteins. The resultant increase in free phenytoin may lead to toxicity. Phenytoin levels and clinical status should be monitored.

Topiramate

See previous discussion under "Hyperammonemia."

PATIENT-CENTERED CARE ACROSS THE LIFE SPAN

Antiepileptic Drugs

Life Stage	Considerations or Concerns
Children	Currently approved AEDs are approved for children, with the exception of eslicarbazepine. Although approved for pediatric use, prescribing information for many AEDs mentions that inadequate studies have been done in younger children.
Pregnant women	Valproate is classified as FDA Pregnancy Risk Category X. It should not be prescribed for pregnant women. Carbamazepine, phenytoin, phenobarbital, and topiramate are FDA Pregnancy Risk Category D drugs. Fetal harm has been documented in humans for these drugs. The remaining drugs are FDA Pregnancy Risk Category C drugs. Fetal harm has been documented in animal studies but not in humans. The lack of documented harm in humans often reflects a lack of studies rather than positive outcomes. Canadian labeling prohibits the prescribing of vigabatrin to pregnant women. The risk to a fetus from uncontrolled seizures is greater than the risk from AEDs. Therefore patients with major seizure disorders should continue to take AEDs throughout pregnancy. To minimize fetal risk, the lowest effective dosage should be determined and maintained, and just one drug should be used whenever possible. To reduce the risk for neural tube defects that can occur with AEDs, pregnant patients should take supplemental folic acid before conception and throughout pregnancy. A much higher than typical dose of 2-5 mg/day is advocated by some specialists and was previously the standard in the UK; however, subsequent animal studies found that high dose folic acid could cause brain damage. The most recent recommendations by the American Academy of Neurology and the American Epilepsy Society recommend the same 0.4 mg/daily dosage currently recommended for all pregnant women. To increase data on pregnancy outcomes, pregnant women taking AEDs are encouraged to enroll in the North American AED Pregnancy Registry at www.aedpregnancyregistry.org.
Breastfeeding Women	Manufacturers advise carefully weighing the benefits of breastfeeding over the risks for adverse effects in the infant. Of note, for women taking vigabatrin, Canadian labeling contraindicates breastfeeding.
Older adults	Beers Criteria list carbamazepine, oxcarbazepine, and phenobarbital among the drugs deemed possibly inappropriate for adults 65 years and older. Additionally, the Pharmacy Quality Alliance identifies phenobarbital as a high-risk medication for patients 56 years and older. Because elderly patients are at increased risk for adverse events (e.g., falls because of sedation), cautious prescribing of all AEDs, often at lower initial doses, is advisable.

Carbapenem Antibiotics

Two carbapenem antibiotics—meropenem and imipenem/cilastatin—can reduce plasma levels of valproic acid. Breakthrough seizures have occurred. Of note, increasing the dosage of valproic acid may be insufficient to overcome this effect. Accordingly, meropenem and imipenem/cilastatin should be avoided in patients taking valproic acid.

Ethosuximide

Therapeutic Use

Ethosuximide [Zarontin] is the drug of choice for absence seizures, the only indication it has. Absence seizures are eliminated in 60% of patients, and, in newly diagnosed patients, practical control is achieved in 80% to 90%.

Mechanism of Action

Ethosuximide suppresses neurons in the thalamus that are responsible for generating absence seizures. The specific mechanism is inhibition of low-threshold calcium currents, known as T currents. Ethosuximide does not block sodium channels and does not enhance GABA-mediated neuronal inhibition.

Pharmacokinetics

Ethosuximide is well absorbed after oral administration. Therapeutic plasma levels range between 40 and 100 mcg/mL. The drug is eliminated by a combination of hepatic metabolism and renal excretion. Its half-life is 60 hours in adults and 30 hours in children. Ethosuximide does not induce drug-metabolizing enzymes.

Adverse Effects and Drug Interactions

Ethosuximide is generally devoid of significant adverse effects and interactions. During initial treatment, it may cause drowsiness, dizziness, and lethargy. These diminish with continued use. Nausea and vomiting may occur and can be reduced by administering the drug with food. Rare but serious reactions include systemic lupus erythematosus, leukopenia, aplastic anemia, and SJS.

Dosage Considerations

Ethosuximide has a long half-life. This allows dosing to be done just once a day; however, dosing twice a day is better tolerated.

Because absence seizures occur many times each day, monitoring the clinical response rather than plasma drug levels is the preferred method for dosage determination. Dosage should be increased until seizures have been controlled or until adverse effects become too great.

Phenobarbital

Phenobarbital, one of our oldest AEDs, is effective and inexpensive, and it can be administered just once a day. Unfortunately, certain side effects—lethargy, depression, learning impairment—can be significant. Hence, although phenobarbital was used widely in the past, it has largely been replaced by newer drugs that are equally effective but better tolerated.

Phenobarbital belongs to the barbiturate family. However, in contrast to most barbiturates, which produce generalized depression of the CNS, phenobarbital is able to suppress seizures at doses that produce only moderate disruption of CNS function. Because it can reduce seizures without causing sedation, phenobarbital is classified as an *anticonvulsant barbiturate* (to distinguish it from most other barbiturates, which are employed as sedatives or "sleeping pills").

The basic pharmacology of the barbiturates is discussed in Chapter 27. Discussion here is limited to the use of phenobarbital for seizures.

Mechanism of Antiseizure Action

Phenobarbital suppresses seizures by potentiating the effects of GABA. Specifically, the drug binds to GABA receptors, causing the receptors to respond more intensely to GABA itself.

Pharmacokinetics

Phenobarbital is administered orally, and absorption is complete. Elimination occurs through hepatic metabolism and renal excretion. Phenobarbital has a long half-life—about 4 days. As a result, once-daily dosing is adequate for most patients. In addition to permitting once-daily dosing, the long half-life has another consequence: 2 to 3 weeks are required for plasma levels to reach plateau. (Recall that, in the absence of a loading dose, an interval equivalent to four half-lives is required to reach plateau.)

Therapeutic Uses

Epilepsy

Phenobarbital is effective against partial seizures and generalized tonic-clonic seizures but not absence seizures. Intravenous phenobarbital can be used for generalized convulsive SE, but other antiseizure drugs are preferred.

Sedation and Induction of Sleep

Like other barbiturates, phenobarbital can be used for sedation and to promote sleep at night. These applications are discussed in Chapter 27.

Adverse Effects

Neuropsychological Effects

Drowsiness is the most common CNS effect. During the initial phase of therapy, sedation develops in practically all patients. With continued treatment, tolerance to sedation develops. Some children and older patients experience paradoxical responses: instead of becoming sedated, they may become irritable and hyperactive. Cognitive deficits may occur in children. Depression may occur in adults. Older adult patients may experience agitation and confusion.

Physical Dependence

Like all other barbiturates, phenobarbital can cause physical dependence. However, at the doses employed to treat epilepsy, significant dependence is unlikely.

Exacerbation of Intermittent Porphyria

Phenobarbital and other barbiturates can increase the risk for acute intermittent porphyria. Accordingly, barbiturates are absolutely contraindicated for patients with a history of this disorder.

Use in Pregnancy

Use of phenobarbital during pregnancy poses a significant risk for major fetal malformations. Women who take phenobarbital during pregnancy or become pregnant while taking the drug should be informed of the potential risk to the fetus.

Like phenytoin, phenobarbital can decrease synthesis of vitamin K–dependent clotting factors and can thereby cause bleeding tendencies in newborns. The risk for neonatal bleeding can be decreased by administering vitamin K to the mother for 1 month before delivery and during delivery and to the infant immediately after delivery.

Other Adverse Effects

Like phenytoin, phenobarbital can interfere with the metabolism of vitamins D and K. Disruption of vitamin D metabolism can cause rickets and osteomalacia.

Toxicity

When taken in moderately excessive doses, phenobarbital causes nystagmus and ataxia. Severe overdose produces generalized CNS depression; death results from depression of respiration. Barbiturate toxicity and its treatment are discussed in Chapter 27.

Drug Interactions

Induction of Drug-Metabolizing Enzymes

Phenobarbital induces hepatic drug-metabolizing enzymes and can thereby accelerate the metabolism of other drugs, causing a loss of therapeutic effects. This is of particular concern with oral contraceptives and warfarin.

CNS Depressants

Being a CNS depressant itself, phenobarbital can intensify CNS depression caused by other drugs (e.g., alcohol, benzodiazepines, opioids). Severe respiratory depression and coma can result. Patients should be warned against combining phenobarbital with other drugs that have CNS-depressant actions.

Valproic Acid

Valproic acid is an AED that has been used in combination with phenobarbital. By competing with phenobarbital for drug-metabolizing enzymes, valproic acid can increase plasma levels of phenobarbital by approximately 40%. Hence, when this combination is used, the dosage of phenobarbital must be reduced.

Drug Withdrawal

When phenobarbital is withdrawn, dosage should be reduced gradually because abrupt withdrawal can precipitate SE. Patients should be warned of this danger and instructed not to discontinue phenobarbital too quickly.

Dosage Considerations

Because phenobarbital has a long half-life, several weeks are required for drug levels to reach plateau. If plateau must be reached sooner, a loading dose schedule can be employed. For example, doses that are twice normal can be given for 4 days. Alternatively, a dose of 10 to 20 mg/kg can be administered and repeated in 20 minutes, as needed. The administration rate should not exceed 60 mg/minute. Unfortunately, these large doses are likely to produce substantial CNS depression.

Primidone

Primidone [Mysoline] is active against all major seizure disorders except absence seizures. The drug is nearly identical in structure to phenobarbital. As a result, the pharmacology of both agents is very similar.

Pharmacokinetics

Primidone is readily absorbed after oral dosing. In the liver, much of the drug undergoes conversion to two active metabolites: phenobarbital and phenylethylmalonamide. Seizure control is produced by primidone itself and by its metabolites. Therapeutic plasma levels range from 5 to 12 mcg/mL. Levels above 15 mcg/mL are considered toxic.

Therapeutic Uses

Primidone is effective against tonic-clonic, simple partial, and complex partial seizures. The drug is not active against absence seizures.

As a rule, primidone is employed in combination with another AED, usually phenytoin or carbamazepine. Primidone is never taken together with phenobarbital because phenobarbital is an active metabolite of primidone, so concurrent use would be irrational.

Adverse Effects

Sedation, ataxia, and dizziness are common during initial treatment but diminish with continued drug use. Like phenobarbital, primidone can cause confusion in older adults and paradoxical hyperexcitability in children. A sense of acute intoxication can occur shortly after dosing. As with phenobarbital, primidone is absolutely contraindicated for patients with acute intermittent porphyria. Serious adverse reactions (acute psychosis, leukopenia, thrombocytopenia, systemic lupus erythematosus) can occur but are rare.

Drug Interactions

Drug interactions for primidone are similar to those for phenobarbital. Primidone can induce hepatic drug-metabolizing enzymes and can thereby reduce the effects of oral contraceptives, warfarin, and other drugs. In addition, primidone can intensify responses to other CNS depressants.

NEWER ANTIEPILEPTIC DRUGS

The group of newer AEDs has 15 members. Although most newer AEDs have not been compared directly with the traditional AEDs (or with each other, for that matter), all of these drugs appear equally effective.

Do the newer AEDs have properties that make them appealing? Certainly. As a group, they are better tolerated than the traditional AEDs and may pose a smaller risk to the developing fetus. Furthermore, only one—oxcarbazepine—induces drug-metabolizing enzymes to a significant degree, and hence interactions with other drugs, including other AEDs, are relatively minor.

The subject of approved indications for the newer AEDs requires comment. When these drugs were introduced, FDA-approved indications were limited to *adjunctive* therapy of certain seizure disorders. None of these drugs was approved for *monotherapy* because clinical trials were limited to patients who were refractory to traditional AEDs. When the trials were conducted, rather than switching patients from a traditional AED to the experimental AED, the experimental AED was *added* to the existing regimen. Hence, when the trials were completed, all we knew for sure was that the new AED was effective when used together with an older AED. We had no data on use of the newer AED alone. As a result, the FDA had no option but to approve the new drug for adjunctive therapy. Since being released, several of the newer AEDs have received FDA approval for monotherapy.

To help prescribers be more comfortable with the newer AEDs, two organizations—the American Academy of Neurology (AAN) and American Epilepsy Society (AES)—convened a panel to evaluate the efficacy and tolerability of these drugs. For some of the newer AEDs, the AAN/AES panel recommended uses not yet approved by the FDA. These recommendations, along with FDA-approved indications, are discussed here.

Oxcarbazepine

Actions and Uses

Oxcarbazepine [Oxtellar XR, Trileptal], a derivative of carbamazepine, is approved for adjunctive therapy of partial seizures in adults and children. Antiseizure effects result from blockade of voltage-sensitive sodium channels in neuronal membranes, an action that stabilizes hyperexcitable neurons and thereby suppresses seizure spread. The drug does not affect neuronal GABA receptors.

Pharmacokinetics

Oxcarbazepine is well absorbed both in the presence and absence of food. In the liver, the drug undergoes rapid conversion to a 10-monohydroxy metabolite (MHD), its active form. MHD has a half-life of 9 hours and undergoes excretion in the urine.

Adverse Effects

The most common adverse effects are dizziness, drowsiness, double vision, nystagmus, headache, nausea, vomiting, and ataxia. Patients should avoid driving and other hazardous activities, unless the degree of drowsiness is low.

Clinically significant *hyponatremia* (sodium concentration below 125 mmol/L) develops in 2.5% of patients. Signs include nausea, drowsiness, headache, and confusion. If oxcarbazepine is combined with other drugs that can decrease sodium levels (especially diuretics), monitoring of sodium levels may be needed.

Like carbamazepine, oxcarbazepine can cause *serious skin reactions,* including SJS and TEN. There is 30% cross sensitivity among patients with hypersensitivity to carbamazepine. Accordingly, patients with a history of severe reactions to either drug should probably not use the other.

Oxcarbazepine has not caused the severe hematologic abnormalities seen with carbamazepine. Accordingly, routine monitoring of blood counts is not required.

Oxcarbazepine has been associated with serious *multiorgan hypersensitivity reactions.* Although manifestations vary, patients typically present with fever and rash, associated with one or more of the following: lymphadenopathy, hematologic abnormalities, pruritus, hepatitis, nephritis, hepatorenal syndrome, oliguria, arthralgia, or asthenia. If this reaction is suspected, oxcarbazepine should be discontinued.

Drug Interactions

Oxcarbazepine induces some drug-metabolizing enzymes and inhibits others. It does not induce enzymes that metabolize other AEDs. However, it does induce enzymes that metabolize *oral contraceptives* and can thereby render them less effective. Accordingly, women should employ an alternative birth control method.

Oxcarbazepine inhibits the enzymes that metabolize phenytoin and can thereby raise phenytoin levels. Toxicity can result. Phenytoin levels should be monitored and dosage adjusted accordingly.

Drugs that induce drug-metabolizing enzymes (e.g., phenytoin, phenobarbital, carbamazepine) can reduce levels of MHD, the active form of oxcarbazepine. Accordingly, dosage of oxcarbazepine may need to be increased.

Alcohol can intensify CNS depression caused by oxcarbazepine, so it should be avoided.

As noted, oxcarbazepine should be used with caution in patients taking *diuretics* and other drugs that can lower sodium levels.

Lamotrigine

Therapeutic Uses

Lamotrigine [Lamictal] has a broad spectrum of antiseizure activity. The drug is FDA approved for (1) adjunctive therapy of partial seizures in adults and children older than 2 years, (2) adjunctive therapy of generalized seizures associated with Lennox-Gastaut syndrome in adults and children older than 2 years, (3) adjunctive therapy of primary generalized tonic-clonic seizures in adults and children older than 2 years, and (4) monotherapy of partial seizures in patients at least 13 years old who are converting from another AED. In addition, the AAN/AES guidelines recommend using lamotrigine for absence seizures. Lamotrigine is also FDA approved for long-term maintenance therapy of bipolar disorder (see Chapter 26). Investigational uses include myoclonic, absence, and temporal lobe seizures.

Mechanism of Action

Benefits derive mainly from blocking sodium channels and partly from blocking calcium channels. Both actions decrease release of glutamate, an excitatory neurotransmitter.

Pharmacokinetics

Administration is oral, and absorption is nearly complete, both in the presence and absence of food. Blood levels peak 1.5 to 5 hours after dosing and decline with a half-life of 24 hours. The drug undergoes hepatic metabolism followed by renal excretion.

Drug Interactions

The half-life is dramatically affected by drugs that induce or inhibit hepatic drug-metabolizing enzymes. Enzyme inducers (e.g., carbamazepine, phenytoin, phenobarbital) decrease the half-life of lamotrigine to 10 hours, whereas valproate (an enzyme inhibitor) increases the half-life to about 60 hours. Lamotrigine itself is not an inducer or inhibitor of drug metabolism.

Estrogens can lower lamotrigine levels, whereas lamotrigine may lower progestin levels. This can create unique concerns for the provider caring for a woman of childbearing age who wants to take oral contraceptives.

Adverse Effects

Common side effects include dizziness, diplopia (double vision), blurred vision, nausea, vomiting, and headache. Of much greater concern, patients may develop life-threatening rashes, including SJS and TEN. Deaths have occurred. The incidence of severe rash is about 0.8% in patients younger than

16 years and 0.3% in adults. Concurrent use of valproic acid increases this risk. If a rash develops, lamotrigine should be withdrawn immediately.

BLACK BOX WARNING: LAMOTRIGINE [LAMICTAL]

Lamotrigine may cause serious skin reactions such as SJS and TEN. Fatalities have been reported.

Very rarely, patients experience aseptic meningitis (inflammation of the meninges in the absence of bacterial infection). Patients who develop symptoms of meningitis—headache, fever, stiff neck, nausea, vomiting, rash, sensitivity to light—should undergo immediate evaluation to determine the cause. Treatable causes should be managed as indicated. If no clear cause other than lamotrigine is identified, discontinuation of lamotrigine should be considered.

Risk for suicide may be greater than with most other AEDs. Screen patients for suicidality before starting treatment, and monitor for suicidality during the treatment course.

Gabapentin

Therapeutic Uses

Gabapentin [Neurontin] has a broad spectrum of antiseizure activity. However, its only FDA-approved use in epilepsy is adjunctive therapy of partial seizures (with or without secondary generalization). The AAN/AES guidelines also recommend the drug for monotherapy of partial seizures. Gabapentin also has approval for treating postherpetic neuralgia. Interestingly, more than 80% of prescriptions are written for off-label uses, including relief of neuropathic pain (other than postherpetic neuralgia), prophylaxis of migraine, treatment of fibromyalgia, and relief of postmenopausal hot flashes. However, benefits in these disorders are modest, at best. Gabapentin does not appear effective in bipolar disorder.

Two forms of gabapentin are *not currently indicated* for management of epilepsy and, therefore, should not be confused with the form of gabapentin known as Neurontin. These are gabapentin ER [Gralise], which is approved for management of postherpetic neuralgia, and gabapentin enacarbil [Horizant], a prodrug form of gabapentin approved for treatment of moderate to severe restless legs syndrome. Owing to differences in pharmacokinetics, these forms of gabapentin are *not interchangeable with each other or with Neurontin.*

Mechanism of Action

Gabapentin's precise mechanism of action is unknown. The drug is an analog of GABA, but does not directly affect GABA receptors. Rather, it may enhance GABA release, thereby increasing GABA-mediated inhibition of neuronal firing.

Pharmacokinetics

Gabapentin is rapidly absorbed after oral dosing and reaches peak plasma levels in 2 to 3 hours. Absorption is not affected by food. However, as the dosage gets larger, the percentage absorbed gets smaller because, at high doses, the intestinal transport system for uptake of the drug becomes saturated. Gabapentin is not metabolized and is excreted intact in the urine. Its half-life is 5 to 7 hours.

Drug Interactions

Unlike most AEDs, gabapentin is devoid of significant interactions. It doesn't induce or inhibit drug-metabolizing enzymes and doesn't affect the metabolism of other drugs. As a result, gabapentin is well suited for combined use with other AEDs.

Adverse Reactions

Gabapentin is very well tolerated. The most common side effects are somnolence, dizziness, ataxia, fatigue, nystagmus, and peripheral edema. These are usually mild to moderate and often diminish with continued drug use. Patients should avoid driving and other hazardous activities until they are confident they are not impaired.

Pregabalin

Pregabalin [Lyrica], an analog of GABA, is much like gabapentin. Like gabapentin, pregabalin is used for seizures and neuropathic pain. In addition, pregabalin is approved for fibromyalgia. Pregabalin has very few interactions with other drugs, but adverse effects are common, especially dizziness and sleepiness. In contrast to most other antiseizure agents, pregabalin is regulated under the Controlled Substances Act.

Therapeutic Uses

Pregabalin has four approved indications: neuropathic pain associated with diabetic neuropathy, postherpetic neuralgia, adjunctive therapy of partial seizures, and fibromyalgia.

Mechanism of Action

Although the precise mechanism of action has not been established, we do know that pregabalin can bind with calcium channels on nerve terminals and can thereby inhibit calcium influx, which in turn can inhibit release of several neurotransmitters, including glutamate, norepinephrine, and substance P. Reduced transmitter release may underlie seizure control and relief of neuropathic pain. Although pregabalin is an analog of GABA, the drug does not bind with GABA receptors or with benzodiazepine receptors and hence does not work by mimicking or enhancing the inhibitory actions of GABA.

Pharmacokinetics

Pregabalin is well absorbed after oral dosing. Plasma levels peak in 1.5 hours. Food reduces the rate of absorption but not the extent. Oral bioavailability is 90% or greater. Pregabalin does not bind with plasma proteins but does cross the blood-brain and placental barriers. Elimination is renal, 98% as unchanged drug. Metabolism is negligible. The half-life is 6.3 hours.

Adverse Effects

Pregabalin can cause a variety of adverse effects. The most common are dizziness and somnolence, which often persist as long as the drug is being taken. Blurred vision may develop during early therapy but resolves with continued drug use. About 8% of patients experience significant weight gain (7% or more of body weight in just a few months). Other adverse effects include difficulty thinking, headache, peripheral edema, and dry mouth.

Postmarketing reports indicate a risk for hypersensitivity reactions, including life-threatening angioedema, characterized by swelling of the face, tongue, lip, gums, throat, and larynx. Patients should discontinue pregabalin immediately at the first sign of angioedema or any other hypersensitivity reaction (blisters, hives, rash, dyspnea, wheezing).

In clinical trials, three patients developed rhabdomyolysis (muscle breakdown). However, it is not clear that pregabalin was the cause. Nonetheless, patients should be instructed to report signs of muscle injury (pain, tenderness, weakness). If rhabdomyolysis is diagnosed, or even suspected, pregabalin should be withdrawn.

Abuse Potential and Physical Dependence

In clinical trials, 4% to 12% of patients reported euphoria as a side effect. When given to recreational users of sedative-hypnotic drugs, pregabalin produced subjective effects perceived as similar to those of diazepam [Valium]. On the basis of these data, the Drug Enforcement Agency has classified pregabalin under Schedule V of the Controlled Substances Act.

Abrupt discontinuation can cause insomnia, nausea, headache, diarrhea, and other symptoms that suggest physical dependence. To avoid withdrawal symptoms, pregabalin should be discontinued slowly, over 1 week or more.

Possible Reproductive Toxicity

At this time, pregabalin is classified in FDA Pregnancy Risk Category C: animal studies show a risk for fetal harm, but no controlled studies in women have been done. The reason for this designation is that *data on human reproduction are lacking. When given to pregnant female rats and rabbits, pregabalin caused fetal growth delay, fetal death, structural abnormalities (e.g., skeletal and visceral malformation), and impaired function of the nervous system and reproductive system. Given this, choice of a different AED is recommended for pregnant women.*

When given to male rats before and during mating with untreated females, pregabalin decreased sperm counts and motility, decreased fertility, reduced fetal weight, and caused fetal abnormalities. Men using the drug should be informed about the possibility of decreased fertility and male-mediated teratogenicity. Use of a condom is recommended for men taking pregabalin who have sex with women who may become pregnant.

Use in Breastfeeding

We do not know with certainty whether pregabalin is excreted in breast milk. Until additional data are available, it is best for the patient to either stop nursing or stop taking pregabalin unless it is determined that the benefits of breastfeeding outweigh the risks of pregabalin exposure to the infant.

Drug Interactions

Alcohol, opioids, benzodiazepines, and other CNS depressants may intensify the depressant effects of pregabalin. Accordingly, such combinations should be avoided.

Extensive studies have failed to show pharmacokinetic interactions with any other drugs. Pregabalin does not inhibit cytochrome P450 isoenzymes. Whether it can induce these isoenzymes is unknown. Pregabalin does not interact with oral contraceptives and does not alter the kinetics of any antiseizure drugs studied (carbamazepine, lamotrigine, phenobarbital, phenytoin, topiramate, valproic acid, and tiagabine).

Levetiracetam

Actions and Uses

Levetiracetam [Keppra] is a unique agent that is chemically and pharmacologically different from all other AEDs. How levetiracetam acts is unknown; however, we know that it does not bind to receptors for GABA or any other known neurotransmitter. In the United States the drug is approved for adjunctive therapy of (1) myoclonic seizures in adults and adolescents 12 years and older, (2) partial-onset seizures in adults and children 4 years and older, and (3) primary generalized tonic-clonic seizures in adults and children 6 years and older. Unlabeled uses include migraine, bipolar disorder, and new-onset pediatric epilepsy. In Europe, the drug is approved for monotherapy of partial seizures, for which it is highly effective.

Pharmacokinetics

After oral dosing, levetiracetam undergoes rapid and complete absorption both in the presence and absence of food. Metabolism is minimal and not mediated by hepatic cytochrome P450 isoenzymes. Levetiracetam is excreted in the urine, largely (66%) unchanged.

Adverse Effects

Adverse effects are generally mild to moderate. The most common are drowsiness and asthenia (lack of strength, weakness). Neuropsychiatric symptoms (agitation, anxiety, depression, psychosis, hallucinations, depersonalization) occur in less than 1% of patients. In contrast to other AEDs, levetiracetam does not impair speech, concentration, or other cognitive functions.

Unlike most other AEDs, levetiracetam does not interact with other drugs. It does not alter plasma concentrations of oral contraceptives, warfarin, digoxin, or other AEDs. These benefits are primarily attributable to the fact that levetiracetam is not metabolized by P450 isoenzymes.

Topiramate

Actions and Uses

Topiramate [Topamax] is another broad-spectrum antiseizure agent. The drug is FDA approved for (1) adjunctive treatment of adults and children 2 years and older with partial seizures, primary generalized tonic-clonic seizures, and seizures associated with Lennox-Gastaut syndrome; (2) monotherapy of adults and children 10 years and older with partial seizures or primary generalized tonic-clonic seizures; and (3) prophylaxis of migraine in adults (see Chapter 23). Seizure reduction occurs by four mechanisms: (1) potentiation of GABA-mediated inhibition, (2) blockade of voltage-dependent sodium channels, (3) blockade of receptors for glutamate, an excitatory neurotransmitter, and (4) inhibition of carbonic anhydrase. Unlabeled uses include bipolar disorder, cluster headaches, neuropathic pain (including the pain of diabetic neuropathy), infantile spasms, essential tremor, binge-eating disorder, bulimia nervosa, and weight loss. Studies also show promise for management of alcohol and cocaine dependence.

Pharmacokinetics

With oral administration, absorption is rapid and not affected by food. Plasma levels peak 2 hours after dosing. Most of the drug is eliminated unchanged in the urine.

Adverse Effects

Although topiramate is generally well tolerated, it can cause multiple adverse effects. Common effects include somnolence, dizziness, ataxia, nervousness, diplopia, nausea, anorexia, and weight loss. Cognitive effects (confusion, memory difficulties, altered thinking, reduced concentration, difficulty finding words) can occur, but the incidence is low at recommended dosages. Kidney stones and paresthesias occur rarely.

Topiramate can cause metabolic acidosis. The drug inhibits carbonic anhydrase and thereby increases renal excretion of bicarbonate, which causes plasma pH to fall. Hyperventilation is the most characteristic symptom. Mild to moderate metabolic acidosis develops in 30% of adult patients, but severe acidosis is rare. Risk factors include renal disease, severe respiratory disorders, diarrhea, and a ketogenic diet. Prolonged metabolic acidosis can lead to kidney stones, fractures, and growth delay. Serum bicarbonate should be measured at baseline and periodically thereafter. Advise patients to inform the prescriber if they experience hyperventilation and other symptoms (fatigue, anorexia). If metabolic acidosis is diagnosed, topiramate should be given in reduced dosage or discontinued.

Topiramate can cause hypohidrosis (reduced sweating), thereby posing a risk for hyperthermia. Significant hyperthermia is usually associated with vigorous activity and an elevated environmental temperature.

There have been case reports of angle-closure glaucoma. Left untreated, this rapidly leads to blindness. Patients should be informed about symptoms of glaucoma (ocular pain, unusual redness, sudden worsening or blurring of vision) and instructed to seek immediate attention if these develop. Fortunately, topiramate-induced glaucoma is rare.

Topiramate is classified in FDA Pregnancy Risk Category D and hence should be used only if the benefits of maternal seizure control are deemed to outweigh the risk to the fetus. Women using topiramate should use an effective form of birth control or should switch to a safer antiseizure drug if pregnancy is intended.

Risk for suicide may be greater than with most other AEDs. Screen patients for suicidality before starting treatment and monitor for suicidality during the treatment course.

Drug Interactions

Phenytoin and carbamazepine can decrease levels of topiramate by about 45%. Topiramate may increase levels of phenytoin.

Tiagabine

Actions and Uses

Tiagabine [Gabitril] is FDA approved only for adjunctive therapy of partial seizures in patients at least 12 years old. The drug blocks reuptake of GABA by neurons and glia. As a result, the inhibitory influence of GABA is intensified, and seizures are suppressed. Off-label uses include management of generalized anxiety disorder, multiple sclerosis, neuropathic pain, posttraumatic stress disorder, psychosis, and spasticity. Recent studies show promise for use of tiagabine in migraine prophylaxis as well as management of bipolar disorder and insomnia. However, owing to a risk for seizures (see later), such off-label use is discouraged.

Pharmacokinetics

Tiagabine has uncomplicated kinetics. Administration is oral. Absorption is rapid and nearly complete. Food reduces the rate of absorption but not the extent. Plasma levels peak about 45 minutes after dosing. In the blood, tiagabine is highly (96%) bound to plasma proteins. Elimination is by hepatic metabolism followed by excretion in the bile and, to a lesser extent, the urine. The serum half-life is 7 to 9 hours.

Adverse Effects

Tiagabine is generally well tolerated. Common adverse effects are dizziness, somnolence, asthenia, nausea, nervousness, and tremor. Like most other AEDs, tiagabine can cause dose-related cognitive effects (e.g., confusion, abnormal thinking, trouble concentrating).

Tiagabine has caused seizures in some patients—but only in those using the drug off-label (i.e., those using the drug for a condition other than epilepsy). A few patients have developed SE, which can be life threatening. In most cases, seizures occurred soon after starting tiagabine or after increasing the dosage. Because of seizure risk, off-label use of tiagabine usually should be avoided. Why are people without epilepsy at risk? Possibly because they are not taking AEDs. Remember, tiagabine is approved only for adjunctive use with other AEDs. It may be that these drugs protect against tiagabine-induced seizures. Because people without epilepsy take tiagabine by itself, they are not protected from seizure development.

Drug Interactions

Tiagabine does not alter the metabolism or serum concentrations of other AEDs. However, levels of tiagabine can be decreased by phenytoin, phenobarbital, and carbamazepine—all of which induce drug-metabolizing enzymes.

Zonisamide

Actions and Uses

Zonisamide [Zonegran] is approved only for adjunctive therapy of partial seizures in adults. The drug belongs to the same chemical family as the sulfonamide antibiotics, but lacks antimicrobial activity. In animal models, zonisamide suppresses focal seizure activity and spread. The underlying mechanism appears to be blockade of neuronal sodium channels and calcium channels. This drug is sometimes used off-label for management of bipolar disorder, migraine prophylaxis, and Parkinson disease.

Pharmacokinetics

Zonisamide undergoes rapid absorption from the GI tract. Bioavailability is nearly 100%, in both the presence and absence of food. In the blood, zonisamide is extensively bound to erythrocytes. As a result, its concentration in erythrocytes is 8 times higher than in plasma. Zonisamide is metabolized in the liver by the 3A4 isoenzyme of cytochrome P450 (CYP3A4). Excretion occurs in the urine. Thirty percent is excreted unchanged, with the remainder in the form of metabolites. The plasma half-life is 63 hours.

Adverse Effects

The most common adverse effects are drowsiness, dizziness, anorexia, headache, and nausea. Metabolic acidosis is also common. Like most other AEDs, zonisamide can impair speech, concentration, and other cognitive processes. Because the drug can reduce alertness and impair cognition, patients should avoid driving and other hazardous activities until they know how the drug affects them.

Zonisamide can have severe psychiatric effects. During clinical trials, 2.2% of patients either discontinued treatment or were hospitalized because of severe depression; 1.1% attempted suicide.

Like all other sulfonamides, zonisamide can trigger hypersensitivity reactions, including some that are potentially fatal (e.g., SJS, TEN, fulminant hepatic necrosis). Accordingly, zonisamide is contraindicated for patients with a history of sulfonamide hypersensitivity. Patients who develop a rash should be followed closely because rash can evolve into a more serious event. If severe hypersensitivity develops, zonisamide should be withdrawn immediately. Fortunately, serious reactions and fatalities are rare.

Zonisamide has adverse effects on the kidneys. In clinical trials, about 4% of patients developed nephrolithiasis (kidney stones). The risk can be reduced by drinking 6 to 8 glasses of water a day (to maintain hydration and urine flow). Patients should be informed about signs of kidney stones (sudden back pain, abdominal pain, painful urination, bloody or dark urine) and instructed to report them immediately. In addition to nephrolithiasis, zonisamide can impair glomerular filtration. Because of its effects on the kidney, zonisamide should be used with caution in patients with kidney disease.

Like topiramate, zonisamide inhibits carbonic anhydrase and can thereby cause metabolic acidosis. The condition develops in up to 90% of children and 43% of adults, usually early in treatment. Risk is increased by renal disease, respiratory disease, diarrhea, and following a ketogenic diet. Metabolic acidosis can delay growth in children, and, over time, can lead to kidney stones and fractures in all patients. Advise patients to report hyperventilation and other signs of metabolic acidosis (e.g., fatigue, anorexia). Determine plasma bicarbonate at baseline and periodically thereafter. If metabolic acidosis is diagnosed, zonisamide should be discontinued or given in reduced dosage.

Rarely, zonisamide causes hypohidrosis (decreased sweating) and hyperthermia (elevation of body temperature). Pediatric patients may be at special risk. In warm weather, hypohidrosis may lead to heat stroke and subsequent hospitalization. Patients should be monitored closely for reduced sweating and increased body temperature.

Drug and Food Interactions

Levels of zonisamide can be affected by agents that induce or inhibit CYP3A4. Inducers of CYP3A4—including St. John's wort (an herbal supplement used for depression) and several AEDs (e.g., phenytoin, phenobarbital, carbamazepine)—can accelerate the metabolism of zonisamide and can thereby reduce the drug's half-life (to as little as 27 hours). Conversely, inhibitors of CYP3A4—including grapefruit juice, azole antifungal agents (e.g., ketoconazole), and several protease inhibitors (e.g., ritonavir)—can slow the metabolism of zonisamide and thereby prolong and intensify its effects.

Felbamate

Felbamate [Felbatol] is an effective AED with a broad spectrum of antiseizure activity. Unfortunately, the drug has potentially fatal adverse effects: aplastic anemia and liver failure. Accordingly, use is restricted to patients with severe epilepsy refractory to all other therapy.

Mechanism of Action

Felbamate increases seizure threshold and suppresses seizure spread. The underlying mechanism is unknown. Unlike some AEDs, such as phenobarbital and benzodiazepines, felbamate does not interact with GABA receptors and does not enhance the inhibitory actions of GABA.

Pharmacokinetics

Felbamate is well absorbed after oral dosing, both in the presence and absence of food. Plasma levels peak in 1 to 4 hours. The drug readily penetrates to the CNS. Although therapeutic plasma levels have not been established, levels of 20 to 120 mcg/mL have been measured during clinical trials. Felbamate is eliminated in the urine, primarily unchanged. Its half-life is 14 to 23 hours.

Therapeutic Uses

Felbamate is approved for (1) adjunctive or monotherapy in adults with partial seizures (with or without generalization) and (2) adjunctive therapy in children with Lennox-Gastaut syndrome. However, because of toxicity, use of the drug is very limited.

Adverse Effects

Felbamate can cause aplastic anemia and liver damage. Because of the risk for liver failure, felbamate should not be used by patients with preexisting liver dysfunction. In addition, patients taking the drug should be monitored for indications of liver injury.

BLACK BOX WARNING: FELBAMATE [FELBATOL]

Felbamate has been associated with an increased risk for aplastic anemia. Associated fatality rates have been estimated at 20% to 30%; however, rates up to 70% have been attributed to this drug.

The most common adverse effects are GI disturbances (anorexia, nausea, vomiting) and CNS effects (insomnia, somnolence, dizziness, headache, diplopia). These occur more frequently when felbamate is combined with other drugs.

Drug Interactions

Felbamate can alter plasma levels of other AEDs, and vice versa. Felbamate increases levels of phenytoin and valproic acid. Levels of felbamate are increased by valproic acid and reduced by phenytoin and carbamazepine. Increased levels of phenytoin and valproic acid (and possibly felbamate) could lead to toxicity; reduced levels of felbamate could lead to therapeutic failure. Therefore, to keep levels of these drugs within the therapeutic range, their levels should be monitored and dosages adjusted accordingly.

Lacosamide

Actions and Uses

Lacosamide [Vimpat] is indicated for add-on therapy of partial-onset seizures in patients 17 years and older. Benefits appear to derive from slow inactivation of sodium channels, resulting in stabilization of hyperexcitable neuronal membranes and subsequent inhibition of repetitive firing. In patients with refractory partial-onset seizures, adding lacosamide to the regimen reduced seizure frequency by 50% or more in roughly 40% of those treated. Compared with other drugs for partial-onset seizures, lacosamide has two advantages. First, it has few drug interactions. Second, it can be administered IV as well as orally.

Pharmacokinetics

Lacosamide undergoes complete absorption after oral administration, and hence oral doses produce the same effect as an equivalent IV dose. Drug levels peak 1 to 4 hours after oral dosing and then decline with a half-life of 13 hours. Elimination is by a combination of hepatic metabolism and renal excretion.

Adverse Effects

Lacosamide is generally well tolerated. The most common adverse effects are dizziness, headache, diplopia, and nasopharyngitis. Other effects include vomiting, fatigue, incoordination, blurred vision, tremor, somnolence, and cognitive changes (e.g., impaired memory, confusion, attention disruption). Lacosamide can prolong the PR interval, so it should be used with caution in patients with cardiac conduction problems and in those taking other drugs that prolong the PR interval. About 1% of patients experience euphoria. As a result, lacosamide is classified as a Schedule V drug under the Controlled Substances Act. Like other AEDs, lacosamide carries a small risk for suicidal thoughts or behavior.

Drug Interactions

Lacosamide has few drug interactions. In clinical trials, it had little effect on plasma levels of other AEDs; however, carbamazepine, fosphenytoin, phenytoin, and phenobarbital may decrease the serum concentration of lacosamide. As noted, lacosamide should be used with caution in patients taking other drugs that can prolong the PR interval (e.g., beta blockers, calcium channel blockers).

Rufinamide

Actions and Uses

Rufinamide [Banzel] is approved as add-on therapy for seizures associated with Lennox-Gastaut syndrome, a severe form of childhood epilepsy. Like some other AEDs (e.g., phenytoin, carbamazepine), rufinamide appears to suppress seizure activity by prolonging the inactive state of neuronal sodium channels. In clinical trials, the drug reduced seizure frequency and severity.

Pharmacokinetics

Rufinamide is well absorbed after oral dosing, especially in the presence of food. Plasma levels peak in 4 to 6 hours. Elimination is by enzymatic conversion to inactive products, followed by excretion in the urine. Of note, inactivation does not involve cytochrome P450 isoenzymes. The plasma half-life is 6 to 10 hours.

Adverse Effects

Adverse effects differ somewhat between children and adults. In children, the most common adverse effects are somnolence, vomiting, and headache. In adults, the most common effects are dizziness, fatigue, nausea, and somnolence. Rufinamide can reduce the QT interval on the electrocardiogram, so it should not be used by patients with familial short QT syndrome. Like all other AEDs, rufinamide may increase suicidal thoughts and behavior.

Drug Interactions

Four AEDs—carbamazepine, phenobarbital, phenytoin, and primidone—can significantly reduce levels of rufinamide. Because rufinamide is not metabolized by P450 isoenzymes, induction of cytochrome P450 cannot be the mechanism. One AED—valproic acid—can increase rufinamide levels by up to 70%. Rufinamide causes mild induction of CYP3A4 and can thereby reduce levels of ethinyl estradiol and norethindrone, common components of oral contraceptives. An alternative form of contraception may be needed. Because rufinamide shortens the QT interval, other drugs that shorten the interval (e.g., digoxin) should be used with caution.

Vigabatrin

Actions and Uses

Vigabatrin [Sabril] has two indications: (1) add-on therapy of complex partial seizures in adults who are refractory to other drugs and (2) monotherapy of infantile spasms in children ages 6 months to 2 years. Vigabatrin is the first drug approved in the United States for infantile spasms, a severe seizure disorder that occurs in children during the first year of life. Benefits in adults and children derive from inhibiting GABA transaminase, the enzyme that inactivates GABA in the CNS. By preventing GABA inactivation, vigabatrin increases GABA availability and thereby enhances GABA-mediated inhibition of neuronal activity. Unfortunately, although vigabatrin is effective, it is also dangerous: The drug can cause permanent loss of vision.

Pharmacokinetics

Vigabatrin is administered by mouth, with or without food. Plasma levels peak in 0.5 to 2 hours. Bioavailability is nearly 100%. The drug undergoes little or no metabolism and is eliminated primarily by renal excretion, with a half-life of 7.5 hours. Monitoring plasma drug levels does not help optimize treatment.

Adverse Effect

Vision Loss

Vigabatrin can cause irreversible damage to the retina, usually manifesting as progressive narrowing of the visual field. Severe damage can produce tunnel vision. Some degree of visual field reduction occurs in 30% or more of patients. Damage to the central part of the retina can reduce visual acuity. Some patients experience retinal damage within days to weeks of treatment onset, whereas others may use the drug for months to years before damage occurs.

BLACK BOX WARNING: VIGABATRIN [SABRIL]

Vigabatrin can cause permanent loss of peripheral vision. Vision should be tested at baseline, then at 4 weeks, and then every 3 months as long as therapy continues.

To reduce the extent of damage, vision should be tested at baseline and every 3 months thereafter. If vision loss is detected, vigabatrin should be discontinued. Stopping will not reverse damage that has already occurred but may limit development of further damage. Unfortunately, even with periodic testing, some patients will develop severe vision loss.

Owing to the risk for vision loss, vigabatrin is available only through a restricted use program, known as SHARE (Support, Help, and Resources for Epilepsy). The goal is to monitor for vision damage and discontinue the drug as soon as possible when damage is detected. SHARE requires registration by prescribers, pharmacists, adult patients, and parents/guardians of young patients. In addition, the program requires that adult and pediatric patients undergo regular vision testing.

Other Adverse Effects

In clinical trials, the most common adverse effects in adults (who received vigabatrin plus other AEDs) were headache, somnolence, fatigue, dizziness, convulsions, increased weight, visual field defects, and depression. Like other AEDs, vigabatrin can promote suicidal thoughts and behavior. Among children, the most common adverse effects were somnolence, bronchitis, and otitis media.

Drug Interactions

The risk for retinal damage is increased by combining vigabatrin with other drugs that can directly damage the retina (e.g., hydroxychloroquine) or with drugs that can promote glaucoma (e.g., glucocorticoids, tricyclic antidepressants). Vigabatrin can reduce levels of phenytoin (by inducing CYP2C9, the 2C9 isoenzyme of cytochrome P450) and can increase levels of clonazepam (by a mechanism that is unknown).

Ezogabine

Ezogabine [Potiga] is a first-in-class potassium channel opener. The drug is approved for adjunctive treatment of partial-onset seizures. Ezogabine activates voltage-gated potassium channels in the neuronal membrane and thereby facilitates potassium efflux. As a result, repetitive neuronal firing and related seizure activity are reduced. Unfortunately, ezogabine also activates potassium channels in the bladder epithelium and thereby promotes urinary hesitancy or urinary retention, a unique side effect among the AEDs. Because of its effects on the bladder, ezogabine should be used with caution (if at all) in patients with preexisting voiding difficulty. The drug can impart a red-orange color to urine. This effect is harmless and unrelated to urinary retention. The most common adverse reactions are somnolence, dizziness, fatigue, confusion, vertigo, tremor, incoordination, double vision, memory impairment, and reduced strength. In addition, ezogabine can cause hallucinations and other symptoms of psychosis. There have been no reports of rash, vision impairment, liver damage, or adverse hematologic effects. Ezogabine has the potential for abuse and is under review for possible regulation as a controlled substance. Like all other AEDs, ezogabine may increase the risk for suicidal thinking or behavior. In contrast to many AEDs, ezogabine has few interactions with other drugs.

Eslicarbazepine

Actions and Uses

Eslicarbazepine [Aptiom] is approved for management of partial seizures. It may be used as either monotherapy or as an adjunct to ongoing therapy. The mechanism of action appears to be related to *blockade of sodium channels.*

Pharmacokinetics

This prodrug is metabolized to the active eslicarbazepine metabolite on first-pass metabolism. As a result, bioavailability is high (>90%). Peak time is 1 to 4 hours with a half-life of 13 to 20 hours. Excretion is primarily in the urine.

Adverse Effects

Most of eslicarbazepine's adverse effects are related to actions on the CNS. These include dizziness and sedation. More than 10% have developed headache and diplopia.

Drug Interactions

Eslicarbazepine is a CYP2C19 inhibitor and a CYP3A4 inducer. This is the mechanism behind many of the interactions with this drug.

When prescribed with phenytoin, eslicarbazepine can increase phenytoin levels and phenytoin can decrease eslicarbazepine levels. Carbamazepine and phenobarbital can also decrease levels of eslicarbazepine.

Other significant interactions may occur with statins, hormonal contraceptives, and warfarin. Eslicarbazepine can lower levels of all these drugs. Dosage adjustments may be required, and alternate forms of birth control may need to be considered.

Perampanel

Actions and Uses

Perampanel is approved for adjunctive therapy for treatment of both tonic-clonic seizures and partial seizures. Its antiepileptic effects are the result of AMPA *glutamate antagonism.*

Pharmacokinetics

When taken on an empty stomach, absorption is rapid and peak time is 0.5 to 2.5 hours. (Peak time is delayed by 2–3 hours if taken with meals.) Approximately 95% of perampanel is protein bound. Multiple isoenzymes are involved in the metabolism of perampanel, including CYP3A4/5, CYP1A2, and CYP2B6. Excretion is primarily by feces, with about 20% by urine.

Adverse Effects

Atypical anger and aggression have occurred in some patients taking perampanel. This may occur in as many as 20% of patients taking the drug.

BLACK BOX WARNING: PERAMPANEL [FYCOMPA]

Perampanel has been associated with serious psychiatric reactions. These include anger, aggression, hostility, violence, and even homicidal ideation.

Other than hostility, the most common adverse effects are dizziness, drowsiness, fatigue, and headache. Nausea, vomiting, abdominal discomfort, and weight gain may also occur.

Drug Interactions

Perampanel can decrease the effectiveness of hormonal contraceptives, particularly progestins. It can enhance the effect of CNS depressants, thus increasing risks related to sedation and, if significant, respiratory drive.

Phenytoin, carbamazepine, and oxcarbazepine can decrease perampanel levels by 50% or more through hepatic enzyme induction. *Care must be undertaken to adjust for this when making adjustments in therapy.*

Maternal and fetal or infant bleeding risks are also a concern. *Phenobarbital, phenytoin, carbamazepine,* and *primidone* reduce levels of vitamin K–dependent clotting factors by inducing hepatic enzymes, increasing the risk for bleeding. To reduce the risk, some resources, including product labeling, recommend that pregnant patients be given vitamin K before delivery. The most recent guidelines of the American Academy of Neurology and the American Epilepsy Society, however, conclude that the evidence is insufficient to support vitamin K administration in the pregnant patient. They also do not recommend vitamin K supplementation in neonates born to these women beyond that recommended for all newborns. For additional information, see http://www.neurology.org/content/73/2/126.full.pdf.

For women of childbearing age who are not pregnant, it is essential to consider interactions of AEDs with oral contraceptives. Eight AEDs decrease the effectiveness of oral contraceptives: carbamazepine, eslicarbazepine, lamotrigine, oxcarbazepine, phenytoin, phenobarbital, rufinamide, and topiramate. Four of these—carbamazepine, phenytoin, phenobarbital, and topiramate—are associated with harm to the human fetus. If it is necessary to prescribe any of these drugs, it is important to advise the patient of the risks and the need for additional contraceptives if pregnancy is not desired.

Management of Generalized Convulsive Status Epilepticus

Convulsive SE is defined as a continuous series of tonic-clonic seizures that lasts for at least 20 to 30 minutes. Consciousness is lost during the entire attack. Tachycardia, elevation of blood pressure, and hyperthermia are typical. Metabolic sequelae include hypoglycemia and acidosis. If SE persists for more than 20 minutes, it can cause permanent neurologic injury (cognitive impairment, memory loss, worsening of the underlying seizure disorder) and even death. Generalized convulsive SE is a medical emergency that requires immediate treatment. Management of SE is discussed in Chapter 89.

PRESCRIBING AND MONITORING CONSIDERATIONS

Implications That Apply to All Antiepileptic Drugs

Therapeutic Goal

The goal of treatment is to minimize or eliminate seizure events, thereby allowing the patient to live a normal or nearly normal life.

Baseline Data

Before initiating treatment, it is essential to know the type of seizure involved (e.g., absence, generalized tonic-clonic) and how often seizure events occur.

Administration Considerations

Dosage Determination

Dosages are often highly individualized and difficult to establish. Clinical evaluation of therapeutic and adverse effects is essential to establish a dosage that is both safe and effective. For several AEDs (especially those used to treat tonic-clonic seizures), knowledge of plasma AED levels can facilitate dosage adjustment.

Promoting Adherence

Seizure control requires rigid adherence to the prescribed regimen; nonadherence is a major cause of therapeutic failure. Monitoring plasma AED levels can motivate adherence and facilitate assessment of nonadherence.

Ongoing Monitoring and Interventions

Evaluating Therapeutic Effects

Teach the patient (or a family member) to maintain a seizure frequency chart, indicating the date, time, and nature of all seizure events. The prescriber can use this record to evaluate treatment, make dosage adjustments, and alter drug selections.

Minimizing Danger From Uncontrolled Seizures

Potentially hazardous activities (e.g., driving, operating dangerous machinery) must be restricted until seizure control is achieved. Also, because seizures may recur after they are largely under control, patients need to carry some form of identification (e.g., Medic Alert bracelet) to aid in diagnosis and treatment if a seizure occurs.

Minimizing Adverse Effects

CNS Depression. Most AEDs depress the CNS. Signs of CNS depression (sedation, drowsiness, lethargy) are most prominent during the initial phase of treatment and decline with continued drug use. Until this effect declines, patients should avoid driving and other hazardous activities. Until then, to minimize adverse CNS effects, use low initial doses and give the largest portion of the daily dose at bedtime.

Withdrawal Seizures. Abrupt discontinuation of AEDs can lead to SE. Consequently, medication should be withdrawn slowly (over 6 weeks to several months). Patients will need to take precautions not to run out of medications. Alerting patients of the need for follow-up visits prior to time for medication refills may be helpful.

Usage in Pregnancy. In most cases, the risk from uncontrolled seizures exceeds the risk from medication, and hence women with major seizure disorders should continue to take AEDs during pregnancy. However, the lowest effective dosage should be employed, and, if possible, only one drug should be used. One AED—valproic acid—should be avoided: the drug is highly teratogenic and can decrease the IQ of children exposed to it in utero. To reduce the risk for neural tube defects, pregnant patients taking any AED should be prescribed at least .04 mg of folic acid daily. Ideally, this should be started prior to becoming pregnant.

Suicidal Thoughts and Behavior. The AEDs pose small risk for suicidal thoughts and behavior. Screen for suicidality before starting treatment. Involve families or significant others in care if AEDs are required for patient with depression for whom suicide is a risk factor and assess for these concerns at every clinical encounter.

Minimizing Adverse Interactions

CNS Depressants. Drugs with CNS-depressant actions (e.g., alcohol, antihistamines, barbiturates, opioids) will intensify the depressant effects of AEDs, thereby posing a serious risk. Avoid prescribing drugs with CNS-depressant properties, including opioids, barbiturates, and antihistamines, unless absolutely necessary. When required, minimum effective doses should be used.

AEDs interact with many other drugs, as well. While some of the most important have been mentioned in this chapter, it is not feasible to list them all. Therefore, always consult product labeling or use a medication interaction program to identify any possible interactions prior to prescribing additional drugs.

Phenytoin

Nursing implications for phenytoin include those presented here as well as those presented earlier under "Implications that Apply to All Antiepileptic Drugs."

Identifying High-Risk Patients

Intravenous phenytoin is *contraindicated* for patients with sinus bradycardia, sinoatrial block, second- or third-degree atrioventricular block, or Stokes-Adams syndrome.

Administration Considerations

Intravenous

To minimize the risk for severe reactions (e.g., cardiovascular collapse), infuse phenytoin slowly (no faster than 50 mg/min).

Do not mix phenytoin solutions with other drugs.

To minimize venous inflammation at the injection site, flush the needle or catheter with saline immediately after completing the phenytoin infusion.

Ongoing Monitoring and Interventions

Minimizing Adverse Effects

Many adverse effects can be managed by the patient. See the Patient Education box for suggestions to include when giving medication instructions.

Dermatologic Reactions. Phenytoin can cause a morbilliform rash that may rarely progress to SJS or TEN. If a rash develops, phenytoin should be discontinued for safety reasons and another drug prescribed. The risk of SJS/TEN may be increased by a genetic variation known as HLA-B*1502, seen primarily in patients of Asian descent.

Minimizing Adverse Interactions

Warfarin and Oral Contraceptives. Phenytoin can decrease the effects of warfarin and oral contraceptives (as well as other drugs) by inducing hepatic drug-metabolizing enzymes. Dosages of warfarin and oral contraceptives may need to be increased.

Carbamazepine

Nursing implications for carbamazepine include those presented here as well as those presented earlier under "Nursing Implications that Apply to All Antiepileptic Drugs."

Therapeutic Goal

Carbamazepine is used to treat partial seizures (simple and complex) and tonic-clonic seizures.

Baseline Data

Obtain complete blood counts before treatment.

Identifying High-Risk Patients

Carbamazepine is *contraindicated* for patients with a history of bone marrow depression or adverse hematologic reactions to other drugs. Screen Asian patients for the HLA-B*1502 gene variation, which increases the risk for SJS or TEN.

Ongoing Evaluation and Interventions

Minimizing Adverse Effects

CNS Effects. Carbamazepine can cause headache, visual disturbances (nystagmus, blurred vision, diplopia), ataxia, vertigo, and unsteadiness. To minimize these effects, initiate therapy with low doses and have the patient take the largest part of the daily dose at bedtime.

Hematologic Effects. Carbamazepine can cause leukopenia, anemia, thrombocytopenia, and, very rarely, fatal aplastic anemia. To reduce the risk for serious hematologic

Patient Education

ANTIEPILEPTIC DRUGS

To promote adherence, educate patients about the importance of taking AEDs exactly as prescribed. Inform them that, after a safe and effective dosage has been established, small deviations in dosage can lead to toxicity or to loss of seizure control.

Inform patients about the dangers of abrupt drug withdrawal and instruct them never to discontinue drug use without consulting the prescriber. Advise patients who are planning a trip to carry extra medication to ensure an uninterrupted supply in the event they become stranded where medication is unavailable. Explain the need to obtain refills on time so that they do not run out of drugs.

Teach the patient (or a family member) to maintain a seizure frequency chart, indicating the date, time, and nature of all seizure events. They should bring this with them to all clinic appointments.

Advise patients to avoid potentially hazardous activities (e.g., driving, operating dangerous machinery) until seizure control is achieved. It may be necessary to explain laws concerning this risk. Also, because seizures may recur after they are largely under control, advise patients to carry some form of identification (e.g., Medic Alert bracelet) to aid in diagnosis and treatment if a seizure occurs.

Forewarn patients about CNS depression and advise them to avoid driving and other hazardous activities if CNS depression is significant. To prevent additive CNS depressant effects, warn patients against using alcohol and other CNS depressants.

To reduce the risk for neural tube defects, advise women to take folic acid supplements before and throughout pregnancy.

Educate patients, families, and caregivers about signs that may precede suicidal behavior (e.g., increased anxiety, agitation, mania, or hostility) and advise them to report these immediately.

Phenytoin

Instruct patients to shake the phenytoin oral suspension before dispensing to provide consistent dosing.

Inform patients that excessive doses of phenytoin can produce sedation, ataxia, diplopia, and interference with cognitive function. Instruct them to notify the prescriber if these occur.

Inform patients that phenytoin often promotes overgrowth of gum tissue. To minimize harm and discomfort, teach them proper techniques of brushing, flossing, and gum massage. You may let them know that some studies recommend 0.4-0.5 mg of folic acid daily, though this is not a proven benefit.

Carbamazepine

Inform patients taking carbamazepine (and rarely, phenytoin) that these drugs can cause a measles-like rash that may progress to much more serious conditions: SJS or TEN. Instruct patients to notify the prescriber immediately if a rash develops.

Advise patients taking carbamazepine about manifestations of low RBC, WBC, and platelet counts (pallor, weakness, fever, sore throat, easy bruising, petechiae) and instruct them to notify the prescriber if these occur.

Instruct patients taking carbamazepine (and other drugs metabolized by CYP3A4 isoenzymes) not to drink grapefruit juice.

Valproic Acid

Advise patients to take valproic acid with meals and instruct them to ingest tablets and capsules intact, without crushing or chewing.

Inform patients taking valproic acid about signs and symptoms of liver injury (reduced appetite, malaise, nausea, abdominal pain, jaundice) and instruct them to notify the prescriber if these develop.

For patients taking valproic acid, teach the signs of pancreatitis (abdominal pain, nausea, vomiting, anorexia) and instruct them to get an immediate evaluation if these develop.

Phenobarbital

Inform parents that children taking phenobarbital may become irritable and hyperactive and instruct them to notify the prescriber if these behaviors occur.

effects, (1) obtain complete blood counts at baseline and periodically thereafter, (2) avoid carbamazepine in patients with preexisting hematologic abnormalities, and (3) assess for signs and symptoms of low cell counts (fever, sore throat, pallor, weakness, infection, easy bruising, petechiae) at each clinic appointment and follow up with appropriate laboratory testing if they occur.

Birth Defects. Carbamazepine can cause neural tube defects. Use in pregnancy only if the benefits of seizure suppression outweigh the risks to the fetus.

Severe Skin Reactions. Carbamazepine can cause SJS or TEN, especially among patients with HLA-B*1502, a genetic variation seen almost exclusively in patients of Asian descent. To reduce risk, the FDA recommends that patients of Asian descent be tested for HLA-B*1502. If SJS or TEN develops, carbamazepine should be discontinued. Because HLA-B*1502 may also increase the risk for SJS or TEN in response to phenytoin, phenytoin should not be used as an alternative to carbamazepine in patients with the mutation.

Minimizing Adverse Interactions

Interactions Due to Induction of Drug Metabolism. Carbamazepine can decrease responses to other drugs by inducing hepatic drug-metabolizing enzymes. Effects on oral contraceptives and warfarin are of particular concern. Patients using these drugs will require increased dosages to maintain therapeutic responses.

Phenytoin and Phenobarbital. These drugs can decrease responses to carbamazepine by inducing drug-metabolizing enzymes (beyond the degree of induction caused by carbamazepine itself). Dosage of carbamazepine may need to be increased.

Grapefruit Juice. Grapefruit juice can increase levels of carbamazepine. It will be important not only to instruct patients of this but also to include this in the dietary orders of hospitalized patients.

Valproic Acid

Nursing implications for valproic acid include those presented here as well as those presented earlier under "Implications that Apply to All Antiepileptic Drugs."

Therapeutic Goal

Valproic acid is used to treat all major seizure disorders: tonic-clonic, absence, myoclonic, atonic, and partial (simple, complex, and secondarily generalized).

Baseline Data

Obtain baseline tests of liver function.

Identifying High-Risk Patients

Valproic acid is *contraindicated* for patients with significant hepatic dysfunction and for children younger than 3 years who are taking other AEDs. Avoid valproic acid during pregnancy.

Administration Considerations

Valproic acid should be taken with meals. Patients should swallow tablets and capsules intact, without crushing or chewing.

Ongoing Monitoring and Interventions

Minimizing Adverse Effects

Gastrointestinal Effects. Nausea, vomiting, and indigestion are common. These can be reduced by using an enteric-coated formulation (see Table 19.4) and by taking valproic acid with meals.

Hepatotoxicity. Rarely, valproic acid has caused fatal liver injury. To minimize risk, (1) don't use valproic acid in conjunction with other drugs in children younger than 3 years, (2) don't use valproic acid in patients with preexisting liver dysfunction, (3) evaluate liver function at baseline and periodically thereafter, (4) assess patients for signs and symptoms of liver injury (reduced appetite, malaise, nausea, abdominal pain, jaundice) at each clinic visit and, (5) use valproic acid in the lowest effective dosage.

Pancreatitis. Valproic acid can cause life-threatening pancreatitis. Assess patients for signs of pancreatitis (abdominal pain, nausea, vomiting, anorexia) at each encounter. If pancreatitis is diagnosed, valproic acid should be withdrawn.

Pregnancy-Related Harm. Valproic acid may cause neural tube defects and other congenital malformations, especially when taken during the first trimester. In addition, the drug can reduce the IQ of children exposed to it in utero. Valproic acid is classified in FDA Pregnancy Risk Category D and should be avoided by women of childbearing potential—unless it is the only AED that will work.

Hyperammonemia. Combining valproic acid with topiramate poses a risk of hyperammonemia so these should never be prescribed together as dual therapy. If this should occur (e.g. if prescribed by another provider) and symptoms develop (vomiting, lethargy, altered level of consciousness or cognitive function), blood ammonia should be measured. If the level is excessive, either valproic acid or topiramate should be withdrawn.

Minimizing Adverse Interactions

Antiepileptic Drugs. Valproic acid can elevate plasma levels of phenytoin and phenobarbital. Levels of phenobarbital and phenytoin should be monitored and their dosages adjusted accordingly.

Carbapenem Antibiotics. Meropenem and imipenem/cilastatin can reduce plasma levels of valproic acid. Breakthrough seizures have occurred. These antibiotics should be avoided in patients taking valproic acid.

Phenobarbital

Nursing implications that apply to the antiseizure applications of phenobarbital include those presented here and those presented earlier under "Implications that Apply to All Antiepileptic Drugs." Nursing implications that apply to the barbiturates as a group are summarized in Chapter 33.

Therapeutic Goal

Oral phenobarbital is used for partial seizures (simple and complex) and tonic-clonic seizures. Intravenous therapy is used for convulsive SE.

Identifying High-Risk Patients

Phenobarbital is *contraindicated* for patients with a history of acute intermittent porphyria.

Use with *caution* during pregnancy.

Administration Considerations

Oral

A loading schedule may be employed to initiate treatment. Monitor for excessive CNS depression when these large doses are used.

Intravenous

Rapid IV infusion can cause severe adverse effects. Perform infusions slowly.

Ongoing Monitoring and Interventions

Minimizing Adverse Effects

Neuropsychological Effects. Phenobarbital may cause cognitive deficits in children. It may also cause paradoxical excitement in both children and elderly patients. Avoid its use in these populations, if possible. Assess pediatric and geriatric patients taking this drug for hyperactivity or irritable behavior.

Exacerbation of Intermittent Porphyria. Phenobarbital can exacerbate acute intermittent porphyria, so it is absolutely contraindicated for patients with a history of this disorder.

Minimizing Adverse Interactions

Interactions Caused by Induction of Drug Metabolism. Phenobarbital induces hepatic drug-metabolizing enzymes and can thereby decrease responses to drugs metabolized by those enzymes. Effects on *oral contraceptives* and *warfarin* are a particular concern; their dosages should be increased.

Valproic Acid. Valproic acid increases blood levels of phenobarbital. To avoid toxicity, reduce phenobarbital dosage.

CHAPTER

20

Drugs for Muscle Spasm and Spasticity

Jacqueline Rosenjack Burchum, DNSc, FNP-BC, CNE

In this chapter we consider two groups of drugs that cause skeletal muscle relaxation. One group is used for localized muscle spasm. The other is used for spasticity. With only one exception (dantrolene), these drugs produce their effects through actions in the central nervous system (CNS). As a rule, the drugs used to treat spasticity do not relieve acute muscle spasm, and the drugs used to treat acute muscle spasm do not relieve spasticity. Hence the two groups are not interchangeable.

DRUG THERAPY OF MUSCLE SPASM: CENTRALLY ACTING MUSCLE RELAXANTS

Muscle spasm is defined as involuntary contraction of a muscle or muscle group. Muscle spasm is often painful and interferes with muscle function. Spasm can result from a variety of causes, including epilepsy, hypocalcemia, acute and chronic pain syndromes, and trauma (localized muscle injury). Discussion here is limited to spasm resulting from muscle injury.

Treatment of spasm involves physical measures as well as drug therapy. Physical measures include immobilization of the affected muscle, application of cold compresses, whirlpool baths, and physical therapy. For drug therapy, two groups of medicines are used: (1) analgesic antiinflammatory agents (e.g., aspirin) and (2) centrally acting muscle relaxants. The analgesic antiinflammatory agents are discussed in Chapter 55. The centrally acting muscle relaxants are discussed later in this chapter.

The family of centrally acting muscle relaxants consists of nine drugs: baclofen, carisoprodol, chlorzoxazone, cyclobenzaprine, diazepam, metaxalone, methocarbamol, orphenadrine, and tizanidine. All have similar pharmacologic properties, so we will consider these agents as a group.

Mechanism of Action

For most centrally acting muscle relaxants, the mechanism of spasm relief is unclear. In laboratory animals, high doses can depress spinal motor reflexes. However, these doses are much higher than those used in humans. Hence many investigators believe that relaxation of spasm results primarily from the *sedative properties* of these drugs and not from specific actions exerted on CNS pathways that control muscle tone.

Two drugs—diazepam and tizanidine—are thought to relieve spasm by enhancing presynaptic inhibition of motor neurons in the CNS. Diazepam promotes presynaptic inhibition by enhancing the effects of gamma-aminobutyric acid (GABA), an inhibitory neurotransmitter. Tizanidine promotes inhibition by acting as an agonist at presynaptic $alpha_2$ receptors.

Therapeutic Use

The centrally acting muscle relaxants are used to relieve localized spasm resulting from muscle injury. These agents can decrease local pain and tenderness and can increase range of motion. Benefits of treatment equal those of aspirin and the other analgesic antiinflammatory drugs. Because there are no studies to indicate the superiority of one centrally acting muscle relaxant over another, drug selection is based largely on risks versus benefits and patient response. With the exception of baclofen and diazepam, the central muscle relaxants are not useful for treating spasticity or other muscle disorders resulting from CNS pathology.

Adverse Effects

CNS Depression

All of the centrally acting muscle relaxants can produce generalized depression of the CNS. *Drowsiness, dizziness,* and *lightheadedness* are common. Patients should be warned not to participate in hazardous activities (e.g., driving) if CNS depression is significant. In addition, they should be advised to avoid alcohol and all other CNS depressants.

Hepatic Toxicity

Chlorzoxazone [Lorzone, Parafon Forte DSC], *tizanidine* [Zanaflex], and *metaxalone* [Skelaxin] can cause liver damage. Liver function should be assessed before starting treatment and periodically thereafter. If liver injury develops, these drugs should be discontinued. If the patient has preexisting liver disease, these drugs should be avoided.

Physical Dependence

Chronic, high-dose therapy can cause physical dependence, manifesting as a potentially life-threatening abstinence syndrome if these drugs are abruptly withdrawn. Accordingly, withdrawal should be done slowly.

Other Adverse Effects

Carisoprodol, chlorzoxazone, cyclobenzaprine, metaxalone, methocarbamol, orphenadrine, and tizanidine have significant anticholinergic properties and hence may cause dry mouth, blurred vision, photophobia, elevated heart rate, urinary retention, and constipation. Methocarbamol may turn urine brown, black, or dark green; patients should be forewarned of this harmless effect. Tizanidine can cause dry mouth, hypotension, hallucinations, and psychotic symptoms. Carisoprodol can be hazardous to patients predisposed to intermittent porphyria, so it is contraindicated for this group.

Patient Education

CENTRALLY ACTING SKELETAL MUSCLE RELAXANTS

Inform patients about possible depressant effects such as drowsiness, lightheadedness, and fatigue. Advise them to avoid driving and other hazardous activities if significant impairment occurs. If they must be taken by older patients, it is essential to explain about the increased risk of falls. Teach patients and family members home safety measures to decrease fall risk such as ensuring adequate lighting and avoiding scatter rugs. Let patients know that CNS depressant effects are worsened by intake of other CNS depressants, including alcohol and first generations antihistamines. Warn patients against abrupt discontinuation to avoid withdrawal reactions.

Dosage and Administration

All centrally acting skeletal muscle relaxants can be administered orally (Table 20.1). In addition, two agents—methocarbamol and diazepam—can be administered by intramuscular and intravenous injection.

DRUGS FOR SPASTICITY

The term *spasticity* refers to a group of movement disorders of CNS origin. These disorders are characterized by heightened muscle tone, spasm, and loss of dexterity. The most common causes are multiple sclerosis and cerebral palsy. Other causes include traumatic spinal cord lesions and stroke. Spasticity is managed with a combination of drugs and physical therapy.

Three drugs—baclofen, diazepam, and dantrolene—can relieve spasticity. Two of these—baclofen and diazepam—act in the CNS. In contrast, dantrolene acts directly on skeletal muscle. With the exception of baclofen and diazepam, the drugs employed to treat muscle spasm (i.e., the centrally acting muscle relaxants) are not effective against spasticity.

TABLE 20.1 ■ Drugs for Muscle Spasm

Name	Preparation	Usual Adult Oral Dosage	Administration
Baclofen [Lioresal, Gablofen]	10-mg, 20-mg tablets	Initial: 5 mg 3 times/day. May increase to 15-20 mg 3 or 4 times/day	May be taken with or without food
Carisoprodol [Soma]	250-mg, 350 mg tablets	250-350 mg 3 times/day and at bedtime	May be taken with or without food
Chlorzoxazone [Lorzone, Parafon Forte DSC]	Lorzone: 375-mg, 750-mg tablets (scored) Parafon Forte DSC: 500-mg tablets (scored)	500-750 mg 3 or 4 times/day	May be taken with or without food
Cyclobenzaprine [Fexmid]	Fexmid: 7.5-mg tablets Generic: 5-mg, 7.5-mg, 10-mg tablets	5-10 mg 3 times/day	May be taken with or without food; however, taking with food may decrease GI distress
Cyclobenzaprine ER [Amrix]	15-mg, 30-mg ER capsule	15 or 30 mg once every 24 hours	Swallow tablets whole.
Dantrolene [Dantrium]	25-mg, 50-mg, 100-mg capsules	The initial adult dosage is 25 mg once, then 100 mg 3 to 4 times a day.	Capsules may be opened and sprinkled on food.
Diazepam [Valium]	Valium: 2-mg, 5-mg, 10-mg (scored) tablets Diazepam Intensol oral concentrated solution: 5 mg/mL Generic oral solution: 1 mg/mL	2-10 mg 3 or 4 times/day	Taking with food is recommended. Oral concentrate should be measured by specially designed dropper (included with the medication) and then mixed with drinks or soft foods such as applesauce or pudding.
Metaxalone [Metaxall, Skelaxin]	Metaxall: 800-mg (scored) tablets Skelaxin: 800-mg (scored) tablets	800 mg 3 or 4 times/day	May be taken with or without food; however, bioavailability may be increased if given with food, resulting in increased CNS depression.
Methocarbamol [Robaxin, Robaxin-750]	Robaxin: 500-mg (scored) tablets Robaxin-750: 750-mg tablets	1-1.5 g 4 times/day	May be crushed and mixed with food.
Orphenadrine [Norflex]	100-mg ER tablet	100 mg twice a day	Do not crush ER tablet.
Tizanidine [Zanaflex]	4-mg tablet (scored) 2-mg, 4-mg, 6-mg capsules	Initial: 2 mg every 6-8 hours May increase to 8 mg every 6-8 hours (Maximum, 36 mg/day)	Capsules may be opened and sprinkled on food; however, absorption is increased. This should be considered when selecting the strength to prescribe for those with difficulty swallowing whole capsules.

ER, extended release; GI, gastrointestinal.

Baclofen

Mechanism of Action

Baclofen [Lioresal, Gablofen] acts within the spinal cord to suppress hyperactive reflexes involved in regulation of muscle movement. The precise mechanism of reflex attenuation is unknown. Because baclofen is a structural analog of the inhibitory neurotransmitter GABA, it may act by mimicking the actions of GABA on spinal neurons. Baclofen has no direct effects on skeletal muscle.

Therapeutic Use

Baclofen can reduce spasticity associated with multiple sclerosis, spinal cord injury, and cerebral palsy—but not with stroke. The drug decreases flexor and extensor spasms and suppresses resistance to passive movement. These actions reduce the discomfort of spasticity and allow increased performance. Because baclofen has no direct muscle relaxant action, and hence does not decrease muscle strength, baclofen is preferred to dantrolene when spasticity is associated with significant muscle weakness. Baclofen does not relieve the spasticity of Parkinson disease or Huntington chorea.

Adverse Effects

The most common side effects involve the CNS and gastrointestinal tract. Serious adverse effects are rare.

CNS Effects

Baclofen is a CNS depressant and hence frequently causes *drowsiness, dizziness, weakness,* and *fatigue.* These responses are most intense during the early phase of therapy and diminish with continued drug use. CNS depression can be minimized with doses that are small initially and then gradually increased. Patients should be cautioned to avoid alcohol and other CNS depressants because baclofen will potentiate the depressant actions of these drugs.

Overdose can produce *coma* and *respiratory depression.* Because there is no antidote to baclofen overdose, treatment is supportive and should be instituted immediately.

Withdrawal

Although baclofen does not appear to cause physical dependence, abrupt discontinuation has been associated with adverse reactions. Abrupt withdrawal of *oral* baclofen can cause visual hallucinations, paranoid ideation, and seizures. Accordingly, withdrawal should be done slowly (over 1 to 2 weeks). (Although not typically ordered by nonphysician providers, it is interesting to note that a black box warning alerts providers against abrupt withdrawal of *intrathecal* baclofen. Potential reactions include high fever, altered mental status, exaggerated rebound spasticity, and muscle rigidity that, in rare cases, has advanced to rhabdomyolysis, multiple organ system failure, and death.)

Other Adverse Effects

Baclofen frequently causes nausea, constipation, and urinary retention. Patients should be warned about these possible reactions.

> **Patient Education**
>
> **BACLOFEN**
>
> Tell patients about possible depressant effects such as drowsiness, lightheadedness, and fatigue and warn them to avoid hazardous activities such as driving. Caution patients to avoid other CNS depressants because these drugs will intensify the depressant effects of baclofen. Baclofen frequently causes nausea, constipation, and urinary retention. Patients should be warned about these possible reactions and provided with interventions to manage these conditions. It is also important to warn patients that abrupt discontinuation may cause psychiatric symptoms such as visual hallucinations, paranoia, and seizures.

Diazepam

Diazepam [Valium] is a member of the benzodiazepine family. Although diazepam is the only benzodiazepine labeled for treating spasticity, other benzodiazepines have been used off-label. The basic pharmacology of the benzodiazepines is discussed in Chapter 27.

Actions

Like baclofen, diazepam acts in the CNS to suppress spasticity. Beneficial effects appear to result from mimicking the actions of GABA at receptors in the spinal cord and brain. Diazepam does not affect skeletal muscle directly. Because diazepam has no direct effects on muscle strength, the drug is preferred to dantrolene when muscle strength is marginal.

Adverse Effects

Sedation is common when treating spasticity. To minimize sedation, initial doses should be low. Other adverse effects are discussed in Chapter 27.

Dantrolene

Mechanism of Action

Unlike baclofen and diazepam, which act within the CNS, dantrolene [Dantrium] acts directly on skeletal muscle. The drug relieves spasm by suppressing release of calcium from the sarcoplasmic reticulum, and hence the muscle is less able to contract. Fortunately, therapeutic doses have only minimal effects on contraction of smooth muscle and cardiac muscle.

Therapeutic Uses

> **Patient Education**
>
> **DANTROLENE**
>
> Inform patients about possible depressant effects (drowsiness, dizziness, lightheadedness, fatigue) and advise them to avoid driving and other hazardous activities if significant impairment occurs. Inform patients about signs of liver dysfunction (e.g., jaundice, abdominal pain, malaise) and instruct them to seek medical attention if these develop. Warn patients to avoid CNS depressants (e.g., alcohol, benzodiazepines, opioids, antihistamines) because these drugs will intensify depressant effects of dantrolene.

Spasticity
Dantrolene can relieve spasticity associated with multiple sclerosis, cerebral palsy, and spinal cord injury. Unfortunately, because dantrolene suppresses spasticity by causing a generalized reduction in the ability of skeletal muscle to contract, treatment may be associated with a significant reduction in strength. As a result, overall function may be reduced rather than improved. Accordingly, care must be taken to ensure that the benefits of therapy (reduced spasticity) outweigh the harm (reduced strength). If beneficial effects do not develop within 45 days, dantrolene should be stopped.

Adverse Effects

Hepatic Toxicity
Dose-related liver damage is the most serious adverse effect. The incidence is 1 in 1000. Deaths have occurred. Hepatotoxicity is most common in women older than 35 years. By contrast, liver injury is rare in children younger than 10 years. To reduce the risk for liver damage, liver function tests (LFTs) should be performed at baseline and periodically thereafter. If LFTs indicate liver injury, dantrolene should be withdrawn. Because of the potential for liver damage, dantrolene should be administered in the lowest effective dosage and for the shortest time necessary.

Other Adverse Effects
Muscle weakness, drowsiness, and diarrhea are the most common side effects. Muscle weakness is a direct extension of dantrolene's pharmacologic action. Other effects may include anorexia, nausea, vomiting, and acne-like rash.

BLACK BOX WARNING: DANTROLENE

Fatal hepatotoxicity has occurred, especially at higher doses, even with short-term therapy. The lowest effective dose should be used. Because patients may be asymptomatic, baseline liver function tests should be obtained followed by frequent monitoring of these levels throughout therapy.

PRESCRIBING AND MONITORING CONSIDERATIONS FOR DRUGS USED TO TREAT MUSCLE SPASM: CENTRALLY ACTING SKELETAL MUSCLE RELAXANTS

Except where noted, the nursing implications summarized here apply to all centrally acting muscle relaxants used to treat muscle spasm.

Therapeutic Goal
These drugs are used to relieve signs and symptoms of muscle spasm.

Baseline Data
For patients taking dantrolene, metaxalone, and tizanidine, obtain baseline LFTs.

Identifying High-Risk Patients
Avoid *chlorzoxazone, metaxalone,* and *tizanidine* in patients with liver disease.

Measures to Enhance Therapeutic Effects
The treatment plan should include appropriate physical measures (e.g., immobilization of the affected muscle, application of cold compresses, whirlpool baths, and physical therapy).

Ongoing Monitoring and Interventions

Minimizing Adverse Effects

CNS Depression
All central muscle relaxants cause CNS depression. Depressant effects may include drowsiness, lightheadedness, and fatigue. These may be dangerous if the patient must engage in hazardous activities (e.g. truck-driving or construction). If necessary for treatment of older adults, fall precautions should be instituted.

Hepatic Toxicity
Chlorzoxazone, metaxalone, and *tizanidine* can cause liver damage. Obtain LFTs before treatment and periodically thereafter. If liver damage develops, discontinue treatment. Avoid these drugs in patients with preexisting liver disease.

Minimizing Adverse Interactions

CNS Depressants
CNS depressants potentiate the depressant effects of centrally acting skeletal muscle relaxants. Common CNS depressants include alcohol, benzodiazepines, opioids, and first generation antihistamines. Avoid prescribing additional CNS depressants unless benefits exceed risks.

Avoiding Withdrawal Reactions
Central muscle relaxants can cause physical dependence. To avoid an abstinence syndrome, withdraw gradually.

Baclofen

Therapeutic Goal
Baclofen is used to relieve signs and symptoms of spasticity.

Baseline Data
Assess for spasm, rigidity, pain, range of motion, and dexterity. Obtain baseline LFTs.

Administration Considerations
Patients with muscle spasm may be unable to self-medicate. Provide assistance if needed.

Ongoing Monitoring and Interventions

Evaluating Therapeutic Effects
Monitor for reductions in rigidity, muscle spasm, and pain and for improvements in dexterity and range of motion.

Minimizing Adverse Effects
CNS Depression. Baclofen is a CNS depressant. Depressant effects such as drowsiness and fatigue prohibit engagement in activities that require mental alertness.

Minimizing Adverse Interactions
CNS Depressants. Additive effects will occur if taken with other CNS depressants. Carefully weigh the risks of prescribing to patients who take other CNS depressants

Avoiding Withdrawal Reactions

Baclofen. Abrupt withdrawal can cause visual hallucinations, paranoid ideation, and seizures. Tapering drug dosage when discontinuing baclofen can prevent these effects.

Dantrolene

The prescribing implications summarized here apply only to the use of dantrolene for spasticity.

Therapeutic Goal

Dantrolene is used to relieve signs and symptoms of spasticity.

Baseline Data

Assess for spasm, rigidity, pain, range of motion, and dexterity. Obtain baseline LFTs.

Identifying High-Risk Patients

Dantrolene is *contraindicated* for patients with active liver disease (e.g., cirrhosis, hepatitis).

Administration Considerations

Patients with muscle spasm may be unable to self-medicate. Provide assistance if needed.

Ongoing Monitoring and Interventions

Monitoring

Therapeutic Effects. Monitor for reductions in rigidity, spasm, and pain and for improvements in dexterity and range of motion.

Adverse Effects. Monitor LFTs and assess for reduced muscle strength.

Minimizing Adverse Effects

CNS Depression. Dantrolene is a CNS depressant. Depressant effects such as drowsiness, lightheadedness, and fatigue pose a danger if patients engage in hazardous activities.

Hepatic Toxicity. Dantrolene is hepatotoxic. Assess liver function at baseline and periodically thereafter. If signs of liver dysfunction develop, withdraw dantrolene.

Muscle Weakness. Dantrolene can decrease muscle strength. Evaluate muscle function to ensure that benefits of therapy (decreased spasticity) are not outweighed by reductions in strength.

Minimizing Adverse Interactions

CNS Depressants. CNS depressants (e.g., alcohol, benzodiazepines, opioids, antihistamines) will intensify depressant effects of dantrolene. Carefully weigh benefits versus risks if the patient will be taking other CNS depressants.

Diazepam

Prescribing implications for diazepam and other benzodiazepines are covered in Chapter 27.

PATIENT-CENTERED CARE ACROSS THE LIFE SPAN

Muscle Relaxants

Life Stage	Considerations or Concerns
Children	Baclofen, dantrolene, and diazepam are approved for infants and children. Metaxalone is approved for children aged 13 years and older. Cyclobenzaprine is approved for children aged 15 years and older. Carisoprodol is approved for children aged 16 years and older. Chlorzoxazone, orphenadrine, and tizanidine are not approved for children. Methocarbamol is restricted for use in children aged 16 years and older unless it is being prescribed for tetanus.
Pregnant women	Methocarbamol is Pregnancy Risk Category B. Adverse effects have not occurred in animal studies. Diazepam is Pregnancy Risk Category D. Teratogenic effects have occurred in humans. For the remaining drugs in this chapter, except for chlorzoxazone, animal studies have demonstrated adverse effects; therefore they are Pregnancy Risk Category C. Inadequate studies have been conducted with chlorzoxazone; therefore it is not recommended for pregnant women.
Breastfeeding women	Breastfeeding is not recommended when taking these drugs.
Older adults	Carisoprodol, chlorzoxazone, cyclobenzaprine, diazepam, metaxalone, methocarbamol, and orphenadrine are identified in the Beers Criteria as a potentially inappropriate medication to be avoided in patients 65 years and older because of anticholinergic effects and/or sedation. However, baclofen, dantrolene, and tizanidine also have a high incidence of sedation. Older patients taking any drug in this chapter are at increased risk for falls and subsequent injury.

UNIT VI
Drugs for Pain

CHAPTER 21
Local Anesthetics

Laura D. Rosenthal, DNP, ACNP, FAANP

Local anesthetics are drugs that suppress pain by blocking impulse conduction along axons. Conduction is blocked only in neurons located near the site of administration. The great advantage of local anesthesia, compared with inhalation anesthesia, is that pain can be suppressed without causing generalized depression of the entire nervous system. Local anesthetics carry much less risk than do general anesthetics.

We begin the chapter by considering the pharmacology of the local anesthetics as a group. After that, we discuss three prototypic agents: procaine, lidocaine, and cocaine. We conclude by discussing specific routes of anesthetic administration.

BASIC PHARMACOLOGY OF THE LOCAL ANESTHETICS

Classification

There are two major groups of local anesthetics: *esters* and *amides*. The ester-type anesthetics, represented by *chloroprocaine* [Nesacaine], contain an ester linkage in their structure. In contrast, the amide-type agents, represented by *lidocaine* [Xylocaine], contain an amide linkage. The ester-type agents and amide-type agents differ in two important ways: (1) method of inactivation and (2) promotion of allergic responses. Contrasts between the esters and amides are shown in Table 21.1.

Mechanism of Action

Local anesthetics stop axonal conduction by *blocking sodium channels* in the axonal membrane. Recall that propagation of an action potential requires movement of sodium ions from outside the axon to the inside. This influx takes place through specialized sodium channels. By blocking axonal sodium channels, local anesthetics prevent sodium entry and thereby block conduction.

Selectivity of Anesthetic Effects

Local anesthetics are nonselective modifiers of neuronal function. That is, they will block action potentials in all neurons to which they have access. The only way to achieve selectivity is by delivering the anesthetic to a limited area.

Although local anesthetics can block traffic in all neurons, blockade develops more rapidly in some neurons than in others. Specifically, small, nonmyelinated neurons are blocked more rapidly than large, myelinated neurons. Because of this differential sensitivity, some sensations are blocked sooner than others. Specifically, perception of pain is lost first, followed in order by perception of cold, warmth, touch, and deep pressure.

The effects of local anesthetics are not limited to sensory neurons: these drugs also block conduction in motor neurons.

> **Patient Education**
>
> **SELF-INFLICTED INJURY**
>
> Because anesthetics eliminate pain, and because pain can be a warning sign of complications, patients recovering from anesthesia must be protected from inadvertent harm until the anesthetic wears off. Caution the patient against activities that might result in unintentional harm.

Time Course of Local Anesthesia

Ideally, local anesthesia would begin promptly and would persist no longer (or shorter) than needed. Unfortunately, although onset of anesthesia is usually rapid (Tables 21.2 and 21.3), duration of anesthesia is often less than ideal. In some cases, anesthesia persists longer than needed. In others, repeated administration is required to maintain anesthesia of sufficient duration.

Onset of local anesthesia is determined largely by the molecular properties of the anesthetic. Before anesthesia can occur, the anesthetic must diffuse from its site of administration to its sites of action within the axon membrane. Anesthesia is delayed until this movement has occurred. The ability of an anesthetic to penetrate the axon membrane is determined by three properties: *molecular size, lipid solubility,* and *degree of ionization at tissue pH.* Anesthetics of small size, high lipid solubility, and low ionization cross the axon membrane rapidly. In contrast, anesthetics of large size, low lipid solubility, and high ionization cross slowly. Obviously, anesthetics that penetrate the axon most rapidly have the fastest onset.

Termination of local anesthesia occurs as molecules of anesthetic diffuse out of neurons and are carried away in the blood. The same factors that determine onset of anesthesia (molecular size, lipid solubility, degree of ionization) also help determine duration. In addition, *regional blood flow* is an important determinant of how long anesthesia will last. In areas where blood flow is high, anesthetic is carried away quickly, and effects terminate with relative haste. In regions where blood flow is low, anesthesia is more prolonged.

TABLE 21.1 ▪ Contrasts Between Ester and Amide Local Anesthetics

Property	Ester-Type Anesthetics	Amide-Type Anesthetics
Characteristic chemistry	Ester bond	Amide bond
Representative agent	Procaine	Lidocaine
Incidence of allergic reactions	Low	Very low
Method of metabolism	Plasma esterases	Hepatic enzymes

Use With Vasoconstrictors

Local anesthetics are frequently administered in combination with a vasoconstrictor, usually *epinephrine*. The vasoconstrictor decreases local blood flow and thereby delays systemic absorption of the anesthetic. Delaying absorption has two benefits: It *prolongs anesthesia* and *reduces the risk for toxicity*. Because absorption is slowed, less anesthetic is used and a more favorable balance is established between the rate of entry of anesthetic into circulation and the rate of its conversion into inactive metabolites.

It should be noted that absorption of the vasoconstrictor itself can result in systemic toxicity (e.g., palpitations, tachycardia, nervousness, hypertension). If adrenergic stimulation from absorption of epinephrine is excessive, symptoms can be controlled with alpha- and beta-adrenergic antagonists.

Pharmacokinetics

Absorption and Distribution

Although administered for local effects, local anesthetics do get absorbed into the blood and become distributed to all parts

TABLE 21.2 ▪ Topical Local Anesthetics: Trade Names, Indications, and Time Course of Action

			Indications		Time Course of Action*	
Chemical Class	Generic Name	Trade Name	Skin	Mucous Membranes	Peak Effect (min)	Duration (min)
Amides	Dibucaine	Nupercainal	✓		<5	15-45
	Lidocaine†	Xylocaine, Lidoderm, others	✓	✓	2-5	15-45
Esters	Benzocaine	Many names	✓	✓	<5	15-45
	Cocaine	Generic only	✓	✓	1-5	30-60
	Tetracaine†	None‡	✓	✓	3-8	30-60
Others	Dyclonine	Sucrets (spray)		✓	<10	<60
	Pramoxine	Tronolane, others	✓		3-5	—

*Based primarily on application to mucous membranes.
†Also administered by injection.
‡For application to the skin, tetracaine is available only in combination products, such as Cetacaine.

TABLE 21.3 ▪ Injectable Local Anesthetics: Trade Names and Time Course of Action

			Time Course of Action*	
Chemical Class	Generic Name	Trade Name	Onset (min)	Duration (hr)
Amides	Lidocaine†	Xylocaine	<2	0.5-1
	Bupivacaine	Marcaine	5	2-4
	Mepivacaine	Carbocaine	3-5	0.75-1.5
	Prilocaine	Citanest	<2	≥1
	Ropivacaine	Naropin	10-30‡	0.5-6‡
Esters§	Chloroprocaine	Nesacaine	6-12	0.5
	Tetracaine†	Pontocaine	≤15	2-3

*Values are for *infiltration* anesthesia in the absence of epinephrine (epinephrine prolongs duration twofold to threefold).
†Also administered topically.
‡Values are for epidural administration (without epinephrine).
§Because of the risk for allergic reactions, the ester anesthetics are rarely administered by injection.

of the body. The rate of absorption is determined largely by blood flow to the site of administration.

Metabolism

The process by which a local anesthetic is metabolized depends on the class—ester or amide—to which it belongs. *Ester-type* local anesthetics are metabolized in the blood by enzymes known as *esterases.* In contrast, *amide-type* anesthetics are metabolized by enzymes in the *liver.* For both types of anesthetic, metabolism results in inactivation.

The balance between rate of absorption and rate of metabolism is clinically significant. If a local anesthetic is absorbed more slowly than it is metabolized, its level in blood will remain low, and systemic reactions will be minimal. Conversely, if absorption outpaces metabolism, plasma drug levels will rise, and the risk for systemic toxicity will increase.

Adverse Effects

Adverse effects can occur locally or distant from the site of administration. Local effects are less common.

Central Nervous System

When absorbed in sufficient amounts, local anesthetics cause central nervous system (CNS) excitation followed by depression. During the excitation phase, *seizures* may occur. If needed, excessive excitation can be managed with an intravenous benzodiazepine (diazepam or midazolam). Depressant effects range from *drowsiness* to *unconsciousness* to *coma.* Death can occur secondary to *depression of respiration.* If respiratory depression is prominent, mechanical ventilation with oxygen is indicated.

Cardiovascular System

When absorbed in sufficient amounts, local anesthetics can affect the heart and blood vessels. In the heart, these drugs suppress excitability in the myocardium and conducting system and thereby can cause *bradycardia, heart block, reduced contractile force,* and *even cardiac arrest.* In blood vessels, anesthetics relax vascular smooth muscle; the resultant vasodilation can cause *hypotension.*

Allergic Reactions

An array of hypersensitivity reactions, ranging from *allergic dermatitis* to *anaphylaxis,* can be triggered by local anesthetics. These reactions, which are relatively uncommon, are much more likely with the *ester-type* anesthetics (e.g., chloroprocaine) than with the amides. Patients allergic to one ester-type anesthetic are likely to be allergic to all other ester-type agents. Fortunately, cross-hypersensitivity between the esters and amides has not been observed. Therefore the amides can be used when allergies contraindicate use of ester-type anesthetics. Because they are unlikely to cause hypersensitivity reactions, the amide-type anesthetics have largely replaced the ester-type agents when administration by injection is required.

Methemoglobinemia

Topical *benzocaine* can cause methemoglobinemia, a blood disorder in which hemoglobin is modified such that it cannot release oxygen to tissues. If enough hemoglobin is converted to methemoglobin, death can result. Methemoglobinemia has been associated with benzocaine liquids, sprays, and gels. Most cases were in children younger than 2 years treated with benzocaine gel for teething pain. Because of this risk, topical benzocaine should not be used in children younger than 2 years without the advice of a health care professional, and should be used with caution in older children and adults when applied to mucous membranes of the mouth.

PROPERTIES OF INDIVIDUAL LOCAL ANESTHETICS

Chloroprocaine

Chloroprocaine [Nesacaine] is the prototype of the ester-type local anesthetics. The drug is not effective topically and must be given by injection. Administration in combination with epinephrine delays absorption. Although chloroprocaine is readily absorbed, systemic toxicity is rare because plasma esterases rapidly convert the drug to inactive, nontoxic products. Being an ester-type anesthetic, procaine poses a greater risk for allergic reactions than do the amide-type anesthetics. Individuals allergic to chloroprocaine should be considered allergic to all other ester-type anesthetics, but not to the amides.

Prototype Drugs

LOCAL ANESTHETICS

Ester-Type Local Anesthetics

Chloroprocaine

Amide-Type Local Anesthetics

Lidocaine

Preparations and Dosage

Drug	Forms	Usual Adult Doses
Chloroprocaine [Nesacaine]	Injection 1% to 3%	Inject small volumes subcutaneously until the entire area is anesthetized. Maximal dose of 80 mL 1% strength
Lidocaine [Xylocaine]	Injection 0.5% to 5%	Inject small volumes subcutaneously until the entire area is anesthetized. Maximal dose of 30 mL 1% strength
Cocaine oronasolaryngeal	Solution 4% and 10%	1 mg/kg topically once. Alt: 1-2 mL of solution per nostril once

Lidocaine

Lidocaine, introduced in 1948, is the prototype of the amide-type agents. One of today's most widely used local anesthetics, lidocaine can be administered topically and by injection. Anesthesia with lidocaine is more rapid, more intense, and more prolonged than an equal dose of procaine. Effects can be extended by coadministration of epinephrine. Allergic reactions are rare, and individuals allergic to ester-type anesthetics are not cross-allergic to lidocaine. If plasma levels of lidocaine climb too high, CNS and cardiovascular toxicity can result. Inactivation is by hepatic metabolism.

In addition to its use in local anesthesia, lidocaine is employed to treat dysrhythmias (see Unit XXII on drugs for acute care). Control of dysrhythmias results from suppression of cardiac excitability secondary to blockade of cardiac sodium channels.

Cocaine

Cocaine was our first local anesthetic. It is an ester-type anesthetic. In addition to causing local anesthesia, cocaine has pronounced effects on the sympathetic and central nervous systems. These sympathetic and CNS effects are due largely to blocking the reuptake of norepinephrine by adrenergic neurons.

Anesthetic Use

Cocaine is an excellent local anesthetic. Administered topically, the drug is employed for anesthesia of the ear, nose, and throat. Anesthesia develops rapidly and persists for about 1 hour. Unlike other local anesthetics, cocaine causes intense vasoconstriction (by blocking norepinephrine uptake at sympathetic nerve terminals on blood vessels). Accordingly, the drug should not be given in combination with epinephrine or any other vasoconstrictor. Despite its ability to constrict blood vessels, cocaine is readily absorbed after application to mucous membranes. Significant effects on the brain and heart can result. The drug is inactivated by plasma esterases and liver enzymes.

CNS Effects

Cocaine produces generalized CNS stimulation. Moderate doses cause euphoria, talkativeness, reduced fatigue, and increased sociability and alertness. Excessive doses can cause seizures. Excitation is followed by CNS depression. Respiratory arrest and death can result.

Although cocaine does not seem to cause substantial physical dependence, psychological dependence can be profound. The drug is subject to widespread abuse and is classified under Schedule II of the Controlled Substances Act. Cocaine abuse is discussed in Chapter 33.

Cardiovascular Effects

Cocaine stimulates the heart and causes vasoconstriction. These effects result from (1) central stimulation of the sympathetic nervous system and (2) blockade of norepinephrine uptake in the periphery. Stimulation of the heart can produce *tachycardia* and potentially fatal *dysrhythmias.* Vasoconstriction can cause *hypertension.* Cocaine presents an especially serious risk to individuals with cardiovascular disease (e.g., hypertension, dysrhythmias, angina pectoris).

Other Local Anesthetics

In addition to the drugs discussed previously, several other local anesthetics are available. These agents differ with respect to indications, route of administration, mode of elimination, duration of action, and toxicity.

The local anesthetics can be grouped according to route of administration: topical versus injection. (Very few agents are administered by both routes, primarily because the drugs that are suitable for topical application are usually too toxic for parenteral use.) Table 21.2 lists the topically administered local anesthetics along with trade names and time course of action. Table 21.3 presents equivalent information for the injectable agents.

CLINICAL USE OF LOCAL ANESTHETICS

Local anesthetics may be administered *topically* (for surface anesthesia) and *by injection* (for infiltration anesthesia, nerve block anesthesia, intravenous regional anesthesia, epidural anesthesia, and spinal anesthesia). The uses and hazards of these anesthesia techniques are discussed next.

Topical Administration

Surface anesthesia is accomplished by applying the anesthetic directly to the skin or a mucous membrane. The agents employed most commonly are *lidocaine, tetracaine,* and *cocaine.*

Therapeutic Uses

Local anesthetics are applied to the *skin* to relieve pain, itching, and soreness of various causes, including infection, thermal burns, sunburn, diaper rash, wounds, bruises, abrasions, plant poisoning, and insect bites. Application may also be made to *mucous membranes* of the nose, mouth, pharynx, larynx, trachea, bronchi, vagina, and urethra. In addition, local anesthetics may be used to relieve discomfort associated with hemorrhoids, anal fissures, and pruritus ani.

Systemic Toxicity

Topical anesthetics applied to the skin can be absorbed in amounts sufficient to produce serious or even life-threatening effects. Cardiac toxicity can result in bradycardia, heart block, or cardiac arrest. CNS toxicity can result in seizures, respiratory depression, and coma. Obviously, the risk for toxicity increases with the amount absorbed, which is determined primarily by (1) the amount applied, (2) skin condition, and (3) skin temperature. Accordingly, to minimize the amount absorbed, and thereby minimize risk, patients should do the following:

- Apply the smallest amount needed.
- Avoid application to large areas.
- Avoid application to broken or irritated skin.
- Avoid strenuous exercise, wrapping the site, and heating the site, all of which can accelerate absorption by increasing skin temperature.

Administration by Injection

Injection of local anesthetics carries significant risk and requires special skills. Injections are usually performed by an anesthesiologist. Because severe systemic reactions may occur, equipment for resuscitation should be immediately available. Also, an intravenous line should be in place to permit rapid treatment of toxicity. Inadvertent injection into an artery or vein can cause severe toxicity. To ensure the needle is not in a blood vessel, it should be aspirated before injection. After administration, the patient should be monitored for cardiovascular status, respiratory function, and state of consciousness. To reduce the risk for toxicity, local anesthetics should be administered in the lowest effective dose.

Infiltration Anesthesia

Infiltration anesthesia is achieved by injecting a local anesthetic directly into the immediate area of surgery or manipulation. Anesthesia can be prolonged by combining the anesthetic with epinephrine. The agents employed most frequently for infiltration anesthesia are lidocaine and bupivacaine.

Nerve Block Anesthesia

Nerve block anesthesia is achieved by injecting a local anesthetic into or near nerves that supply the surgical field, but at a site distant from the field itself. This technique has the advantage of producing anesthesia with doses that are smaller than those needed for infiltration anesthesia. Drug selection is based on required duration of anesthesia. For shorter procedures, lidocaine or mepivacaine might be used. For longer procedures, bupivacaine would be appropriate.

CHAPTER

22

Opioid Analgesics, Opioid Antagonists, and Nonopioid Centrally Acting Analgesics

Laura D. Rosenthal, DNP, ACNP, FAANP

Analgesics are drugs that relieve pain without causing loss of consciousness. In this chapter, we focus mainly on the opioid analgesics, the most effective pain relievers available. The opioid family, whose name derives from *opium,* includes such widely used agents as morphine, fentanyl, codeine, and oxycodone [OxyContin].

OPIOID ANALGESICS

Introduction to the Opioids

Terminology

An *opioid* is any drug, natural or synthetic, that has actions similar to those of morphine. The term *opiate* is more specific and applies only to compounds present in opium (e.g., morphine, codeine).

Endogenous Opioid Peptides

The body has three families of peptides—*enkephalins, endorphins,* and *dynorphins*—that have opioid-like properties. Although we know that endogenous opioid peptides serve as neurotransmitters, neurohormones, and neuromodulators, their precise physiologic role is not fully understood. Endogenous opioid peptides are found in the central nervous system (CNS) and in peripheral tissues.

Opioid Receptors

There are three main classes of opioid receptors, designated *mu, kappa,* and *delta.* From a pharmacologic perspective, mu receptors are the most important because opioid analgesics act primarily by activating mu receptors, although they also produce weak activation of kappa receptors. As a rule, opioid analgesics do not interact with delta receptors. In contrast to opioid analgesics, endogenous opioid peptides act through all three opioid receptors, including delta receptors. Important responses to activation of mu and kappa receptors are shown in Table 22.1.

Mu Receptors

Responses to activation of mu receptors include analgesia, respiratory depression, euphoria, and sedation. In addition, mu activation is related to physical dependence.

A study in genetically engineered mice underscores the importance of mu receptors in drug action. In this study, researchers studied mice that lacked the gene for mu receptors. When these mice were given morphine, the drug had no effect. It did not produce analgesia or physical dependence, and it did not reinforce social behaviors that are thought to indicate subjective effects. Hence, at least in mice, mu receptors appear both necessary and sufficient to mediate the major actions of opioid drugs.

Kappa Receptors

As with mu receptors, activation of kappa receptors can produce analgesia and sedation. In addition, kappa activation may underlie psychotomimetic effects seen with certain opioids.

Classification of Drugs That Act at Opioid Receptors

Drugs that act at opioid receptors are classified on the basis of how they affect receptor function. At each type of receptor, a drug can act in one of three ways: as an *agonist, partial agonist,* or *antagonist.* Based on these actions, drugs that bind opioid receptors fall into three major groups: (1) pure opioid agonists, (2) agonist-antagonist opioids, and (3) pure opioid antagonists. The actions of drugs in these groups at mu and kappa receptors are shown in Table 22.2.

Pure Opioid Agonists

The pure opioid agonists activate mu receptors and kappa receptors. By doing so, the pure agonists can produce analgesia, euphoria, sedation, respiratory depression, physical dependence, constipation, and other effects. The pure agonists can be subdivided into two groups: *strong opioid agonists* and *moderate to strong opioid agonists.* Morphine is the prototype of the strong agonists. Codeine is the prototype of the moderate to strong agonists.

Agonist-Antagonist Opioids

Three agonist-antagonist opioids are available in oral (PO) form: pentazocine, butorphanol, and buprenorphine. The actions of these drugs at mu and kappa receptors are shown in Table 22.2. When administered alone, the agonist-antagonist opioids produce analgesia. However, if given to a patient who is taking a pure opioid agonist, these drugs can *antagonize* analgesia caused by the pure agonist. Pentazocine [Talwin] is the prototype of the agonist-antagonists.

TABLE 22.1 ■ Important Responses to Activation of Mu and Kappa Receptors

	Receptor Type	
Response	**Mu**	**Kappa**
Analgesia	✓	✓
Respiratory depression	✓	
Sedation	✓	✓
Euphoria	✓	
Physical dependence	✓	
Decreased gastrointestinal motility	✓	✓

TABLE 22.2 ■ Drug Actions at Mu and Kappa Receptors

	Receptor Type	
Drugs	**Mu**	**Kappa**
PURE OPIOID AGONISTS		
Morphine, codeine, meperidine, and other morphine-like drugs	Agonist	Agonist
AGONIST-ANTAGONIST OPIOIDS		
Pentazocine, nalbuphine, butorphanol	Antagonist	Agonist
Buprenorphine	Partial agonist	Antagonist
PURE OPIOID ANTAGONISTS		
Naloxone, naltrexone, others	Antagonist	Antagonist

Pure Opioid Antagonists

The pure opioid antagonists act as antagonists at mu and kappa receptors. These drugs do not produce analgesia or any of the other effects caused by opioid agonists. Their principal use is reversal of respiratory and CNS depression caused by overdose with opioid agonists. In addition, one of these drugs—methylnaltrexone—is used to treat opioid-induced constipation. Naloxone [Narcan] is the prototype of the pure opioid antagonists.

Prototype Drugs

OPIOID ANALGESICS AND ANTAGONISTS

Pure Opioid Agonists
Morphine

Agonist-Antagonist Opioids
Pentazocine

Pure Opioid Antagonists
Naloxone

BASIC PHARMACOLOGY OF THE OPIOIDS

Morphine

Morphine is the prototype of the strong opioid analgesics and remains the standard by which newer opioids are measured. Morphine has multiple pharmacologic effects, including analgesia, sedation, euphoria, respiratory depression, cough suppression, and suppression of bowel motility.

Overview of Pharmacologic Actions

Morphine has multiple pharmacologic actions. In addition to relieving pain, the drug causes drowsiness and mental clouding, reduces anxiety, and creates a sense of well-being. Through actions in the CNS and periphery, morphine can cause respiratory depression, constipation, urinary retention, orthostatic hypotension, emesis, miosis, cough suppression, and biliary colic. With prolonged use, the drug produces tolerance and physical dependence.

Individual effects of morphine may be beneficial, detrimental, or both. For example, analgesia is clearly beneficial, whereas respiratory depression and urinary retention are clearly detrimental. Certain other effects, such as sedation and reduced bowel motility, may be beneficial or detrimental, depending on the circumstances of drug use.

Therapeutic Use: Relief of Pain

The principal indication for morphine is relief of moderate to severe pain. The drug can relieve postoperative pain, pain of labor and delivery, and chronic pain caused by cancer and other conditions.

Morphine relieves pain without causing loss of consciousness. The drug is more effective against constant, dull pain than against sharp, intermittent pain. However, even sharp pain can be relieved by large doses. The ability of morphine to cause mental clouding, sedation, euphoria, and anxiety reduction can contribute to relief of pain.

The use of morphine and other opioids to relieve pain is discussed further in this chapter and in Chapter 83.

Adverse Effects

Respiratory Depression

Respiratory depression is the most serious adverse effect. At equianalgesic doses, all of the pure opioid agonists depress respiration to the same extent. Death after an overdose is almost always from respiratory arrest. Opioids depress respiration primarily through activation of mu receptors, although activation of kappa receptors also contributes.

The time course of respiratory depression begins up to 90 minutes after PO ingestion. With prolonged use of opioids, tolerance develops to respiratory depression. Huge doses that would be lethal to a nontolerant individual have been taken by opioid addicts without noticeable effect. Similarly, tolerance to respiratory depression develops during long-term clinical use of opioids (e.g., in patients with cancer). Certain patients, including the very young, older adults, and those with respiratory disease (e.g., asthma, emphysema), are especially sensitive to respiratory depression and hence must be monitored closely. Outpatients should be informed about the risk for respiratory depression and instructed to notify the prescriber if respiratory distress occurs.

Patient Education

RESPIRATORY DEPRESSION

Respiratory depression is increased by concurrent use of other drugs with CNS-depressant actions (e.g., alcohol, barbiturates, benzodiazepines). Accordingly, these drugs should be avoided. Outpatients should be warned against use of alcohol and all other CNS depressants.

Pronounced respiratory depression can be reversed with naloxone [Narcan], an opioid antagonist. However, dosing must be carefully titrated because excessive doses will completely block the analgesic effects of morphine, causing pain to return.

BLACK BOX WARNING: OPIOIDS

Opioid medications can cause respiratory arrest in both opioid-naïve and opioid-tolerant patients. Monitor for respiratory depression, especially during new-onset therapy or after escalation of dose.

Constipation

Opioids promote constipation through actions in the CNS and gastrointestinal (GI) tract. Specifically, by activating mu receptors in the gut, these drugs can suppress propulsive intestinal contractions, intensify nonpropulsive contractions, increase the tone of the anal sphincter, and inhibit secretion of fluids into the intestinal lumen. As a result, constipation can develop after a few days of opioid use. Potential complications of constipation include fecal impaction, bowel perforation, rectal tearing, and hemorrhoids.

Opioid-induced constipation can be managed with a combination of pharmacologic and nonpharmacologic measures. The goal is to produce a soft, formed stool every 1 to 2 days. Principal nondrug measures are physical activity and increased intake of fiber and fluids (for prevention) and enemas (for treatment). Most patients also require *prophylactic drugs:* a stimulant laxative, such as senna, is given to counteract reduced bowel motility; a stool softener, such as docusate [Colace], plus polyethylene glycol (an osmotic laxative) can provide additional benefit. If these prophylactic drugs prove inadequate, the patient may need *rescue therapy* with a strong osmotic laxative, such as lactulose or sodium phosphate. As a last resort, patients may be given *methylnaltrexone* [Relistor], an oral drug that blocks mu receptors in the intestine. As discussed later in the chapter, methylnaltrexone can't cross the blood-brain barrier and hence does not reverse opioid-induced analgesia.

Because of their effects on the intestine, opioids are highly effective for treating diarrhea. In fact, antidiarrheal use of these drugs preceded analgesic use by centuries. The impact of opioids on intestinal function is an interesting example of how an effect can be detrimental (constipation) or beneficial (relief of diarrhea) depending on who is taking the medication. Opioids employed specifically to treat diarrhea are discussed in Chapter 64.

Orthostatic Hypotension

Morphine-like drugs lower blood pressure by blunting the baroreceptor reflex and by dilating peripheral arterioles and veins. Peripheral vasodilation results primarily from morphine-induced release of histamine.

Patient Education

HYPOTENSION

Hypotension is mild in the recumbent patient but can be significant when the patient stands up. Patients should be informed about symptoms of hypotension (lightheadedness, dizziness) and instructed to sit or lie down if they occur. Also, patients should be informed that hypotension can be minimized by moving slowly when changing from a supine or seated position to an upright position. Patients should be warned against walking if hypotension is substantial. Hospitalized patients may require ambulatory assistance. Hypotensive drugs can exacerbate opioid-induced hypotension.

Urinary Retention

Morphine can cause urinary hesitancy and urinary retention. Three mechanisms are involved. First, morphine increases tone in the bladder sphincter. Second, morphine increases tone in the detrusor muscle, thereby elevating pressure within the bladder, causing a sense of urinary urgency. Third, in addition to its direct effects on the urinary tract, morphine may interfere with voiding by suppressing awareness of bladder stimuli. To reduce discomfort, patients should be encouraged to void every 4 hours. Urinary hesitancy or retention is especially likely in patients with benign prostatic hypertrophy. Drugs with anticholinergic properties (e.g., tricyclic antidepressants, antihistamines) can exacerbate the problem.

In addition to causing urinary retention, morphine may decrease urine production largely by decreasing renal blood flow, and partly by promoting release of antidiuretic hormone.

Emesis

Morphine promotes nausea and vomiting through direct stimulation of the chemoreceptor trigger zone of the medulla. Emetic reactions are greatest with the initial dose and then diminish with subsequent doses. Nausea and vomiting are uncommon in recumbent patients but occur in 15% to 40% of ambulatory patients, suggesting a vestibular component. Nausea and vomiting can be reduced by pretreatment with an antiemetic (e.g., prochlorperazine) and by having the patient remain still.

Euphoria and Dysphoria

Euphoria is defined as an exaggerated sense of well-being. Morphine often produces euphoria when given to patients in pain. Although euphoria can enhance pain relief, it also contributes to the drug's potential for abuse. Euphoria is caused by activation of mu receptors.

In some individuals, morphine causes *dysphoria* (a sense of anxiety and unease). Dysphoria is uncommon among patients in pain but may occur when morphine is taken in the absence of pain.

Sedation

When administered to relieve pain, morphine is likely to cause drowsiness and some mental clouding. Although these effects can complement analgesic actions, they can also be detrimental. Outpatients should be warned about CNS depression and advised to avoid hazardous activities (e.g., driving) if sedation is significant. Sedation can be minimized by taking smaller doses more often or using opioids that have short half-lives.

Neurotoxicity

Opioid-induced neurotoxicity can cause delirium, agitation, myoclonus, hyperalgesia, and other symptoms. Primary risk factors are renal impairment, preexisting cognitive impairment, and prolonged, high-dose opioid use. Management consists of hydration and dose reduction. For patients who must take opioids long term, opioid rotation (periodically switching from one opioid to another) may reduce neurotoxicity development.

Pharmacokinetics

With oral morphine therapy, duration of action depends on the formulation. For example, with immediate-release (IR) tablets, effects last 4 to 5 hours, whereas with extended-release (ER) capsules, effects last 24 hours.

To relieve pain, morphine must cross the blood-brain barrier and enter the CNS. Because the drug has poor lipid solubility, it does not cross the barrier easily. Consequently, only a small fraction of each dose reaches sites of analgesic action. Because the blood-brain barrier is not well developed in infants, these patients generally require lower doses than do older children and adults.

Morphine is inactivated by hepatic metabolism. When taken by mouth, the drug must pass through the liver on its way to the systemic circulation. Much of an oral dose is inactivated during this first pass through the liver. In patients with liver disease, analgesia and other effects may be intensified and prolonged. Accordingly, it may be necessary to reduce the dosage or lengthen the dosing interval.

Tolerance and Physical Dependence

With continuous use, morphine can cause tolerance and physical dependence. These phenomena, which are generally inseparable, reflect cellular adaptations that occur in response to prolonged opioid exposure.

Tolerance

Tolerance can be defined as a state in which a larger dose is required to produce the same response that could formerly be produced with a smaller dose. Alternatively, tolerance can be defined as a condition in which a particular dose now produces a smaller response than it did when treatment began. Because of tolerance, dosage must be increased to maintain analgesic effects.

Tolerance develops to many—but not all—of morphine's actions. With prolonged treatment, tolerance develops to *analgesia, euphoria,* and *sedation.* As a result, with long-term therapy, an increase in dosage may be required to maintain these desirable effects. Fortunately, as tolerance develops to these therapeutic effects, tolerance also develops to *respiratory depression.* As a result, the high doses needed to control pain in the tolerant individual are not associated with increased respiratory depression.

Very little tolerance develops to *constipation* and *miosis.* Even in highly tolerant addicts, constipation remains a chronic problem, and constricted pupils are characteristic.

Cross-tolerance exists among the opioid agonists (e.g., oxycodone, methadone, fentanyl, codeine, heroin). Accordingly, individuals tolerant to one of these agents will be tolerant to all the others. No cross-tolerance exists between opioids and general CNS depressants (e.g., barbiturates, ethanol, benzodiazepines, general anesthetics).

Physical Dependence

Physical dependence is defined as a state in which an abstinence syndrome will occur if drug use is abruptly stopped. Opioid dependence results from adaptive cellular changes that occur in response to the continuous presence of these drugs. Although the exact nature of these changes is unknown, it is clear that, after these compensatory changes have taken place, the body requires the continued presence of opioids to function normally. If opioids are withdrawn, an abstinence syndrome usually will follow.

The intensity and duration of the opioid abstinence syndrome depends on two factors: the half-life of the drug being used and the degree of physical dependence. With opioids that have relatively short half-lives (e.g., morphine), symptoms of abstinence are intense but brief. In contrast, with opioids that have long half-lives (e.g., methadone), symptoms are less intense but more prolonged. With any opioid, the intensity of withdrawal symptoms parallels the degree of physical dependence.

For individuals who are highly dependent, the abstinence syndrome can be extremely unpleasant. Initial reactions include yawning, rhinorrhea, and sweating. Onset occurs about 10 hours after the final dose. These early responses are followed by anorexia, irritability, tremor, and "gooseflesh"—hence the term *cold turkey.* At its peak, the syndrome manifests as violent sneezing, weakness, nausea, vomiting, diarrhea, abdominal cramps, bone and muscle pain, muscle spasm, and kicking movements—hence the term *kicking the habit.* Giving an opioid at any time during withdrawal rapidly reverses all signs and symptoms. Left untreated, the morphine withdrawal syndrome runs its course in 7 to 10 days. It should be emphasized that, although withdrawal from opioids is unpleasant, the syndrome is rarely dangerous. In contrast, withdrawal from general CNS depressants (e.g., barbiturates, alcohol) can be lethal (see Chapter 27).

To minimize the abstinence syndrome, opioids should be withdrawn gradually. When the degree of dependence is moderate, symptoms can be avoided by administering progressively smaller doses over 3 days. When the patient is highly dependent, dosage should be tapered more slowly—over 7 to 10 days. With a proper withdrawal schedule, withdrawal symptoms will resemble those of a mild case of flu—even when the degree of dependence is high.

It is important to note that physical dependence is rarely a complication when opioids are taken *acutely* to treat pain. Hospitalized patients receiving morphine 2 to 3 times a day for up to 2 weeks show no significant signs of dependence. If morphine is withheld from these patients, no significant signs of withdrawal can be detected. The issue of physical dependence as a clinical concern is discussed further later in the chapter.

Infants exposed to opioids in utero may be born drug dependent. If the infant is not provided with opioids, an abstinence syndrome will ensue. Signs of withdrawal include excessive crying, sneezing, tremor, hyperreflexia, fever, and diarrhea. The infant can be weaned from drug dependence by administering dilute paregoric in progressively smaller doses.

Cross-dependence exists among pure opioid agonists. As a result, any pure agonist will prevent withdrawal in a patient who is physically dependent on any other pure agonist.

Abuse Liability

Morphine and the other opioids are subject to abuse, largely because of their ability to cause pleasurable experiences (e.g., euphoria and sedation). Physical dependence contributes to abuse: when dependence exists, the ability of opioids to ward off withdrawal serves to reinforce their desirability in the mind of the abuser.

The abuse liability of the opioids is reflected in their classification under the Controlled Substances Act. (The provisions of this act are discussed in Chapter 30.) As shown in Table 22.3, morphine and all other strong opioid agonists are classified under Schedule II. This classification reflects a moderate to high abuse liability. The agonist-antagonist opioids have a lower abuse liability and hence are classified under Schedule IV (butorphanol, pentazocine) or Schedule III (buprenorphine), or have no classification at all. Health care personnel who prescribe, dispense, and administer opioids must adhere to the procedures set forth in the Controlled Substances Act.

TABLE 22.3 ▪ Interactions of Morphine-Like Drugs With Other Drugs

Interacting Drugs	Outcome of the Interaction
ADVERSE INTERACTIONS	
CNS depressants	Increased respiratory depression and sedation
Barbiturates	
Benzodiazepines	
Alcohol	
General anesthetics	
Antihistamines	
Phenothiazines	
Agonist-antagonist opioids	Precipitation of a withdrawal reaction
Anticholinergic drugs	Increased constipation and urinary retention
Atropine-like drugs	
Antihistamines	
Phenothiazines	
Tricyclic antidepressants	
Hypotensive agents	Increased hypotension
Monoamine oxidase inhibitors	Hyperpyrexic coma
BENEFICIAL INTERACTIONS	
Amphetamines	Increased analgesia and decreased sedation
Antiemetics	Suppression of nausea and vomiting
Naloxone	Suppression of symptoms of opioid overdose
Dextromethorphan	Increased analgesia; possible reduction in tolerance

Fortunately, abuse is rare when opioids are employed to treat pain. The issue of abuse as a clinical concern is addressed in depth later in the chapter.

Precautions

Some patients are more likely than others to experience adverse effects. Common sense dictates that opioids be used with special caution in these people. Conditions that can predispose patients to adverse reactions are discussed next.

Decreased Respiratory Reserve

Because morphine depresses respiration, it can further compromise respiration in patients with impaired pulmonary function. Accordingly, the drug should be used with caution in patients with asthma, emphysema, kyphoscoliosis, chronic cor pulmonale, and extreme obesity. Caution is also needed in patients taking other drugs that can depress respiration (e.g., barbiturates, benzodiazepines, general anesthetics).

Other Precautions

Infants and *older-adult patients* are especially sensitive to morphine-induced respiratory depression. In patients with *inflammatory bowel disease,* morphine may cause toxic megacolon or paralytic ileus. Because morphine and all other opioids are inactivated by liver enzymes, effects may be intensified and prolonged in patients with *liver impairment.* Severe hypotension may occur in patients with preexisting *hypotension* or *reduced blood volume.* In patients with *benign prostatic hypertrophy,* opioids may cause acute urinary retention; repeated catheterization may be required.

Drug Interactions

The major interactions between morphine and other drugs are shown in Table 22.3. Some interactions are adverse, and some are beneficial.

Toxicity

Clinical Manifestations

Opioid overdose produces a classic triad of signs: *coma, respiratory depression,* and *pinpoint pupils.* Coma is profound, and the patient cannot be aroused. Respiratory rate may be as low as 2 to 4 breaths/minute. Although the pupils are constricted initially, they may dilate as hypoxia sets in (secondary to respiratory depression). Hypoxia may cause blood pressure to fall. Prolonged hypoxia may result in shock. When death occurs, respiratory arrest is almost always the immediate cause.

Treatment

Treatment consists primarily of *ventilatory support* and giving an *opioid antagonist.* Naloxone [Narcan] is the traditional antagonist of choice. The pharmacology of the opioid antagonists is discussed later.

Preparations

Morphine Alone

Morphine sulfate, by itself, is available in eight nonparenteral formulations:

- IR tablets (15 and 30 mg)
- Controlled-release tablets (15, 30, 60, 100, and 200 mg) sold as *MS Contin*
- ER tablets (20, 30, 50, 60, 80, and 100 mg)
- Sustained-release capsules (10, 20, 30, 40, 50, 60, 70, 80, 100, 130, 150, and 200 mg) sold as *Kadian* and *Morphine SR* 🍁

- ER capsules (10, 30, 45, 60, 75, 90, 100, 120, and 200 mg) sold as *M-Eslon* ♣
- Standard oral solution (10 and 20 mg/5 mL) sold as *MSIR*
- Concentrated oral solution (100 mg/5 mL) sold as *MSIR*
- Rectal suppositories (5, 10, 20, and 30 mg) sold as *Statex* ♣

Morphine and Naltrexone [Embeda]

In 2010, the U.S. Food and Drug Administration (FDA) approved Embeda, a fixed-dose combination of morphine and naltrexone, an opioid antagonist (see later). The product is designed to discourage morphine abuse. Embeda capsules are filled with tiny pellets that have an outer layer of ER morphine and an inner core of naltrexone. When the capsules are swallowed intact, only the morphine is absorbed. However, if the pellets are crushed, the naltrexone will be absorbed too, thereby blunting the effects of the morphine. As a result, potential abusers cannot get a quick high by crushing the pellets to release all of the morphine at once. However, abusers can still get high by simply taking a large dose. Embeda capsules are more expensive than other ER morphine products and should be prescribed only when abuse appears likely.

Alcohol can accelerate release of morphine from Embeda pellets. As a result, the entire dose can be absorbed quickly—rather than over 24 hours—thereby causing a potentially fatal spike in morphine blood levels. Accordingly, patients should be warned against alcohol consumption.

Embeda capsules are available in six morphine/naltrexone strengths: 20 mg/0.8 mg, 30 mg/1.2 mg, 50 mg/2 mg, 60 mg/2.4 mg, 80 mg/3.2 mg, and 100 mg/4 mg. Dosing is done once or twice daily. Patients can swallow Embeda capsules whole, or they can open the capsules and sprinkle the pellets on applesauce, which must be ingested without chewing.

Dosage and Administration

General Guidelines

Dosage must be individualized. High doses are required for patients with a low tolerance to pain or with extremely painful disorders. Patients with sharp, stabbing pain need higher doses than patients with dull pain. Older adults generally require lower doses than younger adults. Neonates require relatively low doses because their blood-brain barrier is not fully developed. For all patients, dosage should be reduced as pain subsides. Outpatients should be warned not to increase dosage without consulting the prescriber.

Routes and Dosages

Oral

Oral dosing is generally reserved for patients with chronic, severe pain, such as that associated with cancer. Because oral morphine undergoes extensive metabolism on its first pass through the liver, oral doses are usually higher than parenteral doses. A typical dosage is 10 to 30 mg repeated every 4 hours as needed. However, oral dosing is highly individualized, and some patients may require 75 mg or more. Controlled-release formulations may be administered every 8 to 12 hours, and the ER formulation [Kadian] is given every 12 to 24 hours. Patients should be instructed to swallow these products intact, without crushing or chewing. Also, warn patients using Kadian or Embeda capsules not to drink alcohol, which can accelerate release of morphine from these products.

Other Strong Opioid Agonists

In an effort to produce a strong analgesic with a low potential for respiratory depression and abuse, pharmaceutical scientists have created many new opioid analgesics. However, none of the newer pure opioid agonists can be considered truly superior to morphine; these drugs are essentially equal to morphine with respect to analgesic action, abuse liability, and the ability to cause respiratory depression. Also, to varying degrees, they all cause sedation, euphoria, constipation, urinary retention, cough suppression, hypotension, and miosis. However, despite their similarities to morphine, the newer drugs do have unique qualities. Hence one agent may be more desirable than another in a particular clinical setting. With all of the newer pure opioid agonists, toxicity can be reversed with an opioid antagonist (e.g., naloxone). Important differences between morphine and the newer strong opioid analgesics are discussed later. Table 22.4 shows dosages, routes, and time courses for morphine and the newer agents.

Fentanyl

Fentanyl [Duragesic, Abstral, Actiq, Fentora, Onsolis, Lazanda, Subsys] is a strong opioid analgesic with a high milligram potency (about 100 times that of morphine). Eight formulations are available for administration by four different routes: parenteral, transdermal, transmucosal, and intranasal. Depending on the route, fentanyl may be used for surgical analgesia, chronic pain control, and control of breakthrough pain in patients taking other opioids. All preparations are regulated under Schedule II of the Controlled Substances Act.

Fentanyl, regardless of route, has the same adverse effects as other opioids: respiratory depression, sedation, constipation, urinary retention, and nausea. Of these, respiratory depression is the greatest concern. Signs of toxicity can be reversed with an opioid antagonist (e.g., naloxone).

Fentanyl is metabolized by CYP3A4 (the 3A4 isoenzyme of cytochrome P450), and hence fentanyl levels can be increased by CYP3A4 inhibitors (e.g., ritonavir, ketoconazole). Patients taking these inhibitors should be closely monitored for severe respiratory depression and other signs of toxicity.

Transdermal System

The fentanyl transdermal system [Duragesic] consists of a fentanyl-containing patch that is applied to the skin of the upper torso. The drug is slowly released from the patch and absorbed through the skin, reaching effective levels in 24 hours. Levels remain steady for another 48 hours, after which the patch should be replaced. If a new patch is not applied, effects will nonetheless persist for several hours, owing to continued absorption of residual fentanyl remaining in the skin.

Transdermal fentanyl is indicated only for persistent severe pain in patients who are already opioid tolerant. Use in nontolerant patients can cause fatal respiratory depression. The patch should not be used in children younger than 2 years or in anyone younger than 18 years who weighs less than 110 pounds. Also, the patch should not be used for postoperative pain, intermittent pain, or pain that responds to a less powerful analgesic.

Like other strong opioids, fentanyl overdose poses a risk for fatal respiratory depression. If respiratory depression develops, it may persist for hours after patch removal, owing to continued absorption of fentanyl from the skin.

Fentanyl patches are available in five strengths, which deliver fentanyl to the systemic circulation at rates of 12.5, 25, 50, 75, and 100 mcg/hour. The smallest effective patch should be used. If a dosage greater than 100 mcg/hour is required, a combination of patches can be applied. After placing a fentanyl patch, it must not be exposed to direct heat (e.g., heating pads, hot baths, electric blankets) because doing so can accelerate fentanyl release, as can fever, sunbathing, and strenuous exercise. Because full analgesic effects can take up to 24 hours to develop, PRN therapy with a short-acting opioid may be required until the patch takes effect. As with other long-acting opioids, if breakthrough pain occurs, supplemental dosing with a short-acting opioid is indicated. For

TABLE 22.4 ▪ Clinical Pharmacology of Pure Opioid Agonists

Drug and Route*	Equianalgesic Dose (mg)†	Time Course of Analgesic Effects		
		Onset (min)	Peak (min)	Duration (hr)
Codeine				
PO	200	30-45	60-120	4-6
Fentanyl				
Transdermal	—	Delayed	24-72	72
Transmucosal‡	—	10-15	20	1-2
Nasal spray	—	10-15	15-20	1-2
Hydrocodone				
PO	30	10-30	30-60	4-6
Hydromorphone				
PO (IR)	7.5	30	90-120	4
PO (ER)	7.5	—	360-480	18-24
Levorphanol				
PO	4	10-60	90-120	6-8
Meperidine				
PO	300	15	60-90	2-4
Methadone				
PO	20	30-60	90-120	4-6§
Morphine				
PO (IR)	30	—	60-120	4-5
PO (ER)	30	—	420	8-12
Oxycodone				
PO (IR)	20	15-30	60	3-4
PO (CR)	20	—	120-180	Up to 12
Oxymorphone				
PO (IR)	10	—	—	4-6
PO (ER)	10	—	—	Up to 12
Rectal	10	15-30	120	3-6
Tapentadol				
PO	100	45-60	90-120	4-8

*IM administration should be avoided whenever possible.
†Dose in milligrams that produces a degree of analgesia equivalent to that produced by a 10-mg IM dose of morphine.
‡Data are for the Actiq lozenge on a stick.
§With repeated doses, methadone's duration of action may increase up to 48 hours.
CR, controlled release; ER, extended release; IR, immediate release.

most patients, patches can be replaced every 72 hours, although some may require a new patch in 48 hours. Used or damaged patches should be folded in half with the medication side touching and flushed down the toilet. Unused patches should be stored out of reach of children.

Transmucosal

Fentanyl for transmucosal administration is available in four formulations: lozenges on a stick [Actiq], buccal tablets [Fentora], sublingual spray [Subsys], and sublingual tablets [Abstral]. All five products are approved only for *breakthrough cancer pain in patients at least 18 years old who are already taking opioids around-the-clock and have developed some degree of tolerance,* defined as needing, for 1 week or longer, at least: 60 mg of oral morphine a day, or 30 mg of oral oxycodone a day, or 25 mg of oral oxymorphone a day, or 8 mg of oral hydromorphone a day, or 25 mcg of fentanyl per hour, or an equianalgesic dose of another opioid. Transmucosal fentanyl must not be used for acute pain, postoperative pain, headache, or athletic injuries. Furthermore, it is essential to appreciate that the dose of fentanyl in these formulations is sufficient to kill nontolerant individuals—especially children. Accordingly, these products must be stored in a secure, child-resistant location.

All fentanyl transmucosal formulations are regulated as Schedule II products. Owing to risks of misuse, abuse, and overdose, all transmucosal fentanyl products are available only through a restricted distribution program, called the Transmucosal Immediate Release Fentanyl Risk Evaluation and Mitigation Strategy (TIRF REMS) Access program. The patient must enroll in this program to receive these products, and they are available only through pharmacies enrolled in the TIRF REMS program.

Adverse effects of transmucosal fentanyl are like those of other opioid preparations. The most common are dizziness, anxiety, confusion, nausea, vomiting, constipation, dyspnea, weakness, and headache. The biggest concerns are respiratory depression and shock.

Because of differences in bioavailability, *transmucosal fentanyl products are not interchangeable on a microgram-for-microgram basis.* For example, a 100-mcg buccal tablet produces about the same fentanyl blood level as does a

200-mcg lozenge. Accordingly, if a patient switches from one transmucosal product to another, dosage of the new product must be titrated to determine a strength that is safe and effective.

Lozenge on a Stick

The fentanyl lozenge on a stick [Actiq]—also known as oral transmucosal fentanyl citrate (OTFC)—consists of a raspberry-flavored lozenge on a plastic handle and looks much like a lollipop.

To administer the unit, patients place it between the cheek and the lower gum and actively suck it. Periodically, the unit should be moved from one side of the mouth to the other. Consumption of the entire lozenge should take 15 minutes. As the patient sucks, some of the drug is absorbed directly and rapidly through the oral mucosa, and some is swallowed and absorbed slowly from the GI tract. Analgesia begins in 10 to 15 minutes, peaks in 20 minutes, and persists 1 to 2 hours.

Dosing should begin with a 200-mcg unit. If breakthrough pain persists, the patient can take another 200-mcg unit 15 minutes after finishing the first one (i.e., 30 minutes after starting the first). Unit size should be gradually increased until an effective dose is determined. If the patient needs more than 4 units/day, it may be time to give a higher dose of his or her long-acting opioid.

To promote safe and effective use of the Actiq system, the manufacturer provides an Actiq Welcome Kit as well as a Child Safety Kit with the initial drug supply. The kit contains educational materials and safe storage containers for unused, partially used, and completely used units.

Buccal Tablets

Fentanyl buccal tablets [Fentora] are available in five strengths: 100, 200, 400, 600, and 800 mcg. Patients should place the tablet above a rear molar between the cheek and the gum and let it dissolve in place, usually in 15 to 30 minutes. Remaining fragments should be swallowed with a glass of water. Patients should not split, chew, suck, or swallow the tablets. The initial dose is 100 mcg. If 100 mcg is inadequate, another 100 mcg can be taken in 30 minutes. During each subsequent episode, dosage may be gradually increased, if needed, until an effective dose is established.

Sublingual Spray

Fentanyl sublingual spray [Subsys] is available in doses of 100, 200, 400, 600, 800, 1200, and 1600 mcg/spray. Individual doses of Subsys are supplied in single-use spray units. After the medication is dispensed under the tongue, the spray unit must be disposed of in a disposal bag provided by the manufacturer. The initial dose should be 100 mcg. If pain is not relieved by 30 minutes after the first dose, one additional dose may be administered. Use should be limited to four doses per day.

Sublingual Tablets

Fentanyl sublingual tablets [Abstral] are available in six strengths: 100, 200, 300, 400, 600, and 800 mcg. Each strength is a different color and shape. Patients should place the tablet on the floor of the mouth directly under the tongue and allow it to dissolve completely. If the mouth is dry, it should be moistened with water before dosing. Tablets must not be chewed, sucked, or swallowed. Patients should not eat or drink until the tablet is gone.

The initial dose is 100 mcg. If 100 mcg is inadequate, another 100 mcg can be taken in 30 minutes. No more than two doses should be used for any pain episode, and patients should wait at least 2 hours before dosing again. With each subsequent episode, the dose should be titrated until a safe and effective dose is identified.

Intranasal

Fentanyl nasal spray [Lazanda] is much like transmucosal fentanyl. Like transmucosal fentanyl, Lazanda is indicated only for breakthrough cancer pain in patients at least 18 years old who are already taking opioids around-the-clock and have developed some degree of tolerance. The spray must not be used for acute pain, postoperative pain, headache, or athletic injuries. Because of differences in bioavailability, Lazanda is not interchangeable with other fentanyl products on a microgram-for-microgram basis. Adverse effects are like those of other opioid preparations. The biggest concerns are respiratory depression and shock. As with the transmucosal products, the dose of fentanyl in Lazanda can be fatal to nontolerant individuals, so the spray must be stored in a secure, child-resistant location.

Intranasal fentanyl is supplied in 5-mL bottles that have a metered-dose nasal spray pump. Each bottle contains enough solution for 8 sprays. Two strengths are available: 100 or 400 mcg/spray. Dosing starts with 100 mcg. If needed, dosage can be titrated upward at subsequent pain episodes as follows: 200 mcg (100 mcg in each nostril), 400 mcg (400 mcg in 1 nostril), and then 800 mcg (400 mcg in 2 nostrils). Patients should allow at least 2 hours between doses. If more than 5 days elapse since the last dose, the bottle should be discarded and replaced with a new one.

BLACK BOX WARNING: FENTANYL

Products containing fentanyl can cause fatal respiratory depression. Many of these products are only available through restricted distribution programs secondary to misuse and abuse.

Meperidine

Meperidine [Demerol] shares the major pharmacologic properties of morphine. With oral administration, analgesia is strong. Meperidine was once considered a first-line drug for relief of moderate to severe pain. Now, use of meperidine has declined significantly for several reasons. First, the drug has a short half-life, so dosing must be repeated at short intervals. Second, meperidine interacts adversely with a number of drugs. Third, with continuous use, there is a risk for harm owing to accumulation of a toxic metabolite. Accordingly, routine use of the drug should be avoided. However, meperidine may still be appropriate for patients who can't take other opioids and for patients with drug-induced rigors or postanesthesia shivering.

Meperidine can interact with monoamine oxidase inhibitors (MAOIs) to cause excitation, delirium, hyperpyrexia, and convulsions. Coma and death can follow. The underlying mechanism appears to be excessive activation of serotonin receptors owing to meperidine-induced blockade of serotonin reuptake. Clearly, the combination of meperidine with an MAOI should be avoided. Other drugs that increase serotonin availability (e.g., tricyclic antidepressants, selective serotonin reuptake inhibitors [SSRIs]) may also pose a risk.

Repeated dosing results in accumulation of normeperidine, a toxic metabolite that can cause dysphoria, irritability, tremors, and seizures. To avoid toxicity, treatment should not exceed 48 hours, and the dosage should not exceed 600 mg/24 hours.

Meperidine is available in tablets (50 and 100 mg) and a syrup (10 mg/mL) for oral use, and in solution (10, 25, 50, 75, and 100 mg/mL) for intravenous (IV), intramuscular (IM), or subcutaneous (subQ) injection. The usual adult dosage is 50 to 150 mg (IM, subQ, or PO) repeated every 3 to 4 hours as needed—up to a maximum of 600 mg/day. The usual dosage for children is 1 to 1.8 mg/kg (IM, subQ, or PO) repeated every 3 to 4 hours as needed. As noted, prolonged use must be avoided.

Methadone

Methadone [Diskets, Dolophine, Methadose] has pharmacologic properties very similar to those of morphine. The drug is effective orally and has a long duration of action. Repeated dosing can result in accumulation. Methadone is used to relieve pain and to treat opioid addiction. Use of methadone for pain control has risen dramatically. The use of methadone in drug-abuse treatment programs is discussed in Chapter 33.

Because methadone can cause QT prolongation, all patients should receive an electrocardiogram (ECG) before treatment, 30 days later, and

Patient Education

METHADONE TOXICITY

To reduce risk for methadone toxicity, patients should be warned against taking more methadone than was prescribed and should be cautioned to avoid other CNS depressants, such as benzodiazepines, alcohol, and other opioids.

Methadone is supplied in IR tablets (5, 10, and 40 mg) and in solution (1, 2, and 10 mg/mL) for oral use, and in solution (10 mg/mL) for IM and subQ injection. In addition, the drug is available in dispersible 40-mg tablets for detoxification and maintenance of opioid addicts. Initial oral analgesic doses for adults range from 2.5 to 20 mg repeated every 8 to 12 hours as needed annually thereafter. If the QT interval exceeds 500 msec, stopping methadone or reducing the dosage should be considered.

BLACK BOX WARNING: METHADONE

Methadone prolongs the QT interval and hence may pose a risk for potentially fatal dysrhythmia. Torsades de pointes has developed in patients taking 65 to 400 mg/day. To reduce risk, methadone should be used with great caution—if at all—in patients with existing QT prolongation or a family history of long QT syndrome and in those taking other QT-prolonging drugs. In addition, methadone causes severe respiratory depression that can be potentially fatal.

Hydromorphone, Oxymorphone, and Levorphanol

Basic Pharmacology

All three drugs are strong opioid agonists with pharmacologic actions like those of morphine, and all three are indicated for moderate to severe pain. Dosages and time courses are shown in Table 22.4. Adverse effects include respiratory depression, sedation, cough suppression, constipation, urinary retention, nausea, and vomiting. Of note, hydromorphone may cause less nausea than morphine. Toxicity can be reversed with an opioid antagonist (e.g., naloxone). All three drugs are Schedule II agents.

BLACK BOX WARNING: HYDROMORPHONE AND OXYMORPHONE

Hydromorphone and oxymorphone have high abuse potential and can cause fatal respiratory depression, especially when used in combination with other sedating agents such as alcohol. Long-acting forms of oxymorphone should be prescribed only by a provider with additional education regarding chronic pain.

Preparations, Dosage, and Administration

Hydromorphone. Hydromorphone [Dilaudid, Exalgo, Jurnista ♣] is available in six formulations:

- IR tablets (2, 4, and 8 mg) sold as *Dilaudid*
- ER tablets (8, 12, 16, 32, and 64 mg) sold as *Exalgo* and *Jurnista* ♣
- Oral liquid (1 mg/mL) sold as *Dilaudid*
- Rectal suppositories (3 mg) sold as *Dilaudid*

With the IR tablets, the usual adult dosage is 2 mg every 4 to 6 hours. With the ER tablets, dosage is based on how much opioid was being used before switching to the ER tablets. With the oral liquid, the usual adult dosage is 2.5 to 10 mg every 3 to 6 hours. With the rectal suppositories, the usual dosage is 3 mg every 6 to 8 hours.

Oxymorphone. Oxymorphone [Opana] is available in three formulations:

- IR tablets (5 and 10 mg) sold as *Opana*
- ER tablets (5, 7.5, 10, 15, 20, 30, and 40 mg) sold as *Opana ER*

All oxymorphone tablets should be taken on an empty stomach because dosing with food can produce excessive peak levels. Also, alcohol should be avoided because it can increase blood levels of oral oxymorphone. For oral therapy in opioid-naïve patients, the usual initial dosage is 10 to 20 mg every 4 to 6 hours (using IR tablets) or 5 mg every 12 hours (using ER tablets).

Levorphanol

Levorphanol is available in 2-mg oral tablets. The usual adult oral dosage is 2 mg, repeated in 6 to 8 hours as needed.

Moderate to Strong Opioid Agonists

The moderate to strong opioid agonists are similar to morphine in most respects. Like morphine, these drugs produce analgesia, sedation, and euphoria. In addition, they can cause respiratory depression, constipation, urinary retention, cough suppression, and miosis. Differences between the moderate to strong opioids and morphine are primarily quantitative: the moderate to strong opioids produce less analgesia and respiratory depression than morphine and have a somewhat lower potential for abuse. As with morphine, toxicity from the moderate to strong agonists can be reversed with naloxone.

Codeine

Codeine is indicated for relief of mild to moderate pain. The drug is usually administered by mouth. Side effects are dose limiting. As a result, although taking codeine can produce significant pain relief, the degree of pain relief that can be achieved *safely* is quite low—much lower than with morphine. When taken in its usual analgesic dose (30 mg), codeine produces about as much pain relief as 325 mg of aspirin or 325 mg of acetaminophen.

For analgesic use, codeine is formulated alone and in combination with nonopioid analgesics (either aspirin or acetaminophen). Because codeine and nonopioid analgesics relieve pain by different mechanisms, the combinations can produce greater pain relief than either agent alone. Codeine alone is classified under Schedule II of the Controlled Substances Act. The combination preparations are classified under Schedule III. Although codeine is classified along with morphine in Schedule II, the abuse liability of codeine appears to be significantly lower.

Codeine is an extremely effective cough suppressant and is widely used for this action. The antitussive dose (10 mg) is lower than analgesic doses. Codeine is formulated in combination with various agents to suppress cough. These mixtures are classified under Schedule V.

BLACK BOX WARNING: CODEINE

In the liver, about 10% of each dose of codeine undergoes conversion to *morphine,* the active form of codeine. The enzyme responsible is CYP2D6 (the 2D6 isoenzyme of cytochrome P450). Among ultrarapid metabolizers, who carry multiple copies of the *CYP2D6* gene, codeine is unusually effective and has led to death in some children. Severe toxicity can also develop in breastfed infants whose mothers are taking codeine. The cause is high levels of morphine in breast milk, owing to ultrarapid codeine metabolism.

Preparations, Dosage, and Administration

Codeine is available in tablets (15, 30, and 60 mg) and in solution (30 mg/5 mL).

The usual analgesic dosage for adults is 15 to 60 mg every 3 to 6 hours (up to a maximum of 120 mg/24 hr). The usual analgesic dosage for children 1 year and older is 0.5 mg/kg every 4 to 6 hours (up to a maximum of 60 mg/24 hr).

Oxycodone

Oxycodone [OxyContin, Roxicodone, OxyIR ♣, Targiniq ER, Xartemis XR] has analgesic actions equivalent to those of codeine. Administration is oral. Oxycodone is available by itself in IR tablets (5, 10, 15, 20, and 30 mg), IR capsules (5 mg), controlled-release tablets (10, 15, 20, 30, 40, 60, and 80 mg), and oral solutions (1 and 20 mg/mL). In addition, the drug is available in combination with aspirin (as Percodan), acetaminophen (as Percocet, Roxicet, others), and ibuprofen (as Combunox). All formulations are classified under Schedule II.

BLACK BOX WARNING: OXYCODONE

Like oxymorphone and hydromorphone, oxycodone has a high potential for abuse and can cause fatal respiratory depression. Long-acting forms of oxycodone should be prescribed only by providers with additional education regarding chronic pain.

Oxycodone is metabolized by CYP3A4, so drugs that induce or inhibit CYP3A4 can alter oxycodone levels. Specifically, drugs that induce CYP3A4 (e.g., carbamazepine, phenytoin, rifampin) can lower oxycodone levels and thereby compromise pain relief. Conversely, drugs that inhibit CYP3A4 (e.g., clarithromycin, azole antifungal drugs, HIV protease inhibitors) can raise oxycodone levels and thereby pose a risk for toxicity.

Controlled-release oxycodone [OxyContin] is a long-acting analgesic designed to relieve moderate to severe pain around-the-clock for an extended time. Dosing is done every 12 hours—not PRN. If breakthrough pain occurs, supplemental dosing with a short-acting analgesic is indicated.

Owing to increasing reports of OxyContin abuse, safety warnings have been strengthened, and, in 2010, the product was reformulated. The new formulation bears the imprint OP; the old formulation bears the imprint OC. Reformulation occurred because abusers could crush the OxyContin OC tablets and then "snort" the resulting powder, or dissolve the powder in water and inject it intravenously. Both practices allowed *immediate* absorption of the entire dose and thereby produced blood levels that were much higher than those produced when the tablets were ingested whole and absorbed gradually. The result was an intense "high" coupled with a risk for fatal respiratory depression. Compared with the old tablets, OxyContin OP tablets are much harder to crush into a powder. And if exposed to water or alcohol, the tablets form a thick gel, rather than a solution that can be drawn into a syringe and injected.

To minimize risk, patients should swallow OxyContin tablets whole, without breaking, crushing, or chewing. Furthermore, the 80-mg formulation must be reserved for patients who are already opioid tolerant. As with all other opioids, concerns about abuse and addiction should not interfere with using OxyContin to manage pain. Rather, the drug must simply be prescribed appropriately and then used as prescribed.

A new formulation of oxycodone (agonist) paired with naloxone (antagonist), marketed as *Targiniq ER*, was approved in 2014 for treatment of chronic pain. Because *Targiniq ER* contains naloxone, an opioid antagonist, patients are deterred from abusing the drug because crushing the tablets will cause symptoms of opioid withdrawal. As with other long-acting opioids, *Targiniq ER* can cause fatal respiratory depression and should only be prescribed by providers with additional education regarding chronic pain.

Hydrocodone

Hydrocodone has analgesic actions equivalent to those of codeine. The drug is taken orally to relieve pain and to suppress cough. The usual IR dosage is 5 mg. New ER products [Zohydro ER, Hysingla ER] contain only hydrocodone and are taken every 12 to 24 hours. IR hydrocodone is combined with acetaminophen or ibuprofen. For cough suppression, the drug is combined with antihistamines and nasal decongestants. All of these products are currently classified under Schedule II. Trade names for combination products containing hydrocodone include *Vicodin, Vicoprofen,* and *Lortab.*

BLACK BOX WARNING: HYDROCODONE

All forms of hydrocodone contain a black box warning. Products that contain acetaminophen [Vicodin] are associated with hepatotoxicity. The ER forms of hydrocodone can cause fatal respiratory depression and should only be prescribed by providers with additional education regarding chronic pain.

Tapentadol

Actions and Uses

Tapentadol [Nucynta] is indicated for oral therapy of moderate to severe pain—acute or chronic—in patients aged 18 years and older. Analgesic effects are equivalent to those of oxycodone. Like other opioids, tapentadol can cause CNS depression and respiratory depression and has a significant potential for abuse. However, the drug differs from other opioids in two important ways. First, in addition to activating mu opioid receptors, tapentadol blocks reuptake of norepinephrine, similar to tramadol, discussed later. Second, tapentadol causes less constipation than traditional opioids.

Pharmacokinetics

Tapentadol is administered PO, and plasma levels peak about 1.5 hours after dosing. Because of extensive first-pass metabolism, bioavailability is only 32%. The drug is eliminated primarily by renal excretion. Its half-life is approximately 4 hours.

Adverse Effects

The most common adverse effects are nausea, vomiting, headache, dizziness, and drowsiness. Like other opioids, tapentadol can cause respiratory depression and hence should be avoided in patients with preexisting respiratory depression and in those with acute or severe asthma. As noted, the drug causes less constipation than other opioids. Nonetheless, tapentadol is contraindicated for patients with paralytic ileus. As discussed later, tramadol, a drug similar to tapentadol, poses a risk for seizures. To date, seizures have not been reported with tapentadol. Nonetheless, caution should be exercised in patients with a history of seizure disorders. Owing to its abuse potential, tapentadol is classified as a Schedule II substance. Patients should be monitored for abuse and addiction. Tapentadol is classified in FDA Pregnancy Risk Category C, indicating that no adequate studies in pregnant patients have been performed.

Drug Interactions

The depressant effects of tapentadol can add to those of other agents (e.g., alcohol, opioids, barbiturates, benzodiazepines) and can thereby increase the risk for respiratory depression, sedation, and even coma. Because tapentadol can increase serum levels of norepinephrine (by blocking norepinephrine uptake), combined use with an MAOI might result in hypertensive crisis (see Chapter 25). Accordingly, tapentadol should not be used within 14 days of taking an MAOI. Package labeling says that a life-threatening serotonin syndrome could result from combining tapentadol with an SSRI (e.g., fluoxetine), a serotonin and norepinephrine reuptake inhibitor (e.g., venlafaxine), a tricyclic antidepressant (e.g., amitriptyline), or a serotonin agonist (e.g., eletriptan). However, in clinical trials, combined use with an SSRI had no ill effects. Tapentadol neither inhibits nor induces P450 enzymes, and hence clinically relevant interactions involving the cytochrome P450 system seem unlikely.

Preparations, Dosage, and Administration

Tapentadol is available in two formulations: IR tablets (50, 75, and 100 mg), sold as Nucynta, and ER tablets (50, 100, 150, 200, and 250 mg), sold as Nucynta ER. The IR tablets are indicated only for moderate to severe acute pain. The ER tablets are indicated only for moderate to severe chronic pain, and then only in patients who require continuous, around-the-clock treatment with an opioid analgesic. Dosages are as follows:

- *IR tablets:* The recommended dosage is 50, 75, or 100 mg every 4 to 6 hours. When initiating treatment, a second dose can be given 1 hour after the first. The maximum dosage on the first day is 700 mg. The maximum dosage on all subsequent days is 600 mg. In patients with moderate hepatic impairment, the dosage should be no more than 50 mg every 8 hours. In patients with severe hepatic or renal impairment, tapentadol should not be used.

- *ER tablets:* The initial dosage is 50 mg twice a day, and the maximum dosage is 250 mg twice a day. For patients with moderate hepatic impairment, the initial dosage is 50 mg once a day, and the maximum dosage is 100 mg once a day. As with the IR tablets, the ER tablets should not be used in patients with severe hepatic or renal impairment.

Agonist-Antagonist Opioids

Compared with pure opioid agonists, the agonist-antagonists have a low potential for abuse, produce less respiratory depression, and generally have less powerful analgesic effects. If given to a patient who is physically dependent on a pure opioid agonist, these drugs can precipitate withdrawal. The clinical pharmacology of the agonist-antagonists is shown in Table 22.5.

Pentazocine

Actions and Uses

Pentazocine [Talwin] was the first agonist-antagonist opioid available and can be considered the prototype for the group. The drug is indicated for mild to moderate pain. Pentazocine is much less effective than morphine against severe pain.

Pentazocine acts as an *agonist* at kappa receptors and as an *antagonist* at mu receptors. By activating kappa receptors, the drug produces analgesia, sedation, and respiratory depression. However, unlike the respiratory depression caused by morphine, *respiratory depression caused by pentazocine is limited:* beyond a certain dose, no further depression occurs. Because it lacks agonist actions at mu receptors, pentazocine produces little or no euphoria. In fact, at supratherapeutic doses, pentazocine produces unpleasant reactions (anxiety, strange thoughts, nightmares, hallucinations). These psychotomimetic effects may result from activation of kappa receptors. Because of its subjective effects, pentazocine has a low potential for abuse and is classified between Schedule II and Schedule IV depending on the state regulations.

If administered to a patient who is physically dependent on a pure opioid agonist, pentazocine can precipitate withdrawal. Recall that mu receptors mediate physical dependence on pure opioid agonists and that pentazocine acts as an antagonist at these receptors. By blocking access of the pure agonist to mu receptors, pentazocine will prevent receptor activation, thereby triggering withdrawal. Accordingly, *pentazocine and other drugs that block mu receptors should never be administered to a person who is physically dependent on a pure opioid agonist.* If a pentazocine-like agent is to be used, the pure opioid agonist must be withdrawn first.

Physical dependence can occur with pentazocine, but symptoms of withdrawal are generally mild (e.g., cramps, fever, anxiety, restlessness). Treatment is rarely required. As with pure opioid agonists, toxicity from pentazocine can be reversed with naloxone.

TABLE 22.5 ▪ Clinical Pharmacology of Opioid Agonist-Antagonists

Drug and Route	Equianalgesic Dose (mg)*	Time Course of Analgesic Effects: Onset (min)	Peak (min)	Duration (hr)
Butorphanol				
Intranasal	2-3	Within 15	60-120	4-5
Pentazocine				
PO	—	15–30	60-90	3†

*Dose in milligrams that produces a degree of analgesia equivalent to that produced by a 10-mg IM dose of morphine.
†Duration may increase greatly in patients with liver disease.

Preparations, Dosage, and Administration

Pentazocine is available in combination with naloxone for oral therapy.

Oral. For oral therapy, pentazocine is available as pentazocine/naloxone (50 mg/0.5 mg) [Talwin NX]. The usual dosage is 1 tablet every 3 to 4 hours but may be increased to 2 tablets every 3 to 4 hours if needed, for a daily maximum of 12 tablets (600 mg pentazocine).

Butorphanol

Butorphanol [Stadol, Stadol NS] has actions similar to those of pentazocine. The drug is an agonist at kappa receptors and an antagonist at mu receptors. Analgesic effects are less than those of morphine. As with pentazocine, there is a "ceiling" to respiratory depression. The drug can cause psychotomimetic reactions, but these are rare. Butorphanol increases cardiac work and should not be given to patients with myocardial infarction. Physical dependence can occur, but symptoms of withdrawal are relatively mild. The drug may induce a withdrawal reaction in patients physically dependent on a pure opioid agonist. Butorphanol has a low potential for abuse and is regulated as a Schedule IV substance. Toxicity can be reversed with naloxone.

Butorphanol is administered by nasal spray (primarily to treat migraine). The usual intranasal dosage is 1 mg (1 spray from the metered-dose spray device) repeated in 60 to 90 minutes if needed. The two-dose sequence may then be repeated every 3 to 4 hours as needed.

Buprenorphine

Basic Pharmacology

Buprenorphine [Belbuca, Bunavail, Butrans, Suboxone] differs significantly from other opioid agonist-antagonists. The drug is a partial agonist at mu receptors and an antagonist at kappa receptors. Analgesic effects are like those of morphine, but significant tolerance has not been observed. Although buprenorphine can depress respiration, severe respiratory depression has not been reported. Like pentazocine, buprenorphine can precipitate a withdrawal reaction in persons physically dependent on a pure opioid agonist. Physical dependence on buprenorphine develops, but symptoms of abstinence are delayed: Peak responses may not occur until 2 weeks after the final dose was taken. Although pretreatment with naloxone can prevent toxicity from buprenorphine, naloxone cannot readily reverse toxicity that has already developed. (Buprenorphine binds very tightly to its receptors and hence cannot be readily displaced by naloxone.) Buprenorphine is classified as a Schedule III substance. In addition to its use for analgesia, buprenorphine is used to treat opioid addiction (see Chapter 33).

Buprenorphine prolongs the QT interval, posing a risk for potentially fatal dysrhythmias. Accordingly, the drug should not be used by patients with long QT syndrome or a family history of long QT syndrome, or by patients using QT-prolonging drugs (e.g., quinidine, amiodarone).

The risk for adverse effects may be increased by coexisting conditions, including psychosis, alcoholism, adrenocortical insufficiency, and severe liver or renal impairment.

Preparations

Buprenorphine is available in five formulations, four which are discussed here: transdermal patch, buccal film, sublingual tablets, and a sublingual film. The patch and buccal film are approved for pain management. The sublingual products are approved only for opioid addiction—but are used off-label for pain management.

Transdermal Patch. The buprenorphine patch, sold as Butrans, is indicated for moderate to severe chronic pain in patients who need continuous analgesia for an extended time. The patch is applied once every 7 days. Three strengths are available, delivering 5, 7.5, 10, 15, or 20 mcg/hour. The lowest strength is used for opioid-naïve patients, or for those using an opioid in low dosage (e.g., oral morphine, 30 mg/day). Dosage may be titrated to the next higher strength after a minimum of 72 hours. Breakthrough pain can be managed with acetaminophen, a nonsteroidal antiinflammatory drug, or a short-acting opioid.

Patches are applied to eight sites: upper outer arm, upper front of chest, upper side of chest, and upper back—on the right and left sides of the body. The site should be rotated when a new patch is applied, and no site should be reused within 21 days. The site should be hairless, or nearly so. If needed, hair can be removed by clipping, not by shaving. The site may be cleaned, but only with water, not with soaps, alcohol, or abrasives. No lotion or oil should be applied. Patches should not be cut or exposed to heat, including heating pads, heated waterbeds, hot baths, saunas, heat lamps, or extended sunshine. If a patch falls off during the 7-day dosing interval, a new patch should be applied, but at a different site. If patch use is stopped, opioids should not be given for 24 hours.

Sublingual Tablets and Sublingual Film. Buprenorphine is available in three sublingual formulations. One formulation, tablets, contains buprenorphine alone (2 or 8 mg). The other two formulations, tablets and films marketed as Suboxone, contain a mixture of buprenorphine/naloxone (2 mg/0.5 mg, 4 mg/1 mg, 8 mg/2 mg, or 12 mg/3 mg). All three sublingual formulations are approved only for managing opioid addiction. However, they are also used off-label for analgesia. For opioid addiction, dosing is done once a day. For pain management, dosing is done 3 or 4 times a day. The use of these sublingual products is restricted in the United States. To prescribe Suboxone or Subutex, a provider must undergo training and register for appropriate access. Use of these products for opioid addiction is discussed further in Chapter 40.

Buccal Film. A new form of buprenorphine [Belbuca] was approved in 2015 for management of chronic pain. The film is applied to the inside of the cheek every 12 hours. Because it is used for treatment of around-the-clock chronic pain, it has the potential to cause life-threatening respiratory depression. Belbuca should only be prescribed by providers with additional education regarding chronic pain.

PRESCRIBING OPIOIDS FOR CHRONIC, NONCANCER PAIN

The amount of prescription opioids has risen steeply since 1990. Efforts to improve pain management have led to a 10-fold increase in opioid prescriptions, accompanied by a substantial increase in abuse, serious injuries, and deaths. In 2013, accidental overdose with prescription opioids resulted in 16,235 fatalities.

In patients with chronic pain of nonmalignant origin, opioids can reduce discomfort, improve mood, and enhance function. Accordingly, pain experts now recommend that opioids not be withheld from people with chronic pain. Nonetheless, because of concerns about addiction, tolerance, adverse effects, diversion to street use, and regulatory action, physicians, physician assistants, and nurse practitioners are often reluctant to prescribe these drugs. To some degree, all of these concerns are legitimate. However, patients still have a right to effective treatment. Hence there is a need to balance patients' rights with prescribers' concerns. Before the creation of the Centers for Disease Control and Prevention (CDC) pain guidelines in 2016 (Box 22.1), the American Academy of Pain Medicine and the American Pain Society also issued guidelines for using opioids in patients with chronic noncancer pain. Provisions include the following:

- Using opioids only after nonopioid analgesics or more conservative methods have failed
- Discussing the benefits and risks of long-term opioids with the patient
- When possible, using only one prescriber and one pharmacy
- Ensuring comprehensive follow-up to assess efficacy and side effects of treatment and to monitor for signs of opioid abuse
- Stopping opioids after an attempt at opioid rotation has produced inadequate benefit
- Fully documenting the entire process

CLINICAL USE OF OPIOIDS

Prescribing Guidelines

Pain Assessment

Assessment is an essential component of pain management. Pain and current functional status should be evaluated at every patient appointment. Assessment should include documentation of where the pain is located, what type of pain is present (e.g., dull, sharp, stabbing), how the pain changes with time, what makes the pain better, what makes it worse, and how much the pain impairs the patient's ability to function. In addition, you should assess for psychological factors that can reduce pain threshold (anxiety, depression, fear, anger).

Patient Education

It is crucial that the patient understand the risks and benefits of using opioids to treat chronic, noncancer pain. The provider should discuss goals of care regarding pain and function. Treatment goals set by the patient and provider should be realistic. These goals should be revisited at each patient appointment. If the risks begin to outweigh the benefits of opioid therapy, a new plan should be developed.

Initiating Therapy

Nonpharmacologic therapy and nonopioid therapy should be used to treat chronic pain before starting opioid therapy. If these modalities are not successful in improving patient pain and function, opioid therapy can be considered. Although research is lacking regarding the safest way to initiate opiate therapy in the patient with chronic pain, there is a small amount of evidence to suggest that starting patients on ER or long-acting medications before starting with IR medications may lead to increases in medication overdose. Therefore current recommendations suggest initiating therapy with IR medications first. In addition, use of nonopioid, adjuvant medications should continue to maximize pain control and patient function. The CDC has included a checklist for providers initiating opioid therapy. This can be found at http://stacks.cdc.gov/view/cdc/38025.

Dosage Determination

Providers should start with the lowest effective dosage for the patient. "Standard" doses cannot be relied on as appropriate for all patients. For example, if a "standard" 10-mg dose of morphine were employed for all adults, only 70% would receive adequate relief; the other 30% would be undertreated. Not all patients have the same tolerance for pain, and hence some need larger doses than others for the same disorder. Some conditions hurt more than others. Older-adult patients metabolize opioids slowly and therefore require lower doses than younger adults. Because the blood-brain barrier of newborns is poorly developed, these patients are especially sensitive to opioids; therefore they generally require smaller

BOX 22.1 ▪ CDC GUIDELINES FOR SAFE OPIATE PRESCRIBING

Determining When to Initiate or Continue Opioids for Chronic Pain

1. Nonpharmacologic therapy and nonopioid pharmacologic therapy are preferred for chronic pain. Clinicians should consider opioid therapy only if expected benefits for both pain and function are anticipated to outweigh risks to the patient. If opioids are used, they should be combined with nonpharmacologic therapy and nonopioid pharmacologic therapy, as appropriate.
2. Before starting opioid therapy for chronic pain, clinicians should establish treatment goals with all patients, including realistic goals for pain and function, and should consider how therapy will be discontinued if benefits do not outweigh risks. Clinicians should continue opioid therapy only if there is clinically meaningful improvement in pain and function that outweighs risks to patient safety.
3. Before starting and periodically during opioid therapy, clinicians should discuss with patients known risks and realistic benefits of opioid therapy and patient and clinician responsibilities for managing therapy.

Opioid Selection, Dosage, Duration, Follow-Up, and Discontinuation

4. When starting opioid therapy for chronic pain, clinicians should prescribe immediate-release opioids instead of extended-release/long-acting (ER/A) opioids.
5. When opioids are started, clinicians should prescribe the lowest effective dosage. Clinicians should use caution when prescribing opioids at any dosage, should carefully reassess evidence of individual benefits and risks when increasing dosage to ≥50 morphine milligram equivalents (MME)/day, and should avoid increasing dosage to ≥90 MME/day or carefully justify a decision to titrate dosage to ≥90 MME/day.
6. Long-term opioid use often begins with treatment of acute pain. When opioids are used for acute pain, clinicians should prescribe the lowest effective dose of immediate-rdease opioids and should prescribe no greater quantity than needed for the expected duration of pain severe enough to require opioids. Three days or less will often be sufficient; more than seven days will rarely be needed.
7. Clinicians should evaluate benefits and harms with patients within 1 to 4 weeks of starting opioid therapy for chronic pain or of dose escalation. Clinicians should evaluate benefits and harms of continued therapy with patients every 3 months or more frequently. If benefits do not outweigh harms of continued opioid therapy, clinicians should optimize other therapies and work with patients to taper opioids to lower dosages or to taper and discontinue opioids.

Assessing Risk and Addressing Harms of Opioid Use

8. Before starting and periodically during continuation of opioid therapy, clinicians should evaluate risk factors for opioid-related harms. Clinicians should incorporate into the management plan strategies to mitigate risk, including considering offering naloxone when factors that increase risk for opioid overdose, such as history of overdose, history of substance use disorder, higher opioid dosages (≥50 MME/day), or concurrent benzodiazepine use, are present.
9. Clinicians should review the patient's history of controlled substance prescriptions using state prescription drug monitoring program (PDMP) data to determine whether the patient is receiving opioid dosages or dangerous combinations that put him or her at high risk for overdose. Clinicians should review PDMP data when starting opioid therapy for chronic pain and periodically during opioid therapy for chronic pain, ranging from every prescription to every 3 months.
10. When prescribing opioids for chronic pain, clinicians should use urine drug testing before starting opioid therapy and consider urine drug testing at least annually to assess for prescribed medications as well as other controlled prescription drugs and illicit drugs.
11. Clinicians should avoid prescribing opioid pain medication and benzodiazepines concurrently whenever possible.
12. Clinicians should offer or arrange evidence-based treatment (usually medication-assisted treatment with buprenorphine or methadone in combination with behavioral therapies) for patients with opioid use disorder.

All recommendations are category A (apply to all patients outside of active cancer treatment, palliative care, and end-of-life care) except recommendation 10 (designated category B, with individual decision making required); see full guideline for evidence ratings.

From Dowell D, Haegerich TM, Chou R. CDC recommendations for prescribing opioids for chronic pain—United States, 2016. MMWR Recomm Rep 2016;65(1):1-49.

doses (on a milligram-per-kilogram basis) than do older infants and young children.

To minimize physical dependence and abuse, opioid analgesics should be administered in the lowest effective dosages for the shortest time needed. Be aware, however, that larger doses are needed for patients who have more intense pain and for those who have developed tolerance. As pain diminishes, opioid dosage should be reduced. As soon as possible, the patient should be switched to a nonopioid analgesic, such as aspirin or acetaminophen.

Avoiding a Withdrawal Reaction

When opioids are administered in high doses for 20 days or more, clinically significant physical dependence may develop. Under these conditions, abrupt withdrawal will precipitate an abstinence syndrome. To minimize symptoms of abstinence, opioids should be withdrawn slowly, tapering the dosage over 3 days. If the degree of dependence is especially high, as can occur in opioid addicts, dosage should be tapered over 7 to 10 days.

Physical Dependence, Abuse, and Addiction as Clinical Concerns

The objective of the following discussion is to dispel concerns about dependence, abuse, and addiction in the medical patient so that these concerns do not result in undermedication and needless suffering.

Definitions

Before we can discuss the clinical implications of physical dependence, abuse, and addiction, we need to define these terms.

Physical Dependence

As noted, physical dependence is a state in which an abstinence syndrome will occur if the dependence-producing drug is abruptly withdrawn. *Physical dependence is NOT the same as addiction.*

Abuse

Abuse can be broadly defined as *drug use that is inconsistent with medical or social norms.* By this definition, abuse is determined primarily by the reason for drug use and by the setting in which that use occurs—and not by the pharmacologic properties of the drug itself. For example, whereas it is *not* considered abuse to administer 20 mg of morphine in a hospital to relieve pain, it *is* considered abuse to administer the same dose of the same drug on the street to produce euphoria. The concept of abuse is discussed at length in Chapter 30.

Addiction

Addiction is defined by the American Society of Addiction Medicine as *a disease process characterized by continued use of a psychoactive substance despite physical, psychological, or social harm.* Note that nowhere in this definition is addiction equated with physical dependence. In fact, physical dependence is not even part of the definition. The concept of addiction is discussed further in Chapter 30.

Although physical dependence is not required for addiction to occur, physical dependence *can* contribute to addictive behavior. If an individual has already established a pattern of compulsive drug use, physical dependence can reinforce that pattern. For the individual with a marginal resolve to discontinue opioid use, the desire to avoid symptoms of withdrawal may be sufficient to promote continued drug use. However, in the presence of a strong desire to become drug free, physical dependence, by itself, is insufficient to motivate continued addictive behavior.

For the purpose of this discussion, the population can be divided into two groups: individuals who are prone to drug abuse and individuals who are not. One source estimates that about 8% of the population is prone to drug abuse, whereas the other 92% is not. Individuals who are prone to drug abuse have a tendency to abuse drugs inside the hospital and out. Nonabusers, on the other hand, will not abuse drugs in a clinical setting or anywhere else. Withholding analgesics from abuse-prone individuals is not going to reverse their tendency to abuse drugs. Conversely, administering opioids to non–abuse-prone persons will not convert them into abusers.

If a patient who did not formerly abuse opioids does abuse these drugs after therapeutic exposure, you should not feel responsible for having created an addict. That is, if a patient tries to continue opioid use after no longer indicated, it is probable that the patient was abuse prone before you met him or her. The only action that might have prevented opioid abuse by such a patient would have been to withhold opioids entirely—an action that may not have been reasonable.

Balancing the Need to Provide Pain Relief With the Desire to Minimize Abuse

Although concerns about opioid abuse in the clinical setting are small, they cannot be dismissed entirely. You are still obligated to administer opioids with discretion in an effort to minimize abuse. The first step is to identify patients at risk for abuse by using a screening tool, such as *NIDA-Modified ASSIST,* available at www.drugabuse.gov/nidamed/screening/nmassist.pdf. When nonabusers say they need more pain relief, believe them and provide it. In contrast, when a likely abuser requests more analgesic, some healthy skepticism is in order. When there is doubt as to whether a patient is abuse prone or not, logic dictates giving the patient the benefit of the doubt and providing the medication.

The second step is to become familiar with the state prescription drug monitoring program (PDMP). This database contains information regarding all scheduled medications prescribed to a patient, including who prescribed them and the amount prescribed. Providers should carefully review the patient's history with controlled substances and check the PDMP both at initiation of opioid therapy as well as periodically during the course of treatment. Evaluation of the database allows providers to assess for medication combinations that may promote dangerous side effects.

Finally, the provider should consider obtaining a urine drug test for controlled substances, including illicit drugs, before initiation of therapy and at least annually after that. Patients taking multiple medications, including those like benzodiazepines, other opiates, or heroin, may be at increased risk for fatal overdose. Providers that receive unexpected results can use this opportunity to educate the patient or change the patient's treatment plan.

REMS to Reduce Opioid-Related Morbidity, Mortality, and Abuse

In 2011, the FDA introduced a new Risk Evaluation and Mitigation Strategy (REMS) for ER and long-acting prescription opioids. The objective is to reduce injuries and death from prescription opioids and to reduce abuse.

The central component is education for prescribers (e.g., physicians, nurse practitioners, physician assistants) and patients. Training for prescribers focuses on patient selection, balancing the risks and benefits of opioids, monitoring treatment, and recognizing opioid misuse, abuse, and addiction. In addition, prescribers are taught how to counsel patients on the safe use of opioids and are given written instructions for their patients. When patients have a prescription filled, the pharmacy provides a Medication Guide.

The REMS program does have limitations. First, prescriber participation is *voluntary,* not mandatory. Prescribers who chose not to accept training may do so. Second, the REMS does not apply to all opioids. With the exception of transmucosal fentanyl and sublingual buprenorphine, IR products are largely exempt because they are considered safer than long-acting and ER products. Yes, IR products can cause death. However, the risk is much higher with long-acting and ER products because the dose of opioid is much greater than it is in IR products. Products currently covered by the REMS include the following:

- Buprenorphine, transdermal [Butrans] and sublingual [Suboxone]
- Fentanyl, transdermal [Duragesic] and transmucosal [Abstral, Actiq, Fentora,, Subsys]
- Hydrocodone [Hysingla ER, Zohydro ER]
- Hydromorphone [Exalgo]
- Methadone [Dolophine]
- Morphine [Avinza, Kadian, MS Contin]
- Morphine/naltrexone [Embeda]
- Oxycodone [OxyContin, Targiniq ER, Xartemis ER]
- Oxymorphone [Opana ER]

Cancer-Related Pain

Treating chronic pain of cancer differs substantially from treating acute pain of other disorders. When treating cancer pain, the objective is to maximize comfort. Psychological and physical dependence are minimal concerns. Patients should be given as much medication as needed to relieve pain. In the words of one pain specialist, "No patient should wish for death because of the physician's reluctance to use adequate amounts of opioids." With proper therapy, cancer pain can be effectively managed in about 90% of patients. Cancer pain is discussed fully in Chapter 83.

OPIOID ANTAGONISTS

Opioid antagonists are drugs that block the effects of opioid agonists. Principal uses are treatment of opioid overdose, relief of opioid-induced constipation, reversal of postoperative opioid effects (e.g., respiratory depression, ileus), and management of opioid addiction. Four pure antagonists are available and three are discussed here: naloxone [Narcan], methylnaltrexone [Relistor], and naltrexone [ReVia, Vivitrol].

Naloxone

Mechanism of Action

Naloxone [Narcan] is a structural analog of morphine that acts as a competitive antagonist at opioid receptors, thereby blocking opioid actions. Naloxone can reverse most effects of the opioid agonists, including respiratory depression, coma, and analgesia.

Pharmacologic Effects

When administered in the absence of opioids, naloxone has no significant effects. If administered before giving an opioid, naloxone will block opioid actions. If administered to a patient who is already receiving opioids, naloxone will reverse analgesia, sedation, euphoria, and respiratory depression. If administered to an individual who is physically dependent on opioids, naloxone will precipitate an immediate withdrawal reaction.

Pharmacokinetics

Naloxone was traditionally restricted for use in the inpatient setting. Now with new legislation, naloxone is available for use by patients and families in the outpatient setting to help prevent opioid-related deaths from accidental overdose. After IM or subQ injection, effects begin within 2 to 5 minutes and persist several hours. Elimination is by hepatic metabolism. The half-life is approximately 2 hours. Naloxone cannot be used orally because of rapid first-pass inactivation.

PATIENT-CENTERED CARE ACROSS THE LIFE SPAN

Opioid Analgesics

Life Stage	Patient Care Concerns
Infants	Regular use of opioids during pregnancy can cause physical dependence in the fetus, resulting in withdrawal after delivery.
Children	Adequately assess pain with a standardized pain scale. Aspirin, as an adjuvant to opioids, should be avoided because of risk for Reye syndrome. There remains lack of research regarding best practice in treatment of chronic noncancer pain in children.
Pregnant women	Taking opioids in early pregnancy can increase the risk for congenital heart defects, spina bifida, and gastroschisis.
Breastfeeding women	Limited data suggest small amounts of opioids are excreted in breast milk. This can result in infant drowsiness.
Older adults	Persistent pain is often undertreated in the frail older-adult population. The American Geriatrics Association recommends that providers consider treating moderate to severe uncontrolled pain with opiates after a trial of acetaminophen.

Therapeutic Uses

Reversal of Opioid Overdose

Naloxone is the drug of choice for treating overdose with a pure opioid agonist. The drug reverses respiratory depression, coma, and other signs of opioid toxicity. Naloxone can also reverse toxicity from agonist-antagonist opioids (e.g., pentazocine, nalbuphine). However, the doses required may be higher than those needed to reverse poisoning by pure agonists.

Dosage must be carefully titrated when treating toxicity in opioid addicts because the degree of physical dependence in these individuals is usually high and hence an excessive dose of naloxone can transport the patient from a state of poisoning to one of acute withdrawal. Accordingly, treatment should be initiated with a series of small doses rather than one large dose. Because the half-life of naloxone is shorter than that of most opioids, repeated dosing is required until the crisis has passed. If the patient received a dose of naloxone by a friend or family member for a suspected overdose, the patient should be transported by emergency providers to the nearest emergency department for further evaluation.

In some cases of accidental poisoning, there may be uncertainty as to whether unconsciousness is due to opioid overdose or to overdose with a general CNS depressant (e.g., barbiturate, alcohol, benzodiazepine). When uncertainty exists, naloxone is nonetheless indicated. If the cause of poisoning is a barbiturate or another general CNS depressant, naloxone will be of no benefit—but neither will it cause any harm.

Other Opioid Antagonists

Methylnaltrexone

Actions and Therapeutic Use

Methylnaltrexone [Relistor] and naloxegol [Movantik] are selective mu opioid antagonists indicated for opioid-induced constipation in patients with chronic pain who are taking opioids continuously and who have not responded to standard laxative therapy. Benefits derive from blocking mu opioid receptors in the GI tract. Both drugs work in the periphery and hence do not block opioid receptors in the CNS. Accordingly, the drugs do not decrease analgesia and cannot precipitate opioid withdrawal.

Pharmacokinetics

Methylnaltrexone is rapidly absorbed after subQ injection, reaching peak plasma levels within 30 minutes. Naloxegol can be taken orally on a daily basis and has a slightly longer half-life (6 to 11 hours) than methylnaltrexone. Methylnaltrexone undergoes minimal metabolism and is excreted in the urine (50%) and feces (50%), primarily as unchanged drug. The terminal half-life is 8 hours. Naloxegol is metabolized in the liver and largely excreted in the feces (68%).

Adverse Effects, Precautions, and Drug Interactions

Methylnaltrexone and naloxegol are generally well tolerated. The most common adverse effects are *abdominal pain, flatulence, nausea, dizziness,* and *diarrhea.* In the event of severe or persistent diarrhea, these drugs should be discontinued. In patients with known or suspected mechanical GI obstruction, methylnaltrexone and naloxegol should be avoided. No significant drug interactions have been reported with methylnaltrexone. Naloxegol should be used with caution in patients taking CYP3A4 inhibitors.

Preparations, Dosage, and Administration

Methylnaltrexone [Relistor] is available in solution (12 mg/0.6 mL) for subQ injection into the upper arm, abdomen, or thigh. Because defecation can occur rapidly, a bathroom should be immediately available. Dosing is usually done once every 48 hours, and should not exceed once every 24 hours. Dosage in patients without cancer is 12 mg SC daily. In palliative care patients, dosage is based on weight as follows: 8 mg for patients from 38 kg to under 62 kg (84 lb to <136 lb); 12 mg for patients 62 to 114 kg (136 to 251 lb); and 0.15 mg/kg for patients under 38 kg or over 114 kg. In patients with severe renal impairment, defined as creatinine clearance below 30 mL/minute, dosage should be reduced by 50%. Methylnaltrexone should be stored at room temperature and protected from light.

Naltrexone

Naltrexone [ReVia, Vivitrol], given PO or IM, is a pure opioid antagonist used for opioid and alcohol abuse. In opioid abuse, the goal is to prevent euphoria if the abuser should take an opioid. Because naltrexone can precipitate a withdrawal reaction in persons who are physically dependent on opioids, candidates for treatment must be rendered opioid free before naltrexone is started. Although naltrexone can block opioid-induced euphoria, the drug does not prevent craving for opioids. As a result, many addicts fail to comply with treatment. Therapy with naltrexone has been considerably less successful than with methadone, a drug that eliminates craving for opioids while blocking euphoria. Use of naltrexone for alcohol dependence and opioid addiction is discussed in Chapters 31 and 33, respectively.

When dosage is excessive, naltrexone can cause hepatocellular injury. Accordingly, the drug is contraindicated for patients with acute hepatitis or liver failure. Warn patients about the possibility of liver injury and advise them to discontinue the drug if signs of hepatitis develop.

Intramuscular administration can cause injection-site reactions, which are sometimes severe. Moderate reactions include pain, tenderness, induration, swelling, erythema, bruising, and pruritus. Severe reactions—cellulitis, hematoma, abscess, necrosis—can cause significant scarring and may require surgical intervention.

Naltrexone is available in two formulations: (1) 50-mg tablets, marketed as ReVia, for oral dosing; and (2) an ER suspension (380 mg/vial), marketed as Vivitrol, for IM dosing. For oral therapy, a typical dosing schedule consists of 100 mg on Monday and Wednesday and 150 mg on Friday. Alternatively, the drug can be administered daily in 50-mg doses. For IM dosing, the usual regimen is 380 mg once a month.

NONOPIOID CENTRALLY ACTING ANALGESIC—TRAMADOL

Tramadol [Ultram, Ultram ER, Ryzolt, Rybix ODT] is a moderately strong analgesic with a low potential for dependence, abuse, or respiratory depression. The drug relieves pain through a combination of opioid and nonopioid mechanisms.

Tramadol [Ultram] relieves pain by mechanisms largely or completely unrelated to opioid receptors. This drug causes little or no respiratory depression, physical dependence, or abuse.

Mechanism of Action

Tramadol is an analog of codeine that relieves pain in part through weak agonist activity at mu opioid receptors. However, it seems to work primarily by blocking uptake of norepinephrine and serotonin, thereby activating monoaminergic spinal inhibition of pain. Naloxone, an opioid antagonist, only partially blocks tramadol's effects.

Therapeutic Use

Tramadol is approved for moderate to moderately severe pain. The drug is less effective than morphine and no more effective than codeine combined with aspirin or acetaminophen. Analgesia begins 1 hour after oral dosing, is maximum at 2 hours, and continues for 6 hours.

Pharmacokinetics

Tramadol is administered by mouth and reaches peak plasma levels in 2 hours. Elimination is by hepatic metabolism and renal excretion. The half-life is 5 to 6 hours.

Adverse Effects

Tramadol has been used by millions of patients, and serious adverse effects have been rare. Respiratory depression is minimum at recommended doses. The most common side effects are sedation, dizziness, headache, dry mouth, and constipation. Seizures have been reported in more than 280 patients and hence the drug should be avoided in patients with epilepsy and other neurologic disorders. Severe allergic reactions occur rarely. Although generally very safe, tramadol can be fatal in overdose, especially when combined with another CNS depressant.

Drug Interactions

Tramadol can intensify responses to CNS depressants (e.g., alcohol, benzodiazepines) and therefore should not be combined with these drugs.

By inhibiting uptake of norepinephrine, tramadol can precipitate a hypertensive crisis if combined with a monoamine oxidase inhibitor. Accordingly, the combination is absolutely contraindicated.

By inhibiting uptake of serotonin, tramadol can cause serotonin syndrome in patients taking drugs that enhance serotonergic transmission. Among these are SSRIs, serotonin and norepinephrine reuptake inhibitors, tricyclic antidepressants, MAOIs, and triptans. If these drugs must be combined with tramadol, the patient should be monitored carefully, especially during initial therapy and times of dosage escalation.

Abuse Liability

Abuse liability is very low, and hence tramadol is classified as Schedule IV under the Controlled Substances Act. There have been reports of abuse, dependence, withdrawal, and intentional overdose, presumably for subjective effects. Consequently, tramadol should not be given to patients with a history of drug abuse, and the recommended dosage should not be exceeded.

Warning: Suicide

Tramadol can be a vehicle for suicide. When taken alone, and especially when combined with another CNS depressant, tramadol can cause severe respiratory and CNS depression. Deaths have occurred, primarily in patients with a history of emotional disturbance, suicidal ideation or behavior, or misuse of alcohol or other CNS depressants. To reduce risk, tramadol should not be prescribed for patients who are suicidal or addiction prone and should be used with caution in patients who are depressed, taking sedatives or antidepressants, or prone to excessive alcohol use.

Preparations, Dosage, and Administration

Tramadol is available alone and in combination with acetaminophen. Tramadol alone is available in three formulations: (1) 50-mg IR tablets, sold as Ultram; (2) 50-mg orally disintegrating tablets (ODTs), sold as Rybix ODT; and (3) ER tablets (100, 200, and 300 mg), sold as Ultram ER, ConZip, and Ryzolt. Dosages are as follows:

- *IR tablets* [Ultram] and *ODTs* [Rybix ODT]. The recommended adult dosage is 50 to 100 mg every 4 to 6 hours as needed, up to a maximum of 400 mg/day. In patients with significant renal or hepatic impairment, the dosing interval should be increased to 12 hours, and the total daily dose should not exceed 200 mg (with renal impairment) or 100 mg (with hepatic impairment). Inform patients that the ODTs should be placed on the tongue until dissolved (about 1 minute), and then swallowed, with or without water.
- *ER tablets* [Ultram ER, ConZip, Ryzolt]. For patients who are not currently taking IR tramadol, the dosage is 100 mg once a day initially, then titrated every 5 days in 100-mg increments to a maximum of 300 mg once a day. For patients currently taking IR tramadol, the initial once-daily dosage should equal the total daily dosage of IR tramadol (rounded *down* to the nearest 100 mg). Dosage can then be titrated up or down as needed. ER tramadol should not be used by patients with severe hepatic or renal impairment.

Tramadol combined with acetaminophen [Ultracet] is indicated for short-term therapy of acute pain. Each tablet contains 37.5 mg tramadol and 325 mg acetaminophen. The recommended dosage is 2 tablets every 4 to 6 hours (but should not exceed 8 tablets/day). Treatment should not exceed 5 days.

CHAPTER

23 Drugs for Headache

Laura D. Rosenthal, DNP, ACNP, FAANP

Headache is a common symptom that can be triggered by a variety of stimuli, including stress, fatigue, acute illness, and sensitivity to alcohol. Many people experience mild, episodic headaches that can be relieved with over-the-counter medications, such as aspirin, acetaminophen [Tylenol, others], and ibuprofen [Motrin, Advil, others]. For these individuals, medical intervention is unnecessary. In contrast, some people experience severe, recurrent, debilitating headaches that are frequently unresponsive to aspirin-like drugs. For these individuals, medical attention is merited. In this chapter, we focus on severe forms of headache—specifically, migraine, cluster, and tension-type headaches.

When attempting to treat headache, we must differentiate between headaches that have an identifiable underlying cause (e.g., severe hypertension; hyperthyroidism; tumors; infection; disorders of the eyes, ears, nose, sinuses, and throat) and headaches that have no identifiable cause (e.g., migraine and cluster headaches). If there is a clear cause, it should be treated directly (Table 23.1).

As we consider drugs for headache, keep three basic principles in mind. First, antiheadache drugs may be used in two ways: to abort an ongoing attack or to prevent an attack from occurring. Second, not all patients with a particular type of headache respond to the same drugs. Hence therapy must be individualized. Third, several of the drugs employed to treat severe headaches (e.g., ergotamine, opioids) can cause physical dependence. Accordingly, every effort should be made to keep dependence from developing. If dependence does develop, a withdrawal procedure is needed.

MIGRAINE HEADACHE

Characteristics, Pathophysiology, and Overview of Treatment

Characteristics

Migraine headache is characterized by throbbing head pain of moderate to severe intensity that may be unilateral (60%) or bilateral (40%). Most patients also experience nausea and vomiting, along with neck pain and sensitivity to light and sound. Physical activity intensifies the pain. During a prolonged attack, patients develop *hyperalgesia* (augmented responses to painful stimuli) and *allodynia* (painful responses to normally innocuous stimuli). Migraines usually develop in the morning after arising. Pain increases gradually and lasts 4 to 72 hours (median duration, 24 hours). On average, attacks occur 1.5 times a month. Precipitating factors include anxiety, fatigue, stress, menstruation, alcohol, weather changes, and tyramine-containing foods.

Migraine has two primary forms: migraine *with aura* and migraine *without aura.* In migraine with aura, the headache is preceded by visual symptoms (flashes of light, a blank area in the field of vision, zigzag patterns). Of the two forms, migraine without aura is more common, affecting about 70% of people with migraine.

Migraine afflicts 36 million people in the United States and more than 10% of the population worldwide. The headaches are more common and more severe in females, with a lifetime incidence of 43%, compared with 18% in males. About 65% of people with migraine are women in their late teens, 20s, or 30s. With some women, migraine attacks are worse during menstruation but subside during pregnancy and cease after menopause, indicating a hormonal component to the attacks. A family history of the disease is typical.

Migraine is highly debilitating. An attack can prevent participation in social and leisure activities and can result in lost productivity at home, school, and work. According to the World Health Organization, disability caused by a severe migraine attack equals that caused by quadriplegia, psychosis, or dementia.

Pathophysiology

Migraine headache is a *neurovascular* disorder that involves *dilation* and *inflammation* of intracranial blood vessels. Headache generation begins with neural events that trigger vasodilation. Vasodilation then leads to pain, which leads to further neural activation, thereby amplifying pain-generating signals. Neurons of the trigeminal vascular system, which innervate intracranial blood vessels, are key components.

The exact cause of migraine pain is not completely understood—although vasodilation and inflammation are clearly involved. Available data suggest that two compounds—*calcitonin gene–related peptide* (CGRP) and *serotonin* (5-hydroxytryptamine [5-HT])—play important roles. The role of CGRP is to *promote migraine,* and the role of 5-HT is to *suppress* migraine. Data that implicate CGRP as a cause of migraine include the following:

- Plasma levels of CGRP rise during a migraine attack.
- Stimulation of neurons of the trigeminal vascular system promotes release of CGRP, which in turn promotes vasodilation and release of inflammatory neuropeptides.
- Dosing with sumatriptan, a drug that relieves migraine, lowers elevated levels of CGRP.
- Sumatriptan can suppress release of CGRP from cultured trigeminal neurons.

Data that support a protective role for 5-HT include the following:

- Plasma levels of 5-HT drop by 50% during a migraine attack.

TABLE 23.1 ■ Diagnosis and Treatment of Headache

DIAGNOSIS

Evaluate type of headache with detailed history and physical examination
Assess functional impairment
Rule out causes for concern

Migraine Treatment	Cluster Headache Treatment	Tension-Type Headache Treatment
Select treatment based on severity and functional impairment	Determine acute treatment	Determine acute treatment
MILD	Oxygen	Acetaminophen
	Sumatriptan	Aspirin
Aspirin or aspirin combinations	Determine prophylactic treatment	NSAIDs
Triptans	Verapamil	Determine prophylactic treatment
MODERATE	Corticosteroids	Amitriptyline
Dihydroergotamine (DHE)	Lithium	Patient education and lifestyle
Ergotamine	Patient education and lifestyle modifications	
NSAID combination products		
SEVERE		
Metoclopramide		
Triptans		
Ergotamine or DHE		
NSAIDs (Ketorolac)		
PROPHYLAXIS		
Beta blockers		
Tricyclic antidepressants		
Antiepileptics		
Consider hormonally related migraine in females		
NSAIDs		
Triptans		
Prophylaxis with estrogen		
Patient education and lifestyle modifications		

Adapted from Diagnosis and Treatment of Headache. ICHI Health Care Guideline, 11th ed. January 2013.

- Depletion of 5-HT with reserpine can precipitate an attack in migraine-prone individuals.
- Administration of 5-HT or sumatriptan, both of which activate 5-HT receptors, can abort an ongoing attack.

Overview of Treatment

Drugs for migraine are employed in two ways: to abort an ongoing attack and to prevent attacks from occurring. Drugs used to abort an attack fall into two groups: nonspecific analgesics (aspirin-like drugs and opioid analgesics) and migraine-specific drugs (serotonin$_{1B/1D}$ receptor agonists [triptans] and ergot alkaloids). Drugs employed for prophylaxis include beta blockers (e.g., propranolol), tricyclic antidepressants (e.g., amitriptyline), and antiepileptic drugs (e.g., divalproex).

Nondrug measures can help. Patients should try to control or eliminate triggers and should maintain a regular pattern of eating, sleeping, and exercise because, in people with migraine, the brain seems to have a low tolerance for the ups and downs of life. When an attack has begun, the migraineur should retire to a dark, quiet room. Placing an ice pack on the neck and scalp can help.

Abortive Therapy

The objective of abortive therapy is to eliminate headache pain and suppress associated nausea and vomiting. Treatment should commence at the earliest sign of an attack. Because migraine causes gastrointestinal (GI) disturbances (nausea, vomiting, and gastric stasis), oral therapy may be ineffective after an attack has begun. Hence, for treatment of an established attack, a drug that can be administered by injection, nasal spray, or rectal suppository may be best. As noted, two types of drugs are used: nonspecific analgesics and migraine-specific agents. Representative drugs are listed in Table 23.2.

Drug selection depends on the intensity of the attack. For mild to moderate symptoms, an *aspirin-like drug* (e.g., aspirin, naproxen) may be sufficient. For moderate to severe symptoms, patients should take a *migraine-specific drug,* such as a serotonin$_{1B/1D}$ agonist, or—less frequently used—an ergot alkaloid (ergotamine or dihydroergotamine). If these agents fail to relieve pain, an *opioid analgesic* (e.g., butorphanol) may be needed. Note that opioids should be reserved for treatment in patients with migraines resistant to all other treatments.

Use of abortive medications (both nonspecific and migraine specific) should be limited to 1 or 2 days a week. More frequent use can lead to *medication overuse headache* (MOH), also known as drug-induced headache or drug-rebound headache (see section on MOH).

Antiemetics are important adjuncts to migraine therapy. By reducing nausea and vomiting, these drugs can (1) make the patient more comfortable and (2) permit therapy with oral antimigraine drugs. Two antiemetics—*metoclopramide* [Reglan] and *prochlorperazine* (formerly available as *Compazine*)—are used most often. Of the two, metoclopramide is preferred. In addition to suppressing nausea and vomiting, metoclopramide can reverse gastric stasis caused by the attack

TABLE 23.2 ▪ Migraine Headache: Drugs for Abortive Therapy

Nonspecific Analgesics	Usual Dosage
ASPIRIN-LIKE DRUGS	
Nonsteroidal antiinflammatory drugs (e.g., aspirin, naproxen, diclofenac)	Per specific drug instructions
Acetaminophen + aspirin + caffeine [Excedrin Migraine]	2 caplets (250 mg/250 mg/65 mg) once at onset
Opioid Analgesics	
Butorphanol nasal spray	1 spray (1 mg) in one nostril; may repeat in 60 min
MIGRAINE-SPECIFIC DRUGS	See Table 23.3
Selective Serotonin$_{1B/1D}$ Receptor Agonists (Triptans)	
Almotriptan [Axert]	
Eletriptan [Relpax]	
Frovatriptan [Frova]	
Naratriptan [Amerge]	
Rizatriptan [Maxalt]	
Sumatriptan [Imitrex, Sumavel DosePro, Zecuity]	
Zolmitriptan [Zomig]	
Ergot Alkaloids	
Dihydroergotamine intranasal spray [Migranal]	1 spray (0.5 mg) each nostril and repeat in 15 minutes
Ergotamine sublingual [Ergomar]	1 tablet (2 mg) under tongue at onset; may administer 1 additional tablet at 30-min intervals ×2.
Ergotamine + caffeine [Cafergot, Migergot]	1-2 tablets (1 mg/100 mg) at onset; may administer 1 additional tablet at 30-min intervals ×4.

and can thereby facilitate absorption of oral antimigraine drugs. Like metoclopramide, prochlorperazine suppresses nausea and vomiting. However, because of its anticholinergic actions, prochlorperazine can make gastric stasis even worse.

Analgesics

Aspirin-Like Drugs

Aspirin, acetaminophen, naproxen, diclofenac, and other aspirin-like analgesics can provide adequate relief of mild to moderate migraine attacks. In fact, when combined with metoclopramide (to enhance absorption), aspirin may work as well as sumatriptan, a highly effective antimigraine drug. Moreover, the combination of aspirin plus metoclopramide costs less than sumatriptan and causes fewer adverse effects.

Acetaminophen should be used only in combination with other drugs, not alone. One effective combination, marketed as *Excedrin Migraine,* consists of acetaminophen, aspirin, and caffeine.

Opioid Analgesics

Opioid analgesics are reserved for severe migraine that has not responded to first-line medications. This is because of the potential for abuse as well as MOH. The recommended agent is *butorphanol nasal spray* [Stadol NS].

Serotonin$_{1B/1D}$ Receptor Agonists (Triptans)

The serotonin$_{1B/1D}$ receptor agonists, also known as *triptans,* are first-line drugs for terminating a migraine attack. These agents relieve pain by constricting intracranial blood vessels and suppressing release of inflammatory neuropeptides. All are well tolerated. Rarely, they cause symptomatic coronary vasospasm. Table 23.3 presents the clinical pharmacology of the triptans.

Sumatriptan

Sumatriptan [Imitrex, Sumavel DosePro] was the first triptan available and will serve as our prototype for the group. The drug can be administered by mouth, nasal inhalation, or subcutaneous (subQ) injection. Additionally, an iontophoretic transdermal system [Zecuity] was approved in 2013.

Mechanism of Action. Sumatriptan, an analog of 5-HT, causes selective activation of 5-HT$_{1B}$ and 5-HT$_{1D}$ receptors (5-HT$_{1B/1D}$ receptors). The drug has no affinity for 5-HT$_2$ or 5-HT$_3$ receptors, nor does it bind to adrenergic, dopaminergic, muscarinic, or histaminergic receptors. Binding to 5-HT$_{1B/1D}$ receptors on intracranial blood vessels causes vasoconstriction. Binding to 5-HT$_{1B/1D}$ receptors on sensory nerves of the trigeminal vascular system suppresses release of CGRT, a compound that promotes release of inflammatory neuropeptides. As a result, sumatriptan reduces release of inflammatory neuropeptides and thereby diminishes perivascular inflammation. Both actions—vasoconstriction and decreased perivascular inflammation—help relieve migraine pain.

Therapeutic Use. Sumatriptan is taken to abort an ongoing migraine attack. The drug relieves headache and associated symptoms (nausea, neck pain, photophobia, phonophobia). In clinical trials, sumatriptan gave complete relief to most patients. Beneficial effects begin about 15 minutes after subQ or intranasal dosing and 30 to 60 minutes after oral dosing. Complete relief occurs in 40% to 60% of patients 2 hours after subQ dosing, in 30% to 60% of patients 2 hours after intranasal dosing, in 18% of patients 2 hours after transdermal dosing, and in 50% to 60% of patients 4 hours after oral dosing. Unfortunately, headache returns in about 40% of patients within 24 hours. In comparison, the 24-hour recurrence rate with dihydroergotamine is only 14%. In patients who respond to subQ sumatriptan, subsequent administration of oral sumatriptan can delay recurrence but does not prevent it. In addition to migraine, sumatriptan is approved for cluster headaches.

Pharmacokinetics. With oral or intranasal dosing, bioavailability is low (about 15%). The transdermal system has even lower bioavailability (about 6%), whereas with subQ dosing, bioavailability is high (97%). As a result, oral and intranasal doses are considerably higher than subQ and transdermal doses. Sumatriptan undergoes extensive hepatic metabolism, primarily by monoamine oxidase (MAO), followed by excretion in the urine. The half-life is short—about 2.5 hours.

Adverse Effects. Sumatriptan is generally well tolerated. Most side effects are transient and mild. Coronary vasospasm is the biggest concern.

CHEST SYMPTOMS. About 50% of patients experience unpleasant chest symptoms, usually described as "heavy

TABLE 23.3 ▪ Clinical Pharmacology of the Triptans

Generic Name [Trade Name]	Route	Onset (min)	Duration	Half-Life (hr)	Dosage	Contraindicated Drugs: SSRIs, SNRIs, Triptans, Ergots	Contraindicated Drugs: MAOIs	Contraindicated Drugs: CYP3A4 Inhibitors	Comments
Sumatriptan									
[Imitrex]	Oral	30-60	Short	2.5	25, 50, or 100 mg; may repeat in 2 hr (max. 200 mg/24 hr)	✓	✓		First triptan available and best understood. Available in three fast-acting formulations: nasal spray, an autoinjector for subQ dosing (using a needle), and a needle-free device for subQ dosing [Sumavel DosePro].
[Imitrex]	Nasal spray	15-20			5 or 20 mg; may repeat in 2 hr (max. 40 mg/24 hr)				
[Imitrex]	SubQ, with needle	10-15			6 mg; may repeat in 1 hr (max. 12 mg/24 hr)				
[Sumavel DosePro]	SubQ, needle-free	10			6 mg; may repeat in 1 hr (max. 12 mg/24 hr)				
Almotriptan [Axert]	Oral	30-120	Short	3-4	6.25 or 12.5 mg; may repeat in 2 hr (max. 25 mg/24 hr)	✓			Incidence of chest discomfort (pain, tightness, pressure) is lower than with other triptans. Decrease dosage if combined with a CYP3A4 inhibitor.
Eletriptan [Relpax]	Oral	60	Short	4	20 or 40 mg; may repeat in 2 hr (max. 40 mg/24 hr)	✓		✓	Bioavailability increased by high-fat meal. Good balance between fast onset and long duration.
Frovatriptan [Frova]	Oral	120-180	Long	26	2.5 mg; may repeat in 2 hr	✓			Slowest onset, longest half-life, and lowest rate of headache recurrence. Decrease dose if combined with propranolol.
Naratriptan [Amerge]	Oral	60-180	Intermediate	6	1 or 2.5 mg; may repeat in 4 hr (max. 5 mg/24 hr)	✓			Slower onset and longer duration than most triptans.
Rizatriptan [Maxalt, Maxalt MLT]	Oral	30-120	Short	2-3	5 or 10 mg; may repeat in 2 hours (max. 30 mg/24 hr)	✓	✓		May be the most consistently effective triptan. Decrease dose if combined with propranolol. Available in melt-in-the-mouth wafers [Maxalt MLT] that can be taken without water.
Zolmitriptan									
[Zomig, Zomig ZMT]	Oral	45	Short	3	2.5 or 5 mg; may repeat in 2 hr (max. 10 mg/24 hr)	✓	✓		Available in a fast-acting nasal spray, and in melt-in-the-mouth wafers [Zomig ZMT] that can be taken without water.
[Zomig]	Nasal spray	15			5 mg; may repeat in 2 hr (max. 10 mg/24 hr)				
[Zecuity]	Transdermal	60	Short	3.1	6.5 mg patch; may repeat in 4 hours (max. two patches in 24 hours.)	✓	✓		Newest form of sumatriptan approved for transdermal use in 2013. Requires use of a metal transdermal system that cannot get wet.

CYP3A4, the 3A4 isozyme of cytochrome P450; MAOIs, monoamine oxidase inhibitors; SNRIs, serotonin and norepinephrine reuptake inhibitors; SSRIs, selective serotonin reuptake inhibitors; subQ, subcutaneous.

arms" or "chest pressure" rather than pain. These symptoms are transient and *not* related to ischemic heart disease. Possible causes are pulmonary vasoconstriction, esophageal spasm, intercostal muscle spasm, and bronchoconstriction. Patients should be forewarned of these symptoms and reassured that they are not dangerous.

CORONARY VASOSPASM. Very rarely, sumatriptan and other triptans can cause angina secondary to coronary vasospasm. Electrocardiographic changes have been observed in patients with coronary artery disease (CAD) or Prinzmetal (vasospastic) angina. To reduce the risk for angina, avoid sumatriptan in patients with risk factors for CAD until CAD has been ruled out. These patients include postmenopausal women, men older than 40 years, smokers, and patients with hypertension, hypercholesterolemia, diabetes, or a family history of CAD. Owing to the risk for coronary vasospasm, sumatriptan is contraindicated for patients with a history of ischemic heart disease, myocardial infarction (MI), uncontrolled hypertension, or other heart disease.

TERATOGENESIS. *Sumatriptan should be avoided during pregnancy.* When given daily to pregnant rabbits, the drug was embryolethal at blood levels only 3 times higher than those achieved with a 6-mg subQ injection in humans (a typical dose). Accordingly, unless the prescriber directs otherwise, women should be instructed to avoid the drug if they are pregnant or think they might be, if they are trying to become pregnant, or if they are not using an adequate form of contraception. Sumatriptan is classified in U.S. Food and Drug Administration (FDA) Pregnancy Risk Category C.

OTHER ADVERSE EFFECTS. Mild reactions include *vertigo, malaise, fatigue,* and *tingling sensations.* Transient pain and redness may occur at sites of subQ injection. The intranasal formulation tastes bad and may irritate the nose and throat.

Drug Interactions

ERGOT ALKALOIDS AND OTHER TRIPTANS. Sumatriptan, other triptans, and ergot alkaloids (e.g., ergotamine, dihydroergotamine) all cause vasoconstriction. Accordingly, if one triptan is combined with another or with an ergot alkaloid, excessive and prolonged vasospasm could result. Therefore sumatriptan should not be used within 24 hours of an ergot derivative or another triptan.

MONOAMINE OXIDASE INHIBITORS. Monoamine oxidase inhibitors (MAOIs) can suppress hepatic degradation of sumatriptan, causing its plasma level to rise. Toxicity can result. Accordingly, sumatriptan should not be combined with an MAOI and should not be used within 2 weeks of stopping an MAOI.

SELECTIVE SEROTONIN REUPTAKE INHIBITORS (SSRIs) AND SEROTONIN/NOREPINEPHRINE REUPTAKE INHIBITORS (SNRIs). As discussed in Chapter 25, the SSRIs (e.g., fluoxetine [Prozac]) and SNRIs (e.g., duloxetine [Cymbalta]) indirectly activate serotonin receptors in the brain (by increasing the availability of serotonin at brain synapses). If receptor activation is excessive, serotonin syndrome can occur. Signs and symptoms include altered mental status (agitation, confusion, disorientation, anxiety, hallucinations, poor concentration) as well as incoordination, myoclonus, hyperreflexia, excessive sweating, tremor, and fever. Deaths have occurred. Because the triptans *directly* activate serotonin receptors, and the SSRIs and SNRIs *indirectly* activate serotonin receptors, you can see how combining these drugs could lead to excessive receptor activation. Accordingly, these combinations should not be used.

Zolmitriptan. Zolmitriptan [Zomig, Zomig ZMT] is indicated for terminating an ongoing migraine attack. The drug is similar to sumatriptan with regard to mechanism, efficacy, time course, side effects, and interactions. Zolmitriptan is formulated for oral and intranasal use. Effects from intranasal administration begin in 15 minutes, compared with 45 minutes for the oral products. However, although the nasal spray is faster, it does have two drawbacks: it tastes bad (albeit not as bad as sumatriptan nasal spray), and only one strength (5 mg/spray) is available. If a smaller dose is needed, an oral formulation must be used. Regardless of the formulation, about 65% of patients respond within 2 hours. If headache persists, dosing can be repeated 2 hours after the initial dose. The maximum dose per 24 hours is 10 mg. Headache recurs in 8% to 32% of patients. Adverse effects are generally mild and transient. Like sumatriptan, zolmitriptan causes harmless, transient chest discomfort. Of much greater concern, the drug can cause coronary vasospasm and hence is contraindicated for patients with ischemic heart disease, prior MI, or uncontrolled hypertension. Like sumatriptan, zolmitriptan should not be administered within 24 hours of an ergot alkaloid or another triptan or within 2 weeks of stopping an MAOI. To avoid serotonin syndrome, zolmitriptan should not be combined with an SSRI or SNRI.

Naratriptan. Naratriptan [Amerge] is indicated for oral therapy of an ongoing migraine attack. Compared with most other triptans, naratriptan has a slower onset and longer duration. Because effects persist, the 24-hour migraine recurrence rate may be reduced. Like other triptans, naratriptan causes transient chest discomfort. Also like other triptans, the drug can cause coronary vasospasm and hence is contraindicated for patients with ischemic heart disease, prior MI, or uncontrolled hypertension. To avoid excessive vasospasm, naratriptan should not be administered within 24 hours of an ergot alkaloid or another triptan. Like other triptans, naratriptan should not be combined with an SSRI or SNRI, owing to the risk for serotonin syndrome. In contrast to some triptans, naratriptan can be used safely with an MAOI.

Rizatriptan. Rizatriptan [Maxalt, Maxalt MLT] may be the most consistently effective triptan for terminating an ongoing migraine attack. The drug is similar to sumatriptan with regard to mechanism, efficacy, time course, side effects, and interactions. Adverse effects are generally mild and transient. Like other triptans, rizatriptan causes harmless, transient chest discomfort. Also like other triptans, the drug can cause coronary vasospasm and hence is contraindicated for patients with ischemic heart disease, prior MI, or uncontrolled hypertension. To avoid excessive vasospasm, rizatriptan should not be administered within 24 hours of an ergot alkaloid or another triptan, or within 2 weeks of stopping an MAOI. Like other triptans, rizatriptan should not be combined with an SSRI or SNRI, owing to the risk for serotonin syndrome. Propranolol can raise levels of rizatriptan, and hence a dosage reduction may be needed. Rizatriptan may harm the developing fetus: in rats, the drug increased perinatal mortality, reduced learning capacity, and decreased preweaning and postweaning weight. However, postmarketing studies suggest that, in humans, rizatriptan may not increase the risk for congenital anomalies or spontaneous abortion. Because these studies were done on small populations, the drug should be used with caution in pregnant patients until further research is completed.

Almotriptan. Almotriptan [Axert] is indicated for oral therapy of an ongoing migraine attack. The drug is similar to sumatriptan with regard to mechanism, efficacy, and time course—and is better tolerated. Adverse effects are minimal. Like other triptans, almotriptan can cause harmless, transient chest discomfort—but the incidence is very low (only 0.3%). Also like other triptans, the drug can cause coronary vasospasm and hence is contraindicated for patients with ischemic heart disease, prior MI, or uncontrolled hypertension. Almotriptan is metabolized by CYP3A4 (the 3A4 isozyme of cytochrome P450), and thus a dosage reduction is recommended if the drug is combined with a potent CYP3A4 inhibitor (e.g., ketoconazole, itraconazole, clarithromycin, ritonavir). To avoid excessive vasospasm, almotriptan should not be administered within 24 hours of an ergot alkaloid or another triptan. Like other triptans, almotriptan should not be combined with an SSRI or SNRI, owing to a risk for serotonin syndrome. In contrast to some triptans, almotriptan can be combined safely with an MAOI.

Frovatriptan. Frovatriptan [Frova] is indicated for oral therapy of an ongoing migraine attack. The drug is similar to other triptans with regard to mechanism and side effects—but is less effective and has very different kinetics. Effects begin slowly but are sustained—thanks to the drug's long half-life (26 hours). Although the number of patients responding at 2 hours is low (37% to 46%), rates of headache recurrence are low too (7% to 23%)—lower than with any other triptan. Adverse effects are mild and transient. Like sumatriptan, frovatriptan can cause harmless, transient chest discomfort. In addition, the drug can cause coronary vasospasm and hence is contraindicated for patients with ischemic heart disease, prior MI, or uncontrolled hypertension. To avoid excessive vasospasm, frovatriptan should not be administered within 24 hours of an ergot alkaloid or another triptan. However, it can be used concurrently with an MAOI. Like other triptans, frovatriptan should not be combined with an SSRI or SNRI, owing to the risk for serotonin syndrome.

Eletriptan. Eletriptan [Relpax] is indicated for oral therapy of an ongoing migraine attack. The drug is at least as effective as oral sumatriptan and may have a faster onset. Like other triptans, eletriptan can cause transient chest discomfort. Also like other triptans, it can cause coronary vasospasm and hence is contraindicated for patients with ischemic heart disease, prior MI, or uncontrolled hypertension. To avoid excessive vasospasm, eletriptan should not be administered within 24 hours of an ergot alkaloid or another triptan. However, the drug may be used concurrently with an MAOI because eletriptan is not broken down by MAO. Eletriptan is metabolized in the liver by CYP3A4, and thus strong inhibitors of CYP3A4 (e.g., ketoconazole, itraconazole, clarithromycin, ritonavir) may cause toxicity by raising eletriptan levels. Accordingly, eletriptan should not be used within 72 hours of these drugs. Eletriptan levels may also be raised by verapamil, a moderate CYP3A4 inhibitor used for migraine prophylaxis; caution is advised. Like other triptans, eletriptan should not be combined with an SSRI or SNRI, owing to the risk for serotonin syndrome.

Prototype Drugs

DRUGS FOR MIGRAINE HEADACHE

Nonsteroidal Antiinflammatory Drugs
Aspirin

Selective Serotonin Receptor Agonists
Sumatriptan

Ergot Alkaloids
Ergotamine

Ergot Alkaloids

Ergotamine

Mechanism of Antimigraine Action. Ergotamine has complex actions, and the precise mechanism by which it aborts migraine is unknown. Ergotamine can alter transmission at serotonergic, dopaminergic, and alpha-adrenergic junctions. Current evidence suggests that antimigraine effects are related to agonist activity at subtypes of serotonin receptors, specifically 5-HT_{1B} and 5-HT_{1D} receptors. Additional evidence indicates that ergotamine can block inflammation associated with the trigeminal vascular system, perhaps by suppressing release of CGRP. Relief may also be related to vascular effects. In cranial arteries, ergotamine acts directly to promote constriction and reduce the amplitude of pulsations. In addition, the drug can affect blood flow by depressing the vasomotor center.

Therapeutic Uses. Ergotamine is used as a second-line drug used for stopping an ongoing migraine attack in patients who have not responded to a triptan. Owing to the risk for dependence (see later), ergotamine should not be taken daily on a long-term basis.

Pharmacokinetics. Administration may be oral, sublingual, or rectal. Bioavailability with oral and sublingual administration is low. Bioavailability with rectal administration is higher. Although the half-life of ergotamine is only 2 hours, pharmacologic effects can still be observed 24 hours after dosing. Ergotamine undergoes metabolism by CYP3A4, followed by excretion in the bile.

Adverse Effects. Ergotamine is well tolerated at usual therapeutic doses. The drug can stimulate the chemoreceptor trigger zone, causing *nausea and vomiting* in about 10% of patients, thereby augmenting nausea and vomiting caused by the migraine itself. Concurrent treatment with metoclopramide or a phenothiazine antiemetic (e.g., prochlorperazine) can help reduce these responses. Other common side effects include *weakness in the legs, myalgia, numbness and tingling in the fingers and toes, angina-like pain,* and *tachycardia or bradycardia.*

Overdose. Acute or chronic overdose can cause serious toxicity referred to as *ergotism.* In addition to the adverse effects seen at therapeutic doses, overdose can cause ischemia secondary to constriction of peripheral arteries and arterioles: the extremities become cold, pale, and numb; muscle pain develops; and gangrene may eventually result. Patients should be informed about these responses and instructed to seek immediate medical attention if they develop. The risk for ergotism is highest in patients with sepsis, peripheral vascular disease, and renal or hepatic impairment. Management consists of discontinuing ergotamine, followed by measures to maintain circulation (treatment with anticoagulants and with intravenous (IV) nitroprusside, phentolamine, or nitroglycerin as appropriate).

Drug Interactions

Triptans. Ergotamine should not be combined with triptans (e.g., sumatriptan, zolmitriptan) because a prolonged vasospastic reaction could occur. To avoid this problem, dosing with ergotamine and serotonin agonists should be separated by at least 24 hours.

Physical Dependence. Regular daily use of ergotamine, even in moderate doses, can cause physical dependence. The withdrawal syndrome is characterized by headache, nausea, vomiting, and restlessness. That is, withdrawal resembles a migraine attack. Patients who experience these symptoms are likely to resume taking the drug, thereby perpetuating the cycle of dependence. Hospitalization may be required to break the cycle. To avoid dependence, dosage and duration of treatment must be restricted (see dosing guidelines later).

Contraindications. Ergotamine is contraindicated for patients with hepatic or renal impairment, sepsis (gangrene has resulted), CAD, peripheral vascular disease, and uncontrolled hypertension and for those taking potent inhibitors of CYP3A4. In addition, the drug should not be taken during pregnancy because it can promote uterine contractions and hence might cause fetal harm or abortion. In fact, because of its effects on the uterus, ergotamine is classified in FDA Pregnancy Risk Category X: the risk of use by pregnant patients clearly outweighs any possible benefits. Warn women of childbearing age to avoid pregnancy while using this drug.

Dihydroergotamine

Therapeutic Uses

Parenteral dihydroergotamine [D.H.E. 45, Migranal]—given by the intramuscular (IM), IV, or subQ route—is a second-line drug for terminating a migraine attack. The drug also may be given by intranasal spray. A formulation for oral inhalation is undergoing review by the FDA. Intranasal dihydroergotamine is less effective than intranasal sumatriptan but is associated with a lower rate of migraine recurrence.

Pharmacologic Effects

The actions of dihydroergotamine are similar to those of ergotamine. Like ergotamine, dihydroergotamine alters transmission at serotonergic, dopaminergic, and alpha-adrenergic junctions. In contrast to ergotamine, dihydroergotamine causes little nausea and vomiting, no physical dependence, and minimal peripheral vasoconstriction (when used alone). Diarrhea, however, is prominent.

Pharmacokinetics

Dihydroergotamine may be administered parenterally or by nasal spray—but not by mouth (owing to extensive first-pass metabolism). In the liver, the drug is metabolized by CYP3A4. An active metabolite (8′-hydroxydihydroergotamine) contributes to therapeutic effects. The half-life of dihydroergotamine plus the active metabolite is about 21 hours.

BLACK BOX WARNING: ERGOTAMINE AND DIHYDROERGOTAMINE

Potent inhibitors of CYP3A4 can raise ergotamine to dangerous levels, posing a risk for intense vasospasm. Cerebral and/or peripheral ischemia can result. Accordingly, concurrent use with CYP3A4 inhibitors is contraindicated.

Other Abortive Agents

Sumatriptan and Naproxen

Sumatriptan and naproxen (a nonsteroidal antiinflammatory drug) are available in a fixed-dose combination under the trade name Treximet. In clinical trials, the combination was better than either agent alone at relieving the pain of a migraine attack. In addition, the combination effectively reduced nausea and sensitivity to both light and sound. Presumably, the superior benefits of the combination derive from attacking migraine by multiple mechanisms: naproxen reduces pain and inflammation, whereas sumatriptan causes vasoconstriction and inhibits release of inflammatory neuropeptides.

BLACK BOX WARNING: TREXIMET

Treximet increases the risk for serious GI bleeding and other potentially fatal adverse events, including stomach or intestinal perforation.

Preventive Therapy

In 2012, the American Academy of Neurology and the American Headache Society published new guidelines on the pharmacologic treatment for prevention of migraines, the *Evidence-Based Guideline Update: Pharmacologic Treatment for Episodic Migraine Prevention in Adults.* Prophylactic therapy can reduce the frequency, intensity, and duration of migraine attacks and can improve responses to abortive drugs. Preventive treatment is indicated for patients who have frequent attacks (three or more a month), attacks that are especially severe, or attacks that do not respond adequately to abortive agents. Preferred drugs for prophylaxis include propranolol, divalproex, and amitriptyline. All three are effective and well tolerated, and with all three, benefits take 4 to 6 weeks to develop. Major preventive agents are listed in Table 23.4.

TABLE 23.4 ▪ Migraine Headache: Drugs for Preventive Therapy

Drugs	Usual Daily Dosage (mg)
BETA-ADRENERGIC BLOCKING AGENTS	
Propranolol [Inderal]	80-240
Metoprolol [Lopressor]	50-200
ANTIEPILEPTIC DRUGS	
Divalproex [Depakote ER]	500-1000
Topiramate [Topamax]	Initiate with 25 nightly for 1 week. Advance to 25 twice daily for additional week Third week increase to 25 am and 50 pm. Final dosing 50 PO twice daily
TRICYCLIC ANTIDEPRESSANTS	
Amitriptyline [Elavil]	25-150 at bedtime
ESTROGENS (FOR MENSTRUALLY ASSOCIATED MIGRAINE)	
Estrogen gel	1.5 × 7 days starting 2 days before the expected attack
Estrogen patch [Alora, Climara, Vivelle-Dot]	0.01 daily × 7 days starting 2 days before the expected attack

Beta Blockers

Beta blockers are first-line drugs for migraine prevention. Of the available beta blockers, *propranolol* is used most often, although *metoprolol* is now deemed as effective as propranolol. Treatment can reduce the number and intensity of attacks in 70% of patients. Benefits take a few weeks to develop. The most common side effects are extreme tiredness and fatigue, which occur in about 10% of patients. In addition, the drug can exacerbate symptoms of asthma and might promote depression. If rizatriptan is used for abortive therapy, its dosage must be reduced. In addition to propranolol and metoprolol, three other beta blockers—*timolol, atenolol,* and *nadolol*—can help prevent migraine attacks. In contrast, beta blockers that possess intrinsic sympathomimetic activity (e.g., acebutolol, pindolol) are *not* effective. The basic pharmacology of the beta blockers is discussed in Chapter 14.

Antiepileptic Drugs

Several drugs that were developed for epilepsy can reduce migraine attacks. Proof of efficacy is strongest for divalproex [Depakote ER] and topiramate [Topamax]. Gabapentin [Neurontin] and tiagabine [Gabitril] appear promising, although extensive proof of efficacy is lacking.

Divalproex

Divalproex [Depakote ER], employed first for epilepsy and later for bipolar disorder (manic-depressive illness), is now approved for prophylaxis of migraine too. The drug is a form of valproic acid (see Chapter 19). Divalproex reduces the incidence of attacks by 50% or more in 30% to 50% of patients. However, when attacks do occur, their intensity and duration are not diminished. In patients with migraine, the most common side effect is nausea. Other side effects include fatigue, weight gain, tremor, bone loss, and reversible hair loss.

BLACK BOX WARNING: DIVALPROEX

Potentially fatal pancreatitis and hepatitis can occur. In addition, divalproex can cause neural tube defects in the developing fetus, and hence is contraindicated (Category X) during pregnancy.

Topiramate

Topiramate [Topamax], originally developed for epilepsy, was approved for migraine prophylaxis in 2004. Benefits take several weeks to develop and appear equal to those of beta blockers, tricyclic antidepressants, or divalproex. However, topiramate costs much more than these drugs. In clinical trials, topiramate reduced migraine frequency by at least 50% in 83% of adolescents and about 50% of adults. The drug also reduced the need for rescue medication. Unfortunately, side effects are common, especially paresthesias, fatigue, and cognitive dysfunction (psychomotor slowing, word-finding difficulty, impairment of concentration and memory). Other side effects include metabolic acidosis and moderate weight loss (owing to anorexia, nausea, and diarrhea). To minimize side effects, dosage should be low initially and then gradually increased. The basic pharmacology of topiramate is discussed in Chapter 19.

Tricyclic Antidepressants

Tricyclic antidepressants can prevent migraine and tension-type headaches in some patients. The underlying mechanism has not been established but may involve inhibiting reuptake of serotonin, making more of the transmitter available for action. The tricyclic agent used most often is *amitriptyline* [Elavil]. Because amitriptyline is effective in patients who are not depressed, it would seem that benefits do not depend on elevation of mood. Like other tricyclic antidepressants, amitriptyline can cause hypotension and anticholinergic effects (dry mouth, constipation, urinary retention, blurred vision, tachycardia). Excessive doses can cause dysrhythmias. The basic pharmacology of amitriptyline is discussed in Chapter 25.

Estrogens and Triptans for Menstrually Associated Migraine

Menstrually associated migraine is defined as migraine that routinely occurs within 2 days of the onset of menses. An important trigger is the decline in estrogen levels that precedes menstruation. For many women, menstrually associated migraine can be prevented by taking estrogen supplements, which compensate for the premenstrual estrogen drop. Topical preparations—estrogen gel and estrogen patches [e.g., Divigel, Climara]—work well.

Perimenstrual triptans can also help. For example, frovatriptan, naratriptan, and zolmitriptan can reduce the frequency, intensity, and duration of menstrually associated migraine. Dosing is done for 6 days each month, beginning 2 days before the expected onset of menses.

In addition, naproxen sodium at a dosage of 550 mg twice daily, given 6 days before to 7 days after menses, has demonstrated effectiveness in the prevention of migraine.

Other Drugs for Prophylaxis

Botulinum Toxin

In 2010, the FDA approved injections of botulinum toxin A [Botox] for prevention of headaches in adults with chronic migraine (defined as having 15 or more headache days per month), but not for patients with less frequent headaches. Treatment consists of 31 injections, made into muscles of the scalp, neck, and upper back. Treatment is expensive, and benefits are modest: on average, patients experience about 2 fewer headache days a month.

BLACK BOX WARNING: BOTULINIM TOXIN

Botulinum toxin can spread from the site of injection and produce muscle weakness, difficulty with respiration, and swallowing difficulties that can be life threatening.

Angiotensin-Converting Enzyme Inhibitors (ACEIs) and Angiotensin II Receptor Blockers (ARBs)

For prophylaxis of migraine, ACEIs and ARBs are considered third-line drugs. Benefits are limited to a 25% reduction in migraine days. Side effects include hyperkalemia, hypotension, volume depletion, and angioedema. When used during pregnancy, these drugs can injure the developing fetus. How ACEIs and ARBs reduce migraine attacks is unknown, although it is thought that they may stabilize blood vessels and alter sympathetic activity. The basic pharmacology of these drugs is discussed in Chapter 36.

Supplements

Riboflavin. Riboflavin (vitamin B_2) can reduce the number and severity of migraine attacks, but benefits are modest and develop slowly. In one study, patients with migraine with frequent attacks took 400 mg of riboflavin a day. After 3 months, the number of attacks was decreased by 37%. In addition, the average duration of each attack also declined. Side effects were minimal.

Coenzyme Q-10. In two studies, daily therapy with coenzyme Q-10 (CoQ-10) produced a significant reduction in the occurrence of migraine attacks when compared with placebo. Subjects took 150 mg of CoQ-10 each morning or 100 mg 3 times daily. After 3 months, the number of days on which headaches occurred declined by at least 50% in 61% and 47% of study participants, respectively. However, although headache frequency declined, headache intensity was not affected. CoQ-10 was well tolerated.

Butterbur. Extracts made from the root of *Petasites hybridus*, a plant whose common name is butterbur, can reduce the frequency of migraine attacks. In a double-blind, placebo-controlled trial, about 1 in 5 patients taking 75 mg of extract twice daily experienced a 50% or greater reduction in migraine frequency. The only side effects were mild GI symptoms (e.g., nausea, burping, stomach pain). However, butterbur root contains pyrrolizidine alkaloids, which, if not removed during processing, can cause liver damage and cancer. In the study noted, the preparation employed, sold as Petadolex, was pyrrolizidine free.

CLUSTER HEADACHES

Characteristics

Cluster headaches occur in a series or "cluster" of attacks. Each attack lasts 15 minutes to 2 hours and is characterized by severe, throbbing, unilateral pain in the orbital-temporal area (i.e., near the eye). A typical cluster consists of one or two such attacks every day for 2 to 3 months. An attack-free interval of months to years separates each cluster. Along with headache, patients usually experience lacrimation, conjunctival redness, nasal congestion, rhinorrhea, ptosis (drooping eyelid), and miosis (constriction of the pupil)—all on the same side as the headache. Although related to migraine, cluster headaches differ in several ways: (1) they are not preceded by an aura, (2) they do not cause nausea and vomiting, (3) they can be more debilitating, (4) they are less common and occur mostly in males (5:1 ratio), (5) they are not associated with a family history of attacks, and (6) management is different.

Drug Therapy

Prophylaxis

Primary therapy is directed at prophylaxis. Effective agents include glucocorticoids (prednisone and dexamethasone), verapamil, and lithium. High-dose prednisone (40 to 80 mg/day) or dexamethasone (4 mg twice daily) acts rapidly, producing results in 48 hours. However, because long-term use of glucocorticoids carries serious risks (see Chapter 56), treatment should stop in 1 to 2 months. Verapamil is a first-line agent for preventing chronic cluster headache. This drug is effective, easy to use, and safe. Lithium is considered a second-line drug for prophylaxis. The drug is effective but can cause multiple adverse effects, and dosing is difficult. To ensure therapeutic effects and minimize toxicity, blood levels of lithium must be monitored; the target range is 0.4 to 0.8 mEq/L. With all of these drugs, prophylactic therapy should be limited to the cluster cycle and then discontinued when the current cycle is over. Drugs for prophylaxis are listed in Table 23.5.

Treatment

If an attack occurs despite preventive therapy, it can be aborted with sumatriptan or oxygen. Sumatriptan (6 mg subQ) is the treatment of choice for cluster headaches. Inhaling 100% oxygen (7 to 10 L/min for 15 to 20 minutes) is also highly effective and has virtually no adverse effects. In the past, ergot preparations (e.g., intravenous dihydroergotamine, sublingual ergotamine) were commonly used. However, their use today is limited because modern trials are small in population and lack evidence that these drugs work any better at relieving cluster headaches than placebo.

TENSION-TYPE HEADACHE

Characteristics

Tension-type headaches are the most common headache type. These headaches are characterized by moderate, nonthrobbing pain, usually located in a "headband" distribution. Headache is often associated with scalp tingling and a sense of tightness or pressure in the head and neck. Precipitating factors include eye strain, aggravation, frustration, and life's daily stresses. Depressive symptoms (sleep disturbances, including early and frequent awakening) are often present. Tension headaches may be episodic or chronic. By definition, chronic tension-type headaches occur 15 or more days per month for at least 6 months.

TABLE 23.5 ▪ Drugs Used for Prophylaxis of Cluster Headache

Drug*	Usual Daily Dosage (mg)
CALCIUM CHANNEL BLOCKERS	
Verapamil [Calan, others]	240-420
NEUROSTABILIZERS	
Divalproex [Depakote]	500-1500
Lithium [Lithobid]	600-1200†
Topiramate [Topamax]	50-200
NONSTEROIDAL ANTIINFLAMMATORY DRUGS	
Indomethacin	100-150
Naproxen	1000-1500
GLUCOCORTICOIDS	
Dexamethasone	8
Prednisone	40-80
ERGOT ALKALOIDS	
Ergotamine	1.2

*None of the drugs listed is approved by the FDA for cluster headache prophylaxis.
†Dosage is adjusted on the basis of serum lithium levels.

Treatment

An acute attack of mild to moderate intensity can be relieved with a nonopioid analgesic: acetaminophen or a nonsteroidal antiinflammatory drug (e.g., aspirin, ibuprofen, naproxen). An analgesic-sedative combination (e.g., aspirin-butalbital) may also be used. However, because of their potential for dependence and abuse, these combinations should be reserved for acute therapy of episodic attacks; they are inappropriate for patients with chronic daily headaches.

For prophylaxis, amitriptyline [Elavil], a tricyclic antidepressant, is the drug of choice. Dosing at bedtime will help relieve any depression-related sleep disturbances in addition to protecting against headache. Amitriptyline can cause anticholinergic side effects (e.g., dry mouth, constipation) and poses a risk for cardiotoxicity at high doses (see Chapter 25).

In addition to receiving drugs, patients should be taught how to manage stress. Instruction should include cognitive coping skills and information on relaxation techniques (e.g., massage, hot baths, biofeedback, deep muscle relaxation).

MEDICATION OVERUSE HEADACHE

MOH is a chronic headache that develops in response to frequent use of headache medicines and that resolves days to weeks after the overused drug is withdrawn. The stage for MOH is set when headache drugs are taken too often, especially if the dosage is high. Discontinuing the medication brings on the MOH, which causes the patient to resume taking medicine—setting up a repeating cycle of MOH, followed by medication use and discontinuation, followed by another MOH, and so on. One reason the cycle gets established is that patients don't realize that the drugs they're taking to *treat* headache can, if taken too often, become the *cause* of headache. Failing to recognize MOH for what it is, patients take more and more medicine to make their headaches go away, but only succeed in making MOH worse.

Almost all of the medicines used for abortive headache therapy can cause MOH: analgesics (aspirin-like drugs, opioids), triptans, ergotamine (but not dihydroergotamine), and caffeine.

The treatment for MOH is to stop taking all headache medicines. Unfortunately, when medication is withdrawn, headaches increase for a while. Their duration and intensity depend on the drug that was overused. With triptans, withdrawal headaches are relatively mild and often resolve in a few days. In contrast, with analgesics or ergots, withdrawal headaches are more intense and may persist for 2 weeks or more.

Several measures can *decrease the risk* for developing MOH. The most important is to limit the use of abortive medicines. If possible, patients should take these drugs no more than 2 or 3 times a week—and doses should be no higher than actually needed. Alternating headache medicines may help, too, because this would limit exposure to any one drug. If headaches begin to occur more than 2 or 3 times a month, prophylactic therapy should be tried. Implementing nondrug measures—stress reduction, avoidance of triggers, getting sufficient sleep, relaxation techniques, and biofeedback—can reduce the need for headache medicines and decrease exposure to drugs that cause MOH.

UNIT VII
Psychotherapeutic Drugs

CHAPTER 24

Antipsychotic Agents and Their Use in Schizophrenia

Laura D. Rosenthal, DNP, ACNP, FAANP

The antipsychotic agents are a chemically diverse group of compounds used for a broad spectrum of psychotic disorders. Specific indications include schizophrenia, delusional disorders, bipolar disorder, depressive psychoses, and drug-induced psychoses. As a rule, antipsychotics should not be used to treat dementia-related psychosis in older adults, owing to a risk for increased mortality.

Since their introduction in the early 1950s, the antipsychotic agents have catalyzed revolutionary change in the management of psychotic illnesses. Before these drugs were available, psychoses were largely untreatable and patients were fated to a life of institutionalization. With the advent of antipsychotic medications, many patients with schizophrenia and other severe psychotic disorders have been able to leave psychiatric hospitals and return to the community. Others have been spared hospitalization entirely. For those who must be institutionalized, antipsychotic drugs have at least reduced suffering.

The antipsychotic drugs fall into two major groups: (1) *first-generation antipsychotics* (FGAs), also known as *conventional antipsychotics*; and (2) *second-generation antipsychotics* (SGAs), also known as *atypical antipsychotics.* Both groups are equally effective. All of the FGAs produce strong blockade of dopamine in the central nervous system (CNS). As a result, they all can cause serious movement disorders, known as *extrapyramidal symptoms* (EPSs). The SGAs produce moderate blockade of receptors for dopamine and much stronger blockade of receptors for serotonin. Because dopamine receptor blockade is only moderate, the risk for EPSs is lower than with the FGAs. However, although the SGAs carry a reduced risk for EPSs, they carry a significant risk of *metabolic effects*—weight gain, diabetes, and dyslipidemia—that can cause cardiovascular events and early death.

SCHIZOPHRENIA: CLINICAL PRESENTATION AND ETIOLOGY

Clinical Presentation

Schizophrenia is a chronic psychotic illness characterized by disordered thinking and a reduced ability to comprehend reality. Symptoms usually emerge during adolescence or early adulthood. In the United States about 3.2 million people are affected.

Three Types of Symptoms

Symptoms of schizophrenia can be divided into three groups: positive symptoms, negative symptoms, and cognitive symptoms. Positive and negative symptoms are shown in Table 24.1.

Positive Symptoms and Negative Symptoms

Positive symptoms can be viewed as an exaggeration or distortion of normal function, whereas negative symptoms can be viewed as a loss or diminution of normal function. Positive symptoms include hallucinations, delusions, agitation, tension, and paranoia. Negative symptoms include lack of motivation, poverty of speech, blunted affect, poor self-care, and social withdrawal. Positive and negative symptoms respond equally to FGAs and SGAs.

Cognitive Symptoms

Cognitive symptoms include disordered thinking, reduced ability to focus attention, and prominent learning and memory

TABLE 24.1 ■ Positive and Negative Symptoms of Schizophrenia

Positive Symptoms	Hallucinations Delusions Disordered thinking Disorganized speech Combativeness Agitation Paranoia
Negative Symptoms	Social withdrawal Emotional withdrawal Lack of motivation Poverty of speech Blunted affect Poor insight Poor judgment Poor self-care

Prototype Drugs

ANTIPSYCHOTIC AGENTS

Traditional Antipsychotics
Chlorpromazine (a low-potency agent)
Haloperidol (a high-potency agent)

Atypical Antipsychotic
Clozapine

difficulties. Subtle changes may appear years before symptoms become florid, when thinking and speech may be completely incomprehensible to others. Cognitive symptoms may respond equally to FGAs and SGAs.

Acute Episodes

During an acute schizophrenic episode, delusions (fixed false beliefs) and hallucinations are frequently prominent. Delusions are typically religious, grandiose, or persecutory. Auditory hallucinations, which are more common than visual hallucinations, may consist of voices arguing or commenting on one's behavior. The patient may feel controlled by external influences. Disordered thinking and loose association may render rational conversation impossible. Affect may be blunted or labile. Misperception of reality may result in hostility and lack of cooperation. Impaired self-care skills may leave the patient disheveled and dirty. Patterns of sleeping and eating are usually disrupted.

Residual Symptoms

After florid symptoms (e.g., hallucinations, delusions) of an acute episode remit, less vivid symptoms may remain. These include suspiciousness, poor anxiety management, and diminished judgment, insight, motivation, and capacity for self-care. As a result, patients frequently find it difficult to establish close relationships, maintain employment, and function independently in society. Suspiciousness and poor anxiety management contribute to social withdrawal. Inability to appreciate the need for continued drug therapy may cause nonadherence, resulting in relapse and perhaps hospital readmission.

Long-Term Course

The long-term course of schizophrenia is characterized by episodic acute exacerbations separated by intervals of partial remission. As the years pass, some patients experience progressive decline in mental status and social functioning. However, many others stabilize, or even improve. Maintenance therapy with antipsychotic drugs reduces the risk for acute relapse but may fail to prevent long-term deterioration.

Etiology

Although there is strong evidence that schizophrenia has a biologic basis, the exact etiology is unknown. Genetic, perinatal, neurodevelopmental, and neuroanatomic factors may all be involved. Possible primary defects include excessive activation of CNS receptors for dopamine and insufficient activation of CNS receptors for glutamate. Although psychosocial stressors can precipitate acute exacerbations in susceptible patients, they are not considered causative.

FIRST-GENERATION (CONVENTIONAL) ANTIPSYCHOTICS

The FGAs have been in use for decades, and their pharmacology is well understood. Accordingly, it seems appropriate to begin with these drugs, even though their use has greatly declined. Because the pharmacology of the FGAs and SGAs is very similar, when you understand the FGAs, you will know a great deal about the SGAs as well.

Group Properties

In this section we discuss pharmacologic properties shared by all FGAs. Much of our attention focuses on adverse effects. Of these, extrapyramidal side effects are of particular concern. Because of these neurologic side effects, the FGAs are also known as *neuroleptics*.

Classification

The FGAs can be classified by potency or chemical structure. From a clinical viewpoint, classification by potency is more helpful.

Classification by Potency

First-generation antipsychotics can be classified as *low potency, medium potency,* or *high potency* (Table 24.2). The low-potency drugs, represented by chlorpromazine, and the high-potency drugs, represented by haloperidol, are of particular interest.

It is important to note that, although the FGAs differ from one another in potency, they all have the same ability to relieve symptoms of psychosis. Recall that the term *potency* refers only to the size of the dose needed to elicit a given response; potency implies nothing about the maximal effect a drug can produce. Hence, when we say that haloperidol is more potent than chlorpromazine, we only mean that the dose of haloperidol required to relieve psychotic symptoms is smaller than the required dose of chlorpromazine. We do not mean that haloperidol can produce greater effects. When administered in therapeutically equivalent doses, both drugs elicit an equivalent antipsychotic response.

If low-potency and high-potency neuroleptics are equally effective, why distinguish between them? The answer is that, although these agents produce identical *antipsychotic* effects, they differ significantly in *side effects.* Hence, by knowing the potency category to which a particular neuroleptic belongs, we can better predict its undesired responses. This knowledge is useful in drug selection and providing patient care and education.

Chemical Classification

The FGAs fall into four major chemical categories (Table 24.3). One of these categories, the phenothiazines, has three subgroups. Drugs in all groups are equivalent with respect to antipsychotic actions, and hence chemical classification is not emphasized in this chapter.

TABLE 24.2 ▪ Antipsychotic Drugs: Relative Potency and Incidence of Selected Side Effects

Drug	Trade Name	Equivalent Oral Dose (mg)*	Incidence of Side Effects: Extrapyramidal Effects[†]	Sedation	Orthostatic Hypotension	Anticholinergic Effects	Metabolic Effects: Weight Gain, Diabetes Risk, Dyslipidemia	Significant QT Prolongation	Prolactin Elevation	Metabolized by CYP3A4
FIRST-GENERATION (CONVENTIONAL) ANTIPSYCHOTICS										
Low Potency										
Chlorpromazine	generic only	100	Moderate	High	High	Moderate	Moderate	Yes	Low	—
Thioridazine	generic only	100	Low	High	High	High	Moderate	Yes	Low	—
Medium Potency										
Loxapine	Loxitane	13	Moderate	Moderate	Low	Low	Low	No	Moderate	—
Perphenazine	generic only	8	Moderate	Moderate	Low	Low	—	No	Low	—
High Potency										
Fluphenazine	generic only	1	Very high	Low	Low	Low	—	No	Moderate	—
Haloperidol	Haldol	2	Very high	Low	Low	Low	Moderate	Yes	Moderate	—
Pimozide	Orap	1	High	Moderate	Low	Moderate	—	Yes	Moderate	—
Thiothixene	Navane	2	High	Low	Moderate	Low	Moderate	No	Moderate	—
Trifluoperazine	generic only	1	High	Low	Low	Low	—	No	Moderate	—
SECOND-GENERATION (ATYPICAL) ANTIPSYCHOTICS										
Aripiprazole	Abilify	2	Very low	Low	Low	None	None/low	No	Low	Yes
Asenapine	Saphris	4	Moderate	Moderate	Moderate	Low	Low	Yes	Low	Slightly
Brexpiprazole	Rexulti	2	Very low	Very low	Low	None	Low	No	Low	Yes
Cariprazine	Vraylar	1.5	Very low	Moderate	Low	Low	Moderate	No	No	Yes
Clozapine	Clozaril, FazaClo, Versacloz	75	Very low	High	Moderate	High	High	No	Low	Yes
Iloperidone	Fanapt	4	Very low	Moderate	Moderate	Moderate	Moderate	Yes	Low	Yes
Lurasidone	Latuda	10	Moderate	Moderate	Low	None	None/low	No	Low	Yes
Olanzapine	Zyprexa	3	Low	Moderate	Moderate	Moderate	High	No	Low	No
Paliperidone	Invega	2	Moderate	Low	Low	None	Moderate	Yes	High	Slightly
Quetiapine	Seroquel	95	Very low	Moderate	Moderate	None	Moderate/high	Yes	Low	Yes
Risperidone	Risperdal	1	Moderate	Low	Low	None	Moderate	No	High	No
Ziprasidone	Geodon, Zeldox ♣	20	Low	Moderate	Moderate	None	None/low	Yes	Low	Yes

*Doses listed are the therapeutic equivalent of 100 mg of oral chlorpromazine.

[†]Incidence here refers to *early* extrapyramidal reactions (acute dystonia, parkinsonism, akathisia). The incidence of *late* reactions (tardive dyskinesia) is the same for all traditional antipsychotics.

TABLE 24.3 ▪ Antipsychotic Drugs: Routes and Dosages

Chemical Group and Generic Name	Trade Name	Availability	Usual Total Daily Dose for Schizophrenia (mg)*
Chlorpromazine	generic only	10-, 25-, 50-, 100-, 200-mg tablets	300–1000
Thioridazine	generic only	10-, 15-, 25-, 50-, 100-, 150-, 200-mg tablets	300–800
Fluphenazine	generic only	1-, 2.5-, 5-, 10-mg tablets 2.5-mg/mL elixir 5-mg/mL oral concentrate	5–20
Perphenazine	generic only	2-, 4-, 8-, 16-mg tablets	12–64
Trifluoperazine	generic only	1-, 2-, 5-, 10-mg tablets	15–50
Thiothixene	generic only	1-, 2-, 5-, 10-, 20-mg capsules	15–50
Haloperidol	Haldol	0.5-, 1-, 2-, 5-, 10-, 20-mg tablets 2-mg/mL liquid	6–40
Loxapine	Loxitane	5-, 10-, 25-, 50-mg capsules	30–100
Aripiprazole	Abilify	2-, 5-, 10-, 15-, 20-, 30-mg tablets 1-mg/mL oral solution 10-, 15-mg orally disintegrating tablets	10–30
Asenapine	Saphris	5-, 10-mg sublingual tablets	10–20
Brexpiprazole	Rexulti	0.25-, 0.5-, 1-, 2-, 3-, 4-mg tablets	2–4
Cariprazine	Vraylar	1.5-, 3-, 4.5-, 6-mg capsules	1.5–6
Clozapine	Clozaril, FazaClo, Versacloz	12.5-, 25-, 50-, 100-, 200-mg tablets 50-mg/mL oral suspension 12.5-, 25-, 100-, 150-, 200-mg orally disintegrating tablets	150–600
Iloperidone	Fanapt	1-, 2-, 4-, 6-, 8-, 10-, 12-mg tablets	12–24
Lurasidone	Latuda	20-, 40-, 60-, 80-, 120-mg tablets	40–160
Olanzapine	Zyprexa	2.5-, 5-, 7.5-, 10-, 15-, 20-mg tablets 5-, 10-, 15- ,20-mg orally disintegrating tablets	5–30
Paliperidone	Invega	1.5-, 3-, 6-, 9-mg extended release tablets	3–12
Quetiapine	Seroquel	25-, 50-, 100-, 200-, 300-, 400-mg immediate release tablets 50-, 100-, 200-, 300-, 400- mg extended-release tablets	300–750
Risperidone	Risperdal	0.25-, 0.5-, 1-, 2-, 3-, 4-mg film-coated tablets 1-mg/mL oral solution 0.5-, 1-, 2-, 3-, 4-mg orally disintegrating tablets	2–8
Ziprasidone	Geodon, Zeldox 🍁	20-, 40-, 60-, 80-mg capsules	8–160

*Higher doses may be given for acute symptom management or in patients with refractory symptoms.

Two chemical categories—*phenothiazines* and *butyrophenones*—deserve attention. The phenothiazines were the first modern antipsychotic agents. Chlorpromazine, our prototype of the low-potency neuroleptics, belongs to this family. The butyrophenones stand out because they are the family to which haloperidol belongs. Haloperidol is the prototype of the high-potency FGAs.

Mechanism of Action

The FGAs block a variety of receptors within and outside the CNS. To varying degrees, they block receptors for dopamine, acetylcholine, histamine, and norepinephrine. There is little question that blockade at these receptors is responsible for the major *adverse effects* of the antipsychotics. However, because the etiology of psychotic illness is unclear, the relationship of receptor blockade to *therapeutic effects* can only be guessed. The current dominant theory suggests that FGA drugs suppress symptoms of psychosis by blocking dopamine$_2$ (D_2) receptors in the mesolimbic area of the brain. In support of this theory is the observation that all of the FGAs produce D_2 receptor blockade. Furthermore, there is a close correlation between the clinical potency of these drugs and their potency as D_2 receptor antagonists.

Therapeutic Use: Schizophrenia

Schizophrenia is the primary indication for antipsychotic drugs. These agents effectively suppress symptoms during acute psychotic episodes and, when taken chronically, can greatly reduce the risk for relapse. Initial effects may be seen in 1 to 2 days, but substantial improvement usually takes 2 to 4 weeks, and full effects may not develop for several months. Positive symptoms may respond somewhat better than negative symptoms or cognitive dysfunction. All of the FGA agents are equally effective, although individual patients may respond better to one FGA than to another. Consequently, selection among these drugs is based primarily on their side effect profiles, rather than on therapeutic effects. It must be noted that antipsychotic drugs do not alter the underlying pathology of schizophrenia. Hence, treatment is not curative—it offers only symptomatic relief. Management of schizophrenia is discussed later in the chapter.

Neuroleptics may be employed acutely to help manage patients with bipolar disorder going through a severe manic phase. Neuroleptic medications are also used to treat Tourette syndrome, a rare inherited disorder characterized by severe motor tics, barking cries, grunts, and outbursts of obscene language. Additional applications include suppression of emesis through dopamine receptor blockade, relief of symptoms caused by Huntington chorea, and treatment of organic mental syndromes.

Adverse Effects

The antipsychotic drugs block several kinds of receptors and produce an array of side effects, including a variety of undesired effects. However, these drugs are generally very safe; death from overdose is practically unheard of. Among the many side effects FGAs can produce, the most troubling are the extrapyramidal reactions—especially tardive dyskinesia (TD).

Extrapyramidal Symptoms

EPSs are movement disorders resulting from effects of antipsychotic drugs on the extrapyramidal motor system. The extrapyramidal system is the same neuronal network whose malfunction is responsible for the movement disorders of Parkinson disease (PD). Although the exact cause of EPSs is unclear, blockade of D_2 receptors is strongly suspected.

Four types of EPS occur. They differ with respect to time of onset and management. Three of these reactions—acute dystonia, parkinsonism, and akathisia—occur early in therapy and can be managed with a variety of drugs. The fourth reaction—TD—occurs late in therapy and has no satisfactory treatment. Characteristics of EPSs are shown in Table 24.4.

The *early* reactions occur *less frequently* with *low-potency* agents (e.g., chlorpromazine) than with high-potency agents (e.g., haloperidol). In contrast, the risk for TD is equal with all FGAs.

For many patients, EPSs are uncomfortable, disturbing, and sometimes dangerous. Some manifestations of EPSs, such as TD, are irreversible. It is crucial to monitor patients treated with antipsychotic medications for evidence of EPSs.

Acute Dystonia

Acute dystonia can be both disturbing and dangerous. The reaction develops within the first few days of therapy and frequently within hours of the first dose. Typically, the patient develops severe spasm of the muscles of the tongue, face, neck, or back. Oculogyric crisis (involuntary upward deviation of the eyes) and opisthotonus (tetanic spasm of the back muscles causing the trunk to arch forward while the head and lower limbs are thrust backward) may also occur. Severe cramping can cause joint dislocation. Laryngeal dystonia can impair respiration.

Intense dystonia is a crisis that requires rapid intervention. Initial treatment consists of an anticholinergic medication (e.g., benztropine, diphenhydramine) administered by the intramuscular (IM) or intravenous (IV) route. As a rule, symptoms resolve within 5 minutes of IV dosing and within 15 to 20 minutes of IM dosing.

It is important to differentiate between acute dystonia and psychotic hysteria. Misdiagnosis of acute dystonia as hysteria could result in giving bigger antipsychotic doses, thereby causing the acute dystonia to become even worse.

Parkinsonism

Antipsychotic-induced parkinsonism is characterized by bradykinesia, mask-like facies, drooling, tremor, rigidity, shuffling gait, cogwheeling, and stooped posture. Symptoms develop within the first month of therapy and are indistinguishable from those of idiopathic PD.

Neuroleptics cause parkinsonism by blocking dopamine receptors in the striatum. Because idiopathic PD is also due to reduced activation of striatal dopamine receptors (see Chapter 21), it is no wonder that PD and neuroleptic-induced parkinsonism share the same symptoms.

Neuroleptic-induced parkinsonism is treated with some of the drugs used for idiopathic PD. Specifically, centrally acting *anticholinergic drugs* (e.g., benztropine, diphenhydramine) and *amantadine* [Symmetrel] may be employed. Levodopa and direct dopamine agonists (e.g., bromocriptine) should be avoided because these drugs activate dopamine receptors and might thereby counteract the beneficial effects of antipsychotic treatment.

Use of antiparkinsonism drugs should not continue indefinitely. Antipsychotic-induced parkinsonism tends to resolve spontaneously, usually within months of its onset. Accordingly, antiparkinsonism drugs should be withdrawn after a few months to determine whether they are still needed.

If parkinsonism is severe, switching to an SGA is likely to help. As discussed later, the risk for parkinsonism with SGAs is much lower than with FGAs.

Akathisia

Akathisia is characterized by pacing and squirming brought on by an uncontrollable need to be in motion. This profound

TABLE 24.4 ▪ Extrapyramidal Side Effects of Antipsychotic Drugs

Type of Reaction	Time of Onset	Features	Management
EARLY REACTIONS			
Acute dystonia	A few hours to 5 days	Spasm of muscles of tongue, face, neck, and back; opisthotonus	Anticholinergic drugs (e.g., benztropine) IM or IV
Parkinsonism	5–30 days	Bradykinesia, mask-like facies, tremor, rigidity, shuffling gait, drooling, cogwheeling, stooped posture	Anticholinergics (e.g., benztropine, diphenhydramine), amantadine, or both. For severe symptoms, switch to a second-generation antipsychotic.
Akathisia	5–60 days	Compulsive, restless movement; symptoms of anxiety, agitation	Reduce dosage or switch to a low-potency antipsychotic. Treat with a benzodiazepine, beta blocker, or anticholinergic drug.
LATE REACTION			
Tardive dyskinesia	Months to years	Oral-facial dyskinesias, choreoathetoid movements	Best approach is prevention; no reliable treatment. Discontinue all anticholinergic drugs. Give benzodiazepines. Reduce antipsychotic dosage. For severe TD, switch to a second-generation antipsychotic.

IM, intramuscular; IV, intravenous; TD, tardive dyskinesia.

sense of restlessness can be very disturbing. The syndrome usually develops within the first 2 months of treatment. Like other early EPSs, akathisia occurs most frequently with high-potency FGAs.

Three types of drugs have been used to suppress symptoms: *beta blockers, benzodiazepines,* and *anticholinergic drugs.* Although these drugs can help, reducing antipsychotic dosage or switching to a low-potency FGA may be more effective.

It is important to differentiate between akathisia and exacerbation of psychosis. If akathisia were to be confused with anxiety or psychotic agitation, it is likely that antipsychotic dosage would be increased, thereby making akathisia more intense.

Tardive Dyskinesia

TD, the most troubling EPS, develops in 15% to 20% of patients during long-term therapy with FGAs. The risk is related to duration of treatment and dosage size. For many patients, symptoms are irreversible.

TD is characterized by involuntary choreoathetoid (twisting, writhing, worm-like) movements of the tongue and face. Patients may also present with lip-smacking movements, and their tongues may flick out in a "fly catching" motion. One of the earliest manifestations of TD is slow, worm-like movement of the tongue. Involuntary movements that involve the tongue and mouth can interfere with chewing, swallowing, and speaking. Eating difficulties can result in malnutrition and weight loss. Over time, TD produces involuntary movements of the limbs, toes, fingers, and trunk. For some patients, symptoms decline after a dosage reduction or drug withdrawal. For others, TD is irreversible.

The cause of TD is complex and incompletely understood. One theory suggests that symptoms result from excessive *activation* of dopamine receptors. It is postulated that, in response to chronic receptor blockade, dopamine receptors of the extrapyramidal system undergo a functional change such that their sensitivity to activation is increased. Stimulation of these "supersensitive" receptors produces an imbalance in favor of dopamine and thereby produces abnormal movement. In support of this theory is the observation that symptoms of TD can be reduced (temporarily) by *increasing* antipsychotic dosage, which increases dopamine receptor blockade. (Because symptoms eventually return even though antipsychotic dosage is kept high, dosage elevation cannot be used to treat TD.)

There is no reliable management for TD. Measures that may be tried include gradually withdrawing anticholinergic drugs, giving benzodiazepines, and reducing the dosage of the offending FGA. For patients with severe TD, switching to an SGA may help because SGAs are less likely to promote TD.

Because TD has no reliable means of treatment, prevention is the best approach. Antipsychotic drugs should be used in the lowest effective dosage for the shortest time required. After 12 months, the need for continued therapy should be assessed. If drug use must continue, a neurologic evaluation should be done at least every 3 months to detect early signs of TD. For patients with chronic schizophrenia, dosage should be tapered periodically (at least annually) to determine the need for continued treatment.

Other Adverse Effects

Neuroleptic Malignant Syndrome. Neuroleptic malignant syndrome (NMS) is a rare but serious reaction that carries a 4% risk for mortality—down from 30% in the past, thanks to early diagnosis and intervention. Primary symptoms are "lead pipe" rigidity, sudden high fever (temperature may exceed 41°C), sweating, and autonomic instability, manifested as dysrhythmias and fluctuations in blood pressure. Level of consciousness may rise and fall, the patient may appear confused or mute, and seizures or coma may develop. Death can result from respiratory failure, cardiovascular collapse, dysrhythmias, and other causes. NMS is more likely with high-potency FGAs than with low-potency FGAs.

Treatment consists of supportive measures, drug therapy, and immediate withdrawal of antipsychotic medication. Hyperthermia should be controlled with cooling blankets and antipyretics (e.g., aspirin, acetaminophen). Hydration should be maintained with fluids. Benzodiazepines may relieve anxiety and help reduce blood pressure and tachycardia. Two drugs—*dantrolene* and *bromocriptine*—may be especially helpful. Dantrolene is a direct-acting muscle relaxant (see Chapter 20). In patients with NMS, this drug reduces rigidity and hyperthermia. Bromocriptine is a dopamine receptor agonist (see Chapter 17) that may relieve CNS toxicity.

Resumption of antipsychotic therapy carries a small risk for NMS recurrence. The risk can be minimized by (1) waiting at least 2 weeks before resuming antipsychotic treatment, (2) using the lowest effective dosage, and (3) avoiding high-potency agents. If a second episode occurs, switching to an SGA may help.

Anticholinergic Effects. First-generation agents produce varying degrees of muscarinic cholinergic blockade (see Table 24.2) and can elicit the full spectrum of anticholinergic responses (dry mouth, blurred vision, photophobia, urinary hesitancy, constipation, tachycardia). Patients should be informed about these responses and taught how to minimize danger and discomfort. As indicated in Table 24.2, anticholinergic effects are more likely with low-potency FGAs than with high-potency FGAs. Anticholinergic effects and their management are discussed in detail in Chapter 14.

Orthostatic Hypotension. Antipsychotic drugs promote orthostatic hypotension by blocking $alpha_1$-adrenergic receptors on blood vessels. Alpha-adrenergic blockade prevents compensatory vasoconstriction when the patient stands, thereby causing blood pressure to fall. Hypotension is more likely with low-potency FGAs than with the high-potency FGAs (see Table 24.2). Tolerance to hypotension develops in 2 to 3 months.

Patient Education

HYPOTENSION AND SEDATION

Patients should be informed about signs of hypotension (lightheadedness, dizziness) and advised to sit or lie down if these occur. In addition, patients should be informed that hypotension can be minimized by moving slowly when assuming an erect posture. Patients should be warned against participating in hazardous activities (e.g., driving) until sedative effects diminish.

Sedation. Sedation is common during the early days of treatment but subsides within a week or so. Neuroleptic-induced sedation is thought to result from blockade of histamine-1 (H_1) receptors in the CNS. Daytime sedation can be minimized by giving the entire daily dose at bedtime.

Neuroendocrine Effects. Antipsychotics increase levels of circulating *prolactin* by blocking the inhibitory action of dopamine on prolactin release. Elevation of prolactin levels promotes *gynecomastia* (breast growth) and *galactorrhea* in up to 57% of women. Up to 97% of women experience menstrual irregularities. Gynecomastia and galactorrhea can also occur in males. Because prolactin can promote growth of prolactin-dependent carcinoma of the breast, neuroleptics should be avoided in patients with this form of cancer. (It should be noted that, although FGAs can promote the growth of cancers that already exist, there is no evidence that FGAs actually *cause* cancer.)

Seizures. First-generation agents can reduce seizure threshold, thereby increasing the risk for seizure activity. The risk for seizures is greatest in patients with seizure disorders. These patients should be monitored, and, if loss of seizure control occurs, the dosage of their antiseizure medication must be increased.

Sexual Dysfunction. First-generation agents can cause sexual dysfunction in women and men. In women, these drugs can suppress libido and impair the ability to achieve orgasm. In men, FGAs can suppress libido and cause erectile and ejaculatory dysfunction; the incidence is 25% to 60%. Drug-induced sexual dysfunction can make treatment unacceptable to sexually active patients, thereby leading to poor adherence. A reduction in dosage or switching to a high-potency FGA may reduce adverse sexual effects. Patients should be counseled about possible sexual dysfunction and encouraged to report any problems.

Agranulocytosis. Agranulocytosis is a rare but serious reaction. Among the FGAs, the risk is highest with chlorpromazine and certain other phenothiazines. Because agranulocytosis severely compromises the ability to fight infection, a white blood cell (WBC) count should be done whenever signs of infection (e.g., fever, sore throat) appear. If agranulocytosis is diagnosed, the neuroleptic should be withdrawn. Agranulocytosis will then reverse.

Severe Dysrhythmias. Four FGAs—*chlorpromazine, haloperidol, thioridazine,* and *pimozide*—pose a risk for fatal cardiac dysrhythmias. The mechanism is prolongation of the QT interval, an index of cardiac function that can be measured with an electrocardiogram (ECG). Drugs that prolong the QT interval increase the risk for torsades de pointes, a dysrhythmia than can progress to fatal ventricular fibrillation. To reduce the risk for dysrhythmias, patients should undergo an ECG and serum potassium determination before treatment and periodically thereafter. In addition, they should avoid other drugs that cause QT prolongation, as well as drugs that can increase levels of these four FGAs.

BLACK BOX WARNING: OLDER-ADULT PATIENTS WITH DEMENTIA

When used off-label to treat older-adult patients with dementia-related psychosis, all antipsychotics (FGAs and SGAs) about double the rate of mortality. Most deaths result from heart-related events (e.g., heart failure, sudden death) or from infection (mainly pneumonia). Because antipsychotics are not approved for treating dementia-related psychosis, and because doing so increases the risk for death, such use is not recommended.

Signs of Withdrawal and Extrapyramidal Symptoms in Neonates. In 2011, the U.S. Food and Drug Administration (FDA) notified healthcare professionals that neonates exposed to antipsychotic drugs (first or second generation) during the third trimester of pregnancy may experience EPSs and signs of withdrawal. Symptoms include tremor, agitation, sleepiness, difficulty feeding, severe breathing difficulty, and altered muscle tone (increased or decreased). Fortunately, the risk appears low. Neonates who present with EPSs or signs of withdrawal should be monitored. Some will recover within hours or days, but others may require prolonged hospitalization. Despite the risk to the infant, women who become pregnant should not discontinue their medication without consulting the prescriber.

Dermatologic Effects. Drugs in the phenothiazine class can sensitize the skin to ultraviolet light, thereby increasing the risk for severe sunburn. Phenothiazines can also produce pigmentary deposits in the skin as well as the cornea and lens of the eye.

Patient Education

SUN EXPOSURE AND DERMATITIS

Patients should be warned against excessive exposure to sunlight and advised to apply a sunscreen and wear protective clothing. Handling antipsychotics can cause contact dermatitis in patients and healthcare workers. Dermatitis can be prevented by avoiding direct contact with these drugs.

Physical and Psychological Dependence

Development of physical and psychological dependence is rare. Patients should be reassured that addiction and dependence are not likely.

Although physical dependence is minimal, abrupt withdrawal of FGAs *can* precipitate a mild abstinence syndrome. Symptoms, which are related to chronic cholinergic blockade, include restlessness, insomnia, headache, gastric distress, and sweating. The syndrome can be avoided by withdrawing FGAs gradually.

Drug Interactions

Anticholinergic Drugs

Drugs with anticholinergic properties will intensify anticholinergic responses to neuroleptics. Patients should be advised to avoid all drugs with anticholinergic actions, including antihistamines and certain over-the-counter sleep aids.

Central Nervous System Depressants

Neuroleptics can intensify CNS depression caused by other drugs. Patients should be warned against using alcohol and all other drugs with CNS-depressant actions (e.g., antihistamines, benzodiazepines, barbiturates).

Levodopa and Direct Dopamine Receptor Agonists

Levodopa (a drug for PD) may counteract the antipsychotic effects of neuroleptics. Conversely, neuroleptics may counteract the therapeutic effects of levodopa. These interactions occur because levodopa and neuroleptics have opposing effects on receptors for dopamine: levodopa activates dopamine receptors, whereas neuroleptics cause receptor blockade. Like levodopa, the direct dopamine receptor agonists (e.g., bromocriptine) activate dopamine receptors and hence have interactions with neuroleptics identical to those of levodopa.

Toxicity

First-generation antipsychotics are very safe; death by overdose is extremely rare. With chlorpromazine, for example, the therapeutic index is about 200. That is, the lethal dose is 200 times the therapeutic dose.

Overdose produces hypotension, CNS depression, and extrapyramidal reactions. Extrapyramidal reactions can be treated with antiparkinsonism drugs. Hypotension can be treated with IV fluids plus an alpha-adrenergic agonist (e.g., phenylephrine). There is no specific antidote to CNS depression. Excess drug should be removed from the stomach by gastric lavage. Emetics cannot be used because their effects would be blocked by the antiemetic action of the neuroleptic.

Properties of Individual Agents

All of the FGAs are equally effective at alleviating symptoms of schizophrenia, although individual patients may respond better to one FGA than to another. Differences among these agents relate primarily to side effects (see Table 24.2). Because the high-potency agents produce fewer side effects than the low-potency agents, high-potency agents are used more often.

High-Potency Agents

Compared with the low-potency FGAs, the high-potency FGAs cause more early EPSs but cause less sedation, orthostatic hypotension, and anticholinergic effects. Because they cause fewer side effects, high-potency agents are generally preferred for initial therapy.

Haloperidol

Actions and Uses. Haloperidol [Haldol], a member of the *butyrophenone* family, is the prototype of the high-potency FGAs. Principal indications are schizophrenia and acute psychosis. In addition, haloperidol is a preferred agent for Tourette syndrome. The drug can also be used to control severe behavior problems in children (e.g., combative, explosive hyperexcitability unrelated to any immediate provocation), but only as a last resort. Haloperidol is used more than other FGAs.

Pharmacokinetics. Haloperidol may be administered by the oral (PO) or IM route. Oral bioavailability is about 60%. Hepatic metabolism is extensive. Parent drug and metabolites are excreted in the urine.

Adverse Effects. As indicated in Table 24.2, early extrapyramidal reactions (acute dystonia, parkinsonism, akathisia) occur frequently, whereas sedation, hypotension, and anticholinergic effects are uncommon. Note that the incidence of these reactions is opposite to that seen with the low-potency agents. However, the incidence of TD is the same as with all other FGAs. Neuroendocrine effects—galactorrhea, gynecomastia, menstrual irregularities—are seen occasionally. NMS, photosensitivity, convulsions, and impotence are rare.

Haloperidol can prolong the QT interval and hence may pose a risk for *serious dysrhythmias,* especially when given by the IV route or in high doses. The drug should be used with caution in patients with dysrhythmia risk factors, including long QT syndrome, hypokalemia or hyperkalemia, or a history of dysrhythmias, heart attack, or severe heart failure. Combined use with other QT-prolonging drugs (e.g., amiodarone, erythromycin, quinidine) should be avoided.

Other High-Potency Agents

Fluphenazine. Fluphenazine is a high-potency agent indicated for schizophrenia and other psychotic disorders. The drug belongs to the piperazine subclass of phenothiazines. As with other high-potency agents, the most common adverse effects are early EPSs: acute dystonia, parkinsonism, and akathisia. The risk for TD equals that of other FGAs. Effects seen occasionally include sedation, orthostatic hypotension, anticholinergic effects, gynecomastia, galactorrhea, and menstrual irregularities. NMS, convulsions, and agranulocytosis are rare.

Trifluoperazine. Trifluoperazine is a high-potency agent used for schizophrenia and other psychotic disorders. The drug belongs to the piperazine subclass of phenothiazines. The most common adverse effects are early extrapyramidal reactions (acute dystonia, parkinsonism, akathisia). Effects seen occasionally include sedation, orthostatic hypotension, anticholinergic effects, gynecomastia, galactorrhea, menstrual irregularities, and TD. NMS, convulsions, and agranulocytosis are rare.

Thiothixene. Thiothixene is a high-potency agent approved only for schizophrenia. The most common adverse effects are early extrapyramidal reactions (acute dystonia, parkinsonism, akathisia) and anticholinergic effects. Side effects seen occasionally include galactorrhea, gynecomastia, menstrual irregularities, sedation, orthostatic hypotension, and TD. Agranulocytosis, NMS, and convulsions are rare.

Medium-Potency Agents

Loxapine

Loxapine [Loxitane, Adasuve] is a medium-potency agent indicated only for schizophrenia. The side effect profile is similar to that of fluphenazine. Adasuve, approved in December 2012, is used for acute treatment of agitation associated with schizophrenia. Adasuve is available as a 10-mg inhaled powder. Only one inhalation is recommended in a 24-hour period. Because of its potential to cause fatal bronchospasm, Adasuve is restricted to patients enrolled in the Risk Evaluation and Mitigation Strategy (REMS) program.

Perphenazine

Perphenazine is a medium-potency agent used for schizophrenia and other psychotic disorders. Its side-effect profile is like that of fluphenazine.

Low-Potency Agents

Chlorpromazine

Chlorpromazine, formerly available as Thorazine, was the first modern antipsychotic medication. None of the newer FGAs is superior at relieving symptoms of psychotic illnesses. Chlorpromazine is a low-potency FGA and belongs to the phenothiazine family.

Therapeutic Uses. Principal indications are schizophrenia and other psychotic disorders. Additional psychiatric indications are schizoaffective disorder and the manic phase of bipolar disorder. Other uses include suppression of emesis, relief of intractable hiccups, and control of severe behavior problems in children.

Pharmacokinetics. Chlorpromazine may be administered PO, IM, or IV. After oral administration, the drug is well absorbed but undergoes extensive first-pass metabolism. As a result, oral bioavailability is only 30%. When chlorpromazine is given by the IM or IV route, peak plasma levels are 10 times those achieved with an equal PO dose. Excretion is renal, almost entirely as metabolites.

Adverse Effects. The most common adverse effects are sedation, orthostatic hypotension, and anticholinergic effects (dry mouth, blurred vision, urinary retention, photophobia, constipation, tachycardia). Neuroendocrine effects (galactorrhea, gynecomastia, menstrual irregularities) are seen on occasion. Photosensitivity reactions are possible, and patients should be advised to minimize unprotected exposure to sunlight. Because chlorpromazine is a low-potency neuroleptic, the risk for early extrapyramidal reactions (dystonia, akathisia, parkinsonism) is relatively low. However, the risk for TD is the same as with all other FGAs. Chlorpromazine lowers seizure threshold. Accordingly, patients with seizure disorders should be especially diligent about taking antiseizure medication. Like haloperidol, chlorpromazine can prolong the QT interval, and hence may pose a risk for fatal dysrhythmias, especially in patients with dysrhythmia risk factors (e.g., long QT syndrome, hypokalemia, hyperkalemia, history of cardiac dysrhythmias). Agranulocytosis and NMS occur rarely.

Drug Interactions. Chlorpromazine can intensify responses to CNS depressants (e.g., antihistamines, benzodiazepines, barbiturates) and anticholinergic drugs (e.g., antihistamines, tricyclic antidepressants, atropine-like drugs).

Thioridazine

Thioridazine is a low-potency FGA that prolongs the QT interval and hence can cause fatal cardiac dysrhythmias. Because of this danger, the drug should be reserved for treating schizophrenia in patients who have not responded to safer agents. The most common adverse effects are sedation, orthostatic hypotension, anticholinergic effects, weight gain, and inhibition of ejaculation. Effects seen occasionally include extrapyramidal reactions (dystonia, parkinsonism, akathisia, TD), neuroendocrine effects (galactorrhea, gynecomastia, menstrual irregularities), and photosensitivity reactions. NMS, convulsions, agranulocytosis, and pigmentary retinopathy occur rarely. Principal interactions are with anticholinergic drugs and CNS depressants.

BLACK BOX WARNING: PROLONGATION OF QTC INTERVAL

Thioridazine causes dose-related prolongation of QTc interval that may cause torsades de pointes–type arrhythmias and sudden death. Restrict use to schizophrenia resistant to standard antipsychotic drugs.

SECOND-GENERATION (ATYPICAL) ANTIPSYCHOTICS

The SGAs, also known as *atypical antipsychotics,* were introduced in the 1990s and quickly took over 90% of the market, owing to the perception of superior efficacy and greater safety. However, neither initial perception has held up. Thanks to two large, government-sponsored studies, one in the United States and the other in Great Britain, we now know that, in most cases, SGAs and FGAs are equally effective. As for major side effects, the SGAs *are* less likely to cause EPSs, including TD. However, the SGAs carry an even greater risk of their own, namely, serious metabolic effects—weight gain, diabetes, and dyslipidemia—that can lead to cardiovascular events and premature death. Furthermore, like the FGAs, the SGAs can cause sedation and orthostatic hypotension and can increase the risk for death when used to treat dementia-related psychosis in older adults. Finally, even though SGAs have no clear clinical advantage over FGAs, the SGAs cost 10 to 20 times as much.

In addition to their use in schizophrenia, all of the SGAs are approved for bipolar disorder (see Chapter 26).

Clozapine

Clozapine [Clozaril, FazaClo, Versacloz] was the first SGA and will serve as our prototype for the group—even though other SGAs are now used more widely. This drug is our most effective agent for schizophrenia, the only indication it has.

BLACK BOX WARNING: AGRANULOCYTOSIS

Clozapine can cause life-threatening agranulocytosis. Its use should be reserved for patients who have not responded to safer alternatives.

Mechanism of Action

Antipsychotic effects result from blockade of receptors for dopamine and serotonin (5-hydroxytryptamine [5-HT]). Like the FGAs, clozapine blocks D_2 dopamine receptors, but its affinity for these receptors is relatively low. In contrast, the drug produces strong blockade of 5-HT_2 serotonin receptors. Combined blockade of D_2 receptors and 5-HT_2 receptors is thought to underlie therapeutic effects. Low affinity for D_2 receptors may explain why SGAs cause fewer EPSs than do the FGAs. In addition to blocking receptors for dopamine and serotonin, clozapine blocks receptors for norepinephrine (alpha$_1$), histamine, and acetylcholine.

Therapeutic Use

Schizophrenia

Clozapine is approved for relieving general symptoms of schizophrenia and for reducing suicidal behavior in patients with schizophrenia or schizoaffective disorder who are at chronic suicide risk. The drug is highly effective and often works when all other antipsychotics have failed. Like the FGAs, clozapine improves positive, negative, and cognitive symptoms of schizophrenia. Because the incidence of EPSs with clozapine is low, the drug is well suited for patients who have experienced severe EPSs with an FGA.

Pharmacokinetics

Clozapine is rapidly absorbed after oral administration. Plasma levels peak in 3.2 hours. About 95% of the drug is bound to plasma proteins. Clozapine undergoes extensive metabolism by hepatic cytochrome P450 (CYP) isoenzymes (CYP1A2, CYP2D6, and CYP3A4), followed by excretion in the urine and feces. The half-life is approximately 12 hours.

Adverse Effects and Interactions

Common adverse effects include sedation and weight gain (from blocking H_1 receptors); orthostatic hypotension (from blocking alpha-adrenergic receptors); and dry mouth, blurred vision, urinary retention, constipation, and tachycardia (from blocking muscarinic cholinergic receptors). Neuroendocrine effects (galactorrhea, gynecomastia, amenorrhea) and interference with sexual function are minimal. Compared with the FGAs, clozapine carries a low risk for extrapyramidal effects, including TD.

Agranulocytosis

Clozapine produces agranulocytosis in 1% to 2% of patients. The overall risk for death is about 1 in 5000. The usual cause is gram-negative septicemia. Agranulocytosis typically occurs during the first 6 months of treatment, and the onset is usually gradual. Why agranulocytosis occurs is unknown.

Because of the risk for fatal agranulocytosis, monitoring of the WBC count *and* absolute neutrophil count (ANC) is mandatory. Before starting clozapine, both the total WBC count and ANC must be in the normal range (i.e., WBC count of 3500/mm^3 or greater and ANC of 2000/mm^3 or greater). During treatment, the WBC count and ANC must be monitored weekly until the healthcare provider thinks a decrease in intervals is appropriate. Additional testing may be completed when considering the possibility of neutropenia, when adding other antipsychotics, or when clinically indicated. If the total WBC count falls below 3000/mm^3 or if the ANC falls below 1500/mm^3, treatment should be interrupted. When subsequent *daily* monitoring indicates that counts have risen above these values, clozapine can be resumed. If the total WBC count falls below 2000/mm^3 or if the ANC falls below

1000/mm^3, clozapine should be permanently discontinued. Blood counts should be monitored for 4 weeks after drug withdrawal.

Patients should be informed about the risk for agranulocytosis and told that clozapine will not be dispensed if the blood tests have not been done. Also, patients should be informed about early signs of infection (fever, sore throat, fatigue, mucous membrane ulceration) and instructed to report these immediately.

Metabolic Effects: Weight Gain, Diabetes, and Dyslipidemia

Clozapine and the other SGAs can cause a group of closely linked metabolic effects—obesity, diabetes, and dyslipidemia—all of which increase the risk for cardiovascular events. As indicated in Table 24.2, risk is highest with clozapine and olanzapine and lowest with aripiprazole, lurasidone, and ziprasidone.

Weight gain is the metabolic effect of greatest concern because it seems to underlie development of diabetes and dyslipidemia. Among patients taking clozapine, weight gain can be significant. Patients should be informed about the possibility. Body mass index should be measured at baseline, at every visit for 6 months, and every 3 months thereafter. In addition, waist circumference should be measured at baseline and annually thereafter. If significant weight gain occurs, it can be managed with a combination of lifestyle measures and *metformin,* an oral drug used for diabetes. In one study, metformin was more effective than lifestyle measures, and the combination of metformin plus lifestyle measures was more effective than either intervention alone. Antipsychotic drugs promote weight gain through blockade of H_1 receptors in the brain; they also cause decrease in body temperature, which decreases energy expenditure.

Clozapine and all other SGAs can cause *new-onset diabetes.* Patients taking these drugs have developed typical diabetes symptoms, including hyperglycemia, polyuria, polydipsia, polyphagia, and dehydration. In extreme cases, hyperglycemia has led to ketoacidosis, hyperosmolar coma, and even death. Because of diabetes risk, fasting blood sugar should be measured before starting clozapine, 12 weeks later, and annually thereafter. Patients with documented diabetes at treatment onset should be monitored for worsening of glucose control. All patients should be informed about symptoms of diabetes and instructed to report them. If diabetes develops, it can be managed with insulin or an oral antidiabetic drug, such as metformin. Discontinuing clozapine is also an option. However, if the drug has produced control of psychotic symptoms, continuing clozapine and treating the diabetes would seem preferable.

Dyslipidemia associated with clozapine and other SGAs can manifest as increased total cholesterol, low-density lipoprotein (LDL) cholesterol, and triglycerides, along with decreased high-density lipoprotein (HDL) cholesterol. This lipid profile increases the risk for atherosclerosis and coronary heart disease. To monitor effects on lipids, a fasting lipid profile should be obtained at baseline and every 6 months thereafter. A fasting lipid profile should be obtained more frequently for patients on high-risk medications, including clozapine and olanzapine.

Seizures

Generalized tonic-clonic convulsions occur in 3% of patients. The risk for seizures is dose related. Patients should be warned not to drive or to participate in other potentially hazardous activities if a seizure has occurred. Patients with a history of seizure disorders should use the drug with great caution.

Extrapyramidal Symptoms

Although the risk for EPSs with SGAs is relatively low, it is not zero. Hence, like the FGAs, clozapine and other SGAs can cause parkinsonism, acute dystonia, akathisia, and TD.

BLACK BOX WARNING: MYOCARDITIS

Very rarely, clozapine has been associated with myocarditis (inflammation of the heart muscle), which can be fatal. If a patient develops signs and symptoms (e.g., unexplained fatigue, dyspnea, tachypnea, chest pain, palpitations), clozapine should be withheld until myocarditis has been ruled out. If myocarditis is diagnosed, clozapine should not be used again.

Orthostatic Hypotension

Clozapine can cause orthostatic hypotension, sometimes with fainting. Rarely, collapse is severe and accompanied by respiratory or cardiac arrest, or both. Hypotension is most likely during initial dosage titration, especially if dosage escalation is rapid.

Effects in Older-Adult Patients With Dementia

Like the FGAs, the SGAs about double the rate of mortality when used off-label to treat dementia-related psychosis in older adults. Accordingly, because SGAs are not approved for this use, and because they pose a risk to these patients, it is clear that SGAs should not be prescribed for this condition.

Drug Interactions

Because it can cause agranulocytosis, clozapine is contraindicated for patients taking other drugs that can suppress bone marrow function, including many anticancer drugs.

Drugs that induce cytochrome P450 isoenzymes (e.g., phenytoin, rifampin) can lower clozapine levels, and drugs that inhibit P450 isoenzymes (e.g., ketoconazole, erythromycin) can raise clozapine levels. These inducers and inhibitors should be used with caution.

Other Second-Generation Antipsychotics

Risperidone

Risperidone [Risperdal, Risperdal Consta] is a rapid-acting drug originally approved for schizophrenia and then later approved for acute bipolar mania. In patients with schizophrenia, risperidone improves positive symptoms, negative symptoms, and cognitive function. Like other SGAs, it causes fewer EPSs than FGAs. Risperidone is structurally unrelated to clozapine.

Mechanism of Action

We know that risperidone binds to multiple receptors, but we do not know with certainty how clinical benefits are produced. Risperidone is a powerful antagonist at 5-HT_2 receptors and a less powerful antagonist at D_2 receptors. Antagonism at both sites probably underlies therapeutic effects. Risperidone does not block cholinergic receptors but does block H_1 receptors as well as alpha-adrenergic receptors.

Pharmacokinetics

Absorption is rapid and not affected by food. Plasma levels peak about 1 hour after oral dosing. Much of each dose is metabolized to 9-hydroxyrisperidone, whose activity equals that of risperidone itself. Parent drug and metabolite are excreted primarily in the urine. The effective half-life is 24 hours. In patients with hepatic or renal dysfunction, the half-life is prolonged.

Therapeutic Effects

Risperidone relieves positive and negative symptoms of schizophrenia and improves cognitive function. Significant improvement may be seen in 1 week. In patients with severe TD, risperidone may have an antidyskinetic effect.

Adverse Effects

Side effects are generally infrequent and mild and only rarely require discontinuation of treatment. The incidence of EPSs is very low at the recommended dosage. However, at dosages above 10 mg/day, there is a dose-related increase in EPSs. With the long-acting IM formulation, the incidence of EPSs is substantial (about 25%). Risperidone increases prolactin levels, but symptoms (gynecomastia, galactorrhea) are uncommon. Like most other SGAs, risperidone can cause metabolic effects: weight gain, diabetes, and dyslipidemia. Adverse effects that have led to drug discontinuation include agitation, dizziness, somnolence, and fatigue. Excessive doses have caused sedation, difficulty concentrating, and disruption of sleep.

Preparations, Dosage, and Administration

Paliperidone. Paliperidone [Invega, Invega Sustenna] is approved for acute therapy of schizoaffective disorder and for acute and maintenance therapy of schizophrenia. The drug is the active metabolite of risperidone (9-hydroxyrisperidone) and hence has the same adverse and therapeutic effects as risperidone. The two drugs differ primarily in that paliperidone is not extensively metabolized and has no significant kinetic interactions with other drugs. Also, in contrast to risperidone, paliperidone is dosed just once a day and does not require initial dosage titration. Paliperidone can prolong the QT interval and hence should not be combined with other QT-prolonging drugs.

Olanzapine. Olanzapine [Zyprexa] is an SGA approved for (1) schizophrenia, (2) maintenance therapy of bipolar disorder, (3) acute agitation associated with schizophrenia and bipolar mania, and (4) treatment-resistant major depression (in combination with fluoxetine). In addition, olanzapine is used off-label to suppress nausea and vomiting in cancer patients. The drug is similar to clozapine in structure and actions but carries little or no risk for agranulocytosis (although it can cause leukopenia and neutropenia). The risk for metabolic effects is higher than with most other SGAs.

Mechanism of Action. Olanzapine blocks receptors for serotonin, dopamine, histamine, acetylcholine, and norepinephrine. Therapeutic effects are believed to result from blocking 5-HT_2 and D_2 receptors. Adverse effects result in part from blocking receptors for histamine, acetylcholine, and norepinephrine.

Pharmacokinetics. Olanzapine is well absorbed after oral administration. Food does not alter the rate or extent of absorption. Plasma levels peak 6 hours after dosing and decline with a half-life of 30 hours. Hepatic metabolism is extensive.

Therapeutic Uses

Schizophrenia. In patients with schizophrenia, olanzapine is at least as effective as haloperidol or risperidone and produces fewer EPSs than either drug. Comparative trials with clozapine reveal that olanzapine is not inferior to clozapine in patients previously refractory to treatment. Interestingly, olanzapine can relieve psychosis induced by drugs taken for PD, without reversing antiparkinsonism effects.

Bipolar Disorder. Olanzapine is approved for monotherapy of acute mania in patients with bipolar disorder. Benefits appear equal to those of lithium, a drug of choice for this condition (see Chapter 26).

Adverse Effects with Oral Olanzapine. Regarding serious adverse effects, olanzapine is a mixed blessing: the drug carries a low risk for EPSs but carries a high risk for metabolic effects. Acute EPSs are minimal when olanzapine is used at the recommended dosage. Among the SGAs, olanzapine (along with clozapine) poses the highest risk for serious metabolic effects: weight gain, diabetes, and dyslipidemia—all of which can lead to adverse cardiovascular events and premature death. Like all other antipsychotic drugs, olanzapine can increase mortality in older-adult patients with dementia-related psychosis.

Olanzapine can cause leukopenia and neutropenia and can thereby increase the risk for infection. Accordingly, for patients at high risk—including those with preexisting low WBC counts and those with a history of drug-induced leukopenia or neutropenia—complete blood counts should be conducted often during the first few months of treatment. If the ANC falls below 1000/mm3, olanzapine should be discontinued, and the patient should be monitored for fever and other signs of infection. Neutrophil counts should be monitored until they return to normal.

Mild effects are relatively common. Olanzapine causes somnolence in 26% of patients, presumably by blocking H1 receptors. Blockade of muscarinic receptors causes constipation and other anticholinergic effects. Alpha_1-adrenergic blockade causes orthostatic hypotension. After an overdose, the signs and symptoms may include slurred speech, ataxia, nystagmus, hypotension, respiratory depression, and drowsiness.

Adverse Effects With Long-Acting IM Olanzapine. Overdose with the long-acting IM depot preparation of olanzapine [Zyprexa Relprevv] is dangerous. Principal concerns are CNS depression (ranging from mild sedation to coma) and delirium (confusion, disorientation, agitation, anxiety). Patients may also experience EPSs, joint pain, ataxia, aggression, dizziness, weakness, hypertension, and convulsions. Symptoms typically develop within 1 to 3 hours of dosing but may also develop later. After the injection, patients should be observed by a healthcare provider for at least 3 hours and should be warned against driving and other hazardous activities for the remainder of the day.

Ziprasidone. Ziprasidone [Geodon, Zeldox ♣] is an SGA indicated for schizophrenia and acute bipolar mania. In patients with schizophrenia, ziprasidone can improve positive symptoms, negative symptoms, and cognitive function while causing fewer EPSs than FGAs. Like some other SGAs, ziprasidone can cause significant prolongation of the QT interval and can thereby cause potentially fatal dysrhythmias.

Mechanism of Action. Ziprasidone blocks multiple receptor types, including D_2, 5-HT_2, H_1, and alpha-adrenergic receptors. In addition, it blocks reuptake of two transmitters: serotonin and norepinephrine. As with other SGAs, therapeutic effects are believed to result from blockade of D_2 and 5-HT_2 receptors. Blockade of serotonin and norepinephrine uptake may provide antidepressant effects.

Pharmacokinetics. Oral ziprasidone is well absorbed, especially in the presence of food. Binding to plasma proteins is extensive. Ziprasidone undergoes hepatic metabolism, primarily by CYP3A4, followed by excretion in the urine and feces. The elimination half-life is about 7 hours.

Adverse Effects. Ziprasidone is generally well tolerated. The most common side effects are somnolence (perhaps from H_1 blockade), orthostatic hypotension (perhaps from alpha-adrenergic blockade), and rash (the side effect most responsible for discontinuing the drug). EPSs are seen in about 5% of patients. Like other SGAs, ziprasidone can promote weight gain, diabetes, and dyslipidemia. However, the risk is low. Like other antipsychotic drugs, ziprasidone may increase mortality in older-adult patients with dementia-related psychosis.

Like olanzapine, ziprasidone can cause leukopenia and neutropenia and can thereby increase the risk for infection. For patients at high risk (e.g., those with preexisting low WBC counts, those with a history of drug-induced leukopenia or neutropenia), complete blood counts should be conducted often during the first few months of treatment. If the ANC falls below $1000/\text{mm}^3$, ziprasidone should be discontinued, and the patient should be monitored for fever and other signs of infection. Neutrophil counts should be monitored until they return to normal.

Ziprasidone prolongs the QT interval and thereby poses a risk for torsades de pointes, a dysrhythmia that can progress to fatal ventricular fibrillation. QT prolongation is greater than with haloperidol but less than with thioridazine. Because of QT prolongation, ziprasidone should not be given to patients with risk factors for torsades de pointes, the most important being hypokalemia, hypomagnesemia, bradycardia, congenital QT prolongation, and a history of dysrhythmias, myocardial infarction, or severe heart failure.

Drug Interactions. Ziprasidone should not be combined with other drugs that prolong the QT interval. Among these are tricyclic antidepressants, thioridazine, several antidysrhythmic drugs (e.g., amiodarone, dofetilide, quinidine), and certain antibiotics (e.g., clarithromycin, erythromycin, moxifloxacin).

Drugs that induce CYP3A4 (e.g., rifampin, phenytoin) can accelerate the metabolism of ziprasidone and may thereby decrease its levels. Conversely, drugs that inhibit CYP3A4 (e.g., ketoconazole) may increase ziprasidone levels.

Quetiapine

Actions and Uses. Quetiapine [Seroquel] is an SGA indicated for schizophrenia, major depression, and acute episodes of mania and depression in patients with bipolar disorder. In patients with schizophrenia, the drug can improve positive symptoms, negative symptoms, and cognitive function. Like other SGAs, quetiapine produces strong blockade of 5-HT_2 receptors and weaker blockade of D_2 receptors. Blockade of both receptor types is believed responsible for beneficial effects. In addition to blocking receptors for serotonin and dopamine, quetiapine blocks H_1 receptors and alpha-adrenergic receptors, but does not block receptors for acetylcholine.

Pharmacokinetics. Quetiapine is well absorbed after oral administration. The drug undergoes extensive hepatic metabolism, mainly by CYP3A4, followed by excretion in the urine and feces. The half-life is 6 hours.

Adverse Effects. Quetiapine carries a moderate risk for serious metabolic effects (i.e., weight gain, diabetes, and dyslipidemia). As with other SGAs, the risk for EPSs is low at therapeutic doses. Despite structural similarity to clozapine, quetiapine does not pose a risk for agranulocytosis. Common side effects include sedation (from H_1 blockade) and orthostatic hypotension (from alpha blockade). Like other antipsychotics, quetiapine increases the risk for death in older-adult patients with dementia-related psychosis.

Cataracts are a concern. Cataracts developed in dogs fed 4 times the maximal human dose for 6 or 12 months. Lens changes have also developed in patients; quetiapine may have been the cause. Because quetiapine may pose a risk for cataracts, the manufacturer recommends examining the lenses for cataracts at baseline and every 6 months thereafter.

Like ziprasidone, quetiapine can prolong the QT interval, thereby posing a risk for torsades de pointes. Accordingly, quetiapine should not be given to patients with risk factors for torsades de pointes (e.g., hypokalemia, hypomagnesemia, bradycardia, congenital QT prolongation, or a history of dysrhythmias, myocardial infarction, or severe heart failure) or to patients taking drugs that prolong the QT interval.

BLACK BOX WARNING: SUICIDALITY WITH QUETIAPINE

Quetiapine is associated with an increased risk for suicidality in children, adolescents, and your adults with major psychiatric disorders.

Drug Interactions. Metabolism of quetiapine is accelerated by drugs that induce CYP3A4 (e.g., phenytoin, rifampin). As a result, a larger dose of quetiapine may be needed to maintain antipsychotic effects. Conversely, drugs that inhibit CYP3A4 (e.g., ketoconazole, itraconazole, fluconazole, erythromycin) may increase levels of quetiapine and may thereby cause toxicity. Caution is advised. As noted, quetiapine should not be combined with other drugs that prolong the QT interval.

Aripiprazole

Contrasts With Other SGAs. Aripiprazole [Abilify, Abilify Discmelt, Abilify Maintena, Aristada] is the first representative of a unique class of antipsychotic drugs, referred to by some as dopamine system stabilizers (DSSs). Approved indications are schizophrenia, acute bipolar mania, major depressive disorder, agitation associated with schizophrenia or bipolar mania, and irritability associated with autism spectrum disorder. Aripiprazole has a more favorable safety profile than any other SGA but may be less effective than some. In patients with schizophrenia, aripiprazole is like other SGAs: it improves cognitive function, positive symptoms, and negative symptoms while posing a low risk for EPSs and TD. In contrast to other SGAs, aripiprazole is unlikely to cause significant metabolic effects, hypotension, or prolactin release and poses no risk for anticholinergic effects or dysrhythmias. However, like all other antipsychotics, the drug may increase mortality in older-adult patients with dementia-related psychosis.

Mechanism of Action. Like other antipsychotic drugs, aripiprazole can affect multiple receptor types. It blocks H_1, 5-HT_2, and $alpha_1$ receptors, and has mixed effects on 5-HT_1 and D_2 receptors. The drug does not block cholinergic receptors.

As with other SGAs, therapeutic effects are believed to result from interaction with dopamine and serotonin receptors. However, the nature of the interaction differs: whereas other SGAs act as pure antagonists at dopamine and serotonin receptors, aripiprazole acts as a partial agonist at 5-HT1 and D2 receptors and as a pure antagonist only at 5-HT2 receptors. Because aripiprazole is a partial agonist at 5-HT1 and D2 receptors, net effects on receptor activity will depend on how much transmitter (dopamine or serotonin) is present. Specifically, at synapses where transmitter concentrations are low, aripiprazole will bind to receptors and thereby cause moderate activation. Conversely, at synapses where transmitter concentrations are high, aripiprazole will compete with the transmitter for receptor binding and hence will reduce receptor activation. Because of this ability to modulate the activity of dopamine receptors—rather than simply cause receptor activation or blockade—aripiprazole has been dubbed a DSS. Researchers suggest that dopamine system stabilization explains why aripiprazole can improve positive and negative symptoms of schizophrenia while having little or no effect on the extrapyramidal system or prolactin release.

Pharmacokinetics. Aripiprazole is well absorbed after oral administration, both in the presence and absence of food. Plasma levels peak 3 to 5 hours after dosing. Protein binding in blood is high—more than 99%. In the liver, aripiprazole undergoes metabolism by CYP3A4 and CYP2D6. Aripiprazole and its active metabolite—dehydroaripiprazole—have prolonged half-lives: 75 hours and 94 hours, respectively. Because elimination is slow, (1) dosing can be done once a day and (2) about 14 days (four half-lives) are required to achieve steady-state (plateau) plasma drug levels.

Adverse Effects. Aripiprazole is generally well tolerated. The most common side effects are headache, agitation, nervousness, anxiety, insomnia, nausea, vomiting, dizziness, and somnolence. The incidence of EPSs is very low. Only a few cases of NMS have been reported. Among the SGAs, aripiprazole (along with ziprasidone) poses the lowest risk for weight gain, diabetes, and dyslipidemia. Although aripiprazole can block $alpha_1$-adrenergic receptors, the incidence of orthostatic hypotension is low (1.9% vs. 1% in patients on placebo). Aripiprazole does not prolong the QT interval and hence does not pose a risk of dysrhythmias. Also, the drug has little or no effect on prolactin levels and hence does not cause gynecomastia or galactorrhea. Like other antipsychotic drugs, aripiprazole may increase mortality in older-adult patients with dementia-related psychosis.

BLACK BOX WARNING: SUICIDALITY WITH ARIPIPRAZOLE

Aripiprazole is associated with an increased risk for suicidality in children, adolescents, and your adults with major psychiatric disorders.

Drug Interactions. Drugs that induce CYP3A4 (e.g., barbiturates, carbamazepine, phenytoin, rifampin) can accelerate metabolism of aripiprazole and can thereby reduce its blood level. Conversely, drugs that inhibit CYP3A4 (e.g., ketoconazole, itraconazole, fluconazole, erythromycin) can increase aripiprazole levels, as can drugs that inhibit CYP2D6 (e.g., quinidine, fluoxetine, paroxetine).

Brexpiprazole

Contrasts With Other SGAs. Aripiprazole [Abilify, Abilify Discmelt, Abilify Maintena, Aristada] is the first representative of a unique class of antipsychotic drugs, referred to by some as DSSs. Approved indications are schizophrenia, acute bipolar mania, major depressive disorder, agitation associated with schizophrenia or bipolar mania, and irritability associated with autism spectrum disorder. Aripiprazole has a more favorable safety profile than any other SGA but may be less effective than some. In patients with schizophrenia, aripiprazole is like other SGAs: it improves cognitive function, positive symptoms, and negative symptoms while posing a low risk for EPSs and TD. In contrast to other SGAs, aripiprazole is unlikely to cause significant metabolic effects, hypotension, or prolactin release and poses no risk for anticholinergic effects or dysrhythmias. However, like all other antipsychotics, the drug may increase mortality in older-adult patients with dementia-related psychosis.

Mechanism of Action. Like other antipsychotic drugs, aripiprazole can affect multiple receptor types. It blocks H_1, 5-HT_2, and $alpha_1$ receptors and has mixed effects on 5-HT_1 and D_2 receptors. The drug does not block cholinergic receptors.

As with other SGAs, therapeutic effects are believed to result from interaction with dopamine and serotonin receptors. However, the nature of the interaction differs: whereas other SGAs act as pure antagonists at dopamine and serotonin receptors, aripiprazole acts as a partial agonist at 5-HT1 and D2 receptors and as a pure antagonist only at 5-HT2 receptors. Because aripiprazole is a partial agonist at 5-HT1 and D2 receptors, net effects on receptor activity will depend on how much transmitter (dopamine or serotonin) is present. Specifically, at synapses where transmitter concentrations are low, aripiprazole will bind to receptors and thereby cause moderate activation. Conversely, at synapses where transmitter concentrations are high, aripiprazole will compete with the transmitter for receptor binding and hence will reduce receptor activation. Because of this ability to modulate the activity of dopamine receptors—rather than simply cause receptor activation or blockade—aripiprazole has been dubbed a DSS. Researchers suggest that dopamine system stabilization explains why aripiprazole can improve positive and negative symptoms of schizophrenia while having little or no effect on the extrapyramidal system or prolactin release.

Pharmacokinetics. Aripiprazole is well absorbed after oral administration, both in the presence and absence of food. Plasma levels peak 3 to 5 hours after dosing. Protein binding in blood is high—more than 99%. In the liver, aripiprazole undergoes metabolism by CYP3A4 and CYP2D6. Aripiprazole and its active metabolite—dehydroaripiprazole—have prolonged half-lives: 75 hours and 94 hours, respectively. Because elimination is slow, (1) dosing can be done once a day and (2) about 14 days (four half-lives) are required to achieve steady-state (plateau) plasma drug levels.

Adverse Effects. Aripiprazole is generally well tolerated. The most common side effects are headache, agitation, nervousness, anxiety, insomnia, nausea, vomiting, dizziness, and somnolence. The incidence of EPSs is very low. Only a few cases of NMS have been reported. Among the SGAs, aripiprazole (along with ziprasidone) poses the lowest risk for weight gain, diabetes, and dyslipidemia. Although aripiprazole can block $alpha_1$-adrenergic receptors, the incidence of orthostatic hypotension is low (1.9% vs. 1% in patients on placebo). Aripiprazole does not prolong the QT interval and hence does not pose a risk for dysrhythmias. Also, the drug has little or no effect on prolactin levels and hence does not cause gynecomastia or galactorrhea. Like other antipsychotic drugs, aripiprazole may increase mortality in older-adult patients with dementia-related psychosis.

BLACK BOX WARNING: SUICIDALITY WITH BREXPIPRAZOLE

Brexpiprazole is associated with an increased risk for suicidality in children, adolescents, and your adults with major psychiatric disorders.

Drug Interactions. Drugs that induce CYP3A4 (e.g., barbiturates, carbamazepine, phenytoin, rifampin) can accelerate metabolism of aripiprazole and can thereby reduce its blood level. Conversely, drugs that inhibit CYP3A4 (e.g., ketoconazole, itraconazole, fluconazole, erythromycin) can increase aripiprazole levels, as can drugs that inhibit CYP2D6 (e.g., quinidine, fluoxetine, paroxetine).

Cariprazine. Cariprazine [Vraylar] is an antipsychotic medication whose exact mechanism is unknown. It is thought to act much like aripiprazole, through partial agonist activity at $5\text{-}HT_1$ and D_2 receptors, and as a pure antagonist only at $5\text{-}HT_2$ receptors. Approved indications are schizophrenia, acute bipolar mania, or treatment of mixed episodes associated with bipolar I disorder.

Pharmacokinetics. Plasma levels of cariprazine peak 3 to 6 hours after dosing. Protein binding in blood is high—more than 90%. In the liver, aripiprazole undergoes metabolism by CYP3A4 and CYP2D6. Cariprazine has two major active metabolites, desmethyl cariprazine (DCAR) and didesmethyl cariprazine (DDCAR). Although the drug itself has a shorter half-life of 2 to 4 days, DDCAR has a half-life of approximately 1 to 3 weeks. Availability and dosing of cariprazine is located in Table 24.2.

Brexpiprazole. Brexpiprazole [Rexulti], an additional SGA, was approved in 2015 for the treatment of schizophrenia and as an adjunct drug to antidepressants for the treatment of major depressive disorder (MDD). Like aripiprazole and cariprazine, brexpiprazole is thought to work on both serotonin and dopamine receptors.

Pharmacokinetics. Peak plasma concentrations of brexpiprazole occur about 4 hours after oral ingestion. It is highly protein bound. Brexpiprazole is metabolized by CYP3A4 and CYP2D6 and is excreted largely unchanged in both the urine and feces. Availability and dosing of brexpiprazole are located in Table 24.2.

Asenapine

Therapeutic Use. Asenapine [Saphris] is an SGA indicated for (1) acute and maintenance therapy of schizophrenia in adults and (2) acute monotherapy or acute adjunctive therapy (with lithium or valproate) of manic or mixed manic episodes associated with bipolar disorder. In clinical trials, benefits appeared modest. Asenapine is formulated as a sublingual tablet to allow absorption directly across the oral mucosa. The drug carries a low risk for weight gain, diabetes, or dyslipidemia and has few interactions with other agents. Because of its unique properties, asenapine is well suited for patients who (1) have difficulty swallowing or (2) cannot tolerate the metabolic side effects of some other SGAs.

Mechanism of Action. Asenapine can block D_2, $5\text{-}HT_2$, H_1, and alpha-adrenergic receptors but has little effect on muscarinic receptors. As with other SGAs, clinical benefits appear to result from blockade of D_2 and $5\text{-}HT_2$ receptors. Blockade of H_1 and alpha-adrenergic receptors contributes to side effects.

Pharmacokinetics. When asenapine is swallowed and absorbed from the intestine, it undergoes extensive first-pass metabolism, making bioavailability very low (<2%). In contrast, when the drug is administered sublingually, it gets absorbed directly across the oral mucosa and thereby avoids first-pass metabolism. As a result, bioavailability is relatively high (about 35%). Before elimination in the urine, the drug undergoes metabolism by hepatic CYP1A2. The half-life is about 24 hours.

Adverse Effects. Asenapine is generally well tolerated. The risk for anticholinergic effects, prolactin elevation, and metabolic effects (weight gain, diabetes, dyslipidemia) is low. Blockade of H_1 receptors can promote drowsiness, and blockade of alpha-adrenergic receptors can promote hypotension. In clinical trials, higher doses were associated with EPSs. Asenapine can prolong the QT interval and hence should be avoided by patients with risk factors for QT prolongation, including use of other drugs that can prolong the QT interval. Asenapine has local anesthetic properties and hence can numb the mouth when the sublingual tablets dissolve. Like other antipsychotic drugs, asenapine may increase mortality in older-adult patients with dementia-related psychosis. Rarely, patients have experienced severe allergic reactions, including angioedema and life-threatening anaphylaxis.

Drug Interactions. Asenapine is largely devoid of significant drug interactions. In theory, drugs such as fluvoxamine (Luvox), which strongly inhibit CYP1A2, can increase serum levels of asenapine.

Iloperidone

Actions and Therapeutic Use. Iloperidone [Fanapt] is a chemical relative of risperidone. As with other SGAs, benefits derive from blocking D_2 and $5\text{-}HT_2$ receptors. In clinical trials, efficacy equaled that of risperidone and haloperidol. Iloperidone is better tolerated than some other SGAs but still carries a significant risk for weight gain, hypotension, and QT effects.

Pharmacokinetics. Iloperidone is administered by mouth, and plasma levels peak 2 to 4 hours after dosing. Metabolism is by two hepatic cytochrome P450 isoenzymes: CYP2D6 and CYP3A4. The elimination half-life is 18 to 37 hours.

Adverse Effects. The most common adverse effects are dry mouth, somnolence, fatigue, nasal congestion, and orthostatic hypotension, which can be severe during initial therapy. The incidence of EPSs is very low. Iloperidone carries a low risk for diabetes and dyslipidemia but can cause significant weight gain. The drug prolongs the QT interval and hence poses a risk for serious dysrhythmias. Like other antipsychotic drugs, iloperidone may increase mortality in older-adult patients with dementia-related psychosis.

Drug Interactions. Strong inhibitors of CYP2D6 (e.g., paroxetine) or CYP3A4 (e.g., ketoconazole) can increase levels of iloperidone and can thereby increase QT prolongation. Accordingly, in patients taking such inhibitors, dosage of iloperidone should be reduced. Iloperidone should not be combined with other drugs that prolong the QT interval.

Lurasidone

Actions and Therapeutic Use. Lurasidone [Latuda] is indicated for treatment of schizophrenia and bipolar disorder. In clinical trials, dosages of 20, 40, 80, and 120 mg/day were clearly superior to placebo. As with other SGAs, benefits derive from blocking D_2 and $5\text{-}HT_2$ receptors.

Pharmacokinetics. Administration is oral, and food greatly increases absorption. Plasma levels peak 1 to 3 hours after dosing. Protein binding in blood is high (about 99%). Lurasidone is metabolized in the liver, primarily by CYP3A4, and then excreted in the feces (80%) and urine (9%). The half-life is 18 hours.

Adverse Effects. In clinical trials, the most common adverse events were somnolence, akathisia, parkinsonism, nausea, agitation, and anxiety. Lurasidone does not cause anticholinergic effects or orthostatic hypotension, nor does it prolong the QT interval, and the risk for metabolic effects (diabetes, weight gain, dyslipidemia) is low. Like other antipsychotic drugs, lurasidone may increase mortality in older-adult patients with dementia-related psychosis.

Drug Interactions. Because lurasidone is metabolized by CYP3A4, its levels can be increased by CYP3A4 inhibitors and reduced by CYP3A4 inducers. Accordingly, use of the drug with strong inhibitors (e.g., ketoconazole) or strong inducers (e.g., rifampin) of CYP3A4 is contraindicated.

DEPOT ANTIPSYCHOTIC PREPARATIONS

Depot antipsychotics are long-acting, injectable formulations used for long-term maintenance therapy of schizophrenia. The objective is to prevent relapse and maintain the highest possible level of functioning. As a rule, the rate of relapse is lower with depot therapy than with oral therapy. Depot preparations are valuable for all patients who need long-term treatment—not just for patients who have difficulty with adherence. There is no evidence that depot preparations pose an increased risk for side effects, including NMS and TD. In fact, because depot therapy permits a reduction in the total drug burden (the dose per unit time is lower than with oral therapy), the risk for TD is actually reduced.

Eight depot preparations are currently available: *haloperidol decanoate* [Haldol Decanoate], *fluphenazine decanoate* (generic only), *risperidone microspheres* [Risperdal Consta], *paliperidone palmitate* [Invega Sustenna, Invega Trinza], *aripiprazole* [Abilify Maintena, Aristada], and *olanzapine pamoate* [Zyprexa Relprevv]. After the injection, active drug is slowly absorbed into the blood. Because of this slow, steady absorption, plasma levels remain relatively constant between doses. The dosing interval is 2 to 4 weeks. Typical maintenance dosages are shown in Table 24.5.

MANAGEMENT OF SCHIZOPHRENIA

Drug Therapy

Drug therapy of schizophrenia has three major objectives: (1) suppression of acute episodes, (2) prevention of acute exacerbations, and (3) maintenance of the highest possible level of functioning.

Drug Selection

Like all other drugs, antipsychotics should be selected on the basis of effectiveness, tolerability, and cost. Currently, SGAs are prescribed 10 times more often than FGAs, but that may change. When the SGAs were introduced, available data suggested they were more effective than FGAs and also safer. However, we now know otherwise. A comparative effectiveness review compared FGAs with SGAs in the treatment of schizophrenia in adults. In 113 studies, clozapine was more effective than chlorpromazine in treating the core illness of schizophrenia. Yet when looking at functional outcomes, quality of life, and adverse events, there was no difference between the FGAs and SGAs. Regarding serious side effects, SGAs were initially thought to be safer than FGAs because SGAs pose a lower risk for EPSs. However, over time, it became clear that SGAs posed a serious risk of their own: potentially fatal metabolic effects. Hence, rather than being *free* of serious side effects, the SGAs simply substituted a new serious effect for the old one. As for cost, FGAs are much cheaper. In summary, here's what we know:

- Most FGAs and SGAs are equally effective, except for clozapine, which is more effective than the rest.
- Whereas FGAs pose a greater risk for EPSs, SGAs pose a significant risk for metabolic effects, which may be more detrimental than EPSs.
- FGAs cost much less than SGAs.

Given this information, which drug should we choose? That's still hard to answer. With regard to efficacy and safety, no single agent is clearly superior to the others. So we're back to our initial selection criteria: efficacy, safety, and cost. For a patient who is treatment resistant, a trial with clozapine might be reasonable. For a patient with a history of diabetes or dyslipidemia, an FGA might be a good choice, as might aripiprazole or ziprasidone, two SGAs with a low risk for metabolic effects. If there's no clinical reason to select an SGA over an FGA, cost considerations would suggest choosing an FGA.

Dosing

Dosing with antipsychotics is highly individualized. Older-adult patients require relatively small doses—typically 30% to 50% of those for younger patients. Poorly responsive patients may need larger doses. However, very large doses should generally be avoided because huge doses are probably no more effective than moderate doses and will increase the risk for side effects.

Dosage size and timing are likely to change over the course of therapy. During the initial phase, antipsychotics should be administered in divided daily doses. After an effective dosage has been determined, the entire daily dose can often be given at bedtime. Because antipsychotics cause sedation, bedtime dosing helps promote sleep while decreasing daytime drowsiness. Doses used early in therapy to gain rapid control of behavior are often very high. For long-term therapy, the dosage should be reduced to the lowest effective amount.

TABLE 24.5 ▪ Depot Antipsychotic Preparations

Generic Name [Trade Name]	Availability	Route	Typical Maintenance Dosage
Haloperidol decanoate [Haldol Decanoate]	50 mg/mL and 100 mg/mL	IM	50–200 mg every 4 weeks
Fluphenazine decanoate (generic only)	25 mg/mL	IM, subQ	12.5–50 mg every 2 weeks
Risperidone microspheres [Risperdal Consta]	12.5-, 25-, 37.5, 50-mg microspheres in 2-mL diluent	IM	25–50 mg every 2 weeks
Paliperidone palmitate [Invega Sustenna] [Invega Trinza]	39-, 79-, 117-, 156-, 234-mg prefilled syringes 273-, 410-, 546-, or 819-mg prefilled syringes	IM	117 mg every 4 weeks 273–819 mg every 12 weeks to be started after stable on Sustenna
Olanzapine pamoate [Zyprexa Relprevv]	210-, 300-, 405-mg in single-use vials	IM	150–300 mg every 2 weeks *or* 405 mg every 4 weeks
Aripiprazole [Abilify Maintena]	7.5-mg/mL single-use vials	IM	400 mg every 4 weeks
Aripiprazole lauroxil [Aristada]	441-, 662-, 882-mg single-use prefilled syringe	IM	441 mg every 4 weeks *or* 882 mg every 6 weeks

IM, intramuscular; subQ, subcutaneous.

Routes

Oral

Oral dosing is preferred for most patients. Antipsychotics are available in tablets, capsules, and liquids for oral use.

The liquid formulations require special handling. These preparations are concentrated and must be diluted before use. Dilution may be performed with a variety of fluids, including milk, fruit juices, and carbonated beverages. Some oral liquids are light sensitive and must be stored in amber or opaque containers. Liquid formulations of *phenothiazines* can cause contact dermatitis; nurses and patients should take care to avoid skin contact with these preparations.

Sublingual

One SGA—*asenapine* [Saphris]—is administered as a sublingual tablet designed to be absorbed through the oral mucosa (to avoid first-pass hepatic metabolism). This route has the additional advantage of preventing "cheeking" because doing so will simply cause the drug to be absorbed as intended.

Intramuscular

Intramuscular injection is generally reserved for patients with severe, acute schizophrenia and for long-term maintenance. Depot preparations are given every 2 to 4 weeks (see Table 24.5).

Inhaled

Loxapine [Adasuve] is a formula used for acute treatment of agitation associated with schizophrenia. Adasuve is available as a 10-mg inhaled powder. Only one inhalation is recommended in a 24-hour period.

Initial Therapy

With adequate dosing, symptoms begin to resolve within 1 to 2 days. However, significant improvement takes 1 to 2 weeks, and a full response may not be seen for several months.

Some symptoms resolve sooner than others. During the first week, the goal is to reduce agitation, hostility, anxiety, and tension and to normalize patterns of sleeping and eating. Over the next 6 to 8 weeks, symptoms should continue to steadily improve. The goals over this interval are increased socialization and improved self-care, mood, and formal thought processes. Of the patients who have not responded within 6 weeks, 50% are likely to respond by the end of 12 weeks.

Maintenance Therapy

Schizophrenia is a chronic disorder that usually requires prolonged treatment. The purpose of long-term therapy is to reduce the recurrence of acute florid episodes and to maintain the highest possible level of functioning. Unfortunately, although long-term treatment can be very effective, it also carries a risk for adverse effects, especially TD.

After control of an acute episode, antipsychotic therapy should continue for at least 12 months. Withdrawal of medication before this time is associated with a 55% incidence of relapse, compared with only 20% in patients who continue drug use. Accordingly, patients must be convinced to continue therapy for the entire 12-month course, even though they may be symptom free and consider themselves "cured."

After 12 months, an attempt may be made to discontinue drug use, provided symptoms have been absent for this period of time. Drug continuation past 12 months may be needed to maintain patient stability. About 25% of patients do not need drugs beyond this time. To avoid a withdrawal reaction, dosage should be tapered gradually. It is important that medication not be withdrawn at a time of stress (e.g., when the patient is being discharged after hospitalization). If relapse occurs after withdrawal, treatment should be reinstituted. For many patients, resumption of therapy controls symptoms and prevents further deterioration.

When long-term therapy is conducted, dosage should be adjusted with care. To reduce the risk for TD and other adverse effects, a minimal effective dosage should be established. Annual attempts should be made to lower the dosage or to discontinue treatment entirely.

Long-acting (depot) antipsychotics are especially well suited for prolonged treatment. Depot therapy has three major advantages over oral therapy: (1) the relapse rate may be lower, (2) drug levels are more stable between doses, and (3) the total dose per unit time is lower, thereby reducing the risk for adverse effects, including TD. In the United States only a small number of patients receive depot therapy. The low rate is based in large part on the widely held (but unfounded) perception that depot therapy is for patients who suffer recurrent relapse because of persistent nonadherence with oral therapy.

Promoting Adherence

Poor adherence is a common cause of therapeutic failure and underlies a significant proportion of hospital readmissions. Adherence can be difficult to achieve because treatment is prolonged and because patients may fail to appreciate the need for therapy, or they may be unwilling or unable to take medicine as prescribed. In addition, side effects can discourage adherence. Adherence can be enhanced in the following ways:

- Encouraging family members to oversee medication management
- Establishing a good therapeutic relationship with the patient and family
- Using an IM depot preparation (e.g., fluphenazine decanoate, haloperidol decanoate) for long-term therapy

Patient Education

IMPORTANCE OF FOLLOWING DOSAGE INSTRUCTIONS

Provide patients with written and verbal instructions on dosage size and timing and encourage them to take their medicine exactly as prescribed. Inform patients and their families that antipsychotics must be taken on a regular schedule to be effective and hence should not be used PRN. Educate patients about side effects of treatment and teach them how to minimize undesired responses. Assure patients that antipsychotic drugs do not cause addiction.

Nondrug Therapy

Although drugs can be of great benefit in schizophrenia, medication alone does not constitute optimal treatment. The acutely ill patient needs care, support, and protection; a period of hospitalization may be essential. Counseling can offer the patient and family insight into the nature of schizophrenia and can facilitate adjustment and rehabilitation. Although conventional psychotherapy is of little value in reducing symptoms of schizophrenia, establishing a good therapeutic relationship can help promote adherence and can help the prescriber evaluate the patient, which in turn can facilitate dosage adjustment and drug selection. Behavioral therapy can help reduce stress. Vocational training in a sheltered environment offers the hope of productivity and some measure of independence. Ideally, the patient will be provided with a comprehensive therapeutic program to complement the benefits of medication. Unfortunately, ideal situations don't always exist, leaving many patients to rely on drugs as their sole treatment modality.

CHAPTER

25 Antidepressants

Laura D. Rosenthal, DNP, ACNP, FAANP

Our principal focus in this chapter is drugs used to treat major depression. In addition, we consider four somatic (nondrug) therapies. We begin by discussing depression itself and the basic approach to treatment. After that, we discuss the antidepressant drugs and the somatic therapies.

MAJOR DEPRESSION: CLINICAL FEATURES, PATHOGENESIS, AND TREATMENT OVERVIEW

Depression is the most common psychiatric disorder. In the United States about 30% of the population will experience some form of depression during their lives. At any given time, about 1 in every 8 adults in the United States is depressed. The incidence in women is twice that in men. The risk for suicide among depressed people is high. Unfortunately, depression is underdiagnosed and undertreated: although 50% of depressed individuals seek help, only 20% receive adequate treatment. This is especially sad in that treatment can help many people: about 30% of those given antidepressants achieve full remission; another 20% to 30% achieve at least a 50% reduction in symptom severity.

Clinical Features

The principal symptoms of major depression are *depressed mood* and *loss of pleasure or interest in all or nearly all of one's usual activities and pastimes.* Associated symptoms include insomnia (or sometimes hypersomnia); anorexia and weight loss (or sometimes hyperphagia and weight gain); mental slowing and loss of concentration; feelings of guilt, worthlessness, and helplessness; thoughts of death and suicide; and overt suicidal behavior. For a diagnosis to be made, symptoms must be present most of the day, nearly every day, for at least 2 weeks.

It is important to distinguish between major depression and normal grief or sadness. Whereas major depression is an illness, grief or sadness is not. Rather, grief and sadness are appropriate reactions to a major life stressor (e.g., death of a loved one, loss of a job). In most cases, grief and sadness resolve spontaneously over several weeks and do not require medical intervention. However, if symptoms are unusually intense, and if they fail to resolve within an appropriate time, a major depressive episode may have been superimposed. If this occurs, treatment is indicated.

Pathogenesis

The etiology of major depression is complex and incompletely understood. For some individuals, depression seems to descend "out of the blue"; otherwise healthy people—unexpectedly and without apparent cause—find themselves feeling profoundly depressed. For many others, depressive episodes are brought on by stressful life events, such as bereavement, loss of a job, or childbirth. Because depression does not occur in everyone, it would appear that some people are more vulnerable than others. Factors that may contribute to vulnerability include genetic heritage, a difficult childhood, and chronic low self-esteem.

Clinical observations made in the 1960s led to formulation of the *monoamine-deficiency hypothesis of depression,* which asserts that depression is caused by a functional deficiency of monoamine neurotransmitters (norepinephrine, serotonin, or both). Findings that support the hypothesis include (1) induction of depression with reserpine, a drug that depletes monoamines from the brain; (2) induction of depression with inhibitors of tyrosine hydroxylase, an enzyme needed for monoamine transmitter synthesis; and (3) relief of depression with drugs that intensify monoamine-mediated neurotransmission. Although these observations lend support to the monoamine-deficiency hypothesis, it is clear that the hypothesis is too simplistic. However, despite its shortcomings, the monoamine-deficiency hypothesis does provide a useful conceptual framework for understanding antidepressant drugs.

Treatment Overview

Depression can be treated with three major modalities: (1) pharmacotherapy, (2) depression-specific psychotherapy (e.g., cognitive behavioral therapy or interpersonal psychotherapy), and (3) somatic therapies, such as electroconvulsive therapy and transcranial magnetic stimulation. For patients with mild to moderate depression, drug therapy and psychotherapy can be equally effective. For those with more severe depression, a combination of drug therapy and psychotherapy is better than either intervention alone. Electroconvulsive therapy can be used when a rapid response is needed or when drugs and psychotherapy have not worked. For all patients, aerobic exercise and resistance training can improve mood.

DRUGS USED FOR DEPRESSION

Drugs are the primary therapy for major depression. However, benefits are limited mainly to patients with *severe* depression. In patients with *mild to moderate* depression, antidepressants have little or no beneficial effect.

Available antidepressants are listed in Table 25.1. As indicated, these drugs fall into five major classes: selective serotonin reuptake inhibitors (SSRIs), serotonin-norepinephrine reuptake inhibitors (SNRIs), tricyclic antidepressants (TCAs),

Prototype Drugs

ANTIDEPRESSANTS

Selective Serotonin Reuptake Inhibitor
Fluoxetine

Serotonin-Norepinephrine Reuptake Inhibitor
Venlafaxine

Tricyclic Antidepressant
Imipramine

Monoamine Oxidase Inhibitor
Phenelzine

Atypical Antidepressant
Bupropion

monoamine oxidase inhibitors (MAOIs), and atypical antidepressants. All of these classes are equally effective, as are the individual drugs within each class. Hence differences among these drugs relate mainly to side effects and drug interactions.

Basic Considerations

In this section we consider basic issues that apply to all antidepressant drugs. The information on suicide risk is especially important.

Time Course of Response

With all antidepressants, symptoms resolve slowly. Initial responses develop in 1 to 3 weeks. Maximal responses may not be seen until 12 weeks. Because therapeutic effects are delayed, antidepressants cannot be used PRN. Furthermore, a therapeutic trial should not be considered a failure until a drug has been taken for at least 1 month without success.

Drug Selection

Because all antidepressants have nearly equal efficacy, selection among them is based largely on tolerability and safety. Additional considerations are drug interactions, patient preference, and cost. The usual drugs of first choice are the SSRIs, SNRIs, bupropion, and mirtazapine. Older antidepressants—TCAs and MAOIs—have more adverse effects and are less well tolerated than the first-line agents and hence are generally reserved for patients who have not responded to the first-line drugs.

In some cases, the side effects of a drug, when matched to the right patient, can actually be beneficial. Here are some examples:

- For a patient with fatigue, choose a drug that causes central nervous system (CNS) stimulation (e.g., fluoxetine, bupropion).
- For a patient with insomnia, choose a drug that causes substantial sedation (e.g., mirtazapine).
- For a patient with sexual dysfunction, choose bupropion, a drug that enhances libido.
- For a patient with chronic pain, choose duloxetine or a TCA, drugs that can relieve chronic pain.

Managing Treatment

After a drug has been selected for initial treatment, it should be used for 4 to 8 weeks to assess efficacy. As a rule, dosage should be low initially (to reduce side effects) and then gradually increased (see Table 25.1). If the initial drug is not effective, we have four major options:

- Increase the dosage.
- Switch to another drug in the same class.
- Switch to another drug in a different class.
- Add a second drug, such as lithium or an atypical antidepressant.

After symptoms are in remission, treatment should continue for at least 4 to 9 months to prevent relapse. To this end, patients should be encouraged to take their drugs even if they are symptom free and hence feel that continued dosing is unnecessary. When antidepressant therapy is discontinued, dosage should be gradually tapered over several weeks because abrupt withdrawal can trigger withdrawal symptoms.

BLACK BOX WARNING: SUICIDE RISK WITH ANTIDEPRESSANT DRUGS

Patients with depression often think about or attempt suicide. During treatment with antidepressants, especially early on, the risk for suicide may actually *increase.* Concerns about antidepressant-induced suicide apply mainly to children, adolescents, and adults younger than 25 years.

To reduce the risk for suicide, patients taking antidepressant drugs should be observed closely for suicidality, worsening mood, and unusual changes in behavior. Close observation is especially important during the first few months of therapy and whenever antidepressant dosage is changed (either increased or decreased). Ideally, the patient or caregiver should meet with the prescriber at least weekly during the first 4 weeks of treatment, then biweekly for the next 4 weeks, then once 1 month later, and periodically thereafter. Phone contact may be appropriate between visits. In addition, family members or caregivers should monitor the patient *daily,* being alert for symptoms of decline (e.g., anxiety, agitation, panic attacks, insomnia, irritability, hostility, impulsivity, hypomania, and, of course, emergence of suicidality). If these symptoms are severe or develop abruptly, the patient should see his or her prescriber immediately.

Because antidepressant drugs can be used to *commit* suicide, prescriptions should be written for the smallest number of doses consistent with good patient management. What should be done if suicidal thoughts emerge during drug therapy, or if depression is persistently worse while taking drugs? One option is to switch to another antidepressant. However, as noted, the risk for suicidality appears equal with all antidepressants. Another option is to stop antidepressants entirely. However, this option is probably unwise because the long-term risk for suicide from untreated depression is much greater than the long-term risk associated with antidepressant drugs. If the risk for suicide appears high, temporary hospitalization may be the best protection.

Selective Serotonin Reuptake Inhibitors

The SSRIs were introduced in 1987 and have since become our most commonly prescribed antidepressants, accounting

TABLE 25.1 ▪ Antidepressant Classes and Adult Dosages

Generic Name	Trade Name	Availability	Initial Dose*,† (mg/day)	Maintenance Dose* (mg/day)
SELECTIVE SEROTONIN REUPTAKE INHIBITORS (SSRIS)				
Citalopram	Celexa	10 mg/5 mL oral solution 10-, 20-, 40-mg tablets	20	20–40
Escitalopram	Lexapro, Cipralex ♣	5 mg/5 mL oral solution 5-, 10-, 20-mg tablets	10	10–20
Fluoxetine	Prozac, Sarafem, Selfemra	20 mg/5 mL oral solution 10-, 20-, 60-mg tablets 90-mg delayed release tablets 10-, 20-, 40-mg capsules	20	20–80
Fluvoxamine‡	Luvox	25-, 50-, 100-mg tablets 100-, 150-mg controlled-release capsules	50	100–300
Paroxetine	Paxil, Pexeva	10 mg/5 mL oral solution 10-, 20-, 30-, 40-mg tablets 12.5-, 25-, 37.5-mg controlled-release tablets	12.5–20	20–50
Sertraline	Zoloft	20 mg/mL oral solution 25-, 50-, 100-mg tablets	50	50–200
SEROTONIN-NOREPINEPHRINE REUPTAKE INHIBITORS (SNRIS)				
Desvenlafaxine	Pristiq	50-, 100-mg extended-release tablets	50	50–100
Duloxetine	Cymbalta	20-, 30-, 60-mg delayed-release tablets	40–60	60–120
Levomilnacipran	Fetzima	20-, 40-, 80-, 120-mg capsules	20 mg	40–120
Venlafaxine	Effexor XR	25-, 37.5-, 50-, 75-, 100-mg tablets 37.5-, 75-, 150-, 225-mg extended-release tablets 37.5-, 75-, 150-mg extended-release capsules	37.5–75	75–375
TRICYCLIC ANTIDEPRESSANTS (TCAS)				
Amitriptyline	generic only	10-, 25-, 50-, 75-, 100-, 125-, 150-mg tablets	25–50	100–300
Clomipramine‡	Anafranil	25-, 50-, 75-mg tablets	25	100–250
Desipramine	Norpramin	10-, 25-, 50-, 75-, 100-, 150-mg tablets	25–50	100–300
Doxepin	Sinequan§	10 mg/mL oral solution 10-, 25-, 50-, 75-, 100-, 150-mg tablets	50	75–300
Imipramine	Tofranil	10-, 25-, 50-mg tablets 75-, 100-, 125-, 150-mg capsules	25–50	100–200
Maprotiline	generic only	25-, 50-, 75-mg tablets	75	100–225
Nortriptyline	Aventyl, Pamelor	10 mg/5 mL oral solution 10-, 25-, 50-, 75-mg tablets	75–100	50–150
Protriptyline	Vivactil	5-, 10-mg tablets	15–40	20–60
Trimipramine	Surmontil	10-mg tablets	75–100	75–200
MONOAMINE OXIDASE INHIBITORS (MAOIS)				
Isocarboxazid	Marplan	10-mg tablets	10–20	30–60
Phenelzine	Nardil	15-mg tablets	45	60–90
Selegiline (transdermal)	Emsam	6-, 9-, 12-mg/24 hr transdermal patches	6	6–12
Tranylcypromine	Parnate	10-mg tablets	10–30	30–60
ATYPICAL ANTIDEPRESSANTS				
Amoxapine	generic only	25-, 50-, 100-, 150-mg tablets	100	200–400
Bupropion	Wellbutrin, others	75-, 100-mg tablets 100-, 150-, 200-, 300-mg sustained-release tablets	200	300–450
Mirtazapine	Remeron	7.5-, 15-, 30-, 45-mg tablets 15-, 30-, 45-mg orally disintegrating tablets	15	15–45
Nefazodone	generic only	50-, 100-, 150-, 200-, 250-mg tablets	200	300–600
Trazodone	generic only	50-, 100-, 150-, 300- mg tablets	150	150–600
Trazodone ER	Oleptro	150-, 300-mg extended-release tablets	150	150–375
Vilazodone	Viibryd	10-, 20-, 40-mg tablets	10	40

*Doses listed are *total daily doses.* Depending on the drug and the patient, the total dose may be given in a single dose or in divided doses.
†Initial doses are employed for 4 to 8 weeks, the time required for most symptoms to respond. Dosage is gradually increased as required.
‡Fluvoxamine and clomipramine are not approved for major depression.
§Doxepin is also available in a low-dose formulation, sold as Silenor, for treating insomnia.

for more than $3 billion in annual sales. These drugs are indicated for major depression as well as several other psychological disorders (Table 25.2). Characteristic side effects are nausea, agitation and insomnia, and sexual dysfunction (especially anorgasmia). Like all other antidepressants, SSRIs may increase the risk for suicide. Compared with the TCAs and MAOIs, SSRIs are equally effective, better tolerated, and much safer. Death by overdose is extremely rare.

Fluoxetine

Fluoxetine [Prozac, Prozac Weekly], the first SSRI available, will serve as our prototype for the group. At one time, this drug was the most widely prescribed antidepressant in the world.

Mechanism of Action

The mechanism of action of fluoxetine and the other SSRIs is depicted in Fig. 25.1. As shown, SSRIs selectively block neuronal reuptake of serotonin (5-hydroxytryptamine [5-HT]), a monoamine neurotransmitter. As a result of reuptake blockade, the concentration of 5-HT in the synapse increases, causing increased activation of postsynaptic 5-HT receptors. This mechanism is consistent with the theory that depression stems from a *deficiency* in monoamine-mediated transmission—and hence should be relieved by drugs that can intensify monoamine effects.

It is important to appreciate that blockade of 5-HT reuptake, by itself, cannot fully account for therapeutic effects. Clinical responses to SSRIs (relief of depressive symptoms) and the biochemical effect of the SSRIs (blockade of 5-HT reuptake) do not occur in the same time frame. That is, whereas SSRIs block 5-HT reuptake within hours of dosing, relief of depression takes several weeks to fully develop. This delay suggests that therapeutic effects are the result of adaptive cellular changes that take place in response to prolonged reuptake blockade. Fluoxetine and the other SSRIs do not block reuptake of dopamine or norepinephrine (NE). In contrast to the TCAs (see later), fluoxetine does not block cholinergic, histaminergic, or alpha$_1$-adrenergic receptors. Furthermore, fluoxetine produces CNS excitation rather than sedation.

Therapeutic Uses

Fluoxetine is used primarily for major depression. In addition, the drug is approved for bipolar disorder (see Chapter 26), obsessive-compulsive disorder (see Chapter 28), panic disorder (see Chapter 28), bulimia nervosa, and premenstrual dysphoric disorder (see Chapter 48).

Pharmacokinetics

Fluoxetine is well absorbed after oral administration, even in the presence of food. The drug is widely distributed and highly bound to plasma proteins. Fluoxetine undergoes extensive hepatic metabolism, primarily by CYP2D6 (the 2D6 isoenzyme of cytochrome P450). The major metabolite—norfluoxetine—is active, and later undergoes metabolic inactivation, followed by excretion in the urine. The half-life of fluoxetine is 2 days, and the half-life of norfluoxetine is 7 days. Because the effective half-life is prolonged, about 4 weeks are required to produce steady-state plasma drug levels—and about 4 weeks are required for washout after dosing stops.

Adverse Effects

Fluoxetine is safer and better tolerated than TCAs and MAOIs. Death from overdose with fluoxetine alone has not been reported. In contrast to TCAs, fluoxetine does not block receptors for histamine, NE, or acetylcholine and hence does not cause sedation, orthostatic hypotension, anticholinergic effects, or cardiotoxicity. The most common side effects are sexual dysfunction, nausea, headache, and manifestations of CNS stimulation, including nervousness, insomnia, and anxiety. Weight gain can also occur.

Sexual Dysfunction. Fluoxetine causes sexual problems (impotence, delayed or absent orgasm, delayed or absent ejaculation, decreased sexual interest) in nearly 70% of men and women. The underlying mechanism is unknown.

TABLE 25.2 ▪ Therapeutic Uses of Selective Serotonin Reuptake Inhibitors and Serotonin-Norepinephrine Reuptake Inhibitors

	Therapeutic Use*								
Drug	Major Depression	OCD	Panic Disorder	Social Phobia	GAD	PTSD	PMDD	Bulimia Nervosa	Chronic Pain Disorders[†]
Citalopram [Celexa]	A	U	U	U	U	U	U		
Escitalopram [Lexapro]	A	A	U		A	U			
Fluoxetine [Prozac]	A	A	A	U	U	U	A	A	
Fluvoxamine [Luvox]	U	A	U	A	U	U	U	U	
Paroxetine [Paxil]	A	A	A	A	A	A	A		
Sertraline [Zoloft]	A	A	A	A	U	A	A		
Desvenlafaxine [Pristiq]	A		U	U	U				U
Duloxetine [Cymbalta]	A				A				A
Levomilnacipran [Fetzima]	A				U				U
Venlafaxine [Effexor]	A		A		A				U

*A, approved use; U, unlabeled use.

[†]Chronic musculoskeletal pain, neuropathic pain, or fibromyalgia.

GAD, generalized anxiety disorder; OCD, obsessive-compulsive disorder; PMDD, premenstrual dysphoric disorder; PTSD, posttraumatic stress disorder.

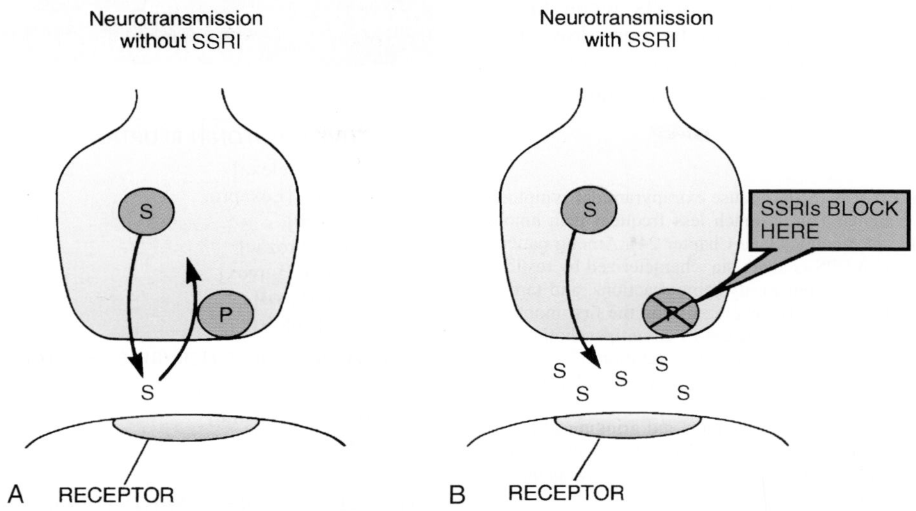

Figure 25.1 ■ Mechanism of action of selective serotonin reuptake inhibitors (SSRIs). **A,** Under drug-free conditions, the actions of serotonin are terminated by active uptake of the transmitter back into the nerve terminals from which it was released. **B,** By inhibiting the reuptake pump for serotonin, the SSRIs cause the transmitter to accumulate in the synaptic space, thereby intensifying transmission. (P, reuptake pump; S, serotonin.)

Sexual dysfunction can be managed in several ways. In some cases, reducing the dosage or taking "drug holidays" (e.g., discontinuing medication on Fridays and Saturdays) can help. Another solution is to add a drug that can overcome the problem. Among these are yohimbine, buspirone [BuSpar], and three atypical antidepressants: bupropion [Wellbutrin, others], nefazodone, and mirtazapine [Remeron]. Drugs such as sildenafil [Viagra] can also help: In *men,* these drugs improve erectile dysfunction as well as arousal, ejaculation, orgasm, and overall satisfaction; in *women,* they can improve delayed orgasm. If all of these measures fail, the patient can try a different antidepressant. Agents that cause the least sexual dysfunction are the same three atypical antidepressants just mentioned.

Sexual problems often go unreported, either because patients are uncomfortable discussing them or because patients don't realize their medicine is the cause. Accordingly, patients should be informed about the high probability of sexual dysfunction and told to report any problems so that they can be addressed.

Weight Gain. Like many other antidepressants, fluoxetine and other SSRIs cause weight gain. When these drugs were first introduced, we thought they caused weight *loss.* During the first few weeks of therapy patients lose weight, perhaps because of drug-induced nausea and vomiting. However, with long-term treatment, the lost weight is regained. Furthermore, about one third of patients continue gaining weight. Although the reason is unknown, a good possibility is decreased sensitivity of 5-HT receptors that regulate appetite.

Serotonin Syndrome. By increasing serotonergic transmission in the brainstem and spinal cord, fluoxetine and other SSRIs can cause serotonin syndrome. This syndrome usually begins 2 to 72 hours after treatment onset. Signs and symptoms include altered mental status (agitation, confusion, disorientation, anxiety, hallucinations, poor concentration) as well as incoordination, myoclonus, hyperreflexia, excessive sweating, tremor, and fever. Deaths have occurred. The syndrome resolves spontaneously after discontinuing the drug. The risk for serotonin syndrome is increased by concurrent use of MAOIs and other drugs (see later section "Drug Interactions").

Patient Education

WITHDRAWAL SYNDROME

Abrupt discontinuation of SSRIs can cause a withdrawal syndrome. Symptoms include dizziness, headache, nausea, sensory disturbances, tremor, anxiety, and dysphoria. These begin within days to weeks of the last dose and then persist for 1 to 3 weeks. Resumption of drug use will make symptoms subside. The withdrawal syndrome can be minimized by tapering the dosage slowly.

Neonatal Effects From Use in Pregnancy. Use of fluoxetine and other SSRIs late in pregnancy poses a small risk for two adverse effects in the newborn: (1) *neonatal abstinence syndrome* (NAS) and (2) *persistent pulmonary hypertension of the newborn* (PPHN). NAS is characterized by irritability, abnormal crying, tremor, respiratory distress, and possibly seizures. The syndrome can be managed with supportive care and generally abates within a few days. PPHN, which compromises tissue oxygenation, carries a significant risk for death, and, among survivors, a risk for cognitive delay, hearing loss, and neurologic abnormalities. Treatment measures include providing ventilatory support, giving oxygen and nitric oxide (to dilate pulmonary blood vessels), and giving intravenous (IV) sodium bicarbonate (to maintain alkalosis) and dopamine or dobutamine (to increase cardiac output and thereby maintain pulmonary perfusion). Infants exposed to SSRIs late in gestation should be monitored closely for NAS and PPHN.

Teratogenesis. The risk for birth defects when taking fluoxetine and other SSRIs appears to be very low. Two SSRIs—*paroxetine* and *fluoxetine*—may cause septal heart defects. But even with these agents, the absolute risk is very low.

Extrapyramidal Side Effects. SSRIs cause extrapyramidal symptoms (EPSs) in about 0.1% of patients. This is much less frequent than among patients taking antipsychotic medications (see Chapter 24). Among patients taking SSRIs, the most common EPS is akathisia, characterized by restlessness and agitation. However, parkinsonism, dystonic reactions, and tardive dyskinesia can also occur. EPSs typically develop during the first month of treatment. The risk is increased by concurrent use of an antipsychotic drug. The underlying cause of SSRI-induced EPSs may be alteration of serotonergic transmission within the extrapyramidal system. For a detailed discussion of EPSs, refer to Chapter 24.

Bruxism. SSRIs may cause bruxism (clenching and grinding of teeth). However, because bruxism usually occurs during sleep, the condition often goes unrecognized. Sequelae of bruxism include headache, jaw pain, and dental problems (e.g., cracked fillings).

SSRIs may cause bruxism by inhibiting release of dopamine, a neurotransmitter that suppresses activity in certain muscles, including those of the jaw. By decreasing dopamine availability, SSRIs could release these muscles from inhibition, and excessive activity could result. This same mechanism may be responsible for SSRI-induced EPSs.

Bruxism can be managed by reducing the SSRI dosage. However, this may cause depression to return. Other options include switching to a different class of antidepressant, use of a mouth guard, and treatment with low-dose buspirone.

Bleeding Disorders. Fluoxetine and other SSRIs can increase the risk for bleeding in the gastrointestinal (GI) tract and at other sites by impeding platelet aggregation. Platelets require 5-HT for aggregation, but can't make it themselves, and hence must take 5-HT up from the blood; by blocking 5-HT uptake, SSRIs suppress aggregation. The SSRIs cause a threefold increase in the risk for GI bleeding. However, the absolute risk is still low (about 1%). Caution is advised in patients with ulcers or a history of GI bleeding, in patients older than 60 years, and in patients taking nonsteroidal antiinflammatory drugs (NSAIDs) or anticoagulants.

Hyponatremia. Fluoxetine can cause hyponatremia (serum sodium <135 mEq/L), probably by increasing secretion of antidiuretic hormone. Most cases involve older-adult patients taking thiazide diuretics. Accordingly, when fluoxetine is used in older-adult patients, sodium should be measured at baseline and periodically thereafter.

Other Adverse Effects. Fluoxetine may cause dizziness and fatigue; patients who experience intense dizziness and fatigue should be warned against driving and other hazardous activities. Skin rash, which can be severe, has occurred in 4% of patients; in most cases, rashes readily respond to drug therapy (antihistamines, glucocorticoids) or to withdrawal of fluoxetine. Other common reactions include diarrhea and excessive sweating.

Drug Interactions

MAOIs and Other Drugs That Increase the Risk for Serotonin Syndrome. MAOIs increase 5-HT availability and hence greatly increase the risk for serotonin syndrome. Accordingly, use of MAOIs with SSRIs is *contraindicated.* Because MAOIs cause *irreversible* inhibition of monoamine oxidase (MAO; see later), their effects persist long after dosing stops. Therefore MAOIs should be withdrawn at least 14 days before starting an SSRI. Because fluoxetine and its active metabolite have long half-lives, at least 5 weeks should elapse between stopping fluoxetine and starting an MAOI. For other SSRIs, at least 2 weeks should elapse between treatment cessation and starting an MAOI.

Other drugs that increase the risk for serotonin syndrome include the serotonergic drugs listed in Table 25.3, drugs that inhibit CYP2D6 (and thereby raise fluoxetine levels), tramadol (an analgesic), and linezolid (an antibiotic that inhibits MAO).

TABLE 25.3 ■ Drugs That Promote Activation of Serotonin Receptors

Drug	Mechanism
SELECTIVE SEROTONIN REUPTAKE INHIBITORS (SSRIS)	
Citalopram [Celexa] Escitalopram [Lexapro, Cipralex ♣] Fluoxetine [Prozac] Fluvoxamine [Luvox] Paroxetine [Paxil] Sertraline [Zoloft]	Block 5-HT reuptake and thereby increase 5-HT in the synapse
SEROTONIN/NOREPINEPHRINE REUPTAKE INHIBITORS (SNRIS)	
Desvenlafaxine [Pristiq] Duloxetine [Cymbalta] Venlafaxine [Effexor XR] Levomilnacipran [Fetzima]	Same as SSRIs
TRICYCLIC ANTIDEPRESSANTS (TCAS)	
Amitriptyline Clomipramine [Anafranil] Desipramine [Norpramin] Doxepin [Sinequan] Imipramine [Tofranil] Trimipramine [Surmontil]	Same as SSRIs
MONOAMINE OXIDASE INHIBITORS (MAOIS)	
Isocarboxazid [Marplan] Phenelzine [Nardil] Selegiline [Emsam]	Inhibit neuronal breakdown of 5-HT by MAO and thereby increase stores of 5-HT available for release
ATYPICAL ANTIDEPRESSANTS	
Mirtazapine [Remeron]	Promotes release of 5-HT
Nefazodone	Same as SSRIs
Trazodone [Oleptro]	Same as SSRIs
ANALGESICS	
Meperidine [Demerol]	Same as SSRIs *and* MAOIs
Methadone [Dolophine]	Same as SSRIs *and* MAOIs
Tramadol [Ultram]	Same as SSRIs
TRIPTAN ANTIMIGRAINE DRUGS	
Almotriptan [Axert] Eletriptan [Relpax] Frovatriptan [Frova] Rizatriptan [Maxalt] Sumatriptan [Imitrex] Zolmitriptan [Zomig]	Cause direct activation of serotonin receptors
OTHERS	
St. John's wort	Same as SSRIs *and* MAOIs
Linezolid [Zyvox]	Same as MAOIs

5-HT, 5-hydroxytryptamine (serotonin); MAO, monoamine oxidase.

Tricyclic Antidepressants and Lithium. Fluoxetine can elevate plasma levels of TCAs and lithium. Exercise caution if fluoxetine is combined with these agents.

Antiplatelet Drugs and Anticoagulants. Antiplatelet drugs (e.g., aspirin, NSAIDs) and anticoagulants (e.g., warfarin) increase the risk for GI bleeding. Exercise caution if fluoxetine is combined with these drugs.

The risk for bleeding with *warfarin* is compounded by a pharmacokinetic interaction. Because fluoxetine is highly bound to plasma proteins, it can displace other highly bound drugs. Displacement of warfarin is of particular concern. Monitor responses to warfarin closely.

Drugs That Are Substrates for or Inhibitors of CYP2D6. Fluoxetine and most other SSRIs are inactivated by CYP2D6. Accordingly, drugs that inhibit this enzyme can raise SSRI levels, thereby posing a risk for toxicity.

In addition to being a substrate for CYP2D6, fluoxetine itself can inhibit CYP2D6. As a result, fluoxetine can raise levels of other drugs that are CYP2D6 substrates. Among these are TCAs, several antipsychotics, and two antidysrhythmics: propafenone and flecainide. Combined use of fluoxetine with these drugs should be done with caution.

Other Selective Serotonin Reuptake Inhibitors

In addition to fluoxetine, five other SSRIs are available: citalopram [Celexa], escitalopram [Lexapro, Cipralex ♣], fluvoxamine [Luvox], paroxetine [Paxil, Pexeva], and sertraline [Zoloft]. All five are similar to fluoxetine. Antidepressant effects equal those of TCAs. Characteristic side effects are nausea, insomnia, headache, nervousness, weight gain, sexual dysfunction, hyponatremia, GI bleeding, and NAS and PPHN (in infants who were exposed to these drugs late in gestation). Serotonin syndrome is a potential complication with all SSRIs, especially if these agents are combined with MAOIs or other serotonergic drugs. The principal differences among the SSRIs relate to duration of action. Patients who experience intolerable adverse effects with one SSRI may find a different SSRI more acceptable. As with fluoxetine, withdrawal should be done slowly. In contrast to the TCAs, the SSRIs do not cause hypotension or anticholinergic effects and, with the exception of fluvoxamine, do not cause sedation. When taken in overdose, these drugs do not cause cardiotoxicity. Therapeutic uses for individual SSRIs are shown in Table 25.2.

Sertraline

Sertraline [Zoloft] is much like fluoxetine: both drugs block reuptake of 5-HT, both relieve symptoms of major depression, both cause CNS stimulation rather than sedation, and both have minimal effects on seizure threshold and the electrocardiogram (ECG). Sertraline is indicated for major depression, panic disorder, obsessive-compulsive disorder, posttraumatic stress disorder, premenstrual dysphoric disorder, and social anxiety disorder. Sertraline is slowly absorbed after oral administration. Food increases the extent of absorption. In the blood, the drug is highly bound (99%) to plasma proteins. Sertraline undergoes extensive hepatic metabolism followed by elimination in the urine and feces. The plasma half-life is approximately 1 day.

Common side effects include headache, tremor, insomnia, agitation, nervousness, nausea, diarrhea, weight gain, and sexual dysfunction. Treatment may also increase the risk for suicide. Because of the risk for serotonin syndrome, sertraline must not be combined with MAOIs and other serotonergic drugs (see Table 25.3). MAOIs should be withdrawn at least 14 days before starting sertraline, and sertraline should be withdrawn at least 14 days before starting an MAOI. Because of a risk for pimozide-induced dysrhythmias, sertraline (which raises pimozide levels) and pimozide should not be combined. Like fluoxetine and other SSRIs, sertraline poses a risk for hyponatremia, GI bleeding, and NAS and PPHN when used late in pregnancy.

Fluvoxamine

Like other SSRIs, fluvoxamine [Luvox] produces powerful and selective inhibition of 5-HT reuptake. The drug is approved for obsessive-compulsive disorder, major depressive disorder, bulimia, and panic disorder. Fluvoxamine is rapidly absorbed from the GI tract, in both the presence and absence of food. The drug undergoes extensive hepatic metabolism followed by excretion in the urine. The half-life is about 15 hours.

Common side effects include nausea, vomiting, dry mouth, headache, constipation, weight gain, and sexual dysfunction. In contrast to other SSRIs, fluvoxamine has moderate sedative effects, although it nonetheless can cause insomnia. Some patients have developed abnormal liver function tests. Accordingly, liver function should be assessed before treatment and weekly during the first month of therapy. Like other SSRIs, fluvoxamine interacts adversely with MAOIs and other serotonergic drugs, and hence these combinations must be avoided. As with other SSRIs, fluvoxamine poses a risk for hyponatremia, GI bleeding, and NAS and PPHN in infants exposed to the drug in utero.

Paroxetine

Like other SSRIs, paroxetine [Paxil, Paxil CR, Pexeva] produces powerful and selective inhibition of 5-HT reuptake. The drug is indicated for major depression, obsessive-compulsive disorder, social anxiety disorder, panic disorder, generalized anxiety disorder, posttraumatic stress disorder, premenstrual dysphoric disorder, and postmenopausal vasomotor symptoms (hot flashes). Paroxetine is well absorbed after oral administration, even in the presence of food. The drug is widely distributed and highly bound (95%) to plasma proteins. Concentrations in breast milk equal those in plasma. The drug undergoes hepatic metabolism followed by renal excretion. The half-life is about 20 hours.

Side effects are dose dependent and generally mild. Early reactions include nausea, somnolence, sweating, tremor, and fatigue. These tend to diminish over time. After 5 to 6 weeks, the major complaints are headache, weight gain, and sexual dysfunction. Like fluoxetine, paroxetine causes signs of CNS stimulation (increased awakenings, reduced time in rapid-eye-movement sleep, insomnia). In contrast to TCAs, paroxetine has no effect on heart rate, blood pressure, or the ECG—but does have some antimuscarinic effects. Like other SSRIs, paroxetine interacts adversely with MAOIs and other serotonergic drugs, and hence these combinations must be avoided. Also, like other SSRIs, paroxetine can increase the risk for GI bleeding and can cause hyponatremia (especially in older-adult patients taking thiazide diuretics). As with other SSRIs, use late in pregnancy can result in NAS and PPHN. In addition, paroxetine, but not other SSRIs (except possibly fluoxetine), poses a small risk for cardiovascular birth defects, primarily ventricular septal defects. Because of this risk, the drug is classified by the U.S. Food and Drug Administration as Pregnancy Risk Category D. Like all other antidepressants, paroxetine may increase the risk for suicide, especially in children and young adults.

Citalopram

Citalopram [Celexa] is very similar to fluoxetine and the other SSRIs. Benefits derive from selective blockade of 5-HT reuptake. The drug does not block receptors for acetylcholine, NE, or histamine. Its only approved indication is major depression. Citalopram is rapidly absorbed from the GI tract, in both the presence and absence of food. Plasma levels peak about 4 hours after dosing. The drug undergoes hepatic metabolism followed by excretion in the urine and feces. The half-life is about 35 hours.

The most common adverse effects are nausea, somnolence, dry mouth, and sexual dysfunction. Additional side effects include weight gain, tachycardia, postural hypotension, headache, paresthesias, hyponatremia, and increased risk for GI bleeding. Large doses are teratogenic in animals. Citalopram enters breast milk in amounts sufficient to cause somnolence, reduced feeding, and weight loss in the infant. Use late in pregnancy can result in NAS and PPHN in the infant. Like all other antidepressants, citalopram may increase the risk for suicide, especially in children and young adults.

Citalopram prolongs the QT interval and hence may pose a risk for fatal dysrhythmias, especially when the dosage exceeds 40 mg/day. Risk is increased in patients with heart disease, long QT syndrome, and low blood levels of potassium and magnesium. Because of the risk for serotonin syndrome, citalopram should not be combined with MAOIs or other serotonergic drugs. Allow at least 14 days to pass between stopping an MAOI and starting citalopram, or vice versa.

Escitalopram

Escitalopram [Lexapro, Cipralex ♣] is the S-isomer of citalopram [Celexa], which is a 50 : 50 mixture of S- and R-isomers. The S-isomer (escitalopram) is responsible for antidepressant effects. The R-isomer has no antidepressant actions but does contribute to side effects. Accordingly, escitalopram retains the therapeutic benefits of citalopram but may be better tolerated. Otherwise, the pharmacology of the two drugs is largely the same. Escitalopram is approved for major depression and generalized anxiety disorder and has additional indication for treatment of obsessive-compulsive disorder in Canada. Like citalopram and other SSRIs, escitalopram is generally well tolerated. In clinical trials, the most common side effects were nausea, insomnia, somnolence, sweating, and fatigue. In addition, 9% of males reported ejaculatory disorders. However, the true incidence of sexual

PATIENT-CENTERED CARE ACROSS THE LIFE SPAN

Antidepressants

Life Stage	Patient Care Concerns
Infants	Use of SSRIs in late pregnancy poses a small risk for NAS, characterized by abnormal crying, irritability, tremor, and possible seizures.
Children/adolescents	Antidepressants may increase the risk for suicide, especially during the early phase of treatment.
Pregnant women	Use of SSRIs late in pregnancy may promote PPHN.
Breast-feeding women	Antidepressants are generally safe in breastfeeding women. Sertraline has been shown to be especially safe.
Older adults	Treatment with SSRIs or SNRIs is generally safe, providing less medication interaction and smaller side-effect profiles.

NAS, neonatal abstinence syndrome; PPHN, persistent pulmonary hypertension of the newborn; SNRI, serotonin-norepinephrine reuptake inhibitor; SSRI, selective serotonin reuptake inhibitor.

dysfunction may be higher because the incidence of sexual problems reported during clinical trials is usually considerably lower than the incidence seen in actual practice. As with other SSRIs, combined use with MAOIs and other serotonergic drugs increases the risk for serotonin syndrome. At least 14 days should separate use of MAOIs and escitalopram. Like citalopram and other SSRIs, escitalopram increases the risk for hyponatremia and GI bleeding and, when used late in pregnancy, may cause NAS or PPHN in the newborn. Like all other antidepressants, this drug can increase the risk for suicide, especially in children and young adults.

Serotonin-Norepinephrine Reuptake Inhibitors

Four drugs—venlafaxine, desvenlafaxine, duloxetine, and levomilnacipran—block neuronal reuptake of serotonin and NE, with minimal effects on other transmitters or receptors. Pharmacologic effects are similar to those of the SSRIs, although the SSRIs may be better tolerated. The SNRIs are indicated for major depression as well as other disorders (see Table 25.2).

Venlafaxine

Venlafaxine [Effexor XR], the first SNRI available, is approved for major depression, generalized anxiety disorder, social anxiety disorder, and panic disorder. The drug produces powerful blockade of NE and 5-HT reuptake and weak blockade of dopamine reuptake. The relationship of these actions to therapeutic effects is uncertain. Venlafaxine does not block cholinergic, histaminergic, or alpha$_1$-adrenergic receptors. Despite impressions that venlafaxine may be superior to SSRIs, when compared directly in clinical trials, the drugs were about equally effective—and SSRIs are probably safer.

Venlafaxine is well absorbed after oral administration, in both the presence and absence of food. In the liver, much of each dose is converted to desvenlafaxine, an active metabolite. The half-life is 5 hours for the parent drug and 11 hours for the active metabolite.

Venlafaxine can cause a variety of adverse effects. The most common is nausea (37%–58%), followed by headache, anorexia, nervousness, sweating, somnolence, and insomnia. Dose-dependent weight loss may occur secondary to anorexia. Venlafaxine can also cause dose-related sustained diastolic hypertension; blood pressure should be monitored. Sexual dysfunction may occur too. Some patients experience sustained mydriasis, which can increase the risk for eye injury in those with elevated intraocular pressure or glaucoma. Like the SSRIs, venlafaxine can cause hyponatremia, especially in older-adult patients taking diuretics. Like all other antidepressants, venlafaxine may increase the risk for suicide, especially in children and young adults.

Combined use of venlafaxine with MAOIs and other serotonergic drugs (see Table 25.3) increases the risk for serotonin syndrome, a potentially fatal reaction. If the clinical situation demands, venlafaxine may be cautiously combined with an SSRI or another SNRI. However, combined use with an MAOI is contraindicated. Accordingly, MAOIs should be withdrawn at least 14 days before starting venlafaxine. When switching from venlafaxine to an MAOI, venlafaxine should be discontinued 7 days before starting the MAOI.

As with the SSRIs, use of venlafaxine late in pregnancy can result in a neonatal withdrawal syndrome, characterized by irritability, abnormal crying, tremor, respiratory distress, and possibly seizures. Symptoms, which can be managed with supportive care, generally abate within a few days.

Abrupt discontinuation can cause an intense withdrawal syndrome. Symptoms include anxiety, agitation, tremors, headache, vertigo, nausea, tachycardia, and tinnitus. Worsening of pretreatment symptoms may also occur. Withdrawal symptoms can be minimized by tapering the dosage over 2 to 4 weeks. Warn patients not to stop venlafaxine abruptly.

Desvenlafaxine

Desvenlafaxine [Pristiq, Khedezla] is the major active metabolite of venlafaxine. Accordingly, the actions and adverse effects of both drugs are similar. Like venlafaxine, desvenlafaxine is a strong inhibitor of 5-HT and NE reuptake and does not block cholinergic, histaminergic, or alpha$_1$-adrenergic receptors. At this time, desvenlafaxine is approved only for major depression, in contrast to venlafaxine, which is approved for major depression, generalized anxiety disorder, panic disorder, and social phobia.

Desvenlafaxine is well absorbed after oral administration, in both the presence and absence of food. Plasma levels peak about 7.5 hours after dosing. The drug undergoes some hepatic metabolism and is excreted in the urine as metabolites and parent drug. The elimination half-life is 11 hours.

Adverse effects are like those of venlafaxine. The most common are nausea, headache, dizziness, insomnia, diarrhea, dry mouth, sweating, and constipation. Sexual effects include erectile dysfunction and decreased libido. Like all other antidepressants, desvenlafaxine may increase the risk for suicide in children and young adults. Some neonates exposed to the drug in utero have required prolonged hospitalization, respiratory support, and tube feeding. Additional concerns include hyponatremia, sustained hypertension, serotonin syndrome, bleeding, seizures, and withdrawal symptoms if the drug is discontinued abruptly.

As with venlafaxine, combining desvenlafaxine with another serotonergic drug increases the risk for serotonin syndrome. Combined use with an SSRI or another SNRI may be done cautiously. In contrast, combined use with an MAOI is contraindicated. Accordingly, MAOIs should be withdrawn at least 14 days before starting desvenlafaxine, and desvenlafaxine should be withdrawn at least 7 days before starting an MAOI.

Duloxetine

Mechanism of Action and Therapeutic Uses

Duloxetine [Cymbalta] was the second SNRI approved for major depression. The drug is a powerful inhibitor of 5-HT and NE reuptake and a much weaker inhibitor of dopamine reuptake. Duloxetine does not bind with receptors for NE, serotonin, dopamine, acetylcholine, or histamine and does not inhibit MAO.

Data on the antidepressant effects of duloxetine are limited. Clinical trials have shown that duloxetine is clearly superior to placebo: treatment reduces depressive symptoms and may also reduce physical pain associated with depression (e.g., backache). Furthermore, benefits may develop quickly, in some cases within 2 weeks of starting treatment. Limited studies have compared duloxetine to SSRIs (fluoxetine and escitalopram) as well as to venlafaxine and desvenlafaxine. There does not appear to be any difference in efficacy when treating depression with duloxetine. In addition, duloxetine seems less well tolerated than the other medications commonly used to treat depression. As a result, there is no basis for choosing duloxetine over other antidepressants.

Pharmacokinetics

Duloxetine is well absorbed after oral dosing. Food reduces the rate of absorption but not the extent. In the blood, duloxetine is highly (90%) bound to albumin. The drug undergoes extensive hepatic metabolism, primarily by the CYP2D6 and CYP1A2 isoenzymes of cytochrome P450. Metabolites are excreted in the urine (70%) and feces (20%). The elimination half-life is 12 hours. In patients with severe renal impairment, levels of duloxetine and its metabolites are greatly increased, and in those with severe hepatic impairment, the half-life is greatly prolonged. Accordingly, duloxetine is not recommended for patients with severe renal or hepatic dysfunction.

Adverse Effects

Duloxetine is generally well tolerated. In clinical trials, the most common adverse effects were nausea, dry mouth, insomnia, somnolence, constipation, reduced appetite, fatigue, increased sweating, and blurred vision. Duloxetine can cause a small increase in blood pressure, and hence blood pressure should be measured at baseline and periodically thereafter. Duloxetine promotes mydriasis and thus should not be used by patients with uncontrolled narrow-angle glaucoma.

Liver toxicity is a concern. Elevation of serum transaminases, indicating liver damage, occurs in about 1% of patients. There have been reports of hepatitis, hepatomegaly, cholestatic jaundice, and elevation of transaminases to more than 20 times the upper limit of normal. To reduce risk, duloxetine should not be given to patients with preexisting liver disease or to those who drink alcohol heavily.

As with venlafaxine, abrupt cessation of treatment can cause a withdrawal syndrome. Symptoms include nausea, vomiting, dizziness, headache, nightmares, and paresthesias. To minimize risk, duloxetine should be withdrawn slowly. Like all other antidepressants, duloxetine may increase the risk for suicide, especially in children and young adults.

Effects in Pregnancy and Lactation

Animal studies indicate that duloxetine interferes with fetal and postnatal development, causing reduced fetal weight, decreased postnatal survival, and neurologic disturbances. Use of duloxetine late in pregnancy can also lead to withdrawal syndrome in the infant. The drug is excreted in the milk of lactating rats. Two studies are currently recruiting pregnant and/or lactating women to examine these effects further. One completed study found duloxetine in the breast milk of six lactating women who received 40 mg twice daily for 3.5 days; the daily infant dose was minimal. However, until the larger studies are completed, use of duloxetine during pregnancy and lactation is not recommended.

Drug Interactions

The combination of duloxetine with heavy alcohol consumption greatly increases the risk for liver damage. Accordingly, duloxetine should not be prescribed to patients with substantial alcohol intake.

Like venlafaxine and other drugs that block 5-HT reuptake, duloxetine can cause serotonin syndrome if combined with an MAOI or any other serotonergic drug. MAOIs should be withdrawn at least 14 days before starting duloxetine, and duloxetine should be withdrawn at least 5 days before starting an MAOI.

Drugs that inhibit CYP1A2 or CYP2D6 can increase duloxetine levels and may thereby cause toxicity. Inhibitors of CYP1A2 include cimetidine [Tagamet], fluvoxamine [Luvox], and ciprofloxacin [Cipro]. Inhibitors of CYP2D6 include fluoxetine [Prozac], paroxetine [Paxil], and quinidine.

Duloxetine is a moderate inhibitor of CYP2D6 and hence may raise levels of drugs that are extensively metabolized by this enzyme. Among these are certain TCAs (e.g., amitriptyline, nortriptyline), type IC antidysrhythmics (propafenone [Rythmol] and flecainide [Tambocor]), and phenothiazines, including thioridazine. Interaction with thioridazine is of special concern owing to a risk for serious ventricular dysrhythmias. Accordingly, the two drugs should not be combined.

Levomilnacipran

Levomilnacipran [Fetzima] is an SNRI approved for major depressive disorder in 2013. In clinical studies, patients taking levomilnacipran showed significant clinical improvement in depressive symptoms. Side effects were similar to those of the other SNRIs, including erectile dysfunction, constipation, and nausea.

Tricyclic Antidepressants

The first TCA—imipramine—was introduced to psychiatry in the late 1950s. Since then, the ability of TCAs to relieve depressive symptoms has been firmly established. For decades, TCAs were drugs of first choice for depression. However, owing to the development of safer alternatives, especially the SSRIs, use of TCAs has greatly declined. The most common adverse effects are sedation, orthostatic hypotension, and anticholinergic effects. The most dangerous effect is cardiac toxicity. When taken in overdose, TCAs can readily prove lethal. Like all other antidepressants, TCAs may increase the risk for suicide. Because all of the TCAs have similar properties, we will discuss these drugs as a group, rather than focusing on a representative prototype.

Chemistry

The structure of imipramine, a representative TCA, is very similar to the structure of the phenothiazine antipsychotics. Because of this similarity, TCAs and phenothiazines have several actions in common. Specifically, both groups produce varying degrees of *sedation, orthostatic hypotension,* and *anticholinergic effects.*

Mechanism of Action

The TCAs block neuronal reuptake of two monoamine transmitters: NE and 5-HT. As a result, TCAs increase the concentration of these transmitters at CNS synapses and thereby intensify their effects. As indicated in Table 25.4, some TCAs block reuptake of NE *and* 5-HT, whereas others only block reuptake of NE. As with the SSRIs, biochemical effects (blockade of transmitter reuptake) occur within hours, whereas therapeutic effects (relief of depression) develop over several weeks. This delay suggests that antidepressant effects are due to adaptive changes brought on by prolonged reuptake blockade, and not to reuptake blockade directly.

Pharmacokinetics

The half-lives of TCAs are long and variable. Because their half-lives are long, TCAs can usually be administered in a single daily dose. Because their half-lives are variable, TCAs require individualization of dosage.

Therapeutic Uses

Depression

TCAs are effective agents for major depression. These drugs can elevate mood, increase activity and alertness, decrease morbid preoccupation, improve appetite, and normalize sleep patterns. Despite their efficacy, TCAs are generally considered second-line drugs, owing to the development of safer and better tolerated alternatives.

Fibromyalgia Syndrome

Fibromyalgia syndrome is a chronic disorder characterized by diffuse musculoskeletal pain, profound fatigue, disturbed sleep, and cognitive dysfunction. TCAs are the most effective drugs we have for reducing symptoms.

Other Uses

TCAs can benefit patients with neuropathic pain (see Chapter 83), chronic insomnia (see Chapter 27), attention-deficit/hyperactivity disorder (see Chapter 29), and panic disorder or obsessive-compulsive disorder (see Chapter 28).

Adverse Effects

The most common adverse effects are orthostatic hypotension, sedation, and anticholinergic effects. The most serious adverse effect is cardiotoxicity. These effects occur because, in addition to blocking reuptake of NE and 5-HT, TCAs cause

TABLE 25.4 ▪ Antidepressants: Adverse Effects and Impact on Neurotransmitters

	Transmitters Affected[a]	Agitation/ Insomnia	Anticholinergic Activity	Sedation	Hypotension	Seizure Risk	Cardiac Toxicity	Weight Gain	Sexual Dysfunction	Other Side Effects
SELECTIVE SEROTONIN REUPTAKE INHIBITORS (SSRIS)										
Citalopram	5-HT	++	0/+		0	0/+	0	+	+++	GI bleeding, hyponatremia, NAS and PPHN in newborns. Citalopram may cause dysrhythmias.[c]
Escitalopram	5-HT	++	0/+	0/+	0	0/+	0	+	+++	
Fluoxetine	5-HT	++	0	[b]	0	0/+	0/+	+	+++	
Fluvoxamine	5-HT	++	0/+	0/+	0	0/+		+	+++	
Paroxetine	5-HT	++	0/+	[b]	0	0/+	0	+	+++	
Sertraline	5-HT	++	0	[b]	0	0/+	0	+	+++	
SEROTONIN-NOREPINEPHRINE REUPTAKE INHIBITORS (SNRIS)										
Desvenlafaxine	NE, 5-HT	++	0	0	0	0/+	0/+	0	++	
Duloxetine	NE, 5-HT	++	0	0	0/+	0/+	0/+	0/+	+	Hepatotoxicity
Venlafaxine	NE, 5-HT	++	0	0	0	0/+	0/+	0	+++	
Levomilnacipran	NE, 5-HT	++	0	0	0	[d]	0/+	0	++	Hyponatremia
TRICYCLIC ANTIDEPRESSANTS (TCAS)										
Amitriptyline	NE, 5-HT	0/+	++++	+++	++	++	+++	+++	++	
Clomipramine	NE, 5-HT	+	++	++	++	+++	+++	++	++	
Doxepin	NE, 5-HT	0/+	++	+++	++	++	+++	+++	++	
Imipramine	NE, 5-HT	+	++	++	++	++	+++	++	++	
Trimipramine	NE, 5-HT	0/+	+++	+++	++	++	+++	++	++	
Desipramine	NE	+	+	[b]	+	+++	+++	+	++	
Maprotiline	NE	+	++	++	+	+++	++	+	++	
Nortriptyline	NE	+	+	+	+	+	++	++	++	
Protriptyline	NE	++	++	[b]	+	++	+++	+	++	
MONOAMINE OXIDASE INHIBITORS (MAOIS)										
Isocarboxazid	NE, 5-HT, DA	++	0	+	+	0	0	+	++	Hypertensive crisis from tyramine in food[e]
Phenelzine	NE, 5-HT, DA	++	0	+	+	0	0	+	++	
Selegiline	NE, 5-HT, DA	++	0	0	0	0	0	0	+	
Tranylcypromine	NE, 5-HT, DA	++	0	[b]	+	0	0	+	++	
ATYPICAL ANTIDEPRESSANTS										
Amoxapine	NE, ↓DA[f]	0/+	+	+	+	++	++	+	++	Parkinsonism
Bupropion	DA	++	0/+	[b]	0	+++	0	0	[g]	Seizures
Mirtazapine	NE, 5-HT	0/+	0/+	++++	0/+	0	0	++++	0	
Nefazodone	5-HT	0/+	0/+	++	0	0	0/+	0/+	0/+	
Trazodone	5-HT	0/+	0/+	++++	+	0	0/+	+	+[h]	Priapism
Vilazodone	5-HT	++	0	++	0	0	0	0	++	Bleeding, hyponatremia

[a]All of the antidepressants *increase* synaptic activity of the transmitters indicated—with the exception of amoxapine, which increases activity of NE, but *blocks* receptors for DA. The TCAs, SSRIs, SNRIs, amoxapine, bupropion, nefazodone, and trazodone decrease transmitter reuptake; vilazodone blocks transmitter reuptake and directly activates 5-HT receptors; MAOIs block transmitter breakdown; and mirtazapine promotes transmitter release.
[b]Produces moderate *stimulation,* not sedation.
[c]NAS, neonatal abstinence syndrome; PPHN, persistent pulmonary hypertension of the newborn.
[d]Levomilnacipran was not tested in patients with seizure disorders.
[e]Hypertensive crisis is not a risk with low-dose (6 mg/day) transdermal selegiline, and possibly not with higher doses.
[f]Amoxapine blocks *reuptake* of NE and blocks *receptors* for DA.
[g]Bupropion may increase sexual desire.
[h]Trazodone can cause priapism (persistent painful erection).
DA, dopamine; 5-HT, 5-hydroxytryptamine (serotonin); NE, norepinephrine.

Patient Education

ORTHOSTATIC HYPOTENSION

Patients should be informed that they can minimize orthostatic hypotension by moving slowly when assuming an upright posture. In addition, patients should be instructed to sit or lie down if symptoms (dizziness, lightheadedness) occur.

direct blockade of receptors for histamine, acetylcholine, and NE. Adverse effects of individual agents are shown in Table 25.4.

Orthostatic Hypotension

Orthostatic hypotension is the most serious of the common adverse responses to TCAs. Hypotension is due in large part to blockade of alpha$_1$-adrenergic receptors on blood vessels.

Anticholinergic Effects

The TCAs block muscarinic cholinergic receptors and can thereby cause an array of anticholinergic effects (dry mouth, blurred vision, photophobia, constipation, urinary hesitancy, and tachycardia). Patients should be informed about possible anticholinergic responses and instructed in ways to minimize discomfort. A detailed discussion of anticholinergic effects and their management is presented in Chapter 122.

Diaphoresis

Despite their anticholinergic properties, TCAs often cause diaphoresis (sweating). The mechanism of this paradoxical effect is unknown.

Sedation

Sedation is a common response to TCAs. The cause is blockade of histamine receptors in the CNS. Patients should be advised to avoid hazardous activities if sedation is prominent.

Cardiac Toxicity

Tricyclics can adversely affect cardiac function. However, in the absence of an overdose or preexisting cardiac impairment, serious effects are rare. The TCAs affect the heart by (1) decreasing vagal influence on the heart (secondary to muscarinic blockade) and (2) acting directly on the bundle of His to slow conduction. Both effects increase the risk of dysrhythmias. To minimize risk, all patients should undergo ECG evaluation before treatment and periodically thereafter. Risk for cardiac toxicity may be higher with desipramine than with other TCAs.

Seizures

TCAs lower seizure threshold and thereby increase seizure risk. Exercise caution in patients with seizure disorders.

BLACK BOX WARNING: SUICIDE RISK WITH TRICYCLIC ANTIDEPRESSANTS

Tricyclic antidepressants and all other antidepressants may increase the risk for suicide in depressed patients, especially during the early phase of treatment. The risk for antidepressant-induced suicide is greatest among children, adolescents, and young adults.

Drug Interactions

Monoamine Oxidase Inhibitors

The combination of a TCA with an MAOI can lead to *severe hypertension,* owing to excessive adrenergic stimulation of the heart and blood vessels. Excessive adrenergic stimulation occurs because (1) inhibition of MAO causes accumulation of NE in adrenergic neurons and (2) blockade of NE reuptake by the tricyclics decreases NE inactivation. Because of the potential for hypertensive crisis, combined therapy with TCAs and MAOIs is generally avoided.

Direct-Acting Sympathomimetic Drugs

Tricyclics *potentiate* responses to direct-acting sympathomimetics (i.e., drugs such as epinephrine and dopamine that produce their effects by direct interaction with adrenergic receptors). Because TCAs block uptake of these agents into adrenergic nerve terminals, they prolong the presence of these agents in the synaptic space.

Indirect-Acting Sympathomimetic Drugs

TCAs *decrease* responses to indirect-acting sympathomimetics (i.e., drugs such as ephedrine and amphetamine that promote release of transmitter from adrenergic nerves). TCAs block uptake of these agents into adrenergic nerves, thereby preventing them from reaching their site of action within the nerve terminal.

Anticholinergic Agents

Because TCAs have anticholinergic actions of their own, they will intensify the effects of other anticholinergic medications. Consequently, patients receiving TCAs should be advised to avoid all other drugs with anticholinergic properties, including antihistamines and certain over-the-counter sleep aids.

CNS Depressants.

CNS depression caused by TCAs will add with CNS depression caused by other drugs. Accordingly, patients should be warned against taking all other CNS depressants, including alcohol, antihistamines, opioids, and barbiturates.

Toxicity

Overdose with a TCA can be life threatening. The lethal dose is only 8 times the average therapeutic dose. To minimize the risk for death by suicide, acutely depressed patients should be given no more than a 1-week supply of their TCA at a time.

Clinical Manifestations

Symptoms result primarily from anticholinergic and cardiotoxic actions. The combination of cholinergic blockade and direct cardiotoxicity can produce *dysrhythmias,* including tachycardia, intraventricular blocks, complete atrioventricular block, ventricular tachycardia, and ventricular fibrillation. Responses to peripheral muscarinic blockade include hyperthermia, flushing, dry mouth, and dilation of the pupils. CNS symptoms are prominent. Early responses are confusion, agitation, and hallucinations. Seizures and coma may follow.

Treatment

Absorption of ingested drug can be reduced with gastric lavage followed by administration of activated charcoal within 2 hours of ingestion. Intravenous administration of sodium bicarbonate is recommended to control dysrhythmias caused by cardiac toxicity. Dysrhythmias should not be treated with procainamide or quinidine because these drugs cause cardiac depression.

Dosage and Routes of Administration

All TCAs can be administered by mouth. Dosages for individual TCAs are shown in Table 25.1. General guidelines for dosing are discussed later.

Initial doses of TCAs should be low (e.g., 75 mg of imipramine a day for adult outpatients). Low initial doses minimize adverse reactions and thereby help promote adherence. High initial doses are both undesirable and unnecessary. High doses are undesirable in that they pose an increased risk for adverse reactions. They are unnecessary in that onset of therapeutic effects is delayed regardless of dosage, and hence aggressive initial dosing offers no benefit.

Because of interpatient variability in TCA metabolism, dosing is highly individualized. As a rule, dosage is adjusted on the basis of clinical response. However, if there is no observable response, plasma drug levels can be used as a guide. After an effective dosage has been established, most patients can take their entire daily dose at bedtime; the long half-lives of the TCAs make divided daily doses unnecessary. Once-a-day dosing at bedtime has three advantages: (1) it's easy, and hence facilitates adherence; (2) it promotes sleep by causing maximal sedation at night; and (3) it reduces the intensity of side effects during the day. If bedtime dosing causes residual sedation in the morning, dosing earlier in the evening can help. Although once-a-day dosing is generally desirable, not all patients can use this schedule. Older adults, for example, can be especially sensitive to the cardiotoxic actions of the tricyclics. As a result, if the entire daily dose were taken at one time, effects on the heart might be intolerable.

Preparations and Drug Selection

Preparations. In the United States nine TCAs are available (see Tables 25.1 and 25.4). All nine are equally effective. Principal differences among these drugs concern side effects (see Table 25.4).

Drug Selection. Selection among TCAs is based on side effects. For example, if the patient is experiencing insomnia, a drug with prominent sedative properties (e.g., doxepin) might be selected. Conversely, if daytime sedation is undesirable, a less sedating agent (e.g., desipramine) might be preferred. Older-adult patients with glaucoma or constipation and males with benign prostatic hypertrophy can be especially sensitive to anticholinergic effects. Hence, for these patients, a drug with weak anticholinergic properties (e.g., nortriptyline) would be appropriate.

Monoamine Oxidase Inhibitors

The MAOIs are second- or third-choice antidepressants for most patients. Although these drugs are as effective as the SSRIs and TCAs, they are more hazardous. The greatest concern is hypertensive crisis, which can be triggered by eating foods rich in tyramine. At this time, MAOIs are drugs of choice only for atypical depression. Three MAOIs—isocarboxazid [Marplan], phenelzine [Nardil], and tranylcypromine [Parnate]—are administered orally, and one—selegiline [Emsam]—is administered by transdermal patch.

Oral Monoamine Oxidase Inhibitors

Mechanism of Action

Before discussing the MAOIs, we need to discuss MAO itself. MAO is an enzyme found in the liver, the intestinal wall, and terminals of monoamine-containing neurons. The function of MAO in neurons is to convert monoamine neurotransmitters—NE, 5-HT, and dopamine—into inactive products. In the liver and intestine, MAO serves to inactivate tyramine and other biogenic amines in food. In addition, these enzymes inactivate biogenic amines administered as drugs.

The body has two forms of MAO, named MAO-A and MAO-B. In the brain, MAO-A inactivates NE and 5-HT, whereas MAO-B inactivates dopamine. In the intestine and liver, MAO-A acts on dietary tyramine and other compounds. All of the MAOIs used for depression are *nonselective.* That is, at *therapeutic* doses, they inhibit both MAO-A and MAO-B. One agent—selegiline (used for depression *and* Parkinson disease)—is selective for MAO-B at the low doses used for Parkinson disease, but is nonselective at the higher doses used for depression.

Antidepressant effects of the MAOIs result from inhibiting MAO-A in nerve terminals (Fig. 25.2). By inhibiting intraneuronal MAO-A, these drugs increase the amount of NE and 5-HT available for release, and thereby intensify transmission at noradrenergic and serotonergic junctions.

Note that antidepressant effects of the MAOIs cannot be fully explained by MAO inhibition alone. The biochemical action of MAOIs (inhibition of MAO) takes place rapidly, whereas the clinical response to MAOIs (relief of depression) develops slowly. In the interval between initial inhibition of MAO and relief of depression, secondary neurochemical events must be taking place. These secondary events, which have not been identified, are ultimately responsible for the beneficial response to treatment.

The MAOIs can act on MAO in two ways: reversibly and irreversibly. All of the MAOIs in current use cause *irreversible* inhibition. Because recovery from irreversible inhibition requires synthesis of new MAO molecules, effects of the irreversible inhibitors persist for about 2 weeks after drug withdrawal. In contrast, recovery from reversible inhibition is more rapid, occurring in 3 to 5 days.

Therapeutic Uses

Depression. MAOIs are equal to SSRIs and TCAs for relieving depression. However, because MAOIs can be hazardous, they are generally reserved for patients who have not responded to SSRIs, TCAs, and other safer drugs. Nonetheless, there *is* one group of patients—those with *atypical depression*—for whom MAOIs are the treatment of choice. As with other antidepressants, beneficial effects do not reach their peak for several weeks.

Adverse Effects

CNS Stimulation. MAOIs cause direct CNS stimulation (in addition to exerting antidepressant effects). Excessive stimulation can produce anxiety, insomnia, agitation, hypomania, and even mania.

Orthostatic Hypotension. Despite their ability to increase the NE content of peripheral sympathetic neurons, the MAOIs *reduce blood pressure* when administered in usual therapeutic doses. Patients should be informed about signs of hypotension (dizziness, lightheadedness) and advised to sit or lie down if

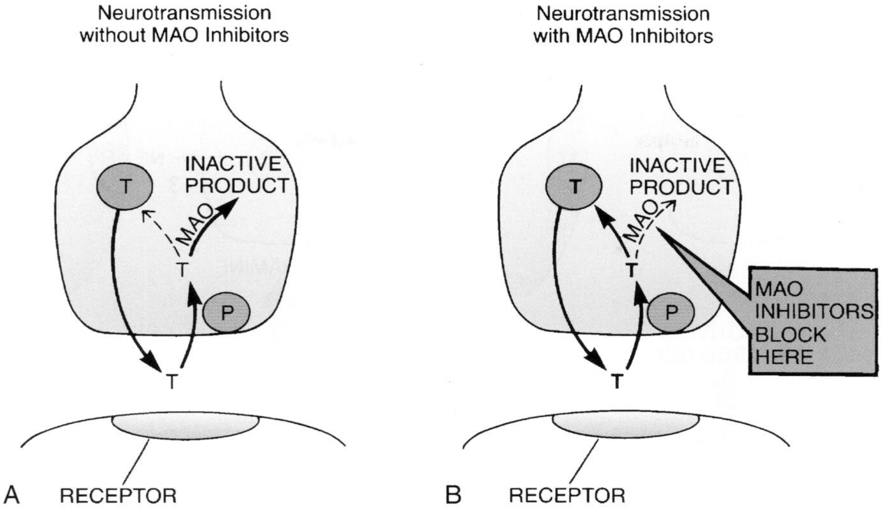

Figure 25.2 ■ Mechanism of action of monoamine oxidase inhibitors (MAOIs). **A,** Under drug-free conditions, much of the norepinephrine or serotonin that undergoes reuptake into nerve terminals becomes inactivated by monoamine oxidase (MAO). Inactivation helps maintain an appropriate concentration of transmitter within the terminal. **B,** MAOIs prevent inactivation of norepinephrine and serotonin, thereby increasing the amount of transmitter available for release. Release of supranormal amounts of transmitter intensifies transmission. (P, reuptake pump; T, transmitter [norepinephrine or serotonin].)

these occur. Also, they should be informed that hypotension can be minimized by moving slowly when assuming an erect posture.

MAOIs reduce blood pressure through actions in the CNS. The following sequence has been proposed: (1) Inhibition of MAO increases the NE content of neurons within the vasomotor center. (2) When NE is released, it binds to postsynaptic alpha receptors on neurons within the vasomotor center, thereby *decreasing* the firing rate of sympathetic nerves that control vascular tone. (3) This reduction in sympathetic activity results in vasodilation, causing blood pressure to fall.

Hypertensive Crisis From Dietary Tyramine. Although the MAOIs normally produce *hypotension,* they can be the cause of severe *hypertension* if the patient eats food that is rich in *tyramine,* a substance that promotes the release of NE from sympathetic neurons. Hypertensive crisis is characterized by severe headache, tachycardia, hypertension, nausea, vomiting, confusion, and profuse sweating—possibly leading to stroke and death.

Before considering the mechanism by which hypertensive crisis is produced, let's consider the effect of dietary tyramine under drug-free conditions. In the absence of MAO inhibition, dietary tyramine is not a threat. Much of the tyramine in food is metabolized by MAO in the intestinal wall. Furthermore, as shown in Fig. 25.3A, any dietary tyramine that gets through the intestinal wall intact will then pass directly to the liver through the hepatic portal circulation. When in the liver, tyramine is immediately inactivated by MAO there. Hence, as long as intestinal and hepatic MAO is functioning, dietary tyramine is prevented from reaching the general circulation and therefore is devoid of adverse effects.

In the presence of MAOIs, the picture is very different: Dietary tyramine can produce a life-threatening hypertensive crisis. Three steps are involved (Fig. 25.3B). First, inhibition of *neuronal* MAO augments NE levels within the terminals of sympathetic neurons that regulate cardiac function and vascular tone. Second, inhibition of *intestinal* and *hepatic* MAO allows dietary tyramine to pass directly through the intestinal wall and liver and then enter the systemic circulation intact. Third, on reaching peripheral sympathetic nerves, tyramine stimulates the release of the accumulated NE, thereby causing massive vasoconstriction and intense stimulation of the heart. Hypertensive crisis results. To reduce the risk for tyramine-induced hypertensive crisis, the following precautions must be taken:

- MAOIs must not be dispensed to patients considered incapable of rigid adherence to dietary restrictions.
- Before an MAOI is dispensed, the patient must be fully informed about the hazard of ingesting tyramine-rich foods.
- The patient must be given a detailed list of foods and beverages to avoid.
- The patient should be instructed to avoid all drugs not specifically approved by the prescriber.

Patient Education

HYPERTENSIVE CRISIS

Patients should be informed about the symptoms of hypertensive crisis (headache, tachycardia, palpitations, nausea, vomiting, sweating) and instructed to seek immediate medical attention if these develop.

In addition to tyramine, several other dietary constituents (e.g., caffeine, phenylethylamine) can precipitate hypertension in patients taking MAOIs. Foods that contain these compounds are listed in Table 25.5. Patients should be instructed to avoid them.

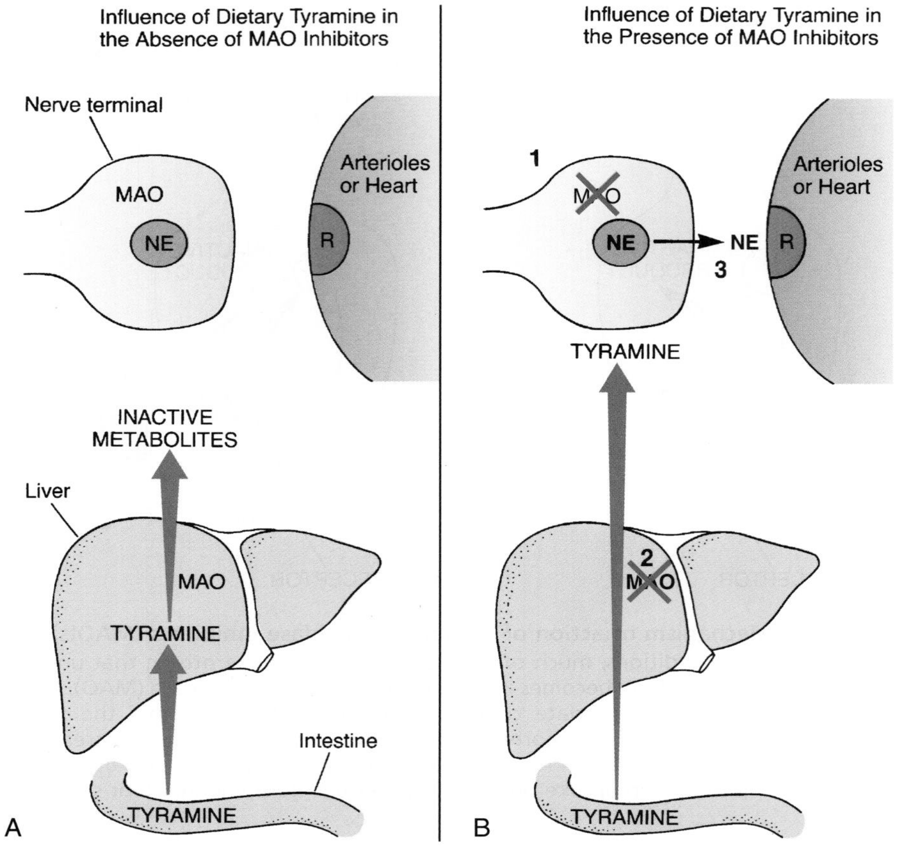

Figure 25.3 ▪ Interaction between dietary tyramine and monoamine oxidase inhibitors (MAOIs).

A, In the absence of MAOIs, much of ingested tyramine is inactivated by monoamine oxidase (MAO) in the intestinal wall (not shown in the figure). Any dietary tyramine that is not metabolized in the intestinal wall is transported directly to the liver, where it undergoes immediate inactivation by hepatic MAO. No tyramine reaches the general circulation. **B,** Three events occur in the presence of MAOIs: (1) Inhibition of neuronal MAO raises levels of norepinephrine in sympathetic nerve terminals. (2) Inhibition of intestinal and hepatic MAO allows dietary tyramine to pass through the intestinal wall and liver to enter the systemic circulation intact. (3) On reaching peripheral sympathetic nerve terminals, tyramine promotes the release of accumulated norepinephrine stores, thereby causing massive vasoconstriction and excessive stimulation of the heart. (NE, norepinephrine; R, receptor for norepinephrine.)

TABLE 25.5 ▪ Foods That Can Interact With Monoamine Oxidase Inhibitors

FOODS THAT CONTAIN TYRAMINE

Category	Foods With High Tyramine Content	Foods With Little or No Tyramine
Vegetables	Avocados, especially if overripe; fermented bean curd; fermented soybean; soybean paste	Most vegetables
Fruits	Figs, especially if overripe; bananas, in large amounts	Most fruits
Meats	Meats that are fermented, smoked, or otherwise aged; spoiled meats; liver, unless very fresh	Meats that are known to be fresh (exercise caution in restaurants; meat may not be fresh)
Sausages	Fermented varieties: bologna, pepperoni, salami, others	Nonfermented varieties
Fish	Dried or cured fish; fish that is fermented, smoked, or otherwise aged; spoiled fish	Fish that is known to be fresh; vacuum-packed fish, if eaten promptly or refrigerated only briefly after opening
Milk, milk products	Practically all cheeses	Milk, yogurt, cottage cheese, cream cheese
Foods with yeast	Yeast extract (e.g., Marmite, Bovril)	Baked goods that contain yeast
Beer, wine	Some imported beers, Chianti wine	Major domestic brands of beer, most wines
Other foods	Protein dietary supplements; soups (may contain protein extract); shrimp paste; soy sauce	

FOODS THAT CONTAIN NONTYRAMINE VASOPRESSORS

Food	Comments
Chocolate	Contains phenylethylamine, a pressor agent; large amounts can cause a reaction
Fava beans	Contain dopamine, a pressor agent; reactions are most likely with overripe beans
Ginseng	Headache, tremulousness, and manic-like reactions have occurred
Caffeinated beverages	Caffeine is a weak pressor agent; large amounts may cause a reaction

Drug Interactions

The MAOIs can interact with many drugs to cause potentially harmful results. Accordingly, *patients should be instructed to avoid all medications*—prescription drugs and over-the-counter drugs—that have not been specifically approved by the prescriber.

Indirect-Acting Sympathomimetic Agents. Indirect-acting sympathomimetics (e.g., ephedrine, amphetamine) are drugs that promote the release of NE from sympathetic nerves. In patients taking MAOIs, these drugs can produce *hypertensive crisis.* The mechanism is the same as that described for tyramine. Patients should be instructed to avoid all sympathomimetic drugs, including ephedrine, methylphenidate, amphetamines, and cocaine. Sympathomimetic agents may be present in cold remedies, nasal decongestants, and asthma medications; all of these should be avoided unless approved by the prescriber.

Interactions Secondary to Inhibition of Hepatic MAO. Inhibition of MAO in the liver can decrease the metabolism of several drugs, including epinephrine, NE, and dopamine. These drugs must be used with caution because their effects will be more intense and prolonged.

Tricyclic Antidepressants. The combination of a TCA with an MAOI may produce hypertensive episodes or hypertensive crisis. As a result, this combination of antidepressants is not employed routinely. However, although potentially dangerous, the combination can benefit certain patients. If concurrent use is employed, caution must be exercised.

Serotonergic Drugs. Combining MAOIs with SSRIs and other serotonergic drugs (see Table 25.3) poses a risk for serotonin syndrome. Accordingly, these combinations should be avoided.

Antihypertensive Drugs. Combined use of MAOIs and antihypertensive agents may result in excessive lowering of blood pressure.

Transdermal MAOI: Selegiline

Transdermal selegiline [Emsam] is the first and only transdermal treatment for major depression. Selegiline inhibits MAO-A as well as MAO-B. Like other MAOIs, selegiline should be reserved for patients who have not responded to preferred antidepressant drugs.

The pharmacology of transdermal selegiline is much like that of the oral MAOIs, but with one important difference: the risk for hypertensive crisis from dietary tyramine is much lower than with oral dosing. With transdermal dosing, selegiline enters the systemic circulation without first passing through the GI tract. As a result, it can achieve therapeutic levels in the CNS while preserving activity of MAO-A in the intestinal wall and liver. Therefore dietary tyramine will be destroyed before it can promote NE release in the periphery. Clinical trials have shown that restricting dietary tyramine is unnecessary with low-dose selegiline (24 mg/24 hours). However, owing to a lack of data, tyramine restriction *is* recommended at higher selegiline doses. Furthermore, with *all* doses of selegiline, sympathomimetic drugs (e.g., phenylephrine, ephedrine, pseudoephedrine, amphetamines) are still able to promote NE release and hence must be avoided, just as with *oral* MAOIs.

Two drugs—carbamazepine [Tegretol] and oxcarbazepine [Trileptal]—can significantly raise levels of selegiline. Accordingly, these drugs are contraindicated.

The most common adverse reaction is localized rash, which develops in about one third of patients. Rash can be managed with topical glucocorticoids.

Atypical Antidepressants

Bupropion

Actions and Uses

Bupropion [Wellbutrin, Budeprion, Aplenzin] is a unique antidepressant similar in structure to amphetamine. Like amphetamine, bupropion has stimulant actions and suppresses appetite. Antidepressant effects begin in 1 to 3 weeks. The mechanism by which depression is relieved is unclear but may be related to blockade of dopamine or NE reuptake. The drug does not affect serotonergic, cholinergic, or histaminergic transmission and does not inhibit MAO. In contrast to SSRIs, bupropion does not cause weight gain or sexual dysfunction. In fact, it appears to *increase* sexual desire and pleasure, so bupropion has been used to counteract sexual dysfunction in patients taking SSRIs and heighten sexual interest in women with hypoactive sexual desire disorder. Because of its efficacy and side-effect profile, bupropion is a good alternative to SSRIs for patients who cannot tolerate SSRIs. Bupropion has two antidepressant indications: (1) major depressive disorder and (2) *prevention* of seasonal affective disorder (SAD). In addition to its use in depression, bupropion, marketed as Zyban and Buproban, is approved as an aid to quit smoking (see Chapter 32). Unlabeled uses include relief of neuropathic pain, treatment of depressive episodes in bipolar disorder, and management of attention-deficit/hyperactivity disorder.

Pharmacokinetics

Bupropion is administered orally. With the immediate-release tablets, plasma levels peak about 2 hours after dosing. Bioavailability is low: in animals, only 5% to 20% of each dose reaches the systemic circulation. Bupropion undergoes extensive hepatic metabolism, primarily by CYP2B6. The elimination half-life ranges from 8 to 24 hours.

Adverse Effects

Bupropion is generally well tolerated but can cause seizures. The most common adverse effects are agitation, headache, dry mouth, constipation, weight loss, GI upset, dizziness, tremor, insomnia, blurred vision, and tachycardia. In addition, bupropion carries a small risk for causing psychotic symptoms, including hallucinations and delusions. Accordingly, the drug should not be used in patients with psychotic disorders. Like other antidepressants, bupropion may increase the risk for suicide in children, adolescents, and young adults. In contrast to many other antidepressants, bupropion does *not* cause adverse sexual effects.

Seizures are the side effect of greatest concern. At doses greater than 450 mg/day, bupropion produces seizures in about 0.4% of patients. Seizure risk can be reduced by *avoiding* the following:

- Doses above 450 mg/day
- Rapid dosage titration (see later)
- Bupropion in patients with seizure risk factors, such as head trauma, preexisting seizure disorder, CNS tumor, and use of other drugs that lower seizure threshold

- Bupropion in patients with anorexia nervosa or bulimia, which seem to increase seizure risk
- Drugs that inhibit CYP2B6, which can elevate bupropion levels

Drug Interactions

As noted, drugs that inhibit CYP2B6 (e.g., sertraline, fluoxetine, paroxetine) can elevate bupropion levels, thereby increasing the risk for seizures. Combined use with these drugs should be avoided.

MAOIs can increase the risk for bupropion toxicity. Accordingly, patients should discontinue MAOIs at least 2 weeks before starting bupropion.

Mirtazapine

Mirtazapine [Remeron] is the first representative of a new class of antidepressants. Benefits appear to result from increased *release* of 5-HT and NE. The mechanism is blockade of presynaptic alpha$_2$-adrenergic receptors that serve to inhibit release. In addition to promoting transmitter release, mirtazapine is a powerful blocker of two serotonin receptor subtypes: 5-HT$_2$ and 5-HT$_3$. The contribution of this effect is unclear. Mirtazapine blocks histamine receptors and thus promotes sedation and weight gain. Antidepressant effects equal those of SSRIs and may develop faster.

Mirtazapine is well absorbed after oral dosing and reaches peak plasma levels in 2 hours. The drug undergoes extensive hepatic metabolism followed by excretion in the urine (75%) and feces (25%). The elimination half-life is 20 to 40 hours.

Mirtazapine is generally well tolerated. Somnolence is the most prominent adverse effect, occurring in 54% of patients. Weight gain, increased appetite, and elevated cholesterol are also common. Sexual dysfunction is minimal. Reversible agranulocytosis was reported in early trials but was not confirmed in later clinical experience. Blockade of muscarinic receptors is moderate, and hence anticholinergic effects are mild. Mirtazapine-induced somnolence can be exacerbated by alcohol, benzodiazepines, and other CNS depressants. Accordingly, these agents should be avoided. Mirtazapine should not be combined with MAOIs.

Other Atypical Antidepressants

Nefazodone

Nefazodone is a novel drug indicated only for depression. Neuropharmacologic actions include blockade of 5-HT$_2$ receptors and alpha$_1$-adrenergic receptors, and weak inhibition of NE and 5-HT reuptake. The contribution of these actions to therapeutic effects is unknown. Life-threatening liver failure is the adverse effect of greatest concern.

Nefazodone is rapidly and completely absorbed after oral administration. Food delays absorption and decreases bioavailability by 20%. Plasma drug levels peak about 1 hour after oral dosing. In the liver, nefazodone undergoes conversion to three active metabolites. The effective half-life of the parent drug and metabolites is 11 to 24 hours.

Nefazodone is generally well tolerated. The most common side effects are sedation, headache, somnolence, dry mouth, nausea, constipation, dizziness, blurred vision, and other visual disturbances. Weight gain and sexual dysfunction are minimal.

Drugs that block reuptake of 5-HT, NE, or both can cause serious reactions if combined with an MAOI. Accordingly, nefazodone and MAOIs must not be combined. If the patient has been taking an MAOI, it should be discontinued at least 2 weeks before starting nefazodone. Conversely, when switching from nefazodone to an MAOI, nefazodone should be discontinued at least 7 days before starting the MAOI.

Nefazodone inhibits hepatic drug-metabolizing enzymes and can thereby raise levels of other drugs, including certain antihistamines, benzodiazepines, and digoxin.

BLACK BOX WARNING: LIVER FAILURE WITH NEFAZODONE

Nefazodone can cause life-threatening liver failure. However, the incidence is extremely low: only 1 case leading to death or liver transplantation for every 250,000 to 300,000 patient-years. As a rule, nefazodone should not be given to patients with preexisting liver disease. Patients who develop signs of liver injury (e.g., nausea, anorexia, abdominal pain, malaise, jaundice) should seek immediate medical attention. If laboratory tests confirm hepatocellular injury, nefazodone should be withdrawn.

Trazodone

Trazodone [Oleptro] is a second-line agent for depression. The drug is not very effective when used alone but, because of its pronounced sedative effects, can be a helpful adjunct for patients with antidepressant-induced insomnia. Trazodone produces selective (but moderate) blockade of 5-HT reuptake. Antidepressant effects take several weeks to develop.

Common side effects are sedation, orthostatic hypotension, and nausea. In contrast to the tricyclic agents, trazodone has minimal anticholinergic actions. Accordingly, trazodone may be useful for older-adult patients and other individuals for whom the anticholinergic effects of the TCAs may be intolerable.

Trazodone prolongs the QT interval and hence poses a risk for dysrhythmias. In postmarketing reports, the drug has been associated with tachycardia, premature ventricular contractions, and potentially fatal torsades de pointes. Fortunately, these reports have been rare. To reduce the risk for dysrhythmias, trazodone should be used with caution in patients with hypokalemia, hypomagnesemia, congenital long QT syndrome, and other cardiac disorders.

Trazodone can cause priapism (prolonged, painful erection). In some cases, surgical intervention has been required. Priapism itself or the procedures required for relief can result in permanent impotence. Patients should be instructed to notify their prescriber or to go to an emergency department if persistent erection occurs. Overdose with trazodone is considered safer than with TCAs or MAOIs. Death from overdose with trazodone alone has not been reported (although death has occurred after overdose with trazodone in combination with another CNS depressant).

Drugs that inhibit CYP3A4 (the 3A4 isoenzyme of cytochrome P450) can decrease metabolism of trazodone and thereby increase its concentration. Toxicity may result. Accordingly, if trazodone is combined with a strong CYP3A4 inhibitor (e.g., ketoconazole, ritonavir), dosage of trazodone should be reduced.

Vilazodone

Vilazodone [Viibryd] works by two mechanisms. First, like the SSRIs, vilazodone selectively blocks serotonin reuptake. Second, vilazodone causes direct activation of serotonin receptors (by acting as a partial agonist). No other antidepressant combines both actions. The drug is more effective than a placebo, but is not more effective than fluoxetine or citalopram—and causes more GI side effects.

Vilazodone is administered by mouth, and food greatly enhances absorption. Plasma levels peak 4 to 5 hours after dosing. In the blood, the drug is highly (96%–99%) protein bound. Vilazodone undergoes extensive hepatic metabolism—mainly by CYP3A4—followed by excretion in the urine.

The most common adverse effects are diarrhea, nausea, dizziness, and insomnia. Sexual dysfunction is also relatively common: Vilazodone reduces libido in males and females; causes abnormal orgasms in males and females; and also causes delayed ejaculation and erectile dysfunction. Like the SSRIs, vilazodone poses a risk for serotonin syndrome, hyponatremia, and abnormal bleeding. Like all other antidepressants, vilazodone may increase suicidality. On the positive side, vilazodone appears to carry little or no risk for seizures, hypotension, weight gain, cardiotoxicity, hepatotoxicity, or anticholinergic effects.

Drug interactions are a concern. The risk for serotonin syndrome is increased by MAOIs and other serotonergic drugs (see Table 25.3). Use of MAOIs with vilazodone is contraindicated, and other serotonergic drugs should be used with caution, if at all. Vilazodone levels can be raised by drugs that inhibit CYP3A4 (e.g., ketoconazole, ritonavir) and lowered by drugs that induce CYP3A4 (e.g., rifampin, isoniazid, barbiturates). A dosage adjustment may be needed. The risk for bleeding is increased by anticoagulants (e.g., warfarin) and by drugs that impede platelet function (e.g., aspirin, NSAIDs).

Amoxapine

Amoxapine is chemically related to the antipsychotic agent loxapine and has both antidepressant and neuroleptic properties. Antidepressant effects are equivalent to those of the TCAs. Because it can cause serious side effects, amoxapine should be reserved for patients with psychotic depression.

Amoxapine is generally well tolerated. Anticholinergic and sedative effects are moderate. After overdose, the risk for seizures is greater than with TCAs. Exercise caution in patients with seizures.

Like loxapine and the other antipsychotics, amoxapine can block receptors for dopamine. As a result, the drug can cause extrapyramidal side effects (e.g., parkinsonism, akathisia). Because of the risk for tardive dyskinesia (an extrapyramidal effect that develops with prolonged use of dopamine antagonists), long-term use of amoxapine should generally be avoided.

Nonconventional Drugs for Depression

St. John's Wort

St. John's wort (Hypericum perforatum) is an herbal product used for oral therapy of depression. For patients with mild to moderate major depression, the product is superior to placebo and may equal the TCAs. However, for patients with severe depression, there is no convincing proof of efficacy. Adverse effects are generally mild, but interactions with conventional drugs are a concern. St. John's wort can decrease the effects of many drugs by (1) inducing cytochrome P450 drug-metabolizing enzymes and (2) inducing P-glycoprotein, a transport protein that exports drugs into the intestinal lumen and urine. In addition, the herb can intensify serotonergic neurotransmission and hence poses a risk for serotonin syndrome if combined with other serotonergic drugs. The pharmacology of St. John's wort is discussed further in Chapter 67.

S-Adenosylmethionine

S-adenosylmethionine (SAMe) is a naturally occurring compound present in high concentration in the brain, liver, adrenal glands, and pineal gland. In the brain, SAMe serves as a methyl donor for the synthesis of neurotransmitters (NE, 5-HT, dopamine) and cell membranes. In patients with severe depression, levels of SAMe in the cerebrospinal fluid (CSF) are reduced. When these patients are given oral or parenteral SAMe, there is a rise in CSF levels of SAMe and a corresponding improvement in depressive symptoms. When compared directly with TCAs, SAMe was more effective and better tolerated. In treatment-resistant patients receiving SSRIs, adding SAMe to the regimen was associated with moderate symptomatic improvement and did not increase the risk for serotonin syndrome. Although studies to date are encouraging, experience with SAMe is limited, and hence there are insufficient data to recommend SAMe for routine use. In the United States SAMe is available without prescription as an enteric-coated dietary supplement.

PERIPARTUM DEPRESSION

Most women (about 80%) experience depressive symptoms after giving birth. For most, the symptoms are mild and transient, reflecting a condition sometimes called the "baby blues." For others, symptoms are severe and persistent, reflecting true postpartum depression, a condition that merits rapid medical attention.

An estimated 60% to 70% of women experience depression postpartum, and in 50% of these depression begins *before* delivery—hence the term *peripartum depression.* Symptoms include tearfulness, sadness, nervousness, irritability, and anxiety, along with difficulty eating and sleeping. The new mother may feel overwhelmed, vulnerable, weak, and alone. She may cry for no clear reason. Her self-esteem and self-confidence may decline, and she may feel unqualified to care for her baby. Fortunately, all of these symptoms pass quickly: they develop a few days after delivery and are gone by day 10. Because these symptoms are so common, they're considered a normal postpartum event. Treatment is neither necessary nor recommended.

True peripartum depression is different. The condition is much less common than the "baby blues" but much more serious. Left untreated, peripartum depression lasts for months and is likely to become worse as time passes. The condition is detrimental to the mother, and it can adversely affect the child, preventing secure attachment and impairing cognitive, emotional, and behavioral development. Immediate intervention is indicated.

True peripartum depression is an episode of major depression that starts in the weeks before or just after giving birth. Otherwise, the diagnostic criteria are the same as for all other episodes of major depression. According to the *Diagnostic and Statistical Manual of Mental Disorders, Fifth Edition* (DSM-5), for a depressive episode to qualify as having peripartum onset, symptoms must begin within *4 weeks* of delivery. However, most clinicians who study the disorder use a different criterion: to them, depression is considered postpartum if it begins within *3 months* of delivery—not just within 4 weeks.

Who is likely to suffer peripartum depression? Sometimes the condition occurs in first-time mothers, and sometimes it doesn't strike until a second, third, or fourth child is born. Among first-time mothers, the incidence is between 8% and 15% (about 1 in 8). For women with a history of the disorder, the risk increases to 33% (1 in 3). In addition to a prior history of the disorder, risk factors include a history of depression unrelated to childbirth, history of premenstrual dysphoric disorder (i.e., severe premenstrual syndrome), and major stress related to family, work, or residence (e.g., death of a loved one, loss of a job, moving away from a familiar town or city).

The underlying cause of peripartum depression is unknown, but several factors are thought to contribute. Heading the list is the sharp drop in estrogen and progesterone levels that occurs after delivery. (Levels of these hormones increase 10-fold during pregnancy and return to baseline after the placenta is expelled.) However, because hormone levels fall in all women, but only some get peripartum depression, other factors—physical, emotional, and social—must be involved. The birthing process may leave women feeling weak and fatigued. Caring for a baby, who needs round-the-clock attention and feeding, exacerbates tiredness and exhaustion. Emotional and social factors may also play a role. Feelings of loss are common: women experience loss of freedom, loss of control, and even loss of identity. Stress increases substantially, owing to increased workload and responsibilities, coupled with feelings of self-doubt and inadequacy, and compounded by a self-imposed (albeit highly unrealistic) expectation to be a "perfect" parent. Stress can be made even worse by financial insecurity and inadequate support from one's partner, family, and friends. Thyroid insufficiency may also contribute: Levels of thyroid hormone often decline after delivery, causing symptoms that can mimic depression. Accordingly, thyroid levels should be checked and, if indicated, replacement therapy should be implemented.

Screening for peripartum depression should be contemplated in all women, although evidence is lacking regarding universal screening. Women with multiple risk factors should be strongly considered. Screening can be accomplished with a quick test: the Edinburgh Postnatal Depression Scale.

Treatment of peripartum depression is much like treatment of major depression unrelated to pregnancy. The goals are to normalize mood and to optimize maternal and social functioning. The principal treatment modalities are psychotherapy and antidepressant drugs, both of which can be effective. In addition, the woman should be encouraged to nurture herself in the following ways:

- Reduce isolation (by going out for at least a short time each day)
- Ensure adequate rest (by doing only what's really needed and letting the rest go)
- Spend time alone with her partner

Other beneficial measures include joining a support group for new mothers and recruiting family members and friends to assist with household and baby-related chores.

Although antidepressants are clearly appropriate, there are few published data to guide selection. In one study of women with postpartum depression, fluoxetine [Prozac], an SSRI, was compared with psychotherapy. Both treatments were equally effective, and both were superior to placebo. Efficacy has also been demonstrated for sertraline [Zoloft], venlafaxine [Effexor], and certain TCAs. For initial therapy, an SSRI is an attractive choice because these drugs are effective and well tolerated and present little risk for toxicity if taken in overdose. However, if a woman has responded to an antidepressant from a different class in the past, that drug should be tried first. To minimize side effects, dosage should be low initially (50% of the usual starting dosage) and then gradually increased. To reduce the risk for relapse, treatment should continue for at least 6 months after symptoms have resolved. Unfortunately, even then the relapse rate is high: between 50% and 85% of patients experience at least one more depressive episode. With each succeeding episode, the risk for another recurrence increases. Accordingly, long-term prophylactic therapy should be considered.

Which antidepressants can be taken safely while breastfeeding? All of these drugs can be detected in breast milk—but levels of some are lower (safer) than levels of others. Sertraline, for example, appears safe. Studies show that drug activity in breastfed infants is extremely low, and no adverse reactions have been observed. The TCAs (e.g., nortriptyline, desipramine) also appear safe: levels are too low for detection in breastfed infants, and follow-up studies have found no developmental deficits. In contrast to sertraline and the TCAs, fluoxetine appears unsafe: the drug and its metabolites reach therapeutic levels in breastfed infants; potential consequences include colic and impaired weight gain. Infants of breastfeeding mothers on antidepressants should be monitored closely for these side effects.

SOMATIC (NONDRUG) THERAPIES FOR DEPRESSION

Nondrug therapies are reserved for patients with severe depression that has not responded to drugs or psychotherapy. Of the four treatments discussed next, electroconvulsive therapy (ECT) appears most effective.

Electroconvulsive Therapy

ECT is a valuable tool for treating depression. This procedure is safe and effective, and benefits develop more rapidly than with drugs or psychotherapy. Accordingly, ECT is especially appropriate when a rapid response is necessary. Candidates for ECT include (1) severely depressed, suicidal patients; (2) older-adult patients at risk for starvation because of depression-induced lack of appetite; and (3) patients who have not responded to antidepressant drugs (50%–60% will respond to ECT).

A single treatment consists of delivering an electrical shock to the scalp that is sufficient to induce a generalized seizure lasting 20 to 30 seconds. Success requires a series of these treatments, typically 2 to 3 per week for a total of 6 to 12 treatments.

Thanks to the adjunctive use of drugs, ECT is much less dramatic and traumatic than in the past. Before the delivery of electroshock, patients are treated with two drugs: a *short-acting neuromuscular blocker* (succinylcholine) and a *short-acting intravenous anesthetic* (e.g., propofol, etomidate, methohexital). The neuromuscular blocker prevents shock-induced seizure movements, which are both hazardous and unnecessary for a therapeutic response. The IV anesthetic prevents conscious awareness of the ECT procedure (without interfering with beneficial actions). Patients may also receive an anticholinergic drug (e.g., glycopyrrolate) to minimize bradycardia and salivation.

ECT can terminate an ongoing depression episode, but a single series of treatments cannot prevent recurrence. Accordingly, some patients are now given "maintenance" treatments, at weekly or monthly intervals. In one study, the relapse rate at 6 months in the absence of maintenance was 73%, compared with only 8% when maintenance ECT was used. Maintenance with antidepressant drugs (e.g., lithium plus amitriptyline) is another option but is significantly less effective than maintenance with ECT.

ECT is very safe. There are no absolute contraindications to its use. The principal adverse effect is amnesia, primarily for events immediately surrounding treatment. However, patients may also experience some loss of older memories, but these usually return within 6 months. There is also transient impairment of cognitive function. Minor adverse effects, which occur immediately after treatment, include nausea, headache, confusion, and muscle discomfort.

Transcranial Magnetic Stimulation

Like ECT, transcranial magnetic stimulation (TMS) is reserved for patients with major depression that has not responded to antidepressant drugs. Magnetic stimulation is accomplished using the *NeuroStar TMS System,* a device that employs an insulated magnetic coil, placed against the scalp, to deliver pulsed magnetic fields to the left dorsolateral prefrontal cortex. The magnetic fields induce electrical currents in the brain, which in turn cause neuronal depolarization and other changes in brain activity. A full course of treatment consists of daily 40-minute sessions for 6 weeks or so. Trial results have been inconsistent. In some trials, TMS was just as effective as ECT, but in other trials, TMS was less effective. How safe is TMS? The procedure is generally well tolerated. Principal adverse effects are transient headaches and scalp discomfort. Patients may also experience eye pain, toothache, muscle twitching, and seizures. Cognitive changes have not been reported.

Vagus Nerve Stimulation

In 2005, the U.S. Food and Drug Administration approved the Vagus Nerve Stimulation (VNS) Therapy System for adjunctive, long-term therapy of patients with *treatment-resistant depression* (TRD), which the manufacturer defines as major depression that has not responded to at least four different antidepressant drugs. The VNS Therapy System—an implanted device that delivers electrical pulses to the vagus nerve—was first developed to treat drug-resistant seizure disorders. In the course of that research, mood elevation was observed in some patients. A trial was then conducted in patients with TRD. However, the results were equivocal. Newer small studies show possible promise in patients with severe, refractory depression. The mechanism by which VNS alleviates depression (if it really does) is unknown. The principal side effects of VNS are hoarseness, voice alteration, cough, and dyspnea, all of which tend to diminish over time. The cost of the VNS system, along with surgical implantation and calibration, is about $25,000.

Light Therapy

Exposure to bright light is an effective treatment of SAD and of nonseasonal major depression. The more intense the light, the greater the response. Light can be beneficial alone and can enhance the response to antidepressant drugs. How does light relieve depression? Possibly by enhancing serotonergic neurotransmission. Light therapy is attractive owing to low cost and low risk.

CHAPTER

26 Drugs for Bipolar Disorder

Laura D. Rosenthal, DNP, ACNP, FAANP

Our topic for this chapter is *bipolar disorder* (BPD), formerly known as *manic-depressive illness.* The disease afflicts an estimated 3.7% of the adult population—more than 6.7 million Americans. The mainstays of therapy are lithium and divalproex sodium (valproate), drugs that can stabilize mood. Many patients also receive an antipsychotic agent, and some may require an antidepressant. BPD is a chronic condition that requires lifelong treatment.

CHARACTERISTICS OF BIPOLAR DISORDER

BPD is a severe biologic illness characterized by recurrent fluctuations in mood. Typically, patients experience alternating episodes in which mood is abnormally elevated or abnormally depressed—separated by periods in which mood is relatively normal. Symptoms usually begin in adolescence or early adulthood but can occur before adolescence or as late as the fifth decade of life. In the absence of treatment, episodes of mania or depression generally persist for several months. As time passes, manic and depressive episodes tend to recur more frequently. Although the precise etiology of BPD is unknown, it is clear that symptoms are caused by altered brain physiology—not by a character flaw or an unstable personality.

Types of Mood Episodes Seen in Bipolar Disorder

Patients with BPD may experience four types of mood episodes: pure manic, hypomanic, major depressive, and mixed.

Pure Manic Episode (Euphoric Mania)

Manic episodes are characterized by persistently heightened, expansive, or irritable mood—typically associated with hyperactivity, excessive enthusiasm, and flight of ideas. Manic individuals display overactivity at work and at play and have a reduced need for sleep. Mania produces excessive sociability and talkativeness. Extreme self-confidence, grandiose ideas, and delusions of self-importance are common. Manic individuals often indulge in high-risk activities (e.g., questionable business deals, reckless driving, gambling, sexual indiscretions), giving no forethought to the consequences. In severe cases, symptoms may resemble those of paranoid schizophrenia (hallucinations, delusions, bizarre behavior).

Hypomanic Episode (Hypomania)

Hypomania can be viewed as a mild form of mania. As in mania, mood is persistently elevated, expansive, or irritable. However, symptoms are not severe enough to cause marked impairment in social or occupational functioning, or to require hospitalization. Psychotic symptoms are absent.

Major Depressive Episode (Depression)

A major depressive episode is characterized by depressed mood and loss of pleasure or interest in all or nearly all of one's usual activities and pastimes. Associated symptoms include disruption of sleeping and eating patterns; difficulty concentrating; feelings of guilt, worthlessness, and helplessness; and thoughts of death and suicide. The characteristics of major depression are discussed further in Chapter 25.

Mixed Episode

In a true mixed episode, patients experience symptoms of mania and depression simultaneously. Patients may be agitated and irritable (as in mania) but may also feel worthless and depressed. The combination of high energy and depression puts them at significant risk for suicide.

Patterns of Mood Episodes

Among people with BPD, mood episodes can occur in a variety of patterns. Contrary to popular belief, not all patients alternate repeatedly between mania and depression. Some experience repeated episodes of mania, and some experience repeated episodes of depression (with an occasional episode of mania). Mood may be normal between episodes of mania and depression, or it may be slightly elevated (hypomania) or slightly depressed (dysphoria).

Mood episodes can vary greatly with respect to how often they occur and how long they last. A single episode may last for days, weeks, months, or more than a year. In the absence of treatment, episodes of mania or hypomania typically last a few months, whereas episodes of major depression typically last at least 6 months. On average, people with BPD experience only four episodes during the first 10 years of their illness. However, some people cycle much more rapidly, experiencing many episodes every year.

On the basis of mood episode type and frequency, BPD can be subdivided into two major categories:

- *Bipolar I disorder*—patients experience manic or mixed episodes, and usually depressive episodes too.
- *Bipolar II disorder*—patients experience hypomanic or depressive episodes, but not manic or mixed episodes.

Etiology

Theories regarding the etiology of BPD continue to evolve. In the past, there was general agreement that BPD was due primarily to an imbalance in neurotransmitters. Today, researchers suspect the real cause may be disruption of neuronal growth and survival. First, neuroimaging studies have shown an association between prolonged mood disorders and atrophy of specific brain regions—especially the subgenual prefrontal cortex, an area involved in emotionality. Second, mood-stabilizing drugs can prevent or reverse neuronal atrophy in patients with BPD, apparently by influencing signaling pathways that regulate neuronal growth and survival.

Prototype Drugs

MOOD-STABILIZING DRUGS FOR BIPOLAR DISORDER

Lithium
Carbamazepine
Valproic acid

TREATMENT OF BIPOLAR DISORDER

Drug Therapy

Types of Drugs Employed

The American Psychiatric Association (APA) and the Veterans Administration both published treatment guidelines for bipolar disorder in 2010. These guidelines discussed both pharmacologic and nonpharmacologic treatments for BPD. To begin, BPD is treated with three major groups of drugs: mood stabilizers, antipsychotics, and antidepressants. In addition, benzodiazepines are frequently used for sedation.

Mood Stabilizers

Mood stabilizers are drugs that (1) relieve symptoms during manic and depressive episodes, (2) prevent recurrence of manic and depressive episodes, and (3) do not worsen symptoms of mania or depression, or accelerate the rate of cycling. The principal mood stabilizers are *lithium* and two drugs originally developed for epilepsy: *divalproex sodium* (valproate) and *carbamazepine.* These drugs are the mainstays of treatment. The pharmacology of lithium and the antiepileptic drugs is discussed later.

Antipsychotics

In patients with BPD, antipsychotic drugs are given to help control symptoms during severe manic episodes, even if psychotic symptoms are absent. Although antipsychotics can be used alone, they are usually employed in combination with a mood stabilizer. For reasons discussed later, the second-generation antipsychotics (e.g., olanzapine, risperidone) are generally preferred to the first-generation agents (e.g., haloperidol).

Antidepressants

Antidepressants may be needed during a depressive episode. However, in patients with BPD, antidepressants are *always* combined with a mood stabilizer because of the long-held belief that, when used alone, antidepressants may elevate mood so much that a hypomanic or manic episode will result. However, a systematic review published in 2014 indicates that the risk for inducing mania may be much lower than previously thought. These data suggest that use of a selective serotonin reuptake inhibitor (SSRI) may be reasonable for the short-term treatment of bipolar depression. Nonetheless, the current guidelines suggest continuing the traditional practice of using an antidepressant only if a mood stabilizer is being used as well.

Although antidepressants have been studied extensively in patients with major depression, research is still lacking in patients with BPD. At this time, there are insufficient data on which to base drug selection. Even so, experts do have their preferences. Among clinicians with extensive experience in BPD, the following are considered antidepressants of choice: *bupropion* [Wellbutrin], *venlafaxine* [Effexor XR], and the SSRIs, such as fluoxetine [Prozac] and sertraline [Zoloft]. One thing we do know is that use of tricyclic antidepressants (TCAs) appears to promote more incidence of mania, and therefore TCAs are not recommended in treatment of BPD. The pharmacology of these drugs is discussed in Chapter 25.

Drug Selection

Acute Therapy: Manic Episodes

Two mood stabilizers—lithium and valproate—are preferred drugs for acute management of manic episodes. The choice between them is based on clinical presentation (e.g., euphoric mania, mania with psychosis, rapid-cycling BPD). As shown in Table 26.1, valproate is preferred to lithium in most cases. In fact, the only exception is euphoric mania, for which lithium is the drug of choice. If the patient does not respond adequately to lithium or valproate alone, the drugs may be used together. Responses to mood stabilizers develop slowly, taking 2 or more weeks to become maximal.

If needed, an antipsychotic agent or a benzodiazepine may be added to the regimen. These adjuvants can help relieve symptoms (e.g., insomnia, anxiety, agitation) until the mood stabilizer takes full effect. For patients with mild mania, a

TABLE 26.1 ▪ Initial Treatment of First Manic Episode

		Preferred Drugs*	
Clinical Presentation	**Preferred Strategy**	**Mood Stabilizers**	**Antipsychotics**
Euphoric mania	Mood stabilizer alone	Valproate or **lithium**	
Dysphoric mania or true mixed mania	Mood stabilizer alone	**Valproate** or lithium	
Mania with psychosis	Mood stabilizer plus an antipsychotic	**Valproate** or lithium	Olanzapine or risperidone
Rapid cycling (currently manic)	Mood stabilizer alone	**Valproate**	

*Drugs of choice, if established, are presented in **bold type.**
Valproate = divalproex sodium.

benzodiazepine (e.g., lorazepam [Ativan]) may be adequate. For patients with severe mania or with symptoms of psychosis, an antipsychotic is preferred; olanzapine or risperidone would be a good choice.

Acute Therapy: Depressive Episodes

Depressive episodes may be treated with a mood stabilizer alone or with a mood stabilizer *plus* an antidepressant—but *never* with an antidepressant alone (because hypomania or mania might result). If depression is mild, monotherapy with a mood stabilizer (lithium or lamotrigine) may be sufficient. If the mood stabilizer is inadequate, an antidepressant can be added, although benefits may be limited. *Symbyax,* a combination drug containing both olanzapine and fluoxetine, was shown to be beneficial in the short-term treatment of BPD in a small study. Preferred antidepressants are bupropion, venlafaxine, or an SSRI.

Long-Term Preventive Treatment

The purpose of long-term therapy is to prevent recurrence of both mania and depression. As a rule, one or more mood stabilizers are employed. Drug selection is based on what worked acutely. For example, if the patient responded to acute therapy with lithium alone, then lithium alone should be tried long term. Other long-term options include valproate alone, and valproate plus lithium. More recently, antipsychotic agents have been employed for long-term maintenance, either as monotherapy or in combination with a mood stabilizer.

Promoting Adherence

Poor patient adherence can frustrate attempts to treat a manic episode. Patients may resist treatment because they fail to see anything wrong with their thinking or behavior. Furthermore, the experience is not necessarily unpleasant. In fact, individuals going through a manic episode may well enjoy it. As a result, to ensure adherence, short-term hospitalization may be required. To achieve this, collaboration with the patient's family may be needed. Because hospitalization per se won't guarantee success, lithium administration should be directly observed to ensure that each dose is actually taken.

Patient Education

ADHERENCE TO LONG-TERM THERAPY

After an acute manic episode has been controlled, long-term prophylactic therapy is indicated, making adherence an ongoing issue. To promote adherence, the patient and family should be educated about the nature of BPD and the importance of taking medication as prescribed. Family members can help ensure adherence by overseeing medication use and by urging the patient to visit his or her prescriber or a psychiatric clinic if a pattern of nonadherence develops.

Nondrug Therapy

Education and Psychotherapy

Ideally, BPD should be treated with a combination of drugs and adjunctive psychotherapy (individual, group, or family); drug therapy alone is not optimal. BPD is a chronic illness that requires supportive therapy and education for the patient and family. Counseling can help patients cope with the sequelae of manic episodes, such as strained relationships, reduced self-confidence, and a sense of shame regarding uncontrolled behavior. Certain life stresses (e.g., moving, job loss, bereavement, childbirth) can precipitate a mood change. Therapy can help reduce the destabilizing effect of these events. Patients should be taught to recognize early symptoms of mood change and encouraged to contact their primary clinician immediately if these develop. Additional measures by which patients can help themselves include the following:

- Maintaining a stable sleep pattern
- Maintaining a regular pattern of activity
- Avoiding alcohol and psychoactive street drugs
- Enlisting the support of family and friends
- Taking steps to reduce stress at work
- Keeping a mood chart to monitor progress

Electroconvulsive Therapy

Electroconvulsive therapy (ECT) is an effective intervention that can be lifesaving in patients with severe mania or severe depression. However, ECT is not a treatment of first choice. It should be reserved for patients who have not responded adequately to drugs. Candidates for ECT include patients with psychotic depression, severe nonpsychotic depression, severe mania, and rapid-cycling BPD. Details of ECT are discussed in Chapter 25.

MOOD-STABILIZING DRUGS

As noted, mood stabilizers are drugs that can relieve an acute manic or depressive episode and can prevent symptoms from recurring—all without aggravating mania or depression and without accelerating cycling. The agents used most often are lithium, valproate, and carbamazepine.

Lithium

Lithium [Lithobid, Carbolith ♣] can stabilize mood in patients with BPD. Beneficial effects were first described in 1949 by John Cade, an Australian psychiatrist. Because of concerns about toxicity, lithium was not approved for use in the United States until 1970. Lithium has a low therapeutic index. As a result, toxicity can occur at blood levels only slightly greater than therapeutic levels. Accordingly, monitoring lithium levels is mandatory.

Chemistry

Lithium is a simple inorganic ion that carries a single positive charge. In the periodic table of elements, lithium is in the same group as potassium and sodium. Not surprisingly, lithium has properties in common with both elements. Lithium is found naturally in animal tissues but has no known physiologic function.

Therapeutic Uses

BPD

Lithium is a drug of choice for controlling acute manic episodes in patients with BPD and for long-term prophylaxis against recurrence of mania or depression. In manic patients, lithium reduces euphoria, hyperactivity, and other symptoms but does not cause sedation. Antimanic effects begin 5 to 7 days after treatment onset, but full benefits may not develop for 2 to 3 weeks. In the past, lithium was considered the drug of choice for all patients experiencing an acute manic episode, regardless of clinical presentation. Today, however, lithium is reserved primarily for patients with classical (euphoric) mania, and valproate is generally preferred for all other patients (see Table 26.1). However, more recent data show that lithium is superior to valproate at preventing suicide in patients with BPD, and hence use of lithium is likely to increase.

Mechanism of Action

Although lithium has been studied extensively, the precise mechanism by which it stabilizes mood is unknown. In the past, research focused on three aspects of brain neurochemistry: (1) altered distribution of certain ions (calcium, sodium, magnesium) that are critical to neuronal function; (2) altered synthesis and release of norepinephrine, serotonin, and dopamine; and (3) effects on second messengers (e.g., cyclic adenosine monophosphate, phosphatidylinositol), which mediate intracellular responses to neurotransmitters. Unfortunately, this research has failed to provide a definitive explanation of how lithium works. Current neurochemical research suggests that lithium may work by (1) altering glutamate uptake and release, (2) blocking the binding of serotonin to its receptors, or (3) inhibiting glycogen synthase kinase-3 beta.

There has been growing interest in the neurotrophic and neuroprotective actions of lithium. As noted earlier, there is evidence that symptoms of BPD may result from neuronal atrophy in certain brain areas. In animal studies, "therapeutic" doses of lithium doubled the level of neurotrophic Bcl-2 proteins. In addition, lithium has been shown to facilitate regeneration of damaged optic nerves. In patients with BPD taking lithium long term, volume of the subgenual prefrontal cortex is greater than in untreated patients. Furthermore, lithium can increase total gray matter in regions known to atrophy in BPD, including the prefrontal cortex, hippocampus, and caudate nucleus. All of these studies suggest that the benefits of lithium may result at least in part from an ability to protect against neuronal atrophy or promote neuronal growth.

Pharmacokinetics

Absorption and Distribution

Lithium is well absorbed after oral administration. The drug distributes evenly to all tissues and body fluids.

Excretion

Lithium has a short half-life owing to rapid renal excretion. Because of its short half-life (and high toxicity), the drug must be administered in divided daily doses. Large, single daily doses cannot be used, even when a slow-release preparation is prescribed. Because lithium is excreted by the kidneys, it must be employed with great care in patients with renal impairment.

Renal excretion of lithium is affected by blood levels of sodium. Specifically, lithium excretion is *reduced* when levels of sodium are *low* because the kidney processes lithium and sodium in the same way. Hence, when the kidney senses that sodium levels are inadequate, it retains lithium in an attempt to compensate. Because of this relationship, in the presence of low sodium, lithium can accumulate to toxic levels. Accordingly, it is important that sodium levels remain normal. Patients should be instructed to maintain normal sodium intake. Because diuretics promote sodium loss, these agents must be employed with caution. Also, sodium loss secondary to diarrhea can be sufficient to cause lithium accumulation. The patient should be told about this possibility.

Dehydration will cause lithium retention by the kidneys, posing the risk for accumulation to dangerous levels. Potential causes of dehydration include hot weather and diarrhea. Counsel patients to maintain adequate hydration.

Monitoring Plasma Lithium Levels

Measurement of plasma lithium levels is an essential component of treatment. *Lithium levels must be kept below 1.5 mEq/L; levels greater than this can produce significant toxicity.* For *initial* therapy of a manic episode, lithium levels should range from 0.6 to 1.2 mEq/L. When the desired therapeutic effect has been achieved, the dosage should be reduced to produce *maintenance* levels of 0.4 to 1 mEq/L. Blood for lithium determinations should be drawn in the morning, 12 hours after the evening dose. During maintenance therapy, lithium levels should be measured every 3 to 6 months.

Adverse Effects

The adverse effects of lithium can be divided into two categories: (1) effects that occur at excessive lithium levels and (2) effects that occur at therapeutic lithium levels. In the subsequent discussion, adverse effects produced at excessive lithium levels are considered as a group. Effects produced at therapeutic levels are considered individually.

Adverse Effects That Occur When Lithium Levels Are Excessive

Certain toxicities are closely correlated with the concentration of lithium in blood. As indicated in Table 26.2, mild responses (e.g., fine hand tremor, gastrointestinal [GI] upset, thirst, muscle weakness) can develop at lithium levels that are still

TABLE 26.2 ▪ Toxicities Associated With Excessive Plasma Level of Lithium

Plasma Lithium Level (mEq/L)	Signs of Toxicity
Less than 1.5	Nausea, vomiting, diarrhea, thirst, polyuria, lethargy, slurred speech, muscle weakness, fine hand tremor
1.5–2	Persistent GI upset, coarse hand tremor, confusion, hyperirritability of muscles, ECG changes, sedation, incoordination
2–2.5	Ataxia, giddiness, high output of dilute urine, serious ECG changes, fasciculations, tinnitus, blurred vision, clonic movements, seizures, stupor, severe hypotension, coma, death (usually secondary to pulmonary complications)
More than 2.5	Symptoms may progress rapidly to generalized convulsions, oliguria, and death

ECG, electrocardiogram; GI, gastrointestinal.

within the therapeutic range (i.e., less than 1.5 mEq/L). When plasma levels exceed 1.5 mEq/L, more serious toxicities appear. At drug levels higher than 2.5 mEq/L, death can occur. Patients should be informed about early signs of toxicity and instructed to interrupt lithium dosing if these appear. In adherent patients, the most common cause of lithium accumulation is sodium depletion.

To keep lithium levels within the therapeutic range, plasma drug levels should be monitored routinely. Levels should be measured every 2 to 3 days at the beginning of treatment and every 3 to 6 months during maintenance therapy.

Treatment of acute overdose is primarily supportive; there is no specific antidote. The severely intoxicated patient should be hospitalized. Hemodialysis is an effective means of lithium removal and should be considered whenever drug levels exceed 2.5 mEq/L.

BLACK BOX WARNING: LITHIUM TOXICITY

Lithium toxicity is closely related to serum lithium levels and can occur at doses close to therapeutic levels. Facilities for prompt and accurate serum lithium determinations should be available before initiating therapy

Adverse Effects That Occur at Therapeutic Levels of Lithium

Early Adverse Effects. Several responses occur early in treatment and then usually subside. *GI effects* (e.g., nausea, diarrhea, abdominal bloating, anorexia) are common but transient. About 30% of patients experience *transient fatigue, muscle weakness, headache, confusion,* and *memory impairment. Polyuria* and *thirst* occur in 30% to 50% of patients and may persist.

Tremor. Patients may develop a fine hand tremor, especially in the fingers, that can interfere with writing and other motor skills. Lithium-induced tremor can be augmented by stress, fatigue, and certain drugs (antidepressants, antipsychotics, caffeine). Tremor can be reduced with a beta blocker (e.g., propranolol) and by measures that reduce peak levels of lithium (i.e., dosage reduction, use of divided doses, or use of a sustained-release formulation).

Polyuria. Polyuria occurs in 50% to 70% of patients taking lithium chronically. In some patients, daily urine output may exceed 3 L. Lithium promotes polyuria by antagonizing the effects of antidiuretic hormone. To maintain adequate hydration, patients should be instructed to drink 8 to 12 glasses of fluids daily. Polyuria, nocturia, and excessive thirst can discourage patients from adhering to the regimen.

Lithium-induced polyuria can be reduced with *amiloride* [Midamor], a potassium-sparing diuretic. Amiloride appears to help by reducing the entry of lithium into epithelial cells of the renal tubule. Polyuria can also be reduced with a thiazide diuretic. However, because thiazides can lower levels of sodium (see Chapter 35), and would thereby increase lithium retention, amiloride is preferred.

Renal Toxicity. Chronic lithium use has been associated with degenerative changes in the kidney. The risk for renal injury can be reduced by keeping the dosage low and, when possible, avoiding long-term lithium therapy. Kidney function should be assessed before treatment and once a year thereafter.

Goiter and Hypothyroidism. Lithium can reduce incorporation of iodine into thyroid hormone and can inhibit thyroid hormone secretion. With long-term use, the drug can cause *goiter* (enlargement of the thyroid gland). Although usually benign, lithium-induced goiter is sometimes associated with *hypothyroidism.* Treatment with thyroid hormone (levothyroxine) or withdrawal of lithium will reverse both goiter and hypothyroidism. Levels of thyroid hormones—triiodothyronine (T_3) and thyroxine (T_4)—and levels of thyroid-stimulating hormone (TSH) should be measured before giving lithium and annually thereafter.

Teratogenesis. Lithium may—or may not—be a teratogen. In older studies, lithium appeared to have significant teratogenic effects: drug use during the first trimester of pregnancy was associated with an 11% incidence of birth defects (usually malformations of the heart). However, in more recent studies, lithium showed little or no teratogenic potential. Nonetheless, lithium is still classified in U.S. Food and Drug Administration Pregnancy Risk Category D. To minimize any potential fetal risk, *lithium should be avoided during the first trimester of pregnancy,* and unless the benefits of therapy clearly outweigh the risks, it should be avoided during the remainder of pregnancy as well. Women of childbearing age should be counseled to avoid pregnancy while taking lithium. Also, pregnancy should be ruled out before initiating lithium therapy.

Use in Lactation. Lithium readily enters breast milk and can achieve concentrations that might harm the nursing infant. Consequently, breastfeeding during lithium therapy should be discouraged.

Other Side Effects. Lithium can cause mild, reversible leukocytosis (10,000–18,000 white blood cells/mm^3); complete blood counts with a differential should be obtained before treatment and annually thereafter. Possible dermatologic reactions include psoriasis, acne, folliculitis, and alopecia.

Drug Interactions

Diuretics

Diuretics promote sodium loss and can thereby increase the risk for lithium toxicity. Toxicity can occur because, in the presence of low sodium, renal excretion of lithium is reduced, causing lithium levels to rise.

Nonsteroidal Antiinflammatory Drugs (NSAIDs)

NSAIDs can increase lithium levels by as much as 60%. By suppressing prostaglandin synthesis in the kidney, NSAIDs can increase renal reabsorption of lithium (and also sodium), causing lithium levels to rise. NSAIDs known to increase lithium levels include ibuprofen [Motrin, others], naproxen [Naprosyn], piroxicam [Feldene], indomethacin [Indocin], and celecoxib [Celebrex]. Interestingly, aspirin (the prototype NSAID) and sulindac [Clinoril] do *not* increase lithium levels. Accordingly, if a mild analgesic is needed, aspirin or sulindac would be a good choice.

Anticholinergic Drugs

Anticholinergics can cause urinary hesitancy. Coupled with lithium-induced polyuria, this can result in considerable discomfort. Accordingly, patients should avoid drugs with prominent anticholinergic actions (e.g., antihistamines, phenothiazine antipsychotics, TCAs).

Dosage and Administration

Dosing

Lithium dosing is highly individualized. Dosage adjustments are based on plasma drug levels and clinical response (Table 26.3).

Plasma levels should be kept within the therapeutic range. Levels between 0.6 and 1.2 mEq/L are generally appropriate for *acute therapy* of manic episodes. For *maintenance therapy,* lithium levels should range from 0.4 to 1 mEq/L. (Levels of 0.6–0.8 mEq/L are effective for most patients.) To avoid serious toxicity, *lithium levels should not exceed 1.5 mEq/L.*

Knowledge of plasma drug levels is not the only guide to lithium dosing; the clinical response is at least as important. Accordingly, when evaluating lithium dosage, we must not forget to look at the patient. Laboratory tests are all well and good, but they are not a substitute for clinical assessment. For example, if blood levels of lithium appear proper but clinical evaluation indicates toxicity, there is no question as to what should be done: reduce the dosage—despite the apparent acceptability of the dosage as reflected by plasma lithium levels.

BLACK BOX WARNING: LIFE-THREATENING ADVERSE REACTIONS TO LITHIUM

Lithium is associated with hepatotoxicity and pancreatitis, including fatalities, usually during the first 6 months of treatment. Children younger than 2 years and patients with mitochondrial disorders are at higher risk.

Lithium is linked to increased fetal risk, particularly neural tube defects, other major malformations, and decreased IQ.

Antiepileptic Drugs

Three antiepileptic drugs—divalproex sodium, carbamazepine, and lamotrigine—can suppress mania and depression and can stabilize mood in patients with BPD (Table 26.4). The efficacy of these agents is firmly established. In fact, one drug—divalproex sodium—is so effective that it has replaced lithium as the drug of choice for many patients. The basic pharmacology of the antiepileptic drugs and their use in seizure disorders is discussed in Chapter 19. Discussion here focuses on their use in BPD.

Divalproex Sodium (Valproate)

Divalproex sodium[1] [Depakote, Epival ♣], or simply valproate, was the first antiseizure agent approved for BPD. Valproate can control symptoms in acute manic episodes and can help prevent relapse into mania. However, the drug is less effective at treatment and prevention of depressive episodes. As with lithium, benefits appear to result at least in part from neurotrophic and neuroprotective effects. In patients with BPD, valproate compares favorably with lithium: both drugs are highly effective, and valproate works faster and has a higher therapeutic index and a more desirable side-effect profile. However, lithium *is* superior in two important respects. First, lithium is better at reducing the risk for suicide. And second, lithium is more effective at preventing relapses. Nonetheless, because of its rapid onset, safety, and overall efficacy, valproate has become a first-line treatment for BPD.

[1]As discussed in Chapter 19, divalproex sodium [Depakote] is a mixture of valproic acid [Depakene, Depacon, Stavzor] and its sodium salt [Depakene]. Only divalproex sodium is approved for BPD, although all three preparations have identical actions.

TABLE 26.3 ▪ Lithium Preparations

Formulation	Lithium Content*	Trade Name	Usual Adult Dose
Capsules	4.06 mEq lithium (150 mg Li_2CO_3)	generic only	300 mg PO three or four times daily
	8.12 mEq lithium (300 mg Li_2CO_3)	Carbolith ♣	300 mg PO three or four times daily
	16.24 mEq lithium (600 mg Li_2CO_3)	generic only	600 mg PO twice daily
Oral solution	Lithium citrate 8 mEq/5 mL (300 mg Li_2CO_3)	generic only	300 mg PO three or four times daily
Immediate-release tablets	8.12 mEq lithium (300 and 450 mg Li_2CO_3)	generic only	300 mg PO three or four times daily
Slow-release tablets	8.12 mEq lithium (300 and 450 mg Li_2CO_3)	Lithobid	600 mg PO twice daily

*Lithium content is expressed in two ways: milliequivalents (mEq) of lithium ion, and milligrams (mg) of lithium carbonate.
PO, oral administration.

TABLE 26.4 ▪ Antiepileptic Drugs Used in Bipolar Disorder

Drug	Trade Name(s)	Availability	Usual Initial Dose	Usual Maintenance Dose/Day
Divalproex sodium	Depakote Depakote ER	125-, 250-, 500-mg DR tablets 125-mg DR capsules 250-, 500-mg ER tablets	250 mg PO three times daily or 500 mg PO at every bedtime	1000–2500 mg
Carbamazepine	Equetro	100-, 200-, 300-mg ER tablets	200 mg PO twice daily	Gradually increase to max dose of 1600
Lamotrigine	Lamictal Lamictal XR	25-, 100-, 150-, 200-mg tablets 25-, 50-, 100-, 200-mg oral dissolving tablets 25-, 50-, 100-, 200-, 250-, 300-mg ER tablets 2-, 5-, 25-mg chewable tablets	25–50 mg PO daily	Gradually increase to 200 mg

DR, delayed release; ER, extended release; PO, oral administration; XR, extended release.

Although valproate has a higher therapeutic index than lithium and is generally better tolerated, it *can* cause serious toxicity. Of greatest concern are rare cases of thrombocytopenia, pancreatitis, and liver failure—all of which require immediate drug withdrawal. In addition, valproate is a teratogen and hence should not be used during pregnancy. GI disturbances (nausea, vomiting, diarrhea, dyspepsia, indigestion) are common. Despite causing GI distress, valproate frequently causes weight gain, a serious and chronic complication of treatment.

Carbamazepine

Carbamazepine [Tegretol, Equetro, others] is approved for treatment and prevention of manic episodes in patients with BPD. Like valproate, carbamazepine appears less effective at treatment and prevention of depression. For treatment of acute manic episodes, the dosage should be low initially (200 mg twice daily) and then gradually increased. The maximal dosage is 1600 mg/day. The target trough plasma level is 4 to 12 mcg/mL. Neurologic side effects (visual disturbances, ataxia, vertigo, unsteadiness, headache) are common early in treatment but generally resolve despite continued drug use. Hematologic effects (leukopenia, anemia, thrombocytopenia, aplastic anemia) are relatively uncommon but can be severe. Accordingly, complete blood counts, including platelets, should be obtained at baseline and periodically thereafter. Carbamazepine induces cytochrome P450 isoenzymes and can thereby accelerate its own metabolism and the metabolism of other drugs (e.g., oral contraceptives, warfarin, valproate, TCAs). To maintain efficacy, dosages of carbamazepine and these other drugs should be increased as needed.

Drug products containing carbamazepine are available under four trade names: *Carbatrol, Equetro, Epitol,* and *Tegretol.* Carbamazepine formulations with any of these names can be used for BPD. However, only one product—Equetro—is actually *approved* for BPD.

BLACK BOX WARNING: SERIOUS ADVERSE REACTIONS TO CARBAMAZEPINE

Serious and sometimes fatal dermatologic reactions, including toxic epidermal necrolysis (TEN) and Stevens-Johnson syndrome (SJS), have been reported during treatment with carbamazepine.

Aplastic anemia and agranulocytosis have also been reported in association with the use of carbamazepine.

Lamotrigine

Lamotrigine [Lamictal] is indicated for long-term maintenance therapy of BPD. The goal is to prevent affective relapses into mania or depression. Lamotrigine may be used alone or in combination with other mood-stabilizing agents. Side effects include headache, dizziness, double vision, and, rarely, life-threatening rashes (Stevens-Johnson syndrome, toxic epidermal necrolysis).

BLACK BOX WARNING: SERIOUS ADVERSE REACTIONS TO LAMOTRIGINE

Serious and sometimes fatal dermatologic reactions, including toxic epidermal necrolysis (TEN) and Stevens-Johnson syndrome (SJ), have been reported during treatment with lamotrigine.

ANTIPSYCHOTIC DRUGS

In patients with BPD, antipsychotic drugs are used *acutely* to control symptoms during manic episodes, and *long term* to help stabilize mood. These drugs benefit patients with or without psychotic symptoms. Although antipsychotics can be used alone, they are usually employed in combination with a mood stabilizer, typically lithium or valproate.

As discussed in Chapter 24, the antipsychotic drugs fall into two major groups: first-generation antipsychotics (conventional antipsychotics) and second-generation antipsychotics (atypical antipsychotics). Compared with the conventional agents, the atypical agents carry a lower risk for extrapyramidal side effects, including tardive dyskinesia. Accordingly, the atypical agents are preferred for BPD.

Six atypical antipsychotics—*olanzapine* [Zyprexa], *quetiapine* [Seroquel], *risperidone* [Risperdal], *aripiprazole* [Abilify], *cariprazine* [Vraylar], and *ziprasidone* [Geodon]—are approved for BPD. (Another one—*clozapine* [Clozaril]—although highly effective in BPD, is not used owing to a risk for agranulocytosis.) All of these drugs are effective against acute mania, when used alone or combined with lithium or valproate. Currently, only four atypical agents—aripiprazole, olanzapine, quetiapine, and ziprasidone—are approved for long-term use to prevent recurrence of mood episodes. Dosages for patients with BPD are shown in Table 26.5.

Pharmacology of the antipsychotics is presented in Chapter 24.

BLACK BOX WARNING: INCREASED MORTALITY IN OLDER ADULTS

Elderly patients with dementia-related psychosis treated with antipsychotic drugs are at an increased risk for death.

TABLE 26.5 ▪ Adult Oral Dosages for Atypical Antipsychotics Used in Bipolar Disorder

Drug	Dosage
Aripiprazole [Abilify]	*Acute Mania:* Start with 15 mg once daily and increase to 30 mg once daily if needed. Do not exceed 30 mg daily.
Cariprazine [Vraylar]	*Acute Mania:* Start with 1.5 mg once daily and increase to 3–6 mg daily.
Olanzapine [Zyprexa]	*Acute Mania:* Start with 10–15 mg once daily. Increase in 5-mg/day increments, as indicated. The effective range is 5–20 mg once daily. *Maintenance Therapy:* The effective range is 5–20 mg once daily.
Olanzapine/fluoxetine [Symbyax]	*Depressive Episodes:* Start with 6 mg olanzapine/25 mg fluoxetine once daily in the evening. The effective range for antidepressant effects is olanzapine 6–12 mg and fluoxetine 25–50 mg.

Continued

TABLE 26.5 ▪ Adult Oral Dosages for Atypical Antipsychotics Used in Bipolar Disorder—cont'd

Drug	Dosage
Quetiapine [Seroquel]	*Acute Mania (with normal liver function):* Give in two divided doses as follows: 100 mg on day 1, 200 mg on day 2, 300 mg on day 3, and 400 mg on day 4. If needed, increase to 600 mg on day 5 and 800 mg on day 6. *Acute Mania (with liver impairment):* Give 25 mg on day 1, then increase by 25–50 mg/day until symptoms are controlled or side effects are intolerable, whichever comes first. *Depressive Episodes:* Give once-daily doses at bedtime as follows: 50 mg on day 1, 100 mg on day 2, 200 mg on day 3, and 300 mg on day 4; if needed, increase to 400 mg on day 5, and 600 mg on day 8.
Risperidone, short-acting [Risperdal]	*Acute Mania:* Start with 2–3 mg once daily; increase to a maximum of 6 mg once daily, if needed.
Risperidone, long-acting [Risperdal Consta]	*Maintenance Therapy:* Start with 25 mg intramuscularly (IM) every 2 weeks. After at least 4 weeks, dosage may be increased to 37.5 mg IM every 2 weeks, and after at least 4 more weeks, increased again to 50 mg IM every 2 weeks.
Ziprasidone [Geodon]	*Acute Mania:* On day 1, give 80 mg (in two divided doses with food). On day 2, increase to 60 or 80 mg twice daily. Based on tolerability and efficacy, adjust dosage within the range of 40–80 mg twice daily. *Maintenance Therapy:* The effective range is 15–30 mg daily.

CHAPTER

27 Sedative-Hypnotic Drugs

Laura D. Rosenthal, DNP, ACNP, FAANP

The sedative-hypnotics are drugs that depress central nervous system (CNS) function. With some of these drugs, CNS depression is more generalized than with others. The sedative-hypnotics are used primarily for two common disorders: anxiety and insomnia. Agents given to relieve anxiety are known as *antianxiety agents* or *anxiolytics*. Agents given to promote sleep are known as *hypnotics*. The distinction between antianxiety effects and hypnotic effects is often a matter of dosage: typically, sedative-hypnotics relieve anxiety in low doses and induce sleep in higher doses. Hence a single drug may be considered both an antianxiety agent and a hypnotic agent, depending on the reason for its use and the dosage employed.

There are three major groups of sedative-hypnotics: barbiturates (e.g., secobarbital), benzodiazepines (e.g., diazepam), and benzodiazepine-like drugs (e.g., zolpidem). The barbiturates were introduced in the early 1900s, the benzodiazepines in the 1950s, and the benzodiazepine-like drugs in the 1990s. Although barbiturates were widely used as sedative-hypnotics in the past, they are rarely used for this purpose today, having been replaced by the newer drugs.

Before the benzodiazepines became available, anxiety and insomnia were treated with barbiturates and other *general CNS depressants*—drugs with multiple undesirable qualities. First, these drugs are powerful respiratory depressants that can readily prove fatal in overdose. As a result, they are "drugs of choice" for suicide. Second, because they produce subjective effects that many individuals find desirable, most general CNS depressants have a high potential for abuse. Third, with prolonged use, most of these drugs produce significant tolerance and physical dependence. And fourth, barbiturates and some other CNS depressants induce synthesis of hepatic drug-metabolizing enzymes and can thereby decrease responses to other drugs. Because the benzodiazepines are just as effective as the general CNS depressants, but do not share their undesirable properties, the benzodiazepines are clearly preferred to the general CNS depressants for treating anxiety and insomnia.

We begin by discussing the basic pharmacology of the sedative-hypnotics and end by discussing their use in insomnia. Use of these drugs for anxiety disorders is addressed in Chapter 28.

BENZODIAZEPINES

Benzodiazepines, along with the newer benzodiazepine receptor agonists, are drugs of first choice for anxiety and insomnia. In addition, these drugs are used to induce general anesthesia and to manage seizure disorders, muscle spasm, and withdrawal from alcohol.

Benzodiazepines were introduced in the late 1950s and remain important today. Perhaps the most familiar member of the family is diazepam [Valium]. The most frequently prescribed members are lorazepam [Ativan] and alprazolam [Xanax, Xanax XR, Niravam].

Because all of the benzodiazepines produce nearly identical effects, we will consider the family as a group, rather than selecting a representative member as a prototype.

Overview of Pharmacologic Effects

Practically all responses to benzodiazepines result from actions in the CNS. Benzodiazepines have few direct actions outside the CNS. All of the benzodiazepines produce a similar spectrum of responses. However, because of pharmacokinetic differences, individual benzodiazepines may differ in clinical applications.

Central Nervous System

All beneficial effects of benzodiazepines, and most adverse effects, result from depressant actions in the CNS. With increasing dosage, effects progress from sedation to hypnosis to stupor.

Benzodiazepines depress neuronal function at multiple sites in the CNS. They *reduce anxiety* through effects on the limbic system, a neuronal network associated with emotionality. They *promote sleep* through effects on cortical areas and on the sleep-wakefulness "clock." They *induce muscle relaxation* through effects on supraspinal motor areas, including the cerebellum. Two important side effects—*confusion* and *anterograde amnesia*—result from effects on the hippocampus and cerebral cortex.

Cardiovascular System

When taken *orally,* benzodiazepines have almost no effect on the heart and blood vessels. In contrast, when administered *intravenously,* even in therapeutic doses, benzodiazepines can produce profound hypotension and cardiac arrest.

Respiratory System

In contrast to the barbiturates, the benzodiazepines are weak respiratory depressants. When taken alone in therapeutic doses, benzodiazepines produce little or no depression of respiration—and with toxic doses, respiratory depression is moderate at most. With oral therapy, clinically significant respiratory depression occurs only when benzodiazepines are combined with other CNS depressants (e.g., opioids, barbiturates, alcohol).

Although benzodiazepines generally have minimal effects on respiration, they can be a problem for patients with respiratory disorders. In patients with chronic obstructive pulmonary disease, benzodiazepines may worsen hypoventilation and hypoxemia. In patients with obstructive sleep apnea (OSA), benzodiazepines may exacerbate apneic episodes. In patients who snore, benzodiazepines may convert partial airway obstruction into OSA.

Molecular Mechanism of Action

Benzodiazepines *potentiate the actions of gamma-aminobutyric acid* (GABA), an inhibitory neurotransmitter found throughout the CNS. These drugs enhance the actions of GABA by binding to specific receptors in a supramolecular structure known as the GABA receptor–chloride channel complex. Note that benzodiazepines do not act as direct GABA agonists—they simply intensify the effects of GABA.

Because benzodiazepines act by amplifying the actions of endogenous GABA, rather than by directly mimicking GABA, there is a limit to how much CNS depression benzodiazepines can produce. This explains why benzodiazepines are so much safer than the barbiturates—drugs that can directly mimic GABA. Because benzodiazepines simply potentiate the inhibitory effects of endogenous GABA, and because the amount of GABA in the CNS is finite, there is a built-in limit to the depth of CNS depression the benzodiazepines can produce. In contrast, because the barbiturates are direct-acting CNS depressants, maximal effects are limited only by the amount of barbiturate administered.

Pharmacokinetics

Absorption and Distribution

Most benzodiazepines are well absorbed after oral administration. Because of their high lipid solubility, benzodiazepines readily cross the blood-brain barrier to reach sites in the CNS.

Metabolism

Most benzodiazepines undergo extensive metabolic alterations. With few exceptions, the *metabolites are pharmacologically active.* As a result, responses produced by administering a particular benzodiazepine often persist long after the parent drug has disappeared. Hence there may be a poor correlation between the plasma half-life of the parent drug and duration of pharmacologic effects. Flurazepam, for example, whose plasma half-life is only 2 to 3 hours, is converted into an active metabolite with a half-life of 50 hours. Hence giving flurazepam produces long-lasting effects, even though flurazepam itself is gone from the plasma in 8 to 12 hours (about four half-lives).

In patients with liver disease, metabolism of benzodiazepines may be reduced, thereby prolonging excretion and intensifying responses. Because certain benzodiazepines (oxazepam, temazepam, and lorazepam) undergo very little metabolic alteration, they may be preferred for patients with hepatic impairment.

Time Course of Action

Benzodiazepines differ significantly from one another with respect to time course. Specifically, they differ in onset and duration of action and in their tendency to accumulate with repeated dosing.

Because all benzodiazepines have essentially equivalent pharmacologic actions, selection among them is based largely on differences in time course. For example, if a patient needs medication to accelerate falling asleep, a benzodiazepine with a rapid onset (e.g., triazolam) would be indicated. However, if medication is needed to prevent waking later in the night, a benzodiazepine with a slower onset (e.g., estazolam) would be preferred. For treatment of anxiety, a drug with an intermediate duration is desirable. For treatment of any benzodiazepine-responsive condition in older adults, a drug such as lorazepam, which is not likely to accumulate with repeated dosing, is generally preferred.

Therapeutic Uses

The benzodiazepines have three principal indications: (1) anxiety, (2) insomnia, and (3) seizure disorders. In addition, they are used as preoperative medications and to treat muscle spasm and withdrawal from alcohol. Although all benzodiazepines share the same pharmacologic properties and therefore might be equally effective for all applications, not every benzodiazepine is actually employed for all potential uses. The principal factors that determine the actual applications of a particular benzodiazepine are (1) the pharmacokinetic properties of the drug itself and (2) research and marketing decisions of pharmaceutical companies. Specific applications of individual benzodiazepines are shown in Table 27.1.

Anxiety

Benzodiazepines are drugs of first choice for acute anxiety. Although all benzodiazepines have anxiolytic actions, only six are marketed for this indication (see Table 27.1). Anxiolytic effects result from depressing neurotransmission in the limbic system and cortical areas. Use of benzodiazepines to treat anxiety disorders is discussed in Chapter 28.

Insomnia

Benzodiazepines are also used in the treatment of insomnia. These drugs decrease latency time to falling asleep, reduce awakenings, and increase total sleeping time. The role of benzodiazepines in managing insomnia is discussed in depth later.

Seizure Disorders

Four benzodiazepines—diazepam, clonazepam, lorazepam, and clorazepate—are employed for seizure disorders. Antiseizure applications are discussed in Chapter 19.

Muscle Spasm

One benzodiazepine—diazepam—is used to relieve muscle spasm and spasticity (see Chapter 20). Effects on muscle tone are secondary to actions in the CNS. Diazepam cannot relieve spasm without causing sedation.

Alcohol Withdrawal

Diazepam and other benzodiazepines may be administered to ease withdrawal from alcohol (see Chapter 31). Benefits derive from cross-dependence with alcohol, which enables benzodiazepines to suppress symptoms brought on by alcohol abstinence.

Adverse Effects

Benzodiazepines are generally well tolerated, and serious adverse reactions are rare. In contrast to barbiturates and other general CNS depressants, benzodiazepines are remarkably safe.

Central Nervous System Depression

When taken to promote sleep, benzodiazepines cause drowsiness, lightheadedness, incoordination, and difficulty concentrating.

TABLE 27.1 ▪ Applications of the Benzodiazepines

	Approved Applications						
Generic Name [Trade Name]	**GAD**	**Insomnia**	**Seizures**	**Muscle Spasm, Spasticity**	**Alcohol Withdrawal**	**Anesthesia Induction or Preanesthesia**	**Anxiety**
Alprazolam [Xanax, Xanax XR, Niravam]	✓						✓
Chlordiazepoxide [Librium]	✓				✓		
Clonazepam [Klonopin, Rivotril 🍁]			✓				✓
Clorazepate [Tranxene-T]	✓		✓		✓		
Diazepam [Valium, Diastat AcuDial]	✓		✓	✓	✓	✓	
Estazolam (generic only)		✓					
Flurazepam (generic only)		✓					
Lorazepam [Ativan]	✓	✓	✓		✓	✓	✓
Midazolam [Versed]						✓*	
Oxazepam (generic only)	✓				✓		
Temazepam [Restoril]		✓					
Triazolam [Halcion]		✓					

*Midazolam, in conjunction with an opioid analgesic, is also used to produce *conscious sedation,* a semiconscious state suitable for minor surgeries and endoscopic procedures.
GAD, generalized anxiety disorder.

When these effects occur at bedtime, they are generally inconsequential. However, if sedation and other manifestations of CNS depression persist beyond waking, interference with daytime activities can result.

Anterograde Amnesia

Benzodiazepines can cause anterograde amnesia (impaired recall of events that take place after dosing). Anterograde amnesia has been especially troublesome with *triazolam* [Halcion]. If patients complain of forgetfulness, the possibility of drug-induced amnesia should be evaluated.

Sleep Driving and Other Complex Sleep-Related Behaviors

Patients taking benzodiazepines in sleep-inducing doses may carry out complex behaviors and then have no memory of their actions. Reported behaviors include sleep driving, preparing and eating meals, and making phone calls. Although these events can occur with normal doses, they are more likely when doses are excessive and when benzodiazepines are combined with alcohol and other CNS depressants. Because of the potential for harm, benzodiazepines should be withdrawn if sleep driving is reported. To minimize withdrawal symptoms, dosing should be tapered slowly, rather than discontinued abruptly.

Paradoxical Effects

When employed to treat anxiety, benzodiazepines sometimes cause paradoxical responses, including insomnia, excitation, euphoria, heightened anxiety, and rage. If these occur, the benzodiazepine should be withdrawn.

Respiratory Depression

Benzodiazepines are weak respiratory depressants. Death from overdose with oral benzodiazepines alone has never been documented. Hence, in contrast to the barbiturates, benzodiazepines present little risk as vehicles for suicide. It must be emphasized, however, that although respiratory depression with *oral* therapy is rare, benzodiazepines can cause severe respiratory depression when administered *intravenously.* In addition, substantial respiratory depression can result from combining oral benzodiazepines with other CNS depressants (e.g., alcohol, barbiturates, opioids).

Abuse

Benzodiazepines have a lower abuse potential than barbiturates and most other general CNS depressants. The behavior pattern that constitutes "addiction" is uncommon among people who take benzodiazepines for therapeutic purposes. When asked about their drug use, individuals who regularly abuse drugs rarely express a preference for benzodiazepines over barbiturates. Because their potential for abuse is low, the benzodiazepines are classified under Schedule IV of the Controlled Substances Act. This contrasts with the barbiturates, most of which are classified under Schedule III.

Use in Pregnancy and Lactation

Benzodiazepines are highly lipid soluble and can readily cross the placental barrier. Use of benzodiazepines during the first trimester of pregnancy is associated with an increased risk for congenital malformations, such as cleft lip, inguinal hernia, and cardiac anomalies. Use near term can cause CNS depression in the neonate. Because they may represent a risk to the fetus, most benzodiazepines are classified in U.S. Food and Drug Administration (FDA) Pregnancy Risk Category D. Four of these drugs—estazolam, flurazepam, temazepam, and triazolam—are in Category X. Women of childbearing age should be warned about the potential for fetal harm and instructed to discontinue benzodiazepines if pregnancy occurs.

Benzodiazepines enter breast milk with ease and may accumulate to toxic levels in the breastfed infant. Accordingly, these drugs should be avoided by nursing mothers.

Other Adverse Effects

Occasional reactions include weakness, headache, blurred vision, vertigo, nausea, vomiting, epigastric distress, and diarrhea. Neutropenia and jaundice occur rarely. Rarely, benzodiazepines may cause severe allergic reactions, including angioedema and anaphylaxis.

Drug Interactions

Benzodiazepines undergo very few important interactions with other drugs. Unlike barbiturates, benzodiazepines do not induce hepatic drug-metabolizing enzymes. Hence benzodiazepines do not accelerate the metabolism of other drugs.

Central Nervous System Depressants

The CNS-depressant actions of benzodiazepines add to those of other CNS depressants (e.g., alcohol, barbiturates, opioids). Hence, although benzodiazepines are very safe when used alone, they can be extremely hazardous in combination with other depressants. Combined overdose with a benzodiazepine plus another CNS depressant can cause profound respiratory depression, coma, and death. Patients should be warned against use of alcohol and all other CNS depressants.

Tolerance and Physical Dependence

Tolerance

With prolonged use of benzodiazepines, tolerance develops to some effects but not to others. No tolerance develops to anxiolytic effects, and tolerance to hypnotic effects is generally low. In contrast, significant tolerance develops to antiseizure effects. Patients tolerant to barbiturates, alcohol, and other general CNS depressants show some cross-tolerance to benzodiazepines.

Physical Dependence

Benzodiazepines can cause physical dependence—but the incidence of *substantial* dependence is low. When benzodiazepines are discontinued after short-term use at therapeutic doses, the resulting withdrawal syndrome is generally mild and often goes unrecognized. Symptoms include anxiety, insomnia, sweating, tremors, and dizziness. Withdrawal from long-term, high-dose therapy can cause more serious reactions, such as panic, paranoia, delirium, hypertension, muscle twitches, and seizures. Symptoms of withdrawal are usually more intense with benzodiazepines that have a short duration of action. With one agent—*alprazolam* [Xanax, Xanax XR, Niravam]—dependence may be a greater problem than with other benzodiazepines. Because the benzodiazepine withdrawal syndrome can resemble an anxiety disorder, it is important to differentiate withdrawal symptoms from the return of the original symptoms of anxiety.

The intensity of withdrawal symptoms can be minimized by discontinuing treatment gradually. Doses should be slowly tapered over several weeks or months. Substituting a benzodiazepine with a long half-life for one with a short half-life is also helpful. Patients should be warned against abrupt cessation of treatment. After discontinuation of treatment, patients should be monitored for 3 weeks for indications of withdrawal or recurrence of original symptoms.

Acute Toxicity

Oral Overdose

When administered in excessive dosage by mouth, benzodiazepines rarely cause serious toxicity. Symptoms include drowsiness, lethargy, and confusion. Significant cardiovascular and respiratory effects are uncommon. If an individual known to have taken an overdose of benzodiazepines does exhibit signs of serious toxicity, it is probable that another drug was taken, too.

Preparations, Dosage, and Administration

Preparations and dosages for insomnia are presented later in the chapter. Preparations and dosages of benzodiazepines used for other disorders are presented in Chapters 19, 20, and 28.

Routes

All benzodiazepines can be administered orally. When used for sedation or induction of sleep, benzodiazepines are almost always administered by mouth.

Oral

Patients should be advised to take oral benzodiazepines with food if gastric upset occurs. Also, they should be instructed to swallow sustained-release formulations intact, without crushing or chewing. Patients should be warned not to increase the dosage or discontinue therapy without consulting the prescriber.

For treatment of insomnia, benzodiazepines should be given on an intermittent schedule (e.g., 3 or 4 days a week) in the lowest effective dosage for the shortest duration required. This will minimize physical dependence and associated drug-dependency insomnia.

Prototype Drugs

SEDATIVE-HYPNOTIC DRUGS

Benzodiazepine
Triazolam

Benzodiazepine-Like Drugs
Zolpidem
Zaleplon

Barbiturate
Secobarbital

Melatonin Receptor Agonist
Ramelteon

BENZODIAZEPINE-LIKE DRUGS

Three benzodiazepine-like drugs are available: zolpidem, zaleplon, and eszopiclone. All three are preferred agents for insomnia. They are not indicated for anxiety. These drugs are structurally different from benzodiazepines, but nonetheless share the same mechanism of action: they all act as *agonists at the benzodiazepine receptor site* on the GABA receptor–chloride channel complex. Like the benzodiazepines, these drugs have a low potential for tolerance, dependence, and abuse and are classified as Schedule IV substances.

Zolpidem

Zolpidem [Ambien, Ambien CR, Edluar, Intermezzo, Zolpimist], our most widely used hypnotic, is approved only for short-term management of insomnia. However, although approval is limited to short-term use, many patients have taken the drug long term with no apparent tolerance or increase in adverse effects. All zolpidem formulations have a rapid onset and hence can help people who have difficulty falling asleep. In addition, the extended-release formulation—Ambien CR—can help people who have difficulty maintaining sleep.

Although structurally unrelated to the benzodiazepines, zolpidem binds to the benzodiazepine receptor site on the GABA receptor–chloride channel complex and shares some properties of the benzodiazepines. Like the benzodiazepines, zolpidem can reduce sleep latency and awakenings and can prolong sleep duration. The drug does not significantly reduce time in rapid eye movement (REM) sleep and causes little or no rebound insomnia when therapy is discontinued. In contrast to the benzodiazepines, zolpidem lacks anxiolytic, muscle relaxant, and anticonvulsant actions because zolpidem doesn't bind with all benzodiazepine receptors. Rather, binding is limited to the benzodiazepine-1 subtype of benzodiazepine receptors.

Zolpidem is rapidly absorbed after oral dosing. Plasma levels peak in 2 hours. The drug is widely distributed, although levels in the brain remain low. Zolpidem is extensively metabolized to inactive compounds that are excreted in the bile, urine, and feces. The elimination half-life is 2.4 hours.

Zolpidem has a side-effect profile like that of the benzodiazepines. *Daytime drowsiness and dizziness* are most common, and these occur in only 1% to 2% of patients. Like the benzodiazepines, zolpidem has been associated with *sleep driving* and other *sleep-related complex behaviors.* At therapeutic doses, zolpidem causes little or no respiratory depression. Safety in pregnancy has not been established. According to the FDA, zolpidem may pose a small risk for anaphylaxis and angioedema.

Short-term treatment is not associated with significant tolerance or physical dependence. Withdrawal symptoms are minimum or absent. Similarly, the abuse liability of zolpidem is low. Accordingly, the drug is classified under Schedule IV of the Controlled Substances Act.

Like other sedative-hypnotics, zolpidem can intensify the effects of other CNS depressants. Patients should be warned against combining zolpidem with alcohol and all other drugs that depress CNS function.

Zaleplon

Zaleplon [Sonata] is the first representative of a new class of hypnotics, the pyrazolopyrimidines. The drug is approved only for short-term management of insomnia, but prolonged use does not appear to cause tolerance. Like zolpidem, zaleplon binds to the benzodiazepine-1 receptor site on the GABA receptor–chloride channel complex, enhancing the depressant actions of endogenous GABA. In contrast to zolpidem, zaleplon has a very rapid onset and short duration of action and hence is good for helping patients fall asleep, but not for maintaining sleep.

Zaleplon is rapidly and completely absorbed after oral dosing. However, because of extensive first-pass metabolism, bioavailability is only 30%. A large or high-fat meal can delay absorption substantially. Plasma levels peak about 1 hour after administration and then rapidly decline, returning to baseline in 4 to 5 hours. Zaleplon is metabolized by hepatic aldehyde oxidase before excretion in the urine. Its half-life is just 1 hour.

Because of its kinetic profile, zaleplon is well suited for people who have trouble falling asleep, but not for people who can't maintain sleep. The drug can also help people who need a sedative-hypnotic in the middle of the night: because of its short duration, zaleplon can be taken at 3:00 AM without causing residual daytime sedation.

Zaleplon is well tolerated. The most common side effects are headache, nausea, drowsiness, dizziness, myalgia, and abdominal pain. Like the benzodiazepines, zaleplon has been associated with rare cases of sleep driving and other complex sleep-related behaviors. Respiratory depression has not been observed. Physical dependence is minimum, the only sign being mild rebound insomnia the first night after drug withdrawal. Next-day sedation and hangover have not been reported. Like the benzodiazepines, zaleplon has a low potential for abuse and hence is classified as a Schedule IV drug.

Eszopiclone

Eszopiclone [Lunesta], like zaleplon and zolpidem, binds selectively with the benzodiazepine-1 receptor on the GABA receptor–chloride channel complex and thereby enhances the depressant actions of endogenous GABA.

Eszopiclone is approved for treating insomnia, with no limitation on how long it can be used. This contrasts with zaleplon and zolpidem, which are approved for short-term use only. Does this mean that eszopiclone is safer than the other two drugs, or less likely to promote tolerance? Not necessarily. It only means that the manufacturer of eszopiclone conducted a prolonged (6-month) study, whereas the manufacturers of the other two drugs did not. In that prolonged study, eszopiclone reduced sleep latency and nighttime awakening, increased total sleep time and sleep quality, had no significant effect on sleep architecture, and showed no indication of tolerance.

Eszopiclone is rapidly absorbed after oral dosing, reaching peak blood levels in 1 to 2 hours. The drug undergoes extensive hepatic metabolism, primarily by CYP3A4 (the 3A4 isoenzyme of cytochrome P450). The resulting inactive (or weakly active) metabolites are excreted in the urine. The elimination half-life is 6 hours.

Eszopiclone is generally well tolerated. The most common adverse effect is a bitter aftertaste, reported by 17% of patients dosed with 2 mg and 34% of those dosed with 3 mg. Other common effects are headache, somnolence, dizziness, and dry mouth. Rebound insomnia may occur on the first night after discontinuing the drug. Like the benzodiazepines and the other benzodiazepine-like drugs, eszopiclone has been associated with cases of sleep driving and other sleep-related complex behaviors. Rarely, eszopiclone may cause anaphylaxis or angioedema. Eszopiclone has a low potential for abuse and hence is classified as a Schedule IV drug.

RAMELTEON: A MELATONIN AGONIST

Ramelteon [Rozerem] is a relatively new hypnotic with a unique mechanism of action: activation of receptors for melatonin. The drug is approved for treating chronic insomnia characterized by difficulty with sleep onset, but not with sleep maintenance. Long-term use is permitted. Of the major drugs for insomnia, ramelteon is the only one not regulated as a controlled substance.

Therapeutic Use

Ramelteon has a rapid onset (about 30 minutes) and short duration and hence is good for inducing sleep but not maintaining sleep. There are no significant residual effects on the day after dosing. Nor is there any rebound insomnia when treatment is stopped after 35 consecutive nights of use. When approving the drug, the FDA put no limit on how long it may be used.

Mechanism of Action

Ramelteon activates receptors for melatonin—specifically the MT_1 and MT_2 subtypes, which are key mediators of the normal sleep-wakefulness cycle. Sleep promotion derives primarily from activating MT_1 receptors. (Under physiologic conditions, activation of MT_1 receptors by endogenous melatonin induces sleepiness.) Ramelteon does not activate MT_3 receptors, which help regulate numerous systems unrelated to sleep. Selectivity for MT_1 and MT_2 receptors explains why ramelteon is superior to melatonin itself for treating insomnia. Ramelteon does not bind with the GABA receptor–chloride channel complex, or with receptors for neuropeptides, benzodiazepines, dopamine, serotonin, norepinephrine, acetylcholine, or opioids.

Pharmacokinetics

Absorption is rapid and nearly complete, although food can reduce both the rate and extent of absorption. Despite generally good absorption, the absolute bioavailability of ramelteon is very low—only 1.8%, owing to extensive first-pass metabolism, primarily by hepatic CYP1A2 (the 1A2 isoenzyme of cytochrome P450). Much of each dose is converted to an active metabolite, designated M-II, that contributes to therapeutic effects. The half-lives of the parent drug and active metabolite average 2 to 5 hours. In patients with hepatic impairment, elimination is delayed and drug levels can rise. Renal impairment does not affect drug levels.

Adverse Effects

Ramelteon is very well tolerated. In clinical trials, the incidence of adverse effects was nearly identical to that of placebo. The most common side effects are somnolence, dizziness, and fatigue. According to the FDA, ramelteon may share the ability of benzodiazepines to cause sleep driving and other sleep-related complex behaviors. Very rarely, patients have reported hallucinations, agitation, and mania.

Ramelteon can increase levels of prolactin and reduce levels of testosterone. As a result, the drug has the potential to cause amenorrhea, galactorrhea, reduced libido, and fertility problems. If these occur, the prescriber should be consulted.

Postmarketing reports indicate a small risk for severe allergic reactions. Rarely, patients have experienced angioedema of the tongue, glottis, or larynx. Some patients also experienced dyspnea and throat constriction, suggestive of anaphylaxis. Patients who experience these symptoms should discontinue ramelteon and never use it again.

Physical Dependence and Abuse

There is no evidence that taking ramelteon leads to physical dependence or abuse. As a result, ramelteon is the first FDA-approved sleep remedy that is not regulated under the Controlled Substances Act.

Drug Interactions

Fluvoxamine [Luvox], a strong inhibitor of CYP1A2, can increase levels of ramelteon more than 50-fold. Accordingly, the combination should be avoided. Weaker inhibitors of CYP1A2 should be used with caution. Alcohol can intensify sedation and hence should be avoided.

Precautions

Ramelteon should be used with caution by patients with moderate hepatic impairment and should be avoided by those with severe hepatic impairment. Because ramelteon promotes sedation, patients should be advised to avoid dangerous activities, such as driving or operating heavy machinery.

Use in Pregnancy and Breastfeeding

Effects during human pregnancy have not been studied. Until more is known, prudence dictates avoiding the drug during pregnancy (or at least using it with caution). Ramelteon is not recommended for use by nursing mothers.

BARBITURATES

The barbiturates have been available for more than 100 years. These drugs cause relatively nonselective depression of CNS function and are the prototypes of the general CNS depressants. Because they depress multiple aspects of CNS function, barbiturates can be used for daytime sedation, induction of sleep, suppression of seizures, and general anesthesia. Barbiturates cause tolerance and dependence, have a high abuse potential, and are subject to multiple drug interactions. Moreover, barbiturates are powerful respiratory depressants that can be fatal in overdose. Because of these undesirable properties, barbiturates are used much less than in the past, having been replaced by newer and safer drugs—primarily the benzodiazepines and benzodiazepine-like drugs (e.g., zolpidem). However, although their use has declined greatly, barbiturates still have important applications in seizure control and anesthesia. Moreover, barbiturates are valuable from an instructional point of view: by understanding these prototypic agents, we gain an understanding of the general CNS depressants as a group, along with an appreciation of why barbiturates are no longer used for anxiety and insomnia.

Classification

Duration of action influences the clinical applications of barbiturates. The ultrashort-acting agents (e.g., methohexital) are used for induction of anesthesia. The short- to intermediate-acting agents (e.g., secobarbital) are used as sedatives and hypnotics. The long-acting agents (e.g., phenobarbital) are used primarily as antiseizure drugs.

Mechanism of Action

Like benzodiazepines, barbiturates bind to the GABA receptor–chloride channel complex. By doing so, these drugs can (1) enhance the inhibitory actions of GABA and (2) directly mimic the actions of GABA.

Because barbiturates can directly mimic GABA, there is no ceiling to the degree of CNS depression they can produce. Hence, in contrast to the benzodiazepines, these drugs can readily cause death by overdose. Although barbiturates can cause general depression of the CNS, they show some selectivity for depressing the reticular activating system (RAS), a neuronal network that helps regulate the sleep-wakefulness cycle. By depressing the RAS, barbiturates produce sedation and sleep.

Pharmacologic Effects

Central Nervous System Depression

Most effects of barbiturates—both therapeutic and adverse—result from generalized depression of CNS function. With increasing dosage, responses progress from sedation to sleep to general anesthesia.

Most barbiturates can be considered nonselective CNS depressants. The main exception is phenobarbital, a drug used to control seizures. Seizure control is achieved at doses that have minimal effects on other aspects of CNS function.

Cardiovascular Effects

At hypnotic doses, barbiturates produce modest reductions in blood pressure and heart rate. In contrast, toxic doses can cause profound hypotension and shock. At high doses, barbiturates depress the myocardium and vascular smooth muscle, along with all other electrically excitable tissues.

Induction of Hepatic Drug-Metabolizing Enzymes

Barbiturates stimulate synthesis of hepatic microsomal enzymes, the principal drug-metabolizing enzymes of the liver. As a result, barbiturates can accelerate their own metabolism and the metabolism of many other drugs by promoting synthesis of porphyrin. Porphyrin is then converted into heme, which in turn is incorporated into cytochrome P450, a key component of the hepatic drug-metabolizing system.

Tolerance and Physical Dependence

Tolerance

When barbiturates are taken regularly, tolerance develops to many—but not all—of their CNS effects. Specifically, tolerance develops to sedative and hypnotic effects and to other effects that underlie barbiturate abuse. However, even with chronic use, very little tolerance develops to toxic effects.

In the tolerant user, doses must be increased to produce the same intensity of response that could formerly be achieved with smaller doses. Hence individuals who take barbiturates for prolonged periods—be it for therapy or recreation—require steadily increasing doses to achieve the effects they desire.

It is important to note that very little tolerance develops to respiratory depression. Because tolerance to respiratory depression is minimum, and because tolerance does develop to therapeutic effects, with continued treatment, the lethal (respiratory-depressant) dose remains relatively constant while the therapeutic dose climbs higher and higher (Fig. 27.1). As tolerance to therapeutic effects increases, the therapeutic dose grows steadily closer to the lethal dose—a situation that is clearly hazardous.

As a rule, tolerance to one general CNS depressant bestows tolerance to all other general CNS depressants. Hence there is cross-tolerance among barbiturates, alcohol, benzodiazepines, general anesthetics, and certain other agents. Tolerance to barbiturates and the other general CNS depressants does not produce significant cross-tolerance with opioids (e.g., morphine).

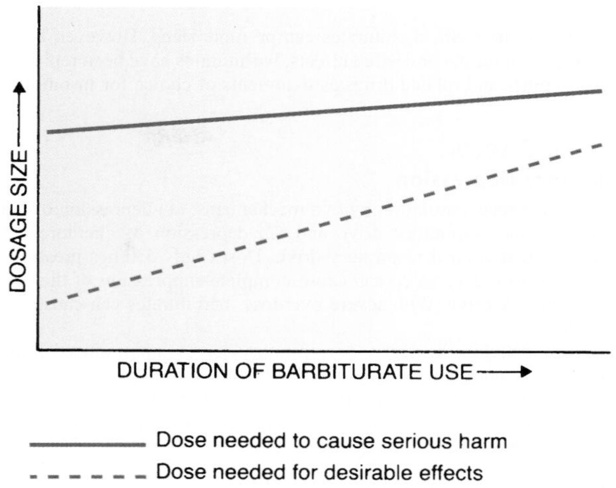

Figure 27.1 ■ Development of tolerance to the toxic and subjective effects of barbiturates.
With prolonged barbiturate use, tolerance develops. However, less tolerance develops to toxic effects than to desired effects. Consequently, as duration of use increases, the difference between the dose producing desirable effects and the dose producing toxicity becomes progressively smaller, thereby increasing the risk for serious harm.

Physical Dependence

Prolonged use of barbiturates results in physical dependence, a state in which continued use is required to avoid an abstinence syndrome. Physical dependence results from adaptive neurochemical changes that occur in response to chronic drug exposure.

Individuals who are physically dependent on barbiturates exhibit cross-dependence with other general CNS depressants. Because of cross-dependence, a person physically dependent on barbiturates can prevent withdrawal symptoms by taking any other general CNS depressant (e.g., alcohol, benzodiazepines). As a rule, cross-dependence exists among all of the general CNS depressants. However, there is no significant cross-dependence with opioids.

The general CNS-depressant abstinence syndrome can be severe. Abrupt withdrawal from general CNS depressants is more dangerous than withdrawal from opioids. Although withdrawal from opioids is certainly unpleasant, the risk for serious injury is low. In contrast, the abstinence syndrome associated with general CNS depressants can be fatal.

The following description illustrates how dangerous withdrawal from general CNS depressants can be. Early reactions include weakness, restlessness, insomnia, hyperthermia, orthostatic hypotension, confusion, and disorientation. By the third day, seizures may develop. Approximately 75% of patients experience psychotic delirium (a state similar to alcoholic delirium tremens). In extreme cases, these symptoms may be followed by exhaustion, cardiovascular collapse, and death. The entire abstinence syndrome evolves over approximately 8 days. Symptom intensity can be greatly reduced by withdrawing barbiturates and other general CNS depressants slowly.

A long-acting barbiturate (e.g., phenobarbital) may be administered to facilitate the withdrawal process. Because of cross-dependence, phenobarbital can substitute for other CNS depressants and can thereby suppress symptoms of withdrawal. Because phenobarbital is eliminated from the body slowly, treatment permits a gradual transition from a drug-dependent state to a drug-free state. When phenobarbital is given to aid withdrawal, its dosage should be reduced gradually over 10 days to 3 weeks.

Therapeutic Uses

Seizure Disorders

Phenobarbital is used for seizure disorders (see Chapter 19). This drug suppresses seizures at doses that are essentially nonsedative.

Insomnia

By depressing the CNS, barbiturates can promote sleep. However, because they can cause multiple undesired effects, barbiturates have been replaced by benzodiazepines and related drugs as treatments of choice for insomnia.

Adverse Effects

Respiratory Depression

Barbiturates reduce ventilation by two mechanisms: (1) depression of brainstem neurogenic respiratory drive and (2) depression of chemoreceptive mechanisms that control respiratory drive. Doses only 3 times greater than those needed to induce sleep can cause complete suppression of the neurogenic respiratory drive. With severe overdose, barbiturates can cause apnea and death.

For most patients, the degree of respiratory depression produced at therapeutic doses is not significant. However, in older-adult patients and those with respiratory disease, therapeutic doses can compromise respiration substantially. Combining a barbiturate with another CNS depressant intensifies respiratory depression.

Suicide

Barbiturates have a low therapeutic index. Accordingly, overdose can readily cause death. Because of their toxicity, the barbiturates are frequently employed as vehicles for suicide and hence should not be dispensed to patients with suicidal tendencies.

Abuse

Barbiturates produce subjective effects that many individuals find desirable. As a result, they are popular drugs of abuse. The barbiturates that are most prone to abuse are those in the short- to intermediate-acting group (e.g., secobarbital). Individual barbiturates within the group are classified under Schedule III of the Controlled Substances Act, reflecting their high potential for abuse. Although barbiturates are frequently abused in nonmedical settings, they are rarely abused during medical use.

Acute Toxicity

Acute intoxication with barbiturates is a medical emergency: left untreated, overdose can be fatal. Poisoning is often the result of attempted suicide, although it can also occur by accident (usually in children and drug abusers). Because acute toxicity from barbiturates and other general CNS depressants is very similar, the discussion that follows applies to all of these drugs.

Symptoms

Acute overdose produces a classic triad of symptoms: respiratory depression, coma, and pinpoint pupils. (Pupils may later dilate as hypoxia caused by respiratory depression sets in.) The three classic symptoms are frequently accompanied by hypotension and hypothermia. Death is likely to result from pulmonary complications and renal failure.

Treatment

Proper management requires an intensive care unit. With vigorous treatment, most patients recover fully.

Treatment has two main objectives: (1) removal of barbiturate from the body and (2) maintenance of an adequate oxygen supply to the brain. Oxygenation can be maintained by keeping the airway patent and giving oxygen.

Administration

Oral administration is employed for daytime sedation and to treat insomnia. Patients should be warned not to increase their dosage or discontinue treatment without consulting the prescriber. Dosages should be reduced for older-adult patients. When terminating therapy, the dosage should be gradually tapered.

MANAGEMENT OF INSOMNIA

Insomnia can be defined as an inability to sleep well. Some people have difficulty falling asleep, some have difficulty maintaining sleep, some are troubled by early morning awakening, and some have sleep that is not refreshing. Insomnia is transient for some people and chronic for others. In any given year, about 30% of Americans experience intermittent insomnia, and about 10% experience chronic insomnia. In the United States the direct costs of insomnia total about $16 billion a year, including the costs of testing, prescriber visits, and hypnotic drugs.

As a result of sleep loss, insomniacs experience daytime drowsiness along with impairment of mood, memory, coordination, and the ability to concentrate and make decisions. Chronic insomnia is a major risk factor for automotive and industrial accidents, marital and social problems, major depression, coronary heart disease, and metabolic and endocrine dysregulation.

Loss of sleep is often the result of a medical condition. Psychiatric disorders often disturb sleep, and pain can keep anyone awake. Sleep is frequently lost owing to concern regarding impending surgery and other procedures.

Basic Principles of Management

Cause-Specific Therapy

Treatment is highly dependent on the cause of insomnia. Accordingly, if therapy is to succeed, the underlying reason for sleep loss must be determined. To make this assessment, a thorough history is required.

When the cause of insomnia is a known medical disorder, primary therapy should be directed at the underlying illness; hypnotics should be employed only as adjuncts. For example, if pain is the reason for lost sleep, analgesics should be prescribed. If insomnia is secondary to major depression, antidepressants are the appropriate treatment. If anxiety is the cause of insomnia, the patient should receive an anxiolytic.

Nondrug Therapy

For many insomniacs, nondrug measures may be all that is needed to promote sleep. For some individuals, avoidance of naps and adherence to a regular sleep schedule is sufficient. For others, decreased consumption of caffeine-containing beverages (e.g., coffee, tea, cola drinks) may fix the problem. Still others may benefit from restful activity as bedtime nears. If environmental factors are responsible for lack of sleep, the patient should be taught how to correct them or compensate for them. All patients should be counseled about sleep fitness (also known as sleep hygiene). Rules for sleep fitness are shown in Box 27.1.

Research has shown that *cognitive behavioral therapy* is *superior* to drug therapy for both short-term and long-term management of chronic insomnia in older adults. Cognitive and behavioral interventions include sleep restriction, control of the bedroom environment, progressive relaxation, and education about sleep hygiene. The American Academy of Sleep Medicine considers these interventions both effective and reliable and hence recommends them as first-line therapy for chronic insomnia, even if drug therapy is also employed.

Therapy With Hypnotic Drugs

Hypnotics should be used only when insomnia cannot be managed by other means. Hence, before resorting to drugs, we should implement nondrug measures, and we should treat any pathology that may underlie inadequate sleep.

Drug therapy of transient insomnia should be short term (just 2–3 weeks). The patient should be reassessed on a regular basis to determine whether drug therapy is still needed.

BOX 27.1 ■ RULES FOR SLEEP FITNESS

- Establish a regular time to go to bed and a regular time to rise—even on weekends. This will help reset your biologic clock.
- Sleep only as long as needed to feel refreshed. Too much time in bed causes fragmented and shallow sleep. In contrast, restricting time in bed helps consolidate and deepen sleep.
- Insulate your bedroom against light and sounds that disturb your sleep (e.g., install carpeting and insulated curtains).
- Keep your bedroom temperature moderate. High temperature may disturb sleep.
- Exercise daily, but not later than 7:00 PM. Regular exercise helps deepen sleep.
- Schedule outdoor time at the same time each day.
- Avoid daytime naps. Staying awake during the day helps you sleep at night.
- Avoid caffeine, especially in the evening.
- Avoid consuming too much fluid in the evening so as to minimize nighttime trips to the bathroom.
- Avoid alcohol in the evening. Although alcohol can help you fall asleep, it causes sleep to be fragmented.
- Avoid tobacco; it disturbs sleep (and shortens your life, too).
- Try having a light snack near bedtime because hunger can disturb sleep—but don't eat heavily.
- Relax before bedtime with soft music, mild stretching, yoga, or pleasurable reading.
- Avoid bright light—including television, computers, and video games—before going to bed.
- Leave your problems outside the bedroom. Reserve time earlier in the evening to work on problems and to plan tomorrow's activities.
- Reserve your bedroom for sleeping and sex. This will help condition your brain to see the bedroom as a place where sleep happens. Don't eat, read, or watch TV in bed.
- If you don't fall asleep within 20 minutes or so, get up and do something relaxing (e.g., read, listen to music, watch TV), and then return to bed when you feel drowsy. Repeat as often as required.
- Don't look at the clock if you wake up during the night. If necessary, turn its face away from the bed.

Escalation of dosage should be avoided. A need for increased dosage suggests development of tolerance. If hypnotic effects are lost in the course of treatment, it is preferable to interrupt therapy rather than elevate dosage. Interruption will allow tolerance to decline, thereby restoring responsiveness to treatment.

In certain patients, hypnotics must be employed with special caution. Patients who snore heavily and those with respiratory disorders have reduced respiratory reserve, which can be further compromised by the respiratory-depressant actions of hypnotics. Hypnotic agents are generally contraindicated for use during pregnancy; these drugs have the potential to cause fetal harm, and their use is rarely an absolute necessity.

Patients taking hypnotics should be forewarned that residual CNS depression may persist the next day. Although CNS depression may not be pronounced, it may still compromise intellectual or physical performance.

When hypnotics are employed, care must be taken to prevent *drug-dependency insomnia,* a condition that can lead to inappropriate prolongation of therapy. Drug-dependency insomnia is a particular problem with older hypnotics (e.g., barbiturates) and develops as follows:

1. Insomnia motivates treatment with hypnotics.
2. With continuous drug use, low-level physical dependence develops.
3. Upon cessation of treatment, a mild withdrawal syndrome occurs and disrupts sleep.
4. Failing to recognize that the inability to sleep is a manifestation of drug withdrawal, the patient becomes convinced that insomnia has returned and resumes drug use.
5. Continued drug use leads to heightened physical dependence, making it even more difficult to withdraw medication without producing another episode of drug-dependency insomnia.

To minimize drug-dependency insomnia, hypnotics should be employed judiciously. That is, they should be used in the lowest effective dosage for the shortest time required.

Major Hypnotics Used for Treatment

Insomnia can be treated with prescription drugs, nonprescription drugs, and alternative medicines. Among the prescription drugs, benzodiazepines and the benzodiazepine-like drugs (zolpidem, zaleplon, and eszopiclone) are drugs of choice. Older sedative-hypnotics, such as barbiturates, are rarely used. Nonprescription drugs and alternative medicines are much less effective than the first-choice drugs and hence should be reserved for people whose insomnia is mild.

As shown in Table 27.2, hypnotic drugs differ with respect to onset and duration of action and hence differ in their applications. Drugs with a rapid onset (e.g., zolpidem) are good for patients who have difficulty falling asleep, whereas drugs with a long duration (e.g., estazolam) are good for patients who have difficulty maintaining sleep. Drugs such as flurazepam, which have both a rapid onset and long duration, are good for patients with both types of sleep problems.

Benzodiazepines

Only four benzodiazepines are marketed specifically for use as hypnotics (see Table 27.2). However, any benzodiazepine with a short to intermediate onset could be employed.

Benzodiazepines have multiple desirable effects on sleep: they decrease the interval to sleep onset, decrease the number of awakenings, and increase total sleeping time. In addition, they impart a sense of deep and refreshing sleep. With most benzodiazepines, tolerance to hypnotic actions develops slowly, allowing them to be used nightly for several weeks without a noticeable loss in hypnotic effects. Furthermore, with most benzodiazepines, treatment does not significantly

TABLE 27.2 ▪ Major Drugs for Insomnia

	Time Course		Use in Insomnia		Bedtime Dosage (mg)	
Drug	**Onset (min)**	**Duration**	**DFA***	**DMS**	**Younger Adult**	**Older Adult**
BENZODIAZEPINES						
Triazolam [Halcion]	15–30	Short	✓		0.125–0.25	0.125
Flurazepam[†](generic only)	30–60	Long	✓	✓	15–30	15
Estazolam (generic only)	15–60	Intermediate		✓	1–2	0.5–1
Temazepam [Restoril]	45–60	Intermediate		✓	15–30	7.5–15
BENZODIAZEPINE-LIKE DRUGS						
Eszopiclone [Lunesta]	30	Intermediate	✓	✓	2–3	1–2
Zolpidem						
Extended-release tablets [Ambien CR]	30	Intermediate	✓	✓	12.5	6.25
Immediate-release tablets [Ambien]	30	Short	✓		10	5
Sublingual [Intermezzo]	30	Short	✓	✓	1.75 for females and 3.5 for males	1.75
Sublingual [Edluar]	30	Short	✓		10	5
Oral spray [Zolpimist]	30	Short	✓		5–10	5
Zaleplon [Sonata]	15–30	Ultrashort	✓		5–10	5
MELATONIN RECEPTOR AGONIST						
Ramelteon [Rozerem]	30	Short	✓		8	8

*DFA, difficulty falling asleep; DMS, difficulty maintaining sleep.
[†]Because of its long duration, this drug is not generally recommended

reduce the amount of time spent in REM sleep, and withdrawal is not associated with significant rebound insomnia.

Two agents—*triazolam* [Halcion] and *flurazepam*—can be considered prototypes of the benzodiazepines used to promote sleep. Triazolam has a rapid onset and short duration, making it a good choice for patients who have difficulty falling asleep (compared with difficulty maintaining sleep). Flurazepam has a delayed onset and more prolonged duration, making it an effective agent for patients who have difficulty maintaining sleep. However, because flurazepam has a relatively long half-life, the drug is likely to cause daytime drowsiness and hence is not used widely today. Triazolam has a much shorter half-life than flurazepam, which is both good news and bad news. The good news is that, because it leaves the body rapidly, triazolam does not cause daytime sedation. The bad news is that, because triazolam is rapidly cleared, treatment is associated with two problems: (1) tolerance to hypnotic effects can develop quickly—in 11 to 18 days, which is much faster than with other benzodiazepines; and (2) triazolam causes more rebound insomnia than other benzodiazepines.

Benzodiazepine-Like Drugs: Zolpidem, Zaleplon, and Eszopiclone

Zolpidem [Ambien, Ambien CR, Edluar, Intermezzo, Zolpimist], zaleplon [Sonata], and eszopiclone [Lunesta] are drugs of first choice for insomnia. All three drugs have the same mechanism as the benzodiazepines—and all three are as effective as the benzodiazepines, and may be safer for long-term use. Furthermore, whereas benzodiazepines are contraindicated during pregnancy, the benzodiazepine-like drugs are not (although use during pregnancy should be discouraged). All three drugs have a rapid onset and hence can help people with difficulty *falling* asleep. Also, with zolpidem and eszopiclone, effects persist long enough to help people who have difficulty *staying* asleep. In contrast, effects of zaleplon fade too rapidly to help people with trouble staying asleep. However, zaleplon is great for people who wake up in the middle of the night. Owing to its ultrashort duration, zaleplon can be taken a few hours before rising and still not cause drowsiness during the day. Of the three drugs, only eszopiclone has been proved effective for long-term use. However, even though long-term studies for zaleplon and zolpidem are lacking, it seems likely that they too would retain efficacy when taken long term. The pharmacology of the benzodiazepine-like drugs was discussed previously.

Ramelteon

Ramelteon [Rozerem] is a melatonin agonist approved for long-term therapy of insomnia. The drug has a rapid onset and short duration and hence is good for inducing sleep, but not maintaining sleep. Ramelteon does not cause tolerance or dependence and is not regulated as a controlled substance. The pharmacology of ramelteon was discussed previously.

OTHER HYPNOTICS

Antidepressants

Trazodone

Trazodone [Oleptro] is an atypical antidepressant with strong sedative actions. The drug can decrease sleep latency and prolong sleep duration and does not cause tolerance or physical dependence. Trazodone is especially useful for treating insomnia resulting from use of antidepressants that cause significant CNS stimulation (e.g., fluoxetine [Prozac], bupropion [Wellbutrin]). Principal adverse effects are daytime grogginess and postural hypotension. (Hypotension results from alpha-adrenergic blockade.) The basic pharmacology of trazodone is presented in Chapter 25.

Doxepin

Doxepin is an old tricyclic antidepressant (TCA) with strong sedative actions. In 2010 the FDA approved a new low-dose formulation for treating patients who have trouble staying asleep. The new formulation (3- and 6-mg tablets) is sold as Silenor. In clinical trials of adults with chronic insomnia, Silenor increased total sleep time and maintained the effect for more than 12 weeks. These benefits probably derive from blocking receptors for histamine. The initial dosage for patients 65 years and older is 3 mg, taken within 30 minutes of bedtime. The initial dosage for patients younger than 65 years is 6 mg. Both dosages are much lower than the dosages used for depression (75–150 mg/day).

In the low doses used for sleep maintenance, doxepin is well tolerated. The most common adverse effects are sedation, nausea, and upper respiratory infection. In the high doses used for depression, doxepin can cause hypotension, dysrhythmias, and anticholinergic effects (e.g., dry mouth, constipation, urinary retention, blurred vision). Owing to the risk for anticholinergic effects, Silenor is contraindicated for patients with untreated narrow-angle glaucoma or severe urinary retention. In addition, Silenor is contraindicated for patients who have taken a monoamine oxidase inhibitor within the past 2 weeks. Unlike the benzodiazepines and benzodiazepine-like drugs, Silenor has little or no potential for abuse and hence is not regulated under the Controlled Substances Act. Accordingly, the drug may be especially appropriate when drug abuse is a concern.

The basic pharmacology of doxepin and other TCAs is presented in Chapter 25.

Antihistamines

Two antihistamines—diphenhydramine [Nytol, Sominex, others] and doxylamine [Unisom]—are FDA approved for use as "sleep aids" and can be purchased without a prescription. These drugs are less effective than benzodiazepines and benzodiazepine-like drugs, and tolerance develops quickly (in 1–2 weeks). Daytime drowsiness and anticholinergic effects (e.g., dry mouth, blurred vision, urinary hesitancy, constipation) are common.

Alternative Medicines

Of the alternative medicines employed to promote sleep, only one—melatonin—appears moderately effective). Melatonin is a hormone the helps regulate our circadian clock, the time-keeping mechanism that controls our sleep-wakefulness cycle. Principal uses for melatonin are insomnia and jet lag. Of note, melatonin is the only hormone that can be purchased without a prescription. The compound is available in health-food stores, vitamin shops, and even airport newsstands.

Melatonin is produced by the pineal gland, a structure located at the base of the brain. Secretion is suppressed by environmental light and stimulated by darkness. Normally, secretion is low during the day, begins to rise around 9:00 PM, reaches a peak between 2:00 AM and 4:00 AM, and returns to baseline by morning. Signals that control secretion travel along a multineuron pathway that connects the retina to the pineal gland.

Several trials indicate that melatonin promotes sleep. For example, doses of 0.3 to 1 mg taken 1 to 2 hours before bedtime can hasten sleep onset and the time to REM sleep, without reducing total time in REM sleep. Melatonin may also ease symptoms of jet lag by resetting the circadian clock to the new time zone. Of all treatments for jet lag, melatonin is the most widely studied. To date, there have been 11 double-blind, placebo-controlled trials. In 8 of these trials, melatonin produced significant benefit. Of the 3 negative studies, two were too small to permit firm conclusions, and one involved subjects whose baseline circadian rhythm may have been inappropriate for evaluation.

When used short term in low doses (e.g., less than 2 mg), melatonin has no observable adverse effects. However, short-term use of large doses can cause hangover, headache, nightmares, hypothermia, and transient depression. In one case, reversible psychosis occurred with a huge daytime dose. Possible adverse effects of long-term use are unknown.

Several others—valerian root, chamomile, passionflower, lemon balm, and lavender—have very mild sedative effects, but proof of benefits in insomnia is lacking.

CHAPTER

28 Management of Anxiety Disorders

Laura D. Rosenthal, DNP, ACNP, FAANP

Anxiety is an uncomfortable state that has both psychological and physical components. The psychological component can be characterized with terms such as *fear, apprehension, dread,* and *uneasiness.* The physical component manifests as tachycardia, palpitations, trembling, dry mouth, sweating, weakness, fatigue, and shortness of breath.

Anxiety is a nearly universal experience that often serves an adaptive function. When anxiety is moderate and situationally appropriate, therapy may not be needed or even desirable. In contrast, when anxiety is persistent and disabling, intervention is clearly indicated.

Anxiety disorders are among the most common psychiatric illnesses. In the United States about 25% of people develop pathologic anxiety at some time in their lives. As a rule, the incidence is higher in women than in men.

In this chapter, we focus on five of the more common anxiety disorders: generalized anxiety disorder, panic disorder, obsessive-compulsive disorder, social anxiety disorder, and posttraumatic stress disorder. Although each type is distinct, they all have one element in common: an unhealthy level of anxiety. In addition, with all anxiety disorders, depression is frequently comorbid.

Fortunately, anxiety disorders often respond well to treatment—either psychotherapy, drug therapy, or both. For most patients, a combination of psychotherapy and drug therapy is more effective than either modality alone.

As indicated in Table 28.1, two classes of drugs are used most: *benzodiazepines* and *selective serotonin reuptake inhibitors* (SSRIs). Benzodiazepines are used primarily for one condition: generalized anxiety disorder (GAD). In contrast, the SSRIs are now used for *all* anxiety disorders. It should be noted that, although SSRIs were developed as antidepressants, they can be very effective against anxiety—whether or not depression is present.

GENERALIZED ANXIETY DISORDER

Characteristics

GAD is a chronic condition characterized by uncontrollable worrying. Of all anxiety disorders, GAD is the least likely to remit. Most patients with GAD also have another psychiatric disorder, usually depression. GAD should not be confused with *situational anxiety,* which is a normal response to a stressful situation; symptoms may be intense, but they are temporary.

The hallmark of GAD is unrealistic or excessive anxiety about several events or activities (e.g., work or school performance) that lasts 6 months or longer. Other psychological manifestations include vigilance, tension, apprehension, poor concentration, and difficulty falling or staying asleep. Somatic manifestations include trembling, muscle tension, restlessness, and signs of autonomic hyperactivity, such as palpitations, tachycardia, sweating, and cold clammy hands.

Treatment

GAD can be managed with nondrug therapy and with drugs. Nondrug approaches include supportive therapy, cognitive behavioral therapy (CBT), biofeedback, and relaxation training. These can help relieve symptoms and improve coping skills in anxiety-provoking situations. When symptoms are mild, nondrug therapy may be all that is needed. However, if symptoms are intensely uncomfortable or disabling, drugs are indicated. In 2015 guidelines for treatment of GAD were published in *American Family Physician.* Current U.S. Food and Drug Administration (FDA)–approved first-line choices for treatment of GAD include benzodiazepines, buspirone, and four antidepressants: venlafaxine, paroxetine, escitalopram,

TABLE 28.1 ▪ First-Line Drugs for Anxiety Disorders

Anxiety Disorder	Benzodiazepines	SSRIs	Others
Generalized anxiety disorder	Alprazolam Chlordiazepoxide Clorazepate Diazepam Lorazepam Oxazepam	Escitalopram Paroxetine	Buspirone Duloxetine Venlafaxine
Panic disorder		Fluoxetine Paroxetine Sertraline	Venlafaxine
Obsessive-compulsive disorder		Citalopram Escitalopram Fluoxetine Fluvoxamine Paroxetine Sertraline	
Social anxiety disorder		Fluvoxamine Paroxetine Sertraline	Venlafaxine
Posttraumatic stress disorder		Fluoxetine Paroxetine Sertraline	Venlafaxine

SSRIs, selective serotonin reuptake inhibitors.

and duloxetine. Although other drugs are recommended for the treatment of GAD, they are currently used off-label. With the benzodiazepines, onset of relief is rapid. In contrast, with buspirone and the antidepressants, onset is delayed. Accordingly, benzodiazepines are preferred drugs for immediate stabilization, especially when anxiety is severe. However, for long-term management, buspirone and the antidepressants are preferred. Because GAD is a chronic disorder, initial drug therapy should be prolonged, lasting at least 12 months and possibly longer. Unfortunately, even after extended treatment, drug withdrawal frequently results in relapse. Hence, for many patients, drug therapy must continue indefinitely.

Benzodiazepines

Benzodiazepines are first-choice drugs for anxiety. Benefits derive from enhancing responses to gamma-aminobutyric acid (GABA), an inhibitory neurotransmitter. Onset of benefits is immediate, and the margin of safety is high. Principal side effects are sedation and psychomotor slowing. Patients should be warned about these effects and informed that they will subside in 7 to 10 days. Because of their abuse potential, benzodiazepines should be used with caution in patients known to abuse alcohol or other psychoactive substances.

Long-term use of benzodiazepines carries a risk for physical dependence. Withdrawal symptoms include panic, paranoia, and delirium. These can be especially troubling for patients with GAD. Furthermore, they can be confused with a return of pretreatment symptoms. Accordingly, clinicians must differentiate between a withdrawal reaction and relapse. To minimize withdrawal symptoms, benzodiazepines should be tapered gradually—over a period of several months. If relapse occurs, treatment should resume.

Of the 12 benzodiazepines available, 6 are approved for anxiety. The agents prescribed most often are alprazolam [Xanax, Xanax XR, Niravam] and lorazepam [Ativan]. However, there is no proof that any one benzodiazepine is clearly superior to the others. Hence, selection among them is largely a matter of prescriber preference. Dosages for anxiety are shown in Table 28.2.

> **Prototype Drugs**
>
> **DRUGS FOR ANXIETY DISRODERS**
>
> **Benzodiazepine**
> Diazepam
>
> **Nonbenzodiazepine-Nonbarbiturate**
> Buspirone

Buspirone

Actions and Therapeutic Use

Buspirone is an anxiolytic drug that differs significantly from the benzodiazepines. Most notably, buspirone is *not* a central nervous system (CNS) depressant. For treatment of anxiety, buspirone is as effective as the benzodiazepines and has two distinct advantages: it has no abuse potential and does not intensify the effects of CNS depressants (benzodiazepines, alcohol, and barbiturates). Its major disadvantage is that anxiolytic effects develop *slowly:* initial responses take a week to appear, and several more weeks must pass before responses peak. Because therapeutic effects are delayed, buspirone is not suitable for PRN use or for patients who need immediate relief. Buspirone has no abuse potential and thus

TABLE 28.2 ▪ Medications Approved for Anxiety Disorders

			Dosage	
Generic Name	**Trade Name**	**Indication**	**Initial**	**Usual Range (mg/day)**
Alprazolam	Xanax, Niravam	GAD	0.25–0.5 mg 3 times/day	0.5–4
	Xanax XR		0.5–1 mg once/day	4
Buspirone	Generic only	GAD	7.5 mg 2 times/day	30–60
Chlordiazepoxide	Librium	GAD	—	15–100
Citalopram	Celexa	OCD	20 mg once/day	40
Clorazepate	Tranxene-T	GAD	—	15–60
Diazepam	Valium	GAD	—	4–40
Duloxetine	Cymbalta	GAD	30–60 mg once/day	30–60
Escitalopram	Lexapro	GAD	10 mg once/day	20
		OCD	10 mg once/day	20
Fluoxetine	Prozac	PD	10 mg once/day	20
		OCD	20 mg once/day	80
Fluvoxamine	Luvox	OCD	50 mg once/day	300
Lorazepam	Ativan	GAD	0.5–1 mg 3 times/day	2–6
Oxazepam	generic only	GAD	—	30–120
Paroxetine	Paxil	GAD	20 mg once/day	20–50
		PD	10 mg once/day	20–40
		OCD	20 mg once/day	60
		SAD	20 mg once/day	20–40
Sertraline	Zoloft	PD	25 mg once/day	50–200
		OCD	50 mg once/day	200
Venlafaxine	Effexor XR	GAD	37.5 mg once/day	75–225

GAD, generalized anxiety disorder; OCD, obsessive-compulsive disorder; PD, panic disorder; SAD, social anxiety disorder.

may be especially appropriate for patients known to abuse alcohol and other drugs.

Because it lacks depressant properties, buspirone is an attractive alternative to benzodiazepines in patients who require long-term therapy but cannot tolerate benzodiazepine-induced sedation and psychomotor slowing. Buspirone is labeled only for *short-term* treatment of anxiety. However, the drug has been taken for as long as a year with no reduction in benefit. Buspirone does not display cross-dependence with benzodiazepines. Hence, when patients are switched from a benzodiazepine to buspirone, the benzodiazepine must be tapered slowly. Furthermore, because the effects of buspirone are delayed, buspirone should be initiated 2 to 4 weeks before beginning benzodiazepine withdrawal. The mechanism by which buspirone relieves anxiety has not been established. The drug binds with high affinity to receptors for serotonin and with lower affinity to receptors for dopamine. Buspirone does not bind to receptors for GABA or benzodiazepines.

Pharmacokinetics

Buspirone is well absorbed after oral administration but undergoes extensive metabolism on its first pass through the liver. Administration with food delays absorption but enhances bioavailability (by reducing first-pass metabolism). The drug is excreted in part by the kidneys, primarily as metabolites.

Adverse Effects

Buspirone is generally well tolerated. The most common reactions are *dizziness, nausea, headache, nervousness, sedation, lightheadedness,* and *excitement.* Furthermore, it poses little or no risk for suicide; huge doses (375 mg/day) have been given to healthy volunteers with only moderate adverse effects (nausea, vomiting, dizziness, drowsiness, miosis).

Drug and Food Interactions

Levels of buspirone can be greatly increased (5- to 13-fold) by *erythromycin* and *ketoconazole.* Levels can also be increased by *grapefruit juice.* Elevated levels may cause drowsiness and subjective effects (dysphoria, feeling "spacey"). Buspirone does not enhance the depressant effects of alcohol, barbiturates, and other general CNS depressants.

Tolerance, Dependence, and Abuse

Buspirone has been used for up to a year without evidence of tolerance, physical dependence, or psychological dependence. No withdrawal symptoms have been observed on termination. There is no cross-tolerance or cross-dependence between buspirone and the sedative-hypnotics (e.g., benzodiazepines, barbiturates). Buspirone appears to have no potential for abuse and hence is not regulated under the Controlled Substances Act.

Antidepressants: Venlafaxine, Paroxetine, Escitalopram, and Duloxetine

At this time, only four antidepressants—venlafaxine [Effexor XR], duloxetine [Cymbalta], paroxetine [Paxil], and escitalopram [Lexapro, Cipralex ♣]—are approved for GAD. Venlafaxine and duloxetine are serotonin-norepinephrine reuptake inhibitors (SNRIs); paroxetine and escitalopram are SSRIs. All four drugs are especially well suited for patients who have depression in addition to GAD. However, they are also effective even when depression is absent. As with buspirone, anxiolytic effects develop slowly: initial responses can be seen in a week, but optimal responses require several more weeks to develop. Because relief is delayed, the antidepressants cannot be used PRN. Compared with benzodiazepines, the antidepressants do a better job of decreasing cognitive and psychic symptoms of anxiety, but are not as good at decreasing somatic symptoms. In contrast to the benzodiazepines, antidepressants have no potential for abuse. However, abrupt discontinuation *can* produce withdrawal symptoms.

Venlafaxine, an SNRI, was the first antidepressant approved for GAD. The drug has been proved effective for both short-term and long-term use. The most common side effect is nausea, which develops in 37% of patients. Fortunately, nausea subsides despite continued treatment. Other common reactions include headache, anorexia, nervousness, sweating, daytime somnolence, and insomnia. In addition, venlafaxine can cause hypertension, although this is unlikely at the doses used in GAD. Combining venlafaxine with a monoamine oxidase inhibitor (MAOI) can result in serious toxicity and hence must be avoided.

Paroxetine and *escitalopram* are the only SSRIs approved for GAD. These drugs are as effective as the benzodiazepines, but less well tolerated. The basic pharmacology of venlafaxine, paroxetine, escitalopram, and duloxetine is discussed in Chapter 25.

PANIC DISORDER

Characteristics

Panic disorder is characterized by recurrent, intensely uncomfortable episodes known as *panic attacks.* A panic attack is an abrupt surge of intense fear or intense discomfort during which four or more of the following are present:

- Palpitations, pounding heart, racing heartbeat
- Sweating
- Trembling or shaking
- Sensation of shortness of breath or smothering
- Feeling of choking
- Chest pain or discomfort
- Nausea or abdominal distress
- Feeling dizzy, unsteady, lightheaded, or faint
- Chills or heat sensations
- Paresthesias (numbness or tingling sensations)
- Derealization (feelings of unreality) or depersonalization (feeling detached from oneself)
- Fear of losing control or going crazy
- Fear of dying

Panic symptoms reach a peak in a few minutes and then dissipate within 30 minutes. Many patients go to an emergency department because they think they are having a heart attack. Some patients experience panic attacks daily; others have only one or two a month. Panic disorder is a common condition that affects 1.6% of Americans at some time in their lives. The incidence in women is 2 to 3 times the incidence in men. Onset of panic disorder usually occurs in the late teens or early 20s.

The underlying cause of panic disorder is unknown. However, malfunction of the brain's "alarm system" is suspected. This malfunction may result from abnormalities in noradrenergic systems, serotonergic systems, or benzodiazepine receptors. Genetic vulnerability also may play a role.

Treatment

Between 70% and 90% of patients with panic disorder respond well to treatment. Two modalities may be employed: drug therapy and CBT. Combining drug therapy with CBT is more effective than either modality alone. As a rule, patients experience rapid and significant improvement. Drug therapy helps suppress panic attacks, whereas CBT helps patients become more comfortable with situations and places they've been avoiding. Additional benefit can be derived from avoiding caffeine and sympathomimetics (which can trigger panic attacks), avoiding sleep deprivation (which can predispose to panic attacks), and doing regular aerobic exercise (which can reduce anxiety).

Drug therapy should continue at least 6 to 9 months. Stopping sooner is associated with a high rate of relapse.

Antidepressants

Panic disorder responds well to all four classes of antidepressants: SSRIs, SNRIs, tricyclic antidepressants (TCAs), and MAOIs. With all four, full benefits take 6 to 12 weeks to develop. Owing to better tolerability, SSRIs are generally preferred. The basic pharmacology of the antidepressants is discussed in Chapter 25.

Selective Serotonin Reuptake Inhibitors

The SSRIs are first-line drugs for panic disorder. At this time, only three SSRIs—fluoxetine [Prozac], paroxetine [Paxil], and sertraline [Zoloft]—are approved for this condition. However, the other SSRIs appear just as effective. The SSRIs decrease anticipatory anxiety, avoidance behavior, and the frequency and intensity of attacks. Furthermore, SSRIs decrease panic attacks regardless of whether the patient is actually depressed. However, if the patient does have coexisting depression, antidepressants will benefit the depression and panic disorder simultaneously. Common side effects include nausea, headache, insomnia, weight gain, and sexual dysfunction. In addition, SSRIs can *increase* anxiety early in treatment.

Venlafaxine

In patients with panic disorder, extended-release venlafaxine [Effexor XR], an SNRI, can induce remission, prevent relapse, and improve quality of life. In clinical trials, efficacy was equal to that of paroxetine, an SSRI. The initial dosage is 37.5 mg/day for 7 days. Daily maintenance doses range between 75 mg and 225 mg. The pharmacology of venlafaxine is discussed in Chapter 25.

Tricyclic Antidepressants

The TCAs (e.g., imipramine [Tofranil], clomipramine [Anafranil]) are second-line drugs for panic disorder. They should be used only after a trial with at least one SSRI has failed. Although TCAs are as effective as SSRIs, they are less well tolerated. The most common side effects are sedation, orthostatic hypotension, and anticholinergic effects: dry mouth, blurred vision, urinary retention, constipation, and tachycardia. Of greater concern, TCAs can cause fatal dysrhythmias if taken in overdose. As with the SSRIs, dosage should be low initially and then gradually increased. For clomipramine, the initial dosage is 25 mg/day, and the target range is 50 to 200 mg/day. For imipramine, the initial dosage is 10 mg/day, and the target range is 100 to 300 mg/day.

MAOIs

Although MAOIs (e.g., phenelzine) are very effective in panic disorder, they are difficult to use. MAOIs can cause significant side effects, including orthostatic hypotension, weight gain, and sexual dysfunction. In addition, they can cause hypertensive crisis if the patient takes certain drugs or consumes foods rich in tyramine. Because of these drawbacks, MAOIs are considered last-line drugs for panic disorder.

Benzodiazepines

Although benzodiazepines are effective in panic disorder, they are now considered second-line drugs because, unlike the SSRIs, benzodiazepines pose a risk for abuse, dependence, and rapid reemergence of symptoms after discontinuation. Of the available benzodiazepines, the agents used most often are alprazolam [Xanax, Niravam], clonazepam [Klonopin, Rivotril ♣], and lorazepam [Ativan]. All three provide rapid and effective protection against panic attacks. These drugs also reduce anticipatory anxiety and phobic avoidance.

OBSESSIVE-COMPULSIVE DISORDER

Characteristics

Obsessive-compulsive disorder (OCD) is a potentially disabling condition characterized by persistent obsessions and compulsions that cause marked distress, consume at least 1 hour a day, and significantly interfere with daily living. An *obsession* is defined as a recurrent, persistent thought, impulse, or mental image that is unwanted and distressing and comes involuntarily to mind despite attempts to ignore or suppress it. Common obsessions include fear of contamination (e.g., acquiring a disease by touching another person), aggressive impulses (e.g., harming a family member), a need for orderliness or symmetry (e.g., personal bathroom items must be arranged in a precise way), and repeated doubts (e.g., did I unplug the iron?). A *compulsion* is a ritualized behavior or mental act that the patient is driven to perform in response to his or her obsessions. In the patient's mind, carrying out the compulsion is essential to prevent some horrible event from occurring (e.g., death of a loved one). If performing the compulsion is suppressed or postponed, the patient experiences increased anxiety. Common compulsions include hand washing, mental counting, arranging objects symmetrically, and hoarding. Patients usually understand that their compulsive behavior is excessive and senseless, but nonetheless are unable to stop.

Treatment

The *2013 Practice Guideline for the Treatment of Patients with Obsessive-Compulsive Disorder,* published by the American Psychiatric Association, indicates that patients with OCD respond to drugs and to behavioral therapy. Optimal treatment consists of both. As a last resort, patients with severe, resistant OCD can be treated with deep brain stimulation.

Behavioral therapy is probably more important in OCD than in any other psychiatric disorder. In the technique employed, patients are exposed to sources of their fears, while being encouraged to refrain from acting out their compulsive rituals. When no dire consequences come to pass, despite the absence of "protective" rituals, patients are able to gradually give up their compulsive behavior. Although this form of therapy causes great anxiety, the success rate is high.

Five drugs are approved for OCD: four SSRIs and one TCA (clomipramine). All five enhance serotonergic transmission. The SSRIs are better tolerated than clomipramine and hence are preferred.

Selective Serotonin Reuptake Inhibitors

The SSRIs are first-line drugs for OCD. Only four SSRIs—fluoxetine [Prozac], fluvoxamine [Luvox], sertraline [Zoloft], and paroxetine [Paxil]—are approved for OCD. However, the remaining two—citalopram [Celexa] and escitalopram [Lexapro, Cipralex ♣]—are also effective. All six reduce symptoms by enhancing serotonergic transmission. They all are equally effective, although individual patients may respond better to one than to another. With all six, beneficial effects develop slowly, taking several months to become maximal. Common side effects include nausea, headache, insomnia, and sexual dysfunction. Weight gain can also occur. Despite this array of side effects, SSRIs are safer than clomipramine and better tolerated.

Therapy of an initial episode should continue for at least 1 year, after which discontinuation can be tried. Withdrawal should be done slowly, reducing the dosage by 25% every 1 to 2 months. Unfortunately, relapse is common; estimates range from 23% to as high as 90%. If relapse continues to occur after three or four attempts at withdrawal, lifelong treatment may be indicated.

SOCIAL ANXIETY DISORDER

Characteristics

Social anxiety disorder is characterized by an intense, irrational fear of situations in which one might be scrutinized by others, or might do something that is embarrassing or humiliating. Exposure to the feared situation almost always elicits anxiety. As a result, the person avoids the situation or, if it can't be avoided, endures it with intense anxiety (manifestations include blushing, stuttering, sweating, palpitations, dry throat, and muscle tension and twitches).

Social anxiety disorder has two principal forms: generalized and performance only. In the generalized form, the person fears nearly all social and performance situations. In the performance-only form, fear is limited to speaking or performing in public.

Social anxiety disorder can be very debilitating. In younger people, it can delay social development, inhibit participation in social activities, impair acquisition of friends, and make dating difficult or even impossible. It can also preclude pursuit of higher education. In older people, it can severely limit social and occupational options.

Social anxiety disorder is one of the most common psychiatric disorders, and *the* most common anxiety disorder. In the United States 13% to 14% of the population is affected at some time in their lives. The disorder typically begins during the teenage years and, left untreated, is likely to continue lifelong.

Treatment

Social anxiety disorder can be treated with psychotherapy, drug therapy, or both. Studies indicate that psychotherapy—both cognitive and behavioral—can be as effective as drugs. However, a combination of psychotherapy *plus* drugs is likely to be more effective than either modality alone.

The SSRIs are considered first-line drugs for most patients. These drugs are especially well suited for patients who fear multiple situations and are obliged to face those situations on a regular basis. Only two SSRIs—paroxetine [Paxil] and sertraline [Zoloft]—are approved for social anxiety disorder, but available data indicate that the other SSRIs are effective too. Initial effects take about 4 weeks to develop; optimal effects are seen in 8 to 12 weeks. Patients should be informed that benefits will be delayed.

Benzodiazepines (e.g., clonazepam [Klonopin, Rivotril ♣], alprazolam [Xanax]) are an option for some patients. These drugs are well tolerated and their benefits are immediate, unlike those of the SSRIs. As a result, benzodiazepines can provide rapid relief and can be used PRN. Accordingly, these drugs are well suited for people whose fear is limited to performance situations, and who must face those situations only occasionally. The usual dosage is 1 to 3 mg/day for clonazepam, and 1 to 6 mg/day for alprazolam.

Propranolol [Inderal] and other beta blockers can benefit patients with performance anxiety. When taken 1 to 2 hours before a scheduled performance, beta blockers can reduce symptoms caused by autonomic hyperactivity (e.g., tremors, sweating, tachycardia, palpitations). Doses are relatively small—only 10 to 80 mg for propranolol.

POSTTRAUMATIC STRESS DISORDER

Characteristics

Posttraumatic stress disorder (PTSD) develops after a *traumatic event* that elicited an immediate reaction of *fear, helplessness,* or *horror.* PTSD has three core symptoms: *re-experiencing* the event, *avoiding reminders* of the event (coupled with generalized emotional numbing), and a persistent state of *hyperarousal.* A traumatic event is one that involves a threat of injury or death or a threat to one's physical integrity. Many events meet this criterion. Among these are physical or sexual assault, rape, torture, combat, industrial explosions, serious accidents, natural disasters, being taken hostage, displacement as a refugee, and terrorist attacks, such as the ones that took place against the World Trade Center and the Pentagon on September 11, 2001. It should be noted that PTSD can affect persons who were only *witnesses* to a traumatic event—not just those who were directly involved.

The epidemiology of PTSD is revealing. In the United States more than 5 million Americans have PTSD in any given year, making PTSD the fourth most common psychiatric disorder. PTSD develops in 5% to 6% of men at some time in their lives, and in 10% to 14% of women. Traumatic events that involve interpersonal violence (e.g., assault, rape, torture) are more likely to cause PTSD than are traumatic events that do not (e.g., car accidents, natural disasters). For example, among rape victims, the incidence of PTSD is 45.9% for women and 65% for men. In contrast, among natural disaster survivors, the incidence is 5.4% for women and 3.7% for men. Combat carries a high risk for PTSD: the disorder develops in up to 40% of soldiers who go to war.

Treatment

PTSD can be treated with psychotherapy and with drugs, as described in a recent evidence-based guideline—*VA/DoD Clinical Practice Guideline for the Management of Post-Traumatic Stress*—released by the Department of Veterans Affairs and Department of Defense in 2010. Two basic types of psychotherapy are recommended: *trauma-focused therapy* and *stress inoculation training.* Trauma-focused therapy uses a variety of cognitive behavioral techniques, including a very effective one known as *exposure therapy,* in which patients repeatedly reimagine traumatic events as a way to make those events lose their power. Stress inoculation training helps patients identify cues that can trigger fear and anxiety and then teaches them techniques to cope with those disturbing reactions.

Regarding drugs, evidence of efficacy is strongest for three SSRIs (fluoxetine, paroxetine, and sertraline) and one SNRI (venlafaxine). Of these four drugs, only two—paroxetine [Paxil] and sertraline [Zoloft]—are approved by the FDA for PTSD. If none of the first-line drugs is effective, the guidelines suggest several alternatives: mirtazapine, a TCA (amitriptyline or imipramine), or an MAOI (phenelzine). Current evidence does *not* support the use of monotherapy with bupropion, buspirone, trazodone, or a benzodiazepine.

CHAPTER

29 Central Nervous System Stimulants and Attention-Deficit/Hyperactivity Disorder

Laura D. Rosenthal, DNP, ACNP, FAANP

CENTRAL NERVOUS SYSTEM STIMULANTS

Central nervous system (CNS) stimulants increase the activity of CNS neurons. Most stimulants act by enhancing neuronal excitation. A few act by suppressing neuronal inhibition. In sufficient doses, all stimulants can cause seizures.

Clinical applications of the CNS stimulants are limited. Currently these drugs have two principal indications: attention-deficit/hyperactivity disorder (ADHD) and narcolepsy.

Please note that CNS stimulants are not the same as antidepressants. The antidepressants act selectively to elevate mood and hence can relieve depression without affecting other CNS functions. In contrast, CNS stimulants cannot elevate mood without producing generalized excitation. Accordingly, the role of stimulants in treating depression is minor.

Our principal focus is on *amphetamines, methylphenidate* [Ritalin, others], and *methylxanthines* (e.g., caffeine). These are by far the most widely used stimulant drugs.

Amphetamines

The amphetamine family consists of amphetamine, dextroamphetamine, methamphetamine, and lisdexamfetamine. All are powerful CNS stimulants. In addition to their CNS actions, amphetamines have significant peripheral actions—actions that can cause cardiac stimulation and vasoconstriction. The amphetamines have a high potential for abuse.

Amphetamine

The term *amphetamine* refers not to a single compound but rather to a 50:50 mixture of dextroamphetamine and levamphetamine.

Lisdexamfetamine

Lisdexamfetamine [Vyvanse] is a prodrug composed of dextroamphetamine covalently linked to L-lysine. After oral dosing, the drug undergoes rapid hydrolysis by enzymes in the intestine and liver to yield lysine and free dextroamphetamine, the active form of the drug. If lisdexamfetamine is inhaled or injected, hydrolysis will not take place and hence the drug is not effective by these routes. Accordingly, it may have a lower abuse potential than other forms of amphetamine.

Methamphetamine

Methamphetamine is simply dextroamphetamine with an additional methyl group.

Mechanism of Action

The amphetamines act primarily by causing release of norepinephrine (NE) and dopamine (DA) and partly by inhibiting reuptake of both transmitters. These actions take place in the CNS and in peripheral nerves. Most pharmacologic effects result from release of NE.

Pharmacologic Effects

Central Nervous System. The amphetamines have prominent effects on mood and arousal. At usual doses, they increase wakefulness and alertness, reduce fatigue, elevate mood, and augment self-confidence and initiative. Euphoria, talkativeness, and increased motor activity are likely. Task performance that had been reduced by fatigue or boredom improves.

Amphetamines can stimulate respiration and suppress appetite and perception of pain. Stimulation of the medullary respiratory center increases respiration. Effects on the hypothalamic feeding center depress appetite. By a mechanism that is not understood, amphetamines can enhance the analgesic effects of morphine and other opioids.

Cardiovascular System. Cardiovascular effects occur secondary to release of NE from sympathetic neurons. Norepinephrine acts in the heart to increase heart rate, atrioventricular conduction, and force of contraction. Excessive cardiac stimulation can cause dysrhythmias. In blood vessels, NE promotes constriction. Excessive vasoconstriction can cause hypertension.

Tolerance. With regular amphetamine use, tolerance develops to elevation of mood, suppression of appetite, and stimulation of the heart and blood vessels. In highly tolerant users, doses up to 1000 mg given intravenously every few *hours* may be required to maintain *euphoric* effects. This compares with *daily* doses of 5 to 30 mg for nontolerant individuals.

Physical Dependence. Chronic amphetamine use produces physical dependence. If amphetamines are abruptly withdrawn from a dependent person, an abstinence syndrome will ensue. Symptoms include exhaustion, depression, prolonged sleep, excessive eating, and a craving for more amphetamine. Sleep patterns may take months to normalize.

Prototype Drugs

CENTRAL NERVOUS SYSTEM STIMULANTS

Amphetamine
Amphetamine sulfate

Amphetamine-Like Drug
Methylphenidate

Methylxanthine
Caffeine

DRUGS FOR ATTENTION-DEFICIT/HYPERACTIVITY DISORDER

CNS Stimulants
Methylphenidate

Nonstimulants
Atomoxetine

Abuse. Because amphetamines can produce euphoria (extreme mood elevation), they have a high potential for abuse. Psychological dependence can occur. (Users familiar with CNS stimulants find the psychological effects of amphetamines nearly identical to those of cocaine.) Because of their abuse potential, all amphetamines, including lisdexamfetamine, are classified under Schedule II of the Controlled Substances Act and must be dispensed accordingly. Whenever amphetamines are used therapeutically, their potential for abuse must be weighed against their potential benefits.

Adverse Effects

CNS Stimulation. Stimulation of the CNS can cause insomnia and restlessness. These effects can occur at therapeutic doses.

Weight Loss. By suppressing appetite, amphetamines can cause weight loss.

Cardiovascular Effects. At recommended doses, stimulants produce a small increase in heart rate and blood pressure. For most patients, these increases lack clinical significance. However, for patients with preexisting cardiovascular disease, stimulants may cause dysrhythmias, anginal pain, or hypertension. Accordingly, amphetamines must be employed with extreme caution in these people. Any patient who develops cardiovascular symptoms while using a stimulant should be evaluated immediately.

Do amphetamines increase the risk for *sudden death*? Probably not. Sudden death in children on these medications is very rare, and evidence is conflicting regarding risk for sudden death. Should children *routinely* receive an electrocardiogram (ECG) before using these drugs? Probably not—despite a 2008 statement from the American Heart Association (AHA) saying it would be reasonable to consider obtaining an ECG in children being evaluated for stimulant therapy of ADHD. The AHA developed this statement because 14 children, 5 with heart defects, died suddenly while using Adderall, a mixture of amphetamine and dextroamphetamine. However, given that millions of children have used the drug, the death rate is no greater than would be expected for a group this size, whether or not Adderall was being used. The bottom line? First, there are conflicting data showing that stimulants increase the risk for sudden death, even in children with heart disease. Second, there are no data showing that limiting the use of stimulants in children with heart defects will protect them from sudden death. And third, there are no data showing that screening for heart disease with an ECG before starting stimulants will be of benefit. Therefore it would seem that *routine* ECGs are unnecessary before starting a child on stimulant therapy, especially if there is no evidence of heart disease. However, if there *is* evidence of heart disease, or evidence of hereditary cardiovascular defects, an ECG might be appropriate.

Psychosis. Excessive amphetamine use produces a state of paranoid psychosis, characterized by hallucinations and paranoid delusions. Amphetamine-induced psychosis looks very much like schizophrenia. Symptoms are thought to result from release of DA. Consistent with this hypothesis is the observation that symptoms can be alleviated with a DA receptor blocking agent (e.g., haloperidol). After amphetamine withdrawal, psychosis usually resolves spontaneously within a week.

In some individuals, amphetamines can unmask latent schizophrenia. For these people, symptoms of psychosis do not clear spontaneously and hence psychiatric care is indicated.

Acute Toxicity.

Symptoms. Overdose produces dizziness, confusion, hallucinations, paranoid delusions, palpitations, dysrhythmias, and hypertension. Death is rare. Fatal overdose is associated with convulsions, coma, and cerebral hemorrhage.

Treatment. Hallucinations can be controlled with chlorpromazine, an antipsychotic drug. An alpha-adrenergic blocker (e.g., phentolamine) can reduce hypertension (by promoting vasodilation). Owing to its ability to block alpha receptors, chlorpromazine helps lower blood pressure. Seizures can be managed with diazepam. Acidifying the urine can accelerate amphetamine excretion.

Therapeutic Uses

Attention-Deficit/Hyperactivity Disorder. The role of amphetamines in ADHD is discussed later.

Narcolepsy. Narcolepsy is a disorder characterized by daytime somnolence and uncontrollable attacks of sleep. By stimulating the CNS, amphetamines can promote arousal and thereby alleviate symptoms.

BLACK BOX WARNING: AMPHETAMINE ABUSE

Amphetamines have a high potential for abuse and dependence. In patients who use amphetamines chronically, withdrawal may occur if use of these medications is suddenly stopped.

Methylphenidate and Dexmethylphenidate

Methylphenidate and dexmethylphenidate are nearly identical in structure and pharmacologic actions. Furthermore, the pharmacology of both drugs is nearly identical to that of the amphetamines.

Methylphenidate

Although methylphenidate [Ritalin, Metadate, Methylin, Concerta, Daytrana, Biphentin ✦] is structurally dissimilar from the amphetamines, the pharmacologic actions of these drugs are essentially the same. Consequently, methylphenidate can be considered an amphetamine in all but structure and name. Methylphenidate and amphetamine share the same mechanism of action (promotion of NE and DA release, and inhibition of NE and DA reuptake), adverse effects (insomnia, reduced appetite, emotional lability), and abuse liability (Schedule II). Like amphetamine, methylphenidate is not a single compound, but rather a 50:50 mixture of dextro and levo isomers. Methylphenidate has two indications: ADHD and narcolepsy.

BLACK BOX WARNING: METHYLPHENIDATE ABUSE

Chronic abuse of methylphenidate can lead to marked tolerance and psychological dependence with varying degrees of abnormal behavior and possible frank psychotic episodes.

Dexmethylphenidate

Dexmethylphenidate [Focalin, Focalin XR], a drug for ADHD, is simply the dextro isomer of methylphenidate. As noted, the dextro isomer accounts for most of the pharmacologic activity of methylphenidate, a 50:50 mixture of dextro and levo isomers. Accordingly, the pharmacology of dexmethylphenidate is nearly identical to that of methylphenidate. The only difference is that the dosage of dexmethylphenidate is one half the dosage of methylphenidate.

Methylxanthines

The methylxanthines are methylated derivatives of xanthine, hence the family name. These compounds consist of a xanthine nucleus with one or more methyl groups attached. Caffeine, the most familiar member of the family, will serve as our prototype.

Caffeine

Caffeine is consumed worldwide for its stimulant effects. In the United States per capita consumption is about 200 mg/day, mostly in the form of coffee. Although clinical applications of caffeine are few, caffeine remains of interest because of its widespread ingestion for nonmedical purposes.

Mechanism of Action

Several mechanisms of action have been proposed. These include (1) reversible blockade of adenosine receptors, (2) enhancement of calcium permeability in the sarcoplasmic reticulum, and (3) inhibition of cyclic nucleotide phosphodiesterase, resulting in accumulation of cyclic adenosine monophosphate (cyclic AMP). Blockade of adenosine receptors appears responsible for most effects.

Pharmacologic Effects

Central Nervous System. In low doses, caffeine decreases drowsiness and fatigue and increases the capacity for prolonged intellectual exertion. With increasing dosage, caffeine produces nervousness, insomnia, and tremors. When administered in very large doses, caffeine can cause convulsions. Despite popular belief, there is little evidence that caffeine can restore mental function during intoxication with alcohol, although it might delay passing out.

Heart. High doses of caffeine stimulate the heart. When caffeinated beverages are consumed in excessive amounts, dysrhythmias may result.

Blood Vessels. Caffeine affects blood vessels in the periphery differently from those in the CNS. In the periphery, caffeine promotes *vasodilation,* whereas in the CNS, caffeine promotes *vasoconstriction.* Constriction of cerebral blood vessels is thought to underlie the drug's ability to relieve headache.

Bronchi. Caffeine and other methylxanthines cause relaxation of bronchial smooth muscle and thereby promote bronchodilation. Theophylline is an especially effective bronchodilator and hence can be used to treat asthma (see Chapter 60).

Kidney. Caffeine is a diuretic. The mechanism underlying increased urine formation is likely related to suppression of antidiuretic hormone in the posterior pituitary.

Reproduction. Caffeine readily crosses the placenta and may pose a risk for birth defects, although that risk appears low. When applied to cells in culture, caffeine can cause chromosomal damage and mutations. However, the concentrations required are much greater than can be achieved by drinking caffeinated beverages. Also, although there is clear proof that caffeine can cause birth defects in animals, studies

PATIENT-CENTERED CARE ACROSS THE LIFE SPAN

Stimulants

Life Stage	Patient Care Concerns
Infants	Caffeine citrate [Cafcit] is used for neonatal apnea. Other CNS stimulants should be avoided in this population.
Children	The stimulant class of drugs for treatment of attention-deficit/hyperactivity disorder (ADHD) has been proved safe and effective for this population. Atomoxetine, a nonstimulant for ADHD, may cause suicidal thinking in children and adolescents.
Pregnant women	Caffeine may pose a small risk for birth defects, although human data are lacking. Methylphenidate and atomoxetine are classified as U.S. Food and Drug Administration Pregnancy Risk Category C because adverse fetal effects have been demonstrated in animal studies.
Breastfeeding women	Stimulants, such as methylphenidate, do not have any reported side effects in the breastfeeding infant. There are limited to no data on the nonstimulants and the effects on breastfeeding infants.
Older adults	Most studies focus on patients older than 65 years because stimulants are often used for treatment of apathy, depression, and fatigue in the older-adult population. Stimulants should be avoided in patients with cardiac disease or glaucoma. Consider a lower starting dose and monitor heart rate, blood pressure, and weight.

have failed to document birth defects in humans. Although caffeine-induced birth defects seem unlikely, caffeine *has* been associated with low birth weight.

According to a meta-analysis reported in 2010, consuming less than 300 mg of caffeine daily does *not* increase the risk for preterm birth. An additional review in 2013 revealed that restricting caffeine consumption during the second and third trimesters of pregnancy did not affect birth weight or length of gestation. Whether higher doses might increase risk is unclear.

Pharmacokinetics

Caffeine is readily absorbed from the gastrointestinal (GI) tract and achieves peak plasma levels within 1 hour. Plasma half-life ranges from 3 to 7 hours. Elimination is by hepatic metabolism.

Therapeutic Uses

Neonatal Apnea. Premature infants may experience prolonged apnea (lasting 15 seconds or more) along with bradycardia. Hypoxemia and neurologic damage may result. Caffeine and other methylxanthines can reduce the number and duration of apnea episodes and can promote a more regular pattern of breathing.

Promoting Wakefulness. Caffeine is used commonly to aid staying awake. The drug is marketed in various over-the-counter preparations [Maximum Strength NoDoz, Vivarin, others] for this purpose. Of course, individuals desiring increased alertness can get just as much caffeine by drinking coffee or some other caffeine-containing beverage.

Acute Toxicity

Caffeine toxicity is characterized by intensification of the responses seen at low doses. Stimulation of the CNS results in excitement, restlessness, and insomnia; if the dosage is very high, seizures may occur. Tachycardia and respiratory stimulation are likely. Sensory phenomena (ringing in the ears, flashing lights) are common. Death from caffeine overdose is rare. When fatalities have occurred, between 5 and 10 g have been ingested.

Miscellaneous Central Nervous System Stimulants

Modafinil

Therapeutic Use

Modafinil [Provigil, Alertec ♣], a unique nonamphetamine stimulant, is approved for promoting wakefulness in patients with excessive sleepiness associated with three disorders: narcolepsy, shift-work sleep disorder (SWSD), and obstructive sleep apnea–hypopnea syndrome (OSAHS). However, although the drug has only three approved uses, most prescriptions (95%) are written for off-label uses, including fatigue, depression, ADHD, jet lag, and sleepiness caused by medications. Investigational uses include ADHD and fatigue associated with multiple sclerosis. The military studied the drug for use in sustaining alertness in helicopter pilots and found it superior to placebo.

In clinical trials, modafinil has been moderately effective. In patients with narcolepsy, modafinil increased wakefulness, but only to about 50% of the level seen in normal people. In contrast, methylphenidate and dextroamphetamine increase wakefulness to about 70% of normal. In patients with SWSD and OSAHS, benefits are about the same as those seen in narcolepsy.

Mechanism of Action

How does modafinil ward off sleep? No one knows. The drug does seem to influence hypothalamic areas involved in maintaining the normal sleep-wakefulness cycle. Also, there is evidence that modafinil inhibits the activity of sleep-promoting neurons (in the ventrolateral preoptic nucleus) by blocking reuptake of norepinephrine.

Pharmacokinetics

Modafinil is rapidly absorbed from the GI tract. Plasma levels peak in 2 to 4 hours. Food decreases the rate of absorption but not the extent. Elimination is by hepatic metabolism followed by renal excretion. The half-life is about 15 hours.

Adverse Effects

Modafinil is generally well tolerated. The most common adverse effects are headache, nausea, nervousness, diarrhea, and rhinitis. Modafinil does not disrupt nighttime sleep. In clinical trials, only 5% of patients dropped out because of undesired effects. Initially, the drug was believed devoid of cardiovascular effects. However, we now know it can increase heart rate and blood pressure, apparently by altering autonomic function. Subjective effects—euphoria; altered perception, thinking, and feeling—are like those of other CNS stimulants. However, modafinil has less abuse potential and hence is regulated as a Schedule IV substance. Physical dependence and withdrawal have not been reported. Modafinil is embryotoxic in laboratory animals and hence should be avoided during pregnancy.

Postmarketing reports link modafinil to rare cases of serious skin reactions, including Stevens-Johnson syndrome, erythema multiforme, and toxic epidermal necrolysis. Patients should be informed about signs of these reactions—swelling or rash, especially in the presence of fever or changes in the oral mucosa—and instructed to discontinue the drug if they develop.

Drug Interactions

Modafinil inhibits some forms of cytochrome P450 (CYP) and induces others. Induction of CYP3A4 (the 3A4 isoenzyme of P450) may accelerate the metabolism of oral contraceptives, cyclosporine, and certain other drugs, thereby causing their levels to decline. Caution is advised.

Preparations, Dosage, and Administration

Modafinil is available in 100- and 200-mg tablets. For patients with narcolepsy or OSAHS, the usual dosage is 200 mg/day, taken as a single dose in the morning. For patients with SWSD, the usual dosage is 200 mg/day, taken as a single dose 1 hour before the shift starts. For patients with severe hepatic impairment, doses should be decreased by 50%. Dosage reduction may also be needed in older adults.

Armodafinil

Armodafinil [Nuvigil] is simply the chemical "mirror image" of modafinil. Armodafinil differs from modafinil in that the R-enantiomer (armodafinil) has a somewhat longer half-life than the S-enantiomer component of modafinil. Otherwise, the two drugs are essentially identical, although armodafinil costs more. Armodafinil has the same indications as modafinil—improving wakefulness in people with narcolepsy, SWSD, and OSAHS—and has similar adverse effects, including the potential for rare but severe skin reactions. Like modafinil, armodafinil is classified as a Schedule IV substance.

ATTENTION-DEFICIT/HYPERACTIVITY DISORDER

Our discussion of ADHD has two parts. We begin by addressing basic concepts in ADHD—specifically, signs and symptoms, etiology, and treatment strategy. After that, we discuss the pharmacology of the drugs used for treatment (Table 29.1).

Basic Considerations

Attention-Deficit/Hyperactivity Disorder in Children

ADHD is the most common neuropsychiatric disorder of childhood, affecting 5% of school-aged children. The incidence in boys is 2 to 3 times the incidence in girls. Symptoms begin between ages 3 and 7 years, usually persist into the teens, and often persist on into adulthood. Most (60%–70%) children respond well to stimulant drugs. Methylphenidate [Ritalin, Concerta, others] is the agent employed most.

TABLE 29.1 ▪ Major Drugs for Attention-Deficit/Hyperactivity Disorder

Drug	Trade Name	Availability	Duration (hr)	Dosing Schedule	Usual Pediatric Maintenance Dosage
STIMULANTS					
Methylphenidate					
Immediate release	Ritalin, Methylin	5-, 10-, 20-mg tablets 2.5-, 5-, 10-mg chewables 5- and 10-mg/mL solution	3–5	2 or 3 times daily	10 mg at 8:00 AM and noon, and 5 mg at 4:00 PM
Sustained release	Ritalin-SR, Metadate ER, Quillivant XR	20-mg tablets 25 mg/5 mL oral suspension	6–8	Once or twice daily	20 or 40 mg in AM plus 20 mg in the early PM if needed
24-hour	Concerta	18-, 27-, 36-, 54-mg tablets. Osmotic-Release Oral System (OROS)	10–12	Once daily	36 mg in the AM
	Metadate CD	10-, 20-, 30-, 40-, 50-, 60-mg capsules containing IR and DR beads	8–12	Once daily	30 mg in the AM
	Ritalin LA	10-, 20-, 30-, 40-mg ER capsules	8–12	Once daily	30 mg in the AM
	Daytrana	10-, 15-, 20-, 30-mg/9-hr transdermal patches	10–12	Once daily	One 15- or 20-mg patch, applied in the AM and removed 9 hr later
Dexmethylphenidate					
Immediate release	Focalin	2.5-, 5-, 10-mg tablets	4–5	Twice daily	10 mg in the AM plus 10 mg in the early PM
Sustained release	Focalin XR	5-, 10-, 15-, 20-, 30-, 35-, 40-mg capsules	12	Once daily	10 mg in the AM
Dextroamphetamine					
Immediate release	Dexedrine, ProCentra	5-, 10-mg tablets 5-mg/mL solution	4–6	Once or twice daily	5 mg in the AM
Sustained release	Dexedrine Spansule	5-, 10-, 15-mg capsules	6–10	Once or twice daily	10 mg at 8:00 AM
Amphetamine Mixture					
Immediate release	Adderall	5-, 7.5-, 10-, 12.5-, 15-, 20-, 30-mg tablets	4–6	Twice daily	5 mg in the AM and 4–6 hr later
Sustained release	Adderall XR	5-, 10-, 15-, 20-, 25-, 30-mg capsules	10–12	Once daily	20 mg in the AM
Lisdexamfetamine					
Sustained release	Vyvanse	20-, 30-, 40-, 50-, 60-, 70-mg capsules	13	Once daily	30 mg in the AM
NONSTIMULANTS					
Atomoxetine	Strattera	10-, 18-, 25-, 40-, 60-, 80-, 100-mg capsules	24	Once or twice daily	80 mg in the AM *or* 40 mg in the AM and early PM
Guanfacine	Intuniv	1-, 2-, 3-, 4-mg ER tablets	24	Once daily	1–4 mg in the AM
Clonidine	Kapvay	0.1-, 0.2-mg ER tablets	24	Twice daily	0.1–0.2 mg in the AM and PM

DR, delayed release; ER, extended release; IR, immediate release.

Signs and Symptoms

ADHD is characterized by *inattention, hyperactivity,* and *impulsivity.* Affected children are fidgety, unable to concentrate on schoolwork, and unable to wait their turn; switch excessively from one activity to another; call out excessively in class; and never complete tasks. To make a diagnosis, symptoms must appear before age 7 years and be present for at least 6 months. Because other disorders—especially anxiety and depression—may cause similar symptoms, diagnosis must be done carefully.

ADHD can be subclassified as predominantly inattentive type, predominantly hyperactive-impulsive type, or combined type, depending on symptom profile.

Etiology

Although various theories have been proposed, the underlying pathophysiology of ADHD is only partially understood. Neuroimaging studies indicate structural and functional abnormalities in multiple brain areas, including the frontal cortex, basal ganglia, brainstem, and cerebellum—regions involved with regulating attention, impulsive behavior, and motor activity. Several theories implicate dysregulation in neuronal pathways that employ NE, DA, and serotonin as transmitters. These theories would be consistent with the effects of atomoxetine (which blocks NE reuptake), imipramine (which blocks NE and serotonin uptake), and stimulant drugs (which promote release of NE and DA and, to some degree, block their uptake). Genetic factors play a significant role.

Management Overview

Multiple strategies may be employed to manage ADHD. In addition to drugs, which are considered first-line treatment, the management program can include family therapy, parent training, and cognitive therapy for the child. Guidelines issued by the American Academy of Pediatrics emphasize the importance of a comprehensive treatment program, involving collaboration among clinicians, families, and educators. For long-term gains, a combination of cognitive therapy and stimulant drugs appears most effective. Of the drugs employed for ADHD, stimulants are most effective and hence are considered agents of choice. The nonstimulants (e.g., atomoxetine, guanfacine, clonidine) are less effective than stimulants and hence are considered second-choice drugs.

Attention-Deficit/Hyperactivity Disorder in Adults

In about 30% to 60% of cases, childhood ADHD persists into adulthood. In the United States about 8 million adults are afflicted, although an estimated 90% are undiagnosed and untreated. Symptoms include poor concentration, stress intolerance, antisocial behavior, outbursts of anger, and inability to maintain a routine. Also, adults with ADHD experience more job loss, divorce, and driving accidents. As in childhood ADHD, therapy with a stimulant drug is the foundation of treatment. Methylphenidate is prescribed most often. About 33% of adults fail to respond to stimulants or cannot tolerate their side effects. For these patients, a trial with a nonstimulant may help. Combining behavioral therapy with drug therapy may be more effective than drug therapy alone.

Drugs Used for Attention-Deficit/Hyperactivity Disorder

Central Nervous System Stimulants

Stimulant drugs are the mainstay of ADHD therapy. Drugs with proven efficacy include *methylphenidate* [Ritalin, Concerta, others], *dexmethylphenidate* [Focalin], *dextroamphetamine-amphetamine mixture* [Adderall], and *lisdexamfetamine* [Vyvanse]. There are no data to support use of one stimulant over another. If one stimulant is ineffective, another should be tried before considering a second-line agent.

The response to stimulants can be dramatic. These drugs can increase attention span and goal-oriented behavior while decreasing impulsiveness, distractibility, hyperactivity, and restlessness. Tests of cognitive function (memory, reading, arithmetic) often improve significantly. Unfortunately, although benefits can be dramatic initially, in children they diminish after 2 to 3 years, as reported in a 2009 paper: *MTA at 8 Years: Prospective Follow-up of Children Treated for Combined-Type ADHD in a Multisite Study.* Nonetheless, stimulant therapy can still buy time to teach children behavioral strategies to help them combat inattention and hyperactivity over the long term.

Although reduction of impulsiveness and hyperactivity with a stimulant may seem paradoxical—it isn't. Stimulants don't suppress rowdy behavior directly. Rather, they improve attention and focus. Impulsiveness and hyperactivity decline because the child is now able to concentrate on the task at hand. It should be noted that stimulants do not create *positive* behavior; they only reduce *negative* behavior. Accordingly, stimulants cannot give a child good study skills and other appropriate behaviors. Rather, these must be learned when the disruptive behavior is no longer an impediment.

Principal adverse effects of the stimulants are *insomnia* and *growth suppression.* Insomnia results from CNS stimulation and can be minimized by reducing the size of the afternoon dose and taking it no later than 4:00 PM. Growth suppression occurs secondary to appetite suppression. Growth reduction can be minimized by administering stimulants during or after meals (which reduces the impact of appetite suppression). In addition, some clinicians recommend taking "drug holidays" on weekends and in the summer (which creates an opportunity for growth to catch up). However, other clinicians argue against this strategy because depriving children of medication during these unstructured times can be hard on them. When stimulants are discontinued, a rebound increase in growth will take place; as a result, adult height may not be affected. Other adverse effects include *headache* and *abdominal pain,* which have an incidence of 10%, and *lethargy* and *listlessness,* which can occur when dosage is excessive.

Nonstimulants

Several nonstimulants are used for ADHD, although only three of them—atomoxetine, guanfacine, and clonidine—are approved by the U.S. Food and Drug Administration (FDA) for this use. The nonstimulants are less effective than the stimulants and hence are considered second-choice drugs. For treatment of ADHD, the nonstimulants may be employed as monotherapy, or as add-on therapy with a stimulant. Unlike the stimulants, the nonstimulants are not regulated as controlled substances.

Atomoxetine, a Norepinephrine Uptake Inhibitor

Description and Therapeutic Effects. Atomoxetine [Strattera] is a unique drug approved for ADHD in children and adults. It was the first *nonstimulant* approved for ADHD, and one of only three drugs approved for ADHD in adults (the others are amphetamine-dextroamphetamine mixture [Adderall XR] and lisdexamfetamine [Vyvanse]). In contrast to the CNS stimulants, atomoxetine has no potential for abuse and hence is not regulated as a controlled substance. As a result, prescriptions can be refilled over the phone, making atomoxetine more convenient than the stimulants. Like the long-acting stimulants, atomoxetine can be administered just once a day.

In clinical trials comparing atomoxetine with placebo in children or adults with ADHD, atomoxetine was clearly superior at reducing symptoms. It should be noted that responses develop slowly: the initial response takes a few days to develop, and the maximal response is seen in 1 to 3 weeks. This contrasts with the CNS stimulants, whose effects are near maximal with the first dose.

Mechanism of Action. Atomoxetine is a *selective inhibitor of NE reuptake* and hence causes NE to accumulate at synapses. Although the precise relationship between this neurochemical action and symptom relief is unknown, it would appear that *adaptive changes* that occur after uptake blockade underlie benefits. Uptake blockade occurs immediately, whereas full therapeutic effects are not seen for at least a week—suggesting that, after uptake blockade occurs, additional processes must take place before benefits can be seen.

Pharmacokinetics. Atomoxetine is rapidly and completely absorbed after oral administration. Plasma levels peak in 1 to 3 hours, depending on whether the drug was taken without or with food. Atomoxetine is metabolized in the liver, primarily by CYP2D6 (the 2D6 isoenzyme of cytochrome P450). For most patients, the half-life is 5 hours. However, for 5% to 10% of patients, the half-life is much longer: 24 hours. These patients have an atypical form of CYP2D6, which metabolizes atomoxetine slowly. Dosage should be reduced in these people.

Adverse Effects. Like the CNS stimulants, atomoxetine is generally well tolerated. In clinical trials, the most common effects were GI reactions (dyspepsia, nausea, and vomiting), reduced appetite, dizziness, somnolence, mood swings, and trouble sleeping. Sexual dysfunction and urinary retention were seen in adults. Severe allergic reactions, including angioneurotic edema, occurred rarely. If allergy develops, patients should discontinue the drug and contact their prescriber immediately.

Atomoxetine may cause *suicidal thinking* in children and adolescents, but not in adults. Fortunately, the incidence is relatively low: about 4 cases per 1000 patients. Risk is greatest during the first few months of treatment. Young patients should be monitored closely for suicidal thinking and behavior and for signs of clinical worsening (e.g., agitation, irritability).

Appetite suppression may result in *weight loss and growth delay.* Among children who took atomoxetine for 18 months or longer, mean height and weight percentiles declined. Because experience with the drug is limited, we don't know if expected adult height will be affected. Nor do we know if "drug holidays" would have an effect on growth.

Atomoxetine poses a small risk for *severe liver injury* that may progress to outright liver failure, resulting in death or the need for a liver transplantation. Patients should be informed about signs of liver injury—jaundice, dark urine, abdominal tenderness, unexplained flu-like symptoms—and instructed to report these immediately. In the event of jaundice or laboratory evidence of liver injury, atomoxetine should be discontinued.

Atomoxetine *may raise or lower blood pressure.* During clinical trials, some patients experienced a small increase in blood pressure and heart rate. Accordingly, atomoxetine should be used with caution by patients with hypertension or tachycardia. During postmarketing surveillance, some patients experienced *hypotension and syncope* (fainting). Patients should be informed of this possibility and advised to sit or lie down if they feel faint.

Drug Interactions. Inhibitors of CYP2D6 can increase levels of atomoxetine and hence must be used with caution. Common examples include paroxetine [Paxil], fluoxetine [Prozac], and quinidine.

Role in ADHD Therapy. Atomoxetine is recommended for treatment of ADHD in cases in which there may be concern for stimulant abuse or there exists a strong aversion to treatment with stimulant medications. Because CNS stimulants are more effective and have a long record of safety and efficacy, it would seem prudent to reserve atomoxetine for patients who are unresponsive to or intolerant of the stimulants. In the absence of a compelling reason, patients doing well on the stimulants shouldn't switch.

Alpha$_2$-Adrenergic Agonists. Two alpha$_2$-adrenergic agonists—guanfacine and clonidine—are approved for ADHD. Both drugs appear less effective than CNS stimulants. Principal side effects are sedation, hypotension, and fatigue. Unlike the CNS stimulants, guanfacine and clonidine are not controlled substances and do not cause anorexia or insomnia. The basic pharmacology of these drugs is discussed in Chapter 15.

GUANFACINE. Available in an extended-release (ER) formulation, sold as *Intuniv,* guanfacine is used for treating children and adolescents with ADHD. In clinical trials, ER guanfacine improved hyperactivity and inattention. Benefits were greater than with placebo, but less than reported with stimulants. Guanfacine activates presynaptic alpha$_2$-adrenergic receptors in the brain. However, we don't know how this action relates to clinical benefits. Principal side effects are somnolence, fatigue, and reduced blood pressure. Effects on blood pressure are most pronounced during initial therapy and whenever dosage is increased. Abrupt discontinuation can cause rebound hypertension. In contrast to the stimulants, guanfacine causes weight gain rather than weight loss, causes somnolence rather than insomnia, and is not regulated under the Controlled Substances Act. Because the drug does not cause anorexia or insomnia, it might be especially good for children who cannot tolerate these effects of stimulants. Guanfacine can also be combined with a stimulant to treat severe ADHD.

Clonidine. ER clonidine [Kapvay] is much like ER guanfacine [Intuniv]. Both drugs are alpha$_2$ agonists, both were developed for hypertension, and both had been used off-label in ADHD for years. In clinical trials of ADHD, ER clonidine was superior to placebo when used alone and provided additional symptom relief when combined with a stimulant. As with guanfacine, principal side effects are somnolence, fatigue, and hypotension. Somnolence can be made worse by alcohol and other CNS depressants. Hypotension can be made worse by antihypertensive agents. Because clonidine can lower blood pressure (and slow heart rate too), blood pressure and heart rate should be measured at baseline, following each dose increase, and periodically thereafter. Like guanfacine, clonidine does not cause anorexia or insomnia and is not a controlled substance.

CHAPTER 30

Drug Abuse I: Basic Considerations

Laura D. Rosenthal, DNP, ACNP, FAANP

Mind-altering drugs have intrigued human beings since the dawn of civilization. Throughout history, people have taken drugs to elevate mood, release inhibitions, distort perceptions, induce hallucinations, and modify thinking. Many of those who take mind-altering drugs restrict use to socially approved patterns. However, many others self-administer drugs to excess. Excessive drug use is our focus in this chapter and the three that follow.

Drug abuse extracts a huge toll on the individual and on society. Tobacco alone kills about 440,000 Americans each year. Alcohol and illicit drugs kill another 100,000. In addition to putting people at risk for death, drug abuse puts them at risk for long-term illness and impairs their ability to fulfill role obligations at home, school, and work. The economic burden of drug abuse is staggering: the combined direct and indirect costs from abusing nicotine, alcohol, and illicit substances are estimated at over $700 *billion* each year.

Drug abuse confronts clinicians in a variety of ways, making knowledge of abuse a necessity. Important areas in which expertise on drug abuse may be applied include (1) diagnosis and treatment of acute toxicity, (2) diagnosis and treatment of secondary medical complications of drug abuse, (3) facilitating drug withdrawal, and (4) providing education and counseling to maintain long-term abstinence.

Our discussion of drug abuse occurs in two stages. In this chapter, we discuss basic concepts in drug abuse. In Chapters 31, 32, and 33, we focus on the pharmacology of specific abused agents and methods of treatment.

DEFINITIONS

Drug Abuse

Drug abuse can be defined as *using a drug in a fashion inconsistent with medical or social norms.* Traditionally, the term also implies drug use that is harmful to the individual or society. As we shall see, although we can give abuse a general definition, deciding whether a particular instance of drug use constitutes "abuse" is often difficult.

Whether or not drug use is considered abuse depends, in part, on the purpose for which a drug is taken. Not everyone who takes large doses of psychoactive agents is an abuser. For example, we do not consider it abuse to take large doses of opioids long term to relieve pain caused by cancer. However, we do consider it abusive for an otherwise healthy individual to take those same opioids in the same doses to produce euphoria.

Abuse can have different degrees of severity. Some people, for example, use heroin only occasionally, whereas others use it habitually and compulsively. Although both patterns of drug use are socially condemned and therefore constitute abuse, there is an obvious quantitative difference between taking heroin once or twice and taking it routinely and compulsively.

Note that, by the previous definition, drug abuse is culturally defined. Because abuse is culturally defined, and because societies differ from one another and are changeable, there can be wide variations in what is labeled abuse. What is defined as abuse can vary from one culture to another. For example, in the United States, moderate consumption of alcohol is not usually considered abuse. In contrast, any ingestion of alcohol may be considered abuse in some Muslim societies. Furthermore, what is defined as abuse can vary from one time to another within the same culture. For example, when a few Americans first experimented with lysergic acid diethylamide (LSD) and other psychedelic drugs, these agents were legal and their use was not generally disapproved. However, when use of psychedelics became widespread, our societal posture changed, and legislation was passed to make the manufacture, sale, and use of these drugs illegal.

As we can see, distinguishing between culturally acceptable drug use and drug use that is to be called abuse is more in the realm of social science than pharmacology. Accordingly, because this is a pharmacology text and not a sociology text, we will not attempt to define just what patterns of drug use do or do not constitute abuse. Instead, we will focus on the pharmacologic properties of abused drugs. Fortunately, we can identify the drugs that tend to be abused and discuss their pharmacology.

Addiction

According to the National Institute on Drug Abuse, addiction is defined as *a chronic, relapsing brain disease that is characterized by compulsive drug seeking and use, despite harmful consequences.* Addiction is a very complex phenomenon that includes social, psychological, genetic, and environmental components. Please note that nowhere in this definition is addiction equated with physical dependence. As discussed later, although physical dependence can contribute to addictive behavior, it is neither necessary nor sufficient for addiction to occur.

Other Definitions

Tolerance results from regular drug use and can be defined as a state in which a particular dose elicits a smaller response than it did with initial use. As tolerance increases, higher and higher doses are needed to elicit desired effects.

Cross-tolerance is a state in which tolerance to one drug confers tolerance to another. Cross-tolerance generally develops among drugs within a particular class, and not between drugs in different classes. For example, tolerance to one opioid (e.g., heroin) confers cross-tolerance to other opioids (e.g., morphine), but not to central nervous system (CNS) depressants, psychostimulants, psychedelics, or nicotine.

Psychological dependence can be defined as an intense subjective need for a particular psychoactive drug.

Physical dependence can be defined as a state in which an abstinence syndrome will occur if drug use is discontinued. Physical dependence is the result of neuroadaptive processes that take place in response to prolonged drug exposure.

Cross-dependence refers to the ability of one drug to support physical dependence on another drug. When cross-dependence exists between drug A and drug B, taking drug A will prevent withdrawal in a patient physically dependent on drug B, and vice versa. As with cross-tolerance, cross-dependence generally exists among drugs in the same pharmacologic family, but not between drugs in different families.

A ***withdrawal syndrome*** is a constellation of signs and symptoms that occurs in physically dependent individuals when they discontinue drug use. Quite often, the symptoms seen during withdrawal are opposite to effects the drug produced before it was withdrawn. For example, discontinuation of a CNS depressant can cause CNS excitation.

DIAGNOSTIC CRITERIA REGARDING DRUGS OF ABUSE

Substance use disorder is best defined as *continued use of a substance despite significant substance-related problems*. There exists a change in brain circuitry that persists despite detoxification. Diagnosis of substance abuse disorder is based on behaviors related to continued use of a substance.

Tolerance and withdrawal are among the criteria established by the American Psychiatric Association (APA) for having a substance use disorder. Please note, however, that tolerance and withdrawal, by themselves, are neither necessary nor sufficient for a substance use disorder to exist. Put another way, the pattern of drug use that constitutes a substance use disorder can exist in persons who are not physically dependent on drugs and who have not developed tolerance. This distinction is extremely important. *Being physically dependent on a drug is not the same as being addicted.* Many people are physically dependent but do not meet the criteria for a substance use disorder. These people are not considered addicts because they do not demonstrate the behavior pattern that constitutes substance dependence. Patients with terminal cancer, for example, are often physically dependent on opioids. However, because their lives are not disrupted by their medication (quite the contrary), their drug use does not meet the criteria for a substance use disorder. Similarly, some degree of physical dependence occurs in all patients who take phenobarbital to control seizure disorders. However, despite their physical dependence, patients with seizure do not carry out stereotypic addictive behavior and therefore do not have a substance use disorder.

Having stressed that physical dependence and addiction are different from each other, we must note that the two states are not entirely unrelated. As discussed later, although physical dependence is not the same as addiction, physical dependence often contributes to addictive behavior.

FACTORS THAT CONTRIBUTE TO DRUG ABUSE

Drug abuse is the end result of a progressive involvement with drugs. Taking psychoactive drugs is usually initiated out of curiosity. From this initial involvement, the user can progress to occasional use. Occasional use can then evolve into compulsive use. Factors that play a role in the progression from experimental use to compulsive use are discussed next.

Reinforcing Properties of Drugs

Reinforcement by drugs can occur in two ways. First, drugs can give the individual an experience that is pleasurable. Cocaine, for example, produces a state of euphoria. Second, drugs can reduce the intensity of unpleasant experiences. For example, drugs can reduce anxiety and stress.

The reinforcing properties of drugs can be clearly demonstrated in experiments with animals. In the laboratory, animals will self-administer most of the drugs that are abused by humans (e.g., opioids, barbiturates, alcohol, cocaine, amphetamines, phencyclidine, nicotine, caffeine). When these drugs are made freely available, animals develop patterns of drug use that are similar to those of humans. Animals will self-administer these drugs (except for nicotine and caffeine) in preference to eating, drinking, and sex. When permitted, they often die of lack of food and fluid. These observations strongly suggest that preexisting psychopathology is not necessary for drug abuse to develop. Rather, these studies suggest that drug abuse results, in large part, from the reinforcing properties of drugs themselves.

Physical Dependence

As defined earlier, *physical dependence* is a state in which an abstinence syndrome will occur if drug use is discontinued. The degree of physical dependence is determined largely by dosage and duration of drug use. Physical dependence is greatest in people who take large doses for a long time. The more physically dependent a person is, the more intense the withdrawal syndrome. Substantial physical dependence develops to the opioids (e.g., morphine, heroin) and CNS depressants (e.g., barbiturates, alcohol). Physical dependence tends to be less prominent with other abused drugs (e.g., psychostimulants, psychedelics, marijuana).

Physical dependence can contribute to compulsive drug use. After dependence has developed, the desire to avoid withdrawal becomes a motivator for continued dosing. Furthermore, if the drug is administered after the onset of withdrawal, its ability to alleviate the discomfort of withdrawal can reinforce its desirability. Please note, however, that although physical dependence plays a role in the abuse of drugs, physical dependence should not be viewed as the primary cause of addictive behavior. Rather, physical dependence is just one of several factors that can contribute to the development and continuation of compulsive use.

Psychological Dependence

Psychological dependence is defined as *an intense subjective need for a drug.* Individuals who are psychologically dependent feel very strongly that their sense of well-being is dependent on continued drug use; a sense of "craving" is felt when the drug is unavailable. There is no question that psychological dependence can be a major factor in addictive behavior. For example, it is psychological dependence—and not physical dependence—that plays the principal role in causing renewed use of opioids by addicts who had previously gone through withdrawal.

Social Factors

Social factors can play an important role in the development of abuse. The desire for social status and approval is a common reason for initiating drug use. Also, because initial drug experiences are frequently unpleasant, the desire for social approval can be one of the most compelling reasons for repeating drug use after the initial exposure. For example, most people do not especially enjoy their first cigarette; were it not for peer pressure, many would quit before they smoked enough for it to become pleasurable. Similarly, initial use of heroin, with its associated nausea and vomiting, is often deemed unpleasant; peer pressure is a common reason for continuing heroin use long enough to develop tolerance to these undesirable effects.

Drug Availability

Drug availability is clearly a factor in the development and maintenance of abuse. Abuse can flourish only in environments where drugs can be readily obtained. In contrast, where procurement is difficult, abuse is minimal. The ready availability of drugs in hospitals and clinics is a major reason for the unusually high rate of addiction among pharmacists, nurses, and physicians.

Vulnerability of the Individual

Some individuals are more prone to becoming drug abusers than others. By way of illustration, let's consider three individuals from the same social setting who have equal access to the same psychoactive drug. The first person experiments with the drug briefly and never uses it again. The second person progresses from experimentation to occasional use. The third goes on to take the drug compulsively. Because social factors, drug availability, and the properties of the drug itself are the same for all three people, these factors cannot explain the three different patterns of drug use. We must conclude, therefore, that the differences must lie in the people: one individual was not prone to drug abuse, one had only moderate tendencies toward abuse, and the third was highly vulnerable to becoming an abuser.

Several psychological factors have been associated with tendencies toward drug abuse. Drug abusers are frequently individuals who are impulsive, have a low tolerance for frustration, and are rebellious against social norms. Other psychological factors that seem to predispose individuals to abusing drugs include depressive disorders, anxiety disorders, and antisocial personality. It is also clear that individuals who abuse one type of drug are likely to abuse other drugs.

There is speculation that some instances of drug abuse may actually represent self-medication to relieve emotional discomfort. For example, some people may use alcohol and other depressants to control severe anxiety. Although their drug use may appear excessive, it may be no more than they need to neutralize intolerable feelings.

Genetics also contribute to drug abuse. Vulnerability to alcoholism, for example, may result from an inherited predisposition.

NEUROBIOLOGY OF ADDICTION

Repeated use of an addictive drug contributes to the transition from voluntary drug use to compulsive use by causing molecular changes in the brain. Each time the drug is taken, it causes changes that promote further drug use. With repeated drug exposure, these changes are reinforced, making drug use increasingly more difficult to control.

Molecular changes occur in the *reward circuit*—a system that normally serves to reinforce behaviors essential for survival, such as eating and reproductive activities. Neurons of the reward circuit originate in the ventral tegmental area of the midbrain and project to the nucleus accumbens. Their major transmitter is *dopamine.* Under normal circumstances, biologically critical behavior, such as sexual intercourse, activates the circuit. The resultant release of dopamine rewards and reinforces the behavior. Like natural positive stimuli, addictive drugs can also activate the circuit and thereby cause dopamine release. In fact, drugs are so effective at activating the circuit that the amount of dopamine released may be 2 to 10 times the amount released by natural stimuli. Ultimately, whether the system is activated by use of drugs or by behavior essential for survival, the outcome is the same: a tendency to repeat the behavior that turned the system on. With repeated activation over time, the system undergoes synaptic remodeling, thereby consolidating changes in brain function. This neural remodeling persists after drug use has ceased.

An important aspect of drug-induced remodeling is a phenomenon known as *downregulation,* which serves to *reduce* the response to drugs. Because drugs release abnormally large amounts of dopamine, the reward circuit is put in a state of excessive activation. In response, the brain (1) produces less dopamine and (2) reduces the number of dopamine receptors. As a result, responses to drugs are reduced. Unfortunately, the ability of natural stimuli to activate the circuit is reduced as well. In the absence of pleasurable feelings from natural stimuli, the abuser is left feeling flat, lifeless, and depressed. The good news is that, when drug use stops, neural remodeling tends to gradually reverse.

PRINCIPLES OF ADDICTION TREATMENT

Drug addiction is a treatable disease of the brain. With therapy, between 40% and 60% of addicts can reduce drug use. The first science-based guide on addiction therapy—*Principles of Drug Addiction Treatment*—was published by the National Institute on Drug Abuse in 1999, and later revised in 2009 and 2012. The guide centers on 13 principles of effective treatment, shown in Box 30.1.

Ideally, the goal of treatment is *complete cessation* of drug use. However, total abstinence is not the only outcome that can be considered successful. Treatment that changes drug use from compulsive to moderate will permit increased productivity, better health, and a decrease in socially unacceptable behavior. Clearly, this outcome is beneficial both to the individual and to society—even though some degree of drug use continues. It must be noted, however, that in the treatment of some forms of abuse, nothing short of total abstinence can be considered a true success. Experience has shown that abusers of *cigarettes, alcohol,* and *opioids* are rarely capable of sustained moderation. Hence, for many of these individuals, abstinence must be complete if there is to be any hope of avoiding a return to compulsive use.

Recovery from addiction is a prolonged process that typically requires multiple treatment episodes because addiction

BOX 30.1 ▪ PRINCIPLES OF DRUG-ADDICTION TREATMENT

1. **Addiction is a complex but treatable disease that affects brain function and behavior.** Drugs of abuse alter brain structure and function, resulting in changes that persist long after drug use has stopped. These persistent changes may explain why former abusers are at the risk for relapse after prolonged abstinence.
2. **No single treatment is appropriate for everyone.** It is critical to match treatment settings, interventions, and services to each patient's problems and needs.
3. **Treatment must be readily available.** Treatment applicants can be lost if treatment is not immediately available or readily accessible. As with other chronic diseases, the earlier treatment is offered in the disease process, the greater the likelihood of positive outcomes.
4. **Effective treatment must attend to multiple needs of the individual, not solely drug use.** In addition to addressing drug use, treatment must address the individual's medical, psychological, social, vocational, and legal problems.
5. **Remaining in treatment for an adequate time is critical.** Treatment duration is based on individual need. Most patients require at least 3 months of treatment to significantly reduce or stop drug use. Additional treatment can produce further progress. As with other chronic illnesses, relapses can occur, signaling a need for treatment to be reinstated or adjusted. Programs should include strategies to prevent patients from leaving prematurely.
6. **Individual and/or group counseling and other behavioral therapies are the most common forms of drug abuse treatment.** In therapy, patients address motivation, build skills to resist drug use, replace drug-using activities with constructive and rewarding activities, and improve problem-solving abilities. Behavioral therapy also addresses incentives for abstinence and facilitates interpersonal relationships. Ongoing group therapy and other peer support programs can help maintain abstinence.
7. **Medication can be an important element of treatment, especially when combined with counseling and other behavioral therapies.** Methadone, buprenorphine, and naltrexone can help persons addicted to opioids. Nicotine replacement therapy (e.g., patches, gum), bupropion, and varenicline can help persons addicted to nicotine. Disulfiram, naltrexone, topiramate, and acamprosate can help persons addicted to alcohol.
8. **Because needs of the individual can change, the plan for treatment and services must be reassessed continually and modified as indicated.** At different times during treatment, a patient may develop a need for medications, medical services, family therapy, parenting instruction, vocational rehabilitation, and social and legal services.
9. **Many drug-addicted individuals also have other mental disorders, which must be addressed.** Because drug addiction often co-occurs with other mental illnesses, patients presenting with one condition should be assessed for other conditions and treated as indicated.
10. **Medically assisted detoxification is only the first stage of addiction treatment and, by itself, does little to change long-term drug use.** Medical detoxification manages the acute physical symptoms of withdrawal—and can serve as a precursor to effective long-term treatment.
11. **Treatment needn't be voluntary to be effective.** Sanctions or enticements coming from the family, employer, or criminal justice system can significantly increase treatment entry, retention, and success.
12. **Drug use during treatment must be monitored continuously because relapses during treatment do occur.** Knowing that drug use is being monitored (e.g., through urinalysis) can help the patient withstand urges to use drugs. Monitoring also can provide early evidence of drug use, thereby allowing timely adjustment of the treatment program.
13. **Treatment programs should provide assessment for HIV/AIDS, hepatitis B and C, tuberculosis, and other infectious diseases, along with counseling to help patients modify behaviors that place them or others at risk.**

HIV/AIDS, human immunodeficiency virus/acquired immunodeficiency syndrome.
Adapted from National Institute on Drug Abuse: Principles of Drug Addiction Treatment: A Research-Based Guide, 3rd ed. (Publication No. 12-4180). Bethesda, MD: National Institutes of Health, 2012.

is a *chronic, relapsing* illness. As such, periods of treatment-induced abstinence will very likely be followed by relapse. This does not mean that treatment has failed. Rather, it simply means that at least one more treatment episode is needed. Eventually, many patients achieve stable, long-term abstinence, along with a more productive and rewarding life.

Because addiction is a complex illness that affects all aspects of life, the treatment program must be comprehensive and multifaceted. In addition to addressing drug use itself, the program should address any related medical, psychological, social, vocational, and legal problems. Obviously, treatment must be tailored to the individual; no single approach works for all people. Multiple techniques are employed. Techniques with proven success include (1) group and individual therapy directed at resolving emotional problems that underlie drug use, (2) substituting alternative rewards for the rewards of drug use, and (3) use of pharmacologic agents to modify the effects of abused drugs. The most effective treatment programs incorporate two or more of these methods. When possible, a specialist in addiction medicine or substance use should be involved in the patient's care.

THE CONTROLLED SUBSTANCES ACT

The *Comprehensive Drug Abuse Prevention and Control Act of 1970,* known informally as the *Controlled Substances Act* (CSA), is the principal federal legislation addressing drug abuse. One objective of the CSA is to reduce the chances that drugs originating from legitimate sources will be diverted to abusers. To accomplish this goal, the CSA sets forth regulations for the handling of controlled substances by manufacturers, distributors, pharmacists, nurses, and physicians. Enforcement of the CSA is the responsibility of the *Drug Enforcement Agency* (DEA), an arm of the U.S. Department of Justice.

Record Keeping

To keep track of controlled substances that originate from legitimate sources, a written record must be made of all transactions involving these agents. Every time a controlled substance is purchased or dispensed, the transfer must be recorded. Physicians, pharmacists, and hospitals must keep an inventory of all controlled substances in stock. This inventory must be reported to the DEA every 2 years. Although not specifically obliged to do so by the CSA, many hospitals use medication dispensing machines that count the controlled substances dispensed during each shift.

Drug Enforcement Agency Schedules

Each drug preparation regulated under the CSA has been assigned to one of five categories: Schedule I, II, III, IV, or V. Drugs in Schedule I have a high potential for abuse and no approved medical use in the United States. In contrast, drugs in Schedules II through V all have approved applications. Assignment to Schedules II through V is based on abuse potential and potential for causing physical or psychological dependence. Of the drugs that have medical applications, those in Schedule II have the highest potential for abuse and dependence. Drugs in the remaining schedules have decreasing abuse and dependence liabilities. Table 30.1 lists the primary drugs that come under the five DEA Schedules.

Scheduling of drugs under the CSA undergoes periodic reevaluation. With increased understanding of the abuse and dependence liabilities of a drug, the DEA may choose to reassign it to a different Schedule. For example, hydrocodone (the opiate in Vicodin) was recently switched from Schedule III to Schedule II.

Prescriptions

The CSA places restrictions on prescribing drugs in Schedules II through V. (Drugs in Schedule I have no approved uses and hence are not prescribed.) Only prescribers registered with the DEA are authorized to prescribe controlled drugs. Regulations on prescribing controlled substances are summarized next.

Schedule II

All prescriptions for Schedule II drugs must be typed or filled out in ink or indelible pencil and signed by the prescriber. Alternatively, prescribers may submit prescriptions using an electronic prescribing procedure. Oral prescriptions may be called in, but only in emergencies, and a written prescription must follow within 72 hours. Prescriptions for Schedule II drugs cannot be refilled. However, a DEA rule issued in 2007 now allows a prescriber to write multiple prescriptions on the same day—for the same patient and same drug—to be filled sequentially for up to a 90-day supply.

Schedules III and IV

Prescriptions for drugs in Schedules III and IV may be oral, written, or electronic. If authorized by the prescriber, these prescriptions may be refilled up to 5 times. Refills must be made within 6 months of the original order. If additional medication is needed beyond the amount provided for in the original prescription, a new prescription must be written.

Schedule V

The same regulations for prescribing drugs in Schedules III and IV apply to drugs in Schedule V. In addition, Schedule V drugs may be dispensed without a prescription provided the following conditions are met: (1) the drug is dispensed by a pharmacist; (2) the amount dispensed is very limited; (3) the recipient is at least 18 years old ; (4) the pharmacist writes and initials a record indicating the date, the name and amount of the drug, and the name and address of the recipient; and (5) state and local laws do not prohibit dispensing Schedule V drugs without a prescription.

Labeling

When drugs in Schedules II, III, and IV are dispensed, their containers must bear this label: *Caution—Federal law prohibits the transfer of this drug to any person other than the patient for whom it was prescribed.*

State Laws

All states have their own laws regulating drugs of abuse. In many cases, state laws are more stringent than federal laws. As a rule, whenever there is a difference between state and federal laws, the more restrictive of the two takes precedence.

TABLE 30.1 ▪ Drug Enforcement Agency Classification of Controlled Substances

Schedule I Drugs	Schedule II Drugs	Schedule III Drugs	Schedule IV Drugs	Schedule V Drugs
Opioids	**Opioids**	**Opioids**	**Opioids**	**Opioids**
Acetylmethadol	Alfentanil	Buprenorphine	Butorphanol	Diphenoxylate plus atropine
Heroin	Codeine	Paregoric	Pentazocine	Pregabalin
Normethadone	Fentanyl	**Cannabinoids**	**Stimulants**	
Many others	Hydrocodone	Dronabinol (THC)	Diethylpropion	
Psychedelics	Hydromorphone	**Stimulants**	Fenfluramine	
Bufotenin	Levorphanol	Benzphetamine	Mazindol	
Diethyltryptamine	Meperidine	Phendimetrazine	Pemoline	
Dimethyltryptamine	Methadone	**Barbiturates**	Phentermine	
Ibogaine	Morphine	Aprobarbital	**Barbiturates**	
d-Lysergic acid diethylamide (LSD)	Opium tincture	Butabarbital	Methohexital	
Mescaline	Oxycodone	Talbutal	Phenobarbital	
3,4-Methylenedioxy-methamphetamine (MDMA)	Oxymorphone	Thiamylal	**Benzodiazepines**	
Psilocin	Remifentanil	Thiopental	Alprazolam	
Psilocybin	Sufentanil	**Miscellaneous Depressants**	Chlordiazepoxide	
Cannabis Derivatives	**Psychostimulants**	Methyprylon	Clonazepam	
Marijuana	Amphetamine	**Anabolic Steroids**	Clorazepate	
Others	Cocaine	Fluoxymesterone	Diazepam	
Gamma-hydroxybutyrate	Dextroamphetamine	Methyltestosterone	Estazolam	
Methaqualone	Methamphetamine	Nandrolone	Flurazepam	
	Methylphenidate	Oxandrolone	Lorazepam	
	Phenmetrazine	Stanozolol	Midazolam	
	Barbiturates	Testosterone	Oxazepam	
	Amobarbital	Many others	Prazepam	
	Pentobarbital	**Others**	Quazepam	
	Secobarbital	Ketamine	Temazepam	
	Miscellaneous Depressants		Triazolam	
	Glutethimide		**Benzodiazepine-like Drugs**	
			Zaleplon	
			Zolpidem	
			Miscellaneous Depressants	
			Chloral hydrate	
			Dichloralphenazone	
			Ethchlorvynol	
			Ethinamate	
			Meprobamate	
			Paraldehyde	

CHAPTER

31

Drug Abuse II: Alcohol

Laura D. Rosenthal, DNP, ACNP, FAANP

Alcohol (ethyl alcohol, ethanol) is the most commonly used and abused psychoactive agent in the United States. Although alcohol does have some therapeutic applications, the drug is of interest primarily for its nonmedical use. When consumed in moderation, alcohol prolongs life and reduces the risk for dementia and cardiovascular disorders. Conversely, when consumed in excess, alcohol diminishes life in both quality and quantity.

In approaching our study of alcohol, we begin by discussing the basic pharmacology of alcohol, and then we discuss alcohol use disorder and the drugs employed for treatment.

BASIC PHARMACOLOGY OF ALCOHOL

Central Nervous System Effects

Acute Effects

Alcohol has two acute effects on the brain: (1) general depression of central nervous system (CNS) function and (2) activation of the reward circuit.

For many years, we believed that alcohol simply dissolved into the neuronal membrane, thereby disrupting the ordered arrangement of membrane phospholipids. However, we now know that alcohol interacts with specific proteins—certain receptors, ion channels, and enzymes—that regulate neuronal excitability. Three target proteins are of particular importance, namely (1) receptors for gamma-aminobutyric acid (GABA), (2) receptors for glutamate, and (3) the 5-HT_3 subset of receptors for serotonin (5-hydroxytryptamine [5-HT]). The *depressant* effects of alcohol result from binding with receptors for GABA (the principal inhibitory transmitter in the CNS) and receptors for glutamate (a major excitatory transmitter in the CNS). When alcohol binds with GABA receptors, it enhances GABA-mediated inhibition, causing widespread depression of CNS activity. When alcohol binds with glutamate receptors, it blocks glutamate-mediated excitation and thereby reduces overall CNS activity. The *rewarding* effects of alcohol result from binding with 5-HT_3 receptors in the brain's reward circuit. When these receptors are activated, they promote release of dopamine, the major transmitter of the reward system. When alcohol binds with these receptors, it enhances serotonin-mediated release of dopamine and intensifies the reward process.

The depressant effects of alcohol are dose dependent. When dosage is low, higher brain centers (cortical areas) are primarily affected. As dosage increases, more primitive brain areas (e.g., medulla) become depressed. With depression of cortical function, thought processes and learned behaviors are altered, inhibitions are released, and self-restraint is replaced by increased sociability and expansiveness. Cortical depression also impairs motor function. As CNS depression deepens, reflexes diminish greatly and consciousness becomes impaired. At very high doses, alcohol produces a state of general anesthesia. (Alcohol can't be used for anesthesia because the doses required are close to lethal.)

Chronic Effects

When consumed chronically and in excess, alcohol can produce severe neurologic and psychiatric disorders. Injury to the CNS is caused by the direct actions of alcohol and by the nutritional deficiencies often seen in chronic heavy drinkers.

Two neuropsychiatric syndromes are common in alcoholics: *Wernicke encephalopathy* and *Korsakoff psychosis.* Both disorders are caused by thiamin deficiency, which results from poor diet and alcohol-induced suppression of thiamin absorption. Wernicke's encephalopathy is characterized by confusion, nystagmus, and abnormal ocular movements. This syndrome is readily reversible with thiamin. Korsakoff psychosis is characterized by polyneuropathy, inability to convert short-term memory into long-term memory, and confabulation (unconscious filling of gaps in memory with fabricated facts and experiences). Korsakoff psychosis is not reversible.

Perhaps the most dramatic effect of long-term excessive alcohol consumption is enlargement of the cerebral ventricles, presumably in response to atrophy of the cerebrum itself. These gross anatomic changes are associated with impairment of memory and intellectual function. With cessation of drinking, ventricular enlargement and cognitive deficits partially reverse, but only in some individuals.

Impact on Cognitive Function

Low to moderate drinking helps preserve cognitive function in older people and may protect against development of dementia.

Effect on Sleep

Although alcohol is commonly used as a sleep aid, it actually disrupts sleep. Drinking can alter sleep cycles, decrease total sleeping time, and reduce the quality of sleep. In addition, alcohol can intensify snoring and exacerbate obstructive sleep apnea.

Other Pharmacologic Effects

Cardiovascular System

When alcohol is consumed acutely and in moderate doses, cardiovascular effects are minor. The most prominent effect is *dilation of cutaneous blood vessels,* causing increased blood flow to the skin. By doing so, alcohol imparts a sensation of warmth—but at the same time promotes loss of heat.

Although the cardiovascular effects of moderate alcohol consumption are unremarkable, chronic and excessive consumption is clearly harmful. Abuse of alcohol results in *direct damage to the myocardium,* thereby increasing the risk for heart failure. Some investigators believe that alcohol may be a major cause of cardiomyopathy in the Western world.

In addition to damaging the heart, alcohol produces a dose-dependent *elevation of blood pressure.* The cause is vasoconstriction in vascular beds of skeletal muscle brought on by increased activity of the sympathetic nervous system. Estimates suggest that heavy drinking may be responsible for 10% of all cases of hypertension.

Not all of the cardiovascular effects of alcohol are deleterious: there is clear evidence that people who drink *moderately* (2 drinks a day or less for men, 1 drink a day or less for women) experience less ischemic stroke, coronary artery disease (CAD), myocardial infarction (MI), and heart failure than do abstainers. It is important to note, however, that *heavy* drinking (5 or more drinks/day) *increases* the risk for heart disease and stroke. Moderate drinking protects against heart disease primarily by raising levels of high-density lipoprotein (HDL) cholesterol. As discussed in Chapter 42, HDL cholesterol protects against CAD, whereas low-density lipoprotein (LDL) cholesterol promotes CAD. Of all the agents that can raise HDL cholesterol, alcohol is one of the most effective known. In addition to raising HDL cholesterol, alcohol may confer protection through four other mechanisms: decreasing platelet aggregation, decreasing levels of fibrinogen (the precursor of fibrin, which reinforces clots), increasing levels of tissue plasminogen activator (a clot-dissolving enzyme), and suppressing the inflammatory component of atherosclerosis. The degree of cardiovascular protection is nearly equal for beer, wine, and distilled spirits. That is, protection is determined primarily by the *amount* of alcohol consumed—not by the particular beverage the alcohol is in. Also, the *pattern* of drinking matters: protection is greater for people who drink moderately 3 or 4 days a week than for people who drink just 1 or 2 days a week. Finally, cardioprotection is greatest for those with an *un*healthy lifestyle: among people who exercise, eat fruits and vegetables, and do not smoke, alcohol has little or no effect on the incidence of coronary events; conversely, among people who lack these behaviors, moderate alcohol intake is associated with a 50% reduction in coronary risk.

Glucose Metabolism

Alcohol has several effects on glucose metabolism that may decrease the risk for type 2 diabetes. For example, alcohol raises levels of adiponectin, a compound that enhances insulin sensitivity. In addition, alcohol suppresses gluconeogenesis, blunts the postprandial rise in blood glucose, and lowers fasting levels of both glucose and insulin.

Bone Health

Alcohol increases bone mineral density, probably by increasing levels of sex hormones.

Respiration

Like all other CNS depressants, alcohol depresses respiration. Respiratory depression from moderate drinking is negligible. However, when consumed in excess, alcohol can cause death by respiratory arrest. The respiratory depressant effects of alcohol are potentiated by other CNS depressants (e.g., benzodiazepines, opioids, barbiturates).

Liver

Alcohol-induced liver damage can progress from fatty liver to hepatitis to cirrhosis, depending on the amount consumed. Acute drinking causes reversible accumulation of fat and protein in the liver. With more chronic drinking, nonviral *hepatitis* develops in about 90% of heavy users. In 8% to 20% of chronic alcoholics, hepatitis evolves into cirrhosis—a condition characterized by proliferation of fibrous tissue and destruction of liver parenchymal cells. Although various factors other than alcohol can cause cirrhosis, alcohol abuse is unquestionably the major cause of *fatal* cirrhosis.

Stomach

Excessive use of alcohol can cause *erosive gastritis.* About one third of alcoholics have this disorder. Two mechanisms are involved. First, alcohol stimulates secretion of gastric acid. Second, when present in high concentrations, alcohol can injure the gastric mucosa directly.

Kidney

Alcohol is a diuretic. It promotes urine formation by inhibiting the release of antidiuretic hormone (ADH) from the pituitary. Because ADH acts on the kidney to promote water reabsorption, thereby decreasing urine formation, a reduction in circulating ADH will increase urine production.

Pancreas

Approximately 35% of cases of acute pancreatitis can be attributed to alcohol, making alcohol the second most common cause of the disorder. Flare-ups typically occur after a bout of heavy drinking. Only 5% of alcoholics develop pancreatitis, and then only after years of overindulgence.

Sexual Function

Alcohol has both psychological and physiologic effects related to human sexual behavior. Although alcohol is not exactly an aphrodisiac, its ability to release inhibitions has been known to motivate sexual activity. Ironically, the physiologic effects of alcohol may frustrate attempts at consummating the activity that alcohol inspired: Objective measurements in males and females show that alcohol significantly decreases our physiologic capacity for sexual responsiveness. In males, long-term use of alcohol may induce *feminization.* Symptoms include testicular atrophy, impotence, sterility, and breast enlargement.

Cancer

Alcohol—even in moderate amounts—is associated with an increased risk for several common cancers. Among these are cancers of the breast, liver, rectum, and aerodigestive tract, which includes the lips, tongue, mouth, nose, throat, vocal cords, and portions of the esophagus and trachea. According to a 2011 study, alcohol causes 10% of all cancers in men and 3% of all cancers in women. The fraction attributable to alcohol is highest for aerodigestive tract cancers (44% in men and 25% in women), somewhat lower for liver cancer (33% and 18%), even lower for colorectal cancer (17% and 4%), and lowest for breast cancer in women (5%). Data suggest that, regarding cancer risk, no amount of alcohol can be considered safe—although risk is lowest with moderate drinking (2 drinks or less a day for men and 1 drink or less a day for women).

Pregnancy

Effects of alcohol on the developing fetus are dose dependent. Risk for fetal injury is greatest with heavy drinking, and much lower with light drinking. Is there some low level of drinking that is *completely* safe? We don't know.

Fetal alcohol exposure can cause structural and functional abnormalities, ranging from mild neurobehavioral deficits to facial malformation and developmental delay. The term *fetal alcohol spectrum disorder* (FASD) is used in reference to the *full range* of outcomes—from mild to severe—that drinking during pregnancy can cause. In contrast, the term *fetal alcohol syndrome* (FAS) is reserved for the most severe cases of FASD, characterized by craniofacial malformations, growth restriction (including microcephaly), and neurodevelopmental abnormalities, manifesting during childhood as cognitive and social dysfunction. In addition to causing FASD and FAS, heavy drinking during pregnancy can result in stillbirth, spontaneous abortion, and giving birth to an alcohol-dependent infant.

Is *light* drinking safe during pregnancy? The data are unclear. Two studies published in 2010 suggest that light drinking may carry little risk. One study, conducted in the United Kingdom, found no clinically relevant behavioral or cognitive problems in 5-year-olds whose mothers consumed 1 to 2 drinks a week during pregnancy. The other study, conducted in Australia, found no link between *low to moderate* alcohol consumption during pregnancy and alcohol-related birth defects (ARBDs), although the same study did show that *heavy* drinking was associated with a fourfold increased risk for an ARBD. These results are consistent with other recent studies, which have failed to show a relationship between occasional or light drinking during pregnancy and abnormalities in newborns or older children. However, because all of these studies were observational, rather than randomized controlled trials, the negative results might be explained by confounding factors, especially educational level, income, or access to prenatal care. Furthermore, because the follow-up time for these studies was relatively short (only 5 years), the long-term effects of light drinking remain unknown.

If there *is* some amount of alcohol that is safe during pregnancy, that amount is very low. Accordingly, despite the studies noted previously, the American College of Obstetricians and Gynecologists (ACOG) and the American Academy of Pediatrics continue to maintain the long-held position that no amount of alcohol can be considered safe during pregnancy. Therefore in the interests of fetal health, all women should be advised to avoid alcohol *entirely* while pregnant or trying to conceive. Having said that, it is important to appreciate that a few drinks early in pregnancy are not likely to harm the fetus. Consequently, if a woman consumed a little alcohol before realizing she was pregnant, she should be reassured that the risk to the fetus—if any—is extremely low.

Lactation

The concentration of alcohol in breast milk parallels the concentration in blood. Recent data indicate that drinking while breastfeeding can adversely affect the infant's feeding and behavior.

Impact on Longevity

The effects of alcohol on life span depend on the amount consumed. *Heavy* drinkers have a higher mortality rate than the population at large. Causes of death include cirrhosis, respiratory disease, cancer, and fatal accidents. The risk for mortality associated with alcohol abuse increases markedly in individuals who consume 6 or more drinks a day.

Interestingly, people who consume *moderate* amounts of alcohol live *longer* than those who abstain—and combining regular exercise with moderate drinking prolongs life even more. Compared with nondrinkers, moderate drinkers have a 30% lower mortality rate, a 50% lower incidence of MI, and a 59% lower incidence of heart failure. According to a study by the American Medical Association, if all Americans were to give up drinking, deaths from heart disease would *increase* by 81,000 a year. Hence, for people who already *are* moderate drinkers, continued moderate drinking would seem beneficial. Conversely, despite the apparent benefits of drinking—and the apparent health disadvantage of abstinence—no one is recommending that abstainers take up drinking. Furthermore, when the risks of alcohol outweigh any possible benefits—such as in pregnancy—then alcohol consumption should be avoided entirely.

Pharmacokinetics

Absorption

Alcohol is absorbed from the stomach and small intestine. About 20% of ingested alcohol is absorbed from the stomach. Gastric absorption is relatively slow and is delayed even further by the presence of food. Absorption from the small intestine is rapid and largely independent of food; about 80% of ingested alcohol is absorbed from this site. Because most alcohol is absorbed from the small intestine, gastric emptying time is a major determinant of individual variation in alcohol absorption.

Distribution

Because alcohol is both nonionic and water soluble, it distributes well to all tissues and body fluids. The drug crosses the blood-brain barrier with ease, allowing alcohol in the brain to equilibrate rapidly with alcohol in the blood. Alcohol also crosses the placenta and hence can affect the developing fetus.

Distribution in body water partly explains why women are more sensitive to alcohol than men. As a rule, women have a lower percentage of body water than men. Hence, when a woman drinks, the alcohol is diluted in a smaller volume of water, causing the concentration of alcohol in tissues and fluids to be relatively high, which causes the effects of alcohol to be more intense.

Metabolism

Alcohol is metabolized in both the liver and stomach. The liver is the primary site. The process begins with conversion of alcohol to acetaldehyde, a reaction catalyzed by *alcohol dehydrogenase.* This reaction is slow and puts a limit on the rate at which alcohol can be inactivated. When formed, acetaldehyde undergoes *rapid* conversion by aldehyde dehydrogenase to acetic acid. Through a series of reactions, acetic acid is then used to synthesize cholesterol, fatty acids, and other compounds.

The kinetics of alcohol metabolism differ from those of most other drugs. With most drugs, as plasma drug levels rise, the amount of drug metabolized per unit time also increases.

This is not true for alcohol: as the alcohol content of blood increases, there is almost no change in the speed of alcohol breakdown. That is, alcohol is metabolized at a relatively *constant rate*—regardless of how much alcohol is present. The average rate at which individuals can metabolize alcohol is about *15 mL (0.5 oz) per hour.*

Because alcohol is metabolized at a slow and constant rate, there is a limit to how much alcohol one can consume without having the drug accumulate. For practical purposes, that limit is about *1 drink per hour.* Consumption of more than 1 drink per hour—be that drink beer, wine, straight whiskey, or a cocktail—will result in alcohol accumulation.

When used on a regular basis, alcohol induces hepatic drug-metabolizing enzymes, thereby increasing the rate of its own metabolism and that of other drugs. As a result, individuals who consume alcohol routinely in high amounts can metabolize the drug faster than people who drink occasionally and moderately.

Males and females differ with respect to activity of alcohol dehydrogenase in the stomach. Specifically, women have lower activity than men. As a result, gastric metabolism of alcohol is significantly less in women. This difference partly explains why women achieve higher blood alcohol levels than men after consuming the same number of drinks.

Tolerance

Chronic consumption of alcohol produces tolerance. As a result, to alter consciousness, people who drink on a regular basis require larger amounts of alcohol than people who drink occasionally. Tolerance to alcohol confers cross-tolerance to general anesthetics, barbiturates, and other general CNS depressants. However, no cross-tolerance develops to opioids. Tolerance subsides within a few weeks after drinking cessation.

Although tolerance develops to many of the effects of alcohol, *very little tolerance develops to respiratory depression.* Consequently, the lethal dose of alcohol for chronic, heavy drinkers is not much bigger than the lethal dose for nondrinkers. Alcoholics may tolerate blood alcohol levels as high as 0.4% (5 times the amount defined by law as intoxicating) with no marked reduction in consciousness. However, if blood levels rise only slightly above this level, death may ensue.

Physical Dependence

Chronic use of alcohol produces physical dependence. If alcohol is withdrawn abruptly, an abstinence syndrome will result. The intensity of the abstinence syndrome is proportional to the degree of physical dependence. Individuals who are physically dependent on alcohol show cross-dependence with other general CNS depressants (e.g., barbiturates, chloral hydrate, benzodiazepines), but not with opioids.

Drug Interactions

Central Nervous System Depressants

The CNS effects of alcohol are additive with those of other CNS depressants (e.g., barbiturates, benzodiazepines, opioids). Consumption of alcohol with other CNS depressants intensifies the psychological and physiologic manifestations of CNS depression and greatly increases the risk for death from respiratory depression.

Nonsteroidal Antiinflammatory Drugs

Like alcohol, aspirin, ibuprofen, and other nonsteroidal antiinflammatory drugs (NSAIDs) can injure the gastrointestinal (GI) mucosa. The combined effects of alcohol and NSAIDs can result in significant gastric bleeding.

Acetaminophen

The combination of acetaminophen [Tylenol, others] with alcohol poses a risk for potentially fatal liver injury. The interaction between alcohol and acetaminophen is discussed further in Chapter 55.

Disulfiram

The combination of alcohol with disulfiram [Antabuse] can cause a variety of adverse effects, some of which are dangerous. These effects, and the use of disulfiram to maintain abstinence, are discussed later.

Antihypertensive Drugs

Because alcohol raises blood pressure, it tends to counteract the effects of antihypertensive medications. However, elevation of blood pressure is significant only when alcohol dosage is high. Conversely, when the dosage is low, alcohol may actually help: among hypertensive men, light to moderate alcohol consumption is associated with reduced risk for both cardiovascular mortality and all-cause mortality.

Acute Overdose

Acute overdose produces vomiting, coma, pronounced hypotension, and respiratory depression. The combination of vomiting and unconsciousness can result in aspiration, which in turn can result in pulmonary obstruction and pneumonia. Alcohol-induced hypotension results from a direct effect on peripheral blood vessels and cannot be corrected with vasoconstrictors (e.g., epinephrine). Hypotension can lead to renal failure (secondary to compromised renal blood flow) and cardiovascular shock, a common cause of alcohol-related death. Although death can also result from respiratory depression, this is not the usual cause.

Because symptoms of acute alcohol poisoning can mimic symptoms of other pathologies (e.g., diabetic coma, skull fracture), a definitive diagnosis may not be possible without measuring alcohol in the blood, urine, or expired air. The smell of "alcohol" on the breath is not a reliable means of diagnosis because the breath odors we associate with alcohol are due to impurities in alcoholic beverages—and not to alcohol itself. Hence, these odors may or may not be present.

Alcohol poisoning is treated like poisoning with all other general CNS depressants. Details of management are discussed in Chapter 27. Alcohol can be removed from the body by gastric lavage and dialysis. Stimulants (e.g., caffeine) should not be given.

Precautions and Contraindications

Alcohol can injure the GI mucosa and should not be consumed by persons with *peptic ulcer disease.* Alcohol is harmful to the liver and should not be used by individuals with *liver disease.* Alcohol should be avoided during *pregnancy* owing to the risk for FASD (including FAS), stillbirth, spontaneous abortion, and neurodevelopmental abnormalities.

Alcohol must be used with caution by patients with *epilepsy.* During alcohol use, the CNS is depressed. When alcohol consumption ceases, the CNS undergoes rebound excitation; seizures can result.

Alcohol causes a dose-related increase in the risk for *breast cancer.* All women—and especially those at high risk—should minimize alcohol consumption. Alcohol also increases the risk for cancer of the liver, rectum, and aerodigestive tract.

Therapeutic Uses

Although our emphasis has been on the nonmedical use of alcohol, it should be remembered that alcohol does have therapeutic applications.

Topical

Topical alcohol can be an effective skin disinfectant.

Local Injection

Injection of alcohol in the vicinity of nerves produces nerve block. This technique can relieve pain from inoperable carcinoma and other causes.

ALCOHOL USE DISORDER

Alcohol use disorder, commonly known as *alcoholism* or *alcohol dependence,* is a chronic, relapsing disorder characterized by impaired control over drinking, preoccupation with alcohol consumption, use of alcohol despite awareness of adverse consequences, and distortions in thinking, especially as evidenced by denial of a drinking problem. The development and manifestations of alcoholism are influenced by genetic, psychosocial, and environmental factors. The disease is progressive and often fatal. In the United States about 8 million adults are alcoholics.

Alcohol use disorder is defined as a problematic pattern of alcohol use leading to clinically significant impairment or distress occurring within a 12-month period. Manifestations of alcohol use disorder can include recurrent alcohol use in situations in which it is physically hazardous; recurrent use resulting in a failure to fulfill major role obligations at work, school, or home; and spending a great deal of time in activities necessary to obtain alcohol, use alcohol, or recover from alcohol.

In the United States, misuse of alcohol is responsible for 6 million nonfatal injuries each year, and 85,000 deaths. Causes of death range from liver disease to automobile wrecks. Fully 45% of all fatal highway crashes are alcohol related. Among teens, alcohol-related crashes are the leading cause of death. Alcohol also causes industrial accidents and is responsible for 40% of industrial fatalities.

Alcohol abuse is a major public health problem, and its consequences are numerous. Alcoholism produces psychological derangements, including anxiety, depression, and suicidal ideation. Malnutrition, secondary to inadequate diet and malabsorption, is common. Poor work performance and disruption of family life reflect the social deterioration suffered by alcoholics. Alcohol abuse during pregnancy can result in FASD (including FAS), stillbirth, and spontaneous abortion. Lastly, chronic alcohol abuse is harmful to the body; consequences include liver disease, cardiomyopathy, and brain damage—not to mention injury and death from accidents.

In 2008, the National Institute on Alcohol Abuse and Alcoholism (NIAAA) updated its document—*Helping Patients Who Drink Too Much: A Clinician*'s *Guide*—that contains clear, concise information on screening, counseling, and treatment of alcohol use disorders. By following this guide, clinicians can help reduce morbidity and mortality among people who drink more than is safe, defined as more than 4 drinks in a day (or 14/week) for men, or more than 3 drinks in a day (or 7/week) for women. Helping patients involves four simple steps:

- Ask about alcohol use.
- Assess for alcohol use disorders, using the Alcohol Use Disorders Identification Test (AUDIT).
- Advise and assist (brief intervention).
- At follow-up: continue support.

This process is founded in part on two lines of evidence. First, we can identify people who misuse alcohol with an easily administered questionnaire, such as AUDIT (Table 31.1). Second, for many people, alcohol consumption can be reduced through brief interventions, such as offering feedback and advice about drinking and about setting goals. Long-term follow-up studies have shown that these simple interventions can decrease hospitalization and lower mortality rates. The guide is available at www.niaaa.nih.gov/guide.

To help individuals who drink too much, the NIAAA created an interactive website, located at rethinkingdrinking.niaaa.nih.gov. Content includes tools to identify and manage problem drinking, plus a calculator for determining the alcohol content of various beverages.

PATIENT-CENTERED CARE ACROSS THE LIFE SPAN

Alcohol

Life Stage	Patient Care Concerns
Infants	See later entry, "Breastfeeding women"
Children/adolescents	Adolescents are more sensitive to alcohol-induced memory impairment than adults, but less sensitive to the motor effects of alcohol. Alcohol exposure during adolescence affects brain functioning during adulthood.
Pregnant women	Use of alcohol while pregnant can cause structural and functional abnormalities in the fetus. These abnormalities are termed *fetal alcohol spectrum disorder* (FASD). It is recommended that pregnant women abstain from alcohol.
Breastfeeding women	The concentration of alcohol in breast milk parallels the concentration in blood. Breastfeeding while consuming alcohol can affect infant behavior.
Older adults	Aging lowers the body's tolerance for alcohol. Many older adults may not metabolize alcohol as efficiently as younger adults. Many older adults take medications that interact with alcohol.

TABLE 31.1 ▪ Screening Instrument: The Alcohol Use Disorders Identification Test (AUDIT)

	0	1	2	3	4	Score
How often do you have a drink containing alcohol?	Never	Monthly or less	2–4 times a month	2–3 times a week	4 or more times a week	
How many drinks containing alcohol do you have on a typical day when you are drinking?	1 or 2	3 or 4	5 or 6	7–9	10 or more	
How often do you have 5 or more drinks on one occasion?	Never	Less than monthly	Monthly	Weekly	Daily or almost daily	
How often during the last year have you found that you were not able to stop drinking once you had started?	Never	Less than monthly	Monthly	Weekly	Daily or almost daily	
How often during the last year have you failed to do what was normally expected of you because of drinking?	Never	Less than monthly	Monthly	Weekly	Daily or almost daily	
How often during the last year have you needed a first drink in the morning to get yourself going after a heavy drinking session?	Never	Less than monthly	Monthly	Weekly	Daily or almost daily	
How often during the last year have you had a feeling of guilt or remorse after drinking?	Never	Less than monthly	Monthly	Weekly	Daily or almost daily	
How often during the last year have you been unable to remember what happened the night before because of your drinking?	Never	Less than monthly	Monthly	Weekly	Daily or almost daily	
Have you or someone else been injured because of your drinking?	No		Yes, but not in the last year		Yes, during the last year	
Has a relative, friend, doctor, or other health care worker been concerned about your drinking or suggested you cut down?	No		Yes, but not in the last year		Yes, during the last year	
Total score						

Instructions to patient: Circle the option that best describes your answer to each question.
Scoring: Record the score (0, 1, 2, 3, or 4) for each response in the blank box at the end of each line, and then add up the total score. The maximum possible is 40. A total score of 8 or more (for men up to age 60 years), or 4 or more (for women, adolescents, and men older than 60 years) is considered a positive screen. For patients with totals near the cut-off points, clinicians may wish to examine individual responses to questions and clarify them during the clinical examination.
Reprinted with permission from the World Health Organization. To reflect standard drink sizes in the United States, the number of drinks in question 3 was changed from 6 to 5.

DRUGS FOR ALCOHOL USE DISORDER

In the United States about 1 million alcoholics seek treatment every year. Although the success rate is discouraging—nearly 50% relapse during the first few months—treatment should nonetheless be tried. The objective is to modify drinking patterns (i.e., to reduce or completely eliminate alcohol consumption). Drugs can help in two ways. First, they can facilitate withdrawal. Second, they can help maintain abstinence after withdrawal has been accomplished.

Drugs Used to Treat the Symptoms of Withdrawal

Management of withdrawal depends on the degree of dependence. When dependence is mild, withdrawal can be accomplished on an outpatient basis without drugs. However, when dependence is great, withdrawal carries a risk for death. Accordingly, hospitalization and drug therapy are indicated. The goals of management are to minimize symptoms of withdrawal, prevent seizures and delirium tremens, and facilitate transition to a program for maintaining abstinence. In theory, any drug that has cross-dependence with alcohol (i.e., any of the general CNS depressants) should be effective. However, in actual practice, benzodiazepines are the drugs of choice. The benefits of benzodiazepines and other drugs used during withdrawal are shown in Table 31.2.

Benzodiazepines

Of the drugs used to facilitate alcohol withdrawal, benzodiazepines are the most effective. Furthermore, they are safe for use in both the inpatient and outpatient settings. In patients with severe alcohol dependence, benzodiazepines can stabilize vital signs, reduce symptom intensity, and decrease the risk for seizures and delirium tremens. Although all benzodiazepines are effective, agents with longer half-lives are generally preferred because they provide the greatest protection against seizures and breakthrough symptoms. The benzodiazepines employed most often are chlordiazepoxide [Librium, others], clorazepate [Tranxene], oxazepam (generic only), and lorazepam [Ativan]. Traditionally, benzodiazepines have been administered around-the-clock on a fixed schedule. However, PRN administration (in response to symptoms) can be just as effective.

Adjuncts to Benzodiazepines

Combining a benzodiazepine with another drug may improve withdrawal outcome. Agents that have been tried include carbamazepine (an antiepileptic drug), clonidine (an alpha$_2$-adrenergic agonist), and atenolol and propranolol

TABLE 31.2 ▪ Drugs Used to Treat the Symptoms of Alcohol Withdrawal

Drug	Benefit During Withdrawal
BENZODIAZEPINES	
Chlordiazepoxide Clorazepate Diazepam Lorazepam Oxazepam	Decrease withdrawal symptoms; stabilize vital signs; prevent seizures and delirium tremens
BETA-ADRENERGIC BLOCKERS	
Atenolol Propranolol	Improve vital signs; decrease craving; decrease autonomic component of withdrawal symptoms
CENTRAL ALPHA$_2$-ADRENERGIC AGONIST	
Clonidine	Decreases autonomic component of withdrawal symptoms
ANTIEPILEPTIC DRUG	
Carbamazepine	Decreases withdrawal symptoms; prevents seizures

(beta-adrenergic blockers). Carbamazepine may reduce withdrawal symptoms and the risk for seizures. Clonidine and the beta blockers reduce the autonomic component of withdrawal symptoms. In addition, the beta blockers may improve vital signs and decrease craving. It should be stressed, however, that these drugs are not very effective as monotherapy. Hence they should be viewed only as adjuncts to benzodiazepines—not as substitutes.

Drugs Used to Maintain Abstinence

After detoxification has been accomplished, the goal is to prevent—or at least minimize—future drinking. The ideal goal is complete abstinence. However, if drinking must resume, keeping it to a minimum is still beneficial because doing so will reduce alcohol-related morbidity.

In trials of drugs used to maintain abstinence, several parameters are used to measure efficacy. These include the following:

- Proportion of patients who maintain complete abstinence
- Days to relapse
- Number of drinking days
- Number of drinks per drinking day

In the United States only three drugs—disulfiram, naltrexone, and acamprosate—are approved for maintaining abstinence. Disulfiram works by causing an unpleasant reaction if alcohol is consumed. Naltrexone blocks the pleasurable effects of alcohol and decreases craving. Acamprosate reduces some of the unpleasant feelings (e.g., tension, dysphoria, anxiety) brought on by alcohol abstinence. Of the three drugs, naltrexone appears most effective. However, even with this agent, benefits are modest.

Owing to the risk for relapse, prolonged treatment is needed. The minimal duration is 3 months. However, continuing for a year or more is not unreasonable. If the first drug fails, clinicians often try a different one.

Disulfiram Aversion Therapy

Therapeutic Effects

Disulfiram [Antabuse] helps alcoholics avoid drinking by causing unpleasant effects if alcohol is ingested. Disulfiram has no applications outside the treatment of alcoholism.

Although disulfiram has been employed for decades, its efficacy is only moderate. In clinical trials, there is emerging evidence that the drug may be only slightly better than placebo at maintaining long-term abstinence; however, long-term studies have not been completed. Disulfiram does decrease the frequency of drinking after relapse has occurred—presumably because of the unpleasant reaction that the patient is now familiar with. Supervised administration of disulfiram may be more effective than when patients self-administer the drug.

Mechanism of Action

Disulfiram disrupts alcohol metabolism by causing *irreversible inhibition of aldehyde dehydrogenase,* the enzyme that converts acetaldehyde to acetic acid. As a result, if alcohol is ingested, *acetaldehyde* will accumulate to toxic levels, producing unpleasant and potentially harmful effects.

Pharmacologic Effects

The constellation of effects caused by alcohol plus disulfiram is referred to as the *acetaldehyde syndrome,* a potentially dangerous event. In its "mild" form, the syndrome manifests as nausea, copious vomiting, flushing, palpitations, headache, sweating, thirst, chest pain, weakness, blurred vision, and hypotension; blood pressure may ultimately decline to shock levels. This reaction, which may last from 30 minutes to several hours, can be brought on by consuming as little as 7 mL of alcohol.

In its most severe manifestation, the acetaldehyde syndrome is life threatening. Possible reactions include marked respiratory depression, cardiovascular collapse, cardiac dysrhythmias, MI, acute congestive heart failure, convulsions, and death. Clearly, the acetaldehyde syndrome is not simply unpleasant; this syndrome can be extremely hazardous and must be avoided.

In the absence of alcohol, disulfiram rarely causes significant effects. Drowsiness and skin eruptions may occur during initial use, but they diminish with time.

Patient Selection

Owing to the severity of the acetaldehyde syndrome, candidates must be carefully chosen. Alcoholics who lack the

Patient Education

DISULFIRAM

Patient education is an extremely important component of therapy. Patients must be thoroughly informed about the potential hazards of treatment, including severe and potentially fatal reactions. Patients should be made aware that the effects of disulfiram will persist about 2 weeks after the last dose, and hence continued abstinence from all sources of alcohol is necessary. This includes cough syrups and alcohol applied to the skin in aftershave and colognes. Individuals using disulfiram should be encouraged to carry identification indicating their status.

determination to stop drinking should not receive disulfiram. In other words, disulfiram must not be administered to alcoholics who are likely to attempt drinking while undergoing treatment.

BLACK BOX WARNING: DISULFIRAM

Disulfiram should never be administered to a patient experiencing alcohol intoxication because this may cause a potentially fatal reaction.

Preparations, Dosage, and Administration

See Table 31.3 for preparations, dosage, and administration.

Naltrexone

Naltrexone [ReVia, Vivitrol] is a pure opioid antagonist that decreases craving for alcohol and blocks alcohol's reinforcing (pleasurable) effects. Alcoholics report that naltrexone decreases their "high." Although the mechanism underlying these effects is uncertain, one possibility is blockade of dopamine release secondary to blockade of opioid receptors. Naltrexone is generally well tolerated. Nausea is the most common adverse effect, followed by headache, anxiety, and sedation. Because naltrexone is an opioid antagonist, the drug will precipitate withdrawal if given to a patient who is opioid dependent. Conversely, if a patient taking naltrexone needs emergency treatment with an opioid analgesic, high doses of the opioid will be required.

Naltrexone was approved for alcoholism on the basis of randomized clinical trials that combined extensive counseling along with the drug. In these trials, naltrexone cut the relapse rate by 50%. Compared with patients taking placebo, those taking naltrexone reported less craving for alcohol, fewer days drinking, fewer drinks per occasion, and reduced severity of alcohol-related problems. In contrast to the original trials, a more recent trial, conducted by the U.S. Department of Veterans Affairs, failed to show any benefit of naltrexone in maintaining abstinence. Why did naltrexone work in the original trials but not in the more recent one? The most likely reason is that the subjects in the two trials were very different: the alcoholic veterans suffered from long-term alcoholism, had little or no social support, and received minimal counseling during the trial, whereas subjects in the earlier studies were younger, had good support systems, and received extensive counseling along with naltrexone. Hence the new study does not prove that naltrexone doesn't work. Rather, it only proves that naltrexone doesn't work for all drinkers, and doesn't work in the absence of adequate counseling. The basic pharmacology of naltrexone is discussed in Chapter 22.

TABLE 31.3 ▪ Preparations, Dosage, and Administration

Drug	Preparations	Usual Adult Dosage
Disulfiram [Antabuse]	250- and 500-mg tablets	Initial dosage 500 mg PO daily for 1–2 wk Maintenance dose 125–500 mg PO daily
Naltrexone [ReVia]	50-mg tablets	50 mg PO daily
Naltrexone [Vivitrol]	Solution for IM injection	380 mg IM every 4 wk
Acamprosate [Campral]	333-mg delayed-release tablets	666 mg PO three times daily, taken with meals

IM, intramuscular; PO, oral administration.

Acamprosate

Therapeutic Use

Acamprosate [Campral] is approved for maintaining abstinence in patients with alcohol dependence after detoxification. Benefits derive from reducing unpleasant feelings (e.g., tension, dysphoria, anxiety) brought on by abstinence. This effect contrasts with the effects of disulfiram (which makes drinking unpleasant) and naltrexone (which blocks the pleasant feelings that alcohol can cause). Acamprosate should be used only as part of a comprehensive management program that includes psychosocial support.

In clinical trials, acamprosate was moderately effective. Compared with patients taking placebo, those taking acamprosate abstained from their first drink longer, had greater rates of complete abstinence, and were abstinent for more total days. Benefits may be related to the degree of alcohol dependence: the greater the dependence, the more likely that acamprosate will help. Among patients who lack psychosocial support, little or no benefit is seen.

Mechanism of Action

Just how acamprosate works is unknown. One theory suggests that acamprosate enhances inhibitory neurotransmission (mediated by GABA) and suppresses excitatory neurotransmission (mediated by glutamate), and thereby restores a balance between these transmitter systems. When given to alcohol-dependent animals, the drug reduces voluntary alcohol intake. Acamprosate is devoid of direct anxiolytic, anticonvulsant, and antidepressant activity, and does not cause alcohol aversion.

Pharmacokinetics

Acamprosate is administered orally, and bioavailability is low (11%). Food reduces absorption even further. The drug has a long half-life (20–33 hours), and hence about 5 days are required for plasma levels to reach a plateau. Acamprosate does not undergo metabolism and is excreted unchanged in the urine.

Adverse Effects

Acamprosate is generally well tolerated. With most adverse effects, the incidence is no greater than with placebo. The principal exception is diarrhea, which occurs in 17% of acamprosate users compared with 10% of those taking placebo. Reports of suicide-related events (suicidal ideation, suicide attempts, completed suicide) are rare but more common than with placebo. Acamprosate can cause fetal malformations in animals (at doses close to those used by humans). Accordingly, it would seem prudent to avoid this drug during pregnancy, especially because alternatives are available. Acamprosate has no potential for dependence or abuse and appears devoid of significant drug interactions.

CHAPTER

32

Drug Abuse III: Nicotine and Smoking

Laura D. Rosenthal, DNP, ACNP, FAANP

Cigarette smoking remains the greatest single cause of preventable illness and premature death. In the United States smoking kills more than 443,000 adults each year—about 1 of every 5 deaths. Around the world, tobacco kills more than 5 million people each year. On average, male smokers die 13.2 years prematurely, and female smokers die 14.5 years prematurely. According to the Centers for Disease Control and Prevention, most deaths result from lung cancer (125,522), heart disease (101,009), and chronic airway obstruction (79,898). Not only do cigarettes kill people who smoke, but also every year, through secondhand smoke, cigarettes kill about 50,000 nonsmoking Americans and about 600,000 nonsmokers worldwide. The direct medical costs of smoking exceed $95 billion a year. Indirect costs, including lost time from work and disability, add up to an additional $97 billion. In the United States the prevalence of smoking among adults fell steadily from 1965 (42%) through the 1980s and 1990s, but decreased only slightly between 2004 (20.9%) and 2013 (19%).

Although tobacco smoke contains many dangerous compounds, nicotine is of greatest concern. Other hazardous components in tobacco smoke include carbon monoxide, hydrogen cyanide, ammonia, nitrosamines, and tar. Tar is composed of various polycyclic hydrocarbons, some of which are proven carcinogens.

Until recently, cigarettes had avoided virtually all federal regulation. However, strong regulations are now in place. Under the *Family Smoking Prevention and Tobacco Control Act,* passed in June 2009, the U.S. Food and Drug Administration (FDA) now has the authority to undertake the following:

- Strengthen advertising restrictions, including the prohibition on marketing to youth
- Require revised and more prominent warning labels
- Require disclosure of all ingredients in tobacco products and restrict harmful additives
- Monitor nicotine yields and mandate gradual nicotine reduction to nonaddictive levels

BASIC PHARMACOLOGY OF NICOTINE

Mechanism of Action

The effects of nicotine result from actions at nicotinic receptors. Whether these receptors are activated or inhibited depends on nicotine dosage. *Low* doses *activate* nicotinic receptors; *high* doses *block* them. The amount of nicotine received from cigarettes is relatively low. Accordingly, cigarette smoking causes receptor *activation.*

Nicotine can activate nicotinic receptors at several locations. Most effects result from activating nicotinic receptors in autonomic ganglia and the adrenal medulla. In addition, nicotine can activate nicotinic receptors in the carotid body, aortic arch, and central nervous system (CNS). As discussed later, actions in the CNS mimic those of cocaine and other highly addictive substances. When present at the levels produced by smoking, nicotine has no significant effect on nicotinic receptors of the neuromuscular junction.

Pharmacokinetics

Absorption of nicotine depends on whether the delivery system is a cigarette, a cigar, or smokeless tobacco. Nicotine in cigarette smoke is absorbed primarily from the lungs. When cigarette smoke is inhaled, between 90% and 98% of nicotine in the lungs enters the blood. Unlike nicotine in cigarette smoke, nicotine in cigar smoke is absorbed primarily from the mouth, as is nicotine in smokeless tobacco.

Nicotine can cross membranes easily and is widely distributed throughout the body. When inhaled in cigarette smoke, nicotine reaches the brain in just 10 seconds.

Nicotine is rapidly metabolized to inactive products. Nicotine and its metabolites are excreted by the kidney. The drug's half-life is 1 to 2 hours.

Pharmacologic Effects

The pharmacologic effects discussed in this section are associated with *low* doses of nicotine. These are the effects caused by smoking cigarettes. Responses to *high* doses are discussed later under "Acute Poisoning."

Cardiovascular Effects

The cardiovascular effects of nicotine result primarily from activating nicotinic receptors in *sympathetic ganglia* and the *adrenal medulla.* Activation of these receptors promotes release of norepinephrine from sympathetic nerves and release of epinephrine (and some norepinephrine) from the adrenals. Norepinephrine and epinephrine act on the cardiovascular system to constrict blood vessels, accelerate the heart, and increase the force of ventricular contraction. The net result is elevation of blood pressure and increased cardiac work. These effects underlie cardiovascular deaths.

Gastrointestinal Effects

Nicotine influences gastrointestinal (GI) function primarily by activating nicotinic receptors in *parasympathetic* ganglia, thereby increasing secretion of gastric acid and augmenting tone and motility of GI smooth muscle. In addition, nicotine can promote vomiting. Nicotine-induced vomiting results from a complex process that involves nicotinic receptors in the aortic arch, carotid sinus, and CNS.

Central Nervous System Effects

Nicotine is a CNS stimulant. The drug stimulates respiration and produces an arousal pattern on an electroencephalograph. Moderate doses can cause tremors, and high doses can cause convulsions.

Nicotine has multiple psychological effects. The drug increases alertness, facilitates memory, improves cognition, reduces aggression, and suppresses appetite. In addition, by promoting release of dopamine, nicotine activates the brain's "pleasure system" located in the mesolimbic area. The effects of nicotine on the pleasure system are identical to those of other highly addictive drugs, including cocaine, amphetamines, and opioids.

Effects During Pregnancy and Lactation

Nicotine exposure during gestation can harm the fetus, and nicotine in breast milk can harm the nursing infant. Nonetheless, because pharmaceutical nicotine is safer than tobacco smoke, it is reasonable to consider using nicotine therapy during pregnancy to help a patient quit smoking.

Tolerance and Dependence

Tolerance

Tolerance develops to some effects of nicotine but not to others. Tolerance does develop to nausea and dizziness, which are common in the novice smoker. In contrast, *very little tolerance develops to the cardiovascular effects:* long-term smokers continue to experience increased blood pressure and increased cardiac work whenever they smoke.

Dependence

Chronic cigarette smoking results in dependence. By definition, this means that individuals who discontinue smoking will experience an abstinence syndrome. Prominent symptoms are craving, nervousness, restlessness, irritability, impatience, increased hostility, insomnia, impaired concentration, increased appetite, and weight gain. Symptoms begin about 24 hours after smoking has ceased and can last for weeks to months. Women report more discomfort than men. Experience has shown that abrupt discontinuation may be preferable to gradual reduction.

Acute Poisoning

Nicotine is highly toxic. Doses as low as 40 mg can be fatal. Toxicity is underscored by the use of nicotine as an insecticide. Common causes of nicotine poisoning include ingestion of tobacco by children and exposure to nicotine-containing insecticides.

Symptoms

The most prominent symptoms involve the cardiovascular, GI, and central nervous systems. Specific symptoms include nausea, salivation, vomiting, diarrhea, cold sweats, disturbed hearing and vision, confusion, and faintness; pulses may be rapid, weak, and irregular. Death results from respiratory paralysis, which is caused by direct effects of nicotine on the muscles of respiration, as well as by effects in the CNS.

Treatment

Management centers on reducing nicotine absorption and supporting respiration; there is no specific antidote to nicotine poisoning. Absorption of ingested nicotine can be reduced by giving activated charcoal. If respiration is depressed, ventilatory assistance is indicated. Because nicotine undergoes rapid metabolic inactivation, recovery from the acute phase of poisoning can occur within hours.

Chronic Toxicity From Smoking

It is now clear that chronic smoking can injure nearly every organ of the body. Smoking causes cardiovascular disease including abdominal aortic aneurysm, chronic lung disease, and cancers of the larynx, cervix, kidney, pancreas, stomach, lung, esophagus, oral cavity, and bladder. Leukemia, cataracts, pneumonia, periodontal disease, and type 2 diabetes are also related to smoking. Smoking during pregnancy increases the risk for low birth weight, preterm labor, stillbirth, miscarriage, spontaneous abortion, perinatal mortality, and sudden infant death. The leading causes of smoking-related death are lung cancer, ischemic heart disease, and chronic airway obstruction.

Prototype Drugs

DRUGS TO AID SMOKING CESSATION

Nicotine-Based Products

Nicotine patch [NicoDerm]
Nicotine gum [Nicorette]
Nicotine lozenge [Nicorette Lozenge]
Nicotine nasal spray [Nicotrol NS]
Nicotine inhaler [Nicotrol Inhaler]

Nicotine-Free Products

Varenicline
Bupropion

PHARMACOLOGIC AIDS TO SMOKING CESSATION

Cigarettes are highly addictive, which makes giving them up very hard. Nonetheless, abstinence *can* be achieved. Every year, about 41% of Americans who smoke make one or more attempts to quit. Of those who try to quit without formal help, only 4% to 7% achieve long-term success. In contrast, when a combination of counseling and drugs is employed, the 6-month abstinence rate approaches 25%. However, even with the aid of counseling and drugs, the first attempt usually fails. In fact, most people try quitting 5 to 7 times before they ultimately succeed. As time without a cigarette increases, the chances of relapse get progressively smaller: Of those who quit for a year, only 15% smoke again; and of those who quit for 5 years, only 3% smoke again.

Long-term smokers should be assured that quitting offers important health benefits. Regardless of how long you have smoked, quitting can reduce the risk for developing a tobacco-related disease, slow the progression of an established tobacco-related disease, and increase life expectancy. These benefits apply not only to people who quit while they are young and healthy, but also to people who quit after age 65 years and to those with established tobacco-related disease. Data from the Nurses' Health Study indicate that former smokers eventually achieve the same disease-risk status as never smokers, even with respect to lung cancer. The risk for chronic obstructive pulmonary disease or death from a heart attack declines to that of never smokers in 20 years, and the risk for lung cancer reaches that of never smokers in 30 years.

Seven drug products have been shown to aid smoking cessation (Table 32.1). Of these seven products, five contain nicotine and two don't. The nicotine-based products—nicotine gum, nicotine lozenge, nicotine patch, nicotine inhaler, and nicotine nasal spray—are employed as nicotine replacement therapy (NRT). The nicotine-free products—sustained-release bupropion (bupropion SR) [Zyban, Buproban] and varenicline [Chantix, Champix ♣]—are taken to decrease nicotine craving and to suppress symptoms of withdrawal. The most effective drug therapies for smoking cessation are varenicline alone and the nicotine patch combined with a short-acting nicotine product (e.g., nasal spray or gum). At this time, we cannot predict who will respond best to a particular product. Accordingly, selection should be based on patient preference, success with a particular product in the past, and side effects.

Interventions for smoking cessation can be found in *Treating Tobacco Use and Dependence: 2008 Update,* a clinical practice guideline issued by the U.S. Public Health Service. As stated in the guideline, tobacco dependence is a chronic condition that warrants repeated intervention until long-term abstinence is achieved. This is the same philosophy that guides treatment of dependence on other highly addictive substances, including cocaine and heroin. Tobacco dependence can be treated with two methods: drugs and counseling. Both methods are effective, but a combination of both is more effective than either one alone. Accordingly, the guidelines recommend that all patients who want to quit be offered (1) at least one smoking cessation drug (bupropion, varenicline, or a nicotine-based product) along with (2) counseling, be it one-on-one, in a group, or over the phone (dial 1-800-QUITNOW in the United States or 1-877-513-5333 in Canada). The overall intervention strategy is summarized in the "5 A's" model for treating tobacco use and dependence:

Ask (screen all patients for tobacco use).
Advise tobacco users to quit.
Assess willingness to make a quit attempt.
Assist with quitting (offer medication and provide or refer to counseling).
Arrange follow-up contacts, beginning within the first week after the quit date.

For additional information on smoking cessation, visit the Internet sites for Canada and the United States listed in Table 32.2.

Nicotine Replacement Therapy

NRT allows smokers to substitute a pharmaceutical source of nicotine for the nicotine in cigarettes—and then gradually withdraw the replacement nicotine. This is analogous to using methadone to wean addicts from heroin.

Five U.S. Food and Drug Administration (FDA)–approved formulations are available: chewing gum, lozenges, transdermal patches, a nasal spray, and an inhaler (see Table 32.1). With the gum, lozenges, patches, and inhaler, blood levels of nicotine rise slowly and remain relatively steady. Because nicotine levels rise slowly, these delivery systems produce less pleasure than cigarettes, but nonetheless do relieve symptoms of withdrawal. With the nasal spray, blood levels of nicotine rise rapidly, much as they do with smoking. Hence the nasal spray provides some of the subjective pleasure that smoking does.

Long-term quit rates are significantly greater with NRT than with placebo—although absolute success rates remain low. For example, the 1-year success with nicotine patches is about 25%, compared with 9% for placebo. Success rates are highest when replacement therapy is combined with counseling.

Nicotine products are classified in FDA Pregnancy Risk Category C (chewing gum, lozenge) or Category D (patch, inhaler, nasal spray). Accordingly, they should generally be avoided during pregnancy. However, because smoking is probably more harmful than NRT, use of NRT during pregnancy is worth consideration.

Nicotine Chewing Gum (Nicotine Polacrilex)

Nicotine chewing gum [Nicorette, others] is composed of a gum base plus nicotine polacrilex, an ion exchange resin to which nicotine is bound. The gum must be chewed to release the nicotine. After release, nicotine is absorbed across the oral mucosa into the systemic circulation. Like other forms of NRT, nicotine gum doubles the cessation success rate.

The most common adverse effects are mouth and throat soreness, jaw muscle ache, eructation (belching), and hiccups. Using optimal chewing technique minimizes these problems.

Patients should be advised to chew the gum slowly and intermittently for about 30 minutes. Rapid chewing can release too much nicotine at one time, resulting in effects similar to those of excessive smoking (e.g., nausea, throat irritation, hiccups). Because foods and beverages can reduce nicotine absorption, patients should not eat or drink while chewing or for 15 minutes before chewing (see Table 32.1).

After 3 months without cigarettes, patients should discontinue nicotine use. Withdrawal should be done gradually. Use of nicotine gum beyond 6 months is not recommended.

Nicotine Lozenges (Nicotine Polacrilex)

The pharmacology of nicotine lozenges [Nicorette Lozenge, Thrive ♣] is very similar to that of nicotine gum. Both products contain nicotine bound to polacrilex. Sucking on the lozenge releases nicotine, which is then absorbed across the oral mucosa into the systemic circulation. Like nicotine gum and other forms of NRT, nicotine lozenges double the cessation success rate.

The most common adverse effects are mouth irritation, dyspepsia, nausea, and hiccups—all of which can be made

TABLE 32.1 ▪ Pharmacologic Aids for Smoking Cessation

Product	Common Side Effects	Advantages	Disadvantages	Preparation	Usual Adult Use	Length of Use
NICOTINE-BASED PRODUCTS						
Nicotine patch [NicoDerm CQ]	Transient itching, burning, and redness under the patch; insomnia	Nonprescription; provides a steady level of nicotine; easy to use; unobtrusive	User cannot adjust dose if craving occurs; nicotine released more slowly than in other products	See table 32.3	See table 32.3	See table 32.3
Nicotine gum [Nicorette, others]	Mouth and throat irritation, aching jaw muscles, dyspepsia	Nonprescription; user controls dose	Unpleasant taste; requires proper chewing technique; cannot eat or drink while chewing the gum; can damage dental work and is difficult for denture wearers to use	2 mg/piece and 4 mg/piece	Low to moderate nicotine dependence: 2 mg >25 cigarettes daily: 4 mg-piece 9–12 pieces a day is reasonable	Use beyond 6 mo is not recommended
Nicotine lozenge [Nicorette Lozenge, Thrive ♣]	Hiccups, dyspepsia, mouth irritation, nausea	Nonprescription; user controls dose; easier to use than nicotine gum	Cannot eat or drink while the lozenge is in the mouth	2 mg/lozenge and 4 mg/lozenge	First cigarette 30 min or more after waking: 2 mg First cigarette within 30 min of waking: 4 mg No more than 5 lozenges every 6 hr or 20 daily	Dosing should decrease over a period of 12 wk Dosing should stop after 12 wk
Nicotine nasal spray [Nicotrol NS]	During 1st week: mouth and throat irritation, rhinitis, sneezing, coughing, teary eyes	User controls dose; fastest nicotine delivery and highest nicotine levels of all nicotine-based products	Prescription required; most irritating nicotine-based product; device visible when used	10 mg within a sealed cartridge	Frequent puffs over 20 min 6–16 cartridges daily	After 3 mo, taper use to complete cessation over additional 2–3 mo
Nicotine inhaler [Nicotrol Inhaler, Nicorette Inhaler ♣]	Mouth and throat irritation, cough	User controls dose; mimics hand-to-mouth motion of smoking	Prescription required; slow onset and low nicotine levels; frequent puffing needed; device visible when used	0.5 mg per activation	One spray per nostril 1–2 times per hour No more than 40 doses per day	Decrease use after 4–6 wk
NICOTINE-FREE PRODUCTS						
Varenicline [Chantix, Champix ♣]	Nausea, sleep disturbances, headaches, abnormal dreams	Easy to use (pill); no nicotine; most effective pharmacologic aid to smoking cessation	Prescription required; may cause neuropsychiatric disturbances, including suicidal thoughts and actions	150 mg tablets	150 mg PO daily × 3 days, 150 mg PO twice daily × 7–12 wk Begin 1–2 wk before smoking cessation	Decrease use after 7-12 weeks
Bupropion [Zyban, Buproban]	Insomnia, dry mouth, agitation	Easy to use (pill); no nicotine; promotes weight loss, which may limit cessation-related weight gain; first-choice drug for smokers with depression	Prescription required; carries a small risk for seizures	0.5- and 1-mg tablets	0.5 mg PO daily × 3 days, 0.5 mg PO twice daily × 3 days, then 1 mg PO twice daily × 12 wk If abstinence is achieved, an additional 12 wk of treatment is warranted Begin 8–35 days before smoking cessation	Decrease use after 12 weeks

TABLE 32.2 ▪ Internet-Based Resources for Smoking Cessation

UNITED STATES

- U.S. Department of Health and Human Services: http://www.surgeongeneral.gov/library/reports/50-years-of-progress/consumer-guide.pdf
- Centers for Disease Control and Prevention: http://www.cdc.gov/tobacco/quit_smoking/
- American Lung Association: http://www.lungusa.org/stop-smoking/

CANADA

- Health Canada: http://www.hc-sc.gc.ca/hc-ps/tobac-tabac/index-eng.php
- The Lung Association: http://www.lung.ca/home-accueil_e.php

TABLE 32.3 ▪ Nicotine Transdermal Systems (Patches)

Trade Name	Surface Area (cm^2)	Hours/Day in Place	Dose Absorbed	Duration of Use: Per Patch Size	Duration of Use: Total
NicoDerm CQ Step 1	30	24	21 mg over 24 hr	First 4–6 wk	8–10 wk
NicoDerm CQ Step 2	20	24	14 mg over 24 hr	Next 2 wk	
NicoDerm CQ Step 3	10	24	7 mg over 24 hr	Next 2 wk	

worse by taking two lozenges at once or by taking several lozenges in immediate succession.

Administration consists of placing the lozenge in the mouth and allowing it to dissolve, which takes 20 to 30 minutes. Users should not eat or drink for 15 minutes before dosing and while the lozenge is in the mouth. Also, they should not chew or swallow the lozenge (Table 32.1).

Nicotine Transdermal Systems (Patches)

Nicotine transdermal systems are nicotine-containing adhesive patches that, after application to the skin, slowly release their nicotine content. The nicotine is absorbed into the skin and then into the blood, producing steady blood levels. Use of the patch about doubles the cessation success rate.

NicoDerm CQ can be purchased without a prescription. As indicated in Table 32.3, the patches come in different sizes. The larger patches release more nicotine.

Nicotine patches are applied once a day to clean, dry, nonhairy skin of the upper body or upper arm. The site should be changed daily and not reused for at least 1 week. NicoDerm CQ patches are left in place for 24 hours and then immediately replaced with a fresh one. Most patients begin with a large patch and then use progressively smaller patches over several weeks. Certain patients (those with cardiovascular disease, those who weigh less than 100 pounds, and those who smoke less than one-half pack of cigarettes a day) should begin with a smaller patch.

Adverse effects are generally mild. Short-lived erythema, itching, and burning occur under the patch in 35% to 50% of users. In 14% to 17% of users, persistent erythema occurs, lasting up to 24 hours after patch removal. Patients who experience severe, persistent local reactions (e.g., severe erythema, itching, edema) should discontinue the patch and contact a physician or nurse practitioner.

Nicotine Inhaler

The nicotine inhaler [Nicotrol Inhaler, Nicorette Inhaler ♣] differs from other NRT products in that it looks much like a cigarette. Puffing on it delivers the nicotine. Because of this delivery method, using the inhaler can substitute for the hand-to-mouth behavior of smoking. In addition to nicotine, the inhaler contains menthol, whose purpose is to create a sensation in the back of the throat reminiscent of that caused by smoke. Like other forms of NRT, the inhaler doubles cessation success rates.

The nicotine inhaler consists of a mouthpiece and a sealed, tubular cartridge. Inside the cartridge is a porous plug containing 10 mg of nicotine. Inserting the cartridge into the mouthpiece breaks the seal. Puffing on the mouthpiece draws air over the plug, and thereby draws nicotine vapor into the mouth. Most of the nicotine is absorbed through the *oral mucosa*—not in the lungs. As a result, blood levels rise slowly and peak 10 to 15 minutes after puffing stops. Blood levels are less than half those achieved with cigarettes. Each cartridge can deliver 300 to 400 puffs (see Table 32.1).

Adverse effects are mild. The most frequent are dyspepsia, coughing, throat irritation, oral burning, and rhinitis. The inhaler should not be used by patients with asthma. Because the cartridges contain dangerous amounts of nicotine, they should be kept away from children and pets.

Nicotine Nasal Spray

Nicotine nasal spray [Nicotrol NS] differs from other NRT formulations in that blood levels of nicotine rise *rapidly* after each administration, thereby closely simulating smoking. Because nicotine levels rise rapidly, the spray provides some of the subjective pleasure associated with cigarettes. As with other forms of NRT, the spray doubles smoking cessation rates (see Table 32.1).

Quitting success with the spray has been good news and bad news. The good news, as reported in one study, is that 27% of users avoided smoking for 1 year—about twice the abstinence rate achieved with placebo. The bad news is that many patients continued to use the spray, being unwilling or unable to give it up. Nonetheless, because the spray delivers nicotine without the additional hazards in cigarettes, using the spray is clearly preferable to smoking.

Adverse effects are mild and temporary. At first, most users experience rhinitis, sneezing, coughing, watering eyes, and nasal and throat irritation. Fortunately, these effects abate in a few days. Nicotine nasal spray should be avoided by patients with sinus problems, allergies, or asthma.

Bupropion SR

Bupropion SR [Zyban, Buproban], an atypical antidepressant, was the first nonnicotine drug approved as an aid to smoking cessation. The drug is structurally similar to amphetamine and, like amphetamine, causes CNS stimulation and suppresses appetite. In people trying to quit cigarettes, bupropion reduces the urge to smoke and reduces some symptoms of nicotine withdrawal (e.g., irritability, anxiety). The drug is effective in the presence and absence of depression. Although the mechanism of action is uncertain, benefits may derive from blocking uptake of norepinephrine and dopamine. For use in depression, bupropion is sold under the trade name Wellbutrin.

Like the NRT products, bupropion SR doubles the cessation success rate. In one trial, patients were given bupropion SR (100, 150, or 300 mg/day) or placebo. At 7 weeks, abstinence rates were 19% with placebo, and 29%, 39%, and 44% with increasing dosages of bupropion SR. At 12 weeks, abstinence rates were lower: 12% with placebo and 20%, 23%, and 23% with increasing dosages of bupropion SR. Combining a nicotine patch with bupropion SR is somewhat more effective than either treatment alone.

Adverse effects are generally mild. The most common are dry mouth and insomnia. High doses (more than 450 mg/day) are associated with a 0.4% risk for seizures. However, at the doses employed for smoking cessation (300 mg/day), seizures have not been reported. Nonetheless, bupropion SR should be avoided in patients with seizure risk factors, such as head trauma, history of seizures, anorexia nervosa, cocaine use, and alcohol withdrawal. Because it suppresses appetite, bupropion SR can cause weight loss. Bupropion SR should not be combined with a monoamine oxidase inhibitor. Nor should it be given to patients taking Wellbutrin, which is just another name for bupropion itself (Table 32.1). The basic pharmacology of bupropion is discussed in Chapter 32.

Varenicline

Varenicline [Chantix, Champix ♣], a partial agonist at nicotinic receptors, is our most effective aid to smoking cessation. In clinical trials, more patients achieved abstinence with varenicline than with bupropion SR or the nicotine patch. Estimated abstinence rates after 6 months were 33.2% with varenicline, 24.2% with bupropion SR, and 23.4% with a nicotine patch. The most common side effect is nausea. The most troubling side effects are psychological changes. Unlike bupropion SR and NRT, varenicline does *not* cause weight loss.

Mechanism of Action

Varenicline acts as a *partial agonist* at a subset of nicotinic receptors—known as $alpha_4beta_2$ nicotinic receptors—whose activation promotes release of dopamine, the compound that mediates the pleasurable effects of nicotine. Compared with nicotine, varenicline binds $alpha_4beta_2$ receptors with greater affinity. Hence, when varenicline is present, access of nicotine to these receptors is blocked. Because varenicline is a partial agonist, receptor binding results in mild activation, which promotes some dopamine release, and thereby helps reduce both nicotine craving and the intensity of withdrawal symptoms. At the same time, the presence of varenicline prevents intense receptor activation by nicotine itself and thereby blocks the reward that nicotine can provide (see Table 32.1).

Pharmacokinetics

Varenicline is readily absorbed from the GI tract, both in the presence and absence of food. Plasma levels peak about 4 hours after dosing. Binding to plasma proteins is low (20%). Metabolism is minimal, and hence most of each dose (92%) is excreted unchanged in the urine. The plasma half-life is 17 to 24 hours. Moderate to severe renal impairment delays excretion and increases varenicline blood levels.

Adverse Effects

In clinical trials, dose-dependent *nausea* was the most common adverse effect, occurring in 30% to 40% of users. Nausea is mild to moderate initially and becomes less severe over time. Other common reactions include sleep disturbances, headaches, abnormal dreams, constipation, dry mouth, flatulence, vomiting, and altered sense of taste. Mild physical dependence develops, but there have been no reports of abuse or addictive behavior. Rarely, varenicline has been associated with seizures, diabetes, dizziness, disturbed vision, and moderate and severe skin reactions, although a causal relationship has not been established.

In 2011, the FDA warned that varenicline can increase the risk for cardiovascular events (e.g., angina pectoris, peripheral edema, hypertension, nonfatal myocardial infarction) in patients with stable cardiovascular disease. After that, a Canadian study revealed a similar risk in patients *without* cardiovascular disease. Fortunately, cardiovascular risk appears to be small—much smaller than the risk posed by smoking. Nonetheless, patients should be warned about cardiovascular risk and instructed to notify the prescriber if they experience new or worsening cardiovascular symptoms and should seek immediate medical attention if symptoms of myocardial infarction appear.

Owing to concerns about unpredictable physical and psychiatric adverse effects, U.S. authorities have banned use of varenicline by truck drivers, bus drivers, airplane pilots, and air traffic controllers.

Preparations, Dosage, and Administration

BLACK BOX WARNING: BUPROPION AND VARENICLINE

Postmarketing reports indicate that both bupropion and varenicline can cause serious *neuropsychiatric effects,* including mood changes, erratic behavior, and suicidality. All patients should be advised to contact their prescriber if they experience a significant change in behavior or mental status. Bupropion and varenicline should be used with caution in patients with a history of psychiatric disease.

Products That Are Not Recommended

According to *Treating Tobacco Use and Dependence: 2008 Update,* there is insufficient proof to recommend the following drugs as aids to smoking cessation: naltrexone, silver acetate, beta blockers, benzodiazepines, and antidepressants other than bupropion SR, including the selective serotonin reuptake inhibitors.

Although not mentioned in the *2008 Update,* electronic cigarettes, or e-cigarettes, should be avoided. E-cigarettes are battery-powered, cigarette-shaped devices that release a puff of vaporized nicotine, sometimes together with flavoring and other chemicals. According to analyses conducted by the FDA, the amount of nicotine per puff can vary widely, and the vapor may contain trace amounts of diethylene glycol and other contaminants. E-cigarettes are promoted on the Internet as aids to quit smoking, but are not FDA approved for this use (or any other use, for that matter). At this writing, the FDA is attempting to regulate e-cigarettes as drug-delivery devices (which seems reasonable) but is meeting resistance from the courts. The bottom line: because the dose of nicotine with e-cigarettes is unpredictable, and because data on safety and efficacy are lacking, the use of e-cigarettes should be discouraged—especially because products of known safety and efficacy are available.

CHAPTER 33

Drug Abuse IV: Major Drugs of Abuse Other Than Alcohol and Nicotine

Laura D. Rosenthal, DNP, ACNP, FAANP

In this chapter, we discuss all of the major drugs of abuse except alcohol (Chapter 31) and nicotine (Chapter 32). As indicated in Table 33.1, abused drugs fall into six major categories: (1) opioids, (2) psychostimulants, (3) depressants, (4) psychedelics, (5) anabolic steroids, and (6) miscellaneous drugs of abuse. The basic pharmacology of many of these drugs is presented in previous chapters, so their discussion here is brief. Agents that have not been addressed previously (e.g., marijuana, *d*-lysergic acid diethylamide [LSD]) are discussed in depth.

TABLE 33.1 ▪ Pharmacologic Categorization of Abused Drugs

Category	Examples
Opioids	Heroin
	Hydromorphone
	Meperidine
	Morphine
	Oxycodone
Psychostimulants	Cocaine
	Dextroamphetamine
	Methamphetamine
	Methylphenidate
Depressants	
Barbiturates	Amobarbital
	Pentobarbital
	Phenobarbital
	Secobarbital
Benzodiazepines	Diazepam
	Flunitrazepam
	Lorazepam
Miscellaneous	Alcohol
	Gamma-hydroxybutyrate
	Meprobamate
	Methaqualone
Psychedelics	Dimethyltryptamine
	LSD
	Mescaline
	Psilocybin
Anabolic steroids	Nandrolone
	Oxandrolone
	Testosterone
Miscellaneous	Dextromethorphan
	Marijuana
	Nicotine
	Nitrous oxide

HEROIN, OXYCODONE, AND OTHER OPIOIDS

The opioids (e.g., heroin, oxycodone, meperidine) are major drugs of abuse. As a result, most opioids are classified as Schedule II substances. The basic pharmacology of the opioids is discussed in Chapter 22.

Patterns of Use

For most abusers, initial exposure to opioids occurs either recreationally (i.e., illicitly) or in the context of pain management in a medical setting. The overwhelming majority of individuals who go on to abuse opioids begin their drug use illicitly. Only an exceedingly small percentage of those exposed to opioids therapeutically develop a pattern of compulsive drug use.

Opioid abuse by health care providers deserves special consideration. It is well established that physicians, nurses, and pharmacists, as a group, abuse opioids to a greater extent than all other groups with similar educational backgrounds. The vulnerability of health care professionals to opioid abuse is primarily due to drug access.

Subjective and Behavioral Effects

Moments after intravenous (IV) injection, heroin produces sensations of pleasure, relaxation, warmth, and thirst. This initial reaction, known as a "rush" or "kick," persists for about 45 seconds. After this, the user experiences a prolonged sense of euphoria. These extended effects, rather than the initial rush, are the primary reason for opioid abuse.

Interestingly, when individuals first use opioids, nausea and vomiting are prominent, and an overall sense of *dysphoria* may be felt. In many cases, were it not for peer pressure, individuals would not continue opioid use long enough to allow these unpleasant reactions to be replaced by a more agreeable experience.

Preferred Drugs and Routes of Administration

In the past, heroin was the most commonly abused opioid drug, but no longer. Prescription opioid analgesics are now abused much more commonly than heroin: in 2014, more than

4.9 million Americans reported past-month abuse of these drugs.

Heroin

Among street users, heroin is the traditional opioid of choice. Because of its high lipid solubility, heroin crosses the blood-brain barrier with ease, causing effects that are both immediate and intense. This combination of speed and intensity sets heroin apart from other opioids. According to the 2014 National Survey on Drug Use and Health, 435,000 Americans 12 years and older reported past-month abuse of heroin. This number has risen secondary to changes made in prescription drugs. Heroin is both cheaper and sometimes easier to obtain than a prescription opiate.

Heroin can be administered in several ways. The order of preference is IV injection, smoking, and nasal inhalation (known as sniffing or snorting). Intravenous injection produces effects with the greatest intensity and fastest onset (7–8 seconds). When heroin is smoked or snorted, effects develop more slowly, peaking in 10 to 15 minutes. Among users who seek addiction treatment, injection is the predominant method of administration. However, because sniffing and smoking are safer and easier than injection, these routes have become increasingly popular.

It should be noted that, when heroin is administered orally or subcutaneously, as opposed to intravenously, its effects cannot be distinguished from those of morphine and other opioids. This observation is not surprising given that, once in the brain, heroin is rapidly converted into morphine, its active form.

Oxycodone

In some parts of the United States, people are abusing the *controlled-release* formulation of oxycodone [OxyContin], an opioid similar to morphine. The controlled-release tablets were designed to provide steady levels of oxycodone over an extended time and are safe and effective when swallowed intact. However, abusers do not ingest the tablets whole. Rather, they crush the tablets and then either snort the powder or dissolve it in water and then inject it intravenously. As a result, the entire dose is absorbed *immediately,* producing blood levels that are dangerously high. Hundreds of deaths have been reported. The risk for respiratory depression and death is greatest in people who have not developed tolerance to opioids.

In an effort to reduce OxyContin abuse, the controlled-release tablets were reformulated in 2010. The new formulation bears the imprint OP, rather than OC, which appeared on the old formulation. Compared with the old tablets, OxyContin OP tablets are much harder to crush into a powder. And if exposed to water or alcohol, the tablets just form a gel, rather than a solution that can be drawn into a syringe and injected. However, there is no evidence that OxyContin OP tablets are less subject to abuse, diversion, overdose, or addiction than the old tablets.

Tolerance and Physical Dependence

Tolerance

With prolonged opioid use, tolerance develops to some pharmacologic effects, but not others. Effects to which tolerance does develop include euphoria, respiratory depression, and nausea. In contrast, little or no tolerance develops to constipation and miosis. Because tolerance to respiratory depression develops in parallel with tolerance to euphoria, respiratory depression does not increase because higher doses are taken to produce desired subjective effects. Persons tolerant to one opioid are cross-tolerant to other opioids. However, there is no cross-tolerance between opioids and general central nervous system (CNS) depressants (e.g., barbiturates, benzodiazepines, alcohol).

Physical Dependence

Long-term use produces substantial physical dependence. The abstinence syndrome resulting from opioid withdrawal is described in Chapter 22. It is important to note that, although the opioid withdrawal syndrome can be extremely unpleasant, it is rarely dangerous.

After the acute abstinence syndrome, which fades in 10 days, opioid addicts may experience a milder but protracted phase of withdrawal. This second phase, which may persist for months, is characterized by insomnia, irritability, and fatigue. Gastrointestinal hyperactivity and premature ejaculation may also occur.

Treatment of Acute Toxicity

Treatment of acute opioid toxicity is discussed in Chapter 22 and summarized here. Overdose produces a classic triad of symptoms: *respiratory depression, coma,* and *pinpoint pupils. Naloxone* [Narcan], an opioid antagonist, is the treatment of choice. This agent rapidly reverses all signs of opioid poisoning. However, dosage must be titrated carefully because if too much is given, the addict will swing from a state of intoxication to one of withdrawal. Owing to its short half-life, naloxone must be readministered every few hours until opioid concentrations have dropped to nontoxic levels, which may take days. Failure to repeat naloxone dosing may result in the death of patients who had earlier been rendered symptom free.

Detoxification

Persons who are physically dependent on opioids experience unpleasant symptoms if drug use is abruptly discontinued. Techniques for minimizing discomfort are presented next.

Methadone Substitution

Methadone, a long-acting oral opioid, is the agent most commonly employed for easing withdrawal. The first step in methadone-aided withdrawal is to substitute methadone for the opioid on which the addict is dependent. Because opioids display cross-dependence with one another, methadone will prevent an abstinence syndrome. After the subject has been stabilized on methadone, withdrawal is accomplished by administering methadone in gradually smaller doses. The resultant abstinence syndrome is mild, with symptoms resembling those of moderate influenza. The entire process of methadone substitution and withdrawal takes about 10 days.

When substituting methadone for another opioid, suppression of the abstinence syndrome requires that methadone dosage be closely matched to the existing degree of physical dependence. Hence, to ensure that methadone dosing is adequate, the extent of physical dependence must be assessed. This can be accomplished by taking a history on the extent of drug use and by observing the patient for symptoms of withdrawal. Of the two approaches, observation is the more reliable. Estimates of drug use based on patient histories may be unreliable because (1) street users don't know the purity of the drugs they have taken, (2) claims of drug use may be inflated in the hope of receiving larger doses of methadone, and (3) addicts from the ranks of the health care professions may report minimal consumption to downplay the extent of abuse. Because information from addicts is not likely to permit accurate assessment of dependence, it is essential to observe the patient to make certain methadone dosage is sufficient to suppress withdrawal.

Uses of methadone for *maintenance therapy* and *suppressive therapy* are discussed separately later.

BLACK BOX WARNING: METHADONE

Methadone can cause life-threatening QT prolongation as well as severe respiratory depression. Because of the long half-life of methadone, it should only be prescribed by health care providers with special training in chronic pain management.

Buprenorphine

Buprenorphine is an agonist-antagonist opioid. Like methadone, buprenorphine can be substituted for the opioid on which an addict is physically dependent and can thereby prevent symptoms of withdrawal. After the addict is stabilized on buprenorphine, the dosage is gradually reduced, thereby keeping symptoms of withdrawal to a minimum. Use of buprenorphine for maintenance therapy is discussed below.

Clonidine-Assisted Withdrawal

Clonidine is a centrally acting alpha$_2$-adrenergic agonist. When administered to an individual physically dependent on opioids, clonidine can suppress some symptoms of abstinence. Clonidine is most effective against symptoms related to autonomic hyperactivity (nausea, vomiting, diarrhea). Modest relief is provided from muscle aches, restlessness, anxiety, and insomnia. Opioid craving is not diminished. The basic pharmacology of clonidine is discussed in Chapter 15.

Drugs for Long-Term Management of Opioid Addiction

Three kinds of drugs are employed for long-term management: *opioid agonists, opioid agonist-antagonists,* and *opioid antagonists.* Opioid agonists (methadone) and agonist-antagonists (buprenorphine) substitute for the abused opioid and are given to patients who are not yet ready for detoxification. In contrast, opioid antagonists (naltrexone) are used to discourage renewed opioid use after detoxification has been accomplished. Drugs used for long-term management of opioid addiction are shown in Table 33.2.

Methadone

In addition to its role in facilitating opioid withdrawal, methadone [Methadose, Diskets] can be used for *maintenance therapy* and *suppressive therapy.* These strategies are employed to modify drug-using behavior in addicts who are not ready to try withdrawal.

Methadone maintenance consists of transferring the addict from the abused opioid to oral methadone. By taking methadone, the addict avoids both withdrawal and the need to procure illegal drugs. Maintenance dosing is done once a day. Maintenance is most effective when done in conjunction with nondrug measures directed at altering patterns of drug use.

Suppressive therapy is done to prevent the reinforcing effects of opioid-induced euphoria. Suppression is achieved by giving the addict progressively larger doses of methadone until a very high dose (120 mg/day) is reached. Building up to this dose creates a high degree of tolerance, and hence no subjective effects are experienced from the methadone itself. Because cross-tolerance exists among opioids, after the

TABLE 33.2 ▪ Drugs for Long-Term Management of Opioid Addiction

Drug	Trade Name	Formulation	Dosing Schedule	CSA Schedule	Comments
OPIOID AGONIST					
Methadone	Methadose, Diskets	Dispersible tablets used to make an oral suspension	Once a day	II	Methadone maintenance may be provided only by Opioid Treatment Programs certified by the federal Substance Abuse and Mental Health Services Administration and approved by the designated state authority.
	Methadose	Concentrated oral liquid	Once a day		
OPIOID AGONIST-ANTAGONIST					
Buprenorphine	Subutex	Sublingual tablet	Once a day	III	Subutex and Suboxone may be prescribed in a primary care setting by any physician or nurse practitioner who has received authorized training and has registered with the Substance Abuse and Mental Health Services Administration.
	Suboxone*	Sublingual tablet	Once a day		
	Suboxone*	Sublingual film	Once a day		
	Bunavail*	Buccal film	Once a day		
OPIOID ANTAGONIST					
Naltrexone	ReVia	Oral tablet	Once a day	NR	Naltrexone is not a controlled substance and hence prescribers do not require special training or certification. Intramuscular naltrexone [Vivitrol] is the only drug approved for opioid addiction that is given monthly, rather than daily. Before receiving naltrexone, patients must undergo opioid detoxification.
	Vivitrol	Extended-release suspension for IM injection	Once a month		

CSA, Controlled Substances Act; IM, intramuscular; NR, not regulated under the CSA.
*In addition to buprenorphine, Suboxone and Bunavail contain naloxone, an opioid antagonist, to discourage intravenous dosing.

patient is tolerant to methadone, taking street drugs, even in high doses, cannot produce significant desirable effects. As a result, individuals made tolerant with methadone will be less likely to seek out illicit opioids.

Use of methadone to treat opioid addicts is restricted to opioid treatment programs approved by the designated state authority and certified by the federal Substance Abuse and Mental Health Services Administration. These restrictions on the nonanalgesic use of methadone are needed to control abuse of methadone, a Schedule II drug with the same abuse liability as morphine and other strong opioids.

The basic pharmacology of methadone is presented in Chapter 22.

Buprenorphine

Buprenorphine [Subutex, Suboxone, Bunavail] is an agonist-antagonist opioid. The drug is a partial agonist at mu receptors and a full antagonist at kappa receptors. Buprenorphine can be used for maintenance therapy and to facilitate detoxification (see earlier). When used for maintenance, buprenorphine alleviates craving, reduces use of illicit opioids, and increases retention in therapeutic programs.

Unlike methadone, which is available only through certified opioid treatment programs, buprenorphine can be prescribed and dispensed in general medical settings, such as primary care offices. Prescribers must receive at least 8 hours of authorized training and must register with the Substance Abuse and Mental Health Services Administration.

Buprenorphine has several properties that make it attractive for treating addiction. Because it is a partial agonist at mu receptors, it has a low potential for abuse—but can still suppress craving for opioids. If the dosage is sufficiently high, buprenorphine can completely block access of strong opioids to mu receptors and can thereby prevent opioid-induced euphoria. With buprenorphine, there is a ceiling to respiratory depression, which makes it safer than methadone. Development of physical dependence is low, and hence withdrawal is relatively mild.

Buprenorphine is currently available in four formulations that are dosed once a day. One formulation—sublingual tablets marketed as *Subutex*—contains buprenorphine *alone.* The other three formulations—sublingual tablets, sublingual films, and buccal film, marketed as *Suboxone* and *Bunavail*—contain buprenorphine *combined with naloxone.* Subutex is used for the first few days of treatment, and then Suboxone is used for long-term maintenance. The newest film, *Bunavail,* is placed on the inside of each cheek and is used for long-term maintenance. The naloxone in Suboxone is there to discourage IV abuse. If taken intravenously, the naloxone in Suboxone will precipitate withdrawal. However, with sublingual administration, very little naloxone is absorbed, and hence, when the drug is administered as intended, the risk for withdrawal is low. Nonetheless, because there *is* a small risk with sublingual Suboxone, treatment is initiated with Subutex, thereby allowing substitution of buprenorphine for the abused opioid. Thereafter, Suboxone is taken for maintenance.

The basic pharmacology of buprenorphine is presented in Chapter 22.

Naltrexone

After a patient has undergone opioid detoxification, naltrexone [ReVia, Vivitrol], a pure opioid antagonist, can be used to discourage renewed opioid abuse. Benefits derive from blocking euphoria and all other opioid-induced effects. By preventing pleasurable effects, naltrexone eliminates the reinforcing properties of opioid use. When the former addict learns that taking an opioid cannot produce the desired response, drug-using behavior will cease. Naltrexone is not a controlled substance, and hence prescribers require no special training or certification.

Naltrexone is available in oral and intramuscular (IM) formulations. The oral formulation, sold as ReVia, is dosed once a day. The IM formulation, sold as Vivitrol, is dosed once a month. At this time, Vivitrol is the only long-acting drug for managing opioid addiction. All other drugs must be taken every day.

The basic pharmacology of naltrexone is presented in Chapter 22.

GENERAL CENTRAL NERVOUS SYSTEM DEPRESSANTS

The family of CNS depressants consists of barbiturates, benzodiazepines, alcohol, and other agents. With the exception of the benzodiazepines, all of these drugs are more alike than different. The benzodiazepines have properties that set them apart. The basic pharmacology of the benzodiazepines, barbiturates, and most other CNS depressants is presented in Chapter 27; the pharmacology of alcohol is presented in Chapter 31. Discussion here is limited to abuse of these drugs.

Barbiturates

The barbiturates embody all of the properties that typify general CNS depressants and hence can be considered prototypes of the group. Depressant effects are dose dependent and range from mild sedation to sleep to coma to death. With prolonged use, barbiturates produce tolerance and physical dependence.

The abuse liability of the barbiturates stems from their ability to produce subjective effects similar to those of alcohol. The barbiturates with the highest potential for abuse have a short to intermediate duration of action. These agents—amobarbital, pentobarbital, and secobarbital—are classified under Schedule II of the Controlled Substances Act. Other barbiturates appear under Schedules III and IV. Despite legal restrictions, barbiturates are available cheaply and in abundance.

Tolerance

Regular use of barbiturates produces tolerance to some effects, but not to others. Tolerance to subjective effects is significant. As a result, progressively larger doses are needed to produce desired psychological responses. Unfortunately, very little tolerance develops to respiratory depression. Consequently, as barbiturate use continues, the dose needed to produce subjective effects moves closer and closer to the dose that can cause respiratory arrest. (Note that this differs from the pattern seen with opioids, in which tolerance to subjective effects and to respiratory depression develop in parallel.) Individuals tolerant to barbiturates show cross-tolerance with other CNS depressants (e.g., alcohol, benzodiazepines, general anesthetics). However, little or no cross-tolerance develops to opioids.

Physical Dependence and Withdrawal Techniques

Chronic barbiturate use can produce substantial physical dependence. Cross-dependence exists between barbiturates and other CNS depressants, but not with opioids. When physical dependence is great, the associated abstinence syndrome can be severe—sometimes fatal. In contrast, the opioid abstinence syndrome, although unpleasant, is rarely life threatening.

One technique for easing barbiturate withdrawal employs phenobarbital, a barbiturate with a long half-life. Because of cross-dependence, substitution of phenobarbital for the abused barbiturate suppresses symptoms of abstinence. After the patient has been stabilized, the dosage of phenobarbital is gradually tapered off, thereby minimizing symptoms of abstinence.

Acute Toxicity

Overdose with barbiturates produces a triad of symptoms: *respiratory depression, coma,* and *pinpoint pupils*—the same symptoms that accompany opioid poisoning. Treatment is directed at maintaining respiration and removing the drug; endotracheal intubation and ventilatory assistance may be required. Details of management are presented in Chapter 27. Barbiturate overdose has no specific antidote. Naloxone, which reverses poisoning by opioids, is not effective against poisoning by barbiturates.

Benzodiazepines

Benzodiazepines differ significantly from barbiturates. Benzodiazepines are much safer than the barbiturates, and overdose with *oral* benzodiazepines *alone* is rarely lethal. However, the risk for death is greatly increased when oral benzodiazepines are combined with other CNS depressants (e.g., alcohol, barbiturates) or when benzodiazepines are administered intravenously. If severe overdose occurs, signs and symptoms can be reversed with *flumazenil* [Romazicon, Anexate ♣], a benzodiazepine antagonist. As a rule, tolerance and physical dependence are only moderate when benzodiazepines are taken for legitimate indications but can be substantial when these drugs are abused. In patients who develop physical dependence, the abstinence syndrome can be minimized by withdrawing benzodiazepines very slowly—over a period of months. The abuse liability of the benzodiazepines is much lower than that of the barbiturates. As a result, all benzodiazepines are classified under Schedule IV of the Controlled Substances Act. Benzodiazepines are discussed in Chapter 27.

PSYCHOSTIMULANTS

Discussion here focuses on two CNS stimulants that have a high potential for abuse: cocaine and methamphetamine. Because of their considerable abuse liability, these drugs are classified as Schedule II agents.

Cocaine

Cocaine is a stimulant extracted from the leaves of the coca plant. The drug has CNS effects similar to those of the amphetamines. In addition, cocaine can produce local anesthesia as well as vasoconstriction and cardiac stimulation. Among abusers, a form of cocaine known as "crack" is used widely. Crack is extremely addictive, and the risk for lethal overdose is high.

According to the National Survey on Drug Use and Health, cocaine use has declined. In 2014, 1.8 million Americans 12 years and older reported using cocaine in any form, compared with 5.5 million in 2005.

Forms

Cocaine is available in two forms: *cocaine hydrochloride* and *cocaine base* (alkaloidal cocaine, freebase cocaine, "crack"). Cocaine base is heat stable, whereas cocaine hydrochloride is not. Cocaine hydrochloride is available as a white powder that is frequently diluted ("cut") before sale. Cocaine base is sold in the form of crystals ("rocks") that consist of nearly pure cocaine. Cocaine base is widely known by the street name "crack," a term inspired by the sound the crystals make when heated.

Routes of Administration

Cocaine *hydrochloride* is usually administered *intranasally.* The drug is "snorted" and absorbed across the nasal mucosa into the bloodstream. A few users (about 5%) administer cocaine hydrochloride intravenously. Cocaine hydrochloride cannot be smoked because it is unstable at high temperature.

Cocaine *base* is administered by *smoking,* a process referred to as "freebasing." Smoking delivers large amounts of cocaine to the lungs, where absorption is very rapid. Subjective and physiologic effects are equivalent to those elicited by IV injection.

Subjective Effects and Addiction

At usual doses, cocaine produces euphoria similar to that produced by amphetamines. In a laboratory setting, individuals familiar with the effects of cocaine are unable to distinguish between cocaine and amphetamine. Cocaine causes euphoria through inhibition of neuronal reuptake of dopamine and thereby increases activation of dopamine receptors in the brain's reward circuit.

As with many other psychoactive drugs, the intensity of subjective responses depends on the rate at which plasma drug levels rise. Because cocaine levels rise relatively slowly with intranasal administration, and almost instantaneously with IV injection or smoking, responses produced by intranasal cocaine are much less intense than those produced by the other two routes.

When crack cocaine is smoked, desirable subjective effects begin to fade within minutes and are often replaced by dysphoria. In an attempt to avoid dysphoria and regain euphoria, the user may administer repeated doses at short intervals. This use pattern—termed *binging*—can rapidly lead to addiction.

Acute Toxicity: Symptoms and Treatment

Overdose is frequent, and deaths have occurred. Mild overdose produces agitation, dizziness, tremor, and blurred vision. Severe overdose can produce hyperpyrexia, convulsions, ventricular dysrhythmias, and hemorrhagic stroke. Angina pectoris and myocardial infarction may develop secondary to coronary artery spasm. Psychological manifestations of overdose include severe anxiety, paranoid ideation, and hallucinations (visual, auditory, and/or tactile). Because cocaine has a short half-life, symptoms subside in 1 to 2 hours.

Although there is no specific antidote to cocaine toxicity, most symptoms can be controlled with drugs. Intravenous *diazepam* or *lorazepam* can reduce anxiety and suppress seizures. *Diazepam* may also alleviate hypertension and dysrhythmias because these result from increased central sympathetic activity. If hypertension is severe, it can be corrected with IV *nitroprusside.* Dysrhythmias associated with prolonging the QT interval may respond to *hypertonic sodium bicarbonate.* Although beta blockers can suppress dysrhythmias, they might further compromise coronary perfusion (by preventing $beta_2$-mediated coronary vasodilation). Reduction of thrombus formation with aspirin can lower the risk for myocardial ischemia. Hyperthermia should be reduced with external cooling.

Chronic Toxicity

When administered intranasally on a long-term basis, cocaine can cause atrophy of the nasal mucosa and loss of sense of smell. In extreme cases, necrosis and perforation of the nasal septum occur. Nasal pathology results from local ischemia secondary to chronic vasoconstriction. Injury to the lungs can occur from smoking cocaine base.

Tolerance, Dependence, and Withdrawal

In animal models, regular administration of cocaine results in *increased* sensitivity to the drug, not tolerance. Whether this holds true for humans is not clear.

The degree of physical dependence produced by cocaine is in dispute. Some observers report little or no evidence of withdrawal after cocaine discontinuation. In contrast, others report symptoms similar to those associated with amphetamine withdrawal: dysphoria, craving, fatigue, depression, and prolonged sleep.

Treatment of Cocaine Addiction

Although achieving complete abstinence from cocaine is extremely difficult, treatment *can* greatly reduce cocaine use. For the cocaine addict, psychosocial therapy is the cornerstone of treatment. This therapy is directed at motivating users to commit to a drug-free life, and then helping them work toward that goal. A combination of individual therapy and group drug counseling is most effective, producing a 70% reduction in cocaine use at 12-month follow-up.

Can medication help with cocaine addiction? To date, no drug has been proved broadly effective in treating cocaine abuse. However, ongoing work with two agents is encouraging:

- *Anticocaine vaccine*—Subjects receiving the vaccine develop antibodies that bind with cocaine and thereby render the cocaine inactive. The higher the antibody titer, the greater the reduction in cocaine use. The vaccine has been tested in mice. Human testing may start in 2016.
- *Disulfiram* [Antabuse]—Subjects receiving a combination of disulfiram plus cognitive behavioral therapy reduced their cocaine use from 2 or 3 times daily to 0.5 times daily. Disulfiram is the same drug discussed in Chapter 31 for treating alcohol abuse.

Methamphetamine

The basic pharmacology of the amphetamine family is discussed in Chapter 29. Discussion here is limited to abuse of methamphetamine.

Description and Routes

Methamphetamine is a white, crystalline powder that readily dissolves in water or alcohol. The drug may be swallowed, "snorted," smoked, or injected intravenously. Owing to its potential for abuse, methamphetamine is classified as a Schedule II drug.

Patterns of Use

Methamphetamine use is declining. According to the 2014 National Survey on Drug Use and Health, use of methamphetamine by Americans 12 years and older continues to decline.

Subjective and Behavioral Effects

As discussed in Chapter 29 amphetamines act primarily by increasing the release of norepinephrine and dopamine, and partly by reducing the reuptake of both transmitters. By doing so, methamphetamine produces arousal and elevation of mood. Euphoria is likely, and talkativeness is prominent. A sense of increased physical strength and mental capacity occurs. Self-confidence rises. Users feel little or no need for food and sleep.

Adverse Psychological Effects

All amphetamines can produce a psychotic state characterized by delusions, paranoia, and auditory and visual hallucinations, making patients look like they have schizophrenia. Although psychosis can be triggered by a single dose, it occurs more commonly with long-term abuse. Methamphetamine-induced psychosis usually resolves spontaneously after drug withdrawal. If needed, an antipsychotic agent (e.g., haloperidol) can be given to suppress symptoms.

Adverse Cardiovascular Effects

Because of its sympathomimetic actions, methamphetamine can cause vasoconstriction and excessive stimulation of the heart, leading to hypertension, angina pectoris, and dysrhythmias. Overdose may also cause cerebral and systemic vasculitis and renal failure. Changes in cerebral blood vessels can lead to stroke. Vasoconstriction can be relieved with an alpha-adrenergic blocker (e.g., phentolamine). Cardiac stimulation can be reduced with a mixed alpha and beta blocker (e.g., labetalol).

Other Adverse Effects

By suppressing appetite, methamphetamine can cause significant weight loss. Use during pregnancy increases the risk for preterm birth, hypertension, placental abruption, intrauterine growth restriction, and neonatal death. Heavy use can promote severe tooth decay, known informally as "meth mouth." Causes include reduced salivation, grinding and clenching of the teeth, increased consumption of sugary drinks, and neglect of oral hygiene. Lastly, methamphetamine can cause direct injury to dopaminergic nerve terminals in the brain, leading to prolonged deficits in cognition and memory.

Tolerance, Dependence, and Withdrawal

Long-term use results in tolerance to mood elevation, appetite suppression, and cardiovascular effects. Although physical dependence is only moderate, psychological dependence can be intense. Methamphetamine withdrawal can produce dysphoria and a strong sense of craving. Other symptoms include fatigue, prolonged sleep, excessive eating, and depression. Depression can persist for months and is a common reason for resuming drug use.

Treatment

Methamphetamine addiction responds well to cognitive behavioral therapy. One such approach, known as the Matrix Model, combines group therapy, individual therapy, family education, drug testing, and encouragement to participate in non–drug-related activities. At this time, no medications are approved for treatment. However, encouraging results have been achieved with two drugs: *bupropion* [Wellbutrin, Zyban], currently approved for major depression and smoking cessation, and *modafinil* [Provigil, Alertec ♣], a nonamphetamine stimulant currently approved for narcolepsy, shift-work sleep disorder, and obstructive sleep apnea–hypopnea syndrome. An additional drug, ibudilast, is in clinical trials. Preliminary results indicate that ibudilast may dampen cravings for methamphetamine and improve cognitive functioning.

MARIJUANA AND RELATED PREPARATIONS

Marijuana is the most commonly used illicit drug in the United States. More than 95 million Americans have tried it at least once. In 2014 nearly 22 million Americans 12 years and older used marijuana. Among youth, rates of daily marijuana use are the highest since the 1970s. Results of the 2012 *Monitoring the Future* survey show that 10.4% of 8th-graders and 25.5% of 10th-graders reported using marijuana in the past year. Marijuana use among 12th-graders has risen to 35.1%.

Cannabis sativa, the Source of Marijuana

Marijuana is prepared from *Cannabis sativa,* the Indian hemp plant—an unusual plant in that it has separate male and female forms. Psychoactive compounds are present in all parts of the male and female plants. However, the greatest concentration of psychoactive substances is found in the flowering tops of the female plants.

The two most common *Cannabis* derivatives are *marijuana* and *hashish.* Marijuana is a preparation consisting of leaves and flowers of male and female plants. Alternative names for marijuana include *grass, weed, pot,* and *dope.* The terms *joint* and *reefer* refer to marijuana cigarettes. Hashish is a dried preparation of the resinous exudate from female flowers. Hashish is considerably more potent than marijuana.

Psychoactive Component

The major psychoactive substance in *Cannabis sativa* is delta-9-tetrahydrocannabinol (THC), an oily chemical with high lipid solubility.

The THC content of *Cannabis* preparations is variable. The highest concentrations are found in the flowers of the female plant. The lowest concentrations are in the seeds. Depending on growing conditions and the strain of the plant, THC in marijuana preparations may range from 1% to 11%.

Mechanism of Action

Psychological effects of THC result from activating specific cannabinoid receptors in the brain. The endogenous ligand for these receptors appears to be *anandamide,* a derivative of arachidonic acid unique to the brain. The concentration of cannabinoid receptors is highest in brain regions associated with pleasure, memory, thinking, concentration, appetite, sensory perception, time perception, and coordination of movement.

There is evidence that marijuana may act in part through the same reward system as opioids and cocaine. Both heroin and cocaine produce pleasurable sensations by promoting release of dopamine in the brain's reward circuit. In rats, intravenous THC also causes dopamine release. Interestingly, release of dopamine by THC is blocked by naloxone, a drug that blocks the effects of opioids. This suggests that THC causes release of dopamine by first causing release of endogenous opioids.

Pharmacokinetics

Administration by Smoking

When marijuana or hashish is smoked, about 60% of the THC content is absorbed. Absorption from the lungs is rapid. Subjective effects begin in minutes and peak 10 to 20 minutes later. Effects from a single marijuana cigarette may persist for 2 to 3 hours. Termination results from metabolism of THC to inactive products.

Oral Administration

When marijuana or hashish is ingested, practically all of the THC undergoes absorption. However, most is inactivated on its first pass through the liver. Hence only 6% to 20% of absorbed drug actually reaches the systemic circulation. Because of this extensive first-pass metabolism, oral doses must be 3 to 10 times greater than smoked doses to produce equivalent effects. With oral dosing, effects are delayed and prolonged: responses begin in 30 to 50 minutes and persist up to 12 hours.

Behavioral and Subjective Effects

Marijuana produces three principal subjective effects: *euphoria, sedation,* and *hallucinations.* This set of responses is unique to marijuana; no other psychoactive drug causes all three. Because of this singular pattern of effects, marijuana is in a class by itself.

Effects of Low to Moderate Doses

Responses to low doses of THC are variable and depend on several factors, including dosage size and route, setting of drug use, and expectations and previous experience of the user. The following effects are common: euphoria and relaxation; gaiety and a heightened sense of the humorous; increased sensitivity to visual and auditory stimuli; enhanced sense of touch, taste, and smell; increased appetite and ability to appreciate the flavor of food; and distortion of time perception such that short spans seem much longer than they really are. In addition to these effects, which might be considered pleasurable (or at least innocuous), moderate doses can produce undesirable responses. Among these are impairment of short-term memory; decreased capacity to perform multistep tasks; slowed reaction time and impairment of motor coordination (which can make driving dangerous); altered judgment and decision making (which can lead to high-risk sexual behavior); temporal disintegration (inability to distinguish between past, present, and future); depersonalization (a sense of strangeness about the self); decreased ability to perceive the emotions of others; and reduced interpersonal interaction.

High-Dose Effects

In high doses, marijuana can have serious adverse psychological effects. The user may experience hallucinations, delusions, and paranoia. Euphoria may be displaced by intense anxiety, and a dissociative state may occur in which the user feels "outside of himself or herself." In extremely high doses, marijuana can produce a state resembling toxic psychosis, which may persist for weeks. Because of the widespread use of marijuana, psychiatric emergencies caused by the drug are relatively common.

Not all users are equally vulnerable to the adverse psychological effects of marijuana. Some individuals experience ill effects only at extremely high doses. In contrast, others routinely experience adverse effects at moderate doses.

Effects of Chronic Use

Chronic, excessive use of marijuana is associated with a behavioral phenomenon known as an *amotivational syndrome,* characterized by apathy, dullness, poor grooming, reduced interest in achievement, and disinterest in the pursuit of conventional goals. The precise relationship between marijuana and development of the syndrome is not known, nor is it certain what other factors may contribute. Available data do not suggest that the amotivational syndrome is due to organic brain damage.

Role in Schizophrenia

Marijuana use is associated with an increased risk for schizophrenia. In young people with no history of psychotic symptoms, marijuana increases the risk for symptom occurrence. In people who already have symptoms, marijuana may prolong symptom persistence. In the stabilized schizophrenic person, marijuana may precipitate an acute psychotic episode.

Physiologic Effects

Cardiovascular Effects

Marijuana produces a dose-related increase in heart rate. Increases of 20 to 50 beats/minute are typical. However, rates up to 140 beats/minute are not uncommon. Pretreatment with propranolol prevents marijuana-induced tachycardia but does not block the drug's subjective effects. Marijuana causes orthostatic hypotension and pronounced reddening of the conjunctivae. These responses apparently result from vasodilation.

Respiratory Effects

When used *acutely,* marijuana produces *bronchodilation.* However, when smoked chronically, the drug causes airway constriction. In addition, chronic use is closely associated with development of bronchitis, sinusitis, and asthma. Lung cancer is another possible outcome. Animal studies have shown that tar from marijuana smoke is a more potent carcinogen than tar from cigarettes.

Effects on Reproduction

Research in animals has shown multiple effects on reproduction. In males, marijuana decreases spermatogenesis and testosterone levels. In females, the drug reduces levels of follicle-stimulating hormone, luteinizing hormone, and prolactin.

Multiple effects may be seen in babies and children who were exposed to marijuana in utero. Some babies present with trembling, altered responses to visual stimuli, and a high-pitched cry. Preschoolers may have a decreased ability to perform tasks that involve memory and sustained attention. Schoolchildren may exhibit deficits in memory, attentiveness, and problem solving.

Altered Brain Structure

Long-term marijuana use is associated with structural changes in the brain. Specifically, the volumes of the hippocampus and amygdala are reduced by an average of 12% and 7.1%, respectively. We don't know if volume reduction is due to reduced cell size, reduced synaptic density, or loss of glial cells or neurons. Interestingly, hippocampal volume loss occurs primarily in the left hemisphere.

Tolerance and Dependence

When taken in extremely high doses, marijuana can produce tolerance and physical dependence. Neither effect, however, is remarkable. Some tolerance develops to the cardiovascular, perceptual, and motor effects of marijuana. Little or no tolerance develops to subjective effects.

To demonstrate physical dependence on marijuana, the drug must be given in very high doses—and even then the degree of dependence is only moderate. Symptoms brought on by abrupt discontinuation of high-dose marijuana include irritability, restlessness, nervousness, insomnia, reduced appetite, and weight loss. Tremor, hyperthermia, and chills may occur too. Symptoms subside in 3 to 5 days. With moderate marijuana use, no withdrawal symptoms occur.

Therapeutic Use

In the United States there are no approved medical uses for marijuana. However, there *are* U.S. Food and Drug Administration (FDA)–approved uses for two *purified* cannabinoids: THC and dronabinol, an analog of THC. A third cannabinoid preparation—nabiximols—is approved in Canada.

Approved Uses for Cannabinoids

Suppression of Emesis

Intense nausea and vomiting are common side effects of cancer chemotherapy. In certain patients, these responses can be suppressed more effectively with cannabinoids than with traditional antiemetics (e.g., prochlorperazine, metoclopramide). At this time, two cannabinoids—*dronabinol* [Marinol] and *nabilone* [Cesamet]—are available for antiemetic use. Dronabinol, a synthetic form of THC, is a Schedule III drug. Nabilone, a THC derivative, is a schedule II drug. Dosage forms and dosages are presented in Chapter 64

Appetite Stimulation

Dronabinol is FDA approved for stimulating appetite in patients with AIDS. By relieving anorexia, treatment may prevent or reverse loss of weight.

Relief of Neuropathic Pain

In 2005, Canadian regulators approved *nabiximols* [Sativex ♣], administered by oral spray, for treating neuropathic pain caused by multiple sclerosis (MS). Nabiximols is a mixture of two cannabinoids: THC and cannabidiol. Because the cannabinoids in Sativex are absorbed through the oral mucosa, the product has a rapid onset (like smoked marijuana) while being devoid of the dangerous tars in marijuana smoke. In the United States nabiximols is under study for treating intractable cancer pain. However, the drug is not yet approved in the United States and cannot be legally imported, owing to its current classification as a Schedule I substance.

Unapproved Uses for Cannabinoids

Glaucoma

In patients with glaucoma, smoking marijuana may reduce intraocular pressure. Unfortunately, marijuana may also reduce blood flow to the optic nerve. We don't know if the drug improves vision.

Multiple Sclerosis

Whether smoked or ingested, marijuana appears to reduce spasticity and tremor of MS. Oral cannabinoids may also reduce urge incontinence. As discussed earlier, cannabinoids can reduce neuropathic pain of MS.

Medical Research on Marijuana

Proponents of making marijuana available by prescription argue that smoked marijuana can reduce chronic pain, suppress nausea caused by chemotherapy, improve appetite in patients with AIDS, lower intraocular pressure in patients with glaucoma, and suppress spasticity associated with MS and spinal cord injury. However, the evidence supporting most of these claims is weak—largely because federal regulations had effectively barred marijuana research.

In 1999, two developments opened the doors to marijuana research. First, an expert panel, convened by the National Academy of Sciences Institute of Medicine, recommended that clinical trials on marijuana proceed. Because smoking marijuana poses a risk for lung cancer and other respiratory disorders, the panel also recommended development of a rapid-onset nonsmoked delivery system. In response to this report and to pressure from scientists and voters, the government created new guidelines that loosened restraints on marijuana research. Under the guidelines, researchers will be allowed to purchase marijuana directly from the federal government. (On behalf of the government, the University of Mississippi maintains a plot of marijuana on 1.8 closely guarded acres.) The only catch is that all proposed research must be approved by the FDA, the National Institute on Drug Abuse, and the Drug Enforcement Agency (DEA). Despite these formidable obstacles, at least one institute—the Center for Medicinal Cannabis Research at the University of California—has begun coordinating and supporting research on medical marijuana. Trials will focus on HIV-related cachexia, neuropathic pain, nausea and vomiting associated with cancer chemotherapy, and muscle spasticity associated with MS and other diseases.

Legal Status of Medical Marijuana

United States

Twenty-three states[a] and the District of Columbia have enacted laws that eliminate criminal penalties for medical use of marijuana, and more states are considering doing the same. Because of the new state laws, patients can now possess and use small amounts of marijuana for medical purposes. In most of these states, qualified patients must have a debilitating medical condition plus documentation from their physician that medical use of marijuana "may be of benefit."

What about federal marijuana regulations? Because marijuana is classified by the Drug Enforcement Agency (DEA) as a Schedule I substance, physicians still cannot *prescribe* the drug—all they can do is *suggest* it may be of benefit. Furthermore, in 2005, the U.S. Supreme Court ruled that DEA legislation trumps the new state laws, and hence people who use or provide medical marijuana can still be prosecuted under federal law, even in states where medical marijuana has been legalized. In a (delayed) response to this ruling, the Department of Justice, in 2009, instructed U.S. attorneys not to use federal resources to prosecute people whose actions comply with state laws that allow medical marijuana use. Hence, although patients may be breaking federal law, the Department of Justice will not prosecute them.

Canada

Medical use of marijuana has been legal in Canada since 2001, when the Marijuana Medical Access Regulations took effect. Patients with documentation from a physician can get their marijuana through Health Canada, or they can get a license to grow their own. Marijuana supplies for Health Canada are grown and distributed by Prairie Plant Systems.

Comparison of Marijuana With Alcohol

In several important ways, responses to marijuana and alcohol are quite different. Whereas increased hostility and aggression are common sequelae of alcohol consumption, aggressive behavior is rare among marijuana users. Although loss of judgment and control can occur with either drug, these losses are greater with alcohol. For the marijuana user, increased appetite and food intake are typical. In contrast, heavy drinkers often suffer nutritional deficiencies. Lastly, whereas marijuana can cause toxic psychosis, dissociative phenomena, and paranoia, these severe acute psychological reactions rarely occur with alcohol.

[a]Alaska, Arizona, California, Colorado, Connecticut, Delaware, Hawaii, Illinois, Maine, Maryland, Massachusetts, Michigan, Minnesota, Montana, Nevada, New Hampshire, New Jersey, New Mexico, New York, Oregon, Rhode Island, Vermont, and Washington.

Synthetic Marijuana

Synthetic cannabis blends showed up on the market in the early 2000s. They became popular because of their availability and their lack of traces in drug tests. They were initially legal because they were thought to contain blends of natural herbs sprayed with chemicals that mimic the effects of THC. These chemicals come in two classes: THC analogs and other compounds.

Although synthetic marijuana was once thought harmless, the American Association of Poison Control Centers reported more than 7000 calls regarding synthetic marijuana in 2015 alone. In addition, several deaths and many episodes of florid psychosis and toxicity are possibly related to synthetic marijuana use. Side effects include hypertension, nausea, vomiting, anxiety, agitation, paranoid behavior, hallucinations, and catatonic state. By 2011, the FDA had placed many of these chemicals on the controlled substances list as Schedule I drugs, making them illegal to possess. However, more than 500 compounds exist; therefore synthetic marijuana is still available. Many organizations, including the U.S. military, have banned all similar compounds.

PSYCHEDELICS

The psychedelics are a fascinating drug family for which LSD can be considered the prototype. Other family members include mescaline, dimethyltryptamine (DMT), psilocin, and salvia. The psychedelics are so named because of their ability to produce what has been termed a *psychedelic state.* Individuals in this state show an increased awareness of sensory stimuli and are likely to perceive the world around them as beautiful and harmonious; the normally insignificant may assume exceptional meaning, the "self" may seem split into an "observer" and a "doer," and boundaries between "self" and "nonself" may fade, producing a sense of unity with the cosmos.

Psychedelic drugs are often referred to as *hallucinogens* or *psychotomimetics.* These names reflect their ability to produce hallucinations as well as mental states that resemble psychoses.

Although psychedelics can cause hallucinations and psychotic-like states, these are not their most characteristic effects. The characteristic that truly distinguishes the psychedelics from other agents is their *ability to bring on the same types of alterations in thought, perception, and feeling that otherwise occur only in dreams.* In essence, the psychedelics seem able to activate mechanisms for dreaming without causing unconsciousness.

d-Lysergic Acid Diethylamide

History

The first person to experience LSD was a Swiss chemist named Albert Hofmann. In 1943, 5 years after LSD was first synthesized, Hofmann accidentally ingested a minute amount of the drug. The result was a dream-like state accompanied by perceptual distortions and vivid hallucinations. The high potency and unusual actions of LSD led to speculation that it might provide a model for studying psychosis. Unfortunately, that speculation did not prove correct: extensive research has shown that the effects of LSD cannot be equated with idiopathic psychosis. With the realization that LSD did not produce a "model psychosis," medical interest in the drug declined. Not everyone, however, lost interest; during the 1960s, nonmedical experimentation flourished. This widespread use caused substantial societal concern, and, by 1970, LSD had been classified as a Schedule I substance. Nonetheless, street use of LSD continues.

Mechanism of Action

LSD acts at multiple sites in the brain and spinal cord. However, effects are most prominent in the cerebral cortex and the locus coeruleus. Effects are thought to result from activation of serotonin-2 receptors. This concept has been reinforced by the observation that *ritanserin,* a selective blocker of serotonin-2 receptors, can prevent the effects of LSD in animals.

Time Course

LSD is usually administered orally but can also be injected or smoked. With oral dosing, initial effects can be felt in minutes. Over the next few hours, responses become progressively more intense, and then subside 8 to 12 hours later.

Subjective and Behavioral Effects

Responses to LSD can be diverse, complex, and changeable. The drug can alter thinking, feeling, perception, sense of self, and sense of relationship with the environment and other people. LSD-induced experiences may be sublime or terrifying. Just what will be experienced during any particular "trip" cannot be predicted.

Perceptual alterations can be dramatic. Colors may appear iridescent or glowing, kaleidoscopic images may appear, and vivid hallucinations may occur. Sensory experiences may merge so that colors seem to be heard and sounds seem to be visible. Afterimages may occur, causing current perceptions to overlap with preceding perceptions. The LSD user may feel a sense of wonderment and awe at the beauty of commonplace things.

LSD can have a profound influence on affect. Emotions may range from elation, good humor, and euphoria to sadness, dysphoria, and fear. The intensity of emotion may be overwhelming.

Thoughts may turn inward. Attitudes may be reevaluated and old values assigned new priorities. A sense of new and important insight may be felt. However, despite the intensity of these experiences, enduring changes in beliefs, behavior, and personality are rare.

Physiologic Effects

LSD has few physiologic effects. Activation of the sympathetic nervous system can produce tachycardia, elevation of blood pressure, mydriasis, piloerection, and hyperthermia. Neuromuscular effects (tremor, incoordination, hyperreflexia, and muscular weakness) may also occur.

Tolerance and Dependence

Tolerance to LSD develops rapidly. Substantial tolerance can be seen after just three or four daily doses. Tolerance to subjective and behavioral effects develops to a greater extent than to cardiovascular effects. Cross-tolerance exists with mescaline and psilocybin, but not with DMT. Because DMT is similar to LSD, the absence of cross-tolerance is surprising. There is no cross-tolerance with amphetamines or THC. On cessation of LSD use, tolerance rapidly fades. Abrupt withdrawal of LSD is not associated with an abstinence syndrome. Hence there is no evidence for physical dependence.

Toxicity

Toxic reactions are primarily psychological. LSD has never been a direct cause of death, although fatalities have occurred from accidents and suicides.

Acute panic reactions are relatively common and may be associated with a fear of disintegration of the self. Such "bad trips" can usually be managed by a process of "talking down" (providing emotional support and reassurance in a nonthreatening environment). Panic episodes can also be managed with an antianxiety agent, such as diazepam. Neuroleptics (e.g., haloperidol, chlorpromazine) may actually intensify the experience, and hence their use is questionable.

A small percentage of former LSD users experience episodic visual disturbances, referred to as *flashbacks* by users and *hallucinogen persisting perception disorder* (HPPD) by clinicians. These disturbances may manifest as geometric pseudohallucinations, flashes of color, or positive afterimages. Visual disturbances may be precipitated by several factors, including marijuana use, fatigue, stress, and anxiety. Phenothiazines exacerbate these experiences rather than providing relief. HPPD appears to be caused by permanent changes in the visual system.

In addition to panic reactions and visual disturbances, LSD can cause other adverse psychological effects. Depressive episodes, dissociative reactions, and distortions of body image may occur. When an LSD experience has been intensely terrifying, the user may be left with persistent residual fear. The drug may also cause prolonged psychotic reactions. In contrast to acute effects, which differ substantially from symptoms of schizophrenia, prolonged psychotic reactions mimic schizophrenia faithfully.

Potential Therapeutic Uses

LSD has no recognized therapeutic applications. The drug has been evaluated in subjects with alcoholism, opioid addiction, and psychiatric disorders, including depression, anxiety, and obsessive-compulsive disorder. In addition, LSD has been studied as a possible means of promoting psychological well-being in patients with terminal cancer. With the possible exception of some psychiatric disorders (e.g., depression, anxiety), LSD has proved either ineffective or impractical.

Salvia

Salvia divinorum is a hallucinogenic herb native to southern Mexico and to Central and South America. Its primary psychoactive component is *salvinorin A,* a potent activator of kappa opioid receptors. The genus *Salvia,* a part of the mint family, is commonly known as sage—hence the colorful street names for *S. divinorum:* Magic Mint, Diviner's Sage, and Sage of the Seers. Salvia is legal in some states, illegal in others, and not yet regulated under the Controlled Substances Act.

Salvia is used extensively in the United States, primarily by teens and young adults. In 2011, 5.9% of high school seniors reported using the drug in the past year. About 1.8 million Americans older than 12 years report having used salvia at least once in their lives.

How is salvia administered? Among Mexican Indians, the traditional method is to chew the leaves or drink a liquid extract. In contrast, recreational users usually smoke the dried leaves, either in a pipe or rolled in a joint. When the smoke is inhaled, salvinorin A undergoes rapid absorption from the lungs. As a result, psychological effects begin quickly (in less than 1 minute) and then quickly fade (typically in 5–10 minutes).

Like other psychedelic drugs, salvia induces a dream-like state of unreality. Users may lose awareness of their own bodies and of the room they are in. They may feel they are floating, traveling through time and space, or merging with or transforming into objects. Some feel they are being twisted or pulled. There may be a sense of overlapping realities and of being in several places at once. Speech may become slurred, and sentences may lack fluent structure. Uncontrollable laughter may break out. Possible physical effects include chills, dizziness, nausea, incoordination, and bradycardia. Whether saliva poses long-term health risks has not been studied. However, we do know that Mexican Indians have used the drug for generations, with no apparent ill effects.

Mescaline, Psilocin, Psilocybin, and Dimethyltryptamine

In addition to LSD and salvia, the family of psychedelic drugs includes mescaline, psilocin, psilocybin, DMT, and several related compounds. Some psychedelics are synthetic, and some occur naturally. DMT and LSD represent the synthetic compounds. Mescaline, a constituent of the peyote cactus, and psilocin and psilocybin, constituents of "magic mushrooms," represent compounds found in nature.

The subjective and behavioral effects of the miscellaneous psychedelic drugs are similar to those of LSD. Like LSD, these drugs can elicit modes of thought, perception, and feeling that are normally restricted to dreams. In addition, they can cause hallucinations and induce mental states that resemble psychosis.

The miscellaneous psychedelics differ from LSD with respect to potency and time course. LSD is the most potent of the psychedelics, producing its full spectrum of effects at doses as low as 0.5 mcg/kg. Psilocin and psilocybin are 100 times less potent than LSD, and mescaline is 4000 times less potent than LSD. Whereas the effects of LSD are prolonged (responses may last 12 or more hours), the effects of mescaline and DMT are shorter: responses to mescaline usually fade within 8 to 12 hours, and responses to DMT fade within 1 to 2 hours.

None of these psychedelics is approved for medical use. The use of psilocybin in patients with terminal cancer and obsessive-compulsive disorder is under investigation.

DEXTROMETHORPHAN

Dextromethorphan (DXM) is a cough suppressant widely available in over-the-counter cough and cold remedies (see Chapter 61). At the low doses needed for cough suppression, DXM is devoid of psychological effects. However, at doses 5 to 10 times higher, DXM can cause euphoria, disorientation, paranoia, and altered sense of time, as well as visual, auditory, and tactile hallucinations. These effects are produced by dextrorphan, a metabolite of DXM that blocks receptors for *N*-methyl-D-aspartate. Note that this is the same mechanism used by phencyclidine and ketamine. Many of the products that contain DXM also contain other drugs, including acetaminophen, antihistamines, phenylephrine, and pseudoephedrine. Therefore, when excessive doses are taken, users are subject to toxicity from these compounds as well as from DXM itself. The principal users of DXM are adolescents and teenagers. Between 1999 and 2004, reports of DXM abuse in these groups rose 10-fold. Many products contain DXM, including Coricidin HBP Cough & Cold, Robitussin DM, and Vicks NyQuil Cough Syrup.

3,4-METHY LENEDIOXYMETHAMPHETAMINE (MDMA, ECSTASY)

MDMA, also known as "ecstasy," is a complex drug with stimulant and psychedelic properties. The drug is structurally related to methamphetamine (a stimulant) and mescaline (a hallucinogen). Low doses produce mild LSD-like psychedelic effects; higher doses produce amphetamine-like stimulant effects. These effects result from (1) blocking reuptake of serotonin and (2) promoting the release of serotonin, dopamine, and norepinephrine. Although MDMA can produce effects that are clearly pleasurable, it can also be dangerous; the biggest concerns are neurotoxicity, seizures, excessive cardiovascular stimulation, and hyperthermia and its sequelae. MDMA is classified as a Schedule I drug.

Time Course and Dosage

MDMA is usually dosed orally, but may also be snorted, injected, or inserted as a rectal suppository. With oral administration, effects begin in 20 minutes, peak in 2 to 3 hours, and persist 4 to 5 hours. The usual dose is 100 mg or less.

Who Uses MDMA and Why?

MDMA is used primarily by adolescents and young adults in cities, in the suburbs, and in rural areas. According to a survey conducted in 2014, 0.9% of 8th-graders, 2.3% of 10th-graders, and 3.6% of 12th-graders had used MDMA in the past year.

Why do people take MDMA? Because it makes them feel very good. The drug can elevate mood, increase sensory awareness, and heighten sensitivity to music. It can also facilitate interpersonal relationships: users report a sense of closeness with others, lowering of defenses, reduced anxiety, enhanced communication, and increased sociability.

Adverse Effects

MDMA is not free of risks. The drug can injure serotonergic neurons, stimulate the heart, and raise body temperature to a dangerous level. In addition, it can cause neurologic effects (e.g., seizures, spasmodic jerking, jaw clenching, teeth grinding) and a host of adverse psychological effects (e.g., confusion, anxiety, paranoia, panic attacks, visual hallucinations, and suicidal thoughts and behavior). Every year, MDMA is associated with several thousand admissions to emergency departments, mainly because of seizures.

MDMA can damage serotonergic neurons, perhaps irreversibly. When administered to rats and primates in doses only 2 to 4 times greater than those that produce hallucinations in humans, MDMA causes *irreversible destruction of serotonergic neurons,* resulting in passivity and insomnia. At least three lines of evidence suggest that MDMA is also neurotoxic in humans. First, MDMA causes dose-related impairment of memory, a brain function mediated in part by serotonin. Memory impairment persists long after MDMA was last taken. Second, the cerebrospinal fluid of long-term MDMA users contains abnormally low concentrations of serotonin metabolites, suggesting a loss of serotonergic neurons. And third, using positron emission tomography to study former MDMA users, researchers demonstrated decreased binding of a ligand selective for the serotonin transporter, indicating damage to serotonergic neurons. In this study, reductions in ligand binding correlated with the extent of MDMA use, and not with the duration of abstinence.

MDMA can cause hyperthermia in association with dehydration, hyponatremia, and rhabdomyolysis. Treatment consists of rapid cooling, rehydration, and administering dantrolene [Dantrium], a drug that relaxes skeletal muscle, thereby reducing heat generation and the risk for rhabdomyolysis. The risk for hyperthermia and dehydration could be greatly reduced by providing ample fluids at dance parties known as "raves" and other events where MDMA is likely to be used.

Because of its amphetamine-like actions, MDMA can increase heart rate, blood pressure, and myocardial oxygen consumption. Remarkably, the increases in heart rate and blood pressure equal those produced by maximal doses of dobutamine, a powerful adrenergic agonist (see Chapter 13). Cardiovascular stimulation poses a special risk to users with heart disease.

Potential Medical Use

Despite its potential for adverse effects, MDMA also has the potential for therapeutic good, owing largely to its ability to decrease feelings of fear and defensiveness and promote feelings of love, trust, and compassion. Small clinical trials of MDMA for treatment of posttraumatic stress disorder and in patients with severe anxiety related to terminal cancer were promising, revealing reduced fear of death and decreased anxiety in patients taking MDMA.

INHALANTS

The inhalants are a diverse group of drugs that have one characteristic in common: administration by inhalation. These drugs can be divided into anesthetics and organic solvents.

Anesthetics

Provided that dosage is modest, anesthetics produce subjective effects similar to those of alcohol (euphoria, exhilaration, loss of inhibitions). The anesthetics that have been abused most are *nitrous oxide* ("laughing gas") and *ether.* One reason for the popularity of these drugs is ease of administration:

both agents can be used without exotic equipment. For nitrous oxide, ready availability also promotes use: small cylinders of the drug, marketed for aerating whipping cream, can be purchased without restriction.

Organic Solvents

A wide assortment of solvents have been inhaled to induce intoxication. These compounds include *toluene, gasoline, lighter fluid, paint thinner, nail-polish remover, benzene, acetone, chloroform,* and *model-airplane glue.* These agents are used primarily by children and the very poor—people who, because of age or insufficient funds, lack access to more conventional drugs of abuse. In recent years, use of inhalants by young children and teens has been rising.

Administration

Solvents are administered by three processes, referred to as "bagging," "huffing," and "sniffing." Bagging is performed by pouring solvent in a bag and inhaling the vapor. Huffing is performed by pouring the solvent on a rag and inhaling the vapor. Sniffing is performed by inhaling the solvent directly from its container.

Acute Pharmacologic Effects

The acute effects of organic solvents are somewhat like those of alcohol (euphoria, impaired judgment, slurred speech, flushing, CNS depression). In addition, these compounds can cause visual hallucinations and disorientation with respect to time and place. High doses can result in sudden death. Possible causes include anoxia, respiratory depression, vagal stimulation (which slows heart rate), and dysrhythmias.

Chronic Toxicity

Prolonged use is associated with multiple toxicities. For example, chloroform is toxic to the heart, liver, and kidneys, and toluene can cause severe brain damage and bone marrow depression. Many solvents can damage the heart; fatal dysrhythmias have occurred secondary to drug-induced heart block.

Management

Management of acute toxicity is strictly supportive. The objective is to stabilize vital signs. We have no antidotes for volatile solvents.

ANABOLIC STEROIDS

Many athletes take anabolic steroids (androgens) to enhance athletic performance. The principal benefit is increased muscle mass and strength. Because of the massive doses that are employed, the risk for adverse effects is substantial. With long-term steroid use, an addiction syndrome develops. Because of their abuse potential, most androgens are now classified as Schedule III drugs. The basic pharmacology of androgens and their abuse by athletes are discussed in Chapter 50.

UNIT IX

Drugs that Affect the Heart, Blood Vessels, Blood, and Blood Volume

CHAPTER 34

Review of Hemodynamics

Laura D. Rosenthal, DNP, ACNP, FAANP

Hemodynamics is the study of the movement of blood throughout the circulatory system, along with the regulatory mechanisms and driving forces involved. Concepts introduced here reappear throughout the chapters on cardiovascular drugs, so we urge you to review these now. Because this is a pharmacology text, and not a physiology text, discussion is limited to hemodynamic factors that have particular relevance to the actions of drugs.

OVERVIEW OF THE CIRCULATORY SYSTEM

The circulatory system has two primary functions: (1) delivery of oxygen, nutrients, hormones, electrolytes, and other essentials to cells and (2) removal of carbon dioxide and metabolic wastes from cells. In addition, the system helps fight infection.

The circulatory system has two major divisions: the *pulmonary circulation* and the *systemic circulation.* The pulmonary circulation delivers blood to the lungs. The systemic circulation delivers blood to all other organs and tissues. The systemic circulation is also known as the *greater circulation* or *peripheral circulation.*

Components of the Circulatory System

The circulatory system is composed of the *heart* and *blood vessels.* The heart is the pump that moves blood through the arterial tree. The blood vessels have several functions:

- *Arteries* transport blood under high pressure to tissues.
- *Arterioles* are control valves that regulate local blood flow.
- *Capillaries* are the sites for exchange of fluid, oxygen, carbon dioxide, nutrients, hormones, and wastes.
- *Venules* collect blood from the capillaries.
- *Veins* transport blood back to the heart. In addition, veins serve as a major reservoir for blood.

Arteries and veins differ with respect to distensibility (elasticity). Arteries are very muscular and hence do not readily stretch. As a result, large increases in arterial pressure (AP) cause only small increases in arterial diameter. Veins are much less muscular and hence are 6 to 10 times more distensible. As a result, small increases in venous pressure cause large increases in vessel diameter, which produce a large increase in venous volume.

Distribution of Blood

The adult circulatory system contains about 5 L of blood, which is distributed throughout the system. As indicated in Fig. 34.1, 9% is in the pulmonary circulation, 7% is in the heart, and 84% is in the systemic circulation. Within the systemic circulation, however, distribution is uneven: most (64%) of the blood is in veins, venules, and venous sinuses; the remaining 20% is in arteries (13%) and arterioles or capillaries (7%). The large volume of blood in the venous system serves as a reservoir.

What Makes Blood Flow?

Blood moves within vessels because the force that drives flow is greater than the resistance to flow. As shown in Fig. 34.2, the force that drives blood flow is the pressure gradient between two points in a vessel. Blood will flow from the point where pressure is higher toward the point where pressure is lower. Resistance to flow is determined by the diameter and length of the vessel and by blood viscosity. From a pharmacologic viewpoint, the most important determinant of resistance is vessel diameter: the larger the vessel, the smaller the resistance. Accordingly, when vessels dilate, resistance declines, causing blood flow to increase—and when vessels constrict, resistance rises, causing blood flow to decline. To maintain adequate flow when resistance rises, blood pressure must rise as well.

How Does Blood Get Back to the Heart?

As indicated in Fig. 34.3, pressure falls progressively as blood moves through the systemic circulation. Pressure is 120 mm Hg when blood enters the aorta, 30 mm Hg when blood enters capillaries, and only 18 mm Hg when blood leaves capillaries, and then drops to negative values (0 to −5 mm Hg) in the right

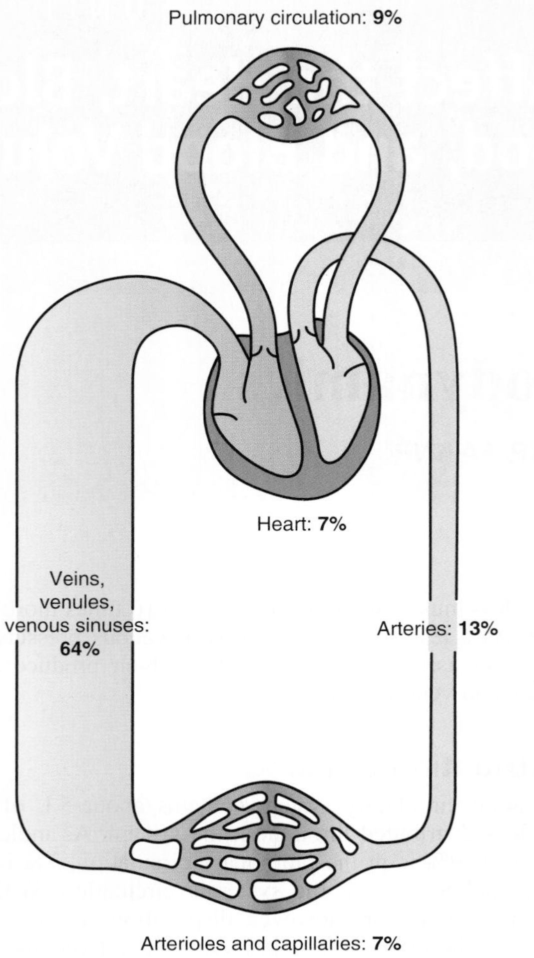

Figure 34.1 ■ Distribution of blood in the circulatory system.
A large percentage of the blood resides in the venous system.

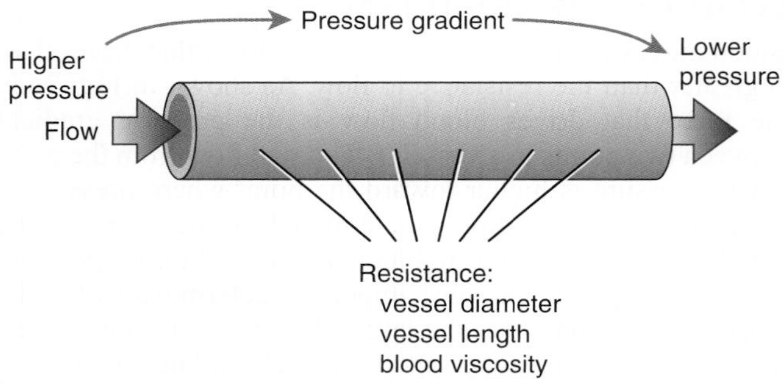

Figure 34.2 ■ Forces that promote and impede flow of blood.
Blood flows from the point of higher pressure toward the point of lower pressure. Resistance to flow is determined by vessel diameter, vessel length, and blood viscosity.

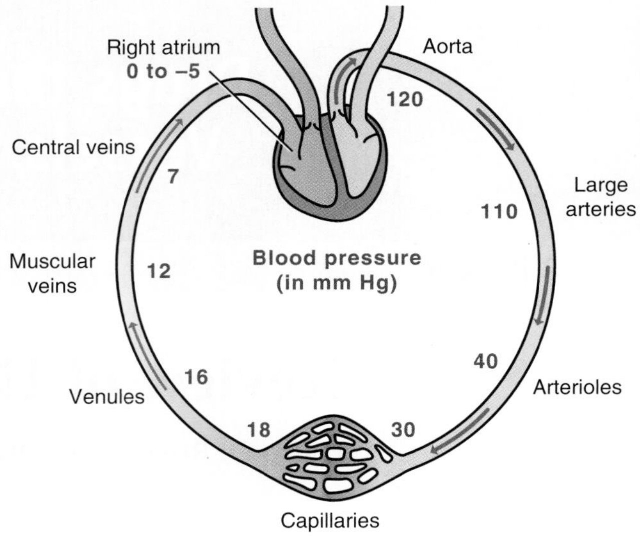

Figure 34.3 ■ Distribution of pressure within the systemic circulation.
Pressure is highest when blood leaves the left ventricle, falls to only 18 mm Hg as blood exits capillaries, and reaches negative values within the right atrium.

atrium. (Negative atrial pressure is generated by expansion of the chest during inspiration.)

Given that pressure is only 18 mm Hg when blood leaves capillaries, we must ask, "How does blood get back to the heart?" In addition to the small pressure head in venules, three mechanisms help ensure venous return. First, negative pressure in the right atrium helps "suck" blood toward the heart. Second, constriction of smooth muscle in the venous wall increases venous pressure, which helps drive blood toward the heart. Third, and most important, the combination of venous valves and skeletal muscle contraction constitutes an auxiliary "venous pump." As shown in Fig. 34.4A, the veins are equipped with a system of one-way valves. When skeletal muscles contract (Fig. 34.4B), venous blood is squeezed toward the heart—the only direction the valves will permit.

REGULATION OF CARDIAC OUTPUT

In the average adult, cardiac output is about 5 L/minute. Hence, every minute, the heart pumps the equivalent of all the blood in the body. In this section, we consider the major factors that determine how much blood the heart pumps.

Determinants of Cardiac Output

The basic equation for cardiac output is:

$$CO = HR \times SV$$

where CO is cardiac output, HR is heart rate, and SV is stroke volume. According to the equation, an increase in HR or SV will increase CO, whereas a decrease in HR or SV will decrease CO. For the average person, heart rate is about 70 beats/minute and stroke volume is about 70 mL. Multiplying these, we get 4.9 L/minute—the average value for CO.

Heart Rate

Heart rate is controlled primarily by the autonomic nervous system (ANS). Rate is increased by the sympathetic branch acting through beta$_1$-adrenergic receptors in the sinoatrial (SA) node. Rate is decreased by the parasympathetic branch

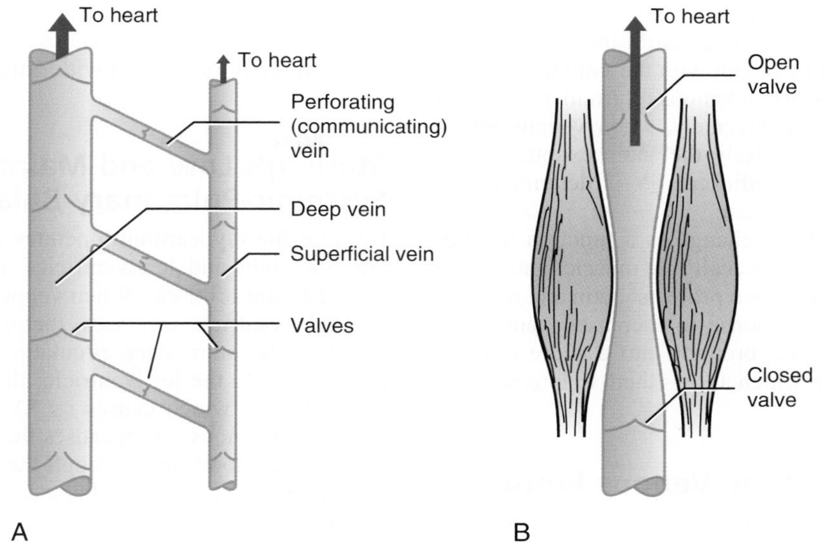

Figure 34.4 ■ Venous valves and the auxiliary venous "pump."
A, Veins and their one-way valves in the leg. The configuration of these valves ensures that blood will move toward the heart. **B,** Contraction of skeletal muscle pumps venous blood toward the heart.

acting through muscarinic receptors in the SA node. Parasympathetic impulses reach the heart through the vagus nerve.

Stroke Volume

Stroke volume is determined largely by three factors: (1) myocardial contractility, (2) cardiac afterload, and (3) cardiac preload. *Myocardial contractility* is defined as the force with which the ventricles contract. Contractility is determined primarily by the degree of cardiac dilation, which in turn is determined by the amount of venous return. The importance of venous return in regulating contractility and SV is discussed separately later. In addition to regulation by venous return, contractility can be increased by the sympathetic nervous system, acting through beta$_1$-adrenergic receptors in the myocardium.

Preload

Preload is formally defined as the amount of tension (stretch) applied to a muscle before contraction. In the heart, stretch is determined by ventricular filling pressure, that is, the *force of venous return:* the greater filling pressure is, the more the ventricles will stretch. Cardiac preload can be expressed as either *end-diastolic volume* or *end-diastolic pressure.* As discussed later, an increase in preload will increase SV, whereas a decrease in preload will reduce SV. Frequently, the terms *preload* and *force of venous return* are used interchangeably—although they are not truly equivalent.

Afterload

Afterload is formally defined as the load against which a muscle exerts its force (i.e., the load a muscle must overcome in order to contract). For the heart, afterload is the *arterial pressure* that the left ventricle must overcome to eject blood. Common sense tells us that, if afterload increases, SV will decrease. Conversely, if afterload falls, SV will rise. Cardiac afterload is determined primarily by the degree of peripheral resistance, which in turn is determined by constriction and dilation of arterioles. That is, when arterioles constrict, peripheral resistance rises, causing AP (afterload) to rise as well. Conversely, when arterioles dilate, peripheral resistance falls, causing AP to decline.

Starling's Law of the Heart

Starling's law states that the force of ventricular contraction is proportional to muscle fiber length (up to a point). Accordingly, as fiber length (ventricular diameter) increases, there is a corresponding increase in contractile force (Fig. 34.5).

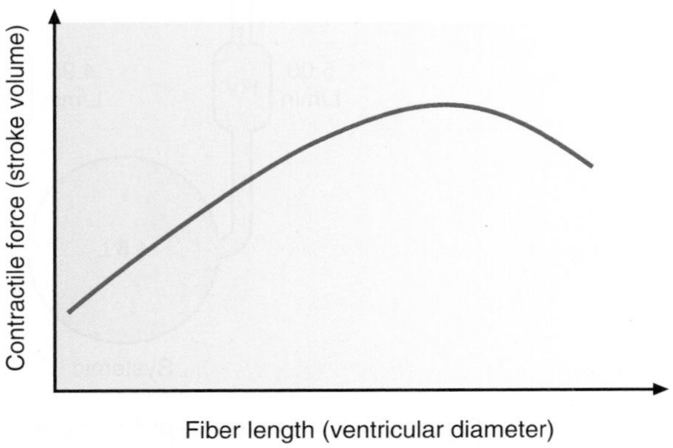

Figure 34.5 ■ The Starling relationship between myocardial fiber length and contractile force.
An increase in fiber length produces a corresponding increase in contractile force. Fiber length increases as the ventricles enlarge during filling. Increased contractile force is reflected by increased stroke volume.

Because of this built-in mechanism, when more blood enters the heart, more is pumped out. As a result, the healthy heart is able to precisely match its output with the volume of blood delivered by veins. That is, when venous return increases, CO increases correspondingly. Conversely, when venous return declines, CO declines to precisely the same extent. Hence, under normal, nonstressed conditions, SV is determined by factors that regulate venous return.

Why does contractile force change as a function of fiber length (ventricular diameter)? Recall that muscle contraction results from the interaction of two proteins: actin and myosin. As the heart stretches in response to increased ventricular filling, actin and myosin are brought into a more optimal alignment with each other, which allows them to interact with greater force.

Factors That Determine Venous Return

Having established that venous return is the primary determinant of SV (and hence CO), we need to understand the factors that determine venous return. With regard to pharmacology, the most important factor is *systemic filling pressure* (i.e., the force that returns blood to the heart). The normal value for filling pressure is 7 mm Hg. This value can be raised to 17 mm Hg by constriction of veins. Filling pressure can also be raised by an increase in blood volume. Conversely, filling pressure, and hence venous return, can be lowered by venodilation or by reducing blood volume. Blood volume and venous tone can both be altered with drugs.

In addition to systemic filling pressure, three other factors influence venous return: (1) the auxiliary muscle pumps discussed previously, (2) resistance to flow between peripheral vessels and the right atrium, and (3) right atrial pressure, elevation of which will impede venous return. None of these factors can be directly influenced with drugs.

Starling's Law and Maintenance of Systemic-Pulmonary Balance

Because the myocardium operates in accord with Starling's law, the right and left ventricles always pump exactly the same amount of blood. When venous return increases, SV of the right ventricle increases, thereby increasing delivery of blood to the pulmonary circulation, which in turn delivers more blood to the left ventricle; this increases filling of the left ventricle, which causes *its* SV to increase. Because an increase in venous return causes the output of *both* ventricles to increase, blood flow through the systemic and pulmonary circulations is always in balance, as long as the heart is healthy.

In the failing heart, Starling's law breaks down. That is, force of contraction no longer increases in proportion to increased ventricular filling. As a result, blood backs up behind the failing ventricle (Fig. 34.6). In this example, output of the left ventricle is 1% less than the output of the right ventricle, which causes blood to back up in the pulmonary circulation. In only 20 minutes, this small imbalance between left and right ventricular output shifts a liter of blood from the systemic circulation to the pulmonary circulation. In less than 40 minutes, death from pulmonary congestion would ensue. This example underscores the importance of systemic-pulmonary balance, and the critical role of Starling's mechanism in maintaining it.

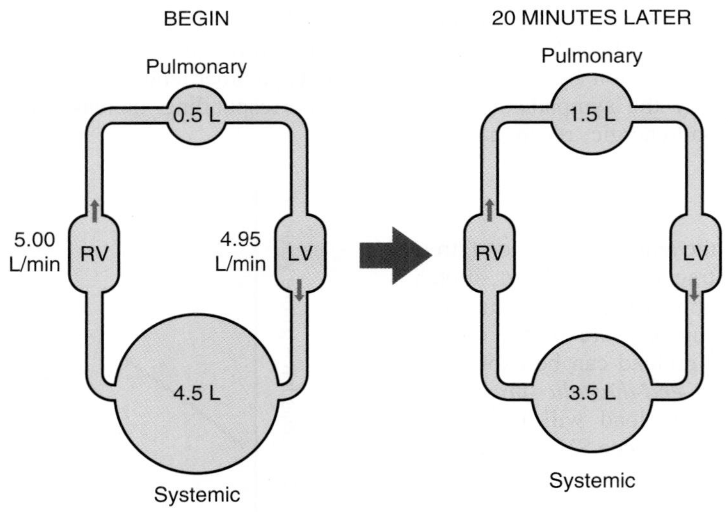

Figure 34.6 ▪ Systemic-pulmonary imbalance that develops when the output of the left and right ventricles is not identical.
In this example, the output of the left ventricle (LV) is 1% less than the output of the right ventricle (RV). Hence, while the right ventricle pumps 5000 mL/min, the left pumps only 4950 mL/min—50 mL/min less than the right side. This causes blood to back up in the pulmonary circulation. After 20 minutes, 1000 mL of blood has shifted from the systemic circulation to the pulmonary circulation. Death would ensue in less than 40 minutes. Numbers in the pulmonary and systemic circulations indicate volume of blood in liters.

REGULATION OF ARTERIAL PRESSURE

Arterial pressure is the driving force that moves blood through the arterial side of the systemic circulation. The general formula for AP is:

$$AP = PR \times CO$$

where AP is arterial pressure, PR is peripheral resistance, and CO is cardiac output. Accordingly, an increase in PR or CO will increase AP, whereas a decrease in PR or CO will decrease AP. Peripheral resistance is regulated primarily through constriction and dilation of arterioles. Cardiac output is regulated by the mechanisms discussed previously. Regulation of AP through processes that alter PR and CO is discussed later.

Overview of Control Systems

Under normal circumstances, AP is regulated primarily by three systems: the ANS, the renin-angiotensin-aldosterone system (RAAS), and the kidneys. These systems differ greatly with regard to timeframe of response. The ANS acts in two ways: (1) it responds rapidly (in seconds or minutes) to acute changes in blood pressure and (2) it provides steady-state control. The RAAS responds more slowly, taking hours or days to influence AP. The kidneys are responsible for long-term control and hence may take days or weeks to adjust AP.

Arterial pressure is also regulated by a fourth system: a family of natriuretic peptides. These peptides come into play primarily under conditions of volume overload.

Steady-State Control by the Autonomic Nervous System

The ANS regulates AP by adjusting CO and PR. Sympathetic tone to the heart increases HR and contractility, thereby increasing CO. In contrast, parasympathetic tone slows the heart, and thereby reduces CO. As discussed in Chapter 13, constriction of blood vessels is regulated exclusively by the sympathetic branch of the ANS; blood vessels have no parasympathetic innervation. Steady-state sympathetic tone provides a moderate level of vasoconstriction. The resultant resistance to blood flow maintains AP. Complete elimination of sympathetic tone would cause AP to fall by 50%.

Rapid Control by the Autonomic Nervous System: the Baroreceptor Reflex

The baroreceptor reflex serves to maintain AP at a predetermined level. When AP changes, the reflex immediately attempts to restore AP to the preset value.

The reflex works as follows. Baroreceptors (pressure sensors) in the aortic arch and carotid sinus sense AP and relay this information to the vasoconstrictor center of the medulla. When AP changes, the vasoconstrictor center compensates by sending appropriate instructions to arterioles, veins, and the heart. For example, when AP drops, the vasoconstrictor center causes (1) constriction of nearly all arterioles, thereby increasing PR; (2) constriction of veins, thereby increasing venous return; and (3) acceleration of HR (by increasing sympathetic impulses to the heart and decreasing parasympathetic impulses). The combined effect of these responses is to restore AP to the preset level. When AP rises too high, opposite responses occur: the reflex dilates arterioles and veins and slows the heart.

The baroreceptor reflex is poised for rapid action—but not for sustained action. When AP falls or rises, the reflex acts within seconds to restore the preset pressure. However, when AP *remains* elevated or lowered, the system resets to the new pressure within 1 to 2 days. After this, the system perceives the new (elevated or reduced) pressure as "normal" and ceases to respond.

Drugs that lower AP will trigger the baroreceptor reflex. For example, if we administer a drug that dilates arterioles, the resultant drop in PR will reduce AP, causing the baroreceptor reflex to activate. The most noticeable response is *reflex tachycardia.* The baroreceptor reflex can temporarily negate efforts to lower AP with drugs.

The Renin-Angiotensin-Aldosterone System

The RAAS supports AP by causing (1) constriction of arterioles and veins and (2) retention of water by the kidneys. Vasoconstriction is mediated by a hormone named *angiotensin II.* Water retention is mediated in part by *aldosterone* through retention of sodium. Responses develop in hours (vasoconstriction) to days (water retention). The RAAS and its role in controlling blood pressure are discussed in Chapter 36.

Renal Retention of Water

When AP remains low for a long time, the kidneys respond by retaining water, which in turn causes AP to rise. Pressure rises because fluid retention increases blood volume, which increases venous pressure, which increases venous return, which increases CO, which increases AP. Water retention is a mechanism for maintaining AP over long periods (weeks, months, years).

Reduction in AP causes the kidneys to retain water because low AP reduces renal blood flow (RBF), which in turn reduces glomerular filtration rate (GFR). Because less fluid is filtered, less urine is produced, and therefore more water is retained. Low AP activates the RAAS, causing levels of angiotensin II and aldosterone to rise. Angiotensin II causes constriction of renal blood vessels and thereby further decreases RBF and GFR. Aldosterone promotes renal retention of sodium, which causes water to be retained along with it.

Postural Hypotension

Postural hypotension, also known as *orthostatic hypotension,* is a reduction in AP that can occur when we move from a supine or seated position to an upright position. The cause of hypotension is pooling of blood in veins, which decreases venous return, which in turn decreases CO. Between 300 and 800 mL of blood can pool in veins when we stand, causing CO to drop by as much as 2 L/minute. When we stand, gravity increases the pressure that blood exerts on veins. Because veins are not very muscular, they are unable to retain their shape when pressure increases, and hence they stretch. The resultant increase in venous volume allows blood to pool.

Two mechanisms help overcome postural hypotension. One is the system of auxiliary venous pumps, which promote venous return. In fact, in healthy individuals, these auxiliary pumps usually prevent postural hypotension from occurring in the first place. When postural hypotension does occur, the baroreceptor reflex can restore AP by (1) constricting veins and arterioles and (2) increasing HR.

What would happen if we gave a drug that promoted dilation of veins (or prevented them from constricting)? In patients taking drugs that interfere with venoconstriction, postural hypotension is more intense and more prolonged. Hypotension is more intense because venous pooling is greater. Hypotension is more prolonged because there is no venoconstriction to help reverse venous pooling. As with drugs that reduce AP by dilating arterioles, drugs that reduce AP by relaxing veins can trigger the baroreceptor reflex and can thereby cause reflex tachycardia.

Natriuretic Peptides

Natriuretic peptides serve to protect the cardiovascular system in the event of volume overload, a condition that increases preload, and thereby increases CO and AP. Volume overload is caused by excessive retention of sodium and water. Natriuretic peptides work primarily by (1) reducing blood volume and (2) promoting dilation of arterioles and veins. Both actions lower AP.

The family of natriuretic peptides has three principal members: *atrial natriuretic peptide* (ANP), *B-* or *brain natriuretic peptide* (BNP), and *C-natriuretic peptide* (CNP). ANP is produced by myocytes of the atria; BNP is produced by myocytes of the ventricles (and to a lesser extent by cells in the brain, where BNP was discovered); and CNP is produced by cells of the vascular endothelium. When blood volume is excessive, all three peptides are released. (Release of ANP and BNP is triggered by stretching of the atria and ventricles, which occurs because of increased preload.)

ANP and BNP have similar actions. Both peptides reduce blood volume and increase venous capacitance and thereby reduce cardiac preload. Three processes are involved. First, ANP and BNP shift fluid from the vascular system to the extravascular compartment; the underlying mechanism is increased vascular permeability. Second, these peptides act on the kidney to cause diuresis (loss of water) and natriuresis (loss of sodium). Third, they promote dilation of arterioles and veins, in part by suppressing sympathetic outflow from the central nervous system. In addition to these actions, ANP and BNP help protect the heart during the early phase of heart failure by suppressing both the RAAS and sympathetic outflow and by inhibiting proliferation of myocytes. Although CNP shares some actions of ANP and BNP, its primary action is to promote vasodilation.

CHAPTER

35 Diuretics

Laura D. Rosenthal, DNP, ACNP, FAANP

Diuretics have two major applications: (1) treatment of hypertension and (2) mobilization of edematous fluid associated with heart failure, cirrhosis, or kidney disease. In addition, because of their ability to maintain urine flow, diuretics are used to prevent renal failure.

REVIEW OF RENAL ANATOMY AND PHYSIOLOGY

Understanding the diuretic drugs requires a basic knowledge of the anatomy and physiology of the kidney. Therefore let's review these topics before discussing the diuretics themselves.

Anatomy

The basic functional unit of the kidney is the *nephron.* As indicated in Fig. 35.1, the nephron has four functionally distinct regions: (1) the *glomerulus,* (2) the *proximal convoluted tubule,* (3) the *loop of Henle,* and (4a, 4b) the *distal convoluted tubule.* All nephrons are oriented within the kidney such that the upper portion of the loop of Henle is located in the renal cortex and the lower end of the loop descends toward the renal *medulla.* Without this orientation, the kidney could not produce concentrated urine.

In addition to the nephrons, the *collecting ducts* (the tubules into which the nephrons pour their contents) play a critical role in kidney function. The final segment of the distal convoluted tubule (4b) plus the collecting duct into which it empties (5) can be considered a single functional unit: the *distal nephron.*

Physiology

Overview of Kidney Functions

The kidney serves three basic functions: (1) cleansing of extracellular fluid (ECF) and maintenance of ECF volume and composition; (2) maintenance of acid-base balance; and (3) excretion of metabolic wastes and foreign substances (e.g., drugs, toxins). Of the three, maintenance of ECF volume and composition is the one that diuretics affect most.

The Three Basic Renal Processes

Effects of the kidney on ECF are the net result of three basic processes: (1) *filtration,* (2) *reabsorption,* and (3) *active secretion.* To cleanse the entire ECF, a huge volume of plasma must be filtered. Furthermore, to maintain homeostasis, practically everything that has been filtered must be reabsorbed—leaving behind only a small volume of urine for excretion.

Filtration

Filtration occurs at the *glomerulus* and is the first step in urine formation. Virtually all small molecules (electrolytes, amino acids, glucose, drugs, metabolic wastes) that are present in plasma undergo filtration. In contrast, cells and large molecules (lipids, proteins) remain behind in the blood. The most prevalent constituents of the filtrate are sodium ions and chloride ions. Bicarbonate ions and potassium ions are also present, but in smaller amounts.

The filtration capacity of the kidney is very large. Each minute the kidney produces 125 mL of filtrate, which adds up to 180 L/day. Because the total volume of ECF is only 12.5 L, the kidneys can process the equivalent of all the ECF in the body every 100 minutes. Hence, the ECF undergoes complete cleansing about 14 times each day.

Be aware that filtration is a *nonselective process* and therefore cannot regulate the composition of urine. Reabsorption and secretion—processes that display a significant degree of selectivity—are the primary determinants of what the urine ultimately contains. Of the two, reabsorption is by far the more important.

Reabsorption

More than 99% of the water, electrolytes, and nutrients that are filtered at the glomerulus undergo reabsorption. This conserves valuable constituents of the filtrate while allowing wastes to undergo excretion. Reabsorption of solutes (e.g., electrolytes, amino acids, glucose) takes place by way of *active transport.* Water then follows passively along the osmotic gradient created by solute reuptake. Specific sites along the nephron at which reabsorption takes place are discussed later. Diuretics work primarily by interfering with reabsorption.

Active Tubular Secretion

The kidney has two major kinds of "pumps" for active secretion. These pumps transport compounds from the plasma into the lumen of the nephron. One pump transports *organic acids,* and the other transports *organic bases.* Together, these pumps can promote the excretion of a wide assortment of molecules, including metabolic wastes, drugs, and toxins. The pumps for active secretion are located in the *proximal convoluted tubule.*

Processes of Reabsorption That Occur at Specific Sites Along the Nephron

Because most diuretics act by disrupting solute reabsorption, to understand the diuretics, we must first understand the major processes by which nephrons reabsorb filtered solutes. Because sodium and chloride ions are the predominant solutes

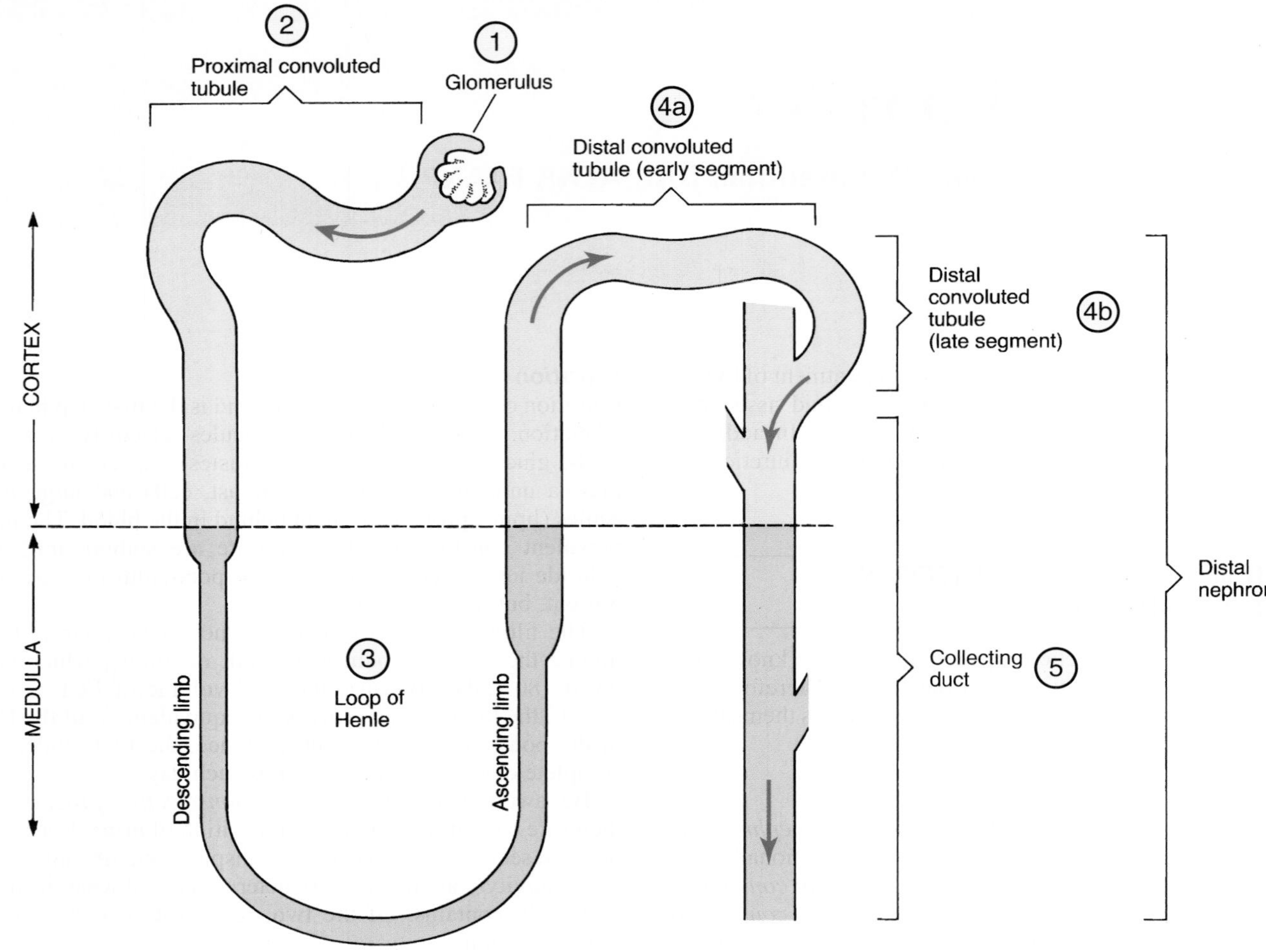

Figure 35.1 ■ Schematic representation of a nephron and collecting duct.

in the filtrate, reabsorption of these ions is of greatest interest. As we discuss reabsorption, numeric values are given for the percentage of solute reabsorbed at specific sites along the nephron. Bear in mind that these values are only approximate. Fig. 35.2 depicts the sites of sodium and chloride reabsorption, indicating the amount of reabsorption that occurs at each site.

Proximal Convoluted Tubule

The proximal convoluted tubule (PCT) has a high reabsorptive capacity. *A large fraction (about 65%) of filtered sodium and chloride is reabsorbed at the PCT.* In addition, essentially all of the bicarbonate and potassium in the filtrate is reabsorbed here. As sodium, chloride, and other solutes are actively reabsorbed, water follows passively. Because solutes and water are reabsorbed to an equal extent, the tubular urine remains isotonic (300 mOsm/L). By the time the filtrate leaves the PCT, sodium and chloride are the only solutes that remain in significant amounts.

Loop of Henle

The *descending limb* of the loop of Henle is freely permeable to water. Hence, as tubular urine moves down the loop and passes through the hypertonic environment of the renal medulla, water is drawn from the loop into the interstitial space. This process decreases the volume of the tubular urine and causes the urine to become concentrated (tonicity increases to about 1200 mOsm/L).

Within the thick segment of the *ascending limb* of the loop of Henle, about *20% of filtered sodium and chloride is reabsorbed* (see Fig. 35.2). Because, unlike the descending limb, the ascending limb is not permeable to water, water must remain in the loop as reabsorption of sodium and chloride takes place. This process causes the tonicity of the tubular urine to return to that of the original filtrate (300 mOsm/L).

Distal Convoluted Tubule (Early Segment)

About 10% of filtered sodium and chloride is reabsorbed in the early segment of the distal convoluted tubule. Water follows passively.

Distal Nephron: Late Distal Convoluted Tubule and Collecting Duct

The distal nephron is the site of two important processes. The first involves exchange of sodium for potassium and is under the influence of aldosterone. The second determines the final concentration of the urine and is regulated by antidiuretic hormone (ADH). Although sodium-potassium exchange is

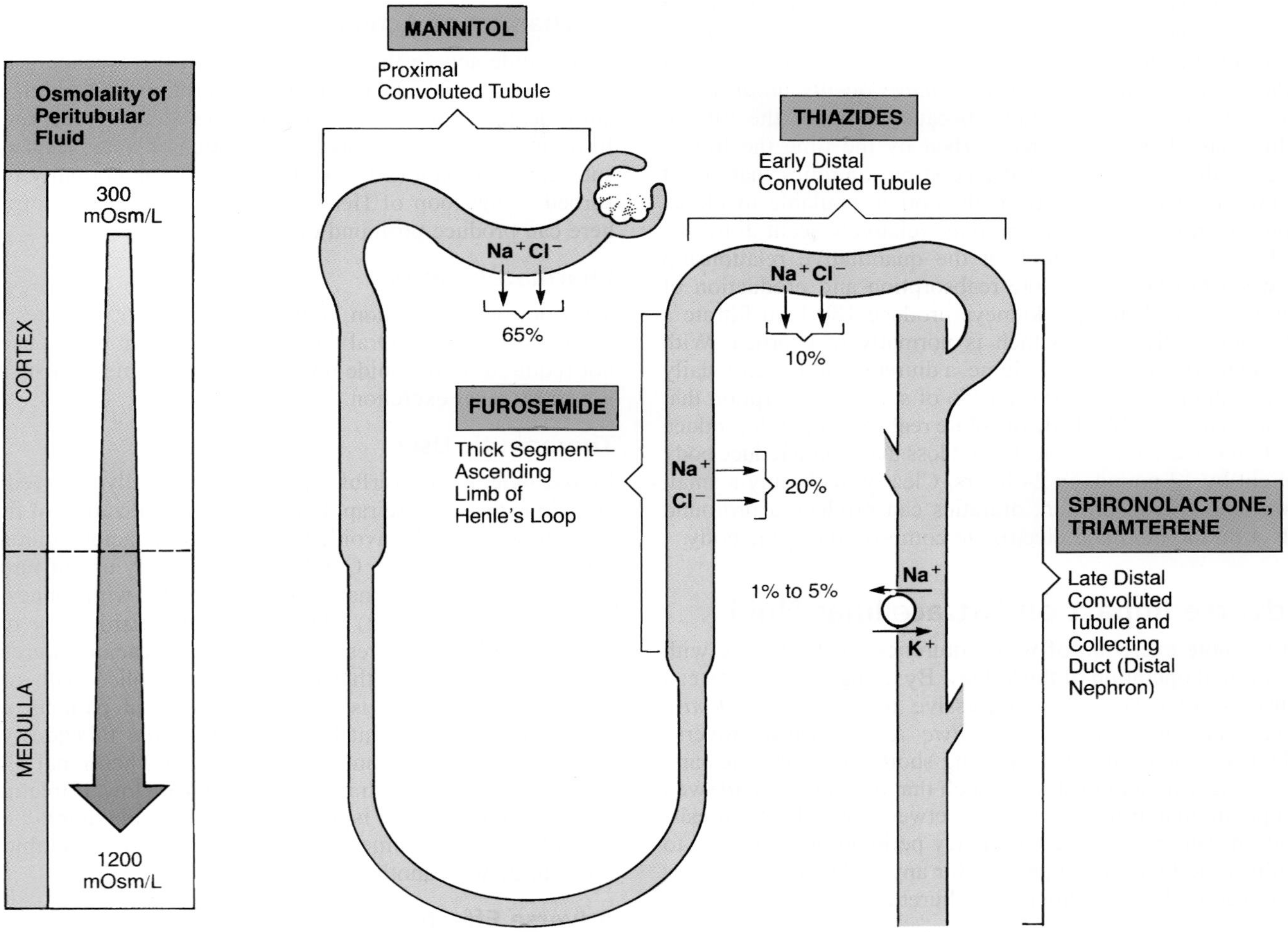

Figure 35.2 ▪ Schematic diagram of a nephron showing sites of sodium absorption and diuretic action. The percentages indicate how much of the filtered sodium and chloride are reabsorbed at each site.

discussed in more detail, we will not continue discussion of ADH because it has little to do with the actions of diuretics.

Sodium-Potassium Exchange

Aldosterone, the principal mineralocorticoid of the adrenal cortex, stimulates reabsorption of sodium from the distal nephron. At the same time, aldosterone causes potassium to be secreted. Although not directly coupled, these two processes—sodium retention and potassium excretion—can be viewed as an exchange mechanism. This exchange is shown in Fig. 35.2. Aldosterone promotes sodium-potassium exchange by stimulating cells of the distal nephron to synthesize more of the pumps responsible for sodium and potassium transport.

Prototype Drugs

DIURETICS

Loop Diuretic

Furosemide

Thiazide Diuretic

Hydrochlorothiazide

Potassium-Sparing Diuretics

Spironolactone
Triamterene

INTRODUCTION TO DIURETICS

How Diuretics Work

Most diuretics share the same basic mechanism of action: blockade of sodium and chloride reabsorption. By blocking the reabsorption of these prominent solutes, diuretics create osmotic pressure within the nephron that prevents the passive reabsorption of water. Hence diuretics cause water and solutes to be retained within the nephron and thereby promote the excretion of both.

The increase in urine flow that a diuretic produces is directly related to the amount of sodium and chloride reabsorption that it blocks. Accordingly, drugs that block solute reabsorption to the greatest degree produce the most profound diuresis. Because the amount of solute in the nephron becomes progressively smaller as filtrate flows from the proximal tubule to the collecting duct, *drugs that act early in the nephron have the opportunity to block the greatest amount of solute reabsorption. As a result, these agents produce the greatest diuresis.* Conversely, because most of the filtered solute has already been reabsorbed by the time the filtrate reaches the distal parts of the nephron, diuretics that act at distal sites have very little reabsorption available to block. Consequently, such agents produce relatively scant diuresis.

It is instructive to look at the quantitative relationship between blockade of solute reabsorption and production of diuresis. Recall that the kidneys produce 180 L of filtrate a day, practically all of which is normally reabsorbed. With filtrate production at this volume, a diuretic will increase daily urine output by 1.8 L for each 1% of solute reabsorption that is blocked. A 3% blockade of solute reabsorption will produce 5.4 L of urine a day—a rate of fluid loss that would reduce body weight by 12 pounds in 24 hours. Clearly, with only a small blockade of reabsorption, diuretics can produce a profound effect on the fluid and electrolyte composition of the body.

Adverse Impact on Extracellular Fluid

To promote excretion of water, diuretics must interfere with the normal operation of the kidney. By doing so, diuretics can cause *hypovolemia* (from excessive fluid loss), *acid-base imbalance,* and *altered electrolyte levels.* These adverse effects can be minimized by using short-acting diuretics and by timing drug administration such that the kidney is allowed to operate in a drug-free manner between periods of diuresis. Both measures will give the kidney periodic opportunities to readjust the ECF to compensate for any undesired alterations produced under the influence of diuretics.

Classification of Diuretics

There are four major categories of diuretic drugs: (1) *loop diuretics* (e.g., furosemide); (2) *thiazide diuretics* (e.g., hydrochlorothiazide); (3) *osmotic diuretics* (e.g., mannitol); and (4) *potassium-sparing diuretics.* The last group, the potassium-sparing agents, can be subdivided into *aldosterone antagonists* (e.g., spironolactone) and *nonaldosterone antagonists* (e.g., triamterene).

In addition to the four major categories of diuretics, there is a fifth group: the *carbonic anhydrase inhibitors.* Although the carbonic anhydrase inhibitors are classified as diuretics, these drugs are employed primarily to lower intraocular pressure (IOP) and not to increase urine production. Consequently, the carbonic anhydrase inhibitors are discussed in Chapter 84.

LOOP DIURETICS

The loop agents are the most effective diuretics available. These drugs produce more loss of fluid and electrolytes than any other diuretics. They are known as *loop diuretics* because their site of action is in the loop of Henle.

Furosemide

Furosemide [Lasix] is the most frequently prescribed loop diuretic and will serve as our prototype for the group.

Mechanism of Action

Furosemide acts in the thick segment of the ascending limb of the loop of Henle to block reabsorption of sodium and chloride (see Fig. 35.2). By blocking solute reabsorption, furosemide prevents passive reabsorption of water. Because a substantial amount (20%) of filtered NaCl is normally reabsorbed in the loop of Henle, interference with reabsorption here can produce profound diuresis.

Pharmacokinetics

With oral administration, diuresis begins in 60 minutes and persists for 8 hours. Oral therapy is used when rapid onset is not required. Furosemide undergoes hepatic metabolism followed by renal excretion.

Therapeutic Uses

Furosemide is a powerful drug that is generally reserved for situations that require rapid or massive mobilization of fluid. This drug should be avoided when less efficacious diuretics (thiazides) will suffice. Conditions that justify use of furosemide include (1) pulmonary edema associated with congestive heart failure (CHF); (2) edema of hepatic, cardiac, or renal origin that has been unresponsive to less efficacious diuretics; and (3) hypertension that cannot be controlled with other diuretics. Furosemide is especially useful in patients with severe renal impairment because, unlike the thiazides (see later), the drug can promote diuresis even when renal blood flow and glomerular filtration rate (GFR) are low. If treatment with furosemide alone is insufficient, a thiazide diuretic may be added to the regimen. There is no benefit to combining furosemide with another loop diuretic.

Adverse Effects

Hyponatremia, Hypochloremia, and Dehydration

Furosemide can produce excessive loss of sodium, chloride, and water. Severe dehydration can result. Signs of evolving dehydration include dry mouth, unusual thirst, and oliguria. Impending dehydration can also be anticipated from excessive loss of weight. If dehydration occurs, furosemide should be withheld.

The risk for dehydration and its sequelae can be minimized by initiating therapy with low doses, adjusting the dosage carefully, and monitoring weight loss every day.

Hypotension

Furosemide can cause a substantial drop in blood pressure. At least two mechanisms are involved: (1) loss of volume and (2) relaxation of venous smooth muscle, which reduces venous return to the heart. Signs of hypotension include

> **Patient Education**
>
> **HYPOTENSION**
>
> Patients should be taught to monitor their blood pressure and instructed to notify the prescriber if it drops substantially. Also, patients should be informed about symptoms of postural hypotension (dizziness, lightheadedness) and advised to sit or lie down if these occur. Patients should be taught that postural hypotension can be minimized by rising slowly.

dizziness, lightheadedness, and fainting. If blood pressure falls precipitously, furosemide should be discontinued. Because of the risk for hypotension, blood pressure should be monitored routinely.

Hypokalemia
Potassium is lost through increased secretion in the distal nephron. If serum potassium falls below 3.5 mEq/L, fatal dysrhythmias may result. As discussed later under "Drug Interactions," loss of potassium is of special concern for patients taking digoxin, a drug for heart failure. Hypokalemia can be minimized by consuming potassium-rich foods (e.g., dried fruits, nuts, spinach, potatoes, bananas), taking potassium supplements, or using a potassium-sparing diuretic.

Ototoxicity
Rarely, loop diuretics cause hearing impairment. With furosemide, deafness is transient. With ethacrynic acid (another loop diuretic), irreversible hearing loss may occur. The ability to impair hearing is unique to the loop diuretics. Diuretics in other classes are not ototoxic. Because of the risk for hearing loss, caution is needed when loop diuretics are used in combination with other ototoxic drugs (e.g., aminoglycoside antibiotics).

Hyperglycemia
Elevation of plasma glucose is a potential, albeit uncommon, complication of furosemide therapy. Hyperglycemia appears to result from inhibition of insulin release. Increased glycogenolysis and decreased glycogen synthesis may also contribute. When furosemide is taken by a diabetic patient, he or she should be especially diligent about monitoring blood glucose content.

Hyperuricemia
Elevation of plasma uric acid is a frequent side effect of treatment. For most patients, furosemide-induced hyperuricemia is asymptomatic. However, for patients predisposed to gout, elevation of uric acid may precipitate a gouty attack. Patients should be informed about symptoms of gout (tenderness or swelling in joints) and instructed to notify the prescriber if these develop.

Use in Pregnancy
When administered to pregnant laboratory animals, loop diuretics have caused maternal death, abortion, fetal resorption, and other adverse effects. There are no definitive studies on loop diuretics during human pregnancy. However, given the toxicity displayed in animals, prudence dictates that pregnant patients use these drugs only if absolutely required.

Impact on Lipids, Magnesium, and Calcium
Furosemide reduces high-density lipoprotein (HDL) cholesterol and raises low-density lipoprotein (LDL) cholesterol and triglycerides. Although these undesirable effects by themselves can increase the risk for coronary heart disease, they are more than balanced by the beneficial effects of the diuretic therapy on the heart. That is, despite adverse effects on lipids, loop diuretics reduce the risk for coronary mortality by 25%.

Furosemide increases urinary excretion of magnesium, posing a risk for magnesium deficiency. Symptoms include muscle weakness, tremor, twitching, and dysrhythmias.

Furosemide increases urinary excretion of calcium. This action has been exploited to treat hypercalcemia.

Drug Interactions

Digoxin
In the presence of low potassium, the risk for serious digoxin-induced toxicity (ventricular dysrhythmias) is greatly increased. Because loop diuretics promote potassium loss, use of these drugs in combination with digoxin can increase the dysrhythmia risk. This interaction is unfortunate in that most patients who take digoxin for heart failure must also take a diuretic. To reduce the risk for toxicity, potassium levels should be monitored routinely, and, when indicated, potassium supplements or a potassium-sparing diuretic should be given.

Ototoxic Drugs
The risk for furosemide-induced hearing loss is increased by concurrent use of other ototoxic drugs—especially aminoglycoside antibiotics (e.g., gentamicin). Accordingly, combined use of these drugs should be avoided.

Potassium-Sparing Diuretics
The potassium-sparing diuretics (e.g., spironolactone, triamterene) can help counterbalance the potassium-wasting effects of furosemide, thereby reducing the risk for hypokalemia.

Lithium
In patients with low sodium, excretion of lithium is reduced. Hence, by lowering sodium levels, furosemide can cause lithium to accumulate to toxic levels. Accordingly, lithium levels should be monitored, and, if they climb too high, lithium dosage should be reduced.

Antihypertensive Agents
The hypotensive effects of furosemide add with those of other hypotensive drugs. To avoid excessive reduction of blood pressure, patients may need to reduce or eliminate use of other hypotensive medications.

Nonsteroidal Antiinflammatory Drugs (NSAIDs)
Aspirin and other NSAIDs can attenuate the diuretic effects of furosemide. The mechanism appears to be inhibition of prostaglandin synthesis in the kidney. Part of the diuretic effect of furosemide results from increasing renal

PATIENT-CENTERED CARE ACROSS THE LIFE SPAN

Diuretics

Life Stage	Patient Care Concerns
Infants	See later entry, "Breastfeeding women"
Children/adolescents	Diuretics can be used safely in children, just in smaller doses. Side-effect profiles are similar to those in adults.
Pregnant women	Animal studies revealed that furosemide can cause maternal death, abortion, and fetal resorption. Risks and benefits must be considered for administration during pregnancy.
Breastfeeding women	Furosemide may decrease breast milk production through excessive diuresis. Data are lacking regarding transmission of drug from mother to infant through breast milk.
Older adults	Diuretics are the most common cause of adverse medication reactions and interactions in older adults. Monitor closely for dehydration and cardiac dysrhythmias.

blood flow, which is thought to occur through a prostaglandin-mediated process. By inhibiting prostaglandin synthesis, NSAIDs prevent the increase in renal blood flow and thereby partially blunt diuretic effects.

Other Loop Diuretics

In addition to furosemide, three other loop diuretics are available: ethacrynic acid [Edecrin], torsemide [Demadex], and bumetanide [Burinex ♣, generic only in United States]. All three are much like furosemide. They all promote diuresis by inhibiting sodium and chloride reabsorption in the thick ascending limb of the loop of Henle. All are approved for edema caused by heart failure, chronic renal disease, and cirrhosis, but only torsemide, like furosemide, is also approved for hypertension. All can cause ototoxicity, hypovolemia, hypotension, hypokalemia, hyperuricemia, hyperglycemia, and disruption of lipid metabolism—specifically, reduction of HDL cholesterol and elevation of LDL cholesterol and triglycerides. Lastly, they all share the same drug interactions: their effects can be blunted by NSAIDs, they can intensify ototoxicity caused by aminoglycosides, they can increase cardiotoxicity caused by digoxin, and they can cause lithium to accumulate to toxic levels. Routes, dosages, and time courses are shown in Table 35.1.

BLACK BOX WARNING: LOOP DIURETICS

All loop diuretics can cause profound diuresis with water and electrolyte depletion.

THIAZIDES AND RELATED DIURETICS

The thiazide diuretics have effects similar to those of the loop diuretics. Like the loop diuretics, thiazides increase renal excretion of sodium, chloride, potassium, and water. In addition, thiazides elevate plasma levels of uric acid and glucose. The principal difference between the thiazides and loop diuretics is that the maximal diuresis produced by the thiazides is considerably lower than the maximal diuresis produced by the loop diuretics. In addition, whereas loop diuretics can be effective even when urine flow is decreased, thiazides cannot.

Hydrochlorothiazide

Hydrochlorothiazide is the most widely used thiazide diuretic and will serve as our prototype for the group. Because of its use in hypertension, hydrochlorothiazide is one of our most widely used drugs.

Mechanism of Action

Hydrochlorothiazide promotes urine production by blocking the reabsorption of sodium and chloride in the *early segment of the distal convoluted tubule* (see Fig. 35.2). Retention of sodium and chloride in the nephron causes water to be retained as well, thereby producing an increased flow of urine. Because only 10% of filtered sodium and chloride is normally reabsorbed at the site where thiazides act, the maximal urine flow these drugs can produce is lower than with the loop diuretics.

The ability of thiazides to promote diuresis is dependent on adequate kidney function. These drugs are ineffective when GFR is low (less than 15–20 mL/min). Hence, in contrast to the loop diuretics, thiazides cannot be used to promote fluid loss in patients with severe renal impairment.

Pharmacokinetics

Diuresis begins about 2 hours after oral administration. Effects peak within 4 to 6 hours and may persist up to 12 hours. Most of the drug is excreted unchanged in the urine (Table 35.2).

TABLE 35.1 ▪ Loop Diuretics: Routes, Time Course, and Dosage

		Time Course			
Drug	Availability	Onset (min)	Duration (hr)	Dosage (mg)	Doses/Day
Furosemide [Lasix]	20-, 40-, 80-mg tablets 40 mg/5mL solution	Within 60	6–8	20–80	1–2
Ethacrynic acid [Edecrin]		Within 30	6–8	50–100	1–2
Bumetanide [Burinex ♣, generic only in United States]		30–60	4–6	0.5–2	1
Torsemide [Demadex]		Within 60	6–8	5–20	1

TABLE 35.2 ▪ Thiazides and Related Diuretics: Dosages and Time Course of Effects

			Time Course		
Generic Name	Trade Name	Availability	Onset (hr)	Duration (hr)	Optimal Oral Adult Dosage (mg/day)
THIAZIDES					
Chlorothiazide	Diuril	250-, 500-mg tablets	1–2	6–12	500–1000
Hydrochlorothiazide	Microzide	12.5-mg capsules 12.5-, 25-, 50-, 100-mg tablets	2	6–12	12.5–25
Methyclothiazide	Enduron	5-mg tablets	2	24	2.5–5
RELATED DRUGS					
Chlorthalidone	Thalitone	25-, 50-, 100-mg tablets	2	24–72	50–100
Indapamide	Lozide ♣, generic only in the United States	1.25-, 2.5-mg tablets	1–2	Up to 36	2.5–5
Metolazone	Zaroxolyn	2.5-, 5-, 10-mg tablets	1	12–24	2.5–20

Therapeutic Uses

Essential Hypertension

The primary indication for hydrochlorothiazide is hypertension, a condition for which thiazides are often drugs of first choice. For many hypertensive patients, blood pressure can be controlled with a thiazide alone, although many other patients require multiple-drug therapy. The role of thiazides in hypertension is discussed in Chapter 39.

Edema

Thiazides are preferred drugs for mobilizing edema associated with mild to moderate heart failure. They are also given to mobilize edema associated with hepatic or renal disease.

Protection Against Postmenopausal Osteoporosis

Thiazides promote tubular reabsorption of calcium and may thereby decrease the risk for osteoporosis in postmenopausal women. Here's how. Before menopause, estrogen from the ovaries acts on renal tubules to promote calcium reabsorption. When menopause occurs, estrogen levels drop, allowing renal excretion of calcium to increase. The resultant decrease in circulating calcium promotes mobilization of calcium from bone and thereby increases the risk for osteoporosis. Because thiazides promote renal calcium retention, they may counteract the calcium loss associated with menopause and may thereby help preserve bone integrity.

Adverse Effects

The adverse effects of thiazide diuretics are similar to those of the loop diuretics. In fact, with the exception that thiazides are not ototoxic, the adverse effects of the thiazides and loop diuretics are nearly identical.

Hyponatremia, Hypochloremia, and Dehydration

Loss of sodium, chloride, and water can lead to hyponatremia, hypochloremia, and dehydration. However, because the diuresis produced by thiazides is moderate, these drugs have a smaller effect on sodium, chloride, and water than do the loop diuretics. To evaluate fluid and electrolyte status, electrolyte levels should be determined periodically, and the patient should be weighed on a regular basis.

Hypokalemia

Like the loop diuretics, the thiazides can cause hypokalemia from excessive potassium excretion. As noted, potassium loss is of particular concern for patients taking digoxin. Potassium levels should be measured periodically, and, if serum potassium falls below 3.5 mEq/L, treatment with potassium supplements or a potassium-sparing diuretic should be instituted. Hypokalemia can be minimized by eating potassium-rich foods.

Hyperglycemia

Like the loop diuretics, the thiazides can elevate plasma levels of glucose. Significant hyperglycemia develops only in diabetic patients, who should be especially diligent about monitoring blood glucose. To maintain normal glucose levels, the diabetic patient may require larger doses of insulin or an oral hypoglycemic drug.

Hyperuricemia

The thiazides, like the loop diuretics, can cause retention of uric acid, thereby elevating plasma uric acid. Although hyperuricemia is usually asymptomatic, it may precipitate gouty arthritis in patients with a history of the disorder. Plasma levels of uric acid should be measured periodically.

Impact on Lipids and Magnesium

Thiazides can increase levels of LDL cholesterol, total cholesterol, and triglycerides. Thiazides increase excretion of magnesium, sometimes causing magnesium deficiency. Symptoms include muscle weakness, tremor, twitching, and dysrhythmias.

Drug Interactions

The important drug interactions of the thiazides are nearly identical to those of the loop diuretics. By promoting potassium loss, thiazides can increase the risk for toxicity from *digoxin.* By lowering blood pressure, thiazides can augment the effects of other *antihypertensive drugs.* By promoting sodium loss, thiazides can reduce renal excretion of *lithium,* thereby causing the drug to accumulate, possibly to toxic levels. *NSAIDs* may blunt the diuretic effects of thiazides. By counterbalancing the potassium-wasting effects of the thiazides, the *potassium-sparing diuretics* can help prevent excessive potassium loss. In contrast to the loop diuretics, the thiazides can be combined with *ototoxic agents* without an increased risk for hearing loss.

POTASSIUM-SPARING DIURETICS

The potassium-sparing diuretics can elicit two potentially useful responses. First, they produce a modest increase in urine production. Second, they produce a substantial *decrease in potassium excretion.* Because their diuretic effects are limited, the potassium-sparing drugs are rarely employed alone to promote diuresis. However, because of their marked ability to decrease potassium excretion, these drugs are often used to counteract potassium loss caused by thiazide and loop diuretics.

There are two subcategories of potassium-sparing diuretics: *aldosterone antagonists* and *nonaldosterone antagonists.* In the United States only one aldosterone antagonist—spironolactone—is used for diuresis. Two nonaldosterone antagonists—triamterene and amiloride—are currently employed.

Spironolactone

Mechanism of Action

Spironolactone [Aldactone] blocks the actions of aldosterone in the distal nephron. Because aldosterone acts to promote sodium uptake in exchange for potassium secretion (see Fig. 35.2), inhibition of aldosterone has the opposite effect: *retention of potassium and increased excretion of sodium.* The diuresis caused by spironolactone is scanty because most of the filtered sodium load has already been reabsorbed by the time the filtrate reaches the distal nephron.

The effects of spironolactone are delayed, taking up to 48 hours to develop (Table 35.3). Recall that aldosterone acts by stimulating cells of the distal nephron to synthesize the proteins required for sodium and potassium transport. By preventing aldosterone's action, spironolactone blocks the synthesis of *new* proteins, but does not stop existing transport proteins from doing their job. Therefore effects are not visible until the existing proteins complete their normal life cycle—a process that takes 1 or 2 days.

BLACK BOX WARNING: SPIROLONACTONE

Spironolactone has been shown to be tumorigenic in rats. Avoid unnecessary use.

TABLE 35.3 ▪ Potassium-Sparing Diuretics: Names, Dosages, and Time Course of Effects

Generic Name	Trade Name	Availability	Time Course		Usual Adult Dosage (mg/day)
			Onset (hr)	Duration (hr)	
Spironolactone	Aldactone	25-, 50-, 100-mg tablets	24–48	48–72	25–200
Triamterene	Dyrenium	50-, 100-mg capsules	2–4	12–16	50–300
Amiloride	Midamor	5-mg tablets	2	24	5–20

Therapeutic Uses

Hypertension and Edema

Spironolactone is used primarily for hypertension and edema. Although it can be employed alone, the drug is used most commonly in combination with a thiazide or loop diuretic. The purpose of spironolactone in these combinations is to counteract the potassium-wasting effects of the more powerful diuretics. Spironolactone also makes a small contribution to diuresis.

Heart Failure

In patients with severe heart failure, spironolactone reduces mortality and hospital admissions. Benefits derive from protective effects of aldosterone blockade in the heart and blood vessels (see Chapter 40).

Adverse Effects

Hyperkalemia

The potassium-sparing effects of spironolactone can result in hyperkalemia, a condition that can produce fatal dysrhythmias. Although hyperkalemia is most likely when spironolactone is used alone, it can also develop when spironolactone is used in conjunction with potassium-wasting agents (thiazides and loop diuretics). If serum potassium rises above 5 mEq/L, or if signs of hyperkalemia develop (e.g., abnormal heart rhythm), spironolactone should be discontinued and potassium intake restricted.

Endocrine Effects

Spironolactone is a steroid derivative with a structure similar to that of steroid hormones (e.g., progesterone, estradiol, testosterone). As a result, spironolactone can cause a variety of endocrine effects, including *gynecomastia, menstrual irregularities, impotence, hirsutism,* and *deepening of the voice.*

Benign and Malignant Tumors

When given long term to rats in doses 25 to 250 times those used in humans, spironolactone has caused benign adenomas of the thyroid and testes, malignant mammary tumors, and proliferative changes in the liver. The risk for tumors in humans from use of normal doses is unknown.

Drug Interactions

Thiazide and Loop Diuretics

Spironolactone is frequently combined with thiazide and loop diuretics. The goal is to counteract the potassium-wasting effects of the more powerful diuretic.

Agents That Raise Potassium Levels

Because of the risk for hyperkalemia, caution must be employed when combining spironolactone with potassium supplements, salt substitutes (which contain potassium chloride), or another potassium-sparing diuretic. In addition, three groups of drugs—angiotensin-converting enzyme (ACE) inhibitors, angiotensin receptor blockers, and direct renin inhibitors—can elevate potassium levels (by suppressing aldosterone secretion) and hence should be combined with spironolactone only when clearly necessary.

Triamterene

Mechanism of Action

Like spironolactone, triamterene [Dyrenium] disrupts sodium-potassium exchange in the distal nephron. However, in contrast to spironolactone, which reduces ion transport *indirectly* through blockade of aldosterone, triamterene is a *direct inhibitor of the exchange mechanism itself.* The net effect of inhibition is a decrease in sodium reabsorption and a reduction in potassium secretion. Hence sodium excretion is increased while potassium is conserved. Because it inhibits ion transport directly, triamterene acts much more quickly than spironolactone. Initial responses develop in hours, compared with days for spironolactone. As with spironolactone, diuresis with triamterene is minimal.

Therapeutic Uses

Triamterene can be used alone or in combination with other diuretics to treat *hypertension* and *edema.* When used alone, triamterene produces mild diuresis. When combined with other diuretics (e.g., furosemide, hydrochlorothiazide), triamterene augments diuresis and helps counteract the potassium-wasting effects of the more powerful diuretic. It is the latter effect for which triamterene is principally employed.

Adverse Effects

Hyperkalemia

Excessive potassium accumulation is the most significant adverse effect. Hyperkalemia is most likely when triamterene is used alone but can also occur when the drug is combined with thiazides or loop diuretics. Caution should be employed when triamterene is used in conjunction with another potassium-sparing diuretic or with potassium supplements or salt substitutes. In addition, caution is needed if the drug is combined with an ACE inhibitor, angiotensin receptor blocker, or direct renin inhibitor.

BLACK BOX WARNING: TRIAMTERENE AND AMILORIDE

Triamterene and amiloride carry a risk for hyperkalemia that is potentially fatal if uncorrected. Monitor potassium levels at treatment start, at dose change, and during illness affecting renal function.

Other Adverse Effects

Relatively common side effects include *nausea, vomiting, leg cramps,* and *dizziness.* Blood dyscrasias occur rarely.

Amiloride

Pharmacologic Properties

Amiloride has actions similar to those of triamterene. Both drugs inhibit potassium loss by direct blockade of sodium-potassium exchange in the distal nephron. Also, both drugs produce only modest diuresis. Although it can be employed alone as a diuretic, amiloride is used primarily to counteract potassium loss caused by more powerful diuretics (thiazides, loop diuretics). The major adverse effect is hyperkalemia. Accordingly, concurrent use of other potassium-sparing diuretics or potassium supplements must be monitored closely. Caution is needed if the drug is combined with an ACE inhibitor, angiotensin receptor blocker, or direct renin inhibitor.

CHAPTER

36 Drugs Acting on the Renin-Angiotensin-Aldosterone System

Laura D. Rosenthal, DNP, ACNP, FAANP

In this chapter we consider four families of drugs: angiotensin-converting enzyme (ACE) inhibitors, angiotensin II receptor blockers (ARBs), direct renin inhibitors (DRIs), and aldosterone antagonists. With all four groups, effects result from interfering with the renin-angiotensin-aldosterone system (RAAS). The ACE inhibitors, available since the 1980s, have established roles in the treatment of hypertension, heart failure, and diabetic nephropathy; in addition, these drugs are indicated for myocardial infarction (MI) and prevention of cardiovascular events in patients at risk. Indications for ARBs are limited to hypertension, heart failure, diabetic nephropathy, and prevention of cardiovascular events in patients at risk. The aldosterone antagonist eplerenone has only two indications: hypertension and heart failure; spironolactone is also used to prevent diuretic-induced hypokalemia and treat hyperaldosteronism. Current indications for DRIs are limited to hypertension. We begin by reviewing the physiology of the RAAS, and then we discuss the drugs that affect it.

PHYSIOLOGY OF THE RENIN-ANGIOTENSIN-ALDOSTERONE SYSTEM

The RAAS plays an important role in regulating blood pressure, blood volume, and fluid and electrolyte balance. In addition, the system appears to mediate certain pathophysiologic changes associated with hypertension, heart failure, and MI. The RAAS exerts its effects through angiotensin II and aldosterone.

Types of Angiotensin

Before considering the physiology of the RAAS, we need to introduce the angiotensin family, which consists of angiotensin I, angiotensin II, and angiotensin III. All three compounds are small polypeptides. Angiotensin I is the precursor of angiotensin II (Fig. 36.1) and has only weak biologic activity. In contrast, angiotensin II has strong biologic activity. Angiotensin III, which is formed by degradation of angiotensin II, has moderate biologic activity.

Actions of Angiotensin II

Angiotensin II participates in all processes regulated by the RAAS. The most prominent actions of angiotensin II are vasoconstriction and stimulation of aldosterone release. Both actions raise blood pressure. In addition, angiotensin II (as well as aldosterone) can act on the heart and blood vessels to cause pathologic changes in their structure and function.

Vasoconstriction

Angiotensin II is a powerful vasoconstrictor. The compound acts directly on vascular smooth muscle (VSM) to cause contraction. Vasoconstriction is prominent in arterioles and less so in veins. As a result of angiotensin-induced vasoconstriction, blood pressure rises. In addition to its direct action on blood vessels, angiotensin II can cause vasoconstriction indirectly by acting on (1) sympathetic neurons to promote norepinephrine release, (2) the adrenal medulla to promote epinephrine release, and (3) the central nervous system to increase sympathetic outflow to blood vessels.

Release of Aldosterone

Angiotensin II acts on the adrenal cortex to promote synthesis and secretion of aldosterone, whose actions are discussed later. The adrenal cortex is highly sensitive to angiotensin II, and hence angiotensin II can stimulate aldosterone release even when angiotensin II levels are too low to induce vasoconstriction. Aldosterone secretion is enhanced when sodium levels are low and when potassium levels are high.

Alteration of Cardiac and Vascular Structure

Angiotensin II may cause pathologic structural changes in the heart and blood vessels. In the heart, it may cause *hypertrophy* and *remodeling*. In hypertension, angiotensin II may be responsible for increasing the thickness of blood vessel walls. In atherosclerosis, it may be responsible for thickening the intimal surface of blood vessels. And in heart failure and MI, it may be responsible for causing cardiac hypertrophy and fibrosis. Known effects of angiotensin II that could underlie these pathologic changes include the following:

- Increased migration, proliferation, and hypertrophy of VSM cells
- Increased production of extracellular matrix by VSM cells
- Hypertrophy of cardiac myocytes
- Increased production of extracellular matrix by cardiac fibroblasts

Actions of Aldosterone

Regulation of Blood Volume and Blood Pressure

After being released from the adrenal cortex, aldosterone acts on distal tubules of the kidney to cause retention of sodium

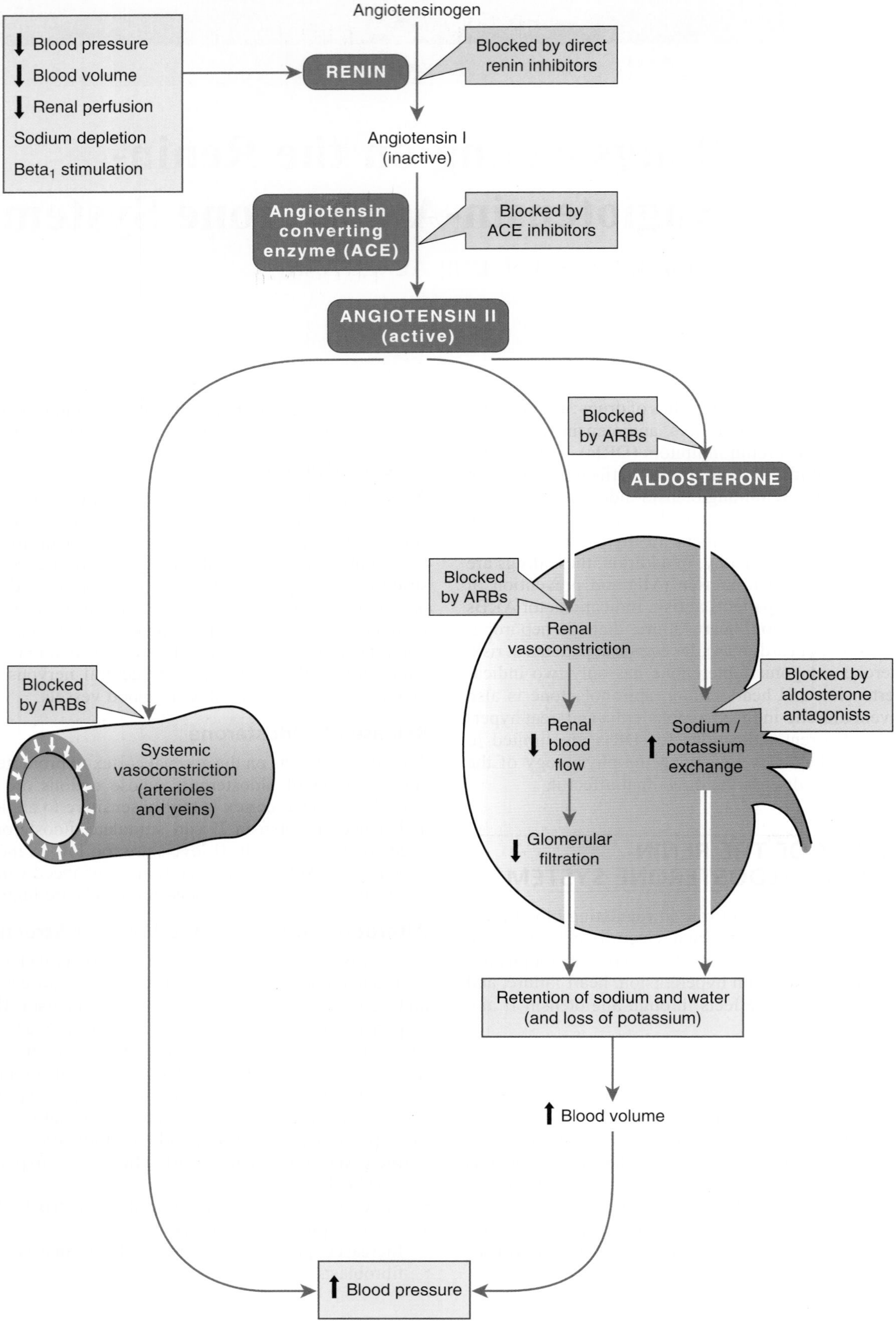

Figure 36.1 ■ Regulation of blood pressure by the renin-angiotensin-aldosterone system.

In addition to the mechanisms depicted, angiotensin II can raise blood pressure by (1) acting on the distal nephron to promote reabsorption of sodium and (2) increasing vasoconstriction by three mechanisms: promoting release of norepinephrine from sympathetic nerves; promoting release of epinephrine from the adrenal medulla; and acting in the central nervous system to increase sympathetic outflow to blood vessels. (ARBs, angiotensin receptor blockers.)

and excretion of potassium and hydrogen. Because retention of sodium causes water to be retained as well, aldosterone increases blood volume, which causes blood pressure to rise.

Pathologic Cardiovascular Effects

Until recently, knowledge of aldosterone's actions was limited to effects on the kidney. Now, however, we know that aldosterone can cause more harmful effects. Like angiotensin II, aldosterone can promote cardiac remodeling and fibrosis. In addition, aldosterone can activate the sympathetic nervous system and suppress uptake of norepinephrine in the heart, thereby predisposing the heart to dysrhythmias. Also, aldosterone can promote vascular fibrosis (which decreases arterial compliance), and it can disrupt the baroreceptor reflex. These adverse effects appear to be limited to states such as heart failure, in which levels of aldosterone can be extremely high.

Formation of Angiotensin II by Renin and Angiotensin-Converting Enzyme

Angiotensin II is formed through two sequential reactions. The first is catalyzed by renin, the second by ACE.

Renin

Renin catalyzes the formation of *angiotensin I* from *angiotensinogen.* This reaction is the rate-limiting step in angiotensin II formation. Renin is produced by juxtaglomerular cells of the kidney and undergoes controlled release into the bloodstream, where it cleaves angiotensinogen into angiotensin I.

Regulation of Renin Release

Because renin catalyzes the rate-limiting step in angiotensin II formation, and because renin must be released into the blood in order to act, the factors that regulate renin release regulate the rate of angiotensin II formation.

Release of renin can be triggered by multiple factors (see Fig. 36.1). Release *increases* in response to a *decline* in blood pressure, blood volume, plasma sodium content, or renal perfusion pressure. Reduced renal perfusion pressure is an especially important stimulus for renin release and can occur in response to (1) stenosis of the renal arteries, (2) reduced systemic blood pressure, and (3) reduced plasma volume (brought on by dehydration, hemorrhage, or chronic sodium depletion). For the most part, these factors increase renin release through effects exerted locally in the kidney. However, some of these factors may also promote renin release through activation of the sympathetic nervous system. (Sympathetic nerves increase secretion of renin by causing stimulation of $beta_1$-adrenergic receptors on juxtaglomerular cells.)

Release of renin is *suppressed* by factors opposite to those that cause release. That is, renin secretion is inhibited by elevation of blood pressure, blood volume, and plasma sodium content. Hence, as blood pressure, blood volume, and plasma sodium content increase in response to renin release, further release of renin is suppressed. In this regard, we can view release of renin as being regulated by a classical negative feedback loop.

Angiotensin-Converting Enzyme (Kinase II)

ACE catalyzes the conversion of angiotensin I (inactive) into angiotensin II (highly active). ACE is located on the luminal surface of all blood vessels. The vasculature of the lungs is especially rich in the enzyme. Because ACE is abundant, conversion of angiotensin I into angiotensin II occurs almost instantaneously after angiotensin I has been formed. ACE is a relatively nonspecific enzyme that can act on a variety of substrates in addition to angiotensin I.

Nomenclature regarding ACE can be confusing and requires comment. As just noted, ACE can act on several substrates. When the substrate is angiotensin I, we refer to the enzyme as ACE. However, when the enzyme is acting on other substrates, we refer to it by different names. Of importance to us, when the substrate is a hormone known as *bradykinin,* we refer to the enzyme as *kinase II.* So, please remember, whether we call it ACE or kinase II, we're talking about the same enzyme.

Regulation of Blood Pressure by the Renin-Angiotensin-Aldosterone System

The RAAS is poised to help regulate blood pressure. Factors that lower blood pressure turn the RAAS on; factors that raise blood pressure turn it off. However, although the RAAS does indeed contribute to blood pressure control, its role in *normovolemic, sodium-replete* individuals is only modest. In contrast, the system can be a major factor in maintaining blood pressure in the presence of *hemorrhage, dehydration,* or *sodium depletion.*

The RAAS, acting through angiotensin II, raises blood pressure through two basic processes: vasoconstriction and renal retention of water and sodium. Vasoconstriction raises blood pressure by increasing total peripheral resistance;

PATIENT-CENTERED CARE ACROSS THE LIFE SPAN

RAAS Inhibitors

Life Stage	Patient Care Concerns
Infants	Captopril and enalapril have been used in infants safely for management of hypertension (HTN).
Children/adolescents	Some ACE inhibitors and ARBs are approved for use in children older than 6 years for treatment of HTN.
Pregnant women	Animal studies revealed that drugs that block the RAAS should be avoided in pregnancy, especially in the second and third trimesters. ACE inhibitors, ARBs, and DRIs are classified in FDA Pregnancy Risk Category D.
Breastfeeding women	Data are lacking regarding effects on the infant when breastfeeding. Caution is advised.
Older adults	The SCOPE and LIFE trials revealed a 25% decrease in stroke in patients 55 to 80 years old using losartan compared with atenolol. A 20% decreased risk for new-onset diabetes was seen with candesartan compared with placebo.

retention of water and sodium raises blood pressure by increasing blood volume. Vasoconstriction occurs within minutes to hours of activating the system and hence can raise blood pressure quickly. In contrast, days, weeks, or even months are required for the kidney to raise blood pressure by increasing blood volume.

Angiotensin II acts in two ways to promote renal retention of water. First, by constricting renal blood vessels, angiotensin II reduces renal blood flow and thereby reduces glomerular filtration. Second, angiotensin II stimulates release of aldosterone from the adrenal cortex. Aldosterone then acts on renal tubules to promote retention of sodium and water and excretion of potassium.

Tissue (Local) Angiotensin II Production

In addition to the traditional RAAS that we've been discussing, in which angiotensin II is produced in the blood and then carried to target tissues, angiotensin II is produced in individual tissues. This permits discrete, local effects of angiotensin II independent of the main system. Interference with local production of angiotensin II may underlie some effects of the ACE inhibitors.

It is important to note that some angiotensin II is produced by pathways that *do not involve* ACE. As a result, drugs that inhibit ACE cannot completely block angiotensin II production.

Prototype Drugs

DRUGS ACTING ON THE RAAS SYSTEM

Angiotensin-Converting Enzyme (ACE) Inhibitor
Captopril

Angiotensin II Receptor Blocker
Losartan

Direct Renin Inhibitor
Aliskiren

Aldosterone Antagonist
Eplerenone

ANGIOTENSIN-CONVERTING ENZYME INHIBITORS

The ACE inhibitors are important drugs for *treating* hypertension, heart failure, diabetic nephropathy, and MI. In addition, they are used to *prevent* adverse cardiovascular events in patients at risk. Their most prominent adverse effects are cough, angioedema, first-dose hypotension, and hyperkalemia. For all of these agents, beneficial effects result largely from suppressing formation of angiotensin II. Because the similarities among ACE inhibitors are much more striking than their differences, we will discuss these drugs as a group, rather than selecting a prototype to represent them.

Mechanism of Action and Overview of Pharmacologic Effects

As shown in Fig. 36.2, ACE inhibitors produce their beneficial effects and adverse effects by (1) reducing levels of angiotensin II (through inhibition of ACE) and (2) increasing levels of bradykinin (through inhibition of kinase II). By reducing levels of angiotensin II, ACE inhibitors can dilate blood vessels (primarily arterioles and to a lesser extent veins), reduce blood volume (through effects on the kidney), and, importantly, prevent or reverse pathologic changes in the heart and blood vessels mediated by angiotensin II and aldosterone. Inhibition of ACE can also cause hyperkalemia and fetal injury. Elevation of bradykinin causes vasodilation (secondary to increased production of prostaglandins and nitric oxide) and can also promote cough and angioedema.

Pharmacokinetics

Regarding pharmacokinetics, the following generalizations apply:

- Nearly all ACE inhibitors are administered *orally.* The only exception is enalaprilat (the active form of enalapril), which is given intravenously.
- Except for captopril and moexipril, all oral ACE inhibitors can be administered with food.

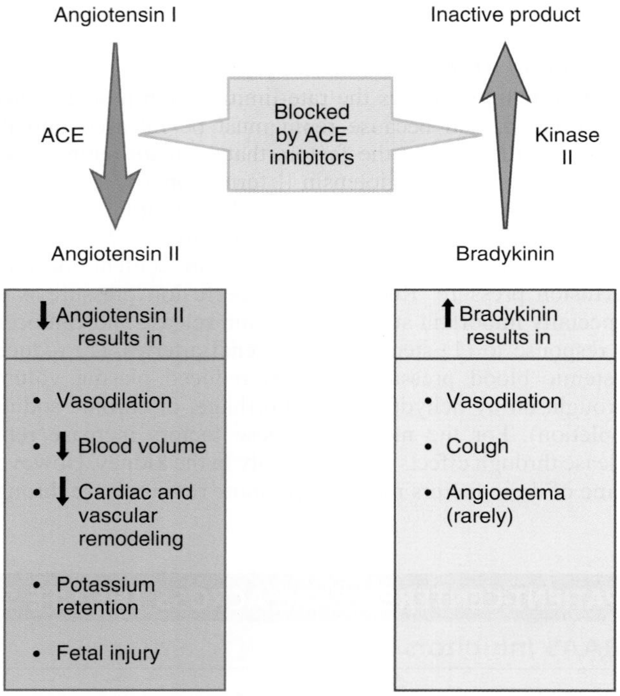

Figure 36.2 ■ Overview of ACE inhibitor actions and pharmacologic effects.
Angiotensin-converting enzyme (ACE) and *kinase II* are two names for the same enzyme. When angiotensin II is the substrate, we call the enzyme ACE; when bradykinin is the substrate, we call it kinase II. Inhibition of this enzyme decreases *production* of angiotensin II (thereby *reducing* angiotensin II levels) and decreases *breakdown* of bradykinin (thereby *increasing* bradykinin levels).

- With the exception of captopril, all ACE inhibitors have prolonged half-lives and hence can be administered just once or twice a day. Captopril is administered 2 or 3 times a day.
- With the exception of lisinopril, all ACE inhibitors are *prodrugs* that must undergo conversion to their active form in the small intestine and liver. Lisinopril is active as given.
- All ACE inhibitors are *excreted by the kidneys.* As a result, nearly all can accumulate to dangerous levels in patients with kidney disease and hence *dosages must be reduced in these patients.* Only one agent—fosinopril—does not require a dosage reduction.

Therapeutic Uses

When the ACE inhibitors were introduced, their only indication was hypertension. Today, they are also used for heart failure, acute MI, left ventricular (LV) dysfunction, and diabetic and nondiabetic nephropathy. In addition, they can help prevent MI, stroke, and death in patients at high risk for cardiovascular events. It should be noted that no single ACE inhibitor is approved for all of these conditions (Table 36.1). However, given that all ACE inhibitors are very similar, it seems likely that all may produce similar benefits.

Hypertension

All ACE inhibitors are approved for hypertension. These drugs are especially effective against malignant hypertension and hypertension secondary to renal arterial stenosis. They are also useful against essential hypertension of mild to moderate intensity—although maximal benefits may take several weeks to develop.

In patients with essential hypertension, the mechanism underlying blood pressure reduction is not fully understood. *Initial* responses are proportional to circulating angiotensin II levels and are clearly related to reduced formation of that compound. (By lowering angiotensin II levels, ACE inhibitors dilate blood vessels and reduce blood volume; both actions help lower blood pressure.) However, with *prolonged* therapy, blood pressure often undergoes additional decline. During this phase, there is no relationship between reductions in blood pressure and reductions in *circulating* angiotensin II. It may

TABLE 36.1 ▪ ACE Inhibitors: Approved Indications and Adult Dosages

Generic Name	Trade Name	Approved Indications	Availability	Starting Dosage*	Usual Maintenance Dosage*
Benazepril	Lotensin	Hypertension	5-, 10-, 20-, 40-mg tablets	10 mg once/day	20–80 mg/day in 1 or 2 doses
Captopril	Capoten	Hypertension	12.5-, 25-, 50-, 100-mg tablets	25 mg 2 or 3 times/day	25–50 mg 2 or 3 times/day
		Heart failure		6.25–12.5 mg 3 times/day	50 mg 3 times/day
		LVD after MI		12.5 mg 3 times/day	50 mg 3 times/day
		Diabetic nephropathy		25 mg 3 times/day	25 mg 3 times/day
Enalapril	Vasotec	Hypertension	2.5-, 5-, 10-, 20-mg tablets	2.5–5 mg once/day	10–40 mg/day in 1 or 2 doses
		Heart failure		2.5 mg twice/day	10–20 mg twice/day
		Asymptomatic LVD		2.5 mg twice/day	10 mg twice/day
Fosinopril	Monopril	Hypertension	10-, 20-, 40-mg tablets	10 mg once/day	20–40 mg/day in 1 or 2 doses
		Heart failure		5–10 mg once/day	20–40 mg once/day
Lisinopril	Prinivil, Zestril	Hypertension	2.5-, 5-, 10-, 20-, 30-, 40-mg tablets	10 mg once/day	10–40 mg once/day
		Heart failure		2.5–5 mg once/day	20–40 mg once/day
		Acute MI		5 mg once/day	10 mg once/day
Moexipril	Univasc	Hypertension	7.5-, 15-mg tablets	7.5 mg once/day	7.5–30 mg/day in 1 or 2 doses
Perindopril	Aceon, Coversyl ♣	Hypertension	2-, 4-, 8-mg tablets	4 mg once/day	4–8 mg/day in 1 or 2 doses
		Stable CAD		4 mg once/day	8 mg once/day
Quinapril	Accupril	Hypertension	5-, 10-, 20-, 40-mg tablets	10–20 mg/day	20–80 mg/day in 1 or 2 doses
		Heart failure		5 mg twice/day	20–40 mg twice/day
Ramipril	Altace	Hypertension	1.25-, 2.5-, 5-, 10-mg capsules	2.5 mg once/day	2.5–20 mg/day in 1 or 2 doses
		Heart failure after MI		1.25–2.5 mg twice/day	5 mg twice/day
		Prevention of MI, stroke, and death in people at high risk for CVD		2.5 mg/day for 1 wk	10 mg once/day
Trandolapril	Mavik	Hypertension	1-, 2-, 4-mg tablets	1 mg once/day	2–4 mg once/day
		Heart failure after MI		1 mg once/day	4 mg once/day
		LVD after MI		1 mg once/day	4 mg once/day

*For all ACE inhibitors except fosinopril, dosage must be reduced in patients with significant renal impairment.
ACE, angiotensin-converting enzyme; CAD, coronary artery disease; CVD, cardiovascular disease; LVD, left ventricular dysfunction; MI, myocardial infarction.

be that the delayed response is due to reductions in *local* angiotensin II levels—reductions that would not be revealed by measuring angiotensin II in the blood.

ACE inhibitors offer several advantages over most other antihypertensive drugs. In contrast to the sympatholytic agents, ACE inhibitors do not interfere with cardiovascular reflexes. Hence exercise capacity is not impaired, and orthostatic hypotension is minimal. In addition, these drugs can be used safely in patients with bronchial asthma, a condition that precludes the use of beta$_2$-adrenergic antagonists. ACE inhibitors do not promote hypokalemia, hyperuricemia, or hyperglycemia—side effects seen with thiazide diuretics. Furthermore, they do not induce lethargy, weakness, or sexual dysfunction—responses that are common with other antihypertensive agents. Most important, *ACE inhibitors reduce the risk for cardiovascular mortality caused by hypertension.* The only other drugs proved to reduce hypertension-associated mortality are beta blockers and diuretics (see Chapter 39).

Heart Failure

ACE inhibitors produce multiple benefits in heart failure. By lowering arteriolar tone, these drugs improve regional blood flow, and, by reducing cardiac afterload, they increase cardiac output. By causing venous dilation, they reduce pulmonary congestion and peripheral edema. By dilating blood vessels in the kidney, they increase renal blood flow and thereby promote excretion of sodium and water. This loss of fluid has two beneficial effects: (1) it helps reduce edema, and (2) by lowering blood volume, it decreases venous return to the heart and thereby reduces right-heart workload. Lastly, by suppressing aldosterone and reducing local production of angiotensin II in the heart, ACE inhibitors may prevent or reverse pathologic changes in cardiac structure. Although only seven ACE inhibitors are approved for heart failure (see Table 36.1), both the American Heart Association and the American College of Cardiology have concluded that the ability to improve symptoms and prolong survival is a class effect. The use of ACE inhibitors in heart failure is discussed further in Chapter 40.

Myocardial Infarction

ACE inhibitors can reduce mortality after acute MI (heart attack). In addition, they decrease the chance of developing overt heart failure. Treatment should begin as soon as possible after infarction and should continue for at least 6 weeks. In patients who develop overt heart failure, treatment should continue long term. As for patients who do not develop heart failure, there are no data to indicate whether continued treatment would be beneficial. At this time, only three ACE inhibitors—captopril, lisinopril, and trandolapril—are approved for patients with MI.

Diabetic and Nondiabetic Nephropathy

ACE inhibitors can benefit patients with diabetic nephropathy, the leading cause of end-stage renal disease in the United States. In patients with overt nephropathy, as indicated by proteinuria of more than 500 mg/day, ACE inhibitors can slow progression of renal disease. In patients with less advanced nephropathy (30–300 mg proteinuria/day), ACE inhibitors can delay onset of overt nephropathy. These benefits were first demonstrated in patients with type 1 diabetes (insulin-dependent diabetes mellitus) and were later demonstrated in patients with type 2 diabetes (non–insulin-dependent diabetes mellitus). More recently, ACE inhibitors have been shown to provide similar benefits in patients with nephropathy unrelated to diabetes.

The principal protective mechanism appears to be reduction of glomerular filtration pressure. ACE inhibitors lower filtration pressure by reducing levels of angiotensin II, a compound that can raise filtration pressure by two mechanisms. First, angiotensin II raises systemic blood pressure, which raises pressure in the afferent arteriole of the glomerulus (Fig. 36.3). Second, it constricts the efferent arteriole, thereby generating back-pressure in the glomerulus. The resultant increase in filtration pressure promotes injury. By reducing levels of angiotensin II, ACE inhibitors lower glomerular filtration pressure and thereby slow development of renal injury.

At this time, the only ACE inhibitor approved for nephropathy is captopril. However, the American Diabetes Association considers benefits in diabetic nephropathy to be a class effect and hence recommends choosing an ACE inhibitor based on its cost and likelihood of patient adherence.

Can ACE inhibitors be used for *primary prevention* of diabetic nephropathy? No. This conclusion is based on the *Renin-Angiotensin System Study* (RASS), which evaluated the effects of an ACE inhibitor—*enalapril* [Vasotec]—and an ARB—*losartan* [Cozaar]—in patients with type 1 diabetes who did not have hypertension or any signs of early kidney disease. Both drugs failed to protect the kidney: compared with patients receiving placebo, those receiving enalapril or losartan developed the same degree of microalbuminuria (an early sign of kidney damage), the same decline in kidney function, and the same changes in glomerular structure (as shown by microscopic analysis of kidney biopsy samples). Hence, although ACE inhibitors may slow progression of established nephropathy, they do not protect against early kidney damage.

Prevention of Myocardial Infarction, Stroke, and Death in Patients at High Cardiovascular Risk

One ACE inhibitor—*ramipril* [Altace]—is approved for reducing the risk for MI, stroke, and death (from cardiovascular causes) in patients at *high* risk for a major cardiovascular

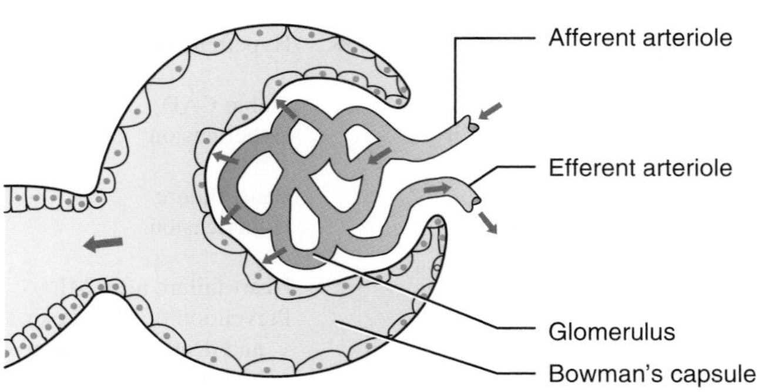

Figure 36.3 ■ Elevation of glomerular filtration pressure by angiotensin II.

Angiotensin II increases filtration pressure by (1) increasing pressure in the afferent arteriole (secondary to increasing systemic arterial pressure) and (2) constricting the efferent arteriole, thereby generating back-pressure in the glomerulus.

event—high risk being defined by (1) a history of stroke, coronary artery disease, peripheral vascular disease, or diabetes, combined with (2) at least one other risk factor, such as hypertension, high low-density lipoprotein cholesterol, low high-density lipoprotein cholesterol, or cigarette smoking. Ramipril was approved for this use based on results of the *Heart Outcomes Prevention Evaluation* (HOPE) trial, a large study in which patients at high cardiovascular risk took either ramipril (10 mg/day) or placebo. Follow-up time was 5 years. The combined end point of MI, stroke, or death from cardiovascular causes was significantly lower in the ramipril group (14% vs. 18%)—a 22% reduction in risk. Possible mechanisms underlying benefits include reduced vascular resistance and protection of the heart, blood vessels, and kidneys from the damage that angiotensin II and aldosterone can cause over time.

Like ramipril, *perindopril* [Aceon, Coversyl ♣] can reduce morbidity and mortality in patients at risk for major cardiovascular events. Benefits were demonstrated in the *EURopean trial On reduction of cardiac events with Perindopril in stable coronary Artery disease* (EUROPA). Patients in EUROPA were at lower risk than those in HOPE.

Can ACE inhibitors other than ramipril and perindopril also reduce cardiovascular risk? Possibly. However, at this time there is insufficient evidence to say for sure.

Diabetic Retinopathy

The RASS trial showed that at least one ACE inhibitor—*enalapril*—can reduce the risk for diabetic retinopathy in *some* patients. Specifically, in patients with *type 1 diabetes* who do not have hypertension, nephropathy, or established retinopathy, enalapril prevented or slowed development of retinal change. However, in patients with type 1 diabetes and *established* retinopathy, enalapril had no benefit. In patients with *type 2 diabetes,* enalapril had no benefit, regardless of retinopathy status.

Adverse Effects

ACE inhibitors are generally well tolerated. Some adverse effects (e.g., first-dose hypotension, hyperkalemia) are due to a reduction in angiotensin II, whereas others (cough, angioedema) are due to elevation of bradykinin.

First-Dose Hypotension

A precipitous drop in blood pressure may occur after the first dose of an ACE inhibitor. This reaction is caused by widespread vasodilation secondary to abrupt lowering of angiotensin II levels. First-dose hypotension is most likely in patients with severe hypertension, in patients taking diuretics, and in patients who are sodium depleted or volume depleted. To minimize the first-dose effect, initial doses should be low. Also, diuretics should be temporarily discontinued, starting 2 to 3 days before starting an ACE inhibitor. Blood pressure should be monitored for several hours after the first dose of an ACE inhibitor. If hypotension develops, the patient should assume a supine position. If necessary, blood pressure can be raised with an infusion of normal saline.

Cough

All ACE inhibitors can cause persistent, dry, irritating, nonproductive cough. Severity can range from a scratchy throat to severe hacking cough. The underlying cause is accumulation of bradykinin secondary to inhibition of kinase II (another name for ACE). Cough occurs in about 10% of patients and is the most common reason for discontinuing therapy. Factors that increase the risk for cough include advanced age, female sex, and Asian ancestry. Cough begins to subside 3 days after discontinuing an ACE inhibitor and is gone within 10 days.

Hyperkalemia

Inhibition of aldosterone release (secondary to inhibition of angiotensin II production) can cause potassium retention by the kidney. As a rule, significant potassium accumulation is limited to patients taking potassium supplements, salt substitutes (which contain potassium), or a potassium-sparing diuretic. For most other patients, hyperkalemia is rare. Patients should be instructed to avoid potassium supplements and potassium-containing salt substitutes unless they are prescribed.

Renal Failure

ACE inhibitors can cause severe renal insufficiency in patients with *bilateral renal artery stenosis or stenosis in the artery to a single remaining kidney.* In patients with renal artery stenosis, the kidneys release large amounts of renin. The resulting high levels of angiotensin II serve to maintain glomerular filtration by two mechanisms: elevation of blood pressure and constriction of efferent glomerular arterioles (see Fig. 36.3). When ACE is inhibited, causing angiotensin II levels to fall, the mechanisms that had been supporting glomerular filtration fail, causing urine production to drop precipitously. Not surprisingly, *ACE inhibitors are contraindicated for patients with bilateral renal artery stenosis (or stenosis in the artery to a single remaining kidney).*

BLACK BOX WARNING: FETAL INJURY

Use of ACE inhibitors during the *second* and *third* trimesters of pregnancy can injure the developing fetus. Specific effects include hypotension, hyperkalemia, skull hypoplasia, pulmonary hypoplasia, anuria, renal failure (reversible and irreversible), and death. Women who become pregnant while using ACE inhibitors should discontinue treatment as soon as possible. Infants who have been exposed to ACE inhibitors during the second or third trimester should be closely monitored for hypotension, oliguria, and hyperkalemia.

Are ACE inhibitors safe *early* in pregnancy? Possibly. Even though an article in the *New England Journal of Medicine* reported that among 209 children exposed to ACE inhibitors during the first trimester, 18 (8.7%) had major congenital malformations, compared with 3.2% of controls, these data contrast with animal studies, which suggest that such malformations are not likely. Furthermore, no mechanism by which ACE inhibitors might disrupt early embryogenesis is known. It is now thought that the malformations attributed to ACE inhibitors are more related to hypertension in pregnancy, not the drug itself. Because there is lack of complete data, however, the U.S. Food and Drug Administration still classifies ACE inhibitors in Pregnancy Risk Category D, and they should be avoided in pregnancy.

Angioedema

Angioedema is a potentially fatal reaction that develops in up to 1% of patients. Symptoms, which result from increased capillary permeability, include giant wheals and edema of the tongue, glottis, lips, eyes, and pharynx. Severe reactions should be treated with subcutaneous epinephrine. If angioedema develops, ACE inhibitors should be discontinued and never used again. Angioedema is caused by accumulation of bradykinin secondary to inhibition of kinase II.

Neutropenia

Neutropenia, with its associated risk for infection, is a rare but serious complication. Neutropenia is most likely in patients with renal impairment and in those with collagen vascular diseases (e.g., systemic lupus erythematosus, scleroderma). These patients should be followed closely. Fortunately, neutropenia is reversible when detected early. If neutropenia develops, ACE inhibitors should be withdrawn immediately. Neutrophil counts should normalize in approximately 2 weeks. In the absence of early detection, neutropenia may progress to fatal agranulocytosis. Patients should be informed about early signs of infection (e.g., fever, sore throat) and instructed to report them immediately. Neutropenia is more common with captopril than with other ACE inhibitors.

Drug Interactions

Diuretics

Diuretics may intensify first-dose hypotension. To prevent this interaction, diuretics should be withdrawn 2 to 3 days before giving an ACE inhibitor. Diuretic therapy can be resumed later if needed.

Antihypertensive Agents

The hypotensive effects of ACE inhibitors are often additive with those of other antihypertensive drugs (e.g., diuretics, sympatholytics, vasodilators, calcium channel blockers). When an ACE inhibitor is added to an antihypertensive regimen, dosages of other drugs may require reduction.

Drugs That Raise Potassium Levels

ACE inhibitors increase the risk for hyperkalemia caused by *potassium supplements and potassium-sparing diuretics.* The risk for hyperkalemia is increased because, by suppressing aldosterone secretion, ACE inhibitors can reduce excretion of potassium. To minimize the risk for hyperkalemia, potassium supplements and potassium-sparing diuretics should be employed only when clearly indicated.

Lithium

ACE inhibitors can cause lithium to accumulate to toxic levels. Lithium levels should be monitored frequently.

Nonsteroidal Antiinflammatory Drugs (NSAIDs)

Aspirin, ibuprofen, and other NSAIDs may reduce the antihypertensive effects of ACE inhibitors.

Preparations, Dosage, and Administration

Except for enalaprilat, all ACE inhibitors are administered orally. Of the oral products, all are available in single-drug formulations. Most are also available in fixed-dose combinations with hydrochlorothiazide, a thiazide diuretic, and one agent—perindopril—is available combined with indapamide (Table 36.2). Two ACE inhibitors—benazepril and trandolapril—are available combined with calcium channel blockers. Except for captopril and moexipril, all oral formulations may be administered without regard to meals; captopril and moexipril should be administered 1 hour before meals. Dosages for all ACE inhibitors (except fosinopril) should be reduced in patients with renal impairment. Dosages for specific indications are shown in Table 36.1.

TABLE 36.2 ▪ ACE Inhibitor Combination Drugs

Generic Name	Trade Name
Benazepril/HCTZ	Lotensin HCT
Benazepril/amlodipine	Lotrel
Captopril/HCTZ	Capozide
Enalapril/HCTZ	Vaseretic
Fosinopril/HCTZ	Monopril-HCT
Lisinopril/HCTZ	Prinzide Zestoretic
Moexipril/HCTZ	Uniretic
Perindopril/indapamide	Coversyl Plus ♣
Perindopril/amlodipine	Prestalia
Quinapril/HCTZ	Accuretic
Ramipril/HCTZ	Altace HCT ♣
Trandolapril/verapamil	Tarka

ACE, angiotensin-converting enzyme.

ANGIOTENSIN II RECEPTOR BLOCKERS

Initially, ARBs were approved only for hypertension. Today, they also are approved for treating heart failure, diabetic nephropathy, and MI and for prevention of MI, stroke, and death in people at high risk for cardiovascular events.

Like the ACE inhibitors, ARBs decrease the influence of angiotensin II. However, the mechanisms involved differ: whereas ACE inhibitors block *production* of angiotensin II, ARBs block the *actions* of angiotensin II. Because both groups interfere with angiotensin II, they both have similar effects. They differ primarily in that ARBs pose a much lower risk for cough or hyperkalemia.

Even though ACE inhibitors and ARBs have very similar effects, these drugs are not clinically interchangeable. We have clear and extensive evidence that ACE inhibitors decrease cardiovascular morbidity and mortality. The evidence for ARBs is less convincing. Accordingly, until more is known, ACE inhibitors are preferred. For patients who cannot tolerate ACE inhibitors, ARBs are an appropriate second choice.

Eight ARBs are available. All eight are very similar—hence we will discuss them as a group, rather than choosing one as a prototype.

Mechanism of Action and Overview of Pharmacologic Effects

ARBs block access of angiotensin II to its receptors in blood vessels, the adrenals, and all other tissues. As a result, ARBs have effects much like those of the ACE inhibitors. By blocking angiotensin II receptors on blood vessels, ARBs cause dilation of arterioles and veins. By blocking angiotensin II receptors in the heart, ARBs can prevent angiotensin II from inducing pathologic changes in cardiac structure. By blocking angiotensin II receptors in the adrenals, ARBs decrease release of aldosterone and can thereby increase renal excretion of sodium and water. Sodium and water excretion is further increased through dilation of renal blood vessels.

In contrast to the ACE inhibitors, ARBs do *not* inhibit kinase II and hence do not increase levels of bradykinin in the lung. As a result, ARBs have a lower risk for cough, the most common reason for stopping ACE inhibitors.

Therapeutic Uses

Hypertension

All ARBs are approved for hypertension. Reductions in blood pressure equal those seen with ACE inhibitors. Evidence that ARBs share the ability of ACE inhibitors to reduce mortality is lacking.

Heart Failure

Currently, only two ARBs—*valsartan* [Diovan] and *candesartan* [Atacand]—are approved for heart failure. In clinical trials, these drugs reduced symptoms, decreased hospitalizations, improved functional capacity, and increased LV ejection fraction. More important, they prolonged survival. Because experience with these drugs is limited, they should be reserved for patients who cannot tolerate ACE inhibitors (because of cough). Although the other ARBs are not yet approved for heart failure, most authorities believe they are effective.

Diabetic Nephropathy

Two ARBs—*irbesartan* [Avapro] and *losartan* [Cozaar]—are approved for managing nephropathy in hypertensive patients with type 2 diabetes. In clinical trials, these drugs delayed development of overt nephropathy and slowed progression of established nephropathy. Benefits are due in part to reductions in blood pressure and in part to mechanisms that have not been determined. How do ARBs compare with ACE inhibitors? Although both groups of drugs can delay progression of nephropathy, only the ACE inhibitors have been shown to reduce mortality. As noted earlier, neither ARBs nor ACE inhibitors are effective for primary prevention of diabetic nephropathy.

Myocardial Infarction

One ARB—*valsartan* [Diovan]—is approved for reducing cardiovascular mortality in post-MI patients with heart failure or LV dysfunction. Approval was based on the results of a major trial—the *Valsartan in Acute Myocardial Infarction Trial* (VALIANT)—that showed that valsartan was as effective as captopril at reducing short-term and long-term mortality in these patients.

Stroke Prevention

One ARB—*losartan* [Cozaar]—is approved for reducing the risk for stroke in patients with hypertension and LV hypertrophy. In clinical studies, stroke prevention with losartan was better than with atenolol (a beta blocker), even though both drugs produced an equivalent decrease in blood pressure. This observation indicates that the benefits of losartan cannot be explained on the basis of reduced blood pressure alone.

Prevention of Myocardial Infarction, Stroke, and Death in Patients at High Cardiovascular Risk

One ARB—*telmisartan* [Micardis]—is approved for reducing the risk for MI, stroke, and death from cardiovascular causes in patients 55 years and older, but only if they are intolerant of ACE inhibitors. (Recall that ramipril, an ACE inhibitor, is also approved for preventing MI, stroke, and death in high-risk patients.) Approval of telmisartan was based on the ONTARGET (Ongoing Telmisartan Alone and in Combination with Ramipril Global Endpoint Trial) study, which showed that telmisartan was similar to ramipril with regard to reducing cardiovascular morbidity and mortality. Of note, combining telmisartan with ramipril was no more effective than either agent alone, but did increase the risk for adverse events. Can other ARBs reduce cardiovascular risk? Possibly, but proof is lacking.

Diabetic Retinopathy

In the RASS study mentioned previously, benefits of the ARB *losartan* [Cozaar] were like those of enalapril: in patients with type 1 diabetes without established retinopathy, losartan slowed the development and progression of retinopathy—but had no benefit in patients with established retinopathy. In patients with type 2 diabetes, the drug offered no benefit at all, regardless of retinopathy status.

Adverse Effects

All of the ARBs are well tolerated. In contrast to ACE inhibitors, ARBs do not cause clinically significant hyperkalemia. Furthermore, because ARBs do not promote accumulation of bradykinin in the lung, they have a lower incidence of cough.

Angioedema

Like the ACE inhibitors, ARBs can cause angioedema, although the incidence may be lower with ARBs. If angioedema occurs, ARBs should be withdrawn immediately and never used again. Severe reactions are treated with subcutaneous epinephrine.

ARBs cause angioedema possibly by increasing bradykinin availability. Unlike ACE inhibitors, ARBs do not inhibit bradykinin breakdown. However, through an indirect mechanism, ARBs may be able to increase local bradykinin synthesis.

About 8% of patients who experience angioedema with an ACE inhibitor will also develop angioedema if given an ARB. Nonetheless, switching to an ARB may be worth the risk for specific patients, namely, those with a disorder for which ARBs are known to improve outcomes (i.e., heart failure, diabetes, and MI).

BLACK BOX WARNING: FETAL HARM

Like the ACE inhibitors, ARBs can injure the developing fetus if taken during the second or third trimester of pregnancy and hence are contraindicated during this period. Also, there is concern that ARBs and ACE inhibitors may harm the fetus earlier in pregnancy and hence should be discontinued as soon as pregnancy is discovered.

Renal Failure

Like the ACE inhibitors, ARBs can cause renal failure in patients with bilateral renal artery stenosis or stenosis in the artery to a single remaining kidney. Accordingly, ARBs must be used with extreme caution in patients with these conditions.

Drug Interactions

The hypotensive effects of ARBs are additive with those of other antihypertensive drugs. When an ARB is added to an antihypertensive regimen, dosages of the other drugs may require reduction.

Preparations, Dosage, and Administration

All ARBs are administered orally, and all may be taken with or without food. All are available alone, and all but azilsartan are also available in fixed-dose combinations with hydrochlorothiazide, a thiazide diuretic (Table 36.3). Dosages for specific indications are shown in Table 36.4.

ALISKIREN, A DIRECT RENIN INHIBITOR

DRIs are drugs that act on renin to inhibit the conversion of angiotensinogen into angiotensin I. By decreasing production of angiotensin I, DRIs can suppress the entire RAAS. Currently, only one DRI—*aliskiren* [Tekturna, Rasilez ♣]—is available.

Blood pressure reduction with aliskiren equals that seen with ACE inhibitors. Aliskiren causes less cough and angioedema than the ACE inhibitors but poses similar risks to the developing fetus.

Mechanism of Action

Aliskiren binds tightly with renin and thereby inhibits the cleavage of angiotensinogen into angiotensin I. Because this reaction is the first and rate-limiting step in the production of angiotensin II and aldosterone, aliskiren can reduce the influence of the entire RAAS. In clinical trials, the drug decreased plasma renin activity by 50% to 80%. Although aliskiren works at an earlier step than either the ACE inhibitors or ARBs, there is no proof that doing so results in superior clinical outcomes.

TABLE 36.3 ▪ ARB Combination Drugs

Generic Name	Trade Name
Azilsartan/chlorthalidone	Edarbyclor
Candesartan/HCTZ	Atacand HCT
Eprosartan/HCTZ	Teveten HCT
Irbesartan/HCTZ	Avalide
Losartan/HCTZ	Hyzaar
Olmesartan/HCTZ	Benicar HCT
	Olmetec Plus ♣
Olmesartan/amlodipine	Azor
Olmesartan/amlodipine/HCTZ	Tribenzor
Telmisartan/HCTZ	Micardis HCT
Telmisartan/amlodipine	Twynsta
Valsartan/HCTZ	Diovan HCT
Valsartan/amlodipine	Exforge
Valsartan/amlodipine/HCTZ	Exforge HCT

ARB, angiotensin II receptor blocker; HCT, hydrochlorothiazide; HCTZ, hydrochlorothiazide.

TABLE 36.4 ▪ Angiotensin II Receptor Blockers: Approved Indications and Adult Dosages

Generic Name	Trade Name	Approved Indications	Availability	Initial Dosage	Maintenance Dosage
Azilsartan	Edarbi	Hypertension	40-, 80-mg tablets	40–80 mg once/day	80 mg once/day
Candesartan	Atacand	Hypertension	4-, 8-, 16-, 32-mg tablets	16 mg once/day	8–32 mg/day in 1 or 2 doses
		Heart failure		4 mg once/day	32 mg once/day
Eprosartan	Teveten	Hypertension	400-, 600-mg tablets	600 mg once/day	400–800 mg/day in 1 or 2 doses
Irbesartan	Avapro	Hypertension	75-, 150-, 300-mg tablets	150 mg once/day	150–300 mg once/day
		Diabetic nephropathy*		300 mg once/day	300 mg once/day
Losartan	Cozaar	Hypertension	25-, 50-, 100-mg tablets	25–50 mg once/day	25–100 mg/day in 1 or 2 doses
		Stroke prevention†		50 mg once/day	50–100 mg once/day
		Diabetic nephropathy*		50 mg once/day	100 mg once/day
Olmesartan	Benicar, Olmetec ♣	Hypertension	5-, 20-, 40-mg tablets	20 mg once/day	20–40 mg once/day
Telmisartan	Micardis	Hypertension	20-, 40-, 80-mg tablets	40 mg once/day	20–80 mg once/day
		Prevention of MI, stroke, and death in people at high risk for CVD but who can't take an ACE inhibitor		80 mg once/day	80 mg once/day
Valsartan	Diovan	Hypertension	40-, 80-, 160-, 320-mg tablets	80–160 mg once/day	80–320 mg once/day
		Heart failure		40 mg twice/day	40–160 mg twice/day
		MI		20 mg twice/day	160 mg twice/day

*In patients with type 2 diabetes.
†In nonblack patients with hypertension and left ventricular hypertrophy.
ACE, angiotensin-converting enzyme; CVD, cardiovascular disease; MI, myocardial infarction.

Therapeutic Use

Aliskiren is approved only for *hypertension.* It may be used alone or in combination with other antihypertensives. In clinical trials, aliskiren reduced blood pressure to the same extent as did ACE inhibitors, ARBs, or calcium channel blockers. Maximal effects developed within 2 weeks. Although aliskiren can reduce blood pressure in hypertensive patients, data are conflicting regarding reduction of negative outcomes (i.e., blindness, stroke, kidney disease, death). The AVOID (Aliskiren in the Evaluation of Proteinuria in Diabetes) study demonstrated a renoprotective effect in diabetic patients when combined with losartan. Yet in the ALTITUDE (Aliskiren Trial in type 2 Diabetes Using Cardiorenal Disease Endpoints) trial, incidence of nonfatal stroke, renal dysfunction, and hypotension led to a premature closure of the study. Given these mixed results, more studies are currently underway. Until the long-term benefits and safety of aliskiren are known, older antihypertensives should be considered first.

Pharmacokinetics

Aliskiren is administered orally, and bioavailability is low (only 2.5%). Dosing with a *high-fat meal* makes availability much lower (about 0.8%). Aliskiren undergoes some metabolism by CYP3A4 (the 3A4 isozyme of cytochrome P450), but the extent of metabolism is not known. About 25% of the drug is eliminated unchanged in the urine. The half-life is about 24 hours.

Adverse Effects

Aliskiren is generally well tolerated. At usual doses, the risk for angioedema, cough, or hyperkalemia is low. At high therapeutic doses, some patients experience diarrhea. Like other drugs that affect the RAAS, aliskiren should be avoided during pregnancy.

Angioedema and Cough

With ACE inhibitors, angioedema and cough result from inhibition of kinase II. Because aliskiren does not inhibit kinase II, the risk for these effects is low. In clinical trials, the incidence of cough was 1.1% with aliskiren, versus about 10% with an ACE inhibitor. Similarly, the incidence of angioedema was 0.06% with aliskiren, versus 1% with an ACE inhibitor. If angioedema does occur, aliskiren should be discontinued immediately.

Gastrointestinal Effects

Aliskiren causes dose-dependent *diarrhea,* seen in 2.3% of patients taking 300 mg/day. Women and older adults are most susceptible. Excessive doses (600 mg/day) are associated with abdominal pain and dyspepsia.

Hyperkalemia

Like the ACE inhibitors, aliskiren rarely causes hyperkalemia when used alone. However, hyperkalemia might be expected if aliskiren were combined with an ACE inhibitor, a potassium-sparing diuretic, or potassium supplements.

BLACK BOX WARNING: FETAL INJURY AND DEATH

Although aliskiren has not been studied in pregnant women, the drug is likely to pose a risk for major congenital malformations and fetal death because the risk for these events is well established with other drugs that suppress the RAAS. Therefore, like the ACE inhibitors and ARBs, aliskiren is contraindicated during the second and third trimesters and should be discontinued as soon as possible when pregnancy occurs.

Drug Interactions

Aliskiren undergoes some metabolism by CYP3A4, but it neither induces nor inhibits the P450 system. In clinical trials, aliskiren had no significant interactions with atenolol, digoxin, amlodipine, or hydrochlorothiazide. However, levels of aliskiren were significantly raised by atorvastatin and ketoconazole (a P450 inhibitor) and significantly lowered by irbesartan. Levels of furosemide were lowered by aliskiren.

Preparations, Dosage, and Administration

Aliskiren is available alone as Tekturna and Rasilez 🍁, in combination with hydrochlorothiazide as Tekturna HCT and Rasilez HCT 🍁, and in combination with amlodipine as Tekamlo. All formulations are indicated for hypertension.

Aliskiren alone [Tekturna, Rasilez 🍁] is available in 150- and 300-mg tablets. The initial dosage is 150 mg once a day. If control of blood pressure is inadequate, dosage may be increased to 300 mg once a day. Daily doses above 300 mg will not increase benefits but will increase the risk for diarrhea. Because high-fat meals decrease absorption substantially, each daily dose should be taken at the same time with respect to meals (e.g., 1 hour before dinner) to achieve a consistent response.

Aliskiren/hydrochlorothiazide [Tekturna HCT, Rasilez HCT 🍁] tablets are available in four strengths—150 mg/12.5 mg, 150 mg/25 mg, 300 mg/12.5 mg, and 300 mg/25 mg—for once-daily dosing. As with Tekturna, each daily dose should be taken at the same time with respect to meals.

Aliskiren/amlodipine [Tekamlo] tablets are available in four strengths—150 mg/5 mg, 150 mg/10 mg, 300 mg/5 mg, and 300 mg/10 mg—for once-daily dosing. As with Tekturna and Tekturna HCT, each daily dose should be taken at the same time with respect to meals.

ALDOSTERONE ANTAGONISTS

Aldosterone antagonists are drugs that block receptors for aldosterone. Two such agents are available: eplerenone and spironolactone. Both drugs have similar structures and actions, and both are used for the same disorders: hypertension and heart failure. They differ, however, in that spironolactone is less selective than eplerenone. As a result, spironolactone causes more side effects.

Eplerenone

Eplerenone [Inspra] is a first-in-class *selective aldosterone receptor blocker.* The drug is used for hypertension and heart failure and has one significant side effect: hyperkalemia.

Mechanism of Action

Eplerenone produces selective blockade of aldosterone receptors, having little or no effect on receptors for other steroid hormones (e.g., glucocorticoids, progesterone, androgens). In the kidney, activation of aldosterone receptors promotes excretion of potassium and retention of sodium and water. Receptor blockade has the opposite effect: retention of potassium and increased excretion of sodium and water. Loss of sodium and water reduces blood volume and hence blood pressure. Blockade of aldosterone receptors at nonrenal sites may prevent or reverse pathologic effects of aldosterone on cardiovascular structure and function.

Therapeutic Use

Hypertension

For treatment of hypertension, eplerenone may be used alone or in combination with other antihypertensive agents. Maximal reductions in blood pressure take about 4 weeks to develop. In clinical trials, reductions in blood pressure were equivalent to those produced by spironolactone and superior to those produced by losartan (an ARB). In patients already using an ACE inhibitor or an ARB, adding eplerenone produced a further reduction in blood pressure.

Although it is clear that eplerenone can lower blood pressure, we have no information on what really matters: the drug's ability to reduce morbidity and mortality in patients with isolated hypertension and lack of LV hypertrophy. Until more is known, eplerenone should be reserved for patients who have not responded to traditional antihypertensive drugs.

Heart Failure

In patients with heart failure, eplerenone can improve symptoms, reduce hospitalizations, and prolong life. Benefits appear to derive from blocking the adverse effects of aldosterone on cardiovascular structure and function. Use of eplerenone in heart failure is discussed in Chapter 40.

Pharmacokinetics

Eplerenone is administered orally, and absorption is not affected by food. Plasma levels peak about 1.5 hours after dosing. Absolute bioavailability is unknown. Eplerenone undergoes metabolism by CYP3A4, followed by excretion in the urine (67%) and feces (32%). The elimination half-life is 4 to 6 hours.

Adverse Effects

Eplerenone is generally well tolerated. The incidence of adverse effects is nearly identical to that of placebo. A few adverse effects—diarrhea, abdominal pain, cough, fatigue, gynecomastia, flu-like syndrome—occur slightly (1%–2%) more often with eplerenone than with placebo.

Hyperkalemia

The greatest concern is hyperkalemia, which can occur secondary to potassium retention. Because of this risk, combined use with potassium supplements, salt substitutes, or potassium-sparing diuretics (e.g., spironolactone, triamterene) is contraindicated. Combined use with ACE inhibitors or ARBs is permissible but should be done with caution. Eplerenone is contraindicated for patients with high serum potassium (above 5.5 mEq/L) and for patients with impaired renal function or type 2 diabetes with microalbuminuria, both of which can promote hyperkalemia. Monitoring potassium levels is recommended for patients at risk (e.g., those taking ACE inhibitors or ARBs).

Drug Interactions

Inhibitors of CYP3A4 can increase levels of eplerenone, thereby posing a risk for toxicity. Weak inhibitors (e.g., erythromycin, saquinavir, verapamil, fluconazole) can double eplerenone levels. Strong inhibitors (e.g., ketoconazole, itraconazole) can increase levels fivefold. If eplerenone is combined with a weak inhibitor, eplerenone dosage should be reduced. Eplerenone should not be combined with a strong inhibitor.

Drugs that raise potassium levels can increase the risk for hyperkalemia. Eplerenone should not be combined with potassium supplements, salt substitutes, or potassium-sparing diuretics. Combining eplerenone with ACE inhibitors or ARBs should be done with caution.

Drugs similar to eplerenone (e.g., ACE inhibitors and diuretics) are known to increase levels of *lithium*. Although the combination of eplerenone and lithium has not been studied, caution is nonetheless advised. Lithium levels should be measured frequently.

Preparations, Dosage, and Administration

Eplerenone [Inspra] is available in 25- and 50-mg tablets. The usual starting dosage is 50 mg once a day, taken with or without food. After 4 weeks, dosage can be increased to 50 mg twice daily (if the hypotensive response has been inadequate). Raising the dosage above 100 mg/day is not recommended because doing so is unlikely to increase the therapeutic response but will increase the risk for hyperkalemia. In patients taking weak inhibitors of CYP3A4, the initial dosage should be reduced by 50% (to 25 mg once a day).

Spironolactone

Spironolactone [Aldactone], a much older drug than eplerenone, blocks receptors for aldosterone but also binds with receptors for other steroid hormones (e.g., glucocorticoids, progesterone, androgens). Blockade of aldosterone receptors underlies beneficial effects in hypertension and heart failure as well as the drug's major adverse effect: hyperkalemia. Binding with receptors for other steroid hormones underlies additional adverse effects: gynecomastia, menstrual irregularities, impotence, hirsutism, and deepening of the voice. The basic pharmacology of spironolactone and its use in heart failure are discussed in Chapters 39 and 40, respectively.

BLACK BOX WARNING: SPIRONOLACTONE

Use of spironolactone is tumorigenic in chronic toxicity studies in rats.

CHAPTER

37 Calcium Channel Blockers

Laura D. Rosenthal, DNP, ACNP, FAANP

Calcium channel blockers (CCBs) are drugs that prevent calcium ions from entering cells. These agents have their greatest effects on the heart and blood vessels. CCBs are used widely to treat hypertension, angina pectoris, and cardiac dysrhythmias. Since 1995, there has been controversy about the safety of CCBs, especially in patients with hypertension and diabetes.

CALCIUM CHANNELS: PHYSIOLOGIC FUNCTIONS AND CONSEQUENCES OF BLOCKADE

Calcium channels are gated pores in the cytoplasmic membrane that regulate entry of calcium ions into cells. Calcium entry plays a critical role in the function of vascular smooth muscle (VSM) and the heart.

Vascular Smooth Muscle

In VSM, calcium channels regulate contraction. When an action potential travels down the surface of a smooth muscle cell, calcium channels open and calcium ions flow inward, thereby initiating the contractile process. If calcium channels are blocked, contraction will be prevented and vasodilation will result.

At therapeutic doses, CCBs act selectively on *peripheral arterioles* and *arteries and arterioles of the heart.* CCBs have no significant effect on veins.

Heart

In the heart, calcium channels help regulate the myocardium, the sinoatrial (SA) node, and the atrioventricular (AV) node. Calcium channels at all three sites are coupled to beta$_1$-adrenergic receptors.

Myocardium

In cardiac muscle, calcium entry has a positive inotropic effect. That is, calcium increases force of contraction. If calcium channels in atrial and ventricular muscle are blocked, contractile force will diminish.

Sinoatrial Node

Pacemaker activity of the SA node is regulated by calcium influx. When calcium channels are open, spontaneous discharge of the SA node increases. Conversely, when calcium channels close, pacemaker activity declines. Hence the effect of calcium channel blockade is to reduce heart rate.

Atrioventricular Node

Impulses that originate in the SA node must pass through the AV node on their way to the ventricles. Because of this arrangement, regulation of AV conduction plays a critical role in coordinating contraction of the ventricles with contraction of the atria.

The excitability of AV nodal cells is regulated by calcium entry. When calcium channels are open, calcium entry increases, and cells of the AV node discharge more readily. Conversely, when calcium channels are closed, discharge of AV nodal cells is suppressed. Hence the effect of calcium channel blockade is to decrease velocity of conduction through the AV node.

Coupling of Cardiac Calcium Channels to Beta$_1$-Adrenergic Receptors

In the heart, calcium channels are coupled to beta$_1$-adrenergic receptors (Fig. 37.1). As a result, when cardiac beta$_1$ receptors are activated, calcium influx is enhanced. Conversely, when beta$_1$ receptors are blocked, calcium influx is suppressed. Because of this relationship, CCBs and beta blockers have identical effects on the heart. That is, they both reduce force of contraction, slow heart rate, and suppress conduction through the AV node.

CALCIUM CHANNEL BLOCKERS: CLASSIFICATION AND SITES OF ACTION

Classification

The CCBs used in the United States belong to three chemical families (Table 37.1). The largest family is the *dihydropyridines,* for which *nifedipine* is the prototype. This family name is encountered frequently and hence is worth remembering. The other two families consist of orphans: *verapamil* is the only *phenylalkylamine,* and *diltiazem* is the only *benzothiazepine.* The drug names are important; the family names are not.

Sites of Action

At therapeutic doses, the dihydropyridines act primarily on arterioles; in contrast, verapamil and diltiazem act on arterioles *and* the heart (see Table 37.1). However, although dihydropyridines don't affect the heart at *therapeutic* doses, *toxic* doses can produce dangerous cardiac suppression (just like verapamil and diltiazem can). The differences in selectivity among CCBs are based on structural differences

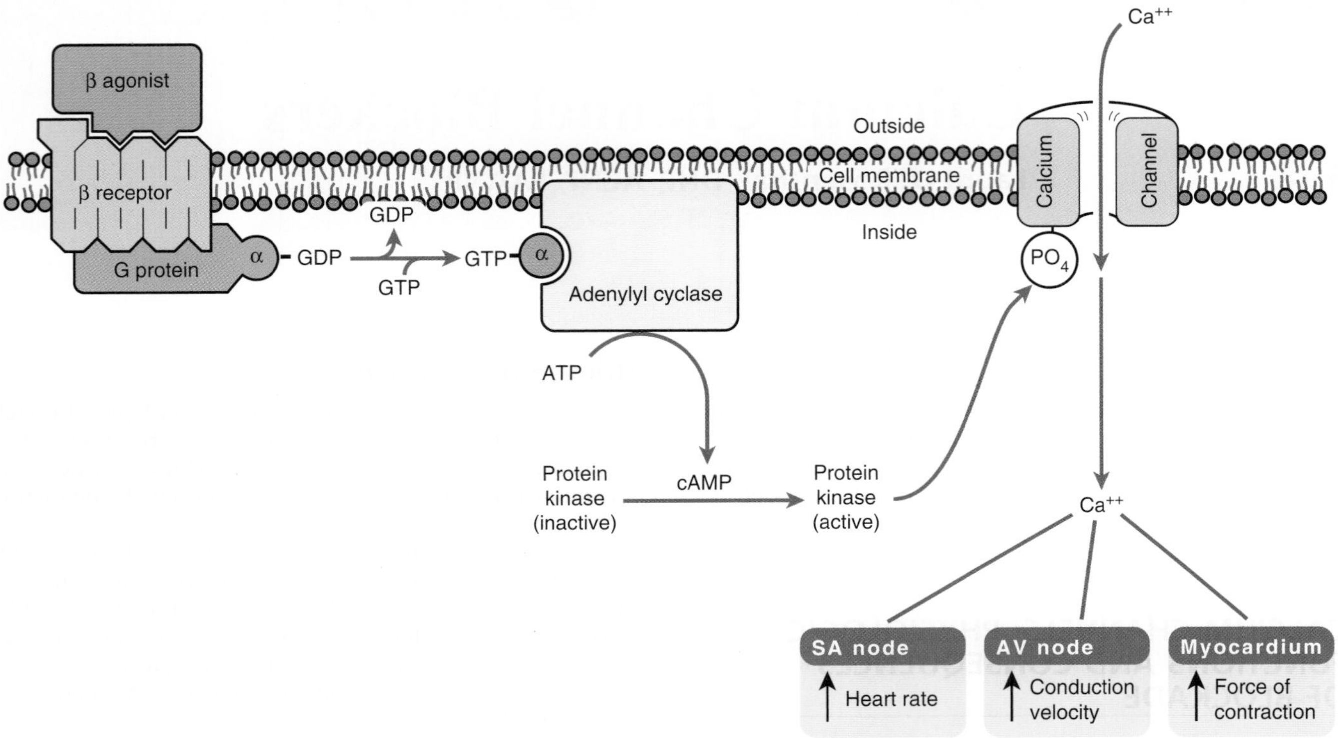

Figure 37.1 ■ Coupling of cardiac calcium channels with beta$_1$-adrenergic receptors. In the heart, beta$_1$ receptors are coupled to calcium channels. As a result, when cardiac beta$_1$ receptors are activated, calcium influx is enhanced. The process works as follows: binding of an agonist (e.g., norepinephrine) causes a conformational change in the beta receptor, which in turn causes a change in G protein, converting it from an inactive state (in which guanosine diphosphate [GDP] is bound to the alpha subunit) to an active state (in which guanosine triphosphate [GTP] is bound to the alpha subunit). (G protein is so named because it binds guanine nucleotides: GDP and GTP.) After activation, the alpha subunit dissociates from the rest of G protein and activates adenylyl cyclase, an enzyme that converts adenosine triphosphate (ATP) to cyclic adenosine monophosphate (cAMP). cAMP then activates protein kinase, an enzyme that phosphorylates proteins—in this case, the calcium channel. Phosphorylation changes the channel such that calcium entry is enhanced when the channel opens. (Opening of the channel is triggered by a change in membrane voltage [i.e., by passage of an action potential].)The effect of calcium entry on cardiac function is determined by the type of cell involved. If the cell is in the SA node, heart rate increases; if the cell is in the AV node, impulse conduction through the node accelerates; and if the cell is part of the myocardium, force of contraction is increased. Because binding of a single agonist molecule to a single beta receptor stimulates the synthesis of many cAMP molecules, with the subsequent activation of many protein kinase molecules, causing the phosphorylation of many calcium channels, this system can greatly amplify the signal initiated by the agonist.

Protoytpe Drugs

CALCIUM CHANNEL BLOCKERS

Agent that Affects the Heart and Blood Vessels

Verapamil

Dihydropyridine: Agent that Acts Mainly on Blood Vessels

Nifedipine

among the drugs themselves and structural differences among calcium channels.

VERAPAMIL AND DILTIAZEM: AGENTS THAT ACT ON VASCULAR SMOOTH MUSCLE AND THE HEART

Verapamil

Verapamil [Calan, Verelan, Covera-HS ♣] blocks calcium channels in blood vessels and in the heart. Major indications

TABLE 37.1 ▪ Calcium Channel Blockers: Classification, Sites of Action, and Indications

		Indications				
Classification	**Sites of Action**	**Hypertension**	**Angina**	**Dysrhythmias**	**Migraine***	**Others**
DIHYDROPYRIDINES						
Nifedipine [Adalat CC, Nifediac, Nifedical, Procardia]	Arterioles	✔	✔		✔	†
Amlodipine [Norvasc]	Arterioles	✔	✔			
Felodipine [Plendil, Renedil] 🍁	Arterioles	✔				
Isradipine [DynaCirc CR]	Arterioles	✔				
Nicardipine [Cardene SR]	Arterioles	✔	✔			
Nimodipine [Nymalize, Nimotop] 🍁	Arterioles				✔	§
Nisoldipine [Sular]	Arterioles	✔				
PHENYLALKYLAMINES						
Verapamil [Calan, Covera-HS 🍁, Verelan]	Arterioles/heart	✔	✔	✔	✔	
BENZOTHIAZEPINES						
Diltiazem [Cardizem, Dilacor XR, Tiazac, others]	Arterioles/heart	✔	✔	✔	✔	

*Investigational use.
†Suppression of preterm labor (investigational use).
§Prophylaxis of neurologic injury after rupture of an intracranial aneurysm.

are angina pectoris, essential hypertension, and cardiac dysrhythmias. Verapamil was the first CCB available and will serve as our prototype for the group.

Hemodynamic Effects

The overall hemodynamic response to verapamil is the net result of (1) direct effects on the heart and blood vessels and (2) reflex responses.

Direct Effects

By blocking calcium channels in the heart and blood vessels, verapamil has five direct effects:

- Blockade at peripheral arterioles causes dilation and thereby reduces arterial pressure.
- Blockade at arteries and arterioles of the heart increases coronary perfusion.
- Blockade at the SA node reduces heart rate.
- Blockade at the AV node decreases AV nodal conduction.
- Blockade in the myocardium decreases force of contraction.

Of the direct effects on the heart, reduced AV conduction is the most important.

Indirect (Reflex) Effects

Verapamil-induced lowering of blood pressure activates the baroreceptor reflex, causing increased firing of sympathetic nerves to the heart. Norepinephrine released from these nerves acts to increase heart rate, AV conduction, and force of contraction. However, because these same three parameters are suppressed by the direct actions of verapamil, the direct and indirect effects tend to neutralize each other.

Net Effect

Because the direct effects of verapamil on the heart are counterbalanced by indirect effects, the drug has little or no net effect on cardiac performance: for most patients, heart rate, AV conduction, and contractility are not noticeably altered. Consequently, the overall cardiovascular effect of verapamil is simply vasodilation accompanied by reduced arterial pressure and increased coronary perfusion.

Pharmacokinetics

Verapamil may be administered orally or intravenously. The drug is well absorbed after oral administration but undergoes extensive metabolism on its first pass through the liver. Consequently, only about 20% of an oral dose reaches the systemic circulation. Effects begin 30 minutes after dosing and peak within 5 hours. Elimination is primarily by hepatic metabolism. Because the drug is eliminated by the liver, doses must be reduced substantially in patients with hepatic impairment.

Therapeutic Uses

Angina Pectoris

Verapamil is used widely to treat angina pectoris. The drug is approved for vasospastic angina and angina of effort. Benefits in both disorders derive from vasodilation. The role of verapamil in angina is discussed in Chapter 43.

Essential Hypertension

Verapamil is a second-line agent for chronic hypertension, used after thiazide diuretics. The drug lowers blood pressure by dilating arterioles. The role of verapamil and other CCBs in hypertension is discussed in Chapter 39.

Cardiac Dysrhythmias

Verapamil, administered intravenously, is used to slow ventricular rate in patients with atrial flutter, atrial fibrillation, and paroxysmal supraventricular tachycardia. Benefits derive from suppressing impulse conduction through the AV node, thereby preventing the atria from driving the ventricles at an excessive rate. Antidysrhythmic applications are discussed in Chapter 41.

Adverse Effects

Common Effects

Verapamil is generally well tolerated. *Constipation* occurs frequently and is the most common complaint. This problem, which can be especially severe in older adults, can be minimized by increasing dietary fluids and fiber. Constipation results from blockade of calcium channels in smooth muscle of the intestine. Other common effects—dizziness, facial flushing, headache, and edema of the ankles and feet—occur secondary to vasodilation.

Cardiac Effects

Blockade of calcium channels in the heart can compromise cardiac function. In the SA node, calcium channel blockade can cause bradycardia; in the AV node, blockade can cause partial or complete AV block; and in the myocardium, blockade can decrease contractility. When the heart is healthy, these effects rarely have clinical significance. However, in patients with certain cardiac diseases, verapamil can seriously exacerbate dysfunction. Accordingly, the drug must be used with special caution in patients with cardiac failure and must not be used at all in patients with sick sinus syndrome or second-degree or third-degree AV block.

Other Effects

In older patients, CCBs have been associated with chronic eczematous eruptions, typically starting 3 to 6 months after treatment onset. If the reaction is mild, switching to a different CCB may help. If the condition is severe, use of verapamil and other CCBs should stop.

Gingival hyperplasia (overgrowth of gum tissue) has been reported.

Drug and Food Interactions

Digoxin

Like verapamil, digoxin suppresses impulse conduction through the AV node. Accordingly, when these drugs are used concurrently, the risk for AV block is increased. Patients receiving the combination should be monitored closely.

Verapamil increases plasma levels of digoxin by about 60%, thereby increasing the risk for digoxin toxicity. If signs of toxicity appear, digoxin dosage should be reduced.

Beta-Adrenergic Blocking Agents

Beta blockers and verapamil have the same effects on the heart: they decrease heart rate, AV conduction, and contractility. Hence, when a beta blocker and verapamil are used together, there is a risk for excessive cardiosuppression. To minimize risk, beta blockers and intravenous (IV) verapamil should be administered several hours apart.

Grapefruit Juice

Grapefruit juice can inhibit the intestinal and hepatic metabolism of many drugs and thus raise their levels. In a case report on verapamil toxicity, consumption of grapefruit juice and verapamil (360 mg over 24 hours) led to a verapamil blood level of 2772 ng/mL—approximately 8 to 24 times higher than would have been achieved without grapefruit juice.

Toxicity

Clinical Manifestations

Overdose can produce severe hypotension and cardiotoxicity (bradycardia, AV block, ventricular tachydysrhythmias).

Treatment

General Measures. Verapamil can be removed from the gastrointestinal tract with gastric lavage followed by activated charcoal. Intravenous (IV) calcium gluconate can counteract both vasodilation and negative inotropic effects, but will not reverse AV block.

Hypotension. Hypotension can be treated with IV norepinephrine, which promotes vasoconstriction (by activating $alpha_1$ receptors on blood vessels) and increases cardiac output (by activating $beta_1$ receptors in the heart). Placing the patient in modified Trendelenburg position (legs elevated) and administering IV fluids may also help.

Bradycardia and AV Block. Bradycardia and AV block can be treated with atropine (an anticholinergic drug that blocks parasympathetic influences on the heart). If pharmacologic measures are inadequate, electronic pacing may be required. Use of glucagon in animal models has improved heart rate through increasing amounts of intracellular cyclic adenosine monophosphate. It has been used successfully in treating human cases of CCB toxicity.

Ventricular Tachydysrhythmias. The preferred treatment is direct-current (DC) cardioversion. Antidysrhythmic drugs (procainamide, lidocaine) may also be tried.

Preparations, Dosage, and Administration

Oral

Verapamil is available in immediate-release (IR) tablets (40, 80, and 120 mg) as Calan; sustained-release (SR) tablets (120, 180, and 240 mg) as Calan SR and Covera-HS ♣; and SR capsules (120, 180, 240, and 360 mg) as Verelan. In addition, verapamil is available as Verelan PM (100-, 200-, and 300-mg capsules), a timed-release formulation that, when administered at bedtime, produces maximal verapamil levels in the morning. The sustained- and timed-release formulations are approved only for hypertension. Instruct patients to swallow these products intact, without crushing or chewing. A fixed-dose combination with trandolapril (an angiotensin-converting enzyme [ACE] inhibitor) is available under the trade name Tarka.

The usual initial dosage for angina pectoris is 80 to 120 mg 3 times a day. The usual initial dosage for essential hypertension is 80 mg 3 times a day (using IR tablets), 180 mg of an SR formulation (administered once a day in the morning with food), or 200 mg of Verelan PM (administered once a day at bedtime). Dosages should be reduced for older-adult patients and for patients with advanced renal or liver disease. Dosages for dysrhythmias are presented in Chapter 41.

Intravenous

Intravenous verapamil is used for dysrhythmias. Because IV verapamil can cause severe adverse cardiovascular effects, blood pressure and the electrocardiogram (ECG) should be monitored and equipment for resuscitation should be immediately available. Intravenous dosages for dysrhythmias are presented in Chapter 41.

Diltiazem

Actions and Uses

Like verapamil, diltiazem [Cardizem, Dilacor XR, Tiazac, others] blocks calcium channels in the heart and blood vessels. As a result, the actions and applications of verapamil and diltiazem are very similar. Diltiazem has the same effects on cardiovascular function as verapamil. Both drugs lower blood pressure through arteriolar dilation, and, because their direct suppressant actions are balanced by reflex cardiac stimulation, both have little net effect on the heart. Like verapamil, diltiazem is used for angina pectoris, essential hypertension, and cardiac dysrhythmias (atrial flutter, atrial fibrillation, and paroxysmal supraventricular tachycardia).

Pharmacokinetics

Oral diltiazem is well absorbed and then extensively metabolized on its first pass through the liver. As a result, bioavailability is only about 50%. Effects begin rapidly (within a few minutes) and peak within half an hour. The drug undergoes nearly complete metabolism before elimination in the urine and feces.

Adverse Effects

Adverse effects are like those of verapamil, except that diltiazem causes less constipation. The most common effects are dizziness, flushing, headache, and edema of the ankles and feet. Like verapamil, diltiazem can exacerbate cardiac dysfunction in patients with bradycardia, sick sinus syndrome, heart failure, or second-degree or third-degree AV block. Like other CCBs, diltiazem may cause chronic eczematous rash in older adults.

PATIENT-CENTERED CARE ACROSS THE LIFE SPAN

Calcium Channel Blockers

Life Stage	Patient Care Concerns
Infants	Verapamil can be used in infants for conversion of certain heart dysrhythmias.
Children/adolescents	Calcium channel blockers are used in children for hypertension, hypertensive emergencies, and hypertrophic cardiomyopathy.
Pregnant women	Calcium channel blockers are classified in U.S. Food and Drug Administration Pregnancy Risk Category C. Risk must be weighed against benefit.
Breastfeeding women	Certain drugs such as verapamil may pose harm to the infant. For other drugs such as nifedipine, data are lacking regarding transmission of drug from mother to infant via breast milk.
Older adults	In older patients, calcium channel blockers have been associated with chronic eczematous eruptions.

Drug and Food Interactions

Like verapamil, diltiazem can exacerbate digoxin-induced suppression of AV conduction and can intensify the cardiosuppressant effects of beta blockers. Patients receiving diltiazem concurrently with digoxin or a beta blocker should be monitored closely for cardiac status. As with verapamil, grapefruit juice can significantly increase levels of diltiazem.

Preparations, Dosage, and Administration

Oral diltiazem is available in IR tablets (30, 60, 90, and 120 mg) as Cardizem, extended-release (ER) tablets (120, 180, 240, 300, 360, and 420 mg) as Cardizem LA, and SR capsules (120, 180, 240, 300, 360, and 420 mg) as Cardizem CD, Cartia XT, Dilacor XR, Dilt-CD, Dilt-XR, Diltia XT, Taztia XT, and Tiazac. The drug is also available in solution (5 mg/mL) for IV administration. The usual initial dosage for hypertension is 180 mg once a day with Cardizem CD, 60 to 120 mg twice a day with Cardizem, and 180 to 240 mg once a day with Cardizem LA or Dilacor XR. Angina pectoris can be treated with IR tablets (30 mg 4 times a day initially and 60 mg 4 times a day for maintenance). Intravenous diltiazem is reserved for dysrhythmias.

DIHYDROPYRIDINES: AGENTS THAT ACT MAINLY ON VASCULAR SMOOTH MUSCLE

All of the drugs discussed in this section belong to the *dihydropyridine* family. At therapeutic doses, these drugs produce significant blockade of calcium channels in blood vessels and minimal blockade of calcium channels in the heart. The dihydropyridines are similar to verapamil in some respects, but quite different in others.

Nifedipine

Nifedipine [Adalat CC, Nifedical XL, Nifediac CC, Procardia, Procardia XL] was the first dihydropyridine available and will serve as our prototype for the group. Like verapamil, nifedipine blocks calcium channels in VSM and thereby promotes vasodilation. However, in contrast to verapamil, nifedipine produces very little blockade of calcium channels in the heart. As a result, nifedipine cannot be used to treat dysrhythmias, does not cause cardiac suppression, and is less likely than verapamil to exacerbate preexisting cardiac disorders. Nifedipine also differs from verapamil in that nifedipine is more likely to cause reflex tachycardia. Contrasts between nifedipine and verapamil are shown in Table 37.2.

TABLE 37.2 ■ Comparisons and Contrasts Between Nifedipine and Verapamil

	Drug	
Property	**Nifedipine**	**Verapamil**
DIRECT EFFECTS ON THE HEART AND ARTERIOLES		
Arteriolar dilation	Yes	Yes
Effects on the Heart		
Reduced automaticity	No	Yes
Reduced AV conduction	No	Yes
Reduced contractile force	No	Yes
MAJOR INDICATIONS		
Hypertension	Yes	Yes
Angina pectoris (classical and variant)	Yes	Yes
Dysrhythmias	No	Yes
ADVERSE EFFECTS		
Exacerbation of		
AV block	No	Yes
Sick sinus syndrome	No	Yes
Heart failure	No	Yes
Effects Secondary to Vasodilation		
Edema (ankles and feet)	Yes	Yes
Flushing	Yes	Yes
Headaches	Yes	Yes
Dizziness	Yes	Yes
Reflex tachycardia	Yes	No
Constipation	No	Yes
DRUG INTERACTIONS		
Intensifies digoxin-induced AV block	No	Yes
Intensifies cardiosuppressant effects of beta blockers	No	Yes
Often combined with a beta blocker to suppress reflex tachycardia	Yes	No

AV, atrioventricular.

Hemodynamic Effects

Direct Effects

The direct effects of nifedipine on the cardiovascular system are limited to blockade of calcium channels in VSM. Blockade of calcium channels in peripheral arterioles causes vasodilation and thus lowers arterial pressure. Calcium channel blockade in arteries and arterioles of the heart increases coronary perfusion. Because nifedipine does not block cardiac calcium channels at usual therapeutic doses, the drug has no *direct* suppressant effects on automaticity, AV conduction, or contractile force.

Indirect (Reflex) Effects

By lowering blood pressure, nifedipine activates the baroreceptor reflex, thereby causing sympathetic stimulation of the heart. Because nifedipine lacks direct cardiosuppressant actions, cardiac stimulation is unopposed, and hence heart rate and contractile force increase.

It is important to note that reflex effects occur primarily with the *immediate-release* formulation of nifedipine, not with the SR formulation. This is because the baroreceptor reflex is turned on only by a *rapid* fall in blood pressure; a gradual decline will not activate the reflex. With the IR formulation, blood levels of nifedipine rise quickly, and hence blood pressure drops quickly and the reflex is turned on. Conversely, with the SR formulation, blood levels of nifedipine rise slowly, so blood pressure falls slowly and the reflex is blunted.

Net Effect

The overall hemodynamic response to nifedipine is simply the sum of its direct effect (vasodilation) and indirect effect (reflex cardiac stimulation). Accordingly, nifedipine (1) lowers blood pressure, (2) increases heart rate, and (3) increases contractile force. Please note, however, that the reflex increases in heart rate and contractile force are transient and occur primarily with the IR formulation.

Pharmacokinetics

Nifedipine is well absorbed after oral administration but undergoes extensive first-pass metabolism. As a result, only about 50% of an oral dose reaches the systemic circulation. With the IR formulation, effects begin rapidly and peak in 30 minutes; with the SR formulation, effects begin in 20 minutes and peak in 6 hours. Nifedipine is fully metabolized before excretion in the urine.

Therapeutic Uses

Angina Pectoris

Nifedipine is indicated for vasospastic angina and angina of effort. The drug is usually combined with a beta blocker to prevent reflex stimulation of the heart, which could intensify anginal pain. Long-term use reduces the rates of overt heart failure, coronary angiography, and coronary bypass surgery—but not rates of stroke, myocardial infarction, or death. The role of nifedipine in angina is discussed in Chapter 43.

Hypertension

Nifedipine is used widely to treat *essential hypertension.* Only the SR formulation should be used. In the past, nifedipine was used for *hypertensive emergencies,* but it has largely been replaced by drugs that are safer. The use of CCBs in essential hypertension is discussed in Chapter 39.

Adverse Effects

Some adverse effects are like those of verapamil; others are quite different. Like verapamil, nifedipine can cause flushing, dizziness, headache, peripheral edema, and gingival hyperplasia and may pose a risk for chronic eczematous rash in older patients. In contrast to verapamil, nifedipine causes very little constipation. Also, because nifedipine causes minimal blockade of calcium channels in the heart, the drug is not likely to exacerbate AV block, heart failure, bradycardia, or sick sinus syndrome. Accordingly, nifedipine is preferred to verapamil for patients with these disorders.

A response that occurs with nifedipine that does not occur with verapamil is *reflex tachycardia.* This response is problematic in that it increases cardiac oxygen demand and can thereby increase pain in patients with angina. To prevent reflex tachycardia, nifedipine can be combined with a beta blocker (e.g., metoprolol).

Immediate-Release Nifedipine

Immediate-release nifedipine has been associated with increased mortality in patients with myocardial infarction and unstable angina. Other IR CCBs have been associated with an increased risk for myocardial infarction in patients with hypertension. However, in both cases, a causal relationship has not been established. Nonetheless, the National Heart, Lung, and Blood Institute has recommended that *immediate-release* nifedipine, especially in higher doses, be used with great caution, if at all. It is important to note that these adverse effects have not been associated with *sustained-release* nifedipine or with any other long-acting CCB.

Drug Interactions

Beta-Adrenergic Blockers

Beta blockers are combined with nifedipine to prevent reflex tachycardia. It is important to note that, whereas beta blockers can *decrease* the adverse cardiac effects of *nifedipine,* they can *intensify* the adverse cardiac effects of *verapamil* and *diltiazem.*

Toxicity

When taken in excessive dosage, nifedipine loses selectivity. Hence toxic doses affect the heart in addition to blood vessels. Consequently, the manifestations and treatment of nifedipine overdose are the same as described previously for verapamil.

Preparations, Dosage, and Administration

Nifedipine is available in IR capsules (10 and 20 mg) as Procardia and in SR tablets (30, 60, and 90 mg) as Adalat CC, Nifedical XL, Nifediac CC, and Procardia XL. Instruct patients to swallow SR tablets whole, without crushing or chewing.

For treatment of angina pectoris, the usual initial dosage is 10 mg 3 times a day. The usual maintenance dosage is 10 to 20 mg 3 times a day. The maximal recommended dosage is 180 mg/day.

For essential hypertension, only the SR tablets are approved. The usual initial dosage is 30 mg once a day.

Other Dihydropyridines

In addition to nifedipine, seven other dihydropyridines are available. All are similar to nifedipine. Like nifedipine, these drugs produce greater blockade of calcium channels in VSM than in the heart.

Nicardipine

At therapeutic doses, nicardipine [Cardene SR] produces selective blockade of calcium channels in blood vessels and has minimal direct effects on the heart. The drug has two indications: essential hypertension and effort-induced angina pectoris. The most common adverse effects are flushing, headache, asthenia (weakness), dizziness, palpitations, and edema of the ankles and feet. As with other CCBs, eczematous rash may develop in older patients. Gingival hyperplasia (overgrowth of gum tissue) has been reported. Like nifedipine, nicardipine can be combined with a beta blocker to promote therapeutic effects and suppress reflex tachycardia. Nicardipine is available in 20- and 30-mg IR capsules (generic only) and in SR capsules (30, 45, and 60 mg) sold as Cardene SR. The usual initial dosage for angina pectoris is 20 mg 3 times a day using the IR capsules. The usual initial dosage for essential hypertension is 20 mg 3 times a day (using IR capsules) or 30 mg twice a day (using SR capsules).

Amlodipine

At therapeutic doses, amlodipine [Norvasc] produces selective blockade of calcium channels in blood vessels, having minimal direct effects on the heart. Approved indications are essential hypertension and angina pectoris (effort induced and vasospastic). Amlodipine is administered orally and absorbed slowly; peak levels develop in 6 to 12 hours. The drug has a long half-life (30–50 hours) and therefore is effective with once-a-day dosing. Principal adverse effects are peripheral and facial edema. Flushing, dizziness, and headache may also occur, as may eczematous rash in older patients. In contrast to other dihydropyridines, amlodipine causes little reflex tachycardia. Amlodipine is available in 2.5-, 5-, and 10-mg tablets. The usual initial dosage for hypertension or angina pectoris is 5 mg once a day. Fixed-dose combinations are also available: amlodipine/benazepril [Lotrel], amlodipine/telmisartan [Twynsta], amlodipine/atorvastatin [Caduet], amlodipine/aliskiren [Tekamlo], amlodipine/olmesartin [Azor], amlodipine/valsartan [Exforge], aliskiren/amlodipine/hydrochlorothiazide [Amturnide], amlodipine/valsartan/hydrochlorothiazide [Exforge HCT], amlodipine/perindopril [Prestalia], and amlodipine/hydrochlorothiazide/olmesartan [Tribenzor].

Isradipine

Like nifedipine, isradipine [DynaCirc CR] produces relatively selective blockade of calcium channels in blood vessels. In the United States the drug is approved only for hypertension. Isradipine is rapidly absorbed after oral administration but undergoes extensive first-pass metabolism. Parent drug and metabolites are excreted in the urine. The most common side effects are facial flushing, headache, dizziness, and ankle edema. Eczematous rash may develop in older patients. In contrast to nifedipine, isradipine causes minimal reflex tachycardia. The drug is available in capsules (2.5 and 5 mg). The usual antihypertensive dosage is 2.5 to 5 mg twice a day.

Felodipine

Felodipine [Plendil ♣, Renedil ♣] produces selective blockade of calcium channels in blood vessels. In the United States the drug is approved only for hypertension. Felodipine is well absorbed after oral administration but undergoes extensive first-pass metabolism. As a result, bioavailability is low—only 20%. Plasma levels peak in 2.5 to 5 hours and then decay with a half-life of 24 hours. Because of its prolonged half-life, felodipine is effective with once-a-day dosing. Characteristic adverse effects are reflex tachycardia, peripheral edema, headache, facial flushing, and dizziness. Eczematous rash may develop in older patients. Gingival hyperplasia has been reported. Felodipine is available in ER tablets (2.5, 5, and 10 mg). The usual dosage for hypertension is 5 to 10 mg once a day. A fixed-dose combination with enalapril (an ACE inhibitor) is also available.

Nimodipine

Nimodipine [Nymalize, Nimotop ♣] produces selective blockade of calcium channels in cerebral blood vessels. The only approved application is prophylaxis of neurologic injury after rupture of an intracranial aneurysm. Benefits derive from preventing cerebral arterial spasm that follows subarachnoid hemorrhage (SAH) and can result in ischemic neurologic injury. Dosing (60 mg every 4 hours) should begin within 96 hours of SAH and continue for 21 days. Nimotop ♣ is available in 30-mg liquid-filled capsules for oral administration and as a 60 mg/20 mL oral solution [Nymalize]. Nimodipine must never be given intravenously, owing to a risk for potentially fatal cardiovascular events.

Nisoldipine

Like nifedipine, nisoldipine [Sular] produces selective blockade of calcium channels in blood vessels; the drug has minimal direct effects on the heart. The only approved indication is hypertension. Nisoldipine is well absorbed after oral administration, but the first-pass effect limits bioavailability to 5%. Plasma levels peak 6 hours after administration. The most common side effects are dizziness, headache, and peripheral edema. Reflex tachycardia may also occur. As with other CCBs, eczematous rash may develop in older patients. Nisoldipine is available in ER tablets (8.5, 17, 20, 25.5, 30, 34, and 40 mg). The dosage for hypertension is 20 to 60 mg once a day.

CHAPTER

38 Vasodilators

Laura D. Rosenthal, DNP, ACNP, FAANP

Vasodilation can be produced with a variety of drugs. What sets vasodilators apart from other drugs that cause vasodilation is their mechanism of action: they act directly on the smooth muscles in arterioles and veins to produce vessel relaxation. Two agents—hydralazine and minoxidil—are introduced here. A third, sodium nitroprusside, is used in emergency situations within inpatient settings. This drug is discussed in Unit XXI on drug therapy in acute care.

In approaching the vasodilators, we begin by considering concepts that apply to the vasodilators as a group. After that we discuss the pharmacology of individual agents.

BASIC CONCEPTS IN VASODILATOR PHARMACOLOGY

Selectivity of Vasodilatory Effects

Vasodilators differ from one another with respect to the types of blood vessels they affect. Both hydralazine and minoxidil produce selective dilation of arterioles. Nitroprusside dilates both arterioles *and* veins.

The selectivity of a vasodilator determines its hemodynamic effects. For example, drugs that dilate *resistance vessels* (arterioles) cause a decrease in cardiac *afterload* (the force the heart works against to pump blood). By decreasing afterload, arteriolar dilators reduce cardiac work while causing cardiac output and tissue perfusion to increase. In contrast, drugs that dilate *capacitance vessels* (veins) reduce the force with which blood is returned to the heart, which reduces ventricular filling. This reduction in filling decreases cardiac *preload* (the degree of stretch of the ventricular muscle before contraction), which in turn decreases the force of ventricular contraction. Hence, by decreasing preload, venous dilators cause a decrease in cardiac work, along with a decrease in cardiac output and tissue perfusion.

Because hemodynamic responses to dilation of arterioles and veins differ, the selectivity of a vasodilator is a major determinant of its effects, both therapeutic and undesired. Undesired effects related to selective dilation of arterioles and veins are discussed later. Therapeutic implications of selective dilation are discussed in Chapters 39, 40, and 43.

Overview of Therapeutic Uses

The vasodilators, as a group, have a broad spectrum of uses. Principal indications are *essential hypertension, hypertensive crisis, angina pectoris, heart failure,* and *myocardial infarction.* The specific applications of any particular agent are determined by its pharmacologic profile. Important facets of that profile are route of administration, site of vasodilation (arterioles, veins, or both), and intensity and duration of effects.

Adverse Effects Related to Vasodilation

Postural Hypotension

Postural (orthostatic) hypotension is defined as a fall in blood pressure brought on by moving from a supine or seated position to an upright position. The underlying cause is relaxation of smooth muscle in *veins.* Because of venous relaxation, gravity causes blood to "pool" in veins, thereby decreasing venous return to the heart. Reduced venous return causes a decrease in cardiac output and a corresponding decrease in blood pressure. Hypotension from venous dilation is minimal in recumbent subjects because, when we are lying down, the effect of gravity on venous return is small.

PHARMACOLOGY OF INDIVIDUAL VASODILATORS

Hydralazine

Cardiovascular Effects

Hydralazine causes selective dilation of arterioles. The drug has little or no effect on veins. Arteriolar dilation results from a direct action on vascular smooth muscle (VSM). The exact mechanism is unknown. In response to arteriolar dilation, peripheral resistance and arterial blood pressure fall. In addition, heart rate and myocardial contractility increase, largely by reflex mechanisms. Because hydralazine acts selectively on arterioles, postural hypotension is minimal.

Pharmacokinetics

Absorption and Time Course of Action

Hydralazine is readily absorbed after oral administration. Effects begin within 45 minutes and persist for 6 hours or longer. With parenteral administration, effects begin faster (within 10 minutes) and last 2 to 4 hours.

Metabolism

Hydralazine is inactivated by a metabolic process known as *acetylation.* The ability to acetylate drugs is genetically determined. Some people are rapid acetylators; some are slow acetylators. The distinction between rapid and slow acetylators can be clinically significant because individuals who acetylate hydralazine slowly are likely to have higher blood levels of the drug, which can result in excessive vasodilation and other undesired effects. To avoid hydralazine accumulation, dosage should be reduced in slow acetylators.

Patient Education

RISK FOR HYPOTENSION WITH VASODILATORS

Vasodilators place patients at increased risk for falls. Patients receiving vasodilators should be informed about symptoms of hypotension (lightheadedness, dizziness) and advised to sit or lie down if these occur. Failure to follow this advice may result in fainting. Patients should also be taught that they can minimize hypotension by avoiding abrupt transitions from a supine or seated position to an upright position.

Therapeutic Uses

Essential Hypertension

Oral hydralazine can be used to lower blood pressure in patients with essential hypertension. The regimen almost always includes a beta blocker and may include a diuretic as well (Table 38.1). Although commonly employed in the past, hydralazine has been largely replaced by newer antihypertensive agents (see Chapter 39).

Heart Failure

As discussed in Chapter 40, hydralazine (usually in combination with isosorbide dinitrate) can be used short term to reduce afterload in patients with heart failure. With prolonged therapy, tolerance to hydralazine develops.

Adverse Effects

Reflex Tachycardia

By lowering arterial blood pressure, hydralazine can trigger reflex stimulation of the heart, thereby causing cardiac work and myocardial oxygen demand to increase. Because hydralazine-induced reflex tachycardia is frequently severe, the drug is usually combined with a beta blocker.

Increased Blood Volume

Hydralazine-induced hypotension can cause sodium and water retention and a corresponding increase in blood volume. A diuretic can prevent volume expansion.

Systemic Lupus Erythematosus–Like Syndrome

Hydralazine can cause an acute rheumatoid syndrome that closely resembles systemic lupus erythematosus (SLE). Symptoms include muscle pain, joint pain, fever, nephritis, pericarditis, and the presence of antinuclear antibodies. The syndrome occurs most frequently in slow acetylators and is rare when dosage is kept below 200 mg/day. If an SLE-like reaction occurs, hydralazine should be discontinued. Symptoms are usually reversible but may take 6 or more months to resolve. In some cases, rheumatoid symptoms persist for years.

Other Adverse Effects

Common responses include headache, dizziness, weakness, and fatigue. These reactions are related to hydralazine-induced hypotension.

Drug Interactions

Hydralazine can be combined with a *beta blocker* to protect against reflex tachycardia and with a *diuretic* to prevent sodium and water retention and expansion of blood volume. Drugs that lower blood pressure will intensify hypotensive responses to hydralazine. Accordingly, if hydralazine is used with other *antihypertensive agents,* care is needed to avoid excessive hypotension. In the treatment of heart failure, hydralazine is usually combined with *isosorbide dinitrate,* a drug that dilates veins.

Minoxidil

Minoxidil produces more intense vasodilation than hydralazine but also causes more severe adverse reactions. Because it is both very effective and very dangerous, minoxidil is reserved for patients with severe hypertension unresponsive to safer drugs.

Cardiovascular Effects

Like hydralazine, minoxidil produces selective dilation of *arterioles.* Little or no venous dilation occurs. Arteriolar dilation decreases peripheral resistance and arterial blood pressure. In response, reflex mechanisms increase heart rate and myocardial contractility. Both responses can increase cardiac oxygen demand and can thereby exacerbate angina pectoris.

Vasodilation results from a direct action on VSM. To relax VSM, minoxidil must first be metabolized to minoxidil sulfate. This metabolite then causes potassium channels in VSM to open. The resultant efflux of potassium hyperpolarizes VSM cells, thereby reducing their ability to contract.

Pharmacokinetics

Minoxidil is rapidly and completely absorbed after oral administration. Vasodilation is maximum within 2 to 3 hours and then gradually declines. Residual effects may persist for 2 days or more. Minoxidil is extensively metabolized. Metabolites and parent drug are eliminated in the urine. The drug's half-life is 4.2 hours.

TABLE 38.1 ▪ Vasodilator Preparations, Dosage, and Administration

Drug	Forms	Usual Adult Doses
Hydralazine	Tablets 10, 25, 50, 100 mg	Low initially 10 mg PO four times daily. Gradually increase. Daily doses >200 mg are associated with increased adverse effects.
Hydralazine/hydrochlorothiazide [Hydra-Zide]	Tablets 25/25 and 50/50 mg	One tablet PO daily. May increase to max of 2 tablets/day.
Hydralazine/isosorbide dinitrate [BiDil]	Tablet 20/37.5 mg	Start with 1 tablet PO three times daily. May increase to max of 6 tablets/day.
Minoxidil	Tablets 2.5 and 10 mg	Initial dose 5 mg PO daily. May increase to max of 100 mg/day.

PO, oral administration.

Therapeutic Uses

The only cardiovascular indication for minoxidil is *severe hypertension.* Because of its serious adverse effects, minoxidil is reserved for patients who have not responded to safer drugs. To minimize adverse responses (reflex tachycardia, expansion of blood volume, pericardial effusion), minoxidil should be used with a beta blocker plus intensive diuretic therapy.

Topical minoxidil [Rogaine, others] is used to promote hair growth in balding men and women (see Chapter 85).

Adverse Effects

Reflex Tachycardia

Blood pressure reduction triggers reflex tachycardia, a serious effect that can be minimized by cotreatment with a beta blocker.

Sodium and Water Retention

Fluid retention is both common and serious. Volume expansion may be so severe as to cause cardiac decompensation. Management of fluid retention requires a loop diuretic (e.g., furosemide) used alone or in combination with a thiazide diuretic. If diuretics are inadequate, dialysis must be employed, or minoxidil must be withdrawn.

Hypertrichosis

About 80% of patients taking minoxidil for 4 weeks or more develop hypertrichosis (excessive growth of hair). Hair growth begins on the face and later develops on the arms, legs, and back. Hypertrichosis appears to result from proliferation of epithelial cells at the base of the hair follicle; vasodilation may also be involved. Hairiness is a cosmetic problem that can be controlled by shaving or using a depilatory. However, many patients find hypertrichosis both unmanageable and intolerable and refuse to continue treatment.

BLACK BOX WARNING: MINOXIDIL

Minoxidil can cause pericardial effusion, occasionally progressing to tamponade, and may exacerbate angina pectoris.

Other Adverse Effects

Minoxidil may cause nausea, headache, fatigue, breast tenderness, glucose intolerance, thrombocytopenia, and skin reactions (rashes, Stevens-Johnson syndrome). In addition, the drug has caused hemorrhagic cardiac lesions in experimental animals.

PATIENT-CENTERED CARE ACROSS THE LIFE SPAN

Vasodilators

Life Stage	Patient Care Concerns
Infants	Hydralazine is used in infants as young as 1 month for management of chronic hypertension.
Children/adolescents	Hydralazine can be used safely in children, just in smaller doses. Side-effect profiles are similar to those of adults.
Pregnant women	Hydralazine and minoxidil are classified in U.S. Food and Drug Administration Pregnancy Risk Category C. Benefits should outweigh the risks.
Breastfeeding women	Data are lacking regarding transmission of drug from mother to infant via breast milk.
Older adults	Monitor for falls because there is increased risk with polypharmacy and associated orthostatic hypotension.

CHAPTER

39 Drugs for Hypertension

Laura D. Rosenthal, DNP, ACNP, FAANP

Hypertension is a common, chronic disorder that affects about 2 million American children, 67 million American adults, and more than 1 billion people worldwide. According to the World Health Organization, hypertension is the leading global risk for mortality, causing 12.8% of all human deaths. Left untreated, hypertension can lead to heart disease, kidney disease, and stroke. Conversely, a treatment program of lifestyle modifications and drug therapy can reduce blood pressure (BP) and the risk for long-term complications. However, although we can reduce symptoms and long-term consequences, we can't cure hypertension. As a result, treatment must continue lifelong, making nonadherence a significant problem. Despite advances in management, hypertension remains undertreated: among Americans with the disease, only 74% undergo treatment, and only 48% take sufficient medicine to bring their BP under control.

In 2014, the *Journal of the American Medical Association* issued revised clinical guidelines on hypertension. This document is titled *2014 Evidence-Based Guidelines for the Management of High Blood Pressure in Adults: Report from the panel members appointed to the Eighth Joint National Committee (JNC 8).* Recommendations in JNC 8 update and simplify those of JNC 7, released in 2003 (see Table 39.1 for comparison). Important changes include creation of similar treatment goals for all hypertensive populations and introduction of new BP thresholds for pharmacologic treatment of hypertension. Throughout this chapter, clinical practice recommendations reflect those in the 2014 hypertension guidelines, except where noted otherwise.[1]

[1]Although the 2014 hypertension guideline is the most influential guideline in the United States, it is not the only authoritative guideline available. Treatment guidelines have been released by several organizations, including the American Society of Hypertension, the Canadian Hypertension Education Program, the European Society of Hypertension in conjunction with the European Society of Cardiology, and the World Health Organization in conjunction with the International Society of Hypertension.

TABLE 39.1 ▪ Comparison of JNC 7 and JNC 8 Guidelines

Condition/ Classification	JNC 7 (mm Hg)	JNC 8 (mm Hg)
Normal (adults <60 yr)	<120/80	<140/90
Diabetes	≤130/80	<140/90
Renal disease	≤130/80	<140/90
Older adult (>60 yr)	<140/90	<150/90

JNC 8, *2014 Evidence-Based Guidelines for the Management of High Blood Pressure in Adults: Report from the panel members appointed to the Eighth Joint National Committee*; JNC 7, *The Seventh Report of the Joint National Committee on Prevention, Detection, Evaluation, and Treatment of High Blood Pressure,* 2003.

BASIC CONSIDERATIONS IN HYPERTENSION

In this section, we consider three issues: (1) classification of BP based on values for systolic and diastolic pressure, (2) types of hypertension, and (3) the damaging effects of chronic hypertension.

Classification of Blood Pressure

In 2003, JNC 7 defined four BP categories: normal, prehypertension, stage 1 hypertension, and stage 2 hypertension. This scheme differs significantly from the 2014 hypertension guidelines, which no longer separate hypertension into different categories. In the 2014 hypertension guidelines, in patients 60 years or older, treatment of hypertension should be initiated at a systolic blood pressure (SBP) of ≥150 mm Hg or a diastolic blood pressure (DBP) of ≥90 mm Hg. In patients younger than 60 years, pharmacologic treatment of hypertension should start at an SBP of ≥140 mm Hg or a DBP of ≥90 mm Hg. These guidelines include patients with chronic kidney disease and diabetes. In JNC 7, these patient populations were treated differently. This is no longer the case.

Types of Hypertension

There are two broad categories of hypertension: *primary hypertension* and *secondary hypertension.* Primary hypertension is by far the most common form of hypertensive disease. Less than 10% of people with hypertension have a secondary form.

Primary (Essential) Hypertension

Primary hypertension is defined as hypertension that has no identifiable cause. A diagnosis of primary hypertension is made by ruling out probable specific causes of BP elevation. Primary hypertension is a chronic, progressive disorder. In the absence of treatment, patients will experience a continuous, gradual rise in BP over the rest of their lives.

In the United States primary hypertension affects about 30% of adults. However, not all groups are at equal risk: older people are at higher risk than younger people; black Americans are at higher risk than white Americans; and postmenopausal women are at higher risk than premenopausal women.

Secondary Hypertension

Secondary hypertension is defined as an elevation of BP brought on by an identifiable primary cause. Because secondary hypertension results from an identifiable cause, it may be possible to treat that cause directly, rather than relying on antihypertensive drugs for symptomatic relief. As a result, some individuals can actually be cured. For example, if hypertension occurs secondary to pheochromocytoma, surgical removal of the tumor may produce permanent cure. When cure is not possible, secondary hypertension can be managed with the same drugs used for primary hypertension.

Consequences of Hypertension

Chronic hypertension is associated with increased morbidity and mortality. Left untreated, prolonged elevation of BP can lead to heart disease, renal dysfunction, and stroke. The degree of injury is directly related to the degree of pressure elevation: The higher the pressure, the greater the risk. Among people 40 to 70 years old, the risk for cardiovascular disease is doubled for each 20 mm Hg increase in SBP or each 10 mm Hg increase in DBP—beginning at 115/75 mm Hg and continuing through 185/155 mm Hg. For people older than 50 years, elevated *systolic* BP poses a greater risk than elevated *diastolic* BP. For patients of all ages, hypertension-related deaths result largely from cerebral hemorrhage, renal failure, heart failure, and myocardial infarction (MI).

Unfortunately, despite its potential for serious harm, hypertension usually remains asymptomatic until long after injury has begun to develop. As a result, the disease can exist for years before overt pathology is evident. Because injury develops slowly and progressively, and because hypertension rarely causes discomfort, many people who have the disease don't know it. Furthermore, many who do know it forgo treatment anyway, largely because hypertension doesn't make them feel bad—that is, until it's too late.

MANAGEMENT OF CHRONIC HYPERTENSION

In this section we consider treatments for chronic hypertension. We begin by addressing patient evaluation and other basic issues, after which we discuss the two modes of management: lifestyle modifications and drug therapy.

Basic Considerations

Diagnosis

Diagnosis should be based on several BP readings, not just one. If an initial screen shows that BP is elevated (but does not represent an immediate danger), measurement should be repeated on two subsequent office visits. At each visit, two measurements should be made, at least 5 minutes apart. The patient should be seated in a chair—not on an examination table—with his or her feet on the floor. High readings should be confirmed in the contralateral arm. If the mean of all readings shows that SBP is indeed greater than 140 mm Hg or that DBP is greater than 90 mm Hg, a diagnosis of hypertension can be made.

Ideally, diagnosis would be based on *ambulatory blood pressure monitoring* (ABPM) because office-based measurements are often abnormally high, causing individuals to be diagnosed with hypertension when they don't really have it. By contrast, when BP is measured with ABPM, false-positive diagnoses can be avoided. Accordingly, some experts recommend that office-based measurements be used only for *screening* and that treatment be postponed until the diagnosis is confirmed using ABPM. In this way, the risks and expense of unnecessary treatment will be avoided.

Benefits of Lowering Blood Pressure

Multiple clinical trials have demonstrated unequivocally that, when the BP of hypertensive individuals is lowered, morbidity is decreased and life is prolonged. Treatment reduces the incidence of stroke by 35% to 40%, MI by 20% to 25%, and heart failure by more than 50%. Although reductions in morbidity are not as dramatic, they are nonetheless significant: among patients with stage 1 hypertension plus additional cardiovascular risk factors, one death would be prevented for every 11 patients who reduced SBP by 12 mm Hg for a period of 10 years—and among those with hypertension plus cardiovascular disease or target-organ damage, one death would be prevented for every 9 patients who achieved a sustained 12 mm Hg reduction in pressure.

Patient Evaluation

Evaluation of patients with hypertension has two major objectives. Specifically, we must assess for (1) identifiable causes of hypertension and (2) factors that increase cardiovascular risk. To aid evaluation, diagnostic tests are required.

Hypertension With a Treatable Cause

As discussed previously, some forms of hypertension result from a treatable cause, such as Cushing syndrome, pheochromocytoma, and use of oral contraceptives. Patients should be evaluated for these causes and managed appropriately. In many cases, direct treatment of the underlying cause can control BP, eliminating the need for further antihypertensive therapy.

Factors that Increase Cardiovascular Risk

Two types of factors—existing target-organ damage and major cardiovascular risk factors—increase the risk for cardiovascular events in people with hypertension. When these factors are present, aggressive therapy is indicated. Accordingly, to select appropriate interventions, we must identify patients with the following types of *target-organ damage:*

- Heart disease
- Left ventricular hypertrophy
- Angina pectoris
- Prior MI
- Prior coronary revascularization
- Heart failure
- Stroke or transient ischemic attack
- Chronic kidney disease
- Peripheral arterial disease
- Retinopathy

We also must identify patients with the following *major cardiovascular risk factors* (other than hypertension):

- Cigarette smoking
- Physical inactivity
- Dyslipidemia
- Diabetes
- Microalbuminuria
- Advancing age (>55 years for men, >65 years for women)
- Family history of premature cardiovascular disease

Diagnostic Tests

The following tests should be done in all patients: electrocardiogram; complete urinalysis; hemoglobin and hematocrit; and blood levels of sodium, potassium, calcium, creatinine, glucose, uric acid, triglycerides, and cholesterol (total, low-density lipoprotein, and high-density lipoprotein cholesterol).

Treatment Goals

The ultimate goal in treating hypertension is to reduce cardiovascular and renal morbidity and mortality. Hopefully, this can be accomplished without decreasing quality of life with the drugs employed. For patients younger than 60 years, the goal is to maintain SBP below 140 mm Hg and DBP below 90 mm Hg. For patients 60 years and older, the goal is to maintain SBP below 150 mm Hg and DBP below 90 mm Hg.

Therapeutic Interventions

We can reduce BP in two ways: we can implement healthy lifestyle changes, and we can treat with antihypertensive drugs. For all patients, a combination of lifestyle changes and drugs is indicated. Lifestyle changes and drug therapy are discussed in detail next.

Lifestyle Modifications

Lifestyle changes offer multiple cardiovascular benefits with little cost and minimal risk. When implemented before hypertension develops, they may actually prevent hypertension. When implemented after hypertension has developed, they can lower BP, possibly decreasing or eliminating the need for drugs. Lastly, lifestyle modifications can decrease other cardiovascular risk factors. Accordingly, all patients should be strongly encouraged to adopt a healthy lifestyle. Key components are discussed here.

Sodium Restriction

Reducing sodium chloride (salt) intake can lower BP in people with hypertension and can help prevent overt hypertension in those with prehypertension. In addition, salt restriction can enhance the hypotensive effects of drugs. However, the benefits of sodium restriction are both small and short lasting: over time, BP returns to its original level, despite continued salt restriction. Nonetheless, the Department of Health and Human Services *2015–2020 Dietary Guidelines for Americans* recommends that all people with hypertension consume no more than 2300 mg of sodium a day. To facilitate salt restriction, patients should be given information on the salt content of foods.

Experts disagree about the relationship between salt intake and BP in *normotensive* patients. In particular, they disagree as to whether a high-salt diet *causes* hypertension. For people with normal BP, a low-salt diet may be considered healthy or unnecessary, depending on the expert you consult.

The DASH Eating Plan

Two studies have shown that we can reduce BP by adopting a healthy diet, known as the Dietary Approaches to Stop Hypertension (DASH) eating plan. This diet is rich in fruits, vegetables, and low-fat dairy products and low in total fat, saturated fats, and cholesterol. In addition, the plan encourages intake of whole-grain products, fish, poultry, and nuts and recommends minimal intake of red meat and sweets. Details are available online at https://www.nhlbi.nih.gov/health/health-topics/topics/dash.

Alcohol Restriction

Excessive alcohol consumption can raise BP and create resistance to antihypertensive drugs. Accordingly, patients should limit alcohol intake: most men should consume no more than 1 ounce/day; women and lighter weight men should consume no more than 0.5 ounce/day. (One ounce of ethanol is equivalent to about two mixed drinks, two glasses of wine, or two cans of beer.)

Aerobic Exercise

Regular aerobic exercise (e.g., walking, swimming, bicycling) can reduce BP by about 10 mm Hg. In addition, exercise reduces the risk for cardiovascular disease and reduces all-cause mortality. In normotensive people, exercise decreases the risk for developing hypertension. Accordingly, patients should be encouraged to develop an exercise program if they have not already done so. An activity as simple as brisk walking 30 to 45 minutes most days of the week is beneficial.

Smoking Cessation

Smoking is a major risk factor for cardiovascular disease. Each time a cigarette is smoked, BP rises. In patients with hypertension, smoking can reduce the effects of antihypertensive drugs. Clearly, all patients who smoke should be strongly encouraged to quit. (Pharmacologic aids to smoking cessation are discussed in Chapter 32.) As a rule, use of nicotine replacement products (e.g., nicotine gum, nicotine patch) does not elevate BP. The cardiovascular benefits of quitting become evident within 1 year.

Weight Loss

Weight loss can reduce BP in 60% to 80% of overweight hypertensive individuals and can enhance responses to antihypertensive drugs. Consequently, a program of weight management and exercise is recommended for patients who are overweight.

Maintenance of Potassium and Calcium Intake

Potassium has a beneficial effect on BP. In patients with hypertension, potassium can lower BP. In normotensive people, high potassium intake helps protect against hypertension, whereas low intake elevates BP. For optimal cardiovascular effects, all adults older than 14 years should take in 4700 mg of potassium a day. Preferred sources are fresh fruits and vegetables. If hypokalemia develops secondary to diuretic therapy, dietary intake may be insufficient to correct the problem. In this case the patient may need to use a potassium supplement, a potassium-sparing diuretic, or a potassium-containing salt substitute.

Although adequate calcium is needed for overall good health, the effect of calcium on BP is only modest. In epidemiologic studies, high calcium intake is associated with a reduced incidence of hypertension. Among patients with hypertension, a few may be helped by increasing calcium intake. To maintain good health, calcium intake should be 1300 mg/day for adults older than 14 years.

Drug Therapy

Drug therapy, together with lifestyle modifications, can control BP in all patients with chronic hypertension. The decision to use drugs should be the result of collaboration between prescriber and patient. We have a wide assortment of antihypertensive drugs. Consequently, for most patients, it should be possible to establish a program that is effective and yet devoid of objectionable side effects.

Prototype Drugs

DRUGS FOR HYPERTENSION

Diuretics

Hydrochlorothiazide
Spironolactone

Beta-Adrenergic Blocker

Metoprolol

Inhibitors of the Renin-Angiotensin-Aldosterone System

Captopril (angiotensin-converting enzyme inhibitor)
Losartan (angiotensin II receptor blocker)
Aliskiren (direct renin inhibitor)
Eplerenone (aldosterone antagonist)

Calcium Channel Blockers

Verapamil
Nifedipine

Review of Blood Pressure Control

Before discussing the antihypertensive drugs, we need to review the major mechanisms by which BP is controlled. This information will help you understand the mechanisms by which drugs lower BP.

Principal Determinants of Blood Pressure

The principal determinants of BP are shown in Fig. 39.1. As indicated, arterial pressure is the product of cardiac output and peripheral resistance. An increase in either will increase BP.

Cardiac Output. Cardiac output is influenced by four factors: (1) heart rate, (2) myocardial contractility (force of contraction), (3) blood volume, and (4) venous return of blood to the heart. An increase in any of these will increase cardiac output, thereby causing BP to rise. Conversely, a decrease in these factors will make BP fall. Hence, to reduce BP, we might give a beta blocker to reduce cardiac output, or a diuretic to reduce blood volume, or a venodilator to reduce venous return.

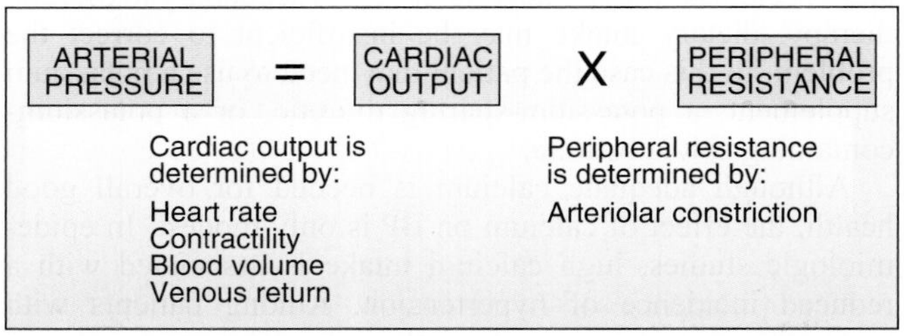

Figure 39.1 ▪ Primary determinants of arterial blood pressure.

Peripheral Vascular Resistance. Vascular resistance is increased by arteriolar constriction. Accordingly, we can reduce BP with drugs that promote arteriolar dilation.

Systems that Help Regulate Blood Pressure

Having established that BP is determined by heart rate, myocardial contractility, blood volume, venous return, and arteriolar constriction, we can now examine how these factors are regulated. Three regulatory systems are of particular significance: (1) the sympathetic nervous system, (2) the renin-angiotensin-aldosterone system (RAAS), and (3) the kidney.

Sympathetic Baroreceptor Reflex. The sympathetic nervous system employs a reflex circuit—the baroreceptor reflex—to keep BP at a preset level. This circuit operates as follows:

1. Baroreceptors in the aortic arch and carotid sinus sense BP and relay this information to the brainstem.
2. When BP is perceived as too low, the brainstem sends impulses along sympathetic nerves to stimulate the heart and blood vessels.
3. BP is then elevated by (a) activation of $beta_1$ receptors in the heart, resulting in increased cardiac output; and (b) activation of vascular $alpha_1$ receptors, resulting in vasoconstriction.
4. When BP has been restored to an acceptable level, sympathetic stimulation of the heart and vascular smooth muscle subsides.

The baroreceptor reflex frequently opposes our attempts to reduce BP with drugs. Opposition occurs because the "set point" of the baroreceptors is high in people with hypertension. That is, the baroreceptors are set to perceive excessively high BP as "normal" (i.e., appropriate). As a result, the system operates to maintain BP at pathologic levels. Consequently, when we attempt to lower BP using drugs, the reduced (healthier) pressure is interpreted by the baroreceptors as below what it should be, and, in response, signals are sent along sympathetic nerves to "correct" the reduction. These signals produce reflex tachycardia and vasoconstriction—responses that can counteract the hypotensive effects of drugs. Clearly, if treatment is to succeed, the regimen must compensate for the resistance offered by this reflex. Taking a *beta blocker,* which will block reflex tachycardia, can be an effective method of compensation. Fortunately, when BP has been suppressed with drugs for an extended time, the baroreceptors become reset at a lower level. Consequently, as therapy proceeds, sympathetic reflexes offer progressively less resistance to the hypotensive effects of medication.

Renin-Angiotensin-Aldosterone System. The RAAS can elevate BP, negating the hypotensive effects of drugs. The RAAS is discussed in Chapter 36 and reviewed briefly here.

The RAAS elevates BP beginning with the release of renin from juxtaglomerular cells of the kidney. These cells release renin in response to reduced renal blood flow, reduced blood volume, reduced BP, and activation of $beta_1$-adrenergic receptors on the cell surface. After its release, *renin* catalyzes the conversion of angiotensinogen into angiotensin I, a weak vasoconstrictor. After this, *angiotensin-converting enzyme*

(ACE) acts on angiotensin I to form *angiotensin II,* a compound that constricts systemic and renal blood vessels. Constriction of systemic blood vessels elevates BP by increasing peripheral resistance. Constriction of renal blood vessels elevates BP by reducing glomerular filtration, which causes retention of salt and water, which in turn increases blood volume and BP. In addition to causing vasoconstriction, angiotensin II causes release of *aldosterone* from the adrenal cortex. Aldosterone acts on the kidney to further increase retention of sodium and water.

Because drug-induced reductions in BP can activate the RAAS, this system can counteract the effect we are trying to achieve. We have five ways to cope with this problem. First, we can suppress renin release with *beta blockers.* Second, we can prevent conversion of angiotensinogen to angiotensin I with a *direct renin inhibitor* (DRI). Third, we can prevent the conversion of angiotensin I into angiotensin II with an *ACE inhibitor.* Fourth, we can block receptors for angiotensin II with an *angiotensin II receptor blocker* (ARB). And fifth, we can block receptors for aldosterone with an *aldosterone antagonist.*

Renal Regulation of Blood Pressure. As discussed in Chapter 34, the kidney plays a central role in long-term regulation of BP. When BP falls, glomerular filtration rate (GFR) falls too, thereby promoting retention of sodium, chloride, and water. The resultant increase in blood volume increases venous return to the heart, causing an increase in cardiac output, which in turn increases arterial pressure. We can neutralize renal effects on BP with *diuretics.*

Antihypertensive Mechanisms: Sites of Drug Action and Effects Produced

As discussed previously, drugs can lower BP by reducing heart rate, myocardial contractility, blood volume, venous return, and the tone of arteriolar smooth muscle. In this section we survey the principal mechanisms by which drugs produce these effects.

The major mechanisms for lowering BP are shown in Fig. 39.2 and Table 39.2. The figure depicts the principal sites at which antihypertensive drugs act. The table shows the effects elicited when drugs act at these sites. The numbering system used in the following text corresponds with the system used in Fig. 39.2 and Table 39.2.

1—Brainstem

Antihypertensive drugs acting in the brainstem suppress sympathetic outflow to the heart and blood vessels, resulting in decreased heart rate, decreased myocardial contractility, and vasodilation. Vasodilation contributes the most to reducing BP. Dilation of arterioles reduces BP by decreasing vascular resistance. Dilation of veins reduces BP by decreasing venous return to the heart.

2—Sympathetic Ganglia

Ganglionic blockade reduces sympathetic stimulation of the heart and blood vessels. Antihypertensive effects result primarily from dilation of arterioles and veins. Ganglionic blocking agents produce such a profound reduction in BP that they are used rarely, and then only for hypertensive emergencies. Because use is so limited, the last one available—mecamylamine—was voluntarily withdrawn from the U.S. market in 2009.

3—Terminals of Adrenergic Nerves

Antihypertensive agents that act at adrenergic nerve terminals decrease the release of norepinephrine, resulting in decreased sympathetic stimulation of the heart and blood vessels. These drugs, known as *adrenergic neuron blocking agents*, are used only rarely. In the United States reserpine is the only drug in this class still on the market.

4—Beta$_1$-Adrenergic Receptors on the Heart

Blockade of cardiac beta$_1$ receptors prevents sympathetic stimulation of the heart. As a result, heart rate and myocardial contractility decline.

5—Alpha$_1$-Adrenergic Receptors on Blood Vessels

Blockade of vascular alpha$_1$ receptors promotes dilation of arterioles and veins. Arteriolar dilation reduces peripheral resistance. Venous dilation reduces venous return to the heart.

6—Vascular Smooth Muscle

Several antihypertensive drugs (see Fig. 39.2) act directly on vascular smooth muscle to cause relaxation. One of these agents—sodium nitroprusside—is used only for hypertensive emergencies. The rest are used for chronic hypertension.

7—Renal Tubules

Diuretics act on renal tubules to promote salt and water excretion. As a result, blood volume declines, causing BP to fall.

Components of the RAAS (8a to 8e)

8a—Beta$_1$ Receptors on Juxtaglomerular Cells. Blockade of beta$_1$ receptors on juxtaglomerular cells suppresses release of renin. The resultant decrease in angiotensin II levels has three effects: peripheral vasodilation, renal vasodilation, and suppression of aldosterone-mediated volume expansion.

8b—Renin. Inhibition of renin decreases conversion of angiotensinogen into angiotensin I and thereby suppresses the entire RAAS. The result is peripheral vasodilation, renal vasodilation, and suppression of aldosterone-mediated volume expansion.

8c—Angiotensin-Converting Enzyme. Inhibitors of ACE suppress formation of angiotensin II. The result is peripheral vasodilation, renal vasodilation, and suppression of aldosterone-mediated volume expansion.

8d—Angiotensin II Receptors. Blockade of angiotensin II receptors prevents the actions of angiotensin II. Hence blockade results in peripheral vasodilation, renal vasodilation, and suppression of aldosterone-mediated volume expansion.

8e—Aldosterone Receptors. Blockade of aldosterone receptors in the kidney promotes excretion of sodium and water and thereby reduces blood volume.

Classes of Antihypertensive Drugs

In this section we consider the principal drugs employed to treat *chronic* hypertension. Drugs for hypertensive emergencies and hypertensive disorders of pregnancy are considered separately.

Diuretics

Diuretics are a mainstay of antihypertensive therapy. These drugs reduce BP when used alone, and they can enhance the effects of other hypotensive drugs. The basic pharmacology of the diuretics is discussed in Chapter 35.

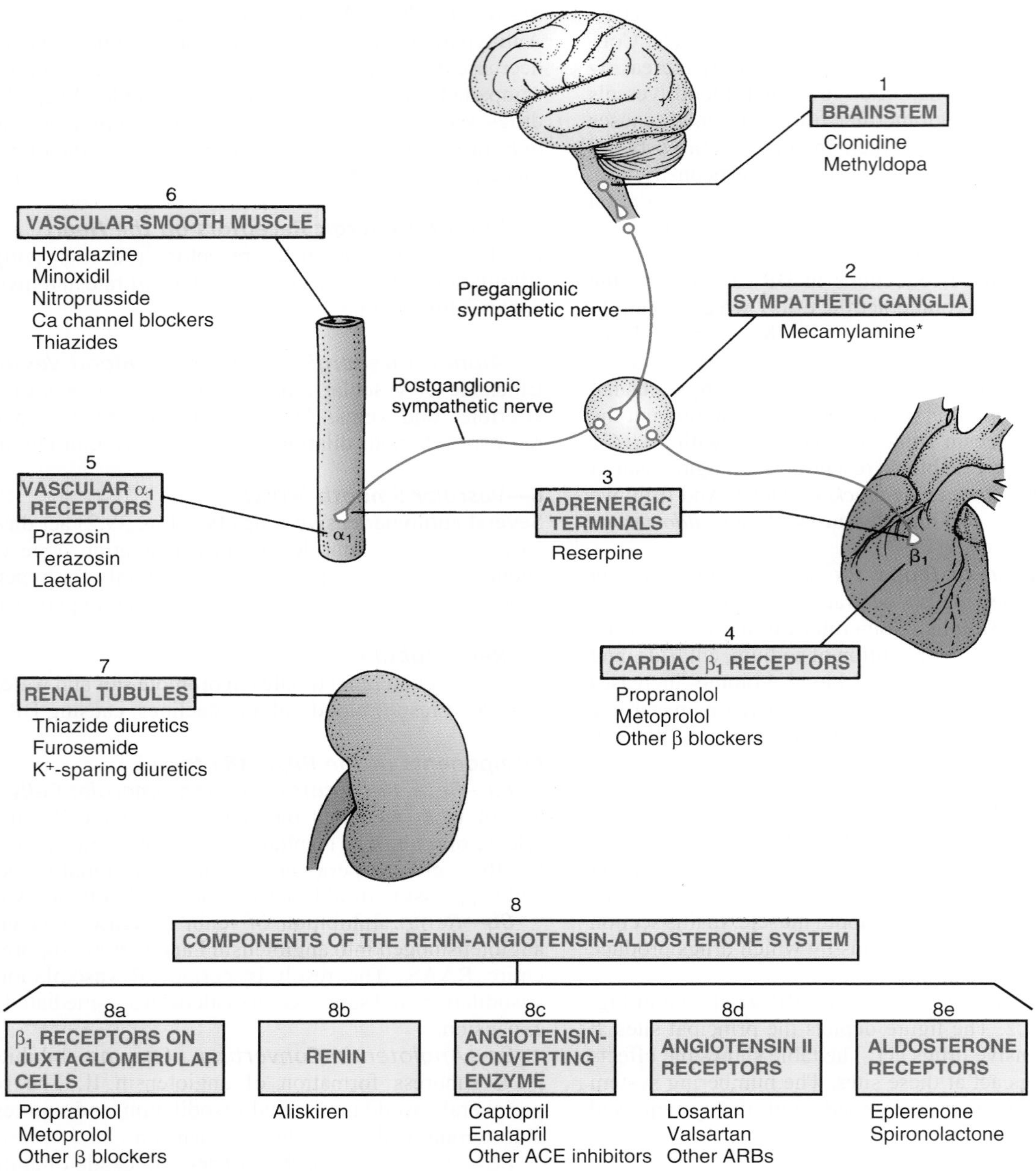

Figure 39.2 ▪ Sites of action of antihypertensive drugs.
Note that some antihypertensive agents act at more than one site: beta (β) blockers act at sites 4 and 8a, and thiazides act at sites 6 and 7. The hemodynamic consequences of drug actions at the sites depicted are shown in Table 39.2. (ACE, angiotensin-converting enzyme; ARB, angiotensin II receptor blocker; *, no longer available in the United States.)

Thiazide Diuretics. Thiazide diuretics (e.g., hydrochlorothiazide, chlorthalidone) are first-line drugs for hypertension. They reduce BP by two mechanisms: reduction of blood volume and reduction of arterial resistance. Reduced blood volume is responsible for initial antihypertensive effects. Reduced vascular resistance develops over time and is responsible for long-term antihypertensive effects. The mechanism by which thiazides reduce vascular resistance has not been determined.

Of the thiazides available, hydrochlorothiazide is used most widely. In fact, hydrochlorothiazide is used more widely than any other antihypertensive drug. Nonetheless, other thiazides, especially chlorthalidone, may be more effective.

The principal adverse effect of thiazides is *hypokalemia.* This can be minimized by consuming potassium-rich foods and using potassium supplements or a potassium-sparing diuretic. Other side effects include *dehydration, hyperglycemia,* and *hyperuricemia.*

TABLE 39.2 ■ Antihypertensive Effects Elicited by Drug Actions at Specific Sites

Site of Drug Action*	Representative Drug	Drug Effects
Brainstem	Clonidine	Suppression of sympathetic outflow decreases sympathetic stimulation of the heart and blood vessels.
Sympathetic ganglia	Mecamylamine†	Ganglionic blockade reduces sympathetic stimulation of the heart and blood vessels.
Adrenergic nerve terminals	Reserpine	Reduced norepinephrine release decreases sympathetic stimulation of the heart and blood vessels.
Cardiac $beta_1$ receptors	Metoprolol	$Beta_1$ blockade decreases heart rate and myocardial contractility.
Vascular $alpha_1$ receptors	Prazosin	$Alpha_1$ blockade causes vasodilation.
Vascular smooth muscle	Hydralazine	Relaxation of vascular smooth muscle causes vasodilation.
Renal tubules	Hydrochlorothiazide	Promotion of diuresis decreases blood volume.
COMPONENTS OF THE RENIN-ANGIOTENSIN-ALDOSTERONE SYSTEM (8A TO 8E)		
8a. $Beta_1$ receptors on juxtaglomerular cells	Metoprolol	$Beta_1$ blockade suppresses renin release, resulting in (1) vasodilation secondary to reduced production of angiotensin II and (2) prevention of aldosterone-mediated volume expansion.
8b. Renin	Aliskiren	Inhibition of renin suppresses formation of angiotensin I, which in turn decreases formation of angiotensin II and thereby reduces (1) vasoconstriction and (2) aldosterone-mediated volume expansion.
8c. Angiotensin-converting enzyme (ACE)	Captopril	Inhibition of ACE decreases formation of angiotensin II and thereby prevents (1) vasoconstriction and (2) aldosterone-mediated volume expansion.
8d. Angiotensin II receptors	Losartan	Blockade of angiotensin II receptors prevents angiotensin-mediated vasoconstriction and aldosterone-mediated volume expansion.
8e. Aldosterone receptors	Eplerenone	Blockade of aldosterone receptors in the kidney promotes excretion of sodium and water and thereby reduces blood volume.

*Site numbers in this table correspond with site numbers in Fig. 39.2.
†No longer available in the United States.

Thiazides are superior to calcium channel blockers (CCBs) and ACE inhibitors as monotherapy and therefore are preferred.

Loop Diuretics. Loop diuretics (e.g., furosemide) produce much greater diuresis than the thiazides. For most individuals with chronic hypertension, the amount of fluid loss that loop diuretics can produce is greater than needed or desirable. Consequently, loop diuretics are not used routinely for hypertension. Rather, they are reserved for (1) patients who need greater diuresis than can be achieved with thiazides and (2) patients with a low GFR (because thiazides won't work when GFR is low). Like the thiazides, the loop diuretics lower BP by reducing blood volume and promoting vasodilation.

Most adverse effects are like those of the thiazides: *hypokalemia, dehydration, hyperglycemia,* and *hyperuricemia.* In addition, loop diuretics can cause *hearing loss.*

Potassium-Sparing Diuretics. The degree of diuresis induced by the potassium-sparing agents (e.g., spironolactone) is small. Consequently, these drugs have only modest hypotensive effects. However, because of their ability to conserve potassium, these drugs can play an important role in an antihypertensive regimen. Specifically, they can balance potassium loss caused by thiazides or loop diuretics. The most significant adverse effect of the potassium-sparing agents is *hyperkalemia.* Because of the risk for hyperkalemia, potassium-sparing diuretics must not be used in combination with one another or with potassium supplements. Also, they should not be used routinely with ACE inhibitors, ARBs, or aldosterone antagonists, all of which promote significant hyperkalemia.

Sympatholytics (Antiadrenergic Drugs)

Sympatholytic drugs suppress the influence of the sympathetic nervous system on the heart, blood vessels, and other structures. These drugs are used widely for hypertension.

There are five subcategories of sympatholytic drugs: (1) beta blockers, (2) $alpha_1$ blockers, (3) alpha/beta blockers, (4) centrally acting $alpha_2$ agonists, and (5) adrenergic neuron blockers.

Beta-Adrenergic Blockers. Like the thiazides, beta blockers (e.g., metoprolol) are widely used antihypertensive drugs. However, despite their efficacy and frequent use, the exact mechanism by which they reduce BP is somewhat uncertain. Beta blockers are less effective in black people than in whites.

The beta blockers have at least four useful actions in hypertension. First, blockade of cardiac $beta_1$ receptors decreases heart rate and contractility, thereby causing cardiac output to decline. Second, beta blockers can suppress reflex tachycardia caused by vasodilators. Third, blockade of $beta_1$ receptors on juxtaglomerular cells of the kidney reduces release of renin and thereby reduces angiotensin II–mediated vasoconstriction and aldosterone-mediated volume expansion. Fourth, long-term use of beta blockers reduces peripheral vascular resistance—by a mechanism that is unknown. This action could readily account for most of their antihypertensive effects.

Three beta blockers have *intrinsic sympathomimetic activity: pindolol, penbutolol, and acebutolol.* That is, they can produce mild activation of beta receptors while blocking receptor activation by strong agonists (e.g., norepinephrine). As a result, heart rate at rest is slowed less than with other beta blockers. Accordingly, if a patient develops symptomatic bradycardia with another beta blocker, switching to one of these may help.

Beta blockers can produce several adverse effects. Blockade of cardiac $beta_1$ receptors can produce *bradycardia, decreased atrioventricular (AV) conduction,* and *reduced contractility.* Consequently, beta blockers should not be used by patients with sick sinus syndrome or second- or third-degree AV block—and must be used with care in patients with heart failure. Blockade of $beta_2$ receptors in the lung can promote *bronchoconstriction*. Accordingly, beta blockers should be used with caution in patients with asthma. If an asthmatic individual must use a beta blocker, a $beta_1$-selective agent (e.g., metoprolol) should be employed. Beta blockers can mask signs of hypoglycemia and therefore must be used with caution in patients with diabetes. Potential side effects of beta blockers include depression, insomnia, bizarre dreams, and sexual dysfunction; however, a review of older clinical trials has shown that the risk is small or nonexistent.

The basic pharmacology of the beta blockers is discussed in Chapter 14.

Alpha₁ Blockers. The $alpha_1$ blockers (e.g., doxazosin, terazosin) prevent stimulation of $alpha_1$ receptors on arterioles and veins, thereby preventing sympathetically mediated vasoconstriction. The resultant vasodilation reduces both peripheral resistance and venous return to the heart.

The most disturbing side effect of alpha blockers is *orthostatic hypotension*. Hypotension can be especially severe with the initial dose. Significant hypotension continues with subsequent doses but is less profound.

The American College of Cardiology (ACC) recommends that alpha blockers *not* be used as first-line therapy for hypertension. In a huge clinical trial known as the Antihypertensive and Lipid-Lowering Treatment to Prevent Heart Attack Trial (ALLHAT), in which doxazosin was compared with chlorthalidone (a thiazide diuretic), patients taking doxazosin experienced 25% more cardiovascular events and were twice as likely to be hospitalized for heart failure. It is not clear whether doxazosin *increased* cardiovascular risk or chlorthalidone *decreased* risk. Either way, the diuretic is clearly preferred to the alpha blocker.

The basic pharmacology of the alpha blockers is discussed in Chapter 14.

Alpha/Beta Blockers: Carvedilol and Labetalol. Carvedilol and labetalol are unusual in that they can block $alpha_1$ receptors as well as beta receptors. Blood pressure reduction results from a combination of actions: (1) $alpha_1$ blockade promotes dilation of arterioles and veins, (2) blockade of cardiac $beta_1$ receptors reduces heart rate and contractility, and (3) blockade of $beta_1$ receptors on juxtaglomerular cells suppresses release of renin. Presumably, these drugs also share the ability of other beta blockers to reduce peripheral vascular resistance. Like other nonselective beta blockers, labetalol and carvedilol can exacerbate bradycardia, AV heart block, and asthma. Blockade of venous $alpha_1$ receptors can produce postural hypotension.

Centrally Acting Alpha₂ Agonists. As discussed in Chapter 15 these drugs (e.g., clonidine, methyldopa) act within the brainstem to suppress sympathetic outflow to the heart and blood vessels. The result is vasodilation and reduced cardiac output, both of which help lower BP. All central $alpha_2$ agonists can cause *dry mouth* and *sedation*. In addition, clonidine can cause severe *rebound hypertension* if treatment is abruptly discontinued. Additional adverse effects of methyldopa are *hemolytic anemia* and *liver disorders*.

Direct-Acting Vasodilators: Hydralazine and Minoxidil

Hydralazine and minoxidil reduce BP by promoting dilation of *arterioles*. Neither drug causes significant dilation of veins. Because venous dilation is minimal, the risk for orthostatic hypotension is low. With both drugs, lowering of BP may be followed by reflex tachycardia, renin release, and fluid retention. Reflex tachycardia and release of renin can be prevented with a beta blocker. Fluid retention can be prevented with a diuretic.

The most disturbing adverse effect of *hydralazine* is a syndrome resembling *systemic lupus erythematosus* (SLE). Fortunately, this reaction is rare at recommended doses. If an SLE-like reaction occurs, hydralazine should be withdrawn. Hydralazine is considered a third-line drug for chronic hypertension.

A less serious effect is excessive hair growth. Because of its capacity for significant side effects, minoxidil is not used routinely for chronic hypertension. Instead, the drug is reserved for patients with severe hypertension that has not responded to safer drugs.

The basic pharmacology of hydralazine and minoxidil is discussed in Chapter 38.

BLACK BOX WARNING: MINOXIDIL

Minoxidil can promote *pericardial effusion* that in some cases progresses to *cardiac tamponade*.

Calcium Channel Blockers

The CCBs fall into two groups: dihydropyridines (e.g., nifedipine) and nondihydropyridines (verapamil and diltiazem). Drugs in both groups promote dilation of arterioles. In addition, verapamil and diltiazem have direct suppressant effects on the heart.

Like other vasodilators, CCBs can cause *reflex tachycardia*. This reaction is greatest with the dihydropyridines and minimal with verapamil and diltiazem. Reflex tachycardia is low with verapamil and diltiazem because of cardiosuppression. Because dihydropyridines do not block cardiac calcium channels, reflex tachycardia with these drugs can be substantial.

Because of their ability to compromise cardiac performance, verapamil and diltiazem must be used cautiously in patients with bradycardia, heart failure, or AV heart block. These precautions do not apply to dihydropyridines.

The immediate-release formulation of *nifedipine* has been associated with increased mortality in patients with MI and unstable angina. As a result, the National Heart, Lung, and Blood Institute has recommended that the use of immediate-release nifedipine be discontinued for treatment of hypertensive emergency.

The basic pharmacology of the CCBs is discussed in Chapter 37.

Drugs that Suppress the RAAS

Because the RAAS plays an important role in controlling BP, drugs that suppress the system—especially the ACE inhibitors—have a significant role in controlling hypertension. The basic pharmacology of these drugs is discussed in Chapter 36.

ACE Inhibitors. The ACE inhibitors (e.g., captopril, enalapril) lower BP by preventing formation of angiotensin II and thereby prevent angiotensin II–mediated vasoconstriction and aldosterone-mediated volume expansion. In hypertensive diabetic patients with renal damage, these actions slow progression of kidney injury. Like the beta blockers, ACE inhibitors are less effective in blacks than in whites. Principal adverse effects are *persistent cough, first-dose hypotension, angioedema,* and *hyperkalemia* (secondary to suppression of aldosterone release). Because of the risk for hyperkalemia, combined use with potassium supplements or potassium-sparing diuretics is generally avoided.

BLACK BOX WARNING: ANGIOTENSIN-CONVERTING ENZYME INHIBITORS

ACE inhibitors can cause serious *fetal harm,* especially during the second and third trimesters of pregnancy, and hence must not be given to pregnant women. ACE inhibitors—along with ARBs and DRIs—are the only antihypertensive drugs specifically contraindicated during pregnancy.

Angiotensin II Receptor Blockers. ARBs lower BP in much the same way as do ACE inhibitors. Like the ACE inhibitors, ARBs prevent angiotensin II–mediated vasoconstriction and release of aldosterone. The only difference is that ARBs do so by blocking the *actions* of angiotensin II, whereas ACE inhibitors block the *formation* of angiotensin II. Both groups lower BP to the same extent. In contrast to ACE inhibitors, ARBs have a low incidence of inducing cough or significant hyperkalemia, but they do cause angioedema.

BLACK BOX WARNING: ANGIONTENSIN II RECEPTOR BLOCKERS

Like the ACE inhibitors, ARBs can cause *fetal harm* and must not be used during pregnancy.

Direct Renin Inhibitors. DRIs act directly on renin to inhibit conversion of angiotensinogen into angiotensin I. As a result, DRIs can suppress the entire RAAS. At this time, only one DRI—*aliskiren* [Tekturna, Rasilez ♣]—is available. Antihypertensive effects equal those of ACE inhibitors, ARBs, and CCBs. Compared with ACE inhibitors, aliskiren causes less hyperkalemia, cough, or angioedema—but poses a similar risk for *fetal harm.* In addition, aliskiren causes *diarrhea* in 2.3% of patients. Also, in patients with type 2 diabetes mellitus, use of aliskiren has demonstrated an increased incidence of renal impairment, hypotension, and hyperkalemia. Because of these findings, use of aliskiren is contraindicated in patients with diabetes mellitus who are also taking an ACE inhibitor or ARB. There are conflicting data regarding reduction of stroke, kidney failure, or MI with use of Aliskiren. Accordingly, until experience with the drug is more extensive, other antihypertensives should be considered first.

BLACK BOX WARNING: DIRECT RENIN INHIBITORS

Like the ACE inhibitors, DRIs can cause *fetal harm* and must not be used during pregnancy.

Aldosterone Antagonists. Aldosterone antagonists lower BP by promoting renal excretion of sodium and water. Only two agents are available: *eplerenone* and *spironolactone.* Both spironolactone and eplerenone promote renal retention of potassium and hence pose a risk for *hyperkalemia.* Accordingly, they should not be given to patients with existing hyperkalemia and should not be combined with potassium-sparing diuretics or potassium supplements. Combined use with ACE inhibitors, ARBs, and DRIs is permissible but must be done with caution. Spironolactone is discussed in Chapter 35, and eplerenone is discussed in Chapter 36.

Fundamentals of Hypertension Drug Therapy

Treatment Algorithm

The basic approach to treating hypertension was published with the new 2014 guidelines in the *Journal of the American Medical Association* and can be found on the JAMA Network at jama.jamanetwork.com/article.aspx?articleid=1791497. As shown in the algorithm at this link, lifestyle changes should be instituted first. If these fail to lower BP enough, drug therapy should be started—and the lifestyle changes should continue. Treatment often begins with a single drug. If needed, another drug may be *added* (if the initial drug was well tolerated but inadequate) or *substituted* (if the initial drug was poorly tolerated). However, before another drug is considered, possible reasons for failure of the initial drug should be assessed. Among these are insufficient dosage, poor adherence, excessive salt intake, and the presence of secondary hypertension. If treatment with two drugs is unsuccessful, a third and even fourth may be added.

Initial Drug Selection

Initial drug selection is determined by the presence or absence of a *compelling indication,* defined as a comorbid condition for which a specific class of antihypertensive drugs has been shown to improve outcomes. Initial drugs for patients with and without compelling indications are discussed next.

Patients Without Compelling Indications. For initial therapy in the absence of a compelling indication, a *thiazide diuretic* is currently recommended for most patients. This preference is based on long-term controlled trials showing conclusively that thiazides can reduce morbidity and mortality in hypertensive patients and are well tolerated and inexpensive too. Other options for initial therapy—*ACE inhibitors, ARBs,* and *CCBs*—equal diuretics in their ability to lower BP. However, they may not be as effective at reducing morbidity and mortality. Accordingly, these drugs should be reserved for special indications and for patients who have not responded to thiazides. Certain other alternatives—*centrally acting sympatholytics* and *direct-acting vasodilators*—are associated with a high incidence of adverse effects and hence are not well suited for initial monotherapy. One last alternative—*$alpha_1$ blockers*—is no longer recommended as first-line therapy. As noted, when the alpha blocker doxazosin was compared with the diuretic chlorthalidone, doxazosin was associated with a much higher incidence of adverse cardiovascular events.

Patients With Compelling Indications. For patients with hypertension plus certain comorbid conditions (e.g., heart failure, diabetes), there is strong evidence that specific antihypertensive drugs can reduce morbidity and mortality. Drugs shown to improve outcomes for six comorbid conditions are indicated in Table 39.3. Clearly, these drugs should be used for initial therapy. If needed, other antihypertensive agents can be added to the regimen. Management of hypertension in patients with diabetes and renal disease—two specific comorbid conditions—is discussed further under "Individualizing Therapy."

TABLE 39.3 ▪ Classes of Antihypertensive Drugs Recommended for Initial Therapy of Hypertension in Patients With Certain High-Risk Comorbid Conditions

High-Risk Comorbid Conditions that Constitute Compelling Indications for the Drugs Checked	Drug Classes Recommended for Initial Therapy of Hypertension					
	Diuretic	Beta Blocker	ACE Inhibitor	ARB	CCB	Aldosterone Antagonist
Heart failure	✔	✔	✔	✔		✔
Post–myocardial infarction		✔	✔			✔
High coronary disease risk	✔	✔	✔		✔	
Diabetes	✔	✔	✔	✔	✔	
Chronic kidney disease			✔	✔		
Recurrent stroke prevention	✔		✔			

ACE, angiotensin-converting enzyme; ARB, angiotensin II receptor blocker; CCB, calcium channel blocker.
Adapted from The seventh report of the Joint National Committee on Prevention, Detection, Evaluation, and Treatment of High Blood Pressure. JAMA 2003;289:2560–2572.

Adding Drugs to the Regimen

Rationale for Drug Selection. When using two or more drugs to treat hypertension, each drug should come from a different class. That is, each drug should have a different mechanism of action. In accord with this guideline, it would be appropriate to combine a beta blocker, a diuretic, and a vasodilator because each lowers BP by a different mechanism. In contrast, it would be inappropriate to combine two thiazide diuretics or two beta blockers or two vasodilators.

Benefits of Multidrug Therapy. Treatment with multiple drugs offers significant benefits. First, by employing drugs that have different mechanisms, we can increase the chance of success: targeting BP control at several sites is likely to be more effective than targeting at one site. Second, when drugs are used in combination, each can be administered in a lower dosage than would be possible if it were used alone. As a result, both the frequency and the intensity of side effects are reduced. Third, when proper combinations are selected, one agent can offset the adverse effects of another. For example, if a vasodilator is used alone, reflex tachycardia is likely. However, if a vasodilator is combined with a beta blocker, reflex tachycardia will be minimal.

Dosing

For each drug in the regimen, *dosage should be low initially and then gradually increased.* For most people with chronic hypertension, the disease poses no immediate threat. Hence there is no need to lower BP rapidly using large doses. Also, when BP is reduced slowly, baroreceptors gradually reset to the new, lower pressure. As a result, sympathetic reflexes offer less resistance to the hypotensive effects of therapy. Finally, because there is no need to drop BP rapidly, and because higher doses carry a higher risk for adverse effects, use of high initial doses would needlessly increase the risk for adverse effects.

Step-Down Therapy

After BP has been controlled for at least 1 year, an attempt should be made to reduce dosages and the number of drugs in the regimen. Of course, lifestyle modifications should continue. When reductions are made slowly and progressively, many patients are able to maintain BP control with less medication—and some can be maintained with no medication at all. If drugs are discontinued, regular follow-up is essential because BP usually returns to hypertensive levels—although it may take years to do so.

Individualizing Therapy

Patients With Comorbid Conditions

Comorbid conditions complicate treatment. Two conditions that are especially problematic—renal disease and diabetes—are discussed here. Preferred drugs for patients with these and other comorbid conditions are shown in Table 39.3. Drugs to avoid in patients with specific comorbid conditions are summarized in Table 39.4.

Renal Disease. Nephrosclerosis secondary to hypertension is among the most common causes of progressive renal disease. Pathophysiologic changes include degeneration of renal tubules and fibrotic thickening of the glomeruli, both of which contribute to renal insufficiency. Nephrosclerosis sets the stage for a downward spiral: renal insufficiency causes water retention, which in turn causes BP to rise higher, which in turn promotes even more renal injury, and so forth. Accordingly, early detection and treatment are essential. To slow progression of renal damage, the most important action is to lower BP. As with other populations, the target BP in patients younger than 60 years is 140/90 mm Hg or lower and is 150/90 mm Hg or lower in patients 60 years and older. Although all classes of antihypertensive agents are effective in nephrosclerosis, ACE inhibitors and ARBs work best. Hence, in the absence of contraindications, all patients should get one of these drugs. In most cases, a diuretic is also used. In patients with advanced renal insufficiency, thiazide diuretics are ineffective, hence a loop diuretic should be employed. Potassium-sparing diuretics should be avoided.

Diabetes. In patients with diabetes, the target BP is the same as with all other populations with special indications (140/90 mm Hg). Preferred antihypertensive drugs are ACE inhibitors, ARBs, CCBs, and diuretics (in low doses). In patients with diabetic nephropathy, ACE inhibitors and ARBs can slow progression of renal damage and reduce albuminuria. In diabetic patients, as in nondiabetic patients, beta blockers and diuretics can decrease morbidity and mortality. Keep in mind, however, that beta blockers can suppress glycogenolysis and mask early signs of hypoglycemia and therefore must be

TABLE 39.4 ▪ Comorbid Conditions that Require Cautious Use or Complete Avoidance of Certain Antihypertensive Drugs

Comorbid Condition	Drugs to Be Avoided or Used With Caution	Reason for Concern
CARDIOVASCULAR DISORDERS		
Heart failure	Verapamil Diltiazem	These drugs act on the heart to decrease myocardial contractility and can thereby further reduce cardiac output.
AV heart block	Beta blockers Labetalol Verapamil Diltiazem	These drugs act on the heart to suppress AV conduction and can thereby intensify AV block.
Coronary artery disease	Hydralazine	Reflex tachycardia induced by hydralazine can precipitate an anginal attack.
Post–myocardial infarction	Hydralazine	Reflex tachycardia induced by hydralazine can increase cardiac work and oxygen demand.
OTHER DISORDERS		
Dyslipidemia	Beta blockers Diuretics	These drugs may exacerbate dyslipidemia.
Renal insufficiency	K^+-sparing diuretics K^+ supplements	Use of these agents can lead to dangerous accumulations of potassium.
Asthma	Beta blockers Labetalol	$Beta_2$ blockade promotes bronchoconstriction.
Depression	Reserpine	Reserpine can cause depression.
Diabetes mellitus	Thiazides Furosemide Beta blockers	Thiazides and furosemide promote hyperglycemia, and beta blockers suppress glycogenolysis and can mask signs of hypoglycemia.
Gout	Thiazides Furosemide	These diuretics promote hyperuricemia.
Hyperkalemia	K^+-sparing diuretics ACE inhibitors Direct renin inhibitors Aldosterone antagonists	These drugs cause potassium accumulation.
Hypokalemia	Thiazides Furosemide	These drugs cause potassium loss.
Collagen diseases	Hydralazine	Hydralazine can precipitate a lupus erythematosus–like syndrome.
Liver disease	Methyldopa	Methyldopa is hepatotoxic.
Preeclampsia	ACE inhibitors ARBs Direct renin inhibitors	These drugs can injure the fetus.

ACE, angiotensin-converting enzyme; ARBs, angiotensin II receptor blockers; AV, atrioventricular.

used with caution. Thiazides and loop diuretics promote hyperglycemia and hence should be used with care.

How do ACE inhibitors compare with CCBs in patients with hypertension and diabetes? In one large study, patients taking nisoldipine (a CCB) had a higher incidence of MI than did patients taking enalapril (an ACE inhibitor). Because the study was not placebo controlled, it was impossible to distinguish between two possible interpretations: (1) the CCB increased the risk for MI or (2) the ACE inhibitor protected against MI. Either way, it seems clear that ACE inhibitors are better than CCBs for patients with hypertension and diabetes.

Patients in Special Populations

Blacks. Hypertension is a major health problem for black adults. Hypertension develops earlier, has a much higher incidence, and is likely to be more severe. As a result, black people face a greater risk for heart disease, end-stage renal disease, and stroke. Compared with the general population, blacks experience a 50% higher rate of death from heart disease, are twice as likely to die of stroke, and are 6 times more likely to experience hypertension-related end-stage renal disease.

With timely treatment, this disparity can be greatly reduced, if not eliminated. We know that blacks and whites respond equally to treatment (although not always to the same drugs). The primary problem is that, among black people, hypertension often goes untreated until after significant organ damage has developed. If hypertension were diagnosed and treated earlier, the prognosis would be greatly improved. Accordingly, it is important that blacks undergo routine monitoring of BP. If hypertension is diagnosed, treatment should begin at once. Because blacks have a high incidence of salt sensitivity and cigarette use, lifestyle modifications are an important component of treatment.

Black people respond better to some antihypertensive drugs than to others. Controlled trials have shown that *diuretics* can decrease morbidity and mortality in blacks. Accordingly, diuretics are drugs of first choice. *CCBs* and *alpha/beta blockers* are also effective. In contrast, monotherapy with *beta blockers* or *ACE inhibitors* is less effective in blacks than in whites. Nonetheless, beta blockers and ACE inhibitors should be used if they are strongly indicated for a comorbid condition. For example, ACE inhibitors should be used in black

PATIENT-CENTERED CARE ACROSS THE LIFE SPAN

Hypertension

Life Stage	Patient Care Concerns
Infants	See later entry, "Breastfeeding women."
Children/adolescents	No data are available on the long-term effects of antihypertensive drugs on growth and development of children. Drugs recommended for treatment of hypertension in children 1–18 years old include ACE inhibitors, diuretics, beta blockers, and calcium channel blockers.
Pregnant women	Drugs of choice in treating pregnant women with mild preeclampsia include labetalol and methyldopa. Magnesium sulfate is used in the prevention of seizures in severe preeclampsia or for treatment of seizures in eclampsia.
Breastfeeding women	Effects of RAAS-blocking drugs have not been studied in breastfeeding. Beta blockers, such as metoprolol, appear safe for the breastfeeding infant. Diuretics appear safe but may suppress lactation.
Older adults	Older adults benefit from SBPs <145 mm Hg. Treatment with ACE inhibitors, diuretics, and/or beta blockers is reasonable. Caution must be taken to avoid overdiuresis when using diuretics in the older-adult population.

ACE, angiotensin-converting enzyme inhibitor; RAAS, renin-angiotensin-aldosterone system: SBP, systolic blood pressure.

patients who have type 1 diabetes with proteinuria. Also, ACE inhibitors should be used in patients with hypertensive nephrosclerosis, a condition for which ACE inhibitors are superior to CCBs. When BP cannot be adequately controlled with a single drug, several two-drug combinations are recommended: an ACE inhibitor plus a thiazide diuretic, an ACE inhibitor plus a CCB, and a beta blocker plus a thiazide.

In 2014, the International Society on Hypertension in Blacks (ISHIB) issued updated guidelines on managing hypertension in black people. Current goals remain consistent with the JNC 8 Guidelines of maintaining BP less than 140/90 mm Hg in this population.

Children and Adolescents. The incidence of secondary hypertension in children is much higher than in adults. Accordingly, efforts to diagnose and treat an underlying cause should be especially diligent. For children with primary hypertension, treatment is the same as for adults—although doses are lower and should be adjusted with care. Because ACE inhibitors and ARBs can cause fetal harm, they should be avoided in girls who are sexually active or pregnant.

Older Adults. By age 65 years, most Americans have hypertension. Furthermore, high BP in this group almost always presents as *isolated systolic hypertension;* DBP is usually normal or low. The good news, as shown in the Hypertension in the Very Elderly Trial (HYVET), is that treatment can reduce the incidence of heart failure, fatal stroke, and all-cause mortality. The bad news is that most older people are not treated.

The new 2014 guidelines advocate for a target BP of less than 150/90 mm Hg in patients 60 years and older. This differs from the 2011 ACC/American Heart Association (AHA) expert consensus document on treatment of hypertension in people 65 years and older, for whom the target *systolic* pressure is below 140 mm Hg (for patients ages 65–79 years) and below 145 mm Hg (for patients 80 years and older). Data supported improved outcomes with tighter BP control in the older adult population are lacking—hence the likely reason for the change in philosophy. Although the newer guidelines may be more lax, they do not serve as a substitute for clinical judgment.

Because cardiovascular reflexes are blunted in older adults, treatment carries a significant risk of orthostatic hypotension. Accordingly, initial doses should be low—about one-half those used for younger adults—and dosage escalation should be done slowly. Drugs that are especially likely to cause orthostatic hypotension (e.g., $alpha_1$ blockers, alpha/beta blockers) should be used with caution.

Minimizing Adverse Effects

Antihypertensive drugs can produce many unwanted effects, including hypotension, sedation, and sexual dysfunction. (Although not stressed previously, practically all antihypertensive drugs can interfere with sexual function.)

The fundamental strategy for decreasing side effects is to tailor the regimen to the sensitivities of the patient. Simply put, if one drug causes effects that are objectionable, a more acceptable drug should be substituted. The best way to identify unacceptable responses is to encourage patients to report them.

Adverse effects caused by exacerbation of comorbid diseases are both predictable and avoidable. We know, for example, that beta blockers can intensify AV block and hence should not be taken by people with these disorders. Other conditions that can be aggravated by antihypertensive drugs are listed in Table 39.4. To help avoid drug-disease mismatches, the medical history should identify all comorbid conditions. With this information, the prescriber can choose drugs that are least likely to make the comorbid condition worse.

High initial doses and rapid dosage escalation can increase the incidence and severity of adverse effects. Accordingly, doses should be low at first and then gradually increased. Remember, there is usually no need to reduce BP rapidly. Hence large initial doses that can produce a rapid fall in BP but also produce adverse effects should be avoided.

Promoting Adherence

The major cause of treatment failure in patients with chronic hypertension is lack of adherence to the prescribed regimen. In this section we consider the causes of nonadherence and discuss some solutions.

Why Adherence Is Often Hard to Achieve

Much of the difficulty in promoting adherence stems from the nature of hypertension itself. Hypertension is a chronic, slowly progressing disease that, through much of its course, is devoid of overt symptoms. Because symptoms are absent, it can be difficult to convince patients that they are ill and need treatment. In addition, because there are no symptoms to relieve, drugs cannot produce an obvious therapeutic response. In the absence of such a response, it can be difficult for patients to believe that their medication is doing anything useful.

Because hypertension progresses very slowly, the disease tends to encourage procrastination. For most people, the adverse effects of hypertension will not become manifest for many years. Realizing this, patients may reason (incorrectly) that they can postpone therapy without significantly increasing risk.

The negative aspects of treatment also contribute to nonadherence. Antihypertensive regimens can be complex and expensive. In addition, treatment must continue lifelong. Lastly, antihypertensive drugs can cause a number of adverse effects, ranging from sedation to hypotension to impaired sexual function. It is difficult to convince people who are feeling good to take drugs that may make them feel worse. Some people may decide that exposing themselves to the negative effects of therapy today is paying too high a price to avoid the adverse consequences of hypertension at some indefinite time in the future.

Ways to Promote Adherence

Patient Education. Adherence requires motivation, and patient education can help provide it. Patients should be taught about the consequences of hypertension and the benefits of treatment. Because hypertension does not cause discomfort, it may not be clear to patients that their condition is indeed serious. Patients must be helped to understand that, left untreated, hypertension can cause heart disease, kidney disease, and stroke. In addition, patients should appreciate that, with proper therapy, the risks for these long-term complications can be minimized, resulting in a longer and healthier life. Lastly, patients must understand that drugs do not cure hypertension—they only control symptoms. Hence, for treatment to be effective, medication must be taken lifelong.

> **Patient Education**
>
> **MONITORING BLOOD PRESSURE**
>
> Patients should be taught the goal of treatment (usually maintenance of BP <140/90–150/90 mm Hg), and they should be taught to monitor and record their BP daily. This increases patient involvement and provides positive feedback that can help promote adherence.

Minimize Side Effects. If we expect patients to comply with long-term treatment, we must keep adverse effects to a minimum. As discussed earlier, adverse effects can be minimized by (1) encouraging patients to report side effects, (2) discontinuing objectionable drugs and substituting more acceptable ones, (3) avoiding drugs that can exacerbate comorbid conditions, and (4) using doses that are low initially and then gradually increased.

Establish a Collaborative Relationship. The patient who feels like a collaborative partner in the treatment program is more likely to comply than is the patient who feels that treatment is being imposed. Collaboration allows the patient to help set treatment goals, create the treatment program, and evaluate progress. In addition, a collaborative relationship facilitates communication about side effects.

Simplify the Regimen. Antihypertensive regimens may consist of several drugs taken multiple times a day. Such complex regimens deter adherence. Therefore, to promote adherence, the dosing schedule should be as simple as possible. After an effective regimen has been established, dosing just once or twice daily should be tried. If an appropriate combination product is available (e.g., a fixed-dose combination of a thiazide diuretic plus an ACE inhibitor), the combination product may be substituted for its components.

Other Measures. Adherence can be promoted by giving positive reinforcement when therapeutic goals are achieved. Involvement of family members can be helpful. Also, adherence can be promoted by scheduling office visits at convenient times and by following up when appointments are missed. For many patients, antihypertensive therapy represents a significant economic burden; devising a regimen that is effective but inexpensive will help.

DRUGS FOR HYPERTENSIVE DISORDERS OF PREGNANCY

Hypertension is the most common complication of pregnancy, with an incidence of about 10%. When hypertension develops, it is essential to distinguish between chronic hypertension and preeclampsia. Chronic hypertension is relatively benign, whereas preeclampsia can lead to life-threatening complications for the patient and the fetus.

Chronic Hypertension

Chronic hypertension, seen in 5% of pregnancies, is defined as hypertension that was present before pregnancy or that developed before the 20th week of gestation. Persistent *severe* hypertension carries a risk to both the patient and the fetus. Potential adverse outcomes include placental abruption, maternal cardiac decompensation, premature birth, fetal growth delay, central nervous system hemorrhage, and renal failure. The goal of treatment is to minimize the risk for hypertension to the patient and fetus while avoiding drug-induced harm to the fetus. With the exception of ACE inhibitors, ARBs, and DRIs, antihypertensive drugs that were being taken before pregnancy can be continued. *ACE inhibitors, ARBs, and DRIs are contraindicated owing to their potential for harm* (fetal growth delay, congenital malformations, neonatal renal failure, neonatal death). When drug therapy is initiated *during* pregnancy, *methyldopa* and *labetalol* are the traditional agents of choice. These drugs have limited effects on uteroplacental and fetal hemodynamics and do not adversely affect the fetus or neonate. Regardless of the drug selected, treatment should not be too aggressive because an excessive drop in BP could compromise uteroplacental blood flow.

According to guidelines issued in 2012 by the American College of Obstetricians and Gynecologists (ACOG), "severe" hypertension requires treatment, whereas "mild" hypertension generally does not. (The ACOG defines severe hypertension as SBP >160 mm Hg or DBP >110 mm Hg, and mild hypertension as SBP 140–159 mm Hg or DBP 90–109 mm Hg.) There is good evidence that treating severe hypertension reduces risk. In contrast, there is little evidence that treating mild hypertension offers significant benefit.

Patients who have chronic hypertension during pregnancy are at increased risk for developing preeclampsia (see later). Unfortunately, reducing BP does *not* lower this risk.

Preeclampsia and Eclampsia

Preeclampsia is a multisystem disorder characterized by the combination of elevated BP (>140/90 mm Hg) and proteinuria (≥300 mg in 24 hours) that develops after the 20th week of gestation. The disorder occurs in about 5% of pregnancies. Rarely, women with preeclampsia develop seizures. If seizures do develop, the condition is then termed *eclampsia.* Risk factors for preeclampsia include black race, chronic hypertension, diabetes, collagen vascular disorders, and previous preeclampsia. The etiology of preeclampsia is complex and incompletely understood.

Preeclampsia poses serious risks for the fetus and mother. Risks for the fetus include intrauterine growth restriction, premature birth, and even death. The mother is at risk for seizures (eclampsia), renal failure, pulmonary edema, stroke, and death.

Management of preeclampsia is based on the severity of the disease, the status of mother and fetus, and the length of gestation. The objective is to preserve the health of the mother and deliver an infant who will not require intensive and prolonged neonatal care. Success requires close maternal and fetal monitoring. Although drugs can help reduce BP, delivery is the only cure.

Management of *mild* preeclampsia is controversial and depends on the duration of gestation. If preeclampsia develops near term, and if fetal maturity is certain, induction of labor is advised. However, if mild preeclampsia develops earlier in gestation, experts disagree about what to do. Suggested measures include bed rest, prolonged hospitalization, treatment with antihypertensive drugs, and prophylaxis with an anticonvulsant. Studies to evaluate these strategies have generally failed to demonstrate benefits from any of them, including treatment with antihypertensive drugs.

The definitive intervention for *severe* preeclampsia is delivery. However, making the choice to induce labor presents a dilemma. Because preeclampsia can deteriorate rapidly, with grave consequences for the patient and fetus, immediate delivery is recommended. However, if the fetus is not sufficiently mature, immediate delivery could threaten its life. Do we deliver the fetus immediately, which would eliminate risk for the patient but present a serious risk for the fetus—or do we postpone delivery, which would reduce risk for the fetus but greatly increase risk for the patient? If the patient elects to postpone delivery, then BP can be lowered with drugs. Because severe preeclampsia can be life threatening, treatment must be done in a tertiary care center to permit close monitoring. The major objective is to prevent maternal cerebral complications (e.g., hemorrhage, encephalopathy). The drug of choice for lowering BP is *labetalol* (20 mg by intravenous [IV] bolus over 2 minutes); dosing may be repeated at 10-minute intervals up to a total of 300 mg.

Because severe preeclampsia can evolve into eclampsia, an antiseizure drug may be given for prophylaxis. *Magnesium sulfate* is the drug of choice. In one study, prophylaxis with magnesium sulfate reduced the risk for eclampsia by 58% and the risk for death by 45%. Dosing is the same as for treating eclampsia.

If eclampsia develops, magnesium sulfate is the preferred drug for seizure control. Initial dosing consists of a 4- to 6-g IV loading dose followed by a continuous IV infusion of 1 to 2 g for the next 24 hours. To ensure therapeutic effects and prevent toxicity, blood levels of magnesium, as well as presence of patellar reflex, should be monitored. The target range for serum magnesium is 4 to 7 mEq/L (the normal range for magnesium is 1.5–2 mEq/L).

When started before 16 weeks of gestation, low-dose *aspirin* reduces the risk for preeclampsia by about 50%. Similarly, *L-arginine* (combined with antioxidant vitamins) can also help. By contrast, several other preparations—magnesium, zinc, vitamin C, vitamin E, fish oil, and diuretics—appear to offer no protection at all.

CHAPTER

40 Drugs for Heart Failure

Laura D. Rosenthal, DNP, ACNP, FAANP

Heart failure is a disease with two major forms: (1) heart failure with left ventricular (LV) systolic dysfunction, now referred to as heart failure with reduced ejection fraction (HFrEF) and (2) diastolic heart failure, also known as heart failure with preserved LV ejection fraction (HFpEF). In this chapter, discussion is limited to the first form. Accordingly, for the rest of this chapter, the term *heart failure* (HF) will be used to denote the first form only.

HF is a progressive, often fatal disorder characterized by ventricular dysfunction, reduced cardiac output, insufficient tissue perfusion, and signs of fluid retention (e.g., peripheral edema, shortness of breath). The disease affects nearly 5 million Americans and, every year, is responsible for 12 to 15 million office visits, 6.5 million hospital days, and about 300,000 deaths. Of those who have HF, 20% are likely to die within 1 year, and 50% within 5 years. HF is primarily a disease of older adults, affecting 4% to 8% of those at age 65 years and more than 9% to 12% of those older than 80 years. Direct and indirect health care costs of HF are estimated at more than $34 billion yearly. With improved evaluation and care, many hospitalizations could be prevented, quality of life could be improved, and life expectancy could be extended.

In the past, HF was commonly referred to as *congestive heart failure*. This term was used because HF frequently causes fluid accumulation (congestion) in the lungs and peripheral tissues. However, because many patients do not have signs of pulmonary or systemic congestion, the term *heart failure* is now preferred.

Drugs recommended for treatment include diuretics, inhibitors of the renin-angiotensin-aldosterone system (RAAS), beta blockers, and digoxin. In this chapter, only digoxin is discussed at length. The other drugs are presented at length in previous chapters, so discussion here is limited to their use in HF.

To understand HF and its treatment, you need a basic understanding of hemodynamics. In particular, you need to understand the role of venous pressure, afterload, and Starling's mechanism in determining cardiac output. You also need to understand the roles of the baroreceptor reflex, the RAAS, and the kidneys in regulating arterial pressure. You can refresh your memory of these concepts by reading Chapter 34.

PATHOPHYSIOLOGY OF HEART FAILURE

HF is a syndrome in which the heart is unable to pump sufficient blood to meet the metabolic needs of tissues. The syndrome is characterized by signs of *inadequate tissue perfusion* (fatigue, shortness of breath, exercise intolerance) and/or signs of *volume overload* (venous distention, peripheral and pulmonary edema). The major underlying causes of HF are chronic hypertension and myocardial infarction. Other causes include valvular heart disease, coronary artery disease, congenital heart disease, dysrhythmias, and aging of the myocardium. In its earliest stage, HF is asymptomatic. As failure progresses, fatigue and shortness of breath develop. As cardiac performance declines further, blood backs up behind the failing ventricles, causing venous distention, peripheral edema, and pulmonary edema. HF is a chronic disorder that requires continuous treatment with drugs.

Cardiac Remodeling

In the initial phase of failure, the heart undergoes remodeling, a process in which the ventricles dilate, hypertrophy, and become more spherical. These alterations in cardiac geometry increase wall stress and reduce LV ejection fraction. Remodeling occurs in response to cardiac injury, brought on by infarction and other causes. The remodeling process is driven primarily by neurohormonal systems, including the sympathetic nervous system (SNS) and the RAAS. In addition to promoting remodeling, neurohormonal factors promote cardiac fibrosis and myocyte death. The net result of these pathologic changes—remodeling, fibrosis, and cell death—is progressive decline in cardiac output. As a rule, cardiac remodeling precedes development of symptoms and continues after they appear. As a result, cardiac performance continues to decline.

Physiologic Adaptations to Reduced Cardiac Output

In response to reductions in cardiac pumping ability, the body undergoes several adaptive changes. Some of these help improve tissue perfusion; others compound existing problems.

Cardiac Dilation

Dilation of the heart is characteristic of HF. Cardiac dilation results from a combination of increased venous pressure (see later) and reduced contractile force. Reduced contractility lowers the amount of blood ejected during systole, causing end-systolic volume to rise. The increase in venous pressure increases diastolic filling, which causes the heart to expand even further.

Because of Starling's mechanism, the increase in heart size that occurs in HF helps improve cardiac output. That is, as the heart fails and its volume expands, contractile force increases, causing a corresponding increase in stroke volume. However, please note that the maximal contractile force that can be developed by the failing heart is considerably lower than the maximal force of the healthy heart. This limitation is reflected in the curve for the failing heart shown in Fig. 40.1.

If cardiac dilation is insufficient to maintain cardiac output, other factors come into play. As discussed later, these are not always beneficial.

Increased Sympathetic Tone

HF causes arterial pressure to fall. In response, the baroreceptor reflex increases sympathetic output to the heart, veins, and arterioles. At the same time, parasympathetic effects on the heart are reduced. The consequences of increased sympathetic tone are summarized here.

- *Increased heart rate.* Acceleration of heart rate increases cardiac output, thereby helping improve tissue perfusion. However, if heart rate increases too much, there will be insufficient time for complete ventricular filling, and cardiac output will fall.
- *Increased contractility.* Increased myocardial contractility has the obvious benefit of increasing cardiac output. The only detriment is an increase in cardiac oxygen demand.
- *Increased venous tone.* Elevation of venous tone increases venous pressure and thereby increases ventricular filling. Because of Starling's mechanism, increased filling increases stroke volume. Unfortunately, if venous pressure is excessive, blood will back up behind the failing ventricles, thereby aggravating pulmonary and peripheral edema. Furthermore, excessive filling pressure can dilate the heart so much that stroke volume will begin to decline.
- *Increased arteriolar tone.* Elevation of arteriolar tone increases arterial pressure, thereby increasing perfusion of vital organs. Unfortunately, increased arterial pressure also means the heart must pump against greater resistance. Because cardiac reserve is minimal in HF, the heart may be unable to meet this challenge, and output may fall.

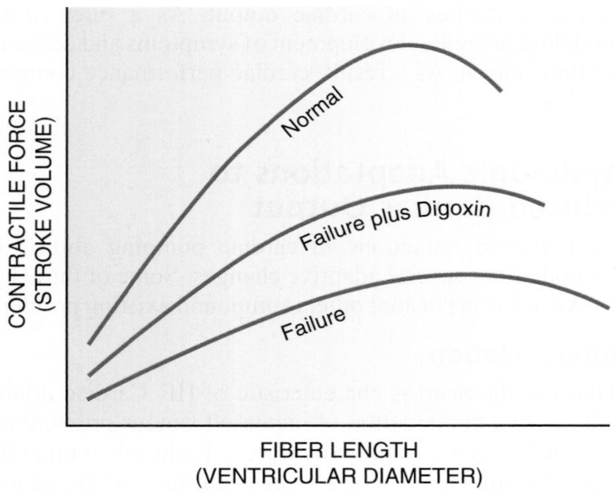

Figure 40.1 ▪ Relationship of ventricular diameter to contractile force.
In the normal heart and the failing heart, increased fiber length produces increased contractile force. However, for any given fiber length, contractile force in the failing heart is much less than in the healthy heart. By increasing cardiac contractility, digoxin shifts the relationship between fiber length and stroke volume in the failing heart toward that in the normal heart.

Water Retention and Increased Blood Volume

Mechanisms

Water retention results from two mechanisms. First, reduced cardiac output causes a reduction in renal blood flow, which in turn decreases glomerular filtration rate (GFR). As a result, urine production is decreased and water is retained.

Second, HF activates the RAAS. Activation occurs in response to reduced blood pressure and reduced renal blood flow. When activated, the RAAS promotes water retention by increasing circulating levels of *aldosterone* and *angiotensin II*. Aldosterone acts directly on the kidneys to promote retention of sodium and water. Angiotensin II causes constriction of renal blood vessels, which decreases renal blood flow and thereby further decreases urine production. In addition, angiotensin II causes constriction of systemic arterioles and veins and thereby increases venous and arterial pressure.

Consequences

As with other adaptive responses to HF, increased blood volume can be beneficial or harmful. Increased blood volume increases venous pressure and thereby increases venous return. As a result, ventricular filling and stroke volume are increased. The resultant increase in cardiac output can improve tissue perfusion. However, as noted, if venous pressure is too high, edema of the lungs and periphery may result. More important, *if the increase in cardiac output is insufficient to maintain adequate kidney function, renal retention of water will progress unabated. The resultant accumulation of fluid will cause severe cardiac, pulmonary, and peripheral edema—and, ultimately, death.*

Natriuretic Peptides

In response to stretching of the atria and dilation of the ventricles, the heart releases two natriuretic peptides: atrial natriuretic peptide (ANP) and B-natriuretic peptide (BNP). As discussed in Chapter 34, these hormones promote dilation of arterioles and veins and also promote loss of sodium and water through the kidneys. Hence they tend to counterbalance vasoconstriction caused by the SNS and angiotensin II, as well as retention of sodium and water caused by the RAAS. However, as HF progresses, the effects of ANP and BNP eventually become overwhelmed by the effects of the SNS and RAAS.

Levels of circulating BNP are an important index of cardiac status in HF patients and thus can be a predictor of long-term survival. High levels of BNP indicate poor cardiac health and can predict a lower chance of survival. Conversely, low levels of BNP indicate better cardiac health and can predict a higher chance of survival. This information can be helpful when assessing the hospitalized patient at discharge: the lower the BNP level, the greater the chances of long-term survival.

The Vicious Cycle of "Compensatory" Physiologic Responses

As discussed previously, reduced cardiac output leads to compensatory responses: (1) cardiac dilation, (2) activation of the SNS, (3) activation of the RAAS, and (4) retention of water and expansion of blood volume. Although these responses represent the body's attempt to compensate for reduced cardiac output, they can actually make matters worse: excessive heart rate can reduce ventricular filling; excessive arterial pressure can lower cardiac output; and excessive venous pressure can cause pulmonary and peripheral edema. Thus, as depicted in Fig. 40.2, the "compensatory" responses can create a self-sustaining cycle of maladaptation that further impairs cardiac output and tissue perfusion. If cardiac output becomes too low to maintain sufficient production of urine, the resultant accumulation of water will eventually be fatal. The actual cause of death is complete cardiac failure secondary to excessive cardiac dilation and cardiac edema.

Signs and Symptoms of Heart Failure

The prominent signs and symptoms of HF are a direct consequence of the pathophysiology just described. Decreased tissue perfusion results in reduced exercise tolerance, fatigue, and shortness of breath; shortness of breath may also reflect pulmonary edema. Increased sympathetic tone produces tachycardia. Increased ventricular filling, reduced systolic ejection, and myocardial hypertrophy result in cardiomegaly (increased heart size). The combination of increased venous tone plus increased blood volume helps cause pulmonary edema, peripheral edema, hepatomegaly (increased liver size), and distention of the jugular veins. Weight gain results from fluid retention.

Classification of Heart Failure Severity

There are two major schemes for classifying HF severity. One scheme, established by the New York Heart Association (NYHA), classifies HF based on the functional limitations it causes. A newer scheme, proposed jointly by the American College of Cardiology (ACC) and the American Heart Association (AHA), is based on the observation that HF is a progressive disease that moves through stages of increasing severity.

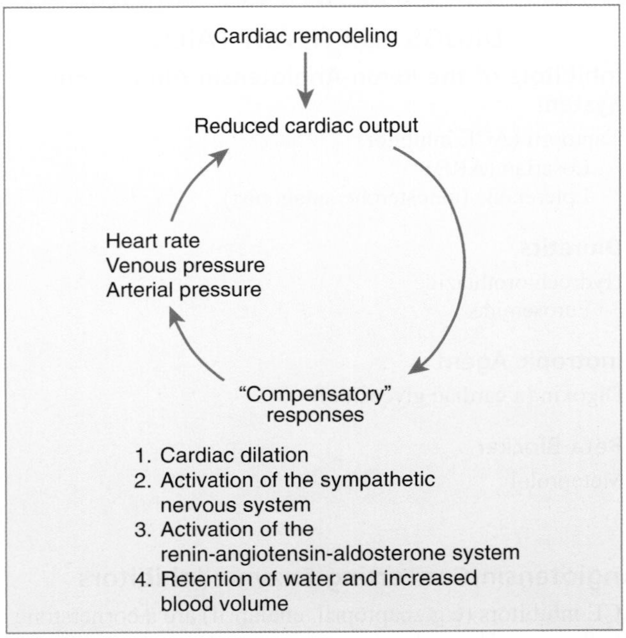

Figure 40.2 ■ The vicious cycle of maladaptive compensatory responses to a failing heart.

The NYHA scheme, which has four classes, can be summarized as follows:

- Class I—no limitation of ordinary physical activity
- Class II—slight limitation of physical activity: normal activity produces fatigue, dyspnea, palpitations, or angina
- Class III—marked limitation of physical activity: even mild activity produces symptoms
- Class IV—symptoms occur at rest

The ACC/AHA scheme, which also has four stages, can be summarized as follows:

- Stage A—at high risk for HF but without structural heart disease or symptoms of HF
- Stage B—structural heart disease but without symptoms of HF
- Stage C—structural heart disease with prior or current symptoms of HF
- Stage D—refractory HF requiring specialized interventions

The ACC/AHA scheme was unveiled in treatment guidelines issued in 2001. The newest version of that document—*2013 ACCF/AHA Guideline for the Management of Heart Failure. Executive Summary: A Report of the American College of Cardiology Foundation/American Heart Association Task Force on Practice Guidelines*—is discussed later under "Management of Heart Failure."

Please note that the ACC/AHA scheme is intended to complement the NYHA scheme, not replace it. The relationship between the two is shown in Fig. 40.3.

OVERVIEW OF DRUGS USED TO TREAT HEART FAILURE

For routine therapy, HF is treated with three types of drugs: (1) diuretics, (2) agents that inhibit the RAAS, and (3) beta blockers. Other agents (e.g., digoxin, dopamine, hydralazine) may be used as well.

Diuretics

Diuretics are first-line drugs for all patients with signs of volume overload or with a history of volume overload. By reducing blood volume, these drugs can decrease venous pressure, arterial pressure (afterload), pulmonary edema, peripheral edema, and cardiac dilation. However, excessive diuresis must be avoided: if blood volume drops too low, cardiac output and blood pressure may fall precipitously, thereby further compromising tissue perfusion. For the most part, benefits of diuretics are limited to symptom reduction. As a rule, these drugs do not prolong survival. The basic pharmacology of the diuretics is discussed in Chapter 35.

Thiazide Diuretics

The thiazide diuretics (e.g., hydrochlorothiazide) produce moderate diuresis. These oral agents are used for long-term therapy of HF when edema is not too great. Because thiazides are ineffective when GFR is low, these drugs cannot be used if cardiac output is greatly reduced. The principal adverse effect of the thiazides is *hypokalemia,* which increases the risk for *digoxin-induced dysrhythmias* (see later).

Loop Diuretics

The loop diuretics (e.g., furosemide) produce profound diuresis. In contrast to the thiazides, these drugs can promote fluid

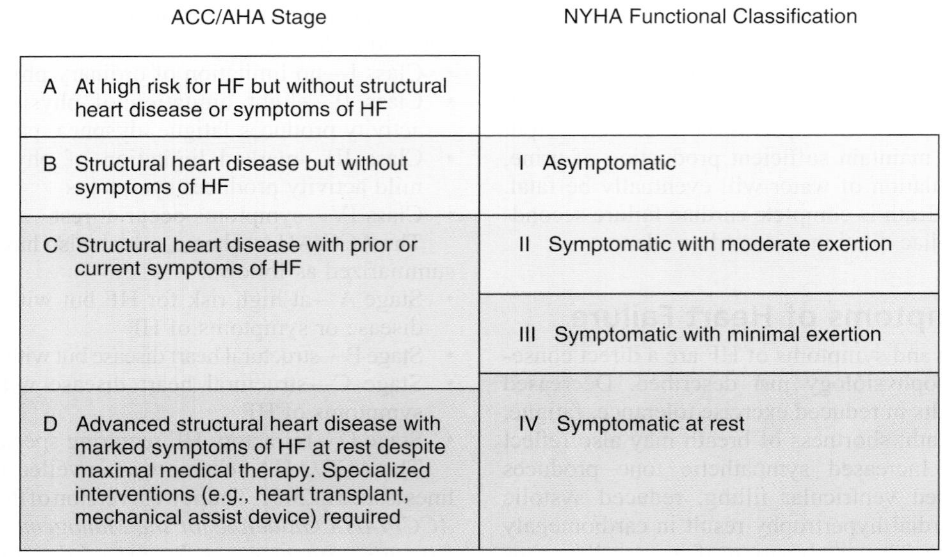
ACC/AHA Stage
NYHA Functional Classification
A At high risk for HF but without structural heart disease or symptoms of HF
B Structural heart disease but without symptoms of HF
I Asymptomatic
C Structural heart disease with prior or current symptoms of HF
II Symptomatic with moderate exertion
III Symptomatic with minimal exertion
D Advanced structural heart disease with marked symptoms of HF at rest despite maximal medical therapy. Specialized interventions (e.g., heart transplant, mechanical assist device) required
IV Symptomatic at rest

Figure 40.3 ■ American College of Cardiology/American Heart Association (ACC/AHA) stages and New York Heart Association (NYHA) functional classification of heart failure.

loss even when GFR is low. Therefore loop diuretics are preferred to thiazides when cardiac output is greatly reduced. Because they can mobilize large volumes of water, and because they work when GFR is low, loop diuretics are drugs of choice for patients with severe HF. Like the thiazides, these drugs can cause *hypokalemia,* thereby increasing the risk for *digoxin toxicity.* In addition, loop diuretics can cause severe *hypotension* secondary to excessive volume reduction.

Potassium-Sparing Diuretics

In contrast to the thiazides and loop diuretics, the potassium-sparing diuretics (e.g., spironolactone, triamterene) promote only scant diuresis. In patients with HF, these drugs are employed to counteract potassium loss caused by thiazide and loop diuretics, thereby lowering the risk for digoxin-induced dysrhythmias. Not surprisingly, the principal adverse effect of the potassium-sparing drugs is *hyperkalemia.* Because *angiotensin-converting enzyme (ACE) inhibitors* and *angiotensin II receptor blockers (ARBs)* also carry a risk for hyperkalemia, caution is needed if these drugs are combined with a potassium-sparing diuretic. Accordingly, when therapy with an ACE inhibitor or ARB is initiated, the potassium-sparing diuretic should be discontinued. It can be resumed later if needed.

One potassium-sparing diuretic—spironolactone—prolongs survival in patients with HF primarily by blocking receptors for aldosterone, not by causing diuresis. This drug and a related agent—eplerenone—are discussed later under "Aldosterone Antagonists."

Drugs That Inhibit the Renin-Angiotensin-Aldosterone System

The RAAS plays an important role both in cardiac remodeling and in the hemodynamic changes that occur in response to reduced cardiac output. Accordingly, agents that inhibit the RAAS can be highly beneficial. Four groups of drugs are available: ACE inhibitors, ARBs, direct renin inhibitors (DRIs), and aldosterone antagonists. Of the four, the ACE inhibitors have been studied most thoroughly in HF. The basic pharmacology of the RAAS inhibitors is presented in Chapter 36.

Prototype Drugs

DRUGS FOR HEART FAILURE

Inhibitors of the Renin-Angiotensin-Aldosterone System

Captopril (ACE inhibitor)
Losartan (ARB)
Eplerenone (aldosterone antagonist)

Diuretics

Hydrochlorothiazide
Furosemide

Inotropic Agent

Digoxin (a cardiac glycoside)

Beta Blocker

Metoprolol

Angiotensin-Converting Enzyme Inhibitors

ACE inhibitors (e.g., captopril, enalapril) are a cornerstone of HF therapy. These drugs can improve functional status and prolong life. In one trial, the 2-year mortality rate for patients taking enalapril was 47% lower than the rate for patients taking placebo. Other large, controlled trials have shown similar benefits. Accordingly, in the absence of specific contraindications, all patients with HF should receive one of these drugs. Although ACE inhibitors can be used alone, they are usually combined with a beta blocker and a diuretic.

ACE inhibitors block production of angiotensin II, decrease release of aldosterone, and suppress degradation of kinins. As a result, they improve hemodynamics and favorably alter cardiac remodeling.

Hemodynamic Benefits

By suppressing production of angiotensin II, ACE inhibitors cause dilation of arterioles and veins, and they decrease release of aldosterone. Resulting benefits in HF are as follows:

- *Arteriolar dilation* improves regional blood flow in the kidneys and other tissues, and, by reducing afterload, it increases stroke volume and cardiac output. Increased renal blood flow promotes excretion of sodium and water.
- *Venous dilation* reduces venous pressure and thereby reduces pulmonary congestion, peripheral edema, preload, and cardiac dilation.
- *Suppression of aldosterone release* enhances excretion of sodium and water while causing retention of potassium.

Interestingly, suppression of angiotensin II production diminishes over time, suggesting that long-term benefits are the result of some other action.

Influence on Cardiac Remodeling

With continued use, ACE inhibitors have a favorable influence on cardiac remodeling. Elevation of kinins is largely responsible. This statement is based in part on the observation that, in experimental models, giving a kinin receptor blocker decreases beneficial effects on remodeling. Also, we know that suppression of angiotensin II production diminishes over time, so reduced angiotensin II cannot fully explain long-term benefits.

Adverse Effects

The principal adverse effects of the ACE inhibitors are *hypotension* (secondary to arteriolar dilation), *hyperkalemia* (secondary to decreased aldosterone release), *intractable cough,* and *angioedema.* In addition, these drugs can cause *renal failure in patients with bilateral renal artery stenosis.* Because of their ability to elevate potassium levels, ACE inhibitors should be used with caution in patients taking potassium supplements or a potassium-sparing diuretic (e.g., spironolactone, triamterene).

BLACK BOX WARNING: RISK WITH ACE INHIBITORS DURING PREGNANCY

Use of ACE inhibitors during pregnancy—especially during the second and third trimesters— can cause *fetal injury.* Accordingly, if pregnancy occurs, these drugs should be discontinued.

Dosage

Adequate dosage is still debated in the literature: higher dosages may be associated with increased survival, but conflicting evidence remains. Results of the Assessment of Treatment with Lisinopril and Survival (ATLAS) trial indicate that the doses needed to increase survival are higher than those needed to produce hemodynamic changes. In contrast to the ATLAS trial, the NETWORK trial and the High Dose Enalapril Study Group did not find a difference in mortality between patients on low-dose or high-dose ACE inhibitors. Treatment with ACE inhibitors should be initiated at low doses and slowly titrated upward if the patient tolerates treatment. Target dosages associated with disease modification are shown in Table 40.1. These dosages should be used unless side effects make them intolerable.

Angiotensin II Receptor Blockers

In patients with HF, the effects of ARBs are similar to those of ACE inhibitors—but not identical. Hemodynamic effects of both groups are much the same. Clinical trials have shown that ARBs improve LV ejection fraction, reduce HF symptoms, increase exercise tolerance, decrease hospitalization, enhance quality of life, and, most important, reduce mortality. However, because ARBs do not increase levels of kinins, their effects on cardiac remodeling are less favorable than those of ACE inhibitors. For this reason, and because clinical experience with ACE inhibitors is much greater than with ARBs, ACE inhibitors are generally preferred. For now, ARBs should be reserved for HF patients who cannot tolerate ACE inhibitors, usually owing to intractable cough. (Because ARBs do not increase bradykinin levels, they do not cause cough.)

Angiotensin Receptor Neprilysin Inhibitor

Sacubitril/Valsartan [Entresto]

Sacubitril/valsartan [Entresto] is a newly approved drug that functions in two different manners. Sacubitril is a new class of drug, called an angiotensin receptor neprilysin inhibitor (ANRI). In simple terms, Entresto increases natriuretic

TABLE 40.1 ▪ Inhibitors of the Renin-Angiotensin-Aldosterone System Used in Heart Failure

Drug	Initial Daily Dose	Maximum Daily Dose
ACE INHIBITORS		
Captopril [Capoten]	6.25 mg 3 times	50 mg 3 times
Enalapril [Vasotec]	2.5 mg twice	10–20 mg twice
Fosinopril [Monopril]	5–10 mg once	40 mg once
Lisinopril [Zestril, Prinivil]	2.5–5 mg once	20–40 mg once
Quinapril [Accupril]	5 mg twice	20 mg twice
Ramipril [Altace]	1.25–2.5 mg once	10 mg once
Trandolapril [Mavik]	1 mg once	4 mg once
ANGIOTENSIN II RECEPTOR BLOCKERS		
Candesartan [Atacand]	4–8 mg once	32 mg once
Losartan [Cozaar]	25–50 mg once	50–100 mg once
Valsartan [Diovan]	20–40 mg twice	160 mg twice
ANGIOTENSIN RECEPTOR NEPRILYSIN INHIBITOR		
Sacubitril/Valsartan [Entresto]	24/26 mg twice	97/103 mg twice
ALDOSTERONE ANTAGONISTS		
Eplerenone [Inspra]	25 mg once	50 mg once
Spironolactone [Aldactone]	12.5–25 mg once	25 mg once or twice

peptides while suppressing the negative effects of the RAAS. As discussed earlier in the chapter, ANP and BNP are important indices of cardiac status in HF patients. Entresto is approved for patients with stages II to IV HF to be used in place of an ACE inhibitor or ARB.

In the PARADIGM-HF study, Entresto was superior to enalapril alone when looking at the overall end points of reduction in hospitalizations, risk for all-cause mortality, and risk for death from cardiovascular causes. In fact, the study was terminated early because of the overwhelmingly positive results.

Because Entresto contains an ARB, the contraindications and side effects are similar. Entresto can cause angioedema, hyperkalemia, and hypotension. Administration should be avoided in pregnancy, as use can cause fetal harm.

Aldosterone Antagonists

In patients with HF, aldosterone antagonists—*spironolactone* [Aldactone] and *eplerenone* [Inspra]—can reduce symptoms, decrease hospitalizations, and prolong life. These benefits were first demonstrated with spironolactone in the Randomized Aldactone Evaluation Study (RALES). Similar results were later obtained with eplerenone. Current guidelines recommend adding an aldosterone antagonist to standard HF therapy, but only in patients with persistent symptoms despite adequate treatment with an ACE inhibitor and a beta blocker.

Aldosterone antagonists work primarily by blocking aldosterone receptors in the heart and blood vessels. To understand these effects, we need to review the role of aldosterone in HF. In the past, researchers believed that all aldosterone did was promote renal retention of sodium (and water) in exchange for excretion of potassium. However, we now know that aldosterone has additional—and more harmful—effects, including the following:

- Promotion of myocardial remodeling (which impairs pumping)
- Promotion of myocardial fibrosis (which increases the risk for dysrhythmias)
- Activation of the SNS and suppression of norepinephrine uptake in the heart (both of which can promote dysrhythmias and ischemia)
- Promotion of vascular fibrosis (which decreases arterial compliance)
- Promotion of baroreceptor dysfunction

During HF, activation of the RAAS causes levels of aldosterone to rise. In some patients, levels reach 20 times normal. As aldosterone levels grow higher, harmful effects increase, and prognosis becomes progressively worse.

Drugs can reduce the effects of aldosterone by either decreasing aldosterone production or blocking aldosterone receptors. ACE inhibitors, ARBs, and DRIs decrease aldosterone production; spironolactone and eplerenone block aldosterone receptors. Although ACE inhibitors and ARBs can reduce aldosterone production, they do not block it entirely. Furthermore, production is suppressed only for a relatively short time. Hence, when ACE inhibitors or ARBs are used alone, detrimental effects of aldosterone can persist. However, when an aldosterone antagonist is added to the regimen, any residual effects are eliminated. As a result, symptoms of HF are improved and life is prolonged.

Aldosterone antagonists have one major adverse effect: *hyperkalemia*. The underlying cause is renal retention of potassium. Risk is increased by renal impairment and by using an ACE inhibitor or ARB. To minimize risk, potassium levels and renal function should be measured at baseline and periodically thereafter. Potassium supplements should be discontinued.

Spironolactone—but not eplerenone—poses a significant risk for *gynecomastia* (breast enlargement) in men, a condition that can be both cosmetically troublesome and painful. In the RALES trial, 10% of males experienced painful breast enlargement.

BLACK BOX WARNING: SPIRONOLACTONE

Spironolactone is associated with tumorigenesis in studies completed on rats.

Direct Renin Inhibitors

As discussed in Chapter 36, DRIs can shut down the entire RAAS. In theory, their benefits in HF should equal those of the ACE inhibitors and ARBs. At this time, only one DRI—*aliskiren* [Tekturna]—is available. In a recent trial, *aliskiren* did not improve outcomes in hospitalized patients with HF. Additional studies on *aliskiren* are being conducted currently. Because of these findings, aliskiren is approved for hypertension, but is not yet approved for HF.

Beta Blockers

The role of beta blockers in HF continues to evolve. Until the mid-1990s, HF was considered an absolute contraindication to these drugs. After all, blockade of cardiac $beta_1$-adrenergic receptors *reduces* contractility—an effect that is clearly detrimental, given that contractility is already compromised in the failing heart. However, it is now clear that, with careful control of dosage, beta blockers can improve patient status. Controlled trials have shown that three beta blockers—*carvedilol* [Coreg], *bisoprolol* [Zebeta], and *sustained-release metoprolol* [Toprol XL]—when added to conventional therapy, can improve LV ejection fraction, increase exercise tolerance, slow progression of HF, reduce the need for hospitalization, and, most important, prolong survival. Accordingly, beta blockers are now recommended as first-line therapy for most patients. These drugs can even be used in patients with severe disease (NYHA class IV), provided the patient is euvolemic and hemodynamically stable. Although the mechanism underlying benefits is uncertain, likely possibilities include protecting the heart from excessive sympathetic stimulation and protecting against dysrhythmias. Because excessive beta blockade can reduce contractility, doses must be very low initially and then gradually increased. Full benefits may not be seen for 1 to 3 months. Among patients with HF, the principal adverse effects are (1) fluid retention and worsening of HF, (2) fatigue, (3) hypotension, and (4) bradycardia or heart block. The basic pharmacology of the beta blockers is discussed in Chapter 14.

Ivabradine (Corlanor)

In 2015, the U.S. Food and Drug Administration approved ivabradine [*Corlanor*] for use in patients with stable, symptomatic HF, LV ejection fraction less than 35% in sinus rhythm, and heart rate greater than 70 beats/minute on maximally tolerated doses of beta blockers, or who have a contraindication to beta blocker use. Because it is new and not included in the current treatment guidelines, we will only discuss ivabradine briefly.

Ivabradine causes a dose-dependent reduction in heart rate by blocking channels responsible for cardiac pacemaker current. Although the drug slows heart rate, it does not possess negative inotropic effects or cause QTc prolongation. When used in recommended doses, heart rate reduction is approximately 10 beats/minutes.

The SHIFT (Systolic Heart failure treatment with the I^f inhibitor ivabradine Trial) study was a randomized, double-blind trial comparing ivabradine to placebo in 6,558 adults. End results revealed use of ivabradine reduced risk of hospitalization for worsening HF or cardiovascular death. Given these findings, ivabradine may be a useful alternative to patients with HF who need additional beta blockade above what is currently available.

Digoxin

Digoxin belongs to a class of drugs known as *cardiac glycosides,* agents best known for their *positive inotropic actions,* that is, their ability to increase myocardial contractile force. By increasing contractile force, digoxin can increase cardiac output. In addition, it can alter the electrical activity of the heart and can favorably affect neurohormonal systems. Unfortunately, although digoxin can reduce symptoms of HF, it does not prolong life. Used widely in the past, *digoxin is considered a second-line agent today.* The pharmacology of digoxin is discussed later.

Vasodilators (Other Than ACE Inhibitors and ARBs)

Isosorbide Dinitrate Plus Hydralazine

For treatment of HF, isosorbide dinitrate (ISDN) and hydralazine are usually combined. The combination represents an alternative to ACE inhibitors or ARBs. However, ACE inhibitors and ARBs are generally preferred.

ISDN [Isordil, others] belongs to the same family as nitroglycerin. Like nitroglycerin, ISDN causes selective dilation of veins. In patients with severe, refractory HF, the drug can reduce congestive symptoms and improve exercise capacity. In addition to its hemodynamic actions, ISDN may inhibit abnormal myocyte growth and thus may delay cardiac remodeling. Principal adverse effects are orthostatic hypotension and reflex tachycardia. The basic pharmacology of ISDN and other organic nitrates is discussed in Chapter 43.

Hydralazine [Apresoline] causes selective dilation of arterioles. By doing so, the drug can improve cardiac output and renal blood flow. For treatment of HF, hydralazine is always used in combination with ISDN because hydralazine by itself is not very effective. Principal adverse effects are hypotension, tachycardia, and a syndrome that resembles systemic lupus erythematosus. The basic pharmacology of hydralazine is discussed in Chapter 38.

BiDil, a fixed-dose combination of hydralazine and ISDN, is approved for treating HF—but only in blacks, making BiDil the first medication approved for a specific ethnic group. Can BiDil help people in other ethnic groups? Probably, but data are lacking: the manufacturer only tested the product in black patients. As discussed in Chapter 6, testing was limited primarily because of regulatory and market incentives, not because there were data suggesting it wouldn't work for others. Of course, now that BiDil is approved, clinicians may prescribe it for anyone they see fit. Each BiDil tablet contains 37.5 mg hydralazine and 20 mg ISDN. The recommended dosage is 1 or 2 tablets 3 times a day.

DIGOXIN, A CARDIAC GLYCOSIDE

Digoxin [Lanoxin] belongs to a family of drugs known as *cardiac glycosides.* These drugs are prepared by extraction from *Digitalis purpurea* (purple foxglove) and *Digitalis lanata* (Grecian foxglove) and hence are also known as *digitalis glycosides.* In the United States digoxin is the only cardiac glycoside available.

Digoxin has profound effects on the mechanical and electrical properties of the heart. In addition, it has important neurohormonal effects. In patients with HF, benefits derive from increased myocardial contractility and from effects on neurohormonal systems.

Digitalis is a dangerous drug because, at doses close to therapeutic, it can cause severe dysrhythmias. Owing to its prodysrhythmic actions, digoxin must be used with respect, caution, and skill.

Digoxin is indicated for HF and for control of dysrhythmias (see Chapter 41). When used for HF, digoxin can reduce symptoms, increase exercise tolerance, and decrease hospitalizations. However, the drug does *not* prolong life. Furthermore, when used by women, it may actually *shorten* life. Because benefits are limited to symptomatic relief, and because the risk for toxicity is substantial, *digoxin is now considered a second-line drug for treating HF.*

Chemistry

Digoxin consists of three components: a steroid nucleus, a lactone ring, and three molecules of digitoxose (a sugar). It is because of the sugars that digoxin is known as a glycoside. The region of the molecule composed of the steroid nucleus plus the lactone ring (i.e., the region without the sugar molecules) is responsible for the pharmacologic effects of digoxin. The sugars only increase solubility.

Mechanical Effects on the Heart

Digoxin exerts a *positive inotropic action* on the heart. That is, the drug *increases the force of ventricular contraction* and can thereby increase cardiac output.

Mechanism of Inotropic Action

Digoxin increases myocardial contractility by inhibiting an enzyme known as *sodium, potassium–adenosine triphosphatase* (Na^+,K^+-ATPase). By way of an indirect process described later, inhibition of Na^+,K^+-ATPase promotes calcium accumulation within myocytes. The calcium then augments contractile force by facilitating the interaction of myocardial contractile proteins: actin and myosin.

To understand how inhibition of Na^+,K^{++}-ATPase causes intracellular calcium to rise, we must first understand the normal role of Na^+,K^+-ATPase in myocytes. That role is shown in Fig. 40.4. As indicated, when an action potential passes along the myocyte membrane (sarcolemma), Na^+ ions and Ca^{++} ions enter the cell, and K^+ ions exit. After the action potential has passed, these ion fluxes must be reversed, so the original ionic balance of the cell can be restored. Na^+,K^+-ATPase is critical to this process. Na^+,K^+-ATPase acts as a "pump" to draw extracellular K^+ ions into the cell while simultaneously extruding intracellular Na^+. The energy required for pumping Na^+ and K^+ is provided by the breakdown of ATP—hence the name Na^+,K^+-ATPase. To complete the normalization of cellular ionic composition, Ca^{++} ions must leave the cell. Extrusion of Ca^{++} is accomplished through an exchange process in which extracellular Na^+ ions are taken into the cell while Ca^{++} ions exit. This exchange of Na^+ for Ca^{++} is a passive (energy-independent) process.

We can now answer the question, how does inhibition of Na^+,K^+-ATPase increase intracellular Ca^{++}? By inhibiting Na^+,K^+-ATPase, digoxin prevents the myocyte from restoring its proper ionic composition following the passage of an action potential. Inhibition of Na^+,K^+-ATPase blocks uptake of K^+ and extrusion of Na^+. Therefore with each successive action potential, intracellular K^+ levels decline and intracellular Na^+ levels rise. It is this rise

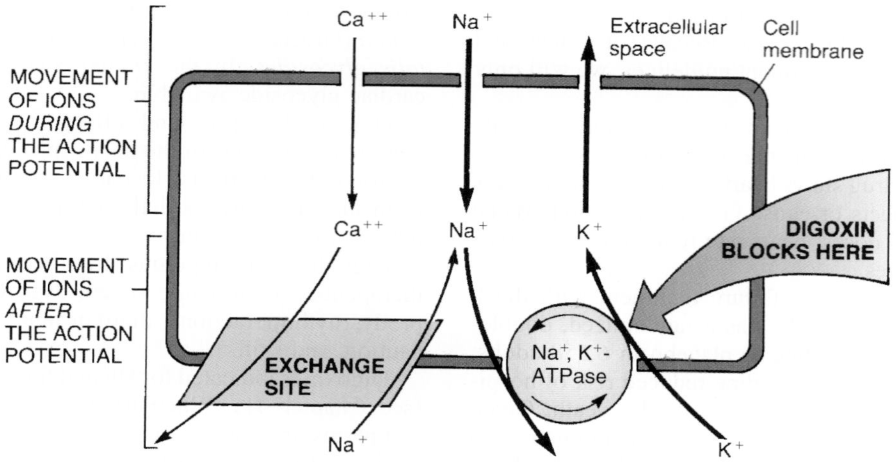

Figure 40.4 ■ Ion fluxes across the cardiac cell membrane.
During the action potential, Na^+ and Ca^{++} enter the cardiac cell and K^+ exits. Following the action potential, Na^+,K^+-ATPase pumps Na^+ out of the cell and takes up K^+. Ca^{++} leaves the cell in exchange for the uptake of Na^+. By inhibiting Na^+,K^+-ATPase, digoxin prevents the extrusion of Na^+, causing Na^+ to accumulate inside the cell. The resulting buildup of intracellular Na^+ suppresses the Na^+-Ca^{++} exchange process, thereby causing intracellular levels of Ca^{++} to rise.

in Na^+ that leads to the rise in intracellular Ca^{++}. In the presence of excess intracellular Na^+, further Na^+ entry is suppressed. Because Na^+ entry is suppressed, the passive exchange of Ca^{++} for Na^+ cannot take place, so Ca^{++} accumulates within the cell.

Relationship of Potassium to Inotropic Action

Potassium ions compete with digoxin for binding to Na^+,K^+-ATPase. This competition is of great clinical significance. Because potassium competes with digoxin, when potassium levels are low, binding of digoxin to Na^+,K^+-ATPase increases. This increase can produce excessive inhibition of Na^+,K^+-ATPase with resultant toxicity. Conversely, when levels of potassium are high, inhibition of Na^+,K^+-ATPase by digoxin is reduced, causing a reduction in the therapeutic response. Because an increase in potassium can impair therapeutic responses, whereas a decrease in potassium can cause toxicity, it is imperative that potassium levels be kept within the normal physiologic range: 3.5 to 5 mEq/L.

Hemodynamic Benefits in Heart Failure

Increased Cardiac Output

In patients with HF, increased myocardial contractility increases cardiac output. By increasing contractility, digoxin shifts the relationship of fiber length to stroke volume in the failing heart toward that in the healthy heart. Consequently, at any given heart size, the stroke volume of the failing heart increases, causing cardiac output to rise.

Consequences of Increased Cardiac Output

As a result of increased cardiac output, three major secondary responses occur: (1) sympathetic tone declines, (2) urine production increases, and (3) renin release declines. These responses can reverse virtually all signs and symptoms of HF. However, they do not correct the underlying problem of cardiac remodeling.

Decreased Sympathetic Tone

By increasing contractile force and cardiac output, digoxin increases arterial pressure. In response, sympathetic nerve traffic to the heart and blood vessels is reduced through the baroreceptor reflex. (Recall that a compensatory *increase* in sympathetic tone had taken place because of HF.)

The decrease in sympathetic tone has several beneficial effects. First, heart rate is reduced, thereby allowing more complete ventricular filling. Second, afterload is reduced (because of reduced arteriolar constriction), thereby allowing more complete ventricular emptying. Third, venous pressure is reduced (because of reduced venous constriction), thereby reducing cardiac distention, pulmonary congestion, and peripheral edema.

Increased Urine Production

The increase in cardiac output increases renal blood flow and thereby increases production of urine. The resultant loss of water reduces blood volume, which in turn reduces cardiac distention, pulmonary congestion, and peripheral edema.

Decreased Renin Release

In response to increased arterial pressure, renin release declines, causing levels of aldosterone and angiotensin II to decline as well. The decrease in angiotensin II decreases vasoconstriction, thereby further reducing afterload and venous pressure. The decrease in aldosterone reduces retention of sodium and water, which reduces blood volume, which in turn further reduces venous pressure.

Summary of Hemodynamic Effects

We can see that, through direct and indirect mechanisms, digoxin has the potential to reverse all of the overt manifestations of HF: cardiac output improves, heart rate decreases, heart size declines, constriction of arterioles and veins decreases, water retention reverses, blood volume declines, peripheral and pulmonary edema decrease, and water weight is lost. In addition, exercise tolerance improves and fatigue is reduced. There is, however, one important caveat: Although digoxin can produce substantial improvement in HF symptoms, it does not prolong life.

Neurohormonal Benefits in Heart Failure

At dosages below those needed for positive inotropic effects, digoxin can modulate the activity of neurohormonal systems. The underlying mechanism is inhibition of Na^+,K^+-ATPase.

In the kidney, digoxin can suppress renin release. By inhibiting Na^+,K^+-ATPase in renal tubules, digoxin decreases tubular absorption of sodium. As a result, less sodium is presented to the distal tubule, so renin release is suppressed.

Through effects on the vagus nerve, digoxin can decrease sympathetic outflow from the central nervous system (CNS). Specifically, by inhibiting Na^+,K^+-ATPase in vagal afferent fibers, digoxin increases the sensitivity of cardiac baroreceptors. As a result, these receptors discharge more readily, thereby signaling the CNS to reduce sympathetic traffic to the periphery.

How important are these effects on renin and sympathetic tone? No one knows for sure. However, they are probably just as important as inotropic effects, and perhaps even more important.

Electrical Effects on the Heart

The effects of digoxin on the electrical activity of the heart are of therapeutic and toxicologic importance. It is because of its electrical effects that digoxin is useful for treating dysrhythmias (see Chapter 41). Ironically, these same electrical effects are responsible for *causing* dysrhythmias, the most serious adverse effect of digoxin.

The electrical effects of digoxin can be bewildering in their complexity. Through a combination of actions, digoxin can alter the electrical activity in noncontractile tissue (sinoatrial [SA] node, atrioventricular [AV] node, Purkinje fibers) as well as in ventricular muscle. In these various regions, digoxin can alter automaticity, refractoriness, and impulse conduction. Whether these parameters are increased or decreased depends on cardiac status, digoxin dosage, and the region involved.

Although the electrical effects of digoxin are many and varied, only a few are clinically significant. These are discussed next.

Mechanisms for Altering Electrical Activity of the Heart

Digoxin alters the electrical properties of the heart by inhibiting Na^+,K^+-ATPase and by enhancing vagal influences on the heart. By inhibiting Na^+,K^+-ATPase, digoxin alters the distribution of ions (Na^+, K^+, Ca^{++}) across the cardiac cell membrane. This change in ion distribution can alter the electrical responsiveness of the cells involved. Because hypokalemia intensifies inhibition of Na^+,K^+-ATPase, hypokalemia intensifies alterations in cardiac electrical properties.

Digoxin acts in two ways to enhance vagal effects on the heart. First, the drug acts in the CNS to increase the firing rate of vagal fibers that innervate the heart. Second, digoxin increases the responsiveness of the SA node to acetylcholine (the neurotransmitter released by the vagus). The net result of these vagotonic effects is (1) decreased automaticity of the SA node and (2) decreased conduction through the AV node.

Effects on Specific Regions of the Heart

In the SA node, digoxin decreases automaticity (by the vagotonic mechanisms just mentioned). In the AV node, digoxin decreases conduction velocity and prolongs the effective refractory period. These effects, which can promote varying degrees of AV block, result primarily from the drug's vagotonic actions. In Purkinje fibers, digoxin-induced inhibition of Na^+,K^+-ATPase results in increased automaticity; this increase can generate ectopic foci that, in turn, can cause ventricular dysrhythmias. In the ventricular myocardium, digoxin acts to shorten the effective refractory period and (possibly) increase automaticity.

Adverse Effects I: Cardiac Dysrhythmias

Dysrhythmias are the most serious adverse effect of digoxin. They result from altering the electrical properties of the heart. Fortunately, when used in the dosages recommended today, dysrhythmias are uncommon.

Digoxin can mimic practically all types of dysrhythmias. AV block with escape beats is among the most common. Ventricular flutter and ventricular fibrillation are the most dangerous.

Because serious dysrhythmias are a potential consequence of therapy, all patients should be evaluated frequently for changes in heart rate and rhythm. If significant changes occur, digoxin should be withheld.

Patient Education

MONITORING HEART RATE

Patients should be taught to monitor their pulses and instructed to report any significant changes in rate or regularity.

Mechanism of Ventricular Dysrhythmia Generation

Digoxin-induced ventricular dysrhythmias result from a combination of four factors:

- Decreased automaticity of the SA node
- Decreased impulse conduction through the AV node
- Spontaneous discharge of Purkinje fibers (caused in part by increased automaticity)
- Shortening of the effective refractory period in ventricular muscle

Increased Purkinje fiber discharge and shortening of the ventricular effective refractory period predispose the ventricles to developing ectopic beats. Potential ectopic beats become manifest because the effects of digoxin on the SA and AV nodes decrease the ability of the normal pacemaker to drive the ventricles, allowing ventricular ectopic beats to take over.

Predisposing Factors

Hypokalemia

The most common cause of dysrhythmias in patients receiving digoxin is hypokalemia secondary to the use of diuretics. Less common causes include vomiting and diarrhea. Hypokalemia promotes dysrhythmias by increasing digoxin-induced inhibition of Na^+,K^+-ATPase, which in turn leads to increased automaticity of Purkinje fibers. Because low potassium can precipitate dysrhythmias, *it is imperative that serum potassium levels be kept within the normal range.* If diuretic therapy causes potassium levels to fall, a potassium-sparing diuretic (e.g., spironolactone) can be prescribed to correct the problem. Potassium supplements may also be used. Patients should be taught to recognize symptoms of hypokalemia (e.g., muscle weakness) and instructed to notify the prescriber if these develop.

Elevated Digoxin Levels

Digoxin has a narrow therapeutic range: drug levels only slightly higher than therapeutic greatly increase the risk for toxicity. Possible causes of excessive digoxin levels include (1) intentional or accidental overdose, (2) increased digoxin absorption, and (3) decreased digoxin elimination.

If digoxin levels are kept within the optimal therapeutic range—now considered to be 0.5 to 0.8 ng/mL—the chances of a dysrhythmia will be reduced. However, it is important to note that careful control over drug levels does not eliminate the risk. As discussed previously, there is only a loose relationship between digoxin levels and clinical effects. As a result, some patients may experience dysrhythmias even when drug levels are within what is normally considered a safe range.

Heart Disease

The ability of digoxin to cause dysrhythmias is greatly increased by the presence of heart disease. Doses of digoxin that have no adverse effects on healthy volunteers can precipitate serious dysrhythmias in patients with HF. The probability and severity of a dysrhythmia are directly related to the severity of the underlying disease. Because heart disease is the reason for taking digoxin, it should be no surprise that people taking the drug are at risk for dysrhythmias.

Diagnosing Digoxin-Induced Dysrhythmias

Diagnosis is not easy, largely because the failing heart is prone to spontaneous dysrhythmias. Hence, when a dysrhythmia occurs, we cannot simply assume that digoxin is the cause: the possibility that the dysrhythmia is the direct result of heart disease must be considered. Compounding diagnostic difficulties is the poor correlation between plasma digoxin levels and dysrhythmia onset. Because of this loose association, the presence of an apparently excessive digoxin level does not necessarily indicate that digoxin is responsible for the problem. Laboratory data required for diagnosis include digoxin level, serum electrolytes, and an electrocardiogram. Ultimately, diagnosis is based on experience and clinical judgment. Resolution of the dysrhythmia after digoxin withdrawal confirms the diagnosis.

Managing Digoxin-Induced Dysrhythmias

With proper treatment, digoxin-induced dysrhythmias can almost always be controlled. Basic management measures are as follows:

- *Withdraw digoxin and potassium-wasting diuretics.* For many patients, no additional treatment is needed. To help ensure that medication is stopped, a written order to withhold digoxin should be made.
- *Monitor serum potassium.* If the potassium level is low or nearly normal, potassium should be replaced. Potassium displaces digoxin from Na^+,K^+-ATPase and thereby helps reverse toxicity. However, if potassium levels are high or if AV block is present, no more potassium should be given. Under these conditions, more potassium may cause complete AV block.
- Some patients may require an antidysrhythmic drug. *Phenytoin* and *lidocaine* are most effective. Quinidine, another antidysrhythmic drug, can cause plasma levels of digoxin to rise and so should not be used.
- Patients who develop bradycardia or AV block can be treated with atropine. (Atropine blocks the vagal influences that underlie bradycardia and AV block.) Alternatively, electronic pacing may be employed.
- When overdose is especially severe, digoxin levels can be lowered using *Fab antibody fragments* [Digibind, Digifab]. After intravenous (IV) administration, these fragments bind digoxin and thereby prevent it from acting. Treatment is expensive: a full neutralizing dose costs $2000 to $3000. *Cholestyramine* and *activated charcoal,* agents that also bind digoxin, can be administered orally to suppress absorption of digoxin from the gastrointestinal (GI) tract.

Adverse Effects II: Noncardiac Adverse Effects

The principal noncardiac toxicities of digoxin concern the GI system and the CNS. Because adverse effects on these systems frequently precede development of dysrhythmias, symptoms involving the GI tract and CNS can provide advance warning of more serious toxicity. Accordingly, patients should be taught to recognize these effects and instructed to notify the prescriber if they occur.

Anorexia, nausea, and *vomiting* are the most common GI side effects. These responses result primarily from stimulation of the chemoreceptor trigger zone of the medulla. Digoxin rarely causes diarrhea.

Fatigue is the most frequent CNS effect. *Visual disturbances* (e.g., blurred vision, yellow tinge to vision, appearance of halos around dark objects) are also relatively common.

Adverse Effects III: Measures to Reduce Adverse Effects

Patient Education

DIGOXIN TOXICITY

Patients should be warned about digoxin-induced dysrhythmias and instructed to take their medication exactly as prescribed. In addition, they should be informed about symptoms of developing toxicity (altered heart rate or rhythm, visual or GI disturbances) and instructed to notify the prescriber if these develop. If a potassium supplement or potassium-sparing diuretic is part of the regimen, it should be taken exactly as ordered.

Drug Interactions

Digoxin is subject to a large number of significant drug interactions. Some are pharmacodynamics, and some are pharmacokinetic. Several important interactions are discussed later. Interactions are shown in Table 40.2.

Diuretics

Thiazide diuretics and *loop diuretics* promote loss of potassium and thereby increase the risk for digoxin-induced dysrhythmias. Accordingly, when digoxin and these diuretics are used concurrently, serum potassium levels must be monitored and maintained within the normal range (3.5–5 mEq/L). If hypokalemia develops, potassium levels can be restored with potassium supplements, a potassium-sparing diuretic, or both.

ACE Inhibitors and ARBs

These drugs can increase potassium levels and can thereby decrease therapeutic responses to digoxin. Exercise caution if

TABLE 40.2 ▪ Drug Interactions With Digoxin

Drug	Effect
PHARMACODYNAMIC INTERACTIONS	
Thiazide diuretics Loop diuretics Succinylcholine	Promote potassium loss and thereby increase the risk for digoxin-induced dysrhythmias
Beta blockers Verapamil Diltiazem	Decrease contractility and heart rate
Sympathomimetics	Increase contractility and heart rate
PHARMACOKINETIC INTERACTIONS	
Cholestyramine Kaolin-pectin Metoclopramide Neomycin Sulfasalazine	Decrease digoxin levels by decreasing digoxin absorption or bioavailability
Aminoglycosides Antacids Azithromycin Clarithromycin Colestipol Erythromycin Omeprazole Tetracycline	Increase digoxin levels by increasing digoxin absorption or bioavailability
Alprazolam Amiodarone Atorvastatin Captopril Diltiazem Nifedipine Nitrendipine Propafenone Quinidine Verapamil	Increase digoxin levels by decreasing excretion of digoxin, altering distribution of digoxin, or both

an ACE inhibitor or ARB is combined with potassium supplements or a potassium-sparing diuretic.

Sympathomimetics

Sympathomimetic drugs (e.g., dopamine, dobutamine) act on the heart to increase the rate and force of contraction. The increase in contractile force can add to the positive inotropic effects of digoxin. These complementary actions can be beneficial. In contrast, the ability of sympathomimetics to increase heart rate may be detrimental in that the risk for a tachydysrhythmia is increased.

Quinidine

Quinidine is an antidysrhythmic drug that can cause plasma levels of digoxin to rise. Quinidine increases digoxin levels by (1) displacing digoxin from tissue binding sites and (2) reducing renal excretion of digoxin. By elevating levels of free digoxin, quinidine can promote digoxin toxicity. Accordingly, concurrent use of quinidine and digoxin should be avoided.

Verapamil

Verapamil, a calcium channel blocker (CCB), can significantly increase plasma levels of digoxin. If the combination is employed, digoxin dosage must be reduced. In addition, verapamil can suppress myocardial contractility and can thereby counteract the benefits of digoxin.

Pharmacokinetics

Absorption

Absorption with digoxin tablets is variable, ranging between 60% and 80%, and can be decreased by certain foods and drugs. Meals high in bran can decrease absorption significantly, as can cholestyramine, kaolin-pectin, and certain other drugs (see Table 40.2). Of note, taking digoxin with meals decreases the rate of absorption but not the extent.

In the past, there was considerable variability in the absorption of digoxin from tablets prepared by different manufacturers. This variability resulted from differences in the rate and extent of tablet dissolution. Because of this variable bioavailability, it had been recommended that patients not switch between different digoxin brands. Today, bioavailability of digoxin in tablets produced by different companies is fairly uniform, making brands of digoxin more interchangeable than in the past. However, given the narrow therapeutic range of digoxin, some authorities still recommend that patients not switch between brands of digoxin tablets—even when prescriptions are written generically—except with the approval and supervision of the prescriber.

Distribution

Digoxin is distributed widely and crosses the placenta. High levels are achieved in cardiac and skeletal muscle, owing largely to binding to Na^+,K^+-ATPase. About 23% of digoxin in plasma is bound to proteins, mainly albumin.

Elimination

Digoxin is eliminated primarily by *renal excretion.* Hepatic metabolism is minimal. Because digoxin is eliminated by the kidneys, renal impairment can lead to toxic accumulation. Accordingly, dosage must be reduced if kidney function declines. Because digoxin is not metabolized to a significant extent, changes in liver function do not affect digoxin levels.

Half-Life and Time to Plateau

The half-life of digoxin is about 1.5 days. Therefore, in the absence of a loading dose, about 6 days (four half-lives) are required to reach plateau. When use of the drug is discontinued, another 6 days are required for digoxin stores to be eliminated.

Single-Dose Time Course

Effects of a single oral dose begin 30 minutes to 2 hours after administration and peak within 4 to 6 hours.

A Note on Plasma Digoxin Levels

Levels above 1 ng/mL offer no additional benefits, but do increase the risk for toxicity. Knowledge of plasma levels can be useful for the following:

- Establishing dosage
- Monitoring compliance
- Diagnosing toxicity
- Determining the cause of therapeutic failure

After a stable blood level has been achieved, routine measurement of digoxin levels can be replaced with an annual measurement. Additional measurements may be useful in the following circumstances:

- Digoxin dosage is changed
- Symptoms of HF intensify

- Kidney function deteriorates
- Signs of toxicity appear
- Drugs that can affect digoxin levels are added to or deleted from the regimen

Although knowledge of digoxin plasma levels can aid the clinician, it must be understood that the extent of this aid is limited. The correlation between plasma levels of digoxin and clinical effects—both therapeutic and adverse—is not very tight: drug levels that are safe and effective for patient A may be subtherapeutic for patient B and toxic for patient C. Because of interpatient variability, knowledge of digoxin levels does not permit precise predictions of therapeutic effects or toxicity. Hence information regarding drug levels must not be relied on too heavily. Rather, this information should be seen as but one factor among several to be considered when evaluating clinical responses.

Preparations, Dosage, and Administration

Preparations

Digoxin is available in three formulations:

- Tablets—0.125 and 0.25 mg
- Pediatric elixir—0.05 mg/mL
- Solution for injection—0.1 and 0.25 mg/mL

Administration

Digoxin can be administered orally and intravenously. Intramuscular administration should be avoided, owing to a risk for tissue damage and severe pain. Before dosing, the rate and regularity of the heartbeat should be determined. If heart rate is less than 60 beats/minute or if a change in rhythm is detected, digoxin should be withheld and the prescriber notified. When digoxin is given intravenously, cardiac status should be monitored continuously for 1 to 2 hours.

Dosage in Heart Failure

Most patients can be treated with initial and maintenance dosages of 0.125 to 0.25 mg/day. Doses above 0.25 mg/day are rarely used or needed. The target plasma drug level is 0.5 to 0.8 ng/mL.

Digitalization

The term digitalization refers to the use of a loading dose to achieve high plasma levels of digoxin quickly. (As noted, 6 days are needed for drug levels to reach plateau if no loading dose is employed.) Although digitalization was common in the past, the practice is now considered both unnecessary and inappropriate in the treatment of chronic HF.

MANAGEMENT OF HEART FAILURE

Our discussion of HF management is based on recommendations in the *2013 ACCF/AHA Guideline for the Management of Heart Failure: Executive Summary A Report of the American College of Cardiology Foundation/American Heart Association Task Force on Practice Guidelines*. These guidelines can be viewed at http://circ.ahajournals.org/content/128/16/1810. As noted earlier, these guidelines approach HF as a progressive disease that advances through four stages of increasing severity. Management for each stage is discussed next and in Fig. 40.5.

These management measures are consistent with those in another guideline—*HFSA 2010 Comprehensive Heart Failure Practice Guideline*—issued by the Heart Failure Society of America (HFSA). In addition to discussing HF with LV systolic dysfunction (i.e., the form of HF that we've been discussing), the HFSA guidelines address other issues, including acutely decompensated HF, HF with preserved LV ejection fraction (diastolic HF), and HF in special populations.

Stage A

By definition, patients in ACC/AHA stage A have no symptoms of HF and no structural or functional cardiac abnormalities—but they do have behaviors or conditions strongly associated with developing HF. Important among these are hypertension, coronary artery disease, diabetes, family history of cardiomyopathy, and a personal history of alcohol abuse, rheumatic fever, or treatment with a cardiotoxic drug (e.g., doxorubicin, trastuzumab).

Management is directed at reducing risk. Hypertension, hyperlipidemia, and diabetes should be controlled, as should ventricular rate in patients with supraventricular tachycardias. An ACE inhibitor or ARB can be useful for patients with diabetes, atherosclerosis, or hypertension. Patients should cease behaviors that increase HF risk, especially smoking and alcohol abuse. (Excessive, chronic consumption of alcohol is a leading cause of cardiomyopathy. In patients with HF, acute alcohol consumption can suppress contractility.) There is no evidence that getting regular exercise can prevent development of HF, although exercise does have other health benefits. Routine use of dietary supplements to prevent structural heart disease is not recommended.

Stage B

Like patients in stage A, those in stage B have no signs or symptoms of HF, but they do have structural heart disease that is strongly associated with development of HF. Among these structural changes are LV hypertrophy or fibrosis, LV dilation or hypocontractility, valvular heart disease, and previous myocardial infarction.

The goal of management is to prevent development of symptomatic HF. The approach is to implement measures that can prevent further cardiac injury, delaying the progression of remodeling and LV dysfunction. Specific measures include all those discussed above for stage A. In addition, treatment with an ACE inhibitor plus a beta blocker is recommended for all patients with a reduced ejection fraction, history of myocardial infarction, or both. For patients who cannot tolerate ACE inhibitors, an ARB may be used instead. As in stage A, there is no evidence that using dietary supplements or getting regular exercise can help prevent progression to symptomatic HF.

Stage C

Patients in stage C have symptoms of HF and also have structural heart disease. As discussed earlier, symptoms include dyspnea, fatigue, peripheral edema, and distention of the jugular veins. Treatment has four major goals: (1) relief of pulmonary and peripheral congestive symptoms, (2) improvement of functional capacity and quality of life, (3) slowing of cardiac remodeling and progression of LV dysfunction, and (4) prolongation of life. Treatment measures include those recommended for stages A and B, plus those discussed subsequently.

Drug Therapy

Drug therapy of HF has changed dramatically over the past 15 to 20 years. Formerly, digoxin was a mainstay of treatment.

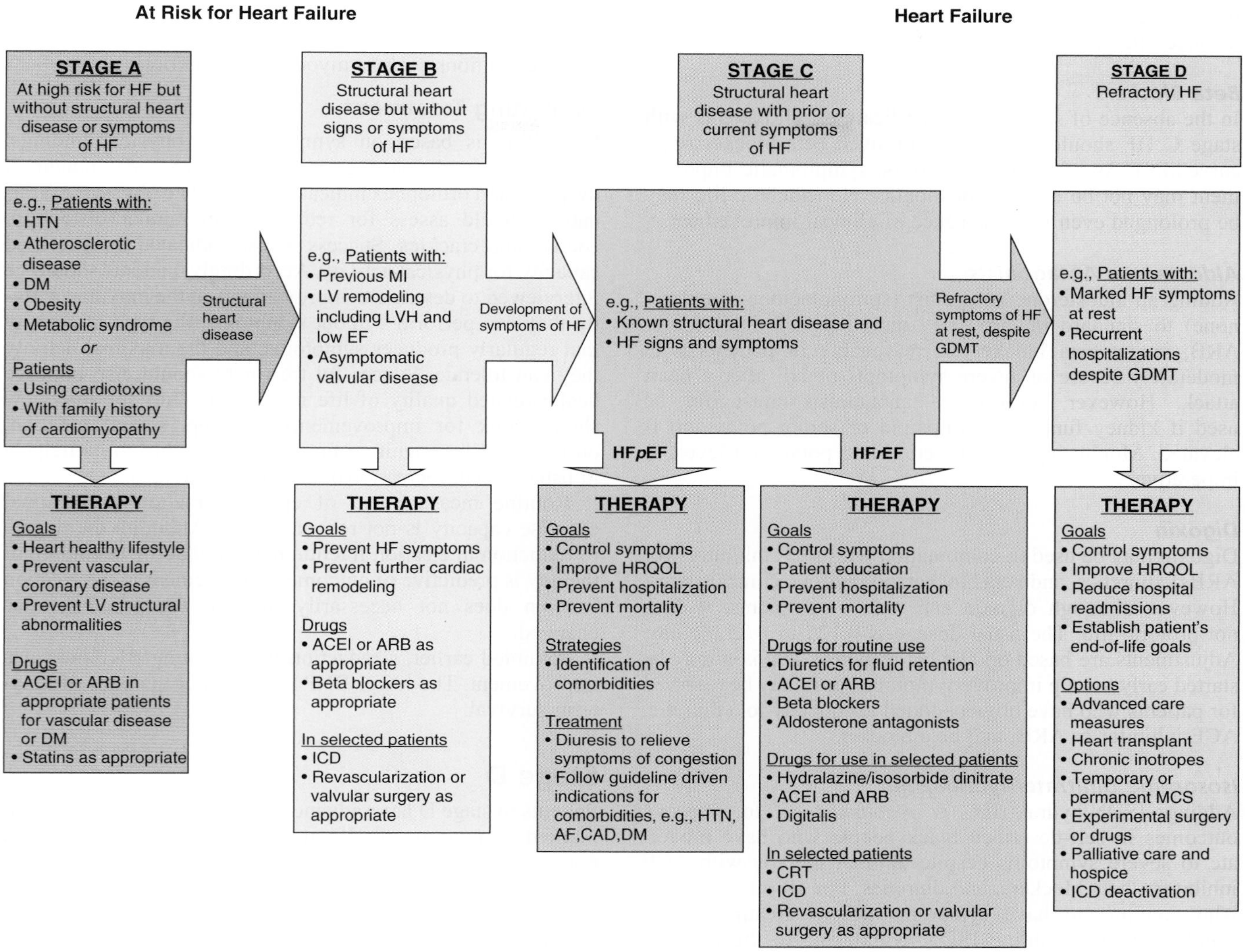

Figure 40.5 ■ Recommended therapies for varying stages of heart failure.
(Adapted from Hunt SA, Abraham WT, Chin MH, et al. 2009 Focused update incorporated into the ACC/AHA 2005 guidelines for the diagnosis and management of heart failure in adults: a report of the American College of Cardiology Foundation/American Heart Association Task Force on Practice Guidelines. J Am Coll Cardiol 2009;53:e1–90)

Today, its role is secondary. First-line therapy now consists of three drugs: a diuretic, an ACE inhibitor or ARB, and a beta blocker. As a rule, digoxin is added only when symptoms cannot be managed with the preferred agents.

Diuretics

All patients with evidence of fluid retention should restrict salt intake and use a diuretic. Diuretics are the only reliable means of correcting fluid overload. Furthermore, these drugs produce symptomatic improvement faster than any other drugs. If renal function is good, a thiazide diuretic will work. However, if renal function is significantly impaired, as it is in most patients, a loop diuretic will be needed. Efficacy of diuresis is best assessed by daily measurement of body weight. After fluid overload has been corrected, diuretic therapy should continue to prevent recurrence. Diuretics should not be used alone. Rather, for most patients, they should be combined with an ACE inhibitor (or ARB) plus a beta blocker. Because aspirin and other nonsteroidal antiinflammatory drugs (NSAIDs) can decrease the effects of diuretics and increase the incidence of acute kidney injury when used in combination with an ACE inhibitor and a diuretic, these agents should be avoided. As noted, although diuretics reduce symptoms, they do not prolong survival.

ACE Inhibitors and ARBs

In the absence of specific contraindications (e.g., pregnancy), all patients with stage C HF should receive an ACE inhibitor. If fluid retention is evident, a diuretic should be used as well. Symptomatic improvement may take weeks or even months to develop. However, even in the absence of symptomatic improvement, ACE inhibitors may prolong life. Dosage should be sufficient to reduce mortality (see Table 40.1). For patients who cannot tolerate ACE inhibitors (owing to intractable cough or angioedema), ARBs remain the recommended alternative.

Beta Blockers

In the absence of specific contraindications, all patients with stage C HF should receive an approved beta blocker (e.g., carvedilol). As with ACE inhibitors, symptomatic improvement may not be evident for months. Nonetheless, life may be prolonged even in the absence of clinical improvement.

Aldosterone Antagonists

Adding an aldosterone antagonist (spironolactone or eplerenone) to standard therapy (i.e., diuretic, ACE inhibitor or ARB, and a beta blocker) is reasonable in patients with moderately severe or severe symptoms of HF after a heart attack. However, aldosterone antagonists must not be used if kidney function is impaired or serum potassium is elevated. Monitoring renal function and potassium levels is imperative.

Digoxin

Digoxin may be used in combination with ACE inhibitors (or ARBs), diuretics, and beta blockers to improve clinical status. However, although digoxin can reduce symptoms, it does not prolong life. The usual dosage is 0.125 to 0.25 mg/day. Adjustments are based on clinical response. Digoxin may be started early to help improve symptoms, or it may be reserved for patients who have not responded adequately to a diuretic, ACE inhibitor or ARB, and beta blocker.

Isosorbide Dinitrate/Hydralazine

Adding ISDN/hydralazine is *recommended* to improve outcomes in self-described black people who have moderate to severe symptoms despite optimal therapy with ACE inhibitors, beta blockers, and diuretics. For all other patients who continue to have symptoms despite treatment with standard therapy, adding ISDN/hydralazine to the regimen is considered *reasonable.* For patients who cannot tolerate ACE inhibitors or ARBs, *substitution* of ISDN/hydralazine is considered reasonable.

Drugs to Avoid

Patients in stage C should avoid three classes of drugs: antidysrhythmics, CCBs, and NSAIDs (e.g., aspirin). Reasons for not using these drugs are as follows:

- *Antidysrhythmic agents*—These drugs have cardiosuppressant and prodysrhythmic actions that can make HF worse. Only two agents—amiodarone [Cordarone] and dofetilide [Tikosyn]—have been proved not to reduce survival.
- *Calcium channel blockers*—These drugs can make HF worse and may increase the risk for adverse cardiovascular events. Only the long-acting dihydropyridine CCBs, such as amlodipine [Norvasc], have been shown not to reduce survival.
- *NSAIDs*—These drugs promote sodium retention and peripheral vasoconstriction. Both actions can make HF worse. In addition, NSAIDs can reduce the efficacy and intensify the toxicity of diuretics and ACE inhibitors. Hence, even though aspirin has beneficial effects on coagulation, it should still be avoided unless clinically indicated for conditions such as myocardial infarction.

Evaluating Treatment

Evaluation is based on symptoms and physical findings. Reductions in dyspnea on exertion, paroxysmal nocturnal dyspnea, and orthopnea indicate success. The physical examination should assess for reductions in jugular distention, edema, and crackles. Success is also indicated by increased capacity for physical activity. Accordingly, patients should be interviewed to determine improvements in the maximal activity they can perform without symptoms, the type of activity that regularly produces symptoms, and the maximal activity they can tolerate. Successful treatment should also improve health-related quality of life in general. Thus the interview should look for improvements in sleep, sexual function, outlook on life, cognitive function, and ability to participate in usual social, recreational, and work activities.

Routine measurement of ejection fraction or maximal exercise capacity is not recommended. Although the degree of reduction in ejection fraction measured at the beginning of therapy is predictive of outcome, improvement in the ejection fraction does not necessarily indicate the prognosis has changed.

As noted earlier, a reduction in circulating BNP indicates improvement. The lower BNP is, the better the odds of long-term survival.

Stage D

Patients in stage D have advanced structural heart disease and marked symptoms of HF at rest, despite treatment with maximal dosages of medications used in stage C. Repeated and prolonged hospitalization is common. For eligible candidates, the best long-term solution is a heart transplantation. An implantable LV mechanical assist device can be used as a "bridge" in patients awaiting a transplant and to prolong life in those who are not transplant eligible.

Management focuses largely on control of fluid retention, which underlies most signs and symptoms. Intake and output should be monitored closely, and the patient should be weighed daily. Fluid retention can usually be treated with a loop diuretic, perhaps combined with a thiazide. If volume overload becomes severe, the patient should be hospitalized and given an IV diuretic. If needed, an IV inotropic agent can be added to increase renal blood flow, thereby enhancing diuresis. Patients should not be discharged until a stable and effective oral diuretic regimen has been established. These drugs are discussed further in Chapter 89.

Beta blockers and ACE inhibitors may be tried, but doses should be low and responses monitored with care. In stage D, beta blockers pose a significant risk for making HF worse, and ACE inhibitors may induce profound hypotension or renal failure.

When severe symptoms persist despite application of all recommended therapies, options for end-of-life care should be discussed with the patient and family.

CHAPTER

41 Antidysrhythmic Drugs

Laura D. Rosenthal, DNP, ACNP, FAANP

A dysrhythmia is defined as *an abnormality in the rhythm of the heartbeat.* In their mildest forms, dysrhythmias have only modest effects on cardiac output. However, in their most severe forms, dysrhythmias can disable the heart so that no blood is pumped at all. Because of their ability to compromise cardiac function, dysrhythmias are associated with a high degree of morbidity and mortality.

There are two basic types of dysrhythmias: *tachydysrhythmias* and *bradydysrhythmias.* In this chapter, we only consider the tachydysrhythmias. This is by far the largest group of dysrhythmias and the group that responds best to drugs. We do not discuss the bradydysrhythmias because they are few in number and are commonly treated with electronic pacing. When drugs are indicated, atropine is usually the agent of choice.

It is important to appreciate that virtually all of the drugs used to treat dysrhythmias can also *cause* dysrhythmias. These drugs can create new dysrhythmias and worsen existing ones. Because of these prodysrhythmic actions, antidysrhythmic drugs should be employed only when the benefits of treatment clearly outweigh the risks.

For two reasons, use of antidysrhythmic drugs is declining. First, research has shown that some of these agents actually *increase* the risk for death. Second, nonpharmacologic therapies—especially implantable defibrillators and radiofrequency ablation—have begun to replace drugs as the preferred treatment for many dysrhythmia types.

A note on terminology: dysrhythmias are also known as *arrhythmias.* Because the term *arrhythmia* denotes an *absence* of cardiac rhythm, whereas *dysrhythmia* denotes an *abnormal* rhythm, dysrhythmia would seem the more appropriate term.

INTRODUCTION TO CARDIAC ELECTROPHYSIOLOGY, DYSRHYTHMIAS, AND THE ANTIDYSRHYTHMIC DRUGS

In this section we discuss background information that will help you understand the actions and uses of antidysrhythmic drugs. We begin by reviewing the electrical properties of the heart and the electrocardiogram (ECG). Next, we discuss how dysrhythmias are generated. After that, we discuss classification of the antidysrhythmic drugs as well as the ability of these drugs to *cause* dysrhythmias. We conclude by discussing the major dysrhythmias and the basic principles that guide antidysrhythmic therapy.

Electrical Properties of the Heart

Dysrhythmias result from alteration of the electrical impulses that regulate cardiac rhythm—and antidysrhythmic drugs control rhythm by correcting or compensating for these alterations. Accordingly, to understand both the generation and treatment of dysrhythmias, we must first understand the electrical properties of the heart. Therefore we begin by reviewing (1) pathways and timing of impulse conduction, (2) cardiac action potentials, and (3) basic elements of the ECG.

Impulse Conduction: Pathways and Timing

For the heart to pump effectively, contraction of the atria and ventricles must be coordinated. Coordination is achieved through precise timing and routing of impulse conduction. In the healthy heart, impulses originate in the sinoatrial (SA) node, spread rapidly through the atria, pass slowly through the atrioventricular (AV) node, and then spread rapidly through the ventricles by way of the His-Purkinje system (Fig. 41.1).

SA Node

Under normal circumstances, the SA node serves as the pacemaker for the heart. Pacemaker activity results from spontaneous phase 4 depolarization (see later). Because cells of the sinus node usually discharge faster than other cells that display automaticity, the SA node normally dominates all other potential pacemakers.

After the SA node discharges, impulses spread rapidly through the atria along the *internodal pathways.* This rapid conduction allows the atria to contract in unison.

AV Node

Impulses originating in the atria must travel through the AV node to reach the ventricles. In the healthy heart, impulses arriving at the AV node are delayed before going on to excite the ventricles. This delay provides time for blood to fill the ventricles before ventricular contraction.

His-Purkinje System

The fibers of the His-Purkinje system consist of specialized conducting tissue. The function of these fibers is to conduct electrical excitation very rapidly to all parts of the ventricles. Stimulation of the His-Purkinje system is caused by impulses leaving the AV node. These impulses are conducted rapidly down the bundle of His, enter the right and left bundle branches, and then distribute to the many fine branches of the Purkinje fibers (see Fig. 41.1). Because impulses travel quickly through this system, all regions of the ventricles are stimulated almost simultaneously, producing synchronized ventricular contraction with resultant forceful ejection of blood.

Cardiac Action Potentials

Cardiac cells can initiate and conduct action potentials, consisting of self-propagating waves of depolarization followed

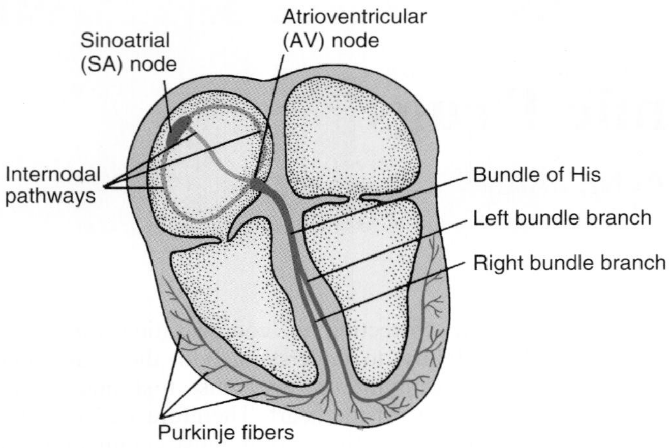

Figure 41.1 ■ Cardiac conduction pathways.

by repolarization. As in neurons, cardiac action potentials are generated by the movement of ions into and out of cells. These ion fluxes take place by way of specific channels in the cell membrane. In the resting cardiac cell, negatively charged ions cover the inner surface of the cell membrane, whereas positively charged ions cover the external surface. Because of this separation of charge, the cell membrane is said to be *polarized.* Under proper conditions, channels in the cell membrane open, allowing positively charged ions to rush in. This influx eliminates the charge difference across the cell membrane, and thus the cell is said to depolarize. After depolarization, positively charged ions are extruded from the cell, causing the cell to return to its original polarized state.

In the heart, two kinds of action potentials occur: *fast potentials* and *slow potentials.* These potentials differ with respect to the mechanisms by which they are generated, the kinds of cells in which they occur, and the drugs to which they respond.

Profiles of fast and slow potentials are depicted in Fig. 41.2. Please note that action potentials in this figure represent the electrical activity of *single cardiac cells.* Such single-cell recordings, which are made using experimental preparations, should not be confused with the ECG, which is made using surface electrodes and thus reflects the electrical activity of the entire heart.

Fast Potentials

Fast potentials occur in fibers of the *His-Purkinje system* and in *atrial and ventricular muscle.* These responses serve to conduct electrical impulses rapidly throughout the heart.

As shown in Fig. 41.2A, fast potentials have five distinct phases, labeled 0, 1, 2, 3, and 4. As we discuss each phase, we focus on its ionic basis and its relationship to the actions of antidysrhythmic drugs.

Phase 0. In phase 0, the cell undergoes *rapid depolarization* in response to *influx of sodium ions.* Phase 0 is important in that the speed of phase 0 depolarization determines the velocity of impulse conduction. Drugs that decrease the rate of phase 0 depolarization (by blocking sodium channels) slow impulse conduction through the His-Purkinje system and myocardium.

Phase 1. During phase 1, rapid (but partial) repolarization takes place. Phase 1 has no relevance to antidysrhythmic drugs.

Phase 2. Phase 2 consists of a prolonged plateau in which the membrane potential remains relatively stable. During this phase, *calcium* enters the cell and promotes contraction of atrial and ventricular muscle. Drugs that reduce calcium entry during phase 2 do *not* influence *cardiac rhythm.* However, because calcium influx is required for contraction, these drugs *can* reduce myocardial contractility.

Phase 3. In phase 3, rapid repolarization takes place. This repolarization is caused by *extrusion of potassium* from the cell. Phase 3 is relevant in that delay of repolarization prolongs the action potential duration and thereby prolongs the effective refractory period (ERP). (The ERP is the time during which a cell is unable to respond to excitation and initiate a new action potential. Therefore extending the ERP prolongs the minimal interval between two propagating responses.) Phase 3 repolarization can be delayed by drugs that block potassium channels.

Phase 4. During phase 4, two types of electrical activity are possible: (1) the membrane potential may remain *stable* (solid line in Fig. 41.2A) or (2) the membrane may undergo *spontaneous depolarization* (dashed line). In cells undergoing spontaneous depolarization, the membrane potential gradually rises until a threshold potential is reached. At this point, rapid phase 0 depolarization takes place, setting off a new action potential. Hence it is phase 4 depolarization that gives cardiac cells *automaticity* (i.e., the ability to initiate an action potential through self-excitation). The capacity for self-excitation makes potential pacemakers of all cells that have it.

Under normal conditions, His-Purkinje cells undergo very slow spontaneous depolarization, and myocardial cells do not undergo any. However, under pathologic conditions, significant phase 4 depolarization may occur in all of these cells, and especially in Purkinje fibers. When this happens, a dysrhythmia can result.

Slow Potentials

Slow potentials occur in cells of the *SA node* and *AV node.* The profile of a slow potential is depicted in Fig. 41.2B. Like fast potentials, slow potentials are generated by ion fluxes. However, the specific ions involved are not the same for every phase.

From a physiologic and pharmacologic perspective, slow potentials have three features of special significance: (1) phase 0 depolarization is slow and mediated by calcium influx, (2) these potentials conduct slowly, and (3) spontaneous phase 4 depolarization in the SA node normally determines heart rate.

Phase 0. Phase 0 (depolarization phase) of slow potentials differs significantly from phase 0 of fast potentials. As we can see from Fig. 41.2, whereas phase 0 of fast potentials is caused by a *rapid influx of sodium,* phase 0 of slow potentials is caused by *slow influx of calcium.* Because calcium influx is slow, the rate of depolarization is slow; and because depolarization is slow, these potentials conduct slowly. This explains why impulse conduction through the AV node is delayed. Phase 0 of the slow potential is of therapeutic significance in that drugs that suppress calcium influx during phase 0 can slow (or stop) AV conduction.

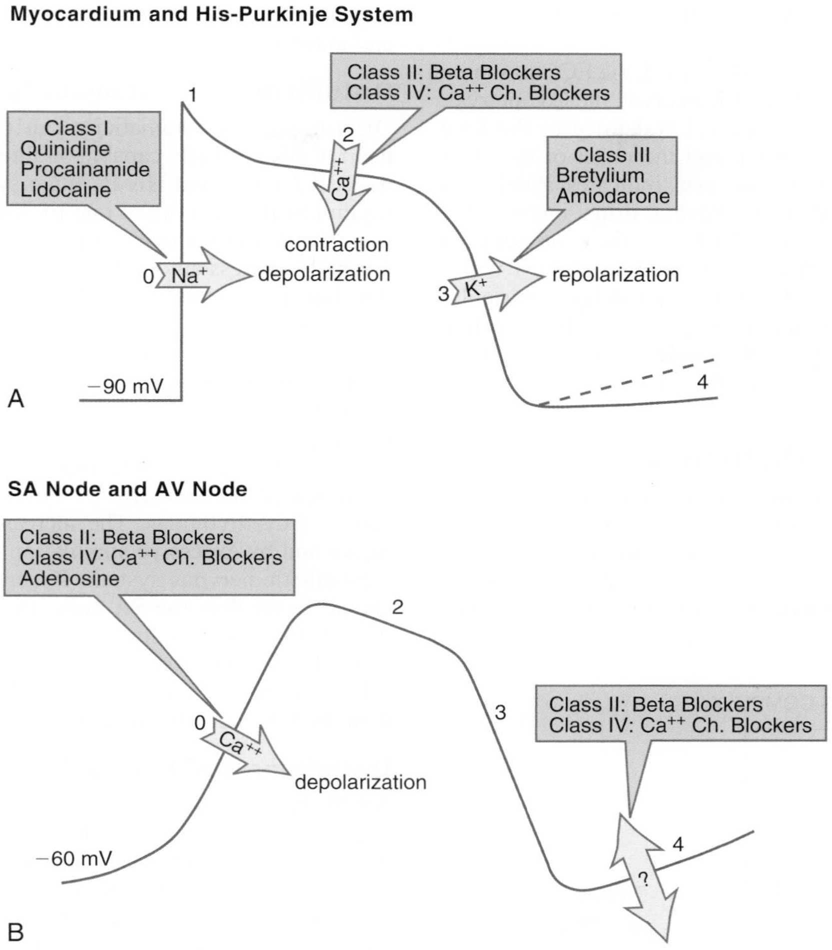

Figure 41.2 ▪ Ion fluxes during cardiac action potentials and effects of antidysrhythmic drugs.

A, Fast potential of the His-Purkinje system and atrial and ventricular myocardium. Blockade of sodium influx by class I drugs slows conduction in the His-Purkinje system. Blockade of calcium influx by beta blockers and calcium channel blockers decreases contractility. Blockade of potassium efflux by class III drugs delays repolarization and thereby prolongs the effective refractory period. **B,** Slow potential of the sinoatrial (SA) node and atrioventricular (AV) node. Blockade of calcium influx by beta blockers, calcium channel blockers, and adenosine slows AV conduction. Beta blockers and calcium channel blockers decrease SA nodal automaticity (phase 4 depolarization); the ionic basis of this effect is not understood.

Phases 2 and 3. Slow potentials lack a phase 1 (see Fig. 41.2B). Phases 2 and 3 of the slow potential are not significant with respect to the actions of antidysrhythmic drugs.

Phase 4. Cells of the SA node and AV node undergo spontaneous phase 4 depolarization. The ionic basis of this phenomenon is complex and incompletely understood.

Under normal conditions, the rate of phase 4 depolarization in cells of the SA node is faster than in all other cells of the heart. As a result, the SA node discharges first and determines heart rate. Hence the SA node is referred to as the cardiac *pacemaker.*

As shown in Fig. 41.2B, two classes of drugs (beta blockers and calcium channel blockers) can suppress phase 4 depolarization. By doing so, these agents can decrease automaticity in the SA node.

The Electrocardiogram

The ECG provides a graphic representation of cardiac electrical activity. The ECG can be used to identify dysrhythmias and monitor responses to therapy. (*Note:* In referring to the electrocardiogram, two abbreviations may be used: EKG and ECG.)

The major components of an ECG are shown in Fig. 41.3. As we can see, three features are especially prominent: the P wave, the QRS complex, and the T wave. The P wave is caused by *depolarization in the atria.* Therefore the P wave corresponds to atrial contraction. The QRS complex is caused by *depolarization of the ventricles,* so the QRS complex corresponds to ventricular contraction. If conduction through the ventricles is slowed, the QRS complex will widen. The T wave is caused by *repolarization of the ventricles,* so this wave is not associated with overt physical activity of the heart.

In addition to the features just described, the ECG has three other components of interest: the PR interval, the QT interval, and the ST segment. The PR interval is defined as the time between the onset of the P wave and the onset of the QRS complex. Lengthening of this interval indicates a delay in conduction through the AV node. Several drugs increase the PR interval. The QT interval is defined as the time between the onset of the QRS complex and completion of the T wave. This interval is prolonged by drugs that delay ventricular repolarization. The ST segment is the portion of the ECG that lies between the end of the QRS complex and the beginning of the T wave. Digoxin depresses the ST segment.

Generation of Dysrhythmias

Dysrhythmias arise from two fundamental causes: *disturbances of impulse formation* (automaticity) and *disturbances of impulse conduction.* One or both of these disturbances underlie all dysrhythmias. Factors that may alter automaticity or conduction include hypoxia, electrolyte imbalance, cardiac surgery, reduced coronary blood flow, myocardial infarction, and antidysrhythmic drugs.

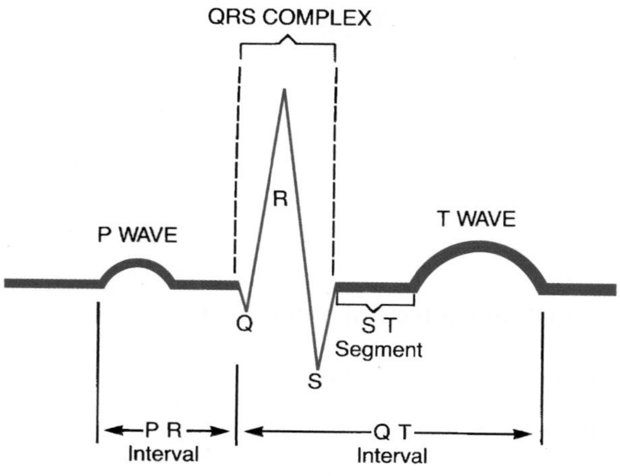

Figure 41.3 ■ The electrocardiogram.

Disturbances of Automaticity

Disturbances of automaticity can occur in any part of the heart. Cells normally capable of automaticity (cells of the SA node, AV node, and His-Purkinje system) can produce dysrhythmias if their normal rate of discharge changes. In addition, dysrhythmias may be produced if tissues that do not normally express automaticity (atrial and ventricular muscle) develop spontaneous phase 4 depolarization.

Altered automaticity in the SA node can produce tachycardia or bradycardia. Excessive discharge of sympathetic neurons that innervate the SA node can augment automaticity to such a degree that sinus tachycardia results. Excessive vagal (parasympathetic) discharge can suppress automaticity to such a degree that sinus bradycardia results.

Increased automaticity of Purkinje fibers is a common cause of dysrhythmias. The increase can be brought on by injury and by excessive stimulation of Purkinje fibers by the sympathetic nervous system. If Purkinje fibers begin to discharge faster than the SA node, they will escape control by the SA node; potentially serious dysrhythmias can result.

Under special conditions, automaticity may develop in cells of atrial and ventricular muscle. If these cells fire faster than the SA node, dysrhythmias will result.

Disturbances of Conduction

AV Block

Impaired conduction through the AV node produces varying degrees of AV block. If impulse conduction is delayed (but not prevented entirely), the block is termed *first degree.* If some impulses pass through the node but others do not, the block is termed *second degree.* If all traffic through the AV node stops, the block is termed *third degree.*

Reentry (Recirculating Activation)

Reentry, also referred to as recirculating activation, is a generalized mechanism by which dysrhythmias can be produced. Reentry causes dysrhythmias by establishing a localized, self-sustaining circuit capable of repetitive cardiac stimulation. Reentry results from a unique form of conduction disturbance.

PATIENT-CENTERED CARE ACROSS THE LIFE SPAN

Antidysrhythmic Drugs

Life Stage	Patient Care Concerns
Infants	See later entry, "Breastfeeding women."
Children/adolescents	Some antidysrhythmic drugs can be used safely in children, just in smaller doses. These include disopyramide, flecainide, and sotalol. Side-effect profiles are similar to those of adults.
Pregnant women	Many of the drugs discussed in this chapter are classified in U.S. Food and Drug Administration Pregnancy Risk Category C or D. Animal studies show adverse fetal effects, and in Category D, there is evidence of human fetal risk. Benefits should outweigh the risks. Dronedarone is classified in Pregnancy Risk Category X.
Breastfeeding women	For most of the drugs discussed in this chapter, data are lacking regarding transmission of drug from mother to infant through breast milk. Breastfeeding is contraindicated in women taking dronederone.
Older adults	Aging alters the absorption, distribution, metabolism, and elimination of antidysrhythmic drugs. Liver and kidney function must be monitored, and antiarrhythmic dosing may need to be adjusted for age. Older-adult patients are also more susceptible to the side effects of many antidysrhythmics, including bradycardia, orthostatic hypotension, urinary retention, and falls.

The mechanism of reentrant activation and the effects of drugs on this process are described next.

In normal impulse conduction, electrical impulses travel down both branches of the Purkinje fiber to cause excitation of the muscle at two locations (Fig. 41.4A). Impulses created within the muscle travel in both directions (to the right and to the left) away from their sites of origin. Those impulses that are moving toward each other meet midway between the two branches of the Purkinje fiber. Because in the wake of both impulses the muscle is in a refractory state, neither impulse can proceed further, so both impulses stop.

In a reentrant circuit (Fig. 41.4B), there is a region of one-way conduction block of one branch of the Purkinje fiber. This region prevents conduction of impulses downward (toward the muscle), but does not prevent impulses from traveling upward. (Impulses can travel back up the block because impulses in muscle are very strong and hence are able to pass the block, whereas impulses in the Purkinje fiber are weaker and so are unable to pass.) A region of one-way block is essential for reentrant activation.

How does one-way block lead to reentrant activation? As an impulse travels down the Purkinje fiber, it is blocked in one branch but continues unimpeded in the other branch. Upon reaching the tip of the second (unblocked) branch, the impulse stimulates the muscle. As described earlier, the impulse in the muscle travels to the right and to the left away from its site of origin. However, in this new situation, as the impulse travels toward the impaired branch of the Purkinje fiber, it meets no impulse coming from the other direction and continues on, resulting in stimulation of the terminal end of the first (blocked) branch. This stimulation causes an impulse to travel backward up the blocked branch of the Purkinje fiber. Because blockade of conduction in that branch is one way (downward only), the impulse can pass upward through the region of block and then back down into the unblocked branch, causing reentrant activation of this branch. Under proper conditions, the impulse will continue to cycle indefinitely, resulting in repetitive ectopic beats.

There are two mechanisms by which drugs can abolish a reentrant dysrhythmia. First, drugs can improve conduction in the sick branch of the Purkinje fiber, and can thereby eliminate the one-way block (Fig. 41.4C). Alternatively, drugs can suppress conduction in the sick branch, thereby converting one-way block into two-way block (Fig. 41.4D).

Classification of Antidysrhythmic Drugs

According to the Vaughan Williams classification scheme, the antidysrhythmic drugs fall into five groups (Table 41.1). There are four major classes of antidysrhythmic drugs (classes I, II, III, and IV) and a fifth group that includes adenosine and

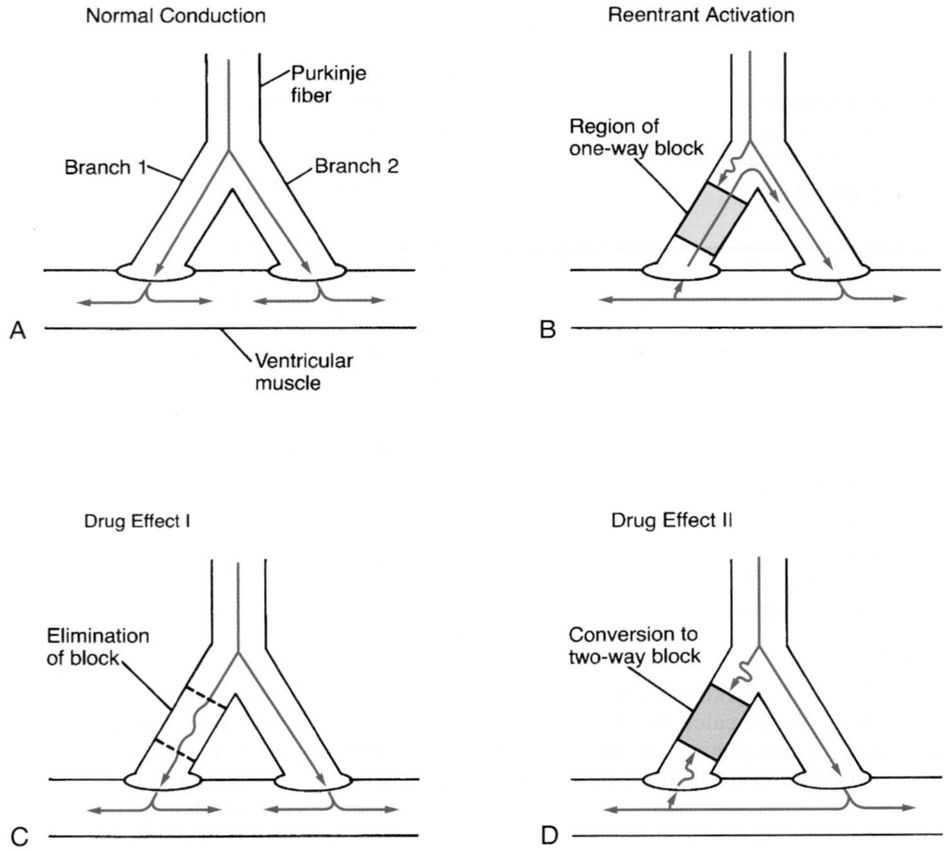

Figure 41.4 ▪ Reentrant activation: mechanism and drug effects.
A, In normal conduction, impulses from the branched Purkinje fiber stimulate the strip of ventricular muscle in two places. Within the muscle, waves of excitation spread from both points of excitation, meet between the Purkinje fibers, and cease further travel. **B,** In the presence of one-way block, the strip of muscle is excited at only one location. Impulses spreading from this area meet no impulses coming from the left and, therefore, can travel far enough to stimulate branch 1 of the Purkinje fiber. This stimulation passes back up the fiber, past the region of one-way block, and then stimulates branch 2, causing reentrant activation. **C,** Elimination of reentry by a drug that improves conduction in the sick branch of the Purkinje fiber. **D,** Elimination of reentry by a drug that further suppresses conduction in the sick branch, thereby converting one-way block into two-way block.

TABLE 41.1 ▪ Vaughan Williams Classification of Antidysrhythmic Drugs

CLASS I: SODIUM CHANNEL BLOCKERS
Class IA
Quinidine
Procainamide [Procan 🍁, generic in United States]
Disopyramide [Norpace, Rythmodan 🍁]
Class IB
Phenytoin [Dilantin]
Mexiletine [Mexitil]
Class IC
Flecainide [Tambocor]
Propafenone [Rythmol, Rythmol SR]
CLASS II: BETA BLOCKERS
Propranolol [Inderal, Inderal LA]
Acebutolol [Sectral]
CLASS III: POTASSIUM CHANNEL BLOCKERS (DRUGS THAT DELAY REPOLARIZATION)
Amiodarone [Cordarone, Pacerone]
Dronedarone [Multaq]
Sotalol [Betapace, Betapace AF]
Dofetilide [Tikosyn]
CLASS IV: CALCIUM CHANNEL BLOCKERS
Verapamil [Calan, Covera 🍁-HS, Verelan]
Diltiazem [Cardizem, Dilacor-XR, Tiazac, others]
OTHER ANTIDYSRHYTHMIC DRUGS
Digoxin [Lanoxin]

digoxin. Membership in classes I through IV is determined by effects on ion movements during slow and fast potentials (see Fig. 41.2).

Class I: Sodium Channel Blockers

Class I drugs block cardiac sodium channels (see Fig. 41.2A). By doing so, these drugs slow impulse conduction in the atria, ventricles, and His-Purkinje system. Class I constitutes the largest group of antidysrhythmic drugs.

Class II: Beta Blockers

Class II consists of beta-adrenergic blocking agents. As suggested by Fig. 41.2, these drugs reduce calcium entry (during fast and slow potentials) and depress phase 4 depolarization (in slow potentials only). Beta blockers have three prominent effects on the heart:

- In the SA node, they reduce automaticity.
- In the AV node, they slow conduction velocity.
- In the atria and ventricles, they reduce contractility.

Cardiac effects of the beta blockers are nearly identical to those of the calcium channel blockers.

Class III: Potassium Channel Blockers (Drugs That Delay Repolarization)

Class III drugs block potassium channels (Fig. 41.2A) and thereby delay repolarization of fast potentials. By delaying repolarization, these drugs prolong both the action potential duration and the effective refractory period.

Class IV: Calcium Channel Blockers

Only two calcium channel blockers—verapamil and diltiazem—are employed as antidysrhythmics. As indicated in Fig. 41.2, calcium channel blockade has the same effect on cardiac action potentials as does beta blockade. Accordingly, verapamil, diltiazem, and beta blockers have nearly identical effects on cardiac function—namely, reduction of automaticity in the SA node, delay of conduction through the AV node, and reduction of myocardial contractility. Antidysrhythmic benefits derive from suppressing AV nodal conduction.

Other Antidysrhythmic Drugs

Adenosine and digoxin do not fit into the four major classes of antidysrhythmic drugs. Both drugs suppress dysrhythmias by decreasing conduction through the AV node and reducing automaticity in the SA node.

Prodysrhythmic Effects of Antidysrhythmic Drugs

Virtually all of the drugs used to treat dysrhythmias have prodysrhythmic (proarrhythmic) effects. That is, *all of these drugs can worsen existing dysrhythmias and generate new ones.* This ability was documented dramatically in the Cardiac Arrhythmia Suppression Trial (CAST), in which use of class IC drugs (encainide and flecainide) to prevent dysrhythmias after myocardial infarction actually *doubled the rate of mortality.* Because of their prodysrhythmic actions, antidysrhythmic drugs should be used only when dysrhythmias are symptomatically significant, and only when the potential benefits clearly outweigh the risks. Applying this guideline, it would be inappropriate to give antidysrhythmic drugs to a patient with nonsustained ventricular tachycardia because this dysrhythmia does not significantly reduce cardiac output. Conversely, when a patient is facing death from ventricular fibrillation, any therapy that might work must be tried. In this case the risk for prodysrhythmic effects is clearly outweighed by the potential benefits of stopping the fibrillation.

Overview of Common Dysrhythmias and Their Treatment

The common dysrhythmias can be divided into two major groups: *supraventricular dysrhythmias* and *ventricular dysrhythmias.* In general, ventricular dysrhythmias are more dangerous than supraventricular dysrhythmias. With either type, intervention is required only if the dysrhythmia interferes with effective ventricular pumping. Treatment often proceeds in two phases: (1) *termination* of the dysrhythmia (with electrical countershock, drugs, or both), followed by (2) *long-term suppression* with drugs. Dysrhythmias can also be treated with an implantable cardioverter-defibrillator (ICD) or by destroying small areas of cardiac tissue using radiofrequency (RF) catheter ablation.

It is important to appreciate that drug therapy of dysrhythmias is highly empiric (i.e., based largely on the response of the patient and not on scientific principles). In practice, this means that, even after a dysrhythmia has been identified, we cannot predict with certainty just which drugs will be effective. Frequently, trials with several drugs are required before control of rhythm is achieved. In the discussion that follows, only first-choice drugs are considered.

Supraventricular Dysrhythmias

Supraventricular dysrhythmias are dysrhythmias that arise in areas of the heart above the ventricles (atria, SA node, AV node). Supraventricular dysrhythmias per se are not especially harmful because dysrhythmic activity within the atria does not significantly reduce cardiac output (except in patients with valvular disorders and heart failure [HF]). Supraventricular tachydysrhythmias *can* be dangerous, however, in that atrial impulses are likely to traverse the AV node, resulting in excitation of the ventricles. If the atria drive the ventricles at an excessive rate, diastolic filling will be incomplete and cardiac output will decline. Hence, when treating supraventricular tachydysrhythmias, the objective is frequently slowing of ventricular rate (by blocking impulse conduction through the AV node) and not elimination of the dysrhythmia itself. Of course, if treatment did abolish the dysrhythmia, this outcome would not be unwelcome. Acute treatment of supraventricular dysrhythmias is accomplished with vagotonic maneuvers, direct-current (DC) cardioversion, and certain drugs: class II agents, class IV agents, adenosine, and digoxin.

Atrial Fibrillation

Atrial fibrillation is the most common sustained dysrhythmia, affecting about 2.6 million people in the United States. The disorder is caused by multiple atrial ectopic foci firing randomly; each focus stimulates a small area of atrial muscle. This chaotic excitation produces a highly irregular atrial rhythm. Depending on the extent of impulse transmission through the AV node, ventricular rate may be very rapid or nearly normal.

In addition to compromising cardiac performance, atrial fibrillation carries a high risk for stroke because, in patients with atrial fibrillation, some blood can become trapped in the atria (rather than flowing straight through to the ventricles), thereby permitting formation of a clot. When normal sinus rhythm is restored, the clot may become dislodged and then may travel to the brain to cause stroke.

Treatment of atrial fibrillation has two goals: improvement of ventricular pumping and prevention of stroke. Pumping can be improved by either (1) restoring normal sinus rhythm or (2) slowing ventricular rate. The preferred method is to slow ventricular rate by *long-term* therapy with a beta blocker (atenolol or metoprolol) or a cardioselective calcium channel blocker (diltiazem or verapamil), both of which impede conduction through the AV node. For patients who elect to restore normal rhythm, options are DC cardioversion, short-term treatment with drugs (e.g., amiodarone, sotalol), or RF ablation of the dysrhythmia source.

To prevent stroke, patients are treated with warfarin or newer anticoagulants. For those undergoing treatment to restore normal sinus rhythm, warfarin should be taken for 3 weeks before the procedure and for 4 weeks after. For those taking an antidysrhythmic drug long term to control ventricular rate, warfarin must be taken long term too. Alternatives to warfarin include three new oral anticoagulants—apixiban [Eliquis], dabigatran [Pradaxa], and rivaroxaban [Xarelto]—and antiplatelet drugs (either aspirin alone or aspirin plus clopidogrel).

Atrial Flutter

Atrial flutter is caused by an ectopic atrial focus discharging at a rate of 250 to 350 times a minute. Ventricular rate is considerably slower, however, because the AV node is unable to transmit impulses at this high rate. Typically, one atrial impulse out of two reaches the ventricles. The treatment of choice is DC cardioversion, which almost always converts atrial flutter to normal sinus rhythm. Cardioversion may also be achieved with intravenous (IV) ibutilide. To prevent the dysrhythmia from recurring, patients may need long-term therapy with drugs—either a class IC agent (flecainide or propafenone) or a class III agent (amiodarone, dronedarone, sotalol, dofetilide).

There are two alternatives to cardioversion: (1) RF ablation of the dysrhythmia focus and (2) control of ventricular rate with drugs. As with atrial fibrillation, ventricular rate is controlled with drugs that suppress AV conduction: verapamil, diltiazem, or a beta blocker.

Like atrial fibrillation, atrial flutter poses a risk for stroke, which can be reduced by treatment with anticoagulants.

Sustained Supraventricular Tachycardia (SVT)

This is usually caused by an AV nodal reentrant circuit. Heart rate is increased to 150 to 250 beats/minute. SVT often responds to interventions that increase vagal tone, such as carotid sinus massage or the Valsalva maneuver. If these are ineffective, an IV beta blocker or calcium channel blocker can be tried. With these drugs, ventricular rate will be slowed even if the dysrhythmia persists. When the dysrhythmia has been controlled, beta blockers and/or calcium channel blockers can be taken orally to prevent recurrence. As a last resort, amiodarone can be used for prevention.

Ventricular Dysrhythmias

In contrast to atrial dysrhythmias, which are generally benign, ventricular dysrhythmias can cause significant disruption of cardiac pumping. Accordingly, the usual objective is to abolish the dysrhythmia. Cardioversion is often the treatment of choice. When antidysrhythmic drugs are indicated, agents in class I or class III are usually employed.

SVT

Ventricular tachycardia arises from a single, rapidly firing ventricular ectopic focus, typically located at the border of an old infarction. The focus drives the ventricles at a rate of 150 to 250 beats/minute. Because the ventricles cannot pump effectively at these rates, immediate intervention is required. Cardioversion is the treatment of choice. If cardioversion fails to normalize rhythm, IV amiodarone should be administered; lidocaine and procainamide are alternatives. For long-term management, drugs (e.g., sotalol, amiodarone) or an ICD may be employed.

Ventricular Fibrillation

Ventricular fibrillation is a life-threatening emergency that requires immediate treatment. This dysrhythmia results from the asynchronous discharge of multiple ventricular ectopic foci. Because many different foci are firing, and because each focus initiates contraction in its immediate vicinity, localized twitching takes place all over the ventricles, making coordinated ventricular contraction impossible. As a result, the pumping action of the heart stops. In the absence of blood flow, the patient becomes unconscious and cyanotic. If heartbeat is not restored rapidly, death soon follows. Electrical countershock (defibrillation) is applied to eliminate fibrillation and restore cardiac function. If necessary, IV lidocaine can be used to enhance the effects of defibrillation. Procainamide may also be helpful. Amiodarone can be used for long-term suppression. As an alternative, an ICD may be employed.

Premature Ventricular Complex (PVC)

PVCs are beats that occur before they should in the cardiac cycle. These beats are caused by ectopic ventricular foci. PVCs may arise from a single ectopic focus or from several foci. In the absence of additional signs of heart disease, PVCs are benign and not usually treated. However, in the presence of acute myocardial infarction, PVCs may predispose the patient to ventricular fibrillation. In this case therapy is required. A beta blocker is the agent of choice.

Digoxin-Induced Ventricular Dysrhythmias

Digoxin toxicity can mimic practically all types of dysrhythmias. Varying degrees of AV block are among the most common. Ventricular flutter and ventricular fibrillation are the most dangerous. Digoxin causes dysrhythmias by increasing automaticity in the atria, ventricles, and His-Purkinje system, and by decreasing conduction through the AV node.

With proper treatment, digoxin-induced dysrhythmias can almost always be controlled. Treatment is discussed in Chapter 40. If antidysrhythmic drugs are required, lidocaine and phenytoin are the agents of choice. In patients with digoxin toxicity, DC cardioversion may bring on ventricular fibrillation. Accordingly, this procedure should be used only when absolutely required.

Torsades de Pointes

Torsades de pointes is an atypical, rapid, undulating ventricular tachydysrhythmia that can evolve into potentially fatal ventricular fibrillation. The main factor associated with development of torsades de pointes is prolongation of the QT interval, which can be caused by a variety of drugs, including class IA and class III antidysrhythmic agents. Acute management consists of IV magnesium plus cardioversion for sustained ventricular tachycardia.

Principles of Antidysrhythmic Drug Therapy

Balancing Risks and Benefits

Therapy with antidysrhythmic drugs is based on a simple but important concept: treat only if there is a clear benefit—and then only if the benefit outweighs the risks. As a rule, this means that intervention is needed only when the dysrhythmia interferes with ventricular pumping.

Treatment offers two potential benefits: reduction of symptoms and reduction of mortality. Symptoms that can be reduced include palpitations, angina, dyspnea, and faintness. For most antidysrhythmic drugs, there is little or no evidence of reduced mortality. In fact, mortality may actually increase.

Antidysrhythmic therapy carries considerable risk. Because of their *prodysrhythmic actions,* antidysrhythmic drugs can exacerbate existing dysrhythmias and generate new ones. Examples abound: toxic doses of digoxin can generate a wide variety of dysrhythmias; drugs that prolong the QT interval can cause torsades de pointes; many drugs can cause ventricular ectopic beats; several drugs (quinidine, flecainide, propafenone) can cause atrial flutter; and one drug—flecainide—can produce incessant ventricular tachycardia. Because of their prodysrhythmic actions, antidysrhythmic drugs can *increase mortality.* Other adverse effects include HF and third-degree AV block (caused by calcium channel blockers and beta blockers), as well as many noncardiac effects, including severe diarrhea (quinidine), a lupus-like syndrome (procainamide), and pulmonary toxicity (amiodarone).

Properties of the Dysrhythmia to Be Considered

Sustained Versus Nonsustained Dysrhythmias

As a rule, nonsustained dysrhythmias require intervention only when they are symptomatic; in the absence of symptoms, treatment is usually unnecessary. In contrast, sustained dysrhythmias can be dangerous, so the benefits of treatment generally outweigh the risks.

Asymptomatic Versus Symptomatic Dysrhythmias

No study has demonstrated a benefit to treating dysrhythmias that are asymptomatic or minimally symptomatic. In contrast, therapy may be beneficial for dysrhythmias that produce symptoms (palpitations, angina, dyspnea, faintness).

Supraventricular Versus Ventricular Dysrhythmias

Supraventricular dysrhythmias are generally benign. The primary harm comes from driving the ventricles too rapidly to allow adequate filling. The goal of treatment is to either (1) terminate the dysrhythmia or (2) prevent excessive atrial beats from reaching the ventricles (using a beta blocker, calcium channel blocker, or digoxin). In contrast to supraventricular dysrhythmias, ventricular dysrhythmias frequently interfere with pumping. Accordingly, the goal of treatment is to terminate the dysrhythmia and prevent its recurrence.

Phases of Treatment

Treatment has two phases: acute and long term. The goal of acute treatment is to terminate the dysrhythmia. For many dysrhythmias, termination is accomplished with DC cardioversion (electrical countershock) or vagotonic maneuvers (e.g., carotid sinus massage), rather than drugs. The goal of long-term therapy is to prevent dysrhythmias from recurring. Quite often, the risks for long-term prophylactic therapy outweigh the benefits.

Long-Term Treatment: Drug Selection and Evaluation

Selecting a drug for long-term therapy is largely empiric. There are many drugs that might be employed, and we usually can't predict which one is going to work. Therefore finding an effective drug is done by trial and error.

Drug selection can be aided with electrophysiologic testing. In these tests, a dysrhythmia is generated artificially by programmed electrical stimulation of the heart. If a candidate drug is able to suppress the electrophysiologically induced dysrhythmia, it may also work against the real thing.

Holter monitoring can be used to evaluate treatment. A Holter monitor is a portable ECG device that is worn by the patient around-the-clock. If Holter monitoring indicates that dysrhythmias are still occurring with the present drug, a different drug should be tried.

Minimizing Risks

Several measures can help minimize risk, including the following:

- Starting with low doses and increasing them gradually
- Using a Holter monitor during initial therapy to detect danger signs—especially QT prolongation, which can precede torsades de pointes
- Monitoring plasma drug levels. Unfortunately, although drug levels can be good predictors of noncardiac toxicity (e.g., quinidine-induced nausea), they are less helpful for predicting adverse cardiac effects

PHARMACOLOGY OF THE ANTIDYSRHYTHMIC DRUGS

As discussed earlier, the antidysrhythmic drugs fall into four main groups—classes I, II, III, and IV—plus a fifth group that includes adenosine and digoxin. The pharmacology of these drugs is presented next and in Table 41.2.

Class I: Sodium Channel Blockers

Class I antidysrhythmic drugs block cardiac sodium channels. By doing so, they decrease conduction velocity in the atria, ventricles, and His-Purkinje system.

There are three subgroups of class I agents. Drugs in all three groups block sodium channels. In addition, class IA agents delay repolarization, whereas class IB agents accelerate repolarization. Class IC agents have pronounced prodysrhythmic actions.

The class I drugs are similar in action and structure to the local anesthetics. In fact, one of these drugs—lidocaine—has both local anesthetic and antidysrhythmic applications. Because of their relationship to the local anesthetics, class I agents are sometimes referred to as *local anesthetic antidysrhythmic agents.*

Class IA Agents

Quinidine

Quinidine is the oldest, best studied, and most widely used class IA drug. Accordingly, quinidine will serve as our prototype for the group. Like other antidysrhythmic agents, quinidine has prodysrhythmic actions.

Chemistry and Source. Quinidine is similar to quinine in structure and actions. The natural source of both drugs is the bark of the South American cinchona tree. Accordingly, these agents are referred to as *cinchona alkaloids.* Like quinine, quinidine has antimalarial and antipyretic properties.

Effects on the Heart. By blocking sodium channels, quinidine *slows impulse conduction* in the atria, ventricles, and His-Purkinje system. In addition, the drug

TABLE 41.2 ▪ Properties of Antidysrhythmic Drugs

Drug	Usual Route	Effects on the ECG	Major Antidysrhythmic Applications
CLASS IA			
Quinidine	PO	Widens QRS, prolongs QT	Broad spectrum: used for long-term suppression of ventricular and supraventricular dysrhythmias
Procainamide	PO	Widens QRS, prolongs QT	Broad spectrum: similar to quinidine, but toxicity makes it less desirable for long-term use
Disopyramide	PO	Widens QRS, prolongs QT	Ventricular dysrhythmias
CLASS IB			
Phenytoin	PO	No significant change	Digoxin-induced ventricular dysrhythmias
Mexiletine	PO	No significant change	Ventricular dysrhythmias
CLASS IC			
Flecainide	PO	Widens QRS, prolongs PR	Maintenance therapy of supraventricular dysrhythmias
Propafenone	PO	Widens QRS, prolongs PR	Maintenance therapy of supraventricular dysrhythmias
CLASS II			
Propranolol	PO	Prolongs PR, bradycardia	Dysrhythmias caused by excessive sympathetic activity; control of ventricular rate in patients with supraventricular tachydysrhythmias
Acebutolol	PO	Prolongs PR, bradycardia	Premature ventricular beats
CLASS III			
Amiodarone	PO, IV	Prolongs QT and PR, widens QRS	Life-threatening ventricular dysrhythmias, atrial fibrillation*
Dronedarone	PO	Prolongs QT and PR, widens QRS	Atrial flutter, atrial fibrillation
Sotalol	PO, IV	Prolongs QT and PR, bradycardia	Life-threatening ventricular dysrhythmias, atrial fibrillation/flutter
Dofetilide	PO	Prolongs QT	Highly symptomatic atrial dysrhythmias
CLASS IV			
Verapamil	PO	Prolongs PR, bradycardia	Control of ventricular rate in patients with supraventricular tachydysrhythmias
OTHERS			
Digoxin	PO, IV	Prolongs PR, depresses ST	Control of ventricular rate in patients with supraventricular tachydysrhythmias

*Amiodarone is widely used for atrial fibrillation, but it is not approved for this use.

Prototype Drugs

ANTIDYSRHYTHMIC DRUGS

Class I: Sodium Channel Blockers

Quinidine (class IA)
Lidocaine (class IB)

Class II: Beta Blocker

Propranolol

Class III: Drug That Delays Repolarization

Amiodarone

Class IV: Calcium Channel Blockers

Verapamil

Others

Digoxin

delays repolarization at these sites, apparently by blocking potassium channels. Both actions contribute to suppression of dysrhythmias.

Quinidine is strongly *anticholinergic* (atropine-like) and blocks vagal input to the heart. The resultant *increase* in SA nodal automaticity and AV conduction can drive the ventricles at an excessive rate. To prevent excessive ventricular stimulation, patients are usually pretreated with digoxin, verapamil, or a beta blocker, all of which suppress AV conduction.

Effects on the ECG. Quinidine has two pronounced effects on the ECG. The drug *widens the QRS complex* (by slowing depolarization of the ventricles) and *prolongs the QT interval* (by delaying ventricular repolarization).

Therapeutic Uses. Quinidine is a broad-spectrum agent active against *supraventricular* and *ventricular dysrhythmias.* The drug's principal indication is long-term suppression of dysrhythmias, including SVT, atrial flutter, atrial fibrillation, and sustained ventricular tachycardia. To prevent quinidine from increasing ventricular rate, patients are usually pretreated with an AV nodal blocking agent (digoxin, verapamil, beta blocker).

BLACK BOX WARNING: QUINIDINE

An analysis of older studies indicates that quinidine may actually *increase* mortality in patients with *atrial flutter* and *atrial fibrillation.*

In addition to its antidysrhythmic applications, quinidine is a drug of choice for severe *malaria* (see Chapter 81).

Pharmacokinetics. Quinidine is rapidly absorbed after oral dosing. Peak responses to quinidine sulfate develop in 30 to 90 minutes; responses to quinidine gluconate develop more slowly, peaking after 3 to 4 hours. Elimination is by hepatic metabolism. Accordingly, patients with liver impairment may require a reduction in dosage. Therapeutic plasma levels are 2 to 5 mcg/mL.

Adverse Effects

DIARRHEA. Diarrhea and other gastrointestinal (GI) symptoms develop in about 33% of patients. These reactions can be immediate and intense, frequently forcing discontinuation of treatment. Gastric upset can be reduced by administering quinidine with food.

CINCHONISM. Cinchonism is characterized by tinnitus (ringing in the ears), headache, nausea, vertigo, and disturbed vision. These can develop with just one dose.

CARDIOTOXICITY. At high concentrations, quinidine can cause severe cardiotoxicity (sinus arrest, AV block, ventricular tachydysrhythmias, asystole). These reactions occur secondary to increased automaticity of Purkinje fibers and reduced conduction throughout all regions of the heart.

As cardiotoxicity develops, the ECG changes. Important danger signals are *widening of the QRS complex* (by 50% or more) and *excessive prolongation of the QT interval.* Notify the prescriber immediately if these changes occur.

ARTERIAL EMBOLISM. Embolism is a potential complication of treating atrial *fibrillation.* During atrial fibrillation, thrombi may form in the atria. When sinus rhythm is restored, these thrombi may be dislodged and cause embolism. To reduce the risk for embolism, anticoagulant therapy is given for 3 to 4 weeks before quinidine and is maintained for an additional 4 weeks. Signs of embolism (e.g., sudden chest pain, dyspnea) should be reported immediately.

OTHER ADVERSE EFFECTS. Quinidine can cause alpha-adrenergic blockade, resulting in vasodilation and subsequent *hypotension.* This reaction is much more serious with IV therapy than with oral therapy. Rarely, quinidine has caused *hypersensitivity reactions,* including fever, anaphylactic reactions, and thrombocytopenia.

Drug Interactions

DIGOXIN. Quinidine can double digoxin levels. The increase is caused by displacing digoxin from plasma albumin and by decreasing digoxin elimination. When these drugs are used concurrently, digoxin dosage must be reduced. Also, patients should be monitored closely for digoxin toxicity (dysrhythmias). Because of its interaction with digoxin, quinidine is a last-choice drug for treating digoxin-induced dysrhythmias.

Other Interactions. Because of its anticholinergic actions, quinidine can intensify the effects of other atropine-like drugs; one possible result is excessive tachycardia. Phenobarbital, phenytoin, and other drugs that induce hepatic drug metabolism can shorten the half-life of quinidine by as much as 50%. Quinidine can intensify the effects of warfarin by an unknown mechanism.

Preparations, Dosage, and Administration.

Preparations. Quinidine is available as two salts: quinidine sulfate and quinidine gluconate. Because these salts have different molecular weights, equal doses (on a milligram basis) do not provide equal amounts of quinidine. A 200-mg dose of quinidine sulfate is equivalent to 275 mg of quinidine gluconate. Quinidine sulfate is available in immediate-release tablets (200 and 300 mg) and sustained-release tablets (300 mg). Quinidine gluconate is available in sustained-release tablets (324 mg) and in solution (80 mg/mL) for parenteral use.

Dosage. The usual dosage of quinidine sulfate is 200 to 300 mg every 6 hours. The usual dosage of quinidine gluconate is 324 to 648 mg every 8 to 12 hours. Dosage is adjusted to produce plasma quinidine levels between 2 and 5 mcg/mL.

Procainamide

Procainamide [Procan ♣] is similar to quinidine in actions and uses. Like quinidine, procainamide is active against a broad spectrum of dysrhythmias. Unfortunately, serious side effects frequently limit its use.

Effects on the Heart and ECG. Like quinidine, procainamide blocks cardiac sodium channels, thereby decreasing conduction velocity in the atria, ventricles, and His-Purkinje system. Also, the drug delays repolarization. In contrast to quinidine, procainamide is only weakly anticholinergic and hence is not likely to increase ventricular rate. Effects on the ECG are the same as with quinidine: widening of the QRS complex and prolongation of the QT interval.

Therapeutic Uses. Procainamide is effective against a broad spectrum of atrial and ventricular dysrhythmias. Like quinidine, the drug can be used for long-term suppression. However, because prolonged therapy is often associated with serious adverse effects, procainamide is less desirable than quinidine for long-term use. In contrast to quinidine, procainamide can be used to terminate ventricular tachycardia and ventricular fibrillation.

Pharmacokinetics. Routes are oral, IV, and intramuscular. Peak plasma levels develop 1 hour after oral dosing. Procainamide has a short half-life and requires more frequent dosing than quinidine.

Elimination is by hepatic metabolism and renal excretion. The major metabolite—N-acetylprocainamide (NAPA)—has antidysrhythmic properties of its own. NAPA is excreted by the kidneys and can accumulate to toxic levels in patients with renal impairment.

Adverse Effects

Systemic Lupus Erythematosus–Like Syndrome. Prolonged treatment with procainamide is associated with severe immunologic reactions. Within a year, about 70% of patients develop antinuclear antibodies (ANAs)—antibodies directed against the patient's own nucleic acids. If procainamide is continued, between 20% and 30% of patients with ANAs go on to develop symptoms resembling those of systemic lupus erythematosus (SLE). These symptoms include pain and inflammation of the joints, pericarditis, fever, and hepatomegaly. When procainamide is withdrawn, symptoms usually slowly subside. If the patient has a life-threatening dysrhythmia for which no alternative drug is available, procainamide can be continued and the symptoms of SLE controlled with a nonsteroidal antiinflammatory drug (e.g., aspirin) or a glucocorticoid. All patients taking procainamide chronically should be tested for ANAs. If the ANA titer rises, discontinuing treatment should be considered.

BLACK BOX WARNING: BLOOD DYSCRASIAS

About 0.5% of patients develop blood dyscrasias, including neutropenia, thrombocytopenia, and agranulocytosis. Fatalities have occurred. These reactions usually develop during the first 12 weeks of treatment. Complete blood counts should be obtained weekly during this time and periodically thereafter. Also, complete blood counts should be obtained promptly at the first sign of infection, bruising, or bleeding. If blood counts indicate bone marrow suppression, procainamide should be withdrawn. Hematologic status usually returns to baseline within 1 month.

Cardiotoxicity. Procainamide has cardiotoxic actions like those of quinidine. Warning signs are QRS widening (more than 50%) and excessive QT prolongation. If these develop, the drug should be withheld and the prescriber informed.

Other Adverse Effects. Like quinidine, procainamide can cause GI symptoms and hypotension. However, these are much less prominent than with quinidine. Procainamide is a derivative of procaine (a local anesthetic); therefore its use is contraindicated in patients with a history of procaine allergy. As with quinidine, arterial embolism may occur during treatment of atrial fibrillation.

Preparations, Dosage, and Administration. Procainamide is available orally in Canada only. It is supplied in capsules (250, 375, and 500 mg) and sustained-release tablets (500, 750, and 1000 mg). The usual maintenance dosage is 50 mg/kg/day in divided doses. The capsules are administered every 3 to 4 hours and the sustained-release tablets every 6 hours. Dosage is adjusted to maintain plasma drug levels between 3 and 10 mcg/mL.

Disopyramide

Disopyramide [Norpace, Rythmodan 🍁] is a class I drug with actions like those of quinidine. However, because of prominent side effects, indications for disopyramide are limited.

Effects on the Heart and ECG. Cardiac effects are similar to those of quinidine. By blocking sodium channels, disopyramide decreases conduction velocity in the atria, ventricles, and His-Purkinje system. In addition, the drug delays repolarization. Anticholinergic actions are greater than those of quinidine. In contrast to quinidine, disopyramide causes a pronounced reduction in contractility. Like quinidine, disopyramide widens the QRS complex and prolongs the QT interval.

Adverse Effects. Anticholinergic responses are most common. These include dry mouth, blurred vision, constipation, and urinary hesitancy or retention. Urinary retention frequently requires discontinuation of treatment.

Because of its negative inotropic effects, disopyramide can cause severe hypotension (secondary to reduced cardiac output) and can exacerbate heart failure. The drug should not be administered to patients with HF or to patients taking a beta blocker. Whenever disopyramide is used, pressor drugs should be immediately available.

Therapeutic Uses. Disopyramide is indicated only for ventricular dysrhythmias (PVCs, ventricular tachycardia, ventricular fibrillation). The drug is reserved for patients who cannot tolerate safer medications (e.g., quinidine, procainamide).

BLACK BOX WARNING: DISOPYRAMIDE

There is increased risk for mortality when using disopyramide to treat non–life-threatening arrhythmias.

Preparations, Dosage, and Administration. Disopyramide [Norpace, Rythmodan 🍁] is available in immediate- and extended-release capsules (100 and 150 mg). An initial loading dose (200–300 mg) is followed by maintenance doses (100–200 mg) every 6 hours.

Class IB Agents

As a group, class IB agents differ from quinidine and the other class IA agents in two respects: (1) whereas class IA agents *delay* repolarization, class IB agents *accelerate* repolarization; and (2) class IB agents have little or no effect on the ECG.

Mexiletine

Mexiletine is an oral analog of lidocaine used for symptomatic ventricular dysrhythmias. Principal indications are PVCs and sustained ventricular tachycardia. Like lidocaine, mexiletine does not alter the ECG. The drug is eliminated by hepatic metabolism, so effects may be prolonged in patients with liver disease or reduced hepatic blood flow. The most common adverse effects are GI (nausea, vomiting, diarrhea, constipation) and neurologic (tremor, dizziness, sleep disturbances, psychosis, convulsions). About 40% of patients find these intolerable. Like other class I agents, mexiletine has prodysrhythmic properties. The dosage is 200 mg every 8 hours. All doses should be taken with food.

BLACK BOX WARNING: MEXILETINE

Mexiletine has been associated with increased risk for mortality when used to treat non–life-threatening arrhythmias.

Class IC Agents

Class IC antidysrhythmics block cardiac sodium channels and thereby reduce conduction velocity in the atria, ventricles, and His-Purkinje system. In addition, these drugs delay ventricular repolarization, causing a small increase in the effective refractory period. All class IC agents can exacerbate existing dysrhythmias and create new ones. Currently, only two class IC agents are available: flecainide and propafenone.

Flecainide

Flecainide [Tambocor] is active against a variety of ventricular and supraventricular dysrhythmias. However, use is restricted largely to maintenance therapy of supraventricular dysrhythmias. Like other class IC agents, flecainide decreases cardiac conduction and increases the effective refractory period. Prominent effects on the ECG are prolongation of the PR interval and widening of the QRS complex. Excessive QRS widening indicates a need for dosage reduction. Flecainide has prodysrhythmic effects. As a result, the drug can intensify existing dysrhythmias and provoke new ones. In patients with asymptomatic ventricular tachycardia associated with acute myocardial infarction, flecainide has caused a twofold increase in mortality. Flecainide decreases myocardial contractility and can thereby exacerbate or precipitate HF. Accordingly, the drug should not be combined with other agents that can decrease contractile force (e.g., beta blockers, verapamil, diltiazem). Elimination is by hepatic metabolism and renal excretion. Flecainide is available in tablets (50, 100, and 150 mg) for oral dosing. Dosage is low initially (50–100 mg every 12 hours) and then gradually increased to a maximum of 400 mg/day.

BLACK BOX WARNING: FLECAINIDE

Because of its potential for serious side effects, flecainide should be reserved for severe ventricular dysrhythmias that have not responded to safer drugs. Patients should be monitored closely.

Propafenone

Propafenone [Rythmol, Rythmol SR] is similar to flecainide in actions and uses. By blocking cardiac sodium channels, the drug decreases conduction velocity in the atria, ventricles, and His-Purkinje system. In addition, it causes a small increase in the ventricular ERP. Prominent effects on the ECG are QRS widening and PR prolongation. Like flecainide, propafenone has prodysrhythmic actions that can exacerbate existing dysrhythmias and create new ones. It is not known whether propafenone, like flecainide, increases mortality in patients with asymptomatic ventricular dysrhythmias after myocardial infarction. Propafenone has beta-adrenergic blocking properties and can thereby decrease myocardial contractility and promote bronchospasm. Accordingly, the drug should be used with caution in patients with HF, AV block, or asthma. Noncardiac adverse effects are generally mild and include dizziness, altered taste, blurred vision, and GI symptoms (abdominal discomfort, anorexia, nausea, vomiting). Propafenone is available in immediate-release tablets (150 and 225 mg) and extended-release capsules (225, 325, and 425 mg). For the immediate-release tablets, the dosage is 150 mg every 8 hours initially, and can be gradually increased to 300 mg every 8 hours. For the extended-release capsules, the dosage is 225 mg every 12 hours initially, and can be gradually increased to 425 mg every 12 hours.

BLACK BOX WARNING: PROPAFENONE

Because of its prodysrhythmic actions, propafenone should be reserved for patients who have not responded to safer drugs.

Class II: Beta Blockers

Class II consists of beta-adrenergic blocking agents. At this time only four beta blockers—propranolol, acebutolol, esmolol, and sotalol—are approved for treating dysrhythmias. One of these drugs—sotalol—also blocks potassium channels, and is discussed under class III. The basic pharmacology of the beta blockers is presented in Chapter 14. Discussion here is limited to their antidysrhythmic use.

Propranolol

Propranolol [Inderal LA] is considered a nonselective beta-adrenergic antagonist, in that it blocks both $beta_1$- and $beta_2$-adrenergic receptors. $Beta_1$ blockade affects the heart, and $beta_2$ blockade affects the bronchi.

Effects on the Heart and ECG

Blockade of cardiac $beta_1$ receptors attenuates sympathetic stimulation of the heart. The result is (1) decreased automaticity of the SA node, (2) decreased velocity of conduction through the AV node, and (3) decreased myocardial contractility. The reduction in AV conduction velocity translates to a prolonged PR interval on the ECG.

It is worth noting that cardiac $beta_1$ receptors are functionally coupled to calcium channels and that $beta_1$ blockade causes these channels to close. Therefore the effects of beta blockers on heart rate, AV conduction, and contractility all result from decreased calcium influx. Because beta blockers and calcium channel blockers both decrease calcium entry, the cardiac effects of these drugs are very similar.

Therapeutic Use

Propranolol is especially useful for treating dysrhythmias caused by excessive sympathetic stimulation of the heart. Among these are sinus tachycardia, severe recurrent ventricular tachycardia, exercise-induced tachydysrhythmias, and paroxysmal atrial tachycardia evoked by emotion or exercise. In patients with supraventricular tachydysrhythmias, propranolol has two beneficial effects: (1) suppression of excessive discharge of the SA node and (2) slowing of ventricular rate by decreasing transmission of atrial impulses through the AV node.

Adverse Effects

Beta blockers are generally well tolerated. Principal adverse effects concern the heart and bronchi. By blocking cardiac $beta_1$ receptors, propranolol can cause *heart failure, AV block,* and *sinus arrest. Hypotension* can occur secondary to reduced cardiac output. In patients with asthma, blocking $beta_2$ receptors in the lung can cause *bronchospasm.* Because of its cardiac and pulmonary effects, propranolol should be used cautiously in patients with asthma and is contraindicated in patients with sinus bradycardia, high-degree heart block, and HF.

Dosage and Administration

Propranolol can be administered orally and, in life-threatening emergencies, by IV injection. Dosages with either route show wide individual variation. Oral dosages range from 10 to 30 mg every 6 to 8 hours. The usual IV dose is 1 to 3 mg injected at a rate of 1 mg/minute.

Acebutolol

Acebutolol [Sectral] is a cardioselective beta blocker approved for oral therapy of PVCs. Adverse effects are like those of propranolol: bradycardia, HF, AV block, and—despite cardioselectivity—bronchospasm. Accordingly, acebutolol should be used cautiously in patients with asthma and is contraindicated in patients with HF, severe bradycardia, and AV block. Acebutolol can also cause adverse immunologic reactions; titers of ANAs may rise, resulting in myalgia, arthralgia, and arthritis. For suppression of PVCs, the initial dosage is 200 mg twice daily. Usual maintenance dosages range from 600 to 1200 mg/day.

Class III: Potassium Channel Blockers

Five class III antidysrhythmics are available: amiodarone, dronedarone, dofetilide, ibutilide, and sotalol (which is also a beta blocker). All five delay repolarization of fast potentials. Hence, all five prolong the action potential duration and ERP. By doing so, they prolong the QT interval. In addition, each drug can affect the heart in other ways, and so they are not interchangeable. Four of the drugs are discussed below. Ibutilide is availiable intravenously only, and is therefore discussed in Chapter 89.

Amiodarone

Amiodarone [Cordarone, Pacerone] is a class III antidysrhythmic agent that has complex effects on the heart. The drug is highly effective against both atrial and ventricular dysrhythmias. Unfortunately, serious toxicities (e.g., lung damage, visual impairment) are common and may persist for months after treatment has stopped. Because of toxicity, amiodarone is *approved* only for life-threatening ventricular dysrhythmias that have been refractory to safer agents. Nonetheless, because of its efficacy, amiodarone is one of our most frequently prescribed antidysrhythmic drugs, used for atrial and ventricular dysrhythmias alike.

Amiodarone is available for oral and IV use. Indications, electrophysiologic effects, time course of action, and adverse effects differ for each route. Accordingly, oral and IV therapy are discussed separately.

BLACK BOX WARNING: PULMONARY TOXICITY

Lung damage—hypersensitivity pneumonitis, interstitial/alveolar pneumonitis, pulmonary fibrosis—is the greatest concern. Symptoms (dyspnea, cough, chest pain) resemble those of HF and pneumonia. Pulmonary toxicity develops in 2% to 17% of patients and carries a 10% risk for mortality. Patients at highest risk are those receiving long-term, high-dose therapy. A baseline chest radiograph and pulmonary function test are recommended. Pulmonary function should be monitored throughout treatment. If lung injury develops, amiodarone should be withdrawn.

Oral Therapy

Therapeutic Use. Although amiodarone is very effective, concerns about toxicity limit its indications. In the United States oral amiodarone is *approved* only for long-term therapy of two life-threatening ventricular dysrhythmias: *recurrent ventricular fibrillation* and *recurrent hemodynamically unstable ventricular tachycardia.* Treatment should be reserved for patients who have not responded to safer drugs.

Amiodarone is our most effective drug for *atrial fibrillation* and is prescribed widely to treat this dysrhythmia—even though it is not approved for this use. The drug is given to convert atrial fibrillation to normal sinus rhythm and to maintain normal sinus rhythm after conversion.

Effects on the Heart and ECG. Amiodarone has complex effects on the heart. Like all other drugs in this class, amiodarone delays repolarization and thereby prolongs the action potential duration and ERP. The underlying cause of these effects may be blockade of potassium channels. Additional cardiac effects include reduced automaticity in the SA node, reduced contractility, and reduced conduction velocity in the AV node, ventricles, and His-Purkinje system. These occur secondary to blockade of sodium channels, calcium channels, and beta receptors. Prominent effects on the ECG are QRS widening and prolongation of the PR and QT intervals. Amiodarone also acts on coronary and peripheral blood vessels to promote dilation.

Pharmacokinetics. Amiodarone is highly lipid soluble and accumulates in many tissues, especially the liver and lungs. The drug is metabolized in the liver by CYP3A4 (the 3A4 isoenzyme of cytochrome P450) and then excreted in the bile. Amiodarone has an extremely long half-life, ranging from 25 to 110 days. Because of its slow elimination, amiodarone continues to act long after dosing has ceased.

Adverse Effects. Amiodarone produces many serious adverse effects. Furthermore, because the drug's half-life is protracted, toxicity can continue for weeks or months after drug withdrawal. To reduce adverse events, the U.S. Food and Drug Administration (FDA) requires that all patients using amiodarone be given a Medication Guide describing potential toxicities.

CARDIOTOXICITY. Amiodarone may cause a paradoxical increase in dysrhythmic activity. In addition, by suppressing the SA and AV nodes, the drug can cause sinus bradycardia and AV block. By reducing contractility, amiodarone can precipitate HF.

THYROID TOXICITY. Amiodarone may cause hypothyroidism or hyperthyroidism. Accordingly, thyroid function should be assessed at baseline and periodically during treatment. Hypothyroidism can be treated with thyroid hormone supplements. Hyperthyroidism can be treated with an antithyroid drug (e.g., methimazole) or thyroidectomy. Discontinuing amiodarone should be considered.

BLACK BOX WARNING: LIVER TOXICITY

Amiodarone can injure the liver. Accordingly, tests of liver function should be obtained at baseline and periodically throughout treatment. If circulating liver enzymes exceed 3 times the normal level, amiodarone should be discontinued. Signs and symptoms of liver injury, which are seen only rarely, include anorexia, nausea, vomiting, malaise, fatigue, itching, jaundice, and dark urine.

OPHTHALMIC EFFECTS. Rarely, amiodarone has been associated with optic neuropathy and optic neuritis, sometimes progressing to blindness. However, a causal relationship has not been established. Patients who develop changes in visual acuity or peripheral vision should undergo ophthalmologic evaluation. If optic neuropathy or neuritis is diagnosed, discontinuation of amiodarone should be considered.

Virtually all patients develop corneal microdeposits. Fortunately, these deposits have little or no effect on vision and so rarely necessitate amiodarone cessation.

TOXICITY IN PREGNANCY AND BREASTFEEDING. Amiodarone crosses the placental barrier and enters breast milk and can thereby harm the developing fetus and breastfeeding infant. Accordingly, pregnancy and breastfeeding should be avoided while using the drug and for several months after stopping it.

DERMATOLOGIC TOXICITY. Patients frequently experience *photosensitivity reactions* (skin reactions triggered by exposure to ultraviolet radiation). To reduce risk, patients should avoid sunlamps and should wear sunblock and protective clothing when outdoors. With frequent and prolonged sun exposure, exposed skin may turn *bluish gray.* Fortunately, this discoloration resolves within months after amiodarone is discontinued.

Other Adverse Effects. Possible *CNS reactions* include ataxia, dizziness, tremor, mood alteration, and hallucinations. *GI reactions* (anorexia, nausea, vomiting) are common.

Drug Interactions. Amiodarone is subject to significant interactions with many drugs. The result can be toxicity or reduced therapeutic effects. Accordingly, combined use with these drugs should be avoided. When it cannot, the patient should be monitored closely. Interactions of concern include the following:

- Amiodarone can *increase* levels of several drugs, including quinidine, procainamide, phenytoin, digoxin, diltiazem,

warfarin, cyclosporine, and three statins: lovastatin, simvastatin, and atorvastatin. Dosages of these agents often require reduction.
- Amiodarone levels can be *increased* by grapefruit juice and by inhibitors of CYP3A4. Toxicity can result.
- Amiodarone levels can be *reduced* by cholestyramine (which decreases amiodarone absorption) and by agents that induce CYP3A4 (e.g., St. John's wort, rifampin).
- The risk for severe dysrhythmias is increased by diuretics (because they can reduce levels of potassium and magnesium) and by drugs that prolong the QT interval, of which there are many.
- Combining amiodarone with a beta blocker, verapamil, or diltiazem can lead to excessive slowing of heart rate.

Dosage. Oral amiodarone [Cordarone, Pacerone] is available in tablets (100, 200, and 400 mg). Treatment should be initiated in a hospital. The following schedule is used for loading: 800 to 1600 mg daily for 1 to 3 weeks, followed by a daily maintenance dosage of 200-600 mg.

Dronedarone

Dronedarone [Multaq] is a derivative of amiodarone. The drug is indicated for oral therapy of *atrial flutter* and *paroxysmal or persistent atrial fibrillation,* but *not* permanent atrial fibrillation. The manufacturer hoped to create a drug with the high efficacy of amiodarone, but with less toxicity. Unfortunately, although dronedarone is somewhat less toxic than amiodarone, it is also less effective. Furthermore, in patients with HF or permanent atrial fibrillation, dronedarone doubles the risk for death. Dronedarone has a much shorter half-life than amiodarone, so adverse effects resolve more quickly.

Effects on the Heart and ECG

Like other class III agents, dronedarone blocks cardiac potassium channels and thereby delays repolarization. In addition, dronedarone can block sodium channels (like class I agents), beta-adrenergic receptors (like class II agents), and calcium channels (like class IV agents). Just how these actions contribute to antidysrhythmic benefits is unclear. Prominent effects on the ECG are PR and QT prolongation and widening of the QRS complex.

Pharmacokinetics

Oral bioavailability is low in the absence of food (4%) and higher in the presence of food (15%). Plasma levels peak 3 to 6 hours after dosing. Dronedarone undergoes extensive metabolism by hepatic CYP3A4, followed by excretion in the feces. The elimination half-life is 13 to 19 hours—much shorter than the 25 to 110 days seen with amiodarone. As a result, steady-state levels are achieved fairly quickly with dronedarone (4–8 days) versus 1 to 5 months with amiodarone.

Adverse Effects

The most common side effects are diarrhea, weakness, nausea, and skin reactions. In contrast to amiodarone, dronedarone does *not* cause significant thyroid toxicity, pulmonary toxicity (e.g., pulmonary fibrosis, pneumonitis), or ocular toxicity (e.g., corneal microdeposits, optic neuropathy)—although it can cause liver toxicity. Dronedarone can increase skin sensitivity to sunlight, but it does not cause the bluish-gray skin discoloration seen with amiodarone. Furthermore, because dronedarone has a much shorter half-life than amiodarone, adverse effects that *do* occur have a much shorter duration.

BLACK BOX WARNING: CARDIAC EFFECTS

In patients with *severe HF,* dronedarone doubles the risk for death, as shown in the ANDROMIDA trial. Accordingly, dronedarone is contraindicated in patients with New York Heart Association (NYHA) class IV HF and in patients with NYHA class II or III HF with recent decompensation that required hospitalization.

In patients with *permanent atrial fibrillation* (as opposed to paroxysmal or persistent atrial fibrillation), dronedarone doubles the risk for death, as shown in the PALLAS trial. Accordingly, dronedarone should not be used in these patients.

Dronedarone reduces SA nodal automaticity and AV nodal conduction, posing a risk for bradycardia and heart block. Accordingly, the drug is contraindicated in patients with sick sinus syndrome or second- or third-degree AV block (unless a pacemaker is in use) and in patients with bradycardia with heart rate less than 50 beats/minute.

Dronedarone prolongs the QT interval (by about 10 msec). Accordingly, the drug should not be used in patients with a QT interval greater than 500 msec or in patients taking drugs or supplements that cause QT prolongation.

Liver Toxicity. Dronedarone has been associated with rare cases of severe liver injury, including two that required liver transplantation. Accordingly, patients should be warned about signs and symptoms of liver injury (e.g., anorexia, nausea, vomiting, malaise, fatigue, itching, jaundice, dark urine) and instructed to contact their provider immediately if these develop. Providers should consider monitoring for liver enzymes in blood, especially during the first 6 months of treatment.

Toxicity in Pregnancy and Breastfeeding. Dronedarone is a proven teratogen and must not be used during pregnancy. In animal studies, doses at or below the mean recommended human dose have produced visceral, skeletal, and external malformations. Accordingly, dronedarone is classified in FDA Pregnancy Risk Category X: risks to the developing fetus clearly outweigh any possible benefit. Women of childbearing age should be counseled about using effective contraception.

We know that dronedarone is excreted in the milk of rats, but information in lactating women is lacking. Nonetheless, owing to the potential risk to nursing infants, dronedarone is contraindicated for use by breastfeeding mothers.

Drug Interactions

Dronedarone is subject to multiple drug interactions, many involving CYP3A4.
- *Strong inhibitors of hepatic CYP3A4* (e.g., ketoconazole, clarithromycin, ritonavir) can make dronedarone accumulate to dangerous levels. Accordingly, concurrent use of these inhibitors is contraindicated. Grapefruit juice, which strongly inhibits *intestinal* CYP3A4, can raise dronedarone levels threefold and so should also be avoided. Moderate inhibitors of hepatic CYP3A4 (e.g., verapamil, diltiazem) should be used with caution.
- *Strong inducers of CYP3A4* (e.g., rifampin, carbamazepine, St. John's wort) can reduce dronedarone levels by as much as 80%, and can thereby greatly reduce dysrhythmia control.

- In addition to being a substrate for CYP3A4, dronedarone can inhibit this enzyme. Accordingly, dronedarone can raise levels of other drugs that are *CYP3A4 substrates*. Substrates with a narrow therapeutic range (e.g., tacrolimus, sirolimus, warfarin) should be used with caution.
- Dronedarone can inhibit CYP2D6 and can thereby increase levels of *CYP2D6 substrates* (e.g., beta blockers, tricyclic antidepressants). Concurrent use of these agents should be done with caution.
- *Beta blockers,* which suppress the SA node and AV conduction, can intensify dronedarone-induced bradycardia and can also increase the risk for AV block.
- Like the beta blockers, two *calcium channel blockers—verapamil* and *diltiazem*—also suppress the SA node and AV conduction and pose the same risk as the beta blockers. In addition, verapamil and diltiazem can inhibit CYP3A4 and can thereby raise dronedarone levels, making the risk for cardiosuppression even greater.
- *Drugs and supplements that prolong the QT interval* (e.g., phenothiazines, tricyclic antidepressants, class I and class III antidysrhythmics) can intensify dronedarone-induced QT prolongation and can thereby increase the risk for torsades de pointes. Accordingly, these drugs are contraindicated for use with dronedarone.

Contraindications

Dronedarone has the following contraindications:

- NYHA class IV HF *or* NYHA class II or III HF with recent decompensation requiring hospitalization
- Liver or lung toxicity related to previous amiodarone use
- Permanent atrial fibrillation
- Second- or third-degree AV block or sick sinus syndrome (except in patients using a pacemaker)
- Bradycardia with heart rate less than 50 beats/minute
- PR interval greater than 280 msec
- QT interval greater than 500 msec
- Use of drugs or supplements that prolong the QT interval
- Use of strong inhibitors of CYP3A4
- Pregnancy
- Breastfeeding
- Severe liver impairment

Preparations, Dosage, and Administration

Dronedarone [Multaq] is supplied in 400-mg tablets for oral dosing. The recommended dosage is 400 mg twice daily, taken with the morning and evening meals. Note that, unlike amiodarone, dronedarone does not require a loading dose.

Sotalol

Actions and Uses

Sotalol [Betapace, Betapace AF] is a beta blocker that also delays repolarization. Hence the drug has combined class II and class III antidysrhythmic properties. Prodysrhythmic properties are pronounced. Sotalol was initially approved only for ventricular dysrhythmias, such as sustained ventricular tachycardia, that are considered life threatening. Later, it was approved for prophylaxis and treatment of atrial flutter and fibrillation, but only if symptoms are severe. The drug is not approved for hypertension or angina pectoris (the primary indications for other beta blockers).

Pharmacokinetics

Sotalol is administered orally and undergoes nearly complete absorption. The drug is excreted unchanged in the urine. Its half-life is 12 hours.

Adverse Effects

At therapeutic doses, sotalol produces substantial beta blockade. It can cause bradycardia, AV block, HF, and bronchospasm. Accordingly, the usual contraindications to beta blockers apply.

BLACK BOX WARNING: SOTOLOL

Sotalol can cause torsades de pointes, a serious dysrhythmia that develops in about 5% of patients. Risk is increased by hypokalemia and by other drugs that prolong the QT interval.

Preparations, Dosage, and Administration

Sotalol is available under two trade names: Betapace and Betapace AF. Betapace (80-, 120-, 160-, and 240-mg tablets) is intended for treating ventricular dysrhythmias. Betapace AF (80-, 120-, and 160-mg tablets) is intended for treating atrial fibrillation and atrial flutter. Although tablets are the same under both trade names, packaging differs: packaging for Betapace provides information specific for treating ventricular dysrhythmias, whereas packaging for Betapace AF provides information specific for treating atrial dysrhythmias. The two should not be interchanged. For both types of dysrhythmias, treatment should start in a hospital. Dosing for both is the same: the initial dosage is 160 mg/day (in two divided doses), and the usual maintenance dosage is 160 to 320 mg/day in two or three divided doses. The dosing interval should be increased in patients with renal impairment.

Dofetilide

Therapeutic Use

Dofetilide [Tikosyn] is an oral class III antidysrhythmic indicated for restoring and maintaining normal sinus rhythm in patients with atrial flutter or atrial fibrillation. The drug causes dose-related QT prolongation and thereby poses a serious risk for torsades de pointes. Accordingly, it should be reserved for patients with highly symptomatic atrial dysrhythmias. Initial treatment requires continuous ECG monitoring in a hospital. Dosage must be carefully titrated on the basis of renal function tests. Dofetilide is available only through authorized hospitals and prescribers.

Effects on the Heart and ECG

Like other class III agents, dofetilide blocks cardiac potassium channels and delays repolarization, prolonging the QT interval. Dofetilide does not affect the PR interval or widen the QRS complex and has no effect on cardiac beta receptors or sodium channels.

Pharmacokinetics

Dofetilide is well absorbed (90%) both in the presence and absence of food. Very little is metabolized. About 80% of each dose is excreted in the urine, primarily unchanged. Renal excretion results largely from active tubular secretion, mediated by cationic pumps (i.e., pumps specific for molecules that are cations). In patients with normal renal function, the drug's half-life is about 10 hours. However, in patients with renal impairment, the half-life is increased. In patients with moderate renal impairment, dosage must be reduced; in patients with severe renal impairment, dofetilide must not be used.

BLACK BOX WARNING

By increasing the QT interval, dofetilide predisposes to torsades de pointes, which can progress to fatal ventricular fibrillation. The risk is directly related to dofetilide blood levels and is increased by hypokalemia and by other drugs that cause QT prolongation. To assess risk, an ECG should be obtained at baseline, and ECG monitoring should be continuous during initial treatment. Dofetilide is contraindicated for patients with a baseline QT interval greater than 440 msec (or greater than 500 msec in patients with ventricular conduction abnormalities).

Drug Interactions

Drugs that are excreted by renal cation pumps can interfere with the excretion of dofetilide, thereby causing its levels to rise. Accordingly, concurrent use of these drugs (e.g., cimetidine, trimethoprim, ketoconazole, prochlorperazine, megestrol) is contraindicated.

Drugs that prolong the QT interval may increase the risk for dysrhythmias and so should be avoided. Among these are class I and class III antidysrhythmics, phenothiazines, tricyclic antidepressants, and some macrolide antibiotics.

Combining verapamil with dofetilide increases the risk for torsades de pointes and should be avoided.

Preparations, Dosage, and Administration

Dofetilide [Tikosyn] is available in capsules (125, 250, and 500 mcg) for oral dosing. Because of the risk for dysrhythmias, treatment must be initiated in a hospital with continuous ECG monitoring for at least 3 days. Because dysrhythmia risk is directly related to plasma drug levels, which in turn are directly related to creatinine clearance (a measure of renal function), creatinine clearance must be monitored. Dosage should be reduced with decreasing creatinine clearance as follows: for patients with normal renal function (creatinine clearance greater than 60 mL/minute), give 500 mcg twice a day; for creatinine clearance 40 to 60 mL/minute, give 250 mcg twice a day; for creatinine clearance 20 to 39 mL/min, give 125 mcg twice a day; and for creatinine clearance below 20 mL/minute, withhold dofetilide. If the QT interval becomes excessively prolonged (greater than 500 msec, or greater than 550 msec in patients with ventricular conduction abnormalities), dosage should be reduced.

Class IV: Calcium Channel Blockers

Only two calcium channel blockers—*verapamil* [Calan, Covera-HS, ♣ Verelan] and *diltiazem* [Cardizem, Dilacor-XR, Tiazac, others]—are able to block calcium channels in the heart. Accordingly, they are the only calcium channel blockers used to treat dysrhythmias. Their basic pharmacology is discussed in Chapter 37. Consideration here is limited to their use against dysrhythmias.

Effects on the Heart and ECG

Blockade of cardiac calcium channels has three effects:

- Slowing of SA nodal automaticity
- Delay of AV nodal conduction
- Reduction of myocardial contractility

Note that these are identical to the effects of beta blockers, which makes sense in that beta blockers promote calcium channel closure in the heart. The principal effect on the ECG is prolongation of the PR interval, reflecting delayed AV conduction.

Therapeutic Uses

Verapamil and diltiazem have two antidysrhythmic uses. First, they can slow ventricular rate in patients with atrial fibrillation or atrial flutter. Second, they can terminate SVT caused by an AV nodal reentrant circuit. In both cases, benefits derive from suppressing AV nodal conduction. With IV administration, effects can be seen in 2 to 3 minutes. Verapamil and diltiazem are not active against ventricular dysrhythmias.

Adverse Effects

Although generally safe, these drugs *can* cause undesired effects. Blockade of cardiac calcium channels can cause *bradycardia, AV block,* and *heart failure.* Blockade of calcium channels in vascular smooth muscle can cause vasodilation, resulting in *hypotension* and *peripheral edema.* Blockade of calcium channels in intestinal smooth muscle can produce *constipation.*

Drug Interactions

Both verapamil and diltiazem can elevate levels of *digoxin,* thereby increasing the risk for digoxin toxicity. Also, because digoxin shares with verapamil and diltiazem the ability to decrease AV conduction, combining digoxin with either drug increases the risk of AV block.

Because verapamil, diltiazem, and *beta blockers* have nearly identical suppressant effects on the heart, combining verapamil or diltiazem with a beta blocker increases the risk for bradycardia, AV block, and HF.

Preparations, Dosage, and Administration

Verapamil

Dosing may be IV or oral. Intravenous therapy is preferred for initial treatment. Oral therapy is used for maintenance.

Verapamil for oral use is available in immediate- and sustained-release tablets. The maintenance dosage is 40 to 120 mg 3 or 4 times a day.

Diltiazem

Like verapamil, diltiazem may be given by IV or PO route. Intravenous therapy is preferred for initial treatment, and oral therapy is used for maintenance.

Diltiazem for oral use is available in immediate-release and extended-release tablets. Maintenance dosing is 120 to 360 mg daily taken in four divided doses.

Other Antidysrhythmic Drugs

Digoxin

Although its primary indication is HF, digoxin [Lanoxin] is also used to treat supraventricular dysrhythmias. The basic pharmacology of digoxin is discussed in Chapter 40. Consideration here is limited to treatment of dysrhythmias.

Effects on the Heart

Digoxin suppresses dysrhythmias by decreasing conduction through the AV node and by decreasing automaticity in the SA node. The drug decreases AV conduction by (1) a direct depressant effect on the AV node and by (2) acting in the CNS to increase vagal (parasympathetic) impulses to the AV node. Digoxin decreases automaticity of the SA node by increasing vagal traffic to the node and by decreasing sympathetic traffic. It should be noted that, although digoxin decreases automaticity in the SA node, it can increase automaticity in Purkinje fibers. The latter effect contributes to dysrhythmias caused by digoxin.

Effects on the ECG

By slowing AV conduction, digoxin prolongs the PR interval. The QT interval may be shortened, reflecting accelerated repolarization of the ventricles. Depression of the ST segment is common. The T wave may be depressed or even inverted. There is little or no change in the QRS complex.

Adverse Effects and Interactions

The major adverse effect is cardiotoxicity (dysrhythmias). Risk is increased by hypokalemia, which can result from concurrent therapy with diuretics (thiazides and loop diuretics). Accordingly, it is essential that potassium levels be kept within the normal range (3.5–5 mEq/L). The most common adverse effects are GI disturbances (anorexia, nausea, vomiting, abdominal discomfort). CNS responses (fatigue, visual disturbances) are also relatively common.

Antidysrhythmic Uses

Digoxin is used only for supraventricular dysrhythmias. The drug is inactive against ventricular dysrhythmias.

Atrial Fibrillation and Atrial Flutter

Digoxin can be used to slow ventricular rate in patients with atrial fibrillation and atrial flutter. Ventricular rate is decreased by reducing the number of atrial impulses that pass through the AV node.

Supraventricular Tachycardia

Digoxin may be employed acutely and chronically to treat SVT. Acute therapy is used to abolish the dysrhythmia. Chronic therapy is used to prevent its return. Digoxin suppresses SVT by increasing cardiac vagal tone and by decreasing sympathetic tone.

Dosage and Administration

Oral therapy is generally preferred. The initial dosage is 1 to 1.5 mg administered in three or four doses over 24 hours. The maintenance dosage is 0.125 to 0.5 mg/day. This dose should be decreased in patients with renal impairment.

CHAPTER

42 Prophylaxis of Atherosclerotic Cardiovascular Disease: Drugs That Help Normalize Cholesterol and Triglyceride Levels

Laura D. Rosenthal, DNP, ACNP, FAANP

Our main topic for the chapter is drugs used to lower cholesterol. Drugs used to lower triglycerides (TGs) are considered as well. Cholesterol plays a role in atherosclerotic cardiovascular disease (ASCVD). ASCVD includes the vessels of the heart as well as the brain. Damage to these vessels can result in myocardial infarction (MI) or stroke. Moderate cardiac ASCVD usually manifests first as anginal pain. Severe cardiac ASCVD sets the stage for acute coronary syndrome (ACS) and MI. In the United States cardiac ASCVD is the leading killer of men and women, causing 386,324 deaths in 2009. According to the American Heart Association, about 16 million Americans have a history of coronary events (angina, MI, or both). More than half of these people are women.

ASCVD begins as a fatty streak in the arterial wall. This is followed by deposition of fibrous plaque. As atherosclerotic plaque grows, it impedes coronary blood flow, causing anginal pain. Worse yet, atherosclerosis encourages formation of thrombi, which can block flow to the brain and heart entirely, thereby causing MI and stroke.

It is important to appreciate that atherosclerosis is not limited to arteries of the heart or brain: Atherosclerotic plaque can develop in any artery and can thereby compromise circulation to any tissue. Furthermore, adverse effects can occur at sites distant from the original lesion: a ruptured lesion can produce a thrombus, which can travel downstream to block a new vessel.

The risk for developing ASCVD is directly related to increased levels of blood cholesterol, in the form of low-density lipoproteins (LDLs). By reducing levels of LDL cholesterol, we can slow progression of atherosclerosis, reduce the risk for serious ASCVD and its potential consequences, and prolong life. The preferred method for lowering LDL cholesterol is modification of diet combined with exercise. Drugs are employed only when diet modification and exercise are insufficient.

We approach our primary topic—cholesterol and its influence on ASCVD—in three stages. First, we discuss cholesterol itself, plasma lipoproteins (structures that transport cholesterol in blood), and the process of atherogenesis. Second, we discuss guidelines for cholesterol screening and management of high cholesterol. Third, we discuss the pharmacology of the cholesterol-lowering drugs, as well as drugs used to lower TGs.

CHOLESTEROL

Cholesterol has several physiologic roles. Of greatest importance, cholesterol is a component of all cell membranes and membranes of intracellular organelles. In addition, cholesterol is required for synthesis of certain hormones (e.g., estrogen, progesterone, testosterone) and for synthesis of bile salts, which are needed to absorb and digest dietary fats. Also, cholesterol is deposited in the stratum corneum of the skin, where it reduces evaporation of water and blocks transdermal absorption of water-soluble compounds.

Some of our cholesterol comes from dietary sources (exogenous cholesterol), and some is manufactured by cells (endogenous cholesterol), primarily in the liver. More cholesterol comes from endogenous production than from the diet. A critical step in hepatic cholesterol synthesis is catalyzed by an enzyme named *3-hydroxy-3-methylglutaryl coenzyme A reductase,* or simply *HMG-CoA reductase.* As discussed later, drugs that inhibit this enzyme—the statins—are our most effective and widely used cholesterol-lowering agents.

An increase in dietary cholesterol produces only a small increase in cholesterol in the blood, primarily because a rise in cholesterol intake inhibits endogenous cholesterol synthesis. Interestingly, an increase in dietary saturated fats produces a substantial (15%–25%) increase in circulating cholesterol because the liver uses saturated fats to make cholesterol. Accordingly, when we want to reduce cholesterol levels, it is more important to reduce intake of saturated fats than to reduce intake of cholesterol itself, although cholesterol intake should definitely be lowered.

PLASMA LIPOPROTEINS

Structure and Function of Lipoproteins

Function

Lipoproteins serve as carriers for transporting lipids—cholesterol and TGs—in blood. Like all other nutrients and metabolites, lipids use the bloodstream to move throughout the body. However, being lipids, cholesterol and TGs are not water soluble and hence cannot dissolve directly in plasma. Lipoproteins provide a means of solubilizing these lipids, thereby permitting transport.

Basic Structure

The basic structure of lipoproteins is depicted in Fig. 42.1. As indicated, lipoproteins are tiny, spherical structures that consist of a *hydrophobic core,* composed of cholesterol and TGs, surrounded by a *hydrophilic shell,* composed primarily of phospholipids. Because the hydrophilic shell completely covers the lipid core, the entire structure is soluble in the aqueous environment of the plasma.

Apolipoproteins

All lipoproteins have one or more *apolipoprotein* molecules embedded in their shell (see Fig. 42.1). Apolipoproteins, which constitute the protein component of lipoproteins, have three functions:

- They serve as recognition sites for cell-surface receptors and thereby allow cells to bind with and ingest lipoproteins.
- They activate enzymes that metabolize lipoproteins.
- They increase the structural stability of lipoproteins.

Classes of Lipoproteins

There are six major classes of plasma lipoproteins. Distinctions among classes are based on size, density, apolipoprotein content, transport function, and primary core lipids (cholesterol or TG). From a pharmacologic perspective, the features of greatest interest are *lipid content, apolipoprotein content,* and *transport function.*

Of the six major classes of lipoproteins, three are especially important in coronary atherosclerosis. These classes are named (1) very-low-density lipoproteins (VLDLs), (2) low-density lipoproteins (LDLs), and (3) high-density lipoproteins (HDLs). Properties of these classes are shown in Table 42.1.

Very-Low-Density Lipoproteins

VLDLs contain mainly *triglycerides* (and some cholesterol), and they account for nearly all of the TGs in blood. The main physiologic role of VLDLs is to *deliver triglycerides* from the liver to adipose tissue and muscle, which can use the TGs as fuel. Each VLDL particle contains one molecule of *apolipoprotein B-100,* which allows VLDLs to bind with cell-surface receptors and thereby transfer their lipid content to cells.

The role of VLDLs in atherosclerosis is unclear. Although several studies suggest a link between elevated levels of VLDLs and development of atherosclerosis, this link has not been firmly established. However, we do know that elevation of TG levels (above 500 mg/dL) increases the risk for *pancreatitis.*

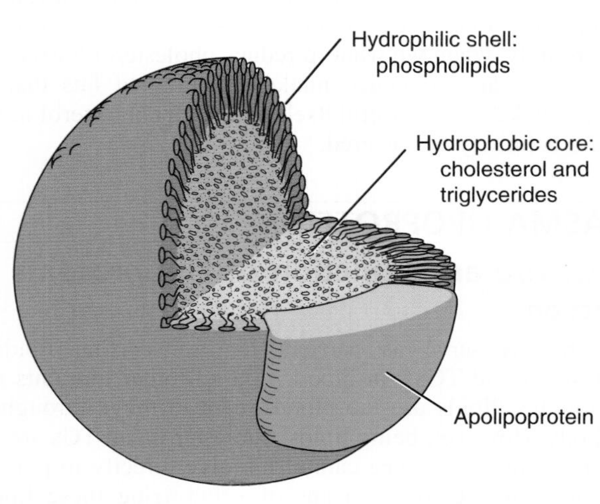

Figure 42.1 ▪ Basic structure of plasma lipoproteins.

Low-Density Lipoproteins

LDLs contain *cholesterol* as their primary core lipid, and they account for the majority (60%–70%) of all cholesterol in blood. The physiologic role of LDLs is *delivery of cholesterol to nonhepatic tissues.* LDLs can be viewed as byproducts of VLDL metabolism, in that the lipids and apolipoproteins that compose LDLs are remnants of VLDL degradation.

Cells that require cholesterol meet their needs through endocytosis (engulfment) of LDLs from the blood. The process begins with binding of LDL particles to LDL receptors on the cell surface. When cellular demand for cholesterol increases, cells synthesize more LDL receptors and thereby increase their capacity for LDL uptake. Accordingly, cells that are unable to make more LDL receptors cannot increase cholesterol absorption. Increasing the number of LDL receptors on cells is an important mechanism by which certain drugs increase LDL uptake and thereby reduce LDL levels in blood.

Of all lipoproteins, LDLs make the greatest contribution to coronary atherosclerosis. The probability of developing ASCVD is directly related to the level of LDLs in blood. Conversely, by reducing LDL levels, we decrease the risk for ASCVD. Accordingly, *when cholesterol-lowering drugs are used, the main goal is to reduce elevated LDL levels.* Multiple studies have shown that, by reducing LDL levels, we can arrest or perhaps even reverse atherosclerosis and can thereby reduce mortality from ASCVD. In fact, for each 1% reduction in the LDL level, there is about a 1% reduction in the risk for a major cardiovascular (CV) event.

TABLE 42.1 ▪ Properties of the Plasma Lipoproteins That Affect Atherosclerosis

Lipoprotein Class	Major Core Lipids	Transport Function	Influence on Atherosclerosis
VLDL	Triglycerides	Delivery of triglycerides to nonhepatic tissues	*Probably contribute* to atherosclerosis
LDL	Cholesterol	Delivery of cholesterol to nonhepatic tissues	*Definitely contribute* to atherosclerosis
HDL	Cholesterol	Transport of cholesterol from nonhepatic tissues back to the liver	*Protect* against atherosclerosis

LDL, low-density lipoprotein; HDL, high-density lipoprotein; VLDL, very-low-density lipoprotein.

High-Density Lipoproteins

Like LDLs, HDLs contain *cholesterol* as their primary core lipid, and they account for 20% to 30% of all cholesterol in the blood. In contrast to LDLs, whose function is delivery of cholesterol to peripheral tissues, HDLs carry cholesterol from peripheral tissues back to the liver. That is, *HDLs promote cholesterol removal.*

The influence of HDLs on ASCVD is dramatically different from that of LDLs. Whereas elevation of LDLs *increases* the risk for ASCVD, elevation of HDLs *reduces* the risk for ASCVD. That is, high HDL levels actively protect against ASCVD.

Low-Density Lipoprotein Versus High-Density Lipoprotein Cholesterol

The previous discussion shows that not all cholesterol in plasma has the same effect on ASCVD. As stated, a rise in cholesterol associated with LDLs increases the risk for ASCVD. In contrast, a rise in cholesterol associated with HDLs lowers the risk. Consequently, when speaking of plasma cholesterol levels, we need to distinguish between cholesterol that is associated with HDLs and cholesterol that is associated with LDLs. To make this distinction, we use the terms *HDL cholesterol* and *LDL cholesterol.* Because LDL cholesterol promotes atherosclerosis, it has been dubbed *bad cholesterol.* Conversely, because HDL seems to protect against atherosclerosis, it is often called *good cholesterol* or *healthy cholesterol.*

ROLE OF LOW-DENSITY LIPOPROTEIN CHOLESTEROL IN ATHEROSCLEROSIS

LDLs initiate and fuel development of atherosclerosis. The process begins with transport of LDLs from the arterial lumen into endothelial cells that line the lumens of blood vessels. From there, they move into the space that underlies the arterial epithelium. When in the subendothelial space, components of LDLs undergo *oxidation.* This step is critical in that oxidized LDLs do the following:

- Attract monocytes from the circulation into the subendothelial space, after which the monocytes are converted to macrophages (which are critical to atherogenesis)
- Inhibit macrophage mobility, thereby keeping macrophages at the site of atherogenesis
- Undergo uptake by macrophages (macrophages do not take up LDLs that have not been oxidized)
- Are cytotoxic and hence can damage the vascular endothelium directly

As macrophages engulf more and more cholesterol, they become large and develop large vacuoles. When macrophages assume this form, they are referred to as *foam cells.* Foam cell accumulation beneath the arterial epithelium produces a *fatty streak,* which makes the surface of the arterial wall lumpy, causing blood flow to become turbulent. Continued accumulation of foam cells can eventually cause rupture of the endothelium, thereby exposing the underlying tissue to the blood. This results in platelet adhesion and formation of microthrombi. As the process continues, smooth muscle cells migrate to the site, synthesis of collagen increases, and there can be repeated rupturing and healing of the endothelium. The end result is a mature atherosclerotic lesion, characterized by a large lipid core and a tough *fibrous cap.* In less mature lesions, the fibrous cap is not strong, and hence the lesions are unstable and more likely to rupture. As a result, arterial pressure and shear forces (from turbulent blood flow) can cause the cap to rupture. Accumulation of platelets at the site of rupture can rapidly cause thrombosis and can thereby cause infarction. Infarction is less likely at sites of mature atherosclerotic lesions. The atherosclerotic process is depicted in Fig. 42.2.

It is important to appreciate that atherogenesis involves more than just deposition of lipids. In fact, atherogenesis is now considered primarily a chronic *inflammatory process.* When LDLs penetrate the arterial wall, they cause mild injury. The injury, in turn, triggers an inflammatory response that includes infiltration of macrophages, T lymphocytes, and other potentially noxious chemicals (e.g., C-reactive protein [CRP]). In the late stage of the disease process, inflammation can weaken atherosclerotic plaque, leading to plaque rupture and subsequent thrombosis.

2013 AMERICAN COLLEGE OF CARDIOLOGY/AMERICAN HEART ASSOCIATION GUIDELINE ON THE TREATMENT OF BLOOD CHOLESTEROL TO REDUCE ATHEROSCLEROTIC CARDIOVASCULAR RISK

It is well established that high levels of cholesterol (primarily LDL cholesterol) cause substantial morbidity and mortality and that aggressive treatment can save lives. Accordingly, periodic cholesterol screening and risk assessment are recommended. If the assessment indicates ASCVD risk, lifestyle changes—especially diet and exercise—should be implemented. If ASCVD risk is high, LDL-lowering drugs should be added to the regimen.

In 1988, the National Cholesterol Education Program (NCEP) began issuing guidelines on cholesterol detection and management. The most recent update was issued in 2001 and amended in 2004, and new guidelines were developed in 2013 in partnership with the American College of Cardiology (ACC) and the American Heart Association (AHA). A summary of the 2013 guidelines—*2013 ACC/AHA Guideline on the Treatment of Blood Cholesterol to Reduce Atherosclerotic Cardiovascular Risk in Adults: A Report of the American College of Cardiology/American Heart Association Task Force on Practice Guidelines*—was published in *the Journal of the American College of Cardiology* and is available at http://circ.ahajournals.org/content/early/2013/11/11/01.cir.0000437738.63853.7a.

Like earlier NCEP guidelines, the 2013 ACC/AHA cholesterol guideline focuses on the role of high cholesterol in ASCVD and stresses the importance of treatment. However, the new guideline focuses specifically on identifying patients who are most likely to benefit from cholesterol-lowering therapy instead of targeting specific cholesterol goals.

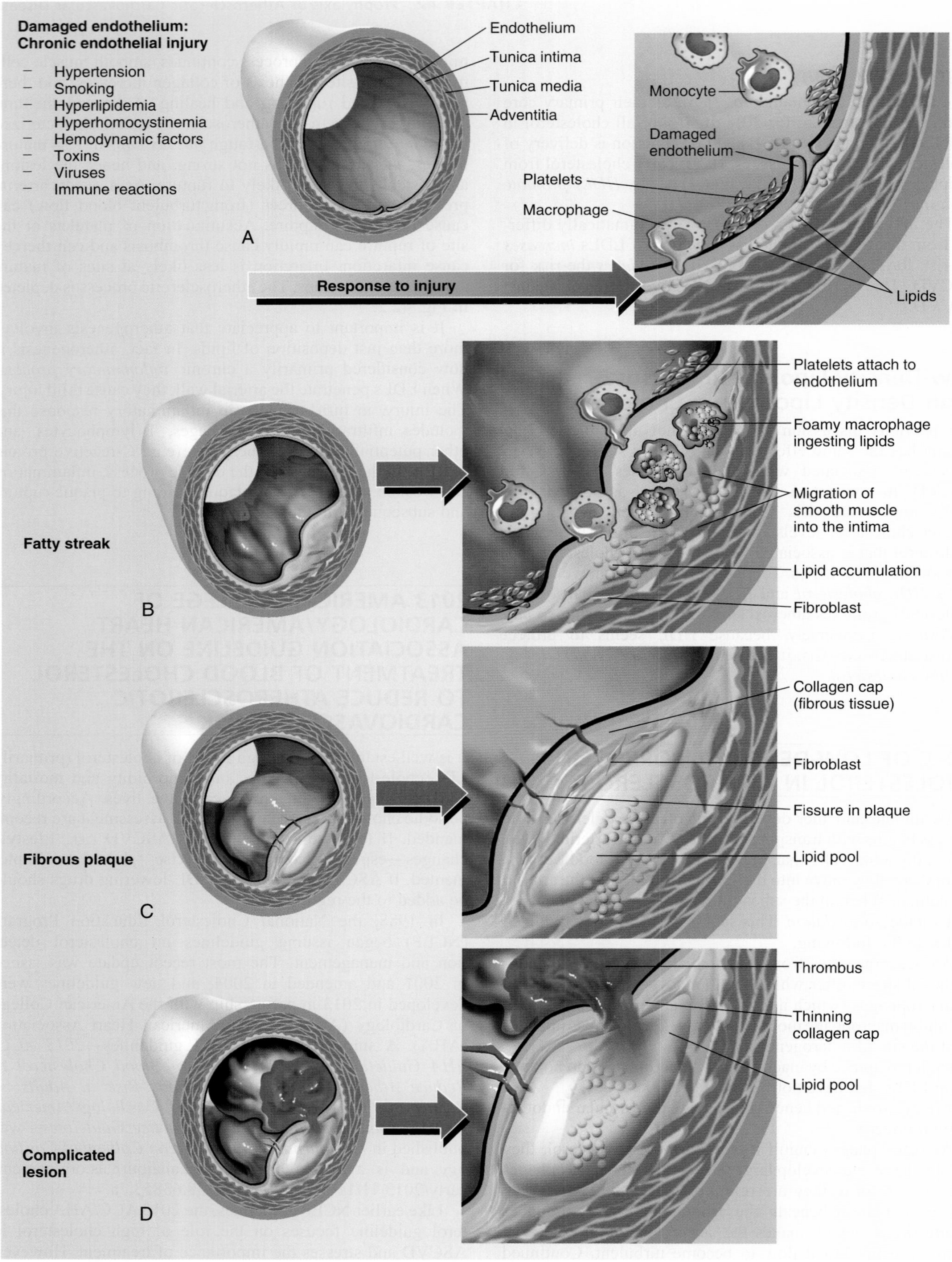

Figure 42.2 ■ **Progression of atherosclerosis.**

A, Damaged endothelium. **B,** Diagram of fatty streak and lipid core formation. **C,** Diagram of fibrous plaque. Raised plaques are visible: some are yellow and some are white. **D,** Diagram of a complicated lesion, showing a thrombus (in red) and collagen (in blue). (From McCance KL, Huether SE: Pathophysiology: The Biologic Basis for Disease in Adults and Children, 7th ed. St. Louis: Elsevier, 2014.)

Cholesterol Screening

Adults

Management of high LDL cholesterol begins with screening, generally done every 5 years for adults older than 20 years. Because the 2013 update only addressed treatment, the ATP III guidelines (*Third Report of the Expert Panel on Detection, Evaluation, and Treatment of High Blood Cholesterol in Adults*) for screening and prevention remain current. ATP III recommends a thorough screening, consisting of total cholesterol, LDL cholesterol, HDL cholesterol, and TGs. Blood for these tests should be drawn after fasting. With the introduction of the new guidelines, patients should be considered for statin treatment if they fall into one of four different risk categories (Box 42.1).

Children and Adolescents

Elevated cholesterol in pediatric patients is a growing concern and is not addressed in the 2013 ACC/AHA blood cholesterol guidelines. However, it is addressed in other guidelines, including one created in 2011 by an expert panel appointed by the National Heart, Lung, and Blood Institute, and endorsed by the American Academy of Pediatrics. This report—*Expert Panel on Integrated Guidelines for Cardiovascular Health and Risk Reduction in Children and Adolescents*—is available at www.nhlbi.nih.gov/guidelines/cvd_ped/summary.htm#chap9.

The guideline recommends lipid screening for *all* children between ages 9 and 11 years, followed by another screen between ages 18 and 21 years. For children with a family history of high cholesterol or heart disease, screening should start sooner: between ages 2 and 8 years. Cholesterol classification for children and adolescents is presented in Table 42.2.

If LDL cholesterol is high, all patients and their families should receive nutritional counseling. In addition, patients should focus on weight control and increased activity, as indicated. Should children use cholesterol-lowering drugs? For two reasons, the answer is, "Probably not." First, these children are in no immediate danger: their risk for developing clinically significant ASCVD in the next 20 years is close to zero. And second, the only data from randomized, controlled trials were in children with familial hypercholesterolemia. No data exist showing that these drugs will improve outcomes when given to children with secondary lipid disorders.

BOX 42.1 ▪ STATIN BENEFIT GROUPS AS DEFINED BY THE 2013 ACC/AHA BLOOD CHOLESTEROL GUIDELINES

- Individuals with clinical ASCVD
- Individuals with primary elevations of LDL cholesterol ≥190 mg/dL
- Individuals 40–75 years of age with diabetes and LDL cholesterol 70–189 mg/dL
- Individuals without clinical ASCVD or diabetes who are 40–75 years of age with LDL cholesterol 70–189 mg/dL and an estimated 10-year ASCVD risk of 7.5% or higher

ASCVD, atherosclerotic cardiovascular disease; LDL, low-density lipoprotein.
From the *2013 ACC/AHA Guideline on the Treatment of Blood Cholesterol to Reduce Atherosclerotic Cardiovascular Risk in Adults: A Report of the American College of Cardiology/American Heart Association Task Force on Practice Guidelines*—available at http://circ.ahajournals.org/content/early/2013/11/11/01.cir.0000437738.63853.7a.

Atherosclerotic Cardiovascular Disease Risk Assessment

Under the 2013 ACC/AHA guidelines, ASCVD risk assessment is directed at determining the patient's *absolute risk for developing clinical coronary disease over the next 10 years.*

TABLE 42.2 ▪ NCEP Classification of Cholesterol Levels for Children and Adolescents*

Category	Total Cholesterol (mg/dL)	LDL Cholesterol (mg/dL)
Acceptable	<170	<110
Borderline	170–199	110–129
Elevated	≥200	≥130

*High-density lipoprotein levels should be greater than or equal to 35 mg/dL, and triglycerides should be less than or equal to 150 mg/dL.
LDL, low-density lipoprotein.
Data from National Cholesterol Education Program: Report of the Expert Panel on Blood Cholesterol Levels in Children and Adolescents. Pediatrics 89(3 Pt 2):525–584, 1992.

PATIENT-CENTERED CARE ACROSS THE LIFE SPAN

Treating Dyslipidemia

Life Stage	Patient Care Concerns
Infants	See later entry "Breastfeeding women."
Children/adolescents	Lovastatin, simvastatin, pravastatin, and atorvastatin are approved for use in children. It is recommended to avoid statin use in children younger than 10 years.
Pregnant women	Statins are classified in FDA Pregnancy Risk Category X. They are contraindicated in pregnancy. Ezetimibe and fibrates are classified in Pregnancy Risk Category C; hence benefit should outweigh risk.
Breastfeeding women	Effects of statins, ezetimibe, and fibrates have not been studied in breastfeeding. Given the possibility of harm, benefit should outweigh risk.
Older adults	In patients 65 years and older, statins, compared with placebo, significantly reduced the risk for MI as well as the risk for stroke by 23.8%. However, the cost-benefit evaluation of treatment in older-adult people should be considered.

The mode of intervention is then determined by the individual's degree of risk.

Factors in Risk Assessment

To assess the ASCVD risk for an individual, we need three kinds of information. Specifically, we need to (1) identify ASCVD risk factors, (2) calculate 10-year ASCVD risk, and (3) identify ASCVD risk equivalents.

Identifying ASCVD Risk Factors

Major risk factors that modify LDL treatment goals include positive risk factors (advancing age, black race, hypertension, cigarette smoking, and low HDL cholesterol) and one negative risk factor (high HDL cholesterol). (LDL itself is not listed because the reason for counting these risk factors is to modify treatment of high LDL.)

We know that diabetes is a very strong predictor of developing ASCVD. Accordingly, we no longer consider diabetes to be a risk *factor.* Instead, for the purpose of risk assessment, diabetes is now considered an ASCVD risk *equivalent.* That is, having diabetes is considered equivalent to having ASCVD as a predictor of a major coronary event.

Calculating 10-Year ASCVD Risk

The 2013 ACC/AHA cholesterol guideline defines high ASCVD risk as 7.5% or greater. Some people are automatically in this risk group—specifically, those with existing ASCVD and those with diabetes. For all other people, 10-year risk must be calculated. The instrument employed most often is the Framingham Risk Prediction Score, which takes five factors into account: age, total cholesterol, HDL cholesterol, smoking status, and systolic blood pressure. These are similar to risk factors noted earlier. Framingham scores can be determined using either (1) the tables for men and women shown in Fig. 42.3 or (2) a web-based risk calculator, such as the one provided by the ACC/AHA at http://tools.cardiosource.org/ASCVD-Risk-Estimator/.

Identifying ASCVD Risk Equivalents

An ASCVD risk equivalent is a condition that poses the same risk for a major coronary event as does established ASCVD (i.e., more than 20% risk for a major event within 10 years). There are two basic ASCVD risk equivalents:

- Diabetes
- The presence of multiple risk factors that confer an ASCVD 10-year risk score ≥7.5%

Identifying an Individual's Atherosclerotic Cardiovascular Disease Risk Category

Under the 2013 ACC/AHA cholesterol guideline, there are four categories of patients who would benefit from statin treatment of cholesterol (see Box 42.1). Category assignment is based on (1) the presence or absence of ASCVD (or an ASCVD risk equivalent, such as diabetes), (2) the number of risk factors the individual has (other than high LDL cholesterol), and (3) the individual's 10-year ASCVD score. Although this assessment sounds complicated, it's not. Let's consider the hypothetical case of Ralph J., and follow along by looking at Fig. 42.3. Mr. J. is 62 years old, hypertensive, and smokes—but, remarkably, his HDL cholesterol is high (above 60 mg/dL). He has no family history of premature ASCVD, does not have ASCVD himself, and does not have diabetes. His 10-year Framingham Risk Prediction Score is 11%. Because his estimated 10-year ASCVD score is greater than 7.5%, Mr. J. should be considered for moderate- to high-intensity drug therapy (Fig. 42.4). This is even easier if you use an online risk assessment tool, such as the ones available at http://www.framinghamheartstudy.org/risk-functions/index.php.

Final Note: Each Type of Dyslipidemia a Patient Has Contributes Independently to Atherosclerotic Cardiovascular Disease Risk

Patients are likely to have more than one type of dyslipidemia—for example, high LDL cholesterol combined with low HDL cholesterol and high TGs—and each of these disorders contributes *independently* to CV risk. This means that fixing just one of these problems will not eliminate the risk posed by the others. Accordingly, to get maximal risk reduction, we must correct all lipid abnormalities that are present.

Treatment of High Low-Density Lipoprotein Cholesterol

Treatment of high LDL cholesterol is based on the individual's ASCVD risk category or the presence of other comorbidities such as diabetes. Treatment may be started with a high-intensity statin or a moderate-intensity statin depending on the patient's risk factors (Table 42.3; see Fig. 42.4). To reduce LDL levels, the 2013 ACC/AHA guideline recommends two forms of intervention: (1) therapeutic lifestyle changes (TLCs) and (2) drug therapy. For some people, cholesterol can be reduced adequately with TLCs alone. Others require TLCs *plus* cholesterol-lowering drugs. Please note that drugs should be used only as an *adjunct* to TLCs—not as a *substitute.*

Therapeutic Lifestyle Changes

Therapeutic lifestyle changes are nondrug measures used to lower LDL cholesterol. TLCs focus on four main issues: diet, exercise, weight control, and smoking cessation. These measures are first-line treatment for LDL reduction and should be implemented before drug therapy. However, TLCs can be a challenge because some people do not eat healthier diets or exercise. Physical conditions such as arthritis can limit attempts at exercise, and economic and time limitations can be a barrier to healthier eating.

The TLC Diet

This diet has two objectives: (1) reducing LDL cholesterol and (2) establishing and maintaining a healthy weight. The central feature of the diet is reduced intake of cholesterol and saturated fats: individuals should limit intake of cholesterol to 200 mg/day or less and intake of saturated fat to 7% or less of total calories. Intake of *trans fats*—found primarily in snack crackers, commercial baked goods, and fried foods—should be minimized. (Many food manufacturers are adding "no trans fat" labels to their product labels, making shopping somewhat easier.)

If the basic TLC diet fails to lower LDL cholesterol adequately, ATP III recommends two additional measures: increased intake of soluble fiber (10–25 g/day; oatmeal is a good source) and increased intake of plant stanols and sterols (2 g/day). Plant stanols and sterols are cholesterol-lowering chemicals found (albeit in very small amounts) in certain

Estimate of 10-year risk for MEN

Age	Points
20–34	−9
35–39	−4
40–44	0
45–49	3
50–54	6
55–59	8
60–64	10
65–69	11
70–74	12
75–79	13

	Points				
Total Cholesterol	Age 20–39	Age 40–49	Age 50–59	Age 60–69	Age 70–79
<160	0	0	0	0	0
160–199	4	3	2	1	0
200–239	7	5	3	1	0
240–279	9	6	4	2	1
≥280	11	8	5	3	1

	Points				
	Age 20–39	Age 40–49	Age 50–59	Age 60–69	Age 70–79
Nonsmoker	0	0	0	0	0
Smoker	8	5	3	1	1

HDL (mg/dL)	Points
≥60	−1
50–59	0
40–49	1
<40	2

Systolic BP (mm Hg)	If Untreated	If Treated
<120	0	0
120–129	0	1
130–139	1	2
140–159	1	2
≥160	2	3

Point Total	10-Year Risk %
<0	<1
0	1
1	1
2	1
3	1
4	1
5	2
6	2
7	3
8	4
9	5
10	6
11	8
12	10
13	12
14	16
15	20
16	25
≥17	≥30

10-Year Risk ______%

Estimate of 10-year risk for WOMEN

Age	Points
20–34	−7
35–39	−3
40–44	0
45–49	3
50–54	6
55–59	8
60–64	10
65–69	12
70–74	14
75–79	16

	Points				
Total Cholesterol	Age 20–39	Age 40–49	Age 50–59	Age 60–69	Age 70–79
<160	0	0	0	0	0
160–199	4	3	2	1	1
200–239	8	6	4	2	1
240–279	11	8	5	3	2
≥280	13	10	7	4	2

	Points				
	Age 20–39	Age 40–49	Age 50–59	Age 60–69	Age 70–79
Nonsmoker	0	0	0	0	0
Smoker	9	7	4	2	1

HDL (mg/dL)	Points
≥60	−1
50–59	0
40–49	1
<40	2

Systolic BP (mm Hg)	If Untreated	If Treated
<120	0	0
120–129	1	3
130–139	2	4
140–159	3	5
≥160	4	6

Point Total	10-Year Risk %
<9	<1
9	1
10	1
11	1
12	1
13	2
14	2
15	3
16	4
17	5
18	6
19	8
20	11
21	14
22	17
23	22
24	27
≥25	≥30

10-Year Risk ______%

Figure 42.3 ■ Tables for calculating Framingham Risk Prediction Scores.
To determine an individual's 10-year risk for developing clinical coronary disease, simply circle the appropriate points for each of the five risk factors considered (age, total cholesterol, smoking status, HDL cholesterol, and systolic blood pressure) and then add up the points. The point total indicates the 10-year risk. For example, a total of 13 points indicates a 10-year risk of 12% for men. (Framingham scores can also be determined using a web-based calculator, such as the one provided by the National Cholesterol Education Program at http://cvdrisk.nhlbi.nih.gov/.)

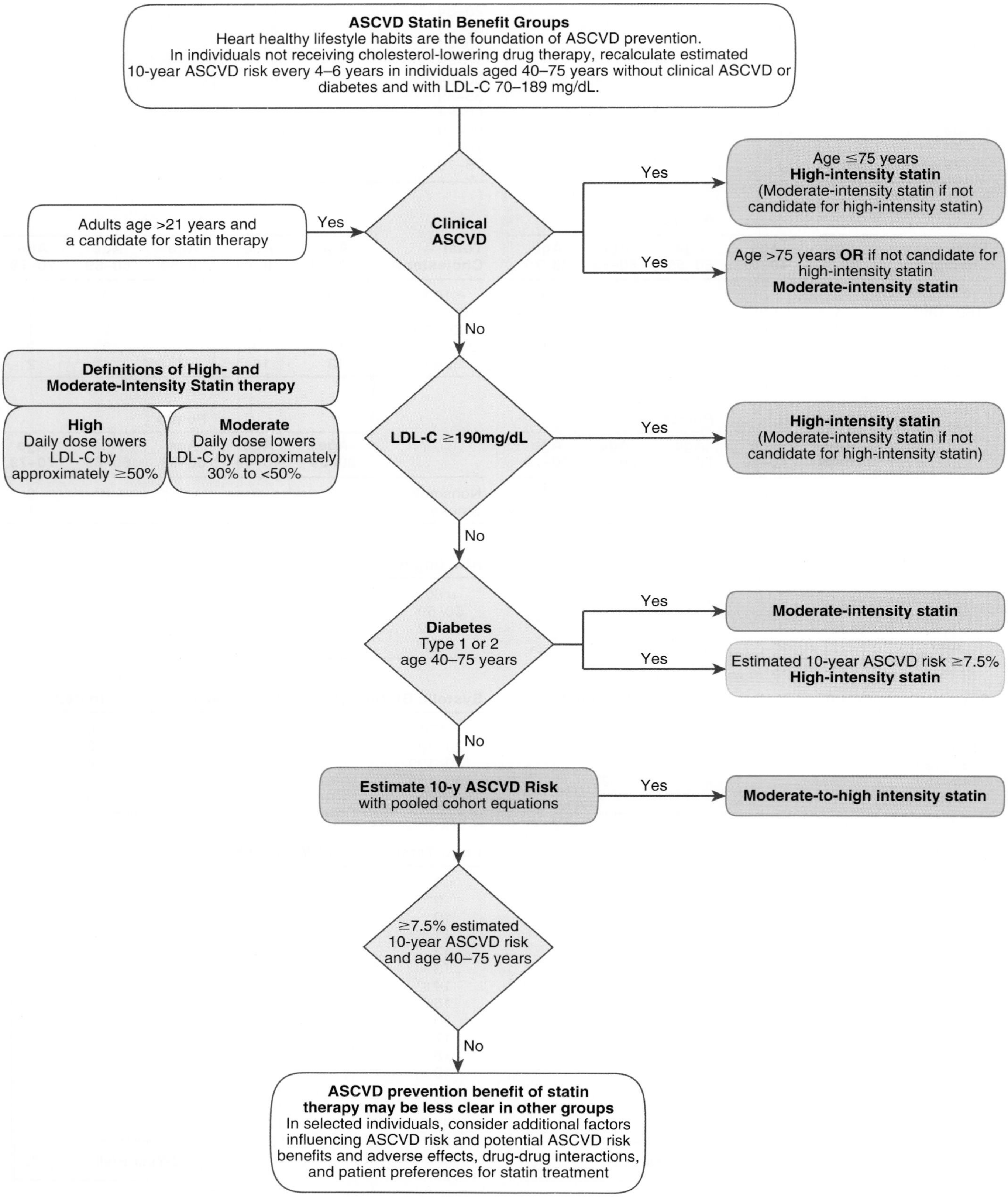

Figure 42.4 ▪ **Recommendations for statin therapy for atherosclerotic cardiovascular disease prevention.**

TABLE 42.3 ■ High-, Moderate-, and Low-Intensity Statin Therapy

High-Intensity Therapy	Moderate-Intensity Therapy	Low-Intensity Therapy
Daily dose lowers LCL-C on average by ≥50%	Daily dose lowers LDL-C on average by ~30% to <50%	Daily dose lowers LDL-C on average by <30%
Atorvastatin: 40–80 mg	Atorvastatin: 10 mg	Simvastatin: 10 mg
Rosuvastatin: 20 mg	Rosuvastatin: 10 mg	Pravastatin: 10–20 mg
	Simvastatin: 20–40 mg	Lovastatin: 20 mg
	Pravastatin: 40 mg	
	Lovastatin: 40 mg	

LDL-C, low-density lipoprotein cholesterol.
Adapted from 2013 ACC/AHA Guideline on the Treatment of Blood Cholesterol to Reduce Atherosclerotic Cardiovascular Risk in Adults: A Report of the American College of Cardiology/American Heart Association Task Force on Practice Guidelines. Available at https://circ.ahajournals.org/content/early/2013/11/11/01.cir.0000437738.63853.7a.full.pdf.

vegetable oils (e.g., canola), nuts (walnuts are a good source), certain fruits, and most beans and many other vegetables. They are also found in some of the cholesterol-lowering margarines, commonly advertised as "buttery spreads" (see later section "Plant Stanol and Sterol Esters").

Exercise

An inactive lifestyle carries an increased risk for ASCVD. Conversely, participating in regular exercise lowers ASCVD risk. Running and swimming, for example, can decrease LDL cholesterol and elevate HDL cholesterol, thereby reducing risk. In addition, exercise can reduce blood pressure, improve overall CV performance, and decrease insulin resistance (important because many people with high cholesterol also have diabetes). Accordingly, ATP III encourages regular physical activity (defined as 30–60 minutes of activity on most days). Improvements in the plasma lipid profile depend more on the total time spent exercising than on the intensity of exercise or improvements in fitness.

Smoking Cessation

Smoking cigarettes raises LDL cholesterol and lowers HDL cholesterol, thereby increasing the risk for ASCVD. Smokers should be strongly encouraged to quit—and nonsmokers should be urged not to start. Drugs to aid smoking cessation are discussed in Chapter 32.

Weight Control

Weight loss can reduce both LDL cholesterol and ASCVD risk. This is especially important for people with metabolic syndrome (see later).

Drug Therapy

Drugs are not the first-line therapy for lowering LDL cholesterol. Rather, drugs should be employed only if TLCs fail to reduce LDL cholesterol to an acceptable level—and then only if the combination of elevated LDL cholesterol and the patient's ASCVD risk category justify drug use. When drugs are used, it is essential that lifestyle modification continues because the beneficial effects of diet and drugs are additive; drugs alone may be unable to achieve the LDL goal. It is important to note that the principal benefit of drug therapy is *primary prevention:* Drugs are much better at preventing or slowing ASCVD than at promoting regression of established coronary atherosclerosis. Furthermore, because LDL cholesterol levels will return to pretreatment values if drugs are withdrawn, *treatment must continue lifelong.* Patients should be made aware of this requirement.

Table 42.4 shows properties of the drug families used to lower LDL cholesterol. The most effective agents are the *HMG-CoA reductase inhibitors* (e.g., atorvastatin [Lipitor]), usually referred to simply as *statins.* A newer class of immunologics called *monoclonal antibodies* can also be used to treat high cholesterol. Lesser used alternatives are *bile acid sequestrants* (e.g., cholestyramine) and *niacin* (nicotinic acid). Although *fibrates* are listed in Table 42.4, these drugs are used primarily to reduce levels of TGs—not LDLs. Treatment is initiated with a single drug, almost always a statin. If the statin is ineffective, a bile acid sequestrant or niacin can be added to the regimen.

In addition to lowering LDL cholesterol, drugs may be used to raise HDL cholesterol. The most effective agents are niacin and the fibrates. However, virtually all of the drugs that we use to lower LDL cholesterol have the added benefit of increasing HDL cholesterol, at least to some degree. This rise of HDL, therefore, can be considered a beneficial "side effect."

Secondary Treatment Targets

Metabolic Syndrome

The term *metabolic syndrome (also known as syndrome X)* refers to a group of metabolic abnormalities associated with an increased risk for ASCVD and type 2 diabetes. The metabolic abnormalities involved are high blood glucose, high TGs, high apolipoprotein B, low HDL, small LDL particles, a prothrombotic state, and a proinflammatory state. Hypertension is both common and important.

According to a joint scientific statement—issued by the International Diabetes Federation Task Force on Epidemiology and Prevention; the National Heart, Lung, and Blood Institute; the American Heart Association; the World Heart Federation; the International Atherosclerosis Society; and the International Association for the Study of Obesity—the metabolic syndrome is diagnosed when three or more of the following are present:

- *High TG levels*—150 mg/dL or higher (or undergoing drug therapy for high TGs)
- *Low HDL cholesterol*—below 40 mg/dL for men or below 50 mg/dL for women (or undergoing drug therapy for reduced HDL)
- *Hyperglycemia*—fasting blood glucose 100 mg/dL or higher (or undergoing drug therapy for hyperglycemia/diabetes mellitus)
- *High blood pressure*—systolic 130 mm Hg or higher and/or diastolic 85 mm Hg or higher (or undergoing drug therapy for hypertension)
- *Waist circumference 40 inches or more for most men or 35 inches or more for most women* (these limits can vary depending on ethnicity, country, or geographic region within a country)

TABLE 42.4 ▪ Drugs Used to Improve Plasma Levels of LDLs, HDLs, and Triglycerides

Drug Class	Effect on LDLs, HDLs, and TGs	Common or Serious Adverse Effects	Contraindications	Clinical Trial Results
HMG-CoA reductase inhibitors (statins)	LDL ↓ 21%–63% HDL ↑ 5%–22% TG ↓ 6%–43%	• Myopathy • Hepatotoxicity	*Absolute:* • Active or chronic liver disease • Pregnancy *Relative:* • Concurrent use of certain drugs*	Reduced major coronary events, stroke, ASCVD deaths, need for coronary procedures, and total mortality
Bile acid sequestrants	LDL ↓ 15%–30% HDL ↑ 3%–5% TG ↓/no change	• GI distress • Constipation • Reduced drug absorption	*Absolute:* • Dysbetalipoproteinemia • TG >400 mg/dL *Relative:* • TG >200 mg/dL	Reduced major coronary events and ASCVD deaths
Niacin (nicotinic acid)	LDL ↓ 14%–17% HDL ↑ 22%–26% TG ↓ 28%–35%	• Flushing • Hyperglycemia • Hyperuricemia • Upper GI distress • Hepatotoxicity	*Absolute* • Chronic liver disease • Gout *Relative:* • Diabetes • Hyperuricemia • Peptic ulcer disease	Reduced major coronary events and, possibly, reduced mortality
Fibrates	LDL ↓ 6%–10%, but may increase if TGs are high HDL ↑ 10%–20% TG ↓ 20%–50%	• Dyspepsia • Gallstones • Myopathy	*Absolute:* • Severe renal disease • Severe liver disease	Reduced major coronary events
Ezetimibe	LDL ↓ 19% HDL ↑ 1%–4% TG ↓ 5%–10%	• Headache • Myalgia, arthralgia, possible myopathy • Abdominal pain, diarrhea	*Absolute:* • Moderate to severe liver injury, especially in patients taking a statin	Effect on coronary events and mortality has not been established
PCSK9 inhibitors	LDL ↓ 50%–60%	• Hypersensitivity reactions • Injection site reactions • Antibody formation	History of hypersensitivity to Repatha or Praluent	Effect on coronary events and mortality has not been established

*Use caution in patients taking niacin, fibrates, and agents that inhibit CYP3A4 (the 3A4 isozyme of P450), including cyclosporine, macrolide antibiotics (e.g., erythromycin), azole antifungal drugs (e.g., ketoconazole), and HIV protease inhibitors (e.g., ritonavir).

↑ = increase, ↓ = decrease; ASCVD, atherosclerotic cardiovascular disease; GI, gastrointestinal; HDL, high-density lipoprotein; LDL, low-density lipoprotein; PCSK9, proprotein convertase subtilisin kexin type 9; TG, triglyceride.

Modified from the Executive Summary of the Third Report of the National Cholesterol Education Program (NCEP) Expert Panel on Detection, Evaluation, and Treatment of High Blood Cholesterol in Adults (Adult Treatment Panel III). JAMA 285:2486–2497, 2001. Data on ezetimibe are from other sources.

Treatment has two primary goals: reducing the risk for atherosclerotic disease and reducing the risk for type 2 diabetes. According to ATP III, basic therapy consists of weight control and increased physical activity, which, together, can reduce all symptoms of the metabolic syndrome. In addition, specific treatment should be directed at lowering blood pressure and TG levels. Patients should take low-dose aspirin to reduce the risk for thrombosis, unless they are at high risk for intracranial bleeds (hemorrhagic stroke).

Although the term *metabolic syndrome* is widely used, there is debate about its clinical relevance. In the CV community, most clinicians believe the term has great utility. By contrast, in the diabetes community, many clinicians feel the term is misleading, in that it implies the existence of a specific disease entity, even though it is defined only by a cluster of risk factors that may or may not have a common underlying cause. Furthermore, they point out that the risk associated with a diagnosis of metabolic syndrome is no greater than the sum of the risks of its components. Accordingly, until there is more proof that the metabolic syndrome actually exists, they believe the term serves no clinical purpose and hence should be avoided. This position was voiced in a joint statement from the American Diabetes Association and the European Association for the Study of Diabetes. The AHA and the National Heart, Lung, and Blood Institute countered with a joint statement of their own, reasserting their belief that the metabolic syndrome is an important clinical entity. Although the two camps disagree about whether the metabolic syndrome is an actual disease, both sides strongly agree that the risk factors that define the syndrome should be identified and treated.

High Triglycerides

High TG levels (above 200 mg/dL) may be an independent risk factor for ASCVD. In clinical practice, high TGs are seen most often in patients with metabolic syndrome. However, high levels may also be associated with inactive lifestyle, cigarette smoking, excessive alcohol intake, type 2 diabetes, certain genetic disorders, and high carbohydrate intake (when carbohydrates account for more than 60% of total caloric intake). In most patients with high TG levels, the first treatment goal is to achieve the original LDL goal.

Dietary modification is always recommended. Statins being taken to lower cholesterol may help lower TGs as well, perhaps to a satisfactory level. However, if TG levels remain unacceptably high, medications specific to TGs—niacin and fibrates—may be needed. Unfortunately, when these drugs are combined with cholesterol-lowering drugs (as they often are), the adverse effects of cholesterol-lowering agents may be intensified.

DRUGS AND OTHER PRODUCTS USED TO IMPROVE PLASMA LIPID LEVELS

As discussed earlier, the lipid abnormality that contributes most to CV disease is high LDL cholesterol. Accordingly, we will focus primarily on drugs for this disorder. Nonetheless, we also need to consider other lipid abnormalities, especially (1) high total cholesterol,[a] (2) low HDL cholesterol, and (3) high TGs.

Some drugs for dyslipidemias are more selective than others. That is, whereas some drugs may improve just one dyslipidemia (e.g., high TGs), others may improve two or more dyslipidemias. The highly selective agents can be useful as add-ons, to "target" a particular lipid abnormality when other medications prove inadequate.

Drugs that lower *LDL cholesterol* levels include HMG-CoA reductase inhibitors (statins), bile acid sequestrants, monoclonal antibodies, niacin, and ezetimibe. All are effective to varying degrees. The HMG-CoA reductase inhibitors—the statins—are more effective than the others, cause fewer adverse effects, are better tolerated, and are more likely to improve clinical outcomes.

As we consider the drugs for lipid disorders, you should be aware of the following: although all of these drugs can improve lipid profiles, not all of them improve clinical outcomes (reduced morbidity and mortality). This leads us to question whether some of the lipid abnormalities are a true cause of pathophysiology and ultimate death, or whether they are simply "associated markers" of some other pathophysiology that we don't yet understand.

Prototype Drugs

LDL CHOLESTEROL– AND TRIGLYCERIDE-LOWERING DRUGS

HMG-CoA Reductase Inhibitor (Statin)

Lovastatin

Bile Acid Sequestrant

Colesevelam

Monoclonal Antibodies (Proprotein Convertase Subtilisin/Kexin Type 9 [PCSK9] Inhibitors)

Alirocumab
Evolocumab

Others

Nicotinic acid
Ezetimibe

[a]Note that total cholesterol is slightly different from the simple sum of LDL cholesterol (LDL-C) plus HDL cholesterol (HDL-C); triglycerides (TGs) also contribute to the value, as in the following equation: total cholesterol = HDL-C + LDL-C + (TG/5) (provided TG levels are below 400 mg/dL).

HMG-CoA Reductase Inhibitors (Statins)

HMG-CoA reductase inhibitors, commonly called *statins,* are the most effective drugs for lowering LDL and total cholesterol. In addition, they can raise HDL cholesterol and lower TGs in some patients. Most important, these drugs have been shown to improve clinical outcomes, including lowering the risk for heart failure, MI, and sudden death. Because of these benefits, and because so many people have ASCVD risks associated with dyslipidemias, statins are among our most widely prescribed drugs—and have earned tens of billions for their makers.

Beneficial Actions

The statins have several actions that can benefit patients with (or at risk for) atherosclerosis. The most obvious and important are reductions of LDL cholesterol.

Reduction of LDL Cholesterol

Statins have a profound effect on LDL cholesterol. Low doses decrease LDL cholesterol by about 25%, and larger doses decrease levels by as much as 63% (Table 42.5). Reductions are significant within 2 weeks and maximum within 4 to 6 weeks. Because cholesterol synthesis normally increases during the night, statins are most effective when given in the evening. If statin therapy is stopped, serum cholesterol will return to pretreatment levels within weeks to months. Therefore treatment should continue lifelong, unless serious adverse effects or specific contraindications (especially pregnancy or muscle damage) arise. The mechanism by which statins reduce cholesterol levels is discussed later.

Elevation of HDL Cholesterol

Statins can increase levels of HDL cholesterol. Recall that low levels of HDL cholesterol (below 40 mg/dL) are an independent risk factor for ASCVD. Hence, by raising HDL cholesterol, statins may help reduce the risk for CV events in yet another way. The objective is to raise levels to 50 mg/dL or more.

Reduction of Triglyceride Levels

Although statins mainly affect cholesterol synthesis and thereby lower LDL cholesterol levels, these drugs may also lower TGs. Just why these "anticholesterol" drugs lower TGs is unknown, but the response has been amply documented. Please note that, although statins may reduce TG levels, they are not actually prescribed for this action. Hence TG reduction is usually a beneficial side effect in patients taking statins to lower their LDL cholesterol. Of note, the ability to lower TGs seems to be short lived, and hence a drug designed to lower TGs (e.g., niacin) eventually may need to be added.

Nonlipid Beneficial CV Actions

There is increasing evidence that statins do more than just alter lipid levels. Specifically, they can promote atherosclerotic plaque stability (by decreasing plaque cholesterol content),

TABLE 42.5 ▪ HMG-CoA Reductase Inhibitors: Selected Aspects of Clinical Pharmacology

Drug	% Change in Serum Lipids*			Effect of CYP3A4 Inhibitors on Statin Levels†	Effect of Renal or Hepatic Impairment on Statin Levels
	LDL-C	HDL-C	TGs		
Atorvastatin [Lipitor]	↓ 25–60	↑ 5–15	↓ 15–50	Moderate ↑	No change with renal disease; significant ↑ with hepatic impairment
Fluvastatin [Lescol, Lescol XL]	↓ 20–40	↑ 2–11	↓ 10–25	None	No change with renal disease; possible ↑ with hepatic impairment
Lovastatin [Altoprev, Mevacor]	↓ 20–40	↑ 5–10	↓ 5–25	Significant ↑	↑ with significant renal impairment; no change with hepatic impairment
Pitavastatin [Livalo]	↓ 40–45	↑ 6–8	↓ 15–30	Little or none	↑ with significant renal impairment; little or no change with hepatic impairment
Pravastatin [Pravachol]	↓ 20–40	↑ 1–15	↓ 10–25	None	Potential ↑ with either renal or hepatic impairment
Rosuvastatin [Crestor]	↓ 30–60	↑ 3–20	↓ 10–40	None	↑ levels with severe renal impairment or hepatic dysfunction
Simvastatin [Zocor]	↓ 25–50	↑ 7–15	↓ 8–40	Significant ↑	Potential ↑ with severe renal or hepatic impairment

*The values were obtained from a variety of studies, and do not reflect dose dependency of drug responses.

†Inhibitors of CYP3A4 (the 3A4 isoenzyme of P450) include itraconazole, ketoconazole, erythromycin, clarithromycin, HIV protease inhibitors, cyclosporine, nefazodone, and substances in grapefruit juice.

↑, increase; ↓, decrease; HDL-C, high-density lipoprotein cholesterol; LDL-C, low-density lipoprotein cholesterol; TGs, triglycerides.

reduce inflammation at the plaque site, slow progression of coronary artery calcification, improve abnormal endothelial function, enhance the ability of blood vessels to dilate, reduce the risk for atrial fibrillation, and reduce the risk for thrombosis by (1) inhibiting platelet deposition and aggregation and (2) suppressing production of thrombin, a key factor in clot formation. All of these actions help reduce the risk for CV events.

Mechanism of Cholesterol Reduction

The mechanism by which statins decrease LDL cholesterol levels is complex and depends ultimately on *increasing the number of LDL receptors on hepatocytes*. The process begins with inhibition of hepatic HMG-CoA reductase, the rate-limiting enzyme in cholesterol biosynthesis. In response to decreased cholesterol production, hepatocytes synthesize more HMG-CoA reductase. As a result, cholesterol synthesis is largely restored to pretreatment levels. However—and for reasons that are not fully understood—inhibition of cholesterol synthesis causes hepatocytes to synthesize more LDL receptors. As a result, hepatocytes are better able to remove more LDLs from the blood. In patients who are genetically unable to synthesize LDL receptors, statins fail to reduce LDL levels, indicating that (1) inhibition of cholesterol synthesis, by itself, is not sufficient to explain cholesterol-lowering effects; and (2) for statins to be effective, synthesis of LDL receptors must increase.

In addition to inhibiting HMG-CoA reductase, statins decrease production of apolipoprotein B-100. As a result, hepatocytes decrease production of VLDLs. This lowers VLDL levels, and TG levels too, because they're the main lipid in VLDLs. Also, statins raise HDL levels by 5% to 22%.

Clinical Trials

Statins slow progression of ASCVD and decrease the risk for stroke, hospitalization, cardiac events, peripheral vascular disease, and death. Benefits are seen in men and women, and in apparently healthy people as well as those with a history of CV events. Hence the statins are useful for both primary and secondary prevention. Furthermore, these drugs can even help people with *normal* LDL levels, in addition to those whose LDL level is high. Statins may also have some added protective effects in people with diabetes.

Secondary Prevention Studies

In patients with evidence of existing ASCVD (angina pectoris or previous MI), statins reduce the risk for death from cardiac causes. This was first demonstrated conclusively in the landmark Scandinavian Simvastatin Survival Study (4S). After 4.9 to 6.3 years of follow-up, the death rate was 12% among patients taking placebo and 8% among those taking simvastatin—a 30% decrease in overall mortality. Benefits were due to a decrease in cardiac-related mortality; deaths from noncardiac causes were the same in both groups.

The Cholesterol and Recurrent Events (CARE) trial demonstrated the ability of statins to reduce the risk for stroke in addition to coronary events. In this study, 4159 people with a history of MI were given pravastatin (40 mg daily) or placebo. After 5 years, the incidence of MI (fatal or nonfatal) was 13.2% in those taking placebo and 10.2% in those taking the drug. Pravastatin also produced a 26% decrease in the risk for stroke.

The Pravastatin or Atorvastatin Evaluation and Infection Therapy (PROVE-IT) trial was the first to show that intensive reductions in LDL with statin therapy provide more CV protection than moderate reductions. In PROVE-IT, 4162 patients with ACS were randomized to either a moderate statin regimen (pravastatin, 40 mg daily) or an intensive statin regimen (atorvastatin, 80 mg daily). The result? LDL levels in the moderate group dropped to 62 mg/dL, compared with 95 mg/dL in the intensive group. Furthermore, not only did intensive therapy produce a greater decrease in LDL cholesterol, it produced a greater reduction in adverse outcomes: after 24 months, the incidence of CV events (death, MI, unstable angina, or revascularization) was only 22.4% in the intensive group compared with 26.3% in the moderate group. These results led the ATP III panel to recommend lower target LDL levels in patients at very high CV risk.

Primary Prevention Studies

Two major studies have demonstrated the ability of statins to reduce mortality in people with no previous history of coronary events. In the first trial—the West of Scotland Coronary Prevention Study (WOSCOPS)—6595 men with high cholesterol were given either pravastatin (40 mg/day) or placebo. During an average follow-up of 4.9 years, 4.1% of those taking placebo died, compared with only 3.2% of those taking the statin. The second trial—the Air Force/Texas Coronary Atherosclerosis Prevention Study (AFCAPS/

TexCAPS)—enrolled 6605 low-risk patients: men and women with average cholesterol levels (221 mg/dL) and no history of CV events. The subjects were randomly assigned to receive lovastatin (20–40 mg/day) or placebo. After an average follow-up of 5.5 years, the incidence of first major coronary events was 5.5% for those taking placebo and 3.5% for those taking the drug—representing a 36% decrease in risk.

Primary Prevention in Patients with Normal Cholesterol Levels

The landmark Heart Protection Study, published in 2002, was the first major trial to demonstrate that statins can reduce the risk for major coronary events in people who have normal levels of cholesterol. This double-blind, placebo-controlled trial enrolled 20,536 high-risk British patients: men and women with diabetes, prior MI, stroke, or prior angioplasty. Some had high levels of LDL and total cholesterol; others had normal levels. Subjects were randomly assigned to receive either simvastatin (40 mg/day) or placebo. After 5 years, the incidence of death was 12.9% in the treatment group, compared with 14.7% in the placebo group. Death from ASCVD was reduced by 18%. In addition, simvastatin reduced the risk for nonfatal MI by 38% and of stroke by 25% and reduced the need for coronary revascularization (e.g., angioplasty) by 30%. Most strikingly, benefits were seen in patients whose LDL cholesterol was normal or low, as well as in those whose levels were high. These data suggest a radical shift in practice. Specifically, they suggest we should treat people at high ASCVD risk—not just those with high cholesterol levels. Obviously, doing so would greatly expand the number of patients receiving statin therapy.

A more recent trial—Justification for the Use of Statins in Prevention: an Intervention Trial Evaluating Rosuvastatin (JUPITER)—reinforced the results of the Heart Protection Study. The study demonstrated that rosuvastatin can reduce the risk for coronary events in people with normal LDL levels but with high levels of CRP and other risk factors for ASCVD.

Prevention in Patients with Diabetes

Results of the Collaborative Atorvastatin Diabetes Study (CARDS) indicate that statin therapy can reduce the risk for CV events in diabetes patients, even if LDL levels are normal. This randomized trial, conducted in Britain and Ireland, enrolled 2838 patients with type 2 diabetes who had no history of CV disease. Half received 10 mg of atorvastatin [Lipitor] daily, and half received a placebo. After a mean of 4 years, the combined incidence of acute coronary events, coronary revascularization, and stroke was only 5.8% in the atorvastatin group, compared with 9% in the placebo group, representing a 36% reduction in risk. These results suggest that statin therapy could benefit most patients with diabetes, regardless of their LDL level.

Therapeutic Uses

When the statins were introduced, they were approved only for hypercholesterolemia (elevated LDL cholesterol levels) in adults. As understanding of their benefits grew, so has the list of indications. Today the statins have nearly a dozen U.S. Food and Drug Administration (FDA)–approved indications and can be prescribed for young patients as well as adults. Indications for individual statins are shown in Table 42.6. Major indications are discussed next.

Hypercholesterolemia

Statins are the most effective drugs we have for lowering LDL cholesterol. In sufficient dosage, statins can decrease LDL cholesterol by more than 60%. For many patients, the treatment goal is to drop LDL cholesterol to below 100 mg/dL. For patients at very high CV risk, a target of 70 mg/dL may be appropriate.

Primary and Secondary Prevention of CV Events

As discussed, statins can reduce the risk for CV events (e.g., MI, angina, stroke) in patients who have never had one (primary prevention), and they can reduce the risk for a subsequent event after one has occurred (secondary prevention). Risk reduction is related to the reduction in LDL: the greater the LDL reduction, the greater the reduction in risk.

Primary Prevention in People With Normal LDL Levels

One agent—*rosuvastatin* [Crestor]—is approved for reducing the risk for CV events in people with *normal* levels of LDL and no clinically evident ASCVD, but who do have an increased risk based on advancing age, high levels of *high-sensitivity C-reactive protein,* and at least one other risk factor for CV disease (e.g., hypertension, low HDL, smoking). Approval for this use was based in large part on results of the JUPITER trial.

TABLE 42.6 ▪ HMG-CoA Reductase Inhibitors: FDA-Approved Indications

Indication	Atorvastatin [Lipitor]	Fluvastatin [Lescol, Lescol XL]	Lovastatin [Altoprev, Mevacor]	Pitavastatin [Livalo]	Pravastatin [Pravachol]	Rosuvastatin [Crestor]	Simvastatin [Zocor]
Primary hypercholesterolemia	✔	✔	✔	✔	✔	✔	✔
Homozygous familial hyperlipidemia	✔					✔	✔
Heterozygous familial hypercholesterolemia in adolescents	✔		✔		✔	✔	✔
Mixed dyslipidemia	✔	✔	✔	✔	✔	✔	✔
Primary dysbetalipoproteinemia	✔				✔	✔	✔
Primary prevention of coronary events	✔		✔		✔	✔*	✔
Secondary prevention of CV events	✔	✔	✔		✔		✔
Increasing HDL cholesterol in primary hypercholesterolemia	✔		✔	✔		✔	✔
Prevention of MI and stroke in type 2 diabetes	✔		✔				
Slowing progression of coronary atherosclerosis		✔	✔		✔	✔	

*Rosuvastatin is approved for primary prevention in patients who have *normal* low-density lipoprotein cholesterol and no clinical evidence of atherosclerotic cardiovascular disease but who do have high levels of C-reactive protein combined with other risk factors for cardiovascular disease.

Post-MI Therapy

Patients who have survived an MI, and who were not on statin therapy at the time of the event, are routinely started on a statin, the rationale being "better late than never." The current trend is to begin statins as soon as the patient is stabilized and able to take oral drugs. Other drugs for MI are discussed in Chapter 88.

Diabetes

Cardiovascular disease is the primary cause of death in people with diabetes. Hence, to reduce mortality, controlling CV risk factors—especially hypertension and high cholesterol—is as important as controlling high blood glucose. The American Diabetes Association recommends a statin for all patients older than 40 years whose LDL cholesterol is greater than 100 mg/dL. The American College of Physicians recommends a statin for (1) all patients with type 2 diabetes plus diagnosed ASCVD—*even if they don't have high cholesterol;* and (2) all adults with type 2 diabetes plus one additional risk factor (e.g., hypertension, smoking, age older than 55 years)—*even if they don't have high cholesterol.* Taken together, these guidelines suggest that most patients with diabetes should receive a statin.

Pharmacokinetics

Statins are administered orally. The amount absorbed ranges between 30% and 90%, depending on the drug. Regardless of how much is absorbed, most of an absorbed dose is extracted from the blood on its first pass through the liver, the principal site at which statins act. Only a small fraction of each dose reaches the systemic circulation. Statins undergo rapid hepatic metabolism followed by excretion primarily in the bile. Only four agents—*lovastatin, pitavastatin, pravastatin,* and *simvastatin*—undergo clinically significant (10%–20%) excretion in the urine.

Three statins—*atorvastatin, lovastatin,* and *simvastatin*—are metabolized by CYP3A4 (the 3A4 isoenzyme of cytochrome P450). As a result, levels of these drugs can be lowered by agents that induce CYP3A4 synthesis and speed up the metabolic inactivation of the statin. More important, statin levels can be increased—sometimes dramatically—by agents that inhibit CYP3A4 (see later).

One agent—*rosuvastatin*—reaches abnormally high levels in people of Asian heritage. At usual therapeutic doses, rosuvastatin levels in these people are about twice those in whites. Accordingly, if rosuvastatin is used by Asians, dosage should be reduced.

Adverse Effects

Statins are generally well tolerated. Side effects are uncommon. Some patients develop headache, rash, or gastrointestinal (GI) disturbances (dyspepsia, cramps, flatulence, constipation, abdominal pain). However, these effects are usually mild and transient. Serious adverse effects—hepatotoxicity and myopathy—are relatively rare. Some statins pose a greater risk than others, as noted subsequently.

Myopathy and Rhabdomyolysis

Statins can injure muscle tissue. *Mild injury* occurs in 5% to 10% of patients. Characteristic symptoms are muscles aches, tenderness, or weakness that may be localized to certain muscle groups or diffuse. Rarely, mild injury progresses to *myositis,* defined as muscle inflammation associated with moderate elevation of creatine kinase (CK), an enzyme released from injured muscle. Release of potassium from muscle may cause blood potassium concentrations to rise. Rarely, myositis progresses to potentially fatal *rhabdomyolysis,* defined as muscle disintegration or dissolution. Release of muscle components leads to marked elevations of blood CK (greater than 10 times the upper limit of normal [ULN]) and elevations of free myoglobin. High levels of CK, in turn, may cause *renal impairment* because excess CK can plug up the glomeruli, thereby preventing normal filtration.

Fortunately, fatal rhabdomyolysis is extremely rare: the overall incidence is less than 0.15 case per 1 million prescriptions. Nonetheless, patients should be informed about the risk for myopathy and instructed to notify the prescriber if unexplained muscle pain or tenderness occurs. How statins cause myopathy is unknown.

Several factors increase the risk for myopathy. Among these are advanced age, small body frame, frailty, multisystem disease (e.g., chronic renal insufficiency, especially associated with diabetes), use of statins in high doses, low vitamin D and coenzyme Q levels, concurrent use of fibrates (which can cause myopathy too), and use of drugs that can raise statin levels (see later). In addition, hypothyroidism increases risk. Accordingly, if muscle pain develops, thyroid function should be assessed. Measurement of CK levels can facilitate diagnosis. Levels should be determined at baseline and again if symptoms of myopathy appear. If the CK level is more than 10 times the ULN, the statin should be discontinued. If the level is less than 10 times the ULN, the statin can be continued, provided myopathy symptoms and the CK level are followed weekly. However, given that weekly blood tests are expensive and inconvenient, it may be best to stop the statin and reevaluate therapy, even when CK levels *are* less than 10 times the ULN. Routine monitoring of CK in asymptomatic patients is unnecessary.

Of the seven statins in current use, *rosuvastatin* [Crestor] poses the highest risk for rhabdomyolysis. But even with this drug, the absolute number of cases is extremely low. With the other statins, the risk is even lower. The risk for serious myopathy is extremely low, whereas the risk for untreated LDL cholesterol is very high. Accordingly, when statins are used to lower cholesterol, the benefits of therapy (reduction of CV events) far outweigh the small risk for myopathy. Additional strategies for management of myalgia include replacement of vitamin D and coenzyme Q and switching statins. Studies reveal that replacement of vitamin D and coenzyme Q can reduce myalgias in patients with low levels. Switching statins can be effective because patients may not have myalgias when taking a different drug, even if it is within the same class.

Hepatotoxicity

Liver injury, as evidenced by elevations in serum transaminase levels, develops in 0.5% to 2% of patients treated 1 year or longer. However, jaundice and other clinical signs are rare. Progression to outright liver failure occurs very rarely. Because of the risk for liver injury, product labeling recommends that liver function tests (LFTs) be done before treatment and then if clinically indicated after starting the drug. If serum transaminase levels rise to 3 times the ULN and remain there, statins should be discontinued. Transaminase levels decline to pretreatment levels after drug withdrawal.

In patients with viral or alcoholic hepatitis, statins should be avoided. However, in patients with the most common cause of hepatitis—nonalcoholic fatty liver disease—statins are acceptable therapy. In fact, in these patients, not only can statins reduce cholesterol levels, they may also decrease liver inflammation, improve LFTs, and reduce steatosis (fatty infiltration in the liver). LFTs should be monitored at baseline and as clinically indicated thereafter. If LFTs climb to 3 times the ULN, statin use should stop.

New-Onset Diabetes

The risk for developing new-onset diabetes while taking a statin is 1 in 500 patients prescribed a statin. Yet many of the patients in these studies had prediabetes before taking a statin. It is unclear whether taking a statin accelerates the advancement from prediabetes to diabetes. Despite the possibility, the CV benefits of taking a statin far outweigh the risk, and management should not change.

Cataracts

An analysis of military health care records between 2003 and 2010 revealed a 27% increase of cataracts in patients who had taken a statin for at least 90 days compared with patients not taking statins. Because this was just one retrospective study in a specific population, more studies are warranted. Until that time, patients should continue taking their statin as prescribed.

Drug Interactions

With Other Lipid-Lowering Drugs

Combining a statin with most other lipid-lowering drugs (except probably the bile acid sequestrants) can increase the incidence and severity of the most serious statin-related adverse events: muscle injury, liver injury, and kidney damage. Increased risk occurs primarily with fibrates (gemfibrozil, fenofibrate), which are commonly combined with statins. The bottom line: when statins are combined with other lipid-lowering agents, use extra caution and monitor for adverse effects more frequently.

With Drugs That Inhibit CYP3A4

Drugs that inhibit CYP3A4 can raise levels of *lovastatin* and *simvastatin* substantially and can raise levels of *atorvastatin* moderately, by slowing their inactivation. Important inhibitors of CYP3A4 include macrolide antibiotics (e.g., erythromycin), azole antifungal drugs (e.g., ketoconazole, itraconazole), HIV protease inhibitors (e.g., ritonavir), amiodarone (an antidysrhythmic drug), and cyclosporine (an immunosuppressant). If these drugs are combined with a statin, increased caution is advised. Some authorities recommend an automatic reduction in statin dosage if these inhibitors are used.

As discussed in Chapter 6, chemicals in grapefruit and grapefruit juice can inhibit CYP3A4. Furthermore, the inhibition may persist for 3 days or more after eating the fruit or drinking its juice. Accordingly, statin users should avoid grapefruits and their juice.

Use in Pregnancy

Statins are classified in FDA Pregnancy Risk Category X: the risks to the fetus outweigh any potential benefits of treatment. Some statins have caused fetal malformation in animal models—but only at doses far higher than those used in humans. To date, teratogenic effects in humans have not been reported. Nonetheless, because statins inhibit synthesis of cholesterol, and because cholesterol is required for synthesis of cell membranes as well as several fetal hormones, concern regarding human fetal injury remains. Moreover, there is no compelling reason to continue lipid-lowering drugs during pregnancy: stopping the statin for 9 months is not going to cause a sudden, dangerous rise in cholesterol levels or risk for ASCVD. Women of childbearing age should be informed about the potential for fetal harm and warned against becoming pregnant. If pregnancy occurs and the patient plans to continue the pregnancy, statins should be discontinued.

Preparations, Dosage, and Administration

Statins are available alone and in fixed-dose combinations. The single-ingredient products are discussed next. The combination products are discussed later in the chapter under the heading "Drug Combinations."

Seven statins are available for use alone: atorvastatin, fluvastatin, lovastatin, pitavastatin, pravastatin, rosuvastatin, and simvastatin. Information on preparations, dosage, and administration is shown in Table 42.7.

Dosing is done once daily, preferably in the *evening* either with the evening meal or at bedtime. Because endogenous cholesterol synthesis increases during the night, statins have the greatest effect when given in the evening.

Drug Selection

Several factors bear on statin selection, including the LDL goal, drug interactions, kidney function, safety in Asian patients, and price.

LDL Goal

If a 30% to 40% reduction in LDL is deemed sufficient, any statin will do. However, if LDL must be lowered by more than 40%, then atorvastatin or simvastatin may be preferred. Furthermore, not only are these two drugs highly effective, clinical experience with them is extensive.

Drug Interactions

Drugs that inhibit CYP3A4 can raise levels of atorvastatin, lovastatin, and simvastatin, thereby increasing the risk for toxicity, especially myopathy and liver injury. Accordingly, in patients taking a CYP3A4 inhibitor, other statins may be preferred.

Kidney Function

For patients with normal renal function, any statin is acceptable. However, for patients with significant renal impairment, atorvastatin and fluvastatin are preferred (because no dosage adjustment is needed).

Safety in Asians

The same dose of *rosuvastatin,* when given to Asian and white subjects, may produce twofold higher blood levels in the Asians. Accordingly, when rosuvastatin is used in Asians, start with the lowest available dosage and monitor diligently.

Niacin (Nicotinic Acid)

Niacin [Niacor, Niaspan] reduces LDL and TG levels—and it increases HDL levels better than any other drug. However,

TABLE 42.7 ▪ HMG-CoA Reductase Inhibitors: Preparations, Dosage, and Administration

Drug	Dosage	Administration With Regard to Meals	Dosage Changes in Special Populations	Preparations
Atorvastatin [Lipitor]	*Initial:* 10 mg at bedtime *Maximum:* 80 mg at bedtime	Take without regard to meals	No changes needed	*Lipitor (tablets):* 10, 20, 40, 80 mg
Fluvastatin [Lescol, Lescol XL]	*Initial:* 20–40 mg at bedtime *Maximum, Lescol:* 40 mg twice a day *Maximum, Lescol XL:* 80 mg at bedtime	Take without regard to meals	Reduce dosage for severe renal impairment	*Lescol (capsules):* 20, 40 mg *Lescol XL (extended-release tablets):* 80 mg
Lovastatin [Altoprev, Mevacor; generics]	*Initial:* 20 mg *Maximum:* 40 mg twice daily or 80 mg at bedtime	Take immediate-release tablets with evening meal to increase absorption. Take extended-release tablets at bedtime.	Reduce dosage for severe renal impairment	*Altoprev (extended-release tablets):* 20, 40, 60 mg *Mevacor and generics (tablets):* 10, 20, 40 mg
Pitavastatin [Livalo]	*Initial:* 2 mg once daily at any time of day *Maximum:* 4 mg once daily	Take without regard to meals	Reduce dosage for moderate to severe renal impairment	*Livalo (tablets):* 1, 2, 4 mg
Pravastatin [Pravachol; generics]	*Initial:* 40 mg at bedtime *Maximum:* 80 mg at bedtime	Take without regard to meals	Reduce dosage for moderate to severe renal impairment	*Pravachol and generics (tablets):* 10, 20, 40, 80 mg
Rosuvastatin [Crestor]	*Initial:* 5–20 mg at bedtime *Maximum:* 40 mg at bedtime	Take without regard to meals	Reduce dosage for severe renal impairment Reduce dosage in Asian patients	*Crestor (tablets):* 5, 10, 20, 40 mg
Simvastatin [Zocor; generics]	*Initial:* 20 mg at bedtime *Maximum:* 40 mg/day (Before 2011, the maximum recommended dosage was higher: 80 mg/day)	Take without regard to meals	Reduce dosage for severe renal impairment	*Zocor and generics (tablets):* 5, 10, 20, 40, 80 mg

despite these favorable effects on lipid levels, niacin does little to improve outcomes, as shown by the AIM-HIGH trial in 2011. Principal adverse effects are intense flushing, GI upset, and liver injury. Niacin is available in three formulations, which differ with respect to onset, duration, and the incidence and severity of side effects.

Effect on Plasma Lipoproteins

Niacin reduces LDL cholesterol by 14% to 17% and TGs by 28% to 35%. In addition, it raises HDL cholesterol by 28% to 35%. Triglyceride levels begin to fall within the first 4 days of therapy. LDL levels decline more slowly, taking 3 to 5 weeks for maximal reductions. Combining niacin with lovastatin can reduce LDL cholesterol by 45% and can raise HDL cholesterol by 41%. Triple therapy (niacin plus a statin plus a bile acid sequestrant) can decrease LDL cholesterol by 70% or more.

Mechanism of Action

The mechanism underlying effects on plasma lipids is not completely understood. We do know that niacin acts in the liver and adipose tissue to inhibit synthesis of TGs and thereby decreases production of VLDLs. Since LDLs are byproducts of VLDL degradation, the fall in VLDL levels causes LDL levels to fall, too. How niacin raises levels of HDL is unclear.

The AIM-HIGH Trial

The AIM-HIGH trial, sponsored by the U.S. National Heart, Lung, and Blood Institute, was designed to answer an important question: does raising HDL cholesterol with niacin reduce the risk for CV events? The study enrolled 3414 patients with low HDL cholesterol, high TGs, and a history of CV disease. Half received simvastatin plus a placebo, and half received simvastatin plus Niaspan (extended-release niacin tablets). After 32 months, Niaspan significantly reduced CV risk factors: compared with patients who took simvastatin alone, patients who took simvastatin plus niacin had higher levels of HDL cholesterol and lower levels of TGs. However, despite these favorable effects on lipid levels, clinical outcomes were not changed: patients who received simvastatin plus niacin had the same incidence of CV events—stroke, fatal or nonfatal MI, hospitalization for ACS, revascularization of coronary arteries—as did those who took simvastatin alone. Clearly, the reduction in *risk factors* with niacin did not reduce *actual risk.* At this time, we don't know if these unexpected results apply to *all* drugs that raise HDL levels, or if they apply only to niacin.

Therapeutic Use

Uses of niacin include mixed elevation of LDLs and TGs and elevation of TGs in combination with low levels of HDLs. One formulation—sold as Niaspan—is approved for raising HDL cholesterol.

Niacin also has a role as a vitamin. The doses employed to correct niacin deficiency are *much* lower than those employed to reduce lipoprotein levels (about 25 mg/day rather than 1–3 g/day). The role of niacin as a vitamin is discussed in Chapter 65.

Adverse Effects

The most frequent adverse reactions involve the skin (flushing, itching) and GI tract (gastric upset, nausea, vomiting, diarrhea). *Intense flushing* of the face, neck, and ears occurs in practically all patients receiving niacin in pharmacologic doses. This reaction diminishes in several weeks and can be attenuated by taking 325 mg of aspirin 30 minutes before each dose. (Aspirin reduces flushing by preventing synthesis of prostaglandins, which mediate the flushing response.) Flushing can also be reduced by using extended-release niacin (e.g., Niaspan) rather than immediate-release niacin (e.g., Niacor).

Niacin is *hepatotoxic*. Severe liver damage has occurred. Liver injury is least likely with Niaspan, the extended-release formulation noted previously. Other long-acting products—sustained-release, controlled-release, or timed-release (e.g., Slo-Niacin) products—should be avoided, owing to increased risk for hepatotoxicity. Because of possible hepatotoxicity, liver function should be assessed before treatment and periodically thereafter.

Niacin can elevate blood levels of uric acid. Exercise caution in patients with gout, and even in patients who have hyperuricemia but no symptoms of gout.

Additional adverse effects are *hyperglycemia* and *gouty arthritis*.

Preparations, Dosage, and Administration

Niacin (niacin) is marketed generically and under several trade names. The drug is available in tablets (immediate-release, timed-release, controlled-release, sustained-release, extended-release) or capsules (timed-release, extended-release, sustained-release).

With immediate-release formulations (prescription Niacor and over-the-counter products), blood levels of niacin climb rapidly. As a result, these products are associated with the highest incidence and severity of facial and upper body flushing, at least for the first few weeks. Thereafter, the intensity of these responses tends to fade. To manage flushing, patients using immediate-release niacin often take prophylactic aspirin. (The need for aspirin is much lower with the long-acting products.) With immediate-release niacin, blood levels of niacin can fall relatively soon. Therefore, to maintain steady blood levels, the total daily dose should be given as two or three divided doses (1–3 g total) rather than as one large dose.

The most popular niacin formulation is Niaspan, an extended-release formulation. After oral dosing, the tablet slowly dissolves, causing blood levels to rise slowly and remain relatively steady. As a result, flushing is minimized, and once-daily dosing (usually 1–3 g) is adequate. The major drawback to Niaspan is that it costs more than other niacin products.

Long-acting niacin [Slo-Niacin] has a longer half-life than other formulations. Although this may seem like a therapeutic advantage (longer lasting high levels of drug), there is an increased risk for hepatotoxicity, and hence this product should be avoided.

Bile Acid Sequestrants

Bile acid sequestrants reduce LDL cholesterol levels. In the past, these drugs were a mainstay of lipid-lowering therapy. Today, they are used primarily as adjuncts to statins. Three agents are available: colesevelam, cholestyramine, and colestipol. Colesevelam is newer than the other two and is better tolerated.

Colesevelam

Colesevelam [Welchol] is the drug of choice when a bile acid sequestrant is indicated. Like the older sequestrants, colesevelam is a nonabsorbable resin that binds (sequesters) bile acids and other substances in the GI tract and thereby prevents their absorption and promotes their excretion. Colesevelam is preferred to the older sequestrants for three reasons: (1) The drug is better tolerated (less constipation, flatulence, bloating, and cramping); (2) It does not reduce absorption of fat-soluble vitamins (A, D, E, and K); and (3) It does not significantly reduce the absorption of statins, digoxin, warfarin, and most other drugs studied.

In addition to its beneficial effects on plasma lipids, colesevelam can help control hyperglycemia in patients with type 2 diabetes. The drug was approved for adjunctive therapy of diabetes in 2008. Diabetes and its management are the subject of Chapter 46.

Effect on Plasma Lipoproteins

The main response to bile acid sequestrants is a reduction in LDL cholesterol. LDL decline begins during the first week of therapy and becomes maximal (about a 20% drop) within about a month. When these drugs are discontinued, LDL cholesterol returns to pretreatment levels in 3 to 4 weeks.

Bile acid sequestrants may increase VLDL levels in some patients. In most cases, the elevation is transient and mild. However, if VLDL levels are elevated before treatment, the increase induced by the bile acid sequestrants may be sustained and substantial. Accordingly, bile acid sequestrants are not drugs of choice for lowering LDL cholesterol in patients with high VLDL levels.

Pharmacokinetics

Bile acid sequestrants are biologically inert. Also, they are insoluble in water, cannot be absorbed from the GI tract, and are not attacked by digestive enzymes. After oral administration, they simply pass through the intestine and are excreted in the feces.

Mechanism of Action

The bile acid sequestrants lower LDL cholesterol through a mechanism that ultimately depends on increasing LDL receptors on hepatocytes. As background, you need to know that bile acids secreted into the intestine are normally reabsorbed and reused. Bile acid sequestrants prevent this reabsorption. After oral dosing, these drugs form an insoluble complex with bile acids in the intestine; this complex prevents the reabsorption of bile acids and thereby accelerates their excretion. Because bile acids are normally reabsorbed, the increase in excretion creates a demand for increased synthesis, which takes place in the liver. Because bile acids are made from cholesterol, liver cells require an increased cholesterol supply to increase bile acid production. The required cholesterol is provided by LDL. To avail themselves of more LDL cholesterol, liver cells increase their number of LDL receptors, thereby increasing their capacity for LDL uptake. The result is an increase in LDL uptake from plasma, which decreases circulating LDL levels. Individuals who are genetically incapable of increasing LDL receptor synthesis are unable to benefit from these drugs.

Therapeutic Use

Colesevelam is indicated as adjunctive therapy to diet and exercise for reducing LDL cholesterol in patients with primary hypercholesterolemia. The drug may be used alone but usually is combined with a statin. On average, colesevelam alone can lower LDL cholesterol by about 20% (the typical range is between 15% and 30%). In contrast, combined therapy with a statin can reduce LDL cholesterol by up to 50%. Similar results can be obtained by combining a sequestrant with niacin.

Adverse Effects

The bile acid sequestrants are not absorbed from the GI tract and hence are devoid of systemic effects. Accordingly, they are safer than all other lipid-lowering drugs.

Adverse effects are limited to the GI tract. *Constipation* is the main complaint. This can be minimized by increasing dietary fiber and fluids. If necessary, a mild laxative may be used. Other GI effects include *bloating, indigestion,* and *nausea.* The older agents—cholestyramine and colestipol—can decrease fat absorption and may thereby *decrease uptake of fat-soluble vitamins.* However, this does not seem to be a problem with colesevelam.

Drug Interactions

The bile acid sequestrants can form insoluble complexes with other drugs. Medications that undergo binding cannot be absorbed and hence are not available for systemic effects. Drugs known to form complexes with the sequestrants include thiazide diuretics, digoxin, warfarin, and some antibiotics. To reduce formation of sequestrant-drug complexes, oral medications that are known to interact should be administered either 1 hour before the sequestrant or 4 hours after.

Preparations, Dosage, and Administration

Colesevelam [Welchol] is supplied in tablets (625 mg) and as a powder (1.875 and 3.75 g) for making an oral suspension. With the tablets, the initial adult dosage is 3 tablets (1.9 g) twice daily or 6 tablets (3.8 g) once daily. With the oral suspension, the initial adult dosage is 1.875 g twice daily or 3.75 g once daily. All doses are taken with food and water. Of note, the dosage for colesevelam is much smaller than that of cholestyramine (4–24 g/day) or colestipol (5–30 g/day).

Older Agents: Cholestyramine and Colestipol

Cholestyramine and colestipol have been available for decades but have been largely replaced by colesevelam because colesevelam is better tolerated, does not impede absorption of fat-soluble vitamins, and has minimal effects on other drugs. Although cholestyramine and colestipol are very safe, they frequently cause constipation, abdominal discomfort, and bloating.

Cholestyramine [Questran, Questran Light, Prevalite] is supplied in powdered form. Instruct patients to mix the powder with fluid because swallowing it dry can cause esophageal irritation and impaction. Appropriate liquids for mixing include water, fruit juices, and soups. Pulpy fruits with a high fluid content (e.g., applesauce, crushed pineapple) may also be used. The dosage range is 4 to 24 g/day.

Colestipol hydrochloride [Colestid] is supplied in granular form (5 g) and in 1-g tablets. The dosage for the granules is 5 to 30 g/day administered in one or more doses. Instruct patients to mix the granules with fluids or pulpy fruits before ingestion. The dosage for the tablets is 2 to 16 g/day administered in one or more doses. Tablets should be swallowed whole and taken with fluid.

Ezetimibe

Ezetimibe [Zetia, Ezetrol ♣] is a unique drug for reducing plasma cholesterol. Benefits derive from blocking cholesterol absorption.

Mechanism of Action and Effect on Plasma Lipoproteins

Ezetimibe acts on cells of the brush border of the small intestine to inhibit dietary cholesterol absorption. The drug also inhibits reabsorption of cholesterol secreted in the bile. Treatment reduces plasma levels of total cholesterol, LDL cholesterol, TGs, and apolipoprotein B. In addition, ezetimibe can produce a small *increase* in HDL cholesterol.

Therapeutic Use

Ezetimibe is indicated as an adjunct to diet modification for reducing total cholesterol, LDL cholesterol, and apolipoprotein B in patients with primary hypercholesteremia. The drug is approved for monotherapy and for combined use with a statin. In clinical trials, ezetimibe alone reduced LDL cholesterol by about 19%, increased HDL cholesterol by 1% to 4%, and decreased TGs by 5% to 10%. When ezetimibe was combined with a statin, the reduction in LDL cholesterol was about 25% greater than with the statin alone. Despite these desirable effects on blood lipids, there is no evidence that ezetimibe reduces atherosclerosis or improves clinical outcomes.

Pharmacokinetics

Ezetimibe is administered orally, and absorption is not affected by food. In the intestinal wall and liver, ezetimibe undergoes extensive conversion to ezetimibe glucuronide, an active metabolite. Both compounds—ezetimibe itself and its main metabolite—are eliminated primarily in the bile. The elimination half-life is about 22 hours.

Adverse Effects

Ezetimibe is generally well tolerated. During clinical trials, the incidence of significant side effects was nearly identical to that seen with placebo. However, during postmarketing surveillance, there have been reports of myopathy, rhabdomyolysis, hepatitis, pancreatitis, and thrombocytopenia. In contrast to the bile acid sequestrants, ezetimibe does not cause constipation and other adverse GI effects.

Drug Interactions

Statins

In patients taking a statin, adding ezetimibe slightly increases the risk for liver damage (as indicated by elevated transaminase levels). If the drugs are combined, transaminase levels should be monitored before starting therapy as well as whenever clinically indicated thereafter. Combining ezetimibe with a statin may also increase the risk for myopathy.

Fibrates

Both ezetimibe and fibrates (gemfibrozil and fenofibrate) can increase the cholesterol content of bile and can thereby increase the risk for gallstones. Both also increase the risk for myopathy. Accordingly, combined use is not recommended.

Bile Acid Sequestrants

Cholestyramine (and possibly colestipol) can significantly decrease the absorption of ezetimibe. To minimize effects on absorption, ezetimibe should be administered at least 2 hours before a sequestrant or more than 4 hours after.

Cyclosporine

Cyclosporine may greatly increase levels of ezetimibe. If the drugs are combined, careful monitoring is needed.

Caution

In patients with hepatic impairment, bioavailability of ezetimibe is significantly increased. At this time, we do not know whether increased availability is harmful. Until more is known, patients with moderate or severe hepatic insufficiency should not be given the drug.

Preparations, Dosage, and Administration

Ezetimibe [Zetia, Ezetrol ♣] is available in 10-mg tablets. The recommended dosage is 10 mg once a day, taken with or without food. If ezetimibe is combined with a statin, both drugs can be taken at the same time. If ezetimibe is combined with a bile acid sequestrant, ezetimibe should be taken 2 hours before the sequestrant or 4 hours after.

Fibric Acid Derivatives (Fibrates)

The fibric acid derivatives, also known as *fibrates,* are the most effective drugs we have for lowering TG levels. In addition, these drugs can raise HDL cholesterol but have little or no effect on LDL cholesterol. Furthermore, there is no proof that fibrates reduce mortality from ASCVD. Fibrates can increase the risk for bleeding in patients taking warfarin (an anticoagulant) and the risk for rhabdomyolysis in patients taking statins. Because of these and other undesired effects, and because mortality is not reduced, fibrates are considered third-line drugs for managing lipid disorders. In the United States three preparations are available: gemfibrozil [Lopid], fenofibrate [Tricor, others], and fenofibric acid [TriLipix, Fibricor], a delayed-release preparation noteworthy for being the first and only fibrate *approved* for use with a statin.

Gemfibrozil

Gemfibrozil [Lopid] decreases TG (VLDL) levels and raises HDL cholesterol levels. The drug does not reduce LDL cholesterol to a significant degree. Its principal indication is hypertriglyceridemia.

Effect on Plasma Lipoproteins

Gemfibrozil decreases plasma TG content by lowering VLDL levels. Maximal reductions in VLDLs range from 40% to 55% and are achieved within 3 to 4 weeks of treatment. Gemfibrozil can raise HDL cholesterol by 6% to 10%. In patients with normal TG levels, the drug can produce a small reduction in LDL levels. However, if TG levels are high, gemfibrozil may actually increase LDL levels.

Mechanism of Action

Gemfibrozil and other fibrates appear to work by interacting with a specific receptor subtype—known as peroxisome proliferator-activated receptor alpha (PPAR alpha)—present in the liver and brown adipose tissue. Activation of PPAR alpha leads to (1) increased synthesis of lipoprotein lipase (LPL) and (2) reduced production of apolipoprotein C-III (an inhibitor of LPL). Both actions accelerate the clearance of VLDLs and thereby reduce levels of TGs. How do fibrates elevate HDL levels? By activating PPAR alpha, fibrates increase production of apolipoproteins A-I and A-II, which in turn facilitates HDL formation.

Therapeutic Use

Gemfibrozil is used primarily to *reduce high levels of plasma triglycerides* (VLDLs). Treatment is limited to patients who have not responded adequately to weight control and diet modification. Gemfibrozil can also reduce LDL cholesterol slightly. However, other drugs (statins, cholestyramine, colestipol) are much more effective.

Gemfibrozil can be used to *raise HDL cholesterol,* although it is not approved for this application. When tested in patients with normal LDL cholesterol and low HDL cholesterol, gemfibrozil reduced the risk for major CV events—but did not reduce *mortality* from ASCVD. Because LDL cholesterol was normal, it appears that benefits were due primarily to elevation of HDL cholesterol, along with reduction of plasma TGs.

Adverse Effects

Gemfibrozil is generally well tolerated. The most common reactions are rash and GI disturbances (nausea, abdominal pain, diarrhea).

Gallstones. Gemfibrozil increases biliary cholesterol saturation, thereby increasing the risk for gallstones. Patients should be informed about manifestations of gallbladder disease (e.g., upper abdominal discomfort, intolerance of fried foods, bloating) and instructed to notify the prescriber at once if these develop. Patients with preexisting gallbladder disease should not take the drug.

Myopathy. Like the statins, gemfibrozil and other fibrates can cause myopathy. Warn patients to report any signs of muscle injury, such as tenderness, weakness, or unusual muscle pain.

Liver Injury. Gemfibrozil is hepatotoxic. The drug can disrupt liver function and may also pose a risk for liver cancer. Periodic tests of liver function are recommended.

Drug Interactions

Gemfibrozil displaces warfarin from plasma albumin, thereby increasing anticoagulant effects. Prothrombin time (international normalized ratio) should be measured frequently to assess coagulation status. Warfarin dosage may need to be reduced.

As noted, gemfibrozil increases the risk for *statin-induced myopathy.* Accordingly, the combination of a statin with gemfibrozil should be used with great caution, if at all.

Preparations, Dosage, and Administration

Gemfibrozil [Lopid] is available in 600-mg tablets. The adult dosage is 600 mg twice a day. Dosing is done 30 minutes before the morning and evening meals.

Fenofibrate

Actions and Uses

Fenofibrate [Tricor, Antara, Lofibra, Triglide, Lipofen, Lipidil ♣] is indicated for hypertriglyceridemia in patients who have not responded to dietary measures. The drug lowers TGs by decreasing levels of VLDLs.

Pharmacokinetics

Fenofibrate is well absorbed from the GI tract, especially in the presence of food. When absorbed, the drug is rapidly converted to fenofibric acid, its active form. In the blood, the drug is 98% protein bound. Elimination is the result of hepatic metabolism followed by renal excretion. The plasma half-life is about 20 hours.

Adverse Effects and Drug Interactions

The most common adverse effects are rash and GI disturbances. Like gemfibrozil, fenofibrate can cause gallstones and liver injury. In animal models, doses 1 to 6 times the maximal human dose caused cancers of the pancreas and liver. Like gemfibrozil, fenofibrate can increase the risk for bleeding with warfarin and the risk for myopathy with statins.

Preparations, Dosage, and Administration

Fenofibrate is available in several formulations that differ with respect to dosage and the impact of food on absorption. Four products are discussed here.

Tricor tablets (48 and 145 mg) are made using NanoCrystal technology to enhance absorption. As a result, dosing can be done with or without food. The dosage range is 48 to 145 mg/day.

Triglide tablets (160 mg), like Tricor tablets, may be administered with or without food. The dosage is 160 mg/day.

Antara capsules (30 and 90 mg), which contain micronized particles, must be administered with food to maximize absorption. The dosage range is 39 to 90 mg/day.

Lofibra capsules (54 and 160 mg) contain micronized particles. Like Antara, Lofibra must be administered with food to maximize absorption. The dosage range is 54 to 160 mg/day.

Fenofibric Acid

Fenofibric acid [TriLipix, Fibricor] is the active metabolite of fenofibrate. Accordingly, the pharmacology of the drug is much like that of the parent compound. Fenofibric acid stands out from other fibrates for being the only group member approved for use with a statin. However, there is no proof that combining the drug with a statin reduces the risk for a major CV event. Furthermore, just like other fibrates, fenofibric acid can cause myopathy, and hence combined use with a statin still poses significant myopathy risk. Therefore the combination must be employed with great care. Fenofibric acid is available in delayed-release capsules (45 and 135 mg, sold as TriLipix; 35 and 105 mg, sold as Fibricor). Daily dosages for hypertriglyceridemia range from 35 to 135 mg. In patients with mild to moderate renal impairment, a low dosage (45 mg/day) should be used. When combined with a statin for patients with mixed dyslipidemias, fenofibric acid should be dosed at 135 mg/day.

MONOCLONAL ANTIBODIES (PROPROTEIN CONVERTASE SUBTILISIN/KEXIN TYPE 9 [PCSK9] INHIBITORS)

Alirocumab [Praluent] and Evolocumab [Repatha] compose a new type of drug class used for patients with high LDL levels, specifically in patients with heterozygous familial hypercholesterolemia or atherosclerotic heart problems who need additional lowering of LDL cholesterol. The PCSK9 inhibitors are indicated as an adjunct to diet modification and maximally tolerated statin therapy for reducing total LDL cholesterol.

Mechanism of Action and Effect on Plasma Lipoproteins

Proprotein convertase subtilisin kexin type 9 (PCSK9) is a protein that binds to low-density lipoprotein receptors (LDLRs) within the liver. LDLR is the primary receptor that clears circulating LDL. When PCSK9 binds to LDLRs, there is an increase in LDL cholesterol because LDLRs cannot clear LDL. By inhibiting PCSK9, we can free up LDLRs and decrease circulating levels of LDL in the blood.

Pharmacokinetics

PCSK9 inhibitors are administered subcutaneously. Because monoclonal antibodies are composed of protein, no specific metabolism studies were conducted. It is thought that the proteins degrade to small peptides and amino acids within the body. Both drugs have a long half-life of 11 to 20 days.

Adverse Effects

Hypersensitivity

Hypersensitivity reactions, including vasculitis, rash, and urticarial requiring hospitalization, have been noted with use of PCSK9 inhibitors.

Immunogenicity

Because this class of drug is composed of protein, there is risk for developing antibodies: 4.8% of patients treated with alirocumab and 0.1% treated with evolocumab developed antibodies to the drug after initiating treatment. These patients also had a higher incidence of injection site reactions compared with patients who did not develop antibodies.

Drug Interactions

Neither drug is noted to have any significant drug interactions.

Preparations, Dosage, and Administration

Alirocumab [Praluent] is available in 75- and 150-mg/mL single-dose prefilled pens and syringes. The recommended dosage is 75 mg subcutaneously every 2 weeks. If the LDL cholesterol response is inadequate, the dose may be increased to 150 mg every 2 weeks. Injection may be administered into the thigh, abdomen, or upper arm.

Evolocumab [Repatha], like alirocumab, is administered subcutaneously every 2 weeks. The recommended dose is 140 mg. Repatha is available in 140-mg/mL single-use prefilled syringes or a 140-mg/mL single-use SureClick autoinjector. Alternate dosing of 420 mg can also be administered every 4 weeks.

Drug Combinations

Simvastatin/Ezetimibe [Vytorin]

Actions and Uses

Simvastatin and ezetimibe are available in fixed-dose combination tablets sold as Vytorin. Vytorin is approved for treatment of mixed dyslipidemia, hypercholesterolemia, and familial hypertriglyceridemia. Because ezetimibe has a different mechanism of action than simvastatin, the combination can lower cholesterol more effectively than simvastatin alone.

With this combination, the dose of simvastatin required to effectively lower cholesterol may be lower than the dose required when simvastatin is used alone. As a result, the risk for statin-related adverse effects can be reduced. Additional benefits of the combination are convenience (take just one pill instead of two) and reduced cost (the combination costs less than both drugs purchased separately).

Despite the advantages of Vytorin, some authorities are concerned that the combination may be less beneficial than simvastatin alone. This concern is based on four facts:

- We have proof that simvastatin alone can decrease adverse outcomes (i.e., MI and other CV events).
- We have no proof that the combination can decrease adverse outcomes of elevated cholesterol (even though it can reduce levels of cholesterol).
- In addition to lowering cholesterol, statins have other beneficial actions (e.g., they often lower elevated TGs).
- When ezetimibe and simvastatin are combined, cholesterol goals can be met using simvastatin in reduced dosage (which is a problem for reasons discussed next).

Because the combination permits a reduction in simvastatin dosage, there is concern that, although the target cholesterol goal may be reached, the reduction in adverse outcomes may be smaller than when cholesterol is lowered using simvastatin alone. Despite concerns, the FDA reviewed the evidence and determined that, although there was no significant change in carotid artery thickness after taking Vytorin, there was a significant decrease in LDL cholesterol in people taking Vytorin, which may decrease CV risk. For this reason, the FDA recommends that patients continue treatment on Vytorin.

Adverse Effects and Drug Interactions

Vytorin is generally well tolerated. However, myopathy is a concern (because both drugs can cause muscle injury). Concurrent use of a fibrate, which can also cause myopathy, increases risk. The risk for myopathy and other adverse effects is also increased by inhibitors of CYP3A4, the enzyme that inactivates simvastatin. Because Vytorin contains a statin, the product is contraindicated for women who are pregnant and for patients with liver disease.

Preparations, Dosage, and Administration

Vytorin tablets contain 10 mg of ezetimibe plus either 10, 20, 40, or 80 mg of simvastatin. The usual starting dosage is 10 mg ezetimibe/20 mg simvastatin each day. Dosing is done once daily, preferably in the evening. The simvastatin dosage can be increased as needed and tolerated.

Atorvastatin/Amlodipine [Caduet]

Atorvastatin and amlodipine (a calcium channel blocker) are available in fixed-dose combination tablets under the trade name Caduet. This is the first single product indicated for dyslipidemia combined with hypertension and/or angina. The combination has one advantage over taking each drug separately: fewer pills to swallow. Eleven amlodipine/atorvastatin combinations are available: 2.5 mg amlodipine with either 10, 20, or 40 mg atorvastatin; 5 mg amlodipine with either 10, 20, 40, or 80 mg atorvastatin; and 10 mg amlodipine with either 10, 20, 40, or 80 mg atorvastatin. Dosage is individualized on the basis of therapeutic response and tolerance of adverse effects. The pharmacology of amlodipine and other calcium channel blockers is discussed in Chapter 37.

Fish Oil

Consuming fatty fish or fish-oil supplements was once associated with a decreased risk for ASCVD and ASCVD-related death. Unfortunately, recent studies have revealed that consuming fish oil provides no advantage in prevention of heart disease in high-risk populations. Yet it is still believed that taking fish oil can reduce the incidence of heart dysrhythmias after MI or heart failure.

Fish oil may be beneficial in prevention of heart dysrhythmias because it contains two "heart healthy" compounds: eicosapentaenoic acid (EPA) and docosahexaenoic acid (DHA). Both compounds are long-chain, omega-3 polyunsaturated fatty acids, with a methyl group at one end and a carboxyl group at the other. They are called omega-3 fatty acids because they have a double bond located three carbons in from the methyl terminus.

How do omega-3 fatty acids help us? The answer is unclear. Benefits of lower doses (850 mg to 1 g) may result from reducing platelet aggregation; reducing thrombosis (by effects on platelets and the vascular endothelium); reducing inflammation (which may help stabilize atherosclerotic plaques); and reducing blood pressure and cardiac dysrhythmias.

Because the evidence is so new regarding lack of benefit in primary prevention of heart disease, the AHA still recommends eating at least two servings of fish a week. Fish with high concentrations of EPA and DHA are preferred. Among these are mackerel, halibut, herring, salmon, albacore tuna, and trout. The goal is to take in, on average, about 1 g of fish oil a day.

Because fish concentrate certain environmental contaminants—especially methylmercury, dioxins, and polychlorinated biphenyls (PCBs)—eating fish carries some risk. Methylmercury can cause heart disease as well as neurologic damage, manifesting as tremor, numbness, tingling, altered vision, and impaired concentration. Exposure in utero or during early childhood can lead to developmental delay, blindness, and seizures. With dioxin and PCBs, carcinogenesis is the major concern. For postmenopausal women, and for men who are middle-aged or older, the benefits of fish outweigh the risks. For women who are pregnant or breastfeeding, fish consumption should be limited to 12 ounces a week, and certain species—swordfish, king mackerel, shark, and golden snapper, all of which may have high levels of methylmercury—should be avoided entirely. Young children should limit fish consumption, too. For people who like salmon, dioxin exposure can be reduced by eating wild salmon, which contains much less dioxin than farm-raised salmon. Exposure to all contaminants can be reduced by using fish-oil supplements, which have much less contamination than fish themselves.

Lovaza

Lovaza is the trade name for the first preparation of omega-3-acid ethyl esters approved by the FDA. The product, available only by prescription, contains a combination of EPA and DHA. Lovaza is approved as an adjunct to dietary measures to reduce very high levels of TGs (500 mg/dL or greater). When used alone, Lovaza can reduce TG levels by 20% to 50%. Combining it with simvastatin produces a further decrease. Because large doses of omega-3 fatty acids can impair platelet function, leading to prolonged bleeding time, the product should be used with care in patients taking anticoagulants or antiplatelet drugs, including aspirin. Lovaza is supplied in 1-g, liquid-filled, soft-gelatin capsules that contain approximately 465 mg of EPA and approximately 375 mg of DHA. The recommended dosage is 4 g/day, taken either all at once (4 capsules) or in two doses (2 capsules twice a day).

Epanova

In 2014, the FDA approved an additional preparation of omega-3-carboxylic acids. Epanova is approved as an adjunct to diet therapy in reducing triglycerides in patients with severe hypertriglyceridemia. Although Epanova has been used to reduce triglyceride levels, its effect on morbidity and mortality has not been determined. Epanova is available in 1-g gelatin capsules. The recommended dose is 2 or 4 g once daily.

Plant Stanol and Sterol Esters

Stanol esters and sterol esters, which are analogs of cholesterol, can reduce intestinal absorption of cholesterol (by 10%) and can thereby reduce levels of LDL cholesterol (by 14%). These compounds do not affect HDL levels or TG levels. ATP III recommends adding plant stanols or sterols to the diet if the basic TLC diet fails to reduce LDL cholesterol to the target level. Where can you get plant stanols and sterols? Two good sources are the Benecol brand of margarine, and soft spreads sold under the trade name Promise.

Estrogen

In postmenopausal women, estrogen therapy (0.625 mg/day) reduces LDL cholesterol by 15% to 25% and increases HDL cholesterol by 10% to 15%. However, despite these beneficial effects on blood lipids, estrogen therapy does little to reduce CV morbidity or mortality in older women. In fact, when estrogen is combined with a progestin for postmenopausal therapy, the risk for MI and other CV events actually goes up. Accordingly, estrogen therapy is no longer recommended for CV protection in postmenopausal women. The risks and benefits of estrogen therapy are discussed in Chapter 48.

Cholestin

Cholestin is the trade name for a dietary supplement that can lower cholesterol levels. The product is made from rice fermented with red yeast. Its principal active ingredient—lovastatin—is identical to the active ingredient in Mevacor, a brand-name, cholesterol-lowering drug. In addition to lovastatin, Cholestin contains at least seven other HMG-CoA reductase inhibitors (statins).

Several clinical trials have demonstrated that Cholestin can lower cholesterol levels, although none has studied its effects on CV events. In a trial conducted at Tufts University School of Medicine, Cholestin reduced total cholesterol by 11.4% and LDL cholesterol by 21% and increased HDL cholesterol by 14.6%. Similarly, in a study conducted at the University of California at Los Angeles Medical School, Cholestin reduced total cholesterol by 16% and LDL cholesterol by 22%. Whether Cholestin also reduces the incidence of ASCVD is unknown.

Information on Cholestin is lacking in four important areas: clinical benefits, adverse effects, drug interactions, and precise mechanism of action. As noted, there are no data on the ability of Cholestin to reduce the risk for MI, stroke, or any other CV event. In contrast, the clinical benefits of prescription statins (lovastatin and all the others) are fully documented. There is little or no information on the adverse effects or drug interactions of Cholestin. In contrast, the safety (and hazards) of prescription statins, as well as their drug interactions, have been studied extensively.

The mechanism by which Cholestin lowers cholesterol levels is only partly understood. The recommended daily dose of Cholestin contains only 5 mg of lovastatin and varying doses of other HMG-CoA reductase inhibitors, compared with 10 mg for the lowest recommended dose of Mevacor. Hence, it seems unlikely that the statins in Cholestin can fully account for the supplement's ability to reduce cholesterol levels. This implies that Cholestin has one or more active ingredients that have not yet been identified. What they are and how they may work is a mystery.

What's the bottom line? Until more is known about Cholestin, stick with statins—medications of proven safety and efficacy. Furthermore, for people with health insurance, using statins is cheaper: most insurers will cover the cost of statins, but will not pay for Cholestin.

CHAPTER

43 Drugs for Angina Pectoris

Laura D. Rosenthal, DNP, ACNP, FAANP

Angina pectoris is defined as sudden pain beneath the sternum, often radiating to the left shoulder, left arm, and jaw. Anginal pain is precipitated when the oxygen supply to the heart is insufficient to meet oxygen demand. Most often, angina occurs secondary to atherosclerosis of the coronary arteries, so angina should be seen as a symptom of a disease and not as a disease in its own right. In the United States more than 10 million people have chronic stable angina; about 500,000 new cases develop annually.

Drug therapy of angina has two goals: (1) prevention of myocardial infarction (MI) and death and (2) prevention of myocardial ischemia and anginal pain. Two types of drugs are employed to decrease the risk for MI and death: cholesterol-lowering drugs and antiplatelet drugs. These agents are discussed in Chapters 42 and 44, respectively.

In this chapter, we focus on antianginal drugs (i.e., drugs that prevent myocardial ischemia and anginal pain). There are three main families of antianginal agents: *organic nitrates* (e.g., nitroglycerin), *beta blockers* (e.g., metoprolol), and *calcium channel blockers* (CCBs; e.g., verapamil). In addition, a fourth agent—*ranolazine*—can be combined with these drugs to supplement their effects. Most of the chapter focuses on the organic nitrates. Beta blockers and CCBs are discussed at length in previous chapters, so consideration here is limited to their use in angina.

DETERMINANTS OF CARDIAC OXYGEN DEMAND AND OXYGEN SUPPLY

Before discussing angina pectoris, we need to review the major factors that determine cardiac oxygen demand and supply.

Oxygen Demand

The principal determinants of cardiac oxygen demand are heart rate, myocardial contractility, and, most important, intramyocardial wall tension. Wall tension is determined by two factors: cardiac preload and cardiac afterload. (Preload and afterload are defined in Chapter 34.) In summary, cardiac oxygen demand is determined by (1) heart rate, (2) contractility, (3) preload, and (4) afterload. Drugs that reduce these factors reduce oxygen demand.

Oxygen Supply

Cardiac oxygen supply is determined by myocardial blood flow. Under resting conditions, the heart extracts nearly all of the oxygen delivered to it by the coronary vessels. Therefore the only way to accommodate an increase in oxygen demand is to increase blood flow. When oxygen demand increases, coronary arterioles dilate; the resultant decrease in vascular resistance allows blood flow to increase. During exertion, coronary blood flow increases fourfold to fivefold. It is important to note that myocardial perfusion takes place only during diastole. Perfusion does not take place during systole because the vessels that supply the myocardium are squeezed shut when the myocardium contracts.

ANGINA PECTORIS: PATHOPHYSIOLOGY AND TREATMENT STRATEGY

Angina pectoris has three forms: (1) *chronic stable angina* (exertional angina), (2) *variant angina* (Prinzmetal or vasospastic angina), and (3) *unstable angina.* Our focus is on stable angina and variant angina. Consideration of unstable angina is discussed in the acute care chapter at the end of your text.

Chronic Stable Angina (Exertional Angina)

Pathophysiology

Stable angina is triggered most often by an increase in physical activity. Emotional excitement, large meals, and cold exposure may also precipitate an attack. Because stable angina usually occurs in response to strain, this condition is also known as *exertional angina* or *angina of effort.*

The underlying cause of exertional angina is coronary artery disease (CAD), a condition characterized by deposition of fatty plaque in the arterial wall. If an artery is only partially blocked by plaque, blood flow will be reduced and angina pectoris will result. However, if complete vessel blockage occurs, blood flow will stop and MI (heart attack) will result.

The effect of CAD on the balance between myocardial oxygen demand and oxygen supply is shown in Fig. 43.1. In both the healthy heart and the heart with CAD, oxygen supply and oxygen demand are in balance during rest. In the presence of CAD, resting oxygen demand is met through dilation of arterioles distal to the partial occlusion. This dilation reduces resistance to blood flow, compensating for the increase in resistance created by plaque.

The picture is very different during exertion. In the healthy heart, as cardiac oxygen demand rises, coronary arterioles dilate, causing blood flow to increase. The increase keeps oxygen supply in balance with oxygen demand. By contrast, in people with CAD, arterioles in the affected region are already fully dilated during rest. Thus, when exertion occurs, there is no way to increase blood flow to compensate for the increase in oxygen demand. The resultant imbalance between oxygen supply and oxygen demand causes anginal pain.

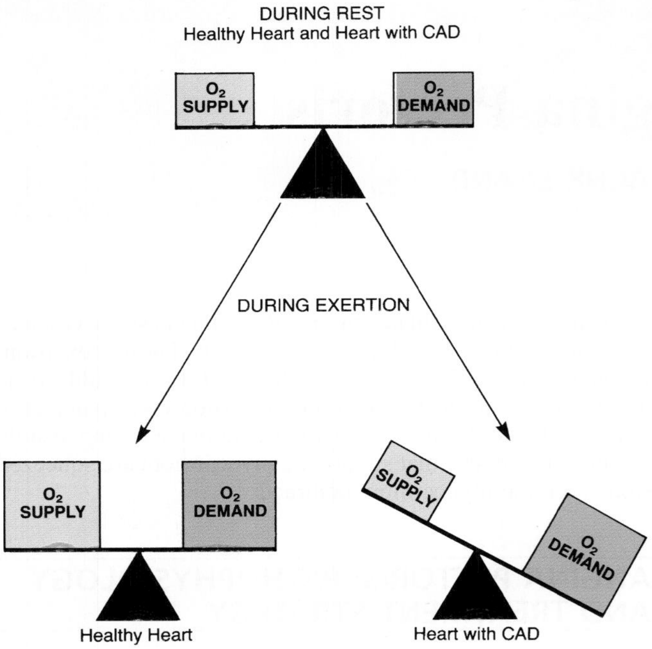

Figure 43.1 ▪ Effect of exertion on the balance between oxygen supply and oxygen demand in the healthy heart and the heart with CAD.
In the healthy heart, O_2 supply and O_2 demand are always in balance; during exertion, coronary arteries dilate, producing an increase in blood flow to meet the increase in O_2 demand. In the heart with CAD, O_2 supply and O_2 demand are in balance only during rest. During exertion, dilation of coronary arteries cannot compensate for the increase in O_2 demand, and an imbalance results.

TABLE 43.1 ▪ Mechanisms of Antianginal Action

	Mechanism of Pain Relief	
Drug Class	**Stable Angina**	**Variant Angina**
Nitrates	*Decrease oxygen demand* by dilating veins, which decreases preload	*Increase oxygen supply* by relaxing coronary vasospasm
Beta blockers	*Decrease oxygen demand* by decreasing heart rate and contractility	Not used
Calcium channel blockers	*Decrease oxygen demand* by dilating arterioles, which decreases afterload (all calcium blockers), and by decreasing heart rate and contractility (verapamil and diltiazem)	*Increase oxygen supply* by relaxing coronary vasospasm
Ranolazine	*Appears to decrease oxygen demand,* possibly by helping the myocardium generate energy more efficiently	Not used

Treatment Strategy

The goal of antianginal therapy is to reduce the intensity and frequency of anginal attacks. Because anginal pain results from an imbalance between oxygen supply and oxygen demand, logic dictates two possible remedies: (1) increase cardiac oxygen supply or (2) decrease oxygen demand. Because the underlying cause of stable angina is occlusion of the coronary arteries, there is little we can do to increase cardiac oxygen supply. Therefore the first remedy is not a real option. Consequently, all we really can do is *decrease cardiac oxygen demand.* As discussed earlier, oxygen demand can be reduced with drugs that decrease heart rate, contractility, afterload, and preload.

Overview of Therapeutic Agents

Stable angina can be treated with three main types of drugs: *organic nitrates, beta blockers,* and *calcium channel blockers.* As noted previously, *ranolazine* can be combined with these drugs for additional benefit. All four groups relieve the pain of stable angina primarily by decreasing cardiac oxygen demand (Table 43.1). Please note that drugs only provide symptomatic relief; they do not affect the underlying pathology. To reduce the risk for MI, all patients with known CAD should receive an antiplatelet drug (e.g., aspirin) unless it is contraindicated. Other measures to reduce the risk for infarction are discussed later in the section "Drugs Used to Prevent Myocardial Infarction and Death."

Nondrug Therapy

Patients should attempt to avoid factors that can precipitate angina. These include overexertion, heavy meals, emotional stress, and exposure to cold.

Risk factors for stable angina should be corrected. Important among these are smoking, hypertension, hyperlipidemia, and a sedentary lifestyle. Patients should be strongly encouraged to quit smoking. Patients with a sedentary lifestyle should be encouraged to establish a regular program of aerobic exercise. Hypertension and hyperlipidemia are major risk factors and should be treated. These disorders are discussed in Chapters 39 and 42, respectively.

Variant Angina (Prinzmetal Angina, Vasospastic Angina)

Pathophysiology

Variant angina is caused by *coronary artery spasm,* which restricts blood flow to the myocardium. Hence, as in stable angina, pain is secondary to insufficient oxygenation of the heart. In contrast to stable angina, whose symptoms occur primarily at times of exertion, variant angina can produce pain at any time, even during rest and sleep. Frequently, variant angina occurs in conjunction with stable angina.

Treatment Strategy

The goal is to reduce the incidence and severity of attacks. In contrast to stable angina, which is treated primarily by reducing oxygen demand, variant angina is treated by *increasing cardiac oxygen supply.* This makes sense in that the pain is caused by a reduction in oxygen supply, rather than by an increase in demand. Oxygen supply is increased with vasodilators, which prevent or relieve coronary artery spasm.

Overview of Therapeutic Agents

Vasospastic angina is treated with two groups of drugs: *calcium channel blockers* and *organic nitrates.* Both relax coronary artery spasm. Beta blockers and ranolazine, which are effective in stable angina, are not effective in variant angina. As with stable angina, therapy is symptomatic only; drugs do not alter the underlying pathology.

ORGANIC NITRATES

The organic nitrates are the oldest and most frequently used antianginal drugs. These agents relieve angina by causing vasodilation. Nitroglycerin, the most familiar organic nitrate, will serve as our prototype.

Prototype Drugs

DRUGS FOR ANGINA PECTORIS

Organic Nitrate
Nitroglycerin

Beta Blockers
Propranolol
Metoprolol

Calcium Channel Blockers
Verapamil
Nifedipine

Drug That Increases Myocardial Efficiency
Ranolazine

Nitroglycerin

Nitroglycerin has been used to treat angina since 1879. The drug is effective, fast acting, and inexpensive. Despite availability of newer antianginal agents, nitroglycerin remains the drug of choice for relieving an acute anginal attack.

Vasodilator Actions

Nitroglycerin acts directly on vascular smooth muscle (VSM) to promote vasodilation. At usual therapeutic doses, the drug acts primarily on *veins.* Dilation of arterioles is only modest.

The biochemical events that lead to vasodilation begin with uptake of nitrate by VSM, followed by conversion of nitrate to its active form: *nitric oxide.* As indicated, conversion requires the presence of *sulfhydryl groups.* Nitric oxide then activates guanylyl cyclase, an enzyme that catalyzes the formation of cyclic guanosine monophosphate (cGMP). Through a series of reactions, elevation of cGMP leads to dephosphorylation of light-chain myosin in VSM. (Recall that, in all muscles, phosphorylated myosin interacts with actin to produce contraction.) As a result of dephosphorylation, myosin is unable to interact with actin, and thus VSM relaxes, causing vasodilation. For our purposes, the most important aspect of this sequence is the conversion of nitrate to its active form—nitric oxide—in the presence of a sulfhydryl source.

Mechanism of Antianginal Effects

Stable Angina

Nitroglycerin decreases the pain of exertional angina primarily by *decreasing cardiac oxygen demand.* Oxygen demand is decreased as follows: by dilating veins, nitroglycerin decreases venous return to the heart and thereby decreases ventricular filling; the resultant decrease in wall tension (preload) decreases oxygen demand.

In patients with stable angina, nitroglycerin does not appear to increase blood flow to ischemic areas of the heart. This statement is based on two observations. First, nitroglycerin does not dilate atherosclerotic coronary arteries. Second, when nitroglycerin is injected directly into coronary arteries during an anginal attack, it does not relieve pain. Both observations suggest that pain relief results from effects of nitroglycerin on peripheral blood vessels—not from effects on coronary blood flow.

Variant Angina

In patients with variant angina, nitroglycerin acts by relaxing or preventing spasm in coronary arteries. Hence the drug *increases oxygen supply.* It does not reduce oxygen demand.

Pharmacokinetics

Absorption

Nitroglycerin is *highly lipid soluble* and crosses membranes with ease. Because of this property, nitroglycerin can be administered by uncommon routes (sublingual, buccal, transdermal) as well as by more conventional routes (oral, intravenous).

Metabolism

Nitroglycerin undergoes *rapid inactivation* by hepatic enzymes (organic nitrate reductases). As a result, the drug has a plasma half-life of only 5 to 7 minutes. When nitroglycerin is administered orally, most of each dose is destroyed on its first pass through the liver.

Adverse Effects

Nitroglycerin is generally well tolerated. Principal adverse effects—headache, hypotension, and tachycardia—occur secondary to vasodilation.

Headache

Initial therapy can produce severe headache. This response diminishes over the first few weeks of treatment. In the meantime, headache can be reduced with aspirin, acetaminophen, or some other mild analgesic.

Orthostatic Hypotension

Relaxation of VSM causes blood to pool in veins when the patient assumes an erect posture. Pooling decreases venous return to the heart, which reduces cardiac output, causing blood pressure to fall. Symptoms of orthostatic hypotension include lightheadedness and dizziness. Patients should be instructed to sit or lie down if these occur. Lying with the feet elevated promotes venous return and can help restore blood pressure.

Reflex Tachycardia

Nitroglycerin lowers blood pressure—primarily by decreasing venous return, and partly by dilating arterioles. By lowering blood pressure, the drug can activate the baroreceptor reflex, causing sympathetic stimulation of the heart. The resultant increase in both heart rate and contractile force increases cardiac oxygen demand, which negates the benefits of therapy. Pretreatment with a beta blocker or verapamil (a CCB that directly suppresses the heart) can prevent sympathetic cardiac stimulation.

Drug Interactions

Hypotensive Drugs

Nitroglycerin can intensify the effects of other hypotensive agents. Consequently, care should be exercised when nitroglycerin is used concurrently with beta blockers, CCBs, diuretics, and all other drugs that can lower blood pressure, including inhibitors of phosphodiesterase type 5 (PDE-5). Also, patients should be advised to avoid alcohol.

Beta Blockers, Verapamil, and Diltiazem

These drugs can suppress nitroglycerin-induced tachycardia. Beta blockers do so by preventing sympathetic activation of beta$_1$-adrenergic receptors on the heart. Verapamil and diltiazem prevent tachycardia through direct suppression of pacemaker activity in the sinoatrial node.

Tolerance

Tolerance to nitroglycerin-induced vasodilation can develop rapidly (over the course of a single day). One possible mechanism is depletion of sulfhydryl groups in VSM: in the absence of sulfhydryl groups, nitroglycerin cannot be converted to nitric oxide, its active form. Another possible mechanism is reversible oxidative injury to mitochondrial aldehyde dehydrogenase, an enzyme needed to convert nitroglycerin into nitric oxide. Patients who develop tolerance to nitroglycerin display cross-tolerance to all other nitrates and vice versa. Development of tolerance is most likely with high-dose therapy and uninterrupted therapy. To prevent tolerance, nitroglycerin and other nitrates should be used in the lowest effective dosages; long-acting formulations (e.g., patches, sustained-release preparations) should be used on an intermittent schedule that allows at least 8 drug-free hours every day, usually during the night. If pain occurs during the nitrate-free interval, it can be managed with sparing use of a short-acting nitrate (e.g., sublingual nitroglycerin) or by adding a beta blocker or CCB to the regimen. Tolerance can be reversed by withholding nitrates for a short time.

Preparations and Routes of Administration

Nitroglycerin is available in several formulations for administration by several routes. This proliferation of dosage forms reflects efforts to delay hepatic metabolism and prolong therapeutic effects.

All nitroglycerin preparations produce qualitatively similar responses; differences relate only to onset and duration of action (Table 43.2). With two preparations, effects begin rapidly (in 1–5 minutes) and then diminish in less than 1 hour. With three others, effects begin slowly but last several hours. Only one preparation—sublingual isosorbide dinitrate tablets—has both a rapid onset and long duration.

TABLE 43.2 ▪ Organic Nitrates: Time Course of Action

Drug and Dosage Form	Onset*	Duration†
NITROGLYCERIN		
Sublingual tablets	Rapid (1–3 min)	Brief (30–60 min)
Translingual spray	Rapid (2–3 min)	Brief (30–60 min)
Oral capsules, SR	Slow (20–45 min)	Long (3–8 hr)
Transdermal patches	Slow (30–60 min)	Long (24 hr)‡
Topical ointment	Slow (20–60 min)	Long (2–12 hr)
ISOSORBIDE MONONITRATE		
Oral tablets, IR	Slow (30–60 min)	Long (6–10 hr)
Oral tablets, SR	Slow (30–60 min)	Long (7–12 hr)
ISOSORBIDE DINITRATE		
Sublingual tablets	Rapid (2–5 min)	Long (1–3 hr)
Oral tablets, IR	Slow (20–40 min)	Long (4–6 hr)
Oral tablets, SR	Slow (30 min)	Long (6–8 hr)
Oral capsules, SR	Slow (30 min)	Long (6–8 hr)

*Nitrates with a *rapid* onset have two uses: (1) termination of an ongoing anginal attack and (2) short-term prophylaxis before anticipated exertion. Of the rapid-acting nitrates, nitroglycerin (sublingual tablet or translingual spray) is preferred to the others for terminating an ongoing attack.
†*Long-acting* nitrates are used for sustained prophylaxis (prevention) of anginal attacks. All cause tolerance if used without interruption.
‡Although patches can release nitroglycerin for up to 24 hours, they should be removed after 12 to 14 hours to avoid tolerance.
IR, immediate release; SR, sustained release.

Applications of specific preparations are based on their time course. Preparations with a *rapid onset* are employed to *terminate an ongoing anginal attack.* When used for this purpose, rapid-acting preparations are administered as soon as pain begins. Rapid-acting preparations can also be used for *acute prophylaxis of angina.* For this purpose, they are taken just before anticipated exertion. *Long-acting preparations* are used to provide *sustained protection* against anginal attacks. To provide protection, they are administered on a fixed schedule (but one that permits at least 8 drug-free hours each day).

Trade names and dosages for nitroglycerin preparations are shown in Table 43.3.

Sublingual Tablets

When administered sublingually, nitroglycerin is absorbed directly through the oral mucosa and into the bloodstream. Hence, unlike orally administered drugs, which must pass through the liver on their way to the systemic circulation, sublingual nitroglycerin bypasses the liver and thereby temporarily avoids inactivation. Because the liver is bypassed, sublingual doses can be low (between 0.3 and 0.6 mg). These doses are about 10 times lower than those required when nitroglycerin is dosed orally.

Effects of sublingual nitroglycerin begin rapidly—in 1 to 3 minutes—and persist up to 1 hour. Because sublingual administration works fast, this route is ideal for (1) terminating an ongoing attack and (2) short-term prophylaxis when exertion is anticipated.

To terminate an acute anginal attack, sublingual nitroglycerin should be administered as soon as pain begins. Administration should not be delayed until the pain has become severe.

TABLE 43.3 ▪ Organic Nitrates: Trade Names and Dosages

Drug and Formulation	Trade Name	Usual Dosage
NITROGLYCERIN		
Sublingual tablets	Nitrostat	0.3–0.6 mg as needed every 5 min for maximum of three doses
Translingual spray	Nitrolingual Pumpspray, NitroMist	1–2 sprays (up to 3 sprays in a 15-min period)
Oral capsules, SR	Nitro-Time	2.5–6.5 mg 3 or 4 times daily; to avoid tolerance, administer only once or twice daily; do not crush or chew
Transdermal patches	Minitran, Nitro-Dur, Transderm Nitro ♣, Trinipatch ♣	1 patch a day; to avoid tolerance, remove after 12–14 hr, allowing 10–12 patch-free hours each day. Patches come in sizes that release 0.1–0.8 mg/hr.
Topical ointment	Nitro-Bid	1–2 inches (7.5–40 mg) every 4–6 hr
Intravenous	Generic only	5 mcg/min initially, then increased gradually as needed (max: 200 mcg/min); tolerance develops with prolonged continuous infusion
ISOSORBIDE MONONITRATE		
Oral tablets, IR	Monoket	20 mg twice daily; to avoid tolerance, take the first dose upon awakening and the second dose 7 hr later
Oral tablets, SR	Imdur	60–240 mg once a day; do not crush or chew
ISOSORBIDE DINITRATE		
Sublingual tablets	Generic only	2.5–5 mg before activities that may cause angina. For acute angina, 2.5–5 mg every 5 min for maximum of three doses. Do not crush or chew
Oral tablets, IR	Isordil Oral Titradose	10–40 mg 2 or 3 times daily; to avoid tolerance, take the last dose no later than 7:00 PM
Oral tablets, SR	Generic only	40 mg every 6–12 hr; to avoid tolerance, take only once or twice daily (at 8:00 AM and 2:00 PM)
Oral capsules, SR	Dilatrate-SR	40 mg every 6–12 hr; to avoid tolerance, take only once or twice daily (at 8:00 AM and 2:00 PM)

IR, immediate release; SR, sustained release.

According to current guidelines, if pain is not relieved in 5 minutes, the patient should call 911 or report to an emergency department because anginal pain that does not respond to nitroglycerin may indicate MI. While awaiting emergency care, the patient can take 1 more tablet, and then a third tablet 5 minutes later.

Patient Education

SUBLINGUAL DRUG ADMINISTRATION

Sublingual administration is unfamiliar to most patients. Accordingly, education is needed. The patient should be instructed to place the tablet under the tongue and leave it there while it dissolves. Nitroglycerin tablets formulated for sublingual use are ineffective if swallowed. To ensure good stability, the tablets should be stored moisture free at room temperature in their original container, which should be closed tightly after each use.

Sustained-Release Oral Capsules

Sustained-release oral capsules are intended for long-term prophylaxis only; these formulations cannot act fast enough to terminate an ongoing anginal attack. Sustained-release capsules contain a large dose of nitroglycerin that is slowly absorbed across the gastrointestinal (GI) wall. In theory, doses are large enough so that amounts of nitroglycerin sufficient to produce a therapeutic response will survive passage through the liver. Because they produce sustained blood levels of nitroglycerin, these formulations can cause tolerance. To reduce the risk for tolerance, these products should be taken only once or twice daily.

Transdermal Delivery Systems

Nitroglycerin patches contain a reservoir from which nitroglycerin is slowly released. After release, the drug is absorbed through the skin and then into the blood. The rate of release is constant and, depending on the patch used, can range from 0.1 to 0.8 mg/hour. Effects begin within 30 to 60 minutes and persist as long as the patch remains in place (up to 14 hours). Patches are applied once daily to a hairless area of skin. The site should be rotated to avoid local irritation.

Tolerance develops if patches are used continuously (24 hours a day every day). Accordingly, a daily "patch-free" interval of 10 to 12 hours is recommended. This can be accomplished by applying a new patch each morning, leaving it in place for 12 to 14 hours, and then removing it in the evening.

Because of their long duration, patches are well suited for sustained prophylaxis. Because patches have a delayed onset, they cannot be used to abort an ongoing attack.

Translingual Spray

Nitroglycerin can be delivered to the oral mucosa using a metered-dose spray device. Each activation delivers a 0.4-mg dose. Indications for nitroglycerin spray are the same as for sublingual tablets: suppression of an acute anginal attack and prophylaxis of angina when exertion is anticipated. As with sublingual tablets, no more than three doses should be administered within a 15-minute interval.

Topical Ointment

Topical nitroglycerin ointment is used for sustained protection against anginal attacks. The ointment is applied to the skin of the chest, back, abdomen, or anterior thigh. (Because nitroglycerin acts primarily by dilating peripheral veins, there is no mechanistic advantage to applying topical nitroglycerin directly over the heart.) After topical application, nitroglycerin is absorbed through the skin and then into the blood. Effects begin in 20 to 60 minutes and may persist up to 12 hours.

Nitroglycerin ointment (2%) is dispensed from a tube, and the length of the ribbon squeezed from the tube determines dosage. (One inch contains about 15 mg of nitroglycerin.) The usual adult dosage is 1 to 2 inches applied every 4 to 6 hours. The ointment should be spread over an area at least 2.5 inches by 3.5 inches and then covered with plastic wrap. Sites of application should be rotated to minimize skin irritation. As with other long-acting formulations, uninterrupted use can cause tolerance.

Discontinuing Nitroglycerin

Long-acting preparations (transdermal patches, topical ointment, sustained-release oral tablets or capsules) should be discontinued slowly. If they are withdrawn abruptly, vasospasm may result.

Summary of Therapeutic Uses

Acute Therapy of Angina

For acute treatment of angina pectoris, nitroglycerin is administered in sublingual tablets and a translingual spray. Both formulations can be used to abort an ongoing anginal attack and to provide prophylaxis in anticipation of exertion.

Sustained Therapy of Angina

For sustained prophylaxis against angina, nitroglycerin is administered in the following formulations: transdermal patches, topical ointment, and sustained-release oral capsules.

Isosorbide Mononitrate and Isosorbide Dinitrate

Both of these drugs have pharmacologic actions identical to those of nitroglycerin. Both drugs are used for angina, both are taken orally, and both produce headache, hypotension, and reflex tachycardia. Differences between them relate only to route of administration and time course of action. Time course determines whether a particular drug or dosage form will be used for acute therapy, sustained prophylaxis, or both. As with nitroglycerin, tolerance can develop to long-acting preparations. To avoid tolerance, the dosing schedule for long-acting preparations should allow at least 12 drug-free hours a day. Time courses are shown in Table 43.2. Trade names and dosages are shown in Table 43.3. A fixed-dose combination of isosorbide dinitrate plus hydralazine is discussed in Chapter 40.

BETA BLOCKERS

Beta blockers (e.g., propranolol, metoprolol) are first-line drugs for *angina of effort,* but are *not* effective against vasospastic angina. When administered on a fixed schedule, beta blockers can provide sustained protection against effort-induced anginal pain. Exercise tolerance is increased, and the frequency and intensity of anginal attacks are lowered. All of the beta blockers appear equally effective. In addition to reducing anginal pain, beta blockers decrease the risk for death, especially in patients with a prior MI.

Beta blockers reduce anginal pain primarily by *decreasing cardiac oxygen demand,* principally through blockade of $beta_1$ receptors in the heart, which decreases heart rate and contractility. Beta blockers reduce oxygen demand further by causing a modest reduction in arterial pressure (afterload). In addition to decreasing oxygen demand, beta blockers help increase oxygen supply. By slowing heart rate, they increase time in diastole and thereby increase the time during which blood flows through myocardial vessels. In patients taking vasodilators (e.g., nitroglycerin), beta blockers provide the additional benefit of blunting reflex tachycardia.

For treatment of stable angina, dosage should be low initially and then gradually increased. The dosing goal is to reduce resting heart rate to 50 to 60 beats/minute and limit exertional heart rate to about 100 beats/minute. Beta blockers should not be withdrawn abruptly because doing so can increase the incidence and intensity of anginal attacks and may even precipitate MI.

Beta blockers can produce a variety of adverse effects. Blockade of cardiac $beta_1$ receptors can produce *bradycardia, decreased atrioventricular (AV) conduction,* and *reduction of contractility.* Consequently, beta blockers should not be used by patients with sick sinus syndrome, heart failure, or second-degree or third-degree AV block. Blockade of $beta_2$ receptors in the lung can promote bronchoconstriction. Accordingly, beta blockers should be used with caution by patients with asthma. If an asthmatic individual absolutely must use a beta blocker, a $beta_1$-selective agent (e.g., metoprolol) should be chosen. Beta blockers can mask signs of hypoglycemia and therefore must be used with caution in patients with diabetes. Rarely, these drugs cause adverse central nervous system effects, including *insomnia, depression,* and *bizarre dreams.*

The basic pharmacology of the beta blockers is discussed in Chapter 14.

CALCIUM CHANNEL BLOCKERS

The CCBs used most frequently are *verapamil, diltiazem,* and *nifedipine* (a dihydropyridine-type calcium channel blocker). Accordingly, our discussion focuses on these three drugs. *All three* can block calcium channels in VSM, primarily in arterioles. The result is arteriolar dilation and reduction of peripheral resistance (afterload). In addition, all three can relax coronary vasospasm. *Verapamil* and *diltiazem* also block calcium channels in the heart and can thereby decrease heart rate, AV conduction, and contractility.

CCBs are used to treat both stable and variant angina. In *variant angina,* these drugs promote relaxation of coronary artery spasm, *increasing cardiac oxygen supply.* In *stable angina,* they promote relaxation of peripheral arterioles; the resultant decrease in afterload *reduces cardiac oxygen demand.* Verapamil and diltiazem can produce modest additional reductions in oxygen demand by suppressing heart rate and contractility.

The major adverse effects of the CCBs are cardiovascular. Dilation of peripheral arterioles lowers blood pressure and can thereby induce *reflex tachycardia.* This reaction is greatest with nifedipine and minimal with verapamil and diltiazem. Because of their suppressant effects on the heart, verapamil and diltiazem must be used cautiously in patients taking beta blockers and in patients with bradycardia, heart failure, or AV block. These precautions do not apply to nifedipine or other dihydropyridines.

The basic pharmacology of the CCBs is discussed in Chapter 37.

RANOLAZINE

Actions and Therapeutic Use

Ranolazine [Ranexa] represents the first new class of antianginal agents to be approved in more than 25 years. In clinical trials, the drug reduced the number of angina episodes per week and increased exercise tolerance. However, these benefits were modest and were smaller in women than in men. Unlike most other antianginal drugs, ranolazine does not reduce heart rate, blood pressure, or vascular resistance. However, it *can* prolong the QT interval and is subject to multiple drug interactions. Ranolazine works by reducing accumulation of sodium and calcium in myocardial cells, which might help the myocardium use energy more efficiently. However, the exact mechanism of action is unknown. Despite limited efficacy, many drug interactions, and a risk for dysrhythmias (see later), ranolazine is now approved as a first-line drug for angina. It may be combined with nitrates, beta blockers, amlodipine (a CCB), and other drugs used for angina treatment.

Pharmacokinetics

Absorption from the GI tract is highly variable, but not affected by food. Plasma levels peak 2 to 5 hours after dosing. In the liver, ranolazine undergoes rapid and extensive metabolism, mainly by CYP3A4 (the 3A4 isoenzyme of cytochrome P450). The drug has a plasma half-life of 7 hours and is excreted in the urine (75%) and feces (25%), almost entirely as metabolites.

Adverse Effects

QT Prolongation

Ranolazine can cause a dose-related increase in the QT interval and may thereby increase the risk for torsades de pointes, a serious ventricular dysrhythmia. Accordingly, the drug is contraindicated for patients with preexisting QT prolongation and for those taking other drugs that can increase the QT interval. In addition, ranolazine is contraindicated for patients at risk for developing high levels of the drug—namely, patients with hepatic impairment or those taking drugs that inhibit CYP3A4. The issue of drug-induced QT prolongation is discussed in Chapter 5.

Elevation of Blood Pressure

In patients with severe renal impairment, ranolazine can raise blood pressure by about 15 mm Hg. Accordingly, blood pressure should be monitored often in these people.

Other Adverse Effects

The most common adverse effects are constipation, dizziness, nausea, and headache.

Drug Interactions

CYP3A4 Inhibitors

Agents that inhibit CYP3A4 can increase levels of ranolazine and can thereby increase the risk for torsades de pointes. Accordingly, moderate or strong CYP3A4 inhibitors should be avoided. Among these agents are grapefruit juice, HIV protease inhibitors (e.g., ritonavir), macrolide antibiotics (e.g., erythromycin), azole antifungal drugs (e.g., itraconazole), and some calcium channel blockers.

QT Drugs

Drugs that prolong the QT interval (e.g., quinidine, sotalol) can increase the risk for torsades de pointes in patients taking ranolazine and hence should be avoided. Chapter 5 presents a comprehensive list of QT drugs.

Calcium Channel Blockers

Most CCBs—but not amlodipine—can inhibit CYP3A4 and thus increase levels of ranolazine. Accordingly, when use of ranolazine plus a CCB is indicated, amlodipine is the only CCB that should be used.

Preparations, Dosage, and Administration

Ranolazine [Ranexa] is formulated in extended-release tablets (500 and 1000 mg) that should be swallowed intact, with or without food. Dosing begins at 500 mg twice daily and may be increased to a maximum of 1000 mg twice daily. Ranolazine may be used in combination with a nitrate, beta blocker, or amlodipine (a CCB), and other drugs for angina.

TREATMENT MEASURES

Guidelines for Management of Chronic Stable Angina

In 1999, three organizations—the American Heart Association (AHA), the American College of Cardiology (ACC), and the American College of Physicians–American Society of Internal Medicine—joined forces to produce the first national guidelines on the management of chronic stable angina. The 1999 guidelines were updated in 2002 and again in 2007. Both updates—*ACC/AHA 2002 Guideline Update for the Management of Patients with Chronic Stable Angina,* and *2007 Chronic Angina Focused Update of the ACC/AHA 2002 Guidelines for the Management of Patients with Chronic Stable Angina*—are available free online at *circ.ahajournals.org.* The following discussion reflects recommendations in these guidelines.

Treatment of stable angina has two objectives: (1) prevention of MI and death, and (2) reduction of cardiac ischemia and associated anginal pain. Although both goals are desirable, prevention of MI and death is clearly more important. If two treatments are equally effective at decreasing anginal pain, but one also decreases the risk for death, then the latter is preferred.

Drugs Used to Prevent Myocardial Infarction and Death

We now have medical treatments that can decrease the risk for MI and death in patients with chronic stable angina. Therapy directed at preventing MI and death is a new paradigm in the management of stable angina, and all practitioners should become familiar with it.

Antiplatelet Drugs

These agents decrease platelet aggregation and thereby decrease the risk for thrombus formation in coronary arteries. The most effective agents are *aspirin* and *clopidogrel.* In patients with stable angina, low-dose aspirin produces a 33% decrease in the risk for adverse cardiovascular events. Benefits of clopidogrel seem equal to those of aspirin, although they are not as well documented. The guidelines recommend that all patients with stable angina take 75 to 162 mg of aspirin daily, unless there is a specific reason not to. Aspirin, clopidogrel, and other antiplatelet drugs are discussed in Chapter 44.

Cholesterol-Lowering Drugs

Elevated cholesterol is a major risk factor for coronary atherosclerosis. Drugs that lower cholesterol can slow the progression of CAD, stabilize atherosclerotic plaques, and even cause plaque regression. Therapies that reduce cholesterol are associated with decreased mortality from coronary heart disease. For example, in patients with established CAD, taking simvastatin can decrease the risk for mortality by 35%. Because of the well-established benefits of cholesterol-lowering therapy, the guidelines recommend that all patients with stable angina receive a cholesterol-lowering drug. The pharmacology of the cholesterol-lowering drugs is discussed in Chapter 42.

Angiotensin-Converting Enzyme (ACE) Inhibitors

There is strong evidence that, in patients with CAD, ACE inhibitors greatly reduce the incidence of adverse outcomes. In the Heart Outcomes Prevention Evaluation (HOPE) trial, for example, ramipril reduced the incidence of stroke, MI, and cardiovascular death. Among one subset of patients—those with diabetes—benefits were particularly striking. Ramipril decreased the risk for stroke by 33%, MI by 22%, and cardiovascular death by 37%. In addition, ramipril reduced the risk for nephropathy, retinopathy, and other microvascular complications of diabetes. Because of these well-documented benefits, the guidelines recommend angiotensin-converting enzyme (ACE) inhibitors for most patients with established CAD, and especially for those with diabetes. The pharmacology of the ACE inhibitors is discussed in Chapter 36.

Antianginal Agents: Drugs Used to Reduce Anginal Pain

The goal of antianginal therapy is to achieve complete (or nearly complete) elimination of anginal pain, along with a return to normal activities. This should be accomplished with a minimum of adverse drug effects.

The basic strategy of antianginal therapy is to provide baseline protection using one or more long-acting drugs (beta blocker, CCB, long-acting nitrate) supplemented with sublingual nitroglycerin when breakthrough pain occurs. A flow plan for drug selection is shown in Fig. 43.2. As indicated, treatment is approached sequentially. Progression from one step to the next is based on patient response. Some patients can be treated with a single long-acting drug, some require two or three, and some require revascularization.

Initial treatment consists of sublingual nitroglycerin plus a long-acting antianginal drug. Beta blockers are the preferred agents for baseline therapy because they can decrease mortality, especially in patients with a prior MI. In addition to providing prophylaxis, beta blockers suppress nitrate-induced reflex tachycardia.

If a beta blocker is inadequate, or if there are contraindications to beta blockade, a long-acting CCB should be added or substituted. Dihydropyridine-type CCBs (e.g., nifedipine) lack cardiosuppressant actions and thus are safer than beta blockers for patients with bradycardia, AV block, or heart failure. When a CCB is to be *combined* with a beta blocker, a dihydropyridine is preferred to verapamil or diltiazem because verapamil and diltiazem will intensify the cardiosuppressant actions of the beta blocker, whereas a dihydropyridine CCB will not.

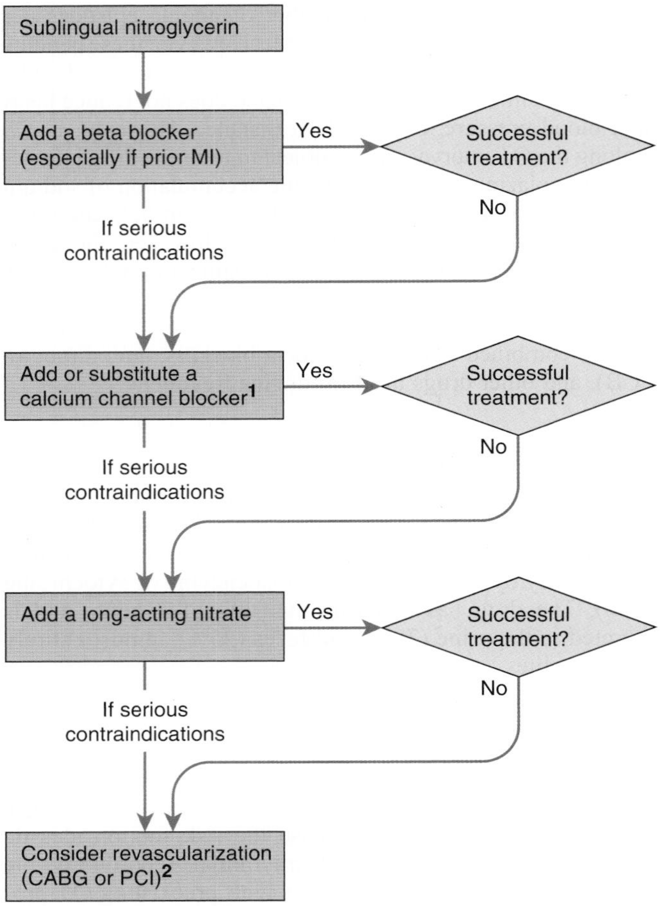

Figure 43.2 ■ Flow plan for antianginal drug selection in patients with chronic stable angina.
(1) Avoid short-acting dihydropyridines. (2) At any point in this process, based on coronary anatomy, severity of angina symptoms, and patient preference, it is reasonable to consider evaluation for coronary revascularization with either percutaneous coronary intervention (PCI) or coronary artery bypass graft (CABG). Unless a patient is documented to have left main, three-vessel, or two-vessel coronary artery disease (CAD) with significant stenosis of the proximal left anterior descending coronary artery, there is no demonstrated survival advantage associated with CABG or PCI in low-risk patients with chronic stable angina. Accordingly, medical therapy should be attempted in most patients before considering PCI or CABG. (Adapted from Gibbons RJ, Chatterjee K, Daley J, et al. ACC/AHA 2002 guideline update for the management of patients with chronic stable angina: a report of the American College of Cardiology/American Heart Association Task Force on Practice Guidelines [Committee to Update the 1999 Guidelines for the Management of Patients with Chronic Stable Angina]. 2002. Available online at circ.ahajournals.org.)

If a CCB is inadequate, or if there are contraindications to calcium channel blockade, a long-acting nitrate (e.g., transdermal nitroglycerin) should be added or substituted. However, because tolerance can develop quickly, these nitrate preparations are less well suited than beta blockers or CCBs for continuous protection.

Note that, as we proceed along the drug-selection flow plan, drugs are *added* to the regimen, resulting in treatment with two or more agents. Combination therapy increases our chances of success because oxygen demand is decreased by multiple mechanisms: beta blockers reduce heart rate and contractility; CCBs reduce afterload (by dilating arterioles); and nitrates reduce preload (by dilating veins).

If combined treatment with a beta blocker, CCB, and long-acting nitrate fails to provide relief, coronary artery bypass graft (CABG) surgery or percutaneous coronary intervention (PCI) may be indicated. Note that these invasive procedures should be considered only after more conservative treatment has been tried.

How should we treat angina in patients who have a coexisting condition? The antianginal drugs employed—nitrates, beta blockers, and CCBs—are the same ones used in patients who have angina alone. However, when selecting among these drugs, we must consider the coexisting disorder as well as the angina. For example, as noted previously, in patients with asthma, CCBs are preferred to beta blockers (because beta blockers promote bronchoconstriction, whereas CCBs do not). Table 43.4 shows more than 20 coexisting conditions and indicates which antianginal agents to use as well as which ones to avoid.

Reduction of Risk Factors

The treatment program should reduce anginal risk factors: smokers should quit; sedentary patients should get aerobic exercise; and patients with diabetes, hypertension, or high cholesterol should receive appropriate therapy.

Smoking

Smoking increases the risk for cardiovascular mortality by 50%. Fortunately, smoking cessation greatly decreases cardiovascular risk. Accordingly, all patients who smoke should be strongly encouraged to quit. Smoking cessation is discussed in Chapter 32.

High Cholesterol

As noted, high cholesterol levels increase the risk of adverse cardiovascular events, and therapies that reduce cholesterol reduce that risk. Accordingly, all patients with high cholesterol levels should receive cholesterol-lowering therapy.

Hypertension

High blood pressure increases the risk for cardiovascular mortality, and lowering blood pressure reduces the risk. Accordingly, all patients with hypertension should receive treatment. Blood pressure should be reduced to 140/90 mm Hg or less. In patients with additional risk factors (e.g., diabetes, heart failure, retinopathy), the target blood pressure is 130/80 mm Hg or less. Management of hypertension is discussed in Chapter 39.

Diabetes

Both type 1 (insulin-dependent) and type 2 (non–insulin-dependent) diabetes increase the risk for cardiovascular mortality. Type 1 increases the risk 3- to 10-fold; type 2 increases the risk 2- to 4-fold. Although there is good evidence that tight glycemic control decreases the risk for microvascular complications of diabetes, there is little evidence to show that tight glycemic control decreases the risk for cardiovascular complications. Nonetheless, it is prudent to strive for optimal glycemic control.

Physical Inactivity

Increased physical activity has multiple benefits. In patients with chronic stable angina, exercise increases exercise

TABLE 43.4 ▪ Choosing Between Beta Blockers and Calcium Channel Blockers for Treating Angina in Patients Who Have a Coexisting Condition

Coexisting Condition	Recommended Treatment (Alternative Treatment)	Drugs to Avoid
MEDICAL CONDITIONS		
Systemic hypertension	Beta blockers (long-acting, slow-release CCBs)	
Migraine or vascular headache	Beta blockers (verapamil or diltiazem)	
Asthma or COPD with bronchospasm	Verapamil or diltiazem	Beta blockers
Hyperthyroidism	Beta blockers	
Raynaud disease	Long-acting, slow-release CCBs	Beta blockers
Type 1 diabetes	Beta blockers, particularly if prior MI, or long-acting, slow-release CCBs	
Type 2 diabetes	Beta blockers or long-acting, slow-release CCBs	
Depression	Long-acting, slow-release CCBs	Beta blockers
Mild peripheral vascular disease	Beta blockers or long-acting, slow-release CCBs	
Severe peripheral vascular disease with ischemia at rest	Long-acting, slow-release CCBs	Beta blockers
CARDIAC DYSRHYTHMIAS AND CONDUCTION ABNORMALITIES		
Sinus bradycardia	Long-acting, slow-release CCBs that do not decrease heart rate	Beta blockers, diltiazem, verapamil
Sinus tachycardia (not due to heart failure)	Beta blockers	
Supraventricular tachycardia	Verapamil, diltiazem, or beta blockers	
AV block	Long-acting, slow-release CCBs that do not slow AV conduction	Beta blockers, diltiazem, verapamil
Rapid atrial fibrillation (with digoxin)	Verapamil, diltiazem, or beta blockers	
Ventricular dysrhythmias	Beta blockers	

Continued

TABLE 43.4 ▪ Choosing Between Beta Blockers and Calcium Channel Blockers for Treating Angina in Patients Who Have a Coexisting Condition—cont'd

Coexisting Condition	Recommended Treatment (Alternative Treatment)	Drugs to Avoid
LEFT VENTRICULAR DYSFUNCTION		
Congestive heart failure		
Mild (LVEF ≥40%)	Beta blockers	
Moderate to severe (LVEF <40%)	Amlodipine or felodipine (nitrates)	Diltiazem, verapamil
Left-sided valvular heart disease		
Mild aortic stenosis	Beta blockers	
Aortic insufficiency	Long-acting, slow-release dihydropyridine CCBs	
Mitral regurgitation	Long-acting, slow-release dihydropyridine CCBs	
Mitral stenosis	Beta blockers	
Hypertrophic cardiomyopathy	Beta blockers, verapamil, diltiazem	Dihydropyridine CCBs, nitrates

AV, atrioventricular; CCB, calcium channel blocker; COPD, chronic obstructive pulmonary disease; LVEF, left ventricular ejection fraction; MI, myocardial infarction.

Adapted from Gibbons RJ, Chatterjee K, Daley J, et al. ACC/AHA 2002 guideline update for the management of patients with chronic stable angina: a report of the American College of Cardiology/American Heart Association Task Force on Practice Guidelines (Committee to Update the 1999 Guidelines for the Management of Patients with Chronic Stable Angina). 2002. Available online at circ.ahajournals.org/.

tolerance and the sense of well-being and decreases anginal symptoms, cholesterol levels, and objective measures of ischemia. Accordingly, the guidelines recommend that patients perform 30 to 60 minutes of a moderate-intensity activity 3 to 4 times a week. Such activities include walking, jogging, cycling, and other aerobic exercises. Exercise by moderate- to high-risk patients should be medically supervised.

Management of Variant Angina

Treatment of vasospastic angina can proceed in three steps. For initial therapy, either a calcium channel blocker or a long-acting nitrate is selected. If either drug alone is inadequate, then combined therapy with a CCB *plus* a nitrate should be tried. If the combination fails to control symptoms, CABG surgery may be indicated. Beta blockers are not effective in vasospastic angina.

CHAPTER

44 Anticoagulant and Antiplatelet Drugs

Laura D. Rosenthal, DNP, ANCP, FAANP

The drugs discussed here are used to prevent formation of thrombi and dissolve thrombi that have already formed. These drugs act in several ways: some suppress coagulation, some inhibit platelet aggregation, and some promote clot degradation. They all interfere with normal hemostasis. As a result, they all carry a significant risk for bleeding.

COAGULATION: PHYSIOLOGY AND PATHOPHYSIOLOGY

Hemostasis

Hemostasis is the physiologic process by which bleeding is stopped. Hemostasis occurs in two stages: (1) formation of a platelet plug, followed by (2) reinforcement of the platelet plug with fibrin. Both processes are set in motion by blood vessel injury.

Stage One: Formation of a Platelet Plug

Platelet aggregation is initiated when platelets come in contact with collagen on the exposed surface of a damaged blood vessel. In response to contact with collagen, platelets adhere to the site of vessel injury. Adhesion initiates platelet *activation,* which in turn leads to massive platelet *aggregation.*

Platelet aggregation is a complex process that ends with formation of *fibrinogen bridges* between *glycoprotein IIb/IIIa (GP IIb/IIIa) receptors* on adjacent platelets (Fig. 44.1). For these bridges to form, GP IIb/IIIa receptors must first undergo activation—that is, they must undergo a configurational change that allows them to bind with fibrinogen. As indicated in Fig. 44.1A, activation of GP IIb/IIIa can be stimulated by multiple factors, including thromboxane A_2 (TXA_2), thrombin, collagen, platelet-activating factor (PAF), and adenosine diphosphate (ADP). Under the influence of these factors, GP IIb/IIIa changes its shape, binds with fibrinogen, and thereby causes aggregation (see Fig. 44.1B). The aggregated platelets constitute a plug that stops bleeding. This plug is unstable, however, and must be reinforced with *fibrin* if protection is to last.

Stage Two: Coagulation

Coagulation is defined as production of *fibrin,* a thread-like protein that reinforces the platelet plug. Fibrin is produced by two convergent pathways (Fig. 44.2), referred to as the *contact activation pathway* (also known as the *intrinsic pathway*) and the *tissue factor pathway* (also known as the *extrinsic pathway*). The two pathways converge at factor Xa, after which they employ the same final series of reactions. In both pathways, each reaction in the sequence amplifies the reaction that follows. Hence, after this sequence is initiated, it becomes self-sustaining and self-reinforcing.

The *tissue factor pathway* is turned on by trauma to the vascular wall, which triggers release of tissue factor,[1] also known as *tissue thromboplastin.* Tissue factor then combines with and thereby activates factor VII, which in turn activates factor X, which then catalyzes the conversion of *prothrombin* (factor II) into *thrombin* (factor IIa). Thrombin then does three things. First, it catalyzes the conversion of fibrinogen into fibrin. Second, it catalyzes the conversion of factor V into *its* active form (Va), a compound that greatly increases the activity of factor Xa, even though it has no direct catalytic activity of its own. Third, thrombin catalyzes the conversion of factor VIII into *its* active form (VIIIa), a compound that greatly increases the activity of factor IXa in the contact activation pathway.

The *contact activation pathway* is turned on when blood makes contact with collagen that has been exposed as a result of trauma to a blood vessel wall. Collagen contact stimulates conversion of factor XII into its active form, XIIa (see Fig. 44.2). Factor XIIa then activates factor XI, which activates factor IX, which activates factor X. After this, the contact activation pathway is the same as the tissue factor pathway. As noted, factor VIIIa, which is produced under the influence of thrombin, greatly increases the activity of factor IXa, even though it has no direct catalytic activity of its own.

Important to our understanding of anticoagulant drugs is the fact that *four coagulation factors—factors VII, IX, X, and II (prothrombin)—require vitamin K for their synthesis.* These factors appear in green boxes in Fig. 44.2. The significance of the vitamin K–dependent factors will become apparent when we discuss warfarin, an oral anticoagulant.

Keeping Hemostasis Under Control

To protect against widespread coagulation, the body must inactivate any clotting factors that stray from the site of vessel injury. Inactivation is accomplished with *antithrombin,* a protein that forms a complex with clotting factors and thereby inhibits their activity. The clotting factors that can be neutralized by antithrombin appear in yellow in Fig. 44.2. As we shall see, antithrombin is intimately involved in the action of *heparin,* an injectable anticoagulant drug.

[1]The term *tissue factor* refers not to a single compound but rather to a complex of several compounds, including a proteolytic enzyme and phospholipids released from tissue membranes.

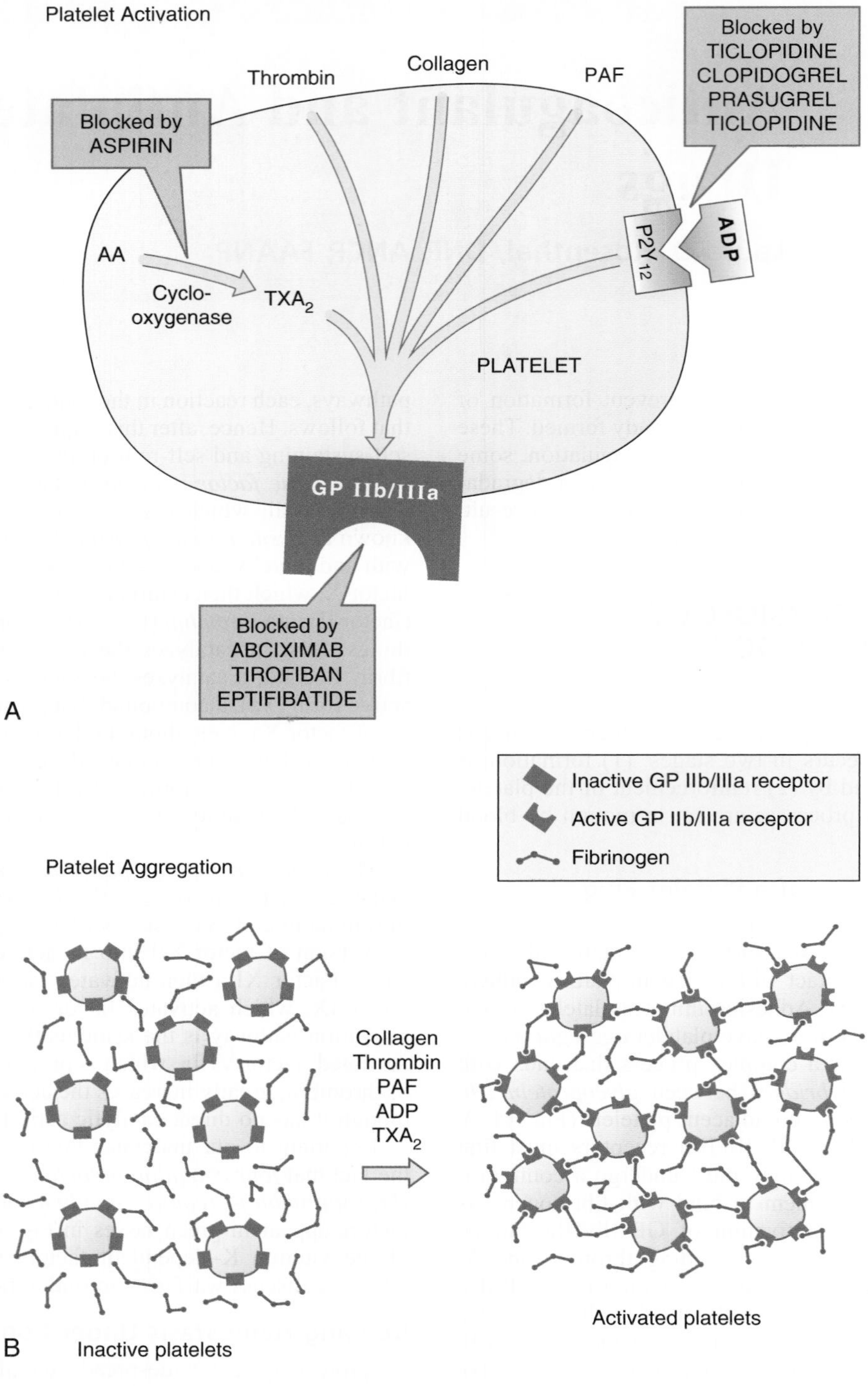

Figure 44.1 ▪ Mechanism of platelet aggregation and actions of antiplatelet drugs. **A,** Multiple factors—thromboxane A_2 (TXA_2), thrombin, collagen, platelet-activating factor (PAF), and adenosine diphosphate (ADP)—promote activation of the glycoprotein (GP) IIb/IIIa receptor. Each platelet has 50,000 to 80,000 GP IIb/IIIa receptors, although only one is shown. **B,** Activation of the GP IIb/IIIa receptor permits binding of fibrinogen, which causes aggregation by forming cross-links between platelets. After aggregation occurs, the platelet plug is reinforced with fibrin (not shown). (AA, arachidonic acid; $P2Y_{12}$, $P2Y_{12}$ ADP receptor.)

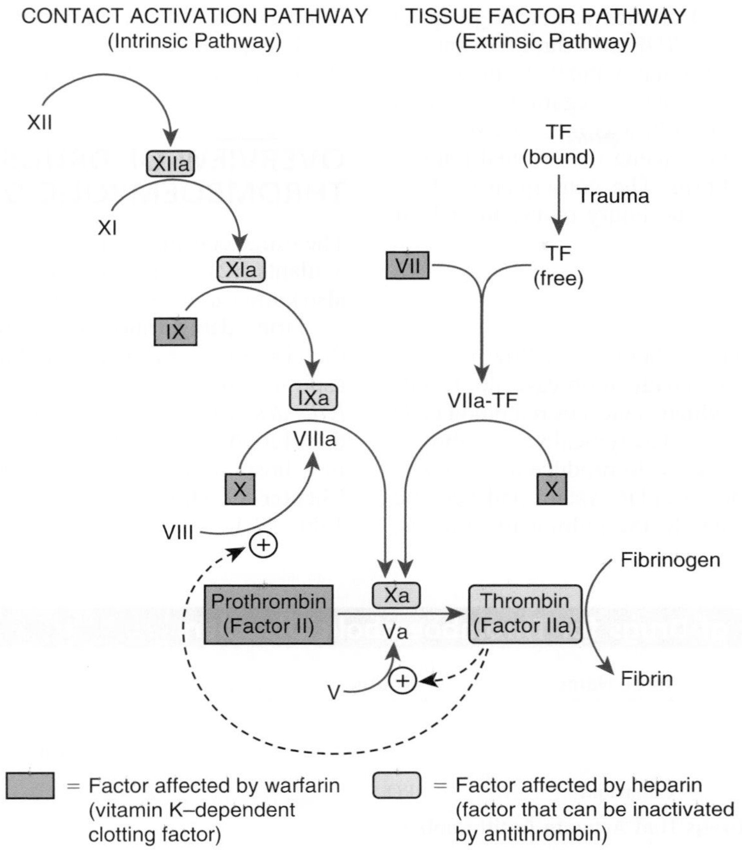

Figure 44.2 ▪ Outline of coagulation pathways showing factors affected by warfarin and heparin.
TF, tissue factor. Common names for factors are shown in roman numerals: V, proaccelerin; VII, proconvertin; VIII, antihemophilic factor; IX, Christmas factor; X, Stuart factor; XI, plasma thromboplastin antecedent; and XII, Hageman factor. The letter "a" after a factor's name (e.g., factor VIIIa) indicates the active form of the factor.

Prototype Drugs

ANTICOAGULANT AND ANTIPLATELET DRUGS

Anticoagulants

Drugs That Activate Antithrombin

Heparin (unfractionated)
Enoxaparin (low-molecular-weight heparin)

Vitamin K Antagonist

Warfarin

Direct Thrombin Inhibitor

Dabigatran

Direct Factor Xa Inhibitors

Rivaroxaban
Apixaban
Edoxaban

Antiplatelet Drugs

Aspirin (cyclooxygenase [COX] inhibitor)
Clopidogrel ($P2Y_{12}$ adenosine triphosphate receptor antagonist)
Vorapaxar (PAR-1 antagonist)

Physiologic Removal of Clots

As healing of an injured vessel proceeds, removal of the clot is eventually necessary. The body accomplishes this with *plasmin,* an enzyme that degrades the fibrin meshwork of the clot. Plasmin is produced through the activation of its precursor, *plasminogen.* The *fibrinolytic drugs* (e.g., alteplase) act by promoting conversion of plasminogen into plasmin.

Thrombosis

A thrombus is a blood clot formed within a blood vessel or within the heart. Thrombosis (thrombus formation) reflects pathologic functioning of hemostatic mechanisms.

Arterial Thrombosis

Formation of an arterial thrombus begins with adhesion of platelets to the arterial wall. (Adhesion is stimulated by damage to the wall or rupture of an atherosclerotic plaque.) After adhesion, platelets release ADP and thromboxane A_2 (TXA_2), and thereby attract additional platelets to the evolving thrombus. With continued platelet aggregation, occlusion of the artery takes place. As blood flow comes to a stop, the coagulation cascade is initiated, causing the original plug to undergo reinforcement with fibrin. The consequence of an arterial thrombus is localized tissue injury owing to lack of perfusion.

Venous Thrombosis

Venous thrombi develop at sites where blood flow is slow. Stagnation of blood initiates the coagulation cascade, resulting in the production of fibrin, which enmeshes red blood cells and platelets to form the thrombus. The typical venous thrombus has a long tail that can break off to produce an *embolus*. Such emboli travel within the vascular system and become lodged at faraway sites, frequently the pulmonary arteries. Hence, unlike an arterial thrombus, whose harmful effects are localized, injury from a venous thrombus occurs secondary to embolization at a site distant from the original thrombus.

OVERVIEW OF DRUGS FOR THROMBOEMBOLIC DISORDERS

The drugs considered fall into three major groups: (1) anticoagulants, (2) antiplatelet drugs, and (3) thrombolytic drugs, also known as fibrinolytic drugs. *Anticoagulants* (e.g., heparin, warfarin, dabigatran) disrupt the coagulation cascade and thereby suppress production of fibrin. *Antiplatelet drugs* (e.g., aspirin, clopidogrel) inhibit platelet aggregation. *Thrombolytic drugs* (e.g., alteplase) promote lysis of fibrin, causing dissolution of thrombi. Because these drugs are used only in a hospital setting, discussion of thrombolytics occurs in Chapter 89. Drugs that belong to these groups are shown in Table 44.1.

TABLE 44.1 ▪ Overview of Drugs for Thromboembolic Disorders

Generic Name	Trade Name	Route	Action	Therapeutic Use
ANTICOAGULANTS			Anticoagulants decrease formation of fibrin	Used primarily to prevent thrombosis in *veins* and the *atria of the heart*
Vitamin K Antagonist				
Warfarin	Coumadin	PO		
Heparin and Its Derivatives: Drugs That Activate Antithrombin				
Heparin (unfractionated)		SubQ, IV		
LMW heparins				
Dalteparin	Fragmin	SubQ		
Enoxaparin	Lovenox	SubQ		
Fondaparinux	Arixtra	SubQ		
Direct Thrombin Inhibitors				
Hirudin Analogs				
Desirudin	Iprivask	SubQ		
Other Direct Thrombin Inhibitors				
Dabigatran	Pradaxa, Pradax ♣	PO		
Direct Factor Xa Inhibitors				
Rivaroxaban	Xarelto	PO		
Apixaban	Eliquis	PO		
Edoxaban	Savaysa	PO		
ANTIPLATELET DRUGS			Antiplatelet drugs suppress platelet aggregation	Used primarily to prevent thrombosis in *arteries*
Cyclooxygenase Inhibitor				
Aspirin		PO		
$P2Y_{12}$ Adenosine Diphosphate Receptor Antagonists				
Clopidogrel	Plavix	PO		
Prasugrel	Effient	PO		
Ticagrelor	Brilinta	PO		
	Generic only	PO		
Protease-Activated Receptor-1 (PAR-1) Antagonists				
Vorapaxar	Zontivity	PO		
Other Antiplatelet Drugs				
Dipyridamole	Persantine	PO		
Cilostazol	Pletal	PO		

LMW, low molecular weight.

Although the anticoagulants and the antiplatelet drugs both suppress thrombosis, they do so by different mechanisms. As a result, they differ in their effects and applications. The *antiplatelet drugs* are most effective at preventing *arterial* thrombosis, whereas *anticoagulants* are most effective against *venous* thrombosis.

ANTICOAGULANTS

By definition, anticoagulants are drugs that *reduce formation of fibrin.* Two basic mechanisms are involved. One anticoagulant—warfarin—inhibits the *synthesis* of clotting factors, including factor X and thrombin. All other anticoagulants inhibit the *activity* of clotting factors: either factor Xa, thrombin, or both.

Anticoagulants are in three pharmacologic classes—vitamin K antagonists, direct factor Xa inhibitors, and direct thrombin inhibitors (see Table 44.1).

Heparin and Its Derivatives: Drugs That Activate Antithrombin

All drugs in this group share the same mechanism of action. Specifically, they greatly enhance the activity of *antithrombin,* a protein that inactivates two major clotting factors: *thrombin* and *factor Xa.* In the absence of thrombin and factor Xa, production of fibrin is reduced, and hence clotting is suppressed.

Our discussion focuses on three preparations: *unfractionated heparin,* the *low-molecular-weight (LMW) heparins,* and *fondaparinux.* Although all three activate antithrombin, they do not have equal effects on thrombin and factor Xa. Specifically, heparin reduces the activity of thrombin and factor Xa more or less equally; the LMW heparins reduce the activity of factor Xa more than they reduce the activity of thrombin; and fondaparinux causes selective inhibition of factor Xa, having no effect on thrombin. Properties of the three preparations are shown in Table 44.2.

Heparin (Unfractionated)

Heparin is a rapid-acting anticoagulant administered only by injection. Heparin differs from warfarin (an oral anticoagulant) in several respects, including mechanism, time course, indications, and management of overdose.

Chemistry

Heparin is not a single molecule, but rather a mixture of long polysaccharide chains, with molecular weights that range from 3000 to 30,000. The active region is a unique pentasaccharide (five-sugar) sequence found randomly along the chain. An important feature of heparin's structure is the presence of many negatively charged groups. Because of these negative charges, heparin is highly polar and hence cannot readily cross membranes.

Mechanism of Anticoagulant Action

Heparin suppresses coagulation by helping antithrombin inactivate clotting factors, primarily thrombin and factor Xa. As shown in Fig. 44.3, binding of heparin to antithrombin produces a conformational change in antithrombin that greatly enhances its ability to inactivate both thrombin and factor Xa. However, the process of inactivating these two clotting factors is distinct. To inactivate thrombin, heparin must simultaneously bind with both thrombin and antithrombin, thereby forming a ternary complex. In contrast, to inactivate factor Xa, heparin binds only with antithrombin; heparin itself does not bind with factor Xa.

By activating antithrombin, and thereby promoting the inactivation of thrombin and factor Xa, heparin ultimately suppresses formation of fibrin. Because fibrin forms the framework of thrombi in *veins,* heparin is especially useful for prophylaxis of *venous thrombosis.* Because thrombin and factor Xa are inhibited as soon as they bind with the heparin-antithrombin complex, the anticoagulant effects of heparin develop *quickly* (within minutes of intravenous [IV] administration). This contrasts with warfarin, whose full effects are not seen for *days.*

Pharmacokinetics

Absorption and Distribution. Because of its polarity and large size, heparin is unable to cross membranes, including those of the gastrointestinal (GI) tract. Consequently, heparin cannot be absorbed if given orally and therefore must be given by injection (IV or subcutaneous [subQ]). Because

TABLE 44.2 ▪ Comparison of Drugs That Activate Antithrombin

Property	Unfractionated Heparin	Low-Molecular-Weight Heparins	Fondaparinux
Molecular weight range	3000–30,000	1000–9000	1728
Mean molecular weight	12,000–15,000	4000–5000	1728
Mechanism of action	Activation of antithrombin, resulting in the inactivation of factor Xa and thrombin	Activation of antithrombin, resulting in preferential inactivation of factor Xa, plus some inactivation of thrombin	Activation of antithrombin, resulting in selective inactivation of factor Xa
Routes	IV, subQ	SubQ only	SubQ only
Nonspecific binding	Widespread	Minimal	Minimal
Laboratory monitoring	aPTT monitoring is essential	No aPTT monitoring required	No aPTT monitoring required
Dosage	Dosage must be adjusted on the basis of aPTT	Dosage is fixed	Dosage is fixed
Setting for use	Hospital	Hospital or home	Hospital or home
Cost	$3/day for heparin itself, but hospitalization and aPTT monitoring greatly increase the real cost	$35/day for LMW heparin (enoxaparin [Lovenox]), but home use and absence of aPTT monitoring greatly reduce the real cost	$59/day for fondaparinux, but home use and absence of aPTT monitoring greatly reduce the real cost

aPTT, activated partial thromboplastin time; LMW, low molecular weight.

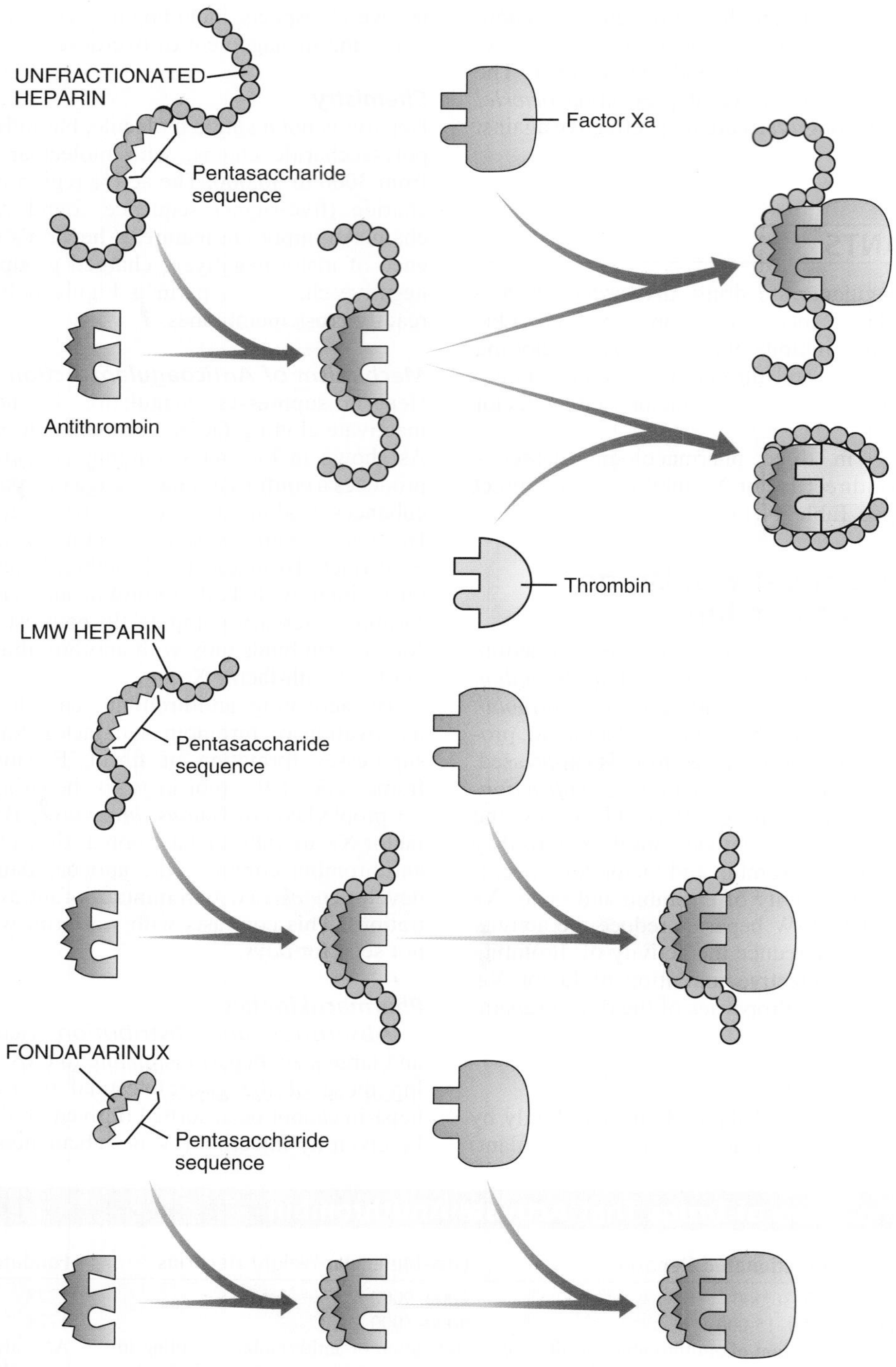

Figure 44.3 ■ Mechanism of action of heparin, low-molecular-weight (LMW) heparins, and fondaparinux.
All three drugs share a pentasaccharide sequence that allows them to bind with—and activate—antithrombin, a protein that inactivates two major clotting factors: thrombin and factor Xa. All three drugs enable antithrombin to inactivate factor Xa, but only heparin also facilitates inactivation of thrombin. *Upper panel:* Unfractionated heparin binds with antithrombin, causing a conformational change in antithrombin that greatly increases its ability to interact with factor Xa and thrombin. When the heparin-antithrombin complex binds with thrombin, heparin changes its conformation so that both heparin and antithrombin come in contact with thrombin. Formation of this ternary complex is necessary for thrombin inactivation. Inactivation of factor Xa is different: it only requires contact between activated antithrombin and factor Xa; contact between heparin and factor Xa is unnecessary. *Middle panel:* LMW heparins have the same pentasaccharide sequence as unfractionated heparin and can bind with and activate antithrombin. However, in contrast to unfractionated heparin, most molecules of LMW heparin can inactivate only factor Xa. They are unable to inactivate thrombin because most molecules of LMW heparin are too small to form a ternary complex with thrombin and antithrombin. *Lower panel:* Fondaparinux is a synthetic pentasaccharide identical in structure to the antithrombin binding sequence found in unfractionated heparin and LMW heparins. Being even smaller than LMW heparins, fondaparinux is too small to form a ternary complex with thrombin and can only inactivate factor Xa.

it cannot cross membranes, heparin does not traverse the placenta and does not enter breast milk.

Protein and Tissue Binding. Heparin binds nonspecifically to plasma proteins, mononuclear cells, and endothelial cells. As a result, plasma levels of free heparin can be highly variable. Because of this variability, intensive monitoring is required (see later).

Metabolism and Excretion. Heparin undergoes hepatic metabolism followed by renal excretion. Under normal conditions, the half-life is short (about 1.5 hours). However, in patients with hepatic or renal impairment, the half-life is increased.

Time Course. Therapy is sometimes initiated with a bolus IV injection, and effects begin immediately. Duration of action is brief (hours) and varies with dosage. Effects are prolonged in patients with hepatic or renal impairment.

Therapeutic Uses

Heparin is a preferred anticoagulant for use during *pregnancy* (because it doesn't cross the placenta) and in situations that require rapid onset of anticoagulant effects, including *pulmonary embolism* (PE) and *massive deep vein thrombosis* (DVT). In addition, heparin is used for patients undergoing *open heart surgery* and *renal dialysis;* during these procedures, heparin serves to prevent coagulation in devices of extracorporeal circulation (heart-lung machines, dialyzers). Low-dose therapy is used to *prevent postoperative venous thrombosis.* Heparin may also be useful for treating *disseminated intravascular coagulation,* a complex disorder in which fibrin clots form throughout the vascular system and in which bleeding tendencies may be present; bleeding can occur because massive fibrin production consumes available supplies of clotting factors. Heparin is also used as an adjunct to thrombolytic therapy of *acute myocardial infarction* (MI).

Adverse Effects

Hemorrhage. All the drugs in this chapter increase the risk for patient bleeding. Bleeding develops in about 10% of patients and is the principal complication of treatment. Hemorrhage can occur at any site and may be fatal. Patients should be monitored closely for signs of blood loss. These include reduced blood pressure, increased heart rate, bruises, petechiae, hematomas, red or black stools, cloudy or discolored urine, pelvic pain (suggesting ovarian hemorrhage), headache or faintness (suggesting cerebral hemorrhage), and lumbar pain (suggesting adrenal hemorrhage). If bleeding develops, heparin should be withdrawn.

The risk for hemorrhage can be decreased in several ways. First, dosage should be carefully controlled so that the activated partial thromboplastin time (see later) does not exceed 2 times the control value. In addition, candidates for heparin therapy should be screened for risk factors (see "Warnings and Contraindications"). Finally, antiplatelet drugs (e.g., aspirin, clopidogrel) should be avoided.

BLACK BOX WARNING: SPINAL OR EPIDURAL HEMATOMA

Heparin and all other anticoagulants pose a risk for spinal or epidural hematoma in patients undergoing spinal puncture or spinal or epidural anesthesia. Pressure on the spinal cord caused by the bleed can result in prolonged or permanent paralysis.

Risk for hematoma is increased by the following:

- Use of an indwelling epidural catheter
- Use of other anticoagulants (e.g., warfarin, dabigatran)
- Use of antiplatelet drugs (e.g., aspirin, clopidogrel)
- History of traumatic or repeated epidural or spinal puncture
- History of spinal deformity, spinal injury, or spinal surgery

Patients should be monitored for signs and symptoms of neurologic impairment. If impairment develops, immediate intervention is needed.

Heparin-Induced Thrombocytopenia (HIT). This is a potentially fatal immune-mediated disorder characterized by reduced platelet counts (thrombocytopenia) and a seemingly paradoxical *increase* in thrombotic events. The underlying cause is development of antibodies against heparin–platelet protein complexes. These antibodies activate platelets and damage the vascular endothelium, thereby promoting both thrombosis and a rapid loss of circulating platelets. Thrombus formation poses a risk for DVT, PE, cerebral thrombosis, and MI. Ischemic injury secondary to thrombosis in the limbs may require amputation of an arm or leg. Coronary thrombosis can be fatal. The primary treatment for HIT is discontinuation of heparin and, if anticoagulation is still needed, substitution of a nonheparin anticoagulant (e.g., argatroban). The incidence of HIT is between 0.2% and 5% among patients who receive heparin for more than 4 days.

HIT should be suspected whenever platelet counts fall significantly or when thrombosis develops despite adequate anticoagulation. Accordingly, to reduce the risk for HIT, patients should be monitored for signs of thrombosis and for reductions in platelets. Platelet counts should be determined frequently (2–3 times a week) during the first 3 weeks of heparin use and monthly thereafter. If severe thrombocytopenia develops (platelet count below 100,000/mm^3), heparin should be discontinued.

Hypersensitivity Reactions. Because commercial heparin is extracted from animal tissues, these preparations may be contaminated with antigens that can promote allergy. Possible allergic responses include chills, fever, and urticaria. Anaphylactic reactions are rare.

Other Adverse Effects. SubQ dosing may produce local irritation and hematoma. Vasospastic reactions that persist for several hours may develop after 1 or more weeks of treatment. Long-term, high-dose therapy may cause osteoporosis.

Warnings and Contraindications

Warnings. Heparin must be used with extreme caution in all patients who have a high likelihood of bleeding. Among these are individuals with hemophilia, increased capillary permeability, dissecting aneurysm, peptic ulcer disease, severe hypertension, or threatened abortion. Heparin must also be used cautiously in patients with severe disease of the liver or kidneys.

Contraindications. Heparin is contraindicated for patients with thrombocytopenia and uncontrollable bleeding. In addition, heparin should be avoided both during and immediately after surgery of the eye, brain, or spinal cord. Lumbar puncture and regional anesthesia are additional contraindications.

Drug Interactions

In heparin-treated patients, platelet aggregation is the major remaining defense against hemorrhage. Aspirin and other drugs that depress platelet function or affect coagulation will weaken this defense and hence must be employed with caution.

Laboratory Monitoring

The objective of anticoagulant therapy is to reduce blood coagulability to a level that is low enough to prevent thrombosis but not so low as to promote spontaneous bleeding. Because heparin levels can be highly variable, achieving this goal is difficult and requires careful control of dosage based on frequent tests of coagulation. The laboratory test employed most commonly is the *activated partial thromboplastin time* (aPTT). The normal value for the aPTT is 40 seconds. At therapeutic levels, heparin *increases* the aPTT by a factor of 1.5 to 2, making the aPTT 60 to 80 seconds. Because heparin has a rapid onset and brief duration, if an aPTT value falls outside the therapeutic range, coagulability can be quickly corrected through an adjustment in dosage: if the aPTT is too long (more than 80 seconds), the dosage should be lowered; conversely, if the aPTT is too short (less than 60 seconds), the dosage should be increased. Measurements of aPTTs should be made frequently (every 4–6 hours) during the initial phase of therapy. When an effective dosage has been established, measuring aPTT once a day will suffice.

Prescription and Preparations

Prescription. Heparin is prescribed in units, not in milligrams. The heparin unit is an index of anticoagulant activity. Heparin dosage is titrated on the basis of laboratory monitoring, and hence dosage can be adjusted as needed based on test results.

Preparations. Heparin sodium is supplied in single-dose vials; multidose vials; and unit-dose, preloaded syringes that have their own needles. Concentrations range from 1000 to 20,000 units/mL.

Dosage and Administration

General Considerations. Heparin is administered by injection only. Two routes are employed: *intravenous* (either intermittent or continuous) and *subcutaneous.* Intramuscular injection causes hematoma and must not be done. Heparin is not administered orally because heparin is too large and too polar to permit intestinal absorption.

Dosage varies by indication. Postoperative prophylaxis of thrombosis, for example, requires relatively small doses. In other situations, such as open heart surgery, much larger doses are needed. The dosages given here are for "general anticoagulant therapy." As a rule, the aPTT should be employed as a guideline for dosage titration; increases in the aPTT of 1.5- to 2-fold are therapeutic. Because heparin is formulated in widely varying concentrations, you must read the label carefully to ensure that dosing is correct.

Low-Molecular-Weight Heparins

Group Properties

LMW heparins are simply heparin preparations composed of molecules that are shorter than those found in unfractionated heparin. LMW heparins are as effective as unfractionated heparin and are easier to use because they can be given using a fixed dosage and don't require aPTT monitoring. As a result, LMW heparins can be used at home, whereas unfractionated heparin must be given in a hospital when administering intravenously. Because of these advantages, LMW heparins are now considered first-line therapy for prevention and treatment of DVT. In the United States two LMW heparins are available: enoxaparin [Lovenox] and dalteparin [Fragmin]. Differences between LMW heparins and unfractionated heparin are shown in Table 44.2.

Production. LMW heparins are made by depolymerizing unfractionated heparin (i.e., breaking unfractionated heparin into smaller pieces). Molecular weights in LMW preparations range between 1000 and 9000, with a mean of 4000 to 5000. In comparison, molecular weights in unfractionated heparin range between 3000 and 30,000, with a mean of 12,000 to 15,000.

Mechanism of Action. Anticoagulant activity of LMW heparin is mediated by the same active pentasaccharide sequence that mediates anticoagulant action of unfractionated heparin. However, because LMW heparin molecules are short, they do not have quite the same effect as unfractionated heparin. Specifically, whereas unfractionated heparin is equally good at inactivating factor Xa *and* thrombin, *LMW heparins preferentially inactivate factor Xa,* being much less able to inactivate thrombin. Why the difference? To inactivate

PATIENT-CENTERED CARE ACROSS THE LIFE SPAN

Anticoagulants

Life Stage	Patient Care Concerns
Infants	Heparin is commonly used in infants needing anticoagulation. Argatroban has been used successfully in infants with HIT. Warfarin is also administered to infants.
Children/adolescents	Many anticoagulants can be used safely in children, just in smaller doses. Side-effect profiles are similar to those of adults.
Pregnant women	Warfarin is classified in FDA Pregnancy Risk Category X and is contraindicated in pregnancy. LMW heparins and unfractionated heparin are commonly used in pregnancy. In pregnant women with HIT, argatroban is a safe alternative.
Breastfeeding women	Data are lacking regarding safety of these medications in breastfeeding. Warfarin and heparin are both safe to use.
Older adults	Atrial fibrillation becomes more common with age. In older adults, benefit must outweigh risk for bleeding secondary to falls, decreased renal function, or polypharmacy.

FDA, U.S. Food and Drug Administration; HIT, heparin-induced thrombocytopenia; LMW, low-molecular-weight.

thrombin, a heparin chain must not only contain the pentasaccharide sequence that activates antithrombin but must also be long enough to provide a binding site for thrombin. This binding site is necessary because inactivation of thrombin requires simultaneous binding of thrombin with heparin and antithrombin (see Fig. 44.3). In contrast to unfractionated heparin chains, most (but not all) LMW heparin chains are too short to allow thrombin binding, and hence LMW heparins are less able to inactivate thrombin.

Therapeutic Use. LMW heparins are *approved* for (1) prevention of DVT after abdominal surgery, hip replacement surgery, or knee replacement surgery; (2) treatment of established DVT, with or without PE; and (3) prevention of ischemic complications in patients with unstable angina, non–Q-wave MI, and ST-elevation MI (STEMI). In addition, these drugs have been used extensively *off-label* to prevent DVT after general surgery and in patients with multiple trauma and acute spinal injury. When used for prophylaxis or treatment of DVT, LMW heparins are at least as effective as unfractionated heparin, and possibly more effective.

Pharmacokinetics. Compared with unfractionated heparin, LMW heparins have higher bioavailability and longer half-lives. Bioavailability is higher because LMW heparins do not undergo nonspecific binding to proteins and tissues and hence are more available for anticoagulant effects. Half-lives are prolonged (up to 6 times longer than that of unfractionated heparin) because LMW heparins undergo less binding to macrophages and hence undergo slower clearance by the liver. Because of increased bioavailability, plasma levels of LMW heparin are highly predictable. As a result, these drugs can be given using a fixed dosage, with no need for routine monitoring of coagulation. Because of their long half-lives, LMW heparins can be given just once or twice a day.

Administration, Dosing, and Monitoring. All LMW heparins are administered by subQ injection. Dosage is sometimes based on body weight, depending on indication. Because plasma levels of LMW heparins are predictable for any given dose, these drugs can be employed using a fixed dosage without laboratory monitoring. This contrasts with unfractionated heparin, which requires dosage adjustments on the basis of aPTT measurements. Because LMW heparins have an extended half-life, dosing can be done once or twice daily. For prophylaxis of DVT, dosing is begun in the perioperative period and continued 5 to 10 days.

Adverse Effects and Interactions. *Bleeding* is the major adverse effect. However, the incidence of bleeding complications is less than with unfractionated heparin. Despite the potential for bleeding, LMW heparins are considered safe for outpatient use. Like unfractionated heparin, LMW heparins can cause immune-mediated *thrombocytopenia.* As with unfractionated heparin, overdose with LMW heparins can be treated with protamine sulfate.

Like unfractionated heparin, LMW heparins can cause *severe neurologic injury,* including permanent paralysis, when given to patients undergoing *spinal puncture* or *spinal or epidural anesthesia.* The risk for serious harm is increased by concurrent use of antiplatelet drugs (e.g., aspirin, clopidogrel) or anticoagulants (e.g., warfarin, dabigatran). Patients should be monitored closely for signs of neurologic impairment.

Cost. LMW heparins cost more than unfractionated heparin (e.g., about $63/day for dalteparin vs. $8/day for unfractionated heparin). However, because LMW heparins can be used at home and don't require aPTT monitoring, the overall cost of treatment is lower than with unfractionated heparin.

Individual Preparations

In the United States two LMW heparins are available: enoxaparin and dalteparin. Additional LMW heparins are available in other countries. Each preparation is unique, so clinical experience with one may not apply fully to the other.

Enoxaparin. Enoxaparin is approved for prevention of DVT after hip and knee replacement surgery or abdominal surgery in patients considered at high risk for thromboembolic complications (e.g., obese patients, those older than 40 years, and those with malignancy or a history of DVT or PE). The drug is also approved for preventing ischemic complications in patients with unstable angina, non–Q-wave MI, or STEMI.

Administration and Dosage. Enoxaparin is administered by deep subQ injection. For patients with normal renal function (or moderate renal impairment), dosages are as follows:

- Prevention of DVT after hip or knee replacement surgery—30 mg every 12 hours starting 12 to 24 hours after surgery and continuing 7 to 10 days.
- Prevention of DVT after abdominal surgery—40 mg once daily, beginning 2 hours before surgery and continuing 7 to 10 days.
- Treatment of established DVT—1 mg/kg every 12 hours
- Patients with unstable angina or non–Q-wave MI—1 mg/kg every 12 hours (in conjunction with oral aspirin, 100–325 mg once daily) for 2 to 8 days.
- Patients with acute STEMI—30 mg/kg by IV bolus plus 1 mg/kg subQ, followed by 1 mg/kg subQ every 12 hours for up to 8 days.

For patients with severe renal impairment, dosage should be reduced.

Dalteparin. Approved indications for dalteparin are prevention of DVT after hip replacement surgery or abdominal surgery in patients considered at high risk for thromboembolic complications, prevention of ischemic complications in patients with unstable angina or non–Q-wave MI, and management of symptomatic venous thromboembolism (VTE). Administration is by deep subQ injection. Dosages are as follows:

- Prevention of DVT after hip replacement surgery—2500 units 1 or 2 hours before surgery, 2500 units that evening (at least 6 hours after the first dose), and then 5000 units once daily for 5 to 10 days.
- Prevention of DVT after abdominal surgery—2500 units once daily for 5 to 10 days, starting 1 to 2 hours before surgery. In high-risk patients, this dose is increased to 5000 units once daily, starting the night before surgery.
- Patients with unstable angina or non–Q-wave MI—120 units/kg (but not more than 10,000 units total) every 12 hours for 5 to 8 days. Concurrent therapy with aspirin (75–165 mg/day) is required.
- Patients with symptomatic VTE—200 units/kg (but not more than 18,000 units total) once daily for 1 month, then 150 units/kg (but not more than 18,000 units total) once daily for months 2 through 6.

Fondaparinux

Actions

Fondaparinux [Arixtra] is a synthetic, subQ anticoagulant that enhances the activity of antithrombin, to cause selective inhibition of factor Xa. The result is reduced production of thrombin and hence reduced coagulation. Note that fondaparinux differs from the heparin preparations, which cause inactivation of thrombin as well as factor Xa.

Fondaparinux is closely related in structure and function to heparin and the LMW heparins. Structurally, fondaparinux is a pentasaccharide identical to the antithrombin-binding region of the heparins. Hence, like the heparins, fondaparinux is able to induce a conformational change in antithrombin, thereby increasing antithrombin's activity—but only against factor Xa, not against thrombin. Why is fondaparinux selective for factor Xa? Because the drug is quite small—even smaller than the LMW heparins. As a result, it is too small to form a complex with both antithrombin and thrombin, and hence cannot reduce thrombin activity (see Fig. 44.3).

Fondaparinux has no effect on prothrombin time, aPTT, bleeding time, or platelet aggregation.

Therapeutic Use

Fondaparinux is approved for (1) preventing DVT after hip fracture surgery, hip replacement surgery, knee replacement surgery, or abdominal surgery; (2) treating acute PE (in conjunction with warfarin); and (3) treating acute DVT (in conjunction with warfarin). The drug is somewhat more effective than enoxaparin (an LMW heparin) at preventing DVT but may cause slightly more bleeding. Anticoagulation may persist for 2 to 4 days after the last dose. Fondaparinux is administered using a fixed dosage and does not require routine laboratory monitoring.

Pharmacokinetics

Fondaparinux is administered by subQ injection. Bioavailability is 100%. Plasma levels peak 2 hours after dosing. The drug is eliminated by the kidneys with a half-life of 17 to 21 hours. The half-life is increased in patients with renal impairment.

Adverse Effects

As with other anticoagulants, bleeding is the biggest concern. The risk is increased by advancing age and renal impairment. Fondaparinux should be used with caution in patients with moderate renal impairment, defined as creatinine clearance (CrCl) of 30 to 50 mL/minute, and avoided in patients with severe renal impairment, defined as CrCl below 30 mL/minute. The drug should also be avoided for prophylactic use in patients weighing less than 50 kg because low body weight increases bleeding risk. After surgery, at least 6 hours should elapse before starting fondaparinux. Aspirin and other drugs that interfere with hemostasis should be used with caution. In contrast to overdose with heparin or LMW heparins, overdose with fondaparinux cannot be treated with protamine sulfate.

Fondaparinux does not promote immune-mediated HIT, although it still can lower platelet counts. During clinical trials, thrombocytopenia developed in 3% of patients. Platelet counts should be monitored, and if they fall below 100,000/mm^3, fondaparinux should be discontinued.

In patients undergoing anesthesia using an epidural or spinal catheter, fondaparinux (as well as other anticoagulants) can cause spinal or epidural hematoma, which can result in permanent paralysis. However, in clinical trials, when fondaparinux was administered no sooner than 2 hours after catheter removal, no hematomas were reported.

Preparations, Dosage, and Administration

Fondaparinux [Arixtra] is available in single-dose, prefilled syringes (2.5, 5, 7.5, and 10 mg). Dosing is done once a day by subQ injection.

For prevention of DVT, the recommended dosage is 2.5 mg once a day, starting 6 to 8 hours after surgery. The usual duration is 5 to 9 days.

For treatment of acute DVT or acute PE, dosage is based on body weight as follows: for patients under 50 kg, 5 mg once daily; for patients 50 to 100 kg, 7.5 mg once daily, and for patients over 100 kg, 10 mg once daily. The usual duration is 5 to 9 days when overlapping with warfarin.

Warfarin, a Vitamin K Antagonist

Warfarin [Coumadin, Jantoven], a vitamin K antagonist, is our oldest *oral* anticoagulant. The drug is similar to heparin in some respects and quite different in others. Like heparin, warfarin is used to prevent thrombosis. In contrast to heparin, warfarin has a delayed onset, which makes it inappropriate for emergencies. However, because it doesn't require injection, warfarin is well suited for long-term prophylaxis. Like heparin, warfarin carries a significant risk for hemorrhage, which is amplified by the many drug interactions to which warfarin is subject.

History

The history of warfarin underscores its potential for harm. Warfarin was discovered after a farmer noticed that his cattle bled after eating spoiled clover silage. The causative agent was identified as bishydroxycoumarin (dicumarol). Research into derivatives of dicumarol led to the synthesis of warfarin. When warfarin was first developed, clinical use was ruled out owing to concerns about hemorrhage. So, instead of becoming a medicine, warfarin was used to kill rats. The drug proved especially effective in this application and remains one of our most widely used rodenticides. Clinical interest in warfarin was renewed after the report of a failed suicide attempt using huge doses of a warfarin-based rat poison. The clinical trials triggered by that event soon demonstrated that warfarin could be employed safely to treat humans.

Mechanism of Action

Warfarin suppresses coagulation by decreasing production of four clotting factors, namely, factors VII, IX, X, and prothrombin. These factors are known as *vitamin K–dependent clotting factors* because an active form of vitamin K is needed to make them. Warfarin works by inhibiting *vitamin K epoxide reductase complex 1* (VKORC1), the enzyme needed to convert vitamin K to the required active form. Because of its mechanism, warfarin is referred to as a *vitamin K antagonist,* a term that is somewhat misleading because it implies antagonism of vitamin K *actions,* not antagonism of vitamin K *activation.* In therapeutic doses, warfarin reduces production of vitamin K–dependent clotting factors by 30% to 50%.

Pharmacokinetics

Absorption, Distribution, and Elimination

Warfarin is readily absorbed after oral dosing. When in the blood, about 99% of warfarin binds to albumin. Warfarin molecules that remain free (unbound) can readily cross membranes, including those of the placenta and milk-producing glands. Warfarin is inactivated in the liver, mainly by CYP2C9, the 2C9 isoenzyme of cytochrome P450. Metabolites are excreted in the urine and feces.

Time Course

Although warfarin acts quickly to inhibit clotting factor *synthesis,* noticeable *anticoagulant effects* are delayed because warfarin has no effect on clotting factors already in circulation. Hence, until these clotting factors decay, coagulation remains unaffected. Because decay of clotting factors occurs with a half-life of 6 hours to 2.5 days (depending on the clotting factor under consideration), initial responses may not be evident until 8 to 12 hours after the first dose. Peak effects take several days to develop.

After warfarin is discontinued, coagulation remains inhibited for 2 to 5 days because warfarin has a long half-life (1.5–2 days). Hence synthesis of new clotting factors remains suppressed, despite stopping dosing.

Therapeutic Uses

Overview of Uses

Warfarin is employed most frequently for long-term prophylaxis of thrombosis. Specific indications are (1) prevention of venous thrombosis and associated PE, (2) prevention of thromboembolism in patients with prosthetic heart valves, and (3) prevention of thrombosis in patients with atrial fibrillation. The drug has also been used to reduce the risk for recurrent transient ischemic attacks (TIAs) and recurrent MI. Because onset of effects is delayed, warfarin is not useful in emergencies. When rapid action is needed, anticoagulant therapy can be initiated with heparin.

Atrial Fibrillation

As discussed in Chapter 41, atrial fibrillation carries a high risk for stroke secondary to clot formation in the atrium. When people have atrial fibrillation, anticoagulant therapy is given long term to prevent clot formation. Until recently, warfarin was the only oral anticoagulant available and hence has been the reference standard for stroke prevention. However, four novel oral anticoagulants (NOACs)—dabigatran [Pradaxa, Pradax ♣], apixaban [Eliquis], edoxaban [Savaysa], and rivaroxaban [Xarelto]—which are much easier to use than warfarin, are likely to replace warfarin as the treatment of choice for many patients.

Monitoring Treatment

The anticoagulant effects of warfarin are evaluated by monitoring *prothrombin time* (PT)—a coagulation test that is especially sensitive to alterations in vitamin K–dependent factors. The average pretreatment value for PT is 12 seconds. Treatment with warfarin prolongs PT.

Traditionally, PT test results had been reported as a *PT ratio,* which is simply the ratio of the patient's PT to a control PT. However, there is a serious problem with this form of reporting: test results can vary widely among laboratories. The underlying cause of variability is thromboplastin, a critical reagent employed in the PT test. To ensure that test results from different laboratories are comparable, results are now reported in terms of an *international normalized ratio* (INR). The INR is determined by multiplying the observed PT ratio by a correction factor specific to the particular thromboplastin preparation employed for the test.

The objective of treatment is to raise the INR to an appropriate value. Recommended INR ranges are shown in Table 44.3. As indicated, an INR of 2 to 3 is appropriate for most patients—although for some patients, the target INR is 2.5 to 3.5. If the INR is below the recommended range, warfarin dosage should be increased. Conversely, if the INR is above the recommended range, dosage should be reduced. Unfortunately, because warfarin has a delayed onset and prolonged duration of action, the INR cannot be altered quickly: after the dosage has been changed, it may take a week or more to reach the desired INR.

INR must be determined frequently during warfarin therapy. PT should be measured daily during the first 5 days of treatment, twice a week for the next 1 to 2 weeks, once a week for the next 1 to 2 months, and every 2 to 4 weeks thereafter. In addition, PT should be determined whenever a drug that interacts with warfarin is added to or deleted from the regimen.

INR can now be monitored at home. Several devices are available, including *CoaguChek* and the *ProTime Microcoagulation System.* These small, hand-held machines are easy to use, provide reliable results, and determine PT and INR values. In addition, the ProTime meter can be programmed by the prescriber with upper and lower INR values appropriate for the individual patient. When this is done, the meter will display either *In Range, INR High,* or *INR Low,* depending on the degree of anticoagulation. Home monitoring is more convenient than laboratory monitoring and gives patients a sense of empowerment. In addition, it improves anticoagulation control. In theory, home monitoring should help reduce bleeding (from excessive anticoagulation) and thrombosis (from insufficient anticoagulation). The CoaguChek meter costs about $1300, and the ProTime meter costs about $2700 to $3500. Each test costs about $10.

TABLE 44.3 ▪ Monitoring Warfarin Therapy: Recommended Ranges of Prothrombin Time–Derived Values

Condition Being Treated	Recommended Ranges	
	Observed PT Ratio*	INR†
Acute myocardial infarction‡	1.3–1.5	2–3
Atrial fibrillation‡	1.3–1.5	2–3
Valvular heart disease‡	1.3–1.5	2–3
Pulmonary embolism	1.3–1.5	2–3
Venous thrombosis§	1.3–1.5	2–3
Tissue heart valves‡	1.3–1.5	2–3
Mechanical heart valves	1.5–2	3–4.5
Systemic embolism		
Prevention	1.3–1.5	2–3
Recurrent	1.5–2	2–3

*Observed prothrombin time (PT) ratio = ratio of patient's PT to a control PT value. In this table, the reagent used to determine the control PT value is one of the preparations of rabbit brain thromboplastin employed in the United States. Had a different preparation of thromboplastin been used, the observed PT ratio could be very different.

†INR (international normalized ratio) is calculated from the observed PT ratio. The INR is equivalent to the PT ratio that would have been obtained if the patient's PT has been compared with a PT value obtained using the International Reference Preparation, a standardized human brain thromboplastin prepared by the World Health Organization. In contrast to PT ratios, INR values are comparable from one laboratory to the next throughout the United States and the rest of the world.

‡For prevention of ischemic stroke and systemic embolism.

§Prophylaxis in high-risk surgery; treatment.

Adverse Effects

Hemorrhage

Bleeding is the major complication of warfarin therapy. Hemorrhage can occur at any site. Patients should be monitored closely for signs of bleeding (reduced blood pressure, increased heart rate, bruises, petechiae, hematomas, red or black stools, cloudy or discolored urine, pelvic pain, headache, and lumbar pain). If bleeding develops, warfarin should be discontinued. Severe overdose can be treated with *vitamin K* (see later). Patients should be encouraged to carry identification (e.g., Medic Alert bracelet) to inform emergency personnel of warfarin use. Of note, compared with warfarin, the newer oral anticoagulants—apixaban, rivaroxaban, and dabigatran—pose a significantly lower risk for serious bleeds.

Several measures can reduce the risk for bleeding. Candidates for treatment must be carefully screened for risk factors (see "Warnings and Contraindications"). INR must be measured frequently. A variety of drugs can potentiate warfarin's effects (see later) and hence must be used with care.

Patient Education

RISK FOR BLEEDING WITH WARFARIN

Patients should be given detailed verbal and written instructions regarding signs of bleeding, dosage size and timing, and scheduling of INR tests. When a patient is incapable of accurate self-medication, a responsible individual must supervise treatment. Patients should be advised to make a record of each dose, rather than relying on memory. A soft toothbrush can reduce gingival bleeding. An electric razor can reduce cuts from shaving.

Warfarin intensifies bleeding during surgery. Accordingly, surgeons must be informed of warfarin use. Patients anticipating elective procedures should discontinue warfarin several days before the appointment. If an emergency procedure must be performed, injection of vitamin K can help suppress bleeding.

Does warfarin increase bleeding during dental surgery? Yes, but not that much. Accordingly, most patients needn't interrupt warfarin for dental procedures, including dental surgery. However, it is important that the INR be in the target range.

Fetal Hemorrhage and Teratogenesis From Use During Pregnancy

Warfarin can cross the placenta and affect the developing fetus. Fetal hemorrhage and death have occurred. In addition, warfarin can cause gross malformations, central nervous system defects, and optic atrophy. Accordingly, *warfarin is classified in U.S. Food and Drug Administration (FDA) Pregnancy Risk Category X: the risks to the developing fetus outweigh any possible benefits of treatment.* Women of childbearing age should be informed about the potential for teratogenesis and advised to postpone pregnancy. If pregnancy occurs, the possibility of termination should be discussed. If an anticoagulant is needed during pregnancy, heparin or LMW heparin, which do not cross the placenta, should be employed.

Use During Lactation

Warfarin enters breast milk. Women should be advised against breastfeeding.

Other Adverse Effects

Adverse effects other than hemorrhage are uncommon. Possible undesired responses include skin necrosis, alopecia, urticaria, dermatitis, fever, GI disturbances, and red-orange discoloration of urine, which must not be confused with hematuria. Long-term warfarin use (more than 12 months) may weaken bones and thereby increase the risk for fractures.

Drug Interactions

General Considerations

Warfarin is subject to a large number of clinically significant adverse interactions—perhaps more than any other drug. As a result of interactions, anticoagulant effects may be reduced to the point of permitting thrombosis, or they may be increased to the point of causing hemorrhage. Patients must be informed about the potential for hazardous interactions and instructed to avoid *all* drugs not specifically approved by the prescriber. This prohibition includes prescription drugs and over-the-counter products.

Interactions between warfarin and other drugs are shown in Table 44.4. As indicated, the interactants fall into three major categories: (1) *drugs that increase anticoagulant effects,* (2) *drugs that promote bleeding,* and (3) *drugs that decrease anticoagulant effects.* The major mechanisms by which anticoagulant effects can be *increased* are (1) displacement of warfarin from plasma albumin, (2) inhibition of the hepatic enzymes that degrade warfarin, and (3) decreased synthesis of clotting factors. The major mechanisms for *decreasing*

TABLE 44.4 ■ Interactions Between Warfarin and Other Drugs

Drug Category	Mechanism of Interaction	Representative Interacting Drugs
Drugs that *increase* the effects of warfarin	Displacement of warfarin from albumin	Aspirin and other salicylates Sulfonamides
	Inhibition of warfarin degradation	Acetaminophen Amiodarone Azole antifungal agents Cimetidine Disulfiram Leflunomide Trimethoprim-sulfamethoxazole
	Decreased synthesis of clotting factors	Certain parenteral cephalosporins, including cefoperazone and cefamandole
Drugs that *promote bleeding*	Inhibition of platelet aggregation	Abciximab Aspirin and other salicylates Cilostazol Clopidogrel Dipyridamole Eptifibatide Prasugrel Ticagrelor Ticlopidine Tirofiban
	Inhibition of clotting factors and/or thrombin	Antimetabolites Apixaban Argatroban Bivalirudin Dabigatran Desirudin Fondaparinux Heparins Rivaroxaban
	Promotion of ulcer formation	Aspirin Glucocorticoids Indomethacin Phenylbutazone
Drugs that *decrease* the effects of warfarin	Induction of drug-metabolizing enzymes	Carbamazepine Phenobarbital Phenytoin Rifampin
	Promotion of clotting factor synthesis	Oral contraceptives Vitamin K_1
	Reduction of warfarin absorption	Cholestyramine Colestipol

anticoagulant effects are (1) acceleration of warfarin degradation through induction of hepatic drug-metabolizing enzymes, (2) increased synthesis of clotting factors, and (3) inhibition of warfarin absorption. Mechanisms by which drugs can *promote bleeding,* and thereby complicate anticoagulant therapy, include (1) inhibition of platelet aggregation, (2) inhibition of clotting factors, and (3) generation of GI ulcers.

The existence of an interaction between warfarin and another drug does not absolutely preclude using the combination. The interaction does mean, however, that the combination must be used with due caution. The potential for harm is greatest when an interacting drug is being added to or withdrawn from the regimen. At these times, PT must be monitored and the dosage of warfarin adjusted to compensate for the effect of removing or adding an interacting drug.

Specific Interacting Drugs

Of the many drugs listed in Table 44.4, a few are especially likely to produce interactions of clinical significance. Four are discussed next.

Heparin. The interaction of heparin with warfarin is obvious: being an anticoagulant itself, heparin directly increases the bleeding tendencies brought on by warfarin. Yet because onset of a therapeutic INR when starting warfarin therapy may take a few days, heparin is often administered alongside warfarin during this time. Combined therapy with heparin plus warfarin must be performed with care.

Aspirin. Aspirin inhibits platelet aggregation. By blocking aggregation, aspirin can suppress formation of the platelet plug that initiates hemostasis. To make matters worse, aspirin can act directly on the GI tract to cause ulcers, thereby initiating bleeding. Therefore, when the antifibrin effects of warfarin are coupled with the antiplatelet and ulcerogenic effects of aspirin, the potential for hemorrhage is significant. Accordingly, patients should be warned specifically against using any product that contains aspirin, unless the provider has prescribed aspirin therapy. Drugs similar to aspirin (e.g., indomethacin, ibuprofen) should be avoided as well.

Nonaspirin Antiplatelet Drugs. Like aspirin, other antiplatelet drugs can increase the risk for bleeding with warfarin. Accordingly, these drugs (e.g., clopidogrel, dipyridamole, ticlopidine, vorapaxar) should be used with caution.

Acetaminophen. In the past, acetaminophen was considered safe for patients taking warfarin. In fact, acetaminophen was routinely recommended as an aspirin substitute for patients who needed a mild analgesic. Now, however, it appears that acetaminophen can increase the risk for bleeding: compared with nonusers of acetaminophen, those who take just 4 regular-strength tablets a day for a week are 10 times more likely to have a dangerously high INR. Unlike aspirin, which promotes bleeding by inhibiting platelet aggregation, acetaminophen is believed to inhibit warfarin degradation, thereby raising warfarin levels. At this time, the interaction between acetaminophen and warfarin has not been proved. Nonetheless, when the drugs are combined, the INR should be monitored closely.

Warnings and Contraindications

Like heparin, warfarin is contraindicated for patients with severe thrombocytopenia or uncontrollable bleeding and for patients undergoing lumbar puncture, regional anesthesia, or surgery of the eye, brain, or spinal cord. Also like heparin, warfarin must be used with extreme caution in patients at high risk for bleeding, including those with hemophilia, increased capillary permeability, dissecting aneurysm, GI ulcers, and severe hypertension, and in women anticipating abortion. In addition, warfarin is contraindicated in the presence of vitamin K deficiency, liver disease, and alcoholism—conditions that can disrupt hepatic synthesis of clotting factors. Warfarin is also contraindicated during pregnancy and lactation.

Vitamin K_1 for Warfarin Overdose

The effects of warfarin overdose can be overcome with vitamin K_1 (phytonadione). Vitamin K_1 antagonizes warfarin's actions and can thereby reverse warfarin-induced inhibition of clotting factor synthesis. (Vitamin K_3—menadione—has no effect on warfarin action.)

As a rule, small doses—2.5 mg by oral administration (PO)—are preferred. Large doses (e.g., 10 mg PO) can cause prolonged resistance to warfarin, thereby hampering restoration of anticoagulation after bleeding is under control.

If vitamin K fails to control bleeding, levels of clotting factors can be raised quickly by infusing fresh whole blood, fresh-frozen plasma, or plasma concentrates of vitamin K–dependent clotting factors.

What About Dietary Vitamin K?

Like medicinal vitamin K, dietary vitamin K can reduce the anticoagulant effects of warfarin. Dietary sources include mayonnaise, canola oil, soybean oil, and green leafy vegetables. Patients do not need to avoid these foods but instead should keep intake of vitamin K constant. If vitamin K intake does increase, then warfarin dosage should be increased as well. Conversely, if vitamin K intake decreases, the warfarin dosage should decrease too.

Contrasts Between Warfarin and Heparin

Although heparin and warfarin are both anticoagulants, they differ in important ways (Table 44.5). Whereas warfarin is given orally, heparin is given by injection. Although both drugs decrease fibrin formation, they do so by different mechanisms: heparin inactivates thrombin and factor Xa, whereas warfarin inhibits synthesis of clotting factors. Heparin and warfarin differ with respect to time course of action: effects of heparin begin and fade rapidly, whereas effects of warfarin begin slowly but persist several days. Different tests are used to monitor therapy: changes in aPTT are used to monitor heparin treatment; changes in PT are used to monitor warfarin. Finally, these drugs differ with respect to management of overdose: protamine is given to counteract heparin; vitamin K_1 is given to counteract warfarin.

Dosage

Basic Considerations

Dosage requirements for warfarin vary widely among individuals, and hence dosage must be tailored to each patient. Traditionally, dosage adjustments have been done empirically (i.e., by trial and error). Dosing is usually begun at 2 to 5 mg/day. Maintenance dosages, which typically range from 2 to 10 mg/day, are determined by the target INR value. For most patients, dosage should be adjusted to produce an INR between 2 and 3.

TABLE 44.5 ▪ Contrasts Between Heparin and Warfarin

	Heparin	Warfarin
Mechanism of action	Activates antithrombin, which then inactivates thrombin and factor Xa	Inhibits synthesis of vitamin K–dependent clotting factors, including prothrombin and factor X
Route	IV or subQ	PO
Onset	Rapid (minutes)	Slow (hours)
Duration	Brief (hours)	Prolonged (days)
Monitoring	aPTT	PT (INR)[†]
Antidote for overdose	Protamine	Vitamin K_1

[†]Test results are reported as an INR (international normalized ratio).
aPTT, activated partial thromboplastin time; PT, prothrombin time.

Genetics and Dosage Adjustment

Patients with variant genes that code for VKORC1 and CYP2C9 are at increased risk for warfarin-induced bleeding and hence require reduced doses. As noted earlier, VKORC1 is the target enzyme that warfarin inhibits, and CYP2C9 is the enzyme that metabolizes warfarin. Variations in VKORC1 increase the enzyme's sensitivity to inhibition by warfarin, and variations in CYP2C9 delay warfarin breakdown. With either variation, effects of warfarin are increased. To reduce the risk for bleeding, the FDA now recommends—but does not require—that patients undergo genetic testing for these variants. Dosage reductions based on this information can be determined using the calculator at www.warfarindosing.org.

Preparations

Warfarin sodium [Coumadin, Jantoven] is available in tablets (1, 2, 2.5, 3, 4, 5, 6, 7.5, and 10 mg) for oral use. In addition, warfarin is available in a formulation for parenteral dosing, which is not commonly done.

Direct Thrombin Inhibitors

The anticoagulants discussed in this section work by direct inhibition of thrombin. Hence they differ from the heparin-like anticoagulants, which inhibit thrombin indirectly (by enhancing the activity of antithrombin). One of the direct thrombin inhibitors—dabigatran—is administered orally; another—desirudin—is administered subcutaneously; and two others—bivalirudin and argatroban—are administered by continuous IV infusion. Only the subQ and PO drugs are suitable for outpatient use.

Dabigatran Etexilate

Dabigatran etexilate [Pradaxa, Pradax ♣] is an *oral* prodrug that undergoes rapid conversion to *dabigatran,* a reversible, direct thrombin inhibitor. Compared with warfarin—our oldest oral anticoagulant—dabigatran has five major advantages: rapid onset; no need to monitor anticoagulation; few drug-food interactions; lower risk for major bleeding; and, because responses are predictable, the same dose can be used for all patients, regardless of age or weight. Contrasts between dabigatran and warfarin are shown in Table 44.6.

Mechanism of Action

Dabigatran is a direct, reversible inhibitor of thrombin. The drug binds with and inhibits thrombin that is free in the blood as well as thrombin that is bound to clots. In contrast, heparin inhibits only free thrombin. By inhibiting thrombin, dabigatran (1) prevents the conversion of fibrinogen into fibrin and (2) prevents the activation of factor XIII and thereby prevents the conversion of soluble fibrin into insoluble fibrin.

Therapeutic Use

Atrial Fibrillation. In the United States dabigatran was first approved for prevention of stroke and systemic embolism in patients with nonvalvular atrial fibrillation. Approval was based on the RE-LY trial, in which more than 18,000 patients were randomized to receive either dabigatran (110 or 150 mg twice daily) or warfarin (dosage adjusted to produce an INR of 2–3). At the lower dabigatran dose (110 mg twice daily), the incidence of bleeding with dabigatran was less than with warfarin, but protection against stroke was less, too. By contrast, at the higher dose (150 mg twice daily), the incidence of bleeding with dabigatran equaled that with warfarin, but the incidence of stroke or embolism was significantly lower. On the basis of these results, the FDA concluded that, for patients with atrial fibrillation, the benefit/risk profile of dabigatran was better at 150 mg twice daily than at 110 mg twice daily, and hence they approved the higher dose for these patients.

Knee or Hip Replacement. Dabigatran is approved for prevention of VTE after knee or hip replacement surgery. The dosage is 220 mg once daily, after an initial dose of 110 mg.

DVT and PE Treatment. In 2014, the FDA approved dabigatran for the treatment of DVT and PE in patients who have been treated with a parenteral anticoagulant for 5 to 10 days and to reduce the risk for recurrent DVT and PE in patients who have been previously treated. The dose for treatment is 150 mg twice daily.

Pharmacokinetics

Dabigatran etexilate is well absorbed from the GI tract, both in the presence and absence of food. (Food delays absorption but does not reduce the extent of absorption.) Plasma levels peak about 1 hour after dosing in the absence of food and 3 hours after dosing in the presence of food. In the blood, plasma esterases rapidly convert dabigatran etexilate to dabigatran, the drug's active form. Protein binding in blood is low (about 35%). Dabigatran is not metabolized by hepatic enzymes. Elimination is primarily renal. The half-life is 13 hours in patients with normal renal function (CrCl 50 mL/min or higher) and increases to 18 hours in patients with moderate renal impairment (CrCl 30–50 mL/min).

Adverse Effects

Bleeding. Like all other anticoagulants, dabigatran can cause bleeding. In the RE-LY trial, about 17% of patients taking 150 mg of dabigatran twice daily experienced bleeding of any intensity, and 3% experienced major bleeding. Patients who develop pathologic bleeding should stop taking the drug. Compared with warfarin, dabigatran is safer, posing a much lower risk for hemorrhagic stroke and other major bleeds.

Because dabigatran is not highly protein bound, dialysis can remove much of the drug (about 60% over 2–3 hours). Because dabigatran is eliminated primarily in the urine, maintaining adequate diuresis is important.

Owing to bleeding risk, dabigatran should be stopped before elective surgery. For patients with normal renal function (CrCl

TABLE 44.6 ▪ Properties of Oral Anticoagulants

	Warfarin [Coumadin]	Rivaroxaban [Xarelto]	Apixaban [Eliquis]	Edoxaban [Savaysa]	Dabigatran Etexilate [Pradaxa, Pradax 🍁]
Mechanism	Decreased synthesis of vitamin K–dependent clotting factors	Inhibition of factor Xa	Inhibition of factor Xa	Inhibition of factor Xa	Direct inhibition of thrombin
INDICATIONS:					
Atrial fibrillation	Yes	Yes	Yes	Yes	Yes
Heart valve replacement	Yes	No	No	No	No
Knee or hip replacement	Yes	Yes	No	No	Yes*
Onset	Delayed (days)	Rapid (hours)	Rapid (hours)	Rapid (hours)	Rapid (hours)
Duration	Prolonged	Short	Short	Short	Short
Antidote available	Yes (oral/parenteral vitamin K)	No	No	No	No
Drug-food interactions	Many	Few	Few	Few	Few
INR testing needed	Yes	No	No	No	No
Dosage	Adjusted based on INR	Fixed	Fixed	Fixed	Fixed
Doses/day	One	One	Two	One	Two
Clinical experience	Extensive	Limited	Limited	Limited	Limited
Advantages, summary	• Decades of clinical experience • Precise dosage timing not critical, owing to long duration • Antidote available for overdose	• Rapid onset • Fixed dosage • No blood tests needed • Less bleeding and hemorrhagic stroke • Few drug-food interactions	Same as rivaroxaban	Same as rivaroxaban	Same as rivaroxaban
Disadvantages, summary	• Delayed onset • Blood tests required • No fixed dosage • Many drug-food interactions	• Dosing on time is important, owing to short duration • No antidote to overdose • Limited clinical experience	Same as rivaroxaban	Same as rivaroxaban	Same as rivaroxaban *plus* gastrointestinal disturbances are common

*Dabigatran etexilate is approved for preventing venous thromboembolism after knee and hip replacement surgery in Canada and Europe, but not in the United States.

50 mL/min or higher), dosing should stop 1 or 2 days before surgery. For patients with renal impairment (CrCl below 50 mL/min), dosing should stop 3 to 5 days before surgery.

GI Disturbances. About 35% of patients experience *dyspepsia* (abdominal pain, bloating, nausea, vomiting) and/or *gastritis-like symptoms* (esophagitis, gastroesophageal reflux disease, gastric hemorrhage, erosive gastritis, hemorrhagic gastritis, GI ulcer). Symptoms of *dyspepsia* can be reduced by taking dabigatran with food and by using an acid-suppressing drug (proton pump inhibitor or histamine-2 receptor blocker). If these measures don't help, patients may try a switch to warfarin, which carries a much lower risk for adverse GI effects.

Drug Interactions

Dabigatran is not metabolized by hepatic P450 enzymes, nor is it an inhibitor or inducer of these enzymes. Accordingly, dabigatran does not have metabolic interactions with other drugs.

Dabigatran etexilate is a substrate for intestinal *P-glycoprotein,* the transporter protein that can pump dabigatran and other drugs back into the intestine. Drugs that inhibit P-glycoprotein can increase dabigatran absorption and blood levels, and drugs that induce P-glycoprotein can decrease dabigatran absorption and blood levels. Combined use with a P-glycoprotein *inhibitor* (e.g., ketoconazole, amiodarone, verapamil, quinidine) could cause bleeding from excessive dabigatran levels, and hence these combinations should be avoided. Combined use with a P-glycoprotein *inducer* appears to be safe, even though it might reduce beneficial effects somewhat.

Bleeding risk is increased by other drugs that impair hemostasis.

Preparations, Dosage, Administration, and Storage

Preparations. Dabigatran etexilate [Pradaxa] is available in three strengths: 75, 110, and 150-mg capsules.

Administration. Dosing may be done with or without food. Patients should swallow the capsules intact. If the capsules are crushed, chewed, or opened, absorption will be increased by 75%, thereby posing a risk for bleeding.

Dosage for Atrial Fibrillation. The usual dosage is 150 mg twice daily. If a dose is missed, it should be taken as soon as possible on the same day. However, if the missed dose cannot be taken at least 6 hours before the next scheduled dose, the missed dose should be skipped.

In patients with significant renal impairment (CrCl 15–30 mL/min), the dosage is 75 mg twice a day. For patients with greater renal impairment (CrCl below 15 mL/min), no dosing recommendation can be made.

Switching From Warfarin to Dabigatran. Discontinue warfarin, wait until the INR falls below 2, and then start dabigatran.

Switching From Dabigatran to Warfarin. Because onset of warfarin's effects is delayed, warfarin should be started before stopping dabigatran, based on CrCl as follows:

- CrCl above 50 mL/min—start warfarin 3 days before stopping dabigatran.
- CrCl 31 to 50 mL—start warfarin 2 days before stopping dabigatran.

- CrCl 15 to 30 mL—start warfarin 1 day before stopping dabigatran.
- CrCl below 15 mL/min—no recommendation can be made.

STORAGE. Dabigatran is unstable, especially when exposed to moisture. To maintain efficacy, the drug must be stored in the manufacturer-supplied bottle, which has a desiccant cap. Patients should open just one bottle at a time and should not distribute dabigatran to any other container, such as a weekly pill organizer. Current labeling says that, after the bottle is opened, dabigatran should be used within 30 days. However, recent evidence indicates that dabigatran capsules maintain efficacy for 4 months, provided they are stored in the original container—away from excessive moisture, heat, and cold—with the cap tightly closed after each use.

Hirudin Analogs

Desirudin

Desirudin [Iprivask] is a direct thrombin inhibitor given by subQ injection. Desirudin is indicated for prevention of DVT in patients undergoing elective hip replacement surgery. In clinical trials, patients experienced fewer thromboembolic events than those given unfractionated heparin or enoxaparin, an LMW heparin.

Desirudin is completely absorbed after subQ injection, achieving peak plasma levels in 1 to 3 hours. Elimination is primarily by renal excretion and partly by proteolytic cleavage. In patients with normal renal function, the elimination half-life is 2 to 3 hours. By contrast, in those with severe renal impairment, the half-life is greatly prolonged (up to 12 hours).

As with other anticoagulants, hemorrhage is the adverse effect of greatest concern. In clinical trials, the incidence of hemorrhage was 30% in the desirudin group compared with 33% in the enoxaparin group and 20% in the heparin group. Less serious effects include wound secretion, injection-site mass, anemia, nausea, and deep thrombophlebitis.

In patients undergoing spinal or epidural anesthesia, desirudin may cause spinal or epidural hematoma, which can result in long-term or even permanent paralysis. Hematoma risk is increased by use of other drugs that impair hemostasis (e.g., nonsteroidal antiinflammatory drugs [NSAIDs], antiplatelet drugs, warfarin, heparin). Patients should be monitored for signs of neurologic impairment and given immediate treatment if they develop.

Desirudin [Iprivask] is administered by deep subQ injection into the thigh or abdominal wall. For patients with normal renal function, the dosage is 15 mg every 12 hours, beginning 5 to 15 minutes before hip surgery (but after induction of regional block anesthesia, if used). For patients with moderate renal impairment (CrCl 30–50 mL/min), dosage is reduced to 5 mg every 12 hours. For those with severe renal impairment (CrCl below 30 mL/min), dosage is reduced to 1.7 mg every 12 hours. For all patients, the usual duration of treatment is 9 to 12 days.

Direct Factor Xa Inhibitors

Rivaroxaban

Actions and Uses

Rivaroxaban [Xarelto] is an *oral* anticoagulant that causes selective inhibition of factor Xa (activated factor X). Unlike fondaparinux, which acts indirectly (see earlier), rivaroxaban binds directly with the active center of factor Xa and thereby inhibits production of thrombin. Compared with warfarin, our oldest oral anticoagulant, rivaroxaban has several advantages: rapid onset, fixed dosage, lower bleeding risk, few drug interactions, and no need for INR monitoring. Rivaroxaban has three approved uses: (1) prevention of DVT and PE after total hip or knee replacement surgery, (2) prevention of stroke in patients with atrial fibrillation, and (3) treatment of DVT and PE unrelated to orthopedic surgery. Contrasts with warfarin are shown in Table 44.6.

Clinical Trials

Knee and Hip Replacement Patients. In a series of trials known as RECORD (Regulation of Coagulation in Orthopedic Surgery to Prevent Deep Vein Thrombosis and Pulmonary Embolism), rivaroxaban was compared with enoxaparin (an LMW heparin) in patients who had undergone hip or knee replacement surgery. Patients who received rivaroxaban (10 mg once daily) were much less likely to experience DVT, VTE, PE, or death compared with patients who received enoxaparin (40 mg once daily or 30 mg twice daily). With both drugs, the incidence of major bleeding episodes was low (0.2%).

Nonvalvular Atrial Fibrillation Patients. In a trial known as ROCKET AF, rivaroxaban was compared with warfarin for preventing stroke in patients with nonvalvular atrial fibrillation (i.e., patients with atrial fibrillation who do not have a prosthetic heart valve or hemodynamically significant valve disease). Rivaroxaban was at least as effective as warfarin and carried the same risk for major hemorrhagic events of all kinds—but had a lower risk for intracranial bleeds and fatal bleeds.

Pharmacokinetics

Rivaroxaban is administered orally, and bioavailability is high (80%–90%). Plasma levels peak 2 to 4 hours after dosing. Protein binding in blood is substantial (92%–95%). Rivaroxaban undergoes partial metabolism by CYP3A4 (the 3A4 isoenzyme of cytochrome P450) and is a substrate for P-glycoprotein, an efflux transporter that helps remove rivaroxaban from the body. Rivaroxaban is eliminated in the urine (36% as unchanged drug) and feces (7% as unchanged drug), with a half-life of 5 to 9 hours. In patients with renal impairment or hepatic impairment, rivaroxaban levels may accumulate.

Adverse Effects

Bleeding. Bleeding is the most common adverse effect and can occur at any site. Patients have experienced epidural hematoma as well as major intracranial, retinal, adrenal, and GI bleeds. Some people have died. Bleeding risk is increased by other drugs that impede hemostasis. How does rivaroxaban compare with warfarin? The risk for hemorrhagic stroke and other major bleeds is significantly lower with rivaroxaban.

In the event of overdose, we have no specific antidote to reverse this drug's anticoagulant effects. However, we *can* prevent further absorption of ingested rivaroxaban with activated charcoal. Treatment with several agents—recombinant factor VIIa, prothrombin complex concentrate (PCC), or activated PCC—can be considered. Preliminary studies of PCC have been promising, but more testing must be completed. Because rivaroxaban is highly protein bound, dialysis is unlikely to remove it from the blood.

Spinal or Epidural Hematoma. Like all other anticoagulants, rivaroxaban poses a risk for spinal or epidural hematoma in patients undergoing spinal puncture or epidural anesthesia. Prolonged or permanent paralysis can result. Rivaroxaban should be discontinued at least 18 hours before removing an epidural catheter; after the catheter is out, another 6 hours should elapse before rivaroxaban is restarted. If a traumatic puncture occurs, rivaroxaban should be delayed for at least 24 hours. Anticoagulant-related spinal or epidural hematoma was discussed further earlier (see "Adverse Effects" under "Heparin").

Drug Interactions. Levels of rivaroxaban can be altered by drugs that inhibit or induce CYP3A4 and P-glycoprotein. Specifically, in patients with *normal renal function,* drugs that inhibit CYP3A4 strongly *and also* inhibit P-glycoprotein (e.g., ketoconazole, itraconazole, ritonavir) can raise rivaroxaban levels enough to increase the risk for bleeding. Similarly, in patients with *renal impairment,* drugs that inhibit CYP3A4 moderately *and also* inhibit P-glycoprotein (e.g., amiodarone, dronedarone, quinidine, diltiazem, verapamil, ranolazine, macrolide antibiotics) can raise rivaroxaban levels enough to increase the risk for bleeding. Conversely, drugs that induce CYP3A4 strongly *and also* induce P-glycoprotein (e.g., carbamazepine, phenytoin, rifampin, St. John's wort) may reduce rivaroxaban levels enough to increase the risk for thrombotic events. Of note, rivaroxaban itself does not inhibit or induce cytochrome P450 enzymes or P-glycoprotein and hence is unlikely to alter the effects of other drugs.

Owing to the risk for bleeding, rivaroxaban should not be combined with other anticoagulants. Concurrent use with antiplatelet drugs and fibrinolytics should be done with caution.

Precautions

Renal Impairment. Renal impairment can delay excretion of rivaroxaban and can thereby increase the risk for bleeding. Accordingly, rivaroxaban should be avoided in patients with *severe* renal impairment, indicated by a CrCl below 30 mL/minute. In patients with moderate renal impairment (CrCl 30–50 mL/min), rivaroxaban should be used with caution. If renal failure develops during treatment, rivaroxaban should be discontinued.

Hepatic Impairment. In clinical trials, rivaroxaban levels and anticoagulation were excessive in patients with moderate hepatic impairment. Accordingly, in patients with moderate or severe hepatic impairment, rivaroxaban should not be used.

Pregnancy. Rivaroxaban appears unsafe in pregnancy. The drug increases the risk for pregnancy-related hemorrhage and may have detrimental effects on the fetus. When pregnant rabbits were given high doses (10 mg/kg or more) during organogenesis, rivaroxaban increased fetal resorption, decreased fetal weight, and decreased the number of live fetuses. However, dosing of rats and rabbits early in pregnancy was not associated with gross fetal malformations. Rivaroxaban is classified in FDA Pregnancy Risk Category C and should be used only if the benefits are deemed to outweigh the risks to the mother and fetus.

Preparations, Dosage, and Administration

Rivaroxaban [Xarelto] is supplied in tablets (10, 15, and 20 mg). Whether dosing is done with food depends on the setting, as discussed later.

Prevention of DVT. The recommended dosage is 10 mg once a day, with or without food, starting 6 to 10 hours after knee or hip replacement surgery. If a dose is missed, it should be taken as soon as possible, and the next dose should be taken as originally scheduled. Treatment duration is 12 days after knee replacement and 35 days after hip replacement.

Nonvalvular Atrial Fibrillation. Dosing is done once a day with the evening meal. For patients with normal renal function, the dosage is 20 mg once daily, and for patients with moderate renal impairment, the dosage is 15 mg once daily. Patients with severe renal impairment should not use this drug.

Treatment of DVT/PE. Dosing is started at 15 mg twice daily for the first 21 days, and then increased to 20 mg daily. Doses should be taken at approximately the same time each day.

Apixaban

Actions and Uses

Apixaban [Eliquis] is an additional *oral* anticoagulant that causes selective inhibition of factor Xa. Apixaban inhibits free and clot-bound factor Xa as well as prothrombinase activity. Apixaban has three approved uses: (1) prevention of stroke and systemic embolism in patients with nonvalvular atrial fibrillation, (2) treatment of DVT and PE, and (3) prophylaxis of DVT in patients undergoing hip or knee replacement.

Pharmacokinetics

Apixaban is administered orally, and bioavailability is moderate (~50%). Plasma levels peak 2 to 4 hours after dosing. Protein binding in blood is substantial (87%). Apixaban undergoes partial metabolism by CYP3A4. Apixaban is eliminated in the urine and feces, with a half-life of 12 hours after repeated dosing. In patients with renal impairment, apixaban levels may accumulate.

Adverse Effects

Bleeding. As with rivaroxaban, bleeding is the most common adverse effect and can occur at any site. Bleeding risk is increased by other drugs that impede hemostasis. How does apixaban compare with warfarin? The risk for hemorrhagic stroke and other major bleeds is significantly lower with apixaban.

In the event of overdose, we have no specific antidote to reverse this drug's anticoagulant effects. Treatment with several agents—recombinant factor VIIa, PCC, or activated PCC—can be considered, but testing has not been completed. Like rivaroxaban, apixaban is highly protein bound. Dialysis is unlikely to remove it from the blood.

Drug Interactions

Levels of rivaroxaban can be altered by drugs that inhibit or induce CYP3A4 and P-glycoprotein. Specifically, in patients with *normal renal function,* drugs that inhibit CYP3A4 strongly *and also* inhibit P-glycoprotein (e.g., ketoconazole, itraconazole, ritonavir) can raise apixaban levels enough to increase the risk for bleeding. Conversely, drugs that induce CYP3A4 strongly *and also* induce P-glycoprotein (e.g., carbamazepine, phenytoin, rifampin, St. John's wort) may reduce apixaban levels enough to increase the risk for thrombotic events.

Precautions

Renal Impairment. Renal impairment can delay excretion of apixaban, increasing the risk for bleeding. In patients with renal impairment, defined as a serum creatinine level greater than or equal to 1.5 mg/dL, apixaban dosing is decreased.

Pregnancy. Studies of apixaban in pregnant patients are lacking. The drug may increase the risk for hemorrhage during pregnancy and delivery. Apixaban is classified in FDA Pregnancy Risk Category B.

Preparations, Dosage, and Administration

Apixaban [Eliquis] is supplied in tablets (2.5 and 5 mg). The recommended dose for most patients with atrial fibrillation is 5 mg taken orally twice daily. In patients with renal impairment, dosing is decreased to 2.5 mg twice daily. For the treatment of DVT, the dose is doubled to 10 mg twice daily. For prophylaxis after orthopedic surgery, the dose is only 2.5 mg twice daily.

Edoxaban

Edoxaban [Savaysa] is a newer *oral* anticoagulant that also causes selective inhibition of factor Xa. Edoxaban has two approved uses: (1) prevention of stroke and systemic embolism in patients with nonvalvular atrial fibrillation and (2) treatment of DVT or PE. Because it is a novel oral anticoagulant, like apixaban and rivaroxaban, edoxaban causes adverse effects and has drug interactions similar to these drugs.

Preparations, Dosage, and Administration

Edoxaban is available in 15-, 30-, and 60-mg tablets. The suggested dose for patients with atrial fibrillation is 60 mg orally daily. Treatment for DVT and PE is weight based. For patients <60 kg, the dose is 30 mg daily. For patients >60 kg, this dose is doubled to 60 mg daily. As with the other NOACs, doses should be decreased in patients with renal impairment.

ANTIPLATELET DRUGS

Antiplatelet drugs suppress platelet aggregation. Because a platelet core constitutes the bulk of an *arterial thrombus,* the principal indication for the antiplatelet drugs is prevention of thrombosis in *arteries.* In contrast, the principal indication for anticoagulants (e.g., heparin, warfarin) is prevention of thrombosis in veins.

There are four major groups of antiplatelet drugs: aspirin (a "group" with one member), $P2Y_{12}$ ADP receptor antagonists, PAR-1 antagonists, and GP IIb/IIIa receptor antagonists. As indicated in Fig. 44.1, aspirin and the $P2Y_{12}$ ADP receptor antagonists affect only one pathway in platelet activation, and hence their antiplatelet effects are limited. In contrast, the GP IIb/IIIa antagonists block the final common step in platelet activation and hence have powerful antiplatelet effects. Properties of the major classes of antiplatelet drugs are shown in Table 44.7. Because GP IIb/IIIa antagonists are given only in the hospital setting, they are discussed further in Chapter 89.

Aspirin

The basic pharmacology of aspirin is discussed in Chapter 55. Consideration here is limited to aspirin's role in preventing arterial thrombosis.

Mechanism of Antiplatelet Action

Aspirin suppresses platelet aggregation by causing *irreversible inhibition of cyclooxygenase,* an enzyme required by platelets to synthesize TXA_2. As noted, TXA_2 is one of the factors that can promote platelet activation. In addition to activating platelets, TXA_2 acts on vascular smooth muscle to promote vasoconstriction. Both actions promote hemostasis. By inhibiting cyclooxygenase, aspirin suppresses both TXA_2-mediated vasoconstriction and platelet aggregation, thereby reducing the risk for arterial thrombosis. Because inhibition of cyclooxygenase by aspirin is irreversible, and because platelets lack the machinery to synthesize new cyclooxygenase, the effects of a single dose of aspirin persist for the life of the platelet (7–10 days).

In addition to inhibiting the synthesis of TXA_2, aspirin can inhibit synthesis of *prostacyclin* by the blood vessel wall. Because prostacyclin has effects that are exactly opposite to those of TXA_2—namely, suppression of platelet aggregation and promotion of vasodilation—suppression of prostacyclin synthesis can partially offset the beneficial effects of aspirin therapy. Fortunately, aspirin is able to inhibit synthesis of TXA_2 at doses that are lower than those needed to inhibit synthesis of prostacyclin. Accordingly, if we keep the dosage of aspirin *low* (325 mg/day or less), we can minimize inhibition of prostacyclin production while maintaining inhibition of TXA_2 production.

Indications for Antiplatelet Therapy

Antiplatelet therapy with aspirin has multiple indications of proven efficacy:

- *Ischemic stroke* (to reduce the risk for death and nonfatal stroke)
- *TIAs* (to reduce the risk for death and nonfatal stroke)
- *Chronic stable angina* (to reduce the risk for MI and sudden death)
- *Unstable angina* (to reduce the combined risk for death and nonfatal MI)
- *Coronary stenting* (to prevent reocclusion)
- *Acute MI* (to reduce the risk for vascular mortality)
- *Previous MI* (to reduce the combined risk for death and nonfatal MI)
- *Primary prevention of MI* (to prevent a first MI in men and in women aged 65 and older)

In all of these situations, prophylactic therapy with aspirin can reduce morbidity, and possibly mortality. Primary prevention of MI is discussed further next.

Primary Prevention of MI

In 2009, the U.S. Preventive Services Task Force (USPSTF) issued updated guidelines on the use of aspirin for primary prevention of MI. The USPSTF recommends the use of aspirin for men ages 45 to 79 years and women ages 55 to 79 years when the potential benefit of a reduction in MI outweighs the potential harm of an increase in GI hemorrhage. Cardiovascular risk is based on five factors—age, gender, cholesterol levels, blood pressure, and smoking status—and can be calculated using an online risk assessment tool, such

TABLE 44.7 ▪ Properties of the Major Classes of Antiplatelet Drugs

	Aspirin, a Cyclooxygenase Inhibitor	$P2Y_{12}$ ADP Receptor Blockers	PAR-1 Antagonists
Representative drug	Aspirin	Clopidogrel [Plavix]	Vorapaxar [Zontivity]
Mechanism of antiplatelet action	Irreversibly inhibits cyclooxygenase and thereby blocks synthesis of thromboxane A_2	Irreversibly blocks receptors for ADP*	Reversibly blocks the PAR-1 expressed on platelets
Route	PO	PO	PO
Duration of effects	Effects persist 7–10 days after the last dose	Effects persist 7–10 days after the last dose*	Effects persist 7–10 days after the last dose
Cost	$3/month	$87/month	$320/month

*ADP receptor blocker—ticagrelor [Brilinta]—causes reversible ADP receptor blockade, so effects wear off faster than with clopidogrel.
ADP, adenosine diphosphate; PAR-1, protease-activated receptor-1.

as those at www.med-decisions.com. Although the optimal aspirin dosage for primary prevention is unknown, low doses (e.g., 81 mg/day) appear as effective as higher ones.

Adverse Effects

Even in low doses, aspirin increases the risk for GI bleeding and hemorrhagic stroke. Among middle-aged people taking aspirin for 5 years, the estimated rate of major GI bleeding episodes is 2 to 4 per 1000 patients, and the rate of hemorrhagic stroke is 0 to 2 episodes per 1000 patients. Use of enteric-coated or buffered aspirin may *not* reduce the risk for GI bleeding. Benefits of treatment must be weighed against bleeding risks. If GI bleeding occurs, adding a proton pump inhibitor (e.g., omeprazole [Prilosec]) to reduce gastric acidity can help.

Dosing

Dosage for preventing cardiovascular (CV) events should be low. Maximal inhibition of platelet cyclooxygenase, and hence maximal effects on platelet function, can be produced in a few days by taking 81 mg/day. Dosages higher than 81 mg/day offer no increase in benefits but do increase the risk for GI bleeding and stroke. Accordingly, for *chronic therapy,* a dosage of 81 mg/day is probably adequate. A higher dosage (e.g., 325 mg/day) is indicated for *initial* treatment of an acute event, such as MI, to establish full antiplatelet effects rapidly—after which 81 mg/day can be taken for maintenance.

$P2Y_{12}$ Adenosine Diphosphate Receptor Antagonists

Drugs in this class block $P2Y_{12}$ ADP receptors on the platelet surface, preventing ADP-stimulated aggregation (see Fig. 44.1). Three $P2Y_{12}$ ADP receptor antagonists are available. Two of them—clopidogrel and prasugrel—cause *irreversible* receptor blockade, and the third—ticagrelor—causes *reversible* receptor blockade. Clopidogrel, prasugrel, and ticagrelor are used for secondary prevention of atherothrombotic events in patients with acute coronary syndrome (ACS), defined as unstable angina or MI. All three drugs are taken orally and can cause serious bleeding.

Clopidogrel

Clopidogrel [Plavix] is an oral antiplatelet drug with effects much like those of aspirin. The drug is taken to prevent stenosis of coronary stents and for secondary prevention of MI, ischemic stroke, and other vascular events.

Antiplatelet Actions

Clopidogrel blocks $P2Y_{12}$ ADP receptors on platelets and thereby prevents ADP-stimulated platelet aggregation. As with aspirin, antiplatelet effects are irreversible and hence persist for the life of the platelet. Effects begin 2 hours after the first dose and plateau after 3 to 7 days of treatment. At the recommended dosage, platelet aggregation is inhibited by 40% to 60%. Platelet function and bleeding time return to baseline 7 to 10 days after the last dose.

Pharmacokinetics

Clopidogrel is rapidly absorbed from the GI tract, both in the presence and absence of food. Bioavailability is about 50%. Clopidogrel is a *prodrug* that undergoes metabolism to its active form, primarily by hepatic CYP2C19 (the 2C19 isoenzyme of cytochrome P450). People with variant forms of the CYP2C19 gene are *poor metabolizers* of clopidogrel and hence may not benefit adequately from the drug.

Therapeutic Use

Clopidogrel is used widely to prevent blockage of coronary artery stents and to reduce thrombotic events—MI, ischemic stroke, and vascular death—in patients with ACS and in those with atherosclerosis documented by recent MI, recent stroke, or established peripheral arterial disease. In patients with ACS, clopidogrel should always be combined with aspirin (75–325 mg once daily).

BLACK BOX WARNING: CLOPIDOGREL

Clopidogrel should not be used in poor metabolizers. Patients with variant forms of the *CYP2C19* gene cannot reliably convert clopidogrel to its active form. When treated with standard dosages of clopidogrel, these poor metabolizers exhibit a higher rate of cardiovascular events compared with normal metabolizers.

Poor metabolizers can be identified by testing a blood or saliva sample for CYP2C19 variants or by simply measuring the platelet response to treatment. Unfortunately, even with this information, the course of action is not clear. Yes, we could give poor metabolizers higher doses—but doses that might be safe and effective have not been established. As an alternative, poor metabolizers could be treated with either prasugrel [Effient] or ticagrelor [Brilinta], two other $P2Y_{12}$ ADP receptor antagonists discussed later.

Adverse Effects

Clopidogrel is generally well tolerated. Adverse effects are about the same as with aspirin. The most common complaints are abdominal pain, dyspepsia, diarrhea, and rash.

Bleeding. Like all other antiplatelet drugs, clopidogrel poses a risk for serious bleeding. However, compared with aspirin, clopidogrel causes less GI bleeding (2% vs. 2.7%) and less intracranial hemorrhage (ICH) (0.4% vs. 0.5%). Owing to bleeding risk, clopidogrel should be discontinued 5 days before elective surgery. If possible, major bleeding should be managed without discontinuing clopidogrel because discontinuation would increase the risk of a thrombotic event.

Patients should be told about the risk for bleeding and warned that they may bruise or bleed more easily and that bleeding will take longer than usual to stop. Also, patients should be informed about signs of bleeding (e.g., blood in the urine, black tarry stools, vomitus that looks like coffee grounds) and instructed to contact the prescriber if these develop. Finally, patients who develop these symptoms should be warned not to stop clopidogrel until the prescriber says they should.

Thrombotic Thrombocytopenic Purpura (TTP). Rarely, patients develop TTP, a potentially fatal condition characterized by thrombocytopenia, hemolytic anemia, neurologic symptoms, renal dysfunction, and fever. Most cases occur during the first 2 weeks of treatment. TTP is a serious disorder that requires urgent treatment, including plasmapheresis.

Drug Interactions

Drugs That Promote Bleeding. Clopidogrel should be used with caution in patients taking other drugs that promote bleeding (e.g., heparin, warfarin, aspirin, and NSAIDs).

PROTON PUMP INHIBITORS (PPIS). Omeprazole [Prilosec, Losec ♣] and other PPIs suppress secretion of gastric acid (see Chapter 62) and hence are often combined with clopidogrel to protect against GI bleeding. Unfortunately, PPIs may also reduce the antiplatelet effects of clopidogrel. PPIs inhibit CYP2C19, the enzyme that converts clopidogrel to its active form. Hence the dilemma: if clopidogrel is used alone, there is a significant risk for GI bleeding; however, if clopidogrel is combined with a PPI to reduce the risk for GI bleeding, antiplatelet effects may be reduced as well. After considering the available evidence, three organizations—the American College of Cardiology, the American Heart Association, and the American College of Gastroenterology—issued a consensus document on the problem. This document concludes that, although PPIs may reduce the antiplatelet effects of clopidogrel somewhat, there is no evidence that the reduction is large enough to be clinically relevant. Accordingly, for patients who have risk factors for GI bleeding (e.g., advanced age, use of NSAIDs or anticoagulants), the benefits of combining a PPI with clopidogrel probably outweigh any risk from reduced antiplatelet effects—and hence combining a PPI with clopidogrel is probably acceptable for these people. Conversely, for patients who lack risk factors for GI bleeding, combined use of clopidogrel with a PPI may reduce the benefits of clopidogrel without offering any meaningful GI protection—and hence combining a PPI with clopidogrel in these patients should probably be avoided. When a PPI *is* used with clopidogrel, pantoprazole [Protonix] would be a good choice because, compared with other PPIs, pantoprazole causes less inhibition of CYP2C19.

CYP2C19 Inhibitors (Other Than PPIs). Like the PPIs, several other drugs can inhibit CYP2C19. Among these are cimetidine, fluoxetine, fluvoxamine, fluconazole, ketoconazole, voriconazole, etravirine, felbamate, and ticlopidine. Because these drugs may reduce the antiplatelet effects of clopidogrel (by reducing its activation), use of alternative drugs is preferred.

Preparations, Dosage, and Administration

Clopidogrel [Plavix] is available in 75-mg tablets. The usual maintenance dosage is 75 mg once a day, taken with or without food. A 300-mg loading dose may be used for some patients. The optimal duration of treatment is unknown. Dosage needn't be changed for older-adult patients or those with renal impairment. Patients being treated for ACS should take daily aspirin (75–325 mg). Clopidogrel should be withdrawn 5 days before elective surgery and then resumed as soon as possible.

Prasugrel

Actions and Uses

Prasugrel [Effient], a close relative of clopidogrel, is an oral antiplatelet drug approved for prevention of thrombotic events in patients with ACS. Like clopidogrel, prasugrel is a prodrug that undergoes conversion to an active metabolite, which then blocks P2Y12 ADP receptors on platelets, causing irreversible inhibition of platelet aggregation. Prasugrel is more effective than clopidogrel and has fewer drug interactions but causes more major bleeding.

Clinical Trial

In a trial known as TRITON-TIMI, prasugrel was compared directly with clopidogrel. The trial enrolled more than 13,000 patients with ACS who were scheduled for coronary angioplasty, also known as percutaneous coronary intervention. The goal with both drugs was to prevent thrombotic complications, including stent restenosis. Patients taking prasugrel experienced fewer thrombotic events but more major bleeding.

Pharmacokinetics

Prasugrel is rapidly absorbed after oral dosing, in both the presence and absence of food. Activation takes place in two steps. The process begins with hydrolysis by esterases in the intestine and ends with conversion to the active metabolite in the liver, primarily by CYP3A4 and CYP2B6, two isoenzymes of cytochrome P450. (Note that activation of prasugrel differs from activation of clopidogrel, which is mediated by CYP2C19.) The entire activation process is fast: plasma levels of the active metabolite peak about 30 minutes after dosing. Elimination of the active form is primarily by hepatic metabolism, followed by excretion in the urine and feces. The active metabolite has a half-life of 7 hours. In patients who weigh less than 60 kg, total exposure to the active metabolite is 30% to 40% higher than in heavier patients. Accordingly, these lighter patients may need a dosage reduction.

Adverse Effects

The principal adverse effect is bleeding, which occurs more often with prasugrel than with clopidogrel. According to results of TRITON-TIMI, among patients not undergoing coronary artery bypass surgery (CABG), the incidence of major bleeding was 2.4% with prasugrel versus 1.8% with clopidogrel, and the incidence of life-threatening bleeding was 0.4% versus 0.1%. Among patients who required CABG surgery, the incidence of major bleeding was greatly increased: 18.8% with prasugrel versus 2.7% with clopidogrel. Accordingly, if CABG surgery is anticipated, prasugrel should not be started. Prasugrel should be avoided by patients at increased risk for bleeding, including patients with active pathologic bleeding, patients older than 75 years, and patients with a history of TIAs or stroke. If possible, major bleeding should be managed without discontinuing prasugrel because discontinuation would increase the risk for a thrombotic event.

Rarely, patients experience hypersensitivity reactions, including potentially life-threatening angioedema. Onset may occur within hours of the first dose, or after 5 to 10 days of treatment.

Data from TRITON-TIMI suggest that prasugrel may increase the risk for cancer. Among patients using the drug, there was a 62% increase in the rate of new and worsening solid tumors. However, we don't know of any plausible mechanism of tumor promotion. The FDA is monitoring for more cancer cases.

Drug Interactions

Other drugs that promote bleeding (e.g., warfarin, heparin, fibrinolytic drugs, chronic NSAIDs) will increase the risk for a serious bleed and hence should be used with great caution. PPIs, which may slow the activation of clopidogrel (by inhibiting CYP2C19), do not prevent the activation of prasugrel. Also, according to the prasugrel package insert, drugs that induce or inhibit CYP3A4 do not have a significant impact on prasugrel activity.

Preparations, Dosage, and Administration

Prasugrel [Effient] is supplied in 5- and 10-mg tablets for oral dosing, with or without food. Treatment consists of a 60-mg loading dose, followed by once-daily 10-mg maintenance doses. For patients who weigh less than 60 kg, maintenance doses may be reduced to 5 mg. All patients should take aspirin daily (80–325 mg).

Ticagrelor

Actions and Uses

Ticagrelor [Brilinta] is a P2Y12 ADP receptor antagonist indicated for prevention of thrombotic events in patients with ACS and to prevent further CV events in patients with history of MI. The drug inhibits platelet aggregation by blocking P2Y12 ADP receptors on the platelet surface. In contrast to clopidogrel and prasugrel, which cause irreversible receptor blockade, ticagrelor causes reversible blockade and hence the effects of ticagrelor wear off faster.

Clinical Trial

In a trial known as PLATO, ticagrelor was compared directly with clopidogrel in patients with recent-onset ACS (within the previous 24 hours). The trial randomized more than 18,000 patients to receive either ticagrelor (180 mg once followed by 90 mg twice daily) or clopidogrel (300 mg once followed by 75 mg once daily). All patients also took a daily aspirin. Compared with clopidogrel, ticagrelor produced a greater reduction in MI, stroke, stent restenosis, and CV death. Unfortunately, these advantages were offset by a greater risk for hemorrhagic events, including fatal intracranial bleeding.

Pharmacokinetics

Ticagrelor is administered by mouth, and food has little effect on absorption. Plasma levels peak 1.5 hours after dosing. Bioavailability is 36%. Unlike clopidogrel and prasugrel, which are prodrugs, ticagrelor is active as administered. In the liver, CYP3A4 converts much of each dose to an active metabolite. Later, the parent drug and active metabolite undergo inactivation by CYP3A4, followed by excretion in the feces (58%) and urine (26%). The elimination half-life is 7 hours for ticagrelor itself and 9 hours for the active metabolite.

Adverse Effects

The most common adverse effects are bleeding and dyspnea. Other adverse effects include headache, cough, dizziness, nausea, noncardiac chest pain, diarrhea, and bradycardia, including ventricular pauses.

Bleeding. Like all other antiplatelet drugs, ticagrelor poses a risk for serious bleeding. In the PLATO study, serious non-CABG bleeding developed in 4.5% of patients taking ticagrelor, compared with 3.8% of patients taking clopidogrel. However, the incidence of CABG-related bleeding was the same with both drugs. Because of bleeding risk, ticagrelor should be discontinued 5 days before elective surgery and then resumed as soon as possible after the surgery is done.

Dyspnea. In the PLATO study, dyspnea developed in 13.8% of patients taking ticagrelor, compared with 7.8% of patients taking clopidogrel. Dyspnea was usually mild to moderate, and often resolved despite continued drug use. Ticagrelor-related dyspnea does not require any specific intervention.

Ventricular Pauses. Ticagrelor can cause ventricular pauses. In the PLATO trial, ventricular pauses were relatively common early in treatment (6% with ticagrelor vs. 3.5% with clopidogrel) but were much less common after 1 month (2.2% with ticagrelor vs. 1.6% with clopidogrel).

BLACK BOX WARNING: ASPIRIN

Aspirin in low doses—75 to 100 mg/day—enhances the effects of ticagrelor. However, higher doses—more than 100 mg/day—actually reduce the benefits of ticagrelor. Accordingly, patients should be warned against taking more than 100 mg of aspirin a day.

Drug Interactions

Drugs That Promote Bleeding. Anticoagulants (e.g., warfarin, heparin, dabigatran), fibrinolytics (e.g., alteplase, reteplase), and antiplatelet drugs (e.g., aspirin, abciximab) will increase the risk for a serious bleed and hence should be used with great caution.

Inhibitors and Inducers of CYP3A4. Because ticagrelor and its active metabolite are eliminated by CYP3A4, drugs that induce CYP3A4 (e.g., rifampin, phenytoin, phenobarbital, carbamazepine) can reduce the therapeutic effects of both compounds, and drugs that inhibit CYP3A4 (e.g., ketoconazole, itraconazole, clarithromycin, telithromycin, ritonavir, saquinavir) can increase the risk for toxicity (by allowing both compounds to accumulate to dangerous levels).

Statins. Ticagrelor inhibits CYP3A4 and can thereby increase levels of simvastatin and lovastatin. To avoid toxicity, dosages of these statins should not exceed 40 mg/day.

Digoxin. Ticagrelor and its active metabolite can inhibit P-glycoprotein, a transport molecule that promotes renal, hepatic, and intestinal elimination of drugs (see Chapter 4). P-glycoprotein inhibition is of particular concern with digoxin, a heart drug with a low margin of safety. To avoid toxicity, digoxin levels should be checked during initial ticagrelor use and whenever ticagrelor dosage is changed.

Contraindications and Precautions

Ticagrelor is contraindicated for patients with active pathologic bleeding, a history of ICH, or severe hepatic impairment. In patients with moderate hepatic impairment, ticagrelor should be used with caution (because levels of ticagrelor itself and its active metabolite could become excessive, thereby increasing the risk for bleeding).

Preparations, Dosage, and Administration

Ticagrelor [Brilinta] is supplied in 90-mg tablets for dosing with or without food. After an initial loading dose (180 mg) combined with 325 mg of aspirin, patients take 90 mg twice daily. Daily aspirin (75–100 mg) should be continued as well. Doses for patients taking ticagrelor for secondary prevention of CV events should take 60 mg twice daily.

Protease-Activated Receptor-1 (PAR-1) Antagonists

Vorapaxar

Uses. Vorapaxar [Zontivity] is approved for use in conjunction with aspirin and/or clopidogrel in the reduction of thrombotic CV events in patients with a history of MI or PAD. When used with other antiplatelet agents, vorapaxar reduces the rate of CV death, MI, stroke, and urgent coronary revascularization.

Mechanism of Action. PAR-1 mediates the effects of thrombin, and these receptors are located on the surface of platelets. By reversibly antagonizing these receptors, vorapaxar inhibits thrombin-induced and thrombin receptor agonist peptide (TRAP)-induced platelet aggregation. Vorapaxar does not work on ADP receptors.

Pharmacokinetics. Vorapaxar is well absorbed after oral administration. Antiplatelet effects begin within 1 hour. The drug undergoes extensive hepatic metabolism followed by excretion in the feces. Vorapaxar has a long half-life (8 days). Effects persist for 7 to 10 days after drug withdrawal (i.e., until new platelets have been synthesized).

Adverse Effects

Bleeding. Like all other antiplatelet drugs, vorapaxar poses a risk for serious bleeding. In the GUSTO study, serious non-CABG bleeding developed in 3% of patients taking vorapaxar. This is similar to the rates seen with ticagrelor in the PLATO trial.

Preparations, Dosage, and Administration. Vorapaxar is available in 2.08-mg tablets. The recommended dosage is 1 tablet daily with or without food. Vorapaxar should be administered with clopidogrel or aspirin because it has not been studied alone in the prevention of thrombotic CV events.

Other Antiplatelet Drugs

Dipyridamole

Dipyridamole [Persantine] suppresses platelet aggregation, perhaps by increasing plasma levels of adenosine. The drug is approved only for prevention of thromboembolism after heart valve replacement. For this application, dipyridamole is always combined with warfarin. The recommended dosage is 75 to 100 mg 4 times a day. A fixed-dose combination of dipyridamole and aspirin is indicated for recurrent stroke (see later).

Dipyridamole Plus Aspirin

Actions and Use. Dipyridamole combined with aspirin is available in a fixed-dose formulation sold as Aggrenox. The product is used to prevent recurrent ischemic stroke in patients who have had a previous stroke or TIA. Both drugs—aspirin and dipyridamole—suppress platelet aggregation. However, because they do so by different mechanisms, the combination is more effective than either drug alone.

Clinical Trial. The benefit of combining aspirin and dipyridamole was demonstrated in the second European Stroke Prevention Study (ESPS-2), a randomized controlled trial that enrolled more than 6000 patients who had suffered a prior ischemic stroke or TIA. Some patients took aspirin alone (25 mg twice daily), some took dipyridamole alone (200 mg twice daily), some took both drugs, and some took placebo. After 24 months, the incidence of fatal or nonfatal ischemic stroke was reduced by 16% with dipyridamole alone, 18% with aspirin alone, and 37% with the combination. Unfortunately, ESPS-2 was tainted by scientific scandal (one investigator, who later resigned, was charged with creating and falsifying data). Although all fraudulent data were discarded before publication, some authorities remain skeptical of the results.

Adverse Effects. The most common adverse effects of the combination are headache, dizziness, and GI disturbances (nausea, vomiting, diarrhea, abdominal pain, dyspepsia). Of course, bleeding is a concern: the product can cause hemorrhage (3.2% vs. 1.5% with placebo), nosebleed (2.4% vs. 1.5%), and purpura (1.4% vs. 0.4%). The aspirin in Aggrenox poses a risk for GI bleeding from peptic ulcers.

Preparations, Dosage, and Administration. Aggrenox capsules contain 25 mg of aspirin and 200 mg of extended-release dipyridamole. The recommended dosage is 2 capsules a day—1 in the morning and 1 at night. The cost is about $317 a month, compared with $3 a month for aspirin alone. It is important to note that the daily dose of aspirin (50 mg) is lower than the dose recommended to prevent MI (at least 80 mg/day). Accordingly, supplemental aspirin may be needed.

Cilostazol

Actions and Therapeutic Use

Cilostazol [Pletal], a platelet inhibitor and vasodilator, is indicated for intermittent claudication. (Intermittent claudication is a syndrome characterized by pain, cramping, and weakness of the calf muscles brought on by walking and relieved by resting a few minutes. The underlying cause is atherosclerosis in the legs.) Cilostazol suppresses platelet aggregation by inhibiting phosphodiesterase type 3 (PDE-3) in platelets, and promotes vasodilation by inhibiting PDE-3 in blood vessels (primarily in the legs). Inhibition of platelet aggregation is greater than with aspirin, ticlopidine, or dipyridamole. Full effects take up to 12 weeks to develop but reverse quickly (within 48 hours) after drug withdrawal.

Adverse Effects

Cilostazol causes a variety of untoward effects. The most common is headache (34%). Others include diarrhea, abnormal stools, palpitations, dizziness, and peripheral edema.

Other drugs that inhibit PDE-3 have increased mortality in patients with heart failure. Whether cilostazol represents a risk is unknown. Nonetheless, heart failure is a contraindication to cilostazol use.

Drug and Food Interactions

Cilostazol is metabolized by hepatic CYP3A4, so cilostazol levels can be increased by CYP3A4 inhibitors (e.g., ketoconazole, itraconazole, erythromycin, fluoxetine, fluvoxamine, nefazodone, sertraline, and grapefruit juice). Metabolism of cilostazol can also be inhibited by omeprazole.

Preparations, Dosage, and Administration

Cilostazol [Pletal] is available in 50- and 100-mg tablets. The usual dosage is 100 mg twice daily, taken 30 minutes before or 2 hours after breakfast and the evening meal. Dosage should be reduced to 50 mg twice daily in patients taking omeprazole and drugs or foods that inhibit CYP3A4.

CHAPTER

45 Drugs for Deficiency Anemias

Laura D. Rosenthal, DNP, ACNP, FAANP

Anemia is defined as a decrease in the number, size, or hemoglobin content of erythrocytes. Causes include blood loss, hemolysis, bone marrow dysfunction, and deficiencies of substances essential for red blood cell (RBC) formation and maturation. Most deficiency anemias result from deficiency of iron, vitamin B_{12}, or folic acid. Accordingly, this chapter focuses on anemias caused by these deficiencies. To facilitate discussion, we begin by reviewing RBC development.

RED BLOOD CELL DEVELOPMENT

RBCs begin developing in the bone marrow and then mature in the blood. As developing RBCs grow and divide, they evolve through four stages (Fig. 45.1). In their earliest stage, RBCs lack hemoglobin and are known as *proerythroblasts*. In the next stage, they gain hemoglobin and are called *erythroblasts*. Both the erythroblasts and the proerythroblasts reside in bone marrow. After the erythroblast stage, RBCs evolve into *reticulocytes* (immature erythrocytes) and enter the systemic circulation. After the reticulocyte stage, circulating RBCs reach full maturity and are referred to as *erythrocytes*.

Development of RBCs requires the cooperative interaction of several factors: bone marrow must be healthy; erythropoietin (a stimulant of RBC maturation) must be present; iron must be available for hemoglobin synthesis; and other factors, including vitamin B_{12} and folic acid, must be available to support synthesis of DNA. If any of these is absent or amiss, anemia will result.

IRON DEFICIENCY

Iron deficiency is the most common nutritional deficiency and the most common cause of nutrition-related anemia. Worldwide, people with iron deficiency number in the hundreds of millions. In the United States about 5% of the population is iron deficient.

Biochemistry and Physiology of Iron

To understand the consequences of iron deficiency as well as the rationale behind iron therapy, we must first understand the biochemistry and physiology of iron. This information is reviewed next.

Metabolic Functions

Iron is essential to the function of hemoglobin, myoglobin (the oxygen-storing molecule of muscle), and a variety of iron-containing enzymes. Most (70%–80%) of the body's iron is present in hemoglobin. A much smaller amount (10%) is present in myoglobin and iron-containing enzymes.

Fate in the Body

The major pathways for iron movement and utilization are shown in Fig. 45.2. In the discussion that follows, the numbers in parentheses refer to the circled numbers in the figure.

Uptake and Distribution

The life cycle of iron begins with (1) uptake of iron into mucosal cells of the small intestine. These cells absorb 5% to 20% of dietary iron. Their maximal absorptive capacity is 3 to 4 mg/day. Iron in the ferrous form (Fe^{++}) is absorbed more readily than iron in the ferric form (Fe^{+++}). Vitamin C enhances absorption, and food reduces absorption.

After uptake, iron can either (2a) undergo storage within mucosal cells in the form of *ferritin* (a complex consisting of iron plus a protein used to store iron) or (2b) undergo binding to *transferrin* (the iron transport protein) for distribution throughout the body.

Utilization and Storage

Iron that is bound to transferrin can undergo one of three fates. Most transferrin-bound iron (3a) is taken up by cells of the bone marrow for incorporation into hemoglobin. Small amounts (3b) are taken up by the liver and other tissues for storage as ferritin. Lastly (3c), some of the iron in plasma is taken up by muscle (for production of myoglobin) and some is taken up by all other tissues (for production of iron-containing enzymes).

Recycling

As Fig. 45.2 depicts, iron associated with hemoglobin undergoes continuous recycling. After hemoglobin is made in bone marrow, iron reenters the circulation (4) as a component of hemoglobin in erythrocytes. (The iron in circulating erythrocytes accounts for about 70% of total body iron.) After 120 days of useful life, RBCs are catabolized (5). Iron released by this process reenters the plasma bound to transferrin (6), and then the cycle begins anew.

Elimination

Excretion of iron is minimal. Under normal circumstances, only 1 mg of iron is excreted each day. At this rate, if none of the lost iron were replaced, body stores would decline by only 10% a year.

Iron leaves the body by several routes. Most excretion occurs through the bowel. Iron in ferritin is lost as mucosal cells slough off, and iron also enters the bowel in bile. Small amounts are excreted in urine and sweat.

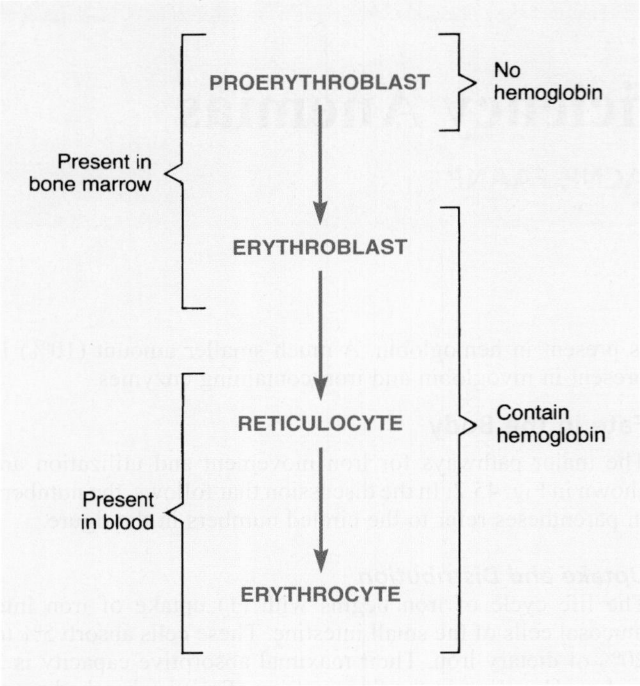

Figure 45.1 ■ Stages of red blood cell development.

Note that, although very little iron leaves the body as a result of excretion (i.e., normal physiologic loss), substantial amounts can leave because of blood loss. Hence menorrhagia, hemorrhage, and blood donations can all cause iron deficiency.

Regulation of Body Iron Content

The amount of iron in the body is regulated through control of intestinal absorption. As noted, most of the iron that enters the body stays in the body. If all dietary iron were readily absorbed, body iron content would rapidly accumulate to a toxic level. However, *excessive buildup is prevented through control of iron uptake: as body stores rise, uptake of iron declines; conversely, as body stores become depleted, uptake increases.* For example, when body stores of iron are high, only 2% to 3% of dietary iron is absorbed. In contrast, when body stores are depleted, as much as 20% may be absorbed.

Daily Requirements

Requirements for iron are determined largely by the rate of erythrocyte production. When RBC production is low, iron needs are low too. Conversely, when RBC production is high, iron needs rise. Accordingly, among infants and children—individuals whose rapid growth rate requires massive RBC synthesis—iron requirements are high (relative to body weight). In contrast, the daily iron needs of adults are relatively low. Adult men need only 8 mg of dietary iron each day. Adult women need considerably more (15–18 mg/day) to replace iron lost through menstruation.

During pregnancy, requirements for iron increase dramatically, owing to (1) expansion of maternal blood volume and (2) production of RBCs by the fetus. In most cases, the iron needs of pregnant women are too great to be met by diet alone. Consequently, iron supplements (about 27 mg/day) are recommended during pregnancy and for 2 to 3 months after delivery.

Table 45.1 shows the recommended dietary allowances (RDAs) of iron as a function of age. The RDA values in the table are about 10 times greater than actual physiologic need because, on average, only 10% of dietary iron is absorbed. Therefore, if physiologic requirements are to be met, the diet must contain 10 times more iron than we need.

Dietary Sources

Iron is available in foods of plant and animal origin. Foods especially rich in iron include egg yolk, brewer's yeast, and wheat germ. Other foods with a high iron content include muscle meats, fish, fowl, cereal grains, beans, and green leafy vegetables. Foods that do not provide much iron include milk and most nongreen vegetables. Because iron can be extracted from cooking utensils, using iron pots and pans can augment dietary iron. Except for individuals who have very high iron requirements (infants, pregnant patients, those undergoing chronic blood loss), the average diet is sufficient to meet iron needs.

Iron Deficiency: Causes, Consequences, and Diagnosis

Causes

Iron deficiency results when there is an imbalance between iron uptake and iron demand. As a rule, the imbalance results from increased demand—not from reduced uptake. The most common causes of increased iron demand are (1) blood volume expansion during pregnancy coupled with RBC synthesis by the growing fetus; (2) blood volume expansion during infancy and early childhood; and (3) chronic blood loss, usually of gastrointestinal (GI) or uterine origin. Rarely, iron deficiency results from reduced iron uptake; potential causes include gastrectomy and sprue.

Consequences

Iron deficiency has multiple effects, the most conspicuous being *iron deficiency anemia.* In the absence of iron for hemoglobin synthesis, red blood cells become *microcytic* and *hypochromic*. The reduced oxygen-carrying capacity of blood results in listlessness, fatigue, and pallor of the skin and mucous membranes. If tissue oxygenation is severely compromised, tachycardia, dyspnea, and angina may result. In addition to causing anemia, iron deficiency impairs myoglobin production and synthesis of iron-containing enzymes. In young children, iron deficiency can cause developmental problems, and in school-aged children, iron deficiency may impair cognition.

Diagnosis

The hallmarks of iron deficiency anemia are (1) the presence of microcytic, hypochromic erythrocytes and (2) the absence of hemosiderin (aggregated ferritin) in bone marrow (Table 45.2). Additional laboratory data that can help confirm a diagnosis include reduced RBC count, reduced reticulocyte hemoglobin content, reduced hemoglobin and hematocrit values, reduced serum iron content, and increased serum iron-binding capacity (IBC).[1]

When a diagnosis of iron deficiency anemia is made, it is imperative that the underlying cause be determined. This is

[1]Serum IBC measures iron binding by transferrin. An *increase* in IBC indicates an increase in the amount of transferrin that is *not* carrying any iron and signals reduced iron availability.

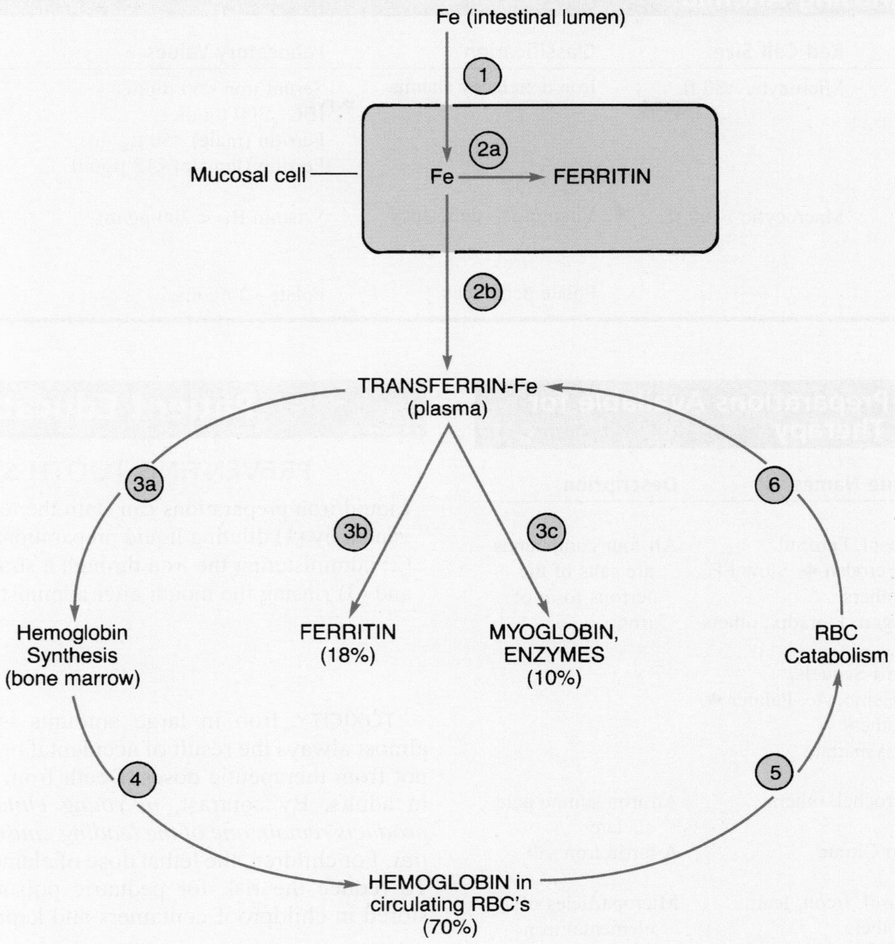

Figure 45.2 ▪ Fate of iron in the body.
Pathways labeled with circled numbers are explained in the text. Values in parentheses indicate percentage of total body stores. Elimination of iron is not shown because most iron is rigidly conserved. Fe, iron; RBC, red blood cell.

TABLE 45.1 ▪ Recommended Dietary Allowances (RDAs) for Iron

Life Stage	Age	RDA for Iron (mg/day)
Infants	7–12 mo	11
Children	1–3 yr	7
	4–8 yr	10
Males	9–13 yr	8
	14–18 yr	11
	≥19 yr	8
Females: nonpregnant, nonlactating	9–13 yr	8
	14–18 yr	15
	19–50 yr	18
	≥51 yr	8
Females: pregnant	14–50 yr	27*
Females: lactating	14–18 yr	10
	19–50 yr	9

*Iron requirements during pregnancy cannot be met through dietary sources alone, so supplements are recommended.

especially true when the suspected cause is GI-related blood loss because GI blood loss may be indicative of peptic ulcer disease or GI cancer, conditions that demand immediate treatment.

Oral Iron Preparations

As shown in Table 45.3, iron for oral therapy is available in multiple forms. Of these, the ferrous salts (especially ferrous sulfate) and carbonyl iron are used most often. Accordingly, the following discussion is limited to these iron preparations.

Ferrous Iron Salts

We have two basic types of iron salts: ferrous salts and ferric salts. Discussion here is limited to the ferrous iron salts because they are absorbed 3 times more readily than the ferric salts and thus are more widely used. Four ferrous iron salts are available: ferrous sulfate, ferrous gluconate, ferrous fumarate, and ferrous aspartate. All four are equally effective, and with all four, GI disturbances are the major adverse effect.

TABLE 45.2 ▪ Diagnosing Anemia

	Red Cell Size	Classification	Laboratory Values	Common Causes
Microcytic anemia	Microcytic <80 fL	Iron deficiency anemia	Serum iron <60 μg/dL IBC <300 μg/dL Ferritin (male) <50 μg/mL Ferritin (female) <12 μg/mL	Poor diet Chronic Blood Loss • Menorrhagia • Colon polyp, • Hemorrhoids
Megaloblastic Anemia	Macrocytic >100 fL	Vitamin B_{12} deficiency	Vitamin B_{12} < 200 pg/mL	Celiac disease Lack of intrinsic factor Enteritis
		Folate deficiency	Folate <2 ng/mL	Low dietary intake

TABLE 45.3 ▪ Iron Preparations Available for Oral Therapy

Iron Preparation	Trade Names	Description
Ferrous iron salts:		
Ferrous sulfate	Feosol, FeroSul, Ferodan ♣, Slow FE, others	All four compounds are salts of the ferrous form of iron
Ferrous gluconate	Fergon, Floradix, others	
Ferrous fumarate	Ferro-Sequels, Hemocyte, Palafer ♣, others	
Ferrous aspartate	FE Aspartate	
Ferrous bisglycinate	Ferrochel, others	An iron–amino acid chelate
Ferric ammonium citrate	Iron Citrate	A ferric iron salt
Carbonyl iron	Feosol, Ircon, Icar, others	Microparticles of elemental iron
Heme-iron polypeptide	Proferrin	Hemoglobin extracted from porcine RBCs
Polysaccharide iron complex	Niferex-150 Forte, Ferrex 150, Triferexx 150 ♣, others	Ferric iron complexed to hydrolyzed starch

Ferrous Sulfate

Indications. Ferrous sulfate is the treatment of choice for iron deficiency anemia. It is also the preferred drug for *preventing* deficiency when iron needs cannot be met by diet alone (e.g., during pregnancy or chronic blood loss). Ferrous sulfate costs less than ferrous gluconate or ferrous fumarate but has equal efficacy and tolerability.

Adverse Effects

GI DISTURBANCES. The most significant adverse effects involve the GI tract. These effects, which are dose dependent, include nausea, heartburn, bloating, constipation, and diarrhea. Gastrointestinal reactions are most intense during initial therapy and become less disturbing with continued drug use. Because of their GI effects, oral iron preparations can aggravate peptic ulcers, regional enteritis, and ulcerative colitis. Accordingly, patients with these disorders should not take iron by mouth. In addition to its other GI effects, oral iron may impart a dark green or black color to stools. This effect is harmless and should not be interpreted as a sign of GI bleeding.

Patient Education

PREVENTING TOOTH STAINING

Liquid iron preparations can stain the teeth. This can be prevented by (1) diluting liquid preparations with juice or water, (2) administering the iron through a straw or with a dropper, and (3) rinsing the mouth after administration.

TOXICITY. Iron in large amounts is toxic. Poisoning is almost always the result of accidental or intentional overdose, not from therapeutic doses. Death from iron ingestion is rare in adults. By contrast, *in young children, iron-containing products remain one of the leading causes of poisoning fatalities.* For children, the lethal dose of elemental iron is 2 to 10 g. To reduce the risk for pediatric poisoning, iron should be stored in childproof containers and kept out of reach.

Symptoms. The effects of iron poisoning are complex. Early reactions include nausea, vomiting, diarrhea, and shock. These are followed by acidosis, gastric necrosis, hepatic failure, pulmonary edema, and vasomotor collapse.

Diagnosis and Treatment. With rapid diagnosis and treatment, mortality from iron poisoning is low (about 1%). Serum iron should be measured and the intestine x-rayed to determine whether unabsorbed tablets are present. Supportive care is the mainstay of treatment. Gastric lavage may be considered in patients with intentional ingestion of large amounts of iron.

If the plasma level of iron is high (above 500 mcg/dL), it should be lowered with parenteral deferoxamine [Desferal]. Deferoxamine adsorbs iron and thereby prevents toxic effects.

Drug Interactions. Interaction of iron with other drugs can alter the absorption of iron, the other drug, or both. *Antacids* reduce the absorption of iron. Coadministration of iron with tetracyclines decreases absorption of both. *Ascorbic acid* (vitamin C) promotes iron absorption but also increases its adverse effects. Accordingly, attempts to enhance iron uptake by combining iron with ascorbic acid offer no advantage over a simple increase in iron dosage.

Preparations. Ferrous sulfate is available in standard tablets and in enteric-coated and sustained-release formulations. The enteric-coated and sustained-release products are designed to reduce gastric disturbances. Unfortunately, although side effects may be lowered, these special formulations have disadvantages. First, iron may be released at variable rates, causing variable and unpredictable absorption. Second, these preparations are expensive. Standard tablets do not share these drawbacks.

Some iron products are formulated with vitamin C. The goal is to improve absorption. Unfortunately, the amount in most products is too low to help: more than 200 mg of vitamin C is needed to enhance the absorption of 30 mg of elemental iron.

Trade names for ferrous sulfate products include *Feosol, FeroSul, Slow FE,* and *Ferodan* ♣.

Dosage and Administration

GENERAL CONSIDERATIONS. Dosing with oral iron can be complicated in that oral iron salts differ with regard to percentage of elemental iron (Table 45.4). Ferrous sulfate, for example, contains 20% iron by weight. In contrast, ferrous gluconate contains only 11.6% iron by weight. Consequently, to provide equivalent amounts of elemental iron, we must use different doses of these iron salts. For example, if we want to provide 100 mg of elemental iron using ferrous sulfate, we need to administer a 500-mg dose. To provide this same amount of elemental iron using ferrous fumarate, the dose would be only 300 mg. In the following discussion, dosage values refer to milligrams of elemental iron, and not to milligrams of any particular iron compound needed to provide that amount of elemental iron.

Food affects therapy in two ways. First, food helps protect against iron-induced GI distress. Second, food decreases iron absorption by 50% to 70%. Therefore we have a dilemma: *Absorption is best* when iron is taken *between* meals, but *GI distress is lowest* when iron is taken *with* meals. As a rule, iron should be administered between meals, maximizing absorption. If necessary, the dosage can be lowered to render GI effects more acceptable.

For two reasons, it may be desirable to take iron *with* food during *initial* therapy. First, because the GI effects of iron are most intense when treatment commences, the salving effects of food can be especially beneficial early on. Second, by reducing GI discomfort during the early phase of therapy, dosing with food can help promote adherence.

USE IN IRON DEFICIENCY ANEMIA. Dosing with oral iron represents a compromise between a desire to replenish lost iron rapidly and a desire to keep GI effects to a minimum. For most adults, this compromise can best be achieved by giving 65 mg 3 times a day, yielding a total daily dose of about 200 mg. Because there is a ceiling to intestinal absorption of iron, doses above this amount provide only a modest increase in therapeutic effect. On the other hand, at dosages greater than 200 mg/day, GI disturbances become disproportionately high. Hence elevation of the daily dose above 200 mg would enhance adverse effects without offering a significant increase in benefits. When treating iron deficiency in infants and children, a typical dosage is 15 mg/kg/day administered in three or four divided doses.

Timing of administration is important: doses should be spaced evenly throughout the day. This schedule gives the bone marrow a continuous iron supply and thereby maximizes RBC production.

Duration of therapy is determined by the therapeutic objective. If correction of anemia is the sole objective, a few months of therapy is sufficient. However, if the objective also includes replenishing ferritin, treatment must continue another 4 to 6 months. It should be noted, however, that drugs are usually unnecessary for ferritin replenishment: in most cases, diet alone can do the job. Accordingly, after anemia has been corrected, pharmaceutical iron can usually be stopped.

PROPHYLACTIC USE. Pregnant women are the principal candidates for prophylactic therapy. A total daily dose of 27 mg, taken between meals, is recommended. Other candidates include infants, children, and women experiencing menorrhagia.

Ferrous Gluconate, Ferrous Fumarate, and Ferrous Aspartate. In addition to ferrous sulfate, three other oral ferrous salts are available: ferrous gluconate [Fergon, Floradix], ferrous fumarate [Ferro-Sequels, Hemocyte, Palafer ♣, others], and ferrous aspartate [FE Aspartate]. Except for differences in percentage of iron content (see Table 45.4), all of these preparations are equivalent. Therefore, when dosage is adjusted to provide equal amounts of elemental iron, ferrous gluconate, ferrous fumarate, and ferrous aspartate produce pharmacologic effects identical to those of ferrous sulfate. All four agents produce equivalent therapeutic responses, and all four cause the same degree of GI distress. Patients who fail to respond to one will not respond to the others. Patients who cannot tolerate the GI effects of one will find the others intolerable, too.

TABLE 45.4 ▪ Commonly Used Oral Iron Preparations

Iron Preparation	Elemental Iron (% by Weight)	Dose Providing 100 mg Elemental Iron
FERROUS IRON SALTS		
Ferrous sulfate	20	500 mg
Ferrous sulfate (dried)	30	330 mg
Ferrous fumarate	33	300 mg
Ferrous gluconate	11.6	860 mg
Ferrous aspartate	16	625 mg
ELEMENTAL IRON		
Carbonyl iron	100	100 mg

Carbonyl Iron

Carbonyl iron is pure, elemental iron in the form of microparticles, which confer good bioavailability. Therapeutic efficacy equals that of the ferrous salts. Because of the microparticles, iron is absorbed slowly, so the risk for toxicity is reduced. Compared with ferrous sulfate, carbonyl iron requires a much higher dosage to cause serious harm. Because of this increased margin of safety, carbonyl iron should pose a reduced risk to children in the event of accidental ingestion.

Carbonyl iron is available in several formulations, including (1) 45-mg tablets, marketed as *Feosol;* (2) 65-mg tablets, marketed as *Ircon;* (3) 90-mg film-coated tablets marketed as *Ferralet 90;* (4) 15-mg chewable tablets, marketed as *Icar;* and (5) a suspension (15 mg/1.25 mL), also marketed as *Icar.* Because these products contain 100% iron, rather than an iron salt, there should be no confusion about dosage: 100 mg of any formulation provides 100 mg of elemental iron. The usual dosage is 100 mg, 3 times a day.

Guidelines for Treating Iron Deficiency

Assessment

Before starting therapy, the cause of iron deficiency must be determined. Without this information, appropriate treatment is impossible. Potential causes of deficiency include pregnancy, bleeding, inadequate diet, and, rarely, impaired intestinal absorption.

The objective is to increase production of hemoglobin and erythrocytes. When therapy is successful, reticulocytes will increase within 4 to 7 days; within 1 week, increases in hemoglobin and the hematocrit will be apparent; and within 1 month, hemoglobin levels will rise by at least 2 g/dL. If these responses fail to occur, the patient should be evaluated for (1) compliance, (2) continued bleeding, (3) inflammatory disease (which can interfere with hemoglobin production), and (4) malabsorption of oral iron.

Routes of Administration

Oral iron is preferred because it is safer than parenteral iron and just as effective. Parenteral iron should be used only when oral iron is ineffective or intolerable. Of the two parenteral routes, the intravenous (IV) route is safer and preferred. These medications are discussed in Chapter 89.

Duration of Therapy

Therapy with oral iron should be continued until hemoglobin levels become normal (about 15 g/dL). This phase of treatment may require 1 to 2 months. After this, continued treatment can help replenish stores of ferritin. However, for most patients, dietary iron alone is sufficient.

Therapeutic Combinations

As a rule, combinations of antianemic agents should be avoided. Combining oral iron with parenteral iron can lead to iron toxicity. Accordingly, use of oral iron should cease before giving iron injections. Combinations of iron with vitamin B_{12} or folic acid should be avoided; as discussed in the following sections, using these combinations can confuse interpretation of hematologic responses.

VITAMIN B_{12} DEFICIENCY

The term *vitamin B_{12}* refers to a group of compounds with similar structures. These compounds are large molecules that contain an atom of cobalt. Because of the cobalt atom, members of the vitamin B_{12} family are known as *cobalamins.*

The most prominent consequences of vitamin B_{12} deficiency are *anemia* and *injury to the nervous system.* Anemia reverses rapidly after vitamin B_{12} administration. Neurologic damage takes longer to repair and, in some cases, may never fully resolve. Additional effects of B_{12} deficiency include GI disturbances and impaired production of white blood cells and platelets.

Biochemistry and Physiology of Vitamin B_{12}

To understand the consequences of vitamin B_{12} deficiency and the rationale behind therapy, we must first understand the normal biochemistry and physiology of B_{12}. This information is reviewed next.

Metabolic Function

Vitamin B_{12} is essential for synthesis of DNA and hence is required for the growth and division of virtually all cells. The mechanism by which the vitamin influences DNA synthesis is depicted in Fig. 45.3. As indicated, vitamin B_{12} helps catalyze the conversion of folic acid to its active form. Active folic acid then participates in several reactions essential for DNA synthesis. Hence *it is by permitting utilization of folic acid that vitamin B_{12} influences cell growth and division*—and it is the absence of usable folic acid that underlies the blood cell abnormalities seen during B_{12} deficiency.

Fate in the Body

Absorption

Efficient absorption of B_{12} requires *intrinsic factor,* a compound secreted by parietal cells of the stomach. After ingestion, vitamin B_{12} forms a complex with intrinsic factor. Upon reaching the ileum, the B_{12}–intrinsic factor complex interacts with specific receptors on the intestinal wall, causing the complex to be absorbed. In the absence of intrinsic factor, absorption of vitamin B_{12} is greatly reduced. However, about 1% of the amount present can still be absorbed by passive diffusion; no intrinsic factor is needed.

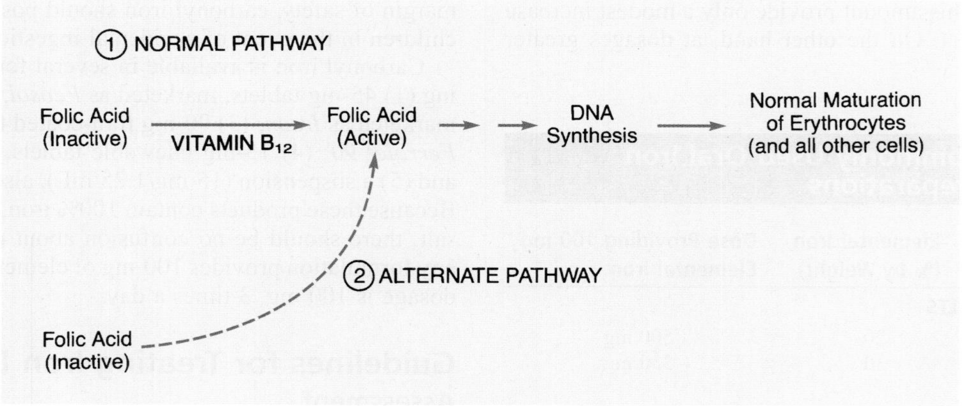

Figure 45.3 ■ Relationship of folic acid and vitamin B_{12} to DNA synthesis and cell maturation.

Folic acid requires activation to be of use. Normally, activation occurs through a vitamin B_{12}-dependent pathway. However, when folic acid is present in large amounts, activation can occur via an alternate pathway, bypassing the need for B_{12}.

Distribution and Storage

After absorption, the vitamin B_{12}–intrinsic factor complex dissociates. Free B_{12} then binds to *transcobalamin II* for transport to tissues. Most vitamin B_{12} goes to the liver and is stored. Total body stores of B_{12} are tiny, ranging from 2 to 3 mg by most estimates.

Elimination

Excretion of vitamin B_{12} takes place very slowly: Each day, about 0.1% of the total body store is lost. Because B_{12} is excreted so slowly, years are required for B_{12} deficiency to develop—even when none of the lost B_{12} is replaced.

Daily Requirements

Because very little vitamin B_{12} is excreted, and because body stores are small to begin with, daily requirements for this vitamin are minuscule. The average adult needs about 2.4 mcg of B_{12} per day. Children need even less.

Dietary Sources

The ability to biosynthesize vitamin B_{12} is limited to microorganisms; higher plants and animals can't make it. The microorganisms that make B_{12} reside in the soil, sewage, and the intestines of humans and other animals. Unfortunately, vitamin B_{12} produced in the human GI tract is unavailable for absorption. Consequently, humans must obtain most of their B_{12} by consuming animal products. Liver and dairy products are especially good sources. Between 10% and 30% of adults older than 50 years are unable to absorb vitamin B_{12} found naturally in foods. Accordingly, these people should meet their requirements by consuming B_{12}-fortified foods or a B_{12}-containing vitamin supplement.

Vitamin B_{12} Deficiency: Causes, Consequences, and Diagnosis

Causes

In most cases, vitamin B_{12} deficiency is the result of *impaired absorption.* Only rarely is insufficient B_{12} in the diet the cause. Potential causes of poor absorption include (1) regional enteritis, (2) celiac disease (a malabsorption syndrome involving abnormalities in the intestinal villi), and (3) development of antibodies directed against the vitamin B_{12}–intrinsic factor complex. In addition, because stomach acid is required to release vitamin B_{12} from foods, the vitamin cannot be absorbed if acid secretion is significantly reduced, as often happens in older adults and in those taking acid-suppressing drugs.

Most frequently, impaired absorption of vitamin B_{12} occurs secondary to a lack of intrinsic factor. The usual causes are atrophy of gastric parietal cells and surgery of the stomach (total gastric resection).

When vitamin B_{12} deficiency is caused by an absence of intrinsic factor, the resulting syndrome is called *pernicious anemia*—a term suggesting a highly destructive or fatal condition. Pernicious anemia is an old term that refers back to the days when, for most patients, vitamin B_{12} deficiency had no effective therapy and the condition was uniformly fatal. Today, vitamin B_{12} deficiency secondary to lack of intrinsic factor can be managed successfully, so the label *pernicious* no longer has its original, ominous connotation.

Consequences

Many of the consequences of B_{12} deficiency result from disruption of DNA synthesis. The tissues affected most are those with a high proportion of cells undergoing growth and division. Accordingly, B_{12} deficiency has profound effects on the bone marrow (the site where blood cells are produced) and the epithelial cells lining the mouth and GI tract.

Megaloblastic Anemia

The most conspicuous consequence of B_{12} deficiency is an anemia in which large numbers of *megaloblasts* (oversized erythroblasts) appear in the bone marrow and in which *macrocytes* (oversized erythrocytes) appear in the blood. These strange cells are produced because of impaired DNA synthesis: lacking sufficient DNA, growing cells are unable to divide; hence, as erythroblasts mature and their division is prevented, oversized cells result. Most megaloblasts die within the bone marrow; only a few evolve into the macrocytes that can be seen in the blood. Because of these unusual cells, the anemia associated with vitamin B_{12} deficiency is often referred to as either *megaloblastic* or *macrocytic* anemia.

Severe anemia is the principal cause of mortality from B_{12} deficiency. Anemia produces peripheral and cerebral hypoxia. Heart failure and dysrhythmias are the usual cause of death.

It is important to note that the hematologic effects of vitamin B_{12} deficiency can be reversed with large doses of *folic acid.* As indicated in Fig. 45.3, when folic acid is present in large amounts, some of it can be activated by an alternate pathway that is independent of vitamin B_{12}. This pathway bypasses the metabolic block caused by B_{12} deficiency, permitting DNA synthesis to proceed.

Neurologic Damage

Deficiency of vitamin B_{12} causes demyelination of neurons, primarily in the spinal cord and brain. A variety of signs and symptoms can result. Early manifestations include paresthesias of the hands and feet and a reduction in deep tendon reflexes. Late-developing responses include loss of memory, mood changes, hallucinations, and psychosis. If vitamin B_{12} deficiency is prolonged, neurologic damage can become permanent.

The precise mechanism by which B_{12} deficiency results in neuronal damage is unknown. We do know, however, that *neuronal damage is not related to effects on folic acid or DNA.* That is, the mechanism that underlies neuronal damage is different from the mechanism that underlies disruption of hematopoiesis. Consequently, although administering large doses of folic acid can correct the hematologic consequences of B_{12} deficiency, folic acid will not improve the neurologic picture.

Other Effects

As noted, vitamin B_{12} deficiency can adversely affect virtually all tissues in which a high proportion of cells are undergoing growth and division. Therefore, in addition to disrupting the production of erythrocytes, lack of B_{12} also prevents the bone marrow from making leukocytes (white blood cells) and thrombocytes (platelets). Loss of these blood elements can lead to infection and spontaneous bleeding. Disruption of DNA synthesis can also suppress division of the cells that form the epithelial lining of the mouth, stomach, and intestine, causing oral ulceration and a variety of GI disturbances.

Diagnosis

When megaloblastic anemia occurs, it may be due to vitamin B_{12} deficiency or other causes, especially a lack of folic acid. Hence, if therapy is to be appropriate, a definitive diagnosis must be made. Two tests are particularly helpful. The first is obvious: measurement of plasma B_{12}. The second procedure, known as the Schilling test, measures vitamin B_{12} absorption.

The combination of megaloblastic anemia plus low plasma vitamin B_{12} plus evidence of B_{12} malabsorption permits a clear diagnosis of vitamin B_{12} deficiency (see Table 45.5).

Vitamin B_{12} Preparations: Cyanocobalamin

Cyanocobalamin is a purified, crystalline form of vitamin B_{12}. This compound is the drug of choice for all forms of B_{12} deficiency.

Adverse Effects

Cyanocobalamin is generally devoid of serious adverse effects. One potential response, *hypokalemia,* may occur as a natural consequence of increased erythrocyte production. Erythrocytes incorporate significant amounts of potassium. Therefore, as large numbers of new erythrocytes are produced, levels of free potassium may fall.

Preparations, Dosage, and Administration

Cyanocobalamin can be given orally, intranasally, and by intramuscular (IM) or subcutaneous (subQ) injection. Most pharmacology texts, including prior editions of this one, will tell you that oral therapy is appropriate only for people who absorb B_{12} well; all other patients (i.e., those with impaired absorption) should use intranasal or parenteral therapy. However, this statement is not correct. Although it *is* true that various conditions—including lack of intrinsic factor, low gastric acidity, and regional enteritis—severely impair B_{12} absorption, these conditions do not prevent absorption entirely. Hence even people with impaired absorption can still be treated orally; the only catch is that doses must be very high. Is there any advantage to oral therapy compared with parenteral therapy? Yes. First, oral therapy is more comfortable. Second, oral therapy is more convenient (because it avoids regular trips to the provider for injections).

TABLE 45.5 ▪ Vitamin B_{12} Deficiency Versus Folic Acid Deficiency

	Vitamin B_{12} Deficiency	Folic Acid Deficiency
Usual cause	Vitamin B_{12} malabsorption from lack of intrinsic factor	Low dietary folic acid
Primary hematologic effect	Megaloblastic anemia	Megaloblastic anemia
Neurologic effect	Damage to brain and spinal cord	None*
Diagnosis	Low plasma vitamin B_{12}; low B_{12} absorption (Schilling test)	Low plasma folic acid
Treatment (usual route)	Cyanocobalamin (PO or IM)	Folic acid (PO)
Usual duration of therapy	Lifelong	Short term

*Folic acid deficiency early in pregnancy can cause neural tube defects in the fetus.
IM, intramuscular; PO, oral administration.

Oral

Oral cyanocobalamin is appropriate for most people with mild to moderate B_{12} deficiency, regardless of the cause. (The principal exception is patients with severe neurologic involvement.) If the B_{12} deficiency is due to malabsorption, dosages must be high—typically 1000 to 10,000 mcg/day. To ensure that absorption has been adequate, B_{12} levels should be measured periodically.

In addition to treating patients with B_{12} deficiency, oral cyanocobalamin can be used as a dietary supplement. The usual dosage is 1000 to 2000 mcg/day.

Three oral formulations are available: standard tablets (100, 500, and 1000 mcg), sublingual tablets (500, 1000, 2500, 5000, and 6000 mcg), and lozenges (50, 100, 250, and 500 mcg).

Parenteral

Parenteral cyanocobalamin (generic only) can be administered by *IM or deep subQ injection. Cyanocobalamin must NOT be given by IV injection.* IM and subQ injections are generally well tolerated, although they occasionally cause pain and other local reactions.

Parenteral administration is indicated for patients with impaired B_{12} absorption—although most of these people can be treated with oral cyanocobalamin instead. If the cause of malabsorption is irreversible (e.g., parietal cell atrophy, total gastrectomy), therapy must continue lifelong. A typical dosing schedule for megaloblastic anemia is 100 mcg IM or deep subQ daily for 6 to 7 days. If there is a positive response after this time, continue to administer 100 mcg every other day for 7 doses, then decrease to every 3 to 4 days for another 2 to 3 weeks. After anemia has been corrected, doses of 100 mcg are administered monthly for life.

Intranasal

Intranasal cyanocobalamin [Nascobal] represents a convenient alternative to IM or subQ injection for people who cannot take cyanocobalamin by mouth. Efficacy of intranasal cyanocobalamin has not been determined for patients with nasal congestion, allergic rhinitis, or upper respiratory infections. Accordingly, until more is known, patients with these disorders should not use this formulation until symptoms subside. Hot foods or liquids can increase nasal secretions, which might flush cyanocobalamin gel from the nose. Accordingly, hot foods should not be eaten within 1 hour before or 1 hour after administering the drug.

Intranasal cyanocobalamin is available in a metered-dose formulation called Nascobal, which delivers 500 mcg/actuation. The dosing schedule is 500 mcg in one nostril once a week.

Guidelines for Treating Vitamin B_{12} Deficiency

Route of B_{12} Administration

As discussed previously, oral therapy can be used for most patients, including those with conditions that impair B_{12} absorption. The major exception is patients with severe neurologic deficits caused by B_{12} deficiency. For these people, parenteral cyanocobalamin is indicated.

Treatment of Moderate B_{12} Deficiency

The primary manifestations of moderate B_{12} deficiency are megaloblasts in the bone marrow and macrocytes in peripheral blood. Moderate deficiency does not cause leukopenia, thrombocytopenia, or neurologic complications. Moderate deficiency can be managed with vitamin B_{12} alone; no other measures are required.

Treatment of Severe B_{12} Deficiency

Severe deficiency produces multiple effects, all of which must be attended to. Unlike mild deficiency, in which erythrocytes are the only blood cells affected, severe deficiency disrupts production of all blood cells. Loss of erythrocytes leads to hypoxia, cerebrovascular insufficiency, and heart failure. Loss of leukocytes encourages infection, and loss of thrombocytes promotes bleeding. In addition to causing serious hematologic deficits, severe B_{12} deficiency has adverse effects on the nervous system and GI tract.

Treatment of severe deficiency involves the following: (1) IM injection of vitamin B_{12} and folic acid (the folic acid accelerates recovery of hematologic deficits); (2) administration of 2 to 3 units of packed RBCs (to correct anemia quickly); (3) transfusion of platelets; and (4) therapy with antibiotics if infection has developed.

After treatment with vitamin B_{12} plus folic acid, recovery from anemia occurs quickly. Within 1 to 2 days, megaloblasts disappear from the bone marrow; within 3 to 5 days, reticulocyte counts become elevated; by day 10, the hematocrit begins to rise; and within 14 to 21 days, the hematocrit becomes normal.

Recovery from neurologic damage is slow and depends on how long the damage had been present. When deficits have been present for only 2 to 3 months, recovery is relatively fast. When deficits have been present for many months or for years, recovery is slow: Months may pass before any improvement is apparent, and complete recovery may never occur.

Long-Term Treatment

For patients who lack intrinsic factor or who suffer from some other permanent cause of vitamin B_{12} malabsorption, lifelong treatment is required. Traditional therapy consists of monthly IM or subQ injections of cyanocobalamin. However, *large* daily oral doses can be just as effective, as can weekly intranasal doses. During prolonged therapy, treatment should be periodically assessed: plasma levels of vitamin B_{12} should be measured every 3 to 6 months, blood samples should be examined for the return of macrocytes, and blood counts should be performed.

Potential Hazard of Folic Acid

Treatment with folic acid can exacerbate the neurologic consequences of B_{12} deficiency. Recall that folic acid, by itself, can reverse the *hematologic* effects of B_{12} deficiency—but will not alleviate *neurologic* deficits. So, by correcting the most obvious manifestation of B_{12} deficiency (anemia), folic acid can mask the fact that deficiency of B_{12} still exists. As a result, *use of folic acid can lead to undertreatment with B_{12} itself* and can thereby permit neurologic damage to progress. Clearly, folic acid is not a substitute for vitamin B_{12}, and vitamin B_{12} deficiency should never be treated with folic acid alone. Whenever folic acid is employed during treatment of vitamin B_{12} deficiency, extra care must be taken to ensure that B_{12} dosage is adequate.

FOLIC ACID DEFICIENCY

In one respect, folic acid deficiency is identical to vitamin B_{12} deficiency: in both states, *megaloblastic anemia* is the most conspicuous pathology. However, in other important ways, folic acid deficiency and vitamin B_{12} deficiency are dissimilar (Table 45.5). Consequently, when a patient presents with megaloblastic anemia, it is essential to determine whether the cause is deficiency of folic acid, vitamin B_{12}, or both.

Physiology and Biochemistry of Folic Acid

Metabolic Function

As noted when we discussed vitamin B_{12}, folic acid (also known as *folate*) is an essential factor for DNA synthesis. Without folic acid, DNA replication and cell division cannot proceed.

To be usable, dietary folic acid must first be converted to an active form. Under normal conditions, activation occurs through a pathway that employs vitamin B_{12} (see Fig. 45.3). However, when large amounts of folate are ingested, some can be activated through an alternate pathway—one that does not employ vitamin B_{12}. Hence, even in the absence of vitamin B_{12}, if sufficient amounts of folic acid are consumed, active folate will be available for DNA synthesis.

Fate in the Body

Folic acid is absorbed in the early segment of the small intestine and then transported to the liver and other tissues, where it is either used or stored.

Folic acid in the liver undergoes extensive enterohepatic recirculation. That is, folate from the liver is excreted into the intestine, after which it is reabsorbed and then returned to the liver through the hepatic-portal circulation. This enterohepatic recirculation helps salvage up to 200 mcg of folate per day. Accordingly, the process is an important way to maintain folate stores.

In contrast to vitamin B_{12}, folic acid is not conserved rigidly: every day, significant amounts are excreted. As a result, if intake of folic acid were to cease, signs of deficiency would develop rapidly (within weeks if body stores were already low).

Daily Requirements

The RDA of folic acid, as set by the Food and Nutrition Board of the Institute of Medicine, is 400 mcg for adult males and for adult females who are neither pregnant nor lactating. RDAs during pregnancy and lactation increase to 600 mcg and 500 mcg, respectively. Although the RDA for adult females is set at 400 mcg, women of childbearing age should consume even more: 400 to 800 mcg of supplemental folate, in addition to the folate in food (see later). Individuals with malabsorption syndromes (e.g., tropical sprue) may require as much as 2000 mcg (2 mg) per day; at these high doses, folate will be taken up in sufficient quantity despite impaired absorption.

Dietary Sources

Folic acid is present in all foods. Good sources include peas, lentils, oranges, whole-wheat products, asparagus, beets, broccoli, and spinach. Also, many grain products (e.g., cereals, bread, pasta, rice, flour) are now fortified with folic acid.

Folic Acid Deficiency: Causes, Consequences, and Diagnosis

Causes

Folic acid deficiency has two principal causes: (1) poor diet (especially in patients who abuse alcohol), and (2) malabsorption secondary to intestinal disease. Rarely, certain drugs may cause folate deficiency.

Alcoholism

Alcoholism, either acute or chronic, may be the most common cause of folate deficiency. Deficiency results for two reasons: (1) insufficient folic acid in the diet and (2) derangement of enterohepatic recirculation secondary to alcohol-induced injury to the liver. Fortunately, with improved diet and reduced alcohol consumption, alcohol-related folate deficiency will often reverse.

Sprue

Sprue is an intestinal malabsorption syndrome that decreases folic acid uptake. Because sprue does not block folate absorption entirely, deficiency can be corrected by giving large doses of folic acid orally.

Consequences

With the important exception that folic acid deficiency does not injure the nervous system, the effects of folate deficiency are identical to those of vitamin B_{12} deficiency. As with B_{12} deficiency, the most prominent consequence of folate deficiency is *megaloblastic anemia.* In addition, like B_{12} deficiency, lack of folic acid may result in leukopenia, thrombocytopenia, and injury to the oral and GI mucosa. Because we already noted that many of the consequences of vitamin B_{12} deficiency result from depriving cells of active folic acid, the similarities between folate deficiency and vitamin B_{12} deficiency should be no surprise.

The Developing Fetus

Folic acid deficiency *very early* in pregnancy can cause neural tube defects (e.g., spina bifida, anencephaly). Accordingly, it is imperative that all women of reproductive age ensure adequate folate levels *before* pregnancy occurs. To accomplish this, the U.S. Preventive Services Task Force now recommends that *all women who may become pregnant consume 400 to 800 mcg of supplemental folic acid each day—in addition to the folate they get from food.*

Other Consequences

As discussed in Chapter 65, folic acid deficiency may increase the risk for colorectal cancer and atherosclerosis.

Folic Acid Preparations

Nomenclature

Two forms of folic acid are available. One form is inactive as administered (but undergoes activation after being absorbed). The second form is active to start with. Both forms have several generic names: the *inactive* form is referred to as *folacin, folate, pteroylglutamic acid,* or *folic acid;* the *active* form is referred to as *leucovorin calcium, folinic acid,* or *citrovorum factor.* The inactive form is by far the most commonly used.

Folic Acid (Pteroylglutamic Acid)

Chemistry

Folic acid is inactive as administered and cannot support DNA synthesis. Activation takes place rapidly after absorption.

Indications

Folic acid has three uses: (1) treatment of megaloblastic anemia resulting from folic acid deficiency; (2) prophylaxis of folate deficiency, especially during pregnancy and lactation; and (3) initial treatment of severe megaloblastic anemia resulting from vitamin B_{12} deficiency.

Adverse Effects

Oral folic acid is nontoxic when used *short term.* Massive dosages (e.g., as much as 15 mg) have been taken with no ill effects. However, as noted in Chapter 65, even moderately large doses (1000 mcg/day), when taken *long term,* may increase the risk for some cancers, including colorectal cancer and cancer of the prostate.

Formulations and Routes of Administration

Folic acid is available in tablets (0.4, 0.8, and 1 mg) for oral use and in a 5-mg/mL solution [Folvite] for IM, IV, or subQ injection. As a rule, injections are reserved for patients with severely impaired GI absorption.

Dosage

For treatment of folate-deficient megaloblastic anemia in adults, the usual oral dosage is 1000 to 2000 mcg/day. After symptoms have resolved, the maintenance dosage is 400 mcg/day. For prophylaxis during pregnancy and lactation, doses up to 1000 mcg/day may be used.

Leucovorin Calcium (Folinic Acid)

Leucovorin calcium is an active form of folic acid used primarily as an adjunct to cancer chemotherapy. Leucovorin is not used routinely to correct folic acid deficiency because folic acid is just as effective and cheaper.

Guidelines for Treating Folic Acid Deficiency

Choice of Treatment Modality

The modality for treating folic acid deficiency should be matched with the cause. If the deficiency is due to poor diet, it should be corrected by dietary measures—not with supplements (except for women who may become pregnant). Ingestion of one serving of a fresh vegetable or one glass of fruit juice a day will often suffice. In contrast, when folate deficiency is the result of malabsorption, diet alone cannot correct the deficiency, so supplemental folate will be needed.

Route of Administration

Oral administration is preferred for most patients. Unlike vitamin B_{12}, folic acid is rarely administered by injection. Even in the presence of intestinal disease, oral folic acid can be effective, provided the dosage is high enough.

Prophylactic Use of Folic Acid

Folic acid should be taken prophylactically only when clearly appropriate. The principal candidates for prophylactic folate are women who might become pregnant and women who are pregnant or lactating. Because folic acid may mask vitamin B_{12} deficiency, indiscriminate use of folate should be avoided.

Treatment of Severe Deficiency

Folic acid deficiency can produce severe megaloblastic anemia. To ensure a rapid response, therapy should be initiated with an IM injection of folic acid and vitamin B_{12}. (Because of the metabolic interrelationship between folic acid and vitamin B_{12}, combining these agents accelerates recovery.) After the initial injection, treatment should be continued with folic acid alone. Folic acid should be given orally in a dosage of 1000 to 2000 mcg/day for 1 to 2 weeks. After this, maintenance doses of 400 mcg/day may be required.

Therapy is evaluated by monitoring the hematologic picture. When treatment has been effective, megaloblasts will disappear from the bone marrow within 48 hours; the reticulocyte count will increase measurably within 2 to 3 days; and the hematocrit will begin to rise in the second week.

UNIT X

Drugs for Endocrine Disorders

CHAPTER 46

Drugs for Diabetes Mellitus

Laura D. Rosenthal, DNP, ACNP, FAANP

DIABETES MELLITUS: BASIC CONSIDERATIONS

The term *diabetes mellitus* is derived from the Greek word for *fountain* and the Latin word for *honey*. The term describes one of the prominent symptoms of untreated diabetes: production of large volumes of glucose-rich urine. Indeed, long ago, the disease we now call diabetes was "diagnosed" by the sweet smell of urine—and, yes, by its sweet taste, too. In this chapter we use the terms *diabetes mellitus* and *diabetes* interchangeably.

Diabetes is primarily a disorder of carbohydrate metabolism. Symptoms mainly result from a deficiency of insulin or from cellular resistance to insulin's actions. The principal sign of diabetes is *sustained hyperglycemia,* which results from impaired glucose uptake by cells and from increased glucose production. When hyperglycemia develops, it can quickly lead to polyuria, polydipsia, ketonuria, and weight loss. Over time, hyperglycemia can lead to heart disease, renal failure, blindness, neuropathy, amputations, impotence, and stroke. There is an often-overlooked point about diabetes: in addition to affecting carbohydrate metabolism, insulin deficiency disrupts metabolism of proteins and lipids. We refer to regulation of blood glucose levels as *glycemic control.*

In the United States diabetes is the most common endocrine disorder and the seventh leading cause of death by disease. According to the 2011 National Diabetes Fact Sheet, compiled by the Centers for Disease Control and Prevention, about 26 million Americans have diabetes, and nearly one fourth of them have not been diagnosed. Another 79 million or so Americans are estimated to have prediabetes and are at increased risk for developing diabetes in the future.

We need to do a better job of diagnosing diabetes and treating it—and we need to do what we can to reduce the risk for developing the disease in the first place. Unfortunately, the risk for developing diabetes is largely genetic, a factor that can't be modified. Nonetheless, we can still reduce risk significantly by adopting a healthy lifestyle, centered on engaging in physical activity and establishing a healthy diet.

Types of Diabetes Mellitus

There are two main forms of diabetes mellitus: type 1 diabetes mellitus (often abbreviated as T1DM) and type 2 diabetes mellitus (often abbreviated as T2DM). Both forms have similar signs and symptoms. Major differences concern etiology, prevalence, treatments, and outcomes (illness severity and deaths). The distinguishing characteristics of type 1 and type 2 diabetes are shown in Table 46.1 and discussed later. Another important form—gestational diabetes—is discussed later under "Diabetes and Pregnancy." Although there are additional forms of diabetes, they are relatively rare and will not be discussed specifically here.

Type 1 Diabetes

Type 1 diabetes accounts for about 5% of all diabetes cases. Between 1.2 million and 2.4 million Americans have this disorder. In the past, type 1 diabetes was called *juvenile-onset diabetes mellitus* or *insulin-dependent diabetes mellitus (IDDM).* These terms have fallen out of favor, however, because type 2 diabetes is becoming more common in children, and many people with type 2 diabetes use insulin to manage their diabetes. Accordingly, the terms *juvenile-onset diabetes mellitus* and *IDDM* are no longer clinically useful. Generally, type 1 diabetes develops during childhood or adolescence, and symptom onset is relatively abrupt. That being said, type 1 diabetes can develop during adulthood.

The primary defect in type 1 diabetes is destruction of pancreatic beta cells—the cells responsible for insulin synthesis and release into the bloodstream. Insulin levels are reduced early in the disease and usually fall to zero later. Beta cell destruction is the result of an autoimmune process (i.e., the patient's immune system inappropriately wages war against its own beta cells). The trigger for this immune response is not entirely known, but genetic, environmental, and infectious factors likely play a role.

Type 2 Diabetes

Type 2 diabetes is the most prevalent form of diabetes, accounting for 90% to 95% of all diagnosed cases. Approximately 22 million Americans have this disease. In the past, type 2 diabetes was called *non–insulin-dependent diabetes mellitus (NIDDM)* or *adult-onset diabetes mellitus.* As discussed previously for type 1 diabetes, these terms are no longer clinically useful because insulin is commonly used by people with type 2 diabetes and type 2 diabetes can occur in all age groups. The disease most commonly begins in middle age and progresses gradually. In contrast to type 1 diabetes,

TABLE 46.1 ▪ Characteristics of Type 1 and Type 2 Diabetes Mellitus

	Type of Diabetes Mellitus	
Characteristics	**Type 1**	**Type 2**
Age of onset	Usually childhood or adolescence	Usually older than 40 years
Speed of onset	Abrupt	Gradual
Family history	Frequently negative	Frequently positive
Prevalence	Approximately 5% of people with diabetes have type 1 diabetes	90%–95% of people with diabetes have type 2 diabetes
Etiology	Autoimmune process	Unknown—but there is a strong familial association, suggesting that heredity is a risk factor
Primary defect	Loss of pancreatic beta cells	Insulin resistance and inappropriate insulin secretion
Insulin levels	Reduced early in the disease and completely absent later	Levels may be low (indicating deficiency), normal, or high (indicating resistance)
Treatment	Insulin replacement is mandatory, along with strict dietary control	Treat with an oral antidiabetic or noninsulin injectable agent and/or insulin, but always in combination with a reduced-calorie diet and appropriate exercise
Blood glucose	Levels fluctuate widely in response to infection, exercise, and changes in caloric intake and insulin dose	Levels are generally more stable than in type 1 diabetes
Symptoms	Polyuria, polydipsia, polyphagia, weight loss	May be asymptomatic initially
Body composition	Usually thin and undernourished at diagnosis	Frequently obese
Ketosis	Common, especially if insulin dosage is insufficient	Uncommon

type 2 diabetes carries little risk for ketoacidosis. However, type 2 diabetes does carry the same long-term risks as type 1 diabetes (see later).

Symptoms of type 2 diabetes usually result from a combination of *insulin resistance* and *impaired insulin secretion.* In contrast to patients with type 1 diabetes, those with type 2 diabetes are capable of insulin synthesis. In fact, early in the disease, insulin levels tend to be normal or slightly elevated, a state known as *hyperinsulinemia.* However, although insulin is still produced, its secretion is no longer tightly coupled to plasma glucose content: release of insulin is delayed, and peak output is subnormal. More important, the target tissues of insulin (liver, muscle, adipose tissue) exhibit insulin resistance: for a given blood insulin level, cells in these tissues are less able to take up and metabolize the glucose available to them. Insulin resistance appears to result from three causes: reduced binding of insulin to its receptors, reduced receptor numbers, and reduced receptor responsiveness. Over time, hyperglycemia leads to diminished pancreatic beta cell function, and hence insulin production and secretion eventually decline as the beta cells work harder to overcome insulin resistance within the tissues.

Although the underlying causes of type 2 diabetes are not entirely known, there is a strong familial association, suggesting that genetics play a role. This possibility was reinforced by a study that implicated the gene for *insulin receptor substrate-2* (IRS-2), a compound that helps mediate intracellular responses to insulin.

Diabetes and Pregnancy

Before the discovery of insulin, virtually all babies born to mothers with severe diabetes died during infancy. Although insulin therapy has greatly improved outcomes, successful management of the diabetic pregnancy remains a challenge. Three factors contribute to the problem. First, the placenta produces hormones that antagonize insulin's actions. Second, production of cortisol, a hormone that promotes hyperglycemia, increases threefold during pregnancy. Both factors increase the body's need for insulin. And third, because glucose can pass freely from the maternal circulation to the fetal circulation, hyperglycemia in the mother will stimulate excessive secretion of insulin in the fetus. The resultant hyperinsulinism can have multiple adverse effects on the fetus.

Successful management of diabetes during pregnancy demands that proper glucose levels be maintained in both the mother and fetus; failure to do so may be teratogenic or may otherwise harm the fetus. Achieving glucose control requires diligence on the part of the mother and her prescriber. Some experts on diabetes in pregnancy advise that blood glucose levels must be monitored 6 to 7 times a day. Insulin dosage and food intake must be adjusted accordingly.

Gestational diabetes is defined as diabetes that appears in the pregnant patient during pregnancy and then subsides rapidly after delivery. Gestational diabetes is managed in much the same manner as any other diabetic pregnancy: blood glucose should be monitored and then controlled with diet and insulin. In most cases, the diabetic state disappears almost immediately after delivery, permitting discontinuation of insulin. However, if the diabetic state persists beyond parturition, it is no longer considered gestational and should be rediagnosed and treated accordingly.

In women taking an oral drug for type 2 diabetes, current practice is to discontinue the oral drug and switch to insulin. The only exception is the oral agent metformin, which is often satisfactory for managing type 2 diabetes in pregnancy. Women who discontinue oral medications can resume oral therapy after delivery.

Diagnosis

Diagnosis of diabetes was once made solely by measuring blood levels of glucose. However, in 2010, the American Diabetes Association (ADA) recommended an alternative test, based on measuring hemoglobin A_{1c}—a test that provides an estimate of glycemic control over the previous 2 to 3 months. For all of these tests, diagnostic values of diabetes are shown in Table 46.2.

Tests Based on Blood Levels of Glucose

Excessive plasma glucose is diagnostic of diabetes. Several tests may be employed: a fasting plasma glucose (FPG) test, a casual plasma glucose test, and an oral glucose tolerance test (OGTT). To make a definitive diagnosis, the patient must be tested on two separate days, and both tests must be positive. Any combination of two tests (e.g., two FPG tests; one FPG test and one OGTT) may be used.

Fasting Plasma Glucose Test

To determine FPG levels, blood is drawn at least 8 hours after the last meal. In normoglycemic individuals, FPG levels are less than 100 mg/dL. If FPG glucose levels are 126 mg/dL or higher, diabetes is present.

Casual Plasma Glucose Test

For this test, blood can be drawn at any time, without regard to meals. Fasting is not required. Of note, the test can be performed in the office, using a finger-stick blood sample and the same type of test device employed by patients at home. A plasma glucose level that is 200 mg/dL or higher suggests diabetes. However, to make a definitive diagnosis, the patient must also display classic signs of diabetes: polyuria, polydipsia, and rapid weight loss. Ketonuria may also be present, but only if blood glucose is extremely high.

Oral Glucose Tolerance Test

This test is often used when diabetes is suspected but could not be definitively diagnosed by measuring fasting or casual plasma glucose levels. The OGTT is performed by giving an oral glucose load (equivalent to 75 g of anhydrous glucose) and measuring plasma glucose levels 2 hours later. In individuals who do not have diabetes, 2-hour glucose levels will be below 140 mg/dL. Diabetes is suggested if 2-hour plasma glucose levels are 200 mg/dL or higher. The OGTT test is more expensive and time consuming than the alternatives and is not used routinely.

TABLE 46.2 ▪ Criteria for the Diagnosis of Diabetes Mellitus

Fasting plasma glucose ≥126 mg/dL*
or
Casual plasma glucose ≥ 200 mg/dL *plus* symptoms of diabetes[†]
or
Oral glucose tolerance test (OGTT): 2-hr plasma glucose ≥200 mg/dL[‡]
or
Hemoglobin A_{1c} 6.5% or higher

**Fasting* is defined as no caloric intake for at least 8 hours.

[†]*Casual* is defined as any time of day without regard to meals. Classical symptoms of diabetes include polyuria, polydipsia, and unexplained weight loss.

[‡]In this OGTT, plasma glucose content is measured 2 hours after ingesting the equivalent of 75 g of anhydrous glucose dissolved in water. The OGTT is not recommended or needed for routine clinical use.

Data from Standards of Medical Care in Diabetes—2014. Diabetes Care 2014;37(Suppl 1):S14-S80.

Hemoglobin A_{1c}

As described later under "Monitoring Treatment," levels of hemoglobin A_{1c}, or simply A_{1c}, reflect average blood glucose levels over the previous 2 to 3 months. Accordingly, if a patient's A_{1c} is high, we know that his or her glucose levels have been high for a relatively long time. In other words, we know that he or she has diabetes. An A_{1c} value of 6.5% or higher is considered diagnostic.

It is important to note that the A_{1c} test is not necessarily accurate in all patients because some people have conditions that can affect hemoglobin levels, thus skewing the results of this test. Among these are pregnancy, chronic kidney or liver disease, recent severe bleeding or blood transfusion, and certain blood disorders, including thalassemia, iron deficiency anemia, and anemia related to vitamin B_{12} deficiency.

Increased Risk for Diabetes (Prediabetes)

Increased risk for diabetes (sometimes referred to as prediabetes) is a state defined by *impaired fasting plasma glucose* (FPG between 100 and 125 mg/dL) or *impaired glucose tolerance* (2-hour OGTT result of 140–199 mg/dL). These values are below those that define diabetes but are too high to be considered normal. People with "prediabetes" are at increased risk for developing type 2 diabetes and cardiovascular disease (CVD)—but not the microvascular complications associated with diabetes (i.e., retinopathy, nephropathy, neuropathy). The risk for CVD can be reduced by dietary modifications, increased physical activity, and, if indicated, use of appropriate drugs to control blood lipids and blood pressure. The risk for progression to diabetes may be reduced by diet and exercise and possibly by certain oral antidiabetic drugs (such as metformin).

It is important to note that many people who meet the criteria for prediabetes never go on to develop diabetes—even if they *don't* modify their lifestyle, and even if they *don't* take antidiabetic drugs. Hence, although prediabetes indicates an increased *risk* for diabetes, it by no means guarantees that diabetes will occur.

Overview of Treatment

The primary goal of treating type 1 or type 2 diabetes is prevention of long-term complications. To minimize complications, treatment must keep glucose levels as close to "normal" as safely possible. In addition, treatment must keep blood pressure and blood lipids within an acceptable range. In both type 1 and type 2 diabetes, proper diet and adequate physical activity are central components of management.

Type 1 Diabetes

Preventing complications of diabetes requires a comprehensive plan directed at glycemic control and reduction of cardiovascular risk factors. Glycemic control is accomplished with an integrated program of diet, self-monitoring of blood glucose (SMBG), physical activity, and insulin replacement. Of importance, glycemic control must be achieved *safely,* that is, adequately controlling glycemia while minimizing the risk for hypoglycemia. An essential component of treatment—education of the patient and his or her caregivers about diet, physical activity, and drugs—is usually left to the nurse and a dietitian or nutritionist.

Dietary Measures

Proper diet, balanced by insulin replacement, is the cornerstone of treatment. Because patients with type 1 diabetes are usually thin, the dietary goal is to maintain weight—not lose it. The ADA recommends that all people with type 1 diabetes be offered intensive insulin therapy education using either a carbohydrate counting or experience-based estimation approach in achieving glycemic control. Although it is widely accepted that such programs are useful for people with type 1 diabetes, studies examining the ideal amount of carbohydrate are largely inconclusive. So how should people with diabetes be advised to eat? Evidence suggests that there is no ideal percentage of calories that should be ingested from carbohydrate, fat, or protein. Accordingly, macronutrient distribution for any given individual should be based on his or her current eating patterns, preferences, and goals.

Physical Activity

Unless specifically contraindicated, regular physical activity should be part of the management program. Physical activity increases cellular responsiveness to insulin and may also increase glucose tolerance. Accordingly, the ADA recommends that patients perform at least 150 minutes of moderate-intensity aerobic activity per week. Because strenuous exercise can produce hypoglycemia, patient and provider must work to establish a safe balance between activity level, caloric intake, and insulin dosage. Unfortunately, although the benefits of physical activity are well established, long-term adherence to a program is often difficult to maintain.

Insulin Replacement

Among patients with type 1 diabetes, survival requires daily dosing with insulin. Before insulin replacement became available, people with type 1 diabetes invariably died within a few years after disease onset. The cause of death was usually ketoacidosis. It is essential to coordinate insulin dosage with carbohydrate intake. If carbohydrate intake is too great or too small with respect to insulin dosage, hyperglycemia or hypoglycemia will result.

Although insulin is the cornerstone to the management of type 1 diabetes, the use of other medications as add-on therapy to insulin is currently under study.

Managing Hypertension and Dyslipidemia

An angiotensin-converting enzyme (ACE) inhibitor (e.g., lisinopril) or an angiotensin II receptor blocker (ARB; e.g., losartan) can reduce the risk for diabetic nephropathy, a long-term consequence of poor glycemic control. These same drugs are preferred agents for managing diabetic hypertension. The current goal, as set by the ADA, is to keep blood pressure at or below 140/90 mm Hg, with lower systolic blood pressure targets (<140 mm Hg) appropriate for some individuals.

To reduce high levels of low-density lipoprotein (LDL) cholesterol, statins (e.g., atorvastatin) are preferred drugs. Not only do statins reduce cardiovascular events in patients with high cholesterol, they reduce cardiovascular events in patients with normal or low cholesterol. Another cholesterol-lowering drug—colesevelam—is discussed separately later because of its recognized role in managing diabetes. See Chapter 42 for a discussion of lipid-lowering therapies.

Type 2 Diabetes

As with type 1 diabetes, preventing long-term complications requires a comprehensive treatment plan. Lifestyle measures (diet and physical activity) and drug therapy are the foundation of glycemic control. Physical activity provides the additional benefit of promoting glucose uptake by muscle, even when insulin levels are low. In addition to glycemic control, the plan should address other factors that can increase morbidity and mortality. Accordingly, all patients should be screened and treated for hypertension, nephropathy, retinopathy, and neuropathy. In addition, dyslipidemias (high LDL cholesterol, low high-density lipoprotein [HDL] cholesterol, and high triglycerides) should be corrected.

Recommendations for glycemic control have changed. Until recently, treatment was started with lifestyle measures *alone;* drugs were added only if these measures failed. Today, treatment is started with lifestyle measures *plus* drug therapy. We no longer wait to use drugs. As a result, glycemic control is established sooner, and the risk for long-term complications is lowered.

Type 2 diabetes can be treated with a variety of oral and injectable drugs. Among the oral drugs, metformin and the sulfonylureas (e.g., glipizide [Glucotrol]) are used most widely. Among the injectable drugs, insulin is used most widely. As type 2 diabetes progresses, less and less insulin is produced. As a result, it is common for people with type 2 diabetes to eventually require insulin therapy.

Given the many drugs available for type 2 diabetes, how does one decide which drugs to use for a given patient? As discussed in a 2015 position statement update—*Management of Hyperglycemia in Type 2 Diabetes, 2015: A Patient-Centered Approach*—issued jointly by the ADA and the European Association for the Study of Diabetes, there are a number of patient-specific considerations that come into play when deciding on a course of treatment. To treat type 2 diabetes, the position statement recommends a four-step approach:

Step 1. At diagnosis, initiate lifestyle changes *plus* metformin.

Step 2. Continue lifestyle changes plus metformin, and *add* a second drug, either a sulfonylurea, a thiazolidinedione, a dipeptidyl peptidase-4 (DPP-4) inhibitor, a sodium-glucose cotransporter 2 (SGLT-2) inhibitor, a glucagon-like peptide-1 (GLP-1) receptor agonist, or basal insulin. The choice of agent is made in light of relative efficacy, hypoglycemia risk, tolerability, weight-related considerations, and cost.

Step 3. Progress from step 2 to a three-drug combination (inclusive of metformin). Again, the choice of regimen used is determined based on drug- and patient-specific considerations.

Step 4. If three-drug combination therapy that includes basal insulin fails to achieve treatment goals after 3 to 6 months, it is recommended to proceed to a more complex insulin regimen, usually in combination with one or more noninsulin medicines.

Treatment should start at step 1 and then progress to steps 2, 3, and 4 if needed.

Determining Appropriate Glycemic Goals

In both type 1 and type 2 diabetes, it is important to determine appropriate glycemic goals for the individual based on his or her lifestyle and other patient-specific considerations. The process of maintaining glucose levels within a normal range, around-the-clock, is often referred to as "tight glycemic control." Maintaining tight glycemic control is difficult but can be worth the trouble, especially for young patients with type 1 diabetes. However, for many patients with type 2 diabetes, the risks of tight control may be greater than the benefits. Table 46.3 shows current recommendations regarding glycemic goals.

Type 1 Diabetes

Benefits

The benefits of tight glycemic control in type 1 diabetes were demonstrated conclusively in the Diabetes Control and Complications Trial (DCCT), in which patients received either *conventional insulin therapy* (one or two injections a day) or *intensive insulin therapy* (four injections a day). After 6.5 years, the patients who received intensive therapy experienced a 50% decrease in clinically significant kidney disease, a 35% to 57% decrease in neuropathy, and a 76% decrease in serious ophthalmic complications. Moreover, onset of ophthalmic problems was delayed, and progression of existing problems was slowed. In addition to reducing these *microvascular* complications, "tight control" decreased *macrovascular* complications: 17-year follow-up data from the DCCT showed a significant reduction in myocardial infarction, coronary revascularization, and angina. Hence, with rigorous control of blood glucose, the high degree of morbidity and mortality traditionally associated with type 1 diabetes can be markedly reduced.

Drawbacks

The greatest concern of intensive therapy and strict glycemic goals is *hypoglycemia.* Because glucose levels are kept relatively low, even a modest overdose with insulin can cause blood glucose to fall too low, so the possibility of hypoglycemia increases. Also, a meal that is skipped or exercise that is too strenuous can do the same. Results of the DCCT showed that, compared with patients using conventional therapy, those using intensive insulin therapy experienced 3 times as many hypoglycemic events requiring the assistance of another person and 3 times as many episodes of hypoglycemia-induced coma or seizures. In addition, patients on intensive insulin therapy experienced greater *weight gain* (about 10 pounds, on average). Other disadvantages are greater inconvenience, increased complexity, and a need for greater patient motivation. Finally, the cost is higher: whereas traditional therapy costs about $1700/year, intensive therapy costs about $4000/year (for multiple daily injections) or $5800 (for continuous infusion with an insulin pump). The cost of test strips for the patient's glucometer adds substantially more to the bill.

TABLE 46.3 ▪ General Glycemic Treatment Targets for Nonpregnant Adults With Diabetes

A_{1c}	<7.0%*
Premeal plasma glucose	70–130 mg/dL*
Peak postmeal plasma glucose	<180 mg/dL*

*Goals should be individualized based on
- Duration of diabetes
- Age/life expectancy
- Comorbid conditions
- Known cardiovascular disease or advanced microvascular complications
- Hypoglycemia unawareness
- Other individualized considerations

Data from the American Diabetes Association.

Type 2 Diabetes

In patients with type 2 diabetes, benefits of tight glycemic control are limited mainly to *microvascular* complications; tight control does little to reduce *macrovascular* complications, as evidenced by studies performed to date. Furthermore, benefits accrue more to younger adults with *recent-onset* disease than to older adults with *well-established* disease. As in type 1 diabetes, tight glycemic control poses a significant risk for *hypoglycemia* and *weight gain.* In addition, tight control may increase the risk for *death.*

The effects of tight glycemic control in type 2 diabetes were demonstrated in four landmark trials:

- United Kingdom Prospective Diabetes Study (UKPDS)
- Action to Control Cardiovascular Risk in Diabetes (ACCORD)
- Action in Diabetes and Vascular Disease: Preterax and Diamicron Modified Release Controlled Evaluation (ADVANCE)
- Veterans Affairs Diabetes Trial (VADT)

These large randomized trials differed in patient populations: whereas the UKPDS trial enrolled younger adults with recent-onset diabetes and no prior cardiovascular events, the ACCORD, ADVANCE, and VADT trials enrolled older adults with long-standing diabetes as well as established CVD or cardiovascular risk factors.

Results of the UKPDS trial, released in 1998, showed a significant reduction in *micro*vascular complications—but little or no reduction in *macro*vascular complications or death. In one branch of the study, nonobese patients were given either intensive therapy or conventional therapy. Mean values for A_{1c} were 7% in the intensive group and 7.9% in the conventional group. Compared with patients in the conventional group, patients in the intensive group had a 12% reduction in total diabetes-related end points (cardiovascular, retinal, and renal damage). However, a reduction in microvascular complications (especially retinal damage) accounted for most of the benefit.

Results of ACCORD, ADVANCE, and VADT were released in 2008. As in the UKPDS trial, tight glycemic control failed to reduce stroke, amputations, all-cause mortality, or mortality from cardiovascular causes. In fact, in the ACCORD trial, intensive therapy was associated with an *increased* risk for death. Tight control also increased the risk for severe hypoglycemia and weight gain. The ADVANCE trial did show a reduction in microvascular outcomes, but the ACCORD trial did not.

Taken together, these four studies suggest that tight glycemic control is most appropriate for younger adults who have recent-onset type 2 diabetes and no cardiovascular complications. Because even short periods of hyperglycemia may increase the risk for complications, optimal therapy should be started as soon as diabetes is diagnosed.

Who should *not* receive intensive therapy? Intensive glycemic control may be inappropriate for patients with the following conditions:

- Long-standing type 2 diabetes
- Advanced microvascular or macrovascular complications
- Extensive comorbid conditions
- A history of severe hypoglycemia
- Limited life expectancy

For these patients, an A_{1c} goal above 7% may be more appropriate than a goal below 7% (see Table 46.3).

Monitoring Treatment

We need monitoring to (1) determine whether glucose levels are being maintained in a safe range, both short term and long term, and (2) guide changes in treatment when the range is not satisfactory or safe. SMBG levels are the standard method for day-to-day monitoring. As mentioned previously, A_{1c} is measured to assess long-term glycemic control.

Self-Monitoring of Blood Glucose

SMBG is recommended for all patients who use insulin. That is, SMBG is recommended for all patients with type 1 diabetes and for all patients with type 2 diabetes receiving insulin. It is additionally used by most patients with type 2 diabetes using other therapies as well. Information on blood glucose concentration provides a guide for "fine-tuning" dosages of insulin and other antidiabetic drugs. The frequency of SMBG for any given patient can vary widely based on the therapies the patient uses and how active he or she is. A patient on metformin monotherapy may only need to check his or her blood sugar once per week, whereas a patient with type 1 diabetes on an intensive insulin regimen may check up to 8 times per day or more. Frequently used target values for blood glucose are 70 to 130 mg/dL before meals and 100 to 140 mg/dL at bedtime.

Monitoring of Hemoglobin A_{1c}

Measurement of hemoglobin A_{1c}—also called *glycosylated hemoglobin* or *glycated hemoglobin*—provides an index of *average glucose levels* over the prior 2 to 3 months. Glucose interacts spontaneously with hemoglobin in red blood cells to form glycosylated derivatives, the most prevalent being A_{1c}. With prolonged hyperglycemia, levels of A_{1c} gradually increase. Because red blood cells have a long life span (120 days), levels of A_{1c} reflect average glucose levels over an extended time. Hence, by measuring A_{1c} every 3 to 6 months, we can get a picture of long-term glycemic control. Please note, however, that measuring A_{1c} tells us nothing about acute, hour-to-hour swings in blood glucose. Accordingly, although measuring A_{1c} is an important part of diabetes management, it is clearly no substitute for SMBG.

Results are usually reported as a *percent of total hemoglobin in blood* (e.g., 7%). In addition, they may be reported as a value for *estimated Average Glucose* (eAG), expressed as mg of glucose/dL of blood (i.e., the same units patients see every day when doing SMBG). Selected A_{1c} values and their eAG equivalents are shown in Table 46.4.

The general goal is to keep the A_{1c} below 7%. Although an A_{1c} goal of below 7% is good for most patients, a less stringent goal (e.g., below 8%) may be appropriate for some patients, such as those with a history of severe hypoglycemia, limited life expectancy, or advanced microvascular or macrovascular complications. According to a 2014 statement issued jointly by the ADA and the European Association for the Study of Diabetes, A_{1c} should be measured every 3 months until the value drops to 7% and at least every 6 months thereafter. As noted previously, a value of 6.5% or greater is considered diagnostic of diabetes.

TABLE 46.4 ▪ Hemoglobin A_{1c} Levels and Their Corresponding eAG Levels*

A_{1c} Level (% of Total Hb)	Corresponding eAG Level	
	mg/dL	mmol/L
6	126	7.0
7	154	8.6
8	183	10.2
9	212	11.8
10	240	13.4
11	269	14.9
12	298	16.5

*The formula to convert from A_{1c} (%) to average glucose concentration equivalents (expressed in mg/dL) is: eAG = (A_{1c} × 28.7) − 46.7.

eAG, estimated average glucose in blood; Hb, hemoglobin.

Data from the American Diabetes Association.

Prototype Drugs

DRUGS FOR DIABETES MELLITUS

Insulin Preparations

Insulin lispro (short duration, rapid acting)
Regular insulin (short duration, slower acting)
NPH insulin (intermediate duration)
Insulin glargine (long duration)

Biguanide

Metformin

Sulfonylurea

Glyburide

Meglitinide (Glinide)

Repaglinide

Thiazolidinedione (Glitazone)

Pioglitazone

Alpha-Glucosidase Inhibitor

Acarbose

Gliptin (Dipeptidyl Peptidase-4 Inhibitor)

Sitagliptin

Sodium-Glucose Cotransporter 2 Inhibitor

Canagliflozin

Incretin Mimetic

Exenatide

INSULIN

Insulin is used to treat all patients with type 1 diabetes and many patients with type 2 diabetes. Our discussion of insulin is divided into three sections: physiology, preparations and administration, and therapeutic use.

Physiology

Structure

The structure of insulin is shown in Fig. 46.1. As indicated, insulin consists of two amino acid chains: the "A" (acidic) chain and the "B" (basic) chain. The A and B chains are linked to each other by two disulfide bridges.

Biosynthesis

Insulin is synthesized in the pancreas by beta cells within the islets of Langerhans. The immediate precursor of insulin is called proinsulin.

Proinsulin consists of insulin itself plus a peptide loop that runs from the A chain to the B chain. This loop is named *connecting peptide* or *C-peptide.* In the final step of insulin synthesis, C-peptide is enzymatically clipped from the proinsulin molecule.

Measurement of plasma C-peptide levels offers a way to assess residual capacity for insulin synthesis. Because commercial insulin preparations lack C-peptide, and because endogenous C-peptide is only present as a byproduct of insulin biosynthesis, the presence of C-peptide in the blood indicates the pancreas is still producing some insulin of its own.

Secretion

The principal stimulus for insulin release is a rise in blood glucose, and the most common cause of glucose elevation is eating a meal, especially one rich in carbohydrates. Under normal conditions, there is tight coupling between rising levels of blood glucose and increased secretion of insulin. Insulin release may also be triggered by amino acids, fatty acids, ketone bodies, and gut hormones such as GLP-1 (more on this later).

The sympathetic nervous system provides additional control of release. Activation of $beta_2$-adrenergic receptors in the pancreas *promotes* secretion of insulin. Conversely, activation of alpha-adrenergic receptors in the pancreas *inhibits* insulin release. Of the two modes of regulation, activation of beta receptors is more important.

Metabolic Actions

The metabolic actions of insulin are primarily *anabolic* (i.e., conservative, constructive). Insulin promotes conservation of energy and buildup of energy stores, such as glycogen. The hormone also promotes cell growth and division.

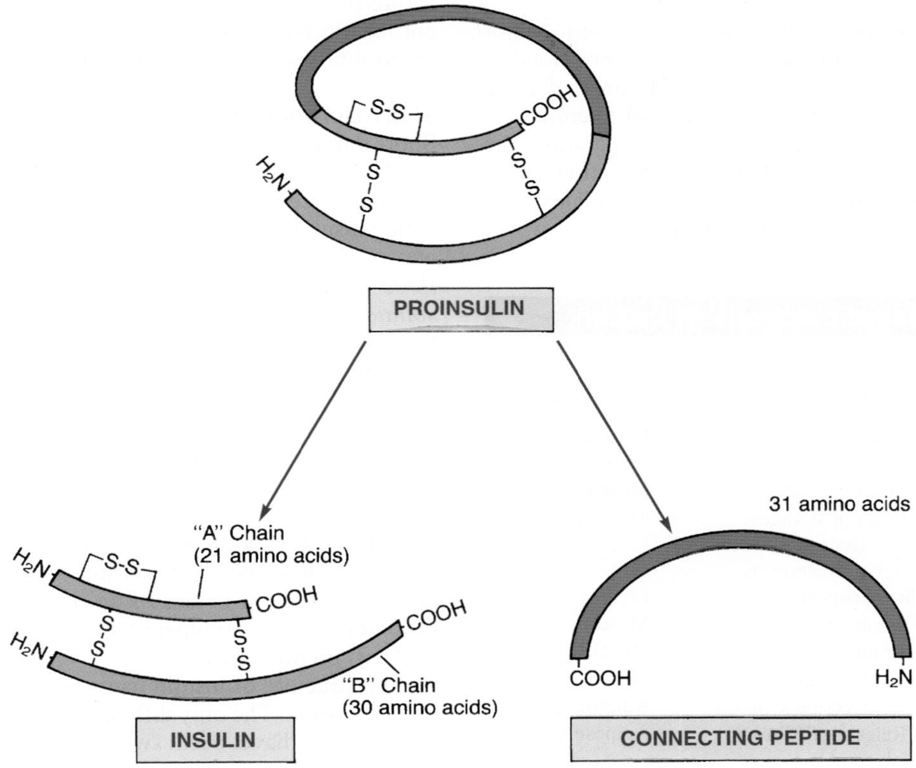

Figure 46.1 ■ Conversion of proinsulin to insulin.
Proinsulin is the immediate precursor of the insulin secreted by our pancreas. Enzymes clip off connecting peptide (C-peptide) to release active insulin, composed of two peptide chains (A and B) connected by two disulfide (S–S) bonds. Because C-peptide arises only from endogenous insulin, its presence in blood indicates that at least some pancreatic insulin is being made.

Insulin acts in two ways to promote anabolic effects. First, it stimulates cellular transport (uptake) of glucose, amino acids, nucleotides, and potassium. Second, insulin promotes synthesis of complex organic molecules. Under the influence of insulin and other factors, glucose is converted into glycogen, amino acids are assembled into proteins, and fatty acids are incorporated into triglycerides. The principal metabolic actions of insulin are shown in Table 46.5.

Metabolic Consequences of Insulin Deficiency

Insulin deficiency puts the body into a *catabolic* mode. Hence, in the absence of insulin, glycogen is converted into glucose, proteins are degraded into amino acids, and fats are converted to glycerol (glycerin) and free fatty acids. These catabolic effects contribute to the signs and symptoms of diabetes. Note that the catabolic effects resulting from insulin deficiency are opposite to the anabolic effects when insulin levels are normal.

Insulin deficiency promotes *hyperglycemia* by three mechanisms: (1) increased glycogenolysis, (2) increased gluconeogenesis, and (3) reduced glucose utilization. *Glycogenolysis,* by definition, generates free glucose by breaking down glycogen. The raw materials that allow increased *gluconeogenesis* are the amino acids and fatty acids produced by metabolic breakdown of proteins and fats. *Reduced glucose utilization* occurs because insulin deficiency decreases cellular uptake of glucose and decreases conversion of glucose to glycogen.

Preparations and Administration

There are many insulin preparations or formulations. Major differences concern time course, appearance (clear or cloudy), concentration, and route of administration. Because of these differences, insulin preparations cannot be used interchangeably. In fact, if a patient is given the wrong preparation, the consequences can be dire. Unfortunately, medication errors with insulins remain all too common, which explains why insulin appears on all lists of "high-alert" agents.

TABLE 46.5 ▪ Metabolic Actions of Insulin

Substance Affected	Insulin Action	Site of Action
Carbohydrates	↑ Glucose uptake	Muscle, adipose tissue
	↑ Glucose oxidation	Muscle
	↑ Glucose storage	Muscle, liver
	↑ Glycogen synthesis	
	↓ Glycogenolysis	
	Gluconeogenesis*	Liver
Amino acids and proteins	↑ Amino acid uptake	Muscle
	↓ Amino acid release	Muscle
	↑ Protein synthesis	Muscle
Lipids	↑ Triglyceride synthesis	Adipose tissue
	↓ Release of FFA and glycerol	Adipose tissue
	↓ Oxidation of FFA to ketoacids†	Liver

*Because of decreased delivery of substrate (fatty acids and amino acids) to the liver.

†Because of decreased delivery of FFA to the liver.

FFA, free fatty acids.

Sources of Insulin

All forms of insulin currently manufactured in the United States are produced using recombinant DNA technology. Some products, referred to as *human insulin,* are identical to insulin produced by the human pancreas. Other products, referred to as *human insulin analogs,* are modified forms of human insulin. The analogs have the same pharmacologic actions as human insulin but have different time courses.

Types of Insulin

There are seven types of insulin: "natural" insulin (also known as regular insulin or native insulin) and six modified insulins. Three of the modified insulins—insulin lispro, insulin aspart, and insulin glulisine—act more rapidly than regular insulin but have a shorter duration of action. The other modified insulins act more slowly than regular insulin but have a longer duration. Two processes are used to prolong insulin effects: (1) complexing natural insulin with a protein and (2) altering the insulin molecule itself. When the insulin molecule has been altered, we refer to the product as a *human insulin analog.*

When classified according to time course, insulin preparations fall into three major groups: short duration, intermediate duration, and long duration (Table 46.6). The short-duration insulins can be subdivided into two groups: rapid acting (insulin lispro, insulin aspart, and insulin glulisine) and slower acting (regular or "natural" insulin). Time courses for different insulin types are shown in Fig. 46.2. Selected properties of insulin types are shown in Table 46.7.

Short Duration: Rapid Acting

Short-duration insulins are administered in association with meals to control the postprandial rise in blood glucose. To provide glycemic control between meals and at night, short-acting insulins must be used in conjunction with an intermediate- or long-acting agent in people with type 1 diabetes. *All three of the rapid-acting insulins are formulated as clear solutions,* and all three require a prescription. For routine therapy, all three are given by the subcutaneous (subQ) route.

Insulin Lispro. Insulin lispro [Humalog] is a rapid-acting analog of regular insulin. Effects begin within 15 to 30 minutes of subQ injection and persist for 3 to 6 hours. Insulin lispro acts faster than regular insulin but has a shorter duration of action. Because of its rapid onset, insulin lispro can be administered immediately before eating, or even after eating. In contrast, regular insulin is generally administered 30 to 60 minutes before meals. The usual route for insulin lispro is subQ by injection or use of an insulin pump. Insulin lispro (100 units/mL) is commercially available in 10-mL vials and as 3-mL prefilled pens.

The structure of insulin lispro is nearly identical to that of natural insulin. The only difference is that the positions of two amino acids have been switched. Because of this switch, molecules of insulin lispro aggregate less than do molecules of regular insulin, which explains why insulin lispro acts more rapidly.

Insulin Aspart. Insulin aspart [NovoLog] is an analog of human insulin with a rapid onset (10–20 minutes) and short duration (3–5 hours). Insulin aspart is very similar to insulin lispro.

TABLE 46.6 ■ Types of Insulin: Time Course of Action After Subcutaneous Injection

Generic Name	Trade Name	Time Course: Onset (min)	Peak (hr)	Duration (hr)
SHORT DURATION: RAPID ACTING				
Insulin lispro	Humalog	15–30	0.5–2.5	3–6
Insulin aspart	NovoLog	10–20	1–3	3–5
Insulin glulisine	Apidra	10–15	1–1.5	3–5
SHORT DURATION: SLOWER ACTING				
Regular insulin	Humulin R, Novolin R	30–60	1–5	6–10
INTERMEDIATE DURATION				
NPH insulin	Humulin N, Novolin N	60–120	6–14	16–24
LONG DURATION				
Insulin glargine	Lantus	70	None*	18–24
Insulin detemir	Levemir	60–120	12–24	Varies†
ULTRALONG DURATION				
Insulin degludec	Tresiba	60	None*	42

*Levels are steady with no discernible peak.
†Duration is dose dependent: at 0.2 units/kg, duration is 12 hours; at 0.4 units/kg, duration is 20 to 24 hours.

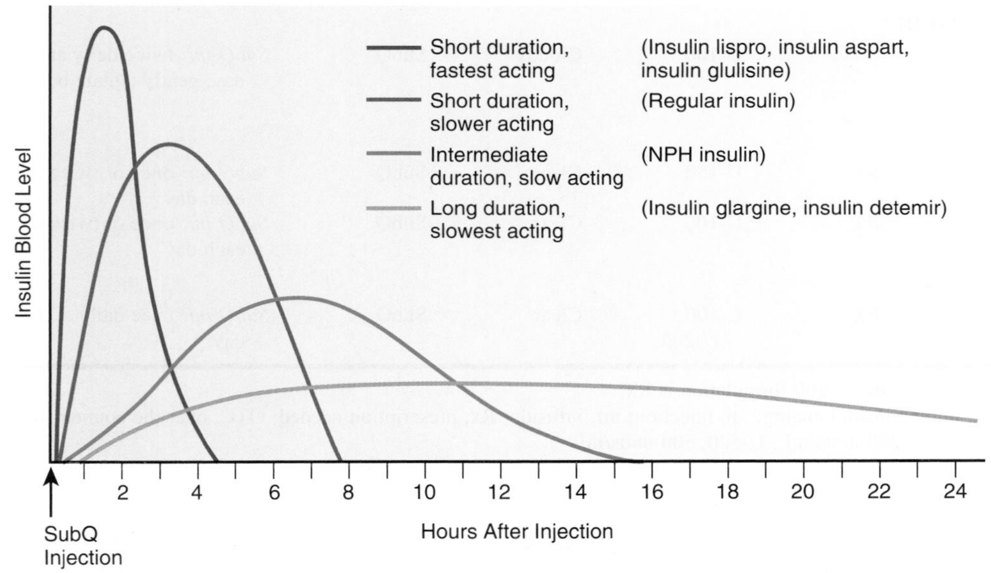

Figure 46.2 ■ Time-effect relationship for different types of insulin after subcutaneous injection.

Insulin aspart (100 units/mL) is supplied in 10-mL vials and 3-mL prefilled pens. Dosing is almost always done by subQ injection or subQ infusion. Because insulin aspart acts rapidly, injections should be made 5 to 10 minutes before meals.

Insulin Glulisine. Like insulin lispro and insulin aspart, insulin glulisine [Apidra] is a synthetic analog of natural human insulin with a rapid onset (10–15 minutes) and short duration (3–5 hours). Owing to its rapid onset, the drug should be administered close to the time of eating. Administration is almost always by subQ injection or continuous subQ infusion. Insulin glulisine (100 units/mL) is available in 10-mL vials and as 3-mL prefilled insulin pens.

Short Duration: Slower Acting

Regular Insulin Injection. Regular insulin [Humulin R, Novolin R] is unmodified human insulin. The product has four approved routes: subQ injection, subQ infusion, IM injection (used rarely), and oral inhalation.

For routine treatment of diabetes, regular insulin can be (1) injected before meals to control postprandial hyperglycemia

TABLE 46.7 ▪ Properties of Insulin Types

Generic Name [Trade Name]	Class	Rx or OTC	Strength	Appearance	Route	Administration Options
SHORT DURATION: RAPID ACTING						
Insulin lispro [Humalog]	HA	Rx	U-100	Clear	SubQ, IV	*SubQ inj:* within 15 min before or just after meals *SubQ inf:* continuous, with bolus just before meals *IV:* approved route, but rarely used
Insulin aspart [NovoLog]	HA	Rx	U-100	Clear	SubQ, IV	*SubQ inj:* 5–10 min before meals *SubQ inf:* continuous, with bolus 5–10 min before meals *IV:* approved route, but rarely used
Insulin glulisine [Apidra]	HA	Rx	U-100	Clear	SubQ, IV	*SubQ inj:* within 15 min before meals or within 20 min after *SubQ inf:* continuous, with bolus 15–20 min before meals *IV:* approved route, but rarely used
SHORT DURATION: SLOWER ACTING						
Regular insulin [Humulin R, Novolin R]	H	OTC*	U-100, U-500	Clear	SubQ, IV, IM	*SubQ inj:* 30 min before meals *SubQ inf:* continuous, with bolus 20–30 min before meals *IV:* for emergencies and glycemic management in the inpatient setting (never use U-500 IV) *IM:* approved route, but rarely used
INTERMEDIATE DURATION						
NPH insulin [Humulin N, Novolin N]	H	OTC	U-100	Cloudy	SubQ	*SubQ inj:* twice daily at the same times each day; gently agitate before use
LONG DURATION						
Insulin glargine [Lantus]	HA	Rx	U-100	Clear	SubQ	*SubQ inj:* once or twice daily at the same time each day
Insulin detemir [Levemir]	HA	Rx	U-100	Clear	SubQ	*SubQ inj:* once or twice daily at the same time each day
ULTRALONG DURATION						
Insulin degludec [Tresiba]	HA	Rx	U-100, U-200	Clear	SubQ	*SubQ inj:* once daily at the same time each day

*U-100 formulations are OTC, the U-500 formulation is Rx.
H, human insulin; HA, human insulin analog; inj, injection; inf, infusion; Rx, prescription needed; OTC, over the counter (no prescription needed); U-100, 100 units/mL; U-200, 200 units/mL; U-500, 500 units/mL

and (2) infused subcutaneously to provide basal glycemic control. After *subQ injection,* molecules of regular insulin form small aggregates at the injection site. As a result, absorption is slightly delayed. Effects begin in 30 to 60 minutes, peak in 1 to 5 hours, and last up to 10 hours. Onset is slower than with the rapid-acting insulins and faster than with the longer acting insulins. Because of this delay, most people using insulin pumps use a rapid-acting insulin analog instead of regular insulin.

Regular insulin is supplied as a clear solution. Two concentrations are available: U-100 (100 units/mL) and U-500 (500 units/mL). Regular insulin [Humulin R] is the only type available in a U-500 strength. U-100 preparations are used by most patients. The U-500 concentration is reserved for patients with extreme insulin resistance. Care should also be taken when using U-500 insulin because insulin syringes are calibrated to be used with U-100 products. Extra caution and education are critical when working with patients using U-500 insulin. Except for the U-500 formulation, all formulations of regular insulin are available without prescription.

Intermediate Duration

Neutral Protamine Hagedorn (NPH) Insulin Suspension. NPH insulin [Humulin N, Novolin N], also known as *isophane insulin,* is prepared by conjugating regular insulin with protamine (a large protein). The presence of protamine decreases the solubility of NPH insulin and thus delays absorption. As a result, onset of action is delayed and duration of action is extended. Because onset is delayed, NPH insulin cannot be administered at mealtime to control postprandial hyperglycemia. Rather, the drug is injected twice or three times daily to provide glycemic control between meals and during the night. Of the longer acting insulins in current use, NPH insulin is the only one suitable for mixing with short-acting insulins. Because protamine is a foreign protein, allergic reactions are possible. NPH insulins are supplied as cloudy suspensions that must be agitated before administration. Administration is by subQ injection only. Like regular insulin, NPH insulins are available without prescription. NPH insulin (100 units/mL) is available in 10-mL vials and in 3-mL prefilled insulin pens.

Long Duration

Insulin Glargine. Insulin glargine [Lantus] is a modified human insulin with a prolonged duration of action (up to 24 hours). The drug is indicated for once-daily subQ dosing to treat adults and children with type 1 diabetes and adults with type 2 diabetes. That being said, some patients require twice-daily administration to achieve a full 24 hours of basal coverage. Dosing may be done any time of day (morning, afternoon, or evening) but should be done at the same time every day, if possible.

Insulin glargine differs from natural human insulin by four amino acids. Hence, when injected subcutaneously, it forms microprecipitates that slowly dissolve and thereby release insulin glargine in small amounts over an extended time. In contrast to other long-acting insulins (e.g., insulin detemir), which cause blood levels to rise to a peak and then fall to a trough, insulin glargine achieves blood levels that are relatively steady.

Insulin glargine is supplied as a *clear solution* in 10-mL vials containing 100 units/mL, and as a prefilled *SoloStar Pen.* The drug should not be mixed with other insulins.

Insulin Detemir. Insulin detemir [Levemir] is a human insulin analog with a slow onset and dose-dependent duration of action. At low doses (0.2 units/kg), effects persist about 12 hours. At higher doses (0.4 units/kg), effects persist for up to 20 to 24 hours. Because of its slow onset and prolonged duration, insulin detemir is used to provide basal glycemic control. It is not given before meals to control postprandial hyperglycemia. Compared with NPH insulin, insulin detemir has a slower onset and longer duration.

Insulin detemir is supplied as a clear, colorless solution (100 units/mL) in 10-mL vials and as a 3-mL *FlexPen.* Dosing is done once or twice daily by subQ injection. Insulin detemir should not be mixed with other insulins and must not be given intravenously. The drug is available by prescription only.

Ultralong Duration

Insulin Degludec. Insulin degludec [Tresiba] is the only human insulin analog with ultralong duration of action. Effects of insulin degludec persist for up to 42 hours. Because of its prolonged duration, insulin degludec is used to provide basal glycemic control. Similarly to insulin glargine, insulin degludec does not have a peak.

Insulin degludec is supplied as a clear, colorless solution in two concentrations of FlexTouch pens (100 units/mL and 200 units/mL). Dosing is done once daily by subQ injection. Insulin degludec should not be mixed with other insulins and must not be given intravenously. The drug is available by prescription only.

Concentration

In the United States insulin is available in two concentrations: 100 units/mL (U-100) and 500 units/mL (U-500). Preparations containing 40 units/mL are available in other countries but not in the United States. U-100 insulins are employed for routine replacement therapy. All insulin types are available in U-100 formulations. Only one product—the *Humulin R* brand of regular insulin—is formulated in the U-500 strength. This product, which is available from the manufacturer by special request, is reserved for emergencies and for patients with severe insulin resistance, generally defined as needing more than 200 units/day.

Patient Education

MIXING INSULINS

Mixing should be done only with insulins of proven compatibility. Of the three longer acting insulins in current use, *only NPH insulin is appropriate for mixing with short-acting insulins* (i.e., regular, lispro, aspart, and glulisine insulins). When a mixture is prepared, the short-acting insulin should be drawn into the syringe first to avoid contaminating the stock vial of the short-acting insulin with NPH insulin.

Commercially available premixed combinations are described in Table 46.8.

Patient Education

INJECTION SITES

The most common sites of subQ injection are the upper arm, thigh, and abdomen (Fig. 46.3). Because rates of absorption vary among sites, patients should make all injections into the same general area (e.g., thigh or abdomen). To reduce the risk for lipodystrophy (see later), injections within the chosen area should be made in different spots, preferably about 1 inch apart. Ideally, each spot should be used only once a month.

Subcutaneous Infusion

Portable Insulin Pumps. These computerized devices deliver a basal infusion of insulin (regular, lispro, aspart, or glulisine) plus bolus doses before each meal. In other words, the pump uses only one type of insulin for both basal and mealtime coverage. The basal infusion is usually about 1 unit/hour and can be programmed to match the patient's metabolic requirements. Basal rates can even be adjusted to different rates throughout the day, depending on the individualized needs of the patient, and are adjustable in some pumps up to $\frac{1}{100}$ of a unit per hour. Mealtime boluses are calculated to match carbohydrate intake and can be adjusted to within $\frac{1}{10}$ of a unit. The pumps are about the size of a small cell phone, weigh only 4 ounces, and are worn on the belt or in a pocket. An infusion set delivers insulin from the pump to a subcutaneous catheter, usually located on the abdomen. The infusion set should be replaced every 1 to 3 days, at which time the catheter is moved to a new infusion site (at least 1 inch away from the old one). Because the pump delivers short-acting insulin, insulin levels will drop quickly if the pump is removed. Accordingly, the pump should remain in place most of the day. However, it can be removed for 1 to 2 hours on special occasions. External insulin pumps cost between $3000 and $5000. Infusion sets, insulin, and glucose monitoring materials add another $300 or more per month to the bill. Aside from expense, the main drawback of the pumps is delivery of too little insulin owing to formation of insulin microdeposits within the tubing.

Implantable Insulin Pumps. These devices are surgically implanted in the abdomen and deliver insulin either intraperitoneally or intravenously. Like external pumps, internal pumps deliver a basal insulin infusion plus bolus doses with meals. Insulin delivery is adjusted by external telemetry. Compared with multiple daily injections, pumps produce superior glycemic control, cause less hypoglycemia and weight gain, and can improve quality of life. As with external pumps, delivery of insulin can be impeded by formation of insulin microprecipitates. Implantable pumps are experimental and not yet available for general use.

TABLE 46.8 ■ Premixed Insulin Combinations*

Description	Trade Name	Time Course		
		Onset (min)	Peak (hr)	Duration (hr)
70% NPH insulin/30% regular insulin	Humulin 70/30	30–60	1.5–16	10–16
	Novolin 70/30	30–60	2–12	10–16
50% NPH insulin/50% regular insulin	Humulin 50/50	30–60	2–12	10–16
70% insulin aspart protamine/30% insulin aspart	NovoLog Mix 70/30	10–20	1–4	15–18
75% insulin lispro protamine/25% insulin lispro	Humalog Mix 75/25	15–30	1–6.5	10–16
50% insulin lispro protamine/50% insulin lispro	Humalog Mix 50/50	15–30	0.8–4.8	10–16

*Use only after the dosages and ratios of the components have been established as correct for the patient.

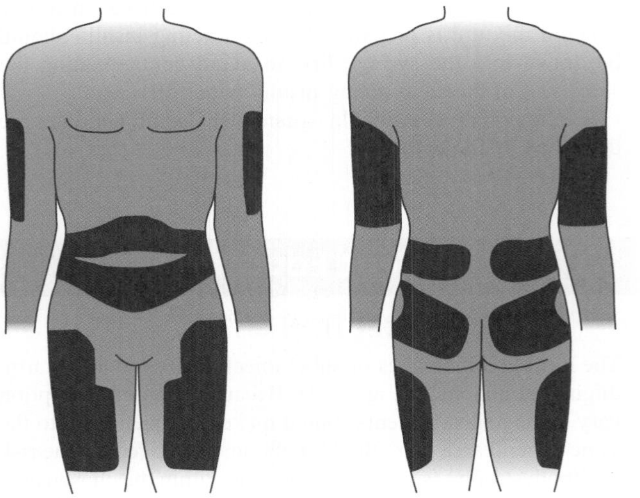

Figure 46.3 ■ Possible sites for subcutaneous injection of insulin.

Inhalation

Inhalation of insulin is an attractive alternative to needle-based dosing. In clinical trials, patient satisfaction with inhaled insulin has been much higher than with insulin injections. One delivery system is currently available for insulin inhalation—Afrezza. This inhaled mealtime insulin product provides good glycemic control with a relatively low incidence of hypoglycemia—and has demonstrated little or no effect on pulmonary function in studies to date. Even though it has not demonstrated effects on pulmonary function, Afrezza is known to cause bronchospasm in patients with chronic lung disease. Therefore there is a Risk Evaluation and Mitigation Strategy (REMS) program in place to protect patients with chronic obstructive pulmonary disease or asthma. Before prescribing Afrezza, the provider should obtain a detailed medical history, physical examination, and spirometry.

Storage

Insulin in *unopened vials* should be stored *under refrigeration* until needed. Vials should not be frozen. When stored unopened under refrigeration, insulin can be used up to the expiration date on the vial.

The vial in current use can be kept at room temperature for up to 1 month without significant loss of activity. Direct sunlight and extreme heat must be avoided. Partially filled vials should be discarded after several weeks if left unused. Injecting insulin stored at room temperature causes less pain than injecting cold insulin and reduces the risk for lipodystrophy.

Mixtures of insulin prepared in *vials* are stable for 1 month at room temperature and for 3 months under refrigeration.

Mixtures of insulin in *prefilled syringes* (plastic or glass) should be stored in a refrigerator, where they will be stable for at least 1 week and perhaps 2 weeks. The syringe should be stored vertically with the needle pointing up to avoid clogging the needle. Before administration, the syringe should be agitated gently to resuspend the insulin.

Therapeutic Use

Indications

The principal indication for insulin is *diabetes mellitus.* Insulin is required by all patients with type 1 diabetes and by many patients with type 2 diabetes. In fact, most of the insulin sold is used by people with type 2 diabetes—largely because type 2 diabetes accounts for 90% to 95% of all cases of diabetes.

Insulin Therapy of Diabetes

Insulin is given to all patients who have type 1 diabetes and to many who have type 2 diabetes. In addition, insulin is the preferred drug to manage gestational diabetes. In treating these disorders, the objective is to prevent complications by keeping blood glucose within an acceptable range. When therapy is successful, both hyperglycemia and hypoglycemia are minimized, and the long-term complications of diabetes are avoided.

Dosage

To achieve optimal glucose control, insulin dosage must be closely matched with insulin needs. If carbohydrate intake is increased, insulin dosage must be increased, too. When a meal is missed or is low in carbohydrates, or when physical activity levels increase, the dosage of insulin must be decreased. Dosing requires additional adjustments to meet specialized needs. For example, insulin needs are *increased* by infection, stress, obesity, the adolescent growth spurt, and pregnancy after the first trimester. Conversely, insulin needs are *decreased* by exercise and during the first trimester of pregnancy. To ensure that insulin dosage is coordinated with insulin requirements, the patient and the health care team must work together to establish an integrated program of nutrition, exercise, insulin replacement therapy, and appropriate blood glucose monitoring.

Total daily dosages may range from 0.1 unit/kg body weight to more than 2.5 units/kg. For patients with type 1 diabetes, initial dosages typically range from 0.5 to 0.6 units/kg/day. For patients with type 2 diabetes, initial dosages typically range from 0.2 to 0.6 units/kg/day.

Dosing Schedules

The schedule of insulin administration helps determine the extent to which glucose control can be achieved. Three dosing schedules are compared here. These example regimens include use of (1) a twice-daily premixed insulin regimen, (2) intensive basal/bolus strategy, and (3) continuous subcutaneous insulin infusion (CSII). Although three example regimens are discussed, it should be noted that practitioners can use available insulin products in a number of ways and combinations to meet patient-specific needs and treatment goals.

Twice-Daily Premixed Regimen. There are several premixed insulin products on the market. As shown in Fig. 46.4A, a twice-daily regimen of such a premixed insulin product can be used to provide both basal and prandial insulin coverage. The advantage of this strategy is that patients only have to give two injections per day. A disadvantage, however, is that if given with breakfast and dinner, there is no mealtime coverage at lunch. Additionally, using a fixed combination does not allow for adjustments of the long-acting or short-acting insulin individually; if the dose is changed, both components are altered.

Intensive Basal/Bolus Strategy. For patients with type 1 diabetes, an intensive basal/bolus strategy is often used. As shown in Fig. 46.4B, this strategy involves the use of a long-acting insulin (such as insulin glargine [Lantus]) in addition to a short-acting insulin (such as regular insulin, insulin aspart, insulin lispro, or insulin glulisine). This insulin dosing strategy allows for very good basal coverage and the ability to dose a short-acting insulin with each meal and as needed to cover snacks or elevated blood glucose levels.

Continuous Subcutaneous Insulin Infusion. CSII is accomplished using a portable infusion pump connected to an indwelling subcutaneous catheter. Four types of insulin may be used: regular, lispro, aspart, and glulisine. To provide a basal level of insulin, the pump is set to infuse insulin continuously at a slow but steady rate. To accommodate insulin needs created by eating, the pump is triggered manually to provide a bolus dose matched in size to the carbohydrate content of each meal. Hence, CSII can adapt to altered insulin needs. Although the use of CSII allows for ease of administration, the use of frequent SMBG is essential to achieve optimal glycemic control. Infusion pumps were discussed earlier in the section on "Subcutaneous Infusion."

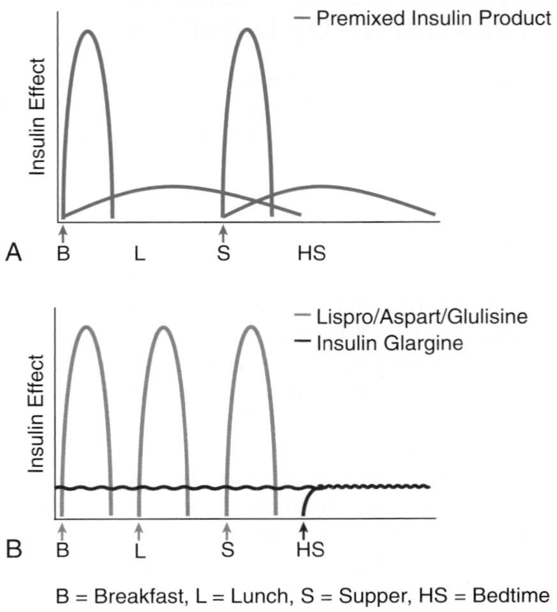

Figure 46.4 ■ Examples of insulin dosing schedules.

Achieving Optimal Glucose Control

As we have seen, the primary requirement for achieving tight glucose control is a method of insulin delivery that permits dosage adjustments that accommodate ongoing variations in insulin needs. Intensive basal/bolus therapy and CSII meet this criterion. In addition to an adaptable method of insulin delivery, achieving tight glucose control requires the following:

- Careful attention to all elements of the treatment program (diet, exercise, insulin replacement therapy)
- Defined glycemic targets
- Self-monitoring of blood glucose in concordance with the patient's individualized management plan
- A high degree of patient motivation
- Extensive patient education

Tight glucose control cannot be achieved without the informed participation of the patient. Accordingly, patients must receive thorough instruction on the following:

- The nature of diabetes
- The importance of optimal glucose control
- The major components of the treatment routine (insulin replacement, SMBG, diet, exercise)
- Procedures for purchasing insulin, syringes, and needles
- The importance of avoiding arbitrary changes between insulins from different manufacturers
- Methods of insulin storage
- Procedures for mixing insulins (if applicable)
- Calculation of dosage adjustments
- Techniques of insulin administration
- Methods for monitoring blood glucose

In the final analysis, responsibility for managing diabetes rests with the patient. The health care team can design a treatment program and provide education and guidance. However, optimal glucose control can only be achieved if the patient is actively involved in his or her own therapy.

Complications of Insulin Treatment

Hypoglycemia

Hypoglycemia (blood glucose below 70 mg/dL) occurs when insulin levels exceed insulin needs. A major cause of insulin excess is overdose. Imbalance between insulin levels and insulin needs can also result from reduced intake of food, vomiting and diarrhea (which reduce absorption of nutrients), excessive consumption of alcohol (which promotes hypoglycemia), unusually intense exercise (which promotes cellular glucose uptake and metabolism), and childbirth (which reduces insulin requirements).

Rapid treatment of hypoglycemia is mandatory: if hypoglycemia is allowed to persist, irreversible brain damage or

Patient Education

HYPOGLYCEMIA

Patients with diabetes and their families should be familiar with the signs and symptoms of hypoglycemia. Establishing whether patients are experiencing hypoglycemia and whether they recognize hypoglycemic symptoms is recommended as a critical component of an encounter with a patient with diabetes. Some symptoms result from activation of the sympathetic nervous system; others arise from a lack of glucose within the CNS. When glucose levels fall *rapidly,* activation of the sympathetic nervous system occurs, resulting in tachycardia, palpitations, sweating, and nervousness. However, if glucose declines *gradually,* symptoms may be limited to those of CNS origin. Mild CNS symptoms include headache, confusion, drowsiness, and fatigue. If hypoglycemia is severe, convulsions, coma, and death may follow.

even death may result. In conscious patients, glucose levels can be restored with a fast-acting oral sugar (e.g., glucose tablets, orange juice, sugar cubes, honey, corn syrup, nondiet soda). However, if the swallowing reflex or the gag reflex is suppressed, nothing should be administered by mouth. In cases of severe hypoglycemia, intravenous (IV) glucose is the preferred treatment. Parenteral *glucagon* is an alternative treatment. (The pharmacology of glucagon is discussed at the end of the chapter.)

In anticipation of hypoglycemic episodes, people with diabetes should always have an oral carbohydrate available (e.g., sugared candy, sugar cubes, glucose tablets). Some prescribers recommend that patients keep glucagon on hand, too—particularly people on insulin therapy. Patients should carry some sort of identification (e.g., a medical alert bracelet) to inform emergency personnel of their condition.

In some patients, hypoglycemia occurs without producing the symptoms noted previously. This is known as *hypoglycemia unawareness.* As a result, the patient remains unaware of hypoglycemia until blood sugar has become dangerously low. Hypoglycemia unawareness is a particular problem among patients practicing tight glucose control. This is because as patients experience more frequent hypoglycemia, they start to have diminished symptoms over time. The risk for dangerous hypoglycemia can be minimized by frequently monitoring blood glucose. Additionally, current recommendations state that treatment goals should be temporarily loosened (such as for several weeks) for people experiencing hypoglycemia unawareness so that they can regain hypoglycemia awareness.

Hypoglycemia can result in coma. The most definitive diagnosis is made by measuring plasma glucose levels: in hypoglycemic coma, glucose levels are very low.

Other Complications

Hypokalemia. Insulin promotes uptake of potassium by cells. Insulin activates a membrane-bound enzyme—Na^+,K^+-ATPase—that pumps potassium into cells and pumps sodium out. Hence, in addition to lowering blood levels of glucose, insulin can lower blood levels of potassium. When insulin dosage is proper, effects on potassium are unremarkable. However, if insulin dosage is excessive, clinically significant hypokalemia can result. Effects on the heart are of greatest concern: hypokalemia can reduce contractility and can cause potentially fatal dysrhythmias.

Lipohypertrophy. Lipohypertrophy (accumulation of subcutaneous fat) can occur when insulin is injected too frequently at the same site. Fat accumulates because insulin stimulates fat synthesis. When use of the site is discontinued, excess fat is eventually lost. Lipohypertrophy can be minimized through systematic rotation of injection sites.

Allergic Reactions. Rarely, patients experience systemic allergic responses. These reactions develop rapidly and are characterized by the widespread appearance of red and intensely itchy welts. Breathing difficulty may develop. If severe allergy develops in a patient who nonetheless must continue insulin use, a desensitization procedure can be performed. This process entails giving small initial doses of human insulin, followed by a series of progressively larger doses.

Drug Interactions

Hypoglycemic Agents

Drugs that lower blood glucose levels can intensify hypoglycemia induced by insulin. Among these drugs are *sulfonylureas, glinides,* and *alcohol* (used acutely or long term in excessive doses). When these drugs are combined with insulin, special care must be taken to ensure as best as possible that blood glucose does not fall too low.

Hyperglycemic Agents

Drugs that raise blood glucose (e.g., *thiazide diuretics, glucocorticoids, sympathomimetics*) can counteract the desired effects of insulin. When these agents are combined with insulin, insulin dosage may need to be increased.

Beta-Adrenergic Blocking Agents

Beta blockers can delay awareness of and response to hypoglycemia by masking signs that are associated with stimulation of the sympathetic nervous system (e.g., tachycardia, palpitations) that hypoglycemia normally causes. Furthermore, because beta blockade impairs glycogenolysis, and because glycogenolysis is one means by which the body can respond to and counteract a fall in blood glucose, beta blockers can make insulin-induced hypoglycemia even worse by preventing the body's natural counterregulatory response.

NONINSULIN MEDICATIONS FOR THE TREATMENT OF DIABETES

The noninsulin medications for the treatment of diabetes fall into two major groups: oral drugs and noninsulin injectable drugs. Their actions and major adverse effects are shown in Table 46.9.

Oral Drugs

There are seven main families of oral antidiabetic drugs: biguanides, sulfonylureas, meglitinides (glinides), thiazolidinediones (glitazones), alpha-glucosidase inhibitors, DPP-4 inhibitors (gliptins), and SGLT-2 inhibitors. These agents are approved for use in type 2 diabetes, but agents such as the SGLT-2 inhibitors are used off-label in combination with insulin for the treatment of type 1 diabetes—with clinical studies in progress. In the past, the oral agents were used only after a program of diet modification and exercise had failed to yield sufficient glycemic control. Today, one oral agent—metformin—is usually started immediately after type 2 diabetes has been diagnosed.

The oral agents work in a variety of ways. Some of them—notably the sulfonylureas, and glinides (collectively

TABLE 46.9 ■ Drugs for Type 2 Diabetes

Class and Specific Agents	Actions	Major Adverse Effects
ORAL DRUGS		
Biguanide		
Metformin [Fortamet, Glucophage, Glumetza, Riomet]	Decreases glucose production by the liver, increases tissue response to insulin	GI symptoms: decreased appetite, nausea, diarrhea Lactic acidosis (rarely)
Second-Generation Sulfonylureas		
Glimepiride [Amaryl] Glipizide [Glucotrol] Glyburide* [DiaBeta, Glynase PresTab]	Promote insulin secretion by the pancreas; may also increase tissue response to insulin	Hypoglycemia Weight gain
Meglitinides (Glinides)		
Nateglinide [Starlix] Repaglinide [Prandin, GlucoNorm ♣]	Promote insulin secretion by the pancreas	Hypoglycemia Weight gain
Thiazolidinediones (Glitazones)		
Pioglitazone [Actos] Rosiglitazone† [Avandia]	Decrease insulin resistance and thereby increase glucose uptake by muscle and adipose tissue and decrease glucose production by the liver	Hypoglycemia, but only in the presence of excessive insulin Heart failure Bladder cancer Fractures (in women) Ovulation and thus possible unintended pregnancy
Alpha-Glucosidase Inhibitors		
Acarbose [Precose, Glucobay ♣] Miglitol [Glyset]	Delay carbohydrate digestion and absorption, thereby decreasing the postprandial rise in blood glucose	GI symptoms: flatulence, cramps, abdominal distention, borborygmus
Dipeptidyl Peptidase-4 (DPP-4) Inhibitors (Gliptins)		
Alogliptin [Nesina] Linagliptin [Tradjenta] Saxagliptin [Onglyza] Sitagliptin [Januvia]	Enhance the activity of incretins (by inhibiting their breakdown by DPP-4) and thereby increase insulin release, reduce glucagon release, and decrease hepatic glucose production	Pancreatitis Hypersensitivity reactions
Sodium-Glucose Cotransporter 2 (SGLT-2) Inhibitors		
Canagliflozin [Invokana] Dapagliflozin [Farxiga]	Increase glucose excretion via the urine by inhibiting SGLT-2 in the kidney tubules, decreasing glucose levels and inducing weight loss by caloric loss through the urine	Genital mycotic infections Orthostasis
Dopamine Agonist		
Bromocriptine [Cycloset]	Activates dopamine receptors in the CNS; how it improves glycemic control is unknown	Orthostatic hypotension Exacerbation of psychosis
NONINSULIN INJECTABLE DRUGS		
Incretin Mimetics		
Exenatide [Byetta] Exenatide extended-release [Bydureon] Liraglutide [Victoza] Albiglutide [Tanzeum]	Lower blood glucose by slowing gastric emptying, stimulating glucose-dependent insulin release, suppressing postprandial glucagon release, and reducing appetite	Hypoglycemia GI symptoms: nausea, vomiting, diarrhea Pancreatitis Renal insufficiency Thyroid cancer? (liraglutide, exenatide extended-release, and albiglutide)
Amylin Mimetics		
Pramlintide [Symlin]	Delays gastric emptying and suppresses glucagon secretion, decreasing the postprandial rise in glucose	Hypoglycemia Nausea Injection-site reactions

*Commonly known as *glibenclamide* outside the United States.

†Owing to a risk for sudden cardiac death, rosiglitazone is available only through a restricted distribution program.

referred to as "insulin secretagogues")—actively drive blood glucose down by increasing insulin release from beta cells of the pancreas. Others—notably metformin (a biguanide), the alpha-glucosidase inhibitors, and SGLT-2 inhibitors—don't drive blood glucose down; rather, they simply modulate the rise in glucose that happens after a meal. This distinction is not just academic: if taken when blood glucose is normal or low, agents that drive glucose down can cause *hypoglycemia.* Hypoglycemia is not a large risk with the drugs that simply impair the postprandial rise in blood glucose.

Biguanides: Metformin

Metformin [Glucophage, Glucophage XR, Fortamet, Glumetza, Riomet], classified chemically as a biguanide, is the drug of choice for initial therapy in most patients with type 2 diabetes. Typically, metformin is started immediately after the diagnosis of type 2 diabetes. The most common side effects are gastrointestinal (GI) disturbances. Lactic acidosis, a potentially fatal complication, is rare.

Mechanism of Action

Metformin lowers blood glucose and improves glucose tolerance in three ways. First, it inhibits glucose production in the liver. Second, it reduces (slightly) glucose absorption in the gut. And third, it sensitizes insulin receptors in target tissues (fat and skeletal muscle) and thereby increases glucose uptake in response to whatever insulin may be available. In contrast to the sulfonylureas (see later), metformin does not stimulate insulin release from the pancreas. As a result, metformin does not actively drive blood glucose levels down and hence poses little if any added risk for hypoglycemia when used alone.

Pharmacokinetics

After oral dosing, metformin is slowly absorbed from the small intestine. Of particular interest, metformin is not metabolized. Rather, it is excreted unchanged by the kidneys. Hence, in the event of renal impairment, metformin can accumulate to toxic levels.

Therapeutic Uses

Glycemic Control. Metformin is used to lower blood sugar in patients with type 2 diabetes. In the past, treatment was reserved for patients who had not responded adequately to a program of diet modification and exercise. Today, however, treatment is usually begun as soon as type 2 diabetes is diagnosed.

Metformin may be used alone or in combination with other agents. When used alone, metformin lowers fasting and postprandial blood glucose levels. When metformin is used as a component of combination therapy, the combination lowers blood sugar more effectively than either drug alone—which is to be expected because other available agents act through different mechanisms.

Metformin is well suited for patients who tend to skip meals. When meals are skipped, blood sugar can drop below a level that is healthy. Because metformin does not lower blood glucose any further, it won't make the situation any worse. In contrast, drugs that actively lower blood glucose, such as the sulfonylureas, can drop a normal or slightly low blood glucose into clinically significant hypoglycemia.

Prevention of Type 2 Diabetes. Data from the Diabetes Prevention Program (DPP), a large study sponsored by the National Institutes of Health, indicate that metformin can delay development of type 2 diabetes in high-risk individuals. The DPP enrolled 3234 people aged 25 to 85 years. All participants had impaired glucose tolerance (as determined by an OGTT), and all were severely overweight. Participants were randomly assigned to one of three protocols: (1) intensive lifestyle changes with the aim of reducing body weight by 7% through moderate exercise (e.g., vigorous walking 30 minutes a day, 5 days a week) combined with a low-fat diet, (2) treatment with metformin (850 mg twice daily), or (3) treatment with placebo. The results? Metformin reduced the risk for developing type 2 diabetes by 31%. However, benefits were limited primarily to younger patients and to those who were most overweight; the drug was relatively ineffective in older patients and those less overweight. It must be stressed, however, that metformin is not a substitute for diet and exercise. In fact, the DPP showed that lifestyle changes are even more effective than metformin: the combination of moderate exercise plus weight loss (5%–7% of initial weight) reduced the average risk for type 2 diabetes by 58%. Benefits were greatest (71%) for people older than 60 years.

Gestational Diabetes. For decades, insulin was considered the preferred, if not the only, antidiabetic drug for managing diabetes during pregnancy, whether the mother had type 1 or type 2 diabetes. Recent clinical studies have compared metformin with insulin in pregnant women with type 2 diabetes. Multiple outcomes were assessed, including glycemic control in the mother, and blood glucose and Apgar scores in the neonate. The result? Outcomes with metformin were essentially the same as those with insulin, the traditional agent for managing gestational diabetes—suggesting that metformin may become an acceptable alternative for many women. (*Note:* The data obtained with metformin do *not* apply to other classes of oral agents, such as the sulfonylureas and glitazones.)

Polycystic Ovary Syndrome (PCOS). PCOS is a combined endocrine-metabolic disorder characterized by androgen excess and insulin resistance. It affects about 5% to 10% of women of reproductive age. Symptoms include irregular periods, anovulation, infertility, acne, and hirsutism. Although not approved for PCOS, metformin can be very helpful. Metformin treatment increases insulin sensitivity and decreases insulin levels, which, through an indirect mechanism, lowers androgen levels. The net result is improved glucose tolerance, improved ovulation, and increased pregnancy rates.

Side Effects

The most common side effects are decreased appetite, nausea, and diarrhea. These generally subside over time. However, in 3% to 5% of patients, *GI side effects* lead to discontinuation of treatment. Therefore the dose of metformin must be titrated up to the target dose to minimize the severity of GI side effects.

Metformin decreases absorption of vitamin B_{12} and folic acid and can thereby cause deficiencies of both. Deficiency of B_{12}, in turn, can contribute to peripheral neuropathy, a common long-term consequence of diabetes. However, there is no proof (yet) that metformin actually makes diabetic neuropathy worse. Likewise, there is no current recommendation about prescribing vitamin B_{12} for patients who are taking the drug. As discussed in Chapter 65, deficiency of folic acid during pregnancy can impair development of the central nervous system (CNS), resulting in neural tube defects, which manifest as anencephaly or spina bifida. Nonetheless, metformin appears to be a safe drug for use during pregnancy.

In contrast to sulfonylureas (see later), metformin does not cause weight gain. In fact, patients maintain or possibly *lose* weight with metformin therapy. As a result, metformin is considered a "weight-neutral" antidiabetic drug, in contrast to several other antidiabetic drugs that tend to increase weight ("weight-positive" drugs). Appetite suppression and weight loss in response to metformin can occur both in the presence and absence of nausea, indicating that reduced food intake because of metformin-induced nausea is not the only reason for weight loss in those patients who lose weight.

BLACK BOX WARNING: METFORMIN

Severe metabolic acidosis can occur with accumulation of metformin. Highest risk occurs in diabetic patients with significant renal impairment.

Metformin and other biguanides inhibit mitochondrial oxidation of lactic acid and can thereby cause lactic acidosis. This condition is a medical emergency and has a mortality rate of about 50%. Fortunately, lactic acidosis is rare (about 3 cases/100,000 patient-years) when metformin is used at recommended doses in patients with good renal function. However, in patients with renal insufficiency, metformin can rapidly accumulate to toxic levels. Accordingly, the drug must never be used by these people. In addition, metformin must be avoided in patients who are prone to increased lactic acid production. Among these are patients with liver disease, severe infection, or a history of lactic acidosis; patients who consume alcohol to excess; and patients with shock and other conditions that can result in hypoxemia.

All patients taking metformin should be informed about early signs of lactic acidosis—hyperventilation, myalgia, malaise, and unusual somnolence—and instructed to report these to the prescriber. Metformin should be withdrawn until lactic acidosis has been ruled out. If lactic acidosis is diagnosed, hemodialysis can correct the condition and remove accumulated metformin.

Because heart failure (HF) can predispose to lactic acidosis, metformin is contraindicated for people with failing hearts. However, in one study, patients with HF who took the drug were *less* likely to die than those who took a sulfonylurea. These data suggest that use of metformin in HF is much safer than previously believed.

Drug Interactions

Alcohol. Like metformin, alcohol can inhibit breakdown of lactic acid, and can thereby intensify lactic acidosis caused by metformin. To minimize risk, patients should avoid consuming alcohol in excess, whether acutely or long term. Discontinuing alcohol entirely would be even safer.

Cimetidine. Cimetidine [Tagamet], a histamine-2 (H_2) blocker used to reduce gastric acidity, can increase the risk for lactic acidosis. Accordingly, if an H_2 blocker is indicated, another member of the family should be used because cimetidine is the only H_2 blocker that poses this risk.

Iodinated Radiocontrast Media. Intravenous radiocontrast media that contain iodine pose a risk for acute renal failure, which could exacerbate metformin-induced lactic acidosis. To reduce risk, patients should discontinue metformin 1 to 2 days before elective radiography. Metformin can then be resumed 48 hours after the procedure, provided laboratory tests show that renal function is normal.

Preparations, Dosage, and Administration

Metformin is available alone in immediate-release (IR) tablets (500, 850, and 1000 mg) as Glucophage; in extended-release (ER) tablets (500, 750, and 1000 mg) as Glucophage XR, Fortamet, and Glumetza; and in an oral solution (500 mg/5 mL) as Riomet. In addition, the drug is available in several fixed-dose combinations with other drugs for type 2 diabetes mellitus (see later).

With the IR tablets and oral solution, the recommended initial dosage is 500 mg twice daily (taken with the morning and evening meals) or 850 mg once daily, taken with a meal. The usual maintenance dosage is 850 mg twice daily. The maximal dosage is 850 mg 3 times a day (for adults) or 2000 mg/day (for children 10–16 years old).

With the ER tablets, dosing is done once daily with the evening meal because this timing may enhance absorption owing to slower GI transit time at night. For previously untreated patients, the initial dosage is 500 mg a day (or 1000 mg once a day using Fortamet). For patients already taking metformin, the total daily dosage remains the same; it's simply taken all at once. The maximal daily dosage is 2000 mg (or 2500 mg using Fortamet).

Sulfonylureas

The sulfonylureas, introduced in the 1950s, were the first oral antidiabetic drugs available. They work by promoting insulin release and hence are only to be used in type 2 diabetes. The sulfonylureas were a major advance in diabetes therapy: for the first time, some patients could be treated with an oral medication, rather than with daily injections of insulin. The major side effects with these drugs are hypoglycemia and weight gain.

The sulfonylureas fall into two groups: *first-generation agents* and *second-generation agents.* Both generations reduce glucose levels to the same extent. How do the generations differ? The second-generation agents are *much more potent* than the first-generation agents, and hence dosages are much lower (as much as 1000 times lower in some cases). More important, with the second-generation agents, *significant drug-drug interactions are less common,* and the outcomes tend to be milder. Because of these differences, the second-generation agents have nearly completely replaced the first-generation agents in clinical practice. Accordingly, our discussion in this chapter is limited to the second-generation agents.

Three second-generation sulfonylureas are currently available (Table 46.10). All have similar actions and side effects, and they all share the same application: treatment of type 2 diabetes.

Mechanism of Action

Sulfonylureas act primarily by stimulating the release of insulin from pancreatic islets. If the pancreas is incapable of insulin synthesis, sulfonylureas will be ineffective—which is why they don't work in patients with type 1 diabetes. With prolonged use, sulfonylureas may increase target cell sensitivity to insulin.

Sulfonylureas promote insulin release by binding with and thereby blocking adenosine triphosphate (ATP)-sensitive potassium channels in the cell membrane. As a result, the membrane depolarizes, thereby permitting influx of calcium, which in turn causes insulin release. The extent of release is glucose dependent and diminishes when plasma glucose declines.

Therapeutic Use

Sulfonylureas are indicated only for type 2 diabetes. These drugs are of no help to patients with type 1 diabetes. Like all other drugs for type 2 diabetes, the sulfonylureas should be used in conjunction with a lifestyle program inclusive of dietary and physical activity interventions. The sulfonylureas may be used alone or together with other antidiabetic drugs.

Adverse Effects

Hypoglycemia. Sulfonylureas cause a dose-dependent reduction in blood glucose and can thereby cause *hypoglycemia.* Importantly, regardless of what the glucose level

TABLE 46.10 ▪ Sulfonylureas: Time Course and Dosage

Generic Name [Trade Name]	Duration (hr)	Dosage*	Approximate Equivalent Dose (mg/24 hr)†
FIRST-GENERATION AGENTS‡			
Tolbutamide [Orinase]	6–12	*Initial:* 1–2 g/day in 1–3 doses *Maximum:* 2–3 g/day in 1–3 doses	1000–1500
Tolazamide (generic only)	12–24	*Initial:* 100–250 mg/day with breakfast *Maximum:* 0.75–1 g/day in 2 doses	250–375
Chlorpropamide (generic only)	24–60	*Initial:* 250 mg/day with breakfast *Maximum:* 750 mg once a day	250–375
SECOND-GENERATION AGENTS			
Glipizide			
Immediate release [Glucotrol]	10–24	*Initial:* 5 mg/day with breakfast *Maximum:* 40 mg/day in 2 doses	10
Sustained release [Glucotrol XL]	24	*Initial:* 5 mg/day with breakfast *Maximum:* 20 mg/day with breakfast	10
Glyburide			
Nonmicronized [DiaBeta]	16–24	*Initial:* 2.5–5 mg day with breakfast *Maximum:* 20 mg/day in 1 or 2 doses	5
Micronized [Glynase PresTab]	12–24	*Initial:* 1.5–3 mg/day with breakfast *Maximum:* 12 mg/day in 1 or 2 doses	3
Glimepiride [Amaryl]	24	*Initial:* 1–2 mg/day with breakfast *Maximum:* 8 mg/day with breakfast	2

*Older adults should use a smaller dose than those noted here.
†These values reflect differences in potency and can be used to estimate what dose to use when switching from one sulfonylurea to another.
‡The first-generation agents are used only rarely.

is—high, normal, or low—sulfonylureas will make it go lower. If the level is high, reducing it will be therapeutic. However, if the level is normal, reducing it will cause mild hypoglycemia. And if the level is already low, reducing it can cause severe hypoglycemia.

Although sulfonylurea-induced hypoglycemia is usually mild, severe and even fatal cases have occurred. Hypoglycemia is sometimes persistent, requiring infusion of dextrose for several days. Hypoglycemic reactions are more likely in patients with kidney or liver dysfunction because sulfonylureas are eliminated by hepatic metabolism and renal excretion and hence may accumulate to dangerous levels when liver or kidney function is impaired. If signs of hypoglycemia develop (fatigue, excessive hunger, profuse sweating, palpitations), the patient should treat the hypoglycemia and notify the prescriber.

Cardiovascular Toxicity. There has been controversy regarding the possibility of adverse cardiovascular reactions to oral antidiabetic drugs. In 1970 the large multicenter University Group Diabetes Program (UGDP) published results indicating that tolbutamide (the first first-generation sulfonylurea available) was linked to an increased risk for mortality from sudden cardiac death. In the UGDP study, cardiac mortality was 2.5 times greater among subjects treated with a combination of diet therapy and tolbutamide than among control subjects who received diet therapy alone. The UGDP study has been criticized on several grounds, including design, patient selection, dosing, and compliance. Subsequent clinical trials, including the UKPDS, failed to confirm the conclusions of the UGDP report. The ADA, which initially endorsed the UGDP study, has since withdrawn its support. Nonetheless, the risk for sudden cardiac death remains a concern—albeit small—and hence appropriate caution should be exercised.

Use in Pregnancy and Lactation. *Sulfonylureas should be avoided during pregnancy.* Although adequate studies in humans are lacking, sulfonylureas are teratogenic in animals. Furthermore, because sulfonylurea therapy during pregnancy often fails to provide good glycemic control, and because even mild hyperglycemia may be hazardous to the fetus, insulin is generally preferred for managing the diabetic pregnancy.

It is especially important to avoid sulfonylureas near term. Newborns exposed to these agents at the time of delivery have experienced severe hypoglycemia lasting as long as 4 to 10 days. Hence, if a sulfonylurea has been taken during pregnancy, it should be discontinued at least 48 hours before the anticipated time of delivery.

Sulfonylureas should not be taken by women who are nursing. These drugs are excreted into breast milk, posing a risk for hypoglycemia to the infant. If a woman wishes to breastfeed, she should substitute insulin for the sulfonylurea.

Drug Interactions

Alcohol. When alcohol is combined with a sulfonylurea (especially a first-generation agent), a disulfiram-like reaction may occur. This syndrome includes flushing, palpitations, and nausea. Disulfiram reactions are discussed in Chapter 31. Also, alcohol can potentiate the hypoglycemic effects of sulfonylureas. Accordingly, patients using the drug must be warned about the risks of alcohol consumption in combination with a sulfonylurea.

Drugs that Can Intensify Hypoglycemia

A variety of drugs, acting by diverse mechanisms, can intensify hypoglycemic responses to most sulfonylureas. Included are nonsteroidal antiinflammatory drugs, sulfonamide antibiotics, alcohol (used acutely in large amounts), and cimetidine. Caution must be exercised when a sulfonylurea is used in combination with these drugs.

Beta-Adrenergic Blocking Agents. Beta blockers can diminish the benefits of sulfonylureas by suppressing insulin release. (Recall that activation of beta receptors is one way to promote insulin release.) In addition, because beta blockers can mask sympathetic responses (primarily tachycardia) to declining blood glucose, use of beta blockers can delay awareness of sulfonylurea-induced hypoglycemia.

Preparations, Dosage, and Administration

This information is shown in Table 46.10.

Meglitinides (Glinides)

Meglitinides—also known as *glinides*—are antidiabetic agents that have the same mechanism as the sulfonylureas: stimulation of pancreatic insulin release. The main difference between the glinides and the sulfonylureas is their pharmacokinetic profile—the glinides are shorter acting and are taken with each meal. Only two glinides are available: repaglinide and nateglinide.

Repaglinide

Actions and Uses. Like the sulfonylureas, repaglinide [Prandin, GlucoNorm ♣] blocks ATP-sensitive potassium channels on pancreatic beta cells and thereby facilitates calcium influx, which leads to increased insulin release. In clinical trials, repaglinide was about as effective as glyburide and glipizide (second-generation sulfonylureas). The drug is approved for type 2 diabetes only. Because repaglinide has the same mechanism as the sulfonylureas, patients who do not respond to sulfonylureas will not respond to this agent either. Repaglinide is approved for monotherapy or combined therapy with metformin or a glitazone.

Pharmacokinetics. Repaglinide undergoes rapid absorption followed by rapid elimination. Blood levels peak within 1 hour of oral dosing and return to baseline about 4 hours later. Elimination results from hepatic metabolism followed by biliary excretion. The drug's half-life is only 1 hour. Blood levels of insulin rise and fall in parallel with levels of repaglinide—and because levels of repaglinide rise and fall quickly, so do blood levels of insulin.

Adverse Effects. Repaglinide is generally well tolerated. The main significant adverse effect is *hypoglycemia.* In patients with liver dysfunction, metabolism of repaglinide may be slowed, and hence the risk for hypoglycemia may be increased. Because of possible hypoglycemia, it is imperative that patients eat no later than 30 minutes after taking the drug.

Drug Interactions. Gemfibrozil [Lopid], a drug used to lower triglyceride levels, can inhibit the metabolism of repaglinide, thereby causing its level to rise. Hypoglycemia can result. If possible, the combination should be avoided. Fenofibrate can be used instead of gemfibrozil.

Preparations, Dosage, and Administration. Repaglinide [Prandin, GlucoNorm ♣] is available in 0.5-, 1-, and 2-mg tablets. Administration must always be associated with a meal. For patients who have not used another oral antidiabetic drug, the initial dosage is 0.5 mg taken 0 to 30 minutes before each meal. Patients who have used another oral antidiabetic drug may take 1 or 2 mg before each meal. The maximal daily dose is 16 mg (4 mg with each meal for up to four meals).

Nateglinide

Basic Pharmacology and Therapeutic Use. The pharmacology of nateglinide [Starlix] is nearly identical to that of repaglinide. Both drugs have the same indication: treatment of type 2 diabetes, either as monotherapy or combined with metformin or a glitazone. They also have the same mechanism of action (promotion of insulin release) and major adverse effect (hypoglycemia), and perhaps the same major drug interaction (elevation of their blood level by gemfibrozil). The two drugs differ primarily with respect to time course. Specifically, nateglinide has a slightly faster onset (30 minutes vs. 1 hour) and a significantly shorter duration (2 hours vs. 4 hours). Because the glinides and sulfonylureas have the same mechanism of action, nateglinide, like repaglinide, will not be effective in patients who have not responded to a sulfonylurea. Nateglinide undergoes extensive metabolism by cytochrome P450 enzymes, followed by rapid and complete excretion, primarily in the urine.

Preparations, Dosage, and Administration. Nateglinide [Starlix] is available in 60- and 120-mg tablets. The initial dosage is 120 mg 3 times a day taken 0 to 30 minutes before a meal. For patients with A_{1c} concentrations close to the target value, the initial dosage is lower: 60 mg 3 times a day taken 0 to 30 minutes before a meal. Please note that dosing must always be associated with a meal. Otherwise, nateglinide-induced insulin release could cause hypoglycemia.

Thiazolidinediones (Glitazones)

The thiazolidinediones, also known as *glitazones* or simply *TZDs,* reduce glucose levels primarily by decreasing insulin resistance. These drugs are not related chemically or functionally to sulfonylureas or biguanides. Their only indication is type 2 diabetes, mainly as an add-on to metformin.

The glitazones have a troubled past and an uncertain future. Rosiglitazone [Avandia] and pioglitazone [Actos] came under scrutiny for their association with myocardial infarction and sudden cardiac death and hence are currently available only under a restricted access program; however, the U.S. Food and Drug Administration (FDA) is considering lifting the restrictions. That leaves pioglitazone as the last TZD on the market. Accordingly, it will be the focus of our discussion about these drugs.

Pioglitazone

Actions and Use. Pioglitazone [Actos] reduces insulin resistance and may also decrease glucose production. The underlying mechanism is activation of a specific receptor type in the cell nucleus, known as the *peroxisome proliferator–activated receptor gamma* (PPAR gamma). By activating PPAR gamma, pioglitazone turns on insulin-responsive genes that help regulate carbohydrate and lipid metabolism. As a result, cellular responses to insulin are increased, thereby promoting (mainly) increased glucose uptake by skeletal muscle and adipose cells and (partly) decreased glucose production by the liver. Because pioglitazone enhances responses to insulin, insulin must be present for the drug to work.

Pioglitazone is approved as an adjunct to diet and exercise to improve glycemic control in adults with type 2 diabetes. The drug can be used as monotherapy but is usually combined with metformin, a sulfonylurea, and/or supplemental insulin. Because insulin is required for pioglitazone to work, the drug is not effective in patients with type 1 diabetes.

Pharmacokinetics. Pioglitazone is well absorbed from the GI tract. Blood levels peak about 2 hours after dosing. Food slows absorption (blood levels peak 3–4 hours after dosing) but does not reduce the extent of absorption. Pioglitazone undergoes conversion to active and inactive metabolites, mainly by CYP2C8 (the 2C8 isoenzyme of cytochrome P450). Metabolites and parent drug are excreted in the feces (mainly) and urine. The half-lives of pioglitazone and its metabolites are 3 to 7 hours and 16 to 24 hours, respectively.

Adverse Effects. Pioglitazone is generally well tolerated. The most common reactions are upper respiratory tract infection, headache, sinusitis, and myalgia.

Although HF can precipitate, for most patients, fluid retention is not clinically significant. However, for patients with HF, especially severe or uncompensated HF, increased fluid

BLACK BOX WARNING: PIOGLITAZONE

Pioglitazone is associated with *heart failure* secondary to renal *retention of fluid.* If HF is diagnosed, pioglitazone should be discontinued or used in reduced dosage.

retention can make HF worse. In these individuals, fluid retention is exacerbated when pioglitazone is used in combination with insulin therapy. Accordingly, pioglitazone should be used with caution in patients with *mild* HF and should be avoided by those with *severe* failure. Patients should be informed about signs of HF (dyspnea, edema, fatigue, rapid weight gain) and instructed to consult the prescriber immediately if these develop. Unlike rosiglitazone, pioglitazone has not been associated with myocardial infarction.

Although TZDs have a low risk for *hypoglycemia* when used as monotherapy, the risk is increased when pioglitazone is combined with insulin or with drugs that inhibit pioglitazone metabolism. Use these combinations with caution.

Pioglitazone can cause *ovulation* in anovulatory premenopausal women, thereby posing a risk for unintended pregnancy. This effect has not been studied in clinical trials, and hence the incidence is unknown. Women should be informed about the potential for ovulation and educated about contraceptive options.

Postmarketing data indicate an increased risk for *bladder cancer,* associated mainly with long-term, high-dose pioglitazone therapy. Package labeling warns against using pioglitazone in patients with active bladder cancer or with a history of bladder cancer. Patients should be informed about signs of bladder cancer (e.g., blood in the urine, worsening urinary urgency, painful urination) and instructed to contact their prescriber if these develop.

Pioglitazone appears to increase the risk for *fractures* in women, but not in men. Most fractures have occurred in the foot, hand, or upper arm, not the spine. Risk appears greater with long-term, high-dose therapy. Fracture risk can be reduced through measures to maintain bone health. Among these are exercise, assuring adequate intake of calcium and vitamin D, and, if indicated, use of drugs for osteoporosis (see Chapter 59).

Although pioglitazone has been associated with rare cases of hepatic failure, a causal relationship has not been established. Nonetheless, serum alanine aminotransferase (ALT), a marker of liver function, should be measured at baseline and periodically thereafter (e.g., every 3–6 months). If ALT levels rise to more than 3 times the upper limit of normal, or if jaundice develops, pioglitazone should be withdrawn. Patients should be informed about symptoms of liver injury (nausea, vomiting, abdominal pain, fatigue, anorexia, dark urine, jaundice) and instructed to notify the prescriber if these develop.

Pioglitazone has mixed effects on *plasma lipids.* One effect—elevation of LDL cholesterol—increases cardiovascular risk. Two other effects—elevation of HDL cholesterol and reduction of triglycerides—reduce cardiovascular risk. The net effect appears to be either (1) a reduction in cardiovascular risk or, at worst, (2) no increase in cardiovascular risk. The HF risk mentioned previously must not be overlooked, however.

Drug Interactions. Like pioglitazone, *insulin* promotes fluid retention, and hence the combination poses an increased risk for HF. Accordingly, using pioglitazone and insulin together should be done with caution.

Drugs that induce or inhibit CYP2C8 can alter pioglitazone levels and can thereby alter the glycemic response. Strong inhibitors of CYP2C8—such as atorvastatin (our most widely used cholesterol-lowering drug) and ketoconazole (an antifungal drug)—can increase pioglitazone levels and prolong its half-life, necessitating a reduction in pioglitazone dosage. Conversely, strong inducers of CYP2C8—such as rifampin (a drug for tuberculosis) and cimetidine (a gastric acid suppressant)—can reduce pioglitazone levels and shorten its half-life, necessitating an increase in pioglitazone dosage.

Preparations, Dosage, and Administration. Pioglitazone [Actos] is available in 15-, 30-, and 45-mg tablets. The initial dosage for monotherapy is 15 or 30 mg once a day, taken with or without food. The maximal dosage is 45 mg once a day for patients not using insulin, but only 30 mg once a day for patients who are using insulin.

Rosiglitazone

Rosiglitazone [Avandia], like pioglitazone, is indicated for the treatment of type 2 diabetes. It is available in 2-, 4-, and 8-mg tablets. The usual dose is 4 to 8 mg per day. Rosiglitazone should be used with caution in patients with hepatic impairment. The provider should monitor liver function tests periodically.

Alpha-Glucosidase Inhibitors

The alpha-glucosidase inhibitors—acarbose and miglitol—act in the intestine to delay absorption of carbohydrates. These drugs are indicated for type 2 diabetes.

Acarbose

Mechanism of Action. Acarbose [Precose, Glucobay ♣] delays absorption of dietary carbohydrates and thereby reduces the rise in blood glucose after a meal. To be absorbed, oligosaccharides and complex carbohydrates must be broken down to monosaccharides by alpha-glucosidase, an enzyme located on the brush border of cells that line the intestine. Acarbose inhibits this enzyme and thereby slows digestion of carbohydrates, which reduces the postprandial rise in blood glucose.

Therapeutic Use. Acarbose is indicated for patients with type 2 diabetes in conjunction with a program of diet modification and exercise. The drug may be used alone or in combination with insulin, metformin, or a sulfonylurea. In clinical trials, 24 weeks of therapy with acarbose alone reduced mean peak postprandial glucose levels by 57 mg/dL, compared with 71 mg/dL for tolbutamide (a sulfonylurea) alone and 85 mg/dL for acarbose plus tolbutamide. In addition to lowering glucose levels after meals, acarbose lowers A_{1c} levels, indicating an overall improvement in glycemic control.

Pharmacokinetics. Acarbose is administered by mouth, and only 2% is absorbed as active drug. As a result, systemic effects are minimal. Because acarbose acts locally in the intestine, lack of absorption is considered beneficial. In the gut, acarbose is converted to inactive products by bacteria and digestive enzymes.

Adverse Effects and Interactions. Acarbose frequently causes *flatulence, cramps, abdominal distention, borborygmus* (rumbling bowel sounds), and *diarrhea.* These responses result from bacterial fermentation of unabsorbed carbohydrates in the colon. Because of the common occurrence of these GI-related side effects, this class of medication is not often used in the United States. In addition to its GI effects, acarbose can decrease absorption of iron, thereby posing a risk for *anemia.*

Hypoglycemia does not occur with acarbose alone but may develop when acarbose is combined with *insulin* or a *sulfonylurea.* When hypoglycemia develops, sucrose cannot be used for oral therapy because acarbose will impede its hydrolysis and thereby delay absorption. Accordingly, in patients taking acarbose, oral therapy of hypoglycemia must be accomplished with glucose itself.

Long-term, high-dose therapy may cause *liver dysfunction.* Asymptomatic elevation of plasma transaminases (which come from damaged liver cells) occurs in about 15% of patients. However, overt jaundice is rare. Liver function tests should be monitored every 3 months for the first year, and periodically thereafter. Liver dysfunction reverses when acarbose is discontinued.

Preparations, Dosage, and Administration. Acarbose [Precose, Glucobay ♣] is available in tablets (25, 50, and 100 mg) to be taken with the first bite of main meals. The recommended initial dosage is 25 mg 3 times a day. Depending on tolerability and postprandial blood glucose levels, the dosage may be increased at 4- to 8-week intervals. The maximal dosage is 50 mg 3 times a day (for patients under 60 kg) and 100 mg 3 times a day (for patients weighing more than 60 kg).

Miglitol

Miglitol [Glyset] is the second alpha-glucosidase inhibitor approved in the United States. Like acarbose, miglitol delays conversion of oligosaccharides and complex carbohydrates to glucose and other monosaccharides and thereby reduces the postprandial rise in blood glucose. In clinical trials, the drug was especially effective among Latinos and African Americans. Hypoglycemia does not occur with miglitol monotherapy but may occur if the drug is combined with insulin or a sulfonylurea. Like acarbose, miglitol causes flatulence, abdominal discomfort, and other GI effects. In contrast to acarbose, miglitol has not been associated with liver dysfunction. As with acarbose therapy, oral sucrose cannot be used to treat hypoglycemia. Rather, oral glucose must be given. Miglitol is available in 25-, 50-, and 100-mg tablets. The initial dosage is 25 mg 3 times daily before meals. The maintenance dosage is 50 or 100 mg 3 times a day.

Dipeptidyl Peptidase-4 Inhibitors (Gliptins)

DPP-4 inhibitors promote glycemic control by enhancing the actions of incretin hormones. Reduction in A_{1c} are modest. Hypoglycemia is uncommon when these drugs are used alone. Pancreatitis and severe hypersensitivity reactions occur rarely.

The ADA considers the DPP-4 inhibitors to be an optional second-line therapy as an add-on to metformin in the treatment of type 2 diabetes. When added to the regimen, the resulting decrease in A_{1c} is about 0.5%. However, for some patients, even this small improvement can be clinically significant.

Sitagliptin

Mechanism of Action. Sitagliptin [Januvia] enhances the actions of *incretin hormones,* endogenous compounds that (1) stimulate glucose-dependent release of insulin and (2) suppress postprandial release of glucagon (a hormone that decreases glucose production in the liver). Both actions help keep blood glucose from climbing too high. How does sitagliptin boost incretin actions? It inhibits DPP-4, an enzyme that inactivates the incretin hormones. As discussed later, another class of drugs—GLP-1 receptor agonists—also boost incretin actions, but by a different mechanism: rather than preventing incretin breakdown, they mimic incretin actions.

Therapeutic Use. Sitagliptin is indicated for type 2 diabetes, either as monotherapy or combined with another antidiabetic drug (e.g., metformin, sulfonylurea, or a glitazone). Like all the other agents for managing diabetes, sitagliptin should be used as an adjunct to diet and exercise.

Pharmacokinetics. Sitagliptin undergoes rapid and nearly complete absorption, both in the presence and absence of food. Blood levels peak about 1 to 4 hours after dosing. Most of the drug is excreted unchanged in the urine. The elimination half-life is about 12 hours.

Adverse Effects and Interactions. Sitagliptin is generally well tolerated. In clinical trials, the most common side effects were upper respiratory tract infection, headache, and inflammation of the nasal passages and throat—at rates similar to those seen with placebo. The incidence of hypoglycemia was about 1.2%, compared with 0.9% with placebo—again a nonsignificant difference.

Rarely, patients have developed *pancreatitis,* including fatal hemorrhagic or necrotizing pancreatitis according to postmarketing reports. Patients should be informed about signs and symptoms of pancreatitis (e.g., severe and persistent abdominal pain, with or without vomiting) and instructed to stop sitagliptin immediately. If pancreatitis is confirmed, sitagliptin should not be resumed. We don't know if patients with a history of pancreatitis are at increased risk, although the FDA recommends cautious use of these agents in such patients.

There have been postmarketing reports of serious *hypersensitivity reactions,* including anaphylaxis, angioedema, and Stevens-Johnson syndrome. However, a causal relationship has not been established. Nonetheless, if a hypersensitivity reaction is suspected, sitagliptin should be discontinued.

Sitagliptin has no known clinically relevant drug interactions and no contraindications, including pregnancy.

Preparations, Dosage, and Administration. Sitagliptin [Januvia] is supplied in film-coated tablets (25, 50, and 100 mg). The usual dosage is 100 mg once daily, taken with or without food. Because sitagliptin is eliminated primarily by renal excretion, dosages should be reduced in patients with renal impairment, as indicated by reduced creatinine clearance. Dosage should be reduced to 50 mg once daily (in moderate renal disease) and 25 mg once daily (in severe renal disease).

Saxagliptin

Actions and Therapeutic Use. Like sitagliptin, saxagliptin [Onglyza] is a DPP-4 inhibitor indicated as an adjunct to diet and exercise to improve glycemic control in adults with type 2 diabetes. Saxagliptin may be used as monotherapy or combined with other antidiabetic agents.

Pharmacokinetics. Saxagliptin is well absorbed, both in the presence and absence of food. Plasma levels peak about 2 hours after dosing. Saxagliptin undergoes conversion to an active metabolite by CYP3A4/5 (the 3A4/5 isoenzyme of cytochrome P450). Parent drug and metabolite are excreted in the urine (75%) and feces (22%). To avoid toxicity, dosage must be reduced in patients taking strong CYP3A4/5 inhibitors (e.g., clarithromycin, ketoconazole, nefazodone, nelfinavir, ritonavir) and in those with significant renal impairment.

Adverse Effects. In clinical trials, the most common adverse effects were upper respiratory infection, urinary tract infection, and headache. Saxagliptin can intensify hypoglycemia caused by a sulfonylurea but causes little or no hypoglycemia when used alone. Like sitagliptin, saxagliptin has been associated with rare cases of pancreatitis and severe hypersensitivity reactions. If symptoms of either develop, saxagliptin should be withdrawn.

Preparations, Dosage, and Administration. Saxagliptin [Onglyza] is supplied in 2.5- and 5-mg tablets for dosing once daily without regard to meals. The usual daily dosage is 5 mg. In patients with mild-to-moderate renal impairment, and in those taking a strong inhibitor of CYP3A4/5, dosage should be reduced to 2.5 mg/day.

Linagliptin

Actions and Therapeutic Use. Linagliptin [Tradjenta] is indicated as an adjunct to diet and exercise to improve glycemic control in adults with type 2 diabetes. As with other gliptins, benefits, which are modest, derive from preserving incretins through inhibition of DPP-4.

Pharmacokinetics. About 30% of each dose is absorbed, both in the presence and absence of food. Plasma levels peak 1.5 hours after dosing. Linagliptin undergoes minimal metabolism. Most of the drug (90%) is excreted unchanged—80% in the feces and 5% in the urine. The effective half-life is 12 hours.

Adverse Effects. Linagliptin is generally well tolerated. The drug has caused hypoglycemia when combined with metformin plus a sulfonylurea, but not when used alone or when combined with just metformin or pioglitazone. Like sitagliptin and saxagliptin, linagliptin has been associated with rare cases of pancreatitis and hypersensitivity reactions. If either of these develop, linagliptin should be withdrawn.

Drug Interactions. Linagliptin is a substrate for P-glycoprotein, a transporter that promotes excretion of linagliptin and other drugs. In theory, drugs that induce P-glycoprotein could reduce levels of linagliptin. Accordingly, the manufacturer recommends that linagliptin not be used with rifampin and other P-glycoprotein inducers.

Preparations, Dosage, and Administration. Linagliptin [Tradjenta] is supplied as 5-mg tablets. The dosage is 5 mg once a day, taken without regard to meals. Unlike dosing with saxagliptin or sitagliptin, dosage needn't be reduced in patients with renal impairment.

Alogliptin

Actions and Therapeutic Use. Alogliptin [Nesina] is indicated as an adjunct to diet and exercise to improve glycemic control in adults with type 2 diabetes. As with other DPP-4 inhibitors, alogliptin improves glycemic control by allowing natural incretin hormones to carry out their glucoregulatory functions for a longer period of time.

Pharmacokinetics. The absolute bioavailability of alogliptin is approximately 100% when administered orally. Alogliptin does not undergo extensive metabolism, with the majority of an oral dose excreted unchanged in the urine; accordingly, this drug is dose-adjusted when used in people with renal impairment, as outlined later. Alogliptin has a terminal half-life of about 20 hours and thus can be administered once daily.

Adverse Effects. As with other DPP-4 inhibitors, alogliptin is generally well tolerated. The most common side effects reported in clinical trials included upper respiratory tract infection and nasopharyngitis. Again, like other agents in this class, hypersensitivity reactions and postmarketing reports of pancreatitis have been noted.

Drug Interactions. Alogliptin is primarily excreted renally, yet no significant drug-drug interactions have been noted with other drugs excreted through the kidneys.

Preparations, Dosage, and Administration. Alogliptin [Nesina] is supplied as 6.25-, 12.5-, and 25-mg tablets. The dosage is 25 mg once daily. Alogliptin is dose-adjusted based on kidney function. Accordingly, the recommended dose is 12.5 mg daily for people with moderate renal impairment, and is 6.25 mg daily for those with significant renal impairment.

Sodium-Glucose Cotransporter 2 Inhibitors

The kidney plays a major role in glucose homeostasis owing to its role in the filtration and reabsorption of glucose in the renal tubules. The transport of glucose from the tubule into the tubular epithelial cells is accomplished by SGLTs. SGLT-2 is a high-capacity, low-affinity transporter expressed chiefly in the kidney that accounts for approximately 90% of glucose reabsorption in the kidney. SGLT-2 inhibitors have been shown to block the reabsorption of filtered glucose, leading to glucosuria. This mechanism of action has proved clinically useful in patients with type 2 diabetes in terms of improving glycemic control. In addition, the glucosuria associated with SGLT-2 inhibition is associated with caloric loss, thus providing a potential benefit of weight loss. Although currently approved agents hold an indication for the management of type 2 diabetes only, these agents are being studied and used off-label in people with type 1 diabetes.

Canagliflozin

Actions and Therapeutic Use. Canagliflozin [Invokana] was the first SGLT-2 inhibitor approved in the United States. By inhibiting SGLT-2 in the kidney, canagliflozin reduces the reabsorption of glucose, thereby increasing urinary glucose excretion. Clinical studies of canagliflozin have shown benefits in terms of improved glycemic control and weight loss.

Pharmacokinetics. The half-life of canagliflozin is approximately 12 hours when taken orally, and thus it can be administered once daily. Peak plasma concentrations are reached within 1 to 2 hours after a given dose.

Adverse Effects. The most common side effects noted with canagliflozin in clinical trials were female genital fungal infections, urinary tract infections, and increased urination. Because SGLT-2 inhibitors increase the amount of sugar present in the urine, the increased risk for such infections is not much of a surprise. In addition, particularly in older adults, use of canagliflozin can lead to postural hypotension and dizziness, particularly if used in combination with diuretics.

Drug Interactions. Coadministration of canagliflozin with UDP-glucuronosyltransferase inducers—such as rifampin, phenytoin, or phenobarbital—can decrease canagliflozin efficacy. Accordingly, if used with such an agent, the 300-mg canagliflozin dose should be considered. Because canagliflozin causes a diuretic effect, the risk for dehydration and hypotension may be increased when used in combination with thiazide and loop diuretics.

Preparations, Dosage, and Administration. Canagliflozin [Invokana] is available as 100- and 300-mg tablets. Canagliflozin is recommended at a starting dose of 100 mg daily taken before the first meal of the day. The dose can be increased to 300 mg once daily, requiring additional glycemic control and an estimated glomerular filtration rate (GFR) of 60 mL/min/1.73 m^2 or greater. Because SGLT-2 inhibitors don't work as well in people with compromised kidney function, canagliflozin is not recommended for people with an estimated GFR below 45 mL/min/1.73 m^2.

Dapagliflozin

Actions and Therapeutic Use. Dapagliflozin [Farxiga] was the second SGLT-2 inhibitor approved in the United States (in 2014). By inhibiting SGLT-2, dapagliflozin suppresses glucose reuptake from tubular urine and thereby increases urinary glucose excretion. As a result, blood levels of glucose decline and weight loss can be seen.

Pharmacokinetics. The half-life of dapagliflozin after oral administration is approximately 13 hours, and thus it can be taken once daily.

Adverse Effects. The most common side effects noted with dapagliflozin in clinical studies were vulvovaginitis and other genital infections, back pain, polyuria, and an increased hematocrit. Orthostasis (particularly if used with diuretics) is possible.

Drug Interactions. Because dapagliflozin induces a diuretic effect in the kidney, the risk for dehydration and hypotension may be increased when used in combination with thiazide and loop diuretics. When used with other antidiabetic agents, patients should also monitor carefully to avoid the possibility of hypoglycemia.

Preparations, Dosage, and Administration. Dapagliflozin [Farxiga] is available as 5- and 10-mg tablets. Dapagliflozin is dosed initially as 5 mg once daily in the morning with or without food. The dose can be subsequently increased to 10 mg once daily, if needed, to achieve desired glycemic control. Because SGLT-2 inhibitors do not work as well in people with diminished kidney function, dapagliflozin is not recommended for use in people with an estimated GFR less than 60 mL/min/1.73 m^2.

Empagliflozin

Actions and Therapeutic Use. Empagliflozin [Jardiance] is approved as an adjunct to diet and exercise in the treatment of type 2 diabetes. Like dapagliflozin, empagliflozin inhibits SGLT-2, therefore suppressing glucose reuptake from tubular urine.

Pharmacokinetics. The half-life of empagliflozin after oral administration is approximately 13 hours, and thus it can be taken once daily.

Adverse Effects. The most common side effects noted with empagliflozin in clinical studies were vulvovaginitis and other genital infections, back pain, polyuria, and an increased hematocrit. Orthostasis (particularly if used with diuretics) is possible.

Drug Interactions. Because empagliflozin induces a diuretic effect in the kidney, the risk for dehydration and hypotension may be increased when used in combination with thiazide and loop diuretics. When used with other antidiabetic agents, patients should also monitor carefully to avoid the possibility of hypoglycemia.

Preparations, Dosage, and Administration. Empagliflozin [Jardiance] is available as 10- and 25-mg tablets. Empagliflozin is dosed initially as 10 mg once daily in the morning with or without food. The dose can be subsequently increased to 25 mg once daily, if needed, to achieve desired glycemic control. Because SGLT-2 inhibitors do not work as well in people with diminished kidney function, dapagliflozin is not recommended for use in people with an estimated GFR less than 45 mL/min/1.73 m^2.

Colesevelam

Colesevelam [Welchol] is best known as a bile-acid sequestrant used to lower plasma cholesterol. However, the drug can also help lower blood glucose.

Accordingly, in 2008, the FDA approved colesevelam to treat type 2 diabetes. Because many patients with diabetes also have high cholesterol, a drug with the potential to treat both disorders is welcome. The pharmacology of colesevelam is discussed in Chapter 42.

Bromocriptine

Bromocriptine, marketed as Cycloset, is now approved as an adjunct to diet and exercise to treat type 2 diabetes. The same drug, marketed as Parlodel, has been available for years to treat Parkinson disease (see Chapter 17) and hyperprolactinemia. In patients with diabetes, bromocriptine may be used as monotherapy or combined with metformin, a sulfonylurea, or other oral antidiabetic drugs. Combined use with insulin has not been studied. Unfortunately, benefits in diabetes are modest: the typical reduction in A_{1c} is only 0.5%.

How does bromocriptine improve glycemic control? The mechanism is unclear. We do know that bromocriptine is a dopamine agonist that can activate dopamine receptors in the brain. By activating these receptors in the hypothalamus, the drug may reverse an abnormal hypothalamic drive that raises plasma levels of glucose, triglycerides, and free fatty acids in insulin-resistant patients.

We also know that, by activating these receptors, bromocriptine can reset circadian rhythms in people with type 2 diabetes. This action, in turn, may reverse some of the metabolic changes associated with insulin resistance.

Principal adverse effects are nausea, drowsiness, and orthostatic hypotension, which can cause dizziness and fainting. Bromocriptine can also exacerbate psychoses. Of note, the drug appears devoid of cardiovascular toxicity.

For treatment of diabetes, bromocriptine [Cycloset] is available in 0.8-mg tablets, which should be taken with food to decrease GI side effects. Dosing is done once daily, within 2 hours of waking in the morning. The daily dosage is 0.8 mg initially, and then increased by 0.8 mg each week until the maximal dose is reached (4.8 mg) or until side effects become intolerable. Although approved, this medication is used very rarely for the treatment of type 2 diabetes.

Oral Combination Products

As noted previously, many patients with type 2 diabetes must take several medications with complementary mechanisms of action to meet glycemic goals. Accordingly, to help minimize the number of pills that patients must take on a daily basis, several oral combination products are commercially available. Because metformin is the recommended first-line agent in combination with lifestyle interventions, most combination products contain metformin with a second antidiabetic agent. Table 46.11 shows combination products available in the United States. Keep in mind, however, that combination products have drawbacks. First, they are often more expensive than taking the components separately. And second, they limit dosing flexibility.

Noninsulin Injectable Agents

In addition to insulin, we now have two additional classes of injectable agents available for the treatment of diabetes. In the amylin mimetic class, pramlintide—the only amylin mimetic currently on the market—is indicated for type 1 *and* type 2 diabetes. The other class of drugs—GLP-1 receptor agonists (or incretin mimetics)—is indicated for type 2 diabetes only, yet these drugs are increasingly being used off-label for people with type 1 diabetes. Because all of these agents are injectable, they are often mistaken for insulin products, but they work very differently than insulin.

TABLE 46.11 ▪ Combination Oral Agents for the Treatment of Type 2 Diabetes

Trade Name	Generic Name
Metaglip	Glipizide-metformin
Glucovance	Glyburide-metformin
Jentadueto	Linagliptin-metformin
Kombiglyze XR	Saxagliptin-metformin
Janumet	Sitagliptin-metformin
Kazano	Alogliptin-metformin
Oseni	Alogliptin-pioglitazone
Duetact	Pioglitazone-glimepiride
ActoPlus Met, ActoPlus Met XR	Pioglitazone-metformin
PrandiMet	Repaglinide-metformin

Glucagon-like Peptide-1 Receptor Agonists

GLP-1 receptor agonists, often referred to as *incretin mimetics,* work by augmenting the effects of the incretin hormone GLP-1. Under physiologic conditions, GLP-1 and other incretins are released from cells of the GI tract after a meal. Incretin mimetics activate receptors for GLP-1 and thereby cause the same effects as endogenous incretins. That is, they slow gastric emptying, stimulate glucose-dependent release of insulin, inhibit postprandial release of glucagon, and suppress appetite. Owing to augmentation of these effects, incretin mimetics are effective in improving glucose control and can induce weight loss. You will recall that DPP-4 inhibitors "boost" the effects of incretin hormones by slowing their degradation by the enzyme DPP-4. GLP-1 receptor agonists, in contrast, are structurally related to the native GLP-1 hormone but are resistant to metabolism by DPP-4. There are currently six GLP-1 receptor agonist products approved in the United States, with multiple other agents currently in development.

Exenatide

Exenatide [Byetta] was the first *incretin mimetic.* The drug is used to improve glucose control in patients with type 2 diabetes. A longer acting formulation of exenatide known as Exenatide Once Weekly [Bydureon] is also currently available and is dosed once weekly (compared with twice daily with Byetta). Nausea is common, and hypoglycemia can occur, particularly if used in combination with a sulfonylurea.

Description and Actions. Exenatide is a synthetic analog of GLP-1, a peptide hormone in the *incretin* family. Exenatide activates receptors for GLP-1 and thereby causes the same effects as endogenous incretins. That is, it slows gastric emptying, stimulates glucose-dependent release of insulin, inhibits postprandial release of glucagon, and suppresses appetite.

Therapeutic Use. Exenatide is indicated as adjunctive therapy to improve glycemic control in patients with type 2 diabetes. In clinical trials, subQ injection of exenatide [Byetta] 5 or 10 mcg twice daily before the two largest meals of the day produced a modest decrease in fasting blood glucose and a large decrease in postprandial blood glucose. Patients did not gain any weight, and many lost weight. In contrast, exenatide ER for injectable suspension [Bydureon] 2 mg given by subQ injection once weekly has a greater effect on fasting glucose as opposed to postprandial blood glucose. These differences are related to the varying pharmacokinetic profiles of these two products.

Pharmacokinetics. For exenatide [Byetta], plasma levels peak 2.1 hours after subQ injection and decline with a half-life of 2.4 hours. Exenatide ER suspension [Bydureon], in contrast, is released slowly from microspheres over approximately 10 weeks, with a peak level of drug reached at about 2 weeks after administration. Exenatide is excreted unchanged in the urine. In patients with mild to moderate renal impairment, clearance is reduced only slightly, and hence no dosage reduction is needed. By contrast, in patients with end-stage renal disease, clearance is reduced significantly, and hence the drug should not be used.

Adverse Effects. Dose-related *hypoglycemia* is common when exenatide is combined with a sulfonylurea (but not when combined with metformin). To minimize hypoglycemia, sulfonylurea dosage may need a reduction. *Gastrointestinal effects*—nausea, vomiting, and diarrhea—are common with exenatide [Byetta]. Exenatide ER suspension [Bydureon] is better tolerated in terms of nausea and vomiting but can result in injection-site irritation and pruritus. In some patients, *antiexenatide antibodies* develop. These antibodies do not cause adverse effects, but they can reduce exenatide's effects.

Exenatide poses a risk for *pancreatitis.* Severe cases have led to pancreatic necrosis, pancreatic hemorrhage, and even death. Patients should be informed about signs and symptoms of pancreatitis—typically severe and persistent abdominal pain, with or without vomiting—and instructed to stop exenatide immediately. If pancreatitis is confirmed, exenatide should not be resumed. Patients with a history of pancreatitis should probably not use this drug.

Exenatide can cause *renal impairment,* sometimes requiring hemodialysis or a kidney transplant. Fortunately, the incidence is low—about 1 case for every 13,000 patients. Risk for renal impairment may be increased by nausea, vomiting, or diarrhea, or any other event that can cause dehydration. Exenatide should be avoided in patients with severe renal impairment and should be used with caution in kidney transplant recipients.

In pregnant animals, doses of exenatide only 3 times the human dose caused *fetal harm,* manifesting as reduced growth and skeletal abnormalities. At this time, the drug is classified in FDA Pregnancy Risk Category C, and hence should be used only if the benefits are believed to outweigh the fetal risk. Furthermore, given the established safety and efficacy of insulin in pregnancy, there seems to be little reason to even try exenatide.

There have been postmarketing reports of serious *hypersensitivity reactions,* including anaphylaxis and angioedema. If severe reaction occurs, patients should stop taking exenatide and seek immediate medical attention.

Drug Interactions. Exenatide delays gastric emptying and hence can slow the absorption of oral drugs, thereby decreasing peak plasma levels and prolonging the time to peak serum levels. Reduced absorption is of particular concern with oral contraceptives and antibiotics, which require high peak concentrations to be maximally effective. To minimize this interaction, give oral drugs at least 1 hour before exenatide.

Preparations, Dosage, and Administration. Exenatide [Byetta] is supplied in prefilled, 60-dose injector pens that deliver 5 or 10 mcg per dose. SubQ injections are made into the thigh, abdomen, or upper arm. The initial dosage is 5 mcg twice daily, administered 0 to 60 minutes before the morning and evening meals—never after the meal. After 1 month, the dosage may be increased to 10 mcg twice daily. If the patient is taking a sulfonylurea, its dosage may need a reduction (to avoid hypoglycemia). If the patient is taking metformin, no dosage reduction is needed. Because of greatly reduced clearance, exenatide should not be used by patients with severe renal impairment. Exenatide ER suspension [Bydureon] is supplied as 2-mg ER powder in single-dose vials or pens for suspension in diluent for injection. SubQ injections are made in the thigh, abdomen, or upper arm.

Liraglutide

Actions and Uses. Liraglutide [Victoza] is an incretin mimetic similar to exenatide. The drug is indicated as an adjunct to diet and exercise to enhance glycemic control in adults with type 2 diabetes. Like exenatide, liraglutide is an analog of human GLP-1 that causes direct activation of GLP-1 receptors and thereby slows gastric emptying, stimulates glucose-dependent insulin release, and inhibits postprandial release of glucagon. Liraglutide is more convenient than exenatide (dosing is done just once a day without regard to meals, rather than twice a day before meals).

Liraglutide can be used alone or combined with other antidiabetic drugs. Most often, the drug is combined with metformin, a sulfonylurea, or another agent. Because sulfonylureas actively drive down blood glucose levels, adding liraglutide to a sulfonylurea regimen increases the risk for hypoglycemia. Reducing the sulfonylurea dosage at the start of liraglutide treatment seems to lower the risk.

Liraglutide has been shown effective as an add-on to rosiglitazone, a drug that is all but gone from use. Although liraglutide has not been studied as an add-on to pioglitazone (the only other glitazone still on the market), it seems likely that liraglutide would be effective with pioglitazone too.

Pharmacokinetics. Pharmacokinetics of liraglutide are unremarkable. Plasma levels peak 8 to 13 hours after subQ dosing. The drug undergoes metabolic breakdown followed by excretion in the urine and feces. The plasma half-life is 13 hours—long enough to permit once-daily dosing.

Adverse Effects. Dose-related GI effects are common, developing in 41% of patients. Specific effects include nausea, diarrhea, and constipation. Hypoglycemia can also occur, especially when liraglutide is combined with a sulfonylurea (but not with metformin).

In clinical trials, 8.6% of patients developed antiliraglutide antibodies. This is surprising, given that liraglutide is nearly identical to human GLP-1, and hence should not be antigenic. In theory, these antibodies could neutralize liraglutide. However, to date, there is no evidence this has happened.

Like exenatide, liraglutide has been associated with rare cases of pancreatitis. If pancreatitis is suspected, liraglutide should be discontinued immediately. If pancreatitis is confirmed, the drug should never be used again. However, if pancreatitis is ruled out, use of liraglutide can resume.

Like exenatide, liraglutide has been associated with rare cases of renal impairment, including new acute renal failure and worsening of chronic renal failure. Most cases occurred in patients who had experienced nausea, vomiting, or diarrhea, or any other event that can cause dehydration. Renal impairment may reverse with supportive treatment and discontinuation of liraglutide and any other potentially causative agents.

There is concern that liraglutide may cause thyroid C-cell tumors, including medullary thyroid carcinoma (MTC). In tests on rodents, clinically relevant doses have caused C-cell tumors. However, there is no proof that liraglutide has caused these tumors in humans.

BLACK BOX WARNING: LIRAGLUTIDE

Liraglutide has been associated with development of thyroid C-cell cancer. The drug is contraindicated in patients with a family history of MTC and in those with multiple endocrine neoplasia syndrome type 2.

Drug Interactions. As noted, combined use with a sulfonylurea can increase the risk for hypoglycemia. Dosage of the sulfonylurea may need a reduction.

Because liraglutide delays gastric emptying, it might delay the absorption of some oral drugs, thereby reducing their peak serum levels and prolonging the time to peak serum levels.

Preparations, Dosage, and Administration. Liraglutide [Victoza] is supplied in prefilled multidose injector pens that deliver 0.6, 1.2, or 1.8 mg/dose. Administration is by subQ injection into the abdomen, thigh, or upper arm. Dosing is done once a day, at any time and independent of meals. The initial dosage is low—0.6 mg once a day—to minimize GI side effects. After 1 week, dosage is increased to 1.2 mg once a day. If that dosage proves inadequate, it can be increased to 1.8 mg once a day.

Albiglutide

Actions and Uses. Albiglutide [Tanzeum] is an incretin mimetic indicated as an adjunct to diet and exercise to enhance glycemic control in adults with type 2 diabetes. Like exenatide ER suspension, albiglutide is administered once weekly by subcutaneous injection. The safety and tolerability profile of albiglutide is likewise similar to that of exenatide ER suspension.

Preparations, Dosage, and Administration. Albiglutide [Tanzeum] is supplied as single-dose pens for administration of 30- and 50-mg doses. Albiglutide is recommended to be initiated at 30-mg once weekly. The dose can be increased to 50-mg once weekly in patients requiring additional glycemic control.

Dulaglutide

Actions and Uses. Like Albiglutide, dulaglutide [Trulicity] is a GLP-1 receptor agonist indicated as an adjunct to diet and exercise to enhance glycemic control in adults with type 2 diabetes. Dulaglutide is administered once weekly by subQ injection. The safety and tolerability profile of albiglutide is likewise similar to that of albiglutide.

Preparations, Dosage, and Administration. Dulaglutide [Trulicity] is supplied as single-dose pens as well as single-dose prefilled syringes. Both pens and syringes are available in 0.75- and 1.5-mg/mL solution. Initiation should be started at 0.75 mg once weekly and can be doubled in patients that need additional control.

Amylin Mimetic: Pramlintide

Pramlintide [Symlin] is the first member of a new class of antidiabetic agents, the amylin mimetics. The drug is used to complement the effects of insulin in patients with type 1 or type 2 diabetes. Severe hypoglycemia is a concern, and nausea is common.

Description and Actions

Pramlintide is a synthetic analog of amylin, a peptide hormone made in the pancreas and coreleased with insulin. Both amylin and pramlintide, which mimics the effects of amylin, reduce postprandial levels of glucose, mainly by delaying gastric emptying and suppressing glucagon secretion. In addition, both agents act in the brain to increase the sense of satiety, helping to lower caloric intake.

Therapeutic Use

Pramlintide is indicated as a supplement to mealtime insulin in patients with type 1 or type 2 diabetes who have failed to achieve glucose control despite optimal insulin therapy. Patients with type 2 diabetes may combine insulin and pramlintide with metformin and/or a sulfonylurea. In clinical trials, adding subQ pramlintide to mealtime insulin decreased postprandial glucose levels, smoothed out glucose fluctuations, and reduced the needed mealtime dose of insulin. Mean reductions in A_{1c} were about 0.39% for those with type 1 diabetes and 0.55% for those with type 2 diabetes.

Pharmacokinetics

Blood levels peak about 20 minutes after subQ injection and decline with a half-life of 49 minutes. Unlike most drugs, pramlintide is metabolized in the kidneys rather than the liver. One active metabolite has been identified.

Adverse Effects

Hypoglycemia is the biggest concern. Pramlintide does not cause hypoglycemia when used alone but poses a risk for severe hypoglycemia when combined with insulin, especially in patients with type 1 diabetes. As a rule, hypoglycemia develops within 3 hours of dosing. To reduce risk, insulin dosage must be decreased, at least initially. Also, pramlintide should not be given to patients who have hypoglycemia unawareness, a history of poor adherence to their insulin regimen, poor adherence to SMBG, or recurrent hypoglycemia needing assistance.

BLACK BOX WARNING: PRAMLINTIDE

Pramlintide poses a risk for severe hypoglycemia when combined with insulin, especially in patients with type 1 diabetes.

Nausea occurs early in therapy and is more common in patients with type 1 diabetes (37%–48%) than type 2 diabetes (28%–30%). The incidence and severity of nausea can be reduced by gradual titration of dosage.

Injection-site reactions—redness, swelling, or itching—may occur but generally resolve within a few days to weeks.

Drug Interactions

By delaying gastric emptying, pramlintide can delay the absorption of oral drugs. Accordingly, oral drugs should be taken 1 hour before injecting pramlintide or 2 hours after. Pramlintide should not be combined with other drugs that slow intestinal motility (e.g., antimuscarinic agents, opioid analgesics) or with drugs that slow the absorption of nutrients (e.g., acarbose, miglitol).

Preparations, Dosage, and Administration

Pramlintide [Symlin] is supplied as prefilled SymlinPens, which should be stored under refrigeration, but not frozen. Pens currently in use, which can be kept cool or at room temperature, should be discarded after 28 days.

Dosing is done before major meals that contain at least 250 kcal or 30 g of carbohydrates. SubQ injections are made into the abdomen or thigh.

In patients with type 1 diabetes, the initial dosage is 15 mcg before meals. If there is no serious nausea for 3 days, dosage can be increased in 15-mcg steps to a maximum of 60 mcg. If 30 mcg causes too much nausea, discontinuation should be considered.

In patients with type 2 diabetes, the initial dosage is 60 mcg before meals. If there is no serious nausea for 3 to 7 days, dosage may be increased to 120 mcg.

In patients with type 1 or type 2 diabetes, the premeal dose of rapid- or short-acting insulin should be decreased by 50% (to reduce the risk for hypoglycemia). When the maintenance dosage of pramlintide is established, the insulin dosage can be titrated upward as needed to achieve desired glycemic control.

GLUCAGON FOR TREATMENT OF SEVERE HYPOGLYCEMIA

Insulin overdose and use of insulin secretagogue medications can cause severe hypoglycemia. The preferred treatment is IV glucose. However, if this option is not available, blood glucose can be restored with glucagon.

Glucagon, a polypeptide hormone produced by alpha cells of the pancreas, has effects on carbohydrate metabolism that are opposite to those of insulin. Specifically, glucagon promotes the breakdown of glycogen to glucose, reduces conversion of glucose to glycogen, and stimulates biosynthesis of glucose. Hence, whereas insulin acts to lower plasma glucose, glucagon causes plasma glucose to rise. In addition to these metabolic effects, glucagon acts on GI smooth muscle to promote relaxation.

Glucagon is used to treat severe hypoglycemia in the ambulatory setting. However, in patients with severe hypoglycemia, IV glucose is preferred because it raises blood glucose immediately, whereas responses to glucagon are somewhat delayed. Accordingly, glucagon should be used only if IV glucose is not an option—such as subQ administration in the home setting before emergency services arrive. When IV glucagon is administered to unconscious patients, the subsequent rise in blood glucose usually restores consciousness in 20 minutes or so. When consciousness is sufficient for swallowing, oral carbohydrates should be given. These will help prevent recurrence of hypoglycemia and will help replenish hepatic glycogen stores.

Glucagon cannot correct hypoglycemia resulting from starvation. Glucagon acts in large part by promoting glycogen breakdown, and people who are starved have little or no glycogen left.

Glucagon is administered parenterally (intramuscularly, subcutaneously, or intravenously). The drug is supplied in powder form and must be reconstituted to a concentration of 1 mg/mL (or less) using the diluent supplied by the manufacturer. A dose of 0.5 to 1 mg is usually effective.

CHAPTER

47 Drugs for Thyroid Disorders

Laura D. Rosenthal, DNP, ACNP, FAANP

Thyroid hormones have profound effects on metabolism, cardiac function, growth, and development. These hormones stimulate the metabolic rate of most cells and increase the force and rate of cardiac contraction. During infancy and childhood, thyroid hormones promote maturation; severe deficiency can produce extreme short stature and permanent mental impairment. Fortunately, most abnormalities of thyroid function can be effectively treated.

We begin our study of thyroid drugs by reviewing thyroid physiology. Next we review the pathophysiology of hypothyroid and hyperthyroid states. Finally, we discuss the agents used for thyroid disorders.

THYROID PHYSIOLOGY

Chemistry and Nomenclature

The thyroid gland produces two active hormones: triiodothyronine (T_3) and thyroxine (T_4, tetraiodothyronine). These hormones have nearly identical structures. The only difference is that T_4 contains four atoms of iodine, whereas T_3 contains three. The biologic effects of T_3 and T_4 are qualitatively similar. However, when compared on a molar basis, T_3 is much more potent.

Preparations of T_3 and T_4 employed clinically, although synthetic, are identical in structure to the naturally occurring hormones. The generic name of synthetic T_3 is *liothyronine,* and the generic name of synthetic T_4 is *levothyroxine.* A fixed-ratio mixture of T_3 plus T_4, known as *liotrix,* is also available.

Synthesis and Fate of Thyroid Hormones

Synthesis

Synthesis of thyroid hormones takes place in four steps (Fig. 47.1). The circled numbers in the figure correspond with these steps:

- *Step 1.* Formation of thyroid hormone begins with the active transport of *iodide* into the thyroid. Under normal conditions, this process produces concentrations of iodide within the thyroid that are 20 to 50 times greater than the concentration of iodide in plasma. When plasma iodide levels are extremely low, intrathyroid iodide content may reach levels that are more than 100 times greater than those in plasma.
- *Step 2.* After uptake, iodide undergoes oxidation to *iodine,* the active form of iodide. Iodide oxidation is catalyzed by an enzyme called *peroxidase.*
- *Step 3.* In this step, activated iodine becomes incorporated into tyrosine residues that are bound to *thyroglobulin,* a large glycoprotein. One tyrosine molecule may receive either one or two iodine atoms, resulting in the production of monoiodotyrosine (MIT) or diiodotyrosine (DIT), respectively.
- *Step 4.* In this final step, iodinated tyrosine molecules are coupled. Coupling of one DIT with one MIT forms T_3 (step 4A); coupling of one DIT with another DIT forms T_4 (step 4B).

Fate

Thyroid hormones are released from the thyroid gland by a proteolytic process. The amount of T_4 released is substantially greater than the amount of T_3 released. However, much of the T_4 that is released undergoes conversion to T_3 by enzymes in peripheral tissues. In fact, conversion of T_4 to T_3 accounts for the majority (about 80%) of the T_3 found in plasma.

More than 99.5% of the T_3 and T_4 in plasma is bound to plasma proteins. Consequently, only a tiny fraction of circulating thyroid hormone is free to produce biologic effects.

Thyroid hormones are eliminated primarily by hepatic metabolism. Because T_3 and T_4 are extensively bound to plasma proteins, metabolism is slow. As a result, the half-lives of these hormones are prolonged—about 1 day for T_3 and 7 days for T_4.

Thyroid Hormone Actions

Thyroid hormones have three principal actions: (1) stimulation of energy use, (2) stimulation of the heart, and (3) promotion of growth and development. Stimulation of energy use elevates the basal metabolic rate, resulting in increased oxygen consumption and increased heat production. Stimulation of the heart increases both the rate and force of contraction, resulting in increased cardiac output and increased oxygen demand. Thyroid effects on growth and development are profound: thyroid hormones are essential for normal development of the brain and other components of the nervous system, and they have a significant effect on maturation of skeletal muscle.

Thyroid hormones produce their effects by modulating the activity of specific genes. Furthermore, it appears that most, if not all, of the effects of thyroid hormones are mediated by T_3, not by T_4. There is good evidence that T_3 penetrates to the cell nucleus and binds with high affinity to nuclear receptors, which in turn bind to specific DNA sequences. The result is modulation of gene transcription, causing production of proteins that mediate thyroid hormone effects. Although T_4 also binds with nuclear receptors, its affinity is low, and gene transcription is not altered. Hence it would seem that T_4 serves only as a source of T_3, having little or no physiologic effects of its own.

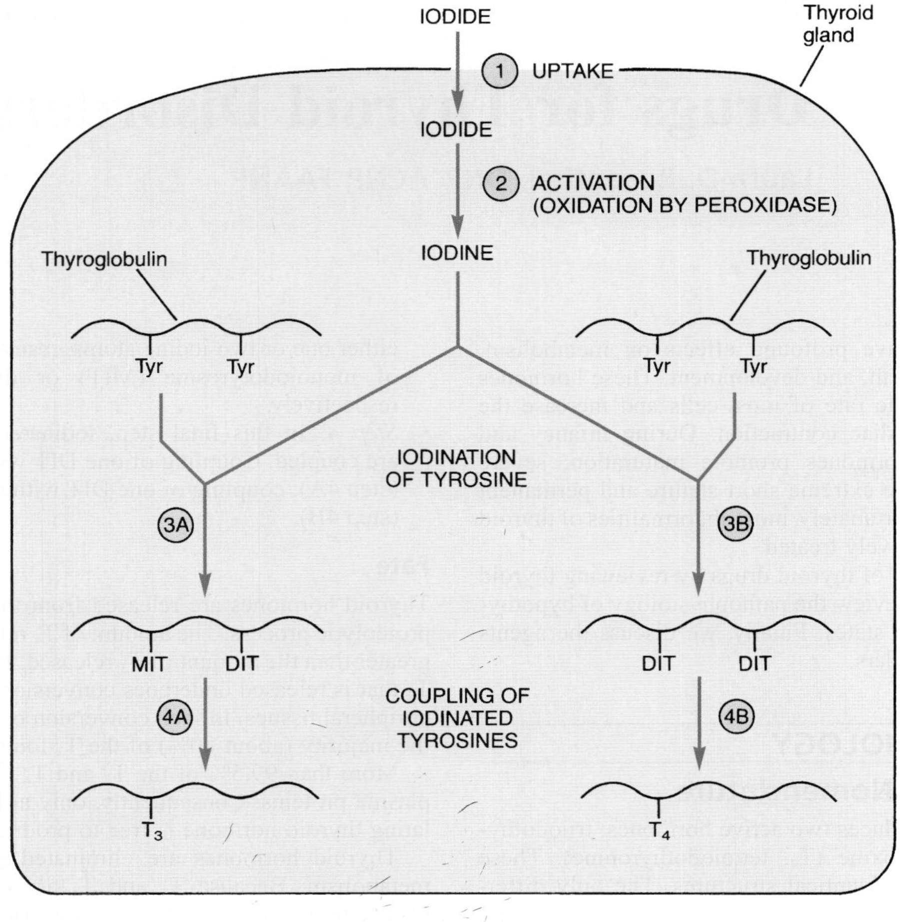

Figure 47.1 ■ Steps in thyroid hormone synthesis.
The reactions at each step (circled numbers) are explained in the text. DIT, diiodotyrosine; MIT, monoiodotyrosine; T_3, triiodothyronine; T_4, thyroxine; Tyr, tyrosine.

Regulation of Thyroid Function by the Hypothalamus and Anterior Pituitary

The functional relationship between the hypothalamus, anterior pituitary, and thyroid is shown in Fig. 47.2. As indicated, thyrotropin-releasing hormone (TRH), secreted by the hypothalamus, acts on the pituitary to cause secretion of thyrotropin (thyroid-stimulating hormone [TSH]). TSH then acts on the thyroid to stimulate all aspects of thyroid function: thyroid size is enlarged, iodine uptake is augmented, and synthesis and release of thyroid hormones are increased. In response to rising plasma levels of T_3 and T_4, further release of TSH is suppressed. The stimulatory effect of TSH on the thyroid, followed by the inhibitory effect of thyroid hormones on the pituitary, constitutes a negative feedback loop.

Effect of Iodine Deficiency on Thyroid Function

When iodine availability is diminished, production of thyroid hormones decreases. The ensuing drop in thyroid hormone levels promotes release of TSH, which acts on the thyroid to increase its size (causing goiter) and ability to concentrate iodine. If iodine deficiency is not too severe, the increased capacity for iodine uptake will restore normal production of T_3 and T_4.

THYROID FUNCTION TESTS

Several laboratory tests can be used to evaluate thyroid function. Three are described here. Values indicating euthyroid (normal), hypothyroid, and hyperthyroid states are shown in Table 47.1.

Serum Thyroid-Stimulating Hormone Test

Serum TSH determinations are used primarily for screening and diagnosis of hypothyroidism and for monitoring replacement therapy in hypothyroid patients.

Measurement of serum TSH is the most sensitive method for diagnosing hypothyroidism because the anterior pituitary is exquisitely sensitive to changes in thyroid hormone levels. As a result, very small reductions in serum T_3 and T_4 can cause a dramatic rise in serum TSH. Therefore even when the degree of hypothyroidism is minimal, it will be reflected by an abnormally high level of TSH. When replacement therapy is instituted, the TSH level should return to normal.

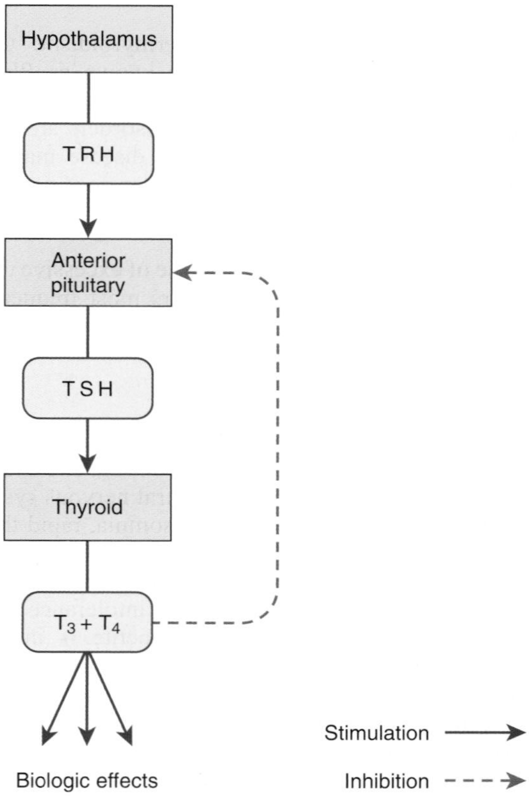

Figure 47.2 ■ Regulation of thyroid function.
Thyrotropin-releasing hormone (TRH) from the hypothalamus stimulates release of thyroid-stimulating hormone (TSH) from the pituitary. TSH stimulates all aspects of thyroid function, including release of triiodothyronine (T_3) and thyroxine (T_4). T_3 and T_4 act on the pituitary to suppress further TSH release.

TABLE 47.1 ■ Serum Values for Thyroid Function Tests*

	Serum Values		
Thyroid Test	**Normal**	**Hypothyroid**	**Hyperthyroid**
Total T_4 (mcg/dL)	4.5–12.5	Under 4.5	Over 12.5
Free T_4 (ng/dL)	0.9–2	Under 0.9	Over 2
Total T_3 (ng/dL)	80–220	Under 80	Over 220
Free T_3 (pg/dL)	230–620	Under 230	Over 620
TSH (microunits/mL)	0.3–6	Over 6	Under 0.3

*Laboratory studies have different reference ranges. These are relative ranges and are not absolute.
T_3, triiodothyronine; T_4, thyroxine; TSH, thyroid-stimulating hormone.

Serum TSH determinations can also be used to distinguish primary hypothyroidism from secondary hypothyroidism. In primary (thyroidal) hypothyroidism, TSH levels are *high*. However, in secondary hypothyroidism (hypothyroidism resulting from anterior pituitary dysfunction), TSH levels are low, normal, or even slightly elevated—despite the presence of low levels of T_3 and T_4.

Serum Thyroxine Test

Testing can measure either *total T_4* (bound plus free) or *free T_4*. Measurement of free T_4 is preferred. The T_4 test can be used to monitor thyroid hormone replacement therapy and to screen for thyroid dysfunction. However, in both cases, measurement of TSH is preferred.

Serum Triiodothyronine Test

As with T_4, we can measure either total or free T_3. Measurement of free T_3 is preferred. This test is useful for diagnosing hyperthyroidism. In this disorder, levels of T_3 often rise sooner and to a greater extent than do levels of T_4. T_3 determinations can also be used to monitor thyroid hormone replacement therapy (all thyroid preparations should increase levels of T_3).

THYROID PATHOPHYSIOLOGY

Hypothyroidism

Hypothyroidism can occur at any age. In adults, mild deficiency of thyroid hormone is referred to simply as *hypothyroidism*. Severe deficiency is called *myxedema*. When hypothyroidism occurs in infants, the resulting condition is called *congenital hypothyroidism*.

Hypothyroidism in Adults

Clinical Presentation

Signs and symptoms of hypothyroidism depend on disease severity. With mild hypothyroidism, symptoms are subtle and may go unrecognized for what they are. In contrast, with moderate to severe disease, characteristic signs and symptoms emerge. The face is pale, puffy, and expressionless. The skin is cold and dry. The hair is brittle, and hair loss occurs. Heart rate and temperature are lowered. The patient may complain of lethargy, fatigue, and intolerance to cold. Mentation may be impaired. Thyroid enlargement may occur if reduced levels of T_3 and T_4 promote excessive release of TSH.

Causes

Hypothyroidism in the adult is usually due to malfunction of the thyroid itself. In iodine-sufficient countries, the principal cause is *chronic autoimmune thyroiditis* (Hashimoto thyroiditis). Other causes are insufficient iodine in the diet, surgical removal of the thyroid, and destruction of the thyroid by radioactive iodine. Adult hypothyroidism may also result from insufficient secretion of TSH and TRH.

Therapeutic Strategy

Hypothyroidism in adults requires replacement therapy with thyroid hormones. In almost all cases, treatment must continue lifelong. Today, the standard replacement regimen consists of *levothyroxine* (T_4) alone. Combined therapy with levothyroxine plus liothyronine (T_3) is an option. However, with only three exceptions, all studies to date indicate that combined T_3/T_4 offers no advantage over T_4 alone. (Remember, when we give T_4, much of it is rapidly converted to T_3, the active form of the hormone.) When replacement doses of T_4 are adequate, they can eliminate all signs and symptoms of thyroid deficiency.

Hypothyroidism During Pregnancy

Maternal hypothyroidism can result in permanent neuropsychological deficits in the child. We have long known that *congenital* hypothyroidism can cause developmental problems (see next section "Hypothyroidism in Infants"). However, it was not until 1999 that researchers demonstrated that *maternal* hypothyroidism—in the absence of fetal hypothyroidism—can decrease IQ and other aspects of neuropsychological function in the child. The effect of maternal hypothyroidism is limited largely to the first trimester, a time during which the fetus is unable to produce thyroid hormones of its own. By the second trimester, the fetal thyroid gland is fully functional, and hence the fetus can supply its own hormones from then on. Therefore to help ensure healthy fetal development, maternal hypothyroidism must be diagnosed and treated very early. Unfortunately, symptoms of hypothyroidism are often nonspecific (e.g., irritability, tiredness, poor concentration), or there may be no symptoms at all. Accordingly, some authorities now recommend routine screening for hypothyroidism as soon as pregnancy is confirmed. If hypothyroidism is diagnosed, replacement therapy should begin immediately.

When women taking thyroid supplements become pregnant, dosage requirements usually increase—often by as much as 50%. The need for increased dosage begins between weeks 4 and 8 of gestation, levels off at about week 16, and then remains steady until parturition. To ensure adequate hormone levels, some authorities increase T_4 dosage by 30% as soon as pregnancy is confirmed. Further adjustments are based on serum TSH levels, which should be monitored closely.

Hypothyroidism in Infants

Clinical Presentation

Hypothyroidism in newborns may be permanent or transient. In either case, congenital hypothyroidism can cause delay in mental development and derangement of growth. In the absence of thyroid hormones, the child develops a large and protruding tongue, potbelly, and dwarfish stature. Development of the nervous system, bones, teeth, and muscles is impaired.

Causes

Congenital hypothyroidism usually results from a failure in thyroid development. Other causes include autoimmune disease, severe iodine deficiency, TSH deficiency, and exposure to radioactive iodine in utero.

Therapeutic Strategy

Hypothyroidism in newborns requires replacement therapy with thyroid hormones. If treatment is initiated within a few days of birth, physical and mental development will be normal. However, if therapy is delayed beyond 3 to 4 weeks, some permanent disability will be evident, although the physical effects of thyroid deficiency will reverse.

In all children, replacement therapy should continue for 3 years, after which it should be stopped for 4 weeks. The objective is to determine whether thyroid deficiency is permanent or transient. If TSH rises, indicating thyroid hormone production is low, we know the deficiency is permanent, so replacement therapy should resume. If TSH and T_4 normalize, we know the deficiency was transient, and hence further replacement therapy is unnecessary.

Hyperthyroidism

There are two major forms of hyperthyroidism: *Graves disease* and *toxic nodular goiter* (also known as *Plummer disease*). Of the two disorders, Graves disease is more common. Signs and symptoms of both disorders are similar. The principal difference is that Graves disease may cause exophthalmos, whereas toxic nodular goiter does not.

Graves Disease

Graves disease is the most common cause of excessive thyroid hormone secretion. This disorder occurs most frequently in women aged 20 to 40 years. The incidence in females is 6 times greater than in males.

Clinical Presentation

Most clinical manifestations result from elevated levels of thyroid hormone. Heartbeat is rapid and strong, and dysrhythmias and angina may develop. The central nervous system is stimulated, resulting in nervousness, insomnia, rapid thought flow, and rapid speech. Skeletal muscles may weaken and atrophy. Metabolic rate is raised, resulting in increased heat production, increased body temperature, intolerance to heat, and skin that is warm and moist. Appetite is increased. However, despite increased food consumption, weight loss occurs if caloric intake fails to match the increase in metabolic rate. Collectively, the above signs and symptoms are referred to as *thyrotoxicosis.*

In addition to thyrotoxicosis, patients with Graves disease often present with *exophthalmos.* The underlying cause is an immune-mediated infiltration of the extraocular muscles and orbital fat by lymphocytes, macrophages, plasma cells, mast cells, and mucopolysaccharides.

Cause

Thyroid stimulation in Graves disease is caused by thyroid-stimulating immunoglobulins (TSIs), which are antibodies produced by an autoimmune process. TSIs increase thyroid activity by stimulating receptors for TSH on the thyroid gland. That is, TSIs mimic the effects of TSH on thyroid function. TSIs are not responsible for exophthalmos.

Treatment

Treatment for Graves disease is directed at decreasing the production of thyroid hormones. Three modalities are employed: (1) surgical removal of thyroid tissue, (2) destruction of thyroid tissue with radioactive iodine, and (3) suppression of thyroid hormone synthesis with an antithyroid drug (methimazole or propylthiouracil). Radiation is the preferred treatment for adults, whereas antithyroid drugs are preferred for younger patients.

Beta blockers and nonradioactive iodine may be used as adjunctive therapy. Beta blockers suppress tachycardia by blocking beta receptors on the heart. Nonradioactive iodine inhibits synthesis and release of thyroid hormones.

Because exophthalmos is not the result of hyperthyroidism per se, this condition is not improved by lowering thyroid hormone production. If exophthalmos is severe, it can be treated with surgery or with high doses of oral glucocorticoids.

Toxic Nodular Goiter (Plummer Disease)

Toxic nodular goiter is the result of a thyroid adenoma. Clinical manifestations are much like those of Graves disease, except exophthalmos is absent. Toxic nodular goiter is a persistent condition that rarely undergoes spontaneous remission. Treatment modalities are the same as for Graves disease. However, if an antithyroid drug is used, symptoms return rapidly when the drug is withdrawn. Accordingly, surgery and radiation, which provide long-term control, are often preferred.

Thyrotoxic Crisis (Thyroid Storm)

Thyrotoxic crisis can occur in patients with severe thyrotoxicosis when they undergo major surgery or develop a severe intercurrent illness (e.g., infection, sepsis). The syndrome is characterized by profound hyperthermia (105° F or even higher), severe tachycardia, restlessness, agitation, and tremor. Unconsciousness, coma, hypotension, and heart failure may ensue. These symptoms are produced by excessive levels of thyroid hormones.

Thyrotoxic crisis can be life-threatening and requires immediate treatment. High doses of potassium iodide or strong iodine solution are given to suppress thyroid hormone release. Methimazole is given to suppress thyroid hormone synthesis. A beta blocker is given to reduce heart rate. Additional measures include sedation, cooling, and giving glucocorticoids and intravenous (IV) fluids.

THYROID HORMONE PREPARATIONS FOR HYPOTHYROIDISM

Thyroid hormones are available as pure, synthetic compounds and as extracts of animal thyroid glands. All preparations have qualitatively similar effects. The synthetic preparations are more stable and better standardized than the animal gland extracts. As a result, the synthetics are preferred to the natural products. Properties of thyroid hormone preparations are shown in Table 47.2.

Levothyroxine (T_4)

Levothyroxine [Levothroid, Synthroid, others] is a synthetic preparation of thyroxine, a naturally occurring thyroid hormone. The structure of levothyroxine is identical to that of the natural hormone. Levothyroxine is the drug of choice for most patients who require thyroid hormone replacement. Consequently, levothyroxine will serve as our prototype for the thyroid hormone preparations.

Prototype Drugs

DRUGS FOR THYROID DISORDERS

Drugs for Hypothyroidism

Levothyroxine (T_4)

Drugs for Hyperthyroidism

Methimazole (a thionamide)

Pharmacokinetics

Absorption

Absorption of oral levothyroxine is reduced by food. Accordingly, to minimize variability in blood levels, levothyroxine should be taken on an empty stomach in the morning, at least 30 to 60 minutes before breakfast.

Conversion to T_3

Much of an administered dose of levothyroxine is converted to T_3 in the body. As a result, levothyroxine can produce nearly normal levels of both T_3 and T_4. Hence, for most patients, there is no need to give T_3 along with levothyroxine.

Half-Life and Plasma Levels

Because levothyroxine is highly protein bound (about 99.97%), the hormone has a prolonged half-life (about 7 days). From a clinical perspective, this long half-life is good news and bad news. The good news is that hormone levels remain fairly steady, even with once-a-day dosing, which makes levothyroxine well suited for lifelong therapy. The bad news is that it takes about 1 month (four half-lives) for plasma levels of levothyroxine to reach plateau (steady state). As a result, onset of full effects is delayed.

Therapeutic Uses

Levothyroxine is indicated for all forms of hypothyroidism, regardless of cause. The drug is used for congenital hypothyroidism, myxedema coma, simple goiter, and primary hypothyroidism in adults and children. Levothyroxine is also used to treat hypothyroidism resulting from insufficient TSH (secondary to pituitary malfunction) and from insufficient TRH (secondary to hypothalamic malfunction). In addition,

TABLE 47.2 ▪ Thyroid Hormone Preparations

Generic Name	Trade Names	Dosage Forms	Approximate Equivalent Dosage*	Description
Levothyroxine	Levothroid, Levoxyl, Synthroid	Tablets, injection	50–60 mcg	Synthetic preparation of T_4 identical to the naturally occurring hormone
Liothyronine	Cytomel, Triostat	Tablets, injection	15–37 mcg	Synthetic preparation of T_3 identical to the naturally occurring hormone
Liotrix	Thyrolar	Tablets	60 mcg	Synthetic T_4 plus synthetic T_3 in a 4:1 fixed ratio
Thyroid	Armour Thyroid, Nature-Throid, Thyroid USP, Westhroid	Tablets, capsules	60 mg	Desiccated animal thyroid glands (rarely used today)

*Approximate dosage needed to produce equivalent effects.
T_3, triiodothyronine; T_4, thyroxine.

levothyroxine is used to maintain proper levels of thyroid hormones after thyroid surgery, irradiation, and treatment with antithyroid drugs.

Adverse Effects

When administered in appropriate dosage, levothyroxine rarely causes adverse effects. With an acute overdose, *thyrotoxicosis* may result. Signs and symptoms include tachycardia, angina, tremor, nervousness, insomnia, hyperthermia, heat intolerance, and sweating. The patient should be informed about these signs and instructed to notify the prescriber if they develop. Chronic overdosage is associated with accelerated bone loss and increased risk for atrial fibrillation, especially in older adults. Loss of bone increases the risk for fractures.

Drug Interactions

Drugs That Reduce Levothyroxine Absorption

Absorption of levothyroxine can be reduced by the following drugs:

- Histamine$_2$ (H_2) receptor blockers (e.g., cimetidine [Tagamet])
- Proton pump inhibitors (e.g., lansoprazole [Prevacid]
- Sucralfate [Carafate]
- Cholestyramine [Questran]
- Colestipol [Colestid]
- Aluminum-containing antacids (e.g., Maalox, Mylanta)
- Calcium supplements (e.g., Tums, Os-Cal)
- Iron supplements (e.g., ferrous sulfate)
- Magnesium salts
- Orlistat [Xenical]

To ensure adequate absorption of levothyroxine, patients should separate administration of levothyroxine and these drugs by 4 hours. As noted earlier, food also reduces absorption.

Drugs That Accelerate Levothyroxine Metabolism

Several drugs can accelerate the metabolism of levothyroxine. Among these are phenytoin [Dilantin], carbamazepine [Tegretol, Carbatrol], rifampin [Rifadin], sertraline [Zoloft], and phenobarbital. Accordingly, to maintain adequate levothyroxine levels, patients taking these drugs may need to increase their levothyroxine dosage.

Warfarin. Levothyroxine accelerates the degradation of vitamin K–dependent clotting factors. As a result, effects of warfarin are enhanced. If thyroid hormone replacement therapy is started in a patient taking warfarin, the dosage of warfarin may need to be reduced.

Catecholamines. Thyroid hormones increase cardiac responsiveness to catecholamines, thereby increasing the risk for catecholamine-induced dysrhythmias. Caution must be exercised when administering catecholamines to patients receiving levothyroxine and other thyroid preparations.

Other Interactions

Levothyroxine can increase requirements for insulin and digoxin. When converting patients from a hypothyroid to a euthyroid state, dosages of insulin and digoxin may need to be increased.

Are Levothyroxine Preparations Interchangeable?

Levothyroxine is available in several brand-name and generic formulations. Whether any of these are interchangeable is in dispute.

Levothyroxine has a narrow therapeutic range, so tight control of plasma drug levels is important. Otherwise, symptoms of hypothyroidism or toxicity will develop. To maintain good control, all pills a patient takes must produce the same levothyroxine levels. Accordingly, if a patient switches from one product to another, the new product must be bioequivalent to the old one.

Whether or not any levothyroxine products—brand-name or generic—are truly equivalent is a point of contention. According to the U.S. Food and Drug Administration (FDA), certain formulations of levothyroxine are therapeutically equivalent to others. For example, the FDA maintains that generic levothyroxine made by Mylan is equivalent to two brand-name products: Levoxyl and Synthroid. However, three medical organizations—the American Association of Clinical Endocrinologists (AACE), The Endocrine Society (TES), and the American Thyroid Association (ATA)—*strongly* disagree, as expressed in a 2004 position statement. They believe the FDA's testing procedure was seriously flawed. First, the FDA only measured blood levels of levothyroxine; they did not measure serum TSH, the favored clinical test for assessing thyroid status. Second, and more important, testing was done in *normal* (euthyroid) volunteers. Hence, when blood levels of levothyroxine were measured, the values reflected the sum of endogenous thyroxine plus levothyroxine contributed by the drug—making it impossible to state with precision how much of the total was truly due to the drug. As a result, conclusions regarding the equivalence of levothyroxine products are questionable. Nonetheless, pharmacists may switch patients from one product to another, often without the knowledge of the patient or prescriber—a practice with the potential for causing toxicity or therapeutic failure.

Given the debate about whether certain levothyroxine products are clinically interchangeable, what should the clinician do? In their position statement, the AACE, TES, and ATA recommend the following:

- Maintain patients on the same brand-name levothyroxine product.
- If a switch *is* made (from one branded product to another, from a branded product to a generic product, or from one generic product to another), retest serum TSH in 6 weeks and adjust the levothyroxine dosage as indicated.
- Advise patients to check with their prescriber before allowing a pharmacist to switch to a different levothyroxine product.

Dosage and Administration I: General Considerations

Routes of Administration

Levothyroxine is almost always administered by mouth. Oral doses should be taken once daily on an empty stomach (to enhance absorption). *Dosing is usually done in the morning, at least 30 to 60 minutes before eating.*

Intravenous administration is used for myxedema coma and for patients who cannot take levothyroxine orally. Intravenous doses are about 50% of the size of oral doses.

Evaluation

The goal of replacement therapy is to provide a dosage that compensates precisely for the existing thyroid deficit. This dosage is determined using a combination of clinical judgment and laboratory tests. When therapy is successful in adults, clinical evaluation should reveal a reversal of the signs and symptoms of thyroid deficiency—and an absence of signs of thyroid excess. Successful therapy of infants is reflected in normalization of intellectual function and normalization of growth and development. Monthly determinations of height provide a good index of success.

Measurement of serum TSH is an important means of evaluation. Successful replacement therapy causes elevated TSH levels to fall. However, TSH will not normalize quickly and often lags behind normalization of serum T_3 and T_4. Hence evaluation should not be done until 6 to 8 weeks after starting treatment. A TSH target of 0.5 to 2 microunits/mL is appropriate for most patients. When an adequate replacement dosage is established, TSH levels will remain suppressed for the duration of treatment.

In some cases serum T_4 must be used to evaluate therapy because TSH secretion remains high in some patients even though levels of thyroid hormones have been restored to normal. When this happens, success is indicated by levels of T_4 in the normal to high-normal range—whether or not TSH values are normal.

Duration of Therapy

For most hypothyroid patients, replacement therapy must be continued for life. Treatment provides symptomatic relief but does not produce cure. Patients must be made fully aware of the chronic nature of their condition. In addition, they should be forewarned that, although therapy will cause symptoms to improve, these improvements do not constitute a reason to interrupt or discontinue drug use.

Dosage and Administration II: Specific Applications

Hypothyroidism in Adults

When calculated on a body weight basis, the average adult dosage is about 1.7 mcg/kg/day. Most patients younger than 50 years can be started on full replacement doses (100–125 mcg/day for a 70-kg adult). For older patients, dosage should be low initially and then gradually increased. A typical starting dosage is 25 to 50 mcg/day. For older adults with coronary heart disease, the starting dosage is even lower—between 12.5 and 25 mcg/day.

Myxedema Coma

Myxedema coma is a rare but serious condition that requires rapid treatment. Levothyroxine is administered intravenously in a dose of 200 to 500 mcg. If required, an additional dose of 100 to 300 mcg can be given 1 day later. Glucocorticoids (e.g., hydrocortisone) are also required.

Congenital Hypothyroidism

In congenital hypothyroidism, thyroid hormone dosage decreases with age. For infants younger than 3 months, the dosage is 10 to 15 mcg/kg/day; for children aged 3 to 5 months, 8 to 10 mcg/kg/day; for children aged 6 to 11 months, 6 to 8 mcg/kg/day; for children aged 1 to 5 years, 5 to 6 mcg/kg/day; and for children aged 6 to 12 years, 4 to 5 mcg/kg/day. In all cases, dosage is adjusted to normalize TSH and free T_4.

Simple Goiter

In simple goiter, the thyroid is enlarged and levels of thyroid hormones are reduced. Thyroid enlargement is caused by TSH that has been released in response to low levels of thyroid hormones. When treating simple goiter, the goal is to provide full replacement doses of thyroid hormones to suppress further TSH release. For many patients, this can be achieved with 100 to 200 mcg of levothyroxine daily.

Liothyronine (T_3)

Liothyronine [Cytomel] is a synthetic preparation of triiodothyronine, a naturally occurring thyroid hormone. The structure of liothyronine is identical to that of thyroid-derived T_3. Because liothyronine is the active form of levothyroxine, the effects of the two drugs are identical.

Contrasts With Levothyroxine

Liothyronine differs from levothyroxine in three important ways: (1) liothyronine has a shorter half-life and shorter duration of action, (2) liothyronine has a more rapid onset, and (3) liothyronine is more expensive. Because of its high price and relatively brief duration of action, liothyronine is less desirable than levothyroxine for long-term use. However, because its effects develop quickly, liothyronine may be superior to levothyroxine in situations that require speedy results, especially myxedema coma.

Evaluation

As with levothyroxine, the dosage of liothyronine is adjusted on the basis of clinical evaluation and laboratory data. Two laboratory tests are useful: free serum T_3 and serum TSH. Because liothyronine is not converted into T_4, plasma levels of T_4 remain low. Hence T_4 levels cannot be used to assess treatment.

Dosage and Administration

The usual route is oral, using Cytomel, although dosing may also be done intravenously, using Triostat. Oral dosage is about 80% of the dosage of levothyroxine. Because of its short half-life, oral liothyronine is taken twice daily, in contrast to levothyroxine, which is taken once daily.

Other Thyroid Preparations

Liotrix

Liotrix [Thyrolar] is a mixture of synthetic T_4 plus synthetic T_3 in a 4 : 1 fixed ratio. (This ratio is similar to the ratio of these hormones in plasma.) The rationale for using liotrix is that the mixture can produce plasma levels of T_4 and T_3 similar to those that occur naturally. However, because levothyroxine alone produces the same ratio of T_4 to T_3, liotrix offers no advantage over levothyroxine for most indications.

Thyroid (Desiccated)

Thyroid [Armour Thyroid, others] consists of desiccated animal thyroid glands. Standardization is based on content of iodine, levothyroxine, and liothyronine. The ratio of levothyroxine to liothyronine is not less than 5 : 1. Thyroid is available in tablets (15–300 mg). For practical purposes, thyroid is obsolete: use is limited to patients who have been taking the preparation for years. Thyroid is rarely prescribed for patients starting therapy today.

DRUGS FOR HYPERTHYROIDISM

Antithyroid Drugs: Thionamides

The thionamide drugs—methimazole and propylthiouracil (PTU)—suppress synthesis of thyroid hormones. These agents can be used long term to treat hyperthyroidism or short term as preparation for subtotal thyroidectomy or therapy with radioactive iodine. Methimazole and PTU are similar in most respects. Primary differences concern pharmacokinetics (Table 47.3) and adverse effects.

TABLE 47.3 ▪ Pharmacokinetics of Methimazole and Propylthiouracil

	Methimazole	Propylthiouracil
Bioavailability	80%–95%	80%–95%
Plasma protein binding	0	75%–80%
Levels in breast milk	Low	Low
Transplacental passage	Higher	Low
Half-life	6–13 hr	1–2 hr
Dosing frequency		
Initial therapy	1–3 times a day	3 or 4 times a day
Maintenance therapy	Once a day	2 or 3 times a day

Methimazole

Methimazole [Tapazole] is a first-line drug for hyperthyroidism. Benefits derive from inhibiting thyroid hormone synthesis. Methimazole is safer and more convenient than PTU and hence is preferred for most patients—except women who are pregnant or breastfeeding, and perhaps patients who are in thyrotoxic crisis.

Mechanism of Action

Therapeutic effects result from blocking synthesis of thyroid hormones. Two mechanisms are involved. First, methimazole prevents the oxidation of iodide, thereby inhibiting incorporation of iodine into tyrosine. Second, methimazole prevents iodinated tyrosines from coupling. Both effects result from inhibiting peroxidase, the enzyme that catalyzes both reactions.

Please note that, although methimazole prevents thyroid hormone synthesis, it does not destroy existing stores of thyroid hormone. Hence, after therapy has begun, it may take 3 to 12 weeks to produce a euthyroid state.

Pharmacokinetics

Methimazole is well absorbed after oral dosing. Binding to plasma proteins is minimal. The drug readily crosses membranes, including those of the placenta. Levels in breast milk are sufficient to affect the nursing infant. The plasma half-life is 6 to 13 hours—long enough to permit once-a-day dosing.

Therapeutic Uses

Methimazole has four applications in hyperthyroidism:

- It can be used as the sole form of therapy for Graves disease.
- It can be employed as an adjunct to radiation therapy until the effects of radiation become manifest.
- It can be given to suppress thyroid hormone synthesis in preparation for thyroid gland surgery (subtotal thyroidectomy).
- It can be given to patients experiencing thyrotoxic crisis.

Adverse Effects

Methimazole is generally well tolerated but should be avoided by women who are pregnant or breastfeeding. Agranulocytosis is the most dangerous toxicity. The reaction is rare (about 3 cases per 10,000 patients) and usually develops during the first 2 months of therapy. Sore throat and fever may be the earliest indications, and patients should be instructed to report these immediately. Because agranulocytosis often develops rapidly, periodic blood counts cannot guarantee early detection. If agranulocytosis occurs, methimazole should be discontinued. Agranulocytosis will then reverse. Treatment with granulocyte colony-stimulating factor (filgrastim [Neupogen]) may accelerate recovery.

Hypothyroidism. When given in high doses, methimazole can convert the patient from a hyperthyroid state to a hypothyroid state. If this occurs, dosage should be reduced. Temporary treatment with thyroid hormone may be required.

Effects in Pregnancy. Methimazole can cause neonatal hypothyroidism, goiter, and even congenital hypothyroidism. Accordingly, the drug should be avoided during the first trimester. Use in the second and third trimesters is considered safe. Compared with methimazole, PTU crosses the placenta poorly, and hence risk to the fetus is low. Accordingly, if a thionamide is needed during the first trimester of pregnancy, PTU is the preferred drug.

Effects in Lactation. Methimazole therapy does not affect thyroid function or intellectual development in breastfed infants with doses up to 20 mg daily.

Preparations, Dosage, and Administration

Methimazole is supplied in tablets (5, 10, 15, and 20 mg) for oral dosing. For treatment of severe disease, doses are high initially (e.g., 30–40 mg once a day) and then decreased for maintenance (5–15 mg once a day). As a rule, treatment continues for 1 to 2 years. When methimazole is discontinued, some 30% to 40% of patients remain euthyroid, indicating remission. Others become hyperthyroid in 1 to 4 weeks, indicating relapse. If relapse occurs, another round of methimazole can be tried. Alternatively, the patient can opt for radiation therapy or surgery.

Propylthiouracil

Like methimazole, PTU suppresses synthesis of thyroid hormones and can be used for Graves disease and other hyperthyroid states. PTU, a much older drug than methimazole, is now considered a second-line treatment.

Contrasts With Methimazole

PTU is much like methimazole but with four significant differences:

- First, and most important, PTU can cause severe liver injury, whereas methimazole does not.
- Second, PTU has a shorter half-life than methimazole (90 minutes vs. 6–13 hours) and hence requires two or three daily doses rather than one.
- Third, PTU crosses the placenta less readily than does methimazole.
- Fourth, PTU blocks conversion of T_4 to T_3 in the periphery, whereas methimazole does not.

Current Role in Treating Hyperthyroidism

Because PTU is more toxic than methimazole and requires more daily doses, methimazole is preferred for most patients. However, there are three groups for whom PTU is preferred:

- Pregnant women, but only during the first trimester. (Methimazole is preferred during the second and third trimesters.)
- Patients experiencing thyroid storm. (Because PTU can block conversion of T_4 to T_3, it may be more effective than methimazole.)
- Patients who are intolerant of methimazole.

Pharmacokinetics

PTU is rapidly absorbed after oral administration. Therapeutic actions begin within 30 minutes. Plasma protein binding is moderate (75%–80%). The half-life is short (about 90 minutes), and hence PTU must be administered 2 or 3 times a day. Transplacental passage is low, as is entry into breast milk.

Adverse Effects

As with methimazole, adverse effects are relatively rare. Nonetheless, severe adverse effects can occur, especially liver injury and agranulocytosis. The most common undesired effect is rash. PTU may also cause nausea, arthralgia, headache, dizziness, and paresthesias.

Adverse Effects Shared With Methimazole

Like methimazole, PTU has caused rare cases of agranulocytosis and can cause hypothyroidism if the dosage is too high. In addition, PTU can harm the developing fetus and the breastfeeding infant.

BLACK BOX WARNING: RISK FOR LIVER INJURY

PTU has caused rare cases of severe liver injury. Transplants have been required, and deaths have occurred. Liver toxicity is unrelated to dosage or duration of treatment. Furthermore, onset is sudden and progression is rapid, and hence performing routine tests of liver function doesn't help.

Preparations, Dosage, and Administration

PTU is available in 50-mg tablets for oral use. Because of its short half-life, PTU requires multiple daily doses.

PATIENT-CENTERED CARE ACROSS THE LIFE SPAN

Thyroid Drugs

Life Stage	Patient Care Concerns
Infants	Thyroid hormone preparation is used to treat hypothyroidism in infants. Treatment should continue for 3 years.
Children/adolescents	Thyroid hormone preparations are used in children and adolescents. Doses are based on clinical response. Antithyroid drugs (methimazole and PTU) are also safe in children. Iodine-131 is not generally used in children.
Pregnant women	Iodine-131 is classified in FDA Pregnancy Risk Category X and is contraindicated in pregnancy. Methimazole should be avoided in the first trimester of pregnancy.
Breastfeeding women	Thyroid hormone preparations and antithyroid medications are generally safe in breastfeeding women.
Older adults	Thyroid gland dysfunction is common in the older adult. This is associated with increased morbidity if not treated. Thyroid hormone preparations and antithyroid medications can be used successfully to treat thyroid dysfunction in the older adult.

Treatment of Graves Disease

High doses (100–300 mg 3 times a day) are used initially. Lower doses (e.g., 50 mg 3 times a day) are used for maintenance. As a rule, treatment continues for 1 to 2 years.

Radioactive Iodine

Physical Properties

Iodine-131 (^{131}I) is a radioactive isotope of stable iodine that emits a combination of beta particles and gamma rays. Radioactive decay of ^{131}I takes place rapidly, with a half-life of 8 days. Hence, after 56 days (seven half-lives), less than 1% of the radioactivity in a dose of ^{131}I remains.

Use in Graves Disease

^{131}I can be used to destroy thyroid tissue in patients with hyperthyroidism. The objective is to produce clinical remission without causing complete destruction of the gland. Unfortunately, delayed hypothyroidism, due to excessive thyroid damage, is a frequent complication.

Effect on the Thyroid

Like stable iodine, ^{131}I is concentrated in the thyroid gland. Destruction of thyroid tissue is produced primarily by emission of beta particles. (The gamma rays from ^{131}I are relatively harmless.) Because beta particles have a very limited ability to penetrate any type of physical barrier, they do not travel outside the thyroid. Hence, damage to surrounding tissue is minimal.

Reduction of thyroid function is gradual. Initial effects become apparent in days or weeks. Full effects develop in 2 to 3 months.

Not all patients respond satisfactorily to a single treatment. About 66% of patients with Graves disease are cured with a single exposure to ^{131}I. Others require two or more treatments.

Advantages and Disadvantages of ^{131}I Therapy

The advantages of ^{131}I treatment are considerable: (1) it has a relatively low cost; (2) patients are spared the risks, discomfort, and expense of thyroid surgery; (3) death from ^{131}I treatment is extremely rare; and (4) no tissue other than the thyroid is injured (patients should be reassured of this).

Treatment with ^{131}I is not without drawbacks. First, the effect of treatment is delayed, taking several months to become maximal. Second, and more important, treatment is associated with a significant incidence of delayed hypothyroidism. Hypothyroidism results from excessive dosage and occurs in up to 90% of patients within the first year after ^{131}I exposure.

Who Should Be Treated and Who Should Not

^{131}I is indicated for adults with hyperthyroidism, as well as patients who have not responded adequately to antithyroid drugs or to subtotal thyroidectomy.

As a rule, very young children are considered inappropriate candidates. The likelihood of delayed hypothyroidism is higher than in adults. Also, there is concern that administration of ^{131}I to young patients may carry a slight risk for cancer. It should be noted, however, that there is no evidence that the use of ^{131}I in Graves disease has ever caused cancer of the thyroid or any other tissue. Although ^{131}I is generally avoided in young children, is it commonly used in postpubertal adolescents and young adults.

^{131}I is *contraindicated in pregnancy and lactation.* Exposure of the fetus to ^{131}I after the first trimester may damage the immature thyroid, and exposure to radiation at any point in fetal life carries a risk for generalized developmental harm. Accordingly, a negative pregnancy test is required before giving ^{131}I. Because ^{131}I enters breast milk, women receiving this agent should not breastfeed.

Dosage

Dosage of ^{131}I is determined by thyroid size and by the rate of thyroidal iodine uptake. For Graves disease, the dosage usually ranges between 4 and 10 millicuries (mCi).

Use in Thyroid Cancer

^{131}I can be used to destroy malignant thyroid cells. However, because most forms of thyroid cancer do not accumulate iodine, only a small percentage of patients are candidates for ^{131}I therapy.

The doses of ^{131}I used to treat cancer are large, ranging from 50 to 150 mCi. These doses are much higher than those used in Graves disease. Because high amounts of radioactivity are involved, body wastes must be disposed of properly. In addition, adverse effects from large doses of ^{131}I can be severe: radiation sickness may occur; leukemia may be produced; and bone marrow function may be depressed, resulting in leukopenia, thrombocytopenia, and anemia. Fortunately, these severe effects are rare.

Diagnostic Use

^{131}I is employed to diagnose a variety of thyroid disorders, including hyperthyroidism, hypothyroidism, and goiter. After ^{131}I administration, the thyroid is scanned for uptake of radioactivity; the amount and location of ^{131}I uptake reveal the extent of thyroid activity. Doses for diagnosis are minuscule (less than 1 microcurie for children and less than 10 microcuries for adults). These tracer doses pose virtually no threat to health. Please note that, although ^{131}I can be used for diagnosis, the preferred isotope is ^{123}I.

Preparations

^{131}I is supplied in capsules and solution for oral administration. Both preparations are odorless and tasteless. Capsules contain between 0.75 and 100 mCi of ^{131}I. Vials of oral solution contain between 3.5 and 150 mCi of ^{131}I.

Nonradioactive Iodine: Lugol Solution

Description

Lugol solution, also known as strong iodine solution, is a mixture containing 5% elemental iodine and 10% potassium iodide. The iodine undergoes reduction to iodide within the gastrointestinal (GI) tract before absorption.

Mechanism of Action

When present in high concentrations, iodide has a paradoxical suppressant effect on the thyroid. Three mechanisms are involved. First, high concentrations of iodide decrease iodine uptake by the thyroid. Second, high concentrations of iodide inhibit thyroid hormone synthesis by suppressing both the iodination of tyrosine and the coupling of iodinated tyrosine residues. Third, high concentrations of iodine inhibit release of thyroid hormone into the blood. All three actions combine to decrease circulating levels of T_3 and T_4.

Unfortunately, the effects of iodide on thyroid function cannot be sustained indefinitely. With long-term iodide administration, suppressant effects become weaker. Accordingly, iodide is rarely used alone for thyroid suppression.

Therapeutic Use

Strong iodine solution can be given to hyperthyroid individuals to suppress thyroid function in preparation for thyroidectomy. Initial effects develop within 24 hours. Peak effects develop in 10 to 15 days. In most cases, plasma levels of thyroid hormone are reduced with methimazole before initiating strong iodine solution. Then strong iodine solution (along with more PTU) is administered for the last 10 days before surgery. In addition to its use before thyroidectomy, strong iodine solution is employed in thyrotoxic crisis.

Adverse Effects

Chronic ingestion of iodine can produce iodism. Signs and symptoms include a brassy taste, a burning sensation in the mouth and throat, soreness of the teeth and gums, frontal headache, coryza (nasal inflammation and sneezing), salivation, and various skin eruptions. All of these fade rapidly after iodine use stops.

Overdose

Iodine is corrosive, so overdose will injure the GI tract. Symptoms include abdominal pain, vomiting, and diarrhea. Swelling of the glottis may cause asphyxiation. Treatment consists of gastric lavage (to remove iodine from the stomach) and giving sodium thiosulfate (to reduce iodine to iodide).

Dosage and Administration

When employed to prepare hyperthyroid patients for thyroidectomy, strong iodine solution is administered in a dosage of 5 to 7 drops 3 times daily for 10 days immediately preceding surgery. Iodine solution should be mixed with juice or some other beverage to mask its unpleasant taste. The dosage for thyrotoxic crisis is 10 drops every 8 hours.

Beta Blockers

Propranolol and other beta blockers can suppress tachycardia and other symptoms of Graves disease. Benefits derive from beta-adrenergic blockade, not from reducing levels of T_3 or T_4. One advantage of beta blockers is that they work quickly, unlike PTU, methimazole, and ^{131}I. Dosages for hyperthyroidism are highly individualized.

Beta blockers are also beneficial in thyrotoxic crisis. In the absence of contraindications (e.g., asthma, heart failure), all patients should receive one immediately. Administration may be oral or IV. The dosage for propranolol is 10 to 40 mg PO every 6 to 8 hours, or 0.5 to 1 mg IV repeated every 4 hours until effects are observed.

The basic pharmacology of beta blockers is discussed in Chapter 47.

UNIT XI
Women's Health

CHAPTER 48

Estrogens and Progestins: Basic Pharmacology and Noncontraceptive Applications

Jacqueline Rosenjack Burchum, DNSc, FNP-BC, CNE

To understand pharmacologic properties of manufactured estrogens and progestins, it is important to first understand properties and actions of the endogenous hormones. We begin this chapter with a discussion of how estrogens and progestins regulate physiologic processes.

Estrogens and progestins (also known as *progestogens*) are hormones with multiple actions. They promote female maturation and help regulate the ongoing activity of female reproductive organs. In addition, they affect bone mineralization and lipid metabolism. The principal endogenous estrogen is estradiol. The principal endogenous progestin is progesterone. Both hormones are produced by the ovaries. During pregnancy, large amounts are produced by the placenta. In addition, small amounts of estrogens and progestins are produced in peripheral tissues.

THE MENSTRUAL CYCLE

Because much of the clinical pharmacology of the estrogens and progestins is related to their actions during the menstrual cycle, understanding the menstrual cycle is central to understanding these hormones. Accordingly, we begin by reviewing the menstrual cycle. The anatomic and hormonal changes that take place during the cycle are shown in Fig. 48.1. As indicated, the first half of the cycle (days 1 through 14) is called the *follicular phase,* and the second half is called the *luteal phase.* One full cycle typically takes approximately 28 days.

Ovarian and Uterine Events

The menstrual cycle consists of a coordinated series of ovarian and uterine events. In the ovary, the following sequence occurs: (1) several ovarian follicles ripen; (2) one of the ripe follicles ruptures, causing ovulation; (3) the ruptured follicle evolves into a corpus luteum; and (4) if fertilization does not occur, the corpus luteum atrophies. As these ovarian events are taking place, parallel events take place in the uterus: (1) while ovarian follicles ripen, the endometrium prepares for nidation (implantation of a fertilized ovum) by increasing in thickness and vascularity; (2) after ovulation, the uterus continues its preparation by increasing secretory activity; and (3) if implantation fails to occur, the thickened endometrium breaks down, causing menstruation, and the cycle begins anew.

The Roles of Estrogens and Progesterone

The uterine changes that occur during the cycle are brought about under the influence of estrogens and progesterone produced by the ovaries. During the first half of the cycle, estrogens are secreted by the maturing ovarian follicles. As suggested by Fig. 48.1, these estrogens act on the uterus to cause proliferation of the endometrium. At midcycle, one of the ovarian follicles ruptures and then evolves into a corpus luteum. For most of the second half of the cycle, estrogens and progesterone are produced by the newly formed corpus luteum. These hormones maintain the endometrium in its hypertrophied state. At the end of the cycle, the corpus luteum atrophies, causing production of estrogens and progesterone to decline. In response to the diminished supply of ovarian hormones, the endometrium breaks down.

The Role of Pituitary Hormones

Two anterior pituitary hormones—follicle-stimulating hormone (FSH) and luteinizing hormone (LH)—play central roles in regulating the menstrual cycle. Precisely timed alterations in the secretion of these hormones are responsible for coordinating the structural and secretory changes that occur throughout the menstrual cycle. During the first half of the cycle, FSH acts on the developing ovarian follicles, causing them to mature and secrete estrogens. The resultant rise in estrogen levels exerts a negative feedback influence on the

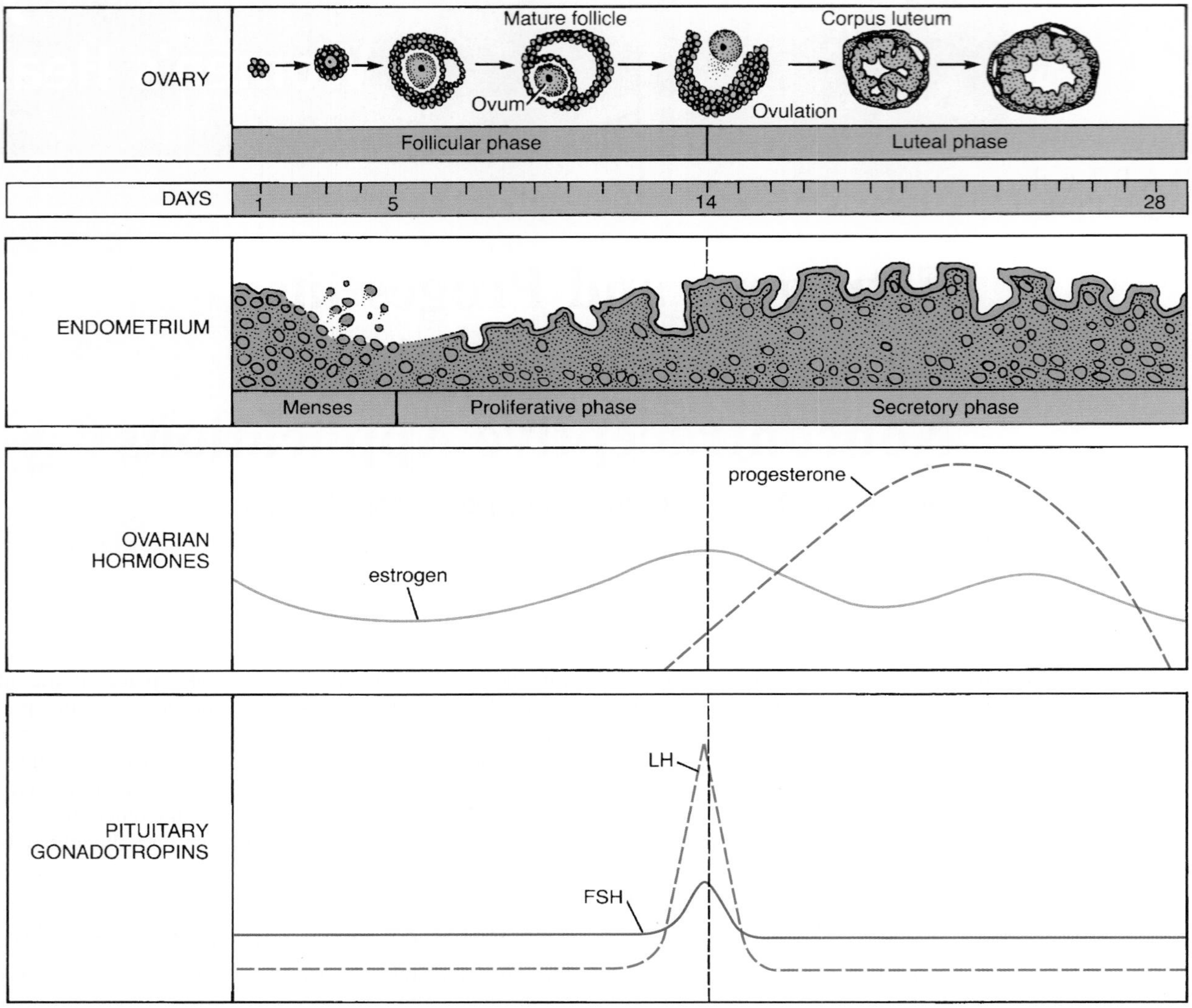

Figure 48.1 ▪ The menstrual cycle: anatomic and hormonal changes. FSH, follicle-stimulating hormone; LH, luteinizing hormone.

pituitary, thereby suppressing further FSH release. At midcycle, LH levels rise abruptly (see Fig. 48.1). This LH surge causes the dominant follicle to swell rapidly, burst, and release its ovum. After ovulation, the ruptured follicle becomes a corpus luteum and, under the influence of LH, begins to secrete progesterone.

ESTROGENS

Biosynthesis and Elimination

Females

In premenopausal women, the ovary is the principal source of estrogen. During the follicular phase of the menstrual cycle, estrogens are synthesized by ovarian follicles; during the luteal phase, estrogens are synthesized by the corpus luteum. The major estrogen produced by the ovaries is *estradiol.* In the periphery, some of the estradiol secreted by the ovaries is converted into *estrone* and *estriol,* hormones that are less potent than estradiol itself. Estrogens are eliminated by a combination of hepatic metabolism and urinary excretion.

During pregnancy, large quantities of estrogens are produced by the placenta. Excretion of these hormones results in high levels of estrogens in the urine.

Males

Estrogen production is not limited to females. In the human male, small amounts of testosterone are converted into estradiol and estrone by the testes. Enzymatic conversion of testosterone in peripheral tissues (e.g., liver, fat, skeletal muscle) results in additional estrogen production.

Mechanism of Action

Like other steroidal hormones (e.g., testosterone, cortisol), estrogen acts primarily through receptors in the cell nucleus, not on the cell surface. Hence, to produce its effects, estrogen must diffuse into cells, migrate to the nucleus, and then bind with an estrogen receptor (ER). The estrogen-ER complex then binds with an estrogen response element on a target gene, altering the rate of gene transcription. It is important to note that not all ERs are found in the nucleus: some ERs are found on cell membranes. Activating these surface receptors produces a rapid response—more rapid than can be produced by activating nuclear receptors.

There are two forms of ERs, termed ER alpha and ER beta. ER alpha is highly expressed in the vagina, uterus, ovaries, mammary glands, vascular epithelium, and hypothalamus. ER beta is expressed in the ovary and prostate and to a lesser extent in the lungs, brain, bones, and blood vessels. Some cells have both types of ER receptor.

Physiologic and Pharmacologic Effects

Effects on Primary and Secondary Sex Characteristics of Females

Estrogens support the development and maintenance of the female reproductive tract and secondary sex characteristics. These hormones are required for the growth and maturation of the uterus, vagina, fallopian tubes, and breasts. In addition, estrogens direct pigmentation of the nipples and genitalia.

Estrogens have a profound influence on physiologic processes related to reproduction. During the follicular phase of the menstrual cycle, estrogens promote (1) ductal growth in the breast, (2) thickening and cornification of the vaginal epithelium, (3) proliferation of the uterine epithelium, and (4) copious secretion of thickened mucus from endocervical glands. In addition, estrogens increase vaginal acidity (by promoting local deposition of glycogen, which is then acted on by lactobacilli and corynebacteria to produce lactic acid). At the end of the menstrual cycle, a decline in estrogen levels can bring on menstruation. However, it is the fall in progesterone levels at the end of the cycle that normally causes breakdown of the endometrium and resultant menstrual bleeding. After menstruation, estrogens promote endometrial restoration.

During pregnancy, the placenta produces estrogen in large amounts. This estrogen stimulates uterine blood flow and growth of uterine muscle. In addition, it acts on the breast to continue ductal proliferation. However, final transformation of the breast for milk production requires the combined influence of estrogen, progesterone, and human placental lactogen.

Metabolic Actions

Endogenous estrogens affect various nonreproductive tissues. Important among these are bone, cardiovascular, and central nervous system (CNS). They also have an important roles glucose homeostasis.

Bone

Estrogens have a positive effect on bone mass. Under normal conditions, bone undergoes continuous remodeling, a process in which bone mineral is resorbed and deposited in equal amounts. The principal effect of estrogens on the process is to block bone resorption, although estrogens may also promote mineral deposition.

During puberty, the long bones grow rapidly under the combined influence of growth hormone, adrenal androgens, and *low* levels of ovarian estrogens. When estrogen levels grow high enough, they promote epiphyseal closure and thereby bring linear growth to a stop.

Cardiovascular Effects

Cardiovascular disease is much less common in premenopausal women. Estrogens have several roles in lowering this risk. For example, estrogen receptors in the vascular smooth muscle respond to activation by decreasing vasoconstriction. Activation of estrogen receptors in vessel endothelium results in the production of nitric oxide, which results in vasodilation and increased perfusion. Estrogens also decrease atherosclerosis through favorable effects on cholesterol levels: levels of low-density lipoprotein (LDL) cholesterol are reduced, whereas levels of high-density lipoprotein (HDL) cholesterol are elevated.

Blood Coagulation

Estrogens both promote and suppress blood coagulation. Estrogens promote coagulation by (1) increasing levels of coagulation factors (e.g., factors II, VII, IX, X, and XII), and (2) decreasing levels of factors that suppress coagulation (e.g., antithrombin). Estrogens suppress coagulation by increasing the activity of factors that promote breakdown of fibrin, a protein that reinforces blood clots. The net effect—increased or decreased coagulation—may be determined by a hereditary defect in one of these targets.

Central Nervous System

In the CNS, estrogens have a neuroprotective effect by defending neurons from the effects of oxidative stress and injury. They also have a role in neuronal growth and repair through stimulation of nerve growth factors. Estrogen-induced synaptic changes, coupled with estrogen-promoted increases in synaptic serotonin, dopamine, and norepinephrine, are thought to preserve cognitive function, enhance short-term memory, and regulate mood. Cerebral perfusion is also enhanced by the release of nitric acid and the resulting vasodilation.

Glucose Homeostasis

Estrogens play an active role in maintaining glucose levels. In conditions that lead to insulin resistance due to impaired transport, estrogen has been shown to increase insulin sensitivity to promote glucose uptake. Estrogens also have a role in insulin secretion and are believed to protect pancreatic islet beta cells from certain types of injury.

Physiologic Alterations Accompanying Menopause

Menopause may occur as the result of surgery (i.e., surgical menopause associated with bilateral oophorectomy) or as the result of declining ovarian function associated with aging. Natural menopause typically begins at about age 51 to 52 years, with 95% of women entering menopause between the ages of 45 and 55 years. During the initial phase, the menstrual cycle becomes irregular, anovulatory cycles may occur, and periods of amenorrhea may alternate with menses. Eventually, ovulation and menstruation cease entirely. Production of ovarian estrogens decreases gradually, coming to a complete stop several years after menstruation has ceased.

Loss of estrogen has multiple effects. Prominent symptoms experienced by the patient include vasomotor symptoms, sleep disturbances, and urogenital atrophy. Additional physiologic changes include bone loss and altered lipid metabolism.

Vasomotor Symptoms

Vasomotor symptoms (hot flashes and night sweats) develop in about 70% of postmenopausal women. Episodes are characterized by sudden skin flushing, sweating, and a sensation of uncomfortable warmth. These episodes can occur at night, resulting in drenching sweats. Severe episodes can cause sleep disturbances, fatigue, and irritability. In most women, hot flashes abate within several months to a few years; in others, they may persist for a decade or more.

Urogenital Atrophy

Of all structures in the body, the urethra and vagina have the highest concentrations of estrogen receptors. Activation of these receptors maintains the functional integrity of the urethra and vaginal epithelium. Hence, when estrogen levels decline during menopause, these structures undergo degenerative change. Atrophy of the urethra causes urge incontinence and urinary frequency. Urethritis and urinary tract infections can also occur. Atrophy of the vaginal epithelium can lead to dryness and pain with intercourse. In addition, alterations in vaginal secretions result in decreased acidity, which can allow the growth of pathogenic bacteria, resulting in vaginal infections.

Mental Changes

Many women report cognitive changes such as difficulty in problem solving and short-term memory loss around the time when menopause begins. Others experience depression or an increase in anxiety. These, also, tended to occur during the time of transition and often compounded sleep disturbances.

Bone Loss

In the absence of estrogen, bone resorption accelerates, leading to a 12% loss of bone density shortly after menopause. Osteoporosis is characterized by bone demineralization, altered bone architecture, and reduced bone strength. Compression fractures of the vertebrae are common and can decrease height and produce a hump. In osteoporotic women, fractures of the hip and wrist can result from minimal trauma.

Altered Lipid Metabolism

Studies have demonstrated slight, but significant, increases in LDL cholesterol with concomitant decreases in HDL cholesterol. These are thought to have a role in the increase in cardiovascular disease that increases after menopause.

Clinical Pharmacology

Now that we have reviewed the effects of endogenous estrogens, let's examine how estrogen preparations are used clinically. We'll begin with a discussion of how these drugs are used.

Therapeutic Uses

Estrogens have contraceptive and noncontraceptive applications. In this chapter, discussion is limited to the noncontraceptive applications. Use of estrogens for contraception is discussed in Chapter 49.

Menopausal Hormone Therapy

Hormone therapy in postmenopausal women is the most common noncontraceptive use of estrogens. When estrogen is used for this purpose, it is usually accompanied by the use of progestins. For this reason, we will cover hormone therapy after the discussion of progestins.

Female Hypogonadism

In the absence of ovarian estrogens, pubertal transformation will not take place. Causes of estrogen deficiency include primary ovarian failure, hypopituitarism, bilateral oophorectomy (removal of both ovaries), and Turner syndrome (a genetic disorder that impairs gonadal function). In girls with estrogen insufficiency, puberty can be induced by giving exogenous estrogens. This treatment promotes breast development, maturation of the reproductive organs, and development of pubic and axillary hair. To simulate normal patterns of estrogen secretion, the regimen should consist of continuous low-dose therapy (for about a year) followed by cyclic administration of estrogen in higher doses. Estrogen therapy for these conditions is typically managed by specialists.

Acne

Estrogens, in the form of oral contraceptives, can help control acne. Treatment is limited to patients at least 14 or 15 years old who want contraception. Use of estrogen for acne is discussed in Chapter 85.

Cancer Palliation

Estrogens are sometimes used for palliative therapy in management of advanced prostate cancer in men and in a select type of metastatic breast cancer in both men and women. This use is directed by an oncologist or other specialist in this field.

Adverse Effects

The principal concerns with estrogen therapy are the potential for endometrial hyperplasia, endometrial cancer, breast cancer, and cardiovascular thromboembolic events. Of these, the potential for endometrial hyperplasia and endometrial cancer can be resolved by prescribing a progestin, if indicated.

Estrogens have been associated with gallbladder disease, jaundice, and headache. Use during menopause may produce or uncover gallbladder disease. Jaundice may develop in women with preexisting liver dysfunction, especially those who experienced cholestatic jaundice of pregnancy. Estrogens can increase the risk for headache, especially migraine.

Nausea is the most frequent undesired response to the estrogens. Fortunately, nausea diminishes with continued use and is rarely so severe as to necessitate treatment cessation. Fluid retention with edema commonly occurs. Most other adverse effects are more of a nuisance (e.g., chloasma, a patchy brown facial discoloration) than a concern.

Contraindications

Estrogens should not be taken by patients with a history of deep vein thrombosis (DVT), pulmonary embolus, or conditions such as stroke or myocardial infarction (MI) that occurred secondary to a thromboembolic event. They should not be prescribed to women who are pregnant or who have vaginal bleeding without a known cause. Patients with a history of liver disease, estrogen-dependent tumors, or breast cancer (except when indicated for management) also should not take estrogens.

Interactions

Estrogens are major substrates of CYP1A2 and CYP3A4. Inducers of these isoenzymes may lower estrogen levels, whereas drugs that are inhibitors may raise estrogen levels. Additionally, they may decrease the effectiveness of some antidiabetic drugs and thyroid preparations. Estrogens can also interact with anticoagulants and other drugs that affect clotting.

Preparations and Routes of Administration

Estrogen is available in conjugated and esterified forms. Esterified estrogens are plant based; conjugated estrogens are natural preparations derived from the urine of pregnant horses. Until mid-2016 synthetic conjugated estrogens A [Cenestin] and B [Enjuvia] were available; however, the manufacturer has withdrawn them from the market. At the time of this writing, there is no generic substitution for these synthetic conjugated estrogens.

Oral

Owing to convenience, the oral route is used more than any other. The most active estrogenic compound—estradiol—is available alone and in combination with progestins.

Transdermal

Transdermal estradiol is available in four formulations:

- Emulsion [Estrasorb]
- Spray [Evamist]
- Gels [EstroGel, Elestrin, Divigel]
- Patches [Alora, Climara, Estraderm, Menostar, Vivelle-Dot, Oesclim ♣]

Application is specific to certain body regions. The emulsion is applied once daily to the top of both thighs and the back of both calves. The spray is applied once daily to the forearm. The gel is applied once daily to one arm, from the shoulder to the wrist or to the thigh (Divigel). The patches are applied to the skin of the trunk (but not the breasts). Rates of estrogen absorption with transdermal formulations range from 14 to 60 mcg/24 hr, depending on the product employed.

Compared with oral formulations, the transdermal formulations have four advantages:

- The total dose of estrogen is greatly reduced (because the liver is bypassed).
- There is less nausea and vomiting.
- Blood levels of estrogen fluctuate less.
- There is a lower risk for DVT, pulmonary embolism, and stroke.

Intravaginal

Estrogens for intravaginal administration are available as tablets, creams, and vaginal rings. The tablets [Vagifem], creams [Estrace Vaginal, Premarin Vaginal], and one of the two available vaginal rings [Estring] are used only for local effects, primarily treatment of vulval and vaginal atrophy associated with menopause. The other vaginal ring [Femring] is used for systemic effects (e.g., control of hot flashes and night sweats) as well as local effects (e.g., treatment of vulval and vaginal atrophy).

Parenteral

Although estrogens are formulated for intravenous (IV) and intramuscular (IM) administration, use of these routes is rare. IV administration is generally limited to acute, emergency control of heavy uterine bleeding.

SELECTIVE ESTROGEN RECEPTOR MODULATORS

Selective estrogen receptor modulators (SERMs) are drugs that activate estrogen receptors in some tissues and block them in others. These drugs were developed in an effort to provide the benefits of estrogen (e.g., protection against osteoporosis, maintenance of the urogenital tract, reduction of LDL cholesterol) while avoiding its drawbacks (e.g., promotion of breast cancer, uterine cancer, and thromboembolism). Four SERMs are available: tamoxifen [Nolvadex-D], toremifene [Fareston], raloxifene [Evista], and bazedoxifene [Duavee]. None of these offers all of the benefits of estrogen, and none avoids all of the drawbacks.

Patient Education

ESTROGEN ADMINISTRATION

Transdermal Patch.

Give the patient the following instructions for using estradiol transdermal patches:

- Apply to an area of clean, dry, intact skin on the abdomen or some other region of the trunk (but not the breasts or waistline) by pressing the patch firmly in place for 10 seconds.
- If the patch falls off, reapply the same patch or, if necessary, apply a new patch.
- Remove the old patch and apply a new patch once or twice weekly according to the product specifications.
- Rotate the application site such that the same site is not used more than once each week.

Transdermal Emulsion.

Instruct the patient to apply the emulsion each morning to the top of both thighs and the back of both calves.

Transdermal Gel.

Instruct the patient to apply the gel once daily after showering to one arm, from the shoulder to the wrist.

Transdermal Spray.

Instruct the patient to apply 1, 2, or 3 sprays once daily to the inner forearm, and then let it dry at least 2 minutes before dressing and at least 30 minutes before washing.

Intravaginal Cream.

Instruct the patient to apply estrogen cream high into the vagina, usually at bedtime, using the applicator provided.

Intravaginal Ring.

Instruct the patient to insert the ring as deeply as possible, and to leave it in place for 3 months, after which it should be removed, and then replaced with a new ring if indicated.

Intravaginal Tablet.

Inform patients that dosing consists of 1 tablet daily for 2 weeks, followed by 1 tablet twice a week thereafter. Instruct patients to insert each tablet as far as comfortably possible using the applicator supplied.

Tamoxifen was the first SERM to be widely used. By blocking estrogen receptors, tamoxifen (and its active metabolite, endoxifen) can inhibit cell growth in the breast. As a result, the drug is used extensively to prevent and treat breast cancer. Unfortunately, blockade of estrogen receptors also produces hot flashes. By activating estrogen receptors, tamoxifen protects against osteoporosis and has a favorable effect on serum lipids. However, receptor activation also increases the risk for endometrial cancer and thromboembolism. The pharmacology of tamoxifen and toremifene (a close relative of tamoxifen) is discussed in Chapter 82.

Raloxifene is very similar to tamoxifen. The principal difference is that raloxifene does not activate estrogen receptors in the endometrium and hence does not pose a risk for uterine cancer. Like tamoxifen, raloxifene protects against breast cancer and osteoporosis, promotes thromboembolism, and induces hot flashes. Raloxifene is approved only for prevention and treatment of osteoporosis and for prevention of breast cancer in high-risk women. Raloxifene is discussed at length in Chapter 59.

In 2013, the U.S. Food and Drug Administration (FDA) approved *Duavee* (conjugated estrogens/bazedoxifene) for prevention of vasomotor symptoms and osteoporosis in postmenopausal women with a uterus. Duavee is the first drug to combine estrogen with an estrogen agonist/antagonist (bazedoxifene). The bazedoxifene component of Duavee reduces the risk for excessive growth of the lining of the uterus that can occur with the estrogen component. Contraindications to taking Duavee are the same as for other estrogen-containing products.

PROGESTINS

Estrogens and progestins are often prescribed together. Before we discuss these uses, it will be helpful to discuss progesterone. As previously mentioned, progesterone is the principal endogenous progestational hormone. As its name implies, progesterone acts before gestation to prepare the uterus for implantation of a fertilized ovum. In addition, progesterone helps maintain the uterus throughout pregnancy.

Biosynthesis

Progesterone is produced by the ovaries *and* the placenta. Ovarian production occurs during the second half of the menstrual cycle. During this period, progesterone is synthesized by the corpus luteum, in response to LH released from the anterior pituitary. If implantation of a fertilized ovum does not occur, progesterone production by the corpus luteum ceases, and menstrual flow begins. However, if implantation *does* take place, the developing trophoblast will produce its own luteotropic hormone—human chorionic gonadotropin (hCG)—that will stimulate the corpus luteum to continue making progesterone. For the first 7 weeks of gestation, the placenta depends entirely on progesterone from the corpus luteum. However, between weeks 7 and 10, production of progesterone is shared between the corpus luteum and placenta. After 10 weeks of gestation, progesterone made by the placenta is sufficient to support pregnancy, and hence ovarian progesterone production declines. Placental synthesis of progesterone and estrogen continues throughout the pregnancy.

Mechanism of Action

As with estrogen, receptors for progesterone are found in the cell nucleus. Hence, to produce an effect, progesterone must diffuse across the cell membrane, migrate to the nucleus, and then bind with a progesterone receptor (PR). The progesterone-PR complex then binds with a progesterone regulatory element on a target gene, thereby rapidly increasing gene transcription. As with estrogen, there are two types of receptors for progesterone, designated PR-A and PR-B. In general, the stimulatory actions of progesterone are mediated by PR-B, whereas inhibitory actions are mediated by PR-A.

Physiologic Effects

Effects During the Menstrual Cycle

Progesterone is secreted during the second half of the menstrual cycle from a proliferative state into a secretory state. If implantation does not occur, progesterone production by the corpus luteum declines. The resultant fall in progesterone levels is the principal stimulus for the onset of menstruation.

In addition to affecting the endometrium, progesterone affects the endocervical glands, breasts, body temperature, respiration, and mood. Under the influence of progesterone, secretions from endocervical glands become scant and viscous. (In contrast, estrogen makes these secretions profuse and watery.) In addition, progesterone causes the epithelium of the breast to divide and grow. Actions in the CNS may cause depression and sleepiness. By increasing the sensitivity of the respiratory center to CO_2, progesterone causes the partial pressure of carbon dioxide (P_{CO_2}) in blood to fall. At midcycle, when ovulation occurs, progesterone raises body temperature by 0.6° C (1° F).

Effects During Pregnancy

As noted, progesterone levels increase during pregnancy. These high levels suppress contraction of *uterine smooth muscle* and thereby help sustain pregnancy. Unfortunately, progesterone also suppresses contraction of *GI smooth muscle,* which leads to prolonged transit time and constipation. In the *breast,* progesterone promotes growth and proliferation of alveolar tubules (acini), the structures that produce milk. Metabolic effects include suppression of arterial P_{CO_2}, altered serum bicarbonate content, and elevation of serum pH. Lastly, progesterone may help suppress the maternal immune system, thereby preventing immune attack on the fetus.

Clinical Pharmacology

Now that we have reviewed the effects of endogenous progesterone, let's examine how progestins are used clinically. We'll begin with a discussion of therapeutic uses.

Therapeutic Uses

Discussion in this chapter is limited to the noncontraceptive uses of progestins. Use for contraception is considered in Chapter 49.

Menopausal Hormone Therapy

The primary noncontraceptive use of progestins is to counteract the adverse effects of estrogen on the endometrium in women undergoing menopausal hormone therapy (HT). This application is discussed later.

Dysfunctional Uterine Bleeding

This condition, characterized by heavy irregular bleeding, occurs when progesterone levels are insufficient to balance the stimulatory influence of estrogen on the endometrium. In the absence of sufficient progesterone, estrogen puts the endometrium in a state of continuous proliferation. Because progesterone is unavailable to induce monthly endometrial breakdown, the excessively proliferative endometrium undergoes spontaneous sloughing at irregular intervals. The result is periodic episodes of severe bleeding.

Treatment has two objectives: the initial goal is cessation of hemorrhage; the long-term goal is to establish a regular monthly cycle. Excessive bleeding can be stopped by administering a progestin for 10 to 14 days. When dosing is stopped, withdrawal bleeding takes place. Bleeding is likely to be profuse and associated with cramping. Giving an oral contraceptive twice daily for 5 to 7 days can help stabilize the endometrium and thereby reduce bleeding duration.

Cyclic therapy is employed to establish a regular monthly cycle. In one regimen, oral dosing is started 10 to 14 days after the onset of each menstrual period and continued for the next 10 days. Alternatively, a progestin can be given for the first 10 days of each month. Both approaches can promote regular endometrial breakdown and menstruation.

Amenorrhea

Progestins can induce menstrual flow in selected women who are experiencing amenorrhea. If endogenous estrogen levels are adequate, treatment with a progestin for 5 to 10 days will be followed by withdrawal bleeding when the progestin is stopped. If estrogen levels are low, it may be necessary to induce endometrial proliferation with an estrogen before giving the progestin.

Endometrial Carcinoma and Hyperplasia

Progestins can provide palliation in women with metastatic endometrial carcinoma, but these drugs do not prolong life. Several months of treatment may be required for a response. Management is by specialists.

Endometrial hyperplasia, a potentially precancerous condition, can be suppressed with progestins. Benefits derive from counteracting the proliferative effects of estrogen. Treatment options include oral therapy with megestrol acetate [Megace] or medroxyprogesterone acetate [Provera] and local delivery of a levonorgestrel using the Mirena IUD.

Other Uses

Progestins are used to support an early pregnancy in women with corpus luteum deficiency syndrome and in women undergoing in vitro fertilization (IVF). One progestin—hydroxyprogesterone acetate [Makena]—is approved for preventing preterm birth in women with a singleton pregnancy and a history of preterm delivery.

Adverse Effects

Up to 20% of patients may experience breast tenderness, headache, abdominal discomfort, arthralgias, and depression. When used continuously for birth control, progestins greatly decrease production of cervical mucus and cause involution of the endometrial layer. Effects on the endometrium lead to spotting, breakthrough bleeding, and irregular menses. Progestins, in combination with estrogen, increase the risk for breast cancer in postmenopausal women.

Preparations and Routes of Administration

Progestins are available in oral, IM, subcutaneous (subQ), intravaginal, intrauterine, and transdermal formulations. Older oral progestins include medroxyprogesterone acetate [Provera], norethindrone [Micronor, Nor-QD, others], norethindrone acetate [Aygestin], megestrol acetate [Megace], levonorgestrel [Plan B One-Step, Next Choice], and a micronized formulation of progesterone [Prometrium]. Newer oral progestins—norgestimate and drospirenone—are available in fixed-dose combinations with estradiol sold as Prefest and Angeliq, respectively. Intramuscular progestins are medroxyprogesterone acetate [Depo-Provera] and progesterone (in oil). Medroxyprogesterone acetate is also available in a formulation for subQ injection [Depo-SubQ Provera 104]. Micronized progesterone for intravaginal use is available as progesterone gel [Crinone] and a vaginal insert [Endometrin]. Transdermal products are limited to norethindrone (formulated with estradiol under the name CombiPatch) and levonorgestrel (formulated with estradiol under the name ClimaraPro). A second-generation progestin—etonogestrel—used for contraception is available by itself as a subQ implant [Nexplanon] and combined with estradiol in a vaginal ring [NuvaRing].

MENOPAUSAL HORMONE THERAPY

Menopausal HT, formerly known as *hormone replacement therapy* (HRT), consists of low doses of estrogen (with or without a progestin) taken to compensate for the loss of estrogen that occurs during menopause. There are two basic regimens for HT: estrogen alone (ET) and estrogen plus a progestin (estrogen/progestin therapy [EPT]). The purpose of estrogen in both regimens is to control menopausal symptoms by replacing estrogen that was lost owing to menopause. The progestin is present for one reason only: to counterbalance estrogen-mediated stimulation of the endometrium, which can lead to endometrial hyperplasia and cancer. (Progestins should not be prescribed for women who have undergone hysterectomy.)

It is typically the vasomotor symptoms that compel most women to seek HT. Hot flashes and the drenching sweats that accompany them can interfere with daily life and cause sleepless nights. Not only are they uncomfortable, but they also may create embarrassing situations, especially for women working with the public when appearances can be important. When vasomotor symptoms are severe, HT can be truly life changing.

Women who take HT often report an improved quality of life as well. In addition to controlling vasomotor symptoms, they report improved sleep, restoration of libido, improved cognition, and enhanced mood. Although there have been insufficient studies to quantify quality-of-life issues, the anecdotal evidence supports this as an added benefit.

From the medical perspective, HT confers three primary benefits: suppression of vasomotor symptoms, prevention of urogenital atrophy, and prevention of osteoporosis and related fractures. For all three, treatment is highly effective. (Unfortunately, the benefits of urogenital atrophy and osteoporosis prevention are not sustained and will decline after HT is withdrawn.)

Given the positive physiologic effects of estrogen and the detrimental physiologic changes that occur with estrogen loss, it might seem logical to prescribe HT for all women experiencing menopause. Indeed, this was once common practice with therapy that began during perimenopause and continued into later years of life. Then, in the early 2000s, data from two landmark studies, the Women's Health Initiative (WHI) and the Heart and Estrogen/progestin Replacement Study and its follow-up (HERS and HERS II), demonstrated that, contrary to popular assumptions, use of HT could increase, rather than prevent, cardiovascular events. Women taking HT in the study also had an increase in thromboembolic events such as DVT and stroke. For women receiving EPT (but not ET), there was a significant increase in the incidence of breast cancer. The reaction in the medical community was strong and swift as many providers stopped prescribing HT altogether and use of HT declined by 80%.

More recently, increased scrutiny of these early studies yielded concerns that have resulted in a reexamination of these risks. Subjects in those studies tended to be older. For example, only 3.5% of women in the WHI study were in the 50- to 54-year age range, which is the age at which most women currently begin HT. Further, the therapy in those studies was at a higher dose, and use was prolonged beyond that of recommended current practice. When WHI data for women aged 50 to 59 years taking HT for less than 10 years were examined, it was discovered that the increase in venous thromboembolic episodes was only between 1.1 to 5 out of 1000 women taking ET and 5.1 to 10 out of 1000 women taking EPT. For women taking ET, there was no increase in coronary heart disease (CHD), and for women taking EPT, CHD increase was 1.1 to 5 out of 1000 women, and venothrombotic episode increase was 5.1 to 10 out of 1000 women. Moreover, when benefits were examined, *for both ET and EPT, 5.1 to 10 out of 1000 women experienced a reduction in overall mortality compared with women not taking HT.*

Subsequent and ongoing research has provided more insight into the relationships of HT to dosage, time of initiation, length of use, and patient age, which were not adequately accounted for in the original reports from these studies. The more informed view of HT has evolved to a more reasoned approach to HT.

Benefits and Risks of Hormone Therapy

As with any drug, prescribing decisions require weighing the benefits and risks. It is important to keep in mind that our understanding of the benefits and risks of HT continues to evolve as current research focuses on the new demographic of younger woman taking HT at lower doses over fewer years.

Prototype Drugs

ESTROGENS AND PROGESTINS

Estrogens

Conjugated estrogens [Premarin]
Estradiol

Progestins

Medroxyprogesterone acetate
Norethindrone

Recognizing that findings based on women older than 60 years taking high-dose, long-term HT for more than a decade could not be generalized to younger women taking low-dose HT for shorter time intervals, The Endocrine Society undertook an extensive review of published research to determine the benefits and risk of HT in women recently menopausal (i.e., less than 10 years postmenopausal) and aged 50 to 59. Significant findings are summarized in Table 48.1. Not included in the table are results of benefits related to the vasomotor and urogenital symptoms because the benefit (90% reduction in symptoms) is firmly established. Also not included are many of the previously assumed risks that were not supported in the data.

Based on these findings, especially considering the benefits of overall mortality, it certainly seems unreasonable to refuse HT for younger women desiring it once individual risks are assessed. Unfortunately, this does not address concerns of older women who have indications for therapy. More studies are needed; however, in the meantime, it is important to recognize that risk for complications increases with age. Further, research findings suggest that use of HT in women older than 65 years may increase the risk for dementia.

TABLE 48.1 ▪ Benefits and Risks of Menopausal Hormone Therapy

	Number of Fewer Cases Per 1000 Women Aged 50–59 Years	
Benefits Over 5 Years	**Estrogen + Progestin (EPT)**	**Estrogen Only (ET)**
Coronary heart disease	0.9	3.8
Osteoporotic fractures	4.9	5.9
Breast cancer	—	1.5
Colorectal cancer	1.2	—
Type 2 diabetes mellitus	11	11
Mortality for all causes	5.3 fewer deaths	5 fewer deaths
	Number of Increased Cases Per 1000 Women Aged 50–59 Years	
Risk Over 5 Years	**Estrogen + Progestin (EPT)**	**Estrogen Only (ET)**
Thromboembolism	5	2
Stroke	1.0	1.2
Breast cancer	6.8	—
Cholecystitis*	9.6	14.2

*Data specific for cholecystitis are based on a larger demographic because data specific to ages 50 to 59 years were not available.

Recommendations on Hormone Therapy Use

When making decisions regarding whether or not to prescribe HT, risk factors for the individual must be inventoried, and the hoped-for benefits should be clearly defined. For women with significant baseline risks (e.g., personal or family history of breast cancer, cardiovascular disease), the risk for harm from HT goes up.

Recently, several expert sources have issued revised recommendations on HT. The recommendations that follow represent a composite of those offered by four groups: the North American Menopause Society, The Endocrine Society, the FDA, and the U.S. Preventive Services Task Force (USPSTF). Fig. 48.2 provides additional guidance.

General Recommendations

To balance benefits and risks, an individual risk profile should be compiled for every woman considering HT. All candidates for HT should be informed of known risks. Women with multiple risk factors should consider alternative therapies. For most women, the benefits of *long-term* HT for disease prevention do not outweigh the risks and hence long-term HT should generally be avoided. Conversely, the benefits of short-term therapy (less than 5 years) to treat menopausal symptoms often *do* justify the risks. To keep risk as low as possible, HT should be used in the lowest dosage and for the shortest time needed to accomplish treatment goals.

Use for Approved Indications

Hormone therapy has only three approved indications:

- Treatment of moderate to severe vasomotor symptoms associated with menopause

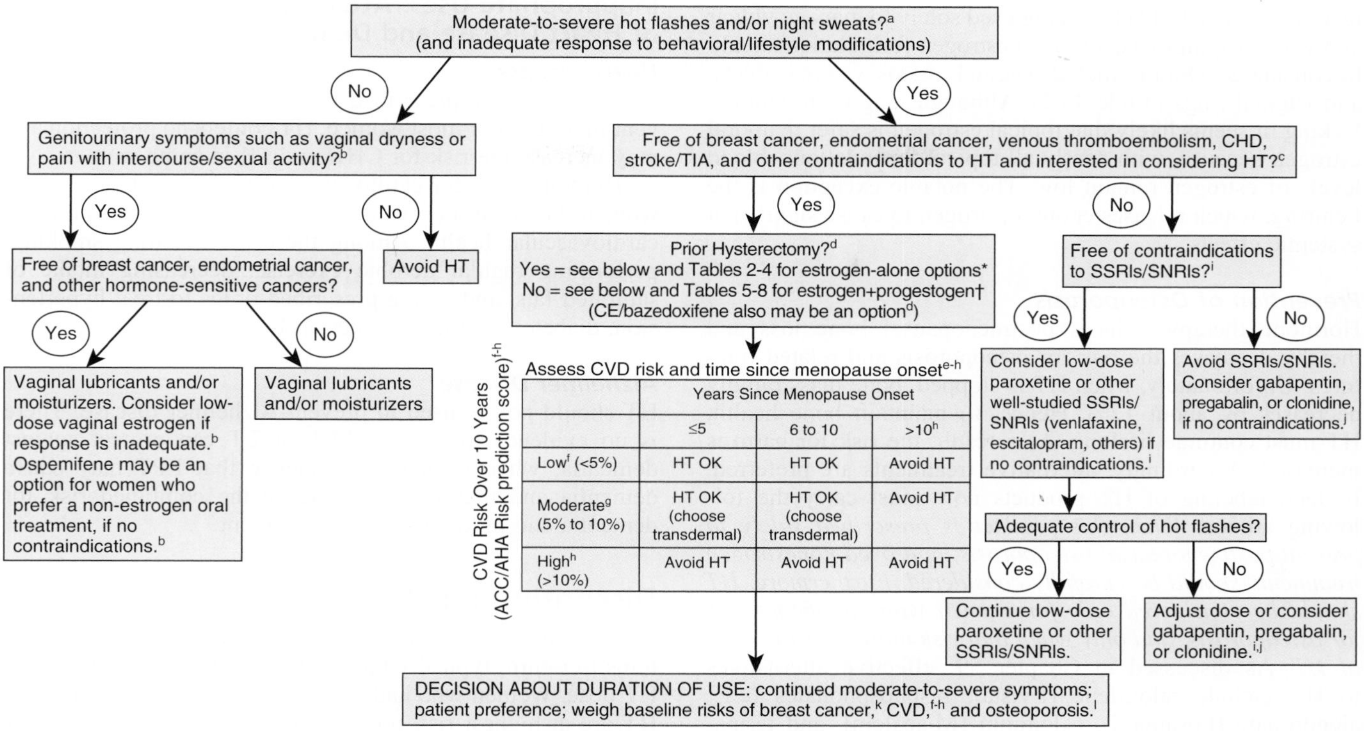

Figure 48.2 ■ Algorithm for menopausal symptom management.
ACC/AHA, American College of Cardiology/American Heart Association; ASCVD, atherosclerotic cardiovascular disease; CE, conjugated estrogens; CHD, coronary heart disease; CVD, cardiovascular disease; EPT, estrogen plus progestogen therapy; ET, estrogen therapy; FDA, U.S. Food and Drug Administration; FSH, follicle stimulating hormone; hCG, human chorionic gonadotropin; HT, menopausal hormone therapy; NAMS, North American Menopause Society; PRL, prolactin; SNRI, serotonin-norepinephrine reuptake inhibitor; SSRI, selective serotonin reuptake inhibitors; TIA, transient ischemic attack; TSH, thyroid-stimulating hormone. (From the North American Menopause Society, http://www.menopause.org/docs/default-source/2014/menopro-app-algorithm-2014.pdf.)

- Treatment of moderate to severe symptoms of vulvar and vaginal atrophy associated with menopause
- Prevention of postmenopausal osteoporosis

Hormone therapy should be restricted to achieving one or more of these goals. With the first two indications, duration of treatment is relatively short (typically 3–4 years), and hence the risk for harm is relatively low—except for women with established heart disease. In contrast, prevention of osteoporosis requires lifelong HT, and hence the risk for harm is higher.

The only indication for long-term *progestin* therapy is protection against endometrial cancer, which could be caused by unopposed estrogen. Accordingly, use of EPT should be limited to women with an intact uterus. For women who have had a hysterectomy, estrogen alone should be used.

Treatment of Vasomotor Symptoms

Hormone therapy is the most effective treatment for vasomotor symptoms (hot flashes, night sweats). To increase safety, the lowest effective dosage should be employed. Furthermore, because vasomotor symptoms subside over time, the need for continued HT should be reassessed at regular intervals.

For women determined to be at too high risk for HT, other options are available, but they are less effective than estrogen. Trials have shown that two antidepressants—*escitalopram* [Lexapro] and *desvenlafaxine* [Pristiq]—can produce a modest but meaningful reduction in both the frequency and severity of hot flashes. Escitalopram is a selective serotonin reuptake inhibitor (SSRI); desvenlafaxine is a serotonin-norepinephrine reuptake inhibitor (SNRI). Other SSRIs and SNRIs are likely to be effective as well. *Paroxetine* [Brisdelle], an SSRI, was approved in 2013 for the treatment of vasomotor symptoms in menopause. Paroxetine is used as an antidepressant and is discussed further in Chapter 25.

By contrast, controlled trials have shown that soy isoflavones do *not* reduce hot flashes. In fact, these preparations may make symptoms worse.

Treatment of Symptoms of Vulvar and Vaginal Atrophy

Estrogen is the most effective treatment for reducing symptoms of menopause-related vulvar and vaginal atrophy, characterized by dryness, irritation, and uncomfortable intercourse. Because systemic estrogen carries significant risks, the FDA recommends that, if HT is being used solely to manage vulvar and vaginal symptoms, a topical estrogen formulation should be considered. Options include vaginal creams, vaginal tablets, and vaginal rings (Table 48.2). Although long-term data are lacking, it seems likely that topical estrogen is safer than oral estrogen because, with nearly all topical formulations, blood levels of estrogen remain low. The notable exception is the Femring, which releases enough estrogen to cause significant systemic effects.

Prevention of Osteoporosis

Hormone therapy reduces postmenopausal bone loss and thereby decreases the risk for osteoporosis and related fractures. Unfortunately, when HT is stopped, bone mass rapidly decreases by about 12%. Hence, to maintain bone health, HT must continue lifelong. As a result, the risk for harm is increased. Accordingly, alternative treatments are preferred. In fact, labeling of HT products now must carry the following advice: *When this product is prescribed solely to prevent postmenopausal osteoporosis, approved nonestrogen treatments should be carefully considered. Furthermore, HT should be considered only for women with significant risk for osteoporosis, and only when that risk outweighs the risks of HT.* As discussed in Chapter 59, effective alternatives to HT include raloxifene [Evista], bisphosphonates (e.g., alendronate [Fosamax]), calcitonin [Miacalcin], and teriparatide [Forteo]. Of course, all women (not to mention men) should practice primary prevention of bone loss by ensuring adequate intake of calcium and vitamin D, performing regular weight-bearing exercise, and avoiding smoking and excessive alcohol use.

TABLE 48.2 ▪ Intravaginal Estrogens for Menopausal Hormone Therapy*

Generic Name	Trade Name	Usual Maintenance Dosage
VAGINAL CREAMS		
Conjugated estrogens	Premarin	Apply 0.5–2 g/day (625 mcg conjugated estrogens/g).†
Estradiol	Estrace	Apply 1–2 g 1–3 times/wk (100 mcg estradiol/g)
VAGINAL RINGS		
Estradiol	Estring	This 2-mg ring releases 7.5 mcg/day for 90 days.
Estradiol acetate	Femring	The 12.4-mg ring releases 50 mcg/day for 90 days.* The 24.8-mg ring releases 100 mcg/day for 90 days.*
VAGINAL TABLETS		
Estradiol hemihydrate	Vagifem	Insert 1 tablet (10 mcg) every day for 2 wk, then 1 tablet twice a week thereafter.

*All intravaginal estrogens are used to treat urogenital atrophy. With one product—Femring—estradiol is absorbed in amounts sufficient to cause systemic effects, both beneficial (e.g., suppression of vasomotor symptoms) and adverse (e.g., increased risk for thrombosis).

†Administer cyclically (3 weeks on and 1 week off). For short-term use only.

Inappropriate Uses: Attempted Prevention of Heart Disease and Dementia

Heart Disease

HT should *not* be prescribed for the express purpose of preventing CHD. For most women, HT confers no protection and may increase the risk for CHD and MI in some women.

To reduce risk for cardiovascular events, postmenopausal women should be counseled about alternative ways to promote cardiovascular health. Among these are avoiding smoking, performing regular aerobic exercise, decreasing intake of saturated fats, and taking prescribed drugs to treat hypertension, diabetes, and high cholesterol.

Alzheimer Disease

HT should not be used to prevent Alzheimer disease. There is no evidence that either EPT or ET can protect against dementia, whereas there *is* evidence that EPT may *cause* dementia and that ET can increase the combined risk for dementia and mild cognitive impairment.

Discontinuing Hormone Therapy

Unfortunately, discontinuation may cause vasomotor symptoms to return; typically this occurs within 4 days of the last HT dose. Women who had severe symptoms before initiating HT are at highest risk for developing intolerable symptoms when they stop.

No firm guidelines exist for stopping HT. There are two basic methods: immediate cessation and tapering slowly. However, there are no controlled studies to indicate which option might result in fewer symptoms. For women who choose to taper slowly, again there are two basic options, referred to as "dose tapering" and "day tapering." With dose tapering, dosing is done every day, but the size of the daily dose is gradually reduced. If intense symptoms return after a dosage reduction, further reductions should be delayed until symptoms improve. With day tapering, the daily dose remains unchanged, but the number of days between doses is gradually increased—starting with dosing every other day, then every third day, and so on. Regardless of which method is used—dose tapering or day tapering—only the dosage of *estrogen* should be lowered. For women on EPT, the *progestin dosage should remain unchanged* because lowering the progestin dosage might permit estrogen to stimulate endometrial growth, thereby posing a risk for endometrial hyperplasia.

Drug Products for Hormone Therapy

Preparations

Preparations for HT are listed in Tables 48.2, 48.3, and 48.4. Dosing may be oral, transdermal, or intravaginal. The oral estrogens employed most often are conjugated equine estrogens [Premarin] (prepared by extraction from pregnant mares' urine), estradiol [Estrace], and estropipate. For transdermal therapy, estradiol is the only estrogen employed, formulated in patches, gels, a spray, and an emulsion. Oral estrogen/progestin combinations include conjugated equine estrogens/medroxyprogesterone acetate [Prempro, Premphase], estradiol/norethindrone acetate [Activella], and ethinyl estradiol/norethindrone [Femhrt]. Combination estrogen/progestin patches are estradiol/norethindrone [CombiPatch] and estradiol/levonorgestrel [ClimaraPro]. Intravaginal products—formulated

TABLE 48.3 ▪ Oral Drugs for Menopausal Hormone Therapy

Generic Name	Trade Name	Usual Dosage
ESTROGENS		
Conjugated estrogens, equine	Premarin	0.3–1.25 mg/day
Esterified estrogens	Menest, Estragen ♣	0.3–2.5 mg/day
Estradiol, micronized	Estrace	0.5–2 mg/day
Estropipate	Generic only	0.75–6 mg/day
PROGESTINS*		
Medroxyprogesterone acetate	Provera	2.5–10 mg
Progesterone (micronized)	Prometrium	200 mg
ESTROGEN/PROGESTIN COMBINATIONS*		
Conjugated estrogens/medroxyprogesterone acetate	Prempro	0.3/1.5, 0.45/1.5, 0.625/2.5, or 0.625/5 mg daily
Conjugated estrogens/medroxyprogesterone acetate	Premphase	*Days 1–14:* 0.625 mg estrogen (alone) daily *Days 15–28:* 0.625/5 mg estrogen/progesterone daily
Estradiol/drospirenone	Angeliq	0.5/0.25 or 1/0.5 mg daily
Estradiol/norethindrone acetate	Activella	0.5/0.1 or 1/0.5 mg daily
Estradiol/norgestimate	Prefest	1 mg estradiol every day; 0.09 mg norgestimate in a repeating cycle of 3 days on and 3 days off
Ethinyl estradiol/norethindrone	Femhrt	2.5 mcg/0.5 mg or 5 mcg/1 mg daily
OTHER ESTROGEN COMBINATIONS		
Esterified estrogens/methyltestosterone	Covaryx	1.25 mg/2.5 mg daily
Esterified estrogens/methyltestosterone	Covaryx HS	0.625/1.25 mg daily
Conjugated estrogens/bazedoxifene†	Duavee	0.45 mg/20 mg twice daily

*Progestins are used to counteract the effects of estrogen on the uterus. The progestins listed can be used when the regimen calls for taking estrogen and progestin separately, rather than using a combination product. In estrogen/progestin regimens, the estrogen is taken daily, and the progestin is taken daily or intermittently (e.g., 14 days on, 14 days off).

†Bazedoxifene is an estrogen antagonist/selective estrogen receptor modulator that acts to reduce excessive growth of the uterine lining that can occur with the estrogen component.

as tablets, creams, and rings—are used primarily to manage symptoms of urogenital atrophy.

Dosing Schedules

Every woman undergoing systemic HT receives an estrogen, and every woman with a uterus also receives a progestin to counteract the stimulant effects of estrogen on the endometrium. Several dosing schedules may be employed. Estrogen and progestin are commonly administered *continuously.* An alternative is to give estrogen continuously but give the progestin cyclically (e.g., on calendar days 15 through 28). However, cyclic progestin has the disadvantage of promoting monthly bleeding, which may explain why most women prefer continuous dosing.

Vaginal estrogens can be given continuously for 1 to 2 weeks, followed by dosing 1 to 3 times per week, titrating the dosing schedule based on symptoms. Estring remains in the vagina for 3 months, after which it is removed and replaced with a new ring.

PRESCRIBING AND MONITORING CONSIDERATIONS

BLACK BOX WARNING: ESTROGEN THERAPY

Endometrial cancer risk is increased in women with a uterus who take unopposed estrogen.

Estrogen may increase the risk for DVT and stroke.

Estrogen is not indicated for cardiovascular disease or dementia and may increase the risk for dementia in women aged 65 years and older.

Estrogens

Preadministration Assessment

Therapeutic Goal

Estrogens are used primarily for contraception (see Chapter 49) and for menopausal HT but only to prevent osteoporosis, suppress vasomotor symptoms, and manage symptoms related to vulvar and vaginal atrophy. Indications unrelated to HT are female hypogonadism, prostate cancer, and dysfunctional uterine bleeding.

Baseline Data

Assessment should include a breast examination, pelvic examination, lipid profile, mammography, and blood pressure measurement. If the indication for HT is vasomotor symptoms, menopause should be verified by a serum FSH level.

Identifying High-Risk Patients

Estrogens are *contraindicated* for patients with estrogen-dependent cancers, undiagnosed abnormal vaginal bleeding, active thrombophlebitis or thromboembolic disorders, or a history of estrogen-associated thrombophlebitis, thrombosis, or thromboembolic disorders. A baseline mammogram can be used to detect breast cancer before prescribing.

Dosing Schedules for Hormone Therapy

Women with an intact uterus should receive estrogen plus progestin, whereas women who have had a hysterectomy should use estrogen alone. In both cases, dosing with oral estrogen is done *daily.* With estrogen plus progestin, the progestin component may be given *daily* or cyclically 10 days per month.

Ongoing Monitoring and Interventions

Monitoring Summary

Because these drugs affect breast and uterine function, the patient should receive a yearly follow-up breast and pelvic examination.

TABLE 48.4 ▪ Transdermal Drugs for Menopausal Hormone Therapy

Generic Name	Trade Name	Strength (mcg absorbed/day)	Application
ESTROGENS			
Transdermal Patches			
Estradiol	Menostar	14	Once weekly
	Climara	25, 37.5, 50, 60, 75, 100	Once weekly
	Alora	25, 50, 75, 100	Twice weekly
	Oesclim ♣	25, 37.5, 50, 75, 100	Twice weekly
	Vivelle-Dot	25, 37.5, 50, 75, 100	Twice weekly
	Estraderm	50, 100	Twice weekly
Topical Emulsion			
Estradiol hemihydrate	Estrasorb	50	Once daily
Transdermal Spray			
Estradiol	Evamist	1.53–4.6 mg is applied*	Once daily
Topical Gel			
Estradiol	EstroGel	0.75 mg is applied*	Once daily
	Elestrin	0.52 or 1.04 mg is applied*	Once daily
	Divigel	0.25, 0.5, or 1 mg is applied*	Once daily
ESTROGEN/PROGESTIN COMBINATIONS			
Transdermal Patches			
Estradiol/norethindrone	CombiPatch	50/140, 50/250	Twice weekly
Estradiol/levonorgestrel	ClimaraPro	45/15	Once weekly

*Application of this dose produces blood levels of estrogen and estrone similar to those seen in the follicular phase of the ovulatory cycle.

Minimizing Adverse Effects

Nausea. Nausea is common early in treatment. Fortunately, this adverse effect diminishes with time.

Endometrial Hyperplasia and Cancer. Menopausal HT with estrogen alone increases the risk for endometrial carcinoma. Adding a progestin lowers this risk to the pretreatment level.

Breast Cancer. Estrogen, combined with a progestin, produces a small increase in the risk for breast cancer in postmenopausal women.

Cardiovascular Events. Estrogen plus a progestin increases the risk for CHD, MI, DVT, pulmonary embolism, and stroke. For women older than 60 years, therapy with estrogen alone carries the same risks. For women aged 50 to 59 years, therapy with estrogen alone increases the risk for DVT, pulmonary embolism, and stroke but may *protect* against CHD and MI.

Effects Resembling Those Caused by Oral Contraceptives. Use of estrogens for noncontraceptive purposes can produce adverse effects similar to those caused by oral contraceptives (e.g., abnormal vaginal bleeding, hypertension, benign hepatic adenoma, reduced glucose tolerance). Nursing implications regarding these effects are summarized in Chapter 49.

Minimizing Adverse Interactions

Review current medications at each visit. Use of a drug interaction application is recommended to identify any potential interactions.

Patient Education

ESTROGENS

Inform the patient that nausea can be reduced by taking estrogens with food and by dosing at night. Explain that nausea diminishes over time.

Remind patients that estrogens present a small risk of breast cancer and endometrial cancer. To minimize risk of undetected breast cancer, remind patients of the need to receive periodic mammograms. Instruct the patient to report any persistent or recurrent vaginal bleeding, so that the possibility of endometrial carcinoma can be evaluated.

To reduce cardiovascular risk, advise women to avoid smoking, perform regular exercise, decrease intake of saturated fats, and take appropriate drugs to treat hypertension, diabetes, and high cholesterol.

PATIENT-CENTERED CARE ACROSS THE LIFESPAN

Estrogens

Life Stage	Considerations or Concerns
Children	Estrogens are not indicated for prepubertal children.
Pregnant women	Estrogens are contraindicated during pregnancy.
Breastfeeding women	Estrogens may they affect infant development and may decrease both the quantity and quality of milk produced.
Older adults	Beers Criteria includes estrogens among those identified as potentially inappropriate for use in geriatric patients.

BLACK BOX WARNING: ESTROGEN AND PROGESTIN THERAPY

Estrogen plus progestin may increase the risk for thromboembolic events such as DVT, stroke, MI, and pulmonary embolism.

Estrogen plus progestin is not indicated for cardiovascular disease or dementia and may increase the risk for dementia in women aged 65 years and older.

Estrogen plus progestin may increase breast cancer risk.

Progestins

Preadministration Assessment

Therapeutic Goal

Progestins are used for contraception (see Chapter 49) and to counteract endometrial hyperplasia that could be caused by unopposed estrogen during HT. Other uses include dysfunctional uterine bleeding, amenorrhea, endometriosis, and support of pregnancy in women with corpus luteum deficiency. Progestins are also used in IVF cycles and to prevent prematurity in women at high risk for preterm birth.

Baseline Data

The physical examination should include breast and pelvic examinations. A pregnancy test is also warranted in most cases.

Identifying High-Risk Patients

Progestins are *contraindicated* in the presence of undiagnosed abnormal vaginal bleeding. *Relative contraindications* include active thrombophlebitis or a history of thromboembolic disorders, active liver disease, and carcinoma of the breast.

Ongoing Monitoring and Interventions

Gynecologic Effects

Progestins can cause breakthrough bleeding, spotting, and amenorrhea. Instruct patients to report any abnormal vaginal bleeding.

PATIENT-CENTERED CARE ACROSS THE LIFESPAN

Progestins

Life Stage	Considerations or Concerns
Children	Progestins are not indicated for prepubertal children.
Pregnant women	High-dose therapy during the first 4 months of pregnancy has been associated with an increased incidence of birth defects (limb reductions, heart defects, masculinization of the female fetus).
Breastfeeding women	Progestins may contribute to neonatal jaundice.
Older adults	Progestins are only indicated if the patient is taking estrogen and has a uterus.

CHAPTER

49 Birth Control

Laura D. Rosenthal, DNP, ACNP, FAANP

Birth control can be accomplished by interfering with the reproductive process at any step from gametogenesis to nidation (implantation of a fertilized ovum). Pharmacologic methods of contraception include oral contraceptives, etonogestrel implants, injectable medroxyprogesterone acetate, intrauterine devices, vaginal rings, and transdermal patches. Nonpharmacologic methods include surgical sterilization (tubal ligation, vasectomy), mechanical devices (condom, diaphragm, cervical cap), and avoiding intercourse during periods of fertility (calendar method, temperature method, cervical mucus method).

Most of this chapter focuses on combination oral contraceptive pills—the most widely used *reversible* form of contraception. Sterilization is used more often, but is not reversible. In preparing to study these agents and other forms of contraception, you should review Chapter 48, paying special attention to information on the menstrual cycle and the physiologic and pharmacologic effects of estrogens and progestins.

EFFECTIVENESS OF BIRTH CONTROL METHODS

The effectiveness of a birth control method can be expressed as the percentage of unplanned pregnancies that occur while using the method. Employing this criterion, Table 49.1 compares the effectiveness of the major birth control methods. As you can see, the most effective methods are Nexplanon, intrauterine devices (IUDs), and sterilization. Oral contraceptives (OCs), Depo-Provera, the contraceptive ring, and the contraceptive patch are close behind. The least reliable methods include barrier methods, periodic abstinence, spermicides, and withdrawal.

Table 49.1 contains two columns of figures, one labeled *theoretical use* and the other *actual use.* The *perfect use* figures represent pregnancy rates when a method of birth control is employed exactly as it should be (i.e., consistently and with proper technique). The *typical use* figures represent pregnancy rates observed in actual practice. The higher pregnancy rates reported in the *typical use* column are largely an indication that methods of birth control are not always used when and as they should be.

SELECTING A BIRTH CONTROL METHOD

The method of contraception chosen most frequently is sterilization: female sterilization (tubal ligation) plus male sterilization (vasectomy) are selected by 37% of birth control users. OCs or male condoms are chosen by most of the remaining birth control users. Diaphragms, periodic abstinence, IUDs, and other techniques account for a small fraction of birth control use.

Several factors should be considered when choosing a method of birth control. Chief among these are *effectiveness, safety,* and *personal preference.* As shown in Table 49.1, the most effective methods are etonogestrel subdermal implants [Nexplanon], intramuscular medroxyprogesterone acetate [Depo-Provera], sterilization, and IUDs. Three other methods—OCs, the contraceptive ring [NuvaRing], and the contraceptive patch [Ortho Evra]—are close behind. The remaining methods—condoms, the sponge, diaphragm, cervical cap, spermicides, and periodic abstinence—must be used in a near-perfect fashion to afford any reasonable level of protection.

When factoring safety into the selection equation, several guidelines apply. Combination OCs should be avoided by women with certain cardiovascular disorders (see later), as well as by women older than 35 years who smoke. For women in these categories, an alternative method (e.g., diaphragm, progestin-only pill, or IUD) is preferable. Although OCs are effective and relatively convenient, they can also cause significant side effects. Accordingly, women who consider the benefit/risk ratio unfavorable should be advised about alternative contraceptive techniques. Women who are not in a mutually monogamous relationship, and hence are at risk for a sexually transmitted disease (STD), should not use an IUD.

Personal preference is a major factor in providing the motivation needed for consistent implementation of a birth control method. Because even the best form of contraception will be less effective if improperly practiced, the importance of personal preference cannot be overemphasized. Practitioners should take pains to educate patients about the contraceptive methods available so that selection and use can be based on understanding.

Additional factors that bear on selecting a birth control method include family planning goals, age, frequency of sexual intercourse, and the individual's capacity for adherence. If family planning goals have already been met, sterilization of either the male or female partner may be desirable. For women who engage in coitus frequently, OCs or a long-term method (e.g., Nexplanon, Depo-Provera, IUD) are reasonable choices. Conversely, when sexual activity is limited, use of a spermicide, condom, or diaphragm may be more appropriate. Because barrier methods combined with spermicides can offer some protection against STDs (as well as providing contraception), these combinations may be of special benefit to individuals who have multiple partners. If adherence is a problem (as it can be with OCs, condoms, and

TABLE 49.1 ▪ Effectiveness of Birth Control Methods

Birth Control Method	Failure Rate* (%) Actual Use†	Theoretical Use‡
No method	85	85
EXTREMELY EFFECTIVE		
Etonogestrel subdermal implant [Nexplanon]	0.05	0.05
Surgical sterilization		
Female: tubal ligation	0.5	0.5
Male: vasectomy	0.15	0.1
Intrauterine devices		
Copper T 380A [ParaGard]	0.8	0.6
Levonorgestrel T [Mirena]	0.2	0.2
VERY EFFECTIVE		
Oral contraceptives		
Combination pills	8	0.3
Progestin-only pills	8	0.3
Intramuscular medroxyprogesterone acetate [Depo-Provera]	3	0.3
Vaginal contraceptive ring [NuvaRing]	8	0.3
Contraceptive patch [Ortho Evra]	8	0.3
EFFECTIVE		
Condoms		
Male	15	2
Female [FC2 Female Condom]	21	5
Diaphragm with spermicide	16	6
LEAST EFFECTIVE		
Contraceptive sponge [Today Sponge]		
Parous	32	20
Nulliparous	16	9
Spermicide alone	29	18
Periodic abstinence	25	3–5
Withdrawal	27	4

*Failure rate: percentage of women who have an unplanned pregnancy during first year of use.

†Actual use: failure rate usually observed in actual practice.

‡Theoretical use: failure rate that would be expected if the birth control method were practiced exactly as it should be.

diaphragms), use of a long-term method (e.g., vaginal contraceptive ring, IUD, Nexplanon, Depo-Provera) can confer more reliable protection.

To help women select the birth control method that suits them best, Planned Parenthood has created a step-by-step computerized selection tool, accessible online at www.plannedparenthood.org/all-access/my-method-26542.htm. This tool accounts for all of the factors noted previously.

ORAL CONTRACEPTIVES

There are two main categories of OCs: (1) those that contain an estrogen *plus* a progestin, known as *combination OCs,* and (2) those that contain just a progestin, known as "minipills" or *progestin-only OCs.* Of the two groups, combination OCs are by far the more widely used.

Combination Oral Contraceptives

Since their introduction in the late 1950s, combination OCs have become one of our most widely prescribed families of drugs. These drugs are both safe and effective, although minor side effects are common.

Prototype Drugs

DRUGS FOR BIRTH CONTROL

Combination Oral Contraceptive
Ethinyl estradiol/norethindrone

Progestin-Only Oral Contraceptive
Norethindrone

Long-Acting Contraceptives
Subdermal etonogestrel implant [Implanon]
Depot medroxyprogesterone acetate [Depo-Provera]

Drugs for Emergency Contraception
Levonorgestrel alone [Plan B One-Step]
Ulipristal acetate [ella]

Mechanism of Action

Combination OCs reduce fertility primarily by *inhibiting ovulation.* The estrogen in combination OCs suppresses release of follicle-stimulating hormone from the pituitary (and thereby inhibits follicular maturation), and progestin in combination OCs acts in the hypothalamus and pituitary to suppress the midcycle luteinizing hormone surge, which normally triggers ovulation. Secondary mechanisms include thickening of the cervical mucus (creating a barrier to the penetration of sperm) and alteration of the endometrium, making it less hospitable for implantation.

Components

Estrogens

Only three estrogens are employed: *ethinyl estradiol, mestranol,* and *estradiol valerate.* Most combination OCs use ethinyl estradiol. A few older products use mestranol, which undergoes conversion to ethinyl estradiol in the body. One new product—*Natazia*—uses estradiol valerate, which undergoes conversion to estradiol in the body.

Progestins

Combination OCs employ eight different progestins, which can be grouped into four generations (Table 49.2). Progestins in all four generations are equally effective. Differences relate to side effects, especially thrombotic events, androgenic effects (acne, hirsutism, dyslipidemia), and hyperkalemia.

Drospirenone, a fourth-generation progestin, has progestational, antiandrogen, and antialdosterone actions. The drug is a structural analog of spironolactone, a potassium-sparing diuretic that blocks receptors for aldosterone. Drospirenone was developed in an effort to reduce fluid retention caused by the estrogen component in combination OCs. (Estrogens promote fluid retention by activating the renin-angiotensin-aldosterone system. Drospirenone reduces fluid retention by blocking aldosterone receptors, thereby preventing retention of sodium and water. As a result, OCs made with drospirenone may cause less bloating, weight gain, and hypertension than other combination

OCs.) The principal concern with drospirenone is venous thromboembolism, which occurs more often than with other progestins. Also, drospirenone can cause hyperkalemia (secondary to renal retention of potassium).

Effectiveness

As shown in Table 49.1, OCs can be very effective. With perfect use, the failure rate is only 0.3%. However, with typical use, the failure rate is significantly higher: about 8%. Among women of higher weight, efficacy is somewhat reduced. Possible reasons include decreased blood levels of the hormones, sequestration in adipose tissue, and altered metabolism. However, even though efficacy of OCs is slightly reduced in higher weight women, these drugs are still more reliable than most of the alternatives.

Overall Safety

Determining the relative safety of combination OCs is complex. Part of the difficulty lies with the fact that much of our information on the adverse effects of OCs was gathered when these agents were employed in higher doses than those employed today. Newer data show that today's OCs, as currently prescribed, are considerably safer than indicated by older studies. An additional complication stems from the fact that the risk for mortality associated with OCs is much smaller than the risk associated with pregnancy and delivery. Keeping the previous provisos in mind, we can make the following observations on OC safety. Of the contraceptive methods available, OCs produce the broadest spectrum of adverse effects, ranging from nausea to menstrual irregularity to rare thromboembolic disorders. However, despite their wide variety of undesired actions, when used by healthy women, OCs produce no greater mortality than any other form of birth control.

TABLE 49.2 ▪ Progestins Used in Combination Oral Contraceptives

Progestins	Comments
FIRST GENERATION	
Ethynodiol diacetate Norethindrone	• Lower risk for thrombosis than with other progestins • Mildly androgenic
SECOND GENERATION	
Levonorgestrel Norgestrel	• Greater risk for thrombosis than with FGPs • More androgenic than FGPs • Prolonged half-life
THIRD GENERATION	
Desogestrel Norgestimate	• Greater risk for thrombosis than with FGPs (especially desogestrel) • Less androgenic than FGPs
FOURTH GENERATION	
Dienogest Drospirenone	For drospirenone *and* dienogest: • Greater risk for thrombosis than with other progestins (especially drospirenone) • Less androgenic than FGPs • Low risk for acne and hirsutism For *drospirenone only:* • Risk for hyperkalemia

FGPs, first-generation progestins.

Adverse Effects

Combination OCs can cause a variety of adverse effects. However, although many types of effects may occur, severe effects are rare. Hence, compared with the serious risks associated with pregnancy and childbirth, the risks of OCs are low. Nonetheless, because OCs are usually taken by women who are healthy, and because OCs represent a potential health hazard (albeit small), we must take steps to minimize risk. To this end, a full medical history should be obtained. If the history reveals an *absolute* contraindication to OC use (Table 49.3), OCs should not be prescribed. In women with *relative* contraindications, OCs should be used with caution. Candidates for OCs undergo a physical examination before starting these agents.

Thromboembolic Disorders

Combination OCs have been associated with an increased risk for venous thromboembolism (VTE), arterial thromboembolism, pulmonary embolism, myocardial infarction (MI), and thrombotic stroke. Among OC users, the *relative* risk for a thrombotic event is 2 to 3 times the risk in nonusers. However, the *absolute* risk is still very small: about 8 to 10 events per 10,000 woman-years of OC use. Furthermore, the risk for thrombosis associated with OCs is considerably lower than the risk associated with pregnancy and delivery. OCs promote thrombosis in part by raising levels of clotting factors. Thrombosis is not due to atherosclerosis.

Until the mid-1990s, we believed that thrombotic events were caused solely by the estrogen in combination OCs. However, it is now clear that the progestin can contribute, too. Two newer progestins—*drospirenone* and *desogestrel*—appear to carry the greatest risk.

Fortunately, the risk for thrombotic events with OCs used today is much lower than with the OCs used in the past because the amount of estrogen in OCs has been reduced. When combination OCs first became available, they contained high doses of estrogens (e.g., 100 mcg ethinyl estradiol).

TABLE 49.3 ▪ Absolute and Relative Contraindications to the Use of Combination Oral Contraceptives

Absolute contraindications	Thrombophlebitis, thromboembolic disorders, cerebral vascular disease, coronary occlusion, *or* a past history of these conditions, *or* a condition that predisposes to these disorders
	Abnormal liver function
	Known or suspected breast cancer
	Undiagnosed abnormal vaginal bleeding
	Known or suspected pregnancy
	Smokers older than 35 years
Relative contraindications	Hypertension
	Cardiac disease
	Diabetes
	History of cholestatic jaundice of pregnancy
	Gallbladder disease
	Uterine leiomyoma
	Epilepsy
	Migraine

Today's OCs contain no more than 50 mcg ethinyl estradiol (and usually less), so the risk for thromboembolism is quite low.

Major factors that increase the risk for thromboembolism are *heavy smoking, a history of thromboembolism,* and *thrombophilias.* Additional risk factors include diabetes, hypertension, cerebrovascular disease, coronary artery disease, and surgery in which immobilization increases the risk for postoperative thrombosis.

In the past, OCs were not recommended for women older than 35 years because earlier studies indicated an increase in the risk for MI for this group. However, reanalysis showed that the risk was limited to older women who smoked. With today's low-estrogen OCs, nonsmokers may continue use until menopause, with no greater risk for MI than among younger women.

Several measures can help minimize thromboembolic phenomena:

- The estrogen dose in OCs should be no greater than required for contraceptive efficacy.
- OCs containing drospirenone or desogestrel should generally be avoided because they may pose a higher risk for developing VTE.
- OCs should not be prescribed for heavy smokers, women with a history of thromboembolism, or women with other risk factors for thrombosis.
- OCs should be discontinued at least 4 weeks before surgery in which postoperative thrombosis might be expected.

Patient Education

THROMBOSIS AND THROMBOEMBOLISM

Women should be informed about the symptoms of thrombosis and thromboembolism (e.g., leg tenderness or pain, sudden chest pain, shortness of breath, severe headache, sudden visual disturbance) and instructed to consult the prescriber if these occur.

What about the cardiovascular risk for *former* OC users? Data from the Women's Health Initiative suggest that use of OCs in the past may *protect* against cardiovascular disease. Among women with a history of OC use, there was an 8% decrease in the overall incidence of cardiovascular disease, including a reduced risk for angina, MI, peripheral vascular disease, transient ischemic attacks, and elevation of cholesterol.

Women with a history of thrombosis should avoid estrogen/progestin products but can still use a progestin-only method. Options include the levonorgestrel intrauterine system [Mirena], medroxyprogesterone acetate injection [Depo-Provera], the etonogestrel subdermal implant [Nexplanon], and the "minipill"—all of which are discussed later.

Cancer

OCs present no known risk for cancer—with the important exception of promoting (not causing) breast cancer growth. The effects of OCs on cancers of the ovaries, endometrium, cervix, and breast have been studied extensively. Effects on three of these cancers are clear: OCs *protect* against ovarian and endometrial cancer and have *no effect* (positive or negative) on cervical cancer, which is caused by human papillomaviruses.

What about breast cancer? Until a decade ago, the question was unresolved: some studies found a link between OC use and breast cancer; others did not. Now we seem to have a definitive answer: OCs do *not* increase the risk for breast cancer for *most* women. This conclusion is based on data from the Women's Contraceptive and Reproductive Experience (Women's CARE) study. This major study, involving more than 9000 women, found no association between present or past use of OCs and the development of breast cancer. This conclusion applied not only to study participants as a whole but also to women in the following subgroups:

- Those who used OCs with high estrogen content
- Those who used OCs for a prolonged time
- Those who began OC use during adolescence
- Those with a first-degree relative with breast cancer

These results should reassure women who are OC users.

However, although this study shows that OCs do not increase risk for *most* women, the results of another large recent study show that OCs *do* increase risk for *some* women, specifically, women who have the *BRCA1* gene mutation. Even without taking OCs, these women have a very high—50% to 80%—lifetime risk for breast cancer. OCs increase this risk by one third. The same study found that OCs do *not* increase risk in women with the *BRCA2* mutation.

It is important to note that, although OCs do not *cause* breast cancer, estrogens can promote the growth of *existing* breast carcinoma. Accordingly, women with this disease should not take OCs.

Hypertension

Combination OCs can cause hypertension, but the risk with today's low-estrogen preparations is very low. OCs raise blood pressure by increasing blood levels of two compounds: angiotensin and aldosterone. If hypertension develops, and if OCs are determined to be the cause, two options are open: (1) discontinue the OC or (2) continue the OC and manage the hypertension with drugs.

Abnormal Uterine Bleeding

By altering the endometrium, OCs may decrease or eliminate menstrual flow. In addition, breakthrough bleeding and spotting may occur, especially with the use of extended-cycle OCs (e.g., Seasonique, Seasonale). Spotting and bleeding can also occur with monthly cycle OCs, most often during the first 3 months when low-estrogen OCs are used. If a period is missed while taking monthly cycle OCs, the possibility of pregnancy should be assessed. After discontinuation of OCs, normal menstruation usually resumes, although the first period may be delayed. Women with a pretreatment history of irregular menses will return to their previous pattern when OCs are discontinued.

Use in Pregnancy and Lactation

OCs have no therapeutic role during pregnancy and hence are *contraindicated for use by pregnant women.* Pregnancy should be ruled out before starting OC use, and, if pregnancy should occur despite OC use, use should stop immediately. Woman should be assured, however, that inadvertent use of OCs during early pregnancy poses no risk for fetal harm. Because OCs have no role in pregnancy—and *not* because they are harmful—these drugs are classified in U.S. Food and Drug Administration (FDA) Pregnancy Risk Category X.

Combination OCs enter breast milk and reduce milk production, especially in the early stages of lactation. In contrast, progestin-only OCs have little or no effect on milk production and hence are preferred for contraception during lactation, at least early on. (Later, when the milk supply is well established, and especially with the addition of solids to the infant's diet, use of combination OCs may resume.)

Stroke in Women With Migraine

When used by women who experience migraine headaches, OCs may increase the risk for thrombotic stroke. However, the absolute increase is low: only 8 cases per 100,000 women at age 20 years, rising to 80 cases per 100,000 women at age 40 years. Because the risk is low, OCs are generally considered safe for women with migraine, provided they are younger than 35 years, don't smoke, and are healthy, and provided their headaches are not preceded by visual changes known as an aura (migraine with aura has a greater risk for stroke than migraine without aura). Migraine and its management are discussed in Chapter 23.

Benign Hepatic Adenoma

Hepatic adenoma is a rare complication seen in women who use OCs that contain *mestranol.* These highly vascular, nonmalignant tumors are usually picked up as incidental findings on a computed tomography scan or magnetic resonance imaging. If hepatic adenoma is diagnosed, discontinuing OCs usually results in spontaneous tumor regression.

Effects Related to Estrogen or Progestin Imbalance

Many of the mild side effects of combination OCs result from an excess or deficiency of estrogen or progestin. Effects that can result from an excess of estrogen include nausea, breast tenderness, and edema. Progestin excess can increase appetite and cause fatigue and depression. A deficiency in either hormone can cause menstrual irregularities. Side effects related to hormonal imbalance are shown in Table 49.4.

Quite often, these effects can be reduced by adjusting the estrogen/progestin balance of an OC regimen. With most women, therapy is initiated with an OC containing 30 to 35 mcg of ethinyl estradiol. If significant nausea occurs, it can be managed by dosing at bedtime or, if needed, switching to an OC with less estrogen. Using less estrogen can also reduce breast discomfort. During the first 3 months of use, spotting and breakthrough bleeding are common and usually resolve on their own. If they don't, they can be managed by increasing the estrogen dosage or by using a product that contains a different progestin. For women who experience androgenic effects (e.g., acne, hirsutism), switching to an OC that has drospirenone or dienogest can help. Other side effects can be reduced by making similar adjustments. When substituting one combination OC for another, the change is best made at the beginning of a new cycle.

Hyperkalemia

Drospirenone, a fourth-generation progestin, promotes renal retention of potassium and can thereby cause hyperkalemia. Accordingly, the drug is inappropriate for women with conditions that predispose to hyperkalemia (e.g., renal insufficiency, adrenal insufficiency, liver disease). Furthermore, drospirenone should be used with caution in women taking other drugs that can elevate serum potassium. Important among these are angiotensin-converting enzyme inhibitors, angiotensin II receptor blockers, potassium-sparing diuretics, potassium supplements, and nonsteroidal antiinflammatory drugs (when taken daily). If women taking these drugs are using a drospirenone-containing OC, potassium levels should be checked during the first cycle of use.

Glucose Intolerance

OCs can elevate blood glucose levels. This diabetogenic effect is caused by the progestin in OCs. Glucose intolerance is most likely in patients who are already diabetic or have experienced gestational diabetes. Because hypoglycemic agents (e.g., insulin) can control glucose elevations induced by OCs, the presence of diabetes does not preclude OC use. Prediabetic women should be monitored for development of hyperglycemia. Glucose intolerance may occur less with OCs that contain desogestrel or norgestimate.

Other Adverse Effects

Rarely, OCs may precipitate gallbladder disease in women who already have gallstones or a history of gallbladder disease. OCs can occasionally cause ocular injury (e.g., retinal vascular occlusion, retinal edema, optic neuropathy). Accordingly, if visual changes occur, OCs should be discontinued until the underlying cause is diagnosed. Combination OCs have been associated with an increased risk for systemic lupus erythematosus, primarily in women who recently began OC use. Rarely, OCs cause melasma, characterized by dark brown patches on the face.

TABLE 49.4 ▪ Side Effects Caused by an Excess of or Deficiency in the Estrogen or Progestin Content of an Oral Contraceptive Regimen

Estrogen		Progestin	
Excess	**Deficiency**	**Excess**	**Deficiency**
Nausea	Early or midcycle breakthrough bleeding	Increased appetite	Late breakthrough bleeding
Breast tenderness	Increased spotting	Weight gain	Amenorrhea
Edema	Hypomenorrhea	Depression	Hypermenorrhea
Bloating		Tiredness	
Hypertension		Fatigue	
Migraine		Hypomenorrhea	
Cervical mucorrhea		Breast regression	
Polyposis		Monilial vaginitis	
		Acne, oily scalp*	
		Hair loss*	
		Hirsutism*	

*Caused by progestins that have strong androgenic activity.

Noncontraceptive Benefits of Oral Contraceptives

OCs decrease the risk for several disorders, including ovarian cancer, endometrial cancer, ovarian cysts, pelvic inflammatory disease (PID), benign breast disease, iron deficiency anemia, and acne. In addition, OCs favorably affect menstrual symptoms: cramps are reduced, menstrual flow is reduced in volume and duration, and menses are more predictable. In women with premenstrual disorder or premenstrual dysphoric disorder, OCs can reduce symptom intensity. In some women with menstrual-associated migraine, OCs can reduce migraine frequency. Surprisingly, OCs may even benefit women with rheumatoid arthritis.

Drug Interactions

Drugs and Herbs that Reduce the Effects of OCs

Products that induce hepatic cytochrome P450 can accelerate OC metabolism and can thereby reduce OC effects. Products that induce P450 include *rifampin* (used for tuberculosis), *ritonavir* (used for HIV infection), several *antiseizure agents* (carbamazepine, phenobarbital, phenytoin, and primidone), and *St. John's wort* (an herb used for depression). Women taking OCs in combination with any of these agents should be alert for indications of reduced OC blood levels, such as breakthrough bleeding or spotting. If these signs appear, it may be necessary to either (1) increase the estrogen dosage of the OC, (2) combine the OC with a second form of birth control (e.g., condom), or (3) switch to an alternative form of birth control.

Drugs Whose Effects Are Reduced by OCs

OCs can decrease the benefits of warfarin and hypoglycemic agents. By increasing levels of clotting factors, OCs can decrease the effectiveness of *warfarin,* an anticoagulant. By increasing levels of glucose, OCs can counteract the benefits of insulin and other hypoglycemic agents used in diabetes. Accordingly, when combined with OCs, warfarin and hypoglycemic agents may require increased dosage.

Drugs Whose Effects Are Increased by OCs

OCs can impair the hepatic metabolism of several agents, including *theophylline, tricyclic antidepressants, diazepam,* and *chlordiazepoxide.* Because of reduced clearance, these drugs may accumulate to toxic levels. If signs of toxicity appear, dosage of these drugs should be reduced.

Preparations

The combination OCs in current use are listed in Table 49.5. As you can see, nearly all of these products contain the same estrogen: ethinyl estradiol. In contrast, eight different progestins are employed. Products are listed in order of increasing estrogen content. The OCs with low estrogen are safer. As a rule, high-estrogen OCs are reserved for women taking drugs that induce P450. Products with unique properties are discussed next.

Beyaz and Safyral

In addition to an estrogen and a progestin, these combination OCs contain levomefolate, a metabolite of folic acid. The purpose is to reduce the risk for fetal neural tube defects—anencephaly and spina bifida—if pregnancy should occur despite contraceptive use. As discussed in Chapter 65, neural tube defects can result if folic acid is low early in pregnancy.

Natazia

Natazia has two unique components: estradiol valerate and dienogest, a fourth-generation progestin. Estradiol valerate is a prodrug that undergoes rapid conversion to estradiol, the predominant endogenous estrogen. Dienogest, which is much like drospirenone (see previous discussion under "Components"), has strong progestational activity and antiandrogenic activity. However, in contrast to drospirenone, dienogest does not cause potassium retention, and hence there is no need to monitor potassium levels. Unlike all other combination OCs, Natazia employs a four-phase dosing schedule, in which the amount of estradiol decreases over the monthly cycle and the amount of progestin (dienogest) increases. Because of this schedule, duration of withdrawal bleeding is shorter than with other combination OCs, and the intensity of bleeding is lighter. In women who normally experience heavy or prolonged menstrual bleeding, Natazia can reduce blood loss.

Dosing Schedules

With only one exception, combination OCs are dosed in a *cyclic pattern.* For most products, each cycle is *28 days long* (see Table 49.5). However, with a few newer products, the cycle is either *extended* (to 91 days) or *continuous* [Amethyst].

28-Day-Cycle Schedules

The 28-day regimens are subdivided into four groups: *monophasic, biphasic, triphasic,* and *quadriphasic (four-phasic).* In a monophasic regimen, the daily doses of estrogen and progestin remain constant throughout the cycle of use. In the other regimens, the estrogen, the progestin, or both change as the cycle progresses. The biphasic, triphasic, and quadriphasic schedules reflect efforts to more closely simulate ovarian production of estrogens and progestins. However, these preparations appear to offer little or no advantage over monophasic OCs.

Most 28-day cycle products are taken in a repeating sequence consisting of 21 days of an active pill followed by 7 days on which either (1) no pill is taken, (2) an inert pill is taken, or (3) an iron-containing pill is taken. The sequence is begun on either (1) the first day of the menstrual cycle or (2) the first Sunday after the onset of menses. With the first option, protection is conferred immediately, and hence no backup contraception is needed. With a Sunday start, which is done to have menses occur on weekdays rather than the weekend, protection may not be immediate, and hence an alternate form of birth control should be used during the first cycle. With both options, each dose should be taken at the same time every day (e.g., with a meal or at bedtime). Successive dosing cycles should commence every 28 days, even if there is breakthrough bleeding or spotting.

Extended-Cycle and Continuous Schedules

Many health care providers recommend taking combination OCs for an extended time, rather than following the traditional 28-day cycle, because doing so decreases episodes of withdrawal bleeding with its associated menstrual pain, premenstrual symptoms, headaches, and other problems. Prolonged use of OCs is possible because these drugs suppress endometrial thickening, and hence monthly bleeding is not required to slough off hypertrophied tissue. At this time, 12 products—*Amethia, Amethia Lo, Camrese, Camrese Lo, Introvale, Jolessa, Quasense, Seasonale, Seasonique, LoSeasonique, Amethyst,* and *Lybrel*—are packaged and marketed for prolonged use. The following regimens are employed:

- *Introvale, Jolessa, Quasense,* and *Seasonale*—active pills for 84 days, then no pills for 7 days

TABLE 49.5 ▪ Composition of Combination Oral Contraceptives

Trade Name	mcg	Estrogen	mg	Progestin
28-DAY-CYCLE ORAL CONTRACEPTIVES				
Monophasic				
Lo Loestrin Fe[a]	10	Ethinyl estradiol	1	Norethindrone
Junel 1/20	20	Ethinyl estradiol	1	Norethindrone
Junel Fe 1/20				
Loestrin 21 1/20				
Loestrin Fe 1/20				
Loestrin 24 Fe[b]				
Microgestin 1/20				
Microgestin Fe 1/20				
Blisovi 24 Fe				
Gildess 1/20				
Gildess Fe 1/20				
Junel Fe 24				
Larin 1/20				
Larin 24 Fe				
Larin Fe 1/20				
Minastrin 1/20				
Minastrin 24 Fe				
Tarina Fe 1/20				
Aviane	20	Ethinyl estradiol	0.1	Levonorgestrel
Lessina				
Lutera				
Orsythia				
Sronyx				
Amethia Lo				
Falmina				
Gianvi[c]	20	Ethinyl estradiol	3	Drospirenone
Loryna				
YAZ[c]				
Beyaz[c,d]				
Nikki				
Vestura				
Generess Fe[e]	25	Ethinyl estradiol	0.8	Norethindrone
Kaitlib Fe				
Altavera	30	Ethinyl estradiol	0.15	Levonorgestrel
Amethia				
Kurvelo				
Levora				
Marlissa				
Portia				
Cryselle	30	Ethinyl estradiol	0.3	Norgestrel
Elinest				
Low-Ogestrel				
Lo/Ovral-28				
Gildess 1.5/30	30	Ethinyl estradiol	1.5	Norethindrone
Gildess Fe 1.5/30				
Junel 1.5/30				
Junel Fe 1.5/30				
Larin 1.5/30				
Loestrin 21 1.5/30				
Loestrin Fe 1.5/30				
Microgestin 1.5/30				
Microgestin Fe 1.5/30				
Apri	30	Ethinyl estradiol	0.15	Desogestrel
Desogen				
Emoquette				
Enskyce				
Reclipsen				
Ocella	30	Ethinyl estradiol	3	Drospirenone
Syeda				
Safyral[d]				
Yasmin				
Zarah				
Alyacen 1/35	35	Ethinyl estradiol	1	Ethynodiol diacetate
Kelnor 1/35				
Zovia 1/35E				
Balziva	35	Ethinyl estradiol	0.4	Norethindrone
Briellyn				
Femcon Fe[e]				
Gildagia				
Ovcon-35[e]				
Philith				
Vyfemla				
Zenchent Fe				
Zeosa				
Zenchent				
Brevicon	35	Ethinyl estradiol	0.5	Norethindrone
Modicon				
Necon 0.5/35				
Nortrel 0.5/35				
Wera				
Cyclafem 1/35	35	Ethinyl estradiol	1	Norethindrone
Dasetta 1/35				
Necon 1/35				
Norinyl 1/35				
Nortrel 1/35				
Ortho-Novum 1/35				
Pirmella 1/35				
Estarylla	35	Ethinyl estradiol	0.25	Norgestimate
Mono-Linyah				
MonoNessa				
Ortho-Cyclen				
Previfem				
Sprintec				
Ogestrel	50	Ethinyl estradiol	0.5	Norgestrel
Zovia 1/50E	50	Ethinyl estradiol	1	Ethynodiol diacetate
Necon 1/50	50	Mestranol	1	Norethindrone
Norinyl 1/50				
Biphasic				
Necon 10/11	35	Ethinyl estradiol	0.5	Norethindrone (phase 1)
	35	Ethinyl estradiol	1	Norethindrone (phase 2)
Azurette	20	Ethinyl estradiol	0.15	Desogestrel (phase 1)
Kariva	10	Ethinyl estradiol	0	Desogestrel (phase 2)
Bekyree				
Kimidess				
Pimtrea				
Viorele				
Triphasic				
Caziant	25	Ethinyl estradiol	0.1	Desogestrel (phase 1)
Cyclessa	25	Ethinyl estradiol	0.125	Desogestrel (phase 2)

Continued

TABLE 49.5 ▪ Composition of Combination Oral Contraceptives—cont'd

Trade Name	mcg	Estrogen	mg	Progestin
Velivet	25	Ethinyl estradiol	0.15	Desogestrel (phase 3)
Aranelle	35	Ethinyl estradiol	0.5	Norethindrone (phase 1)
Leena	35	Ethinyl estradiol	1	Norethindrone (phase 2)
Tri-Norinyl	35	Ethinyl estradiol	0.5	Norethindrone (phase 3)
Ortho-Novum 7/7/7	35	Ethinyl estradiol	0.5	Norethindrone (phase 1)
Necon 7/7/7	35	Ethinyl estradiol	0.75	Norethindrone (phase 2)
Nortrel 7/7/7	35	Ethinyl estradiol	1	Norethindrone (phase 3)
Alyacen 7/7/7				
Cyclafem 7/7/7				
Dasetta 7/7/7				
Pirmella 7/7/7				
Enpresse	30	Ethinyl estradiol	0.05	Levonorgestrel (phase 1)
Trivora	40	Ethinyl estradiol	0.075	Levonorgestrel (phase 2)
Levonest	30	Ethinyl estradiol	0.125	Levonorgestrel (phase 3)
Myzilra				
Ortho Tri-Cyclen Lo	25	Ethinyl estradiol	0.18	Norgestimate (phase 1)
Tri-Lo-Marzia	25	Ethinyl estradiol	0.215	Norgestimate (phase 2)
Tri-Lo-Sprintec	25	Ethinyl estradiol	0.25	Norgestimate (phase 3)
Tri-Lo-Estarylla				
Ortho Tri-Cyclen	35	Ethinyl estradiol	0.18	Norgestimate (phase 1)
TriNessa	35	Ethinyl estradiol	0.215	Norgestimate (phase 2)
Tri-Previfem	35	Ethinyl estradiol	0.25	Norgestimate (phase 3)
Tri-Sprintec				
Tri-Estarylla				
Tri-Linyah				
Estrostep Fe	20	Ethinyl estradiol	1	Norethindrone (phase 1)
Tilia Fe	30	Ethinyl estradiol	1	Norethindrone (phase 2)
Tri-Legest Fe	35	Ethinyl estradiol	1	Norethindrone (phase 3)
Quadriphasic				
Natazia	3	Estradiol valerate	0	Dienogest (phase 1)
	2	Estradiol valerate	2	Dienogest (phase 2)
	2	Estradiol valerate	3	Dienogest (phase 3)
	1	Estradiol valerate	0	Dienogest (phase 4)
Quartette	20	Ethinyl estradiol	0.15	levonorgestrel (phase 1)
	25	Ethinyl estradiol	0.15	levonorgestrel (phase 2)
	30	Ethinyl estradiol	0.15	levonorgestrel (phase 3)
	10	Ethinyl estradiol	0	levonorgestrel (phase 4)
EXTENDED-CYCLE ORAL CONTRACEPTIVES				
Amethia[f]	30	Ethinyl estradiol	0.15	Levonorgestrel
Ashlyna				
Camrese[f]				
Daysee				
Introvale[g]				
Jolessa[g]				
Quasense[g]				
Seasonale[g]				
Setlakin				
Seasonique[f]				
Amethia Lo[f]	20	Ethinyl estradiol	0.1	Levonorgestrel
Camrese Lo[f]				
LoSeasonique[f]				
CONTINUOUS ORAL CONTRACEPTIVE				
Amethyst[h]	20	Ethinyl estradiol	0.09	Levonorgestrel

[a]The cycle for Loestrin Fe is 26 active tablets followed by 2 ferrous fumarate tablets.
[b]The cycle for Loestrin 24 Fe is 24 active tablets followed by 4 ferrous fumarate tablets.
[c]The cycle for Gianvi, YAZ, and Beyaz is 24 active tablets followed by 4 inert tablets.
[d]Each tablet of Beyaz and Safyral contains 0.451 mg levomefolate (a metabolite of folic acid) to help prevent fetal neural tube defects if pregnancy should occur despite contraceptive use.
[e]Generess Fe, Femcon Fe, and Ovcon-35 are the only chewable OCs available (they may also be swallowed whole).
[f]The cycle for Amethia, Amethia Lo, Camrese, Camrese Lo, Seasonique, and LoSeasonique is 84 active tablets followed by 7 low-estrogen tablets (10 mcg ethinyl estradiol).
[g]The cycle for Introvale, Jolessa, Quasense, and Seasonale is 84 active tablets followed by 7 inert tablets.
[h]Amethyst is taken continuously, without interruption.

- *Amethia, Amethia Lo, Camrese, Camrese Lo, Seasonique,* and *LoSeasonique*—active pills for 84 days, then low-dose estrogen pills for 7 days
- *Amethyst*—active pills are taken continuously, with no scheduled interruption

Hence, with Introvale, Jolessa, Quasense, Seasonale, Amethia, Amethia Lo, Camrese, Camrese Lo, Seasonique, and LoSeasonique, withdrawal bleeding occurs just 4 times a year, instead of 13 as with conventional cycles. With Amethyst, withdrawal bleeding occurs only when dosing is finally stopped. However, although these regimens decrease episodes of *scheduled* bleeding, *breakthrough bleeding* can be more common.

It is important to note that there is nothing special about the estrogen/progestin combinations used in these extended-cycle products. Put another way, we could get the same results with other combination OCs, provided they are *monophasic.* To achieve an extended schedule, the user would simply purchase four packets of a 28-day product (each of which contains 21 active pills) and then take the active pills for 84 days straight.

What to Do if Doses Are Missed

The chances of ovulation (and hence pregnancy) from missing one OC dose are small. However, the risk for pregnancy becomes progressively larger with each successive omission.

For products that use a *28-day cycle,* the following recommendations apply:

- If *1 or more pills* are missed in the *first week,* take one pill as soon as possible and then continue with the pack. Use an additional form of contraception for 7 days.
- If *1 or 2 pills* are missed during the *second or third week,* take one pill as soon as possible and then continue with the *active* pills in the pack—but skip the placebo pills and go straight to a new pack once all the active pills have been taken.
- If *3 or more pills* are missed during the *second or third week,* follow the same instructions given for missing 1 or 2 pills, but use an additional form of contraception for 7 days.

Important note: the response to a missed dose of Natazia, as described in the package insert, is more complex than with other combination OCs.

For combination OCs that use an *extended or continuous cycle,* up to 7 days can be missed with little or no increased risk for pregnancy, provided the pills had been taken *continuously for the prior 3 weeks.*

Progestin-Only Oral Contraceptives

Progestin-only OCs, also known as "minipills," contain a progestin but no estrogen. Because they lack estrogen, minipills do not cause thromboembolic disorders, headaches, nausea, or most of the other adverse effects associated with combination OCs. Unfortunately, although slightly safer than combination OCs, the progestin-only preparations are less effective and are more likely to cause irregular bleeding (breakthrough bleeding, spotting, amenorrhea, inconsistent cycle length, variations in the volume and duration of monthly flow). Irregular bleeding is the major drawback of these products and the principal reason that women discontinue them. Eight products are available: *Camila, Errin, Heather, Jolivette, Ortho Micronor, Nor-QD, Jencycla,* and *Nora-BE.* All contain 0.35 mg *norethindrone.*

Contraceptive effects of the minipill result largely from altering cervical secretions. Under the influence of progestins, cervical glands produce a thick, sticky mucus that acts as a barrier to penetration by sperm. Progestins also modify the endometrium, making it less favorable for implantation. Compared with combination OCs, minipills are weak inhibitors of ovulation, and hence this mechanism contributes little to their effects. Unlike combination OCs, whose administration is cyclic, progestin-only OCs are taken continuously. Use is initiated on day 1 of the menstrual cycle, and one pill is taken daily thereafter. A backup contraceptive method should be used for the first 7 days. Dosing should be done at the same time each day.

If one or more doses is missed, the following guidelines apply. If one pill is missed, it should be taken as soon as remembered, and backup contraception should be used for at least 2 days. The pills should be resumed as scheduled on the next day. If two pills are missed, the regimen should be restarted, and backup contraception should be used for at least 2 days. In addition, if two or more pills are missed and no menstrual bleeding occurs, a pregnancy test should be done.

COMBINATION CONTRACEPTIVES WITH NOVEL DELIVERY SYSTEMS

Two combination contraceptives—*a transdermal patch* and a *vaginal ring*—have the same mechanism as combination OCs, but they deliver hormones in novel ways. Like combination OCs, both of these contraceptives contain two hormones—an estrogen and a progestin—that undergo absorption into the systemic circulation and then prevent pregnancy primarily by suppressing ovulation. What's different is how the hormones are delivered: with the patch, the hormones are absorbed through the skin, and with the vaginal ring, the hormones are absorbed through the vaginal mucosa. Otherwise, the pharmacology of these contraceptives is essentially identical to that of combination OCs.

Transdermal Contraceptive Patch

The Ortho Evra and Xulane transdermal contraceptive patches have the same mechanism as combination OCs. Furthermore, these products have the same contraceptive efficacy and the same incidence of breakthrough bleeding and spotting. The principal difference between them lies with their dosing schedules: whereas combination OCs must be taken every day, the patch is applied just once a week. As a result, the patch is more convenient than OCs, and hence adherence is better.

The Ortho Evra and Xulane patches contain 750 mcg of ethinyl estradiol (the estrogen found in most combination OCs) and 6 mg of norelgestromin (the active metabolite of norgestimate, a progestin found in some OCs). Each day, the patch releases 35 mcg of ethinyl estradiol and 150 mcg of norelgestromin. After release, these hormones penetrate the skin, enter capillaries, and undergo distribution throughout the body. Plasma levels plateau 2 days after the first patch is applied.

Application of the patch, which is 1.75 inches square, is done once a week for 3 weeks, followed by 1 week off (to permit normal menstruation). Patches are applied to the lower abdomen, buttocks, upper outer arm, or upper torso (front or back)—but not to the breasts or to skin that is red, cut, or irritated. To enhance adhesion, the skin should be clean, dry, and free of lotions, creams, and oils. In clinical trials, the pregnancy rate was about 1 for every 100 woman-years of patch use. However, among women who weighed 90 kg (198 lb) or more, the pregnancy rate was significantly higher, suggesting the patch may be inappropriate for women in this weight group.

When should patch use begin? For women not currently using OCs, the first patch should be applied during the first 24 hours of the menstrual period. For women switching from OCs, the first patch should be applied on the first day of withdrawal bleeding.

In clinical trials, 4.6% of patches became partially or completely detached. When this occurs, the patch should be reattached or replaced. If the patch has been off less than 24 hours, backup contraception is unnecessary. However, if the patch has been off more than 24 hours, a new cycle should be started, accompanied by backup contraception during the first 7 days.

The most common adverse effects are breast discomfort, headache, local irritation, nausea, and menstrual cramps. Compared with Triphasil (a combination OC), the patch produces a higher incidence of breast discomfort and dysmenorrhea. Contraindications and drug interactions are the same as for combination OCs.

Does the patch cause more VTE than do OCs? Possibly. Three epidemiologic studies have examined the question. In two of the studies, the risk for VTE in women using the patch was double the risk in women using combination OCs. However, in the third study, there was no difference in risk. Of note, women who use the patch are exposed to 60% more estrogen than women who use an OC containing 35 mcg of estrogen. The higher estrogen exposure could increase the risk for VTE.

Vaginal Contraceptive Ring

NuvaRing is a hormonal contraceptive device designed for vaginal insertion. Like combination OCs, the ring contains an estrogen/progestin combination that prevents pregnancy largely by suppressing ovulation. Adverse effects, drug interactions, warnings, and contraindications for the ring are the same as for combination OCs. The ring is made of transparent, flexible material and looks like a very skinny doughnut, with an overall diameter of 2.1 inches and a cross-sectional diameter of ⅛ inch. Insertion is done by the user.

The NuvaRing contains 2.7 mg of ethinyl estradiol and 11.7 mg of etonogestrel (the active metabolite of desogestrel, a progestin found in some OCs). Each day, the ring releases 15 mcg of ethinyl estradiol and 120 mcg of etonogestrel. After release, the hormones penetrate the vaginal mucosa, undergo absorption into the blood, and then distribute throughout the body. Contraception results from systemic effects—not from local effects in the vagina.

One ring is inserted once each month, left in place for 3 weeks, and then removed; a new ring is inserted 1 week later. During the ring-free week, withdrawal bleeding occurs. The new ring should be inserted on schedule, even if bleeding is still ongoing. If a ring is expelled before 3 weeks have passed, it can be washed off in warm water (not hot water) and reinserted. If the expelled ring cannot be reused, a new one should be inserted. If more than 3 hours elapse between ring expulsion and reinsertion, contraceptive effects may be diminished, and hence backup contraception should be used for 7 days.

Initiating ring use is done as follows:

- For women not currently using contraception, ring use should start anytime during days 1 through 5 of the menstrual cycle, even if bleeding is ongoing; backup contraception should be used during the first 7 days.
- For women switching from combination OCs, ring use should start within 7 days of taking the last active OC; no backup contraception is needed.
- For women switching from progestin-only OCs, ring use should start on the same day the last pill is taken, which can be any day of the month; backup contraception should be used during the first 7 days.
- For women switching from Nexplanon, ring use should start on the same day that the implant is removed; backup contraception should be used during the first 7 days.
- For women switching from a levonorgestrel-containing IUD, ring use should start on the same day the IUD is removed; backup contraception should be used during the first 7 days.
- For women switching from intramuscular (IM) progestin injections, ring use should start on the day of the next scheduled injection; backup contraception should be used during the first 7 days.

The most common adverse effects are vaginitis, headaches, upper respiratory infection, leukorrhea, sinusitis, weight gain, and nausea. Common reasons for discontinuing the ring include foreign body sensations, coital problems, ring expulsion, vaginal symptoms, headache, and emotional lability. The risk for serious adverse effects—thrombosis, embolism, and hypertension—is the same as with combination OCs.

LONG-ACTING CONTRACEPTIVES

Subdermal Etonogestrel Implants

A subdermal system [Nexplanon] for delivery of etonogestrel is available for long-term, reversible contraception. As shown in Table 49.1, Nexplanon is among the most effective contraceptives available.

Description

Nexplanon consists of a single 4-cm rod that contains 68 mg of etonogestrel, a synthetic progestin. The rod is implanted subdermally in the groove between the biceps and triceps in the nondominant arm. Etonogestrel then diffuses slowly and continuously, providing blood levels sufficient for contraception for 3 years, after which the rod is removed. If continued contraception is desired, a new rod is implanted.

Mechanism of Action

Etonogestrel suppresses ovulation and thickens cervical mucus. In addition, it causes the endometrium to become involuted and hence hostile to implantation.

Pharmacokinetics

Daily release of etonogestrel is 60 to 70 mcg initially and gradually declines to 25 to 30 mcg over 3 years. Absorbed drug is slowly metabolized by the liver. When the rod is removed, etonogestrel becomes undetectable within 5 to 7 days.

Drug Interactions

Agents that induce hepatic enzymes—such as barbiturates, phenytoin, rifampin, carbamazepine, topiramate, HIV protease inhibitors, and St. John's wort—may reduce the efficacy of Nexplanon. Accordingly, Nexplanon should not be used by women taking these drugs.

Adverse Effect: Irregular Bleeding

In women using Nexplanon, bleeding episodes are irregular and unpredictable. In clinical trials, amenorrhea occurred in 22% of women; infrequent bleeding (less than three bleeding or spotting episodes in 90 days) occurred in 34% of women; frequent bleeding (more than five bleeding or spotting episodes in 90 days) occurred in 7% of women, and prolonged bleeding (more than 14 days of bleeding in 90 days) occurred in 18% of women. Despite effects on bleeding, levels of hemoglobin were unaffected over 3 years. The general pattern of irregular and unpredictable bleeding does not change while using Nexplanon. Bleeding irregularities are the leading reason for discontinuing the device.

Use During Breastfeeding

Nexplanon is safe to use during breastfeeding after the 21st postpartum day. Very little etonogestrel is excreted in breast milk. In a controlled clinical trial, there were no significant effects on the physical or psychomotor development of infants. Also, Nexplanon had no effect on the production or quality of milk, even when implanted just a few days postpartum.

Depot Medroxyprogesterone Acetate

Depot medroxyprogesterone acetate (DMPA), given by IM or subcutaneous (subQ) injection, protects against pregnancy for 3 months or longer by inhibiting secretion of gonadotropins. The drug thereby (1) inhibits follicular maturation and ovulation, (2) thickens the cervical mucus, and (3) causes thinning of the endometrium, making implantation unlikely. When injections are discontinued, return of fertility is delayed (by an average of 9 months).

DMPA is available in two formulations for contraception. One is by IM injection [Depo-Provera], and the other is by subQ injection [Depo-SubQ Provera 104]. Dosages are 150 mg and 104 mg, respectively, injected once every 3 months. To ensure that the recipient is not pregnant, the first dose should be given either (1) during the first 5 days of a normal menstrual period, (2) within the first 5 days postpartum (if not breastfeeding), or (3) at the sixth week postpartum (if exclusively breastfeeding).

Most adverse effects are like those seen with other progestin-only contraceptives. Menstrual disturbances are common; menstruation may be irregular at first and then, after 6 to 12 months, may cease entirely. Mild weight gain (about 3.5 lb) is likely during the first year. Women may also experience abdominal bloating, headache, depression, and decreased libido. However, it is unclear that DMPA is the cause. Although DMPA has produced uterine and mammary cancers in animals, a large-scale study has shown no increase in the risk for cervical, ovarian, or breast cancer in women—and the risk for endometrial cancer is actually reduced.

DMPA poses a risk for reversible bone loss, but this risk does not outweigh the benefits of treatment. During the first 1 to 2 years of DMPA use, bone mineral density (BMD) declines rapidly, at a rate of 1% to 2% per year. However, after this time, the rate of bone loss slows down. Importantly, when DMPA is discontinued, BMD returns to pretreatment levels, typically within 30 months. Whether DMPA-induced bone loss increases the risk for fractures is unclear. While this story was still evolving, the FDA revised the label for DMPA to include a black box warning that recommends against using the drug for more than 2 years. However, in the light of data gathered, this warning appears unwarranted. Accordingly, in 2008, an American College of Obstetricians and Gynecologists committee counseled that practitioners should not let concerns about bone loss deter them from prescribing DMPA or cause them to limit prescriptions to 2 years. In addition, the committee recommended against routine testing of BMD in women on DMPA. When counseling patients about this issue, practitioners should point out that any risk for fracture with DMPA is theoretical, whereas the risks associated with pregnancy are very real.

Intrauterine Devices

IUDs are among the most reliable forms of reversible birth control (see Table 49.1). In addition, the IUDs available today are very safe when used by appropriate patients. Worldwide, more than 85 million women use these devices. However, IUDs are not popular in the United States: among women who use birth control, only 5.5% choose an IUD. Nonuse of IUDs is largely the legacy of the Dalkon Shield, a poorly designed IUD associated with a high rate of pelvic infection.

Four IUDs are available: the copper T 380A [ParaGard] and the levonorgestrel-releasing intrauterine systems Mirena, Liletta, and Skyla. All are extremely effective. IUDs are placed within 7 days of the onset of menses, and a replacement can be inserted during any phase of the menstrual cycle. ParaGard can remain in place for 10 years, Mirena for 5 years, and Liletta and Skyla for 3 years. These devices prevent conception by producing a harmless local inflammatory response that is spermicidal. ParaGard, whose active ingredient is copper, may also inhibit implantation. Mirena, whose active ingredient is levonorgestrel, also causes endometrial involution and thickening of the cervical mucus. Neither device prevents ovulation.

With proper counseling and patient selection, IUDs are very safe. The principal risk is PID secondary to an STD. Accordingly, IUDs should be used only by women with a low risk for STDs—that is, by women who are monogamous and are confident that their partners are, too. The risk for PID is highest during the first 20 days after insertion, with a rate of 9.7 cases per 1000 woman-years of use. One month after insertion, the risk declines to only 1.4 cases per 1000 woman-years of use.

IUDs can cause cramping and alteration of menses. Cramping is most intense upon IUD insertion and can be minimized by applying a topical anesthetic (2% lidocaine intracervical gel) or by premedicating with ibuprofen. With ParaGard, monthly bleeding is increased. With the levonorgestrel IUDs, light spotting and amenorrhea are common.

In addition to providing long-term contraception, IUDs have other uses. Owing to its ability to greatly reduce menstrual bleeding, Mirena is approved for treating menorrhagia (heavy menstrual bleeding) in women who want to use an IUD for contraception. ParaGard can be used for emergency contraception. In one study, the pregnancy rate with postcoital placement was reduced to 0.2%.

SPERMICIDES

Spermicides are chemical surfactants that kill sperm by destroying their cell membrane. These drugs are available in the form of a foam, gel, jelly, suppository, vaginal film, and contraceptive sponge. All formulations can be purchased without a prescription. When used alone, spermicides are only moderately effective (see Table 49.1). Combined use with a diaphragm or condom increases efficacy. As shown in Table 49.6, spermicidal preparations contain either nonoxynol 9 or octoxynol 9.

Spermicides are generally devoid of serious side effects. Studies show no relationship between spermicides and birth defects. However, there is some evidence that nonoxynol 9 may increase the risk for HIV transmission. The apparent mechanism is promotion of vaginal, cervical, anal, and rectal lesions that facilitate HIV penetration to cells. Allergic reactions (to the drug or vehicle) occur in some women.

Correct use is required for contraceptive efficacy. The spermicide must be applied before intercourse, but no more than 1 hour in advance (when used alone). Containers for foam preparations must be shaken thoroughly before each use to ensure dispersal of the spermicide. Suppositories should be inserted at least 10 to 15 minutes before intercourse to allow time for dissolution. Spermicides should be reapplied each time intercourse is anticipated. Douching should be postponed for at least 6 hours after coitus.

The contraceptive sponge [Today Sponge] is a soft, porous, polyurethane disk impregnated with 1000 mg of nonoxynol 9. When inserted to cover the cervix, it protects against conception by (1) releasing spermicide, (2) absorbing seminal fluid, and (3) blocking penetration of sperm. Unlike other spermicide products, which must be reapplied before each act of intercourse, a single sponge is effective for 24 hours, regardless of how often coitus takes place. After 24 hours, the sponge should be removed. The rates of unintended pregnancy with the sponge are high: 16% among typical nulliparous users, and 32% among parous users. The most common adverse effects are vaginal irritation and dryness. The Today Sponge was voluntarily withdrawn in 1995 and then reintroduced in 2005.

EMERGENCY CONTRACEPTION

Emergency contraception (EC) is defined as contraception that is implemented *after* intercourse. Women can use EC to prevent pregnancy after unprotected intercourse, which can result from sexual assault, contraceptive failure (e.g., broken condom), or other reasons. Safe and effective methods of EC have been available for decades. However, products marketed specifically for EC are relatively new.

In the United States nearly 50% of women aged 15 to 44 years report having had at least one unintended pregnancy. Among teenagers, 88% of pregnancies are unintended. Of the 6 million pregnancies that occur each year, about 3.5 million are accidental. Every year, unintended pregnancies lead to 1.4 million abortions and 1.1 million births that women did not

TABLE 49.6 ■ Spermicides

Formulation	Active Ingredient	Trade Name
Foam	Nonoxynol 9 (12.5%)	Delfen Contraceptive
Jelly	Nonoxynol 9 (3%)	Gynol II Extra Strength Contraceptive*
Gel	Nonoxynol 9 (4%)	Conceptrol Disposable Contraceptive
	Nonoxynol 9 (3.5%)	Advantage 24*
	Nonoxynol 9 (2.2%)	K-Y Plus*
	Nonoxynol 9 (2%)	Shur Seal*
	Octoxynol 9 (1%)	Ortho-Gynol Contraceptive*
Suppository	Nonoxynol 9 (2.27%)	Encare
	Nonoxynol 9 (100 mg)	Semicid
Sponge	Nonoxynol 9 (1000 mg)	Today Sponge
Vaginal film	Nonoxynol 9 (28%)	VCF

*Intended for use only in combination with a vaginal diaphragm.

want—at least not yet. Clearly, if EC were used widely, most abortions and unwanted births could be avoided.

EC can be accomplished in two basic ways: Taking an *emergency contraceptive pill* (ECP), also known as a *morning-after pill,* or inserting a copper-T IUD. Taking an ECP is most common. Furthermore, of the three basic types of ECPs—progestin-only pills, ulipristal-containing pills, and estrogen/progestin pills—the progestin-only pills are used most widely.

Progestin-Only Emergency Contraception Pills

Three progestin-only products are available: Plan B One-Step, Next Choice One Dose, and Next Choice. All three contain *levonorgestrel.* These products are packaged and marketed specifically for emergency contraception. This contrasts with the estrogen/progestin products, which are marketed as OCs but can be used off-label for EC.

Plan B One-Step and Next Choice One Dose

Plan B One-Step and Next Choice One Dose consist of a single, high-dose (1.5-mg) tablet of levonorgestrel, a progestin found in many combination OCs. The package insert calls for taking the tablet within 72 hours of unprotected intercourse. However, although early implementation is best, Plan B One-Step, Next Choice One Dose, and other ECPs can still be effective when started up to 5 days after intercourse. Success is indicated by onset of menstrual bleeding in about 21 days.

Plan B One-Step reduces the odds of pregnancy by 89% and Next Choice One Dose prevented 84% of expected pregnancies, which is better than it may seem. In the absence of these two medications, the pregnancy rate from a single act of unprotected intercourse is about 8% (i.e., 8 women in 100 would become pregnant). However, among women using Plan B One-Step or Next Choice One Dose, only 1 and 1.3 in 100 are likely to become pregnant—a reduction of 89% and 84% respectively.

Plan B One-Step and Next Choice One Dose work primarily by delaying or stopping ovulation. Inhibition of fertilization may also contribute. Of note, levonorgestrel is *not* effective after fertilization has occurred.

The major side effects of Plan B One-Step are heavier menstrual bleeding, nausea, abdominal pain, headache, and dizziness. Nausea can be reduced by taking an antiemetic (e.g., prochlorperazine) 1 hour before dosing. Importantly, if pregnancy does occur, having used levonorgestrel will not increase the risk for major congenital malformations, pregnancy complications, or any other adverse pregnancy outcomes.

Does Plan B One-Step or Next Choice One Dose cause abortion? NO! These drugs will not terminate an existing pregnancy and will not harm a fetus if present. Recall that pregnancy is defined as implantation of a fertilized egg. Because Plan B One-Step and Next Choice One Dose act before fertilization and implantation, they cannot be considered abortifacients.

For women aged 15 years and older, Plan B One-Step and Next Choice One Dose are now available over the counter. No prescription is required. However, you do need a government-issued ID to prove your age, and a licensed pharmacist must dispense the drug. For women who are not yet 15 years old, Plan B One-Step is still available, but a prescription is required. Prescriptions can be obtained from private physicians, clinics run by Planned Parenthood, and student health departments at colleges and universities.

Next Choice

Next Choice consists of two 0.75-mg tablets of levonorgestrel (one half the amount in a single Plan B One-Step or Next Choice One Dose tablet). According to the package insert, women should take 1 tablet within 72 hours of intercourse and a second tablet 12 hours later. However, taking both tablets at the same time is just as effective. (This is equivalent to taking one tablet of Plan B One-Step or Next Choice One Step.) As with Plan B One-Step and Next Choice One Dose, these ECPs can still be effective when started up to 5 days after intercourse but are most effective when taken earlier. Adverse effects are similar to those of Plan B One-Step and Next Choice One Dose. If vomiting occurs within 2 hours of dosing, a repeat dose may be required. Like Plan B One-Step, Next Choice can be obtained without a prescription (by women 15 years and older) or with a prescription (by women younger than 15 years).

Ulipristal Acetate Emergency Contraception Pill

Ulipristal acetate [ella] is a drug that acts as an agonist-antagonist at receptors for progestin. Like levonorgestrel, ulipristal acetate prevents conception primarily by suppressing ovulation. Despite this similarity, ulipristal acetate and levonorgestrel differ in two important ways. First, ulipristal acetate remains highly effective when taken up to *5* days (120 hours) after intercourse, whereas levonorgestrel is most effective when taken within *3* days (72 hours) of intercourse. Second, whereas levonorgestrel [Plan B One-Step, Next Choice, Next Choice One Dose] is available without a prescription for women 15 years and older, ulipristal acetate [ella] requires a prescription for all women, regardless of age. The dosage for ulipristal acetate is 1 tablet (30 mg), taken up to 5 days after unprotected intercourse. Principal adverse effects are headache, nausea, dysmenorrhea, and abdominal pain. If vomiting occurs within 3 hours of dosing, an additional dose may be required.

Estrogen/Progestin Emergency Contraception Pills (Yuzpe Regimen)

The *Yuzpe regimen,* first described in 1974 by Professor A. Alfred Yuzpe, consists of two doses of an OC that contains an estrogen (ethinyl estradiol) plus a progestin (levonorgestrel or norgestrel). The first dose should be taken within 72 hours of unprotected intercourse and the second dose 12 hours later. Pregnancy is prevented by interfering with ovulation, fertilization, and implantation. Like other ECPs, this regimen will not cause abortion. Compared with Plan B One-Step, this regimen is less effective (75% vs. 89%) and causes more nausea (50% vs. 13.3%) and vomiting (19% vs. 6%). Combination OCs that can be used for EC are shown in Table 49.5. However, because other ECPs are more effective, better tolerated, and readily available, these alternatives are used infrequently.

Mifepristone as an Emergency Contraception Pill

One drug—*mifepristone (RU 486)*—can prevent pregnancy *or* cause abortion, depending on when it is taken. If mifepristone is taken within 5 days of unprotected intercourse, it will prevent pregnancy from occurring and thus can be considered an ECP. However, if mifepristone is taken after this time, it may terminate pregnancy that has already begun and thus can be considered an abortifacient. When used as an ECP, mifepristone is 100% effective. The drug is available in the United States but is not approved for EC.

The Copper Intrauterine Device

Insertion of a *copper IUD* within 5 days of unprotected intercourse can prevent pregnancy in most women. The method is more than 99.9% effective, allowing less than 1 pregnancy for every 1000 IUD recipients. IUD insertion has the additional benefit of providing ongoing contraception for up to 10 years. Although using an IUD for EC is highly effective, the technique does have drawbacks: the IUD is expensive, not all women are candidates, and obtaining one quickly may be difficult.

DRUGS FOR MEDICAL ABORTION

Mifepristone (RU 486) With Misoprostol

Mifepristone (RU 486) [Mifeprex] is a synthetic steroid that blocks receptors for progesterone and glucocorticoids. In the United States the drug has one approved indication: termination of early intrauterine pregnancy; cotreatment with misoprostol is usually required. Investigational uses include breast cancer, ovarian cancer, meningiomas, Cushing syndrome, uterine fibroids, and endometriosis. In addition, mifepristone is the most effective drug known for emergency contraception, although it is not used routinely for this purpose.

Mifepristone, followed by misoprostol, is a safe and effective alternative to surgery for termination of early pregnancy. Together, these drugs terminate pregnancy in about 95% of women. Principal adverse effects are abdominal pain and vaginal bleeding, which are unavoidable aspects of abortion. There is also a small risk for infection. In contrast to surgical abortion, which is generally unavailable before 8 weeks of gestation, abortion with mifepristone is performed early—within 7 weeks of conception.

Mechanism of Action

Mifepristone acts through blockade of progesterone receptors. Although mifepristone also blocks receptors for glucocorticoids, this action does not contribute to abortion. In the pregnant uterus, the drug has three effects. First, blockade of progesterone receptors leads to decidual breakdown and detachment of the conceptus. Second, mifepristone promotes cervical softening and dilation. Third, mifepristone increases uterine production of prostaglandins and renders the myometrium more responsive to the contractile effects of these prostaglandins. All three effects lead to expulsion of the conceptus. If mifepristone alone fails to induce abortion, the patient is given 400 mcg of oral misoprostol, a synthetic prostaglandin that reinforces uterine contractions induced by mifepristone. The pharmacology of misoprostol is discussed separately later.

Clinical Trials

In a study conducted in France, the abortion success rate with mifepristone/misoprostol was nearly 99%. Success was defined as termination of pregnancy with complete expulsion of the conceptus. All women in the study had amenorrhea for less than 50 days before receiving mifepristone. Dosing was done as follows: each patient received a 600-mg oral dose of mifepristone and, if abortion had not occurred within 48 hours, each was given a 400-mcg dose of oral misoprostol; a second dose of misoprostol (200 mcg) was offered if abortion had not occurred by 4 hours after the first dose. Only 5.5% of the pregnancies terminated before dosing with misoprostol; with the addition of misoprostol, either one or two doses, the cumulative success rate was 98.7%. In the majority of patients (69%), abortion occurred within 4 hours of the first misoprostol dose.

In the United States success with mifepristone/misoprostol has also been good—although not quite as good as in France. In 1999 American researchers reported that the abortion rate with mifepristone/misoprostol declined with increasing duration of gestation. Success was greatest (92%) when gestation was 49 days or less, falling to 83% during days 50 to 56 of gestation and to 77% during days 57 to 63. The dosages employed were the same as in the French study. Why the success rate was lower than in the French study is unknown.

There is good evidence that intravaginal misoprostol is more effective and better tolerated than oral misoprostol. In one study, women received 600 mg of oral mifepristone, followed by 800 mcg of misoprostol, either PO or intravaginally. After intravaginal misoprostol, 95% of conceptuses were expelled without the need for surgery, compared with only 87% after oral misoprostol. With intravaginal dosing, abortion occurred within 4 hours in 93% of patients, compared with 78% of patients receiving oral misoprostol. The incidence of nausea and vomiting with intravaginal dosing was significantly lower than with oral dosing. Intravaginal misoprostol—but not oral misoprostol—has been associated with very rare cases of severe sepsis, one heart attack, and one death (from hemorrhage) after a ruptured ectopic pregnancy. However, a causal relationship between these events and mifepristone/misoprostol has not been established.

Adverse Effects

The most common side effects are bleeding, cramping, nausea, vomiting, diarrhea, and headache. The most serious adverse effects are severe bleeding and sepsis.

Successful abortion necessarily causes abdominal pain (cramping) and bleeding. Nearly all women experience these events. About 80% of patients experience transient cramping, beginning 1 hour after taking misoprostol; most women require an opioid analgesic for relief. Bleeding and spotting typically last 9 to 16 days. However, in some women, bleeding persists for 30 days or more. About 1% of women experience severe bleeding; treatment measures include curettage, uterotonic drugs (e.g., methylergonovine, ergonovine), and infusion of fluids, blood, or both.

Mifepristone/misoprostol has been associated with a few cases of serious bacterial infection, including very rare cases of fatal septic shock. Accordingly, patients and providers should be alert for typical signs of sepsis (sustained fever of 100.4° F or higher, severe abdominal pain, pelvic tenderness). However, in two confirmed cases of sepsis caused by Clostridium sordellii, these signs were absent. Instead, the patients presented with nausea, vomiting, and diarrhea, without fever or abdominal pain. In patients with typical or atypical presentation, the possibility of infection should be evaluated immediately.

The bleeding caused by mifepristone/misoprostol could mask bleeding due to a ruptured ectopic pregnancy. Accordingly, before mifepristone/misoprostol is used, ectopic pregnancy must be ruled out. This is best done by a routine ultrasound examination.

Misoprostol (but not mifepristone), a proven teratogen, can cause Möbius syndrome, a rare fetal anomaly. Hence if the mifepristone/misoprostol fails to induce abortion, performing surgical abortion should be considered.

Contraindications

Major contraindications to mifepristone/misoprostol are ectopic pregnancy, hemorrhagic disorders, or use of anticoagulant drugs. Because mifepristone blocks receptors for glucocorticoids, it should not be used in women with adrenal insufficiency and those on long-term glucocorticoid therapy.

Preparations, Dosage, and Administration

Mifepristone [Mifeprex] is supplied in single-dose packets containing three 200-mg tablets. The dosage is 600 mg taken all at once—followed in 2 days by 400 mcg of misoprostol (if mifepristone did not induce complete abortion by itself). Mifepristone is available only through qualified physicians; it is not sold in pharmacies.

UNIT XII
Men's Health

CHAPTER 50 Androgens

Jacqueline Rosenjack Burchum, DNSc, FNP-BC, CNE

Androgen hormones are produced by the testes, ovaries, and adrenal cortex. The major endogenous androgen is testosterone. Androgens are noted most for their ability to promote expression of male sex characteristics. However, androgens also influence sexuality in females. In addition, androgens have significant physiologic and pharmacologic effects unrelated to sexual expression or function. The primary clinical application of the androgens is management of androgen deficiency in males. Principal adverse effects are virilization and hepatotoxicity.

TESTOSTERONE

Testosterone is the prototype of the androgen hormones. This compound is the principal endogenous androgen in both males and females. In addition to its physiologic role, testosterone is representative of the androgens employed clinically.

Biosynthesis and Secretion

Males

Testosterone is made by Leydig cells of the testes. Daily production in men ranges from 2.5 to 10 mg. Synthesis is promoted by two hormones of the anterior pituitary: follicle-stimulating hormone (FSH) and luteinizing hormone (LH), also known as interstitial cell–stimulating hormone. Production of testosterone is regulated by negative feedback control: rising plasma levels of testosterone act on the pituitary to suppress further release of FSH and LH, thereby decreasing the stimulus for further testosterone formation.

Some of the testosterone present in plasma is produced by the adrenal glands. However, androgenic activity of adrenal origin is much less than that of testicular origin. Hence, in males, adrenal androgens have minimal functional significance.

Testosterone production changes over time. Peak production occurs around age 17 years. Production then remains steady until age 30 or 40 years, after which it slowly declines. By the time a man reaches 80 years, testosterone production is only half what it was in his youth.

Females

In women, preandrogens (precursors of testosterone) are secreted by the adrenal cortex and ovaries. Conversion into testosterone takes place in peripheral tissues. Synthesis of preandrogens by the adrenal glands is regulated by adrenocorticotropic hormone, whereas synthesis of preandrogens by the ovaries is regulated by LH. Daily testosterone production is about 300 mcg (150 mcg from the ovaries and 150 mcg from the adrenal glands). The total is 10 to 40 times less than the amount produced in men. In the event of ovarian or adrenocortical pathology (e.g., adenoma, carcinoma, hyperplasia), secretion of androgens can increase greatly and may be sufficient to produce virilization. At menopause, testosterone production decreases.

Mechanism of Action

Effects of testosterone on its target tissues are mediated by specific receptors located in the cell cytoplasm. After binding of testosterone to its receptor, the hormone-receptor complex migrates to the cell nucleus and then acts on DNA to promote synthesis of specific messenger RNA molecules. These, in turn, serve as templates for production of specific proteins, which then mediate testosterone effects. It should be noted that in some tissues—prostate, seminal vesicles, and hair follicles—androgen receptors do not interact with testosterone itself. Rather, they interact with dihydrotestosterone, a testosterone metabolite.

Physiologic and Pharmacologic Effects

Effects on Sex Characteristics in Males

Pubertal Transformation

Increased production of testosterone promotes the transformations that signal puberty in males. Under the influence of testosterone, the testes enlarge, after which the penis and scrotum enlarge. Pubic and axillary hair appears, and hair on the trunk, arms, and legs assumes adult male patterns. Testosterone stimulates growth of bone and skeletal muscle, causing height and weight to increase rapidly. Testosterone also accelerates epiphyseal closure, causing bone growth to cease within a few years. The larynx enlarges, thereby deepening the voice. Sebaceous glands increase in number, causing the skin to become oily; acne results if the glands become clogged and infected. The final pubertal change is beard development. Several years are required for all of these changes to occur.

Spermatogenesis

Androgens are necessary for production of sperm by the seminiferous tubules and for maturation of sperm as they pass through the epididymis and vas deferens. Androgen deficiency causes sterility.

Effects on Sex Characteristics in Females

Under physiologic conditions, endogenous androgens have only moderate effects in females. Principal among these are promotion of clitoral growth and, perhaps, maintenance of normal libido. However, when production of androgens becomes excessive (e.g., in girls with congenital adrenal hyperplasia), virilization can take place. Virilization can also occur in response to therapeutic use of androgens or to androgen abuse.

Anabolic Effects

Testosterone promotes growth of skeletal muscle. This anabolic effect results from binding of androgens to the same type of receptor that mediates androgen actions in other tissues. Effects in young males, and in females of any age, can be dramatic. In contrast, effects in healthy adult males are modest. The testes of adult males already produce enough testosterone to cause near-maximal stimulation of the musculature, so, in adult males, the increment in muscle mass that can be achieved with exogenous androgens is relatively small.

Erythropoietic Effects

Testosterone promotes synthesis of erythropoietin, a hormone that acts on bone marrow to increase production of erythrocytes. This action of testosterone, together with the high levels of testosterone present in males, explains why men have a higher hematocrit than women. When women are given testosterone, the hematocrit rises and hemoglobin levels increase by an average of 4.3 g/dL. In contrast, because men have high testosterone levels to begin with, the increase in plasma hemoglobin that can be elicited with exogenous androgens is smaller—only 1 g/dL.

CLINICAL PHARMACOLOGY OF THE ANDROGENS

In addition to testosterone, a few other androgens are employed clinically. All of these agents can bind to androgen receptors, and therefore all can elicit similar responses. Major differences among individual androgens pertain to route of administration, pharmacokinetics, adverse effects, and specific applications.

Classification

The androgens used clinically fall into two basic groups: (1) testosterone and testosterone esters, and (2) 17-alpha-alkylated compounds (noted for their hepatotoxicity). Androgens belonging to each group are shown in Table 50.1.

When speaking of testosterone-like compounds, it is traditional to distinguish between "androgens" and "anabolic steroids." However, we will not make this distinction because it is now clear that the receptor type that mediates the androgenic actions of the androgens is the same receptor type that mediates the anabolic actions of these hormones. Consequently, it has not been possible to separate anabolic activity from androgenic activity: virtually all anabolic hormones are also androgenic. Accordingly, rather than creating two categories—androgens *versus* anabolic steroids—and assigning some agents to one category and some to the other, we will refer to all of the testosterone-like drugs as androgens.

Therapeutic Uses

In April 2015, the FDA published a required label change for testosterone (see http://www.fda.gov/Drugs/DrugSafety/ucm436259.htm). The new labeling approves testosterone use only for those patients with confirmed testosterone deficiency due to hypogonadism. The FDA further emphasized that lowered testosterone due to aging did not meet criteria for hypogonadism. The Endocrine Society has published their clinical guidelines for managing testosterone therapy at http://press.endocrine.org/doi/pdf/10.1210/jc.2009-2354. Their algorithm to guide diagnosis of low testosterone due to hypogonadism is included in this article.

Individual androgens differ in their applications. No single androgen is employed for all of the uses discussed here. Specific applications of individual androgens are shown in Table 50.1.

Male Hypogonadism

When a man has hypogonadism, the testes fail to produce adequate amounts of testosterone, so replacement therapy is

TABLE 50.1 ▪ Approved Uses of Individual Androgens

Androgen	Indications			
	Hypogonadism (Male)	Replacement Therapy (Male)	Delayed Puberty (Male)	Catabolic States
TESTOSTERONE AND TESTOSTERONE ESTERS				
Testosterone	✓	✓		
Testosterone cypionate	✓	✓		
Testosterone enanthate	✓	✓		
17-ALPHA-ALKYLATED ANDROGENS				
Fluoxymesterone	✓	✓	✓	
Methyltestosterone	✓	✓	✓	
Oxandrolone				✓

required. Male hypogonadism may be hereditary, or it may result from other causes, including pituitary failure, hypothalamic failure, and primary dysfunction of the testes.

When complete hypogonadism occurs in boys, puberty cannot take place—unless exogenous androgens are supplied. To induce puberty, a long-acting parenteral preparation (*testosterone enanthate* or *testosterone cypionate*) is chosen. Under the influence of these androgens, the normal sequence of pubertal changes occurs: growth is accelerated, the penis enlarges, the voice deepens, and other secondary sex characteristics become expressed. As in normal males, these changes take place over several years.

Replacement Therapy

Androgen replacement therapy is beneficial when testicular failure occurs in adult males. Some studies demonstrate that treatment restores libido, increases ejaculate volume, and supports expression of secondary sex characteristics. However, treatment will not restore fertility. The principal drugs employed for testosterone replacement are testosterone itself and two testosterone esters: testosterone enanthate and testosterone cypionate. Preparations and dosages for replacement therapy are shown in Table 50.2

Delayed Puberty

In some boys, puberty fails to occur at the usual age (i.e., before age 15 years). Most often, this failure reflects a familial pattern of delayed puberty and does not indicate pathology. Puberty can be expected to occur spontaneously, but later than usual. Hence, although androgen therapy can be employed, treatment is not an absolute necessity. However, the psychological pressures of delayed sexual maturation are sometimes greater than a boy can tolerate. In these cases, a limited course of androgen therapy is indicated. Both fluoxymesterone [Androxy] and methyltestosterone [Android, Methitest, Testred] are approved for this purpose.

If delayed puberty is the result of true hypogonadism, long-term replacement therapy is indicated (see later section "Androgen Preparations for Male Hypogonadism").

Replacement Therapy in Menopausal Women

Testosterone replacement therapy can alleviate some menopausal symptoms, especially fatigue, reduced libido, and reduced genital sensitivity. Testosterone is not approved for replacement in women in the United States, although it is approved in the United Kingdom.

TABLE 50.2 ▪ Products for Androgen Replacement Therapy in Hypogonadal Males

Formulation	Drug	Trade Name	Dosage	CSA Schedule	Comments
Oral tablet	Fluoxymesterone	Androxy	5–20 mg once daily	III	These 17-alpha-alkylated androgens are hepatotoxic, and androgenic effects are erratic. Oral therapy is not generally recommended.
	Methyltestosterone	Android, Methitest, Testred	10–50 mg once daily		
Intramuscular injection	Testosterone cypionate	Depo-Testosterone	50–400 mg every 2–4 wk	III	Safe, but require an office visit every 2–4 wk. Blood levels fluctuate widely (high after dosing and low before the next dose) and thereby cause variations in libido, energy, and mood.
	Testosterone enanthate	Delatestryl ♣	50–400 mg every 2–4 wk		
Transdermal patch	Testosterone	Androderm	One patch/day (delivers 2 or 4 mg/24 hr)	III	Applied to the arm, back, abdomen, or thigh, but *not* the scrotum. Causes local irritation.
Transdermal gel	Testosterone	AndroGel, Testim	5–10 g of 1% gel once daily (delivers 50–100 mg/day)	III	Apply AndroGel to upper arm, shoulder, or abdomen, but *not* the scrotum. Apply Testim only to upper arm or shoulder. Apply Fortesta to the front and inner thigh.
		Fortesta	40–70 mg of 2% gel once daily		Easier to use and better tolerated than testosterone patches. Can transfer to others via intimate contact.
Transdermal topical solution	Testosterone	Axiron	60–180 mg once daily	III	Apply to one or both armpits at the same time each morning. Easier to use and better tolerated than testosterone patches. Can transfer to others via skin-to-skin contact.
Nasal Gel	Testosterone	Natesto	11 mg (2 pump actuations) per nostril 3 times a day	III	Natesto nasal gel is delivered by a metered-dose pump. Each actuation of the pump delivers 5.5 mg of testosterone.
Implantable pellets	Testosterone	Testopel	150–450 mg (2–6 pellets) subQ every 3–6 months	III	Implanted subQ. Long lasting. Produce steady blood levels.
Buccal system	Testosterone	Striant	One buccal system (30 mg) every 12 hr	III	Provides fairly steady testosterone levels but may cause mouth or gum irritation.

CSA, Controlled Substances Act; subQ, subcutaneously.

Treatment of Transsexualism

Testosterone is used as masculinizing therapy for patients who are born with a female body but self-identify as male. Anticipated effects are increased hair growth over the face and body, a deepening of the voice, breast tissue atrophy, and cessation of menses. An increase in muscle tissue relative to adipose tissue also occurs. Therapy is highly individualized by specialists in transgender health.

Cachexia

Cachexia is a wasting of the body associated with severe illnesses such as AIDS, severe trauma, and chronic systemic infections. Testosterone levels often decline in these patients, putting them at risk for wasting and loss of muscle mass. Testosterone therapy decreases this risk. Oxandrolone [Oxandrin] is FDA approved for this purpose. Oxandrolone is an anabolic steroid that is a synthetic derivative of testosterone.

BLACK BOX WARNING: OXANDROLONE [OXANDRIN]

Oxandrolone can cause peliosis hepatitis, a condition in which blood-filled cysts form in the liver leading to liver failure or intraabdominal hemorrhage. It can also contribute to the development of highly vascular liver tumors.

An increased risk for atherosclerosis can occur secondary to marked elevations in LDL and decreases in HDL.

Anemias

Androgens are sometimes used in men and women to treat anemias that have been refractory to other therapy. Anemias most likely to respond include aplastic anemia, anemia associated with renal failure, Fanconi anemia, and anemia caused by cancer chemotherapy. Androgens help relieve anemia by promoting synthesis of erythropoietin, the renal hormone that stimulates production of red blood cells and, possibly, white blood cells and platelets. With the emergence of other therapies such as erythropoietin stimulating agents, however, androgens have fallen out of failure for off-label treatment of anemia.

Adverse Effects

Virilization in Women, Girls, and Boys

Virilization is the most common complication of androgen therapy. When taken in high doses by women, androgens can cause acne, deepening of the voice, proliferation of facial and body hair, male-pattern baldness, increased libido, clitoral enlargement, and menstrual irregularities. Clitoral growth, hair loss, and lowering of the voice may be irreversible. Masculinization can also occur in children. Boys may experience growth of pubic hair, penile enlargement, increased frequency of erections, and even priapism (persistent erection). In girls, growth of pubic hair and clitoral enlargement may occur. To prevent irreversible masculinization, androgens must be discontinued when virilizing effects first appear.

Premature Epiphyseal Closure

When given to children, androgens can accelerate epiphyseal closure, thereby decreasing adult height. To evaluate androgen effects on the epiphyses, radiographic examination of the hand and wrist should be performed every 6 months.

Hepatotoxicity

Androgens can cause *cholestatic hepatitis* and other disorders of the liver. Clinical *jaundice* may occur but is rare. Patients receiving androgens should undergo periodic tests of liver function. If jaundice develops, it will reverse after discontinuation of androgen use. Androgens may also be carcinogenic: *hepatocellular carcinoma* has developed in some patients after prolonged use of these drugs.

It must be emphasized that not all androgens are hepatotoxic: liver damage is associated primarily with the *17-alpha-alkylated androgens.* These androgens all share a structural feature in common: an alkyl group substituted on carbon 17 of the steroid nucleus. Because of their capacity to cause liver damage, *the 17-alpha-alkylated compounds should not be used long term.* In contrast to the 17-alpha-alkylated androgens, testosterone and the testosterone esters (testosterone cypionate, testosterone enanthate) are not associated with liver disease.

Effects on Cholesterol Levels

Androgens can lower plasma levels of high-density lipoprotein (HDL) cholesterol ("good cholesterol") and elevate plasma levels of low-density lipoprotein (LDL) cholesterol ("bad cholesterol"). These actions may increase the risk for atherosclerosis and related cardiovascular events.

Prostate Cancer

Androgens do not cause prostate cancer, but they can promote the growth of this cancer after it occurs. Accordingly, androgens are contraindicated for men with diagnosed prostate

PATIENT-CENTERED CARE ACROSS THE LIFESPAN

Androgens

Life Stage	Considerations or Concerns
Children	Androgens can cause virilization in children. They can also accelerate epiphyseal closure, thereby decreasing adult height.
Pregnant women	Androgens are Pregnancy Risk Category X: the ability to cause fetal harm outweighs any possible therapeutic benefit. Potential fetal changes include vaginal malformation, clitoral enlargement, and formation of a structure resembling the male scrotum. Virilization is most likely when androgens are taken during the first trimester. Women who become pregnant while using androgens should be informed about the possible effect on the fetus.
Breastfeeding women	Testosterone is excreted in breast milk. Breastfeeding is contraindicated.
Older adults	Older patients are at an increased risk for thromboembolic conditions such as myocardial infarction or stroke. Beers Criteria identify testosterone and methyltestosterone as potentially inappropriate for patients 65 years and older.

cancer. Men without diagnosed prostate cancer should be monitored for emergence of covert cancer.

Edema

Edema can result from androgen-induced retention of salt and water. This complication is a concern for patients with heart failure and for those with a predisposition to developing edema from other causes. Treatment consists of discontinuing the androgen and giving a diuretic, if needed.

Abuse Potential

As discussed later, androgens are frequently misused (abused) to enhance athletic performance. Because of their abuse potential, nearly all androgens are regulated as Schedule III controlled substances.

Risk for Thromboembolic Events

There have been post-marketing reports of thromboembolic events, including stroke, myocardial infarction, deep vein thrombosis, and pulmonary embolism. These events are believed to be the result of testosterone's erythropoietic effects. While long-term clinical trials are not available and randomized control trials have been inconclusive, the concern was sufficient to prompt the U.S. Food and Drug Administration (FDA) to issue a Testosterone Product Safety Alert in 2014 to address this potential life-threatening concern. (See http://www.fda.gov/Safety/MedWatch/SafetyInformation/SafetyAlertsforHumanMedicalProducts/ucm384225.htm)

Androgen Preparations for Male Hypogonadism

Treatment options for androgen replacement therapy have expanded in recent years. In the past, intramuscular (IM) therapy with a long-acting testosterone ester was the major treatment mode. Today, we have six attractive alternatives: a nasal gel, transdermal patch, transdermal gel, topical solution, buccal tablet, and implantable subcutaneous pellets. All of these formulations are regulated as Schedule III controlled substances.

Oral Androgens

Only two androgens are approved for oral therapy of male hypogonadism. Both drugs—fluoxymesterone and methyltestosterone—are 17-alpha-alkylated androgens and therefore pose a risk for hepatotoxicity. Accordingly, they should not be used long term and hence are not first-line agents.

Transdermal Testosterone

Testosterone is available in three transdermal formulations: patch, gel, and liquid. With all three formulations, testosterone is absorbed through the skin and then slowly absorbed into the blood.

Patches

Testosterone patches [Androderm] are indicated for male hypogonadism. Two strengths are available, delivering 2 mg or 4 mg of testosterone in 24 hours. Patches are applied once daily to the upper arm, thigh, back, or abdomen. The principal adverse effect is rash at the site of application.

Gels

Testosterone is available in four gel formulations, sold as AndroGel, Testim, Fortesta, and Vogelxo. AndroGel contains 1% or 1.62% testosterone; Testim contains 1% testosterone; and Fortesta contains 2% testosterone. Vogelxo is available in both unit-dose tubes and multidose metered pumps. Each unit-dose tube provides 50 mg testosterone. Each actuation of the pump provides 12.5 mg testosterone. All four gels are applied once daily to treat male hypogonadism. After the gel is applied, testosterone is absorbed rapidly into the skin and then slowly into the blood over the next 24 hours. Compared with transdermal patches, the gels have three advantages: they (1) cause less local irritation, (2) can't fall off, and (3) produce more consistent testosterone levels.

> **BLACK BOX WARNING: TESTOSTERONE GEL AND TOPICAL SOLUTION**
>
> Secondary exposure to testosterone gel on uncovered skin and to testosterone gel on unwashed clothing has resulted in virilization in children.

The principal disadvantage of the gels is that testosterone can be transferred to others by skin-to-skin contact. This is possible because only 10% of an applied dose is absorbed; the other 90% remains on the skin after the gel dries. In one study, blood levels of testosterone were doubled in female partners of gel users after 15 minutes of intimate contact that occurred 2 to 12 hours after the gel had been applied. Testosterone transfer is a concern because the drug can cause virilization of female partners and can also cause fetal harm. In children, contact transfer can cause genital enlargement, premature development of pubic hair, advanced bone age, increased libido, and aggressive behavior. In most cases, these effects regress after testosterone exposure stops. To reduce the risk for unintended gel transfer, the following guidelines should be followed:

- Gel users should wash their hands with soap and warm water after every application.
- Gel users should cover the application site with clothing once the gel has dried.
- Gel users should wash the application site before skin-to-skin contact with another person.
- Women and children should avoid skin-to-skin contact with application sites on gel users.
- Women and children who make accidental contact with a gel application site should wash contaminated skin immediately.

AndroGel is supplied in a metered-dose pump that delivers 12.25 mg per actuation (1%) or 20.25 mg per actuation (1.62%) and in unit-dose foil packets containing 20.25 mg of testosterone (of which 2.5 mg becomes absorbed) and 40.5 mg of testosterone (of which 5 mg becomes absorbed). The gel is applied once daily (preferably in the morning) to clean, dry skin of the shoulders, upper arms, or abdomen—but not the genitalia. Instruct patients to squeeze the entire contents of the packet into the palms and then immediately apply the gel to the skin and rub it in. To prevent the transfer of testosterone to others, patients should wash their hands and, after the gel has dried, keep the treated area covered with clothing. Because testosterone can be washed off, patients should wait 5 to 6 hours before showering or swimming. To ensure safe and effective dosing, blood levels of testosterone should be measured 14 days after initiating therapy and periodically thereafter.

Testim is available in 5-g tubes that contain 50 mg of testosterone, of which 10% (5 mg) gets absorbed. It is applied once daily to skin of the shoulders or upper arms, but not to the abdomen or scrotum. As with AndroGel, patients should wash their hands immediately and keep the treated area covered. They should also avoid showering for at least 2 hours. Testosterone levels should be checked after 14 days and periodically thereafter.

Fortesta is supplied in a metered-dose pump that delivers 10 mg of testosterone per actuation. All doses are applied to the front or inner thigh. As with AndroGel, patients should wash their hands immediately and keep the treated area covered. Also, they should avoid swimming or showering for at least 2 hours. Fortesta is a flammable, alcohol-based formulation, and hence patients should avoid flames or smoking until the gel has dried. Testosterone levels should be checked after days 14 and 35 and periodically thereafter.

Vogelxo in the tube formulation is applied in the same manner as Testim. Vogelxo in the metered-dose pump is applied just as Fortesta is applied. For both, the same advice and precautions apply.

Topical Solution

Testosterone topical solution for underarm application [Axiron] is much like the testosterone gels. The principal difference is the application site: Axiron liquid is formulated specifically for application to the axilla, whereas Testim is applied to the shoulder or upper arm, and AndroGel is applied to the shoulder, upper arm, or abdomen. After application, testosterone is absorbed rapidly into the skin and then slowly into the blood. Steady-state levels are reached in 14 days. After application stops, blood levels take 7 to 10 days to decline to baseline.

Axiron is supplied as an alcohol-based solution in a metered-dose pump that delivers 30 mg of testosterone per actuation. Dosing is done by pumping the liquid onto an applicator (supplied with the pump) and then applying the liquid to clean, dry, intact skin of the underarm—and not to anyplace else. Patients should not swim or bathe for 2 hours after application. If an underarm deodorant or antiperspirant is used, it should be applied before applying testosterone (to avoid contaminating the deodorant or antiperspirant dispenser). Because of its alcohol content, Axiron liquid is flammable. Accordingly, users should stay away from flames until the solution has dried.

Axiron is applied to each axilla at the same time every morning. After 14 days or longer, blood levels of testosterone are measured, and dosage is adjusted up or down as indicated.

Like the testosterone gels, testosterone topical solution can be transferred to others through skin-to-skin contact, posing a risk to women and children. Accordingly, the same guidelines noted previously should be followed. That is, Axiron users should wash their hands after every application, cover the application site with clothing after the solution has dried, and wash the application site before anticipated skin-to-skin contact with another person. Women and children should avoid contact with skin where Axiron was applied and should wash contaminated skin if accidental contact with an application site occurs.

Nasal Gel

Testosterone nasal gel [Natesto] is the newest formulation approved for testosterone administration. It comes in a metered-dose pump that sprays 5.5 mg of testosterone each time the pump is actuated.

Because the drug is administered nasally, patients with nasal disorders or abnormalities (e.g., chronic sinusitis, a severely deviated nasal septum) should not take this drug. There has not been adequate testing for interactions with other nasally administered drugs. Currently, only adrenergic agonists (e.g., oxymetazoline nasal spray) are approved for administration with Natesto.

The route of administration can cause localized reactions. These include rhinorrhea, epistaxis, and nasopharyngitis; however, these tend to be modest effects.

Administration instructions are supplied with the drug; however, it is important that the provider be aware of these in order to answer patient questions.

1. The pump should be primed before use and excess gel removed.
2. The patient should blow the nose before administration.
3. The pump is inserted into the nostril with the tip aimed toward the lateral nostril wall.
4. The pump is depressed slowly until it stops.
5. As the tip is withdrawn, it should be wiped against the lateral nostril wall to ensure that any remaining gel is distributed to the nostril.
6. After administration in both nostrils, the nose should be lightly massaged below the nasal bridge.
7. The patient should avoiding blowing or sniffing for at least 1 hour after administration.

Implantable Testosterone Pellets

Testosterone pellets [Testopel] are long-acting formulations indicated for male hypogonadism and delayed puberty. The pellets are implanted subdermally in the hip area or abdominal wall lateral to the umbilicus. Each pellet contains 75 mg of testosterone. The usual dosage is 150 to 450 mg (2–6 pellets) every 3 to 6 months. About one third of the dose is absorbed the first month, one fourth the second month, and one sixth the third month. For patients switching from IM testosterone propionate or IM testosterone enanthate, the recommended dosage is 2 pellets for each 25 mg of IM testosterone used weekly. For example, a patient receiving 75 mg of IM testosterone enanthate each week would switch to 6 pellets every 3 to 4 months.

Testosterone Buccal Tablets

Testosterone buccal tablets [Striant], approved for male hypogonadism, produce steady blood levels of testosterone. Tablets are applied to the gum area just above the incisor tooth, and are designed to stay in place until removed. To ensure good adhesion, tablets should be held in place (with a finger over the lip) for 30 seconds. The recommended dosage is 1 tablet every 12 hours, alternating sides of the mouth with each dose. If a tablet falls out before 8 hours, it should be replaced with a new one for the remainder of the dosing interval. If a tablet falls out after 8 hours, it should be replaced with a new one, and the next scheduled dose should be skipped (i.e., the replacement tablet should remain in place for 16 hours or so). The tablets are not affected by eating, drinking, chewing gum, or brushing teeth. Adverse effects, which are usually transient, include local irritation, bitter taste, and taste distortion. Treatment for up to 1 year has not caused serious gum changes. It has been hypothesized that transfer of testosterone from buccal routes may occur through saliva transfer during kissing.

Intramuscular Testosterone Esters

Two IM testosterone esters are available: testosterone cypionate [Depo-Testosterone] and testosterone enanthate [Delatestryl]. Both drugs are formulated in oil, and both are long acting. After IM injection, these drugs are slowly absorbed and then hydrolyzed to release free testosterone. Unfortunately, these preparations produce testosterone blood levels that vary widely: testosterone levels are higher than normal immediately after dosing and decline to lower than normal before the next dose. As a result, patients may experience significant variations in libido, energy, and mood.

ANDROGEN (ANABOLIC STEROID) ABUSE BY ATHLETES

Many athletes take androgens (anabolic steroids) and androgen precursors to enhance athletic performance. The potential benefits of this practice, although substantial, are accompanied by significant risks. Drugs commonly used by athletes include nandrolone, stanozolol, and methenolone. All of these drugs are regulated as controlled substances, making their use without a prescription illegal.

Who takes steroids? Steroid use is especially prevalent among baseball players, football players, weight lifters, discus throwers, shot-putters, and bodybuilders. These drugs are also used by sprinters and athletes in endurance sports (e.g., cycling, Nordic skiing). Steroids are used by athletes of all ages. This includes professionals as well as athletes in college, high school, and junior high. Use is not limited to males: some females also take them, despite masculinizing effects.

What can anabolic steroids do for the athlete? Exogenous androgens can significantly increase muscle mass and strength in *males and females of all ages when given in sufficiently large doses.* After 10 weeks, one study showed that testosterone treatment produced a 7-pound increase in muscle mass in subjects who did not exercise and a 13-pound increase in subjects who exercised and took the drug. In contrast, exercise in the absence of exogenous testosterone produced only a 4-pound increase in muscle mass. Similar increases were shown in the subjects' ability to bench-press weights. However, the potential for adverse effects of androgens is substantial. Salt and water retention can lead to hypertension. When administered in the high doses used by athletes, androgens suppress release of LH and FSH, resulting in testicular shrinkage, sterility, and gynecomastia. Acne is common. Reduction of HDL cholesterol and elevation of LDL cholesterol may theoretically accelerate development of atherosclerosis. Because most of the androgens that athletes take are 17-alpha-alkylated compounds, hepatotoxicity (cholestatic hepatitis, jaundice, hepatocellular carcinoma) is an ever-present risk. Most recently, androgens have been linked with kidney damage. In females, androgens can cause menstrual irregularities and virilization (growth of facial hair, deepening of the voice, decreased breast size, uterine atrophy, clitoral enlargement, and male-pattern baldness); baldness, growth of facial hair, and voice change may be irreversible. In boys and girls, androgens promote premature epiphyseal closure, reducing attainable adult height. In boys, androgens can induce premature puberty.

What about psychological effects? Androgens are reputed to cause depression, manic episodes, and aggressiveness. There have been very few controlled studies to measure psychological effects of androgens; however, in the controlled studies undertaken, dosages of androgens were less than those typically taken by athletes. Surveys of athletes who engage in anabolic steroid use indicate an association with risky behavior and aggression; however, it is possible that these were inherent traits of the surveyed athletes regardless of steroid use.

Long-term androgen use can lead to an abuse syndrome. Characteristics include preoccupation with androgen use and difficulty in stopping use. When androgens finally are discontinued, an abstinence syndrome can develop similar to that produced by withdrawal of alcohol, opioids, and cocaine.

Because of their abuse potential, anabolic steroids are classified as Schedule III substances under an amendment to the Controlled Substances Act. (Schedule III drugs are defined as those with a low to moderate potential for dependence.) For more information on drug abuse in sports, a good place to start is www.wada-ama.org, the website of the World Anti-Doping Agency. This organization is dedicated to promoting, coordinating, and monitoring the fight against use of anabolic steroids and other banned substances in sports. Other good resources include the United States Anti-Doping Agency (http://www.usada.org) and the National Center for Drug-Free Sport (http://www.drugfreesport.com/index.asp).

PRESCRIBING AND MONITORING CONSIDERATIONS

Preadministration Assessment

Therapeutic Goals

Males

Treatment of hypogonadism is the only FDA approved use of androgens.

Identifying High-Risk Patients

Androgens are *contraindicated* for pregnant women, for men who have prostate cancer or breast cancer, and for enhancing athletic performance.

Administration Considerations

Advise patients to take oral androgens with food if gastrointestinal (GI) upset occurs.

Transdermal Gel and Solution

Advise patients to wash their hands after applying the gel and to cover the site of application with clothing (to prevent transferring testosterone to others). Instruct patients not to shower or swim for several hours (to avoid washing the drug off). Warn users of the topical solution to avoid being near flames until the liquid has evaporated.

Buccal

Instruct patients to apply buccal tablets to the gum just above the upper incisor tooth and to apply pressure (using a finger on the lip) to ensure good adhesion.

Implantable Pellets

Pellets are implanted subdermally (under local anesthesia) in the hip region or in the abdominal wall lateral to the umbilicus.

Nasal

Instruct patients to blow the nose before using, apply to the lateral nostril wall of both nares, massage the nose after administration, and avoid sniffing or blowing for at least 1 hour after administration.

Ongoing Monitoring and Interventions

Minimizing Adverse Effects

Virilization

Virilization may occur in women, girls, and boys. Assess for deepening voice, chest and facial hair, acne and menstrual irregularities at each clinical encounter. Irreversible changes may be avoided if androgens are withdrawn early.

Premature Epiphyseal Closure

Accelerated bone maturation in children can decrease attainable adult height. Monitor effects on epiphyses with radiographs of the hand and wrist twice yearly.

Hepatotoxicity

The *17-alpha-alkylated androgens* can cause cholestatic hepatitis, jaundice, and other liver disorders. Rarely, liver cancer develops. Monitor for signs and symptoms of liver dysfunction such as jaundice, fatigue, and malaise. Obtain periodic tests of liver function. Liver function normalizes after cessation of drug use. Avoid long-term use of 17-alpha-alkylated preparations.

Edema

Salt and water retention may result in edema. Assess for edema and weight gain at each clinical encounter. Treatment consists of androgen withdrawal and, if necessary, use of a diuretic.

Teratogenesis

Androgens can cause masculinization of the female fetus. Rule out pregnancy before androgen use. Ensure that female patients of child-bearing age are using adequate contraception and engaging in consistent use.

Prostate Cancer

Avoid androgens in men with diagnosed prostate cancer. In men without diagnosed prostate cancer, monitor for exacerbation of preexisting but covert prostate cancer.

Injury From Skin-to-Skin Transfer of Topical Testosterone

Topical testosterone—applied as a gel or topical solution—can transfer to others through skin-to-skin contact. It has been hypothesized that transfer of testosterone from buccal routes may occur through saliva transfer during kissing. Transfer of testosterone to women can cause masculinization, as well as fetal harm if the woman is pregnant. Transfer to children can cause genital enlargement (penis or clitoris), premature development of pubic hair, advanced bone age, increased libido, and aggressive behavior.

Patient Education

TOPICAL TESTOSTERONE

To minimize the risk for accidental skin-to-skin transfer, advise users of testosterone gel or testosterone topical solution to (1) wash their hands after every application, (2) cover the application site with clothing after the gel has dried, and (3) wash the application site before anticipated contact with another person. Also, warn women and children to avoid contact with skin where testosterone was applied and advise them to wash contaminated skin if accidental contact with an application site should occur.

Patient Education

ANDROGENS

Tell female patients about signs of virilization (deepening of the voice, acne, changes in body and facial hair, menstrual irregularities). Instruct them to notify the prescriber if these occur.

Apprise patients about the signs of liver dysfunction (yellow tint to skin and eyes, fatigue, loss of appetite, nausea, dark-colored urine, light-colored stools). Advise them to inform the prescriber if these occur.

Inform patients that swelling of the extremities or unusual weight gain may be evidence of salt and water retention. Counsel them to notify the prescriber if these occur.

Remind patients of child-bearing age that this drug can cause fetal malformations. If the patient is capable of becoming pregnant, emphasize the need for consistent use of reliable contraception.

CHAPTER

51 Drugs for Erectile Dysfunction and Benign Prostatic Hyperplasia

Jacqueline Rosenjack Burchum, DNSc, FNP-BC, CNE

ERECTILE DYSFUNCTION

Erectile dysfunction (ED) is defined as a persistent inability to achieve or sustain an erection suitable for satisfactory sexual performance. In the United States ED affects up to 30 million men. ED is commonly associated with chronic illnesses, especially diabetes, hypertension, and depression. Among men with diabetes, the incidence of ED is between 35% and 75%. Some of the drugs that can cause ED are shown in Table 51.1.

The risk for ED increases with advancing age. According to the National Institutes of Health, ED affects approximately 4% of men in their 50s. Just a decade later, 17% of men in their 60s are unable to achieve any erection at all. This total inability to achieve erection affects 47% of men older than 75 years. Fortunately, new advances in medicine can rectify this problem for most patients.

First-line treatments for ED are lifestyle measures (increased exercise, smoking cessation), changing drug regimens to remove the drugs that may cause ED, and drug therapy with sildenafil [Viagra] or another drug in its class. Other interventions include psychotherapy and surgical implantation of a penile prosthesis.

Physiology of Erection

Before discussing drugs for ED, we need to review the physiology of erection. As shown in Fig. 51.1, the process begins with sexual arousal, which increases parasympathetic nerve traffic to the penis, causing local release of nitric oxide. Nitric oxide then activates guanylyl cyclase, an enzyme that makes cyclic guanosine monophosphate (cGMP). Through a series of steps, cGMP promotes relaxation of arterial and trabecular smooth muscle. The resultant arterial dilation increases local blood flow and blood pressure, which, in combination with relaxation of trabecular smooth muscle, causes expansion and engorgement of sinusoidal spaces in the corpus cavernosum. This, in turn, causes venous occlusion and thereby reduces venous outflow. The combination of increased arterial pressure and arterial inflow plus reduced venous outflow causes sufficient engorgement to produce erection. Erection subsides when cGMP is removed by phosphodiesterase type 5 (PDE-5), an enzyme that converts cGMP into guanosine monophosphate.

Oral Drugs for Erectile Dysfunction: PDE-5 Inhibitors

Drugs for ED fall into two major groups: oral agents and nonoral agents. The oral agents—PDE-5 inhibitors—are by far the most common treatments for ED. These will constitute our primary focus. The nonoral agents—papaverine plus phentolamine, alprostadil—are considered briefly. These drugs are summarized in Table 51.2.

Four PDE-5 inhibitors are available: sildenafil, tadalafil, vardenafil, and avanafil. All are considered first-line therapy for ED. Current guidelines recommend that, in the absence of a specific contraindication, all men with ED be offered one of these drugs. Which drug is preferred? Only a few trials have compared them head-to-head, so there is insufficient evidence to recommend one over the others. Accordingly, selection among them should be based on patient preference and prescriber judgment.

Sildenafil

Sildenafil [Viagra] was introduced in 1998 as the first oral treatment for ED. The drug is reliable and easy to use. Benefits derive from enhancing the natural response to sexual stimuli; sildenafil does not cause erection directly. Although sildenafil is generally well tolerated, it can be dangerous for men taking certain vasodilators, specifically alpha-adrenergic blockers, nitroglycerin, and other nitrates used for angina pectoris.

The erection-enhancing effects of sildenafil were discovered by accident. The drug was developed as a cardiac medicine, but benefits were minimal. However, in the course of testing, some men noticed a surprising side effect: their ED had been cured! The rest, as they say, is history. Sildenafil has been wildly popular. First-year sales were the hottest in pharmaceutical history. By now, tens of millions of men in more than 100 countries have used the drug. In addition to ED, sildenafil is approved for pulmonary arterial hypertension (PAH). When used for this purpose, sildenafil is sold as *Revatio.*

Mechanism of Action

Sildenafil causes selective inhibition of PDE-5. By doing so, it increases and preserves cGMP levels in the penis, thereby making the erection harder and longer lasting. Please note that the drug only enhances the normal erectile response to sexual

TABLE 51.1 ■ Some Drugs That Can Cause Sexual/Erectile Dysfunction

Drug Class	Representative Drug	Incidence of SD/ED*
RENAL/CARDIOVASCULAR DRUGS		
Cardiac Glycosides	Digoxin [Lanoxin]	36%
Adrenergic Neuron Blockers	Reserpine	24%–40%
Central $Alpha_2$-Adrenergic Agonists	Methyldopa	20%–30%
Beta Blockers	Propranolol [Inderal]	10%–15%
Thiazide Diuretics	Hydrochlorothiazide	10%–20%
Aldosterone Antagonists	Spironolactone [Aldactone]	4%–30%
CNS DRUGS		
Selective Serotonin Reuptake Inhibitors	Fluoxetine [Prozac]	Up to 70%
Monoamine Oxidase Inhibitors	Isocarboxazid [Marplan]	16%–31%
Tricyclic Antidepressants	Amitriptyline [Elavil]	7%–30%
Antipsychotics	Chlorpromazine [Thorazine]	30%–60%
Mood Stabilizers	Lithium [Lithobid]	5%–50%
Social Lubricant/Intoxicant	Alcohol	50%–75%
UROGENITAL DRUGS		
5-Alpha-Reductase Inhibitors	Finasteride [Proscar]	33%

*Values for sexual dysfunction/erectile dysfunction (SD/ED) incidence are estimates based on patient reports, not on carefully controlled trials.

Patient Education

PDE-5 INHIBITORS

Inform patients that dosing may be done with or without food, although a high-fat meal will delay absorption of avanafil, sildenafil, or vardenafil (but not tadalafil). Be sure to warn them that grapefruit juice should be avoided because this can raise PDE-5 inhibitor levels.

Advise patients to take avanafil approximately 15 to 30 minutes before sexual activity. All other PDE-5 inhibitors should be taken about 1 hour before sexual activity.

Counsel men with preexisting cardiovascular disease regarding the cardiac risk for sexual activity (irrespective of a PDE-5 inhibitor). Advise men who experience symptoms (e.g., anginal pain, lightheadedness) during sex to refrain from further sexual activity and discuss the event with their prescriber.

Warn patients to seek immediate medical attention if an erection lasts more than 4 hours. Prolonged priapism can cause permanent damage.

Advise patients to stop their PDE-5 inhibitor and seek immediate medical attention if they experience sudden loss of vision in one or both eyes or if hearing loss develops.

Instruct patients to avoid nitrates for at least 12 hours after taking avanafil, for at least 24 hours after taking sildenafil or vardenafil, and for at least 48 hours after taking tadalafil.

stimuli (e.g., erotic imagery, fantasies, physical contact). In the absence of sexual stimuli, nothing happens.

Pharmacokinetics

Sildenafil is well absorbed after oral administration. Bioavailability is about 40%. In fasting subjects, plasma levels peak about 1 hour after dosing. A high-fat meal slows absorption, resulting in a peak plasma level in 2 hours (rather than 1) and reducing the peak concentration. Sildenafil is metabolized in the liver, primarily by the 3A4 isoenzyme of cytochrome P450 (CYP3A4). Both the parent drug and its major metabolite (*N*-desmethyl sildenafil) are biologically active. Both compounds are eliminated primarily in the feces (80%) and partly in the urine (13%). For both compounds, the half-life is 4 hours. Clearance of both is delayed in men older than 65 years and in men with hepatic impairment or severe renal insufficiency, causing drug levels to rise higher and persist longer.

Sexual Benefits

In Men With ED. Sildenafil has been evaluated in several thousand men (aged 19–87 years) with ED of organic, psychogenic, or mixed-cause origin. At least some improvement in erection hardness and duration was seen in 70% of men taking the drug, compared with 20% taking placebo. Benefits were dose related and lasted up to 4 hours, although they began to fade after 2 hours. Sildenafil was able to help a wide range of patients, including those with ED resulting from diabetes, spinal cord injury, and transurethral prostate resection, as well as ED of no known physical cause.

In Men Without ED. Despite anecdotal reports to the contrary, sildenafil has little or no effect on erection quality or duration in men who do not have ED. Any apparent benefits in healthy men are likely the result of a placebo response.

In Women. Sildenafil is not approved for use in women and probably won't be. Although several large-scale studies showed the drug is safe in women, they failed to show much enhancement of sexual arousal. Thus the manufacturer decided not to seek U.S. Food and Drug Administration (FDA) approval for treating female hypoactive sexual desire disorder or any other condition in women.

Adverse Effects

Hypotension. At recommended doses, sildenafil produces a small (8.4/5.5 mm Hg) reduction in blood pressure. However, in men taking nitrates or alpha blockers, severe hypotension can develop.

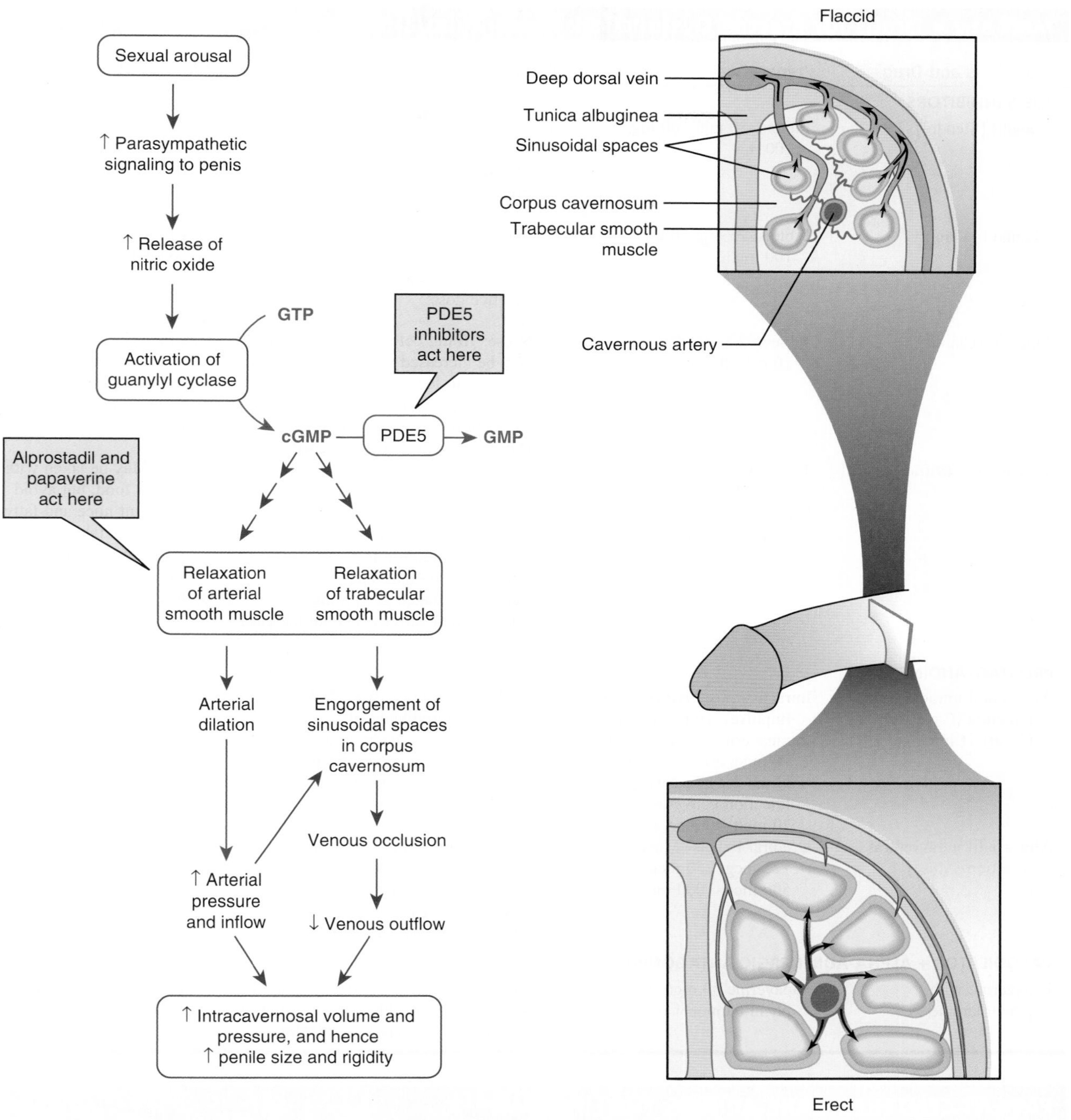

Figure 51.1 ■ **Physiology of penile erection.**
In the flaccid state, there is free outflow of venous blood and restricted inflow of arterial blood. During sexual arousal, cyclic guanosine monophosphate (cGMP) relaxes arterial and trabecular smooth muscle, permitting free inflow of arterial blood and subsequent engorgement of sinusoidal spaces, whose expansion compresses penile veins, restricting blood outflow. The resultant accumulation of blood at elevated pressure increases penile size and rigidity. Removal of cGMP by PDE-5 restores penile smooth muscle to the nonaroused state, and detumescence ensues. (GTP, guanosine triphosphate; PDE-5, phosphodiesterase type 5.)

TABLE 51.2 ■ Drugs for Erectile Dysfunction: Preparation, Dosage, and Administration

Drug Class and Drug	Preparation	Dosage for ED	Administration
PDE-5 INHIBITORS			
Avanafil [Stendra]	Tablets: 50 mg, 100 mg, 200 mg	100 mg taken ± 15 minutes before sexual activity. May be increased to 200 mg, if needed. Decrease to lowest effective dose.	May be taken with or without food, but avoid grapefruit juice. High fat foods delay double the time to onset. Do not take over once a day.
Sildenafil [Viagra]	Tablets: 25 mg, 50 mg, 100 mg	50 mg once daily ± 60 minutes before sexual activity. May be increased to 100 mg, if needed. Decrease to lowest effective dose.	May be taken with or without food, but avoid grapefruit juice. High fat foods may delay onset by as much as 60 minutes. Do not take over once a day.
Tadalafil [Cialis]	Tablets: 2.5 mg, 5 mg, 10 mg, 20 mg	PRN use: 10 mg before sexual activity. May be increased to 20 mg, if needed. Decrease to lowest effective dose. Daily use: 2.5 mg orally once daily; timing unrelated to sexual activity. May increase to 5 mg if needed.	May be taken with or without food, but avoid grapefruit juice. Do not take over once a day. If administered for daily use, take at the same time each day.
Vardenafil [Levitra, Staxyn]	Tablets (Levitra): 2.5 mg, 5 mg, 10 mg, 20 mg Orally Disintegrating Tablets (Staxyn): 10 mg	Levitra: 10 mg taken ± 60 minutes before sexual activity. May be increased to 20 mg, if needed. Decrease to lowest effective dose. Decrease starting dose to 5 mg for patients age 65 and older. Staxyn: 10 mg taken ± 60 minutes before sexual activity. Do not increase dosage.	Levitra: May be taken with or without food, but avoid grapefruit juice and fatty foods. Staxyn: Place tablet on tongue and allow to disintegrate. To not take with food or drink. Both: Do not take over once a day.
PROSTAGLANDIN E_1			
Alprostadil intracavernosal injection [Caverject, Caverject Impulse, Edex]	Intracavernosal Kit (Caverject Impulse): 10 mcg, 20 mcg Intracavernosal Kit (Edex): 10 mcg, 20 mcg, 40 mcg Solution for Intracavernosal Injection (Caverject): 20 mcg, 40 mcg	Typical dosages range from 5–40 mcg. Dosing is individualized; determination is made in the health care setting. Maximum dosing is 60 mcg for Caverject and 40 mcg for Edex.	Patients self-administer injection into the penis. Do not take more than once in 24 hours. Limit total dosing to three times a week.
Alprostadil intraurethral insertion [Muse]	Urethral Pellets (Muse): 125 mcg, 250 mcg, 500 mcg, 1000 mcg	Intraurethral insertion: Initial dosing is 125–250 mcg 5–10 minutes before sexual activity. (Effect lasts 30–60 minutes.) Increase, if needed, to lowest effective dose.	Patients self-insert the pellet into the urethra. Limit use to twice daily.
VASODILATOR + ALPHA-ADRENERGIC ANTAGONIST			
Papaverine with phentolamine	Papaverine 30 mg/mL with phentolamine 1 mg/mL	Dosing is individualized; determination is made in the health care setting. As little as 0.1 mL may be sufficient	Patients self-administer injection into the penis.

PATIENT-CENTERED CARE ACROSS THE LIFE SPAN

Drugs for Erectile Dysfunction

Life Stage	Considerations or Concerns
Children	Safety for PDE-5 inhibitors has not been established. PDE-5 inhibitors are not indicated for children. Alprostadil is indicated for treatment of patent ductus arteriosus in neonates; however, the formulations for ED would not apply.
Pregnant Women	PDE-5 inhibitors are Pregnancy Category B; however, they are not indicated for women and, therefore, should not be taken by pregnant women. Alprostadil urethral pellets and injectable alprostadil or papaverine with phentolamine would not be used by people without a penis. It is recommended that men taking these drugs use a condom if their partner is a pregnant woman.
Breast-Feeding Women	Excretion in breast milk is unknown; however, drugs for erectile dysfunction are not indicated for use in women.
Older Adults	Consider lower dosing when prescribing for older adults age 65 and older.

Priapism. A few cases of priapism (painful erection lasting more than 6 hours) have been reported. If an erection persists more than 4 hours, immediate medical intervention is required. Left untreated, priapism can cause permanent damage of penile tissue. If priapism persists longer than 24 hours, chances are very high that the patient will never be able to have sexual intercourse again. Persistent erection can be relieved by aspirating blood from the corpus cavernosum followed by irrigation with a solution containing a vasoconstrictor (e.g., epinephrine, phenylephrine, metaraminol). If this is unsuccessful, surgery is required.

Nonarteritic Ischemic Optic Neuropathy (NAION). Very rarely, men taking sildenafil have developed NAION, resulting in irreversible blurring or loss of vision. The cause is blockage of blood flow to the optic nerve. In most cases, there were underlying anatomic or vascular risk factors for NAION. Also, although NAION developed during sildenafil use, a direct causal relationship has not been established. Nonetheless, patients with NAION in one eye should not use sildenafil, owing to a potential risk for developing NAION in the other eye.

Sudden Hearing Loss. Very rarely, men taking sildenafil have experienced sudden hearing loss, usually in one ear, sometimes in association with dizziness, vertigo, and tinnitus. Hearing loss may be partial or complete. Hearing returned by the time the loss was reported in one third of cases, but had not returned in the remaining two thirds. To date, a direct causal relationship between sildenafil and hearing loss has not been established. Nonetheless, the drug is suspected because (1) sudden hearing loss is unusual and (2) it developed when sildenafil was taken. Men who experience sudden hearing loss should discontinue the drug—but only if they are taking it for ED; men taking the drug for PAH should continue treatment.

Other Adverse Effects. The most common adverse effects are headache, flushing, and dyspepsia. Sildenafil may also cause nasal congestion, diarrhea, rash, and dizziness. About 3% of patients experience mild transient visual disturbances (blue color tinge to vision, increased sensitivity to light, blurring). In addition, sildenafil may intensify symptoms of obstructive sleep apnea (perhaps by relaxing pharyngeal muscles or dilating pulmonary blood vessels).

Drug Interactions

Nitrates. Both sildenafil and nitrates (e.g., nitroglycerin, isosorbide dinitrate) promote hypotension, and they both do so by increasing cGMP (nitrates increase cGMP formation, and sildenafil slows cGMP breakdown). If these drugs are combined, life-threatening hypotension could result. Therefore *sildenafil is absolutely contraindicated for men taking nitrates.* At least 24 hours should elapse between the last dose of sildenafil and giving a nitrate. If elimination of sildenafil is slowed (owing to a CYP3A4 inhibitor or hepatic or renal impairment), an even longer time should elapse before nitrate use.

Alpha Blockers. Alpha-adrenergic antagonists—including doxazosin [Cardura] and other alpha blockers used for prostatic hyperplasia (see later discussion)—dilate arterioles and can thereby lower blood pressure. Combined use with sildenafil has caused symptomatic postural hypotension. Accordingly, these combinations should be used with caution.

Inhibitors of CYP3A4. Inhibitors of CYP3A4 (e.g., ketoconazole, itraconazole, erythromycin, cimetidine, saquinavir, ritonavir, grapefruit juice) can suppress metabolism of sildenafil, thereby increasing its levels. These combinations should be used with caution.

> **Prototype Drugs**
>
> **DRUGS FOR ERECTILE DYSFUNCTION AND BENIGN PROSTATIC HYPERPLASIA**
>
> **Drugs for Erectile Dysfunction**
>
> **Phosphodiesterase Type 5 Inhibitor**
> Sildenafil
>
> **Nonoral Drugs**
> Papaverine/phentolamine
> Alprostadil
>
> **Drugs for Benign Prostatic Hyperplasia**
>
> **5-Alpha-Reductase Inhibitor**
> Finasteride
>
> **Alpha-Adrenergic Antagonist**
> Tamsulosin

Is Sildenafil Safe for Men With Coronary Heart Disease?

Reports of adverse cardiovascular events, including at least 130 cardiac deaths, raised concern about the safety of sildenafil in men with coronary heart disease (CHD). However, there was a question as to what caused the adverse events: sildenafil or the sexual activity that sildenafil permitted. When attempting to answer this question, researchers made two important observations: First, giving sildenafil to resting men with severe CHD produced no harmful effects on coronary blood flow or any other hemodynamic parameter. Second, in men with stable CHD who were performing exercise, sildenafil had no effect on CHD symptoms, exercise tolerance, or exercise-induced ischemia. Taken together, these results suggest that, in men with CHD, sexual activity—and not sildenafil—is the likely cause of ischemic events. However, even though sildenafil itself appears safe for men with CHD, sexual activity may not be. Accordingly, the drug should be used with caution by men with the following conditions:

- Myocardial infarction, stroke, or life-threatening dysrhythmia within the last 6 months
- Resting hypotension (blood pressure below 90/50 mm Hg)
- Resting hypertension (blood pressure above 170/110 mm Hg)
- Heart failure
- Unstable angina

In addition, *sildenafil should not be used at all by men taking nitroglycerin or any other drug in the nitrate family.*

To reduce the risk for adverse events, candidates for sildenafil therapy should undergo a careful evaluation of cardiovascular function. Those with impaired function should be counseled about the risks posed by sexual activity and all other moderate to intense physical activity.

Vardenafil, Tadalafil, and Avanafil

Vardenafil, tadalafil, and avanafil are very similar to sildenafil. All three drugs inhibit PDE-5, and all three are approved for oral therapy of ED. Vardenafil is unique in that it prolongs the QT interval, and tadalafil is unique in that its effects last 36 hours. Avanafil is unique in that it has the fastest onset of action. Otherwise, the clinical effects of all four PDE-5 inhibitors appear about equal, although some patients may respond better to one than to the others. Properties of all four are shown in Table 51.3.

Vardenafil

Actions and Use. Vardenafil [Levitra, Staxyn], approved in 2003, was the second selective PDE-5 inhibitor released for ED. As with sildenafil, benefits derive from relaxing arterial and trabecular smooth muscle in the penis. Effects begin about 60 minutes after dosing and persist about 4 hours. There is no evidence that vardenafil works faster, longer, or better than sildenafil.

Pharmacokinetics. Oral bioavailability is low (15%) and is decreased further by a high-fat meal. Plasma levels peak about 1 hour after dosing, or after 2 hours if dosing is done with a high-fat meal. Vardenafil undergoes extensive metabolism by hepatic CYP3A4, followed by excretion primarily in the feces. The drug's half-life is 4 to 5 hours.

Adverse Effects. The most common adverse effects are headache, flushing, and rhinitis. Like other PDE-5 inhibitors, vardenafil can lower blood pressure. Like sildenafil, vardenafil can cause visual changes and has been associated with sudden hearing loss and vision loss from NAION.

Vardenafil can prolong the cardiac QT interval and might thereby pose a risk for serious dysrhythmias. However, dysrhythmias have not been reported. Nonetheless, to reduce risk, vardenafil should be used with caution in patients taking other drugs that cause QT prolongation.

Drug Interactions. Vardenafil is contraindicated for use with alpha-adrenergic blockers and with nitroglycerin and other nitrates. Plasma levels can be increased by inhibitors of CYP3A4 (e.g., ketoconazole, ritonavir), and hence such combinations must be used with caution. As noted, caution is needed in patients taking drugs that prolong the QT interval.

Tadalafil

Actions and Uses. Tadalafil [Cialis] was approved mere months after vardenafil. Like sildenafil and vardenafil, the drug is indicated for oral therapy of ED. As with other PDE-5 inhibitors, benefits derive from relaxation of penile arterial and trabecular smooth muscle brought on by accumulation of cGMP. On average, therapeutic levels of the drug are reached by 2 hours after dosing and persist about 36 hours—much longer than with sildenafil or vardenafil. As a result, timing of dosing and sexual activity needn't be tightly coupled. Furthermore, in addition to being approved for PRN dosing (like sildenafil and vardenafil), tadalafil is also approved for daily dosing (but only for men who anticipate sexual activity at least twice a week).

As discussed below, tadalafil is also used for benign prostatic hyperplasia (BPH). In addition, like sildenafil, tadalafil, sold as Adcirca, is used for PAH.

Pharmacokinetics. Absorption rate is variable but unaffected by food. Plasma levels peak 0.5 to 6 hours after dosing and then slowly decline. Tadalafil undergoes metabolism by hepatic CYP3A4, followed by excretion primarily in the feces. The drug's half-life is 17.5 hours.

Adverse Effects. The most common adverse effects are headache, dyspepsia, back pain, myalgia, limb pain, flushing, and nasal congestion. Like other PDE-5 inhibitors, tadalafil can lower blood pressure. Very rarely, the drug alters color vision. A few cases of NAION and sudden hearing loss have been reported, but a causal relationship has not been established. Because tadalafil has a long duration of action, adverse effects may persist for many hours.

Drug Interactions. Tadalafil is contraindicated for use with nitrates or alpha blockers (except tamsulosin [Flomax]). As with sildenafil and vardenafil, CYP3A4 inhibitors can cause levels of tadalafil to rise. To avoid toxicity, men taking CYP3A4 inhibitors should limit tadalafil dosage to 10 mg every 72 hours.

PRN Dosing. The manufacturer does not identify a minimum time between dosing and sexual activity. However, because blood levels peak more slowly than with sildenafil or vardenafil, allowing at least 1 hour for absorption would seem reasonable. Dosage should be reduced in men with moderate renal or hepatic insufficiency. Men with severe hepatic insufficiency should not use the drug. For men taking CYP3A4 inhibitors, the maximal dosage is 10 mg every 72 hours.

Daily Dosing. Daily dosing is recommended only for men who anticipate sexual activity at least twice a week. The medication should be taken at the same time each day.

Avanafil

Actions and Use. Avanafil [Stendra], approved in 2012, is the latest selective PDE-5 inhibitor approved for ED. Actions are the same as for the

TABLE 51.3 ▪ Comparison of PDE-5 Inhibitors

	Drug			
Parameter	**Sildenafil [Viagra]**	**Tadalafil [Cialis]**	**Vardenafil [Levitra, Staxyn]**	**Avanafil [Stendra]**
Date approved	3/27/1998	11/21/2003	8/19/2003	4/28/2012
Dosing schedule	PRN only	PRN *or* once daily	PRN only	PRN
Median time to peak level	1 hr	2 hr	1 hr	30–45 min
Half-life	4 hr	17.5 hr	4–5 hr	5 hr
Duration of action	4 hr	36 hr	4 hr	4 hr
Major mode of metabolism	CYP3A4	CYP3A4	CYP3A4	CYP3A4
DRUG INTERACTIONS				
Nitrates	Contraindicated: Wait 24 hr before giving a nitrate	Contraindicated: Wait 48 hr before giving a nitrate	Contraindicated: Wait 24 hr before giving a nitrate	Contraindicated: Wait 12 hr before giving a nitrate
Alpha blockers	Use with caution	Contraindicated (except for tamsulosin, 0.4 mg once daily)	Contraindicated	Use with caution
CYP3A4 inhibitors	Reduce sildenafil dosage	Reduce tadalafil dosage to no more than 10 mg every 72 hr	Reduce vardenafil dosage	Do not take with strong CYP3A4 inhibitors; reduce dosage with moderate inhibitors
Class I and class III antidysrhythmic drugs	No interaction	No interaction	Vardenafil prolongs the QT interval—avoid class I and class III antidysrhythmics	No interaction

other PDE-5 inhibitors; however, effects begin about 15 minutes after dosing and last about 2 hours.

Pharmacokinetics. Absorption is rapid, with an onset of about 15 minutes. Plasma levels peak about 30 to 45 minutes after dosing in fasting patients, or after 1.25 hours if taken with a high-fat meal. As with other PDE-5 inhibitors, metabolism occurs by hepatic CYP3A4; there is also less metabolism by CYP2C isoenzymes. Excretion is primarily in the feces, with about 20% in the urine. The drug's half-life is approximately 5 hours.

Adverse Effects. Headache is the only adverse effect, occurring in at least 10% of patients. A few patients will experience flushing, nasal congestion, and nasopharyngitis. Like other PDE-5 inhibitors, avanafil can lower blood pressure.

Drug Interactions. Avanafil is contraindicated for use with nitroglycerin and other nitrates. It can increase the hypotensive effects of alcohol and antihypertensive drugs, especially alpha-adrenergic antagonists. A starting dose of 50 mg (the lowest strength available) is recommended if prescribed for patients taking antihypertensive drugs. Plasma levels can be increased when taken with CYP3A4 inhibitors (e.g., ketoconazole, ritonavir, and erythromycin). For this reason, dosing should not exceed 50 mg in 24 hours for patients taking CYP3A4 inhibitors.

Nonoral Drugs for Erectile Dysfunction

Unlike the PDE-5 inhibitors, which are administered orally, the drugs discussed in this section—alprostadil and papaverine/phentolamine—are administered by nonoral routes. Specifically, they are administered either by injection into the penis or by insertion into the urethra. Because of this inconvenient dosing, these drugs are second-line agents for ED.

Alprostadil (Prostaglandin E_1)

Transurethral

Alprostadil pellets [Muse], the only ED drug that is approved for twice-daily use, is inserted into the urethra. Administration is accomplished by loading a pellet into a small plastic applicator, which is then inserted an inch and a half into the urethra. Detailed instructions for insertion are available in the package insert. Both the package insert and a training video are available online at http://www.muserx.com/hcc/about-muse/how-to-use-muse.aspx.

Erection develops 5 to 10 minutes after drug insertion and lasts 30 to 60 minutes. Dosage is determined in the provider's office; the objective is to employ the smallest dose required to produce an erection sufficient for intercourse.

Mechanism of Action

Alprostadil's active ingredient has the same chemical structure as prostaglandin E_1 (PGE_1), which has vasodilating properties. Relaxation of smooth muscle (arterial, venous, and trabecular), causing a rapid inflow of arterial blood. As explained when discussing physiology of erection, the blood fills the vascular sinusoidal spaces of the corpora cavernosa resulting in an erection. Pressure from the engorged penis helps block venous outflow to promote maintenance of the erect state.

Adverse Effects

The most common adverse effect, dull ache in the penis, occurs in 32% of users. Another 12% report urethral burning. Minor bleeding or spotting and testicular pain occur in about 5% of patients. Systemic symptoms are rare when taken as directed and approximate those of placebo use.

Intracavernous

Alprostadil [Caverject, Caverject Impulse, Edex] is also available in a form for direct injection into the corpus cavernosum. A training video demonstrating how to inject the medication plus a link to access written instructions is available online at http://www.caverject.com/how-inject-caverject-impulse.

The response is rapid, and the injections are relatively painless. Optimal dosage is determined in the prescriber's office. The dosing end point is an erection that is sufficient for intercourse but that does not last for more than 1 hour. Injectable alprostadil should be used no more than 3 times a week and not more than once in 24 hours. Acute adverse effects are burning sensations, prolonged erection, and priapism. Penile fibrosis may develop with continued use.

Papaverine Plus Phentolamine

The combination of papaverine (a vasodilator) plus phentolamine (an alpha-adrenergic blocking agent) can provide tumescence when injected directly into the corpus cavernosum. Erection develops within 10 minutes and lasts 2 to 4 hours. In clinical trials, erection suitable for intercourse was produced in 65% to 100% of males with ED of neurologic or vascular origin.

As with the other drugs for ED, papaverine and phentolamine produce erection by increasing arterial inflow to the penis and decreasing venous outflow. Arterial inflow is augmented by alpha-adrenergic blockade (causing arterial dilation) and by the direct relaxant action of papaverine on arterial smooth muscle.

Adverse Effects

Priapism (persistent erection lasting more than 6 hours) occurs in about 10% of patients. Development of painless fibrotic nodules in the corpus is common. Other adverse effects include orthostatic hypotension with dizziness, transient paresthesias, ecchymosis (extravasation of blood into subcutaneous tissue), and difficulty in achieving orgasm or ejaculation.

Papaverine and phentolamine are not approved by the FDA for treatment of erectile dysfunction, and many experts in the field do not recommend their use. As mentioned, there are some significant adverse effects. Also, these drugs come from compounding pharmacies. In light of numerous FDA recalls from compounding pharmacies in recent years, some providers have concerns about safety and quality issues as well.

Clinical Guidelines for Management of Erectile Dysfunction

A number of organizations have published clinical guidelines for management of ED, including the American Urological Association in 2005 (see http://www.auanet.org/education/guidelines/erectile-dysfunction.cfm) and the American College of Physicians in 2011, which did not address transurethral and injectable drugs (see http://www.aafp.org/dam/AAFP/documents/patient_care/clinical_recommendations/acp-hormonaltest-ed.pdf). In 2015 the Canadian Urologic Association developed and published updated clinical guidelines for treatment of erectile dysfunction. These are available at http://www.ncbi.nlm.nih.gov/pmc/articles/PMC4336024/pdf/cuaj-1-2-23.pdf (Fig. 51.2)

BENIGN PROSTATIC HYPERPLASIA

BPH is a common condition that develops in more than 50% of men by age 60 years, and 90% by age 85 years. Although BPH and prostate cancer can coexist, there is no evidence that one predisposes to the other.

Pathophysiology and Overview of Treatment

Pathophysiology

The prostate is a heart-shaped gland that surrounds the male urethra. Its major function is to produce fluids that contribute to ejaculate volume. In healthy men, the prostate is walnut sized and weighs between 4 and 20 g. In men with BPH, prostate mass may reach 50 to 80 g.

BPH is a nonmalignant prostate enlargement caused by excessive growth of epithelial (glandular) cells and smooth muscle cells. Overgrowth of epithelial cells causes *mechanical obstruction* of the urethra, whereas overgrowth of smooth muscle causes *dynamic obstruction* of the urethra. In men with BPH, the ratio of epithelium to smooth muscle varies from 1 : 3 to 4 : 1—in general, the larger the prostate, the higher the percentage of epithelium.

Signs and symptoms of BPH include urinary hesitancy, urinary urgency, increased frequency of urination, dysuria,

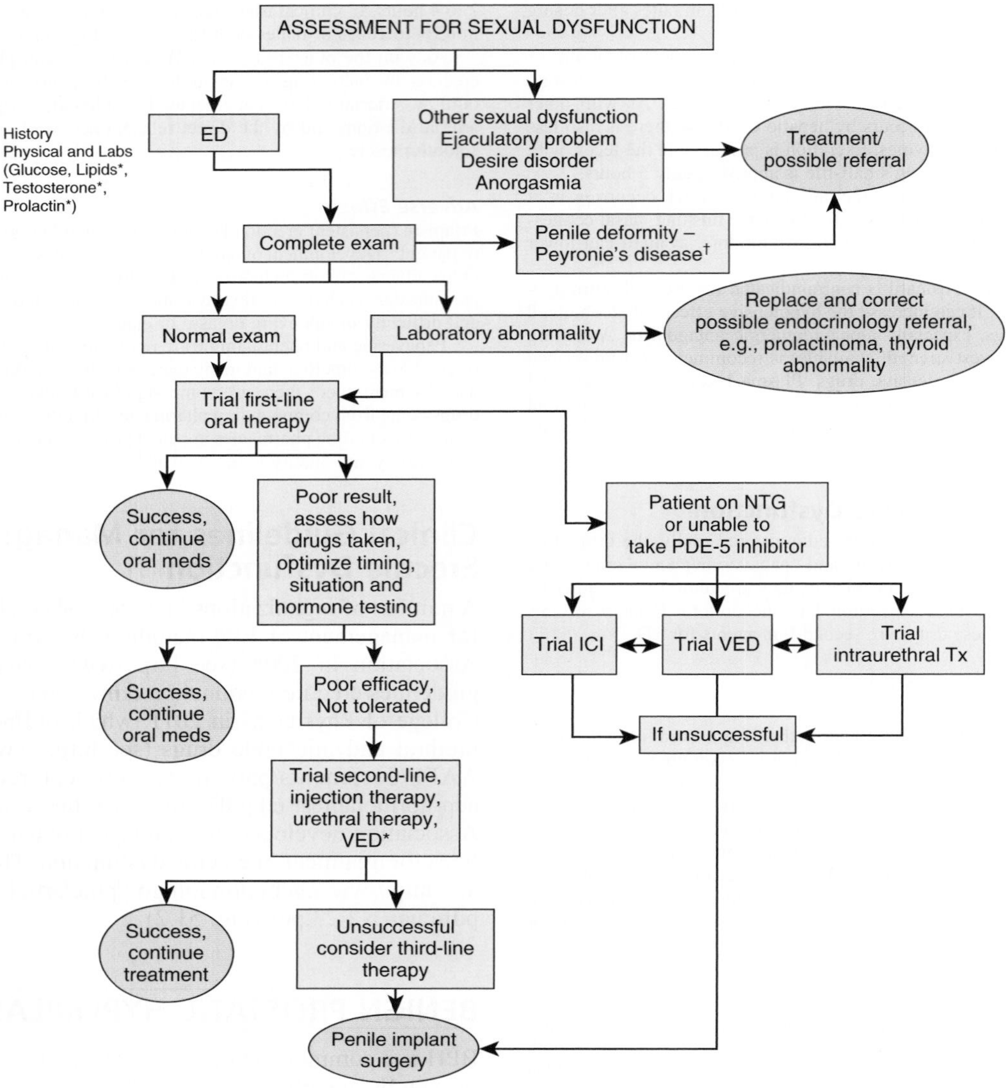

Figure 51.2 ■ **Management of erectile dysfunction.**
(From Bella AJ, Lee JC, Carrier S, et al. 2015 CUA practice guidelines for erectile dysfunction. Can Urol Assoc J 2015;9:23–29; http://www.ncbi.nlm.nih.gov/pmc/articles/PMC4336024/figure/f1-cuaj-1-2-23/; an alternate source is http://www.ncbi.nlm.nih.gov/pmc/articles/PMC4336024/pdf/cuaj-1-2-23.pdf.)

nocturia, straining to void, postvoid dribbling, decreased force and caliber of the urinary stream, and a sensation of incomplete bladder emptying. There is no direct correlation between symptoms and prostate size. Therefore some men with only moderate enlargement may be highly symptomatic, whereas others with substantial enlargement may have no symptoms. Long-term complications of BPH include obstructive nephropathy, bladder stones, and recurrent urinary tract infections.

Treatment Modalities

BPH can be managed in three ways: invasive treatments, drug therapy, and "watchful waiting." Invasive options include transurethral resection of the prostate, laser prostatectomy, transurethral electrovaporization of the prostate, and transurethral microwave therapy. These procedures are most appropriate for men with severe symptoms or complications. Drugs are indicated for men with moderate symptoms. Watchful waiting, which consists of annual reevaluation with reconsideration of management based on results, is appropriate for men with minimal symptoms.

Drug Therapy of Benign Prostatic Hyperplasia (BPH)

BPH can be treated with two major classes of drugs: *5-alpha-reductase inhibitors* and *alpha$_1$-adrenergic antagonists.* With both, the goal is to relieve bothersome urinary symptoms and delay disease progression. The 5-alpha-reductase inhibitors are most appropriate for men with very large prostates (mechanical obstruction), whereas alpha blockers are preferred for men with relatively small prostates (dynamic obstruction). Major drugs for BPH are shown in Table 51.4 and 51.5, and preparation, dosing, and administration of drugs for BPH is provided in Table 51.5.

5-Alpha-Reductase Inhibitors

Two 5-alpha-reductase inhibitors are available: finasteride and dutasteride. Both drugs can reduce prostate size, although several months are required for a noticeable effect. There is no proof that one drug works better than the other.

Finasteride

Finasteride [Proscar] acts in reproductive tissue to inhibit 5-alpha reductase, an enzyme that converts testosterone to dihydrotestosterone (DHT), the active form of testosterone in the prostate. Treatment reduces levels of DHT in blood by 70% (but does not decrease testosterone levels). By decreasing DHT availability, finasteride promotes regression of prostate epithelial tissue and thereby decreases *mechanical obstruction* of the urethra. Because the percentage of epithelial tissue is highest in very large prostates, finasteride is most effective in men whose prostates are highly enlarged. Conversely, the drug confers less benefit if the degree of enlargement is small. Be aware that prostate shrinkage occurs slowly—over a period of 6 to 12 months.

By reducing levels of DHT, finasteride can protect against prostate cancer—but only cancers classified as low grade. Finasteride does not protect against high-grade prostate cancer. In fact, when given to healthy men to prevent prostate cancer, finasteride actually *increased* the likelihood of a high-grade tumor. Accordingly, the Oncologic Drugs Advisory Committee of the FDA recommends against allowing the manufacturer to label finasteride as a drug for prostate cancer prevention.

Finasteride is generally well tolerated. However, in 5% to 10% of patients, it decreases ejaculate volume and libido. In addition, gynecomastia develops in some men.

Finasteride is classified in FDA Pregnancy Risk Category X because it is teratogenic to the male fetus. Finasteride is contraindicated for women who are pregnant or may become pregnant. In addition, because finasteride can be absorbed through the skin, pregnant women should not handle tablets that have been broken or crushed. Men are also advised not to donate blood if taking finasteride or until at least 1 month after stopping the drug to avoid the risk of having a pregnant woman as the blood recipient.

Finasteride decreases serum levels of prostate-specific antigen (PSA), a marker for prostate cancer. The expected decline is 30% to 50%. PSA levels should be determined before treatment and 6 months later. If PSA levels do not fall as expected, the patient should be evaluated for cancer of the prostate.

For treatment of BPH, therapy continues for life. As discussed in Chapter 86, the drug is also available in 1-mg tablets, sold as *Propecia,* for treatment of male-pattern baldness.

Dutasteride

Dutasteride [Avodart] is similar to finasteride in most respects. However, there are two important differences. First, with dutasteride, the reduction in circulating DHT is more complete. And second, dutasteride has an extremely long half-life (about 5 weeks); therefore it takes months to clear the drug after dosing has stopped.

Like finasteride, dutasteride inhibits 5-alpha reductase and thereby suppresses production of DHT. However, whereas finasteride inhibits only the form of 5-alpha reductase found in reproductive tissues, dutasteride also inhibits the form found in the skin and liver. As a result, dutasteride produces a greater reduction in circulating DHT (93% vs. 70%). Whether this translates to a greater clinical response has not been established because dutasteride and finasteride have not been directly compared.

TABLE 51.4 ▪ Drugs for Benign Prostatic Hyperplasia

Generic Name	Trade Name	Actions in BPH	Adverse Effects
5-ALPHA-REDUCTASE INHIBITORS			
Dutasteride Finasteride	Avodart Proscar	Reduce dihydrotestosterone production, which causes the prostate to shrink, which reduces mechanical obstruction of the urethra. May also delay BPH progression. Benefits take months to develop.	Decreased ejaculate volume and libido. Teratogenic to the male fetus.
ALPHA$_1$ BLOCKERS			
Selective Alpha$_{1a}$ Blockers			
Silodosin Tamsulosin	Rapaflo Flomax	Blockade of alpha$_{1a}$ receptors relaxes smooth muscle in the bladder neck, prostate capsule, and prostatic urethra, and thereby decreases dynamic obstruction of the urethra. Benefits develop rapidly.	Abnormal ejaculation (ejaculation failure, reduced ejaculate volume, retrograde ejaculation). Risk of floppy-iris syndrome during cataract surgery.
NONSELECTIVE ALPHA$_1$ BLOCKERS			
Alfuzosin Doxazosin Terazosin	Uroxatral, Xatral ♣ Cardura, Cardura XL Hytrin	Same as the selective alpha$_{1a}$ blockers.	Hypotension, fainting, dizziness, somnolence, and nasal congestion (from blocking alpha$_1$ receptors on blood vessels)
ALPHA$_{1A}$ BLOCKER/5-ALPHA-REDUCTASE INHIBITOR			
Tamsulosin/dutasteride	Jalyn	Combination of the effects of 5-alpha-reductase inhibitors and selective alpha$_{1a}$ blockers	Decreased libido and abnormal ejaculation (ejaculation failure, reduced ejaculate volume, retrograde ejaculation)
Tadalafil	Cialis	Smooth muscle relaxation in the bladder, prostate, and urethra	Hypotension, priapism

TABLE 51.5 ▪ Drugs for BPH: Preparation, Dosage, and Administration

Drug Class and Drug	Preparation	Dosage for BPH	Administration
ALPHA$_1$-ADRENERGIC ANTAGONISTS			
Alfuzosin [Uroxatral, Xatral ♣]	ER Tablet: 10 mg	10 mg once daily	Take 30 minutes after a meal at the same time each day. Swallow capsules whole.
Doxazosin [Cardura, Cardura XL]	IR Tablet: 1 mg, 2 mg, 4 mg, 8 mg (scored) ER Tablet: 4 mg, 8 mg	IR Tablet: 1 mg once daily. May increase gradually to a maximum of 8 mg once daily. ER Tablet: 4 mg once daily. May increase to 8 mg once daily.	With IR tablets, bedtime administration, especially for the first dose, may decrease adverse effects associated with orthostatic hypotension. Administer ER tablets with morning meal. Swallow tablets whole.
Silodosin [Rapaflo]	Capsule: 4 mg, 8 mg	8 mg once daily. Reduce to 4 mg once daily with moderate renal impairment. Contraindicated in severe renal or hepatic impairment.	Take with the same meal each day. Capsules may be opened and sprinkled on soft food but should not be chewed
Terazosin [Hytrin ♣]	Capsule: 1 mg, 2 mg, 5 mg, 10 mg Tablet: 1 mg, 2 mg, 5 mg, 10 mg	Initial: 1 mg once daily Typical: 10 mg once daily Maximum: 20 mg once daily	May be taken with or without food. Bedtime administration recommended
Tamsulosin [Flomax]	Capsule: 0.4 mg	0.4 mg once daily May increase to 0.8 mg daily.	Take 30 minutes after a meal at the same time each day.
5-ALPHA-REDUCTASE INHIBITORS			
Dutasteride [Avodart]	Capsule: 0.5 mg	0.5 mg once a day	May take with or without food. Swallow capsules whole
Finasteride [Proscar]	Tablets: 5 mg	5 mg once a day	May take with or without food.
PDE-5 INHIBITOR			
Tadalafil [Cialis]	Tablets: 2.5 mg, 5 mg, 10 mg, 20 mg	5 mg once a day If taking an alpha blocker, dosing should start at 2.5 mg once a day, and then increase to 5 mg once a day as needed and tolerated.	May be taken with or without food, but avoid grapefruit juice.
COMBINATION PRODUCTS: ALPHA$_1$-ADRENERGIC ANTAGONIST + 5-ALPHA-REDUCTASE INHIBITOR			
Tamsulosin + dutasteride [Jalyn]	Capsule: Tamsulosin 0.4 mg + dutasteride 0.5 mg	1 capsule daily	Take 30 minutes after any meal at the same time each day. Swallow capsules whole.

ER, extended release; IR, immediate release

Dutasteride is generally well tolerated. However, like finasteride, dutasteride reduces ejaculate volume and libido in some men and causes a decline in PSA in all men.

Dutasteride is classified in FDA Pregnancy Risk Category X. It can be absorbed through the skin, so pregnant women should not handle the drug. Men should not donate blood while using dutasteride or for at least 6 months after stopping it to avoid transmission to women through an infusion.

Like finasteride, dutasteride can reduce the likelihood of a low-grade prostate tumor, but it increases the likelihood of a high-grade prostate tumor. Accordingly, the drug should not be used for prostate cancer prevention.

Although many capsules can be opened and sprinkled on food, this is not the case with dutasteride. The capsule contents can be irritating to the oropharyngeal mucosa; therefore the capsule must be swallowed whole with a full glass of water.

Alpha$_1$-Adrenergic Antagonists

Five alpha$_1$ blockers are approved for BPH: *alfuzosin* [Uroxatral, Xatral ♣], *terazosin* [Hytrin], *doxazosin* [Cardura], *silodosin* [Rapaflo], and *tamsulosin* [Flomax]. These drugs have not been directly compared in clinical trials, so we can't say whether one is more effective than the others. However, two newer ones—silodosin and tamsulosin—may be better tolerated. The pharmacology of these drugs is discussed in Chapter 14. Discussion here is limited to their use in BPH.

Mechanism of Action

Blockade of alpha$_1$ receptors relaxes smooth muscle in the bladder neck (trigone and sphincter), prostate capsule, and prostatic urethra, thereby decreasing *dynamic obstruction* of the urethra. Symptomatic improvement and increased urinary flow develop *rapidly.* Because dynamic obstruction is the major contributor to symptoms in patients with relatively mild prostatic enlargement, alpha blockers are preferred to 5-alpha-reductase inhibitors for these men. To maintain benefits, alpha blockers must be taken lifelong. Unlike the 5-alpha-reductase inhibitors, the alpha$_1$ blockers do not reduce prostate size.

Receptor Specificity and Impact on Blood Pressure

The alpha blockers differ regarding specificity of receptor blockade and resultant effect on blood pressure. Specifically, whereas silodosin and tamsulosin are *selective for alpha$_{1a}$ receptors* (the type of alpha$_1$ receptors found in the prostate), alfuzosin, terazosin, and doxazosin are *nonselective alpha$_1$ blockers* and hence block alpha$_1$ receptors in blood vessels as well as alpha$_{1a}$ receptors in the prostate. By blocking alpha$_1$ receptors in blood vessels, the three nonselective agents promote vasodilation and can thereby lower blood pressure. In fact, two of these drugs—doxazosin and terazosin—were developed as antihypertensive agents; their use in BPH came later. Because of their effect on blood pressure, the nonselective alpha$_1$ blockers are especially useful for patients who have hypertension in addition to BPH—but may be dangerous for men with reduced blood pressure. Conversely, because silodosin and tamsulosin have little or no effect on blood pressure, they are of no benefit to men with hypertension—but are preferred if reducing blood pressure would be a problem.

Adverse Effects

The alpha$_1$ blockers are generally well tolerated. For the nonselective agents (alfuzosin, doxazosin, and terazosin), principal adverse effects are hypotension, fainting, dizziness, somnolence, and nasal congestion. Because *silodosin* and *tamsulosin* have minimal effects on vascular smooth muscle, these drugs are less likely to cause hypotension, fainting, dizziness, or nasal congestion. However, silodosin and tamsulosin *can* cause abnormal ejaculation (ejaculation failure, reduced volume, retrograde ejaculation), whereas the nonselective agents do not. In contrast to dutasteride and finasteride, the alpha blockers do not reduce levels of PSA.

For men undergoing cataract surgery, alpha blockade increases the risk for intraoperative *floppy-iris syndrome,* a complication that can increase postoperative pain, delay recovery, and reduce the hoped-for improvement in vision acuity. In severe cases, the syndrome can cause defects to the iris that may lead to blindness. Men anticipating cataract surgery should postpone alpha blocker therapy until after the procedure. Men already taking an alpha blocker should be sure to tell their ophthalmologist.

Drug Interactions

Exercise caution when combining nonselective alpha blockers with other drugs that lower blood pressure; excessive hypotension could result. Drugs of concern include organic nitrates (e.g., nitroglycerin), antihypertensive drugs, and PDE-5 inhibitors used for ED (e.g., sildenafil [Viagra]).

Strong inhibitors of CYP3A4 such as erythromycin, itraconazole, nefazodone, and HIV protease inhibitors (e.g., ritonavir) can dramatically increase levels of alfuzosin and silodosin. Accordingly, alfuzosin and silodosin must not be combined with these drugs.

Use in Women

Tamsulosin and other alpha blockers are being used off-label to treat women with urinary hesitancy or urinary retention associated with bladder outlet obstruction or insufficient contraction of the bladder detrusor muscle. Benefits derive from relaxing smooth muscle in the bladder neck and urethra. Maximal improvement may take several weeks to develop.

Alpha$_1$ Blocker/5-Alpha-Reductase Inhibitor Combination

In clinical trials, combining an alpha blocker with a 5-alpha-reductase inhibitor has been superior to treatment with either agent alone. Because alpha blockers and 5-alpha-reductase inhibitors work by different mechanisms, it is not surprising that combining them can be helpful: the alpha blocker can provide rapid symptomatic relief (by relaxing prostate-related smooth muscle), while, over time, the 5-alpha-reductase inhibitor can provide additional symptomatic relief (by shrinking the prostate) and may also delay disease progression.

Research has demonstrated effectiveness with tamsulosin plus dutasteride and doxazosin plus finasteride. Presumably, other combinations of an alpha blocker with a 5-alpha-reductase inhibitor would also be effective. If a single dose is preferred, tamsulosin plus dutasteride [Jalyn] is available.

Tadalafil, a PDE-5 Inhibitor

Tadalafil [Cialis] is approved for men who have BPH by itself or BPH combined with ED. In men with BPH, tadalafil produces a modest decrease in symptoms (urinary frequency, urinary urgency, straining), but does not improve urine flow rate. Furthermore, only 1 in 6 men benefit. Initial improvement is seen in 2 weeks. How does tadalafil help? Possibly by relaxing smooth muscle in the prostate, bladder, and urethra. Although tadalafil is the only PDE-5 inhibitor approved for ED, other PDE-5 inhibitors can reduce symptoms, too. Owing to the risk for hypotension, tadalafil should be used with caution in men taking an alpha blocker and should be avoided in men taking nitrates.

Other Drugs for Benign Prostatic Hyperplasia

Anticholinergics

Symptoms of overactive bladder (OAB), such as urgency and frequency, are often experienced by men with BPH. Anticholinergic drugs (specifically

PATIENT-CENTERED CARE ACROSS THE LIFE SPAN

Drugs for Benign Prostatic Hyperplasia

Life Stage	Considerations or Concerns
Children	These drugs are not approved for children.
Pregnant Women	The alpha1-adrenergic antagonists are FDA Pregnancy Risk Category B with the exception of doxazosin and terazosin, which are Pregnancy Risk Category C. Finasteride and dutasteride are classified in Pregnancy Risk Category X; they are teratogenic to the male fetus. Because these drugs can be absorbed through the skin, pregnant women should not handle finasteride or dutasteride tablets that have been broken or crushed. Men taking finasteride or dutasteride should not donate blood to avoid the risk of exposing a pregnant recipient. To donate blood after stopping the drug, a wait of at least 1 month is required after stopping finasteride and at least 6 months after stopping dutasteride.
Breast-Feeding Women	It is not known if 5-alpha-reductase inhibitors are excreted in breast milk. Women taking these drugs for off-label uses (e.g. hirsutism) should not breastfeed.
Older Adults	Beers Criteria includes the peripheral alpha-1 blockers doxazosin and terazosin among its listing of potentially inappropriate medications for patients age 65 and older.

antimuscarinics) are helpful when this occurs. Those approved for OAB include darifenacin, fesoterodine, oxybutynin, solifenacin, tolterodine, and trospium. These may be used alone or in combination with an alpha blocker such as tamsulosin to improve urinary symptoms (see Chapter 12).

Botulinum Toxin

Botulinum toxin [Botox, others], a well-known remedy for facial wrinkles, can also help men with BPH. A single injection into the prostate can relieve urinary symptoms for up to 1 year. Benefits derive in part from blocking release of acetylcholine from neurons that innervate urinary tract smooth muscle. However, because the drug also reduces both prostate size and blood levels of PSA, other mechanisms must also be involved.

Complementary and Alternative Medication for Benign Prostatic Hyperplasia

Saw palmetto is an herbal preparation used widely to treat BPH despite numerous randomized control trials (RCTs) that refuted findings of earlier less rigorous studies. In 2012 a Cochrane review of 32 RCTs involving 5666 men found no significant difference between saw palmetto and a placebo, even at doses 2 and 3 times the usual dose.

What about other CAMs? In their latest clinical guidelines, the American Urological Association declined to recommend any dietary supplement or herbal treatment, including saw palmetto, until there is a sufficient body of evidence from rigorous clinical trials to support their use.

Clinical Guidelines for Management of Benign Prostatic Hyperplasia

The American Urological Association updated their clinical guidelines for management of benign prostatic hyperplasia in 2010 (Fig. 51.3). These are available online at https://www.auanet.org/common/pdf/education/clinical-guidance/Benign-Prostatic-Hyperplasia.pdf.

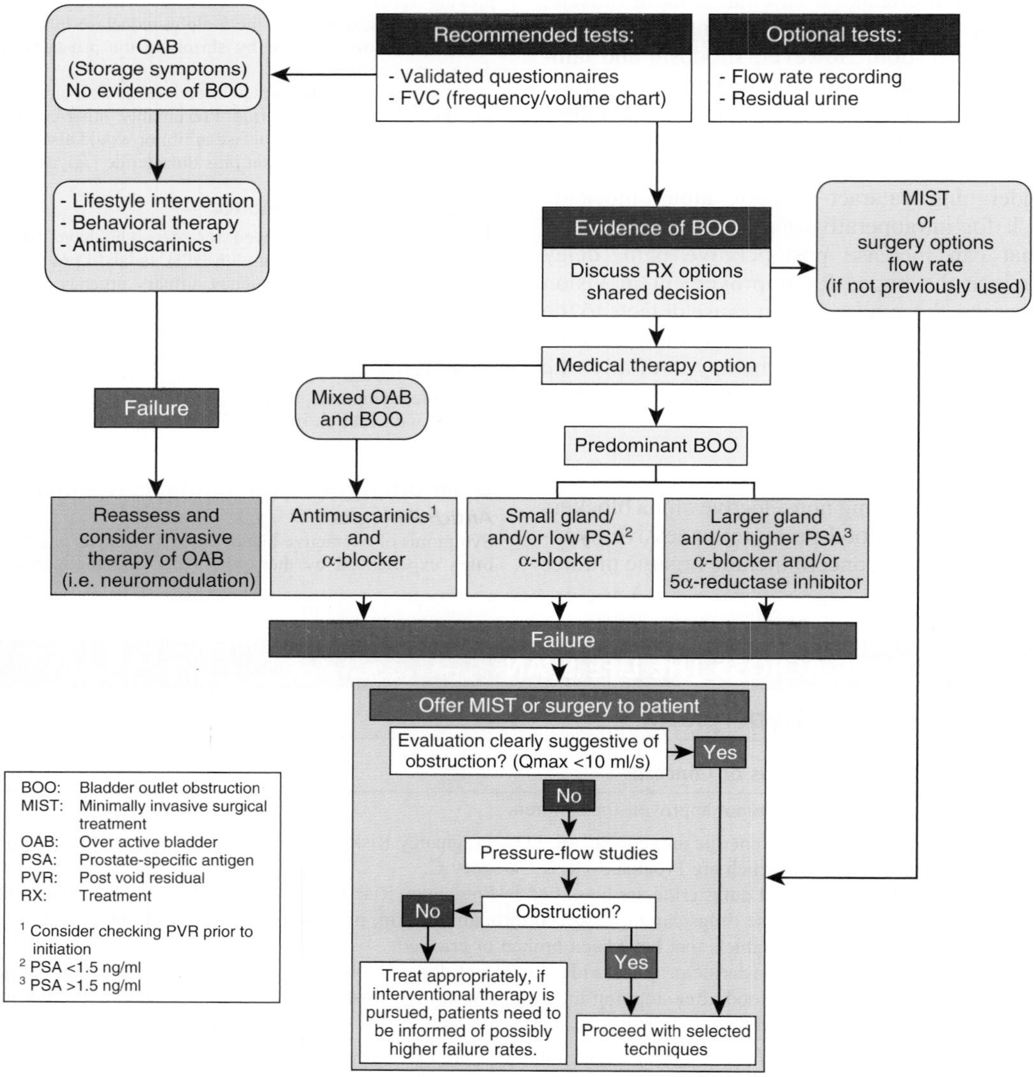

Figure 51.3 ■ Management of symptomatic benign prostatic hyperplasia. OAB, overactive bladder; BOO, bladder outlet. (From https://www.auanet.org/common/pdf/education/clinical-guidance/Benign-Prostatic-Hyperplasia.pdf.)

Prescribing and Monitoring Considerations PDE-5 Inhibitors

The nursing implications that follow pertain only to the use of PDE-5 inhibitors for ED, not for their use in pulmonary arterial hypertension (PAH).

Therapeutic Goal

PDE-5 inhibitors are used to enhance both the hardness and duration of erection in men with ED.

Baseline Data

Evaluate patients for cardiovascular disorders, including stroke, hypotension, hypertension, heart failure, unstable angina, myocardial infarction, and recent history of a severe dysrhythmia.

Identifying High-Risk Patients

PDE-5 inhibitors are *contraindicated* for men taking nitrates (e.g., nitroglycerin) and should generally be avoided by men taking alpha blockers. Avoid *vardenafil*—but not sildenafil or tadalafil—in men taking class I or class III antidysrhythmic drugs.

Use PDE-5 inhibitors with *caution* in men taking CYP3A4 inhibitors and in those with NAION, coronary heart disease, and other cardiovascular disorders.

Administration Considerations

Dosing With Food

These drugs may be taken with or without food. High-fat meals will delay absorption of avanafil, sildenafil, or vardenafil (but not tadalafil). Grapefruit juice may decrease metabolism resulting in a higher than recommended drug level.

Timing of Dose

All PDE-5 inhibitors may be used PRN. Avanafil should be taken approximately 15- to 30 minutes before sexual activity. All other PDE-5 inhibitors should be taken about 1 hour before sexual activity. Only *tadalafil* is approved for daily dosing.

Ongoing Evaluation and Interventions

Minimizing Adverse Effects

Cardiac Risk. For men with preexisting cardiovascular disease, consider carefully the cardiac risk associated with sexual activity before prescribing a PDE-5 inhibitor or any drug for ED.

Priapism. PDE-5 inhibitors can cause priapism, which can result in permanent ED owing to local tissue damage. Treatment, which must be instituted promptly, involves aspiration of blood from the corpus cavernosum followed by irrigation with a vasoconstrictor.

Nonarteritic Ischemic Optic Neuropathy. Very rarely, men taking PDE-5 inhibitors have developed NAION with resultant irreversible blurring of vision or blindness. Monitor for vision changes with each refill.

Sudden Hearing Loss. Very rarely, men taking PDE-5 inhibitors have developed sudden loss of hearing, sometimes associated with dizziness, vertigo, and tinnitus. Monitor for hearing changes with each refill.

Minimizing Adverse Interactions

Nitrates. Combining a PDE-5 inhibitor with a nitrate (e.g., nitroglycerin) can cause a severe drop in blood pressure. Concurrent use of these drugs is contraindicated.

Alpha-Adrenergic Blockers. Combining a PDE-5 inhibitor with an alpha blocker (e.g., doxazosin) can cause a serious drop in blood pressure. To avoid harm, use caution when combining *sildenafil* or *avanafil* with an alpha blocker; do not combine *tadalafil* with any alpha blockers except tamsulosin, and do not combine *vardenafil* with any alpha blockers at all.

Inhibitors of CYP3A4. Agents that inhibit CYP3A4 (e.g., ketoconazole, ritonavir, grapefruit juice) can raise PDE-5 inhibitor levels. To avoid harm, dosage of the PDE-5 inhibitor should be reduced.

Antidysrhythmic Drugs. Avoid prescribing *vardenafil* for men taking class I or class III antidysrhythmic drugs. Vardenafil prolongs the QT interval and can thereby cause a severe dysrhythmia when combined with these agents.

UNIT XIII

Antiinflammatory, Antiallergic, and Immunologic Drugs

CHAPTER 52

Review of the Immune System

Jacqueline Rosenjack Burchum, DNSc, FNP-BC, CNE

The immune system protects us from invading organisms (viruses, bacteria, fungi, and parasites) and can destroy cancer cells before they destroy us. Unfortunately, the immune system does not always act in our best interest: it can attack transplanted organs and tissues and can turn on the cells it normally protects.

To study the immune system, we begin with an overview. After that, we discuss the two major types of specific immune responses: antibody-mediated immunity (humoral immunity) and cell-mediated immunity.

INTRODUCTION TO THE IMMUNE SYSTEM

Our objective in this section is to establish an overview of immune system components and how they function. Much of the information introduced here is amplified later.

Natural Immunity Versus Specific Acquired Immunity

Our bodies can mount two types of immune responses, referred to as *natural immunity* (innate or native immunity) and *specific acquired immunity.* Factors that confer natural immunity include physical barriers (e.g., skin), phagocytic cells, and natural killer cells. All of these factors are present before exposure to a particular infectious agent, and all respond nonspecifically. In contrast, specific acquired immune responses occur only after exposure to a foreign substance. The foreign substances that induce specific responses are called *antigens,* and the objective of the immune response is to destroy them. With each succeeding reexposure to a particular antigen, the specific immune response to that antigen becomes more rapid and more intense. Specific immune responses are possible because certain cells of the immune system (T lymphocytes and B lymphocytes) possess receptors that can recognize individual antigens. Our focus here is on specific acquired immunity, not on natural immunity.

Cell-Mediated Immunity Versus Antibody-Mediated (Humoral) Immunity

Specific acquired immune responses can be classified as either cell mediated or humoral. *Cell-mediated immunity* refers to immune responses in which targets are attacked directly by immune system cells—specifically, cytolytic T cells and macrophages. *Humoral immunity* refers to immune responses that are mediated by *antibodies.* (The term *humoral*—defined as "pertaining to elements dissolved in blood or body fluids"—connotes that antibodies dissolved in the blood.)

Introduction to Cells of the Immune System

Immune responses are mediated by several types of cells, some of which play a bigger role than others. The major actors are the *lymphocytes* (B cells, cytolytic T cells, helper T cells), *macrophages,* and *dendritic cells.* Accessory cells include neutrophils and basophils. With the exception of some dendritic cells, all of the cells involved in the immune response arise from pluripotent stem cells in the bone marrow (Fig. 52.1) and, for at least part of their life cycle, circulate in the blood. Defining characteristics of individual immune system cells are shown in Table 52.1.

B Lymphocytes (B Cells)

B lymphocytes have the job of making *antibodies.* Hence, B cells mediate humoral immunity. As discussed later, antibody specificity is determined by the structure of highly specific receptors found on the surface of B cells. Like all other lymphocytes, B cells circulate in the blood and lymph. B cells are so named because in chickens, where B cells were discovered, these cells are produced in the *bursa of Fabricius,* a structure not found in mammals. In humans and other mammals, B cells are produced in the bone marrow.

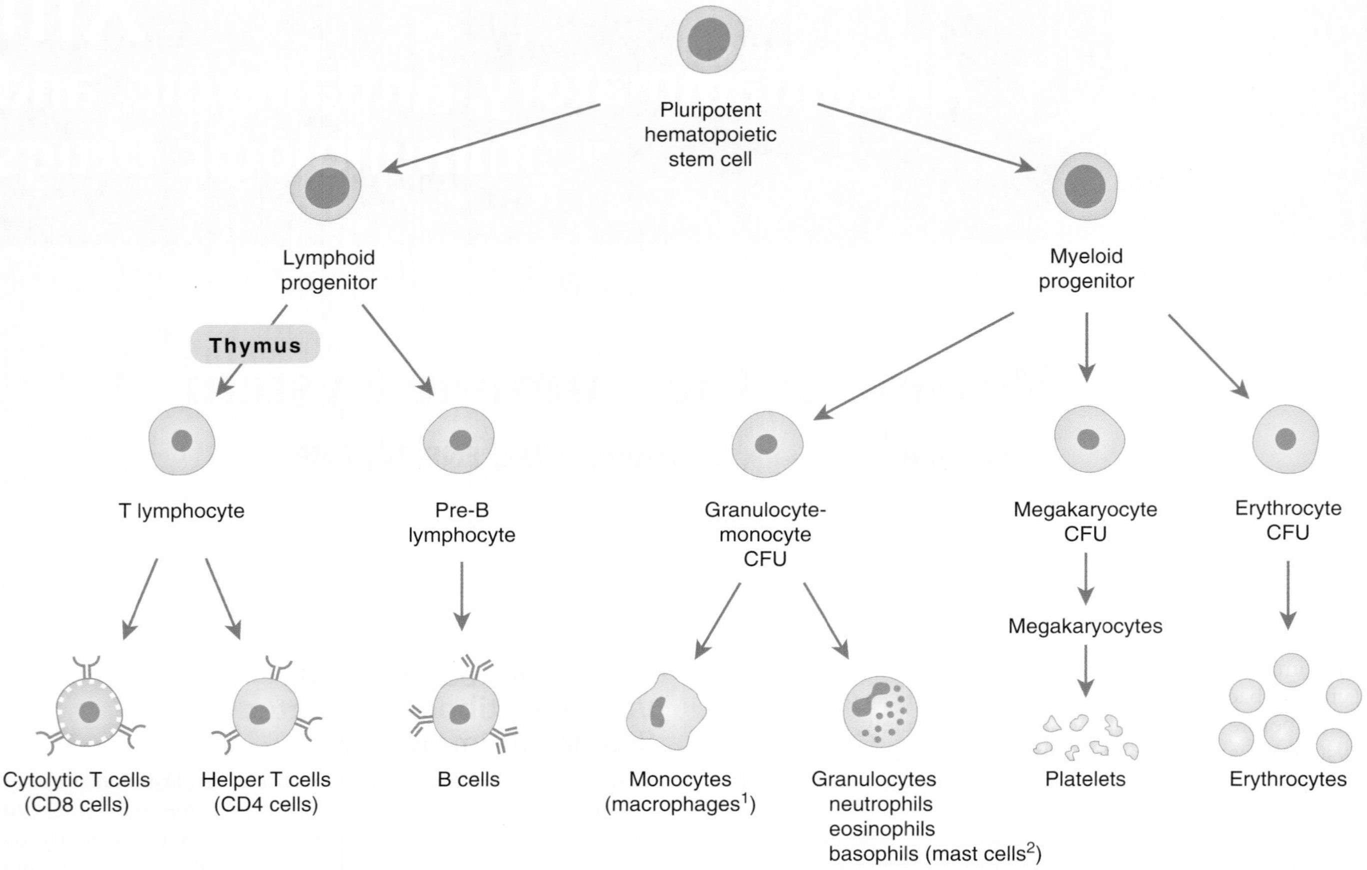

Figure 52.1 ■ Maturation of blood cells.
With the exception of platelets and erythrocytes, all of the mature blood cells shown participate in immune responses. However, only cells of lymphoid origin (cytolytic T cells, helper T cells, B cells) possess receptors that can recognize specific antigens. Monocytes that have moved into tissues are called macrophages. [1]Basophils that have moved into tissues are called mast cells. [2]CFU, colony-forming unit.

Cytolytic T Lymphocytes (Cytolytic T Cells, CD8 Cells)

Cytolytic T cells are key players in cellular immunity. These cells do not produce antibodies. Rather, they attack and kill target cells directly. Specificity of attack is determined by the presence of antigen molecules on the surface of the target cell and specific receptors for that antigen on the surface of the T cell. Cytolytic T cells are also known as *CD8 cells* and *cytotoxic T cells*. The designation "CD8" refers to the presence of cell-surface marker molecules known as *cell differentiation complex 8*. The "T" in T cell stands for thymus, the organ in which cytolytic T cells and helper T cells mature. Like B cells, cytolytic T cells circulate in the blood and lymph.

Helper T Lymphocytes (Helper T Cells, CD4 Cells)

Helper T cells contribute to the immune response in three ways: (1) they have an essential role in antibody production by B cells, (2) they release factors that promote type IV sensitivity reactions, also known as delayed-type hypersensitivity (DTH), and (3) they participate in the activation of cytolytic T cells. Specificity of helper T cells is achieved through highly specific cell-surface receptors that recognize individual antigens. Like other lymphocytes, helper T cells circulate in the blood and lymph. Helper T cells carry CD4 (cell differentiation complex 4) marker molecules on their surface and hence are referred to as *CD4 cells*.

The term *helper* is somewhat misleading in that it connotes a useful but dispensable role. Nothing could be further from reality. Helper T cells are not simply nice to have around, they are absolutely required for an effective immune response. The critical nature of their contribution—and the grim consequences of their absence—are manifested in people with HIV/AIDS: helper T cells are the immune cells that HIV attacks. Because of helper T-cell loss, AIDS patients are at high risk for death from opportunistic infection.

Macrophages

Macrophages begin their existence in the bone marrow, enter the blood as monocytes, and then infiltrate tissues, where they evolve into macrophages. Macrophages are present in all organs and tissues.

The primary function of macrophages is *phagocytosis* (i.e., ingestion of microbes, other foreign material, and cellular debris). In their role as phagocytes, macrophages are the principal scavengers of the body. Although their major job is phagocytosis, macrophages also have an important

TABLE 52.1 ▪ Cells of the Immune System

Cell Type	Synonyms	Primary Immune-Related Actions
MAJOR CELL TYPES		
B lymphocytes	B cells	• Produce antibodies
CTLs	Cytolytic T cells, cytotoxic T cells, CD8 cells	• Lyse target cells
Helper T lymphocytes	Helper T cells, CD4 cells	• Promote proliferation and differentiation of B cells and CTLs • Initiate delayed-type hypersensitivity
Macrophages		• Promote proliferation and differentiation of helper T cells and CTLs by serving as APCs • Participate in delayed-type hypersensitivity • Phagocytize cells tagged with antibodies • Phagocytize cells in the effector stage of delayed-type hypersensitivity
Dendritic cells		• Promote proliferation of CTLs and helper T cells by serving as APCs
ACCESSORY CELLS		
Mast cells		• Mediate immediate hypersensitivity reactions
Basophils		• Mediate immediate hypersensitivity reactions
Neutrophils	Polymorphonuclear leukocytes	• Phagocytize foreign particles (e.g., bacteria), especially those tagged with IgG • Mediate inflammation
Eosinophils		• Attack helminths and foreign particles that have been coated with IgE • Contribute to immediate hypersensitivity reactions

APC, antigen-presenting cell; CTL, cytolytic T lymphocyte; Ig, immunoglobulin.

role in specific acquired immunity, natural immunity, and inflammation.

In specific acquired immunity, macrophages have three functions: (1) they are required for activation of T cells (both helper T cells and cytolytic T cells), (2) they are the final mediators of DTH, and (3) they phagocytize cells that have been tagged with antibodies. Of these three immune-related roles, activation of T cells is arguably the most critical. When performing this function, macrophages are referred to as *antigen-presenting cells* (APCs). Because antigen presentation is an absolute requirement for specific immune responses (see later), you can appreciate how important macrophages are.

Dendritic Cells

Dendritic cells perform the same antigen-presenting task as do macrophages. However, unlike macrophages, dendritic cells do not also serve as scavengers. Dendritic cells are found in lymph nodes and other lymphoid tissues.

Mast Cells and Basophils

These cells mediate immediate hypersensitivity reactions. Mast cells, which are derived from basophils, are concentrated in the skin and other soft tissues. Basophils circulate in the blood. Both cell types release histamine, heparin, and other compounds that cause the symptoms of immediate hypersensitivity. Release of these mediators is triggered when an antigen binds to antibodies on the cell surface. The role of mast cells and basophils in allergic reactions is discussed in Chapter 61.

Neutrophils

Neutrophils, also known as polymorphonuclear leukocytes, phagocytize bacteria and other foreign particles. As discussed later, neutrophils avidly devour cells that have been tagged with antibodies of the immunoglobulin G (IgG) class. Accordingly, neutrophils can be viewed as important effectors in humoral immunity. Neutrophils are also major contributors to inflammation.

Eosinophils

Eosinophils attack and destroy foreign particles that have been coated with antibodies of the IgE class. Their usual target is helminths (parasitic worms). Eosinophils also contribute to tissue injury and inflammation associated with immediate hypersensitivity reactions.

Antibodies

Antibodies are a family of structurally related glycoproteins that mediate humoral immunity. The most characteristic feature of antibodies is their ability to recognize and bind with specific antigens. Alternative names for antibodies are *immunoglobulins* and *gamma globulins*.

All antibodies are produced by B lymphocytes. Some of the antibodies that B cells produce are retained on the surface of the B cell, where they serve as the receptors whereby B cells recognize specific antigens. However, most of the antibodies that B cells produce are secreted from the cell, after which they bind to their specific antigen, thereby initiating the effector phase of humoral immunity. The process of antibody production is discussed in detail later.

All antibodies are composed of units that have the same basic structure. As shown in Fig. 52.2, antibodies have four chains: two heavy chains and two light chains. Disulfide bridges connect the four chains to form a unit. Each heavy chain and each light chain has two regions, one in which the sequence of amino acids is *constant* and one in which the sequence is highly *variable*. The variable regions form the antigen-binding site.

There are five classes of antibodies (immunoglobulins), known as IgA, IgD, IgE, IgG, and IgM. All are constructed from the same basic parts just described. However, the heavy chains differ for each class. Primary functions of the five classes are shown in Table 52.2.

When antibodies are subjected to digestion by papain in the laboratory, they break down into three pieces (see Fig. 52.2). Two of the pieces retain the ability to bind antigen and hence are called *Fab fragments* (fragment, antigen binding). The third piece does not bind antigen and tends to form crystals in the test tube and hence is called the *Fc fragment* (fragment, crystalline).

Antigens

Antigens are molecules that induce specific immune responses and, as a result, become the targets of those responses. By way of analogy, an antigen is like the child who pokes a stick in a hornet's nest, at once triggering a response and becoming its target. An antigen may trigger production of antibodies, cytotoxic T cells, or both—all of which can then attack the antigen.

Most antigens are large molecules. Because antigens are big, the antigen-binding region of the resultant antibodies cannot recognize and bind the entire antigen molecule. Rather, the antibodies recognize and bind selected small portions of the antigen, referred to as *epitopes* or *antigenic determinants.* All antigens have multiple epitopes. As a result, more than one antibody can bind the antigen.

In research and in clinical practice, we may want to generate antibodies to molecules that are too small to induce an immune response. To overcome this obstacle, we can link the small molecule to a larger molecule, usually a protein. When this is done, the small molecule is referred to as a *hapten,* and the large molecule is referred to as a *carrier.* At least some of the resultant antibodies will be selective for the hapten.

TABLE 52.2 ■ Functions of Antibody Classes

Class	Function
IgA	• Located in mucous membranes of the GI tract and lungs and in many secretions, where it serves as the first line of defense against microbes entering the body via these routes • Transferred to infants via breast milk; is not absorbed from the GI tract but does protect the infant against microbes *in* the GI tract
IgD	• Found only on the surface of mature B cells, where it serves as a receptor for antigen recognition (along with IgM)
IgE	• Binds to the surface of mast cells; subsequent binding of antigen to IgE stimulates release of histamine, heparin, and other mediators from the mast cells, thereby causing symptoms of allergy (e.g., hives, hay fever) • Binds to parasitic worms, after which eosinophils bind to IgE and release compounds that lyse the worms
IgG	• Produced in copious amounts in response to antigenic stimulation and hence is the major antibody in blood • Fixes complement and thereby promotes target-cell lysis • Binds target cells and thereby enhances phagocytosis • Transferred across the placenta to the fetal circulation, thereby providing neonatal immunity
IgM	• First class of antibody produced in response to an antigen • Fixes complement and thereby promotes target-cell lysis • Present on the surface of mature B cells, where it serves as a receptor for antigen recognition (along with IgD)

Ig, immunoglobulin.

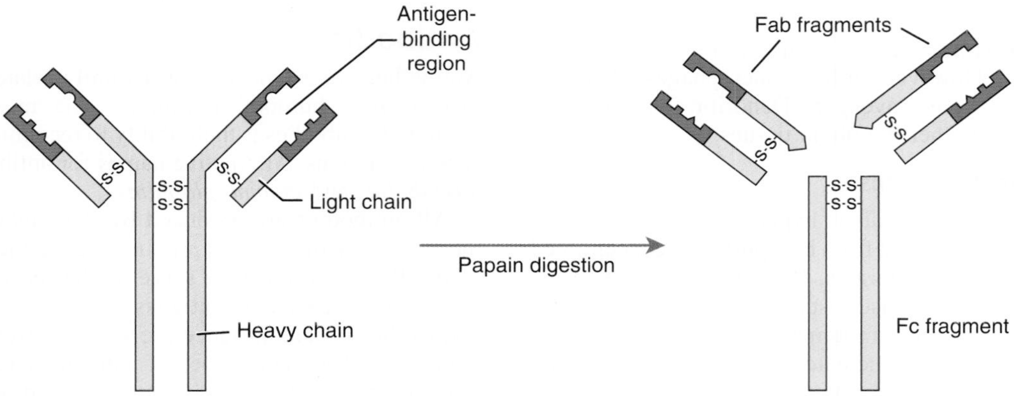

Figure 52.2 ■ Antibody structure.
The basic antibody structure depicting heavy and light chains is shown on the *left.* Variable regions of the heavy and light chains, which form the antigen-binding site, appear in *green.* As shown on the *right,* papain digestion of antibodies produces two types of fragments: Fab fragments, which retain the ability to bind antigen, and Fc fragments, which do not bind antigen and tend to crystallize in the test tube.

Characteristic Features of Immune Responses

Cell-mediated immunity and humoral immunity share five characteristic features: specificity, diversity, memory, time limitation, and selectivity for antigens of nonself origin (i.e., the ability to discriminate between self and nonself).

Specificity

Cell-mediated and humoral immune responses are triggered by specific antigens, and their purpose is to destroy the antigen that triggered the response. The ability to respond to a specific antigen (i.e., the ability to make subtle distinctions among related molecules) is conferred by highly specific receptors on B cells and T cells.

Diversity

Our immune systems can respond to millions of different antigenic determinants. This is possible because our immune systems have millions of clones of B and T lymphocytes—each of which is preprogrammed to recognize a different antigenic determinant. As noted, this ability to discriminate between antigens is the result of having unique cell-surface receptors.

Memory

Exposure to an antigen affects the immune system such that reexposure produces a faster, larger, and more prolonged response compared with the initial exposure (Fig. 52.3). During the initial response, B and T lymphocytes that recognize the antigen undergo proliferation. Most of the new cells participate in the attack against the antigen. However, some of the new cells become *memory cells,* thereby increasing the pool of antigen-specific cells available to respond in the future. Hence, when the antigen is encountered again, the memory cells mobilize and thereby accelerate and intensify the response.

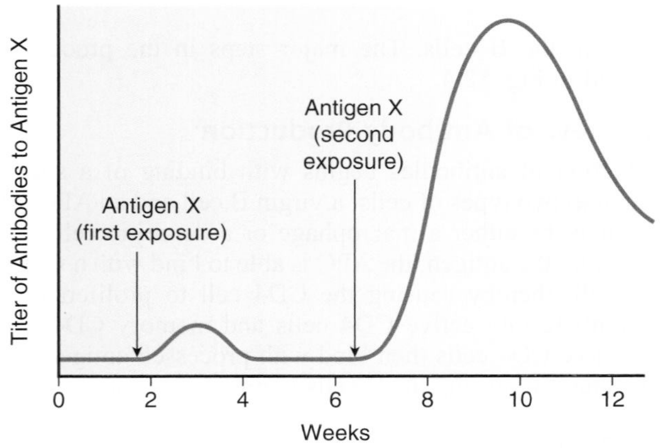

Figure 52.3 ■ Memory and time limitation of immune responses.
After the initial exposure to antigen X, antibody levels rise slowly, peak at a low level, and then decline rapidly. After the second exposure to antigen X, antibody levels rise more rapidly, reach a higher peak, persist longer, and then slowly decline.

Time Limitation

Immune responses don't last indefinitely. They are time limited. The reasons are twofold: First, as the immune response proceeds, it greatly decreases the level of antigen that initiated the response, thereby attenuating the stimulus for continuing. Second, activated B cells and T cells only function for a short time, after which they become quiescent or die. Hence, in the absence of a continuing stimulus to generate more active B cells and T cells, the immune response fades.

Selectivity for Antigens of Nonself Origin

Under normal conditions, our immune systems target only foreign antigens, leaving potentially antigenic molecules on our own cells untouched. Sparing of self is possible because, as T cells develop in the thymus, cells that are able to react with antigens of self origin are eliminated. As discussed later, this discrimination between self and nonself is made possible by *major histocompatibility complex* (MHC) molecules.

When the ability to discriminate between self and nonself fails, our immune systems can attack our own cells. The result is an *autoimmune disease.* There are many diseases of autoimmune origin, including psoriasis, multiple sclerosis, rheumatoid arthritis, myasthenia gravis, type 1 diabetes, systemic lupus erythematosus, two inflammatory bowel diseases (ulcerative colitis and Crohn disease), and two thyroid diseases (Graves disease and Hashimoto thyroiditis).

Phases of the Immune Response

Specific immune responses can be viewed as having three main phases: recognition, activation, and effector.

Recognition Phase

The recognition phase occurs when a mature lymphocyte encounters its matching antigen. All specific immune responses begin with antigen recognition by B cells and T cells. Antigen recognition is possible because of antigen-specific receptors on the lymphocyte surface.

Activation Phase

Antigen recognition activates the lymphocyte, which then undergoes proliferation and differentiation. Some of the daughter cells differentiate into cells that actively participate in the immune response, attacking the source of the antigen. Other daughter cells differentiate into memory cells, thereby preparing the host for a more intense, rapid, and prolonged response in the event of antigen reexposure.

Effector Phase

In this stage, the immune system attempts to eliminate the specific antigen that initiated the response. With cell-mediated or antibody-mediated immunity, several effector mechanisms can be involved. In cell-mediated immunity, antigen-bearing target cells can be lysed by cytolytic T cells, or they can be ingested by macrophages. In antibody-mediated immunity, target cells may be primed for attack by phagocytes or by the complement system.

Major Histocompatibility Complex Molecules

The *major histocompatibility complex* is a group of *genes* that codes for *MHC molecules,* which become expressed on the surface of all cells. MHC molecules are critical to immune system function. They play a key role in the activation of helper and cytotoxic T lymphocytes, they guide cytotoxic T lymphocytes toward target cells, and they provide the basis for distinguishing between self and nonself.

There are two classes of MHC gene products, referred to as *class I MHC molecules* and *class II MHC molecules.* Class I MHC molecules are found on virtually all cells except erythrocytes; class II MHC molecules are found primarily on B cells and APCs (macrophages and dendritic cells). As discussed later, *class I MHC molecules* on the surface of APCs help initiate immune responses by "presenting" antigen to *cytotoxic T cells.* In contrast, *class II MHC molecules* on the surface of APCs help initiate immune responses by presenting antigen to *helper T cells.*

As a rule, the sequence of amino acids in MHC molecules produced by one individual differs from the sequence of amino acids in MHC molecules produced by everyone else. That is, it is rare for two individuals to have MHC molecules that are identical. As a result, MHC molecules from one individual are recognized as foreign (nonself) by the immune systems of nearly everyone else. Hence, when we attempt to transplant organs between individuals who are not identical twins, immune rejection of the transplant is likely. To reduce the risk for rejection, we can treat patients with immunosuppressant drugs.

Cytokines, Lymphokines, and Monokines

The terms *cytokine, lymphokine,* and *monokine* are encountered frequently when discussing the immune system and can be a source of confusion. The term *cytokine* refers to any mediator molecule (other than an antibody) released by *any* immune system cell. A *lymphokine* is simply a cytokine released by a *lymphocyte,* and a *monokine* is simply a cytokine released by a *mononuclear phagocyte* (monocyte or macrophage). Put another way, *cytokine* is a generic term for the whole class of nonantibody mediators released by immune cells, whereas the terms *lymphokine* and *monokine* are more restrictive, referring only to nonantibody mediators released by lymphocytes and mononuclear phagocytes, respectively. Examples of cytokines and their functions are listed in Table 52.3.

TABLE 52.3 ▪ Functions of Selected Cytokines

Cytokine	Function
IL-1	Stimulates lymphocyte progenitor cells
IL-2	Stimulates proliferation and differentiation of helper T cells and cytolytic T cells
IL-3	Stimulates proliferation of bone marrow lineage cells, B cells, and T cells
IL-4	Activates B cells, T cells, and macrophages
IL-5	Stimulates generation of eosinophils
IL-6	Stimulates proliferation of bone marrow cells and plasma cells
IL-7	Stimulates B cells and T cells
IL-8	Attracts neutrophils, B cells, and T cells
IL-9	Stimulates proliferation of mast cells
IL-10	Inhibits some T cells
IL-11	Enhances actions of IL-3
IL-12	Enhances actions of IL-2
Interferon alpha	Activates macrophages, cytolytic T cells, and natural killer cells
Interferon gamma	Activates macrophages and T cells and enhances expression of MHC molecules
Tumor necrosis factor	Kills tumor cells; promotes inflammation
Granulocyte-macrophage colony-stimulating factor	Stimulates proliferation of monocytes, macrophages, and granulocytes (neutrophils, eosinophils, basophils)

IL, interleukin; MHC, major histocompatibility complex.

ANTIBODY-MEDIATED (HUMORAL) IMMUNITY

As noted, there are two types of immune responses: humoral immunity and cell-mediated immunity. In this section, we review humoral immunity, focusing on (1) how antibodies are produced and (2) the mechanisms by which antibodies protect us. Cell-mediated immunity is discussed in the section that follows.

Production of Antibodies

Antibody production requires the cooperative interaction of three types of cells: *B cells,* which actually make the antibodies; *helper T cells* (CD4 cells), which stimulate the B cells; and an *antigen-presenting cell* (either a macrophage or a dendritic cell), which activates the CD4 cells so that they can then help the B cells. The major steps in the process are depicted in Fig. 52.4.

Overview of Antibody Production

Production of antibodies begins with binding of a specific antigen to two types of cells: a virgin B cell and an APC. The APC may be either a macrophage or a dendritic cell. After processing the antigen, the APC is able to bind with a specific CD4 cell, thereby causing the CD4 cell to proliferate and differentiate into active CD4 cells and memory CD4 cells. The active CD4 cells then bind with processed antigen on B cells, thereby causing the B cells to proliferate and differentiate into (1) plasma cells, which manufacture the antibodies and (2) memory B cells, which await the next antigen exposure.

Specific Cellular Events in Antibody Production

B Cells

Participation of B cells in the immune response begins with recognition and binding of a *specific antigen.* The receptor that B cells employ for antigen recognition is actually an antibody (IgD or IgM). For any given B cell, this antibody (receptor) is highly specific for just one antigenic determinant. After the antigen binds the B-cell receptor, the receptor-antigen complex is internalized and the antigen is broken

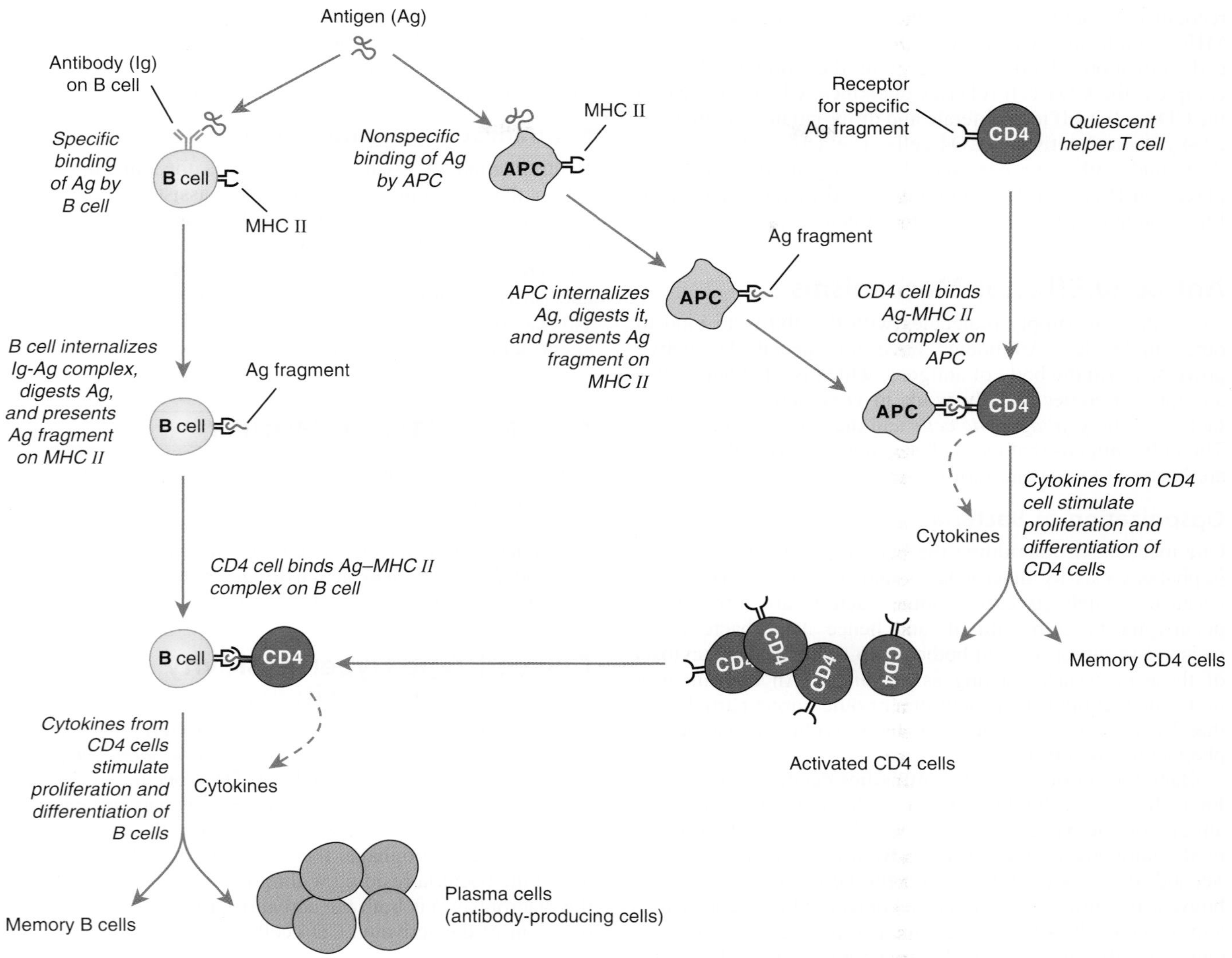

Figure 52.4 ■ Major events in antibody-mediated (humoral) immunity. Humoral immunity requires three types of cells: B cells, antigen-presenting cells (APCs), and helper T cells (CD4 cells). Binding of a CD4 cell with an APC activates the CD4 cell, which then binds with a B cell and releases cytokines, which then stimulate the B cell. Ig, immunoglobulin (antibody); MHC II, class II MHC molecule.

down into small peptide fragments. Each fragment is then complexed with a *class II MHC molecule,* after which the *antigen–MHC II complexes* are transported to the cell surface. (In Fig. 52.4, only one such complex is shown. However, in a real cell, many such complexes, each with a different piece of the antigen, would appear on the cell surface.) The final step of B-cell activation occurs when a CD4 helper T cell recognizes and binds with an antigen–MHC II complex on the B cell. This binding causes the CD4 cell to secrete cytokines, which then stimulate the B cell to proliferate and differentiate into two types of cells: plasma cells and memory B cells. The plasma cells are the cells that make antibodies. The memory cells serve to hasten, intensify, and prolong the immune response if antigen exposure should recur.

Antigen-Presenting Cells

APCs are essential for activation of CD4 helper T cells because CD4 cells cannot recognize antigen that is free in solution. Rather, they can only recognize antigen that has been complexed with an MHC II molecule.

Participation of APCs in the immune response begins with nonspecific binding of antigen to the APC (see Fig. 52.4). Next, as in B cells, the antigen is internalized and broken into fragments, which are then complexed with MHC II molecules and transported to the cell surface, where they are available for interaction with CD4 cells.

Helper T Cells (CD4 Cells)

The job of CD4 cells in humoral immunity is to activate B cells. In the absence of activation by CD4 cells, B cells are unable to proliferate and produce antibodies.

Participation of CD4 cells in the immune response begins when these cells bind with an antigen–MHC II complex on the surface of an APC. Binding is mediated by a receptor on the CD4 cell that is specific for the particular antigen in the antigen–MHC II complex. (As noted, for the CD4 cell to recognize the antigen, the antigen must be complexed with an MHC II molecule, which is why the APC is essential for CD4 cell activation.) Upon binding with the antigen–MHC II complex, the CD4 cell releases cytokines, which then cause the CD4 cell itself to proliferate and differentiate into memory CD4 cells and activated CD4 cells. The activated CD4 cells then bind with their corresponding antigen–MHC II complexes on B cells, release cytokines, and thereby cause proliferation and differentiation of the B cells.

Antibody Effector Mechanisms

Antibodies are simply molecules with the ability to bind to other molecules. Antibodies have no special destructive powers. To rid the body of antigens, which is what antibodies are for, antibodies usually work in conjunction with other factors, namely, *phagocytic cells* and the *complement system.* The only antigens that antibodies can neutralize without help are bacterial toxins and viruses.

Opsonization of Bacteria

One mechanism for ridding the body of pathogenic bacteria is phagocytosis by macrophages and neutrophils. However, because of their structures, some bacteria are difficult for phagocytes to grab hold of, and hence these bacteria are resistant to ingestion. Antibodies help promote phagocytosis of these bacteria by acting as *opsonins.* (An opsonin is a molecule that binds to a bacterium or other target particle and thereby promotes phagocytosis by providing a handle for phagocytes to grab.)

Bacterial opsonization by antibodies occurs in two steps. First, the antigen-binding region of the antibody binds with antigen on the bacterial surface, which leaves the Fc portion of the antibody projecting away from the bacterial surface. Second, phagocytes link up with the Fc portion of the antibody, which brings them in close contact with the bacterium, and hence enables them to commence phagocytosis. Phagocytes are able to bind the Fc fragment because they have high-affinity receptors for Fc on their surface. Most of the antibodies that act as opsonins belong to the IgG class.

Activation of the Complement System

The complement cascade is a complex system consisting of at least 20 serum proteins that, when activated, can cause multiple effects, including cell lysis, opsonization, degranulation of mast cells, and infiltration of phagocytes. The system can be activated in two ways, known as the *classical pathway* and the *alternative pathway.* The classical pathway is activated by *antibodies;* the alternative pathway is not. However, with both pathways, the end results are essentially the same. Consideration here is limited to the classical pathway.

The classical pathway is turned on when C1 (the first component of the complement system) encounters an antigen-antibody complex and then binds with the Fc region of the antibody. C1 will not bind with antibody that is free in solution, and hence free antibodies cannot activate the system. Activation of the complement system triggers a cascade of reactions that amplify the response at each stage. The result is production of compounds that can injure target cells.

Lysis of target cells that have been tagged with antibodies is the most dramatic effect of the complement system. Lysis is caused by cylindrical *membrane attack complexes,* which are formed by the complement cascade. After their insertion into the target-cell membrane, the attack complexes act as pores through which fluid can enter the cell. Fluid influx causes the target cell to swell and then burst.

Neutralization of Viruses and Bacterial Toxins

Neutralization of toxins and viruses is the only protective action that antibodies can perform unassisted. To hurt us, bacterial toxins must first bind with receptors on our cells. Likewise, to infect us, viruses must first bind with cell-surface receptors. By binding with antigenic determinants on toxins and viruses, antibodies make it impossible for toxins and viruses to bind with cellular receptors. As a result, these agents can no longer hurt us.

CELL-MEDIATED IMMUNITY

Cell-mediated immunity has two branches, one mediated by *helper T lymphocytes* (CD4 cells) plus *macrophages,* and one mediated primarily by *cytolytic T lymphocytes* (CD8 cells). In the branch mediated by CD4 cells and macrophages, the result is called *delayed-type hypersensitivity.* In the branch mediated by CD8 cells, the result is *target-cell lysis.*

Delayed-Type Hypersensitivity (Type IV Hypersensitivity)

The object of DTH is to rid the body of bacteria that replicate primarily within macrophages (e.g., *Listeria monocytogenes, Mycobacterium tuberculosis*). For DTH to occur, two cells are needed: an *infected macrophage* and a *CD4 helper T cell.* The macrophage serves to activate the CD4 cell, which in turn activates the macrophage, thereby enabling the macrophage to kill the bacteria residing within. Hence, the same cell (i.e., the macrophage) is both the activator of the CD4 cell and the recipient of the activated CD4 cell's help.

Activation of Helper T Cells

Activation of CD4 cells in DTH is essentially identical to the activation of CD4 cells in humoral immunity. As shown in Fig. 52.5, the process begins when a macrophage becomes infected with intracellular bacteria. As in humoral immunity, the macrophage breaks down the antigen to small peptides, combines each peptide with a class II MHC molecule, and then presents the antigen–MHC II complexes on its surface. In the next step, a CD4 cell binds with an antigen–MHC II complex on the macrophage. As discussed earlier, selectivity of binding is determined by receptors on the CD4 cell that recognize a specific antigen fragment—but only when the fragment is bound to a class II MHC molecule. Binding of the CD4 cell with the APC causes the CD4 cell to release (1) cytokines that cause the CD4 cell itself to proliferate and differentiate into memory cells and (2) mediators of DTH, including interferon gamma and tumor necrosis factor.

Activation of Macrophages

Interferon gamma, released from the activated CD4 cell, is the major stimulus for macrophage activation. In response to interferon gamma, macrophages increase production of lysosomes and reactive oxygen. The reactive oxygen is ultimately responsible for killing bacteria inside the macrophage. In

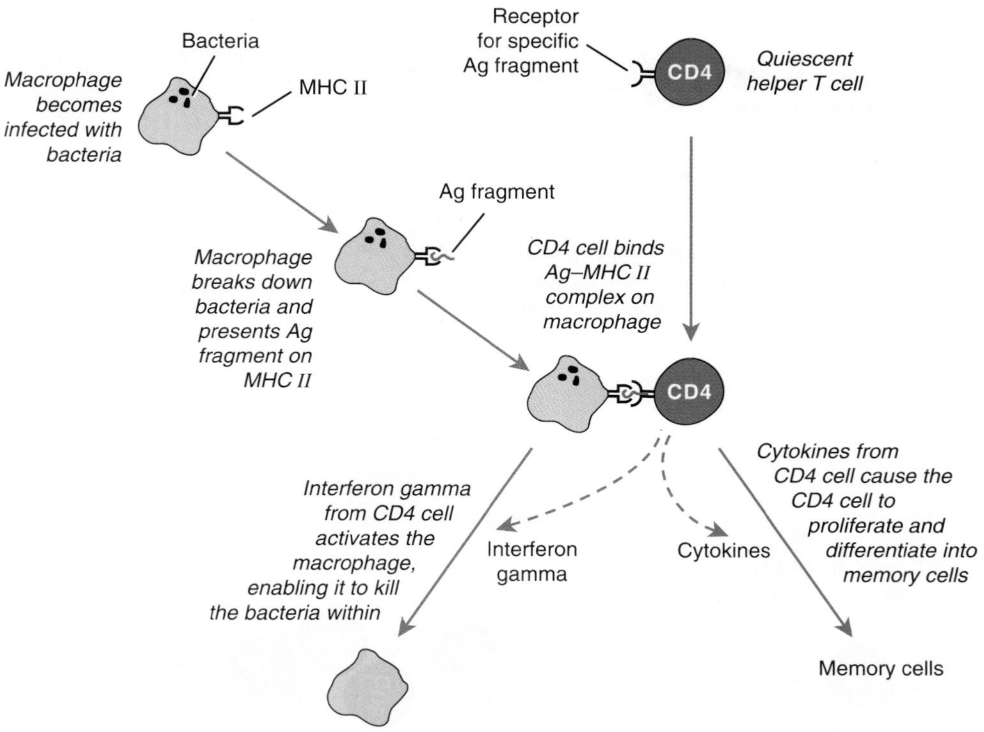

Figure 52.5 ▪ Cell-mediated immunity: delayed-type hypersensitivity (DTH). DTH requires two cells: an infected macrophage and a CD4 cell. Binding of the CD4 cell to the macrophage activates the CD4 cell, which then releases interferon gamma and several cytokines. Interferon gamma activates the macrophage. The cytokines cause the CD4 cell to proliferate and differentiate into memory cells. Ag, antigen; MHC II, class II MHC molecule.

addition to ridding macrophages of bacteria, DTH produces local inflammation.

Cytolytic T Lymphocytes

Cytolytic T lymphocytes (CTLs, CD8 cells) kill other cells. Their principal job is to kill self cells that are infected with viruses, thereby halting viral replication. In addition, CTLs participate in rejection of transplants. Here our discussion is limited to killing virally infected cells.

The process by which CTLs kill other cells has two stages: activation of CTLs, followed by recognition and killing of the target cell. The process is depicted in Fig. 52.6.

Activation of Cytolytic T Cells

Activation of CTLs requires the participation of an *antigen-presenting cell* and a *helper T cell* (CD4 cell). The process is very similar to the activation of CD4 cells discussed earlier. However, there is one important difference: whereas CD4 cells specifically recognize antigen that is bound to a *class II* MHC molecule on an APC, CTLs specifically recognize antigen that is bound to a *class I* MHC molecule on an APC.

In viral infections, activation of CTLs begins with processing of viral antigens by an APC. As shown in Fig. 52.6, the APC combines the antigen with a class I MHC molecule and then presents the antigen–MHC I complex on its surface. Next, a pre-CTL binds to the antigen–MHC I complex. (Like CD4 cells, each pre-CTL has receptors that are specific for a particular antigen–MHC I complex.) Linking of the pre-CTL with the APC primes the pre-CTL for the next stage of activation: stimulation by cytokines (interleukin-2, interferon gamma, and probably others) provided by an activated CD4 cell. (Activation of the CD4 cell, which is not shown in Fig. 52.6, occurs when the CD4 cell encounters an APC that has a viral antigen–MHC II complex.) In response to the cytokines released by the CD4 cell, the pre-CTL undergoes proliferation and differentiation into memory CTLs and activated CTLs.

Recognition of Virally Infected Target Cells

CTLs recognize their targets by the presence of an antigen–MHC I complex. This is the same process by which CTLs recognize APCs. As noted earlier, virtually all cells in the body carry class I MHC molecules. (Class II molecules are limited to APCs and B cells.) Hence, when a cell is infected with a virus, viral antigens form intracellular complexes with MHC I molecules, after which the antigen–MHC I complexes are presented on the cell surface. As shown in Fig. 52.6, activated CTLs recognize the antigen–MHC I complex and hence bind with the target cell. Because only cells that are infected with the virus will bear viral antigens on their class I MHC molecules, attack by CTLs is limited to infected cells; all others are spared.

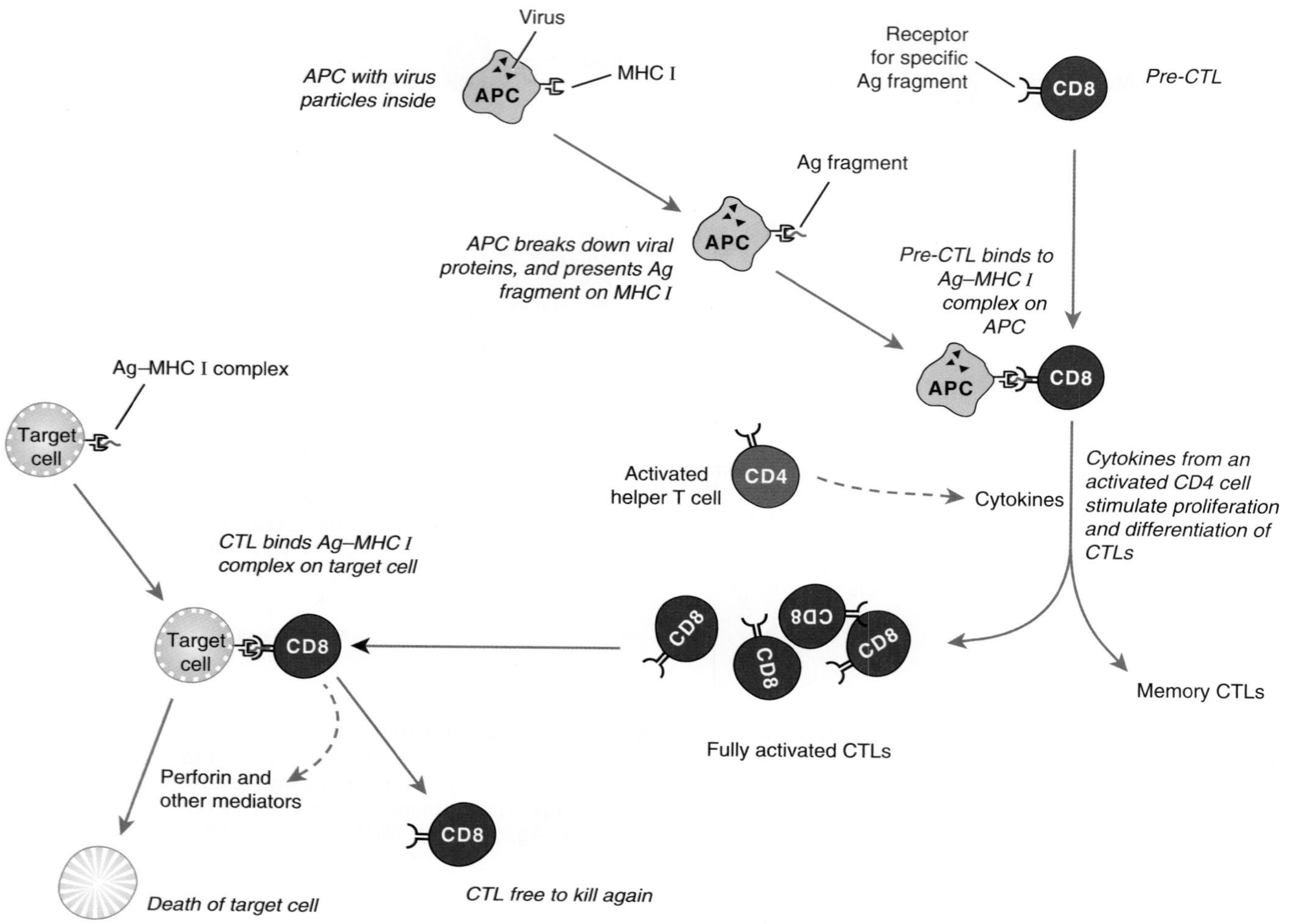

Figure 52.6 ■ Cell-mediated immunity: cytolytic T cells. This branch of cell-mediated immunity requires three types of cells: cytolytic T lymphocytes (CTLs), antigen-presenting cells (APCs), and CD4 cells. Binding of the pre-CTL with the APC begins the activation of the CTL. Stimulation of the CTL by cytokines from the CD4 cell completes the activation of the CTL, which then binds with and kills its target. Activation of the CD4 cells, which is not shown, takes place as depicted in Figs. 52.4 and 52.5. Ag, antigen; MHC I, class I MHC molecule.

Mechanisms of Cell Kill

Binding of a CTL to its target cell causes the CTL to release mediators that kill the target. Two mechanisms of cell kill are involved: *lysis* and *apoptosis* (programmed cell death). The mediator of lysis is called *perforin,* a molecule that forms pores in the target-cell membrane; the resultant influx of fluid causes the cell to swell and then burst. (This mechanism is very similar to one by which the complement system causes cell lysis.) The mediators of apoptosis have not been identified with certainty. However, their effects are very clear. The initial effect is activation of intracellular enzymes that digest the cell's own DNA. This is followed by fragmentation of the nucleus and cell death. Only the target cell is harmed; bystander cells and the CTL itself are not touched. In fact, after releasing its mediators, the CTL disconnects from the doomed target and goes on to seek another target cell.

CHAPTER

53 Childhood Immunization

Laura D. Rosenthal, DNP, ACNP, FAANP

The purpose of immunization is to protect against infectious diseases. Thanks to widespread immunization, the incidence of several infectious diseases has been dramatically reduced, and one disease—smallpox—has been eliminated from the planet. Of all the advances in medicine, none has reduced sickness and death more than immunization.

Experience has shown that the most effective way to reduce vaccine-preventable diseases (VPDs) is to create a highly immune population. Accordingly, universal vaccination is a national goal. Although immunization carries some risk, the risks from failing to vaccinate are much greater. Discussion in this chapter is limited to childhood immunization.

GENERAL CONSIDERATIONS

Definitions

To discuss immunization, we must use special terminology. Accordingly, we begin by defining some terms.

Vaccine

A vaccine is a preparation containing whole or fractionated microorganisms. Administration causes the recipient's immune system to manufacture antibodies directed against the microbe from which the vaccine was made. Most of the preparations discussed in this chapter are vaccines.

Killed Vaccines versus Live Vaccines

There are two major classes of vaccines: killed and live (albeit attenuated). Killed vaccines are composed of whole, killed microbes or isolated microbial components (e.g., the polysaccharide of *Haemophilus influenzae* type b or the surface antigen of hepatitis B). In contrast, live, attenuated vaccines are composed of live microbes that have been weakened or rendered completely avirulent. Live vaccines can be dangerous in recipients who are immunocompromised because these people are unable to mount an effective immune response, even against an avirulent organism.

Toxoid

A toxoid is a bacterial toxin that has been changed to a nontoxic form. Administration causes the recipient's immune system to manufacture antitoxins (i.e., antibodies directed against the natural bacterial toxin). Antitoxins protect against injury from toxins, but do not kill the bacteria that produce them. In this chapter, only two toxoids are considered: tetanus toxoid and diphtheria toxoid.

Vaccination

The terms *vaccination* and *vaccine* derive from *vaccinia,* a virus whose name in turn derives from *vacca* (Latin for cow). At one time, vaccinia virus was used as a vaccine against smallpox. (Vaccinia itself causes cowpox—a mild sickness—and in the process induces synthesis of smallpox antibodies.) Hence, when the term *vaccination* was originally coined, it had the limited meaning of giving vaccinia to generate immunity against smallpox. Today, vaccination refers broadly to giving any vaccine or toxoid.

Immunization: Active versus Passive

Immunization is a more inclusive term than *vaccination,* in that immunization refers to production of both active immunity and passive immunity, whereas vaccination refers to production of active immunity only.

Active immunity develops in response to infection or to administration of a vaccine or toxoid. In either case, the result is endogenous production of antibodies. Active immunity takes weeks or months to develop but is long lasting. Discussion in this chapter is limited almost exclusively to active immunization.

Passive immunity is conferred by giving a patient *preformed* antibodies (immune globulins). Unlike active immunity, passive immunity protects immediately but persists only as long as the antibodies remain in the body.

Specific Immune Globulins

These preparations contain a high concentration of antibodies directed against a specific antigen (e.g., hepatitis B virus). Administration provides immediate passive immunity. These preparations are made from donated blood.

Public Health Effects of Immunization

Widespread vaccination has had a profound effect on public health. In the United States vaccination has greatly reduced the incidence of some infectious diseases (e.g., pertussis, mumps, tetanus) and virtually eliminated five others: diphtheria, smallpox, poliomyelitis, rubella, and measles. With two diseases, results have been even more dramatic: wild-type polio is gone from the Western hemisphere, and smallpox is gone from the planet.

Despite these successes, we still have a long way to go: although our national vaccination rate is at an all-time high, every year 2.1 million children ages 1 to 3 years receive few or no vaccinations. In some parts of the country, more than 50% of children are not current. The consequences of failing to vaccinate can be enormous. For example, between 1989 and 1991, a measles epidemic occurred; 55,000 cases were reported, 11,000 people were hospitalized, and more than 130 people died, half of them young children. In 2014, 667 cases of measles were reported in the United States, the most since the year 2000. The most recent set of outbreaks occurred in 2015, when 189 people contracted measles, many of them exposed at an amusement park in California.

The Childhood Immunization Initiative is directed at preventing disease epidemics. The goal is to eliminate all indigenous cases of diphtheria, measles, rubella, tetanus, and *H. influenzae* type b infection from the United States. The program aims to achieve these goals by improving vaccine delivery systems, increasing community participation, reducing vaccine costs to parents, developing safer and simpler vaccines, and involving more federal agencies in providing vaccines to populations that otherwise might not have access to them. Thanks to these strategies, two of these diseases—diphtheria and rubella—are virtually gone from this country.

From a strictly economic viewpoint, vaccination is a sound investment. On average, we save $14 in future health care costs for every dollar we spend on vaccination.

Reporting Vaccine-Preventable Diseases

Public health officials rely on healthcare providers to report cases of VPDs. Nearly all VPDs that occur in the United States are notifiable. Health care providers should report individual cases to their local or state health department. Each week, the state health departments make a report to the Centers for Disease Control and Prevention (CDC). The information is used to (1) determine whether an outbreak is occurring, (2) evaluate prevention and control strategies, and (3) evaluate the effect of national immunization policies and practices.

Immunization Records

The *National Childhood Vaccine Act* requires a permanent record of each mandated vaccination a child receives. The information should be recorded in either (1) the permanent medical record of the recipient or (2) a permanent office log or file. The following data are required:

- Date of vaccination
- Route and site of vaccination
- Vaccine type, manufacturer, lot number, and expiration date
- Name, address, and title of the person administering the vaccine

The purpose of these records is twofold. First, they help ensure that children receive appropriate vaccinations. Second, they help avoid overvaccination and thereby reduce the risk for possible hypersensitivity reactions. To promote uniformity in record keeping, an official immunization card has been adopted by every state and the District of Columbia.

Adverse Effects of Immunization

Vaccines are generally very safe. Although mild reactions are common, serious events are rare. Many children experience local reactions (discomfort, swelling, and erythema at the injection site). Fever is also common. Very rare but severe effects include *anaphylaxis* (e.g., in response to measles, mumps, and rubella virus vaccine); acute *encephalopathy* (caused by diphtheria and tetanus toxoids and pertussis vaccine); and vaccine-associated *paralytic poliomyelitis* (caused by oral poliovirus vaccine). In 2011 the safety of vaccines was reaffirmed in a lengthy report—*Adverse Effects of Vaccines: Evidence and Causality*—issued by the Institute of Medicine of the National Academies.

Vaccinations can hurt. This pain, in turn, can lead to needle fears, procedural anxiety, and avoiding additional immunizations. Accordingly, minimizing pain is a primary goal. Strategies to reduce pain and anxiety include holding the child upright during the vaccination, applying a topical anesthetic, providing tactile stimulation, performing intramuscular injections rapidly without prior aspiration, and injecting the most painful vaccine last. Pain can be further reduced by use of microneedles, needle-free devices, and intranasal vaccines. What about giving analgesic-antipyretics, such as acetaminophen and ibuprofen? Evidence from a study in Russia indicates that giving these drugs before or shortly after vaccination can reduce the immune response. In addition, studies show that prophylactic administration of antipyretics does not significantly reduce the incidence of fever or pain. Accordingly, routine prophylactic use of these drugs to prevent pain or fever should be discouraged. Yet because there has been only one study regarding immune response and antipyretic agents, the American Academy of Pediatrics (AAP) still condones their use for children who experience pain or fever after the immunization is given.

Immunocompromised children are at special risk from live vaccines. The reason is that, in the absence of an adequate immune response, the viruses or bacteria in these normally safe vaccines are able to multiply in profusion, thereby causing serious infection. Accordingly, live vaccines should generally be avoided in children who are severely immunosuppressed. Causes of immunosuppression include congenital immunodeficiency, HIV infection, leukemia, lymphoma, generalized malignancy, and therapy with radiation, cytotoxic anticancer drugs, and high-dose glucocorticoids.

Some parents are concerned that *thimerosal,* a mercury-based preservative found in some vaccines, might cause *autism.* For two reasons, this concern is unfounded. First, several large, high-quality studies conducted in Denmark, Britain, and the United States have failed to show a causal link between childhood immunization using thimerosal-containing vaccines and development of autism. Second, thimerosal is being phased out of vaccines made here (owing to concerns about mercury exposure, not concerns about autism). At this time, the amount of thimerosal in most routinely used childhood vaccines is either zero or extremely low (less than 0.5 mcg per 0.5-mL dose). The only exceptions are certain flu vaccines, which still contain thimerosal as a preservative. However, even if these flu vaccines are used, total mercury exposure from childhood vaccination will still be well below the limit considered safe by the U.S. Food and Drug Administration (FDA) and the Environmental Protection Agency.

The risk for serious adverse reactions can be minimized by observing appropriate *precautions* and *contraindications.* Table 53.1 lists contraindications that apply to all vaccines. Precautions and contraindications that apply to specific

TABLE 53.1 ▪ Contraindications that Apply to All Vaccines and Conditions Often Incorrectly Regarded as Contraindications

True Contraindications (Vaccine Should not Be Administered)	Not Contraindications (Vaccine May Be Administered)
Anaphylactic reaction to a specific vaccine: contraindicates further doses of that vaccine	Mild to moderate local reaction (soreness, erythema, swelling) after a dose of an injectable vaccine
Anaphylactic reaction to a vaccine component: contraindicates use of all vaccines that contain that substance	Mild acute illness with or without low-grade fever
	Diarrhea
	Current antimicrobial therapy
	Convalescent phase of illnesses
Moderate or severe illnesses with or without a fever	Prematurity (same dosage and indications as for normal, full-term infants)
	Recent exposure to an infectious disease
	Personal or family history of either penicillin allergy or nonspecific allergies

vaccines are discussed in the context of those preparations. Certain conditions, such as diarrhea and mild illness, may be inappropriately regarded as contraindications by some practitioners. As a result, vaccination may be needlessly postponed. Conditions that are often considered contraindications, although they are not, are also listed in Table 53.1.

Practitioners are required to report certain adverse events to the *Vaccine Adverse Event Reporting System* (VAERS). The information is used to help determine whether (1) a particular event that occurs after vaccination is actually caused by the vaccine and (2) what the risk factors might be. In addition to reporting events that they are required to report, practitioners should report all other serious or unusual adverse events, regardless of whether they believe the event was caused by the vaccine. Forms for reporting adverse events can be obtained from the VAERS website (www.vaers.hhs.gov) or by calling 1-800-822-7967.

The *National Vaccine Injury Compensation Program* (NVICP), established by the *National Childhood Vaccine Injury Act*, was created to provide compensation for injury or death resulting from vaccination. The program is intended as an alternative to civil litigation in that negligence need not be proved. As a provision of the law, a table was created listing the vaccines covered by the program and the injuries, disabilities, illness, and conditions—including death—for which compensation may be paid. Compensation may also be paid for injuries not listed in the table, provided that (1) a listed vaccine is involved and (2) causality can be demonstrated. Injuries related to vaccines not listed in the table are not covered under the program. Additional information can be obtained by calling 1-800-338-2382.

Vaccine Information Statements

The National Childhood Vaccine Injury Act requires that Vaccine Information Statements (VISs) be given to all vaccinated patients (or their parents or legal representatives) before certain vaccines are administered. The VISs, produced by the CDC, are one-page, two-sided documents that describe the benefits and risks of specific vaccines. For vaccines that require a series of shots, a VIS must be given *before each dose,* not just the first dose. The VISs are available in more than 30 languages, and can be obtained online at www.cdc.gov/vaccines/pubs/vis/default.htm.

Childhood Immunization Schedule

Each year, the CDC Advisory Committee on Immunization Practices (ACIP), in cooperation with the American Academy of Family Physicians (AAFP) and the AAP, issues revised recommendations for childhood immunization in the United States. You can find the yearly schedule recommendations and catch-up immunization schedule for persons aged 4 months through 18 years, as well as the most recent updates, online at www.cdc.gov/vaccines/. Please note that adult immunization schedules can also be found there.

TARGET DISEASES

Routine childhood vaccination is currently recommended for protection against 16 infectious diseases: diphtheria, tetanus (lockjaw), pertussis (whooping cough), measles, mumps, rubella, invasive *H. influenzae* type b, hepatitis A, hepatitis B, polio, varicella (chickenpox), influenza, invasive pneumococcal disease, meningococcal disease (meningitis), rotavirus gastroenteritis, and genital human papillomavirus infection. In the following discussion, certain VPDs are considered in a group (e.g., measles, mumps, rubella) because vaccination against these VPDs is traditionally done simultaneously using a combination vaccine.

Measles, Mumps, and Rubella

Measles

Measles is a highly contagious viral disease characterized by rash and high fever (103°–105°F). Infection is spread by inhalation of aerosolized sputum or by direct contact with nasal or throat secretions. Initial symptoms include fever, cough, headache, sore throat, and conjunctivitis. Three days later, rash develops. Rash begins at the hairline, spreads to the rest of the body in 36 hours, and then fades in a few days. Secondary infections can result in pneumonia and otitis media (inner-ear infection). However, of the potential complications of measles, encephalitis is by far the most serious. Sequelae of encephalitis include blindness, deafness, and convulsions. Although encephalitis is rare (0.1% incidence), it carries a 10% risk for death.

Mumps

Mumps is a viral disease that primarily affects the parotid glands (the largest of the three pairs of salivary glands). Although mumps can occur in adults, it usually occurs in children aged 5 to 15 years. As a rule, the first symptom is swelling in one of the parotid glands, often accompanied by local pain and tenderness. The patient may also experience fever (100°–104°F). Swelling increases for 2 to 3 days and then fades entirely by day 6 or 7. Swelling in the second parotid gland often develops after swelling in the first but may also occur simultaneously or not at all. Painful *orchitis* (inflammation of the testes) develops in about one third of adult and adolescent males. Acute *aseptic meningitis* develops in about 10% of all patients; symptoms, which resolve completely, include dizziness, headache, and vomiting. In the United States the incidence of reported mumps cases has declined from a high of 212,932 in 1984 to only 1283 in 2014.

Rubella

Rubella, also known as German measles, is a generally mild viral infection. However, if it occurs during pregnancy, the consequences can be severe. Initial symptoms include sore throat, mild fever, and swelling in lymph nodes located behind the ears and in the back of the neck. Shortly after, a rash develops on the face and scalp, spreads rapidly to the torso and arms, and then fades in 2 or 3 days. Arthritis may also develop, mainly in women. In pregnant women, rubella can cause miscarriage, stillbirth, and congenital defects, especially if the disease occurs during the first trimester. Possible birth defects include cataracts, heart disease, developmental delay, and hearing loss. In the United States rubella has been eliminated: since 2002, all cases reported here have been traceable to foreigners who brought the disease from abroad.

Diphtheria, Tetanus, and Pertussis

Diphtheria

Diphtheria is a potentially fatal infection caused by *Corynebacterium diphtheriae,* a gram-positive bacillus. The bacterium colonizes the throat and nasal passages and produces a toxin that spreads throughout the body. Initial symptoms include sore throat, fever, headache, and nausea. Colonization of the airway begins as patches of gray or dirty-yellow membrane that eventually grow together, forming a thick coating. This coating, combined with swelling, can impede swallowing and breathing; in severe cases, a tracheostomy is needed. The toxin produced by *C. diphtheriae* can damage the heart and nerves, resulting in heart failure and paralysis. Diphtheria treatment includes giving diphtheria antitoxin and antibiotics (e.g., erythromycin, penicillin G). In the United States only 37 cases were reported between 1980 and 1992. However, of those infected, about 10% died, mainly children and older adults. There were only two reported cases between 2003 and 2015.

Tetanus (Lockjaw)

Tetanus, also known as lockjaw, is a frequently fatal disease characterized by painful spasm of all skeletal muscles. The cause is a potent endotoxin elaborated by *Clostridium tetani,* a gram-positive bacillus. Infection with *C. tetani* typically results from puncturing the skin with a nail, splinter, or other object that is contaminated with soil, street dust, or animal or human feces. The first symptom is often stiffness of the jaw, hence the name *lockjaw.* As infection progresses, the patient may experience stiff neck, difficulty swallowing, restlessness, irritability, headache, chills, fever, and convulsions. Eventually, spasm develops in muscles of the abdomen, back, neck, and face. The case fatality rate is 21%. The yearly incidence of tetanus peaked at 601 cases in 1948, but was only 26 cases in 2013 and decreased to zero cases in 2014. Treatment options include tetanus antitoxin, a booster dose of tetanus toxoid, and antibiotics (e.g., penicillin G, doxycycline).

Pertussis (Whooping Cough)

Pertussis, also known as *whooping cough* or the *100-day cough,* occurs primarily in infants and young children. The cause is *Bordetella pertussis,* a gram-negative bacillus. Initial symptoms include rhinorrhea, mild fever, and persistent cough. As infection worsens, coughing becomes more intense. The acute phase of the disease can last 4 to 6 weeks. During this time, infants experience difficulty eating, drinking, and breathing. Deaths have occurred. Complications of pertussis include pneumonia, seizures, ear infections, and, rarely, permanent neurologic injury. In the United States reported cases dropped from a high of 265,269 in 1934 to 8483 in 2003. However, the rate of pertussis increased to 32,971 reported cases in 2014. Worldwide, the disease afflicts about 60 million people, and kills 335,000 each year, mainly infants and young children. Azithromycin is the treatment of choice.

Poliomyelitis

Poliomyelitis, also known as polio or infantile paralysis, is a serious disease in which the poliovirus attacks neurons of the central nervous system that control muscle movement. The result is skeletal muscle paralysis, usually in the legs. However, muscles of respiration and muscles of the arms may be affected, too. In about 10% of cases, polio is fatal. The disease is caused by three different polioviruses. Paralytic polio is usually caused by type 1 poliovirus. Polio has no cure. However, proper symptomatic treatment can improve comfort and reduce or prevent some crippling effects. Vaccination against polio has eliminated the disease from the Western hemisphere, except for eight to nine cases annually caused by the vaccine itself. To prevent vaccine-induced polio, use of the live virus vaccine (oral polio vaccine) was discontinued in the United States. The number of cases worldwide was 1315 in 2007—nearly quadruple the 359 cases documented in 2014.

Haemophilus influenzae Type b

Haemophilus influenzae type b is a gram-negative bacterium that can cause meningitis, pneumonia, and serious throat and ear infections. The bacterium is the leading cause of serious illness in children under the age of 5 years, and the most common cause of bacterial meningitis, which has a mortality rate of 5%. Among children who survive meningitis, between 25% and 35% suffer lasting neurologic deficits. As a result of childhood vaccination, the annual incidence of infection has dropped significantly. Of the cases that occurred, almost all were in unvaccinated children. Infection with *H. influenzae* can be treated successfully with antibiotics.

Varicella (Chickenpox)

Varicella (chickenpox) is a common, highly contagious, and potentially serious disease of childhood. The causative organism is varicella-zoster virus, a member of the herpesvirus group. Patients typically develop 250 to 500 maculopapular or vesicular lesions, usually on the face, scalp, or trunk. Other symptoms include fever, malaise, and loss of appetite. Among children, the most common complications are bacterial suprainfection and acute cerebellar ataxia. Reye syndrome and encephalitis develop rarely. Among adults, the most serious common complication is varicella pneumonia. As a rule, symptoms in adults are more severe than in children: hospitalization is 10 times more likely in adults, and death is 20 times more likely. Although adults account for only 2% of varicella cases, they account for 50% of varicella-related deaths. Before varicella vaccine became available, more than 90% of children in the United States got chickenpox by age 11 years, which corresponds to 4 million cases a year. In addition, about 11,000 victims were hospitalized each year, and about 100 died. Since universal vaccination began in 1995, hospitalizations have dropped dramatically: one study indicates that, between 2000 and 2006, an estimated 50,000 hospitalizations were avoided.

Herpes zoster, also known as *shingles* or simply *zoster,* develops in 15% of patients years after childhood chickenpox has resolved. The cause is reactivation of varicella-zoster viruses that had been dormant within sensory nerve roots. Episodes of zoster begin with neurologic pain in the area of skin supplied by the affected nerve roots. Blister-like lesions develop within 3 to 4 days and usually disappear 2 to 3 weeks later. However, in about 14% of patients, neurologic pain persists for a month or more—and in a few cases, pain lasts for years.

Hepatitis B

Hepatitis B is a serious liver infection caused by the hepatitis B virus. Acute infection can cause anorexia, malaise, diarrhea, vomiting, jaundice, pain (in muscles, joints, and stomach), and death. Chronic infection can result in cirrhosis, liver cancer, and death. Each year in the United States, hepatitis B infects 100,000 people, puts 17,000 in the hospital, and kills 5000. Worldwide, 400 million people have chronic hepatitis B, and 1 million die of it annually.

Although hepatitis B is found in virtually all body fluids, only blood, serum-derived fluids, saliva, semen, and vaginal fluids are infectious. The most common modes of transmission are needle-stick accidents, sexual contact with an infected partner, maternal-child transmission during birth, and use of contaminated intravenous equipment or solutions.

Hepatitis B is discussed further in Chapter 78.

Hepatitis A

Hepatitis A is a serious liver infection caused by the hepatitis A virus. In the United States hepatitis A infection is declining. In 2014 there were 1781 reported cases of acute hepatitis A in the United States. Symptoms of hepatitis A include fever, malaise, nausea, jaundice, anorexia, diarrhea, and stomach pain. However, not all infected persons become symptomatic. Among children younger than 6 years, only 30% develop symptoms. In contrast, symptoms are present in most older infected children and adults. When symptoms do occur, they develop rapidly and then usually fade in less than 2 months. However, between 10% and 15% of patients experience prolonged or relapsing disease that persists up to 6 months. During the course of the infection, the virus undergoes replication in the liver, passage into the bile, and then excretion in the feces. As a result, the usual mode of transmission is fecal-oral in the context of close personal contact with an infected person. In addition, hepatitis A can be contracted by ingesting contaminated food or water. Blood-borne transmission is rare. Individuals at risk include household and sexual contacts of infected individuals, international travelers, and people living in areas where hepatitis A is endemic (e.g., American Indian reservations, Alaskan Native villages).

Pneumococcal Infection

In the United States *Streptococcus pneumoniae* (pneumococcus) is the leading bacterial cause of childhood meningitis, sepsis, pneumonia, and otitis media. Among children with pneumococcal meningitis, up to 50% suffer permanent brain damage or hearing loss, and about 10% die. The risk for acquiring pneumococcal infection is highest for children younger than 2 years. Factors that increase infection risk include sickle cell disease, immunodeficiency, asplenia, chronic diseases, attending a group child care center, and being a Native American, African American, or Alaskan Native or a socially disadvantaged person. Worldwide, pneumococcal infection ranks among the leading causes of death from infectious disease. Routine childhood immunization against pneumococcal disease began in 2000. Since then, the incidence of severe pediatric infection has dropped sharply.

Meningococcal Infection

Meningococcal infection is a serious disease caused by *Neisseria meningitidis,* also known as meningococcus. Invasive meningococcal disease is a leading cause of meningitis in American children. Worldwide, most infections are caused by five *N. meningitidis* serogroups—designated A, B, C, Y, and W-135—identified on the basis of antigenic differences in surface polysaccharides. In the United States only three serogroups—B, C, and Y—cause most cases. Meningococcal infection is readily transmitted through direct contact with respiratory secretions from patients and from asymptomatic carriers. Injury results from a meningococcal endotoxin, which is produced so quickly that death can result within hours of infection onset. Although only 1400 to 2800 cases occur here each year, the disease is clearly of great concern, with a fatality rate of 10% to 14% despite antibiotic therapy. Furthermore, of those who survive, 11% to 19% suffer severe and permanent sequelae, including neurologic disability, deafness, developmental delay, and limb amputations. Infection rate is highest during infancy, with a second peak during adolescence and early adulthood. Outbreaks can occur in child care centers, schools, and colleges. Risk factors for acquiring the disease include immunodeficiency, antecedent viral infection, household crowding, chronic underlying disease, active and passive smoking, and anatomic and functional asplenia. A meningococcal vaccine was approved in 1981, but it was not very effective in children. Hence routine childhood immunization was not recommended until 2005, the year a more effective vaccine was introduced.

Influenza

Influenza is a serious infection of the respiratory tract and a major cause of morbidity and mortality worldwide.

Characteristics of the influenza virus and of influenza itself (mode of transmission, symptoms, time course, methods of prevention and treatment) are discussed in Chapter 78.

Rotavirus Gastroenteritis

Rotavirus, which infects the intestinal mucosa, is the most common diarrheal pathogen worldwide. Infection presents initially as upset stomach and vomiting, usually with fever, and then progresses to several days of diarrhea, which can be mild to severe. The combination of vomiting and severe diarrhea can result in life-threatening dehydration. Virtually all children become infected repeatedly within the first 5 years of life. However, the first episode is generally the worst. As a result, severe diarrhea and dehydration are most likely in the very young—children 3 to 35 months old. Before a rotavirus vaccine became available, rotavirus annually infected 2.7 million American children younger than 5 years, resulting in more than 400,000 office visits, 55,000 to 70,000 hospitalizations, and 20 to 60 deaths. Worldwide, annual deaths are estimated in the hundreds of thousands. Infected children shed large amounts of rotavirus in their stool, and hence transmission is usually fecal-oral, resulting from touching the stool or a contaminated object. Rotavirus infection can be prevented with two vaccines: RotaTeq and Rotarix.

Genital Human Papillomavirus Infection

Human papillomavirus (HPV) infection is the cause of virtually all anogenital warts and cervical cancers. Transmission occurs most often by direct genital contact during vaginal or anal intercourse. The types of HPV that infect the anogenital region can also cause cancers of the vulva, vagina, urethra, tongue, tonsils, penis, and anus. Cancer of the anus in men and women who have anal intercourse is now as common as cervical cancer was before the Papanicolaou (Pap) test was introduced. The discussion that follows focuses on the role of HPV in cervical cancer and genital warts. Treatment of genital warts is discussed in Chapter 85.

Genital HPV is the most common sexually transmitted infection. In the United States about 14.1 million people become infected each year. Among sexually active males and females, about 50% will be infected at some time during their life. Fortunately, although HPV infections are common, most are benign and clear spontaneously, usually within a few months to a year. As a result, most men and women never get genital warts, and most women never get precancerous cervical lesions or cervical cancer.

About 100 types of HPV are known to exist, about 40 of which infect the anogenital region. The types of HPV associated with malignancy are referred to as *oncogenic* or *high risk,* whereas the types associated with genital warts are called *low risk.* About 95% of genital warts are caused by just two HPV types, known as HPV-6 and HPV-11. About 70% of cervical cancers are caused by two other types, known as HPV-16 and HPV-18. Fortunately, only 2.2% of women carry high-risk strains.

Worldwide, cervical cancer is the second most common cancer among women. Each year, more than 500,000 cases are diagnosed, and about 280,000 prove fatal. In the United States cervical cancer is less prevalent: total new cases are estimated at 12,000 each year. Why so few deaths in the United States? Because most American women undergo regular Pap tests, which detect precancerous and cancerous changes, allowing early intervention (excision or ablation of the affected tissue) before advanced cancer can develop.

Respiratory Syncytial Virus

Respiratory syncytial virus (RSV), an enveloped virus of the Paramyxoviridae family, was first identified in 1956. In the United States RSV infection is the most common cause of bronchiolitis (inflammation of small airways in the lungs) and pneumonia in children younger than 1 year and the most common cause for hospitalization in children younger than 5 years. Worldwide, it is estimated that RSV is responsible for nearly 7% of deaths in children aged 1 month to 1 year; only malaria kills more children in this age group.

All children are at risk for RSV, but the incidence of severe disease is highest in children born prematurely and in those with cardiopulmonary disease. Children at high risk account for nearly half of RSV-related hospital admissions in the United States. An additional at-risk population is older adults, who often suffer from flu-like symptoms caused by RSV.

SPECIFIC VACCINES AND TOXOIDS

The following discussion is limited to the vaccines and toxoids used for routine childhood immunization. The major preparations employed are listed in Table 53.2. Their adverse effects are shown in Table 53.3. Childhood immunization schedules, catch-up schedules, and recent changes—as recommended by the ACIP, the AAP, and the AAFP—are available online at www.cdc.gov/vaccines/.

Measles, Mumps, and Rubella Virus Vaccine

Description

Measles, mumps, and rubella vaccine (MMR), marketed under the trade name *M-M-R II,* is a combination product composed of three live virus vaccines. Administration induces synthesis of antibodies directed against measles, mumps, and rubella viruses. Immunization with MMR is preferred to immunization with the three vaccines separately.

Efficacy

After a single dose of MMR, an effective response develops in 97% of vaccinated patients within 2 to 6 weeks. A second dose increases protection.

Adverse Effects

Mild

Local soreness, erythema, and swelling may develop soon after vaccination. Within 1 to 2 weeks, some children experience glandular swelling in the cheeks and neck and under the jaw. Transient rash develops in 5% to 15% of vaccinated patients. Fever (103° F or higher) that persists for several days occurs in 5% to 15% of vaccinated patients 5 to 12 days after vaccination. MMR-induced fever poses a small risk for febrile seizures, but these seizures do *not* increase the risk for developing epilepsy. Within 1 to 3 weeks of the first dose, about

TABLE 53.2 ■ Vaccines and Toxoids Available in the United States

Preparation Name (Synonym)	Trade Name	Type of Preparation	Route and Site	Number and Timing
Measles, mumps, and rubella virus vaccine (MMR)	M-M-R II	Live virus	SubQ, in outer aspect of upper arm	Two doses: #1: between 12 and 16 months #2: between 4 and 6 years
Measles, mumps, and rubella, and varicella virus vaccine (MMRV)	ProQuad*	Live virus	SubQ, in anterolateral thigh or outer aspect of upper arm	
Diphtheria and tetanus toxoids and acellular pertussis vaccine (DTaP)	Tripedia, DAPTACEL, Infanrix, Boostrix,[†] Adacel[†]	Toxoids (diphtheria and tetanus) plus inactivated bacteria components (pertussis)	IM, in deltoid or mediolateral thigh	Five doses: #1: 2 months #2: 4 months #3: 6 months #4: between 15 and 18 months #5: between 4 and 6 years Booster every 10 years thereafter starting at age 11 years
Diphtheria and tetanus toxoids and acellular pertussis adsorbed, hepatitis B (recombinant), and inactivated poliovirus vaccine	PEDIARIX	Toxoids (diphtheria and tetanus) plus inactivated bacteria components (pertussis) plus inactive viral antigen (hepatitis B) plus inactivated viruses (poliovirus)	IM, in deltoid or anterolateral thigh	
Tetanus and diphtheria toxoids	Tenivac Decavac	Toxoids	IM, in deltoid or mediolateral thigh	
Haemophilus influenzae type b (Hib) conjugate vaccine	ActHIB, PedvaxHIB, Hiberix, Comvax[‡]	Bacterial polysaccharide conjugated to protein	IM, in midthigh or outer aspect of upper arm	Four doses: #1: 2 months #2: 4 months #3: 6 months #4: between 12 and 15 months
Poliovirus vaccine, inactivated (IPV, Salk vaccine)	IPOL	Inactivated viruses of all three polio serotypes	SubQ, in anterolateral thigh	Four doses: #1: 2 months #2: 4 months #3: between 6 and 18 months #4: between 4 and 6 years
Varicella virus vaccine	Varivax	Live virus	SubQ, in deltoid or anterolateral thigh	Two doses: #1: between 12 and 15 months #2: between 4 and 6 years
Hepatitis A vaccine (HepA)	Havrix, VAQTA	Inactive viral antigen	IM, in deltoid	Two doses: #1: 12 months #2: 6–12 months after
Hepatitis B vaccine (HepB)	Recombivax HB, Engerix-B, Comvax[‡]	Inactive viral antigen	IM, in deltoid or anterolateral thigh	Three doses: #1: within 12 hours of birth #2: between 1 and 2 months #3: after an additional 6 months
Pneumococcal conjugate vaccine (PCV13)	Prevnar 13	Bacterial polysaccharide conjugated to protein	IM, in deltoid or anterolateral thigh	Four doses: #1: 2 months #2: 4 months #3: 6 months #4: between 12 and 15 months

Continued

TABLE 53.2 ▪ Vaccines and Toxoids Available in the United States—Cont'd

Preparation Name (Synonym)	Trade Name	Type of Preparation	Route and Site	Number and Timing
Pneumococcal polysaccharide vaccine (PPV)	Pneumovax 23	Bacterial polysaccharide (unconjugated)	IM, in deltoid or anterolateral thigh	
Influenza vaccine (inactivated)	Fluzone, Fluvirin, others	Inactive viral antigen	IM, in deltoid or anterolateral thigh	Yearly after age 6 months
Influenza vaccine (live)	FluMist	Live virus	Intranasal	Approved after age 2 years
Meningococcal conjugate vaccine (MCV4)	Menactra, Menveo	Bacterial polysaccharide conjugated to protein	IM, in deltoid	Two doses: #1: between 11 and 12 years #2: age 16 years
Meningococcal subgroup B recombinant vaccine	*Bexsero, Trumenba.*	Recombinant protein solution	IM, in deltoid	Two doses: #1: between 11 and 12 years #2: at least 1 month after
Rotavirus vaccine	Rotarix, RotaTeq	Live virus	Oral	RotaTeq Three Doses: #1: 6–12 weeks #2: 4–10 weeks after #3: 4–10 weeks after second doseRotarix Two doses: #1: 6–12 weeks #2: 4 weeks later
Human papillomavirus vaccine	Cervarix, Gardasil Gardasil 9	DNA-free virus-like particles	IM, in deltoid or anterolateral thigh	Three doses: #1: as early as age 11 years #2: 2 months after #3: 6 months after the first dose.

*ProQuad combines two older vaccines: M-M-R II and Varivax.
†Boostrix and Adacel are indicated for *booster* immunization, *not* for the *initial* immunization series. Boostrix is for patients 11 to 18 years old. Adacel is for patients 11 to 64 years old.
‡Comvax is a combination vaccine for immunization against *H. influenzae* type b and hepatitis B.
IM, intramuscular; subQ, subcutaneous.

TABLE 53.3 ▪ Adverse Effects of Some Vaccines and Toxoids

Preparation	Mild Effects	Serious Effects
Measles, mumps, and rubella virus vaccine	Local reactions; rash; fever; swollen glands in cheeks and neck and under the jaw; pain, stiffness, and swelling in joints	Anaphylaxis, thrombocytopenia*
Diphtheria and tetanus toxoids and acellular pertussis vaccine	Local reactions, fever, fretfulness, drowsiness, anorexia, persistent crying	Acute encephalopathy, convulsions, shock-like state
Haemophilus influenzae type b conjugate vaccine	Local reactions, fever, crying, diarrhea, vomiting	None
Varicella virus vaccine	Local reactions, fever, mild varicella-like rash (local or generalized)	None
Hepatitis A vaccine	Local soreness, headache, anorexia, fatigue	Anaphylaxis
Hepatitis B vaccine	Local discomfort, fever	Anaphylaxis
Pneumococcal conjugate vaccine	Local reactions, fever, irritability	None
Influenza vaccine (inactivated)	Local reactions, fever	None
Influenza vaccine (live attenuated)	Runny nose, headache, cough, fever	None
Meningococcal conjugate vaccine	Local reactions, headache, fatigue	None
Rotavirus vaccine	Diarrhea, vomiting, ear infection, runny nose, sore throat	Intussusception (rare)
Human papillomavirus vaccine	Local reactions, fainting	None

*A study showing a connection with autism was disproved.

1% of vaccinated patients experience pain, stiffness, and swelling in one or more joints; these symptoms usually subside in a few days but occasionally persist for a month or more. Fever, soreness, and pain can be reduced with acetaminophen or a nonaspirin, nonsteroidal antiinflammatory drug, such as ibuprofen. However, as noted earlier, these drugs should not be given before vaccination to *prevent* discomfort. Rather, they should be reserved for managing discomfort after it develops.

Severe

Transient thrombocytopenia occurs very rarely (0.0025% incidence). MMR-induced thrombocytopenia is generally benign, but hemorrhage has developed in a few vaccinated patients.

MMR can induce anaphylactic reactions. However, the incidence is extremely low: only 11 certain cases have occurred in more than 70 million vaccinations. In the past, MMR-induced anaphylaxis was thought to result from allergy to eggs (the measles component of the vaccine is produced in chick embryo fibroblasts). However, it now appears that egg allergy is not involved. Rather, the leading suspect is a hydrolysis product of gelatin. Until more is known, authorities recommend that MMR be used with extreme caution in children with a known allergy to gelatin. The ACIP is reconsidering whether caution is still required for children with an allergy to eggs.

The Institute of Medicine and the AAP have organized several panels of independent scientists that have determined that there is no causal link between MMR and development of autism, Crohn disease, or any other serious long-term illness. A 1998 paper by Andrew Wakefield, showing a connection between MMR and "autistic enterocolitis," was withdrawn by the publisher in 2010; 10 of the 13 authors have retracted the findings.

Precautions and Contraindications

MMR is *contraindicated* during pregnancy and should be used with *caution* in children with a history of (1) thrombocytopenia or thrombocytopenic purpura or (2) anaphylactic-like reactions to gelatin, eggs, or neomycin (MMR contains a small amount of this antibiotic).

MMR can be administered to children with *mild febrile illness* (e.g., upper respiratory infection with or without low-grade fever). However, for children with *moderate or severe febrile illness,* vaccination should be postponed until the illness has resolved.

Products that contain *immune globulins* (e.g., whole blood, serum, specific immune globulins) contain antibodies against the viruses in MMR and therefore can inhibit the immune response to the vaccine. Accordingly, in children who have received immune globulins, vaccination with MMR should be postponed for at least 3 to 6 months.

In vaccinated patients who are *immunocompromised,* replication of the viruses in MMR may be much greater than normal. If the immunodeficiency is severe, death may occur. However, of the more than 200 million people who have received MMR in the United States, only 5 such deaths have been reported. Nonetheless, ***children with severe immunodeficiency should NOT be given MMR.*** Severe immunodeficiency may result from immunosuppressive drugs (e.g., glucocorticoids, cytotoxic anticancer drugs), certain cancers (e.g., leukemia, lymphoma, generalized malignancy), and advanced HIV infection. It is important to note, however, that if HIV infection is *asymptomatic,* MMR should be given. In this situation, there is no risk for serious adverse events from MMR, whereas there *is* a risk for severe complications from measles should the disease develop. Vaccination with MMR early in the course of HIV infection is preferred because the immune response to vaccination diminishes as HIV infection progresses.

Diphtheria and Tetanus Toxoids and Acellular Pertussis Vaccine

Preparations

Primary vaccination against diphtheria, tetanus, and pertussis is usually done simultaneously using a combination product composed of diphtheria toxoid, tetanus toxoid, and *acellular* pertussis vaccine (DTaP). This vaccine, which is relatively new, has replaced an older product composed of diphtheria toxoid, tetanus toxoid, and *whole-cell* pertussis vaccine (DTP). DTaP is more effective than DTP and causes fewer and milder side effects. Vaccination with DTaP produces antibodies against diphtheria toxin, tetanus toxin, and *B. pertussis.* DTaP is available under several trade names, including *DAPTACEL* and *Infanrix.*

After children have received a full series of DTaP shots, they will need subsequent booster shots. Two booster products are available: *Tdap* and *Td.* Tdap—sold as *Boostrix* and *Adacel*—is composed of tetanus toxoid, reduced diphtheria toxoid, and acellular pertussis vaccine—and hence boosts protection against all three diseases. By contrast, Td boosts protection against only two diseases: tetanus and diphtheria. Tdap was approved in 2005, whereas the tetanus vaccine has been used in America since the 1940's. Because the incidence of pertussis is on the rise, a booster shot with Tdap, rather than Td, is now recommended for all children 11 to 18 years old. Boosters with Td are given every 10 years thereafter.

Products used for immunization against diphtheria, tetanus, and pertussis are shown in Table 53.4.

Efficacy

Immunization with DTaP reduces the risk for disease by 80% to 90%. Protection begins after the third dose and persists 4 to 6 years (against pertussis) and 10 years (against diphtheria and tetanus).

Adverse Effects

Mild

Mild reactions are common. The reactions seen most often are low fever, fretfulness, drowsiness, anorexia, and local reactions: pain, swelling, and redness. Mild reactions usually develop a few hours to 48 hours after vaccination and then resolve in 1 to 2 days. Ibuprofen can decrease fever and pain. However, as noted earlier, ibuprofen should not be given before vaccination to *prevent* discomfort. It should be reserved for managing discomfort after it develops.

Moderate

Moderate reactions occur less often than mild reactions. Persistent, inconsolable crying lasting 3 hours or longer occurs in 1% of vaccinated patients. Crying is most likely

TABLE 53.4 ▪ Products for Immunization Against Diphtheria, Tetanus, and Pertussis

Symbol	Description	Trade Names	Comments
VACCINES FOR CHILDREN YOUNGER THAN 10 YEARS			
DTaP	Diphtheria toxoid, tetanus toxoid, and acellular pertussis vaccine	DAPTACEL, Infanrix	Used for routine vaccination against diphtheria, tetanus, and pertussis
DT	Diphtheria toxoid and tetanus toxoid	Generic only	Used for children younger than 7 years who should not get pertussis vaccine
VACCINES FOR ADOLESCENTS AND ADULTS			
Tdap	Tetanus toxoid, reduced diphtheria toxoid, and acellular pertussis vaccine, adolescent preparation	Boostrix, Adacel	Used as a *booster* in adolescents and adults to protect against all three diseases
Td	Tetanus toxoid and diphtheria toxoid	Tenivac Decavac	Used as a *booster* for adolescents and adults to protect against tetanus and diphtheria, but not pertussis

with the first dose of DTaP and is not associated with long-term sequelae. Fever (105° F or higher) occurs in 0.3% of vaccinated patients; the pertussis component appears responsible. Approximately 0.06% of vaccinated patients develop convulsions (with or without fever). These seizures have no permanent sequelae and do not increase the risk for subsequent febrile or afebrile seizures. A shock-like state develops in 0.06% of vaccinated patients and has no lasting sequelae.

Severe: Encephalopathy

Very rarely, DTaP causes acute encephalopathy. The incidence is between zero and 10.5 episodes per million doses. Most cases occur within 3 days of vaccination. Some of the children who experience acute encephalopathy develop chronic neurologic dysfunction later in life. However, the contribution of acute encephalopathy to long-term neurologic deficits is unclear.

Precautions and Contraindications

DTaP can be administered to children with *mild febrile illness* (e.g., upper respiratory infection with or without low-grade fever). However, for children with *moderate or severe febrile illness,* administration should be postponed until the illness has resolved.

DTaP is *contraindicated* if a prior vaccination with DTaP produced (1) an immediate anaphylactic reaction or (2) encephalopathy within 7 days of vaccination.

DTaP should be administered with *caution* (if at all) if a prior vaccination with DTaP produced any of the following:

- A shock-like state
- Fever (105° F or higher) occurring within 48 hours of vaccination and not attributable to another identifiable cause
- Persistent, inconsolable crying lasting 3 or more hours and occurring within 48 hours of vaccination
- Seizures (with or without fever) occurring within 3 days of vaccination

Poliovirus Vaccine

Preparations

In the past, two polio vaccines were used in the United States: *oral poliovirus vaccine* (OPV, Sabin vaccine) and *inactivated poliovirus vaccine* (IPV, Salk vaccine). OPV is composed of *live,* attenuated viruses. In contrast, IPV is composed of *inactivated* polioviruses. As discussed later, OPV has *caused* polio in a few children, whereas IPV has not and cannot. Because the benefit-to-risk ratio of IPV is clearly superior, OPV has been withdrawn from the U.S. market. The trade name for IPV is *IPOL.*

Efficacy

Between 97.5% and 100% of children receiving IPV develop antibodies to poliovirus types 1, 2, and 3. Antibodies develop after two or more doses and persist for many years.

Adverse Effects of Inactivated Poliovirus Vaccine

IPV is devoid of serious adverse effects. As with other injected drugs, local soreness may occur. IPV contains trace amounts of streptomycin, neomycin, and bacitracin. Children with an allergy to these drugs should be monitored.

Haemophilus influenzae Type b Conjugate Vaccine

Preparations

Vaccines directed against *H. influenzae* type b (Hib) are prepared by conjugating (covalently binding) a purified capsular polysaccharide (PRP) from *H. influenzae* to either (1) tetanus toxoid or (2) an outer membrane protein (OMP) isolated from *N. meningitidis.* The reason for conjugating PRP to these other compounds is to enhance antigenicity. The vaccines made with OMP—marketed as *PedvaxHIB* and *Comvax*[a] and abbreviated PRP-OMP—elicit a stronger immune response than the vaccines made with tetanus toxoid, marketed as *ActHIB* and *Hiberix.*

Efficacy

Immunization with Hib vaccine decreases the risk for disease by 88% to 98%. When PedvaxHIB is used, protection begins

[a]Comvax is a combination vaccine for immunization against *H. influenzae* type b and hepatitis B.

1 week after the first dose. However, when ActHIB is used, protection is delayed, beginning 1 to 2 weeks after the fourth dose. With both vaccines, protection persists for several years.

Adverse Effects

Hib vaccine is among the safest of all vaccines. Serious adverse effects have not been reported. The few adverse effects that do occur are generally transient and mild. Between 2% and 5% of vaccinated patients develop local reactions (swelling, erythema, warmth, and tenderness). About 1% experience fever (temperature above 101° F), crying, diarrhea, or vomiting.

Varicella Virus Vaccine

Description

Varicella virus vaccine is composed of live, attenuated varicella viruses. Two subcutaneously delivered products are available: varicella vaccine by itself, sold as *Varivax,* and varicella vaccine combined with MMR (MMRV), sold as *ProQuad.*

Efficacy

Varicella vaccine, given as a two-dose series, confers full protection in about 99% of vaccinated patients. Furthermore, among those who get chickenpox despite vaccination, symptoms are always mild: these children develop fewer lesions (less than 50, compared with 250–500 for unvaccinated children), experience less fever, and recover more quickly. In Japan, herpes zoster (shingles) has not been observed in any adult who received varicella vaccine as a child, even if breakthrough chickenpox had occurred.

Adverse Effects

Varicella vaccine is very safe; no serious adverse events have been reported. About 25% of vaccinated patients experience erythema, soreness, and swelling at the injection site; 15% develop fever (temperature above 102° F); and 3% develop a mild, local varicella-like rash, consisting of just a few lesions. About 5% of healthy children develop a sparse, generalized varicella-like rash within a month of the injection. In children with leukemia, the incidence of generalized rash is much higher—about 50%. For all vaccinated patients, rates of fever and rash are higher when MMRV is used than when MMR and varicella vaccine are given separately.

In theory, children receiving the vaccine can transmit vaccine viruses to others. However, among otherwise healthy vaccinated patients, such transmission has not been reported. In contrast, among leukemic children who developed a rash after vaccination, a few cases of viral transmission have occurred. To reduce the risk for transmission, vaccinated patients should temporarily avoid close contact with susceptible, high-risk individuals (e.g., neonates, pregnant women, immunocompromised people).

Precautions and Contraindications

Varicella vaccine is *contraindicated* for pregnant patients, individuals with certain cancers (e.g., leukemia, lymphomas), and individuals with hypersensitivity to neomycin or gelatin, both of which are in the vaccine. In addition, the vaccine should generally be avoided by individuals who are immunocompromised, including those with HIV infection or congenital immunodeficiency and those taking immunosuppressive drugs.

Children receiving the vaccine should avoid aspirin and other salicylates for 6 weeks. This precaution is based on the theoretical risk for developing Reye syndrome: if the child develops chickenpox (albeit a mild case) in response to the vaccine, the very small risk for developing Reye syndrome is somewhat increased by concurrent use of salicylates.

We Need to Vaccinate More Children

Although rates of varicella vaccination have increased, many eligible children still do not get vaccinated. Several misconceptions are responsible: Some parents believe chickenpox is a mild disease, some think the vaccine is not effective (vaccination prevents severe chickenpox in 100% of vaccinated patients), and some think the vaccine is not safe (serious reactions are extremely rare, and proof that the vaccine was the cause is lacking).

The major effect of failure to vaccinate will be felt when today's children grow up. Recall that chickenpox in adults is much more severe than in children: compared with children, adults have a 10- to 20-fold increased risk for serious complications, including death. Because many children are being vaccinated, the overall incidence of chickenpox is on the decline. As a result, children who remain unvaccinated may nonetheless avoid chickenpox and hence may reach adulthood without developing antibodies to the disease. Therefore, if they acquire the disease as adults, it is likely to be severe. The moral to this story is that vaccinating children now not only will protect them from chickenpox during childhood but also will protect them from serious harm when they grow up.

Hepatitis B Vaccine

Preparations

Hepatitis B vaccine (HepB) contains *hepatitis B surface antigen* (HBsAg), the primary antigenic protein in the viral envelope. Administration of HepB promotes synthesis of specific antibodies directed against hepatitis B virus. Because HepB is made from a viral component, rather than from a live virus, it cannot cause disease.

HepB is available in pediatric and adult formulations. The pediatric formulation, marketed as *Recombivax HB,* contains 10 mcg of HBsAg/mL. The adult formulation, marketed as *Engerix-B,* contains 20 mcg of HBsAg/mL. A combination vaccine for adults, marketed as *Twinrix,* protects against hepatitis A *and* hepatitis B. In all three products, the HBsAg is produced in yeast using recombinant DNA technology.

Efficacy

Greater than 85% of vaccinated patients are protected after the second dose of HepB, and more than 90% are protected after the third dose. Although the duration of protection has not been determined with precision, it appears to be at least 5 to 7 years.

Adverse Effects and Contraindications

HepB is one of our safest vaccines. The most common reactions are soreness at the injection site and mild to moderate fever. Acetaminophen or ibuprofen may be used to relieve discomfort, but aspirin should be avoided. The only contraindication to HepB is a prior anaphylactic reaction either to HepB itself or to baker's yeast.

Hepatitis A Vaccine

Preparations

Hepatitis A vaccine (HepA) is prepared from inactivated hepatitis A virus In the United States two products are available: *Havrix* and *VAQTA.*

Efficacy

Immunization with HepA decreases the risk for clinical disease by 94% to 100%. Protective levels of antibodies are seen in 94% to 100% of adults and children 1 month after the first dose and in 100% of vaccinated patients 1 month after the second dose. Protection appears to be long lasting: among vaccinated children who were followed for 7 years, no cases of hepatitis A were detected.

Who Should Be Vaccinated?

Hepatitis A vaccination is recommended for *all* children 12 through 23 months old and for children older than 23 months who live in areas where vaccination programs target older children (owing to increased risk for infection). In addition, HepA is recommended for the following:

- People at least 1 year old traveling to places with high rates of hepatitis A, including Central or South America, Mexico, the Caribbean islands, Africa, Asia (except Japan), and southern or eastern Europe
- People in communities that have frequent outbreaks of hepatitis A
- Men who have sex with men
- People who use illegal drugs
- People with chronic liver disease
- People who receive clotting factor concentrates
- People who work with nonhuman primates or who work with hepatitis A in research laboratories

Adverse Effects

Mild reactions are common. Soreness at the injection site occurs in about 54% of adults and 18% of children. Headache occurs in 14% of adults and 9% of children. Other mild reactions include loss of appetite and malaise. When mild reactions occur, they usually begin 3 to 5 days after vaccination and last only 1 to 2 days.

Pneumococcal Conjugate Vaccine

There are two vaccines for use in prevention of pneumococcal disease; a *13-valent pneumococcal conjugate vaccine* (PCV13), sold as *Prevnar 13,* for prevention of invasive pneumococcal disease in infants and children, and an unconjugated vaccine—*pneumococcal polysaccharide vaccine* (PPSV), sold as *Pneumovax 23*—for adults and high-risk children older than 2 years. PPSV does not work in children younger than 2 years.

Description

PCV13 consists of 13 pneumococcal capsular polysaccharide antigens that have been conjugated to a protein carrier—specifically, CRM197, a nontoxic variant of diphtheria toxin. The protein carrier increases antigenicity, especially in infants. The 13 antigens in the vaccine are from the 13 serotypes of *S. pneumoniae* that cause the majority of invasive pneumococcal infections in American children younger than 6 years. PPSV23, like PCV13, contains polysaccharides, but it covers 23 serotypes of pneumococcal disease.

Efficacy

PCV13 and PPSV23 are highly effective. PCV13 vaccination was 100% effective in preventing invasive disease caused by the *S. pneumoniae* serotypes that the vaccine was designed to protect against. Vaccination was also 89% effective at preventing invasive disease caused by *all* serotypes of *S. pneumoniae.* In addition to preventing invasive pneumococcal disease, vaccination with PCV13 caused a modest reduction in cases of otitis media (see Chapter 86). PPSV23 is most effective in the adult population.

Adverse Effects

Both PCV13 and PPSV23 appear very safe. No serious adverse effects have been reported. About 50% to 70% of vaccinated patients get drowsy after the shot, lose their appetite, or develop erythema or tenderness at the injection site. Mild fever develops in 33%, and a higher fever (temperature above 102.2° F) develops in 5%. About 80% become irritable or fussy.

Who Should Be Vaccinated?

The ACIP recommends vaccinating children in the following groups:

- All children younger than 2 years
- All healthy children between their second and fifth birthdays who have not completed the PCV series
- All children between their second and fifth birthdays who have conditions that put them at high risk for serious pneumococcal disease. In this group are children with sickle cell anemia, injury to the spleen, cochlear implants, chronic heart or lung disease, or immunosuppression of any cause (e.g., diabetes, cancer, liver disease, HIV infection, use of immunosuppressive drugs)

Meningococcal Conjugate Vaccine

In the United States we have two *meningococcal conjugate polysaccharide vaccines* (MCVs): *Menactra* and *Menveo.* Both vaccines protect against the same four meningococcal serotypes—hence their abbreviation *MCV4.* Menactra is indicated for people 9 months to 55 years old, and Menveo is indicated for people 2 to 55 years old.

An unconjugated vaccine—*meningococcal polysaccharide vaccine* (MPSV4) [Menomune]—has been available since the 1970s, but is not very effective in children. Accordingly, MCV4 is currently preferred. MPSV4 is active against the same meningococcal serotypes as MCV4.

There are also two recombinant vaccines directed at serotype B meningococci: *Bexsero* and *Trumenba.* Both are approved for use in patients 10 to 25 years of age.

Description

Menactra is a tetravalent conjugate vaccine directed against four meningococcal serogroups: A, C, Y, and W-135. Each dose consists of 4 mcg of capsular polysaccharide from each of the four serogroups conjugated with 48 mcg of a protein carrier, specifically, diphtheria toxoid. The carrier protein increases immunogenicity.

Menveo is nearly identical to Menactra. However, there are two differences. First, the amount of capsular polysaccharide in each dose of Menveo is greater (10 mcg of polysaccharide from serogroup A, and 5 mcg of polysaccharide from serogroups C, Y, and W-135). Second, in Menveo, the polysaccharides are conjugated to a different diphtheria protein.

Bexsero and *Trumenba* are newer vaccines directed specifically at B subgroups of meningococcal disease. *Bexsero* contains 50 mcg of each NHBA, NadA, fHbp, and PorA proteins found on the surface of meningococci. *Trumenba* is comprised of 60 mcg of each fHBP protein subtypes A and B.

Efficacy

The efficacy of MCV4 at preventing meningococcal disease has not been evaluated in clinical trials. However, we do know the vaccine is highly immunogenic. For example, when 423 adolescents were vaccinated, rates of seroconversion for serogroups A, C, Y, and W-135 were 100%, 99%, 98%, and 99%, respectively, as measured by bactericidal antibody assay. FDA approval of MCV4 was based on its documented immunogenicity and the documented ability of other vaccines to prevent meningococcal infection.

Bexsero was studied in adolescents within Canada, Australia, and the United Kingdom. Composite antibody response rates (fHbo, NadA, PorA) rose from a baseline of 24% to 66% at 11 months after the second dose in the United Kingdom and from 0% to 63% in the Canadian and Australian populations. In a controlled trial completed in the United States with children between the ages of 11 and 18 years, *Trumenba* increased rates of serum antibody titer in adolescents from 0.7% to 83% after the third dose.

Adverse Effects

The most common reactions are local pain, headache, and fatigue. Local redness, swelling, and induration are also common.

Concerns that MCV4 might cause *Guillain-Barré syndrome* (GBS)[b] appear to be unfounded, as shown by two large studies. In one study, there were 99 confirmed cases of GBS among 12,589,910 vaccinated patients. In the other study, there were 5 cases among 889,684 vaccinated patients. In both studies, the incidence of GBS was no higher than would be expected in the absence of vaccination. In light of this information, the CDC and ACIP have removed precautionary language regarding a risk for GBS after meningococcal vaccination.

Who Should Be Vaccinated?

The ACIP recommends routine meningococcal vaccination for all children and adolescents aged 11 through 18 years. Children who were not vaccinated at this time should be vaccinated as soon as possible. Vaccination is also recommended for people at increased risk for meningococcal disease, including the following:

- College freshmen living in dormitories
- U.S. military recruits
- Microbiologists who are routinely exposed to meningococcal bacteria
- Anyone traveling to (or living in) a part of the world where meningococcal disease is common
- Anyone who has an injured spleen or whose spleen has been removed
- Anyone who has an immune disorder known as terminal complement component deficiency
- Anyone who might have been exposed to meningitis during an outbreak
- Persons with persistent complement component deficiency, anatomic or functional asplenia, and certain other risk factors

MCV4 is the preferred vaccine for people 2 to 55 years old in these risk groups, but MPSV4 can be used if MCV4 is not available. Only MPSV4 should be used for adults older than 55 years (not because MPSV4 is more effective, but because it is approved for use in this age group, whereas MCV4 is not). The newer subgroup B vaccines may be used in addition to the MCV4 vaccinations, preferably between the ages of 16 and 18 years. These are only recommended for use in children older than 10 years if they are high risk (functional asplenia, complement deficiency).

For more details on dosing, refer to the Meningococcal Vaccine Information Statement and the Adult Immunization Schedule, available online at www.cdc.gov/vaccines, and to Healthcare Personnel Vaccination Recommendations, available online at www.immunize.org/catg.d/p2017.pdf.

Influenza Vaccine

Annual vaccination against influenza, including the H1N1 subtype, is now recommended for all children between ages 6 months and 18 years (as well as all adults). Properties of intramuscular, intradermal, and intranasal influenza vaccines (composition, efficacy, adverse effects, contraindications, preparations, dosage, route), along with information on adult vaccination, are presented in Chapter 78.

Rotavirus Vaccine

Preparations and Efficacy

In the United States two rotavirus vaccines are available: *RotaTeq* and *Rotarix*. Both contain live, attenuated viruses. To induce a strong immune response, these viruses must replicate within the infant's gut. Accordingly, the vaccine is administered orally. RotaTeq and Rotarix differ in composition and dosing schedule.

RotaTeq is a *pentavalent* vaccine directed against the five most common serotypes of human rotavirus, termed G1, G2, G3, G4, and P1A. In trials in the United States and Finland, RotaTeq prevented 74% of *all* rotavirus gastroenteritis cases and 98% of *severe* cases. Vaccination also reduced the need for diarrhea-related hospitalization by 96%.

Rotarix is a *monovalent* vaccine developed from a rotavirus with the most common serotype found in humans. However,

[b]GBS is a serious neurologic disorder that involves inflammatory demyelination of peripheral nerves. Symptoms include symmetrical weakness in the arms and legs, sensory abnormalities, and paralysis of the muscles of respiration. Most patients eventually recover.

although Rotarix is monovalent, it confers protection against four rotavirus serotypes: G1, G3, G4, and G9. In clinical trials, Rotarix prevented 79% of *all* rotavirus gastroenteritis cases, 90% of *severe* cases, and 96% of diarrhea-related hospitalizations.

Safety

Although generally very safe, both RotaTeq and Rotarix may carry a small risk for *intussusception,* a rare, life-threatening form of bowel obstruction that occurs when the bowel folds in on itself, like a collapsing telescope. Of note, during prelicensure testing in more than 130,000 infants, no cases of intussusception were seen. However, with both vaccines, several cases were reported during postmarketing surveillance. Fortunately, the estimated risk is very low: about 1 case for each 50,000 to 70,000 vaccinated patients.

Who Should Be Vaccinated?

The ACIP recommends that all infants receive rotavirus vaccine, beginning at about age 8 weeks.

Who Should Not Be Vaccinated?

Rotarix, but not RotaTeq, is contraindicated for infants with any uncorrected congenital malformation of the gastrointestinal tract that could predispose to intussusception. Both vaccines are contraindicated for children with a history of intussusception.

Some vaccinated patients with *severe combined immunodeficiency (SCID),* a rare inherited disorder, have developed vaccine-acquired rotavirus infection. Accordingly, these vaccines are contraindicated for infants with SCID. Rotavirus vaccines have not been evaluated in children who are immunocompromised for other reasons. Nonetheless, because these vaccines contain live viruses, it would seem prudent to use them with caution in all immunocompromised infants, regardless of the cause.

Infants with moderate to severe diarrhea or vomiting should probably not be vaccinated until they recover.

Human Papillomavirus Vaccine

Three HPV vaccines are available: *Gardasil, Gardasil 9,* and *Cervarix.* These vaccines differ in composition, indications, and immunogenicity. Gardasil is a quadrivalent vaccine, and Gardasil 9 is a 9-valent vaccine; Cervarix is bivalent. Gardasil protects against cervical, vulvar, and vaginal cancer in females, as well as anal cancer and genital warts in females and males. By contrast, Cervarix only protects against cervical cancer—but the protection may last longer than with Gardasil. Gardasil was the first vaccine licensed in the United States for the specific purpose of protecting against cancer of any type.

Quadrivalent and 9-Valent HPV Vaccines: Gardasil and Gardasil 9

Composition

Gardasil is a quadrivalent vaccine designed to stimulate production of neutralizing antibodies directed at four types of HPV—specifically, types 16 and 18 (which cause 70% of cervical cancers) and types 6 and 11 (which cause 95% of genital warts). Gardasil 9 protects against HPV types 6, 11, 16, 18, 31, 33, 45, 52, and 58. The vaccines consist of *virus-like particles* (VLPs), which are virus-sized, empty spheres composed of viral capsid proteins. To the immune system, VLPs look like the actual virus, and hence VLPs can evoke an immune response. Because VLPs are empty (and hence don't contain viral DNA), VLPs cannot cause infection.

Indications

Gardasil and Gardasil 9 are used to prevent cancers, precancerous lesions, and genital warts in females and males.

Cancers and Precancerous Lesions in Female Patients

Gardasil and Gardasil 9 are indicated for girls and women 9 to 26 years old to prevent the following cancers caused by HPV types 16, 18, 31, 33, 45, 52, and 58:

- Cervical cancer
- Vulvar cancer
- Vaginal cancer

In addition, Gardasil and Gardasil 9 are indicated for prevention of the following precancerous and dysplastic lesions caused by HPV types 6, 11, 16, 18, 31, 33, 45, 52, and 58:

- Cervical adenocarcinoma in situ
- Cervical intraepithelial neoplasia grades 1, 2, and 3
- Vulvar intraepithelial neoplasia grades 2 and 3
- Vaginal intraepithelial neoplasia grades 2 and 3
- Anal intraepithelial neoplasia grades 1, 2, and 3

Genital Warts in Females and Males

Gardasil is indicated for females and males 9 to 26 years old to prevent genital warts caused by HPV types 6 and 11.

Anal Cancer in Females and Males

Gardasil is indicated for females and males 9 to 26 years old to prevent anal cancer and precancerous lesions caused by HPV types 6, 11, 16, 18, 31, 33, 45, 52, and 58.

Efficacy

Gardasil is highly effective, as demonstrated in FUTURE II, a phase 3, randomized, double-blind, placebo-controlled trial. Researchers enrolled 12,167 healthy women, aged 16 to 23 years, and gave them three intramuscular injections of Gardasil or placebo over a 6-month interval. During 2 years of follow-up, Gardasil was nearly 100% effective at preventing precancerous cervical lesions, precancerous vaginal and vulvar lesions, and genital warts caused by HPV types 6, 11, 16, and 18. However, although Gardasil protected against new HPV infection, it didn't eliminate infection that was already present. Furthermore, although Gardasil prevented precancerous cervical lesions, the study period was too short to tell whether vaccination prevents cervical cancer. Nonetheless, given that HPV infection causes more than 99% of cervical cancers, it seems highly likely that protection against this cancer will be conferred. At this time, the estimated duration of protection against HPV is 5 to 10 years. Studies are underway to determine whether and when booster vaccination may be needed.

Is a Pap Test Still Needed?

For two reasons, the answer is a resounding *YES!* First, Gardasil and Gardasil 9 only protect against four and nine types of HPV, respectively, leaving vaccinated patients at risk for cervical cancer caused by other types of HPV. Second, because Gardasil does not eliminate preexisting HPV infection, vaccinated patients remain at risk for cancer from infection that was present before the vaccine was given. Therefore vaccinated women should still undergo routine Pap screening to detect precancerous cervical changes, permitting timely treatment before cancer develops.

Safety

Gardasil appears to be very safe. Injection-site reactions—pain, erythema, swelling, and itching—although common, are mild and short lived. Fainting has occurred in teenage girls, sometimes resulting in hospitalization. However, the incidence of fainting is no greater than with other vaccines. Vaccinated patients who feel faint should sit or lie down to prevent falling.

Who Should Be Vaccinated?

Given that HPV infection is sexually transmitted and that HPV infects males and females, universal vaccination would be required to achieve maximal protection in the community. Accordingly, ACIP now recommends *routine* vaccination for males *and* females with quadrivalent HPV vaccine.

Females: Routine Vaccination

The ACIP recommends routine vaccination for all girls 11 to 12 years old. Why girls this young? Because the vaccine only protects against *acquiring* HPV infection. It can't clear infection that already exists. Therefore vaccination is most beneficial when done before vaccinated patients become sexually active, which is the case for most girls in this age group.

Vaccination with the HPV vaccine remains voluntary, not compulsory, throughout most of the United States. Shortly after Gardasil was approved, bills to make vaccination mandatory were introduced in 24 states. However, as of November 2015, only Kentucky, Rhode Island, Virginia, and the District of Columbia required the vaccine for school attendance. Furthermore, parents in Virginia who object can easily have their daughters opt out. Reasons for objection include expense (about $390 for the three-dose series), concerns about safety and efficacy (because HPV vaccine is relatively new), and concerns that conferring protection against a sexually transmitted infection might encourage promiscuity (a concern that has no basis in fact). Parents who are considering withholding vaccination would do well to ask this question: does protecting my daughter against developing cervical cancer later in life outweigh my concerns about vaccination? If the answer is yes, then vaccination should not be withheld.

Males: Routine Vaccination

ACIP recommends the quadrivalent or 9-valent HPV vaccine for all males 11 to 12 years old. Vaccination of males can help protect them from genital warts and HPV-related cancers and may help prevent spread of HPV to females.

Females and Males: Catch-up Vaccination

ACIP recommends the quadrivalent or 9-valent HPV vaccine for females and males 13 to 21 years old who did not receive the vaccine when they were younger.

Who Should Not Be Vaccinated?

HPV vaccine is not recommended for patients who are pregnant. Those who are breastfeeding may receive the vaccine.

Bivalent HPV Vaccine: Cervarix

Composition and Indications

Cervarix is a bivalent vaccine designed to stimulate production of neutralizing antibodies against two types of HPV—specifically, types 16 and 18, which cause 70% of cervical cancers. In contrast to Gardasil, Cervarix does not confer immunity against HPV types 6 and 11, which cause most cases of genital warts. Accordingly, Cervarix is indicated only for prevention of cervical cancers and precancerous lesions caused by HPV types 16 and 18. Unlike Gardasil, Cervarix is not indicated to prevent vaginal or vulvar cancer in females, or anal cancer or genital warts in females or males.

Efficacy

The efficacy of Cervarix was evaluated in a trial that enrolled about 18,000 girls and women aged 15 through 25 years. Half received Cervarix, and half received a control vaccine (Havrix, a vaccine against hepatitis A). Among subjects who did not have HPV infection when the study began, Cervarix was 93% effective at preventing precancerous lesions caused by HPV types 16 and 18. In addition, the vaccine provided cross-protection against HPV types 31, 33, and 45, the next most common causes of cervical cancer after HPV types 16 and 18. By contrast, Gardasil only confers cross-protection against HPV type 31.

Like Gardasil, Cervarix does not confer 100% protection against cervical cancer and is not active against cancer that began before the vaccine was given. Accordingly, vaccinated women should still undergo routine Pap screens to permit early detection and treatment of precancerous lesions.

Duration of Protection

Protection with Cervarix may last longer than with Gardasil because Cervarix is made with a unique adjuvant, a combination of aluminum hydroxide and monophosphoryl lipid A (derived from the bacterial cell wall). This adjuvant induces a stronger immune response than does the adjuvant in Gardasil (aluminum hydroxyphosphate sulfate).

Safety

Like Gardasil, Cervarix appears very safe. Both vaccines often cause mild reactions, although Cervarix causes more of them. The most common *local* reactions with Cervarix are pain, redness, and swelling. The most common *systemic* reactions are fatigue, headache, myalgia, GI symptoms, arthralgia, fever, and rash. Like Gardasil, Cervarix has been associated with fainting, primarily in teenage girls. Vaccinated patients who feel faint should sit or lie down to prevent falling.

Who Should Be Vaccinated? And How?

The ACIP recommends routine vaccination for all girls 11 to 12 years old. In addition, vaccination is recommended for all girls and women 13 to 26 years old who were not vaccinated when they were younger. The route, site, and immunization schedule are the same as for Gardasil.

Who Should Not Be Vaccinated?

Like Gardasil, Cervarix is not recommended for patients who are pregnant but may be used by those who are breastfeeding.

Respiratory Syncytial Virus Vaccine (Experimental)

Scientists are currently testing experimental vaccines to prevent RSV. In animal tests, an RSV vaccine elicited high levels of RSV-specific antibodies. Recruiting is taking place for multiple trials to assess safety and immunogenicity of new RSV vaccines.

CHAPTER 54

Antihistamines

Laura D. Rosenthal, DNP, ACNP, FAANP

Histamine is a small molecule produced in specialized cells throughout the body. The compound plays an important role in allergic reactions and regulation of gastric acid secretion. The antihistamines, a widely used family of drugs, block histamine actions.

To understand the antihistamines, we must first understand histamine itself. Accordingly, the chapter begins with a discussion of histamine, emphasizing its contribution to allergic responses.

HISTAMINE

Histamine is a locally acting compound with prominent and varied effects. In the vascular system, histamine dilates small blood vessels and increases capillary permeability. In the bronchi, histamine produces constriction of smooth muscle. In the stomach, histamine stimulates secretion of acid. In the central nervous system (CNS), histamine acts as a neurotransmitter. Despite this impressive spectrum of actions, clinical use of histamine is limited to diagnostic procedures. However, although its clinical utility is minimal, histamine is still of great interest owing to its involvement in two common pathologic states: allergic disorders and peptic ulcer disease.

Distribution, Synthesis, Storage, and Release

Distribution

Histamine is present in practically all tissues. Levels are especially high in the skin, lungs, and the gastrointestinal (GI) tract. The histamine content of plasma is low.

Synthesis and Storage

In the periphery, histamine is synthesized and stored in two types of cells: *mast cells* and *basophils*. Mast cells are present in the skin and other soft tissues. Basophils are present in blood. In both mast cells and basophils, histamine is stored in secretory granules.

In the CNS, histamine is produced by neurons with cell bodies in the posterior hypothalamus and with axonal projections to the frontal and temporal cortices and other brain regions.

Release

Release of histamine from mast cells and basophils is produced by allergic and nonallergic mechanisms.

Allergic Release

The initial requirement for allergic release is production of antibodies of the immunoglobulin E class. These antibodies are generated after exposure to specific allergens (e.g., pollens, insect venoms, certain drugs). Once made, the antibodies become attached to the outer surface of mast cells and basophils (Fig. 54.1). When the individual is reexposed to the allergen, the allergen becomes bound by the antibodies. Binding of allergen to adjacent antibodies creates a bridge between those antibodies. By a mechanism that is not fully understood, this bridging process mobilizes intracellular calcium. The calcium, in turn, causes the histamine-containing storage granules to fuse with the cell membrane and disgorge their contents into the extracellular space. Note that allergic release of histamine requires *prior exposure* to the allergen; an allergic reaction cannot occur during initial allergen exposure.

Nonallergic Release

Several agents (certain drugs, radiocontrast media, plasma expanders) can act directly on mast cells to trigger histamine release. With these agents, no prior sensitization is needed. Cell injury can also cause direct release.

Physiologic and Pharmacologic Effects

Histamine acts primarily through two types of receptors, named histamine-1 (H_1) and histamine-2 (H_2). The response produced depends on which of these receptors is involved.

Effects of Histamine-1 Stimulation

Vasodilation

Activation of H_1 receptors causes dilation of small blood vessels (arterioles and venules). Vasodilation is prominent in the skin of the face and upper body, causing the area to become warm and flushed. If extensive vasodilation occurs, total peripheral resistance declines and blood pressure falls.

Increased Capillary Permeability

Activation of H_1 receptors increases capillary permeability. Receptor activation causes capillary endothelial cells to contract, creating openings between these cells through which fluid, protein, and platelets can escape. Escape of fluid and protein into the interstitial space produces edema. If loss of intravascular fluid is substantial, blood pressure may fall.

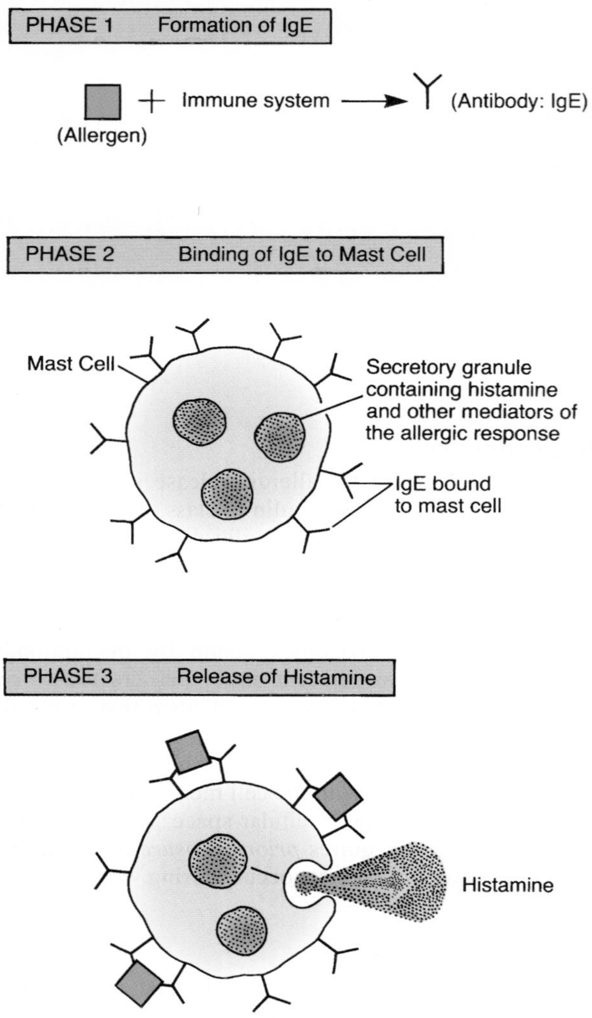

Figure 54.1 ■ Release of histamine by allergen-antibody interaction. (IgE, immunoglobulin E.)

Bronchoconstriction

H_1 activation causes constriction of the bronchi. If histamine is administered to an individual with asthma, severe bronchoconstriction will follow. However, although *exogenous* histamine can induce bronchial constriction, histamine is not the cause of bronchoconstriction that occurs during a spontaneous asthma attack. Consequently, antihistamines are of no use for treating asthma.

CNS Effects

In the CNS, H_1 receptors have a role in cognition, memory, and the cycle of sleeping and waking. In addition, H_1 receptors appear to have a role in seizure suppression, modulation of neurotransmitter release, and regulation of energy and endocrine homeostasis.

Other Effects

Activation of H_1 receptors on sensory nerves produces *itching* and *pain.* H_1 activation also promotes *secretion of mucus.*

Effects of Histamine-2 Stimulation

The major response to activation of H_2 receptors is *secretion of gastric acid.* Histamine acts directly on parietal cells of the stomach to promote acid release. Although acetylcholine and gastrin also help regulate acid release, histamine has a dominant role. We know this because, in the presence of H_2 blockade, acetylcholine and gastrin are unable to elicit acid secretion.

Role of Histamine in Allergic Responses

Allergic reactions are mediated by histamine and other compounds (e.g., prostaglandins, leukotrienes, tryptase). The intensity of an allergic reaction is determined by which mediator is involved. The symptoms of mild allergy (e.g., rhinitis, itching, localized edema) are caused largely by histamine acting at H_1 receptors. As a result, mild allergic conditions (e.g., hay fever, acute urticaria, mild transfusion reactions) are generally responsive to antihistamine therapy.

THE TWO TYPES OF ANTIHISTAMINES: HISTAMINE-1 ANTAGONISTS AND HISTAMINE-2 ANTAGONISTS

Antihistamines fall into two basic categories: H_1 receptor antagonists and H_2 receptor antagonists. The principal use of H_1 blockers is treatment of mild allergic disorders. The principal use of H_2 blockers is treatment of gastric and duodenal ulcers. Because H_2 antagonists do not block H_1 receptors, these drugs are of no use for treating allergies. In this chapter, we focus on H_1 antagonists. The H_2 blockers, which are widely used, are discussed in Chapter 62.

Histamine$_1$ Antagonists

Basic Pharmacology

The H_1 antagonists are the classic antihistamines. Because of its historical use, the term *antihistamines* is still employed as a synonym for the subgroup of histamine antagonists that produce selective H_1 blockade. Here, we continue to use the term *antihistamine* interchangeably with H_1 blocker and H_1 antagonist.

Although all H_1 antagonists available have similar antihistaminic actions, these drugs differ significantly in side effects. Because of these differences, selection of a prototype to represent the group is not feasible. Thus, rather than structuring discussion around one prototypic drug, we discuss the H_1 antagonists collectively. Differences among individual antihistamines are addressed as appropriate.

Classification

The H_1 antagonists fall into two major groups: *first-generation H_1 antagonists* and *second-generation H_1 antagonists.* The principal difference between the groups is that first-generation antihistamines are highly sedating, whereas second-generation antihistamines are not.

Mechanism of Action

H_1 blockers bind selectively to H_1-histaminic receptors, thereby blocking the actions of histamine at these sites. H_1

antagonists do not block H_2 receptors. Also, they do not block release of histamine from mast cells or basophils.

It should be noted that, although interaction of the classic antihistamines with *histaminic* receptors is limited to the H_1 receptor subtype, these drugs can also bind to *nonhistaminic* receptors. Most notably, certain antihistamines can bind to and block *muscarinic* receptors. This action underlies several important side effects.

Pharmacologic Effects

Peripheral Effects

The major therapeutic effects of the H_1 antagonists can be attributed to preventing the actions of histamine at H_1 receptors. In arterioles and venules of the skin, H_1 blockers inhibit the dilator actions of histamine and thereby reduce localized flushing. In capillary beds, the antihistamines prevent histamine-induced increases in permeability and thereby reduce edema. By blocking histamine at sensory nerves, H_1 antagonists reduce itching and pain. Blockade of H_1 receptors in mucous membranes suppresses secretion of mucus.

Effects on the CNS

Antihistamines can cause both excitation and depression of the CNS. At therapeutic doses, antihistamines produce CNS depression: reaction time is slowed, alertness is diminished, and drowsiness is likely. These effects are more pronounced with some antihistamines than with others. With most second-generation antihistamines (e.g., fexofenadine), CNS depression is negligible.

Overdose with antihistamines can produce *CNS stimulation.* Seizures frequently result. Very young children are especially sensitive to CNS stimulation by these drugs.

Other Pharmacologic Effects

Blockade of muscarinic cholinergic receptors by antihistamines can produce typical *anticholinergic* responses. These are discussed later under "Adverse Effects." Several antihistamines can suppress nausea and vomiting, as discussed later under "Motion Sickness."

Therapeutic Uses

All of the H_1 antagonists are useful in treating allergic disorders. Some are also indicated for other conditions (e.g., motion sickness, insomnia).

Mild Allergy

Antihistamines can reduce symptoms of mild allergies. In people with *seasonal allergic rhinitis,* H_1 blockers can reduce sneezing, rhinorrhea, and itching of the eyes, nose, and throat. In patients with *acute urticaria,* these drugs can reduce redness, itching, and edema. The antihistamines can also reduce symptoms of *allergic conjunctivitis* and urticaria associated with *mild transfusion reactions.* In all these conditions, benefits result from H_1 receptor blockade—not from preventing allergen-induced release of histamine from mast cells and basophils. Because mild allergic reactions may be mediated by substances in addition to histamine, antihistamines often fail to produce complete relief.

Motion Sickness

Some antihistamines, such as promethazine [Phenergan] and dimenhydrinate [Dramamine], are labeled for use in motion sickness. Benefits derive from blocking H_1 receptors and muscarinic receptors in the neuronal pathway leading from the vestibular apparatus of the inner ear to the vomiting center of the medulla. Motion sickness and its treatment are discussed in Chapter 64.

Insomnia

The ability of antihistamines to cause drowsiness has been exploited in the treatment of insomnia. Practically every over-the-counter (OTC) sleep aid contains an H_1 antagonist—diphenhydramine or pyrilamine—as its active ingredient. However, although antihistamines can induce sleep when used in sufficient dosage, the doses recommended for OTC preparations are usually too low to be effective.

Adverse Effects

All of the H_1 blockers can produce undesired effects. As a rule, these responses are more of a nuisance than a source of serious discomfort or danger. Frequently, side effects subside with continued drug use. Because individual antihistamines differ in their abilities to produce particular side effects (Table 54.1), adverse responses can be minimized by judicious drug selection.

Sedation

Sedation is the most common side effect of the antihistamines and can lead to serious consequences. For students, sedation

PATIENT-CENTERED CARE ACROSS THE LIFE SPAN

Antihistamines

Life Stage	Patient Care Concerns
Infants	Antihistamines can cause sedation in infants. Although they can be used in small doses in children older than 6 months, caution should be employed.
Children/adolescents	Antihistamines can be used safely in children, just in smaller doses. Side-effect profiles are similar to those of adults. Promethazine is contraindicated in children younger than 2 years because deaths have occurred in this population.
Pregnant women	There has been debate regarding whether antihistamines cause fetal harm when used in pregnancy. Many of these drugs are classified in U.S. Food and Drug Administration Pregnancy Risk Category C and should be avoided unless absolutely necessary.
Breastfeeding women	Occasional, small doses of antihistamines do not appear to cause sedation in infants. Caution should be used.
Older adults	Because antihistamines can cause sedation, smaller doses should be used initially and titrated up if needed. Also, these medications can make glaucoma or benign prostatic hyperplasia worse.

can impair learning and memory. For drivers, sedation greatly increases the risk for an accident. In fact, the degree of impairment seen with antihistamines equals that seen when blood levels of alcohol exceed the legal limit. Worse yet, impairment can occur without feeling tired. Accordingly, patients should exercise extreme caution when driving or performing other hazardous activities. They should also avoid alcohol and other CNS depressants, which will intensify the depressant effects of the H_1 antagonist. Fortunately, tolerance to sedation often develops within a few days or weeks. If a preparation with a long half-life is being used, daytime sedation can be minimized by administering the entire daily dose at night.

The second-generation antihistamines exert little or no sedative effect. First, these drugs are relatively large molecules with low lipid solubility, so they can't cross the blood-brain barrier. Second, these drugs have low affinity to the type of H_1 receptor found in the brain. In contrast, the first-generation antihistamines are relatively small molecules with high lipid solubility and hence can readily cross the blood-brain barrier. In addition, these drugs have a high affinity for H_1 receptors of the CNS.

For patients who experience disabling sedation with a first-generation H_1 antagonist, therapy with a second-generation (nonsedating) antihistamine is likely to help.

Nonsedative CNS Effects

In addition to sedation, antihistamines can cause dizziness, incoordination, confusional states, and fatigue. Older patients are especially sensitive to these actions. In some patients, paradoxical excitation occurs, resulting in insomnia, nervousness, tremors, and even seizures. CNS stimulation is most common in children and after overdose.

Gastrointestinal Effects

Gastrointestinal disturbances are common. Responses include nausea, vomiting, loss of appetite, and diarrhea or constipation. These reactions can be minimized by administering antihistamines with food.

Anticholinergic Effects

The H_1 antagonists possess weak atropine-like properties. These antimuscarinic actions can produce drying of mucous membranes in the mouth, nasal passages, and throat. Cholinergic blockade may also result in urinary hesitancy, constipation, and palpitations. If dry mouth becomes distressing, discomfort can be minimized by using hard sugarless candy and by taking frequent sips of liquid. Antihistamines should be used with caution in patients with asthma because thickening of bronchial secretions may impair breathing. Care is also needed in patients with other conditions that can be made worse by muscarinic blockade (e.g., urinary retention, benign prostatic hyperplasia, hypertension). The second-generation antihistamines are the least anticholinergic.

BLACK BOX WARNING: PROMETHAZINE

Promethazine [Phenergan, Phenadoz] can cause severe respiratory depression, especially in very young patients. Deaths have occurred. Accordingly, the drug is now contraindicated for use in children younger than 2 years and should be used with caution in children older than 2 years.

TABLE 54.1 ▪ Pharmacologic Effects of Histamine-1 Antagonists Used for Parenteral Therapy

Drug	H_1-Blocking Activity	Sedative Effects	Anticholinergic Effects
FIRST-GENERATION AGENTS			
Alkylamines			
Brompheniramine	+++	+	++
Chlorpheniramine	++	+	++
Dexchlorpheniramine	+++	+	++
Ethanolamines			
Clemastine	+ to ++	++	+++
Diphenhydramine	+ to ++	+++	+++
Phenothiazine			
Promethazine*	+++	+++	+++
Piperazine			
Hydroxyzine	++ to +++	+++	++
SECOND-GENERATION (NONSEDATING) AGENTS			
Cetirizine†	+++	+	±
Levocetirizine†	+++	+	±
Fexofenadine	+++	±	±
Loratadine	++ to +++	±	±
Desloratadine	++ to +++	±	±

*Promethazine is contraindicated in children younger than 2 years owing to a risk for fatal respiratory depression. *Parenteral* promethazine can cause severe local tissue injury.

†Cetirizine and levocetirizine have mild sedative effects.

H_1, histamine-1; ±, low to none; +, low; ++, moderate; + + +, high.

Severe Local Tissue Injury

Extravasation of IV *promethazine* can cause severe local tissue injury, including gangrene that requires amputation. Severe injury can also occur with inadvertent perivascular or intraarterial administration, or with administration into or near a nerve. Accordingly, when parenteral dosing is needed, the preferred route is intramuscular; subcutaneous promethazine is contraindicated.

Drug Interactions: Central Nervous System Depressants

Alcohol and other CNS depressants (e.g., barbiturates, benzodiazepines, opioids) can intensify the depressant effects of H_1 antagonists. Patients should be advised against drinking alcoholic beverages. If medications with CNS-depressant properties are combined with H_1 blockers, dosage of the depressant may need to be lowered.

Use in Pregnancy and Lactation

Pregnancy

The margin of safety of antihistamines in pregnancy is unknown. There have been reports of fetal malformation, but direct involvement of H_1 antagonists has not been proved. Given the uncertainty over the safety of these drugs, it is recommended that antihistamines be used only when clearly necessary and only when the benefits of treatment outweigh the potential risks to the fetus. Antihistamines should be avoided late in the third trimester because newborns are particularly sensitive to the adverse actions of these drugs.

Lactation

The H_1 antagonists can be excreted in breast milk, thereby posing a risk to the nursing infant. Because infants, and especially newborns, are unusually sensitive to antihistamines, these drugs should be avoided by women who are breastfeeding. If necessary, small, occasional doses will likely not cause harm.

Acute Toxicity

Although the antihistamines have a large margin of safety, acute poisoning is nonetheless common, owing to the widespread availability of these drugs. CNS effects are prominent, especially anticholinergic reactions. Specific symptoms and treatment are described next.

Symptoms

The anticholinergic actions of H_1 blockers produce symptoms resembling those of atropine poisoning (dilated pupils, flushed face, hyperpyrexia, tachycardia, dry mouth, urinary retention). In children, CNS excitation is prominent, manifesting as hallucinations, incoordination, ataxia, and convulsions. In extreme cases, intoxication progresses to coma, cardiovascular collapse, and death.

Treatment

There is no specific antidote to antihistamine poisoning. Hence, treatment is directed at drug removal and managing symptoms. Absorption can be minimized by giving activated charcoal (to adsorb the drug), followed by a cathartic (to hasten its export from the GI tract). Convulsions can be treated with intravenous benzodiazepines (lorazepam, midazolam). Hyperthermia can be reduced by applying ice packs or by giving sponge baths.

Preparations

As noted previously, the H_1 antagonists can be divided into two major groups: first-generation H_1 antagonists and second-generation H_1 antagonists. The first-generation agents can cause significant sedation. In contrast, the second-generation agents cause little or no sedation. All of the H_1 blockers can be administered by mouth. In addition, some can be given parenterally, by nasal spray, or by rectal suppository. Routes and dosages for individual H_1 antagonists are shown in Table 54.2.

First-Generation Histamine-1 Antagonists

The first-generation antihistamines can be grouped into five major categories (see Table 54.1). These groups differ in antihistaminic efficacy and the ability to cause sedation and muscarinic blockade. Given these differences, it may be possible, through judicious drug selection, to produce effective H_1 blockade while minimizing undesired effects.

Sedation can be a significant problem. Among the first-generation agents, CNS depression is most prominent with the ethanolamines (e.g., diphenhydramine) and phenothiazines (e.g., promethazine) and least prominent with the alkylamines (e.g., chlorpheniramine). For many patients, the alkylamines can provide effective H_1 blockade while causing only a modest reduction in alertness. If sedation remains excessive with an alkylamine, a second-generation agent should be tried.

Most first-generation agents have significant anticholinergic properties. As a result, they can cause dry mouth, urinary hesitancy, and other typical anticholinergic side effects.

Second-Generation (Nonsedating) Histamine-1 Antagonists

Second-generation antihistamines produce much less sedation than first-generation agents because (1) the second-generation agents cross the blood-brain barrier poorly and (2) they have a low affinity for H_1 receptors of the CNS. Synergism with alcohol and other CNS depressants is low. Nonetheless, combined use of CNS depressants and the second-generation agents should be avoided. In addition to lacking sedative effects, the second-generation agents are largely devoid of anticholinergic actions. When these drugs were introduced, they all required a prescription. Now, three agents—cetirizine, fexofenadine, and loratadine—are available over the counter. Because all of these drugs are very similar, initial selection can usually be based on price. If a cheaper agent proves ineffective, a more expensive agent can be tried.

Descriptions that follow are limited to the five second-generation agents that are used for oral therapy. Two other second-generation agents, azelastine [Astelin, Astepro] and olopatadine [Patanase], both used for local effects in the nose, are discussed in Chapter 60.

Fexofenadine. Fexofenadine [Allegra, Allegra Allergy] is approved for oral therapy of seasonal allergic rhinitis and for chronic idiopathic urticaria. Of the second-generation antihistamines now available, fexofenadine appears to offer the best combination of efficacy and safety. In clinical trials, the incidence of drowsiness and other side effects was nearly the same as with placebo. Fexofenadine has a half-life of 14.4 hours and is excreted unchanged in the urine. The drug is available in standard tablets (30, 60, and 180 mg) and a suspension (6 mg/mL), marketed as Allegra Children's Liquid, and in orally disintegrating tablets (30 mg), marketed as Allegra Children's Meltable Tablets. For all formulations, dosage should be reduced in patients with renal impairment.

Certain fruit juices (e.g., apple juice, orange juice, grapefruit juice) can reduce fexofenadine absorption, possibly reducing therapeutic effects. The mechanism is inhibition of organic anion transporting polypeptides, which contribute to absorption of fexofenadine from the GI tract. To ensure

TABLE 54.2 ▪ H_1 Antagonists Used for Systemic Therapy: Trade Names, Routes, and Dosage

Generic Name	Trade Names	Routes	Usual Adult Oral Dosage
FIRST-GENERATION AGENTS			
Alkylamines			
Brompheniramine	Bromfed DM, others	PO	12 mg every 4–6 h
Chlorpheniramine	Chlor-Trimeton, others	PO	4 mg every 4–6 h
Dexchlorpheniramine	Generic only	PO	2 mg every 4–6 h
Ethanolamines			
Clemastine	Tavist Allergy	PO	1.34 mg every 12 h
Diphenhydramine	Benadryl	PO, IV, IM	25–50 mg every 6–8 h
Phenothiazine			
Promethazine*	Phenadoz, Phenergan, others	PO, IV, IM, rectal suppository	12.5–25 mg every 6 h
Piperazine			
Hydroxyzine	Vistaril	PO	25–100 mg every 4–8 h
Piperidine			
Cyproheptadine	Generic only	PO	4 mg every 6–8 h
SECOND-GENERATION (NONSEDATING) AGENTS			
Cetirizine†	Zyrtec, Reactine ♣	PO	5–10 mg every 24 h Children 2–5 yr: 2.5 mg every 24 h
Levocetirizine†	Xyzal	PO	5 mg every 24 h Children 6–11 yr: 2.5 mg every 24 h Children 6 mo–5 yr: 1.25 mg every 24 h
Fexofenadine	Allegra, Allegra ODT	PO	180 mg every 24 h Children 6–11 yr: 30 mg every 12 h Children 6 mo–2 yr: 15 mg every 12 h
Loratadine	Alavert, Claritin	PO	10 mg every 24 h Children 2–5 yr: 5 mg every 24 h
Desloratadine	Clarinex, Clarinex RediTabs, Aerius ♣	PO	5 mg every 24 h Children 6–11 yr: 2.5 mg every 24 h Children 1–5 yr: 1.25 mg every 24h Children 2–11 mo: 1 mg every 24 h

*Promethazine is contraindicated in children younger than 2 years owing to a risk for fatal respiratory depression.
†Cetirizine and levocetirizine have mild sedative effects.

fexofenadine absorption, patients should not drink fruit juices within 4 hours before dosing or 1 to 2 hours after dosing.

Cetirizine. Cetirizine [Zyrtec, Zyrtec ODT, Zyrtec Allergy, Reactine ♣] is indicated for allergic rhinitis and chronic idiopathic urticaria. Administration is oral, and food delays absorption. Cetirizine is eliminated by a combination of hepatic metabolism and renal excretion. Its half-life is 8.3 hours. Although cetirizine is generally well tolerated, it can cause drowsiness, fatigue, and dryness of the mouth, nose, and throat. Cetirizine—and levocetirizine, its active isomer—cause more sedation than the other second-generation antihistamines, but less sedation than the first-generation drugs. Cetirizine is available in standard tablets (5 mg), chewable tablets (5 and 10 mg), orally disintegrating tablets (10 mg), and a syrup (1 mg/mL). Dosage should be reduced in patients with significant hepatic or renal impairment.

Levocetirizine. Levocetirizine [Xyzal] is the levo (active) isomer of cetirizine and shares that drug's indications: allergic rhinitis and chronic idiopathic urticaria. Like cetirizine, levocetirizine is more sedating than the other second-generation antihistamines but less sedating than the first-generation agents. The most common side effects are drowsiness, fatigue, muscle weakness, and dry mouth. Alcohol and other CNS depressants can intensify sedation and hence should be avoided. Levocetirizine is supplied in scored 5-mg tablets and an oral solution (0.5 mg/mL) that can be administered without regard to meals. To minimize sedation, dosing should be done in the evening. Dosing should be reduced in adults with mild to moderate renal impairment, and children with any degree of renal impairment should not use the drug.

Loratadine. Loratadine [Claritin, Alavert, others] is approved only for seasonal allergic rhinitis. Like other second-generation antihistamines, the drug is generally well tolerated. However, in clinical trials, 8% of patients experienced drowsiness, and 12% experienced headache. Loratadine is administered orally, and food delays absorption. The drug undergoes extensive hepatic metabolism and has a half-life of 8 to 28 hours. Loratadine is available in five formulations: a syrup (1 mg/mL), 10-mg liquid-gels, 10-mg standard tablets, 10-mg orally disintegrating tablets [Alavert], and 10-mg rapidly disintegrating tablets [Claritin RediTabs] designed to dissolve on the tongue. For patients with significant hepatic or renal impairment, dosing should be done every other day.

Desloratadine. Desloratadine [Clarinex, Clarinex RediTabs, Aerius ♣] is the major active metabolite of loratadine. The two drugs differ primarily in that desloratadine has a longer half-life (27 hours vs. 8.4 hours). However, although desloratadine has a longer half-life, there is no proof that its effects persist longer. Approved indications are seasonal allergic rhinitis, perennial allergic rhinitis, and chronic idiopathic urticaria. Desloratadine has no significant drug interactions, and at the recommended dosage, the incidence of adverse effects is similar to that of placebo. About 7% of patients metabolize desloratadine very slowly, causing its effects to be more intense. Desloratadine is available in 5-mg standard tablets, 5-mg rapidly disintegrating tablets [Clarinex RediTabs], and a syrup (2.5 mg/5 mL). For patients with liver or renal impairment, the manufacturer recommends reducing the initial dosage to 5 mg every other day.

CHAPTER

55 Cyclooxygenase Inhibitors: Nonsteroidal Antiinflammatory Drugs and Acetaminophen

Laura D. Rosenthal, DNP, ACNP, FAANP

The family of cyclooxygenase inhibitors consists of aspirin and related drugs. Most of these agents have three useful effects: they can suppress inflammation, relieve pain, and reduce fever. In addition, aspirin—and only aspirin—can protect against myocardial infarction (MI) and stroke. All of these effects are produced through one central mechanism: inhibition of cyclooxygenase, the enzyme responsible for synthesis of prostanoids (prostaglandins and related compounds). This same mechanism underlies their principal adverse effects: gastric ulceration, bleeding, and renal impairment. Cyclooxygenase inhibition also underlies MI and stroke, which can occur with most of these drugs, but *not* with aspirin.

MECHANISM OF ACTION

All of the drugs discussed here work by inhibiting *cyclooxygenase* (COX), the enzyme that converts arachidonic acid into *prostanoids: prostaglandins* and related compounds (prostacyclin, thromboxane A_2 [TXA_2]). To understand the drugs that inhibit COX, we must first understand COX itself.

Cyclooxygenase is found in all tissues and helps regulate multiple processes. At sites of tissue injury, COX catalyzes the synthesis of prostaglandin E_2 (PGE_2) and prostaglandin I_2 (PGI_2, also called prostacyclin), which promote inflammation and sensitize receptors to painful stimuli. In the stomach, COX promotes synthesis of PGE_2 and PGI_2, which help protect the gastric mucosa. Three mechanisms are involved: reduced secretion of gastric acid, increased secretion of bicarbonate and cytoprotective mucus, and maintenance of submucosal blood flow. In platelets, COX promotes synthesis of TXA_2, which stimulates platelet aggregation. In blood vessels, COX promotes synthesis of prostacyclin, which causes vasodilation. In the kidney, COX catalyzes synthesis of PGE_2 and PGI_2, which promote vasodilation and thereby maintain renal blood flow. In the brain, COX-derived prostaglandins mediate fever and contribute to perception of pain. In the uterus, COX-derived prostaglandins help promote contractions at term. It is important to appreciate that prostaglandins, prostacyclin, and TXA_2 act *locally;* these compounds do not affect sites distant from where they were made.

Cyclooxygenase has two forms, named cyclooxygenase-1 (COX-1) and cyclooxygenase-2 (COX-2). COX-1 is found in practically all tissues, where it mediates "housekeeping" chores. Important among these are protecting the gastric mucosa, supporting renal function, and promoting platelet aggregation. In contrast, COX-2 is produced mainly at sites of *tissue injury,* where it mediates inflammation and sensitizes receptors to painful stimuli. COX-2 is also present in the *brain* (where it mediates fever and contributes to perception of pain), the *kidneys* (where it supports renal function), *blood vessels* (where it promotes vasodilation), and the *colon* (where it can contribute to colon cancer). Because COX-1 primarily mediates beneficial processes, whereas COX-2 primarily mediates harmful processes, COX-1 has been dubbed the "good COX" and COX-2 the "bad COX." Some important functions of COX-1 and COX-2 are shown in Table 55.1.

Having established the roles of COX-1 and COX-2, we can now predict the effects of drugs that inhibit these enzymes. Inhibition of COX-1 (good COX) results largely in harmful effects:

- Gastric erosion and ulceration
- Bleeding tendencies
- Renal impairment

Inhibition of COX-1 also has one very beneficial effect:

- Protection against MI and stroke (secondary to reduced platelet aggregation)

Inhibition of COX-2 (bad COX) results largely in beneficial effects:

- Suppression of inflammation
- Alleviation of pain
- Reduction of fever
- Protection against colorectal cancer

Inhibition of COX-2 also has two adverse effects:

- Renal impairment
- Promotion of MI and stroke (secondary to suppressing vasodilation)

CLASSIFICATION OF CYCLOOXYGENASE INHIBITORS

The cyclooxygenase inhibitors fall into two major categories: (1) drugs that have antiinflammatory properties and (2) drugs that lack antiinflammatory properties. Agents in the first group are referred to as *nonsteroidal antiinflammatory drugs* (NSAIDs). Representative members include aspirin, ibuprofen [Advil, Motrin, others], naproxen [Aleve, others], and celecoxib [Celebrex]. The second class consists of just one drug: *acetaminophen* [Tylenol, others]. Acetaminophen can reduce pain and fever but cannot suppress inflammation.

The NSAIDs can be subdivided into two groups: (1) *first-generation NSAIDs* (conventional NSAIDs, traditional NSAIDs) and (2) *second-generation NSAIDs* (selective COX-2 inhibitors, coxibs). The first-generation agents inhibit COX-1 *and* COX-2. The second-generation agents inhibit COX-2 only. Because the first-generation agents inhibit both COX isoforms, they are unable to suppress pain and inflammation without posing a risk for serious side effects (gastric ulceration, bleeding, renal impairment). In contrast, because of their selectivity for COX-2, the second-generation NSAIDs, *in theory,* can suppress pain and inflammation while (possibly) causing fewer adverse effects than the first-generation NSAIDs. However, *in reality,* COX-2 inhibitors appear even less safe than the first-generation agents, owing to an increased risk for MI and stroke.

Table 55.2 shows the principal indications and adverse effects of the first-generation NSAIDs, second-generation NSAIDs, and acetaminophen.

FIRST-GENERATION NONSTEROIDAL ANTIINFLAMMATORY DRUGS

The first-generation NSAIDs—a large and widely used group of drugs—inhibit COX-1 and COX-2. In the United States more than 70 million prescriptions are written annually and more than 30 billion tablets are sold over the counter. The traditional NSAIDs are used to treat inflammatory disorders

TABLE 55.1 ▪ Cyclooxygenase-1 and Cyclooxygenase-2: Functions and Effect of Inhibition

Location	COX Isoform	COX Reaction Product	Response to COX Reaction Product	Effect of COX Inhibition
Stomach	COX-1	PGE_2, PGI_2	Gastric protection: Increased bicarbonate secretion Increased mucus production Decreased acid secretion Maintenance of submucosal blood flow	Gastric ulceration
Platelets	COX-1	TXA_2	Platelet aggregation	Bleeding tendencies Protection against MI
Blood vessels	COX-2	Prostacyclin	Vasodilation	Vasoconstriction (which can promote MI)
Kidney	COX-1, COX-2	PGE_2, PGI_2	Maintenance of renal function: Renal vasodilation Maintenance of renal perfusion	Renal impairment
Injured tissue	COX-2	PGE_2	Inflammation Pain	Reduced inflammation Analgesia
Brain	COX-2	Unknown	Fever Pain	Reduced fever Analgesia
Colon/rectum	COX-2	Unknown	Colorectal cancer promotion	Colorectal cancer protection

COX-1, cyclooxygenase-1; COX-2, cyclooxygenase-2; MI, myocardial infarction; PGE_2, prostaglandin E_2; PGI_2, prostaglandin I_2, (prostacyclin); TXA_2, thromboxane A_2.

TABLE 55.2 ▪ Principal Indications and Adverse Effects of the Four Major Types of Cyclooxygenase Inhibitors

	First-Generation NSAIDs: Aspirin	First-Generation NSAIDs: All Others	Second-Generation NSAIDs (Coxibs)	Acetaminophen
INDICATIONS				
Inflammation	Yes	Yes	Yes	No
Pain	Yes	Yes	Yes	Yes
Fever	Yes	Yes	No	Yes
Prevention of MI and stroke	Yes	No	No	No
ADVERSE EFFECTS				
Gastric ulceration	Yes	Yes	Yes*	No
Renal impairment	Yes	Yes	Yes	No
Bleeding	Yes	Yes	No	No
MI and stroke	No	Yes	Yes	No
Liver damage with overdose	No	No	No	Yes

*Despite their selectivity for cyclooxygenase-2, coxibs can still cause gastric ulceration, although it may be less than with other nonsteroidal antiinflammatory drugs (NSAIDs).

(e.g., rheumatoid arthritis, osteoarthritis, bursitis), alleviate mild to moderate pain, suppress fever, and relieve dysmenorrhea. Because they cannot inhibit COX-2 without inhibiting COX-1, first-generation NSAIDs cannot suppress inflammation without posing a risk for serious harm: NSAID-induced ulcers are responsible for more than 100,000 hospitalizations and 7000 to 10,000 deaths each year. Aspirin is the oldest member of the family and prototype for the group.

Prototype Drugs

CYCLOOXYGENASE INHIBITORS (ASPIRIN-LIKE DRUGS)

First-Generation Nonsteroidal Antiinflammatory Drugs (NSAIDs)

Aspirin

Ibuprofen

Second-Generation NSAID (Selective Cyclooxygenase-2 Inhibitor)

Celecoxib

Drug That Lacks Antiinflammatory Actions

Acetaminophen

Aspirin

Aspirin is a highly valuable and effective medication. The drug provides excellent relief of mild to moderate pain, reduces fever, protects against thrombotic disorders, and remains a drug of choice for rheumatoid arthritis and other inflammatory conditions. Despite the introduction of many new NSAIDs, aspirin remains one of the most widely used members of the group and is the standard against which the others must be compared.

Chemistry

Aspirin belongs to a chemical family known as *salicylates.* All members of this group are derivatives of salicylic acid. Aspirin is produced by substituting an acetyl group onto salicylic acid. Because of this acetyl group, aspirin is commonly known as *acetylsalicylic acid,* or simply ASA.

Mechanism of Action

Aspirin is a nonselective inhibitor of cyclooxygenase. Most beneficial effects—reductions of inflammation, pain, and fever—result from inhibiting COX-2. One beneficial effect—protection against MI and ischemic stroke—results from inhibiting COX-1. Major adverse effects—gastric ulceration, bleeding, and renal impairment—result from inhibiting COX-1.

It is important to note that aspirin is an *irreversible* inhibitor of cyclooxygenase. In contrast, all other NSAIDs are *reversible* (competitive) inhibitors. Because inhibition of cyclooxygenase by aspirin is irreversible, duration of action depends on how quickly specific tissues can synthesize new molecules of COX-1 and COX-2. With other NSAIDs, effects decline as soon as drug levels fall.

Pharmacokinetics

Absorption

Aspirin is absorbed rapidly and completely after oral dosing. The principal site of absorption is the small intestine. When administered by rectal suppository, aspirin is absorbed slowly, and blood levels are lower than with oral dosing.

Metabolism

Aspirin has a very short half-life (15–20 minutes) owing to rapid conversion to *salicylic acid,* an *active* metabolite. The rate of inactivation of salicylic acid depends on the amount present: at low therapeutic levels, salicylic acid has a half-life of approximately 2 hours, but at high therapeutic levels, the half-life may exceed 20 hours.

Distribution

Salicylic acid is extensively bound to plasma albumin. At therapeutic levels, binding is between 80% and 90%. Aspirin undergoes distribution to all body tissues and fluids, including breast milk, fetal tissues, and the central nervous system (CNS).

Excretion

Salicylic acid and its metabolites are excreted by the kidneys. Excretion of salicylic acid is highly dependent on urinary pH. Accordingly, by raising the pH of urine from 6 to 8, we can increase the rate of excretion fourfold.

Plasma Drug Levels

Low therapeutic doses of aspirin produce plasma salicylate levels less than100 mcg/mL. Antiinflammatory doses produce salicylate levels of about 150 to 300 mcg/mL. Signs of salicylism (toxicity) begin when plasma salicylate levels exceed 200 mcg/mL. Severe toxicity occurs at levels above 400 mcg/mL.

Therapeutic Uses

Suppression of Inflammation

Aspirin is an initial drug of choice for rheumatoid arthritis, osteoarthritis, and juvenile arthritis. Aspirin is also indicated for other inflammatory disorders, including rheumatic fever, tendinitis, and bursitis. The dosages employed to suppress inflammation are considerably larger than dosages used for analgesia or reduction of fever. The use of aspirin and other NSAIDs to treat arthritis is discussed further in Chapter 57.

The precise mechanisms by which aspirin decreases inflammation have not been established. We do know that prostanoids contribute to several components of the inflammatory process. Hence inhibition of COX-2 provides a partial explanation of antiinflammatory effects. Other possible mechanisms include modulation of T-cell function, suppression of inflammatory cell infiltration, and stabilization of lysosomes.

Analgesia

Aspirin is used widely to relieve mild to moderate pain. The degree of analgesia produced depends on the type of pain. Aspirin is most active against joint pain, muscle pain, and headache. For some forms of postoperative pain, aspirin can be more effective than opioids. However, aspirin is relatively ineffective against severe pain of visceral origin. In contrast to opioid analgesics, aspirin produces neither tolerance nor physical dependence. In addition, aspirin is safer than opioids.

Aspirin relieves pain primarily through actions in the periphery. At sites of injury, prostanoids sensitize pain receptors to mechanical and chemical stimulation. Aspirin reduces pain by inhibiting COX-2, thereby suppressing prostanoid production. In addition to this peripheral mechanism, aspirin works in the CNS to help relieve pain.

Reduction of Fever

Aspirin is a drug of choice for reducing temperature in febrile *adults*. However, because of the risk for Reye syndrome (see later), *aspirin should not be used to treat fever in children.* Although aspirin readily reduces fever, it will not lower normal body temperature, nor will it lower temperature that has become elevated in response to physical activity or to a rise in environmental temperature.

Body temperature is regulated by the hypothalamus, which maintains a balance between heat production and heat loss. Fever occurs when the set point of the hypothalamus becomes elevated, causing the hypothalamus to increase heat production and decrease heat loss. Set-point elevation is triggered by local synthesis of prostaglandins in response to endogenous pyrogens (fever-promoting substances). Aspirin lowers the set point by inhibiting COX-2 and thereby inhibits pyrogen-induced synthesis of prostaglandins.

Dysmenorrhea

Aspirin can provide relief from primary dysmenorrhea. Benefits derive from inhibiting prostaglandin synthesis in uterine smooth muscle. (Prostaglandins promote uterine contraction, so suppression of prostaglandin synthesis relieves cramping.) Some of the newer aspirin-like drugs (e.g., ibuprofen, naproxen) are superior to aspirin for dysmenorrhea. The efficacy of the newer drugs is attributed to a greater ability to inhibit COX in the uterus.

Suppression of Platelet Aggregation

Synthesis of TXA_2 in platelets promotes aggregation. Aspirin suppresses platelet aggregation by causing *irreversible* inhibition of COX-1, the enzyme that makes TXA_2. Because platelets lack the machinery to synthesize new COX-1, the effects of a single dose persist for the life of the platelet (about 8 days).

There is a large body of evidence demonstrating that aspirin, through its antiplatelet actions, can benefit a variety of patients. Accordingly, the U.S. Food and Drug Administration (FDA) recommended wider use of aspirin for antiplatelet effects. Professional labeling now recommends daily aspirin for men and women with the following:

- *Ischemic stroke* (to reduce the risk for death and nonfatal stroke)
- *Transient ischemic attacks* (to reduce the risk for death and nonfatal stroke)
- *Acute MI* (to reduce the risk for vascular mortality)
- *Previous MI* (to reduce the combined risk for death and nonfatal MI)
- *Chronic stable angina* (to reduce the risk of MI and sudden death)
- *Unstable angina* (to reduce the combined risk for death and nonfatal MI)
- *Angioplasty and other revascularization procedures* (in patients who have a preexisting condition for which aspirin is already indicated)

According to a review published in the *Journal of the American Medical Association*—"Aspirin Dose for the Prevention of Cardiovascular Disease"—a dose of 75 to 81 mg/day for these indications is adequate. Higher doses, which are commonly prescribed in these circumstances, offer no greater protection but will increase the risk for gastrointestinal (GI) bleeding.

In addition to these applications, aspirin can be taken by healthy people for *primary prevention* of MI and stroke. However, more recent studies show that aspirin provides less protection against cardiovascular disease than once thought. The potential small benefit must be weighed against the major risk of aspirin use, namely, GI hemorrhage. Hence, to determine the *net* benefit of primary prevention for any man or woman, we must determine his or her individual risk for a GI bleed and compare that risk with his or her individual risk for a cardiovascular event (i.e., the risk for an MI in men, or the risk for ischemic stroke in women).[a] Many organizations, including the American Heart Association (AHA), the American Thoracic Society, and the European Society of Cardiology, recommend against the use of aspirin for primary prevention of cardiovascular disease unless the patient has a 10-year risk greater than 10%.

How do we calculate 10-year risk for a cardiovascular event? Risk for an MI or stroke can be assessed using the calculator at http://cvdrisk.nhlbi.nih.gov/.

Cancer Prevention

Colorectal Cancer. There is good evidence that regular use of aspirin decreases the risk for colorectal cancer, even when the dosage is low. Results from the Nurses' Health Study showed that regular use of *high-dose* aspirin (650 mg/day or more) reduces the risk for colorectal cancer. This dosage is much greater than that used to prevent cardiovascular disease and hence poses a significant risk for bleeding. In fact, for every one or two cancers prevented, high-dose aspirin would cause eight additional serious bleeds. Fortunately, more recent studies indicate that *low-dose* aspirin is effective, too. For example, results of a study reported in *The Lancet* in 2010 indicate that taking low-dose aspirin (75–300 mg/day) for more than 5 years reduces the incidence of colorectal cancer (by 24%) as well as mortality from colon cancer (by 35%). At these low doses, the benefits of cancer protection may well outweigh the risk for possible bleeding and other adverse events.

Aspirin protects against colorectal cancer probably by inhibiting COX-2. In animal models, COX-2 promotes tumor growth and metastases, and inhibition of COX-2 slows tumor growth. In humans, most colorectal cancers express COX-2. Furthermore, protection by aspirin is limited to colon cancers that have high COX-2 levels. Aspirin does not protect against colon cancers with little or no COX-2.

---

[a]Major factors that increase the risk for a GI bleed are use of NSAIDs and a history of ulcers. Major risk factors for an MI are advancing age, diabetes, high total cholesterol, low HDL cholesterol, and smoking. Major risk factors for an ischemic stroke are advancing age, hypertension, diabetes, smoking, atrial fibrillation, left ventricular hypertrophy, and a history of cardiovascular disease.

Other Cancers. Available data suggest that protection may not be limited to colorectal cancer. Results of a meta-analysis reported in *The Lancet*, "Effect of daily aspirin on long-term risk of death due to cancer: analysis of individual patient data from randomised trials," show that daily low-dose aspirin reduces the risk for death from *all* solid tumors (by 34%), but does not reduce the risk for death from hematologic cancers. In addition, *The Lancet* published an additional article in 2012 that analyzed 5 randomized controlled trials. This analysis determined that use of aspirin may also prevent distant metastasis of tumors that already exist. Earlier studies have shown protection against specific cancers. In a study involving men older than 60 years, daily use of aspirin and other NSAIDs was associated with a 50% decrease in the incidence of prostate cancer. In a study involving 2884 women, aspirin appeared to reduce the risk for breast cancer, especially among women with hormone receptor–positive tumors and among those who took 7 or more aspirin tablets a week. In another study, taking aspirin at least 3 times a week for at least 6 months was associated with a 40% reduction in the incidence of ovarian cancer. In contrast to these positive results, results from the Women's Health Study found no protection with low-dose aspirin against cancer of the breast, colon, or any other tissue. The reasons for this discrepancy are not clear. Four additional studies are currently underway to examine various effects of aspirin on cancer prevention.

Adverse Effects

When administered short term in analgesic or antipyretic (fever-reducing) doses, aspirin rarely causes serious adverse effects. However, toxicity is common when treating inflammatory disorders, which require long-term high-dose treatment.

Gastrointestinal Effects

The most common side effects are *gastric distress, heartburn,* and *nausea.* These can be reduced by taking aspirin with food or a full glass of water.

Occult GI bleeding occurs often. In most cases, the amount of blood lost each day is insignificant. However, with chronic aspirin use, cumulative blood loss can produce anemia.

Long-term aspirin—*even in low doses*—can cause life-threatening *gastric ulceration, perforation,* and *bleeding.* Ulcers result from four causes:

- Increased secretion of acid and pepsin
- Decreased production of cytoprotective mucus and bicarbonate
- Decreased submucosal blood flow
- The direct irritant action of aspirin on the gastric mucosa

The first three occur secondary to inhibition of COX-1. Direct injury to the stomach is most likely with aspirin preparations that dissolve slowly: owing to slow dissolution, particulate aspirin becomes entrapped in folds of the stomach wall, causing prolonged exposure to high concentrations of the drug. Because aspirin-induced ulcers are often asymptomatic, perforation and upper GI hemorrhage can occur without premonitory signs. (Hemorrhage is due in part to erosion of the stomach wall and in part to suppression of platelet aggregation.) Factors that increase the risk for ulceration include the following:

- Advanced age
- A history of peptic ulcer disease
- Previous intolerance to aspirin or other NSAIDs
- Cigarette smoking
- History of alcohol abuse (Alcohol intensifies the irritant effects of aspirin and should not be consumed.)

What can we do to *prevent* ulcers? According to an expert panel—convened in 2008 by the American College of Gastroenterology, the AHA, and the American College of Cardiology—prophylaxis with a *proton pump inhibitor* (PPI) is recommended for patients at risk, including those with a history of peptic ulcers, those taking glucocorticoids, and older adults. Proton pump inhibitors (e.g., omeprazole, lansoprazole) reduce ulcer generation by suppressing production of gastric acid. In addition to PPIs, other drugs that may be considered include histamine-2 receptor antagonists (H_2RAs) and misoprostol. COX-2 inhibitors may also be tried instead of traditional NSAIDs because they are thought to produce fewer GI side effects. Because many ulcers are caused by infection with *Helicobacter pylori* (see Chapter 62), the panel recommends that patients with ulcer histories undergo testing and treatment for *H. pylori* before starting long-term aspirin use. *Treatment* of NSAID-induced ulcers is discussed in Chapter 62.

Bleeding

Aspirin promotes bleeding by inhibiting platelet aggregation. Taking just two 325-mg aspirin tablets can double bleeding time for about 1 week. (Recall that platelets are unable to replace aspirin-inactivated cyclooxygenase, and hence bleeding time is prolonged for the life of the platelet.) Because of its effects on platelets, *aspirin is contraindicated for patients with bleeding disorders* (e.g., hemophilia, vitamin K deficiency, hypoprothrombinemia). To minimize blood loss during childbirth and elective surgery, *high-dose* aspirin should be discontinued at least 1 week before these procedures. There is no need to stop aspirin before procedures with a low risk for bleeding (e.g., dental, dermatologic, or cataract surgery). In most cases, use of *low-dose* aspirin to protect against thrombosis should *not* be interrupted for elective surgery and dental procedures. Caution is needed when aspirin is used in conjunction with anticoagulants.

In patients taking daily aspirin, high blood pressure increases the risk for hemorrhagic stroke, even though aspirin protects against ischemic stroke. To reduce risk for hemorrhagic stroke, blood pressure should be 150/90 mm Hg (and preferably lower) before starting daily aspirin.

Renal Impairment

Aspirin can cause acute, reversible impairment of renal function, resulting in salt and water retention and edema. Clinically significant effects are most likely in patients with additional risk factors: advanced age, existing renal impairment, hypovolemia, hepatic cirrhosis, or heart failure. Aspirin impairs renal function by inhibiting COX-1, thereby depriving the kidney of prostaglandins needed for normal function.

Development of renal impairment is signaled by reduced urine output, weight gain despite use of diuretics, and a rapid rise in serum creatinine and blood urea nitrogen. If any of these occurs, aspirin should be withdrawn immediately. In most cases, kidney function then returns to baseline level.

The risk for acute renal impairment can be reduced by identifying high-risk patients and treating them with the smallest dosages possible.

In addition to its acute effects on renal function, aspirin may pose a risk for renal papillary necrosis and other types of renal injury when used long term.

Salicylism

Salicylism is a syndrome that begins to develop when aspirin levels climb just slightly above therapeutic. Overt signs include *tinnitus, sweating, headache,* and *dizziness.* Acid-base disturbance may also occur (see later). If salicylism develops, aspirin should be withheld until symptoms subside. Aspirin should then resume, but with a small reduction in dosage. In some cases, development of tinnitus can be used to adjust aspirin dosage: when tinnitus occurs, the maximal acceptable dose has been achieved. However, this guideline may be inappropriate for older patients because they may fail to develop tinnitus even when aspirin levels become toxic.

Acid-base disturbance results from the effects of aspirin on respiration. When administered in high therapeutic doses, aspirin acts on the CNS to stimulate breathing. The resultant increase in CO_2 loss produces *respiratory alkalosis.* In response, the kidneys excrete more bicarbonate. There is also a subsequent buildup of acids, producing a resultant metabolic acidosis. Thus many patients that present with salicylate toxicity will have a mixed acid-base imbalance.

Reye Syndrome

Use of aspirin in children younger than 18 years is associated with Reye syndrome.

This syndrome is a rare but serious illness of childhood that has a mortality rate of 20% to 30%. Characteristic symptoms are encephalopathy and fatty liver degeneration. Epidemiologic data suggested a relationship between Reye syndrome and use of aspirin by children who have influenza or chickenpox. Although a direct causal link between aspirin and Reye syndrome was never established, the Centers for Disease Control and Prevention recommended that aspirin (and other NSAIDs) be avoided by children and teenagers suspected of having influenza or chickenpox. In response to this recommendation, aspirin was removed from most products intended for children, and aspirin use by children declined sharply. As a result, Reye syndrome essentially vanished: the incidence declined from a high of 555 cases in 1980 to no more than 2 cases per year since 1994. If a child with chickenpox or influenza needs an analgesic-antipyretic, acetaminophen can be used safely.

Adverse Effects Associated With Use During Pregnancy

Aspirin poses risks to the pregnant patient and her fetus. Accordingly, the drug is classified in *FDA Pregnancy Risk Category D: there is evidence of human fetal risk, but the potential benefits from use of the drug during pregnancy may outweigh the potential for harm.* The principal risks to pregnant women are (1) anemia (from GI blood loss) and (2) postpartum hemorrhage. In addition, by inhibiting prostaglandin synthesis, aspirin may suppress spontaneous uterine contractions and may thereby prolong labor.

Aspirin crosses the placenta and may adversely affect the fetus. Because prostaglandins help keep the ductus arteriosus patent, inhibition of prostaglandin synthesis by aspirin may induce premature closure of the ductus arteriosus. Aspirin use has also been associated with low birth weight, stillbirth, renal toxicity, intracranial hemorrhage in preterm infants, and neonatal death.

Hypersensitivity Reactions

Hypersensitivity develops in about 0.3% of aspirin users. Reactions are most likely in adults with a history of asthma, rhinitis, and nasal polyps. Hypersensitivity reactions are uncommon in children. The aspirin hypersensitivity reaction begins with profuse, watery rhinorrhea and may progress to generalized urticaria, bronchospasm, laryngeal edema, and shock. Despite its resemblance to severe anaphylaxis, this reaction is not allergic and is not mediated by the immune system. What *does* cause these reactions? Because individuals who react to aspirin are also sensitive to most other NSAIDs, we believe that the reactions are due to inhibition of COX-1, which triggers production of leukotrienes, which in turn causes bronchospasm, hives, and other signs of hypersensitivity. However, if this *is* the mechanism, it remains unclear why hypersensitivity is limited mainly to adults with the predisposing conditions noted earlier. As with severe anaphylactic reactions, *epinephrine* is the treatment of choice.

Hypersensitivity to aspirin is considered a contraindication to using other drugs with aspirin-like properties. Nonetheless, if an aspirin-like drug must be taken, four such drugs are probably safe. One of these—celecoxib—is selective for COX-2. Another—meloxicam—is somewhat selective for COX-2, but only at low doses. The other two—acetaminophen and salsalate—are only weak inhibitors of COX-1.

Cardiovascular Events

In contrast to all other NSAIDs, aspirin does *NOT* increase the risk for thrombotic events, including MI and ischemic stroke. In fact, when taken in low doses, aspirin *protects* against these events.

Erectile Dysfunction

Daily use of aspirin and other NSAIDs is associated with a 22% increase in the risk for erectile dysfunction, as shown in a study of 80,966 men in California. However, a causal relationship has not been established.

Summary of Precautions and Contraindications

Aspirin is contraindicated in patients with *peptic ulcer disease, bleeding disorders* (e.g., hemophilia, vitamin K deficiency, hypoprothrombinemia), and *hypersensitivity to aspirin itself or other NSAIDs.* In addition, the drug should be used with extreme caution by *pregnant women and by children who have chickenpox or influenza.* Caution should also be exercised when treating *older-adult patients, patients who smoke cigarettes,* and *patients with* H. pylori *infection, heart failure, hepatic cirrhosis, hypovolemia, renal dysfunction, asthma, hay fever, chronic urticaria, nasal polyps,* or *a history of alcoholism.* Aspirin should be withdrawn 1 week before elective surgery or the anticipated date of childbirth.

Drug Interactions

Because of its widespread use, aspirin has been reported to interact with many other medications. However, most of these interactions have little clinical significance. Significant interactions are discussed next.

PATIENT-CENTERED CARE ACROSS THE LIFE SPAN

Nonsteroidal Antiinflammatory Drugs

Life Stage	Patient Care Concerns
Infants	Because of the risk for Reye syndrome, aspirin should be avoided in infants. Acetaminophen and ibuprofen can be used safely in small doses for fever.
Children/adolescents	Because of the risk for Reye syndrome, aspirin should be avoided in children and adolescents. Acetaminophen and ibuprofen can be used safely in small doses for fever.
Pregnant women	NSAIDs may result in premature closure of the ductus arteriosus. Therefore their use is contraindicated in the third trimester of pregnancy.
Breastfeeding women	NSAIDs and acetaminophen appear safe for use in breastfeeding mothers.
Older adults	NSAIDs are the most common drug used to treat chronic pain in older adults. These drugs have been shown to increase hospital admissions in this population. Caution should be used with NSAIDs in older adults.

Anticoagulants: Warfarin, Heparin, and Others

Aspirin's most important interactions are with anticoagulants. Because aspirin suppresses platelet function and can decrease prothrombin production, aspirin can intensify the effects of warfarin, heparin, and other anticoagulants. Furthermore, because aspirin can initiate gastric bleeding, augmenting anticoagulant effects can increase the risk for gastric hemorrhage. Accordingly, the combination of aspirin with anticoagulants must be used with care—even when aspirin is taken in low doses to reduce the risk for thrombotic events.

Glucocorticoids

Like aspirin, glucocorticoids promote gastric ulceration. As a result, the risk for ulcers is greatly increased when these drugs are combined—as may happen when treating arthritis. To reduce the risk for gastric ulceration, patients can be given a PPI or H_2RA for prophylaxis.

Alcohol

Combining alcohol with aspirin and other NSAIDs increases the risk for gastric bleeding. To alert the public to this risk, the FDA now requires that labels for aspirin include the following statement: ***Alcohol Warning:*** *If you consume three or more alcoholic drinks every day, ask your doctor whether you should take aspirin or other pain relievers/fever reducers. Aspirin [and related drugs] may cause stomach bleeding.* A similar label is required for all other NSAIDs and acetaminophen.

Nonaspirin NSAIDs

Ibuprofen, naproxen, and other nonaspirin NSAIDs can reduce the antiplatelet effects of aspirin by blocking access of aspirin to COX-1 in platelets. This interaction is important: in patients taking low-dose aspirin to prevent MI or ischemic stroke, other NSAIDs could negate aspirin's benefits. Because immediate-release aspirin produces complete platelet inhibition about 1 hour after dosing, we can prevent interference by giving aspirin about 2 hours before giving other NSAIDs. Of course, we could eliminate interference entirely by using high-dose aspirin, rather than another NSAID, when conditions call for NSAID therapy.

ACE Inhibitors and ARBs

Like aspirin, angiotensin-converting enzyme (ACE) inhibitors and angiotensin receptor blockers (ARBs) can impair renal function. In susceptible patients, combining aspirin with drugs in either class can increase the risk for acute renal failure. High-dose aspirin should be avoided in patients taking these drugs. However, low-dose aspirin taken for antiplatelet effects should be continued.

Vaccines

Aspirin and other NSAIDs may blunt the immune response to vaccines. Accordingly, these drugs should not be used routinely to prevent vaccination-associated fever and pain.

Acute Poisoning

Aspirin overdose is a common cause of poisoning. Although rarely fatal in adults, aspirin poisoning may be lethal in children. The lethal dose for adults is 20 to 25 g. In contrast, as little as 4000 mg (4 g) can kill a child.

Signs and Symptoms

Initially, aspirin overdose produces a state of compensated respiratory alkalosis—the same state seen in mild salicylism. As poisoning progresses, respiratory excitation is replaced with respiratory depression. Acidosis, hyperthermia, sweating, and dehydration are prominent, and electrolyte imbalance is likely. Stupor and coma result from effects in the CNS. Death usually results from respiratory failure.

Treatment

Aspirin poisoning is an acute medical emergency that requires hospitalization. The immediate threats to life are respiratory depression, hyperthermia, dehydration, and acidosis. Treatment is largely supportive. If respiration is inadequate, mechanical ventilation should be instituted. External cooling (e.g., sponging with tepid water) can help reduce hyperthermia. Intravenous fluids are given to correct dehydration; the composition of these fluids is determined by electrolyte and acid-base status. Slow infusion of bicarbonate is given to reverse acidosis. Several measures (e.g., gastric lavage, giving activated charcoal) can reduce further GI absorption of aspirin. Alkalinization of the urine with bicarbonate accelerates excretion of aspirin and salicylate. If necessary, hemodialysis or peritoneal dialysis can be used to remove salicylates.

Formulations

Aspirin is available in multiple formulations, including plain and buffered tablets, enteric-coated preparations, and tablets used to produce a buffered solution. These different formulations reflect efforts to increase rates of absorption and decrease gastric irritation. For the most part, the clinical utility of the more complex formulations is no greater than that of plain aspirin tablets.

Aspirin Tablets, Plain

All brands are essentially the same with respect to analgesic efficacy, onset, and duration. Some less expensive tablets have greater particle size, which results in slower dissolution and prolonged contact with the gastric mucosa, which increases gastric irritation. When aspirin tablets decompose, they smell like vinegar (acetic acid) and should be discarded.

Aspirin Tablets, Buffered

The amount of buffer in buffered aspirin tablets is too small to produce significant elevation of gastric pH. An equivalent effect on pH can be achieved by taking plain aspirin tablets with food or a glass of water. Buffered aspirin tablets are no different from plain tablets with respect to analgesic effects and gastric distress. Buffered tablets may dissolve faster than plain tablets, resulting in somewhat faster onset.

Buffered Aspirin Solution

A buffered aspirin solution is produced by dissolving effervescent aspirin tablets [Alka-Seltzer] in a glass of water. This solution has considerable buffering capacity owing to its high content of sodium bicarbonate. Effects on gastric pH are sufficient to decrease the incidence of gastric irritation and bleeding. In addition, aspirin absorption is accelerated and peak blood levels are raised. Unfortunately, these benefits come with a price. The sodium content of buffered aspirin solution can be detrimental to individuals on a sodium-restricted diet. Also, absorption of bicarbonate can elevate urinary pH, which will accelerate aspirin excretion. Lastly, this highly buffered preparation is expensive. Because of this combination of benefits and drawbacks, the buffered aspirin solution is well suited for occasional use but is generally inappropriate for long-term therapy.

Enteric-Coated Preparations

Enteric-coated preparations dissolve in the intestine rather than the stomach, thereby reducing gastric irritation. Unfortunately, absorption from these formulations can be delayed and erratic. Patients should be advised not to crush or chew them.

Timed-Release Tablets

Timed-release tablets offer no advantage over plain aspirin tablets. Because the half-life of salicylic acid is long to begin with, and because aspirin produces irreversible inhibition of cyclooxygenase, timed-release tablets cannot prolong effects.

Rectal Suppositories

Rectal suppositories have been employed for patients who cannot take aspirin orally. Absorption can be variable, resulting in plasma drug levels that are insufficient in some patients and excessive in others. Also, rectal irritation can occur. Because of these undesirable properties, aspirin suppositories are not generally recommended.

Dosage and Administration

Aspirin is almost always administered by mouth. Gastric irritation can be minimized by dosing with water or food. Dosage depends on the age of the patient and the condition being treated. Adult and pediatric dosages for major indications are shown in Table 55.3.

TABLE 55.3 ■ Aspirin Dosage

Indication	Adult Dosage	Pediatric Dosage*
Aches and pains, fever	325–650 mg every 4 h as needed	*2–3 yr:* 160 mg *4–5 yr:* 240 mg *6–8 yr:* 325 mg *9–10 yr:* 405 mg *11 yr:* 485 mg *Over 11 yr:* 650 mg All of these doses are administered every 4 h as needed
Acute rheumatic fever	5–8 g/day in divided doses	100 mg/kg/day (initially), then 75 mg/kg/day for 4–6 wk
Rheumatoid arthritis	3.6–5.4 g/day in divided doses	90–130 mg/kg/day in divided doses every 4–6 h
SUPPRESSION OF PLATELET AGGREGATION		
Initial therapy	325 mg once a day	
Chronic therapy	80 mg once a day	

*Owing to the risk for Reye syndrome, aspirin is usually avoided in patients younger than 18 years.

Nonaspirin First-Generation Nonsteroidal Antiinflammatory Drugs

In attempts to produce an aspirin-like drug with fewer GI, renal, and hemorrhagic effects than aspirin, the pharmaceutical industry has produced a large number of drugs with actions much like those of aspirin. In the United States more than 20 nonaspirin NSAIDs are available (Table 55.4). Like aspirin, all other first-generation NSAIDs inhibit both COX-1 and COX-2. However, in contrast to aspirin, which causes *irreversible* inhibition of cyclooxygenase, the other traditional NSAIDs cause *reversible* inhibition. All of these drugs have antiinflammatory, analgesic, and antipyretic properties. In addition, they all can cause gastric ulceration, bleeding, and renal impairment—although the intensity of these effects may be less with some agents. Patients who are hypersensitive to aspirin are likely to experience cross-hypersensitivity with other NSAIDs. For most NSAIDs, safety during pregnancy has not been established, and hence use by pregnant women is discouraged.

The principal indications for the nonaspirin NSAIDs are rheumatoid arthritis and osteoarthritis. In addition, certain NSAIDs are used to treat fever, bursitis, tendinitis, mild to moderate pain, and dysmenorrhea (see Table 55.4).

In contrast to aspirin, the nonaspirin NSAIDs *do not* protect against MI and stroke. In fact, they *increase* the risk for thrombotic events. For the NSAIDs as a group, the increase in cardiovascular risk is relatively low—about 12%. Risk is highest with indomethacin (71%), sulindac (41%), and meloxicam (37%). However, although the increase in risk with these drugs appears high, it pales in comparison with smoking, which increases cardiovascular risk by 200% to 300%. To minimize cardiovascular risk, nonaspirin NSAIDs should be used in the lowest effective dosage for the shortest time needed. Also, these drugs should not be used before coronary artery bypass graft (CABG) surgery or for 14 days after. Other measures to reduce risk are discussed later under "American Heart Association Statement on Cyclooxygenase Inhibitors in Chronic Pain."

Although individual NSAIDs differ chemically, pharmacokinetically, and to some extent pharmacodynamically, all are similar clinically: they all produce essentially equivalent antiinflammatory effects, and they all present a similar risk for serious adverse effects (gastric ulceration, bleeding, renal impairment, MI, and stroke). However, for reasons that are not understood, individual patients may respond better to one agent than another. Furthermore, individual patients may tolerate one NSAID better than another. Therefore to optimize

TABLE 55.4 ■ Clinical Pharmacology of the Oral Nonsteroidal Antiinflammatory Drugs

Drug	Maximal Daily Dosage (mg)	Plasma Half-Life (h)	Major Indications[a]				
			Arthritis	Moderate Pain	Fever	Dysmenorrhea	Bursitis/ Tendinitis
FIRST-GENERATION NSAIDS							
Salicylates							
Aspirin (many trade names)	8000	0.2–0.3	A	A	A		
Magnesium salicylate [Doan's Tablets, others]	4640	2–30[b]	A	A	A		
Sodium salicylate* (generic)	3900	2–30[b]	A	A	A		
Salsalate	3000	2–30[b]	A	A	A		
Propionic Acid Derivatives							
Fenoprofen [Nalfon]	3200	3	A	A			
Flurbiprofen (generic)	300	5.7	A	I	I	I	I
Ibuprofen [Advil, Motrin, others][c]	3200	1.8–2	A	A	A	A	
Ketoprofen (generic)	300	2	A	A		A	
Naproxen [Aleve, others][d]	1375	12–17	A	A	A	A	A
Oxaprozin [Daypro]	1800	42–50	A				
Others							
Diclofenac [Cambia, Cataflam, Voltaren XR, Zipsor, Zorvolex][e]	200	2	A	A		A	
Diflunisal (generic)	1500	11–15	A	A			
Etodolac (generic)	1200	7.3	A	A			I
Indomethacin [Indocin]	200	4.5	A				A
Ketorolac (generic)[f]	40 PO 120 IV	5–6	A[g]				
Meclofenamate (generic)	400	1.3	A	A		A	
Mefenamic acid [Ponstel, Ponstan ♣]	1000	2		A		A	
Meloxicam [Mobic, Mobicox ♣]	15	15–20	A				
Nabumetone (generic)	2000	22	A				
Piroxicam [Feldene]	20	50	A				
Sulindac [Clinoril]	400	7.8	A				A
Tolmetin (generic)	1800	2–7	A				
SECOND-GENERATION NSAIDS (COX-2 INHIBITORS)							
Celecoxib [Celebrex]	800	11	A	A		A	

[a]A, U.S. Food and Drug Administration–approved indication; I, investigational use.
[b]Half-life increases with increasing dosage.
[c]Ibuprofen is also available in two *intravenous* formulations, sold as Caldolor and NeoProfen.
[d]Naproxen is also available in a fixed-dose combination with esomeprazole sold as Vimovo.
[e]Diclofenac is also available in three *topical* formulations, sold as Flector Patch, Pennsaid, and Voltaren Gel, and in a fixed-dose combination with misoprostol sold as Arthrotec.
[f]Ketorolac is also available in an *intravenous* formulation, sold generically, and in an *intranasal* formulation, sold as Sprix.
[g]Ketorolac is approved only for *acute* pain; use should not exceed 5 days.
*Available as a combination pill with methenamine, sold as Cystex.
COX-2, cyclooxygenase-2; IV, intravenous; NSAID, nonsteroidal antiinflammatory drug; PO, oral.

therapy for each patient, trials with more than one NSAID may be needed.

Ibuprofen

Basic Pharmacology

Ibuprofen [Advil, Motrin, Caldolor, others] is the prototype of the propionic acid derivatives. Other members of the family are shown in Table 55.4 and discussed individually below. Like aspirin, ibuprofen inhibits cyclooxygenase and has antiinflammatory, analgesic, and antipyretic actions. The drug is used to treat fever, mild to moderate pain, and arthritis. In addition, ibuprofen appears superior to most other NSAIDs for relief of primary dysmenorrhea, presumably because it produces good inhibition of cyclooxygenase in uterine smooth muscle. In clinical trials, ibuprofen was highly effective at promoting closure of the ductus arteriosus in preterm infants, a condition for which indomethacin is the current treatment of choice.

Ibuprofen is generally well tolerated, and the incidence of adverse effects is low. The drug produces less gastric bleeding than aspirin and less inhibition of platelet aggregation as well. Consequently, ibuprofen is among the safer NSAIDs for use with anticoagulants. Very rarely, ibuprofen has been associated with Stevens-Johnson syndrome, a severe hypersensitivity reaction that causes blistering of the skin and mucous membranes and can result in scarring, blindness, and even death. Like other nonaspirin NSAIDs, ibuprofen may pose a risk for MI and stroke.

Oral Preparations and Dosages

Ibuprofen, by itself, is available in five oral formulations: (1) standard tablets (100, 200, 400, 600, and 800 mg); (2) chewable tablets (50 and 100 mg); (3) capsules (200 mg); (4) a 20-mg/mL oral suspension [Children's Advil, Children's Motrin, PediaCare Fever]; and (5) a 40-mg/mL oral suspension [Advil Pediatric Drops, Motrin Infant's, PediaCare Fever]. Administration with meals or milk can reduce gastric distress.

Dosages for adults are as follows:

- Arthritis—1.2 to 3.2 g/day administered in three or four divided doses
- Primary dysmenorrhea—400 mg every 4 hours as needed
- Mild to moderate pain—400 mg every 4 to 6 hours as needed

Dosages for children are as follows:

- Juvenile arthritis—30 to 40 mg/kg/day in three or four divided doses
- Fever reduction—5 mg/kg every 6 to 8 hours (for temperatures up to 102.5° F) or 10 mg/kg every 6 to 8 hours (for temperatures above 102.5° F) as needed. The total daily dose should not exceed 40 mg/kg.

Oral ibuprofen is also available in three fixed-dose combinations: (1) ibuprofen/oxycodone [Combunox] for short-term oral therapy of moderate to severe pain, (2) ibuprofen/hydrocodone [Vicoprofen] for short-term oral therapy of moderate to severe pain, and (3) ibuprofen/famotidine [Duexis] for treatment of rheumatoid arthritis and osteoarthritis, while reducing the risk for GI ulcers.

Nonacetylated Salicylates: Magnesium Salicylate, Sodium Salicylate, and Salsalate

Similarities to Aspirin

The nonacetylated salicylates are similar to aspirin (an acetylated salicylate) in most respects. Like aspirin, these drugs inhibit COX-1 and COX-2 and are employed to treat arthritis, moderate pain, and fever. The most common adverse effects are GI disturbances. As with aspirin, these drugs should not be given to children with chickenpox or influenza owing to the possibility of precipitating Reye syndrome.

Contrasts With Aspirin

In contrast to aspirin, the nonacetylated salicylates cause little or no suppression of platelet aggregation. As a result, these drugs cannot protect against MI and stroke and may actually increase risk.

Because of its sodium content, sodium salicylate should be avoided in patients on a sodium-restricted diet (e.g., patients with hypertension or heart failure).

Magnesium salicylate may accumulate to toxic levels in patients with chronic renal insufficiency and hence should not be used by these people.

Salsalate is a prodrug that breaks down to release two molecules of salicylate in the alkaline environment of the small intestine. Because the stomach is not exposed to salicylate, salsalate produces less gastric irritation than aspirin.

Preparations, Dosage, and Administration

Magnesium salicylate [Doan's Tablets, others] is supplied in 580-mg caplets and tablets for oral use. The usual dosage is 1090 mg every 6 hours. The maximal dosage is 4640 mg/day, administered in three or four doses.

Sodium salicylate (generic) is supplied in a combination pill with methenamine marketed as Cystex (162.5 mg/162 mg). Dosing is 2 tablets with a full glass of water 4 times a day for treatment of urinary pain.

Salsalate is supplied in capsules (500 mg) and tablets (500 and 750 mg) for oral use. The usual dosage is 3000 mg/day in divided doses.

Fenoprofen

Fenoprofen [Nalfon] belongs to the propionic acid family of NSAIDs. Like other NSAIDs, the drug inhibits synthesis of prostanoids, thereby causing antiinflammatory, analgesic, and antipyretic effects. Fenoprofen is indicated for arthritis and mild to moderate pain. The most common adverse effects are GI disturbances. Fenoprofen is supplied in tablets (600 mg) and capsules (200 and 400 mg). The usual dosage for mild to moderate pain is 200 mg every 4 to 6 hours as needed. The dosage range for rheumatoid arthritis and osteoarthritis is 300 to 600 mg every 6 to 8 hours, but should not exceed 3.2 g/day.

Flurbiprofen

Flurbiprofen is chemically related to ibuprofen and the other derivatives of propionic acid. The drug is approved for arthritis and has been used investigationally for bursitis, tendinitis, moderate pain, fever, and primary dysmenorrhea. The most common adverse effects are GI disturbances (dyspepsia, nausea, diarrhea, abdominal pain). The risk for serious GI effects (ulceration, perforation, hemorrhage) may be greater than with ibuprofen. Like other NSAIDs, flurbiprofen can exacerbate renal impairment and may pose a risk for MI and stroke. The drug is supplied in tablets (50 and 100 mg) for oral use. The usual dosage for rheumatoid arthritis is 200 to 300 mg/day administered in two to four divided doses.

Ketoprofen

Ketoprofen belongs to the propionic acid family of NSAIDs. The drug inhibits synthesis of prostanoids and has antiinflammatory, analgesic, and antipyretic effects. Indications are rheumatoid arthritis, osteoarthritis, mild to moderate pain, and primary dysmenorrhea. The most common adverse effects are dyspepsia, nausea, vomiting, and abdominal pain. Ketoprofen is supplied in immediate-release capsules (50 and 75 mg) and extended-release capsules (100, 150, and 200 mg). The usual dosage for rheumatoid arthritis is 200 to 225 mg/day administered in three or four divided doses. The dosage for moderate pain or primary dysmenorrhea is 25 to 50 mg every 6 to 8 hours as needed.

Naproxen

Actions and Uses

Naproxen [Aleve, Anaprox, Naprelan, Naprosyn], a member of the propionic acid family of NSAIDs, is highly selective for COX-1. The drug has a prolonged half-life and so can be administered less frequently than other propionic acid derivatives (e.g., ibuprofen). Naproxen is approved for arthritis, bursitis, tendinitis, primary dysmenorrhea, fever, and mild to moderate pain. Like other NSAIDs, the drug acts primarily by inhibiting cyclooxygenase.

Adverse Effects

Naproxen is among the better tolerated NSAIDs. The most common adverse effects are GI disturbances. Like other NSAIDs, the drug can compromise renal function and may increase the risk for MI and stroke. However, because naproxen is COX-1 selective, the risk for MI and stroke appears lower than with other traditional NSAIDs. Bleeding time can be prolonged secondary to reversible inhibition of platelet aggregation.

Preparations, Dosage, and Administration

Naproxen is supplied in immediate-release tablets (220, 250, 275, 375, and 500 mg) sold as Aleve, Anaprox, and Naprosyn; a 550-mg double-strength tablet sold as Anaprox DS; delayed-release enteric-coated tablets (375 and 500 mg) sold as EC-Naprosyn; controlled-release tablets (375, 500, and 750 mg) sold as Naprelan; and an oral suspension (25 mg/mL) sold as Naprosyn and Naproxen. For all products, the usual dosage for rheumatoid arthritis is 250 to 500 mg of naproxen twice daily. The dosage for mild to moderate pain is 500 mg initially followed by 250 mg every 6 to 8 hours as needed.

Naproxen/Esomeprazole [Vimovo]

Vimovo is a fixed-dose combination of naproxen plus esomeprazole, a PPI that blocks production of gastric acid (see Chapter 62), and thereby protects against naproxen-induced ulcers. Vimovo delayed-release tablets are available in two naproxen/esomeprazole strengths: 375 mg/20 mg and 500 mg/20 mg. For patients with osteoarthritis, rheumatoid arthritis, or ankylosing spondylitis, the usual dosage is 1 tablet twice daily.

Oxaprozin

Oxaprozin [Daypro] belongs to the propionic acid family of NSAIDs. Approved uses are rheumatoid arthritis and osteoarthritis. As with other NSAIDs, benefits derive from inhibiting synthesis of prostanoids. Like other propionic acid derivatives, oxaprozin is generally well tolerated. The drug has an unusually long half-life (42–50 hours) and hence can be administered just once a day. Oxaprozin is available in 600-mg tablets. The dosage for arthritis is 1200 mg once a day. The maximal dosage is 1800 mg/day.

Diclofenac

Oral

Oral diclofenac [Voltaren XR, Cataflam, Cambia, Zipsor, Zorvolex] is approved for rheumatoid arthritis, osteoarthritis, ankylosing spondylitis, mild pain, primary dysmenorrhea, and migraine. As with other NSAIDs, antiinflammatory, analgesic, and antipyretic effects result from inhibiting cyclooxygenase. Diclofenac is well absorbed after oral administration but undergoes extensive (40%–50%) metabolism on its first pass through the liver. In the blood, about 99.5% of the drug is protein bound, primarily to albumin. Diclofenac is metabolized by the liver and excreted in the urine.

The most common adverse effects are abdominal pain, dyspepsia, and nausea. By impairing renal function, diclofenac can cause fluid retention, which can exacerbate hypertension and heart failure. Diclofenac can cause severe liver injury, even with topical therapy. Accordingly, patients should receive periodic tests of liver function and should be instructed to report manifestations of liver injury (e.g., jaundice, fatigue, nausea). If liver injury is diagnosed, diclofenac should be discontinued.

Diclofenac is supplied in immediate-release tablets (50 mg) as Cataflam, generic enteric-coated delayed-release tablets (25, 50, and 75 mg), extended-release tablets (100 mg) as Voltaren XR, liquid-filled capsules (25 mg) as Zipsor, immediate-release tablets (18 and 35 mg) as Zorvolex, and a powder for oral solution (50 mg) as Cambia. The dosage for rheumatoid arthritis is 150 to 200 mg/day administered in two or three divided doses. The dosage for osteoarthritis is 100 to 150 mg/day administered in two or three divided doses. The Zorvolex dose for mild to moderate pain is 54 to 105 mg/day administered in three divided doses.

Topical

Diclofenac is available in three topical formulations—Voltaren Gel, Flector Patch, and Pennsaid (solution)—for treatment of pain and inflammation. Voltaren Gel is for osteoarthritis, Flector Patch is for minor pain, and Pennsaid is for osteoarthritis of the knee. A fourth topical formulation—Solaraze—is used for actinic keratoses (see Chapter 85). Topical diclofenac is more expensive than oral diclofenac, but also safer: with topical therapy, blood levels are only about 5% of those achieved with oral therapy, and hence the risk for systemic toxicity is low. Efficacy of topical diclofenac appears about equal to that of oral therapy. Whether topical diclofenac shares the drug interactions of oral diclofenac has not been determined.

Voltaren Gel (1% diclofenac sodium) was the first prescription topical NSAID for treating pain and inflammation. Application is done to the knees, elbows, and other amenable joints. For joints of the lower extremity (knees, ankles, feet), the dosage is 4 g of gel applied 4 times a day. For joints of the upper extremity (elbows, wrists, hands), the dosage is 2 g of gel applied 4 times a day. Total body exposure should not exceed 32 g/day. Treated areas should be protected from sunlight (natural or artificial). Local dermatitis is the principal adverse effect.

Flector Patch (1.3% diclofenac epolamine) is the first prescription NSAID patch indicated for pain of strains, sprains, and contusions. One patch is applied over the injury twice a day—but only to skin that is intact. The patch should not be worn while bathing or showering. Local reactions—pruritus, dermatitis, burning—are the principal adverse effects.

Pennsaid is a 1.5% or 2% solution of diclofenac sodium, formulated with 45% dimethyl sulfoxide (DMSO) to facilitate skin penetration. The product has only one indication: osteoarthritis of the knee. Efficacy equals that of oral diclofenac. Application is done 4 times a day. For each application, 40 drops are spread around the entire knee (front, back, and sides). Application-site reactions are common. Among these are dry skin, erythema and induration, pruritus, and contact dermatitis with vesicles. Systemic effects are minimal. Patients may experience a garlicky odor or taste owing to the DMSO. As with Voltaren Gel, the treated area should not be exposed to sunlight, natural or artificial.

Diclofenac/Misoprostol [Arthrotec]

Oral diclofenac, in combination with misoprostol, is available under the trade name Arthrotec. Misoprostol is a prostaglandin analog that can protect against NSAID-induced ulcers. The combination product is approved for patients with rheumatoid arthritis or osteoarthritis who are at high risk for NSAID-induced gastric or duodenal ulcers. In patients with arthritis, the combination is as effective as diclofenac alone and produces significantly less GI ulceration. The most bothersome side effect is diarrhea (caused by misoprostol). Misoprostol can induce uterine contraction, and hence the product is contraindicated for use during pregnancy. Diclofenac/misoprostol is supplied in two strengths: 50 mg/200 mcg and 75 mg/200 mcg. For rheumatoid arthritis or osteoarthritis, the usual dosage is 50 mg/200 mcg 3 or 4 times a day.

Diflunisal

Diflunisal is a derivative of salicylic acid. However, unlike the salicylates, diflunisal is not converted to salicylic acid in the body. The drug is indicated for mild to moderate pain, rheumatoid arthritis, and osteoarthritis. Like other NSAIDs, the drug inhibits prostaglandin synthesis and can cause GI disturbances, suppression of platelet aggregation, and renal impairment and may increase the risk for MI and stroke. Diflunisal has a prolonged half-life (11–15 hours) and hence can be administered only 2 or 3 times a day. Diflunisal is supplied in tablets (250 and 500 mg) for oral use. For treatment of arthritis and mild to moderate pain, the initial dose is 500 to 1000 mg. Maintenance doses of 250 to 500 mg are administered every 8 to 12 hours.

Etodolac

Etodolac is indicated for rheumatoid arthritis, osteoarthritis, and moderate pain. Investigational uses include bursitis and tendinitis. Like other NSAIDs, etodolac produces many of its effects by suppressing the synthesis of prostanoids. The most common adverse effects are dyspepsia, nausea, vomiting, diarrhea, and abdominal pain. Etodolac may cause less gastric ulceration and bleeding than other NSAIDs. The drug is supplied in immediate-release tablets (400 and 500 mg), extended-release tablets (400, 500, and 600 mg), and capsules (200 and 300 mg). The recommended dosage for arthritis is 800 to 1200 mg/day of the extended-release medication or 400 to 1000 mg/day of the immediate-release medication in divided doses. The dosage for moderate pain is 200 to 400 mg every 6 to 8 hours.

Indomethacin

Actions and Uses

Indomethacin [Indocin, Tivorbex] is an effective antiinflammatory agent approved for arthritis, bursitis, tendinitis, and, as discussed in Chapter 58, acute gouty arthritis. Although indomethacin is able to reduce pain and fever, it is not routinely used for these effects, owing to potential toxicity.

Pharmacokinetics

Indomethacin is well absorbed after oral administration and distributes to all body fluids and tissues. The drug is metabolized in the liver. Metabolites and parent drug are excreted in the urine and feces.

Adverse Effects

Untoward effects are seen in 35% to 50% of patients, causing about 20% to discontinue treatment. The most common adverse effect is severe frontal headache, which occurs in 25% to 50% of patients. Other CNS effects (dizziness, vertigo, confusion) are also common. Seizures and psychiatric changes (e.g., depression, psychosis) have occurred. Mild GI reactions (nausea, vomiting, indigestion) develop in 3% to 9% of users. More severe GI effects (ulceration with perforation, hemorrhage) may also occur. Hematologic reactions (neutropenia, thrombocytopenia, aplastic anemia) have occurred but are rare. Indomethacin suppresses platelet aggregation.

Precautions and Contraindications

Because of its adverse effects, indomethacin is generally contraindicated for infants and children younger than 14 years, patients with peptic ulcer disease, and women who are pregnant or breastfeeding. Caution is required in patients with seizures and psychiatric disorders, in patients involved in hazardous activities, and in patients receiving anticoagulant therapy.

Preparations, Dosage, and Administration

Indomethacin [Indocin] is available in immediate-release capsules (25 and 50 mg), extended-release capsules (75 mg), an oral suspension (5 mg/mL), and rectal suppositories (50 mg). For treatment of rheumatoid arthritis, the initial dosage is 25 mg 2 or 3 times a day. The maximal daily dosage is 200 mg. Gastrointestinal reactions can be reduced by dosing with meals.

A new form of indomethacin was recently approved and is available in 20- and 40-mg capsules sold as Tivorbex. Tivorbex is unique because the capsules contain particles that are 20 times smaller than traditional indomethacin particles. This allows for increased dissolution, thus producing an equianalgesic effect at smaller doses and therefore less toxic side effects.

Ketorolac

Actions and Uses

Ketorolac is a powerful analgesic with minimal antiinflammatory actions. Pain relief is equivalent to that produced by morphine and other opioids. Although ketorolac lacks the serious adverse effects associated with opioids (respiratory depression, tolerance, dependence, abuse potential), it nonetheless has serious adverse effects of its own. Accordingly, use should be short term and restricted to managing acute pain of moderate to severe intensity. Ketorolac is not indicated for chronic pain or for minor aches and discomfort. The usual indication is postoperative pain, for which ketorolac can be as effective as morphine. Like other NSAIDs, ketorolac suppresses prostaglandin synthesis. This action is thought to underlie analgesic effects.

Pharmacokinetics

Ketorolac is administered orally and parenterally (intramuscularly or intravenously). The drug is eliminated by hepatic metabolism and urinary excretion. In young adults, ketorolac has a half-life of 4 to 6 hours. The half-life may be prolonged in older adults and in those with renal impairment.

Adverse Effects and Contraindications

Ketorolac can cause all of the adverse effects associated with other NSAIDs, including peptic ulcers, GI bleeding or perforation, prolonged bleeding time, renal impairment, hypersensitivity reactions, suppression of uterine contractions, and premature closure of the ductus arteriosus. Concurrent use with other NSAIDs increases the risk for these effects and hence is contraindicated. Other contraindications include active peptic ulcer disease, history of peptic ulcer disease or recent GI bleeding, advanced renal impairment, confirmed or suspected intracranial bleeding, use before major surgery, history of NSAID hypersensitivity reactions, and use during labor and delivery.

Preparations, Dosage, and Administration

Oral Therapy. Ketorolac is available in 10-mg tablets for oral dosing. Dosing is parenteral initially, followed by oral dosing if needed. Owing to risks associated with prolonged use, treatment (parenteral plus oral) should not exceed 5 days.

Oral ketorolac is indicated only as a follow-up to parenteral therapy. Initial oral doses are based on preceding parenteral doses. The usual oral maintenance dosage is 10 mg every 4 to 6 hours. Combined oral and parenteral treatment should not exceed 5 days.

Intranasal Therapy. Ketorolac [Sprix] is available in a metered-dose spray device (15.75 mg/actuation) for short-term, intranasal treatment of moderate to moderately severe pain. As with oral and parenteral therapy, treatment should not exceed 5 days. Dosage depends on weight, age, and renal function. For patients with normal renal function who weigh more than 50 kg, the usual dosage is 2 sprays (one 15.75-mg spray in each nostril) every 6 to 8 hours as needed. The dosage is lower—one 15.75-mg spray in one nostril every 6 to 8 hours as needed—for older adults and those who have impaired kidney function or weigh less than 50 kg.

Meclofenamate

Meclofenamate is indicated for rheumatoid arthritis, osteoarthritis, mild to moderate pain, and dysmenorrhea. As with other NSAIDs, benefits derive from inhibiting cyclooxygenase. Therapeutic effects are no better than with other NSAIDs, but adverse GI effects are greater: 3% to 9% of patients experience nausea, vomiting, abdominal pain, and cramps; worse yet, 10% to 33% develop diarrhea. Because of this poor benefit-to-risk profile, meclofenamate is not a drug of first choice. Meclofenamate is available in 50- and 100-mg capsules. Dosages are as follows: arthritis, 200 to 400 mg/day in three or four divided doses; moderate pain, 50 mg every 4 to 6 hours; and dysmenorrhea, 100 mg 3 times a day for up to 6 days.

Mefenamic Acid

Mefenamic acid [Ponstel, Ponstan ♣] is indicated for relief of primary dysmenorrhea and moderate pain. The principal adverse effect is diarrhea, which can be severe. Mefenamic acid is supplied in 250-mg capsules. The dosage for primary dysmenorrhea is 500 mg initially followed by 250 mg every 6 hours as needed. The drug should be administered with food or milk to reduce gastric distress. Usual treatment duration is 2 to 3 days.

Nabumetone

Nabumetone is a prodrug that undergoes hepatic conversion to its active form: 6-MNA. In contrast to most traditional NSAIDs, 6-MNA inhibits COX-2 more than COX-1. Although nabumetone has antipyretic, analgesic, and antiinflammatory properties, the drug is approved only for osteoarthritis and rheumatoid arthritis. Principal adverse effects are diarrhea, abdominal cramps, dyspepsia, and nausea. Nabumetone causes much less GI ulceration than other first-generation NSAIDs, possibly because it preferentially inhibits COX-2. Nabumetone is supplied in 500- and 750-mg tablets. Dosing with food increases the rate of absorption. Treatment of arthritis begins with a single 1000-mg dose. After this, the daily dosage is 1500 to 2000 mg administered in one or two doses. Dosage should be reduced in patients with renal impairment.

Piroxicam

Piroxicam [Feldene] has antiinflammatory, analgesic, and antipyretic properties but is approved only for rheumatoid arthritis and osteoarthritis. The drug's most outstanding feature is its long half-life (about 50 hours). Because piroxicam is eliminated so slowly, therapeutic effects can be maintained with once-a-day dosing. In general, piroxicam is better tolerated than aspirin. Undesired effects are seen in 11% to 46% of patients, causing between 4% and 12% to discontinue therapy. Gastrointestinal reactions are most common, occurring in about 20% of patients. The incidence of gastric ulceration is about 1%. Like aspirin, piroxicam inhibits platelet aggregation and prolongs bleeding time. The drug is supplied in 10- and 20-mg capsules for oral use. The usual dosage is 20 mg once a day or 10 mg twice daily.

Sulindac

Sulindac [Clinoril] is a prodrug that undergoes conversion to its active form in the body. The drug is approved for rheumatoid arthritis, osteoarthritis, tendinitis, bursitis, and acute gouty arthritis. Principal adverse effects are abdominal distress, dyspepsia, nausea, vomiting, and diarrhea. Gastric ulceration is less common than with some other NSAIDs. Like other NSAIDs, sulindac causes reversible inhibition of platelet aggregation, prolongs bleeding time, and impairs renal function. The drug is supplied in 150- and 200-mg tablets. The usual dosage is 150 mg administered twice daily with meals. The maximal daily dosage is 400 mg.

Tolmetin

Tolmetin is approved for rheumatoid arthritis and osteoarthritis. The drug has analgesic and antipyretic properties but is not employed to relieve fever or pain unrelated to inflammation. Adverse effects occur in 25% to 40% of patients, causing between 5% and 10% to discontinue treatment. Gastrointestinal effects (nausea, vomiting, indigestion) are most common. Gastric ulceration has occurred, but less frequently than with aspirin. Nonetheless, caution should be exercised in patients with a history of peptic ulcer disease. Hypersensitivity reactions are more common than with aspirin. Effects on the CNS (headache, dizziness, anxiety, drowsiness) are less severe and less frequent than with indomethacin. Unlike most other NSAIDs, tolmetin does not augment the effects of warfarin, an oral anticoagulant. The drug is supplied in tablets (200 and 600 mg) and capsules (400 mg). For rheumatoid arthritis, the initial dosage is 400 mg 3 times a day. The maximal daily dosage is 1.8 g. Gastrointestinal distress can be minimized by dosing with food.

Meloxicam

Meloxicam [Mobic, Vivlodex, Mobicox ♣] can inhibit COX-1 and COX-2 but shows selectivity for COX-2 at low doses. Like other NSAIDs, the drug has analgesic, antiinflammatory, and antipyretic actions. Approved indications are osteoarthritis, rheumatoid arthritis, and pauciarticular/polyarticular-course juvenile rheumatoid arthritis (JRA). For osteoarthritis, meloxicam is as effective as first-generation NSAIDs. Direct comparison with true COX-2 inhibitors (e.g., celecoxib) has not been made. Despite its COX-2 selectivity, meloxicam has a side-effect profile like that of the first-generation NSAIDs. Gastrointestinal effects (abdominal pain, constipation, diarrhea, dyspepsia, flatulence, nausea, and vomiting) occur in 20% to 25% of patients. More serious effects—GI ulceration, bleeding, perforation, and death—have also occurred. Meloxicam does not suppress platelet aggregation. The drug has a long half-life (15–20 hours) and undergoes elimination in the urine (50%) and feces (50%). Meloxicam is available in tablets (7.5 and 15 mg) and an oral solution (7.5 mg/5 mL). Both formulations can be taken with or without food. Because of its long half-life, meloxicam can be administered just once a day. The recommended dose for initial and maintenance therapy of osteoarthritis and rheumatoid arthritis is 7.5 mg/day. For patients with JRA, the recommended daily dosage is 0.125 mg/kg (but no more than 7.5 mg).

Meloxicam is now available in a "Solumatrix" form using "fine particle technology" sold as Vivlodex. Capsules (5 and 10 mg) of Vivlodex contain particles of meloxicam that are 10 times smaller than traditional tablets. This allows for adequate pain control in osteoarthritis at 33% lower doses. Using less drug can decrease the toxic side effects of meloxicam.

BLACK BOX WARNING: FIRST-GENERATION NONSTEROIDAL ANTIINFLAMMATORY DRUGS

All first-generation NSAIDs are associated with increased risk for gastrointestinal bleeding and cardiovascular events that can lead to hospitalization or death.

SECOND-GENERATION NONSTEROIDAL ANTIINFLAMMATORY DRUGS (CYCLOOXYGENASE-2 INHIBITORS, COXIBS)

The COX-2 inhibitors, also known as coxibs, were developed on the theory that selective inhibition of COX-2 should be able to suppress pain and inflammation while posing little or no risk for gastric ulceration. To some degree, theory and reality agree: coxibs are just as effective as traditional NSAIDs at suppressing inflammation and pain, and they pose a somewhat lower risk for GI side effects. However, even with coxibs, patients can develop clinically significant gastroduodenal ulceration and bleeding. Furthermore, like traditional NSAIDs, coxibs can impair renal function and can thereby cause hypertension and edema. Coxibs also increase the risk for MI and stroke.

Celecoxib

Therapeutic Use

Celecoxib [Celebrex] was the first selective COX-2 inhibitor to reach the market. The drug is indicated for osteoarthritis, rheumatoid arthritis, ankylosing spondylitis, juvenile idiopathic arthritis, acute pain, and dysmenorrhea. In addition, celecoxib is used off-label for a rare genetic disorder known as familial adenomatous polyposis, which predisposes to development of colorectal cancer. For patients with arthritis, celecoxib is equal to naproxen (an NSAID) at relieving joint pain, stiffness, and swelling. Owing to concerns about cardiovascular safety, celecoxib is considered a last-choice drug for long-term management of pain (see later under "American Heart Association Statement on Cyclooxygenase Inhibitors in Chronic Pain").

It is important to note that celecoxib does *not* provide the cardiovascular benefits of aspirin because celecoxib does not inhibit COX-1 in platelets and hence does not suppress platelet aggregation.

Mechanism of Action

Celecoxib causes selective inhibition of COX-2, the COX isoform whose products mediate inflammation and pain. At therapeutic doses, celecoxib does not inhibit COX-1, the COX isoform whose products protect the stomach, help maintain renal function, and promote platelet aggregation.

Pharmacokinetics

Celecoxib is well absorbed after oral administration. Plasma levels peak in 3 hours. Binding to plasma proteins is extensive (97%). The drug undergoes hepatic metabolism followed by renal excretion. The half-life is 11 hours.

Adverse Effects

In premarketing trials, celecoxib was well tolerated. The discontinuation rate owing to adverse effects was 7.1% for celecoxib versus 6.1% for placebo. The most common complaints were *dyspepsia* and *abdominal pain.* Celecoxib does not decrease platelet aggregation and hence does not promote bleeding. Possible cardiovascular events are the biggest concern.

Gastroduodenal Ulceration

Because celecoxib does not inhibit COX-1, the isoform of COX that protects the stomach, a low incidence of gastroduodenal ulceration would be expected. Some data support this expectation; others do not. When celecoxib was first approved, conclusions about its safety were based on 6-month data from the Celecoxib Arthritis Safety Study (CLASS), which indicated that celecoxib caused less GI toxicity than conventional NSAIDs (diclofenac, naproxen, ibuprofen). However, longer term (12-month) data from the same study showed *no difference* in GI toxicity between celecoxib and conventional NSAIDs. Other studies have shown that, compared with patients taking conventional NSAIDs, those taking celecoxib had a lower incidence of endoscopically detectable ulcers and a lower incidence of hospitalization for GI bleeding. What's the bottom line? Celecoxib *may* be safer than conventional NSAIDs, especially when used short term. However, convincing data of superior safety are lacking. Like traditional NSAIDs, celecoxib can be combined with a PPI to reduce GI complications.

Cardiovascular Events

There is strong evidence that coxibs, like other nonaspirin NSAIDs, increase the risk for MI, stroke, and other serious cardiovascular events. In the Adenoma Prevention with Celecoxib (APC) trial, patients who took 400 mg or 800 mg of celecoxib a day experienced more major fatal or nonfatal cardiovascular events than did patients who took placebo. To minimize risk, celecoxib should be used in the lowest effective dosage for the shortest time needed. Also, the drug should be avoided in patients with existing heart disease and those who have just undergone CABG surgery, and should be used with caution in patients with cardiovascular risk factors, such as hypertension, diabetes, and dyslipidemia. Other measures to reduce risk are discussed later under "American Heart Association Statement on Cyclooxygenase Inhibitors in Chronic Pain."

Why is the risk for MI and stroke increased? First, because celecoxib does not inhibit COX-1, platelet aggregation is not suppressed. Second, because celecoxib inhibits COX-2 in blood vessels, vasoconstriction is increased. These two factors—unimpeded platelet aggregation and increased vasoconstriction—increase the likelihood of vessel blockage after the process of thrombosis has begun.

Renal Impairment

Like conventional NSAIDs, celecoxib can impair renal function, thereby posing a risk to patients with hypertension, edema, heart failure, or kidney disease. Renal impairment apparently results from inhibiting COX-2.

Sulfonamide Allergy

Celecoxib contains a sulfur molecule and hence can precipitate an allergic reaction in patients allergic to sulfonamides. Accordingly, the drug should be avoided by patients with sulfa allergy.

Use in Pregnancy

Celecoxib and other NSAIDs can cause premature closure of the ductus arteriosus. Accordingly, these drugs are contraindicated during the third trimester of pregnancy.

Drug Interactions

Warfarin

Celecoxib may increase the anticoagulant effects of warfarin and may thereby increase the risk for bleeding. Celecoxib itself does not inhibit platelet aggregation and does not promote bleeding. However, the drug may enhance the anticoagulant effects of warfarin (perhaps by increasing warfarin levels). Celecoxib may be combined with warfarin, but effects of warfarin should be monitored closely, especially during the first few days of treatment.

Other Interactions

Information on the interactions of celecoxib with other drugs is limited. Celecoxib may decrease the diuretic effects of furosemide as well as the antihypertensive effects of ACE inhibitors. Conversely, celecoxib may increase levels of lithium (a drug for bipolar disorder). Levels of celecoxib may be increased by fluconazole (an antifungal drug).

Preparations, Dosage, and Administration

Celecoxib [Celebrex] is available in capsules (50, 100, 200, and 400 mg). To minimize cardiovascular risk, the drug should be used in the lowest effective dosage for the shortest time needed. Approved dosages are as follows:

- *Osteoarthritis*—100 mg twice daily or 200 mg once daily ♣
- *Rheumatoid arthritis*—100 or 200 mg twice daily
- *Acute pain*—On day 1, 400 mg initially plus another 200 mg if needed; on all subsequent days, 200 mg twice daily as needed
- *Primary dysmenorrhea*—Same as for acute pain

ACETAMINOPHEN

Acetaminophen [Tylenol, Ofirmev, many others] is like aspirin in some respects but different in others. Acetaminophen has *analgesic* and *antipyretic* properties equivalent to those of aspirin. However, in contrast to aspirin and the other NSAIDs, *acetaminophen is devoid of clinically useful antiinflammatory and antirheumatic actions.* In addition, acetaminophen does not suppress platelet aggregation, does not cause gastric ulceration, and does not decrease renal blood flow or cause renal impairment. However, acetaminophen overdose can cause severe liver injury. In the United States acetaminophen is used more than any other analgesic.

Mechanism of Action

Differences between the effects of acetaminophen and aspirin are thought to result from selective inhibition of cyclooxygenase, the enzyme needed to make prostaglandins and related compounds. Whereas aspirin can inhibit cyclooxygenase in both the CNS and the periphery, inhibition by acetaminophen is limited to the CNS; acetaminophen has only minimal effects on cyclooxygenase at peripheral sites. By decreasing prostaglandin synthesis in the CNS, acetaminophen is able to reduce fever and pain. The inability to inhibit prostaglandin synthesis outside the CNS may explain the absence of antiinflammatory effects, gastric ulceration, and adverse effects on the kidneys and platelets.

Pharmacokinetics

Acetaminophen is readily absorbed after oral dosing and undergoes wide distribution. Most of each dose is metabolized by the liver, and the metabolites are excreted in the urine. The plasma half-life is approximately 2 hours.

Acetaminophen can be metabolized by two pathways; one is major, and the other is minor (Fig. 55.1). In the major pathway, acetaminophen undergoes conjugation with glucuronic acid and other compounds to form nontoxic metabolites. In the minor pathway, acetaminophen is oxidized by a cytochrome P450–containing enzyme into a highly reactive toxic metabolite: *N*-acetyl-*p*-benzoquinone imine. At therapeutic doses, practically all of the drug is converted to nontoxic metabolites through the major pathway. Only a small fraction is converted into the toxic metabolite through the minor pathway. Furthermore, under normal conditions, the toxic metabolite undergoes rapid conversion to a nontoxic form; glutathione is required for the conversion. In the event of acetaminophen overdose, a larger than normal amount is processed through the minor pathway, and hence a large quantity of the toxic metabolite is produced. As the liver attempts to clear the metabolite, glutathione is rapidly depleted, and further detoxification stops. As a result, the toxic metabolite accumulates, causing damage to the liver (see later).

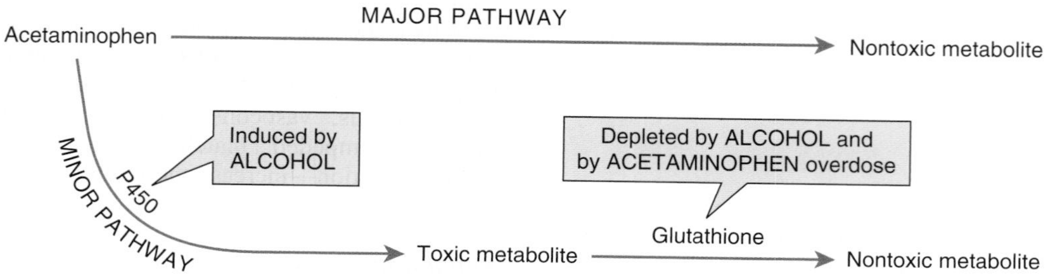

Figure 55.1 ▪ Metabolism of acetaminophen.

Adverse Effects

Adverse effects are extremely rare at therapeutic doses. Acetaminophen does not cause gastric ulceration or renal impairment and does not inhibit platelet aggregation. In addition, there is no evidence linking acetaminophen with Reye syndrome. Individuals who are hypersensitive to aspirin only rarely experience cross-hypersensitivity with acetaminophen. Overdose can cause severe *liver injury* (see later).

Data from the Nurses' Health Study show an association between daily use of *acetaminophen* (500 mg or more/day) and development of *hypertension.* Additional studies that examined a possible relationship between acetaminophen and hypertension in both men and women found conflicting results. Until more data become available, it would be prudent to monitor blood pressure in patients who take acetaminophen daily. The mechanism by which acetaminophen might raise blood pressure is unknown.

Studies have shown an association between acetaminophen and development of *asthma.* However, as with hypertension, a causal relationship has not been established. In fact, regarding asthma, the association may well be the other way around. That is, people may be taking acetaminophen *because* they have respiratory symptoms, rather than having respiratory symptoms because they took acetaminophen. To prove that acetaminophen actually does cause asthma, stronger data are needed.

Rarely, patients experience *anaphylaxis,* a severe hypersensitivity reaction characterized by breathing difficulty associated with swelling of the face, mouth, and throat. If these symptoms develop, patients should seek immediate medical help.

Acetaminophen use has also been associated with Stevens-Johnson Syndrome (SJS), acute generalized exanthematous pustulosis (AGEP), and toxic epidermal necrolysis (TEN). SJS and TEN are characterized by painful rash, blistering of the skin and mucous membranes, and detachment of the epidermis. These are considered medical emergencies because they can result in death. Recovery can take weeks to months. AGEP is characterized by pustular lesions that predominately affect the upper trunk and body folds. AGEP usually resolves within 2 weeks of onset. These reactions can occur at any time, even if the patient has taken acetaminophen previously. If rash appears while taking acetaminophen, the drug should be stopped and the patient should seek medical attention.

Drug and Vaccine Interactions

Alcohol

Regular alcohol consumption increases the risk for liver injury from acetaminophen—but only if acetaminophen dosage is excessive. Three mechanisms are involved. First, alcohol induces synthesis of the P450-containing enzyme in the minor metabolic pathway, thereby increasing production of acetaminophen's toxic metabolite (see Fig. 55.1). Second, stores of glutathione are depleted in chronic alcoholics. As a result, the liver is unable to convert the toxic metabolite to a nontoxic form. Third, chronic alcohol abusers often have preexisting liver damage, which renders them less able to tolerate injury from acetaminophen.

Alcohol in combination with acetaminophen can increase the risk for liver and kidney damage. Although information regarding liver disease and acetaminophen has existed for some time, newer data reveal that even low-dose combinations of alcohol and acetaminophen can lead to renal dysfunction. Authorities recommend that, if you drink alcohol on a regular basis, you should consume no more than 2000 mg of acetaminophen a day (one half the normal maximum).

Although therapeutic doses of acetaminophen may be safe for alcohol drinkers, *high* doses certainly are not. Accordingly, to alert the public to the potential risk of combining alcohol with acetaminophen, the FDA requires that acetaminophen labels bear the following statement: ***Alcohol Warning:*** *If you consume three or more alcoholic drinks every day, ask your doctor whether you should take acetaminophen or other pain relievers/fever reducers.*

Warfarin

There is evidence that acetaminophen may increase the risk for bleeding in patients taking warfarin. This is surprising because, unlike NSAIDs, acetaminophen does not suppress platelet aggregation and so should not promote bleeding. Yes, acetaminophen may inhibit warfarin metabolism, which would cause warfarin levels to rise. Although this interaction has not been proven, caution is advised. Accordingly, for patients taking more than 1 g of acetaminophen daily for several days, responses to warfarin should be monitored closely. Occasional use of acetaminophen is not a concern.

Vaccines

Acetaminophen and other analgesic-antipyretics can blunt the immune response to childhood vaccines. Accordingly, routine use of these drugs to prevent vaccination-associated pain or fever should be discouraged.

Therapeutic Uses

Acetaminophen is indicated for relief of pain and fever. Because acetaminophen is not associated with Reye syndrome, the drug is preferred to NSAIDs for use by children suspected of having chickenpox or influenza. Because it does not cause GI injury, acetaminophen is preferred to NSAIDs for patients with peptic ulcer disease. In addition, acetaminophen may be a safe alternative to aspirin for patients who have experienced aspirin hypersensitivity reactions. Because of its weak antiinflammatory actions, acetaminophen is *not* useful for treating arthritis or rheumatic fever.

Acute Toxicity: Liver Damage

Overdose with acetaminophen can cause severe liver injury and death. The cause is accumulation of the toxic metabolite discussed earlier. In the United States acetaminophen overdose—intentional or unintentional—is the leading cause of acute liver failure, accounting for about 50% of all cases. Risk for liver injury is increased by fasting, chronic alcohol use, and taking more than 4000 mg of acetaminophen a day.

Signs and Symptoms

The principal feature of acetaminophen overdose is *hepatic necrosis.* Severe poisoning can progress to hepatic failure, coma, and death. Early symptoms of poisoning (nausea, vomiting, diarrhea, sweating, abdominal discomfort) belie the severity of intoxication. It is not until 48 to 72 hours after drug ingestion that overt indications of hepatic injury appear.

Treatment

Liver damage can be minimized by giving *acetylcysteine* [Mucomyst ♣, Acetadote], a specific antidote to acetaminophen. Acetylcysteine reduces injury by substituting for depleted glutathione in the reaction that converts the toxic metabolite of acetaminophen to its nontoxic form. When given within 8 to 10 hours of acetaminophen overdose, acetylcysteine is 100% effective at preventing severe liver injury. And even when administered as much as 24 hours after poisoning, it can still provide significant protection. Acetylcysteine may be administered orally or intravenously.

For oral therapy, acetylcysteine is supplied in solution (100 and 200 mg/mL) and should be diluted to 50 mg/mL with water, fruit juice, or a cola beverage. Conventional treatment consists of a loading dose (140 mg/kg) followed by 17 more doses (70 mg/kg) given every 4 hours for 72 hours. However, for most patients, treatment can be stopped after just 20 hours. Oral acetylcysteine has an extremely unpleasant odor and may induce vomiting. If the patient is unable to tolerate oral dosing, acetylcysteine can be administered intravenously or through a nasogastric tube.

Minimizing Risk

Risk for liver failure is very low with normal therapeutic doses (up to 4000 mg/day), except in people who drink alcohol, are undernourished, or have liver disease. Patient education can help reduce injury. Accordingly, you should do the following:

- Inform patients about the risk for liver toxicity.
- Advise patients to consume no more than 4000 mg of acetaminophen a day, including the amount in combination prescription products (e.g., Vicodin, Percocet) as well as over-the-counter products.
- Advise patients who are undernourished (e.g., owing to fasting or illness) to consume no more than 3000 mg of acetaminophen a day. Undernourished people are at risk because they have low stores of glutathione, the cofactor needed to convert the toxic metabolite of acetaminophen to a nontoxic form.
- Advise patients not to drink alcohol while taking acetaminophen.
- Advise patients who won't stop drinking alcohol (more than 3 drinks a day) to take no more than 2000 mg of acetaminophen a day.
- Advise patients with liver disease to ask their prescriber if acetaminophen is safe.

To help reduce overdosage, McNeil Consumer Healthcare, maker of the *Tylenol* brand of acetaminophen, changed the dosing recommendations on Tylenol labels. On the new labels, issued in 2011, the maximal daily dose of *Extra-Strength Tylenol* (500 mg/tablet) is stated as 3000 mg (6 tablets), and the maximal daily dose of *Regular Strength Tylenol* (325 mg/tablet) is stated as 3250 mg (10 tablets). Other manufacturers are expected to make similar changes. Please note, however, that the maximal daily dose recommended by the FDA is still 4000 mg, even though these product labels recommend a lower dose.

Preparations, Dosage, and Administration

Preparations

Numerous acetaminophen-containing products are on the market, including a wide assortment of fixed-dose combinations. The drug is available in rectal suppositories, solution for intravenous dosing, and multiple oral formulations (standard tablets, chewable tablets, effervescent granules, capsules, liquids, elixirs, and solutions). Many products are available over the counter, and many others require a prescription. Furthermore, product strengths vary widely. All these products are mentioned here because they create a significant risk for overdose—either from taking two or more products that both contain acetaminophen or from taking too much of a single-ingredient product (owing to failure to carefully read the label). You should alert patients to these dangers.

Dosage and Administration

Oral. The recommended oral dosage for adults and children older than 12 years is 325 to 650 mg every 4 to 6 hours, up to a maximum of 4000 mg/day. Dosages for younger children are based either on body weight—10 to 15 mg/kg/dose—or on age as follows:

- Up to 3 months—40 mg every 4 hours
- 4 to 11 months—80 mg every 4 hours
- 12 to 23 months—120 mg every 4 hours
- 2 to 3 years—160 mg every 4 hours
- 4 to 5 years—240 mg every 4 hours
- 6 to 8 years—320 mg every 4 to 6 hours
- 9 to 10 years—400 mg every 4 to 6 hours
- 11 years—480 mg every 4 to 6 hours
- 12 years—640 mg every 4 to 6 hours

Rectal. Acetaminophen suppositories [FeverAll, Acephen] are available in four strengths: 80, 120, 325, and 650 mg. The recommended dosage for adults and children over 12 years is 650 mg every 4 to 6 hours, up to a maximum of 3900 mg/day. Dosages for younger children vary with age as follows:

- 3 to 11 months—80 mg every 6 hours
- 12 to 36 months—80 mg every 4 hours
- 3 to 6 years—120 mg every 4 to 6 hours
- 6 to 12 years—325 mg every 4 to 6 hours

AMERICAN HEART ASSOCIATION (AHA) STATEMENT ON CYCLOOXYGENASE INHIBITORS IN CHRONIC PAIN

Because most COX inhibitors—and especially COX-2 inhibitors—increase the risk for MI and stroke, the AHA recommends a stepped-care approach to their use, as discussed in an article titled "Use of Nonsteroidal Anti-inflammatory Drugs: An Update for Clinicians: A Scientific Statement from the American Heart Association." Recommendations in the article apply specifically to managing musculoskeletal pain in patients with or at high risk for cardiovascular disease. However, the recommendations may also apply to patients who lack documented cardiovascular risk. The approach has four basic steps:

Step 1. Begin with nondrug measures. Options include physical therapy, exercise, weight loss, orthotics, and application of heat or cold.

Step 2. If nondrug measures don't work, initiate drug therapy using *acetaminophen* or *aspirin,* which do not increase cardiovascular risk. If these drugs can't control pain, an opioid or tramadol can be tried, but only short term.

Step 3. If step 2 drugs are ineffective or intolerable, try other nonselective NSAIDs, such as naproxen, ibuprofen, or a nonacetylated salicylate (e.g., magnesium salicylate).

Step 4. As a *last resort,* try the selective COX-2 inhibitor celecoxib. Of all the NSAIDs, COX-2 inhibitors pose the greatest risk for cardiovascular harm, and hence celecoxib is a last-choice drug for chronic pain.

Whenever these drugs are employed, patients should use the lowest effective dosage for the shortest time required. During steps 2, 3, and 4, if the patient is considered at high risk for a thrombotic event, low-dose aspirin (81 mg/day) plus a PPI or H_2RA should be *added* to the regimen (except, of course, if high-dose aspirin is already in use).

CHAPTER

56 Glucocorticoids in Nonendocrine Disorders

Jacqueline Rosenjack Burchum, DNSc, FNP-BC, CNE

In the body, the adrenal cortex produces corticosteroids. These include mineralocorticoids, which modulate salt and water balance, and glucocorticoids, which influence carbohydrate metabolism and other processes. The amount of glucocorticoids manufactured by the body is relatively low compared with that of many glucocorticoid drugs. *Physiologic* effects, such as modulation of glucose metabolism, are elicited by *low* doses of glucocorticoids. For example, low (physiologic) doses of glucocorticoids are used to treat adrenocortical insufficiency. In contrast, *pharmacologic* effects (e.g., suppression of inflammation) require *high* doses. In high (pharmacologic) doses, glucocorticoids are used to treat inflammatory disorders (e.g., asthma, rheumatoid arthritis) and certain cancers. High doses are also used to suppress immune responses in organ transplant recipients.

All of the glucocorticoid drugs can produce the same spectrum of therapeutic effects. Differences among individual agents pertain to time course and side effects. Because the similarities among these drugs are much more striking than the differences, we will not focus on a prototypic agent. Instead, we will discuss the glucocorticoids as a group.

REVIEW OF GLUCOCORTICOID PHYSIOLOGY

Physiologic Effects

Physiologic responses can be elicited with low doses of glucocorticoids. At higher doses, these effects are simply more intense. When glucocorticoids are used to treat nonendocrine disorders, physiologic responses occur as side effects.

Metabolic Effects

Glucocorticoids influence the metabolism of carbohydrates, proteins, and fats. The principal effect on carbohydrate metabolism is elevation of blood glucose. Glucocorticoids do this by promoting synthesis of glucose from amino acids, reducing peripheral glucose utilization, and reducing glucose uptake by muscle and adipose tissue. Glucocorticoids also promote storage of glucose in the form of glycogen.

Glucocorticoids have a negative effect on protein metabolism. Specifically, these drugs suppress synthesis of proteins from amino acids and divert amino acids for production of glucose. These actions can reduce muscle mass, decrease the protein matrix of bone, and cause thinning of the skin. Nitrogen balance becomes negative.

The most consistent effect of glucocorticoids on fat metabolism is stimulation of lipolysis (fat breakdown). Long-term, high-dose therapy can cause fat redistribution, resulting in the central obesity (potbelly), rounded face (moon face), and fat pad at the cervical spine (buffalo hump) that characterize Cushing syndrome.

Cardiovascular Effects

Glucocorticoids are required to maintain the functional integrity of the vascular system. When levels of endogenous glucocorticoids are low, capillaries become more permeable, vasoconstriction is suppressed, and blood pressure falls. Glucocorticoids *increase* the number of circulating red blood cells and polymorphonuclear leukocytes and *decrease* counts of lymphocytes, eosinophils, basophils, and monocytes.

Effects During Stress

At times of physiologic stress (e.g., surgery, infection, trauma, hypovolemia), the adrenal glands secrete large quantities of glucocorticoids and epinephrine. Working together, these hormones help maintain blood pressure and blood glucose levels. If glucocorticoid release is insufficient, hypotension and hypoglycemia will occur. If the stress is especially severe, glucocorticoid insufficiency can result in circulatory failure and death.

Effects on Water and Electrolytes

To varying degrees, individual glucocorticoids can exert actions similar to aldosterone, the major mineralocorticoid released by the adrenal glands. Accordingly, glucocorticoids can act on the kidney to promote retention of sodium and water while increasing urinary excretion of potassium. The net result is hypernatremia, hypokalemia, and edema. Fortunately, most of the glucocorticoids employed as drugs have very low mineralocorticoid activity (Table 56.1).

Respiratory System Effects in Neonates

During labor and delivery, the adrenal glands of the full-term infant release a burst of glucocorticoids, which act to hasten maturation of the lungs. In the preterm infant, production of glucocorticoids is low, resulting in a high incidence of respiratory distress syndrome.

Control of Synthesis and Secretion

Synthesis and release of glucocorticoids are regulated by a negative feedback loop. The principal components of the loop

TABLE 56.1 ■ Systemic Glucocorticoids: Half-Lives, Relative Potencies, and Equivalent Doses

Drug	Biologic Half-Life (h)	Relative Mineralocorticoid Potency*	Relative Glucocorticoid (Antiinflammatory) Potency†	Equivalent Antiinflammatory Dose (mg)‡
SHORT ACTING				
Cortisone	8–12	2	0.8	25
Hydrocortisone	8–12	2	1	20
INTERMEDIATE ACTING				
Prednisolone	18–36	1	4	5
Prednisone	18–36	1	4	5
Methylprednisolone	18–36	0	5	4
Triamcinolone	18–36	0	5	4
LONG ACTING				
Betamethasone	36–54	0	20–30	0.75
Dexamethasone	36–54	0	20–30	0.75

*Relative mineralocorticoid activity (sodium and water retention; potassium depletion): 0, very low; 1, moderate; 2, high.
†Glucocorticoid potency values are relative to the potency of hydrocortisone.
‡Approximate *oral* or *intravenous* dose needed to produce equivalent antiinflammatory effects.

are the hypothalamus, anterior pituitary, and adrenal cortex (Fig. 56.1). The loop is turned on when stress or some other stimulus from the central nervous system acts on the hypothalamus to cause release of corticotropin-releasing hormone (CRH). CRH then stimulates the pituitary to release adrenocorticotropic hormone (ACTH), which in turn acts on the adrenal cortex to promote synthesis and release of cortisol (the principal endogenous glucocorticoid). Cortisol has two basic effects: first, it stimulates physiologic responses; second, it acts on the hypothalamus and pituitary to suppress further release of CRH and ACTH. By inhibiting release of CRH and ACTH, cortisol suppresses its own production. As a result, this negative feedback loop keeps glucocorticoid levels within an appropriate range. When glucocorticoids are administered chronically in large doses, the feedback loop remains continuously suppressed. As discussed later, persistent suppression can be dangerous.

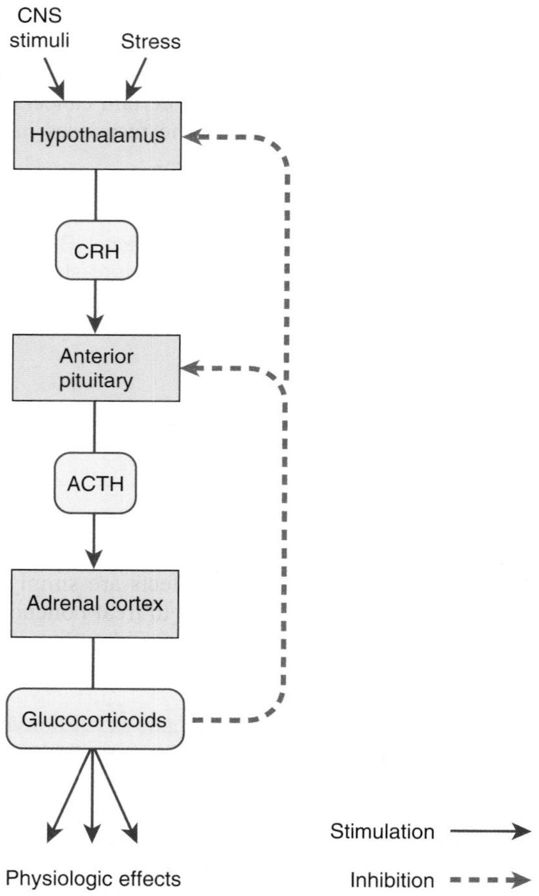

Figure 56.1 ■ Feedback regulation of glucocorticoid synthesis and secretion.
ACTH, adrenocorticotropic hormone; CNS, central nervous system; CRH, corticotropin-releasing hormone.

PHARMACOLOGY OF THE GLUCOCORTICOIDS

Molecular Mechanism of Action

Mechanistically, glucocorticoids differ from most drugs in two ways: (1) glucocorticoid receptors are located *inside* the cell, rather than on the cell surface; and (2) glucocorticoids modulate the production of regulatory proteins, rather than the activity of signaling pathways.

Here's how they do it. First, glucocorticoids penetrate the cell membrane and then bind with receptors in the *cytoplasm,* thereby converting the receptor from an inactive form to an active form. Next, the receptor-steroid complex migrates to the cell *nucleus,* where it binds to chromatin in DNA, thereby altering the activity of target genes. In most cases, activity of the target gene is increased, causing increased transcription of messenger RNA molecules that code for specific regulatory proteins. However, in some cases, activity of the target gene is suppressed, and hence synthesis of certain regulatory proteins declines.

Pharmacologic Effects

When administered in the high doses employed to treat nonendocrine disorders, glucocorticoids produce antiinflammatory and immunosuppressive effects—effects not seen at physiologic doses. Of course, these high doses also produce the physiologic effects seen at low doses.

Effects on Metabolism and Electrolytes

The effects of high-dose therapy on metabolism and electrolytes are like those seen with physiologic doses—but are more intense. With high doses, glucose levels rise, protein synthesis is suppressed, and fat deposits are mobilized. As noted, most glucocorticoids have very little mineralocorticoid activity. Accordingly, these drugs do not usually induce significant sodium retention or potassium loss. However, these effects do occur in some patients and can be hazardous. In all patients, high-dose therapy can inhibit intestinal absorption of calcium, an effect not seen at physiologic doses.

Antiinflammatory and Immunosuppressant Effects

The major clinical applications of the glucocorticoids stem from their ability to suppress immune responses and inflammation. Effects on the immune system and inflammation are interrelated, so we will consider them together.

Before discussing the actions of glucocorticoids, we need to review the process of inflammation. Characteristic symptoms of inflammation are pain, swelling, redness, and warmth. These are initiated by chemical mediators (prostaglandins, histamine, leukotrienes) and are amplified by the actions of lymphocytes and phagocytic cells (neutrophils and macrophages). Prostaglandins and histamine promote several symptoms of inflammation—swelling, redness, and warmth—by causing vasodilation and increasing capillary permeability. Prostaglandins and histamine contribute to pain: histamine stimulates pain receptors directly; prostaglandins sensitize pain receptors to stimulation by histamine and other mediators. Neutrophils and macrophages heighten inflammation by releasing lysosomal enzymes, which cause tissue injury. Lymphocytes, which are important elements of the immune system, intensify inflammation by (1) causing direct cell injury and (2) promoting formation of antibodies that help perpetuate the inflammatory response.

Glucocorticoids act through several mechanisms to interrupt the inflammatory processes. These drugs can inhibit synthesis of chemical mediators (prostaglandins, leukotrienes, histamine), reducing swelling, warmth, redness, and pain. In addition, they suppress infiltration of phagocytes, so damage from lysosomal enzymes is averted. Lastly, glucocorticoids suppress proliferation of lymphocytes and thereby reduce the immune component of inflammation.

It is important to appreciate that the mechanisms by which glucocorticoids suppress inflammation are more diverse than the mechanisms by which nonsteroidal antiinflammatory drugs (NSAIDs) act. As discussed in Chapter 55, NSAIDs suppress inflammation primarily by inhibiting prostaglandin production. The glucocorticoids share this mechanism and act in other ways, too. Because they act by multiple mechanisms, glucocorticoids have much greater antiinflammatory effects than do NSAIDs.

Pharmacokinetics

Absorption

The rate of glucocorticoid absorption depends on the route of administration and the specific glucocorticoid. With oral administration, absorption of all glucocorticoids is rapid and nearly complete. After intramuscular (IM) injection, absorption is rapid with two types of glucocorticoid esters (sodium phosphates and sodium succinates) and relatively slow with other derivatives (e.g., acetates, acetonides). Absorption from local sites of injection (e.g., intraarticular, intralesional) is slower than from IM sites.

Duration of Action

Duration depends on dosage, route, and drug solubility. For glucocorticoids administered orally or intravenously, duration is determined largely by biologic half-life (see Table 56.1). With IM administration, duration is a function of water solubility: highly soluble preparations have a shorter duration than less soluble preparations. For locally administered glucocorticoids, duration is determined by solubility and by the specific site of administration.

Metabolism and Excretion

Glucocorticoids are metabolized primarily by the liver. As a rule, the resulting metabolites are inactive. Excretion of metabolites is renal.

Therapeutic Uses in Nonendocrine Disorders

As has been mentioned, high-dose therapy is required for management of nonendocrine conditions. For some conditions, long-term therapy is required as well. Because prolonged, high-dose therapy can produce serious adverse effects, the potential benefits of treatment must be weighed carefully against the very real risks.

Rheumatoid Arthritis

Glucocorticoids are indicated for adjunctive treatment of acute exacerbations of rheumatoid arthritis. These drugs can reduce inflammation and pain, but do not alter the course of the disease. Because of the risk for serious complications, prolonged systemic use should be avoided when possible.

When arthritis is limited to just a few joints, intraarticular injections may be advantageous. Local injections can be highly effective and cause less toxicity than systemic therapy. Frequently, reductions in pain and inflammation can be so dramatic as to prompt vigorous use of joints that were previously immobile. Because excessive use of diseased joints can cause injury, patients should be warned against overactivity, even though symptoms have eased.

The use of glucocorticoids in rheumatoid arthritis is discussed further in Chapter 57.

Systemic Lupus Erythematosus

Systemic lupus erythematosus (SLE) is a chronic disease similar in many ways to rheumatoid arthritis. However, in SLE, inflammation is not limited to joints. Rather, it occurs throughout the body. Symptoms frequently include pleuritis, pericarditis, and nephritis. A severe episode can be fatal. Fortunately, manifestations of SLE can usually be controlled with prompt and aggressive glucocorticoid therapy.

Inflammatory Bowel Disease

Glucocorticoids are used to treat severe cases of ulcerative colitis and Crohn disease, the two most common forms of inflammatory bowel disease. Administration may be oral or intravenous. Glucocorticoid therapy of these disorders is considered further in Chapter 64.

Miscellaneous Inflammatory Disorders

Glucocorticoids are useful in a variety of inflammatory disorders in addition to those discussed previously. Conditions that respond include bursitis, tendinitis, synovitis, osteoarthritis, gouty arthritis, and inflammatory disorders of the eye.

Allergic Conditions

Glucocorticoids can control symptoms of allergic reactions. Responsive conditions include allergic rhinitis (see Chapter 61), bee stings, and drug-induced allergies. Because glucocorticoid responses are delayed, these drugs have little value as *sole* therapy for severe allergic reactions (e.g., anaphylaxis). For life-threatening allergic reactions, epinephrine is the treatment of choice.

Asthma

Glucocorticoids are the most effective antiasthma agents available. For treatment of asthma, they may be administered orally or by inhalation. Adverse effects are minimal with inhaled glucocorticoids. In contrast, oral therapy can cause serious toxicity and hence should be reserved for patients who have failed to respond to safer treatments (e.g., inhaled glucocorticoids, inhaled cromolyn sodium). The use of glucocorticoids in asthma is discussed at length in Chapter 60.

Dermatologic Disorders

Glucocorticoids are beneficial in a wide variety of skin diseases, including pemphigus, psoriasis, mycosis fungoides, seborrheic dermatitis, contact dermatitis, and exfoliative dermatitis. For mild disease, topical administration is usually adequate. For severe disorders, systemic therapy may be needed. It should be noted that topical glucocorticoids can be absorbed in amounts sufficient to produce systemic toxicity. Topical therapy is discussed further in Chapter 85.

Adverse Effects

The adverse effects discussed next occur in response to *pharmacologic* (as opposed to *physiologic*) doses of glucocorticoids. The intensity of these effects increases with dosage size and treatment duration. These effects are not seen when dosage is physiologic. Furthermore, most are not seen when treatment is brief (a few days or less), even when doses are high.

Adrenal Insufficiency

Prolonged administration of pharmacologic doses of glucocorticoids can suppress production of glucocorticoids by the adrenal glands, resulting in adrenal insufficiency. The mechanism, consequences, and management of adrenal insufficiency are discussed under "Adrenal Suppression."

Osteoporosis

Development

Osteoporosis with resultant fractures is a frequent and serious complication of prolonged systemic glucocorticoid therapy. (Although osteoporosis is likely with prolonged systemic glucocorticoid therapy, it is uncommon when glucocorticoids are inhaled or administered topically.) The ribs and vertebrae are affected most. In some patients on high-dose glucocorticoids, vertebral compression fractures occur within weeks of beginning glucocorticoid use. Patients should be observed for signs of compression fractures (back and neck pain) and for indications of fractures in other bones.

How do glucocorticoids cause bone loss? The most important mechanism is suppression of bone formation by osteoblasts. In addition, glucocorticoids accelerate bone resorption by osteoclasts. Also, these drugs reduce intestinal absorption of calcium, causing hypocalcemia. In response to hypocalcemia, release of parathyroid hormone increases, which increases mobilization of calcium from bone.

Management

Several measures can greatly reduce development of osteoporosis and subsequent fractures. Before glucocorticoid treatment, bone mineral density of the lumbar spine should be measured. This will identify patients at highest risk and provide a baseline for evaluating bone loss during treatment. When appropriate, glucocorticoids should be administered topically or by inhalation because bone loss is less with these routes than with systemic therapy.

PATIENT-CENTERED CARE ACROSS THE LIFE SPAN

Glucocorticoids

Life Stage	Patient Care Concerns
Children	Long-term use of steroid medications can cause inhibition of bone growth. This may result in decreased stature.
Pregnant women	Glucocorticoids are classified in U.S. Food and Drug Administration Pregnancy Risk Category C or D, depending on the specific drug and formulation. Inadequate studies have been conducted in pregnant women; however, studies in animals have demonstrated both teratogenic and physiologic effects. These range from an increased incidence of cleft palate, spontaneous abortion, and low birth weight in nonprimates to impaired postnatal growth, impaired glucose-insulin homeostasis, increased blood pressure, and increased production of cortisol in response to mild stress in primates.
Breastfeeding women	When physiologic doses or low pharmacologic doses are used, the concentration achieved in milk is probably too low to affect the nursing infant. However, when large pharmacologic doses are employed, the amount ingested by the infant may be sufficient to cause growth delay and other adverse effects. Breastfeeding is not recommended for women taking large doses of glucocorticoids.
Older adults	Long-term use of glucocorticoids can cause osteoporosis, adrenal insufficient, and GI ulceration. These may affect older adults disproportionately.

Drugs can help reduce bone loss. All patients should receive *calcium* and *vitamin D* supplements. Sodium restriction combined with a thiazide diuretic can enhance intestinal absorption of calcium and can decrease urinary excretion of calcium. There is solid evidence that a *bisphosphonate* can prevent glucocorticoid-induced bone loss by inhibiting bone resorption by osteoclasts. *Calcitonin* [Miacalcin], which also inhibits osteoclasts, is another option. For patients with significant bone loss, *teriparatide* [Forteo] may be preferred because, unlike bisphosphonates and calcitonin, which only prevent bone *resorption,* teriparatide actively promotes new bone *formation.* In postmenopausal women, *estrogen* therapy is an effective way to reduce bone loss. However, as discussed in Chapter 48, the risks of estrogen therapy generally outweigh the benefits. The roles of calcium, vitamin D, bisphosphonates, calcitonin, teriparatide, and estrogen in the prophylaxis and treatment of osteoporosis are discussed fully in Chapter 59.

Infection

By suppressing host defenses (immune responses and phagocytic activity of neutrophils and macrophages), glucocorticoids can increase susceptibility to infection. The risk for acquiring a new infection is increased, as is the risk for reactivating a latent infection (e.g., tuberculosis). In addition, because suppression of both the immune system and neutrophils reduces inflammation and other manifestations of infection, a fulminant infection may develop without detection. Hence, glucocorticoids not only increase susceptibility to infection but also can mask the presence of an infection as it progresses. To minimize risk for infection, patients should avoid close contact with people who have a communicable disease. If a significant infection occurs, glucocorticoids should be continued only if absolutely necessary, and then only in combination with appropriate antimicrobial or antifungal therapy.

One infection—known as PCP (for *P*neumo*c*ystis *p*neumonia)—deserves special mention. The causative organism is *Pneumocystis jiroveci* (formerly called *Pneumocystis carinii*). PCP, commonly known as an opportunistic infection in people with AIDS, also occurs with alarming frequency in people receiving high doses of glucocorticoids. Accordingly, it has been suggested that PCP prophylaxis be considered for all people taking glucocorticoids long term in high doses.

Glucose Intolerance

Because of their effects on glucose production and utilization, glucocorticoids can increase plasma glucose levels, thereby causing hyperglycemia and glycosuria. Patients with diabetes may need to increase the dosage of hypoglycemic medication. For patients with normal pancreatic function, significant elevation of blood glucose is unlikely. However, because glucocorticoids can unmask latent diabetes, even patients without a diagnosis of diabetes should undergo periodic evaluation of blood glucose levels.

Myopathy

High-dose glucocorticoid therapy can cause myopathy (muscle injury), manifesting as weakness. The proximal muscles of the arms and legs are affected most. Damage to muscle may be sufficient to prevent ambulation. If myopathy develops, glucocorticoid dosage should be reduced. Myopathy then gradually resolves over several months.

Fluid and Electrolyte Disturbance

Because of their mineralocorticoid activity, glucocorticoids can cause sodium and water retention and potassium loss. Retention of water and sodium can cause hypertension and edema. Hypokalemia can predispose to dysrhythmias and toxicity from digitalis. Fortunately, most of the glucocorticoids in current use have minimal mineralocorticoid activity. Therefore serious fluid and electrolyte disturbance is rare. The risk for fluid and electrolyte disturbance can be reduced by (1) using glucocorticoids that have low mineralocorticoid activity, (2) restricting sodium intake, and (3) taking potassium supplements or consuming potassium-rich foods (e.g., potatoes, bananas, citrus fruits). Patients should be informed about signs of fluid retention (e.g., weight gain, swelling of the lower extremities) and advised to contact the prescriber if these develop. Patients should also be alert for signs of hypokalemia (e.g., muscle weakness or fatigue, irregular pulse).

Growth Delay

Glucocorticoids can suppress growth in children. Growth delay is probably the result of reduced DNA synthesis and decreased cell division. To assess effects on growth, height and weight should be measured at regular intervals. Growth suppression can be minimized with alternate-day therapy. This dosing schedule is discussed later.

Psychological Disturbances

Systemic glucocorticoids can cause psychological disturbances. About 60% of patients experience a mild reaction: insomnia, anxiety, agitation, or irritability. Another 6% experience a severe reaction: delirium, hallucinations, depression, euphoria, or mania. Of these, up to one third may become suicidal. Of note, previous psychiatric illness does not seem to predispose patients to psychological reactions—and a history of good mental health does not confer protection.

Psychological reactions are dose and duration dependent. Long-term low-dose therapy is more likely to cause depression. In contrast, short-term high-dose therapy is more likely to cause mania and other psychoses. Cognitive impairment (e.g., distractibility, memory loss) can occur with either dosing pattern.

Psychological effects reverse when glucocorticoids are withdrawn. Delirium and hallucinations usually resolve quickly—within a few days to a week. Mood disturbances (depression, mania) resolve more slowly—over 6 weeks or longer.

Can we use drugs to manage symptoms? Yes. Drugs typically used to manage mood disorders and psychosis have demonstrated success in managing the psychological adverse effects in many patients. Occasionally, though, psychological effects are unresponsive to the usual drugs used to manage these conditions.

Cataracts and Glaucoma

Cataracts are a common complication of long-term glucocorticoid therapy. Risk factors are in dispute; cataract development may be related to age, dosage, or individual susceptibility. To facilitate early detection, patients should undergo an eye examination every 6 months. Also, patients should be advised to contact the prescriber if vision becomes cloudy or blurred.

Oral glucocorticoids can cause open-angle glaucoma. Onset of ocular hypertension develops rapidly and reverses within 2 weeks of glucocorticoid cessation.

Peptic Ulcer Disease

Glucocorticoids have actions that can lead to peptic ulcer disease. By inhibiting prostaglandin synthesis, glucocorticoids can augment secretion of gastric acid and pepsin, inhibit production of cytoprotective mucus, and reduce gastric mucosal blood flow. These actions predispose to gastrointestinal (GI) ulceration. Making matters worse, glucocorticoids can decrease gastric pain, thereby masking ulcer development. As a result, perforation and hemorrhage can occur without warning. The risk for ulceration is increased by concurrent use of other ulcerogenic drugs, such as aspirin and other NSAIDs. To provide early detection of ulcer formation, stools should be periodically checked for occult blood. Patients should be instructed to notify the prescriber if feces become black and tarry. If GI ulceration occurs, glucocorticoids should be slowly withdrawn (unless their continued use is considered essential to support life). Treatment with antiulcer medication is indicated.

Iatrogenic Cushing Syndrome

Long-term glucocorticoid therapy can induce a cushingoid syndrome with symptoms identical to those of naturally occurring Cushing syndrome. Prominent symptoms are hyperglycemia, glycosuria, fluid and electrolyte disturbances, osteoporosis, muscle weakness, cutaneous striations, and lowered resistance to infection. As mentioned earlier, redistribution of fat to the abdomen, face, and posterior neck produces the characteristic "potbelly," "moon face," and "buffalo hump."

Use in Pregnancy and Lactation

Pregnancy

Glucocorticoids can cross the placenta and affect the developing fetus. This may result in multiple risks for the developing fetus. (See box on page 622.) Of particular concern is the risk for fetal adrenal hypoplasia. Therefore, when large doses have been employed, the infant should be assessed for adrenal sufficiency and given replacement therapy if indicated. Whenever glucocorticoids are to be used during pregnancy, the benefits must be carefully weighed against the potential fetal risk.

Lactation

Glucocorticoids enter breast milk placing the nursing infant at risk. (See box on page 622.) Consequently, women receiving high-dose glucocorticoid therapy should be warned against breastfeeding.

Drug Interactions

Interactions Related to Potassium Loss

As noted, glucocorticoids can increase urinary loss of potassium and can thereby induce hypokalemia. Consequently, glucocorticoids must be used with caution when combined with *digoxin* (because hypokalemia increases the risk for digoxin-induced dysrhythmias) and when combined with *thiazide* or *loop diuretics* (because these potassium-depleting diuretics will increase the risk for hypokalemia). When glucocorticoids are given together with any of the previously mentioned drugs, it is advisable to monitor plasma potassium levels and be alert for signs and symptoms of digoxin toxicity and fluid and electrolyte imbalance.

Nonsteroidal Antiinflammatory Drugs

NSAIDs have the same effects on the GI tract as do glucocorticoids. Accordingly, concurrent use of these agents increases the risk for ulceration and GI bleeding.

Insulin and Oral Hypoglycemics

As noted, glucocorticoids promote hyperglycemia. To maintain glycemic control, patients with diabetes may require increased doses of a glucose-lowering drug (insulin or another hypoglycemic agent).

Vaccines

Because of their immunosuppressant actions, glucocorticoids can decrease antibody responses to vaccines. Accordingly, immunization should not be attempted for some vaccines while glucocorticoids are in use. Furthermore, if a live virus vaccine is employed, the immunosuppressant action of glucocorticoids increases the risk for developing viral disease.

Precautions and Contraindications

Contraindications

Glucocorticoids are contraindicated for patients with *systemic fungal infections* and for those receiving *live virus vaccines.*

Precautions

Glucocorticoids must be used with caution in *pediatric patients* and in *women who are pregnant or breastfeeding.* Caution is also required in patients with *hypertension, heart failure, renal impairment, esophagitis, gastritis, peptic ulcer disease, myasthenia gravis, diabetes mellitus, osteoporosis, open-angle glaucoma,* and *infections that are resistant to treatment.* In addition, caution is required during concurrent therapy with *potassium-depleting diuretics, digoxin, insulin, oral hypoglycemics,* and *NSAIDs.*

Adrenal Suppression

Development of Adrenal Suppression

Like cortisol and other endogenous glucocorticoids, the glucocorticoids that we administer as drugs suppress release of CRH from the hypothalamus and ACTH from the anterior pituitary. By doing so, exogenous glucocorticoids inhibit the synthesis and release of endogenous glucocorticoids by the adrenal glands. During long-term therapy, the pituitary loses much of its ability to manufacture ACTH and, in response to the prolonged absence of ACTH, the adrenal glands atrophy and lose their ability to synthesize cortisol and other glucocorticoids. As a result, when prolonged glucocorticoid therapy is discontinued, there is a period during which the adrenal glands are unable to produce glucocorticoids. The time needed for adrenal recovery is highly variable: it may be as short as 5 days or as long as a year. The extent of adrenal suppression and the time required for recovery are determined primarily by the duration of glucocorticoid use; dosage size is less important. Development of adrenal suppression can be minimized through alternate-day dosing (see later).

Adrenal Suppression and Physiologic Stress

Recall that, when stress occurs, the adrenal glands normally secrete large amounts of glucocorticoids. If the stress is sufficiently severe (e.g., trauma, surgery), these glucocorticoids are essential for supporting life. Accordingly, because of adrenal suppression, *it is imperative that patients receiving long-term glucocorticoid therapy be given increased doses at times of stress* (unless the dosage is already very high). Furthermore, *after glucocorticoid use has ceased, supplemental doses are required whenever stress occurs until recovery of adrenal function is complete.* To ensure appropriate care in emergencies, patients should carry an identification card or bracelet to inform emergency personnel of their glucocorticoid needs. In addition, patients should always have an emergency supply of glucocorticoids on hand.

Glucocorticoid Withdrawal

To allow time for recovery of adrenal function, withdrawal of glucocorticoids should be done slowly. The withdrawal schedule is determined by the degree of adrenal suppression. A representative schedule is as follows: (1) taper the dosage to a physiologic range over 7 days; (2) switch from multiple daily doses to single doses administered each morning; (3) taper the dosage to 50% of physiologic values over the next month; and (4) monitor for production of endogenous cortisol and, when basal levels have returned to normal, cease routine glucocorticoid dosing (but be prepared to give supplemental doses at times of stress). As a rule, tapering is unnecessary when oral glucocorticoids have been used for less than 2 to 3 weeks.

In addition to unmasking adrenal insufficiency, stopping glucocorticoids may produce a withdrawal syndrome. Symptoms include hypotension, hypoglycemia, myalgia, arthralgia, and fatigue. In patients being treated for arthritis and certain other disorders, these symptoms may be confused with return of the underlying disease. Discomfort of withdrawal can be minimized by gradual dosage reduction and by concurrent treatment with NSAIDs.

Preparations and Routes of Administration

Preparations

The glucocorticoids employed clinically include hydrocortisone (cortisol) and synthetic derivatives of hydrocortisone. Individual glucocorticoids differ with respect to (1) biologic half-life, (2) mineralocorticoid potency, and (3) glucocorticoid (antiinflammatory) potency (see Table 56.1).

The term *biologic half-life* refers to the time required for glucocorticoids to leave body tissues. In most cases, these drugs are cleared from tissues more slowly than from the blood. Hence the biologic half-life is usually longer than the plasma half-life. When glucocorticoids are administered by mouth or by intravenous (IV) injection, it is the biologic half-life, and not the plasma half-life, that determines duration of action. Because of differences in their biologic half-lives, individual glucocorticoids can be classified as short acting, intermediate acting, or long acting.

Glucocorticoids with high *mineralocorticoid potency* (cortisone, hydrocortisone) can cause significant retention of sodium and water, coupled with depletion of potassium. These effects can be especially hazardous for patients with hypertension or heart failure and for those taking digoxin. Because of the potential dangers of sodium retention and potassium loss, glucocorticoids with high mineralocorticoid activity should not be administered systemically for long periods.

The differences in *glucocorticoid potency* are reflected in the doses required to produce antiinflammatory effects—not mineralocorticoid effects. As with other drugs, potency is relatively unimportant. However, it is important to appreciate that, in order to produce equivalent therapeutic effects, dosages for some glucocorticoids must be much larger than for others.

Routes of Administration

Glucocorticoids can be administered *orally, parenterally* (IV, IM, subcutaneous [subQ]), *topically,* and *intranasally* and by *local injection* (e.g., intraarticular, intralesional) or *inhalation.* Topical application is used for dermatologic disorders (see Chapter 85), inhalation therapy is used for asthma (see Chapter 60), and intranasal therapy is used for allergic rhinitis (see Chapter 61). Because local therapy (topical, intranasal, inhalation, local injection) minimizes systemic toxicity, this form of treatment is preferred to systemic therapy (oral, parenteral). When systemic effects are needed, oral administration is preferred to parenteral. It is important to note that, even when glucocorticoids are administered for local effects, absorption can be sufficient to produce systemic effects. That is, local administration does not eliminate toxicity risk.

Individual glucocorticoids are available as various esters (e.g., prednisolone *acetate,* prednisolone *sodium phosphate*). When glucocorticoids are administered by routes other than oral or IV, the particular ester employed is a major determinant of duration of action. As indicated in Table 56.2, not all esters can be administered by all routes. Therefore, when preparing to give a glucocorticoid, you should verify that the ester ordered is appropriate for the intended route.

Dosage

General Guidelines for Dosing

For most patients, the therapeutic objective is to reduce symptoms to an acceptable level. Complete relief is not usually an appropriate goal.

Dosages are highly individualized and, for any patient with any disorder, dosage must be determined by trial and error. For patients whose disorder is not an immediate threat to life, the dosage should be low initially and then increased gradually until symptoms are under control. In the event of a life-threatening disorder, a large initial dose should be used, and, if a response does not occur rapidly, the dose should be doubled or even tripled. When glucocorticoids are used for a long time, the dosage should be reduced until the smallest effective amount has been established. Prolonged treatment with high doses should be done only if the disorder (1) is life threatening or (2) has the potential to cause permanent disability. During long-term treatment, an increase in dosage will be needed at times of stress unless the dosage is very high to begin with. If disease status changes, appropriate adjustment of dosage must be made.

As noted, abrupt termination of long-term therapy may unmask adrenal insufficiency. To minimize the effects of adrenal insufficiency, glucocorticoid withdrawal should be gradual. Patients must be warned against abrupt discontinuation.

TABLE 56.2 ■ Glucocorticoid Routes of Administration

	Routes of Administration							
	Systemic			Local				
Drug	**PO**	**IM**	**IV**	**IA**	**IB**	**IL**	**IS**	**ST**
Betamethasone	✓							
Betamethasone sodium phosphate		✓	✓	✓		✓		✓
Betamethasone acetate/sodium phosphate		✓		✓		✓	✓	✓
Cortisone acetate	✓	✓						
Dexamethasone	✓							
Dexamethasone sodium phosphate		✓	✓	✓		✓	✓	✓
Hydrocortisone	✓							
Hydrocortisone acetate				✓	✓	✓	✓	✓
Hydrocortisone sodium succinate		✓	✓					
Methylprednisolone	✓							
Methylprednisolone acetate		✓		✓		✓		✓
Methylprednisolone sodium succinate		✓	✓					
Prednisolone	✓							
Prednisolone acetate	✓							
Prednisolone acetate/sodium phosphate		✓		✓	✓		✓	✓
Prednisolone sodium phosphate	✓							
Prednisone	✓							
Triamcinolone acetonide		✓		✓	✓	✓		
Triamcinolone hexacetonide				✓		✓		

IA, intraarticular; IB, intrabursal; IL, intralesional; IM, intramuscular; IS, intrasynovial; IV, intravenous; PO, oral; ST, soft tissue.

Alternate-Day Therapy

In alternate-day therapy, a large dose (of an intermediate-acting glucocorticoid) is given every other morning. This dosing schedule contrasts with traditional therapy, in which multiple smaller doses are administered daily. Benefits of alternate-day therapy are (1) reduced adrenal suppression, (2) reduced risk for growth delay, and (3) reduced toxicity overall. Adrenal insufficiency is decreased because, over the extended interval between doses, plasma glucocorticoids decline to a level that is low enough to permit some production of ACTH, thereby promoting some synthesis of cortisol by the adrenal glands. To allow maximal recovery of endocrine function, doses should be administered before 9:00 AM, and long-acting agents should be avoided. Early morning administration is also helpful in that it mimics (sort of) the burst of glucocorticoids normally released by the adrenal glands at dawn.

Unfortunately, alternate-day therapy does have one drawback: in the long interval between doses, drug levels may fall to a subtherapeutic value, thus permitting flare-up of symptoms. Symptoms are likely to be most intense late on the second day after a dose is given. If symptoms become intolerable, switching to a single daily dose may be sufficient to provide control. As with alternate-day treatment, patients taking single daily doses should administer their medicine before 9:00 AM.

PRESCRIBING AND MONITORING CONSIDERATIONS

Glucocorticoids

The nursing implications here apply to all glucocorticoids, but only to their use for *nonendocrine disorders.* Implications specific to *asthma therapy* are discussed in Chapter 60.

Therapeutic Goal

Glucocorticoids are used to suppress rejection of organ transplants and to treat a variety of inflammatory, allergic, and neoplastic disorders. When treating inflammatory and allergic disorders, the goal is to suppress signs and symptoms to an acceptable level, not to eliminate them.

Baseline Data

Make a full assessment of the specific disorder (e.g., rheumatoid arthritis, asthma, psoriasis) being treated. These data are used to determine the initial dosage and to guide dosage adjustments as treatment proceeds. Document baseline blood pressure and weight. Determine bone mineral density if therapy will be prolonged. Plot height on children to assess for delayed growth. Also, for prolonged or high dose therapy, check serum glucose, electrolytes, and a complete blood count. Following prolonged treatment, HPA axis suppression may be assessed by checking ACTH stimulation test and plasma or urine cortisol testing.

Identifying High-Risk Patients

Glucocorticoids are *contraindicated* for patients with systemic fungal infections and for individuals receiving live virus vaccines.

Use glucocorticoids with *caution* in pediatric patients and in women who are pregnant or breastfeeding. In addition, exercise *caution* in patients with hypertension, open-angle glaucoma, heart failure, renal impairment, esophagitis, gastritis, peptic ulcer disease, myasthenia gravis, diabetes mellitus, osteoporosis, and infections that are resistant to treatment and in patients receiving potassium-depleting diuretics, digoxin, insulin, oral hypoglycemics, or NSAIDs. When these drugs are necessary, dosage adjustments may be required.

Administration Considerations

Routes and Administration

Glucocorticoids are administered orally, parenterally (IV, IM, subQ), topically (to skin and mucous membranes), intranasally, by inhalation, and by local injection (e.g., intraarticular, intralesional). Routes for specific preparations are shown in Table 56.2. (Glucocorticoids administered topically, inhalation, and intranasally are presented in Chapters 85, 60, and 61, respectively.)

Dosage

Dosage is determined empirically. For patients whose disorder does not threaten life, dosage should be low initially and then gradually increased, until the desired response is achieved. For a life-threatening disorder, initial doses should be as large as needed to control symptoms. During prolonged therapy, the dosage should be reduced to the smallest effective amount. Supplemental doses are needed at times of stress, unless the dosage is very high to begin with.

Alternate-Day Therapy

Alternate-day dosing reduces adrenal suppression and other toxicities. Glucocorticoids should be taken before 9:00 AM every other day.

Drug Withdrawal

Glucocorticoids taken chronically must be withdrawn gradually. After termination, supplemental doses are needed during times of stress until adrenal function has recovered fully.

Ongoing Monitoring and Interventions

Evaluating Therapeutic Effects

Evaluate therapy by making periodic comparisons of current signs and symptoms with the pretreatment assessment. Dosage adjustment is based on these evaluations.

Minimizing Adverse Effects

General Measures. First, keep the dosage as low as possible and the duration of treatment as short as possible. Second, use alternate-day therapy if possible. Third, when appropriate, administer glucocorticoids topically, intranasally, by inhalation, or by local injection, rather than systemically.

Adrenal Insufficiency. Long-term therapy suppresses the ability of the adrenal glands to make glucocorticoids. Increase the dosage when stress occurs (e.g., surgery, trauma, infection) unless the dosage is very high to begin with. After termination of therapy, supplemental doses are required at times of stress until adrenal recovery is complete. Expression of adrenal insufficiency can be reduced by withdrawing glucocorticoids gradually. Adrenal insufficiency can be minimized through alternate-day dosing and use of glucocorticoids that have an intermediate duration of action.

Osteoporosis. Glucocorticoid-induced osteoporosis predisposes the patient to fractures, especially of the ribs and vertebrae. Monitor patients for signs of compression fractures (neck or back pain) and for indications of other fractures. Evaluate status with bone densitometry. Several drugs can help prevent osteoporosis. Important among these are calcium supplements, vitamin D supplements, thiazide diuretics (combined with salt restriction), bisphosphonates (e.g., risedronate, zoledronate), teriparatide, and calcitonin. Estrogen therapy can reduce bone loss in postmenopausal women, but the benefits are not likely to outweigh the risks.

Infection. Glucocorticoids increase the risk for morbidity from infection. Warn patients to avoid close contact with persons who have a communicable disease. Treat established infections with appropriate antimicrobial drugs. Glucocorticoids may need to be withdrawn gradually unless they are absolutely required.

Glucose Intolerance. Glucocorticoids can cause hyperglycemia and glycosuria. Patients with diabetes may need to decrease their caloric intake and use higher doses of hypoglycemic medication (insulin or an oral hypoglycemic).

Fluid and Electrolyte Disturbance. Glucocorticoids can cause sodium and water retention and loss of potassium. These effects can be minimized by (1) using glucocorticoids that have low mineralocorticoid activity, (2) restricting sodium intake, and (3) taking potassium supplements or consuming potassium-rich foods (e.g., bananas, citrus fruits).

Growth Delay. Glucocorticoids can suppress growth in children. Evaluate growth by making periodic measurements of height and weight. Alternate-day therapy minimizes effects on growth.

Cataracts and Glaucoma. Cataracts are a common complication of long-term therapy. Open-angle glaucoma may also develop. The patient should be given an eye examination every 6 months.

Peptic Ulcer Disease. Glucocorticoids may increase the risk for ulcer formation and can mask ulcer symptoms. Have stools checked periodically for occult blood. If ulcers develop, glucocorticoids should be slowly withdrawn—unless their continued use is considered essential for life—and antiulcer therapy should be instituted.

Psychological Disturbances. Systemic glucocorticoids can cause psychological disturbances, both mild (insomnia, anxiety, agitation, irritability) and severe (delirium, hallucinations, depression, euphoria, mania). Depression is more likely with low-dose, long-term therapy, whereas psychoses (mania, delirium) are more likely with high-dose, short-term therapy. Psychological disturbances are reversible and usually resolve within days to weeks after drug withdrawal. Depression may respond to a mood stabilizer (e.g., carbamazepine, valproic acid) or a selective serotonin reuptake inhibitor (e.g., fluoxetine [Prozac]). Psychotic symptoms may respond to an atypical antipsychotic. Monitor for suicidal ideation.

Use in Pregnancy and Lactation

Glucocorticoids can induce adrenal hypoplasia in the developing fetus. When large doses have been employed, the newborn should be assessed for adrenal insufficiency and given replacement therapy if indicated.

During high-dose therapy, the glucocorticoid content of breast milk may become high enough to affect the nursing infant. Warn women who are receiving high-dose therapy not to breastfeed.

Other Adverse Effects

Myopathy and *Cushing syndrome* can be minimized by implementing the general measures noted at the beginning of this section. There are no specific measures to prevent these complications.

Minimizing Adverse Interactions

Interactions Related to Potassium Loss. Glucocorticoid-induced potassium loss can be augmented by *potassium-depleting diuretics* (thiazides, loop diuretics) and can increase the risk for toxicity from *digoxin.* If digoxin and glucocorticoids are used concurrently, potassium levels should be monitored. Also, be alert for indications of cardiotoxicity.

Nonsteroidal Antiinflammatory Drugs. NSAIDs can increase the risk for gastric ulceration during glucocorticoid therapy. Exercise caution when this combination is employed.

Insulin and Other Hypoglycemics. Glucocorticoids can elevate blood levels of glucose. Diabetic patients may need to increase their dosage of insulin or other hypoglycemic drugs.

Vaccines. Glucocorticoids can decrease antibody responses to vaccines and can increase the risk for infection from live virus vaccines. Some vaccines should not be given while glucocorticoids are in use.

Patient Education

GLUCOCORTICOIDS

Instruct patients to take their medicine in the morning to mimic natural physiologic timing of hormone release. Administration with milk or a snack may decrease GI distress.

Warn the patient against abrupt discontinuation of treatment when therapy is with high or prolonged dosing. Adrenal suppression may be life-threatening. Withdrawal symptoms may also occur.

Advise the patient to carry identification (e.g., Medic Alert bracelet) to ensure proper dosing in emergencies. Trauma and other emergencies will require higher doses of glucocorticoids to mimic the normal stress response.

Explain that glucocorticoids can increase the risk for infection. Inform patients about early signs of infection (e.g., fever, malaise), and instruct them to call the clinic if these occur.

Educate patients about signs and symptoms of fluid retention (e.g., weight gain, swelling of the lower extremities) and hypokalemia (e.g., muscle weakness, irregular pulses, cramping), and instruct them to notify the prescriber if these develop.

To decrease the risk of cataracts and glaucoma, reinforce the need for eye examinations during therapy. Instruct the patient to call the clinic if vision becomes cloudy or blurred.

Explain that these drugs can cause GI bleeding. It is important to avoid over-the-counter drugs without first checking with the provider. Instruct the patient to call the clinic if stools become black and tarry.

Inform patients about possible psychological reactions, and instruct them to report disturbing symptoms. Explain that dosage adjustments or other medications may be needed to manage these symptoms.

UNIT XIV
Drugs for Bone and Joint Disorders

CHAPTER 57

Drug Therapy of Rheumatoid Arthritis

Jacqueline Rosenjack Burchum, DNSc, FNP-BC, CNE

Rheumatoid arthritis (RA) is an autoimmune, inflammatory disorder that affects about 1% of the American population. Each year, the disease results in more than 9 million physician visits and more than 250,000 hospitalizations. Although RA can develop at any age, initial symptoms usually appear during the third and fourth decades. Among younger patients, the incidence of RA in females is 3 times greater than in males. However, among patients older than 60 years, the incidence in men and women is equal. Rheumatoid arthritis follows a progressive course and can eventually cause joint deformities and functional limitations. In many cases, drug therapy can delay disease progression. In others, benefits are limited to symptomatic relief. Some of the drugs used for RA were introduced in preceding chapters. Additional drugs are introduced here.

PATHOPHYSIOLOGY OF RHEUMATOID ARTHRITIS

Onset of RA is heralded by symmetrical joint stiffness and pain. Symptoms are most intense in the morning and abate as the day advances. Joints become swollen, tender, and warm. For some patients, periods of spontaneous remission occur. For others, injury progresses steadily. In addition to joint injury, RA has systemic manifestations, including fever, weakness, fatigue, weight loss, thinning of the skin, scleritis (inflammation of the sclera), corneal ulcers, vasculitis (which can be severe), and nodules under the skin and periosteum (connective tissue that surrounds all bones).

The progression of joint deterioration is shown in Fig. 57.1. Inflammation begins in the synovium—the membrane that encloses the joint cavity. As inflammation intensifies, the synovial membrane thickens and begins to envelop the articular cartilage. This overgrowth is referred to as *pannus.* Damage to the cartilage is caused by enzymes released from the pannus and by chemicals and enzymes produced by the inflammatory process raging within the synovial space. Ultimately, the articular cartilage undergoes total destruction, resulting in direct contact between bones of the joint, followed by eventual bone fusion. After this, inflammation subsides.

Joint destruction is caused by an autoimmune process in which the immune system mounts an attack against synovial tissue. During the attack, mast cells, macrophages, and T lymphocytes produce cytokines and cytotoxins—compounds that promote inflammation and joint destruction. The cytokines of greatest importance are tumor necrosis factor (TNF), interleukin-1 (IL-1), IL-6, interferon gamma, platelet-derived growth factor, and granulocyte-macrophage colony-stimulating factor. Why the immune system attacks joints is unclear.

OVERVIEW OF THERAPY

Treatment is directed at (1) relieving symptoms (pain, inflammation, and stiffness), (2) maintaining joint function and range of motion, (3) minimizing systemic involvement, and (4) delaying disease progression. To achieve these goals, a combination of pharmacologic and nonpharmacologic measures is used.

Nondrug Measures

Nondrug measures for managing RA include physical therapy, exercise, and surgery. Physical therapy may consist of massage, warm baths, and applying heat to the affected regions. These procedures can enhance mobility and reduce inflammation. A balanced program of rest and exercise can decrease joint stiffness and improve function. However, excessive rest and excessive exercise should be avoided: too much rest will foster stiffness, and too much activity can intensify inflammation.

Orthopedic surgery has made marked advances. For patients with severe disease of the hip or knee, total joint replacement can be performed. When joints of the hands or wrists have been damaged severely, function can be improved through removal of the diseased synovium and repair of ruptured tendons. Plastic implants can help correct deformities.

A complete program of treatment should include patient education and counseling. The patient should be informed about the nature of RA, the possible consequences of joint

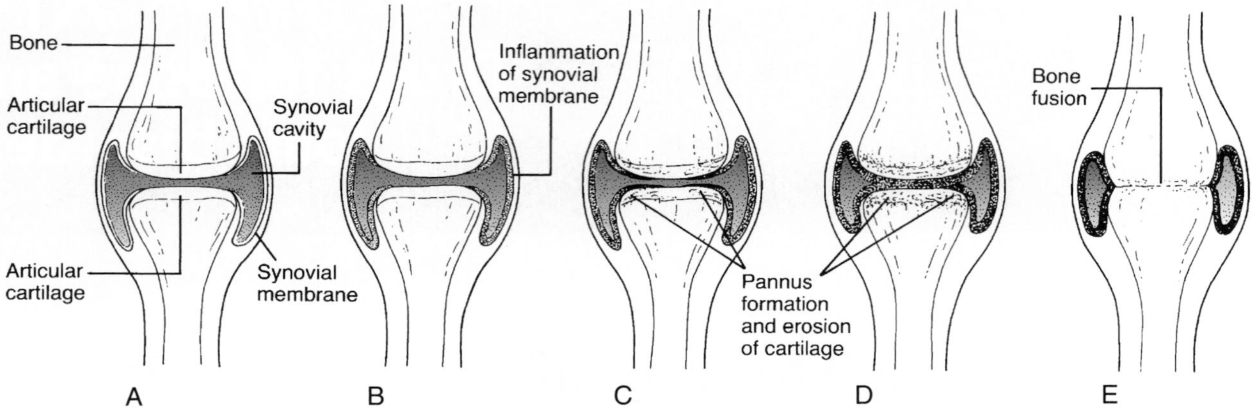

Figure 57.1 ■ Progressive joint degeneration in rheumatoid arthritis.
A, Healthy joint. **B,** Inflammation of synovial membrane. **C,** Onset of pannus formation and cartilage erosion. **D,** Pannus formation progresses, and cartilage deteriorates further. **E,** Complete destruction of joint cavity together with fusion of articulating bones.

degeneration, management measures, and the benefits and limitations of drug therapy. If loss of mobility limits function at home, on the job, or in school, consultation with a social worker, occupational therapist, or specialist in vocational rehabilitation may be appropriate.

Drug Therapy

Antiarthritic drugs can produce symptomatic relief, and some drugs, if started very early in the disease process, can induce protracted remission. However, remission is rarely complete, and the disease typically advances steadily. As a result, drug therapy is chronic and hence success requires patient motivation and cooperation.

Classes of Antiarthritic Drugs

The antirheumatic drugs fall into three major groups:

- Nonsteroidal antiinflammatory drugs (NSAIDs)
- Glucocorticoids
- Disease-modifying antirheumatic drugs (DMARDs)

These major groups differ with respect to time course of effects, toxicity, and ability to slow RA progression.

The NSAIDs provide rapid relief of symptoms but do not prevent joint damage and do not slow disease progression. The NSAIDs are safer than DMARDs and glucocorticoids; thus treatment with NSAIDs requires less vigorous monitoring.

Like the NSAIDs, glucocorticoids provide rapid relief of symptoms. In addition, they can slow disease progression. Unfortunately, although glucocorticoids are effective, with long-term use they can cause serious toxicity. As a result, treatment is usually limited to short courses.

By definition, DMARDs are drugs that reduce joint destruction and slow disease progression. However, benefits develop more slowly than with the NSAIDs. The DMARDs are more toxic than NSAIDs, and therefore close monitoring is required. In the discussion that follows, DMARDs are subdivided into two basic groups—*nonbiologic DMARDs* (traditional DMARDs) and *biologic DMARDs*—based on their molecular size and method of production. The nonbiologic DMARDs are small molecules that are synthesized using conventional chemical techniques. In contrast, the biologic DMARDs are large molecules that are produced through recombinant DNA technology.

Drug Selection

Management of RA is overseen by a rheumatologist or other specialists. DMARDs, in particular, are associated with significant effects and sometimes dangerous risks. Lifespan considerations are a special concern. (See Box 57.1.)

Management of RA is aggressive. Current guidelines recommend starting a DMARD *early*—within 3 months of RA diagnosis for most patients. (See Fig. 57.2.) The aim is to delay joint degeneration. Recall that NSAIDs only provide symptomatic relief; they do not slow disease progression. In contrast, DMARDs may be able to arrest the disease process. By instituting DMARD therapy early—rather than waiting until joint degeneration has advanced to the point at which NSAIDs can no longer control symptoms—it is possible to delay or even prevent serious joint injury.

Because the effects of DMARDs take weeks or months to develop, whereas the effects of NSAIDs are immediate, an NSAID is given until the DMARD has had time to act, after which the NSAID can be withdrawn. As in the past, glucocorticoids are generally reserved for short-course management of symptom flare-ups and to control symptoms until DMARDs take effect. If joint injury progresses despite treatment with an initial DMARD (typically methotrexate), another DMARD can be added or substituted.

You can find detailed information on pharmacologic management of RA in clinical guidelines sponsored by the American College of Rheumatology (ACR). The document, *2015 American College of Rheumatology Guideline for the Treatment of Rheumatoid Arthritis,* is available at http://www.rheumatology.org/Portals/0/Files/ACR%202015%20RA%20Guideline.pdf.

NONSTEROIDAL ANTIINFLAMMATORY DRUGS

The basic pharmacology of the NSAIDs is discussed in Chapter 55. Consideration here is limited to their role in RA.

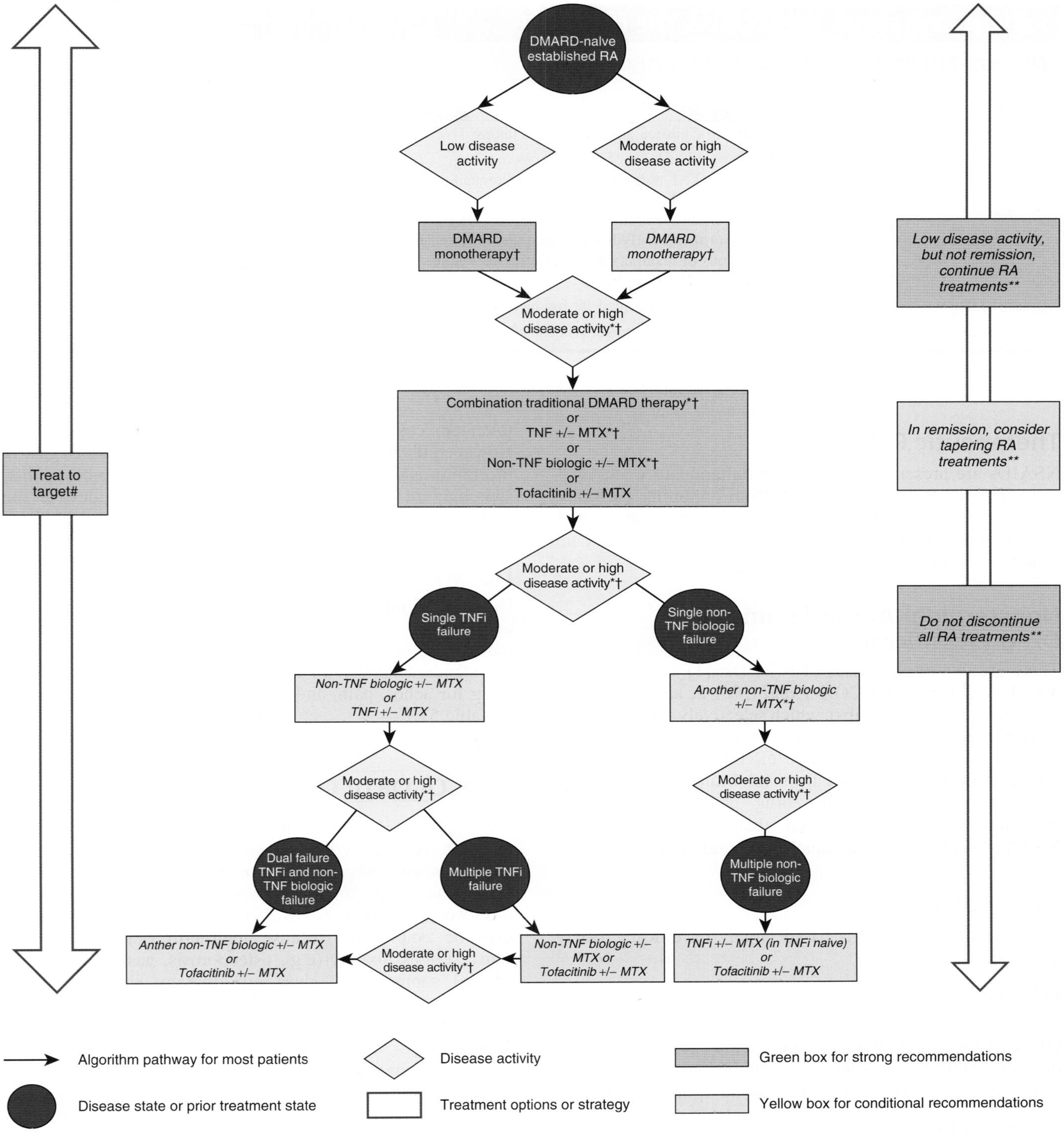

* = consider adding low-dose glucocorticoids (<10 mg/day of prednisone or equivalent) in patients with moderate or high RA disease activity when starting disease-modifying antirheumatic drugs (DMARDs) and in patients with DMARD failure or biologic failure.

† = consider using short-term glucocorticoids (defined as < 3 months treatment) for RA disease flares. Glucocorticoids should be used at the lowest possible dose and for the shortest possible duration to provide the best benefit-risk ratio for the patient.

\# = treatment target should ideally be low disease activity or remission.

** = tapering denotes scaling back therapy (reducing dose or dosing frequency), not discontinuing it and if done, must be conducted slowly and carefully.

Figure 57.2 ▪ Algorithm for rheumatoid arthritis management.
(From 2015 American College of Rheumatology Guidelines for the Treatment of Rheumatoid Arthritis. http://www.rheumatology.org/Portals/0/Files/ACR%202015%20RA%20Guideline.pdf.)

PATIENT-CENTERED CARE ACROSS THE LIFE SPAN

Disease-Modifying Antirheumatic Drugs

Life Stage	Considerations or Concerns
Children	*Biologic DMARDs:* Children and adolescents taking TNF antagonists have developed lymphoma and other malignancies.
Pregnant women	*Biologic DMARDs:* TNF antagonists are FDA Pregnancy Risk Category B. Rituximab and abatacept are Pregnancy Risk Category C. *Nonbiologic DMARDs:* Azathioprine is teratogenic. Both leflunomide and methotrexate can cause fetal death and congenital abnormalities. Hydroxychloroquine may cause fetal ocular toxicity; however, in some conditions such as maternal lupus or malaria, the drug decreases fetal risk associated with the conditions it treats. Sulfasalazine is Pregnancy Risk Category B.
Breastfeeding women	Breastfeeding is not recommended for mothers taking DMARDs.
Older adults	Elderly patients may be at a greater risk for infection secondary to DMARD immunosuppressive effects.

Therapeutic Role

NSAIDs are prescribed for their antiinflammatory and analgesic actions. Both actions result from inhibiting cyclooxygenase (COX). NSAIDs only provide symptomatic relief; they do not slow disease progression. Accordingly, they are usually combined with a DMARD.

Nonsteroidal Antiinflammatory Drug Classification

There are two main classes of NSAIDs: (1) *first-generation NSAIDs,* which inhibit COX-1 *and* COX-2; and (2) *second-generation NSAIDs* (coxibs), which selectively inhibit COX-2. Antiinflammatory and analgesic effects result from inhibiting COX-2, whereas major adverse effects—especially gastroduodenal ulceration—result from inhibiting COX-1. Therefore the selectivity of this drug class results in less gastrointestinal (GI) ulceration than the first-generation NSAIDs, while producing equal therapeutic effects.

Drug Selection

Selection of an NSAID is based largely on efficacy, safety, and cost.

Efficacy

All of the NSAIDs have essentially equal antirheumatic effects. However, individual patients may respond better to one NSAID than to another. Accordingly, it may be necessary to try more than one agent to achieve an optimal response.

Safety and Cost

All prescription-strength NSAIDs carry a boxed warning regarding risk for thrombotic events and GI ulceration and bleeding. Although the risk for GI problems is lessened with COX-2 inhibitors, the risk for thrombotic events may be increased because coxibs inhibit COX-1 to a far lesser degree than traditional NSAIDs. (Recall that COX-1 has a role in the production of thromboxane A_2, which participates in blood clotting.) Selection must balance these factors. Coxibs are more expensive than traditional NSAIDs. If symptoms are controlled with a first-generation NSAID and the drug is well tolerated, cost considerations will dictate using that drug. However, if a first-generation NSAID produces serious gastric ulceration and the patient is at low risk for thrombosis, then switching to celecoxib might be appropriate—despite the increased cost.

Dosage

Dosages employed for antiinflammatory effects are considerably higher than those required for analgesia or fever reduction. For example, treatment of RA may require 5.2 g (16 standard tablets) of aspirin a day, compared with only 2.6 g for aches, pain, and fever. Dosages for RA are shown in Table 57.1.

GLUCOCORTICOIDS

The glucocorticoids are powerful antiinflammatory drugs that can relieve symptoms of severe RA and may also delay disease progression. For patients with generalized symptoms, *oral* glucocorticoids are indicated. However, if only one or two joints are affected, *intraarticular injections* may be employed. Because long-term oral therapy can cause serious toxicity (e.g., osteoporosis, gastric ulceration, adrenal suppression), short-term therapy should be used whenever possible. Most often, glucocorticoids are used for temporary relief until drugs with more slowly developing effects (e.g., methotrexate) can provide control. They may also be employed for flares, which are disease exacerbations that occur in patients whose condition was previously controlled. Long-term therapy should be limited to patients who have failed to respond adequately to all other options. The pharmacology of the glucocorticoids is discussed in Chapter 56.

NONBIOLOGIC (TRADITIONAL) DISEASE-ANTIMODIFYING RHEUMATIC DRUGS

As noted, the nonbiologic DMARDs are small molecules produced using conventional synthetic procedures. With several of these drugs, benefits result from immunosuppression. Unlike

TABLE 57.1 ▪ Nonsteroidal Antiinflammatory Drugs: Oral Dosage for Rheumatoid Arthritis

Generic Name	Trade Name	Daily Dosage
FIRST-GENERATION NSAIDS		
Salicylates		
Aspirin	Multiple trade names	3.6–5.4 g/day in divided doses
Magnesium salicylate	Doan's Extra Strength	650–1160 mg every 6 hours as needed
Salsalate	Generic only	3 g/day (in 2 or 3 doses)
Nonsalicylates		
Diclofenac (salt)	Cambia, Cataflam, Voltaren, Zipsor	Immediate release: 150–200 mg/day (in 3 or 4 doses) Delayed release: 150–200 mg daily (in 2–4 divided doses) Extended release: 100 mg daily or 200 mg daily (in 2 divided doses)
Diclofenac (free acid)	Zorvolex	18–35 mg 3 times a day
Diclofenac/misoprostol	Arthrotec	50 mg diclofenac/200 mcg misoprostol 3 or 4 times daily
Diflunisal	Generic only	250–500 mg twice daily
Etodolac	Generic only	Immediate release: 400 mg 2 times/day *or* 300 mg 2–3 times/day *or* 500 mg 2 times/day Extended release: 400–1000 mg once daily
Fenoprofen	Nalfon	300–600 mg 3 or 4 times/day
Flurbiprofen	Generic only	200–300 mg/day (in 2–4 doses)
Ibuprofen	Motrin, Advil, others	400–800 mg 3 or 4 times/day
Indomethacin	Indocin	25–50 mg 3 times/day
Ketoprofen	Generic only	Immediate release: 150–300 mg/day (in 3 or 4 doses) Extended release: 100–200 mg once a day
Meclofenamate	Generic only	200–400 mg/day (in 3 or 4 doses)
Meloxicam	Mobic, Mobicox 🍁	7.5 mg once a day
Nabumetone	Generic only	1–2 g/day (in 1 or 2 doses)
Naproxen	Naprosyn Naprelan EC-Naprosyn	Immediate release: 250–500 mg twice daily Extended release: 750–1500 mg/daily Delayed release: 375–500 mg twice daily
Naproxen sodium	Aleve, others	250–500 mg twice daily
Naproxen/esomeprazole	Vimovo	375–500 mg (naproxen) twice daily
Oxaprozin	Daypro	1.2 g once a day
Piroxicam	Feldene	10 mg twice daily *or* 20 mg once a day
Sulindac	Clinoril	150–200 mg twice daily
Tolmetin	Generic only	200–600 mg 3 times/day
SECOND-GENERATION NSAIDS (COX-2 INHIBITORS)		
Celecoxib	Celebrex	100–200 mg twice daily

COX, cyclooxygenase; NSAID, nonsteroidal antiinflammatory drug.

the NSAIDs, whose benefits are limited to symptomatic relief, the nonbiologic DMARDs can slow disease progression. These drugs are potentially more harmful than the NSAIDs, and clinical responses develop more slowly. The nonbiologic DMARDs cost much less than the biologic DMARDS, largely because the nonbiologic agents are easier to make.

Methotrexate

Methotrexate [Rheumatrex, Trexall] acts faster than all other DMARDs. Therapeutic effects may develop in 3 to 6 weeks. At least 80% of patients improve with this drug. Benefits are the result of immunosuppression secondary to reducing the activity of B and T lymphocytes. Many rheumatologists consider methotrexate the DMARD of first choice, owing to its efficacy, relative safety, low cost, and extensive use in RA. Major toxicities are hepatic fibrosis, bone marrow suppression, GI ulceration, and pneumonitis. Periodic tests of liver and kidney function are mandatory, as are complete blood cell and platelet counts. Methotrexate can cause fetal death and congenital abnormalities and therefore is contraindicated during pregnancy. Recent data suggest that patients using methotrexate for RA may have a reduced life expectancy, owing to increased deaths from cardiovascular disease, infection, and certain cancers (melanoma, lung cancer, and non-Hodgkin lymphoma). For treatment of RA, methotrexate is administered once a *week,* either orally or by injection. Dosing with folic acid (at least 5 mg/week) is recommended to reduce GI and hepatic toxicity.

BLACK BOX WARNING: METHOTREXATE [RHEUMATREX, TREXALL]

Methotrexate can cause numerous and potentially fatal toxicities of the bone marrow, liver, lungs, and kidneys. Other fatalities have occurred associated with skin reactions and due to hemorrhagic enteritis and gastrointestinal perforation.

Sulfasalazine

Sulfasalazine [Azulfidine, Azulfidine EN-tabs] has been used for decades to treat inflammatory bowel disease. Benefits for RA may result from antiinflammatory and immunomodulatory actions. In patients with RA, sulfasalazine can slow the progression of joint deterioration, sometimes with just 1 month of treatment. Gastrointestinal reactions (nausea, vomiting, diarrhea, anorexia, abdominal pain) are the most common reasons for stopping treatment. These reactions can be minimized by using an enteric-coated formulation and by dividing the daily dosage. Dermatologic reactions (pruritus, rash, urticaria) are also common. Fortunately, serious adverse effects—hepatitis and bone marrow suppression—are rare. To ensure early detection, periodic monitoring for hepatitis and bone marrow function (complete blood counts, platelet counts) should be performed. Because of its structure, sulfasalazine should not be prescribed for patients with sulfa allergy. Sulfasalazine is discussed in Chapter 64.

Leflunomide

Actions and Uses

Leflunomide [Arava] is a powerful immunosuppressant indicated for adults with active RA. In clinical trials, the drug decreased signs and symptoms and slowed disease progression. Compared with methotrexate, leflunomide is about equally effective but is potentially more hazardous and more expensive. Accordingly, the drug is often reserved for second-line use.

Leflunomide is a prodrug that undergoes conversion to its active form—metabolite 1 (M1)—in the body. M1 inhibits dihydroorotate dehydrogenase, a mitochondrial enzyme needed for de novo synthesis of pyrimidines, which in turn are needed for T-cell proliferation and antibody production. In vitro, leflunomide inhibits T-cell proliferation. In animals, it suppresses inflammation.

Pharmacokinetics

After oral dosing, leflunomide is converted to M1 by enzymes in the intestine and liver. Levels of M1 peak in 6 to 12 hours. The active form undergoes further metabolism followed by excretion in the urine and bile. The half-life is prolonged: 16.5 days. As a result, a series of loading doses is needed to achieve steady state quickly.

Adverse Effects

The most common adverse effects occur in at least 10% of patients: diarrhea, respiratory infection, reversible alopecia, and rash. The drug has also been associated with much more serious reactions: pancytopenia, Stevens-Johnson syndrome, and severe hypertension.

Leflunomide is hepatotoxic. Elevation of liver enzymes occurs in about 10% of patients. In postmarketing reports, the drug has been associated with more than 130 cases of severe liver injury, including 14 that were fatal. Liver function should be assessed at baseline, every month for the first 6 months of treatment, and every 6 to 8 weeks thereafter. Leflunomide should be avoided in patients with liver impairment, hepatitis B, or hepatitis C. Patients should be informed about signs of liver injury—abdominal pain, fatigue, dark urine, and jaundice—and advised to report them immediately.

Leflunomide may increase the risk for serious infection. The drug is immunosuppressive and can suppress the bone marrow. Rarely, patients experience sepsis and other severe infections, including tuberculosis. Deaths have occurred. If an infection develops, it may be necessary to interrupt leflunomide use. To reduce risk, platelet counts and blood cell counts should be conducted at baseline, every month for the first 6 months of treatment, and every 6 to 8 weeks thereafter. If evidence of bone marrow suppression is detected, leflunomide should be discontinued. Patients should be screened for tuberculosis before starting this drug.

Leflunomide is carcinogenic in animals but has not been associated with cancer in humans.

Leflunomide and Pregnancy

Leflunomide is contraindicated during pregnancy. Patients who wish to become pregnant must first clear leflunomide from the body. A three-step protocol is followed:

Step 1: Discontinue leflunomide.
Step 2: Take cholestyramine (8 g 3 times a day) for 11 days. (Cholestyramine binds leflunomide and its metabolites in the intestine, accelerating their excretion. Without cholestyramine, safe levels might not be achieved for 2 years.)
Step 3: Verify that plasma drug levels are below 20 mcg/L.

To minimize any risk for fetal injury, men using leflunomide who wish to father a child should undergo the same clearance procedure.

Drug Interactions

Leflunomide can inhibit the metabolism of certain NSAIDs (e.g., ibuprofen, diclofenac), causing their levels to rise. In addition, leflunomide can intensify liver damage from other hepatotoxic drugs (e.g., methotrexate) and hence should not be combined with such agents. Rifampin (a drug for tuberculosis) can raise leflunomide levels by 40%. Conversely, two other agents—cholestyramine and activated charcoal—can rapidly lower leflunomide levels.

Hydroxychloroquine

Hydroxychloroquine [Plaquenil], a drug with antimalarial actions, is considered a preferred DMARD in the 2015 ACR treatment guidelines. How hydroxychloroquine works in RA is unknown. As a rule, the drug is usually combined with methotrexate. By itself, hydroxychloroquine does not slow disease progression, but early use can improve long-term outcomes.

Hydroxychloroquine should be taken with food or milk. Concurrent therapy with antiinflammatory agents (NSAIDs or glucocorticoids) is indicated during the latency period.

Retinal damage, which is rare, is the most serious toxicity. Retinopathy may be irreversible and can produce blindness. Visual loss is directly related to dosage. Low doses may be used in long-term treatment with little risk. When dosage has been excessive, retinal damage may appear after treatment has ceased and may progress in the absence of continued drug use. Patients should undergo a thorough ophthalmologic examination before treatment and every 6 months thereafter. Hydroxychloroquine should be discontinued at the first sign of retinal injury. Patients should be advised to contact the prescriber if any visual disturbance is noted.

Other Nonbiologic Disease-Modifying Antirheumatic Drugs

Several drugs that are FDA approved for RA are used infrequently, largely because of adverse effects. Some (azathioprine, cyclosporine, minocycline, and gold) are no longer recommended; however, they may still be used as a last resort when other drugs fail to meet therapeutic objectives. These drugs are discussed briefly here.

Penicillamine

Penicillamine [Cuprimine, Depen] can relieve symptoms of RA and can delay disease progression. Unfortunately, treatment may be associated with serious toxicity, especially bone marrow suppression and autoimmune disorders. Because it is associated with fatalities, penicillamine use should be restricted to cases where RA is severe and unresponsive to other treatment. Therapeutic effects take 3 to 6 months to develop.

Gold Salts

Gold salts—auranofin [Ridaura]—have been used in RA for decades. Treatment can relieve pain and stiffness and may also delay disease progression. The mechanism underlying these benefits is unknown. Unfortunately, adverse effects are common. Potential reactions include intense pruritus, rashes, stomatitis, kidney damage, severe blood dyscrasias, encephalitis, hepatitis, peripheral neuritis, pulmonary infiltrates, and profound hypotension.

BLACK BOX WARNING: AURANOFIN [RIDAURA]

Gold compounds can cause gold toxicity manifested by serious blood dyscrasias, stomatitis, profuse diarrhea, proteinuria, hematuria, and rash.

Azathioprine

Azathioprine [Imuran] is an older DMARD with immunosuppressive and antiinflammatory actions. Serious toxicities include hepatitis and blood dyscrasias (leukopenia, thrombocytopenia, anemia). The drug may also pose a small risk for malignancy.

Cyclosporine

Cyclosporine [Neoral, Sandimmune], an immunosuppressive drug used to prevent rejection of transplanted organs, can reduce symptoms of RA. Because it can cause kidney damage and other serious adverse effects, cyclosporine should be reserved for severe, progressive RA that has not responded to safer DMARDs. In patients with an inadequate response to methotrexate, adding cyclosporine may produce significant improvement.

Minocycline

Minocycline [Minocin], an antibiotic in the tetracycline family, has been used experimentally in RA management. It can improve morning stiffness, joint pain and tenderness, and activities of daily living. In addition, it may delay disease progression in some patients. The precise mechanism by which it accomplishes this is unknown. The ACR did not include minocycline in the 2015 guidelines because of its infrequent use and the lack of new data since 2012.

Protein A Column [Prosorba]

The Prosorba column, used in combination with plasmapheresis, decreases the titer of circulating immune complexes that promote symptoms of RA. The column contains an adsorbent compound—protein A—that binds to antibodies of the immunoglobulin G (IgG) class and to IgG-antigen complexes. When the patient's plasma is passed through the column, these antibodies and immune complexes are removed. Treatment should be reserved for patients with moderate to severe RA who have been refractory to or intolerant of methotrexate and other DMARDs. The most common adverse effects are transient increases in joint swelling, joint pain, and fatigue.

BIOLOGIC DISEASE-MODIFYING ANTIRHEUMATIC DRUGS

The biologic DMARDs are immunosuppressive drugs that target specific components of the inflammatory process (Table 57.2). These drugs are usually combined with methotrexate.

TABLE 57.2 ▪ Disease-Modifying Antirheumatic Drugs

NONBIOLOGIC (TRADITIONAL) DMARDS	
Major drugs	Methotrexate [Rheumatrex, Trexall]
	Sulfasalazine [Azulfidine]
	Leflunomide [Arava]
	Minocycline [Minocin]
	Hydroxychloroquine [Plaquenil]
Minor drugs	Azathioprine [Imuran]
	Cyclosporine [Neoral, Sandimmune]
	Penicillamine [Cuprimine, Depen]
	Protein A [Prosorba]
	Gold salts:
	Gold sodium thiomalate [Aurolate, Myochrysine]
	Auranofin [Ridaura]
BIOLOGIC DMARDS	
Tumor necrosis factor antagonists	Adalimumab [Humira]
	Certolizumab pegol [Cimzia]
	Etanercept [Enbrel]
	Golimumab [Simponi, Simponi Aria]
	Infliximab [Remicade]
B-lymphocyte–depleting agent	Rituximab [Rituxan]
T-cell activation inhibitor	Abatacept [Orencia]
Interleukin-6 receptor antagonist	Tocilizumab [Actemra]
Interleukin-1 receptor antagonist	Anakinra [Kineret]

DMARD, disease-modifying antirheumatic drug.

Of the biologic agents available, only seven are used routinely. Five of these—etanercept, infliximab, adalimumab, golimumab, and certolizumab pegol—interfere with TNF. One agent—rituximab—promotes destruction of B lymphocytes, and one agent—abatacept—inhibits activation of T lymphocytes. Because these drugs suppress immune function, they all pose a risk for serious infections, and perhaps cancer. As noted, the biologic DMARDs are so named because they are manufactured using recombinant DNA technology, an expensive process that is reflected in the cost of these drugs, which can range from $14,000 to more than $65,000 a year.

Tumor Necrosis Factor Antagonists

The drugs in this group work by neutralizing TNF, an important immune mediator of joint injury in RA. Five TNF antagonists are available. In patients with RA, all five are highly and equally effective. Unfortunately, all five pose a risk for serious infections, including bacterial sepsis, invasive fungal infections, hepatitis B infection, and tuberculosis (TB). Rarely, patients experience severe allergic reactions, heart failure, liver failure, hematologic disorders, neurologic disorders, or cancer. The principal differences among these drugs concern dosing schedule and route of administration.

In addition to their use in RA, these drugs are approved for other inflammatory disorders, including psoriatic arthritis, ankylosing spondylitis, and Crohn disease (Table 57.3).

Etanercept

Etanercept [Enbrel] was the first TNF antagonist available and will serve as our prototype for the group. Like all other TNF antagonists, etanercept is highly effective at reducing RA symptoms and disease progression but may also promote serious infections and other adverse effects.

Prototype Drugs

DRUGS FOR RHEUMATOID ARTHRITIS

Nonsteroidal Antiinflammatory Drugs

Aspirin (a first-generation NSAID)
Celecoxib (a COX-2 inhibitor)

Glucocorticoids

Prednisone

Disease-Modifying Antirheumatic Drugs

Methotrexate (immunosuppressant)
Etanercept (TNF antagonist)

Mechanism of Action

Etanercept suppresses inflammation by neutralizing TNF. As noted earlier, TNF is an important contributor to RA pathophysiology. In patients with RA, TNF binds with receptors on cells in the synovium and thereby stimulates production of chemotactic factors and endothelial adhesion molecules, which in turn promote infiltration of neutrophils and macrophages. The result is inflammation and joint destruction.

How does etanercept neutralize TNF? Etanercept is a large molecule composed of two receptors for TNF that are linked to the Fc component of IgG. The TNF receptors, which are

TABLE 57.3 ▪ Approved Indications for Tumor Necrosis Factor Antagonists

Approved Indications	Etanercept [Enbrel]	Infliximab [Remicade]	Adalimumab [Humira]	Golimumab [Simponi]	Certolizumab [Cimzia]
Rheumatoid arthritis	✓	✓	✓	✓	✓
Ankylosing spondylitis	✓	✓	✓	✓	✓
Juvenile idiopathic arthritis	✓		✓		
Psoriatic arthritis	✓	✓	✓	✓	✓
Plaque psoriasis	✓	✓	✓		
Crohn disease		✓	✓		✓
Ulcerative colitis		✓	✓	✓	

produced through recombinant DNA technology, are identical to the TNF receptors found on human cells. Like the TNF receptors on our cells, etanercept binds tightly with TNF and thereby prevents TNF from interacting with its natural receptors on cells.

Therapeutic Uses

Etanercept is indicated for patients with moderately to severely active RA. In clinical trials, the drug was slightly superior to methotrexate at delaying progression of joint damage, and it suppressed signs and symptoms of RA more rapidly. Among patients who had failed to respond to methotrexate, addition of etanercept for 6 months reduced symptoms in 61%, compared with 27% who continued taking methotrexate alone.

In addition to RA, etanercept is approved for ankylosing spondylitis, plaque psoriasis, psoriatic arthritis, and juvenile idiopathic arthritis.

Pharmacokinetics

Etanercept is administered by subcutaneous (subQ) injection. Plasma levels peak about 3 days after dosing. The drug is cleared from the plasma with a half-life of 115 hours (about 5 days). The mode of elimination is unknown. One hypothesis is that metabolism of the bound TNF-drug complex takes place through peptide or amino acid degradation, after which elimination of metabolites takes place in the bile or urine while amino acids are recycled.

BLACK BOX WARNING: TUMOR NECROSIS FACTOR ANTAGONISTS

Patients taking TNF antagonists (adalimumab, certolizumab pegol, etanercept, golimumab, and infliximab) are at an increased risk for developing serious systemic infections and sepsis.

Children and adolescents taking TNF antagonists have developed lymphoma and other malignancies.

Adverse Effects

Mild Effects. Injection-site reactions—itching, erythema, swelling, pain—occur in 37% of patients but usually subside in a few days. Other mild but less common reactions include headache, rhinitis, dizziness, cough, and abdominal pain.

Serious Infections. Etanercept increases the risk for serious infections, including invasive fungal infections (e.g., histoplasmosis, coccidioidomycosis, candidiasis) and infections caused by *Mycobacterium tuberculosis* and other opportunistic pathogens, such as *Legionella pneumophila* and *Listeria monocytogenes.* Why do these infections develop? Under normal conditions, TNF plays a crucial role in our immune response to infections, especially those caused by *M. tuberculosis* and other intracellular pathogens. Accordingly, when we neutralize TNF with etanercept, the risk for infections goes up. Infection risk is further increased by diabetes, HIV infection, and concurrent use of immunosuppressant drugs, including glucocorticoids and methotrexate.

Tuberculosis is a special concern. When TB develops in patients taking etanercept, the disease is often extrapulmonary and disseminated. To reduce risk, potential users should be tested for latent TB and, if the test is positive, should undergo TB treatment before etanercept is used. During etanercept treatment, patients should be monitored closely for TB development.

Etanercept may promote reactivation of latent infection with hepatitis B virus (HBV). Fatalities have occurred. Candidates for etanercept therapy should be tested for latent HBV, and those who test positive should be monitored closely. If reactivation of HBV infection occurs, etanercept should be stopped and the patient given antiviral drugs.

To reduce infection risk, etanercept should not be given to patients with active infection, including infections that are chronic or localized. Patients who develop a new infection should be monitored closely. Etanercept should be used with caution in patients with a history of recurrent infection or any condition that predisposes them to acquiring infection (e.g., advanced or poorly controlled diabetes). If a severe infection develops, etanercept should be discontinued.

Severe Allergic Reactions. Rarely, etanercept has been associated with severe allergic reactions, including Stevens-Johnson syndrome (SJS), erythema multiforme, and toxic epidermal necrolysis (TEN). The median onset of symptoms in known cases was 28 days after starting etanercept. Patients and providers should be alert for these reactions.

Heart Failure. Etanercept may pose a risk for heart failure. In patients using the drug, existing cases of heart failure have gotten worse, and new cases have developed. Exercise caution in patients with existing heart failure and monitor them closely for disease progression.

Cancer. Etanercept and other TNF antagonists may increase the risk for lymphoma and other malignancies, primarily in children, adolescents, and young adults.

Hematologic Disorders. Etanercept may pose a small risk for hematologic disorders, including neutropenia, thrombocytopenia, and aplastic anemia, which can be fatal. Advise patients who develop signs or symptoms of a blood disorder (persistent fever, bruising, bleeding, pallor) to seek immediate medical attention. If a significant hematologic abnormality is diagnosed, discontinuing etanercept should be considered.

Liver Injury. Rarely, etanercept has been associated with severe liver injury, including acute liver failure. Some patients have required a liver transplant, and some have died. Patients should be informed about symptoms of liver injury—fatigue, yellow skin, yellow eyes, anorexia, right-sided abdominal pain, dark brown urine—and advised to seek medical attention if these develop. If severe liver injury is diagnosed, discontinuation of etanercept should be considered. Etanercept should be used with caution in patients with preexisting liver dysfunction.

CNS Demyelinating Disorders. Etanercept has been associated with rare cases of CNS demyelinating disorders, including multiple sclerosis, myelitis, and optic neuritis. However, a causal relationship has not been established. Nonetheless, caution is advised, especially in patients with a preexisting or recent-onset demyelinating disorder.

Drug Interactions. By neutralizing TNF, etanercept may increase the risk for acquiring or transmitting infection after immunization with a *live virus vaccine.* Accordingly, live virus vaccines should be avoided. In pediatric patients, vaccinations should be up to date before starting the drug.

Immunosuppressant drugs—including glucocorticoids, methotrexate, tocilizumab, anakinra, and abatacept—increase the risk for serious infection. Use these combinations with caution.

Preparations, Dosage, and Administration. Preparation, dosage, and administration of etanercept and other DMARDs are provided in Table 57.4.

Infliximab

Actions and Uses

Infliximab [Remicade], formulated for intravenous (IV) use, was the second TNF antagonist approved for RA. Like etanercept, infliximab binds to and thereby neutralizes TNF. However, the two drugs are structurally different: whereas etanercept is composed of two TNF receptors, infliximab is a TNF antibody.

In patients with RA, infliximab is approved for combined use with methotrexate to reduce symptoms and delay disease progression. Infliximab is also approved for psoriasis (see Chapter 85), psoriatic arthritis, ankylosing spondylitis, and two intestinal disorders: Crohn disease and ulcerative colitis (see Chapter 64).

Adverse Effects

Like etanercept, infliximab has immunosuppressant actions that can increase the risk for serious infection, including bacterial sepsis, invasive fungal infections, HBV infection, and TB. Accordingly, the drug should not be given to patients with chronic infections and should be temporarily withdrawn if an acute infection develops. Patients should receive a TB test and HBV test to rule out latent infection before treatment.

Like other TNF inhibitors, infliximab has been associated with rare cases of heart failure, liver failure, hematologic disorders, neurologic disorders, severe allergic reactions, and cancer.

Infliximab is administered by slow IV infusion. Infusion reactions are common, manifesting as flu-like symptoms, headache, fever, chills, dyspnea, hypotension, skin reactions, and GI disturbance. Rarely, patients experience anaphylaxis. Symptoms can be reduced by pretreatment with an antihistamine, acetaminophen, or a glucocorticoid. Mild reactions can be managed by slowing or interrupting the infusion. If anaphylaxis develops, the infusion should be stopped.

Adalimumab

Like infliximab, adalimumab [Humira] is a monoclonal antibody that binds to and thereby neutralizes TNF. The drug is indicated for adults with moderate to severe RA who have not responded adequately to one or more DMARDs. In these patients, adalimumab can reduce symptoms and slow progression of joint damage. The drug may be used alone or in combination with methotrexate or other DMARDs. In addition to RA, adalimumab is approved for ankylosing spondylitis, juvenile idiopathic arthritis, plaque psoriasis, psoriatic arthritis, ulcerative colitis, and Crohn disease.

Adalimumab is generally well tolerated. The most common side effects are injection-site reactions (rash, erythema, itching, pain, swelling), which develop in about 20% of patients. Like other TNF inhibitors, adalimumab can promote serious infections (e.g., bacterial sepsis, invasive fungal infections, HBV infection, TB) and has been associated with rare cases of heart failure, liver failure, hematologic disorders, neurologic disorders, severe allergic reactions, and cancer.

Golimumab

Golimumab [Simponi, Simponi Aria] is approved for RA—but only in combination with methotrexate. Like infliximab, golimumab is a monoclonal antibody that binds with and thereby neutralizes TNF. In addition to RA, golimumab is approved for treatment of ulcerative colitis, ankylosing spondylitis, and psoriatic arthritis.

In clinical trials, the most common adverse effects were injection-site reactions, upper respiratory tract infections, and nasopharyngitis. However, except for injection-site reactions, the incidence of these adverse effects was only slightly higher than in patients receiving placebo. Like other TNF inhibitors, golimumab can promote serious infections (e.g., bacterial sepsis, invasive fungal infections, HBV infection, TB) and has been associated with rare cases of heart failure, liver failure, hematologic disorders, neurologic disorders, severe allergic reactions, and cancer.

Certolizumab Pegol

Certolizumab pegol [Cimzia] is a monoclonal antibody derivative designed to neutralize TNF. The drug consists of a recombinant humanized Fab antibody fragment that has been covalently bound to polyethylene glycol (PEG). Because of this "pegylation," the drug is eliminated slowly, with a half-life of 17 days. Certolizumab is approved for treatment of adults with moderate to severe RA, Crohn disease, ankylosing spondylitis, and psoriatic arthritis. In patients with RA, the combination of certolizumab plus methotrexate is more effective than certolizumab alone.

Certolizumab can cause serious adverse effects. In clinical trials, the most common events were upper respiratory tract infections, urinary tract infections, and arthralgia. Like other TNF inhibitors, certolizumab can promote serious infections (e.g., bacterial sepsis, invasive fungal infections, HBV infection, TB) and has been associated with rare cases of heart failure, liver failure, hematologic disorders, neurologic disorders, severe allergic reactions, and cancer.

Rituximab, a B-Lymphocyte–Depleting Agent

Actions and Uses

Rituximab [Rituxan] reduces the number of B lymphocytes, cells that play an important role in the autoimmune attack on joints. As a result, rituximab can reduce symptoms of RA and slow disease progression. How does it work? Rituximab is a monoclonal antibody directed against CD20, an antigen found exclusively on the surface of B lymphocytes. When rituximab binds with CD20, the immune system attacks the rituximab–B-cell complex, causing B-cell lysis and death.

Rituximab, in combination with methotrexate, is indicated for IV therapy of adults with moderate to severe RA who have not responded to one or more TNF antagonists. In addition, rituximab is indicated for two inflammatory disorders of blood vessels—Wegener granulomatosis and microscopic polyangiitis—and for two types of cancer: B-cell non-Hodgkin lymphoma and B-cell chronic lymphocytic leukemia.

Adverse Effects

Infusion Reactions

Rituximab can cause severe infusion-related hypersensitivity reactions, beginning within 30 to 120 minutes. The immediate reaction and its sequelae include hypotension, bronchospasm, angioedema, hypoxia, pulmonary infiltrates, myocardial infarction, and cardiogenic shock. Deaths have occurred within 24 hours. To reduce the risk for these events, patients should be premedicated with an antihistamine and acetaminophen and monitored during the infusion. If a severe reaction occurs, management includes giving glucocorticoids, epinephrine, bronchodilators, and oxygen.

Mucocutaneous Reactions

Rituximab has been associated with severe mucocutaneous reactions, including SJS, lichenoid dermatitis, vesiculobullous dermatitis, and TEN. Deaths have occurred. Reaction onset is typically 1 to 3 weeks after rituximab exposure. Patients who experience these reactions should seek immediate medical attention and should not receive rituximab again.

Hepatitis B Reactivation

There have been reports of HBV reactivation, leading to fulminant hepatitis, hepatic failure, and death. Patients at high risk for HBV should be screened before getting rituximab. Asymptomatic carriers should be closely monitored for clinical and laboratory signs of active HBV infection while taking rituximab, and for several months after stopping.

TABLE 57.4 ▪ Disease-Modifying Antirheumatic Drugs: Common Dosages for Rheumatoid Arthritis

Drug Name	Preparation	Dosage	Administration
NONBIOLOGIC (TRADITIONAL) DMARDS			
Methotrexate [Rheumatrex, Trexall]	Tablet: 2.5 mg, 5 mg, 7.5 mg, 10 mg, 15 mg Solution: 25 mg/mL Autoinjector: 15 different dosages ranging from 7.5 mg/0.15 mL to 30 mg/0.6 mL	Oral, subQ, and IM: 7.5 mg weekly initially then adjusted upward until optimal response is achieved or a maximal dose of 20–30 mg/week is reached Optional oral dosing: 10–15 mg/week initially, and then increased by 5 mg/week every 2–4 weeks, up to a maintenance level of 20–30 mg/week	Autoinjectors allow for self-administration. Dosing with folic acid is recommended to reduce GI and hepatic toxicity.
Sulfasalazine [Azulfidine, Azulfidine EN-tabs]	IR tablet: 500 mg (scored) ER tablet: 500 mg	Initial: 0.5–1 g/day Maintenance: 1 g given 2 or 3 times a day	Avoid in patients who are allergic to sulfonamides. Space tablets evenly throughout the day, preferably after meals. Swallow ER tablets whole.
Leflunomide [Arava]	Tablets: 10 mg, 20 mg	Initial: loading doses of 100 mg once a day for 3 days Maintenance: 10–20 mg daily	May be given with or without food
Hydroxychloroquine [Plaquenil]	Tablet: 200 mg	Initially: 400–600 mg/day increased slowly to achieve optimal response over 1–3 months Maintenance: 200–400 mg/day	Take with food or milk
BIOLOGIC DMARDS			
Adalimumab [Humira]	Prefilled syringe: 20 mg/0.4 mL, 40 mg/0.8 mL Autoinjector: 40 mg/0.8 mL	40 mg every 2 weeks If used without methotrexate: 40 mg once a week	Administer subQ in the anterior thigh or abdomen. Rotate sites. Avoid areas where the skin is tender, bruised, red, or indurated.
Certolizumab pegol [Cimzia]	Prefilled syringe: 200 mg/mL	Initial: 400 mg repeated at 2 and 4 weeks Maintenance: 200 mg every 2 weeks or 400 mg every month	Inject subQ into the abdomen or thigh. Two separate injections are needed because of the size of the dose.
Etanercept [Enbrel]	Prefilled syringe: 25 mg/0.5 mL, 50 mg/mL Autoinjector: 50 mg/mL Powder: 25-mg for reconstitution in 1 mL of sterile bacteriostatic water	Adult: 50 mg subQ once a week Children ages 4–17 years: 0.8 mg/kg (up to a maximum of 50 mg) once a week	Inject subQ into the abdomen or anterior thigh. Avoiding areas that are tender, bruised, red, or indurated. Solutions that are discolored or cloudy or contain particles should not be used.
Golimumab [Simponi, Simponi Aria]	Prefilled syringe: 50 mg/0.5 mL, 100 mg/mL Autoinjector: 50 mg/0.5 mL, 100 mg/mL Solution for IV administration: 50 mg/4 mL	SubQ (Simponi): 50 mg once a month IV (Simponi Aria): 2 mg/kg repeated at 4 weeks and then every 8 weeks for maintenance	Inject subQ into the abdomen or anterior thigh. Avoiding areas that are tender, bruised, red, or indurated. IV: Infuse diluted solution over 30 minutes. Do not infuse other medications in the same line.
Infliximab [Remicade]	Powder: 100 mg in single-use vials to be dissolved in 10 mL of sterile water, followed by dilution in 0.9% sodium chloride to a final volume of 250 mL.	Initial: 3 mg/kg repeated at 2 weeks and 6 weeks Maintenance: 3 mg/kg every 8 weeks	IV solutions should be clear and either colorless or pale yellow; discard if discolored or with visible particles.
Rituximab [Rituxan]	Solution: 10 mg/mL in 10-mL and 50-mL vials	Initial: 1000 mg IV infusion repeated in 2 weeks Subsequent treatment: 1000 mg every 24 weeks if needed	Dilute to 1–4 mg/mL for IV infusion. Premedicate with an antihistamine, acetaminophen, and IV corticosteroid 30 minutes before infusion. Start at 50 mg/h and, if no reaction, increase rate to 400 mg/h. Monitor closely for infusion reactions.

TABLE 57.4 ■ Disease-Modifying Antirheumatic Drugs: Common Dosages for Rheumatoid Arthritis—cont'd

Drug Name	Preparation	Dosage	Administration
Abatacept [Orencia]	Prefilled syringe: 125 mg/mL IV: 250-mg powder for reconstitution in sterile water	SubQ: 125 mg weekly, preferably after a single IV loading dose of 10 mg/kg IV for adults <60 kg, give 500 mg; 60–100 kg, give 750 mg; >100 kg, give 1000 mg Repeat at 2 weeks and 4 weeks after first infusion and then repeat every 4 weeks IV for polyarticular juvenile idiopathic arthritis: <75 kg, give 10 mg/kg; 75–100 kg, give 750 mg; >100 kg, give 1000 mg. As in adults, dosing is done on days 0, 14, and 28, and every 4 weeks thereafter.	Reconstitute with gentle swirling motion to minimize foam. Dilute reconstituted solution to a final volume of 100 mL. Discard discolored solution or solutions containing particles. Infuse over 30 minutes. Do not infuse other medications in the same line.
Tocilizumab [Actemra]	Prefilled syringe: 162 mg/0.9 mL IV: 80 mg, 300 mg, and 400 mg as a concentrated solution (20 mg/mL) for dilution in 0.9% sodium chloride to a final volume of 100 mL	SubQ: <100 kg, give 162 mg every 2 weeks; may increase if response suboptimal >100 kg, give 162 mg weekly IV: 4 mg/kg every 4 weeks, given as a single 60-minute IV drip infusion. The dosage can be increased to 8 mg/kg every 4 weeks based on the clinical response. The maximal single dose is 800 mg.	SubQ: Discard if discolored or with visible particles. Rotate injection sites. Avoid areas where the skin is tender, bruised, red, or indurated. IV: Discard solution if discolored or with visible particles. Infuse over 60 minutes. Do not infuse other medications in the same line.
Anakinra [Kineret]	Prefilled syringe: 100 mg/0.67 mL	SubQ: 100 mg once daily	Do not shake before administration. Rotate injection sites. Avoid areas where the skin is tender, bruised, red, or indurated.

ER, extended release; GI, gastrointestinal; IM, intramuscular; IR, immediate release; IV, intravenous; subQ, subcutaneous.

Progressive Multifocal Leukoencephalopathy (PML)

Rituximab has been associated with rare cases of PML, a severe infection of the CNS caused by reactivation of the JC virus, an opportunistic pathogen resistant to all available drugs. Most cases have occurred in patients being treated for non-Hodgkin lymphoma. Patients and prescribers should be alert for any new neurologic signs and symptoms. If PML is diagnosed, rituximab should be discontinued immediately.

Other Adverse Effects

Like other monoclonal antibodies, rituximab can cause a flu-like syndrome, especially during the initial infusion. Symptoms include fever, chills, nausea, vomiting, and myalgia. Rituximab causes transient neutropenia, but this does not appear to increase the risk for infection.

Preparations, Dosage, and Administration

Rituximab [Rituxan] is supplied in solution (10 mg/mL) in 10- and 50-mL single-use vials. The concentrated solution should be diluted in 0.9% sodium chloride or 5% dextrose in water to a final concentration of 1 to 4 mg/mL and then administered by IV infusion. To reduce the risk for infusion reactions, patients should be premedicated with an antihistamine and acetaminophen. Premedication with an IV corticosteroid such as methylprednisolone is also recommended for patients with RA.

Abatacept, a T-Cell Activation Inhibitor

Abatacept [Orencia], a first-in-class T-cell activation inhibitor, reduces symptoms of RA and disease progression. Patients who have not responded adequately to methotrexate or TNF antagonists have experienced significant improvement with this drug. Like other biologic DMARDs, abatacept poses a risk for serious infections and may also pose a small risk for cancer.

Therapeutic Uses

Abatacept has two approved indications: to reduce symptoms and delay disease progression in adults with moderately to severely active RA and to decrease symptoms of moderately to severely active polyarticular juvenile idiopathic arthritis in children 6 years and older. For adult patients with RA, abatacept may be used alone or in combination with most other DMARDs, but not with TNF antagonists or anakinra. For children with juvenile idiopathic arthritis, the drug may be used alone or in combination with methotrexate.

Mechanism of Action

In patients with RA, activated T lymphocytes play a key role in the autoimmune attack on joints. Abatacept prevents T-cell activation. Here's how. For T cells to achieve full activity, they must be stimulated by antigen-presenting cells (APCs). Abatacept—a complex molecule composed of a ligand (cytotoxic T-lymphocyte–associated antigen 4) linked to IgG1—binds with receptors on APCs and thereby prevents the APCs from activating T cells. The results are reduced T-cell proliferation and reduced production of interferon gamma, interleukins, and TNF.

Adverse Effects

Abatacept is generally well tolerated. The most common adverse effects are headache, upper respiratory infection, nasopharyngitis, and nausea.

Because abatacept suppresses immune function, the drug can increase the risk for serious infections. Infections seen most often are pneumonia, cellulitis, bronchitis, diverticulitis, pyelonephritis, and urinary tract infections. Patients should be told about infection risk and advised to report suspected infection immediately. If a serious infection develops, abatacept should be discontinued.

Abatacept may blunt the effect of all vaccines and may increase the risk for infection from live virus vaccines. Before abatacept is given to children, all vaccinations should be up to date. Live virus vaccines should not be used in children or adults during abatacept use and for 3 months after stopping.

Drug Interactions

Abatacept should not be used in conjunction with TNF antagonists. The combination increases the risk for serious infection and offers no benefit over abatacept alone.

Tocilizumab, an Interleukin-6 Receptor Antagonist

In patients with RA, IL-6 helps amplify the autoimmune attack on joints. Accordingly, drugs that block the actions of IL-6 can reduce RA symptoms and disease progression. At this time, tocilizumab is the only drug that works by this mechanism.

Actions and Therapeutic Use

Tocilizumab [Actemra] is a first-in-class IL-6 receptor antagonist. In 2010 the FDA approved tocilizumab for IV therapy of adults with moderately to severely active RA. However, owing to the risk for infection and other serious adverse effects, tocilizumab is indicated only for those patients with RA who have not responded adequately to other DMARDs. In five clinical trials involving more than 4000 patients, tocilizumab was significantly more effective than placebo at reducing joint tenderness and swelling. Tocilizumab may be combined with methotrexate, but not with TNF inhibitors or other DMARDs that increase the risk for infection. In addition to treatment of RA, tocilizumab has also received FDA approval for management of polyarticular juvenile idiopathic arthritis and systemic juvenile idiopathic arthritis.

How does tocilizumab work? The drug is a monoclonal antibody that blocks receptors for IL-6, a proinflammatory cytokine that helps mediate the autoimmune attack against the joints of patients with RA. By blocking IL-6 receptors, tocilizumab prevents IL-6 from promoting injury. Tocilizumab is the first drug to work by this mechanism.

Adverse Effects

The most serious adverse effects are infections, GI perforation, liver injury, and hematologic effects: neutropenia and thrombocytopenia. Other adverse effects include headache, nasopharyngitis, hypertension, and increased cholesterol levels.

Serious Infections

Owing to its immunosuppressant actions, tocilizumab increases the risk for life-threatening infections. Infections seen in clinical trials include TB, invasive fungal infections, and opportunistic infections caused by bacteria, viruses, protozoa, and other pathogens. Before starting tocilizumab, patients should be tested for latent TB and treated as indicated. During tocilizumab therapy, patients should be closely monitored for signs and symptoms of infection. In the event of certain laboratory changes—increased transaminase levels, reduced neutrophil counts, or reduced platelet counts—tocilizumab should be given in reduced dosage or discontinued, depending on the magnitude of the change. Treatment should be interrupted if the patient develops a serious infection.

BLACK BOX WARNING: TOCILIZUMAB [ACTEMRA]

Tocilizumab may cause an increased risk for developing serious and potentially fatal infections.

GI Perforation

In clinical trials, perforation of the colon occurred rarely. Most cases were complications of preexisting diverticulitis (i.e., inflammation of diverticula [small outpouchings] along the colon wall). Patients at high risk for perforation—especially those with diverticulitis—should be closely monitored. Patients should be instructed to contact their prescriber in the event of severe, persistent abdominal pain.

Liver Injury

Tocilizumab can cause liver injury, as indicated by elevation of circulating liver transaminases (aspartate aminotransferase and alanine aminotransferase). Tocilizumab should not be initiated if transaminase levels are more than 2 times the upper limit of normal (ULN). Transaminase levels should be monitored every 4 to 8 weeks during treatment, and if the levels exceed 5 times the ULN, tocilizumab should be discontinued.

Neutropenia and Thrombocytopenia

Tocilizumab can reduce counts of neutrophils and platelets. Neutrophil reduction increases the risk for infection. In clinical trials, reduction of platelets was not associated with increased bleeding. Neutrophil and platelet counts should be determined at baseline and every 4 to 8 weeks during treatment. Tocilizumab should not be initiated if the absolute neutrophil count (ANC) is below 2000/mm^3 or if the platelet count is below 100,000/mm^3. Patients taking tocilizumab should discontinue the drug if the ANC falls below 500/mm^3 or if the platelet count falls below 50,000/mm^3.

Drug Interactions

In general, tocilizumab should not be combined with other strong immunosuppressants, owing to an increased risk for serious infections. Antirheumatic drugs to avoid include the TNF antagonists (e.g., etanercept), T-cell inhibitors (e.g., abatacept), IL-1 antagonists (e.g., anakinra), and drugs that block the CD20 antigen (e.g., rituximab).

Tocilizumab can reduce blood levels of other drugs. Under normal circumstances, IL-6 suppresses the activity of several cytochrome P450 drug-metabolizing isoenzymes. By blocking receptors for IL-6, tocilizumab can negate that suppression and can thereby increase rates of drug metabolism. Drugs whose levels may be diminished include oral contraceptives, warfarin (an anticoagulant), proton pump inhibitors (which reduce gastric acidity), and HMG-CoA reductase inhibitors (which reduce cholesterol levels). Dosages for all of these agents may need to be increased.

Anakinra, an Interleukin-1 Receptor Antagonist

Anakinra [Kineret] reduces symptoms of RA by blocking receptors for IL-1, a proinflammatory cytokine that plays a central role in synovial inflammation and joint destruction. The drug is indicated for patients with moderate to severe RA that has not responded to one or more nonbiologic DMARDs (e.g., methotrexate). It is also approved for treatment of neonatal-onset multisystem inflammatory disease. When administrating this drug, the solution should not be shaken, and injection sites should be rotated.

Like the TNF antagonists, anakinra poses a risk for serious infections. Accordingly, the drug should not be given to patients with active infection and should be stopped if a serious infection develops. Because both anakinra and the TNF antagonists increase infection risk, these drugs should not be combined.

PRESCRIBING AND MONITORING CONSIDERATIONS FOR TUMOR NECROSIS FACTOR ANTAGONISTS

Therapeutic Goal

TNF inhibitors are used to reduce symptoms and delay disease progression in patients with moderate to severe RA.

Identifying High-Risk Patients

TNF inhibitors are *contraindicated* in patients with demyelinating disorders, severe heart failure, and active infections, including TB and HBV infection.

Exercise *caution* in patients who are immunosuppressed (e.g., owing to HIV infection or immunosuppressant drugs) and in those with diabetes, mild heart failure, liver dysfunction, latent TB, latent HBV infection, a history of recurrent infection, and any condition that predisposes to acquiring an infection.

Administration Considerations

Adalimumab, Certolizumab, Etanercept, Golimumab

Teach patients and caregivers how to administer subQ injections, using either a syringe (adalimumab, certolizumab, etanercept, golimumab) or an autoinjector (adalimumab, etanercept, golimumab). Instruct patients to (1) inject medication into the abdomen or anterior thigh, (2) rotate the injection site, and (3) avoid areas where the skin is tender, bruised, red, or indurated.

Ongoing Monitoring and Interventions

Tuberculin skin testing should be carried out before prescribing a TNF antagonist. A chest x-ray is recommended, especially for patients who will receive methotrexate. Baseline laboratory testing should include a complete blood count with white blood cell differential to be followed by a repeat analysis after the first month of therapy and every 3 to 6 months thereafter. Liver function testing should be included for patients with a history of hepatic disease. Pregnancy should be ruled out for women of childbearing age. For patients with or at risk for heart disease, a cardiology consultation is recommended.

Minimizing Adverse Effects

Serious Infections

TNF antagonists increase the risk for serious infections, including invasive fungal infections (e.g., histoplasmosis, coccidioidomycosis, candidiasis), reactivated HBV infection, and infections caused by *M. tuberculosis* and other opportunistic pathogens. Risk is increased by diabetes, HIV infection, and concurrent use of immunosuppressant drugs.

In general, avoid TNF antagonists in patients with active infections and closely monitor those who develop a new infection. Use caution in patients with a history of recurrent infection or any condition that predisposes them to acquiring an infection (e.g., advanced or poorly controlled diabetes). If a severe infection develops, TNF antagonists should be discontinued.

To minimize the risk for TB, test patients for latent TB (using a blood test or tuberculin skin test) and, if the test is positive, treat for TB before starting the TNF antagonist. During TNF antagonist treatment, monitor closely for development of TB.

To minimize the risk for HBV reactivation, test for HBV before starting the TNF antagonist. Closely monitor patients with a positive result. If reactivation of HBV infection occurs, stop the TNF antagonist and treat with antiviral drugs.

Allergic Reactions

Rarely, TNF antagonists have been associated with severe allergic reactions, including SJS, erythema multiforme, and TEN. Monitor for skin rashes and other dermatologic manifestations.

Heart Failure

TNF antagonists may cause new-onset heart failure and may worsen existing heart failure. Exercise caution in patients with mild heart failure and monitor them closely for heart failure progression. Avoid TNF antagonists in patients with severe heart failure.

Cancer

TNF antagonists may increase the risk for lymphoma and other malignancies, primarily in children, adolescents, and young adults. Parents of children should be apprised of this risk.

Hematologic Disorders

TNF antagonists may pose a risk for hematologic disorders, including neutropenia, thrombocytopenia, and aplastic anemia. If a significant hematologic abnormality is diagnosed, discontinuing the TNF antagonist should be considered.

Liver Injury

Rarely, TNF inhibitors have been associated with severe liver injury, including acute liver failure. Some patients have required a liver transplant, and some have died. If severe liver injury is diagnosed, discontinuing the TNF antagonist should be considered. Exercise caution in patients with preexisting liver dysfunction.

CNS Demyelinating Disorders

TNF antagonists have been associated with rare cases of CNS demyelinating disorders, including multiple sclerosis, myelitis, and optic neuritis. Avoid TNF antagonists in patients with a preexisting or recent-onset demyelinating disorder.

Injection-Site Reactions: Adalimumab, Certolizumab, Etanercept, and Golimumab

Injection-site reactions—redness, swelling, itching, pain—are common with these drugs.

Infusion Reactions: Infliximab

Infusion reactions—flu-like symptoms, headache, fever, chills, dyspnea, hypotension, skin reactions, GI disturbance—are common with *infliximab.* To reduce symptoms, pretreat with an antihistamine, acetaminophen, or a glucocorticoid. Manage mild reactions by slowing or interrupting the infusion. In the event of a severe reaction (e.g., anaphylaxis), stop the infusion and do not use infliximab again.

Minimizing Adverse Interactions

Immunosuppressants

Drugs that suppress immune function (e.g., glucocorticoids, methotrexate, tocilizumab, anakinra, abatacept) increase the risk for infections. Use these drugs with caution.

Live Virus Vaccines

TNF antagonists may increase the risk for acquiring or transmitting infection after immunization with a live virus vaccine. Accordingly, live virus vaccines should be avoided.

Patient Education

TUMOR NECROSIS FACTOR INHIBITORS

Inform patients about the risk for infection and other reactions. Instruct them to seek medical attention for signs or symptoms of infection, skin rashes, bruising, bleeding, or pallor. Advise patients to report signs of heart failure such as shortness of breath and orthopnea, fatigue, and edema. Teach patients about symptoms of liver injury—fatigue, yellow skin, yellow eyes, anorexia, right-sided abdominal pain, dark brown urine—and advise them to seek medical attention if these develop. Patients should also know about the increased risk of cancer.

Inform patients and parents of pediatric patients that vaccinations should be current before therapy with a TNF antagonist starts. Once therapy begins, live virus vaccines must be avoided.

Explain to patients receiving adalimumab, certolizumab, etanercept, and golimumab that it is common to have redness, swelling, itching, and discomfort at the injection site. Inform them that symptoms usually subside in a few days, but they should contact the prescriber if the reaction persists.

CHAPTER

58

Drug Therapy of Gout

Jacqueline Rosenjack Burchum, DNSc, FNP-BC, CNE

Gout is a painful inflammatory disorder seen mainly in men. Symptoms result from deposition of uric acid crystals in joints. We begin by discussing the pathophysiology of gout, after which we discuss the drugs used for treatment.

PATHOPHYSIOLOGY OF GOUT

Gout is a recurrent inflammatory disorder characterized by *hyperuricemia* (high blood levels of uric acid) and episodes of *severe joint pain,* typically in the large toe. Hyperuricemia—defined as blood uric acid above 7 mg/dL in men, or 6 mg/dL in women—can occur through two mechanisms: (1) excessive production of uric acid and (2) impaired renal excretion of uric acid. Acute attacks are precipitated by crystallization of sodium urate (the sodium salt of uric acid) in the synovial space. Deposition of urate crystals promotes inflammation by triggering a complex series of events. A key feature of the inflammatory process is infiltration of leukocytes, which, when inside the synovial cavity, phagocytize urate crystals and then break down, causing release of destructive lysosomal enzymes. When hyperuricemia is chronic, large and gritty deposits, known as *tophi,* may form in the affected joint. Also, deposition of urate crystals in the kidney may cause renal damage. Fortunately, when gout is detected and treated early, the disease can be arrested and these chronic sequelae avoided.

OVERVIEW OF DRUG THERAPY

In patients with gout, drugs are used in two ways. First, they are given short term to relieve symptoms of an acute gouty attack. Second, they are given long term to lower blood levels of uric acid.

In patients with infrequent flare-ups (less than three per year), treatment of symptoms may be all that is needed. Nonsteroidal antiinflammatory drugs (NSAIDs) are considered first-line agents for relieving pain of an acute gouty attack. Glucocorticoids are an acceptable option. In the past, colchicine was considered a drug of choice for acute gout—even though it has a poor risk-to-benefit ratio. Today, colchicine is generally reserved for patients who are unresponsive to or intolerant of safer agents.

In patients with chronic gout, tophaceous gout, or frequent gouty attacks (three or more per year), drugs for hyperuricemia are indicated. Three types of drugs may be employed: agents that decrease uric acid production, agents that increase uric acid excretion (*uricosuric* drugs), and agents that convert uric acid to allantoin. A discussion of drugs used to treat gout follows. Drug preparations, dosage, and administration are presented in Table 58.1. Lifespan considerations are provided in Box 58.1.

DRUGS FOR ACUTE GOUTY ARTHRITIS

Nonsteroidal Antiinflammatory Drugs

BLACK BOX WARNING: NONSTEROIDAL ANTIINFLAMMATORY DRUGS

NSAIDs may increase the risk for myocardial infarction, stroke, and other thromboembolic events.

NSAIDs increase the risk for dangerous gastrointestinal adverse effects such as bleeding, ulceration, and perforation.

For acute gouty arthritis, NSAIDs are considered agents of first choice. Compared with colchicine, NSAIDs are better tolerated and their effects are more predictable. Benefits derive from suppressing inflammation. Treatment should start as soon as possible after symptom onset. Most patients experience marked relief within 24 hours; swelling subsides over the next few days. Adverse effects of NSAIDs include gastrointestinal (GI) ulceration, impaired renal function, fluid retention, and increased risk for cardiovascular events. However, because the duration of treatment is brief, the risk for these complications is low. Which NSAID should be used? There is no good evidence that any NSAID is superior to the others for treatment of gout. Commonly used NSAIDs include indomethacin [Indocin] and naproxen [Naprosyn, Anaprox ♣, others]. (See Table 58.1.)

Glucocorticoids

Glucocorticoids (e.g., prednisone), given orally or intramuscularly, are highly effective for relieving an acute gouty attack—although NSAIDs are generally preferred. Candidates for glucocorticoid therapy include patients who are hypersensitive to NSAIDs, patients who have medical conditions that contraindicate use of NSAIDs, and patients with severe gout that is unresponsive to NSAIDs. Because of their effects on carbohydrate metabolism, glucocorticoids should be avoided, when possible, in patients prone to hyperglycemia. For oral therapy, prednisone can be used. For intramuscular (IM) therapy, triamcinolone acetonide can be used. Glucocorticoids are discussed in Chapter 56.

Colchicine

Colchicine [Colcrys, Mitigare] is an antiinflammatory agent with effects specific for gout. In the past, colchicine was considered a first-line drug for

PATIENT-CENTERED CARE ACROSS THE LIFE SPAN

Drugs for Gout

Life Stage	Considerations or Concerns
Children	U.S. labeling for indomethacin recommends using the lowest dose that is effective at the shortest possible duration. Canadian labeling contraindicates its use for patients younger than14 years. When given for gout prophylaxis (as opposed to familiar Mediterranean fever), colchicine is not recommended for patients younger than 16 years. Febuxostat is not recommended for children. Allopurinol may be given to children younger than 6 years for the purpose of treating hyperuricemia associated with cancer therapy. Probenecid has been given to children as young as 2 years for purposes unrelated to gout.
Pregnant women	Although most NSAIDs are FDA Pregnancy Risk Category C, some studies have demonstrated fetal cardiovascular abnormalities and cleft palate after NSAID exposure. Exposure to indomethacin after 30 weeks' gestation has resulted in a number of abnormalities, resulting in a Pregnancy Risk Category of D if taken later in pregnancy. Colchicine is Pregnancy Risk Category C. Of the xanthine oxidase inhibitors, both febuxostat and allopurinol are Pregnancy Risk Category C; however, animal studies with febuxostat have demonstrated an increase in fetal mortality. Probenecid has not been associated with increased fetal risk.
Breastfeeding women	U.S. labeling recommends against breastfeeding by mothers taking indomethacin and naproxen. Canadian labeling contraindicates breastfeeding by mothers taking these drugs. Breastfeeding is not recommended for other drugs taken for gout. For patients taking xanthine oxidase inhibitors, Canadian labeling contraindicates breastfeeding.
Older adults	The Beers Criteria list both indomethacin and naproxen among those drugs considered potentially inappropriate for patients 56 years and older and notes that, of all NSAIDs, indomethacin carries the greatest risk. Colchicine can be dangerous if the older patient has renal impairment.

FDA, U.S. Food and Drug Administration; NSAID, nonsteroidal antiinflammatory drug.

gout. However, owing to the common occurrence of GI toxicity and the availability of safe and effective alternatives, its use has declined.

Therapeutic Use

Colchicine has two applications in gout. First, it can be used short term to treat an acute gouty attack. Second, it can be used long term to prevent attacks from recurring. Colcrys is approved for both uses. Mitigare is approved only for prophylaxis.

Acute Gouty Arthritis

High-dose colchicine can produce dramatic relief of an acute gouty attack. Within hours, patients whose pain had made movement impossible are able to walk. Inflammation disappears completely within 2 to 3 days.

Prophylaxis of Gouty Attacks

When taken during asymptomatic periods, low-dose colchicine can decrease the frequency and intensity of acute flare-ups. Colchicine may also be given for prophylaxis when urate-lowering therapy is initiated because there is a tendency for gouty episodes to increase at this time.

Mechanism of Action

We do not fully understand how colchicine relieves or prevents episodes of gout. We do know that colchicine does not decrease urate production or removal. It may work, at least in part, by inhibiting leukocyte infiltration: in the absence of leukocytes, there is no phagocytosis of uric acid and no subsequent release of lysosomal enzymes. How does colchicine inhibit leukocyte migration? It disrupts microtubules, the structures required for cellular motility. Because microtubules are also required for cell division, colchicine is toxic to any tissue that has a large percentage of proliferating cells. Disruption of cell division in the GI tract and bone marrow underlies major toxicities of the drug.

Pharmacokinetics

Colchicine is readily absorbed after oral dosing, in both the presence and absence of food. Large amounts reenter the intestine through the bile and intestinal secretions and then undergo reabsorption. Final elimination occurs primarily through two processes: metabolism by hepatic CYP3A4 (the 3A4 isoenzyme of cytochrome P450) and renal excretion of intact drug.

Adverse Effects

Gastrointestinal Effects

The most characteristic side effects are nausea, vomiting, diarrhea, and abdominal pain. These responses, which occur during treatment of acute gouty attacks, result from injury to the rapidly proliferating cells of the GI epithelium. With the high doses used in the past, these GI effects developed in nearly all patients. However, with the lower doses used today, GI toxicity is less common but still develops in 25% of patients. If GI symptoms occur, colchicine should be discontinued immediately, regardless of the status of joint pain.

Myelosuppression

Injury to rapidly proliferating cells can suppress bone marrow function and can thereby cause leukopenia, granulocytopenia, thrombocytopenia, and pancytopenia. Accordingly, colchicine should be used with caution in patients with hematologic disorders.

Myopathy

Colchicine can cause rhabdomyolysis (muscle breakdown) during long-term low-dose therapy. Risk is increased in patients with renal and hepatic impairment and in those taking statin drugs (e.g., atorvastatin, simvastatin), which can cause rhabdomyolysis on their own. Patients should be monitored for signs of muscle injury (tenderness, pain, weakness).

Drug Interactions

Statins

As noted, atorvastatin, simvastatin, and other statins can increase the risk for colchicine-induced muscle injury. If possible, combined use of statins and colchicine should be avoided.

Drugs That Can Increase Colchicine Levels

Life-threatening reactions have occurred when combining colchicine with two classes of drugs: P-glycoprotein (PGP) inhibitors and inhibitors of CYP3A4. Recall from Chapter 4 that PGP is a transporter protein that can reduce plasma drug levels through effects in the liver, kidney, and intestine. Hence, by inhibiting PGP, drugs such as cyclosporine and ranolazine can cause colchicine to accumulate to toxic levels. Similarly, by inhibiting

TABLE 58.1 ■ Preparations, Dosages, and Administration of Antigout Drugs

Name	Preparation	Dosage	Administration
NONSTEROIDAL ANTIINFLAMMATORY DRUGS			
Indomethacin [Indocin, Tivorbex]	Indocin: 50-mg rectal suppository, 25 mg/5 mL oral suspension Tivorbex: 20-mg, 40-mg capsule Generic: 25-mg, 50-mg capsule Generic ER: 75-mg capsule	50 mg 3 times daily initially until pain is tolerable, then reduce dosage and continue dosing for 3–5 days	To decrease GI effects, administer with or after meals or with a snack. ER forms should be swallowed whole.
Naproxen [Anaprox ♣, Naprosyn, Naprelan, many others]	Anaprox: 275 mg ♣ Anaprox DS: 550 mg Naprosyn: 500-mg scored tablets EC-Naprosyn: 375-mg, 500-mg enteric-coated tablets Generic: 250-, 375-, 500-mg tablets Naprelan (ER): 375-, 500-, 750-mg controlled-release tablets	Naprosyn: 750 mg initially, then 250 mg every 8 hours until attack subsides Naprosyn ER: 1 tablet initially, then one tablet daily until attack subsides Anaprox: 825 mg initially, then 275 mg every 8 hours until attack subsides	To decrease GI effects, administer with or after meals or with a snack. ER and EC forms should be swallowed whole.
ANTIGOUT ANTIINFLAMMATORY DRUG			
Colchicine [Colcrys, Mitigare]	Colcrys: 0.6-mg scored tablet Mitigare: 0.6-mg capsule	Acute attack (Colcrys only): 1.2 mg at first sign of the flare, followed by 0.6 mg 1 hour later (maximum, 1.8 mg/24 hours) Prophylaxis (Colcrys, Mitigare): 0.6 mg once or twice daily (maximum, 1.2 mg/24 hours)	Administer with or without food. Do not take with grapefruit juice.
GLUCOCORTICOIDS			
Prednisone (oral) [Deltasone]	Deltasone: 20-mg (scored) tablets	30–50 mg once daily or in two divided doses until pain is tolerable; then gradually taper off the drug over 7–10 days	Administer at mealtime or with food to decrease GI upset.
Triamcinolone acetate (IM) [Aristospan, Kenalog]	Aristospan: 20 mg/mL in 1-mL and 5-mL vials Kenalog: 10 mg/mL in 5-mL vial; 40 mg/mL in 1-mL, 5-mL, and 10-mL vials	40–60 mg; may repeat after 1–4 days if flare continues	Shake well to ensure homogeneous suspension of medication, then withdraw into syringe immediately.
XANTHINE OXIDASE INHIBITORS			
Allopurinol [Zyloprim]	100- and 300-mg tablets	Dosages should be individualized to decrease plasma urate to 6 mg/dL.* Chronic tophaceous gout: 100 mg once a day, then increase by 50- to 100-mg increments every few weeks until urate target level is reached. Standard maintenance dose: 300 mg a day up to a maximum of 800 mg/day Secondary hyperuricemia in adults: 100–800 mg/day	May be taken with or without food.
Febuxostat [Uloric]	40-mg and 80-mg tablets	40 mg/day initially, increase to 80 mg/day, if needed	May be taken with or without food
URICOSURIC AGENTS			
Probenecid [generic only]	500-mg tablets	250 mg twice daily for 1 week. The maintenance dosage is 500 mg twice daily.	Administration with food decreases GI upset.
RECOMBINANT URIC ACID OXIDASE			
Pegloticase [Krystexxa]	8 mg/mL	8 mg IV every 2 weeks	Dilute 1 mL in 250 mL NS or ½ NS IV solution and administer over 2 hours. Monitor for infusion reaction.
COMBINATION DRUGS			
Colchicine and probenecid [generic]	Colchicine 0.5 mg + probenecid 500 mg	One tablet daily for 1 week, then 1 tablet twice daily	Do not begin therapy in the presence of an acute gout flare

*Dosage should be reduced in patients with renal disease.
EC, enteric coated; ER, extended release; GI, gastrointestinal; IV, intravenous; NS, normal saline.

CYP3A4, drugs such as ketoconazole, clarithromycin, and the HIV protease inhibitors (e.g., nelfinavir, ritonavir) can cause colchicine levels to rise. Accordingly, combined use of colchicine with strong inhibitors of either PGP or CYP3A4 should generally be avoided and is contraindicated in patients with hepatic or renal impairment.

Precautions and Contraindications

Colchicine should be used with care in older-adult and debilitated patients and in patients with cardiac, renal, hepatic, and GI disease.

As noted, combined use of colchicine with strong inhibitors of PGP or CYP3A4 should generally be avoided. For both acute therapy and long-term prophylaxis, dosage should be adjusted on the basis of liver function, kidney function, and use of interacting drugs. Prescribing information for Mitigare, but not Colcrys, includes contraindications for hepatic or renal impairment.

Colchicine is classified in U.S. Food and Drug Administration Pregnancy Risk Category C. It should be avoided during pregnancy, unless the perceived benefits outweigh the potential risks.

DRUGS FOR HYPERURICEMIA (URATE-LOWERING THERAPY)

Urate-lowering therapy (ULT) is indicated for patients who experience relatively frequent acute gouty attacks. The goal is to promote dissolution of urate crystals, prevent new crystal formation, prevent disease progression, reduce the frequency of acute attacks, and improve quality of life. For most patients, ULT must continue lifelong.

Four drugs—*allopurinol, febuxostat, probenecid,* and *pegloticase*—are used to reduce uric acid levels. Three mechanisms are involved. Allopurinol and febuxostat inhibit uric acid formation. Probenecid accelerates uric acid excretion. Pegloticase converts uric acid to allantoin, a compound that is readily excreted by the kidney. With all four drugs, the goal is to reduce plasma uric acid to 6 mg/dL or less. These drugs lack antiinflammatory and analgesic actions, so they are not useful against an acute gouty attack. The effects of all four drugs on uric acid are shown in Fig. 58.1.

Xanthine Oxidase Inhibitors: Allopurinol and Febuxostat

Two xanthine oxidase inhibitors are now available: allopurinol and febuxostat. Both seem equally effective. Allopurinol has been in use for decades, whereas febuxostat is relatively new. Because experience with allopurinol is more extensive, and febuxostat is much more expensive, allopurinol is often preferred.

Allopurinol

Therapeutic Uses

Allopurinol [Zyloprim] is the current drug of choice for *chronic tophaceous gout.* By reducing blood uric acid levels, allopurinol prevents new tophus formation and causes regression of tophi that have already formed, thereby allowing joint function to improve. Reversal of hyperuricemia also decreases the risk for nephropathy from deposition of urate crystals in the kidney.

Allopurinol can be used for hyperuricemia that develops secondary to cancer chemotherapy and to certain blood dyscrasias, such as polycythemia vera, myeloid metaplasia, and leukemia. Hyperuricemia develops during chemotherapy because, when cells die, breakdown of DNA releases uric acid. To minimize hyperuricemia, allopurinol should be administered before chemotherapy starts.

Mechanism of Action

Allopurinol and its major metabolite (alloxanthine) inhibit *xanthine oxidase* (XO), an enzyme required for uric acid formation. XO catalyzes the final two reactions that lead to formation of uric acid from breakdown products of DNA.

Pharmacokinetics

Allopurinol is well absorbed after oral dosing and then undergoes rapid conversion to alloxanthine, an active metabolite. Alloxanthine is then eliminated slowly by renal excretion. Because alloxanthine has a prolonged

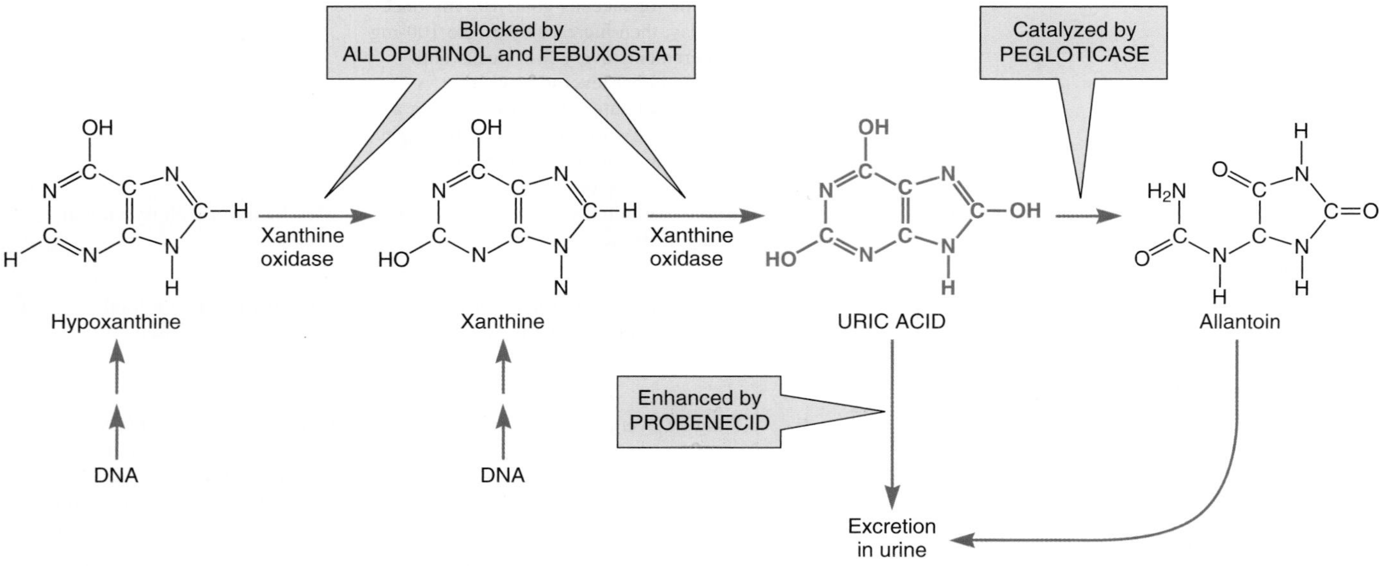

Figure 58.1 ▪ Drugs that lower plasma levels of uric acid.
These drugs lower plasma urate by three mechanisms: allopurinol and febuxostat reduce uric acid formation, pegloticase catalyzes conversion of uric acid to allantoin, and probenecid facilitates uric acid excretion by the kidney.

half-life (about 25 hours), therapeutic effects are long lasting. Consequently, once-a-day dosing is adequate.

Adverse Effects

Allopurinol is generally well tolerated. The most serious toxicity is a rare but potentially fatal hypersensitivity syndrome, characterized by rash, fever, eosinophilia, and dysfunction of the liver and kidneys. If rash or fever develops, allopurinol should be discontinued immediately. Many patients recover spontaneously; others may require hemodialysis or glucocorticoid therapy.

Initial therapy may elicit an acute gouty attack. This can be prevented by giving colchicine (0.6 mg once or twice daily), or a low-dose NSAID (e.g., 25 mg indomethacin twice daily, or 250 mg naproxen twice daily).

Mild side effects seen occasionally include GI reactions (nausea, vomiting, diarrhea, abdominal discomfort) and neurologic effects (drowsiness, headache, metallic taste). Prolonged use (more than 3 years) may cause cataracts; periodic ophthalmic examinations are recommended.

The risk for drug accumulation can be a problem if administered to patients with renal impairment. This can be minimized by decreasing the dosage.

Drug Interactions

Allopurinol can inhibit hepatic drug-metabolizing enzymes, thereby delaying the inactivation of other drugs. This interaction is of particular concern for patients taking warfarin, whose dosage should be reduced. If possible, combined use with mercaptopurine or azathioprine should be avoided because both of these anticancer drugs are substrates for XO and hence could accumulate to toxic levels in the presence of allopurinol. If combined use can't be avoided, then dosages of mercaptopurine and azathioprine should be greatly reduced (by as much as 75%). Theophylline, a drug for asthma, is also a substrate for XO and hence should not be combined with allopurinol. The combination of allopurinol plus ampicillin is associated with a high incidence of rash; if rash develops, allopurinol should be discontinued immediately.

Prototype Drugs

DRUGS FOR GOUT

Xanthine Oxidase Inhibitor
Allopurinol

Uricosuric Agent
Probenecid

Recombinant Uric Acid Oxidase
Pegloticase

Febuxostat

Febuxostat [Uloric] is an alternative to allopurinol. Like allopurinol, febuxostat lowers urate levels by inhibiting XO. As with allopurinol, symptoms of gout may flare during initial therapy. Accordingly, patients should receive prophylactic NSAIDs or colchicine for up to 6 months after starting treatment. Adverse effects of febuxostat, which are uncommon, include liver function abnormalities, nausea, arthralgia, and rash. High doses (80 mg/day) are associated with a small increase in cardiovascular events. Like allopurinol, febuxostat should not be combined with drugs that are substrates for XO, especially theophylline, mercaptopurine, and azathioprine. In contrast to allopurinol, which is eliminated entirely by the kidneys, febuxostat is eliminated by hepatic metabolism, followed by renal excretion. No dosage adjustment is needed for patients with mild to moderate renal or hepatic impairment.

Probenecid, a Uricosuric Agent

Actions and Uses

Probenecid (generic only) acts on renal tubules to inhibit reabsorption of uric acid. As a result, excretion of uric acid is increased and hyperuricemia is reduced. By lowering plasma urate levels, probenecid prevents formation of new tophi and facilitates regression of existing tophi. Probenecid should not be initiated at the beginning of an acute gout attack. The drug may exacerbate acute episodes of gout, and hence treatment should be delayed until the acute attack has been controlled. During the initial months of therapy, probenecid may induce acute attacks of gout. If an attack occurs, the probenecid should be continued; colchicine or indomethacin can be added for relief. In addition to its use in gout, probenecid may be employed to prolong the effects of penicillins and cephalosporins (by delaying their excretion by the kidneys).

Adverse Effects

Probenecid is well tolerated by most patients. Mild *GI effects* (nausea, vomiting, anorexia) occur occasionally. These can be reduced by taking the drug with food. *Hypersensitivity reactions,* usually manifesting as rash, develop in about 4% of patients. *Renal injury* may occur from deposition of urate in the kidney. The risk for kidney damage can be minimized by alkalinizing the urine and consuming 2.5 to 3 L of fluid daily during the first few days of treatment.

Drug Interactions

Aspirin and other *salicylates* interfere with the uricosuric action of probenecid. Accordingly, probenecid should not be used concurrently with these drugs. Probenecid inhibits the renal excretion of several drugs, including *indomethacin* and *sulfonamides;* dosages of these agents may require reduction.

Pegloticase, a Recombinant Form of Uric Acid Oxidase

Therapeutic Use

Pegloticase [Krystexxa] is indicated for intravenous (IV) therapy of chronic gout in patients who have not responded to oral ULT (e.g., allopurinol, probenecid). Although pegloticase is quite effective, the drug costs $6468 and higher for a single 8-mg dose and carries a significant risk for severe adverse effects. Accordingly, pegloticase is considered a treatment of last resort.

Mechanism of Action

How does pegloticase reduce urate levels? The drug is a recombinant form of *uricase* (urate oxidase), an enzyme that catalyzes the conversion of uric acid to allantoin, an inert, water-soluble compound that is readily excreted by the kidney. Uricase is present in nearly all mammals—but not in humans and higher primates.

Adverse Effects

As with other drugs for ULT, patients are likely to experience *gout flare* during the first few months of treatment. To reduce flare intensity, patients should take colchicine or an NSAID during this time.

During premarketing trials, pegloticase triggered *anaphylaxis* in 6.5% of patients. Symptoms include wheezing, perioral or lingual edema, hemodynamic instability, and rash. To reduce risk, patients should be pretreated with an antihistamine and glucocorticoid. Administration should be done in a setting equipped to manage a severe reaction.

BLACK BOX WARNING: PEGLOTICASE [KRYSTEXXA]

Anaphylaxis and infusion reactions may occur. These typically occur within 2 hours after infusion but may be delayed. Administration should take place in health care facilities prepared for management of life-threatening reactions.

Premedicate with an antihistamine and a glucocorticoid and monitored closely during the infusion.

During premarketing trials, *infusion reactions* were seen in 26% to 41% of patients. Symptoms include urticaria, dyspnea, chest discomfort, erythema, and pruritus. These reactions were seen despite pretreatment with an antihistamine, acetaminophen, and an IV glucocorticoid. If a reaction develops, slowing the infusion rate may reduce symptom intensity.

Pegloticase is *contraindicated* for patients with inherited *glucose-6-phosphate dehydrogenase* (G6PD) *deficiency,* owing to a risk for hemolysis and methemoglobinemia. Patients at higher risk (e.g., those of African or Mediterranean ancestry) should be screened for G6PD deficiency before receiving the drug.

PHARMACOLOGIC MANAGEMENT OF GOUT

As we have mentioned, treatment of an acute gout attack or flare varies from prophylactic management to prevent joint and tissue damage and to prevent recurrent gout attacks. In 2012 the American College of Rheumatology (ACR) released guidelines for both situations. These are summarized in the ACR algorithms. (Fig. 58.2 provides guidance for baseline management of gout and Fig. 58.3 details recommendations for an acute gout attack. A third algorithm, Fig. 58.4, illustrates antiinflammatory prophylaxis). The full articles are available online at http://www.rheumatology.org/Practice-Quality/Clinical-Support/Clinical-Practice-Guidelines/Gout.

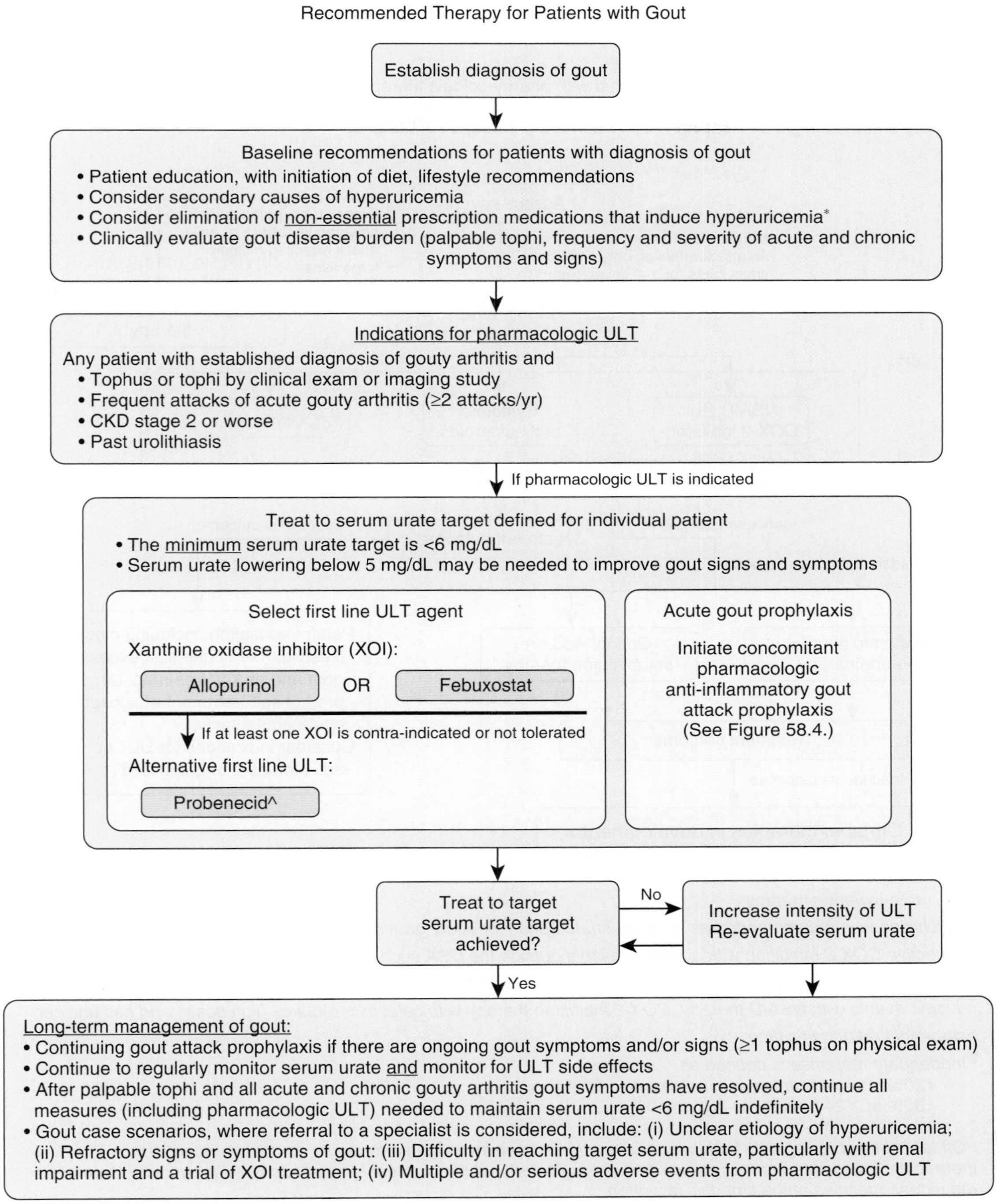
Recommended Therapy for Patients with Gout
Establish diagnosis of gout
Baseline recommendations for patients with diagnosis of gout
• Patient education, with initiation of diet, lifestyle recommendations
• Consider secondary causes of hyperuricemia
• Consider elimination of non-essential prescription medications that induce hyperuricemia*
• Clinically evaluate gout disease burden (palpable tophi, frequency and severity of acute and chronic symptoms and signs)
Indications for pharmacologic ULT
Any patient with established diagnosis of gouty arthritis and
• Tophus or tophi by clinical exam or imaging study
• Frequent attacks of acute gouty arthritis (≥2 attacks/yr)
• CKD stage 2 or worse
• Past urolithiasis
If pharmacologic ULT is indicated
Treat to serum urate target defined for individual patient
• The minimum serum urate target is <6 mg/dL
• Serum urate lowering below 5 mg/dL may be needed to improve gout signs and symptoms
Select first line ULT agent
Xanthine oxidase inhibitor (XOI):
Allopurinol
OR
Febuxostat
If at least one XOI is contra-indicated or not tolerated
Alternative first line ULT:
Probenecid^
Acute gout prophylaxis
Initiate concomitant pharmacologic anti-inflammatory gout attack prophylaxis (See Figure 58.4.)
Treat to target serum urate target achieved?
No
Increase intensity of ULT
Re-evaluate serum urate
Yes
Long-term management of gout:
• Continuing gout attack prophylaxis if there are ongoing gout symptoms and/or signs (≥1 tophus on physical exam)
• Continue to regularly monitor serum urate and monitor for ULT side effects
• After palpable tophi and all acute and chronic gouty arthritis gout symptoms have resolved, continue all measures (including pharmacologic ULT) needed to maintain serum urate <6 mg/dL indefinitely
• Gout case scenarios, where referral to a specialist is considered, include: (i) Unclear etiology of hyperuricemia; (ii) Refractory signs or symptoms of gout: (iii) Difficulty in reaching target serum urate, particularly with renal impairment and a trial of XOI treatment; (iv) Multiple and/or serious adverse events from pharmacologic ULT

*Examples of serum urate-elevating drugs that might be non-essential in a given patient, and potentially replaced by alternative agents that do not elevate serum urate:
- Niacin for management of hyperlipidemia
- Thiazide and loop diuretics for hypertension. However, in discussion, and without a specific vote, the TFP recognized the value of thiazide treatment in many patients with hypertension, and cautioned against imprudent cessation of thiazide treatment to lessen hyperuricemia at the cost of worsened control of blood pressure in difficult to control hypertension.
- Calcineurin inhibition with cyclosporine or tacrolimus, if it is not essential for immune suppression.

^ Probenecid is not recommended as a first line or alternative first line ULT agent if the CrCl is <50

ULT, urate-lowering therapy; CKD, chronic kidney disease; CrCl, creatinine clearance.

Figure 58.2 ■ Baseline recommendations for patients with gout. (Adapted from https://www.rheumatology.org/Portals/0/Files/ACR%20Guidelines%20for%20Management%20of%20Gout_Part%201.pdf.)

Management of an Acute Gout Attack

General Principles:
- Acute gouty arthritis attacks should be treated with pharmacologic therapy
- To provide optimal care, pharmacologic treatment should be initiated within 24 hours of acute gout attack onset
- Ongoing pharmacologic ULT should not be interrupted during an acute gout

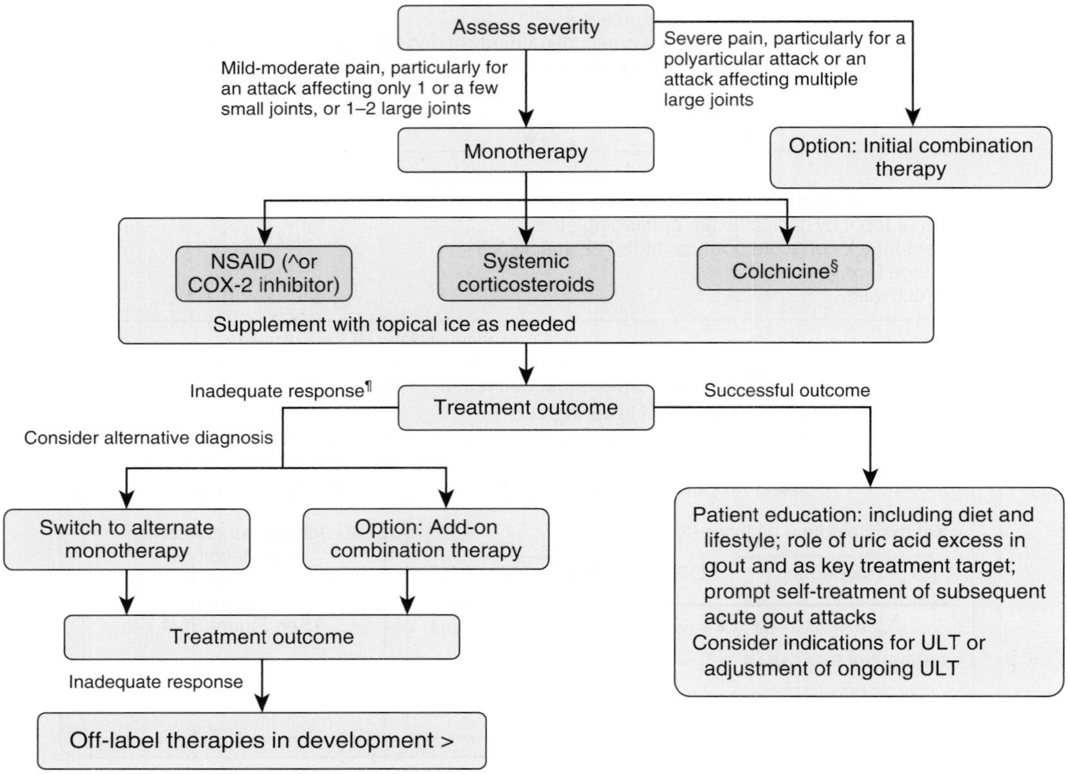

ULT, urate-lowering therapy

§ *Colchicine was recommended as an appropriate option for acute gout if started within 36 hours of symptom onset.*

^ *Selective COX-2 inhibition with agents available outside the USA such as etoricoxib was recommended as an option in patients with GI contra-indications or intolerance to NSAIDs, but selective COX-2 inhibition shares many adverse events with NSAID therapy. COX-2 inhibition therapy with celecoxib requires high doses and has unclear risk-benefit ratio at this time.*

¶ *Inadequate response is defined as*
<20% improvement in pain score within 24 hours or
<50% at ≥ 24 hours

>Off-label use of biologic IL-1 inhibitor treatment has been investigated for acute gout when non-biologic therapeutic categories are ineffective or contra-indicated, but this approach is not approved for gout by medical regulatory agencies at the time this is written.

Figure 58.3 ▪ **Management of an acute gout attack.**
(Adapted from http://www.rheumatology.org/Portals/0/Files/Gout_Part_2_ACR-12.pdf.)

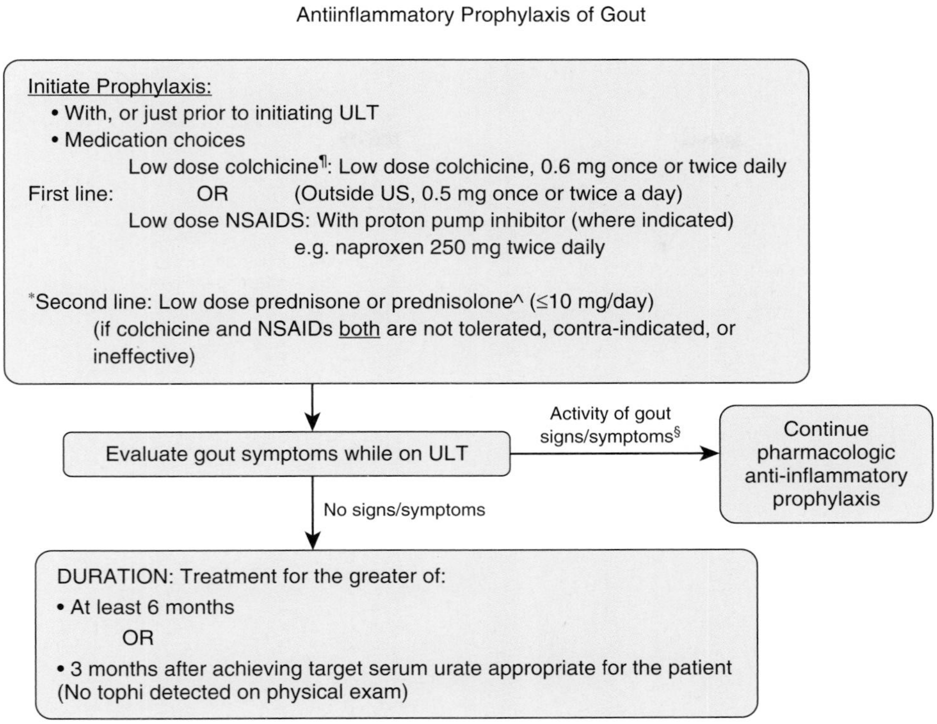

^ *Without specific task force panel (TFP) vote, the TFP advised that this measure requires particular, continued attention to risk-benefit ratio*

§ *Examples include: acute gouty arthritis in the past 3 months, presence of palpable tophus or tophi, chronic tophaceous gouty arthropathy (with chronic synovitis) in the past 3 months*

* *Lack of consensus: Prednisone/prednisolone at doses above 10 mg/day*

¶ *The TFP did not specifically address case scenarios involving renal impairment adjusted colchicine dosing for gout attack prophylaxis*

Pharmacologic antiinflammatory prophylaxis of gout attacks and its relationship to pharmacologic urate-lowering therapy (ULT). The figure provides an algorithm for use of antiinflammatory prophylaxis agents to prevent acute gout attacks. The schematic highlights specific recommendations by the TFP on decision making on the initiation, options, and duration of prophylaxis relative to pharmacologic ULT therapy, relative to achievement of the treatment objectives of ULT. NSAIDs = nonsteroidal antiinflammatory drugs.

Figure 58.4 ▪ Antiinflammatory prophylaxis of gout.
(From http://www.rheumatology.org/Portals/0/Files/Gout_Part_2_ACR-12.pdf.)

CHAPTER

59

Drugs Affecting Calcium Levels and Bone Mineralization

Jacqueline Rosenjack Burchum, DNSc, FNP-BC, CNE

It is difficult to exaggerate the biologic importance of calcium, an element critical to blood coagulation and to the functional integrity of bone, nerve, muscle, and the heart. Because these calcium-dependent processes can be seriously disrupted by alterations in calcium availability, calcium levels must stay within narrow limits. To regulate calcium, the body employs three factors: parathyroid hormone, vitamin D, and calcitonin. When these regulatory mechanisms fail, hypercalcemia or hypocalcemia results.

Our discussion of calcium and related drugs has four parts. First, we review calcium physiology. Second, we discuss the syndromes produced by disruption of calcium metabolism. Third, we discuss the pharmacologic agents used to treat calcium-related disorders. And fourth, we consider osteoporosis, the most common calcium-related disorder.

CALCIUM PHYSIOLOGY

Functions, Sources, and Daily Requirements

Functions

Calcium is critical to the function of the skeletal system, nervous system, muscular system, and cardiovascular system. In the skeletal system, calcium is required for the structural integrity of bone. In the nervous system, calcium helps regulate axonal excitability and transmitter release. In the muscular system, calcium participates in excitation-contraction coupling and contraction. In the cardiovascular system, calcium plays a role in myocardial contraction, vascular contraction, and blood coagulation.

Dietary Sources

Dairy products are good sources of calcium. For example, we can get about 300 mg from 1 cup of milk, 6 ounces of yogurt, or 1.5 ounces of cheese. Good nondairy sources include tofu (240 mg/0.5 cup), broccoli (180 mg/cup), and cooked spinach (240 mg/cup). Additionally, many processed foods are calcium fortified. Examples include fortified orange juice (300 mg/8 oz) and fortified cereals (250–1000 mg/serving). Information on the calcium content of other foods is available at www.ucsfhealth.org/education/calcium_content_of_selected_foods/index.html.

Daily Requirements

In 2010, the Institute of Medicine (IOM) of the National Academies issued updated recommendations in a report titled *Dietary Reference Intakes for Calcium and Vitamin D* (Table 59.1). Are North Americans getting enough calcium? According to the IOM report, some of us get sufficient calcium from our diets. However, there is concern that two groups—adolescent girls and postmenopausal women—may not get enough calcium from diet alone and may need calcium supplements. How much supplemental calcium should be taken? Only enough to make up the difference between what the diet provides (about 600–900 mg/day) and the recommended dietary allowance (RDA). Taking too much supplemental calcium increases the risk for vascular calcification, myocardial infarction, stroke, and kidney stones.

Body Stores

Calcium in Bone

Most calcium in the body (more than 98%) is present in bone. It is important to appreciate that bone—and the calcium it contains—is not static. Rather, bone undergoes continuous remodeling, a process in which old bone is resorbed, after which new bone is laid down (Fig. 59.1). The cells that resorb (break down) old bone are called *osteoclasts*, and the cells that deposit new bone are called *osteoblasts.* Both cell types originate in the bone marrow. In adults, about 25% of trabecular bone (the honeycomb-like material in the center of bones) is replaced each year. In contrast, only 3% of cortical bone (the dense material that surrounds trabecular bone) is replaced each year.

Calcium in Blood

The normal value for total serum calcium is 10 mg/dL (2.5 mmol/L, 5 mEq/L). Of this total, about 50% is bound to proteins and other substances and hence is unavailable for use. The remaining 50% is present as free, ionized calcium—the form that participates in physiologic processes.

Absorption and Excretion

Absorption

Absorption of calcium takes place in the small intestine. Under normal conditions, about one third of ingested calcium is absorbed. Absorption is increased by parathyroid hormone (PTH) and vitamin D. In contrast, glucocorticoids decrease calcium absorption. Also, foods with insoluble fiber and phytic acid, such as whole-grain cereals and wheat bran, and foods containing oxalates, such as spinach, can interfere with calcium absorption.

TABLE 59.1 ■ Daily Calcium Intake by Life-Stage Group

Life-Stage Group*	Calcium Intake (mg/day) AI†	RDA	UL‡
0–6 months	200	—	1000
6–12 months	260	—	1500
1–3 years	—	700	2500
4–8 years	—	1000	2500
9–18 years	—	1300	3000
19–50 years	—	1000	2500
51–70 years			
Males	—	1000	2000
Females	—	1200	2500
Older than 70 years	—	1200	2000

*All values apply to males and females, except in the 51- to 70-year-old group. Calcium requirements do not change during pregnancy or lactation.

†Values for adequate intake (AI) are derived through experimental or observational data that show a mean calcium intake that appears to sustain a desired indicator of health, such as calcium retention in bone, for most members of the population group. AI values are employed for young children because there are insufficient data to derive an RDA.

‡The tolerable upper intake level (UL) is defined as the maximal intake that is not likely to pose a risk for adverse health effects in almost all healthy individuals in a specified group. The UL is not intended to be a recommended level of intake. There is no established benefit to consuming calcium above the recommended dietary allowance (RDA).

Data from the Institute of Medicine of the National Academies: Dietary Reference Intakes for Calcium and Vitamin D. Washington, DC: The National Academies Press, 2010.

Excretion

Calcium excretion is primarily renal. The amount lost is determined by glomerular filtration and the degree of tubular reabsorption. Excretion can be reduced by PTH, vitamin D, and thiazide diuretics (e.g., hydrochlorothiazide). Conversely, excretion can be increased by loop diuretics (e.g., furosemide), calcitonin, and loading with sodium. In addition to calcium lost in urine, substantial amounts can be lost in breast milk.

Physiologic Regulation of Calcium Levels

Blood levels of calcium are tightly controlled. Three processes are involved:

- Absorption of calcium from the intestine
- Excretion of calcium by the kidney
- Resorption or deposition of calcium in bone

Regulation of these processes is under the control of three factors: *parathyroid hormone, vitamin D,* and *calcitonin,* as shown in Table 59.2. Note that preservation of calcium levels in blood takes priority over preservation of calcium in bone. Therefore, if serum calcium is low, calcium will be resorbed from bone and transferred to the blood—even if resorption compromises the structural integrity of bone.

Parathyroid Hormone

Release of PTH is regulated primarily by calcium, acting through calcium-sensing receptors on cells of the parathyroid gland. When calcium levels are *high,* activation of the calcium-sensing receptors is *increased,* causing secretion of PTH to be *suppressed.* Conversely, when calcium levels are

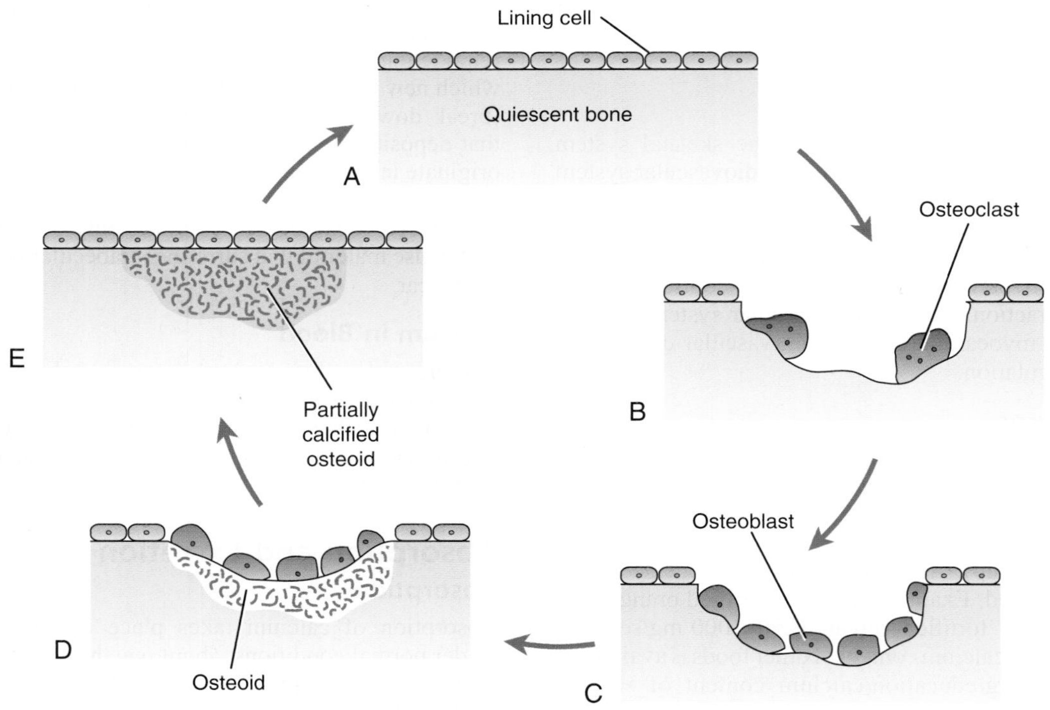

Figure 59.1 ■ Bone remodeling cycle.
A, Quiescent bone with lining cells covering the surface. **B,** Resorption of old bone by multinucleated osteoclasts. **C,** Osteoblasts migrate to the absorption site. **D,** Osteoblasts deposit osteoid, a matrix of collagen and other proteins. **E,** Osteoid undergoes calcification.

TABLE 59.2 ▪ Effects of Parathyroid Hormone, Vitamin D, and Calcitonin on Calcium and Phosphate

	PTH	Vitamin D	Calcitonin
CALCIUM			
Plasma calcium level	Increase	Increase	Decrease
Intestinal calcium absorption	Increase	Increase	No effect
Renal calcium excretion	Decrease	Decrease	Increase
Calcium resorption from bone	Increase	Increase	Decrease
PHOSPHATE			
Plasma phosphate level	Decrease	Increase	

PTH, parathyroid hormone.

low, receptor activation is reduced, causing PTH release to rise. PTH then restores calcium to normal levels by three mechanisms:

- PTH promotes calcium resorption from bone.
- PTH promotes tubular reabsorption of calcium that had been filtered by the kidney glomerulus.
- PTH promotes activation of vitamin D and thereby promotes increased absorption of calcium from the intestine. In addition to its effects on calcium, PTH reduces plasma levels of phosphate.

Vitamin D

Vitamin D is similar to PTH in that both agents increase plasma calcium levels, and they do so by the same mechanisms: (1) increasing calcium resorption from bone, (2) decreasing calcium excretion by the kidney, and (3) increasing calcium absorption from the intestine. Vitamin D differs from PTH in that vitamin D elevates plasma levels of phosphate, whereas PTH reduces levels of phosphate.

Calcitonin

Calcitonin, a hormone produced by the thyroid gland, decreases plasma levels of calcium. Hence, calcitonin acts in opposition to PTH and vitamin D. Calcitonin is released from the thyroid gland when calcium levels in blood rise too high. Calcitonin lowers calcium levels by inhibiting the resorption of calcium from bone and increasing calcium excretion by the kidney. Unlike PTH and vitamin D, calcitonin does not influence calcium absorption.

CALCIUM-RELATED PATHOPHYSIOLOGY

Hypercalcemia

Clinical Presentation

Hypercalcemia is usually asymptomatic. When symptoms are present, they often involve the kidney (damage to tubules and collecting ducts, resulting in polyuria, nocturia, and polydipsia), gastrointestinal (GI) tract (nausea, vomiting, and constipation), and central nervous system (lethargy and depression). Hypercalcemia may also result in dysrhythmias and deposition of calcium in soft tissues. As noted previously, consuming too much supplemental calcium increases the risk for vascular calcification, myocardial infarction, stroke, and kidney stones.

Causes

Hypercalcemia may arise from a variety of causes. Life-threatening elevations in calcium are most often the result of cancer. Hyperparathyroidism is another common cause of severe hypercalcemia. Additional causes include vitamin D intoxication, sarcoidosis, and use of thiazide diuretics.

Treatment

Calcium levels can be lowered with drugs that (1) promote urinary excretion of calcium, (2) decrease mobilization of calcium from bone, (3) decrease intestinal absorption of calcium, and (4) form complexes with free calcium in blood. For severe hypercalcemia, initial therapy consists of replacing lost fluid with intravenous (IV) saline, followed by diuresis using IV saline and a loop diuretic (e.g., furosemide). Other agents for lowering calcium include inorganic phosphates (which promote calcium deposition in bone and reduce calcium absorption); edetate disodium (EDTA, which binds calcium and promotes its excretion); glucocorticoids (which reduce intestinal absorption of calcium); and a group of drugs—calcitonin, bisphosphonates (e.g., pamidronate), and gallium nitrate—that inhibit resorption of calcium from bone. Cinacalcet [Sensipar], a drug that suppresses PTH section, can be used for hypercalcemia associated with hyperparathyroidism.

Hypocalcemia

Clinical Presentation

Hypocalcemia increases neuromuscular excitability. As a result, tetany, convulsions, and spasm of the pharynx and other muscles may occur.

Cause

Hypocalcemia is caused most often by a deficiency of either PTH, vitamin D, or dietary calcium. Other causes include chronic renal failure and long-term use of certain medications, such as magnesium-based laxatives and drugs used to manage osteoporosis (e.g., bisphosphonates and denosumab).

Treatment

Severe hypocalcemia is corrected by infusing an IV calcium preparation, usually calcium gluconate (see Chapter 89). After calcium levels have been restored, an oral calcium salt (e.g., calcium citrate) can be given for maintenance. Vitamin D should be included in the regimen if there is a coexisting deficiency.

Osteomalacia

Osteomalacia results from insufficient vitamin D. In the absence of vitamin D, mineralization of bone is impaired, resulting in bowing of the legs, fractures of the long bones, and kyphosis. In addition, patients may experience diffuse, dull, aching bone pain. Treatment consists of vitamin D replacement therapy.

Osteoporosis

Osteoporosis, the most common disorder of calcium metabolism, is characterized by low bone mass and increased bone fragility. Osteoporosis is discussed at length in a later section.

Paget Disease of Bone

Clinical Presentation

Paget disease of bone is a chronic condition seen most frequently in adults older than 40 years. After osteoporosis, Paget disease is the most common disorder of bone in the United States. The disease is characterized by increased bone resorption and replacement of the resorbed bone with abnormal bone. Increased bone turnover causes elevation in serum alkaline phosphatase (reflecting increased bone deposition) and increased urinary hydroxyproline (reflecting increased bone resorption). It is important to note that alterations in bone homeostasis do not occur evenly throughout the skeleton. Rather, alterations occur locally, most often in the pelvis, femur, spine, skull, and tibia. Although most people with Paget disease are asymptomatic, about 10% experience bone pain and osteoarthritis. Skeletal deformity may also occur. Bone weakness may lead to fractures. Neurologic complications may occur secondary to compression of the spinal cord, spinal nerves, and cranial nerves. If bone associated with hearing is affected, deafness may result.

Treatment

Asymptomatic patients are usually not treated. Mild pain can be managed with analgesics and antiinflammatory agents. When the disease is more severe, a bisphosphonate is the treatment of choice. Benefits derive from suppressing bone resorption.

Hypoparathyroidism

Reductions in PTH usually result from inadvertent removal of the parathyroid glands during surgery on the thyroid gland. Lack of PTH causes hypocalcemia, which in turn may produce paresthesias, tetany, skeletal muscle spasm, laryngospasm, and convulsions. Symptoms can be relieved with calcium supplements and vitamin D.

Hyperparathyroidism

Primary Hyperparathyroidism

Primary hyperparathyroidism usually results from a benign parathyroid adenoma. The resulting increase in PTH secretion causes hypercalcemia and lowers serum phosphate. Hypercalcemia can cause skeletal muscle weakness, constipation (from decreased smooth muscle tone), and central nervous system (CNS) symptoms (lethargy, depression). Hypercalciuria and hyperphosphaturia are also present and may cause renal calculi. Mobilization of calcium and phosphate from bone may produce bone abnormalities. Management of hyperparathyroidism is typically overseen by an endocrinologist. The only definitive treatment for primary hyperparathyroidism is surgical resection of the parathyroid glands. Hypercalcemia can be managed with calcium-lowering drugs, including cinacalcet [Sensipar], a drug that suppresses PTH secretion.

Secondary Hyperparathyroidism

Secondary hyperparathyroidism is a common complication of chronic kidney disease, occurring in nearly all patients undergoing dialysis. The disorder is characterized by high levels of PTH and disturbances of calcium and phosphorus homeostasis. Traditionally, the disorder has been managed with a vitamin D sterol (e.g., paricalcitol) and calcium-containing phosphate-binding agents. However, these treatments frequently make mineral homeostasis worse. Cinacalcet [Sensipar] has been advocated by some experts because of its ability to reduce PTH levels while having a positive effect on calcium and phosphorus; however, others (e.g., the Kidney Disease: Improving Global Outcomes [KDIGO] working group), recommend against its use in the early or predialysis stages of kidney disease.

DRUGS FOR DISORDERS INVOLVING CALCIUM AND BONE MINERALIZATION

Calcium Salts

Calcium salts are available in oral and parenteral formulations for treating hypocalcemic states. These salts differ in their percentages of elemental calcium, which must be accounted for when determining dosage.

Oral formulations are presented here. Information on parenteral calcium preparations are available in Chapter 89.

Therapeutic Uses

Oral calcium preparations are used to treat *mild hypocalcemia.* In addition, calcium salts are taken as *dietary supplements.* As discussed in Chapter 48, calcium supplements may have the added benefit of reducing symptoms of *premenstrual syndrome.* Also, data indicate that calcium supplements can produce a significant, albeit modest, reduction in recurrence of *colorectal adenomas.*

Adverse Effects

When calcium is taken chronically in high doses (3–4 g/day), *hypercalcemia* can result. Hypercalcemia is most likely in patients who are also receiving large doses of vitamin D. Signs and symptoms include GI disturbances (nausea, vomiting, constipation), renal dysfunction (polyuria, nephrolithiasis), and CNS effects (lethargy, depression). In addition, hypercalcemia may cause cardiac dysrhythmias and deposition of calcium in soft tissue. Hypercalcemia can be minimized with frequent monitoring of plasma calcium content.

Drug Interactions

Glucocorticoids (e.g., prednisone) reduce absorption of oral calcium, leading to osteoporosis with long-term use. Calcium reduces absorption of a number of drugs when administered together. These drugs include tetracycline and quinolone antibiotics, thyroid hormone, the anticonvulsant phenytoin, and bisphosphonates. Thiazide diuretics decrease renal calcium excretion and may thereby cause hypercalcemia; however, loop diuretics increase calcium excretion and may cause hypocalcemia.

Food Interactions

Certain foods contain substances that can suppress calcium absorption. One such substance—oxalic acid—is found in spinach, rhubarb, Swiss chard, and beets. Phytic acid, another depressant of calcium absorption, and insoluble fiber, which also hampers absorption, are present in bran and whole-grain cereals. Oral calcium supplements should not be administered with these foods.

Preparations and Dosage

The calcium salts available for oral administration are shown in Table 59.3. Note that the dosage required to provide a particular amount of elemental calcium differs among preparations. Calcium carbonate, for example, has the highest percentage of calcium. Chewable tablets are preferred to standard tablets because of more consistent bioavailability. Bioavailability of calcium citrate appears especially good, owing to high solubility. When calcium supplements are taken, total daily calcium intake (dietary plus supplemental) should equal the values in Table 59.1. To help ensure adequate absorption, no more than 600 mg should be consumed at one time.

Patient Education

CALCIUM SALTS

Individual calcium salts differ with respect to percentage of elemental calcium. As a result, the dose required to provide a specific amount of calcium differs among the salts. Advise patients against switching to a different preparation.

Advise patients to take oral calcium salts with a large glass of water. Dosing with or shortly after meals promotes absorption. Advise patients to avoid taking calcium with foods that can suppress calcium absorption (e.g., spinach, Swiss chard, beets, bran, whole-grain cereals).

Inform patients about signs of hypercalcemia (nausea, vomiting, constipation, frequent urination, lethargy, and depression) and instruct them to notify the prescriber if these occur.

Calcium binds to tetracyclines, thereby reducing tetracycline absorption. Instruct patients to separate administration of these agents by at least 1 hour.

Calcium interferes with absorption of thyroid hormone. Instruct patients to separate administration of these agents by several hours.

Vitamin D

The term *vitamin D* refers to two compounds: *ergocalciferol* (vitamin D_2) and *cholecalciferol* (vitamin D_3). Vitamin D_3 is the form of vitamin D produced naturally in humans when our skin is exposed to sunlight. Vitamin D_2 is a form of vitamin D that occurs in plants. Vitamin D_2 is used as a prescription drug and to fortify foods. Both forms are used in over-the-counter supplements. It is important to note that both forms of vitamin D produce nearly identical biologic effects. Therefore, rather than distinguishing between them, we will use the term *vitamin D* to refer to vitamins D_2 and D_3 collectively.

TABLE 59.3 ■ Oral Calcium Salts

Generic Name	Trade Name	Calcium Content	Dose Providing 1000 mg of Calcium
Calcium acetate	PhosLo, Calphron, Eliphos	25%	4 g
Calcium carbonate	Tums, Rolaids, others	40%	2.6 g
Calcium citrate	Citracal, Cal-Cee	21%	4.8 g
Calcium glubionate	Calcionate	6.6%	15.2 g
Calcium gluconate*	Cal-G	9%	11 g
Calcium lactate	Cal-Lac	13%	7.6 g
Tricalcium phosphate	Posture	39%	2.6 g

*Also available in parenteral form.

Therapeutic Uses

Vitamin D is essential for bone health, owing to its effects on calcium utilization. The primary indications for vitamin D are vitamin D deficiency and associated conditions such as rickets, osteomalacia, and hypoparathyroidism.

Some studies suggest that vitamin D may also protect against diabetes, arthritis, cardiovascular disease, autoimmune disorders, and cancers of the breast, colon, prostate, and ovary. However, according to the IOM report on calcium and vitamin D, the available data are insufficient to support health claims beyond bone health. Until more definitive data are available, the possibility of additional benefits remains open, but not proved.

Physiologic Actions

Vitamin D is an important regulator of calcium and phosphorus homeostasis. Vitamin D increases blood levels of both elements, primarily by increasing their absorption from the intestine and promoting their resorption from bone. In addition, vitamin D reduces renal excretion of calcium and phosphate (although the quantitative significance of this effect is not clear). With usual doses of vitamin D, there is no net loss of calcium from bone. However, vitamin D *can* promote bone decalcification if serum calcium concentrations cannot be maintained by increasing intestinal calcium absorption.

Sources and Daily Requirements

Sources

Vitamin D is obtained through the diet, supplements, and exposure to sunlight. With the exception of shiitake mushrooms and oily fish (e.g., salmon, tuna), natural foods have very little vitamin D. Accordingly, dietary vitamin D is obtained mainly through vitamin D–fortified foods, especially cereals, milk, yogurt, margarine, cheese, and orange juice.

Requirements

In 2010, the IOM issued revised guidelines for vitamin D intake. They now recommend the following:

- For children younger than 1 year, 400 international units (IU)/day
- For all people aged 1 through 70 years, 600 IU/day
- For adults aged 71 years and older, 800 IU/day

These recommendations are based on the assumption that people get very little of their vitamin D from exposure to sunlight.

According to the IOM report, most people in North America have blood levels of vitamin D in the range needed to support good bone health and hence do not need vitamin D supplements. Whether taking supplements would confer other benefits remains to be proved.

Vitamin D Deficiency

Vitamin D deficiency is defined by a serum concentration of 25-hydroxyvitamin D (25-[OH]D) below 20 ng/mL. (Levels above 20 ng/mL are sufficient to maintain bone health.) In actual practice, the target level of 25-(OH)D is usually 30 to 60 ng/mL.

How much vitamin D is needed to *treat deficiency?* In 2011, The Endocrine Society made the following recommendations:

- For children younger than 1 year, 2000 IU/day
- For children aged 1 to 18 years, 4000 IU/day
- For adults 19 years and older, up to 10,000 IU/day

Much higher doses are needed for patients who are obese and for those taking glucocorticoids and other drugs that suppress calcium absorption or that increase calcium excretion.

Screening for vitamin D deficiency is recommended for patients at risk, including those who are pregnant, are obese, or have dark skin (because, compared with light-skinned people, they make less vitamin D in response to sunlight). For others, the U.S. Preventive Services Task Force (USPSTF), in their 2014 update, declined to recommend for or against vitamin D deficiency screening for nonpregnant adults 18 years and older.

Activation of Vitamin D

To affect calcium and phosphate metabolism, vitamin D must first undergo activation. The extent of activation is carefully regulated and is determined by calcium availability: when plasma calcium falls, activation of vitamin D is increased. The pathways for activating vitamins D_2 and D_3 are shown in Fig. 59.2.

Let's begin by focusing on vitamin D_3, the natural human vitamin. Vitamin D_3 (cholecalciferol) is produced in the skin through the action of sunlight on provitamin D_3 (7-dehydrocholesterol). Neither provitamin D_3 nor vitamin D_3 itself possesses significant biologic activity. In the next reaction, enzymes in the liver convert cholecalciferol into calcifediol, which serves as a transport form of vitamin D_3 and possesses only slight biologic activity. In the final step, calcifediol is converted into the highly active calcitriol. This reaction occurs in the kidney and can be stimulated by (1) PTH, (2) a drop in dietary vitamin D, and (3) a fall in plasma levels of calcium.

Vitamin D_2 is activated by the same enzymes that activate vitamin D_3. As we saw with vitamin D_3, only the last compound in the series (in this case 1,25-dihydroxyergocalciferol) has significant biologic activity.

Pharmacokinetics

As a rule, vitamin D is administered orally and then absorbed from the small intestine. Bile is essential for absorption. In the absence of sufficient bile, intramuscular (IM) dosing may be required. In the blood, vitamin D is transported complexed with vitamin D–binding protein. Storage of vitamin D occurs primarily in the liver. As discussed, vitamin D undergoes metabolic activation. Reactions that occur in the liver produce the major transport form of vitamin D. A later reaction (in the kidney) produces the fully active form. Excretion of vitamin D is through the bile. Urinary excretion is minimal.

Viewing Vitamin D as a Hormone

Although referred to as a vitamin, vitamin D has all the characteristics of a hormone. With sufficient exposure to sunlight, the body can manufacture all the vitamin D it needs. Hence, under ideal conditions, external sources of vitamin D appear unnecessary. After its production in the skin, vitamin D travels to other locations (liver, kidney) for activation. Like other hormones, activated vitamin D then travels to various sites in the body (bone, intestine, kidney) to exert regulatory actions. Also like other hormones, vitamin D undergoes feedback regulation: as plasma levels of calcium fall, activation of vitamin D increases; when plasma levels of calcium return to normal, activation of vitamin D declines.

Toxicity (Hypervitaminosis D)

Serious vitamin D toxicity (hypervitaminosis D) can be produced by vitamin D doses that exceed 1000 IU/day (in infants) and 50,000 IU/day (in adults). Poisoning occurs most commonly in children; causes include accidental ingestion by the child and excessive dosing with vitamin D by parents. Doses of potentially toxic magnitude are also encountered clinically. When huge therapeutic doses are used, the margin of safety is small, and patients should be monitored closely for signs of poisoning.

Clinical Presentation

Most signs and symptoms of vitamin D toxicity occur secondary to hypercalcemia. Early symptoms include weakness, fatigue, nausea, vomiting, anorexia, abdominal cramping, and constipation. With persistent and more severe hypercalcemia, kidney function is affected, resulting in polyuria, nocturia, and proteinuria, in addition to neurologic symptoms such as seizures, confusion, and ataxia. Cardiac dysrhythmia and coma may occur. Calcium deposition in soft tissues can damage the heart, blood vessels, and lungs; calcium deposition in the kidneys can cause nephrolithiasis. Very large doses of vitamin D can cause decalcification of bone, resulting in osteoporosis; mobilization of bone calcium can occur despite the presence of high calcium concentrations in blood. In children, vitamin D poisoning can suppress growth for 6 months or longer.

Treatment

Treatment consists of stopping vitamin D intake, reducing calcium intake, and increasing fluid intake. Glucocorticoids may be given to suppress calcium absorption. If hypercalcemia is severe, renal excretion of calcium can be accelerated using a combination of IV saline and furosemide.

Preparations, Dosage, and Administration

There are five preparations of vitamin D. Three of these—ergocalciferol, cholecalciferol, and calcitriol—are identical to forms of vitamin D that occur naturally. The other two—paricalcitol and doxercalciferol—are synthetic derivatives of natural vitamin D. (The naturally occurring preparations are highlighted in green boxes in Fig. 59.2.) Individual vitamin D preparations differ in their clinical applications.

Two forms of vitamin D—vitamin D_3 (cholecalciferol) and vitamin D_2 (ergocalciferol)—are used routinely as dietary supplements. Of the two, vitamin D_3 is preferred because it is more effective than vitamin D_2 at raising blood levels of 25-(OH)D, the active form of vitamin D in the body.

Vitamin D is almost always administered by mouth. Dosage is usually prescribed in international units (IU). (One IU is equivalent to the biologic activity in 0.025 mcg of vitamin D_3.) Daily dosages of vitamin D range from 400 IU (for dietary supplementation) to as high as 500,000 IU (for vitamin D–resistant rickets). Additional information on preparation, dosage, and administration is available in Table 59.4.

Patient Education

VITAMIN D

Instruct the patient to swallow oral preparations intact, without crushing or chewing.

Therapeutic responses to vitamin D require adequate calcium intake. Encourage intake of foods that are high in calcium.

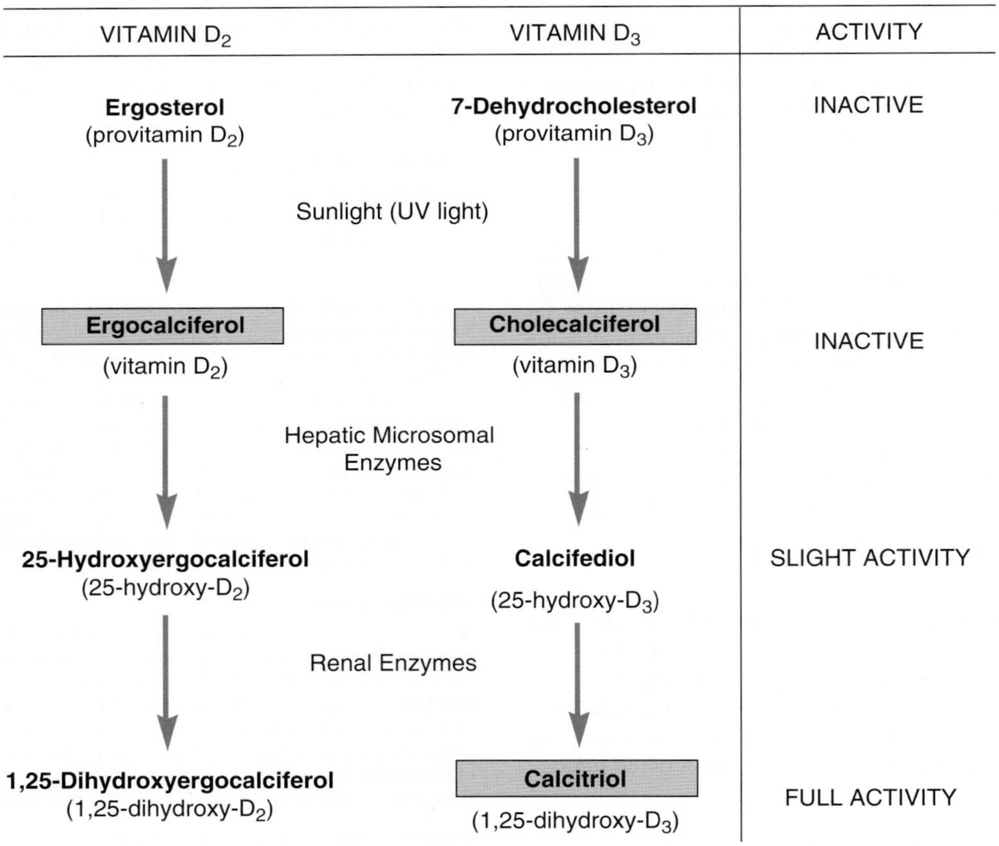

Figure 59.2 ■ Vitamin D activation.
Ergosterol is found in yeasts and fungi. 7-Dehydrocholesterol is present in the skin. *Green boxes* indicate forms of vitamin D used therapeutically.

Calcitonin-Salmon

Calcitonin-salmon [Miacalcin, Fortical], a form of calcitonin derived from salmon, is similar in structure to calcitonin synthesized by the human thyroid. Salmon calcitonin produces the same metabolic effects as human calcitonin but has a longer half-life and greater milligram potency. The drug is usually given by nasal spray but can also be given by injection. Intranasal calcitonin was removed from the Canadian market in 2013 because of an increased risk for malignancy associated with this formulation; however, it remains available in the United States.

Actions

Calcitonin has two principal actions: (1) it inhibits the activity of osteoclasts and thereby decreases bone resorption, and (2) it inhibits tubular resorption of calcium and thereby increases calcium excretion. As a result of decreasing bone turnover, calcitonin decreases alkaline phosphatase in blood and increases hydroxyproline in urine. Preparations and dosages for the different indications are presented in Table 59.5.

Therapeutic Uses

Osteoporosis

Calcitonin-salmon, given by nasal spray or injection, is indicated for *treatment* of established postmenopausal osteoporosis—but not for prevention. Benefits derive from suppressing bone resorption. The treatment program should include supplemental calcium and adequate intake of vitamin D.

Paget Disease of Bone

Calcitonin is helpful in moderate to severe Paget disease and is the drug of choice for rapid relief of pain associated with the disorder. Benefits occur secondary to inhibition of osteoclasts. Neurologic symptoms caused by spinal cord compression may be reduced.

TABLE 59.4 ▪ Indications, Preparation, and Dosage of Vitamin D Preparations

Drug Name	Indications	Preparation	Dosage
Ergocalciferol (vitamin D_2) [Calciferol Drops, Drisdol]	Hypoparathyroidism, vitamin D–resistant rickets, familial hypophosphatemia	Capsules: 50,000 IU Oral solution: 8000 IU/mL	Vitamin D–resistant rickets: 12,000–500,000 IU daily Hypoparathyroidism: 25,000–200,000 IU daily (together with 4 g of calcium lactate 6 times/day)
Cholecalciferol (vitamin D_3) [Delta-D]	Prophylaxis and treatment of vitamin D deficiency	Capsules: 1000, 2000, 5000, 10,000, 25,000, and 50,000 IU Liquid: 400 and 5000 units/mL Tablets: 2000, 3000, 5000, and 50,000 IU	Prophylaxis: varies depending on risk Deficiency: • <1 year old, 2000 IU/day • 1–18 years old, 4000 IU/day • Age 19 years and older, up to 10,000 IU/day
Calcitriol (1,25-Dihydroxy-D_3) [Rocaltrol, Vectical, Calcijex ♣, Silkis ♣]	Hypoparathyroidism and management of hypocalcemia in patients undergoing chronic renal dialysis	Capsules: 0.25 and 0.5 mcg Oral solution: 1 mcg/mL Solution for injection:1 mcg/mL	Dialysis: daily oral doses of 0.5–1 mcg usually adequate Hypoparathyroidism: Initial dosage 0.25 mcg/day administered orally
Doxercalciferol [Hectorol]	Prevention and treatment of secondary hyperparathyroidism in patients undergoing chronic renal dialysis	Capsules: 0.5, 1, and 2.5 mcg*	Dosage carefully tailored to the patient Initial dosing: 10 mcg 3 times weekly administered at dialysis Adjusting dosage: gradually increase to a maximum of 20 mcg 3 times a week
Paricalcitol [Zemplar]	Prevention and treatment of secondary hyperparathyroidism in patients undergoing chronic renal dialysis	Capsules: 1, 2, and 4 mcg*	Initial dosing: 1–2 mcg/dose (with the once-daily schedule) or 2–4 mcg/dose (with the 3-times-weekly schedule) Adjusting dosage: gradually increase every 2–4 weeks based on the PTH level

*Also available for IV administration.
IU, international unit.

TABLE 59.5 ▪ Indications, Preparation, and Dosage of Calcitonin

Drug Name	Indications	Preparation	Dosage
Intranasal salmon calcitonin [Miacalcin, Fortical]	Management of postmenopausal osteoporosis	Metered dose spray device delivers 200 IU per activation	200 IU (1 spray) each day, alternating nares daily
Parenteral salmon calcitonin [Miacalcin]	Postmenopausal osteoporosis, Paget disease of bone, hypercalcemia	2-mL vials containing 200 IU/mL Administration is IM or subQ. Dosages are the same for both routes.	Postmenopausal osteoporosis: 100 IU every other day Paget disease of bone: 100 IU/day initially, followed by 50 IU (daily or 3 times a week) Hypercalcemia: initial dosage is 4 IU/kg every 12 hours; maximal dosage is 8 IU/kg every 6 hours

IM, intramuscular; IU, international unit; subQ, subcutaneous.

Hypercalcemia

Calcitonin can lower plasma calcium levels in patients with hypercalcemia secondary to hyperparathyroidism, vitamin D toxicity, and cancer. Levels of calcium (and phosphorus) are reduced owing to inhibition of bone resorption and increased renal excretion of calcium. Although calcitonin is effective against hypercalcemia, it is not a preferred treatment.

Adverse Effects

With intranasal dosing, nasal dryness and irritation are the most common complaints. As previously mentioned, studies demonstrating an increase in malignancies associated with nasal administration prompted withdrawal of this drug in Canada. After parenteral (IM, subcutaneous [subQ]) administration, about 10% of patients experience nausea, which diminishes with time. An additional 10% have inflammatory reactions at the injection site. Flushing of the face and hands may also occur. When salmon calcitonin is taken for a year or longer, neutralizing antibodies often develop. In some patients, these antibodies bind enough calcitonin to prevent therapeutic effects.

> **Patient Education**
>
> **CALCITONIN SALMON**
>
> Instruct patients using Miacalcin to prime the metered-dose pump by holding the bottle upright and depressing the two white sidearms toward the bottle 6 times, which should produce a faint initial spray. The drug is then administered by placing the nozzle in the nostril and depressing the pump handle.
>
> Teach patients how to inject calcitonin subcutaneously and instruct them to rotate sites of injection.

Bisphosphonates

Bisphosphonates are structural analogs of pyrophosphate, a normal constituent of bone. These drugs undergo incorporation into bone, and then inhibit bone resorption by decreasing the activity of osteoclasts. Principal indications are postmenopausal osteoporosis, osteoporosis in men, glucocorticoid-induced osteoporosis (GIOP), Paget disease of bone, and hypercalcemia of malignancy. Bisphosphonates may also help prevent and treat bone metastases in patients with cancer (see Chapter 82).

Bisphosphonates differ with respect to indications, routes, and dosing schedules. Some bisphosphonates are given by oral (PO) route, some by IV route, and some by both routes. Dosing schedules vary from as often as once a day (with oral agents) to as seldom as once every 2 years (with IV zoledronate). As with many drugs for osteoporosis and similar bone disorders, calcium and vitamin D supplements are recommended if there is inadequate dietary intake.

Four bisphosphonates approved for management of osteoporosis and GIOP are currently available in the United States. These are alendronate [Fosamax, Fosamax Plus D, Binosto], ibandronate [Boniva], risedronate [Actonel, Atelvia], and zoledronate [Reclast, Zometa, Aclasta ♣]. Additional bisphosphonates have been approved for treatment of Paget disease (e.g., tiludronate [Skelid], etidronate [generic only]) or complications of malignancy (e.g., pamidronate [Aredia]); however, because these conditions are typically managed by endocrinologists, rheumatologists, and oncologists, they have been omitted from this chapter.

Alendronate is the most widely used oral bisphosphonate. It will serve as our prototype for the family.

> **Prototype Drugs**
>
> **DRUGS AFFECTING CALCIUM LEVELS AND BONE MINERALIZATION**
>
> **Antiresorptive Agents**
>
> Conjugated equine estrogens [Premarin]
> Raloxifene (selective estrogen receptor modulator)
> Alendronate (bisphosphonate)
> Calcitonin-salmon nasal spray
> Denosumab (RANKL inhibitor)
>
> **Bone-Forming Agent**
>
> Teriparatide

Alendronate

Therapeutic Use

The primary purpose of alendronate is the prevention and treatment of osteoporosis in postmenopausal women, in whom benefits derive from decreasing bone resorption by osteoclasts. It is also approved for treating osteoporosis in men. In this group, the drug increases bone mineral density (BMD), reduces vertebral fractures, and decreases loss of height.

Alendronate is considered a first-choice drug for the prevention and treatment of GIOP, a common complication of glucocorticoid therapy. Studies indicate that alendronate helps restore lost bone and may reduce the risk for fractures in this instance.

It is also a first-line treatment for Paget disease. Continuous daily therapy for 3 months produces a 50% decrease in serum alkaline phosphatase, indicating a substantial reduction in bone turnover. As in osteoporosis, benefits derive from inhibiting bone resorption by osteoclasts.

Pharmacokinetics

Alendronate is administered orally, but bioavailability is very low (only 0.7%). If the drug is taken with solid food, essentially none is absorbed. Even coffee or orange juice can decrease absorption by 60%. Absorption is also decreased by divalent (also known as bivalent) cations—including calcium, magnesium, and iron—which bind with alendronate and all other bisphosphonates. Of the small fraction that undergoes absorption, about 50% is excreted unchanged in the urine; however, the remaining 50% is taken up rapidly by bone. After alendronate has become incorporated into bone, it remains there for years and sometimes decades.

Mechanism of Action

Alendronate suppresses resorption of bone by decreasing both the number and activity of osteoclasts. Several mechanisms are involved. As osteoclasts begin to resorb alendronate-containing bone, they ingest some of the drug, which then acts on the osteoclasts to inhibit their activity. In addition, alendronate reduces the *number* of osteoclasts by (1) acting directly to decrease their recruitment and (2) acting on osteoblasts, which then produce an inhibitor of osteoclast formation.

Adverse Effects

Alendronate is generally well tolerated. Esophagitis is the principal concern. Rarely, the drug causes musculoskeletal pain, ocular inflammation, atypical femur fractures, and osteonecrosis of the jaw (ONJ). The risk for these adverse effects increases with long-term use. Fortunately, because bisphosphonates remain in bone for extensive periods of time, they continue to prevent fractures for years, and possibly for decades, after being discontinued.

Esophagitis. Esophagitis, sometimes resulting in ulceration, is the most serious adverse effect. Fortunately, esophagitis is rare, occurring in only 1 of every 10,000 patients. The cause of injury is prolonged contact with the esophageal mucosa, which can occur if alendronate fails to pass completely through the esophagus. Reasons for incomplete passage include taking the drug with insufficient water, taking the drug in a supine position, lying down after taking the drug, and having a preexisting esophageal disorder that impedes drug passage. Because of the risk for esophagitis, alendronate is contraindicated for patients with esophageal disorders that could prevent successful swallowing and for patients who are unable to sit or stand for at least 30 minutes. If symptoms of esophageal injury occur during treatment (e.g., difficulty swallowing, pain on swallowing, or new or worsening heartburn), patients should be instructed to discontinue alendronate and contact the prescriber.

Atypical Femoral Fractures. Alendronate and other bisphosphonates have been associated with atypical fractures of the femur, which occur with little or no trauma. Why do these fractures occur? One explanation is that excessive suppression of bone turnover reduces bone remodeling, and, as a result, repair of microcracks is suppressed and bone strength is reduced. Fortunately, the absolute risk for atypical fractures is low—about 5 additional cases for every 10,000 patient-years of bisphosphonate use. Risk increases with duration of treatment.

Do the benefits of preventing typical fractures (which are common) outweigh the risk of causing atypical fractures (which are rare)? The answer is clearly "Yes"—but only for women with osteoporosis who are deemed at high risk for a typical fracture. For women without osteoporosis who are at low risk for a typical fracture, the benefits of bisphosphonates may not justify the risks.

What can be done to reduce the risk for an atypical fracture? In 2010, a task force assembled by the American Society for Bone and Mineral Research recommended the following:

- Do not prescribe bisphosphonates for patients considered at low risk for osteoporosis-related fractures.
- Consider alternative treatments, such as raloxifene or teriparatide, for patients with osteoporosis of the spine and normal (or only moderately reduced) BMD of the femoral neck or hip.
- After 5 years of bisphosphonate use, evaluate annually the need for continued treatment.

Esophageal Cancer. Alendronate and other oral bisphosphonates may—or may not—increase the risk for esophageal cancer. Studies have reached conflicting conclusions. If the risk is real, it is small (about 1 additional case for every 1000 patients older than 60 years treated for 5 years) and probably due to esophageal injury caused during oral dosing. Measures that might reduce risk include reducing the dosing frequency (i.e., dosing weekly rather than daily), taking the drug with a full glass of water, and staying upright for 30 to 60 minutes after dosing.

Musculoskeletal Pain. Musculoskeletal pain, sometimes severe, has been reported during postmarketing surveillance. So far, a causal link with alendronate has not been established. Onset may occur shortly after the first dose or months later. Pain can be managed with analgesics, including opioids and ketorolac when pain is severe. In most cases, discomfort gradually resolves after stopping alendronate. Interestingly, among patients who resume alendronate use, only 11% experience a return of pain. If pain does return, patients taking the drug for osteoporosis can switch to a different agent, such as raloxifene, calcitonin-salmon, or teriparatide.

Ocular Problems. Ocular problems are rare but can be serious. Possible effects include conjunctivitis, scleritis, blurred vision, and eye pain. Drug-induced release of inflammatory cytokines may be the cause. Advise patients to report any vision changes or eye pain.

Osteonecrosis of the Jaw. Very rarely, patients have developed ONJ, a potentially severe complication. This is seen mostly with IV bisphosphonates.

Hyperparathyroidism. In patients with Paget disease, alendronate can induce hyperparathyroidism. By inhibiting accelerated bone resorption, alendronate causes blood levels of calcium to fall; in response, secretion of PTH is increased. To prevent hyperparathyroidism, patients should receive calcium supplements.

Atrial Fibrillation. Because an intravenous bisphosphonate (zoledronate) has been associated with rare cases of atrial fibrillation (AF), there has been ongoing concern that oral alendronate may also cause the disorder. In 2008 the U.S. Food and Drug Administration (FDA), based on data from clinical trials, determined there was no significant AF risk with oral formulations of bisphosphonates. Data from more recent research; however, have raised the issue once again. In 2014 the American Journal of Cardiology published a report of findings from a meta-analysis of randomized controlled trials and observational studies that contradicts earlier findings. Those authors assert that there is increased, although low, risk for new-onset AF with both oral and IV bisphosphonates.

Administration

Proper administration is necessary to maximize bioavailability and minimize the risk for esophageal injury. Alendronate absorption is dramatically diminished when taken with food. To maximize bioavailability, alendronate should be taken in the morning before breakfast (i.e., on an empty stomach). No food, including orange juice or coffee, should be consumed for at least 30 minutes after administration. Because minerals such as calcium, magnesium, and iron bind with alendronate and all other bisphosphonates, many experts advise waiting at least 2 hours after administration before taking calcium products, mineral supplements, or antacids.

To minimize the risk for esophagitis, patients should be instructed to do the following:

- Take alendronate with a full glass of water.
- Remain upright (sitting or standing) for at least 30 minutes.
- Avoid chewing or sucking alendronate tablets.

Additional information on preparation and dosage of alendronate and other bisphosphonates is available in Table 59.6.

Risedronate

Actions and Uses

Risedronate [Actonel, Atelvia, Actonel DR] is an oral bisphosphonate approved for postmenopausal osteoporosis, male osteoporosis, GIOP, and Paget disease of bone. As with other bisphosphonates, benefits derive from inhibiting osteoclast-mediated resorption of bone. In postmenopausal women with osteoporosis, risedronate increases BMD and reduces the risk for vertebral and nonvertebral fractures.

Pharmacokinetics

Like other oral bisphosphonates, risedronate is poorly absorbed from the GI tract. Absorption is only 1% under fasting conditions. The effect of food depends on the formulation used. With Actonel (an immediate-release [IR] formulation), food greatly reduces absorption. By contrast, with Atelvia (an enteric-coated, delayed-release [DR] formulation), food does not reduce absorption. In fact, Atelvia should be taken with food to reduce stomach pain. After absorption, most of the drug becomes incorporated into bone. The rest is excreted unchanged in the urine. Risedronate in bone persists for years.

TABLE 59.6 ▪ Indications, Preparation, and Dosage of Bisphosphonates

Drug Name	Indications	Preparation	Dosage
Alendronate [Fosamax, Binosto] Alendronate + vitamin D [Fosamax Plus D]	Prevention and treatment of osteoporosis in postmenopausal women, osteoporosis in men, Paget disease, and GIOP	Tablets (Fosamax): 70 mg Tablets (generic): 5, 10, 35, 40, and 70 mg Effervescent tablet (Binosto): 70 mg Oral solution (generic): 70 mg/75 mL Tablets (Fosamax D): 70 mg alendronate: 2800 IU vitamin D_3, 70 mg alendronate: 5600 IU vitamin D_3	Osteoporosis in postmenopausal women, prevention: 5-mg tablet daily or 35 mg once weekly Osteoporosis in postmenopausal women, treatment: 10-mg tablet daily or 70 mg once weekly Osteoporosis in men: 10-mg tablet once daily or 70 mg once weekly Paget disease: 40 mg once daily for 6 months for men or women GIOP for men, premenopausal women, and postmenopausal women taking estrogen: 5 mg once daily GIOP for postmenopausal women not taking estrogen: 10 mg once daily
Risedronate [Actonel, Atelvia]	IR: Prevention and treatment of osteoporosis in postmenopausal women, osteoporosis in men, prevention or treatment of GIOP, and Paget disease of bone DR: postmenopausal osteoporosis	IR (Actonel): 5, 30, 35, and 100-mg tablets DR: (Atelvia): 35-mg enteric-coated tablets	Postmenopausal osteoporosis, Actonel: 5 mg once daily, 35 mg once weekly, or 150 mg once a month Postmenopausal osteoporosis, Atelvia: 35 mg once weekly Osteoporosis in men, Actonel: 35 mg once a week GIOP, Actonel: 5 mg once daily Paget disease of bone: 30 mg once daily
Ibandronate [Boniva]	Prevention and treatment of postmenopausal osteoporosis	Tablets: 150 mg IV: 3 mg/3 mL prefilled syringes	Prevention and treatment of osteoporosis, tablets: 150 mg once a month on the same day each month Treatment of osteoporosis, IV: 3 mg every 3 months
Zoledronate (zoledronic acid) [Aclasta ♣, Reclast, Zometa]	Aclasta ♣: Treatment of osteoporosis in postmenopausal women, patients >50 years with history of low trauma hip fracture, osteoporosis in men, prevention and treatment of GIOP, and Paget disease of bone Reclast: Prevention and treatment of osteoporosis in postmenopausal women, osteoporosis in men, GIOP, and Paget disease Zometa: hypercalcemia of malignancy	Aclasta ♣: 5 mg/100 mL Reclast: 5 mg/100 mL	Aclasta ♣: For all indications *except Paget disease:* 5 mg IV once a year Paget disease: one 5 mg dose Treatment of postmenopausal osteoporosis: 5 mg once a year Prevention of postmenopausal osteoporosis: 5 mg once every 2 years Osteoporosis in men: 5 mg once a year GIOP: 5 mg once a year, infused over 15 minutes or longer Paget disease: 5 mg (one dose produces extended remission; specific retreatment data not available)

DR, delayed release; GIOP, glucocorticoid-induced osteoporosis; IR, immediate release.

Adverse Effects

The most common adverse effects are arthralgia, diarrhea, headache, rash, nausea, and a flu-like syndrome. Like alendronate, risedronate poses a significant risk for esophagitis and a very small risk for atypical femoral fractures. Ocular problems, and musculoskeletal pain are rare. If risedronate poses a risk for esophageal cancer, ONJ, or AF, the risk is very small.

Administration

Risedronate is supplied in IR tablets sold as Actonel and in enteric-coated DR tablets sold as Atelvia. With the IR tablets, each dose should be taken in the morning before ingesting the first food or fluids of the day (except for water). With the DR tablets, each dose should be taken in the morning after breakfast. (Atelvia is the only oral bisphosphonate that can be taken after eating, rather than before.) With both formulations, dosing should be done with a full glass of water. Also, the patient should be upright when swallowing and should not lie down for at least 30 minutes. Like alendronate, risedronate binds to divalent cations such as calcium, iron, and magnesium; therefore, calcium products, mineral supplements, and antacids should not be administered within 2 hours of administering either risedronate formulation.

Ibandronate

Actions and Uses

Ibandronate [Boniva] is approved for prevention and treatment of postmenopausal osteoporosis. Dosing may be done once a month (PO) or once every 3 months (IV). As with other bisphosphonates, benefits derive from inhibiting osteoclast-mediated resorption of bone. In clinical trials, ibandronate increased BMD in the lumbar spine and other sites and reduced the risk for vertebral fractures. Although comparative studies have not been done, the drug is probably as effective as alendronate and risedronate, the only other bisphosphonates approved for oral therapy of osteoporosis.

Pharmacokinetics

With oral dosing, bioavailability is extremely low—only 0.6%. Food decreases availability by another 90%. After absorption, ibandronate undergoes rapid binding to bone or excretion in the urine. Metabolism, if any, is minimal. The half-life in blood is 10 to 60 hours. However, because of binding to bone, active drug remains in the body for years.

Adverse Effects and Interactions

With oral administration, ibandronate is generally well tolerated. Like other oral bisphosphonates, it can cause adverse GI effects, including esophagitis, dyspepsia, and abdominal pain. Ocular inflammation, atypical fractures, and ONJ are rare. Musculoskeletal pain has not been reported. Whether ibandronate increases the risk for esophageal cancer is unknown. As with other bisphosphonates, divalent cations (e.g., calcium, magnesium, iron) can greatly decrease absorption.

With IV administration, ibandronate and other bisphosphonates can cause renal damage. Intravenous ibandronate should not be used by patients taking other nephrotoxic drugs or by those with severe renal impairment, defined as serum creatinine above 2.3 mg/dL or creatinine clearance less than 30 mL/min. Kidney function should be determined before each dose, and, if severe renal impairment is detected, the dose should be withheld. In addition to causing renal damage, IV ibandronate may cause an acute reaction characterized by fever, joint pain, and myalgia, primarily with the first dose.

Administration

Oral. Oral dosing is done on an empty stomach in the morning. Patients should swallow tablets whole with a full glass of water, while standing or sitting upright. For 60 minutes after dosing, patients must remain upright and must not eat or drink anything, including medications and dietary supplements. IV administration is discussed in Chapter 89.

Intravenous. The risk for renal damage is increased if ibandronate is administered rapidly. Accordingly, ibandronate should be administered by slow IV push over an interval of 15 to 30 seconds.

Zoledronate

Actions and Uses

Zoledronate [Reclast, Zometa, Aclasta ♣], also called zoledronic acid, is an IV bisphosphonate with approved indications for *postmenopausal osteoporosis, osteoporosis in men, Paget disease of bone, glucocorticoid-induced osteoporosis, multiple myeloma or metastatic bone lesions from solid tumors,* and *hypercalcemia of malignancy* (HCM). In addition, the drug is used off-label to prevent bone loss, fractures, and other skeletal-related events (SREs) in patients receiving any of a variety of therapies that create a risk for bone loss. Like other bisphosphonates, zoledronate undergoes incorporation into bone, where it remains for years. When osteoclasts ingest the drug, it inhibits their activity, preventing bone resorption.

For management of postmenopausal osteoporosis, zoledronate differs from all other bisphosphonates in that dosing is done just once a year or once every 2 years. Compared with placebo treatment, once-yearly zoledronate decreases the incidence of vertebral fractures by 70%, hip fractures by 41%, and nonvertebral fractures by 25%. In addition, zoledronate improves BMD and markers of bone metabolism.

Adverse Effects

The most common reaction is transient fever, followed by nausea, constipation, dyspnea, abdominal pain, and bone and joint pain. In addition, zoledronate can cause clinically significant reductions in serum levels of calcium, phosphorus, and magnesium. Accordingly, levels of these elements should be followed and corrected when indicated.

Zoledronate has been associated with bone injury, most often *osteonecrosis of the jaw,* a condition characterized by local bone death and decreased bone strength. The underlying cause is impaired blood perfusion. (Bisphosphonates impair perfusion by inhibiting growth of blood vessels.) Among patients using zoledronate, most cases of ONJ developed after tooth extractions and other dental procedures, which can increase risk by promoting infection. Other risk factors include cancer, cancer chemotherapy, use of systemic glucocorticoids, and poor oral hygiene. To reduce ONJ risk, a dental examination with appropriate preventive dentistry should be conducted before giving zoledronate, especially in patients with ONJ risk factors.

Zoledronate can cause dose-dependent *kidney damage,* which can progress to acute renal failure and, rarely, to death. Risk is increased by the following:

- Chronic renal impairment
- Advanced age
- Dehydration (e.g., secondary to fever, sepsis, diarrhea)
- Use of diuretics (which can cause dehydration)
- Use of nephrotoxic drugs
- Rapid infusion of zoledronate

Owing to the risk for renal failure, zoledronate may be contraindicated in patients with significant renal impairment. When not contraindicated, dosage varies depending on the underlying condition and creatinine clearance. To minimize risk, dosage should be kept low (5 mg or less per infusion), and the infusion should be slow (15 minutes or longer). In addition, the patient should be adequately hydrated before each infusion. To monitor for renal damage, creatinine clearance should be determined at baseline, before each dose, and periodically after each infusion. If renal impairment develops, zoledronate dosage should be reduced.

Rarely, zoledronate has been associated with serious *atrial fibrillation,* resulting in hospitalization. In one trial, the incidence was 1.3%, compared with 0.5% in patients taking placebo. Most cases developed more than 30 days after zoledronate infusion.

Drug Interactions

Risk for renal failure is increased by *diuretics* (which can cause dehydration) and by other *nephrotoxic drugs,* including cyclosporine, amphotericin B, aminoglycoside antibiotics, and the nonsteroidal antiinflammatory drugs (NSAIDs).

Patient Education

BISPHOSPHONATES

To minimize the risk for esophagitis, instruct patients to swallow the tablet whole with a full glass of water while sitting or standing upright. Explain that it is important to remain upright for at least 30 minutes (60 minutes with ibandronate).

Intake of food, even in small amounts, prevents absorption of bisphosphonates. Instruct patients to take these drugs in the morning before eating or drinking anything other than water. (This applies to all oral bisphosphonates except Atelvia, a delayed-release brand of risedronate, which can and should be administered after eating.) After dosing, postpone ingesting anything—including orange juice, coffee, antacids, and calcium, iron, or magnesium supplements—for at least 30 minutes (60 minutes with ibandronate).

Estrogen

The basic pharmacology of estrogen, as well as postmenopausal estrogen therapy, is discussed in Chapter 48. Discussion here focuses on the role of estrogen in osteoporosis.

When estrogen levels decline, either because of natural menopause or surgical removal of the ovaries, osteoclasts increase in number, causing bone resorption to increase dramatically. Estrogen replacement can restore the brake on osteoclast proliferation and can therefore suppress resorption.

Low dose estrogen (e.g., 0.3 mg/day) is recommended for the purpose of osteoporosis prevention. Women with an intact uterus should also receive a progestin (e.g., medroxyprogesterone) to minimize the risk for estrogen-induced endometrial cancer. For women without a uterus, the progestin is unnecessary.

For years, hormone therapy (HT)—estrogen with or without a progestin— had been considered the treatment of choice for preventing postmenopausal bone loss. Today, however, the benefits do not always outweigh the risks. Yes, HT does reduce bone loss and the risk for osteoporotic fractures; however, HT increases the risk for breast cancer, cholecystitis, and thromboembolic events such as myocardial infarction and stroke.

Despite the risks, estrogen is still approved for preventing and treating bone loss after menopause or surgical removal of the ovaries, because treatment reduces the overall risk for fractures by 24%. Estrogen is most effective when initiated immediately after menopause; however, treatment begun later in life can still offer significant protection. If estrogen is discontinued, a period of accelerated bone loss will ensue. For providers and patients who prefer not to use estrogen for prevention and treatment of osteoporosis, we have effective alternatives: raloxifene, bisphosphonates, calcitonin, and teriparatide. Women currently using HT for osteoporosis are encouraged to consider a switch to an alternative drug.

BLACK BOX WARNING: ESTROGEN

Estrogen therapy is associated with an increased risk for endometrial cancer in women with a uterus who take unopposed estrogen, an increased risk for venous thromboembolic events (e.g., deep vein thrombosis and pulmonary embolism). It also may increase the risk for dementia in women 65 years and older.

Raloxifene

Raloxifene [Evista] belongs to a class of agents known as *selective estrogen receptor modulators* (SERMs)—drugs that exert estrogenic effects in some tissues and antiestrogenic effects in others. Like estrogen, raloxifene preserves BMD and reduces plasma levels of cholesterol. However, in contrast to estrogen, which promotes cancer of the breast and endometrium, raloxifene protects against these cancers. Because of its effects on bone, raloxifene is used to prevent and treat postmenopausal osteoporosis. Because of its effects on breast tissue, the drug is used to reduce the risk for breast cancer. Another SERM—tamoxifen—is used to *treat* breast cancer as well as prevent it (see Chapter 82).

Mechanism of Action

Raloxifene and other SERMs are structurally similar to estrogen, so they can bind to estrogen receptors. However, unlike estrogen itself, which functions as an agonist in all tissues, SERMs function as agonists in some tissues and antagonists in others. Hence SERMs can either mimic or block the actions of estrogen, depending on the SERM and the tissue involved. Raloxifene mimics the effects of estrogen on bone, lipid metabolism, and blood clotting and blocks estrogen effects in the breast and endometrium.

Pharmacokinetics

Raloxifene is administered by mouth, and 60% is absorbed. However, owing to extensive first-pass metabolism, absolute bioavailability is below 2%. Excretion is fecal. The drug's half-life is about 28 hours.

Therapeutic Uses

Raloxifene offers significant benefits regarding osteoporosis and breast cancer but also poses a risk for serious thromboembolic events. Accordingly, women must carefully weigh the risks and benefits before choosing this drug.

Postmenopausal Osteoporosis

Raloxifene is used to prevent and treat osteoporosis in postmenopausal women. The drug can preserve or increase BMD, although not as effectively as estrogen. Raloxifene reduces the risk for *spinal* fractures by 55%, but does not reduce the risk for fractures at other sites.

Breast Cancer

Raloxifene protects against estrogen receptor–positive breast cancer. It is approved for reducing the risk for invasive breast cancer in postmenopausal women who either (1) have osteoporosis or (2) are at high risk for breast cancer, even if they don't have osteoporosis.

Adverse Effects and Interactions

Deep Vein Thrombosis and Pulmonary Embolism.

Like estrogen, raloxifene increases the risk for thromboembolic events such as DVT, pulmonary embolism (PE), and stroke. Because inactivity promotes DVT, patients should discontinue raloxifene at least 72 hours before prolonged immobilization (e.g., postsurgical recovery, extended bed rest) and should not resume the drug until full mobility has been restored. Also, patients should minimize periods of restricted activity, as can happen when traveling or revising a pharmacology text. Raloxifene is contraindicated for patients with a history of venous thrombotic events.

BLACK BOX WARNING: RALOXIFENE

Raloxifene is associated with an increased risk for venous thromboembolic events (e.g., deep vein thrombosis and pulmonary embolism) and an increased risk for death from stroke when given to postmenopausal women who have a history or risk for coronary heart disease.

Fetal Harm

Raloxifene is classified in *FDA Pregnancy Risk Category X: the potential for fetal harm outweighs any possible benefits of use during pregnancy.* In animal studies, doses below those used in humans have resulted in abortion, delayed fetal development, decreased neonatal survival, and anatomic abnormalities, including hydrocephaly and uterine hypoplasia. Although use during pregnancy is obviously no concern for postmenopausal patients, it can be a concern for younger women taking the drug to prevent breast cancer.

Comparison With Estrogen

The SERMs were developed in hope of creating a drug with all the benefits of estrogen and none of its drawbacks. Raloxifene partly fulfills this hope. Table 59.7 shows the ways in which estrogen and raloxifene are alike and different.

TABLE 59.7 ■ Comparison of Estrogen and Raloxifene

Drug Target	Estrogen	Raloxifene
Bone	Increases BMD and reduces fracture risk	Increases BMD (but not as much as estrogen) and reduces fracture risk
Breast	Increases risk for breast cancer; causes breast enlargement and pain	Protects against breast cancer; does *not* cause breast enlargement or pain
Endometrium	Increases risk for endometrial cancer	Does *not* promote endometrial cancer and *may* offer protection
Plasma lipids	Lowers LDL cholesterol and raises HDL cholesterol	Lowers LDL cholesterol, but does not raise HDL cholesterol
Menopausal symptoms	Alleviates menopausal symptoms (e.g., hot flashes, vaginal dryness and itching)	Does *not* alleviate menopausal symptoms and may actually increase hot flashes
Menstruation	Causes bleeding in 45% of postmenopausal women	Causes bleeding in 3%–5% of postmenopausal women
Blood clotting	Increases risk for DVT and pulmonary embolism	Increases risk for DVT and pulmonary embolism
Coronary heart disease	Black box warning related to cardiovascular disease	Black box warning related to cardiovascular disease
Developing fetus	Contraindicated during pregnancy because of possible fetal harm	Contraindicated during pregnancy because of possible fetal harm

BMD, bone mineral density; DVT, deep vein thrombosis; HDL, high-density lipoprotein; LDL, low-density lipoprotein.

Preparations, Dosage, and Administration

Raloxifene [Evista] is available in 60-mg oral tablets. The dosage is 60 mg once a day, taken with or without food. Women taking raloxifene to prevent or treat postmenopausal osteoporosis should ensure adequate intake of calcium and vitamin D.

Patient Education

RALOXIFENE

Advise women taking raloxifene for osteoporosis to ensure adequate intake of calcium and vitamin D.

Because raloxifene increases the risk for DVT, PE, and thrombotic stroke, advise patients to discontinue raloxifene at least 72 hours before prolonged immobilization (e.g., postsurgical recovery, extended bed rest) and to resume treatment only after full mobility has been restored. Instruct patients to avoid extended periods of restricted activity, as can happen when traveling.

Bazedoxifene and Estrogen

Bazedoxifene, a SERM, and estrogen are available in a combination tablet (Duavee). It is available as 20 mg bazedoxifene and 0.45 mg conjugated estrogens to be taken once a day for postmenopausal osteoporosis. Additional information regarding this drug is available in Chapter 48.

Teriparatide

Teriparatide [Forteo] is a form of PTH produced by recombinant DNA technology. The drug has three indications:

- Treatment of osteoporosis in postmenopausal women
- Treatment of osteoporosis in men
- Treatment of GIOP

Teriparatide is the only drug for osteoporosis that increases bone formation. (All others decrease bone resorption.) In postmenopausal women with documented osteoporosis, daily subQ injections of teriparatide for 18 months increased BMD of the lumbar spine and femoral neck and reduced the risk for vertebral fractures by 65%. Similar responses are seen in men. Teriparatide-induced increases in BMD are twice those seen with alendronate.

How does teriparatide (PTH) affect bone? The drug has two actions: it (1) increases bone resorption by osteoclasts and (2) increases bone deposition by osteoblasts. The net effect—resorption or deposition—depends on how the drug is administered. When given by continuous IV infusion, which produces a *steady* elevation of serum PTH, teriparatide *decreases* BMD, primarily by accelerating calcium resorption by osteoclasts. In contrast, when given by daily subQ injections, which produce *transient* elevations in serum PTH, the drug *increases* BMD, primarily by increasing bone deposition by osteoblasts.

Adverse effects included nausea, headache, arthralgias, back pain, and leg cramps. Orthostatic hypotension and associated dizziness may occur within 4 hours of injection, so the patient should be in a location where it is possible to lie down, if needed. This adverse effect decreases after the first few doses. Temporary increases in serum levels of calcium, magnesium, and uric acid may occur.

BLACK BOX WARNING: TERIPARATIDE

Teriparatide causes osteosarcoma in animal testing. This may indicate a potential increased risk for osteosarcoma in humans.

Preparations, Dosage, and Administration

Teriparatide [Forteo] is supplied in special prefilled pen injectors that contain 600 mcg/2.4 mL (250 mcg/3 mL in Canada) and are designed to deliver a predetermined amount of drug with each activation. For all indications, the recommended dosage is 20 mcg once daily by subQ injection into the anterior thigh or abdomen. Each pen can be used up to 28 days after the first injection, after which it should be discarded, even if some drug remains. Patients should store the pens cold—2° to 8°C (36°–46°F)—but not frozen, and should take them out of the cold only to make an injection. The cost for each syringe (a 28-day supply) in the United States is more than $2400, so treatment costs can be very expensive.

Denosumab

Therapeutic Uses

Denosumab [Prolia, Xgeva] is a first-in-class receptor activator of nuclear factor kappa-B ligand (RANKL) inhibitor with three indications: (1) treatment of osteoporosis in men and postmenopausal women at high risk for fractures; (2) treatment of bone loss in men and women receiving certain anticancer therapy (e.g., androgen deprivation therapy for prostate cancer and aromatase inhibitor therapy for breast cancer); and (3) prevention of SREs in patients with bone metastases from solid tumors. Dosage is much higher in patients with bone metastases than in patients with osteoporosis, and hence side effects are more severe in patients with bone metastases.

Denosumab is marketed under two trade names: Prolia and Xgeva. *Prolia* is used for men and women with a high risk for fractures or who have bone loss due to anticancer therapy. *Xgeva* is used for bone metastases.

Clinical Trials

Osteoporosis in Postmenopausal Women

Denosumab was tested in a 3-year study that enrolled 7868 postmenopausal women with osteoporosis. Half the women received denosumab (60 mg injected subQ every 6 months), and the other half received placebo injections. All subjects also received at least 1000 mg of calcium daily and at least 400 IU of vitamin D daily. Compared with the women who got placebo injections, those who got denosumab had 68% fewer vertebral fractures, 40% fewer hip fractures, and 20% fewer fractures at other sites (wrist, leg, or shoulder). In a separate 12-month study, denosumab (60 mg subQ every 6 months) increased BMD at multiple sites (lumbar spine, femoral neck, trochanter, radius) more effectively than oral alendronate (70 mg once a week). Taken together, these data suggest that denosumab is equal to bisphosphonates for treating postmenopausal osteoporosis.

Prevention of Skeletal-Related Events in Patients With Bone Metastases

In cancer patients, denosumab is used to prevent (delay) SREs—bone fracture, spinal cord compression, bone pain requiring radiation—after cells from a solid tumor have metastasized to bone. In patients with breast cancer or prostate cancer, denosumab was *superior* to zoledronate at delaying SREs. In patients with other cancers, denosumab was *equal* to zoledronate at delaying SREs.

Mechanism of Action

Denosumab is a monoclonal antibody that decreases the formation and function of osteoclasts and thereby decreases bone resorption and increases BMD and bone strength. What's the underlying mechanism? Denosumab prevents the activation of a receptor known as RANK, found on the surface of osteoclasts and their precursor cells. Under normal conditions, RANK is activated by binding with an endogenous compound known as the *RANK ligand,* or simply RANKL. When activated by RANKL, RANK stimulates the formation and activity of osteoclasts. Denosumab binds with RANKL and thereby prevents RANKL from activating RANK.

Pharmacokinetics

Administration is subQ. Blood levels peak 10 days after a single injection. The elimination half-life is 28 days. Renal impairment does not affect denosumab kinetics. The effect of hepatic impairment has not been studied.

Adverse Effects

In postmenopausal women with osteoporosis, the most common adverse effects are back pain, pain in the extremities, musculoskeletal pain, hypercholesterolemia, and urinary bladder infection. In cancer patients with bone metastases, the most common adverse effects are fatigue, hypophosphatemia, and nausea. In all patients, suppression of bone turnover may delay fracture healing and increase the risk for new fractures and ONJ. The most serious adverse effects—hypocalcemia, infections, skin reactions, and ONJ—are discussed next.

Hypocalcemia

Denosumab can exacerbate preexisting hypocalcemia, presumably by reducing osteoclast activity. If hypocalcemia is present, it must be corrected before starting denosumab. The risk for hypocalcemia is elevated in patients with impaired renal function (including those on dialysis) and patients with other risk factors (e.g., a history of hypoparathyroidism, thyroid surgery, malabsorption syndromes, or excision of the small intestine). The manufacturer recommends monitoring levels of calcium, magnesium, and phosphorus in this at-risk group. To help prevent hypocalcemia when taking denosumab, all patients should take 1000 mg of calcium every day and at least 400 IU of vitamin D every day.

Serious Infections

Denosumab increases the risk for serious infections, although the absolute risk is low. In clinical trials, some patients developed endocarditis, serious skin infections, and infections of the abdomen, urinary tract, and ear. Patients who develop signs of severe infection should seek immediate medical attention. Infection risk is increased in patients who are immunocompromised (e.g., owing to HIV infection or treatment with immunosuppressant drugs).

Dermatologic Reactions

Denosumab increases the risk for dermatitis, eczema, rashes, and other skin reactions. Of note, these are not limited to the injection site. If a severe reaction occurs, discontinuation of denosumab should be considered.

Osteonecrosis of the Jaw

Like the bisphosphonates, denosumab increases the risk for ONJ. Risk is further increased by invasive dental procedures (e.g., tooth extractions, dental implants, oral surgery), and hence these should be conducted before starting denosumab. Patients who develop ONJ should be under the care of a dentist or oral surgeon. Maintaining good oral hygiene reduces ONJ risk.

Prolia: Dosage and Administration

Prolia is indicated for osteoporosis in postmenopausal women and in men at risk for fractures. The drug is supplied in (1) single-use vials containing 1 mL of a 60-mg/mL solution and (2) single-use, prefilled syringes containing 1 mL of a 60-mg/mL solution. The recommended dosage is 60 mg every 6 months, by subQ injection into the upper arm, upper thigh, or abdomen. If a dose is missed, it should be given as soon as possible. Subsequent doses should be given every 6 months thereafter. To prevent hypocalcemia, patients should take 1000 mg of calcium daily plus at least 400 IU of vitamin D daily.

Xgeva: Dosage and Administration

Xgeva is indicated for preventing SREs in patients with bone metastases from solid tumors. The drug is supplied in single-use vials that contain 120 mg denosumab/1.7 mL. The recommended dosage is 120 mg every 4 weeks by subQ injection into the upper arm, upper thigh, or abdomen. As with Prolia, patients should take calcium and vitamin D to prevent hypocalcemia.

Prolia and Xgeva: Storage, Warming, and Inspection

Solutions should be stored under refrigeration and then warmed before use (by standing at room temperature for 15–30 minutes). All preparations should be clear and colorless (or pale yellow). Preparations that have particles or are cloudy or discolored should not be used.

Cinacalcet

Actions and Therapeutic Use

Cinacalcet [Sensipar] is a "calcimimetic" drug approved for primary hyperparathyroidism (caused by parathyroid carcinoma) as well as secondary hyperparathyroidism (caused by chronic kidney disease [CKD]). In both cases, benefits derive from decreasing secretion of PTH. How is secretion suppressed? Recall that extracellular calcium regulates PTH secretion by binding with calcium-sensing receptors on cells of the parathyroid gland, thereby signaling those cells to reduce PTH secretion. Cinacalcet increases the sensitivity of the calcium-sensing receptors to activation by extracellular calcium. As a result, the ability of calcium to suppress PTH release is amplified.

Clinical trials have shown that, in patients with hyperparathyroidism secondary to CKD, cinacalcet decreases serum PTH by 23% to 46% and improves calcium and phosphorus homeostasis. Similarly, in patients with primary hyperparathyroidism, the drug decreases serum PTH and normalizes serum calcium.

Pharmacokinetics

Dosing is oral, and absorption is increased by food. In the blood, cinacalcet is highly bound (93%–97%) to plasma proteins. Cinacalcet undergoes extensive hepatic metabolism, followed by excretion in the urine (80%) and feces (15%). The drug's half-life is 30 to 40 hours.

Adverse Effects

The most common adverse effects are nausea, vomiting, and diarrhea. Because cinacalcet lowers calcium levels, hypocalcemia is an obvious concern. Accordingly, calcium levels should be monitored, and patients should be informed about possible manifestations of hypocalcemia (e.g., cramping, convulsions, myalgias, paresthesias, tetany) and instructed to report them.

Drug Interactions

Cinacalcet is metabolized in part by cytochrome P450 isoenzyme 3A4, so inhibitors of this enzyme (e.g., ketoconazole, itraconazole, erythromycin) can raise cinacalcet levels. If cinacalcet is used with one of these drugs, cinacalcet dosage may need an adjustment.

Monitoring

In patients with parathyroid carcinoma, measure serum calcium within 1 week of the first dose and each dosage change. After a maintenance dosage has been established, measure serum calcium every 2 months.

In patients with secondary hyperparathyroidism, measure serum calcium and phosphorus within 1 week of the first dose and each dosage change, and measure PTH within 4 weeks of the first dose and each dosage change. After a maintenance dosage has been established, measure calcium and phosphorus monthly and PTH every 1 to 3 months.

Preparations, Dosage, and Administration

Cinacalcet [Sensipar] is available in tablets (30, 60, and 90 mg) for oral use. To enhance absorption, the drug should be taken with a meal or shortly after.

In patients with parathyroid carcinoma, the initial dosage is 30 mg twice daily. Then, every 2 to 4 weeks, dosage is increased as follows—60 mg twice daily, 90 mg twice daily, 90 mg 3 times/day, up to a maximum of 90 mg 4 times a day—until the dosing goal (normalization of serum calcium) is achieved.

In patients with secondary hyperparathyroidism, the initial dosage is 30 mg once daily. Then, every 2 to 4 weeks, dosage is increased as follows—60 mg once daily, 90 mg once daily, 120 mg once daily, up to a maximum of 180 mg once daily—until the dosing goal (PTH level between 150 and 300 pg/mL) is achieved.

Drugs for Hypercalcemia

Furosemide

Furosemide, a loop diuretic, promotes renal excretion of calcium. This action is useful for treating hypercalcemic emergencies. In managing such emergencies, isotonic saline (IV) must be given before furosemide. The dosage of furosemide for adults is 80 to 100 mg every 1 to 2 hours as needed, infused no faster than 4 mg/min. To avoid fluid and electrolyte imbalance, urinary losses must be measured and replaced. The basic pharmacology of furosemide is discussed in Chapter 35.

Glucocorticoids

Glucocorticoids reduce intestinal absorption of calcium and can thereby reduce hypercalcemia. For severe hypercalcemia, parenteral glucocorticoid therapy is indicated (e.g., 100–500 mg hydrocortisone sodium succinate IV daily). Because glucocorticoids can produce serious adverse effects when taken chronically, the risks for long-term treatment must be carefully weighed against the benefits. The basic pharmacology of the glucocorticoids is discussed in Chapter 56.

Bisphosphonates

Pamidronate, etidronate, and zoledronate are approved for HCM. The mechanism is suppression of bone resorption by osteoclasts. The pharmacology of these agents is discussed previously.

Inorganic Phosphates

Phosphates reduce plasma levels of calcium and thus can be used to treat hypercalcemia. Suggested mechanisms for reducing plasma calcium include (1) decreased bone resorption, (2) increased bone formation, and (3) decreased intestinal absorption of calcium (secondary to decreased renal activation of vitamin D). Intravenous use of phosphates is hazardous and limited to patients with life-threatening hypercalcemia. Oral administration is considerably safer.

Oral phosphates are used for mild to moderate hypercalcemia. These agents should not be given to patients with renal impairment or elevated serum phosphate. Oral phosphates should not be combined with antacids that contain aluminum, magnesium, or calcium—agents that bind phosphate and thereby prevent its absorption. Initial treatment should provide 1 to 2 g of phosphorus/day. Doses are reduced when serum calcium levels normalize.

Edetate Disodium

EDTA [Endrate] is a chelating agent that binds calcium in the blood. As a result, it can rapidly reduce plasma levels of free calcium. The EDTA-calcium complex is filtered by the glomerulus, but not reabsorbed by kidney tubules, and hence renal excretion of calcium is increased. Although EDTA is highly effective at reducing hypercalcemia, it can be dangerous: EDTA can cause profound hypocalcemia, resulting in tetany, convulsions, dysrhythmias, and possibly death. Severe nephrotoxicity can also occur. Because of its toxicity, EDTA is used only for life-threatening hypercalcemic crisis. The usual adult dose is 40 mg/kg infused over 4 to 6 hours. The total daily dose must not exceed 3 g.

OSTEOPOROSIS

General Considerations

Osteoporosis is a serious medical problem characterized by low bone mass, altered bone architecture, and increased bone fragility. Because of bone fragility, patients are susceptible to fractures from minor traumatic events, such as coughing, rolling over in bed, or falling from a standing position.

Osteoporosis is the most common bone disease in humans. More than 10 million Americans have osteoporosis—80% of them older women—and another 34 million have reduced bone mass, a risk factor for osteoporosis. Every year, osteoporosis leads to 1.5 million fractures. The most common fracture sites are the vertebrae (spine), distal forearm (wrist), and femoral neck (hip). Vertebral fractures can result in loss of height, spinal deformity, chronic back pain, and impaired breathing. Complications from hip fractures are a significant cause of mortality: of the 300,000 Americans who get hip fractures each year, about 50,000 die of complications.

The economic burden of osteoporosis is high. Each year in the United States, osteoporosis-related fractures lead to more than 432,000 hospital admissions, nearly 2.5 million medical office visits, and about 180,000 admissions to nursing homes—at an estimated cost of $17 billion, or $47 million a day.

Bone Mass

In men and women, bone mass changes across the life span. Bone mass peaks in the third decade, remains stable to age 50 years, and then slowly declines—at a rate that is usually less than 1% a year. In addition to this slow, aging-related decline, women go through a phase of *accelerated* bone loss (2%–3% a year) that begins after menopause and continues for several years. In both the slow and accelerated phases of decline, bone is lost because resorption of old bone outpaces deposition of new bone.

Primary Prevention: Calcium, Vitamin D, and Lifestyle

The risk for osteoporosis can be reduced by lifelong implementation of measures that can help maximize bone strength. Specifically, we need to ensure sufficient intake of calcium and vitamin D, and we need to adopt a lifestyle that promotes bone health. Calcium is needed to maximize bone growth early in life and to maintain bone integrity later in life. Vitamin D is needed to ensure calcium absorption. The amount of calcium needed for optimal bone health is indicated in Table 59.1. Note that calcium requirements are greatest for adolescents and teens (1300 mg/day), then drop for younger adults (1000 mg/day), and then rise for older adults (1200 mg/day). If diet alone cannot meet calcium needs, supplements should be employed. Lifestyle measures that promote bone health include the following:

- Performing regular weight-bearing exercise (walking, yoga, dancing, racquet sports, weight lifting, stair climbing)
- Avoiding excessive alcohol
- Avoiding smoking

Diagnosing Osteoporosis and Assessing Fracture Risk

Osteoporosis is diagnosed by measuring BMD, an important predictor of fracture risk. Both the National Osteoporosis Foundation (NOF) and the USPSTF recommend routine BMD testing for *all women* beginning at age 65 years and for *younger postmenopausal women* deemed at increased risk for osteoporotic fractures. In addition, the NOF recommends testing of *all men* age 70 and older. (The USPSTF makes no recommendation regarding men.) BMD testing is not recommended for children or adolescents, nor is routine testing indicated for premenopausal women or healthy young men.

The standard technique for measuring BMD is *dual-energy x-ray absorptiometry* (DEXA). DEXA scans only take a few minutes, and exposure to radiation is minimal—about $\frac{1}{10}$ that of a standard chest radiograph. Results of DEXA scans are reported in terms of *standard deviations* (SD) below mean BMD values in young adults. A BMD value that is 1 SD below the mean indicates 10% bone loss, a value that is 2 SD below the mean indicates 20% bone loss, and so forth. Using this system, the World Health Organization (WHO) has defined *normal* BMD for women as being no more than 1 SD below the mean for young adults. BMD values between 1 SD below the mean and 2.5 SD below the mean define *low bone mass* (also known as *osteopenia*). BMD values 2.5 SD or greater below the mean define *osteoporosis.* To simplify communication, we can talk about DEXA results in terms of a *T-score,* rather than using the phrase *SD above (or below) the mean.* For example, instead of saying that a BMD reading was 2.5 SD below the mean, we can simply say the T-score was −2.5.

PATIENT-CENTERED CARE ACROSS THE LIFE SPAN

Drugs Affecting Bone Mineralization

Life Stage	Patient Care Concerns
Infants, children, and adolescents	With the exception of calcium and vitamin D, these drugs are not recommended for children, except denosumab when taken for bone cancer. In this instance it is advised only for "skeletally mature" adolescents who are 13–17 years old.
Pregnant women	The FDA has assigned a Pregnancy Risk Category of D/X for denosumab (D for Xgeva; X for Prolia). Estrogen and raloxifene are Pregnancy Risk Category X drugs. The remaining drugs are classified in Pregnancy Risk Category C; however, there is a theoretical concern that bisphosphonates could cause harm that has not yet been verified owing to inadequate long-term studies. Nasal spray formulations of calcitonin-salmon are not recommended during pregnancy. Although vitamin D_2 and calcium formulations receiving an assigned Pregnancy Risk Category were given a C classification, this is generally considered to be a concern only if the intake exceeds recommendations. Vitamin D_3 has not been assigned a Pregnancy Risk Category classification.
Breastfeeding women	Estrogen decreases both the quality and quantity of milk and may affect infant growth and development. For the remaining drugs, with the exception of calcium and vitamin D, breastfeeding is not recommended because of inadequate studies.
Older adults	Estrogen meets Beers Criteria (strength of recommendation: strong) for potentially inappropriate use in older patients. Because frail older adults commonly have difficulty swallowing, those who take bisphosphonates may be at an increased risk for esophagitis. Owing to occurrences of low-impact atypical femur fractures in older women who have had long-term bisphosphonate therapy, some orthopedists recommend against continuing bisphosphonate therapy beyond 5 years.

Although loss of bone at one site (e.g., wrist) can predict the risk for fractures at other sites (e.g., hip, spine), it is preferable to measure BMD at specific sites to predict the risk for those sites. Accordingly, a thorough evaluation would include BMD measurements in the wrist, spine, and hip—the sites at which osteoporotic fractures occur most often.

Although we use BMD values to diagnose osteoporosis, it is important to understand that low BMD is not the only predictor of fractures. Other important predictors include a family history of hip fractures, a personal history of fractures, low body mass index, and use of oral glucocorticoids. To account for these risk factors, the WHO developed an important tool, called FRAX, which can assess an *individual*'s 10-year risk for experiencing a fracture. This web-based, interactive program is available online at www.shef.ac.uk/FRAX/. Individual risk is calculated after entering the following data:

- Age
- Gender
- Weight
- Height
- Previous fracture
- Hip fracture in a parent
- Secondary osteoporosis (i.e., malnutrition, hyperthyroidism, diabetes, and other disorders associated with osteoporosis)
- Rheumatoid arthritis
- Glucocorticoid use
- Current smoking
- Alcohol consumption
- Hip BMD

Of note, FRAX is tailored to specific countries and, for the United States, to four specific subgroups: Blacks, Hispanics, Caucasians, and Asians.

Who Should Be Treated?

In 2016, The American Association of Clinical Endocrinologists and the American College of Endocrinology released joint clinical practice guidelines for diagnosis and treatment of postmenopausal osteoporosis. (See https://www.aace.com/files/final-appendix-sept-7.pdf,) According to this document, postmenopausal women and men 50 years and older should be considered for treatment if they present with any of the following:

- A hip fracture or vertebral fracture.
- Osteoporosis (T-score of −2.5 or less at the femoral neck or spine).
- Low bone mass (T-score between −1 and −2.5 at the femoral neck or spine) *plus either* a 10-year probability of a hip fracture of 3% or more *or* a 10-year probability of another major osteoporosis-related fracture of 20% or more, based on a U.S.-adapted FRAX calculation.

Treating Osteoporosis in Women

The objective of osteoporosis treatment is to reduce the occurrence of fractures by maintaining or increasing bone strength. Recommended management is summarized in Fig. 59.3.

Two types of drugs can be used: (1) agents that decrease bone resorption and (2) agents that promote bone formation. Not surprisingly, these are the same drugs previously covered in this chapter. Antiresorptive drugs—estrogen, raloxifene, bisphosphonates, calcitonin, and denosumab—are used most often. These agents do a good job of preventing bone loss by reducing osteoclast activity, but are largely unable to reverse bone mass that has already occurred. Accordingly, antiresorptive drugs are most beneficial when used early—before substantial loss has occurred. With all antiresorptive drugs, success requires a sufficiency of calcium and vitamin D. At this time, teriparatide [Forteo] is the only drug that effectively promotes bone formation. Of the drugs employed for osteoporosis, three agents—teriparatide, denosumab, and zoledronate (a bisphosphonate)—are most likely to reduce fractures.

Treating Osteoporosis in Men

In the United States about 2 million men have aging-related osteoporosis, and another 3 million are at risk. Hip fractures occur in 80,000 American men annually, compared with 269,000 American women. Of the men who get a hip fracture, 36% die within a year. Although rates of osteoporosis and fractures in men are significant, they are still much lower than in women. As discussed, bone mass in men peaks in the third decade and begins progressive decline at about age 50 years. The rate of decline in men is about equal to that in women—except that in men, there is no counterpart to the accelerated phase of bone loss that occurs after menopause. If men and women lose bone mass at similar rates, why do men experience less osteoporosis? The main reason is that bones in men, at their peak, are larger and stronger than bones in women. Hence, after decline begins, male bones can tolerate more loss before fractures are likely. Factors that contribute to the risk for osteoporosis in men include low testosterone, prolonged use of glucocorticoids, white race, calcium deficiency, vitamin D deficiency, smoking, excessive alcohol consumption, and insufficient exercise. As in women, 10-year fracture risk can be assessed using the FRAX calculator developed by the WHO.

Treatment of male osteoporosis is confounded by a paucity of research. (Osteoporosis is one of the few areas of therapeutics in which research in women has greatly exceeded research in men.) At this time, only five drugs—*alendronate* [Fosamax], *risedronate* [Actonel],[a] *zoledronate* [Reclast], *teriparatide* [Forteo], and *denosumab* [Prolia]—are approved for osteoporosis in men. In one study, 2 years of alendronate increased BMD of the lumbar spine and hip and significantly decreased the incidence of vertebral fractures. Benefits with risedronate, zoledronate, and teriparatide are similar. For alendronate, zoledronate, and teriparatide, dosages are the same as those used in women. For risedronate, the only approved dosage is 35 mg once a week. Calcitonin has been tried in men, but proof of efficacy is lacking. If testosterone deficiency underlies osteoporosis, testosterone replacement therapy is indicated, unless the patient has testicular cancer or some other disorder that contraindicates testosterone use. All men should ensure adequate intake of calcium and vitamin D.

[a]The delayed-release formulation of risedronate, sold as *Atelvia,* is not approved for osteoporosis in men, although it *is* approved for osteoporosis in women.

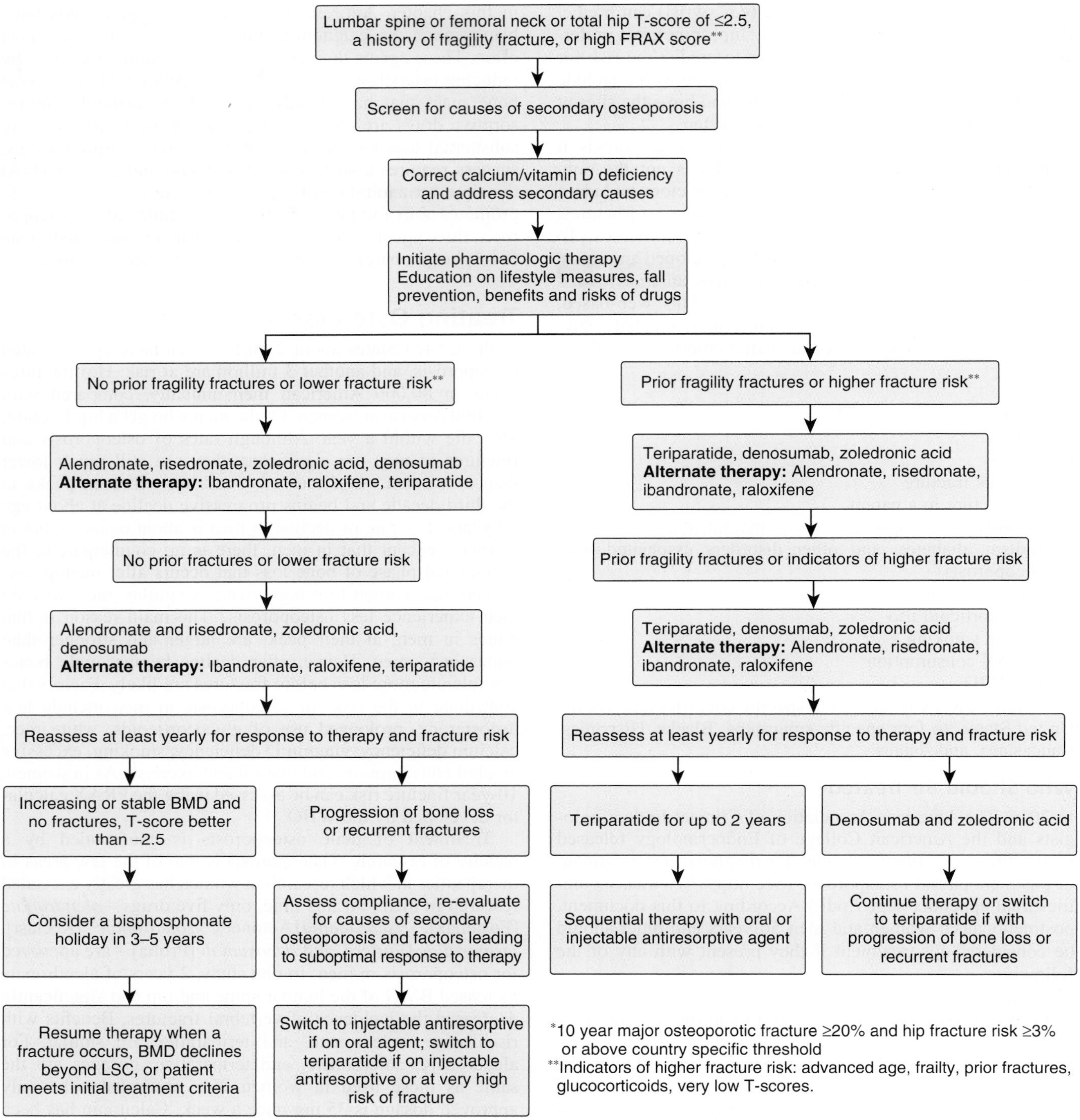

Figure 59.3 ■ Postmenopausal osteoporosis treatment algorithm.
(From: Camacho, P., Petak, S. M., Binkley, N., Clarke, B. L., Harris, S. T., Hurley, D. L. … Watts, N. B. (2016). American Association of Clinical Endocrinologists and American College of Endocrinology clinical practice guidelines for the diagnosis and treatment of postmenopausal osteoporosis – 2016. *Endocrine Practice, 22* (Suppl 4), 1-42. Available at https://www.aace.com/files/final-appendix-sept-7.pdf.)

PRESCRIBING AND MONITORING CONSIDERATIONS

Vitamin D

Assessment

Therapeutic Goals

Goals include treatment of rickets, osteomalacia, and hypoparathyroidism, and prevention of vitamin D deficiency.

Baseline Data

The prescriber may order serum levels of vitamin D, calcium, phosphorus, and alkaline phosphatase as well as a 24-hour urinary calcium determination.

Assess dietary vitamin D and calcium content. (Adjustment may be needed to ensure calcium sufficiency.)

Identifying High-Risk Patients

Vitamin D is *contraindicated* in patients with hypercalcemia, hypervitaminosis D, and malabsorption syndrome.

Exercise *caution* in patients taking digoxin.

Ongoing Monitoring and Interventions

Monitoring Summary

Monitor serum calcium, serum phosphorus, and urinary calcium.

Minimizing Adverse Interactions

Digoxin. Vitamin D–induced hypercalcemia can cause dysrhythmias in patients taking digoxin. Monitor serum calcium and make certain it remains within normal range.

Management of Toxicity. Large therapeutic doses may cause hypervitaminosis D, a syndrome characterized by hypercalcemia, hypercalciuria, decalcification of bone, and deposition of calcium in soft tissues. Monitor serum calcium content; levels should stay below 10 mg/dL. Monitor serum phosphorus and urinary calcium as well. If vitamin D toxicity develops, instruct the patient to discontinue vitamin D immediately, increase fluid intake, and institute a low-calcium diet. In severe cases, calcium excretion can be accelerated with IV saline plus furosemide.

Oral Calcium Salts

Assessment

Therapeutic Goals

Goals include treatment of mild hypocalcemia and supplementation of dietary calcium.

Baseline Data

Obtain a serum calcium level.

Identifying High-Risk Patients

Calcium salts are *contraindicated* for patients with hypercalcemia, renal calculi, and hypophosphatemia.

Administration Considerations

Individual calcium salts differ with respect to percentage of elemental calcium. As a result, the dose required to provide a specific amount of calcium differs among the salts.

Ongoing Monitoring and Interventions

Minimizing Adverse Effects

Prolonged therapy can cause hypercalcemia. Hypercalcemia can be minimized with frequent monitoring of serum calcium.

Minimizing Adverse Interactions

Glucocorticoids. These drugs reduce calcium absorption; increased calcium dosage may be required.

Tetracyclines. Calcium binds to tetracyclines, thereby reducing tetracycline absorption.

Thyroid Hormone. Calcium interferes with absorption of thyroid hormone.

Thiazide Diuretics. Thiazides decrease renal excretion of calcium. A reduction in calcium dosage may be needed to avoid hypercalcemia.

Loop Diuretics. Loop diuretics increase calcium excretion. An increase in calcium dosage may be needed to avoid hypocalcemia.

Calcitonin-Salmon

Assessment

Therapeutic Goals

Goals include treatment of postmenopausal osteoporosis, Paget disease of bone, and hypercalcemia.

Baseline Data

The prescriber may order measurements of serum alkaline phosphatase, calcium, and phosphorus, as well as a 24-hour urinary hydroxyproline.

Identifying High-Risk Patients

Salmon calcitonin is *contraindicated* for patients allergic to this preparation.

Ongoing Monitoring and Interventions

Evaluating Therapeutic Effects

Postmenopausal Osteoporosis. Measurement of BMD should indicate slowing of bone loss (and perhaps a small increase in BMD).

Paget Disease of Bone. Monitor for reductions in bone pain, serum alkaline phosphatase levels, and 24-hour urinary hydroxyproline value.

Hypercalcemia. Monitor for reductions in serum calcium and phosphorus levels.

Bisphosphonates Used for Osteoporosis

Assessment

Therapeutic Goals

Goals include prevention and treatment of osteoporosis.

Baseline Data

Obtain baseline values for BMD in the hip, spine, and wrist. For patients receiving zoledronate, obtain a baseline value for creatinine clearance and assess for adequate hydration.

Identifying High-Risk Patients

Oral bisphosphonates are *contraindicated* for patients with esophageal disorders that can impede swallowing and for patients who cannot sit or stand for at least 30 minutes (60 minutes with ibandronate).

Zoledronate, an IV bisphosphonate, is *contraindicated* for patients with acute renal failure or creatinine clearance below 35 mL/min and should be used with *caution* in patients who are older or dehydrated and in those with chronic renal impairment and those taking other nephrotoxic drugs.

Administration Considerations

Proper administration is needed to maximize absorption and minimize the risk for esophagitis. Patients must be able to sit upright for at least 30 minutes (60 minutes with ibandronate) after taking bisphosphonates. To ensure absorption, bisphosphonates must be taken on an empty stomach; no food should be ingested for at least 30 minutes (60 minutes with ibandronate) after administration.

Ongoing Monitoring and Interventions

Evaluating Therapeutic Effects

Obtain periodic determinations of BMD. If BMD increases, or at least remains constant, treatment is a success. Conversely, a significant decline in BMD indicates failure.

Minimizing Adverse Effects

Esophagitis. Oral bisphosphonates can cause severe esophagitis, sometimes resulting in ulceration. Avoid these drugs in patients with esophageal disorders that could impede swallowing and in patients who are unable to sit or stand for 30 minutes (60 minutes with ibandronate).

Atypical Femoral Fractures. Rarely, long-term bisphosphonate therapy has been associated with atypical fractures of the femur. To reduce risk, prescribers should do the following:

- Use these drugs only when needed (i.e., avoid bisphosphonates in patients considered at low risk for osteoporosis-related fractures).
- Consider alternative treatments, such as raloxifene or teriparatide, for patients with osteoporosis of the spine and normal (or only moderately reduced) BMD of the femoral neck or hip.
- Perform an annual reevaluation of the need for continued therapy in patients who have taken bisphosphonates for 5 years.

Esophageal Cancer. Oral bisphosphonates may (or may not) increase the risk for *esophageal cancer.* Measures that might reduce risk include reducing the dosing frequency (e.g., dosing monthly or weekly rather than daily), taking the drug with a full glass of water, and staying upright for 30 to 60 minutes after dosing.

Musculoskeletal Pain. Rarely, bisphosphonates cause muscle, bone, and joint pain. Severe pain may require an opioid or ketorolac for relief. As a rule, pain gradually diminishes when bisphosphonates are withdrawn. In most cases, pain does not return when bisphosphonates are resumed. If it does resume, osteoporosis should be managed with a different drug (e.g., calcitonin-salmon, teriparatide, raloxifene).

Ocular Problems. Rarely, bisphosphonates cause conjunctivitis, scleritis, blurred vision, eye pain, and other ocular problems. Inquire about vision changes or discomfort at each patient encounter.

Osteonecrosis of the Jaw. ONJ occurs primarily with IV bisphosphonates. To reduce ONJ risk, a dental examination with appropriate preventive dentistry should be conducted before giving bisphosphonates.

Renal Toxicity. Intravenous *zoledronate* can damage the kidney, leading to acute renal failure and possibly death. Exercise caution in patients at increased risk (owing to advanced age, chronic renal impairment, dehydration, or use of diuretics or nephrotoxic drugs). Before dosing, ensure that hydration is adequate and that kidney function is adequate too (creatinine clearance above 35 mL/min). To reduce risk, infuse zoledronate slowly (over 15 minutes or more). Monitor renal function by determining creatinine clearance at baseline, before each dose, and periodically after each infusion. If renal impairment develops, zoledronate dosage should be reduced.

Minimizing Adverse Interactions

Interactions With Zoledronate. Risk for renal failure with zoledronate is increased by use of *diuretics* (which can cause dehydration) and by use of other *nephrotoxic drugs,* including cyclosporine, amphotericin, aminoglycoside antibiotics, and the NSAIDs. Exercise caution in patients using these agents.

Raloxifene

Assessment

Therapeutic Goals

Goals include prevention and treatment of postmenopausal osteoporosis and reducing the risk for invasive breast cancer in postmenopausal women who have osteoporosis or a high risk for breast cancer.

Baseline Data

Obtain baseline values for BMD in the hip, vertebrae, and forearm.

Identifying High-Risk Patients

Raloxifene is *contraindicated* for use by patients who are pregnant or have a history of venous thrombotic events.

Ongoing Monitoring and Interventions

Evaluating Therapeutic Effects

For women taking raloxifene to prevent or treat osteoporosis, obtain periodic determinations of BMD. If BMD increases, or at least remains constant, treatment is a success. Conversely, a significant decline in BMD indicates failure.

Minimizing Adverse Effects

Venous Thromboembolism. Raloxifene increases the risk for DVT, PE, and thrombotic stroke. Do not give raloxifene to patients with a history of venous thrombotic events. Do not prescribe this drug for patients who require prolonged inactivity such as bed rest.

Fetal Harm. Raloxifene can cause fetal harm and must not be used during pregnancy.

Estrogen

Prescribing and monitoring implications for estrogen are summarized in Chapter 48.

UNIT XV
Respiratory Tract Drugs

CHAPTER 60

Drugs for Asthma and Chronic Obstructive Pulmonary Disease

Jacqueline Rosenjack Burchum, DNSc, FNP-BC, CNE

BASIC CONSIDERATIONS

Asthma is a common, chronic disorder that occurs in 1 in 11 children and 1 in 12 adults in the United States. Characteristic signs and symptoms are a sense of breathlessness and tightness in the chest, together with wheezing, dyspnea, and cough. The underlying cause is immune-mediated airway inflammation. In the United States nearly 25.7 million people have the disease, representing an increase of almost 15% since the early 2000s. Each year, the disease kills about 3500 Americans. However, despite these sobering statistics, with proper treatment, most patients can lead full lives with no limitations.

Chronic obstructive pulmonary disease (COPD) is a chronic, progressive, largely irreversible disorder characterized by airflow restrictions and inflammation. In most cases, COPD is preventable; the most common cause is smoking cigarettes. Symptoms include chronic cough, excessive sputum production, wheezing, dyspnea, and poor exercise tolerance. In the United States COPD affects about 24 million people. In the most recent report by the Centers for Disease Control and Prevention, chronic lower respiratory diseases were listed as the third leading cause of death in the United States. Unfortunately, although drug therapy is highly effective in asthma, benefits in COPD are minimal and limited to a small improvement in symptoms. Drug therapy does not slow disease progression, reduce hospitalizations, or prolong life.

Pathophysiology of Asthma

Asthma is a *chronic inflammatory* disorder of the airways. In about 50% of children with asthma and in some adults, airway inflammation results from an immune response to known allergens. In the remaining children and in most adults, the cause of airway inflammation is unknown—although as-yet unidentified allergens are suspected.

Fig. 60.1 depicts the events that lead to inflammation and bronchoconstriction in patients whose asthma is caused by specific allergens. Although this model may not apply completely to all asthma patients, it nonetheless provides a basis for understanding the drugs used for treatment. The inflammatory process begins with binding of allergen molecules (e.g., house dust mite feces) to immunoglobulin E (IgE) antibodies on mast cells. This causes mast cells to release an assortment of mediators, including histamine, leukotrienes, prostaglandins, and interleukins. These mediators have two effects. They act immediately to cause *bronchoconstriction.* In addition, they promote infiltration and activation of inflammatory cells (eosinophils, leukocytes, macrophages). These inflammatory cells then release mediators of their own. The end result is *airway inflammation,* characterized by edema, mucus plugging, and smooth muscle hypertrophy, all of which obstruct airflow. In addition, inflammation produces a state of *bronchial hyperreactivity.* Because of this state, mild trigger factors (e.g., cold air, exercise, tobacco smoke) are able to cause intense bronchoconstriction.

Pathophysiology of Chronic Obstructive Pulmonary Disease

Symptoms of COPD result largely from two pathologic processes: *chronic bronchitis* and *emphysema.* In most cases, both processes are caused by an exaggerated inflammatory reaction to cigarette smoke. Chronic bronchitis—defined by chronic cough and excessive sputum production—results from hypertrophy of mucus-secreting glands in the epithelium of the larger airways. Emphysema is defined as enlargement of the air space within the bronchioles and alveoli brought on by deterioration of the walls of these air spaces. Among individuals with COPD, the relative contribution of these two processes can vary. That is, some patients may suffer primarily from chronic bronchitis, some primarily from emphysema, and some from both disease processes.

Fig. 60.2 depicts the events that lead to inflammation, airway obstruction, and air trapping in patients with COPD. Irritants such as tobacco smoke initiate an inflammatory response in the airways. As a result of the frequent and recurrent irritation and the subsequent response by various leukocytes and inflammatory mediators, pathologic changes result in the bronchial edema and increase in mucus secretion that

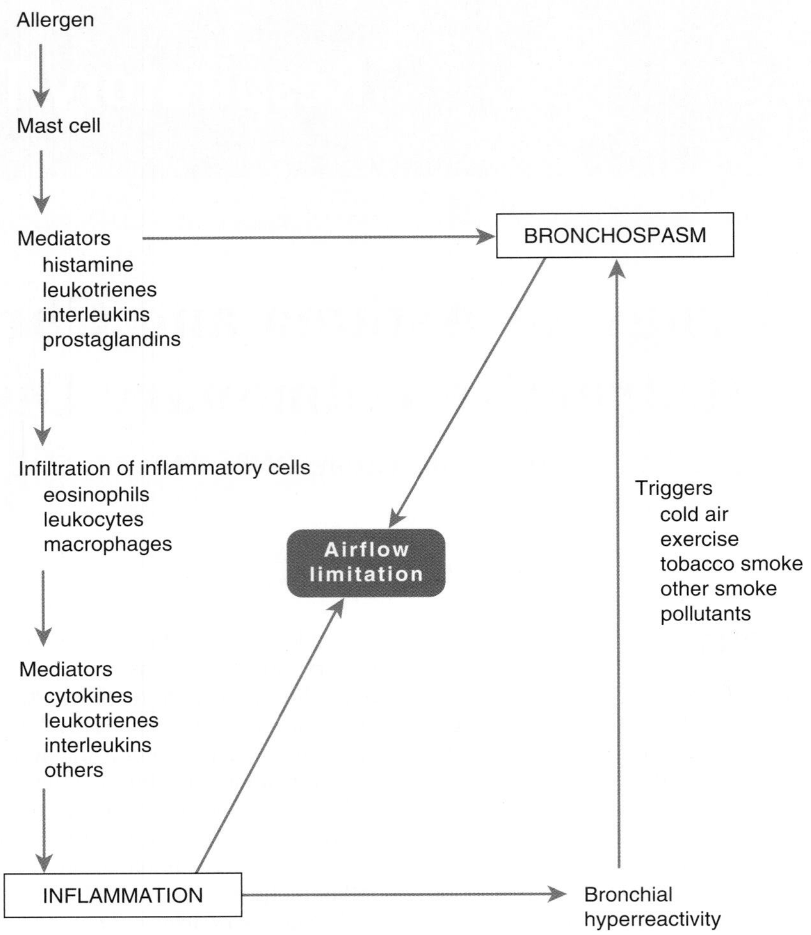

Figure 60.1 ■ Allergen-induced inflammation and bronchospasm in asthma.

characterize chronic bronchitis. Additionally, the continuous inflammation inhibits the production of protease inhibitors, which have a protective role in maintaining alveolar integrity. As a result of the inhibition, the protease enzymes break down elastin, resulting in the destruction of alveolar walls and the decrease in elastic recoil that characterize emphysema. In a small percentage of the population, emphysema results from a genetic alteration that results in alpha-1 antitrypsin deficiency. (Alpha-1 antitrypsin is a protease inhibitor that protects the lungs from enzymatic destruction by proteases.)

Overview of Drugs for Asthma and Chronic Obstructive Pulmonary Disease

The major drugs for asthma and COPD are shown in Table 60.1. They fall into two main pharmacologic classes: *antiinflammatory agents* and *bronchodilators*. The principal antiinflammatory drugs are the *glucocorticoids*. The principal bronchodilators are the *beta$_2$ agonists*. For chronic asthma and stable COPD, glucocorticoids are administered on a fixed schedule, almost always by inhalation. Beta$_2$ agonists may be administered on a fixed schedule for long-term control or as needed (PRN) to manage an acute attack. Like the glucocorticoids, beta$_2$ agonists are usually inhaled.

Prototype Drugs

DRUGS FOR ASTHMA AND CHRONIC OBSTRUCTIVE PULMONARY DISEASE

Antiinflammatory Drugs: Glucocorticoids

Beclomethasone (inhaled)
Prednisone (oral)

Antiinflammatory Drugs: Others

Cromolyn (mast cell stabilizer, inhaled)
Zafirlukast (leukotriene modifier, oral)

Bronchodilators: Beta$_2$-Adrenergic Agonists

Albuterol (inhaled, short acting)
Salmeterol (inhaled, long acting)

Bronchodilators: Methylxanthine

Theophylline

Anticholinergic Drug

Ipratropium

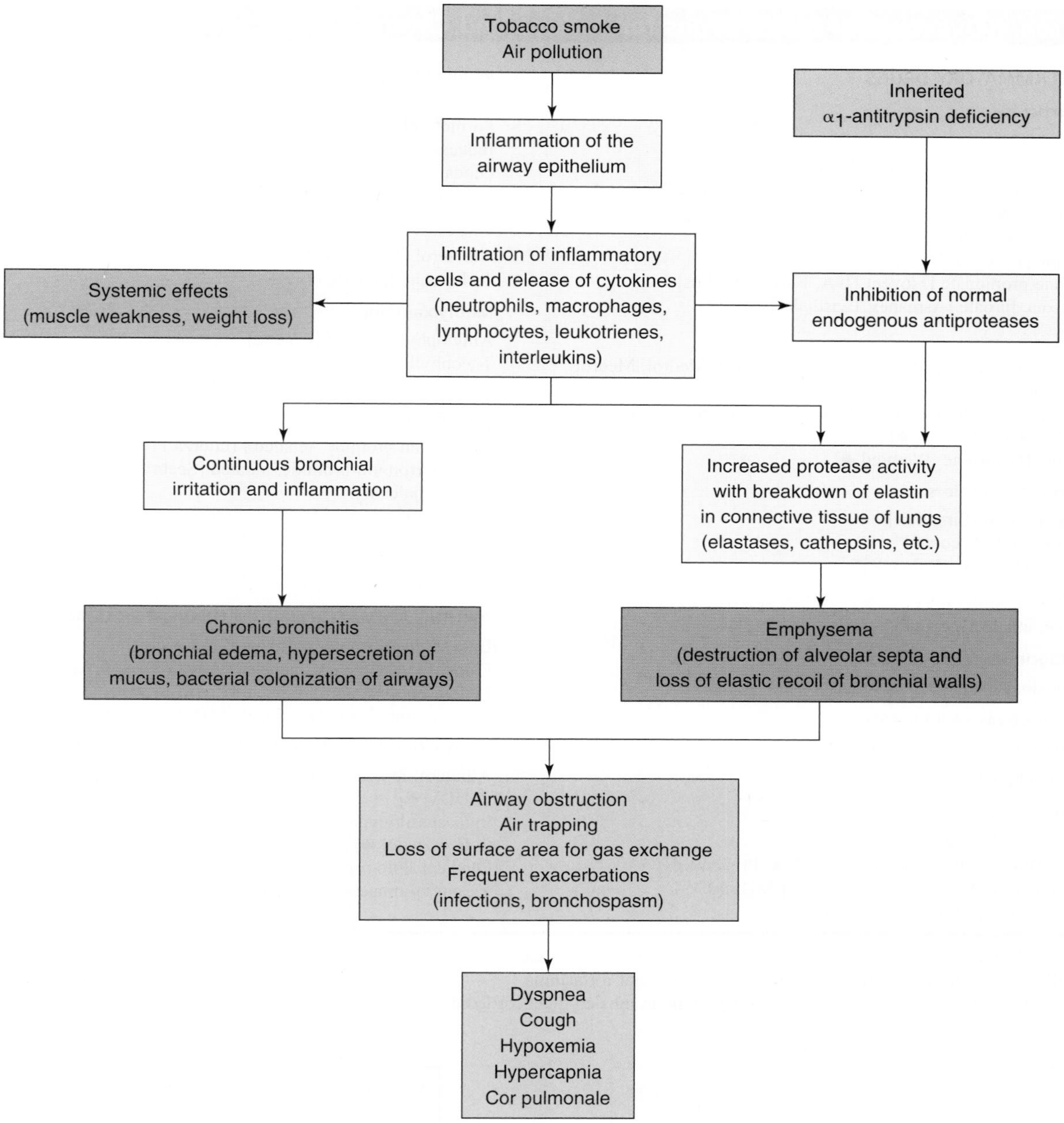

Figure 60.2 ▪ Pathogenesis of chronic bronchitis and emphysema.

Administering Drugs by Inhalation

Most antiasthma drugs can be administered by inhalation. This route has three advantages: (1) therapeutic effects are enhanced by delivering drugs directly to their site of action, (2) systemic effects are minimized, and (3) relief of acute attacks is rapid. Three types of inhalation devices are usually employed: metered-dose inhalers (MDIs), dry-powder inhalers (DPIs), and nebulizers. Some pharmaceutical companies also have developed specialized inhaler devices for their products.

Metered-Dose Inhalers

MDIs are small, hand-held, pressurized devices that deliver a measured dose of drug with each actuation. Dosing is usually accomplished with 1 or 2 inhalations. When 2 inhalations are needed, an interval of at least 1 minute should separate the first inhalation from the second.

When using most MDIs, the patient must begin to inhale before activating the device. This requires hand-breath coordination, making MDIs difficult to use correctly. Accordingly, patients will need a demonstration as well as written and verbal instruction. Even with optimal use, only about 10% of the dose reaches the lungs. About 80% effects the oropharynx and is swallowed, and the remaining 10% is left in the device or exhaled.

Spacers are devices that attach directly to the MDI to increase delivery of drug to the lungs and decrease deposition of drug on the oropharyngeal mucosa (Fig. 60.3). Several

TABLE 60.1 ▪ Overview of Major Drugs for Asthma and Chronic Obstructive Pulmonary Disease

ANTIINFLAMMATORY DRUGS

Glucocorticoids

Inhaled

Beclomethasone dipropionate [QVAR]
Budesonide [Pulmicort Flexhaler, Pulmicort Respules, Pulmicort Turbuhaler 🍁]
Ciclesonide [Alvesco]
Flunisolide [Aerospan]
Fluticasone propionate [Flovent HFA, Flovent Diskus]
Mometasone furoate [Asmanex Twisthaler]

Oral

Methylprednisolone [A-Methapred, Depo-Medrol, Medrol, Medrol Dose-Pak]
Prednisolone [Flo-Pred, Orapred ODT, Millipred, Pediapred, Prelone, Hydeltra TBA 🍁]
Prednisone [Deltasone, Winpred 🍁]

Leukotriene Modifiers

Montelukast, oral [Singulair]*
Zafirlukast, oral [Accolate]*
Zileuton, oral [Zyflo, Zyflo CR]*

Cromolyn

Cromolyn, inhaled [generic]*

IgE Antagonist

Omalizumab, subcutaneous [Xolair]*

Phosphodiesterase-4 Inhibitors

Roflumilast, oral [Daliresp, Daxas 🍁]

BRONCHODILATORS

Beta$_2$-Adrenergic Agonists

Inhaled: Short Acting

Albuterol [ProAir HFA, ProAir RespiClick, Proventil HFA, Ventolin HFA, Airomir 🍁, Apo-Salvent MDI 🍁]
Levalbuterol [Xopenex, Xopenex HFA]

Inhaled: Long Acting‡

Arformoterol [Brovana]†
Formoterol [Foradil Aerolizer, Perforomist, Oxeze Turbuhaler 🍁]‡
Indacaterol [Arcapta Neohaler, Onbrez Breezhaler 🍁]†
Olodaterol [Striverdi Respimat]†
Salmeterol [Serevent Diskus]‡

Oral

Albuterol [VoSpire ER]
Terbutaline (generic only)

Methylxanthines

Aminophylline, oral [generic]
Theophylline, oral [Theo-24, Elixophyllin, Theolair 🍁, Theolair-SR, Pulmophylline, Theo ER 🍁]

Anticholinergics

Aclidinium bromide, inhaled [Tudorza Pressair]†
Glycopyrronium bromide, inhaled [Seebri Neohaler, Seebri Breezhaler 🍁]†
Ipratropium, inhaled [Atrovent HFA]
Tiotropium, inhaled [Spiriva, Spiriva HandiHaler, Spiriva Respimat]
Umeclidinium, inhaled [Incruse Ellipta]†

ANTIINFLAMMATORY/BRONCHODILATOR COMBINATIONS

Budesonide/formoterol, inhaled [Symbicort]
Fluticasone/salmeterol, inhaled [Advair Diskus, Advair HFA]
Fluticasone/vilanterol, inhaled [Breo Ellipta]
Mometasone/formoterol, inhaled [Dulera, Zenhale 🍁]

BETA AGONIST/CHOLINERGIC ANTAGONIST COMBINATIONS

Albuterol/ipratropium, inhaled [Combivent Respimat, Combivent UDV 🍁]†
Indacaterol/glycopyrronium, inhaled [Utibron Neohaler, Ultibro Breezhaler 🍁]†
Olodaterol/tiotropium, inhaled [Stiolto Respimat]†
Vilanterol/umeclidinium, inhaled [Anoro Ellipta]†

*Approved only for asthma, not for chronic obstructive pulmonary disease.
†Approved only for chronic obstructive pulmonary disease, not for asthma.
‡For treatment of asthma, must always be combined with an inhaled glucocorticoid.

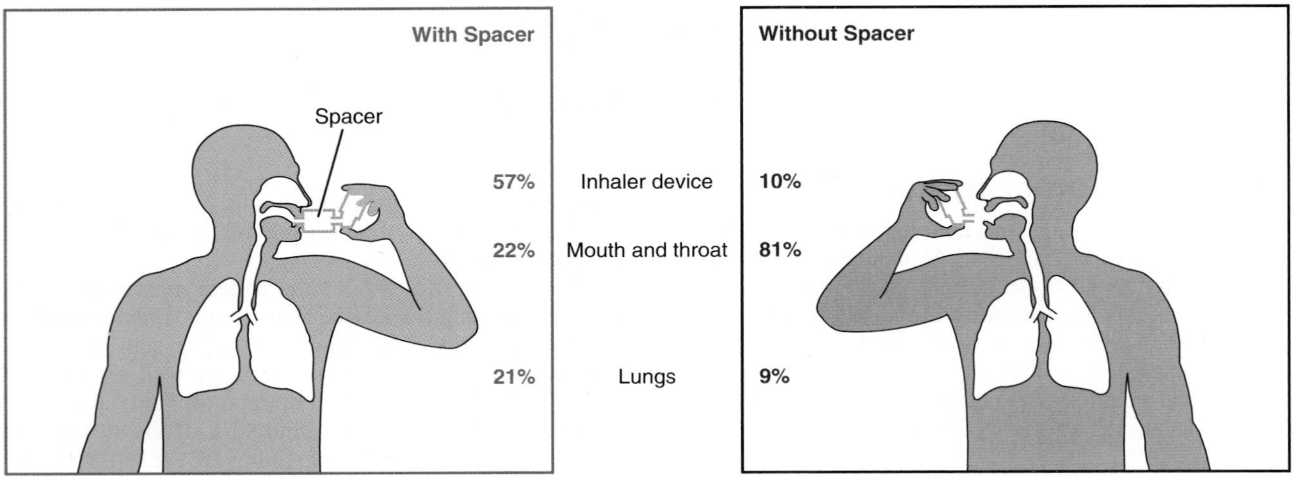

Figure 60.3 ▪ Impact of a spacer device on the distribution of inhaled medication. Note that, when a spacer is used, more medication reaches its site of action in the lungs, and less is deposited in the mouth and throat.

kinds of spacers are available for use with MDIs. Some spacers contain a one-way valve that activates on inhalation, obviating the need for good hand-breath coordination. Some spacers also contain an alarm whistle that sounds off when inhalation is too rapid, thus maximizing effective drug administration. They can also prevent bronchospasm that may occur with sudden intake of an inhaled drug.

Dry-Powder Inhalers

DPIs are used to deliver drugs in the form of a dry, micronized powder directly to the lungs. Unlike MDIs, DPIs are breath activated. As a result, DPIs don't require the hand-breath coordination needed with MDIs, and so DPIs are much easier to use. Compared with MDIs, DPIs deliver more drug to the lungs (20% of the total released vs. 10%) and less to the oropharynx. Also, spacers are not used with DPIs.

Nebulizers

A nebulizer is a small machine used to convert a drug solution into a mist. The droplets in the mist are much finer than those produced by inhalers, resulting in less drug deposit on the oropharynx and increased delivery to the lung. Inhalation of the nebulized mist can be done through a face mask or through a mouthpiece held between the teeth. Because the mist produced by a nebulizer is inhaled with each breath, hand-breath coordination is not a concern. Nebulizers take several minutes to deliver the same amount of drug contained in 1 inhalation from an inhaler, but for some patients, a nebulizer may be more effective than an inhaler. Although nebulizers are usually used at home or in a clinic or hospital, these devices, which weigh less than 10 pounds, are sufficiently portable for use in other locations.

ANTIINFLAMMATORY DRUGS

Antiinflammatory drugs—especially inhaled glucocorticoids—are the foundation of asthma and COPD therapy. These drugs are taken daily for long-term control. Most people with asthma require these drugs for management at some point.

Glucocorticoids

Glucocorticoids (e.g., budesonide, fluticasone) are the most effective drugs available for long-term control of airway inflammation. Administration is usually by inhalation, but may also be intravenous (IV) or oral. Adverse reactions to inhaled glucocorticoids are generally minor, as are reactions to systemic glucocorticoids taken *acutely.* However, when *systemic* glucocorticoids are used *long term,* severe adverse effects are likely. The basic pharmacology of the glucocorticoids is presented in Chapter 56. Discussion here is limited to their use in asthma.

Mechanism of Antiasthma Action

Glucocorticoids reduce asthma symptoms by *suppressing inflammation.* Specific antiinflammatory effects include the following:

- Decreased synthesis and release of inflammatory mediators (e.g., leukotrienes, histamine, prostaglandins)
- Decreased infiltration and activity of inflammatory cells (e.g., eosinophils, leukocytes)
- Decreased edema of the airway mucosa (secondary to a decrease in vascular permeability)

By suppressing inflammation, glucocorticoids reduce bronchial hyperreactivity and decrease airway mucus production. There is also some evidence that glucocorticoids may increase the number of bronchial beta$_2$ receptors as well as their responsiveness to beta$_2$ agonists.

Use in Asthma

Glucocorticoids are used for *prophylaxis* in managing chronic asthma; therefore, dosing must be done on a fixed schedule—not PRN. Because beneficial effects develop slowly, these drugs cannot be used to abort an ongoing attack. Glucocorticoids do not alter the natural course of asthma, even when used in young children; however, they provide significant long term control and management of symptoms.

Inhalation Use

Inhaled glucocorticoids are first-line therapy for management of the inflammatory component of asthma. Most patients with persistent asthma should use these drugs daily. Inhaled

PATIENT-CENTERED CARE ACROSS THE LIFE SPAN

Antiinflammatory Agents

Life Stage	Patient Care Concerns
Children	Inhaled glucocorticoids are the preferred long-term treatment for children of all ages, including infants. Face masks are recommended for administration of inhaled glucocorticoids to children younger than 4 years. Alternative treatments include cromolyn and leukotriene receptor antagonists (e.g., montelukast), but evidence supporting these drugs for asthma management is lower than that supporting inhaled glucocorticoids. Montelukast is the only leukotriene modifier approved for children aged 1–5 years.
Pregnant women	Inhaled glucocorticoids are classified in FDA Pregnancy Risk Category C; however, they are preferred for uncontrolled asthma in pregnant women because uncontrolled asthma is associated with greater fetal risks. Of the leukotriene modifiers, montelukast and zafirlukast are Pregnancy Risk Category B, whereas zileuton is Pregnancy Risk Category C.
Breastfeeding women	Inhaled glucocorticoids are not a contraindication to breastfeeding. Women taking systemic glucocorticoids should not breastfeed.
Older adults	Benefits exceed risk. Inhaled glucocorticoids are much safer than systemic formulations.

glucocorticoids are very effective and are much safer than systemic glucocorticoids.

Oral Use

Oral glucocorticoids may be required for patients with moderate to severe persistent asthma or for management of acute exacerbations of asthma or COPD. Because of their potential for toxicity, these drugs are prescribed only when symptoms cannot be controlled with safer medications (inhaled glucocorticoids, inhaled $beta_2$ agonists). Because the risk for toxicity increases with duration of use, treatment should be as brief as possible.

Adverse Effects

Inhaled Glucocorticoids

These preparations are largely devoid of serious toxicity, even when used in high doses. The most serious concern is adrenal suppression.

The most common adverse effects are *oropharyngeal candidiasis* and *dysphonia* (hoarseness, speaking difficulty). Both effects result from local deposition of inhaled glucocorticoids. To minimize these effects, patients should rinse the mouth with water and gargle after each administration. Using a spacer device can help too. If candidiasis develops, it can be treated with an antifungal drug.

With long-term, high-dose therapy, some *adrenal suppression* may develop, although the degree of suppression is generally low. In contrast, with prolonged use of *oral* glucocorticoids, adrenal suppression can be profound.

Glucocorticoids can *slow* growth in children and adolescents—but these drugs do *not* decrease adult height. *Short-term* studies have shown that inhaled glucocorticoids slow growth; however, *long-term* studies indicate that adult height, although delayed, is not reduced. Less is known regarding whether glucocorticoids suppress growth and development of the brain, lungs, and other organs, in part because having asthma alone can affect organ growth. Because the benefits of inhaled glucocorticoids tend to be much greater than the risks, current guidelines for asthma management recommend these drugs for children while monitoring for evidence of complications.

Long-term use of inhaled glucocorticoids may promote *bone loss*. Fortunately, the amount of loss is much lower than the amount caused by oral glucocorticoids. To minimize bone loss, patients should (1) use the lowest dose that controls symptoms, (2) ensure adequate intake of calcium and vitamin D, and (3) participate in weight-bearing exercise.

There has been concern that prolonged therapy might increase the risk for *cataracts* and *glaucoma*. Although this may be an issue of concern with continuous use of high-dose inhaled glucocorticoids, this problem is not associated with long-term use of low to medium doses of inhaled glucocorticoids.

Oral Glucocorticoids

When used acutely (less than 10 days), even in very high doses, oral glucocorticoids do not cause significant adverse effects. However, prolonged therapy, even in moderate doses, can be hazardous. Potential adverse effects include *adrenal suppression, osteoporosis, hyperglycemia, peptic ulcer disease,* and, in young patients, *growth suppression.*

Patient Education

GLUCOCORTICOIDS

Inform patients that glucocorticoids are intended for preventive therapy—not for aborting an ongoing attack. Instruct patients to administer glucocorticoids on a regular schedule—not PRN.

Instruct patients on the proper use of inhalers. Have patients demonstrate proper technique. If patients are prescribed both a SABA and a glucocorticoid, explain that delivery of glucocorticoids to the bronchial tree can be enhanced by inhaling a SABA 5 minutes before inhaling the glucocorticoid.

Teach patients with chronic asthma to monitor and record PEF, symptom frequency and symptom intensity, nighttime awakenings, effect on normal activity, and SABA use.

Advise patients to rinse their mouth and gargle after dosing to minimize dysphonia and oropharyngeal candidiasis.

Counsel patients to contact the clinic if they develop complications following a change from oral to inhaled glucocorticoids. Wearing a medical alert bracelet is advisable for patients who are at risk of adrenal insufficiency associated with long-term systemic use.

Advise patients to ensure adequate intake of calcium and vitamin D to decrease risk of bone loss. Performing weight-bearing exercise provides additional protection.

Adrenal suppression is of particular concern. As discussed in Chapter 56, prolonged glucocorticoid use can decrease the ability of the adrenal cortex to produce glucocorticoids of its own. This can be life-threatening at times of severe physiologic stress (e.g., surgery, trauma, or systemic infection). Because high levels of glucocorticoids are required to survive severe stress and because adrenal suppression prevents production of endogenous glucocorticoids, *patients must be given increased doses of oral or IV glucocorticoids at times of stress. Failure to do so can prove fatal.*

Compensating for Adrenal Insufficiency

When patients have been on prolonged systemic glucocorticoid therapy, the adrenal glands decrease their endogenous production of glucocorticoids. If systemic therapy is stopped suddenly, as when switching from oral therapy to inhalation therapy, the patient can die. Similarly, during times of severe physical stress when the body would normally produce high levels of glucocorticoids, if the dose of systemic glucocorticoids is not increased to compensate, the patient can die. What important lesson can you take from this? When discontinuing a systemic glucocorticoid, you must be sure it is done gradually to allow the body to resume producing the endogenous hormone. On the other hand, if a patient taking systemic glucocorticoids experiences severe physical stress, such as a motor vehicle crash, or is scheduled for a stressful procedure, such as surgery, you must prescribe additional glucocorticoids to supplement for the endogenous hormone that the patient cannot produce.

Adrenal suppression is also a concern when discontinuing prolonged use of oral glucocorticoids or when transferring from an oral route to an inhaled route. Several months are required for recovery of adrenocortical function, so it is important to decrease the dosage gradually. Throughout this time, all patients—including those switched to inhaled glucocorticoids—must be given supplemental oral or IV glucocorticoids at times of severe stress.

A complete list of contraindications to oral glucocorticoids is presented in the "Prescribing and Monitoring Considerations" section at the end of this chapter.

Preparations, Dosage, and Administration

Inhaled Glucocorticoids

Six glucocorticoids are available for inhalation (Table 60.2). Four are available in MDIs, three are available in DPIs, and one is available in suspension for nebulization. Inhaled glucocorticoids are administered on a regular schedule—not PRN. Pediatric and adult dosages are shown in Table 60.2. The dosage should be kept as low as possible to minimize adrenal suppression, possible bone loss, and other adverse effects.

Nebulized Budesonide

Budesonide suspension [Pulmicort Respules] is the first inhaled glucocorticoid formulated for nebulized dosing. The product is approved for maintenance therapy of persistent asthma in children 1 to 8 years old. Improvement should begin in 2 to 8 days; maximal benefits may take 4 to 6 weeks to develop. Budesonide suspension is available in 2-mL ampules containing 250 or 500 mcg of the drug. Administration is done with a jet nebulizer equipped with a mouthpiece or face mask; ultrasonic nebulizers should not be used. Administration takes 5 to 10 minutes. For children who are not taking an oral glucocorticoid, the initial dosage is 500 mcg/day in one or two doses. For children who are taking an oral glucocorticoid, the initial dosage is 1000 mcg/day in one or two doses. After 1 week, dosage of the oral glucocorticoid should be tapered off.

Oral Glucocorticoids

Methylprednisolone, prednisone, and prednisolone are preferred glucocorticoids for oral therapy of asthma. The dosage is the same regardless of the drug.

When beginning therapy with oral glucocorticoids, dosing initially focuses on bringing symptoms under control. The National Asthma Education and Prevention Program (NAEPP) guidelines recommend an initial burst of 40 to 60 mg administered daily for 3 to 10 days for adults. The initial pediatric dosage is 1 to 2 mg/kg/day for 3 to 10 days. Thereafter, the typical dose is 0.25 to 2 mg/kg daily or every other day for children younger than 12 years and 7.5 to 60 mg daily or every other day for older children and adults. For long-term treatment, alternate-day dosing is recommended to minimize adrenal suppression. After symptoms have been controlled for 3 months, dosages should be decreased gradually to establish the lowest dosage that can keep the patient free of symptoms. As discussed previously, the dosage of oral glucocorticoids must be increased during times of stress.

Leukotriene Modifiers

Leukotrienes modifiers suppress the effects of leukotrienes, which are compounds that promote smooth muscle constriction, blood vessel permeability, and inflammatory responses through direct action as well as through recruitment of eosinophils and other inflammatory cells. In patients with asthma, these drugs can decrease bronchoconstriction and inflammatory responses such as edema and mucus secretion.

Three leukotriene modifiers are currently available: zileuton, zafirlukast, and montelukast. Zileuton blocks leukotriene synthesis; zafirlukast and montelukast block leukotriene receptors. All three drugs are dosed orally. Current guidelines recommend using these agents as second-line therapy (if an inhaled glucocorticoid cannot be used) and as add-on therapy when an inhaled glucocorticoid alone is inadequate. Although generally well tolerated, all of the leukotriene modifiers can cause adverse neuropsychiatric effects, including depression, suicidal thinking, and suicidal behavior.

Zileuton

Zileuton [Zyflo, Zyflo CR], an inhibitor of leukotriene synthesis, is approved for asthma prophylaxis and maintenance therapy in adults and children 12 years and older. Symptomatic improvement can be seen within 1 to 2 hours of dosing. Because effects are not immediate, zileuton cannot be used to abort an ongoing attack. Zileuton is less effective than an inhaled glucocorticoid alone and appears to be less effective than a long-acting inhaled beta$_2$ agonist as adjunctive therapy in patients not adequately controlled with an inhaled glucocorticoid.

Mechanism of Action

Benefits derive from inhibiting 5-lipoxygenase, the enzyme that converts arachidonic acid into leukotrienes. This decreases the amount of leukotrienes available to induce inflammation.

Pharmacokinetics

Zileuton is given orally and undergoes rapid absorption, in both the presence and absence of food. Plasma levels peak 2 to 3 hours after dosing. Zileuton is rapidly metabolized by the liver, and the metabolites are excreted in the urine. Its plasma half-life is 2.5 hours.

Adverse Effects

Zileuton can injure the liver, as evidenced by increased plasma levels of alanine aminotransferase (ALT) activity. A few patients have developed symptomatic hepatitis, which reversed after drug withdrawal. To reduce the risk for serious liver injury, ALT activity should be monitored. The recommended schedule is once a month for 3 months, then every 2 to 3 months for the remainder of the first year, and periodically thereafter.

Postmarketing reports indicate that zileuton and the other leukotriene modifiers can cause adverse neuropsychiatric effects, including depression, anxiety, agitation, abnormal dreams, hallucinations, insomnia, irritability, restlessness, and suicidal thinking and behavior. If these develop, switching to a different medication should be considered.

TABLE 60.2 ▪ Inhaled Glucocorticoids: Formulations and Dosages

		Dosage	
Drug	**Formulation**	**Adults**	**Children**
Beclomethasone dipropionate [QVAR]	MDI: 40 or 80 mcg/inhalation	40–320 mcg twice daily	40–80 mcg twice daily (5–11 years)
Budesonide			
[Pulmicort Flexhaler]	DPI: 90 or 180 mcg/inhalation	360–720 mcg twice daily	180–360 mcg twice daily (6–17 years)
[Pulmicort Respules]	Suspension for nebulization	250–500 mcg once or twice daily *or* 1000 mcg once daily	500–1000 mcg/day (1–8 years)
Ciclesonide [Alvesco]	MDI: 80 or 160 mcg/inhalation	80–320 mcg twice daily	80–320 mcg twice daily (12 years and up)
Flunisolide [Aerospan]	MDI: 80 mcg/inhalation	160–320 mcg twice daily	80–320 mcg twice daily (6–11 years)
Fluticasone propionate			
[Flovent HFA]	MDI: 44, 110, or 220 mcg/inhalation	88–440 mcg twice daily	88 mcg twice daily (4–11 years)
[Flovent Diskus]	DPI: 50, 100, or 250 mcg/inhalation	100–1000 mcg twice daily	50–100 mcg twice daily (4–11 years)
Mometasone furoate [Asmanex Twisthaler]	DPI: 110 or 220 mcg/inhalation	220–440 mcg once or twice daily	110 mcg once daily (4–11 years)

DPI, dry-powder inhaler; MDI, metered-dose inhaler.

Zileuton is metabolized by cytochrome P450, where it acts as an inhibitor of CYP1A2 isoenzymes and can slow metabolism of drug substrates metabolized by this pathway, increasing their levels. Combined use with theophylline can markedly increase theophylline levels, so dosage of theophylline should be reduced. Zileuton can also increase levels of warfarin and propranolol.

Preparations, Dosage, and Administration

Zileuton is available in 600-mg immediate-release tablets, sold as Zyflo, and 600-mg extended-release tablets, sold as Zyflo CR. With the immediate-release tablets, the recommended dosage is 600 mg 4 times a day. With the extended-release tablets, the recommended dosage is two 600 mg tablets twice a day, taken within 1 hour of the morning and evening meals.

Zafirlukast

Zafirlukast [Accolate] was the first representative of a unique group of antiinflammatory agents, the leukotriene receptor antagonists. The drug is approved for maintenance therapy of chronic asthma in adults and children 5 years and older.

Mechanism of Action

Benefits derive in part from reduced infiltration of inflammatory cells, resulting in decreased bronchoconstriction.

Pharmacokinetics

Zafirlukast is administered orally, and absorption is rapid. Food reduces absorption by 40%; therefore, the drug should be administered at least 1 hour before meals or 2 hours after. Zafirlukast undergoes hepatic metabolism followed by fecal excretion. The half-life is about 10 hours but may be as long as 20 hours in older adults.

Adverse Effects

The most common side effects of zafirlukast are headache and gastrointestinal (GI) disturbances, both of which are infrequent. Arthralgia and myalgia may also occur. Like zileuton, zafirlukast can cause depression, suicidal thinking, hallucinations, and other neuropsychiatric effects. A few patients have developed Churg-Strauss syndrome, a potentially fatal disorder characterized by weight loss, flu-like symptoms, and pulmonary vasculitis (blood vessel inflammation). However, in most cases, symptoms developed when glucocorticoids were being withdrawn, suggesting that glucocorticoid withdrawal may be a contributing factor.

Rarely, patients develop clinical signs of liver injury (e.g., abdominal pain, jaundice, fatigue). If these occur, zafirlukast should be discontinued, and liver function tests (especially serum ALT) should be performed immediately. If test results are consistent with liver injury, zafirlukast should not be resumed. Curiously, signs of liver injury have developed mainly in females.

Zafirlukast inhibits several isoenzymes of cytochrome P450 and can suppress metabolism of other drugs, causing their levels to rise. Concurrent use can raise serum theophylline to toxic levels. Theophylline levels should be closely monitored, especially when zafirlukast is started or stopped. Zafirlukast can also raise levels of warfarin (an anticoagulant) and thus may cause bleeding.

Preparations, Dosage, and Administration

Zafirlukast is available in 10- and 20-mg tablets. The dosage for adults and children 12 years and older is 20 mg twice a day. The dosage for children age 5 to 11 years is 10 mg twice a day. Zafirlukast should not be administered with food.

Montelukast

Montelukast [Singulair], a leukotriene receptor blocker, is the most commonly used leukotriene modulator. The drug has three approved indications: (1) prophylaxis and maintenance therapy of asthma in patients at least 1 year old; (2) prevention of exercise-induced bronchospasm (EIB) in patients at least 15 years old; and (3) relief of allergic rhinitis (see Chapter 61). Montelukast cannot be used for quick relief of an asthma attack because effects develop too slowly. For prophylaxis and maintenance therapy of asthma, maximal effects develop within 24 hours of the first dose and are maintained with once-daily dosing in the evening. In clinical trials, montelukast decreased asthma-related nocturnal awakening, improved morning lung function, and decreased the need for a short-acting inhaled beta$_2$ agonist throughout the day. Although montelukast is approved for preventing EIB, a short-acting beta$_2$ agonist is preferred.

Mechanism of Action

Montelukast has a high affinity for leukotriene receptors in the airway and on proinflammatory cells such as eosinophils. By occupying these receptors, the drug blocks receptor activation by the body's leukotrienes.

Pharmacokinetics

Montelukast is rapidly absorbed after oral administration. Bioavailability is about 64%. Blood levels peak 3 to 4 hours after ingestion. The drug is highly bound (more than 99%) to plasma proteins. Montelukast undergoes extensive metabolism by hepatic cytochrome P450 enzymes followed by excretion in the bile. The plasma half-life ranges from 2.7 to 5.5 hours.

Adverse Effects

Montelukast is generally well tolerated. In clinical trials, adverse effects were equivalent to those of placebo. In contrast to zileuton and zafirlukast, montelukast does not seem to cause liver injury. As with zafirlukast, Churg-Strauss syndrome has occurred when glucocorticoid dosage was reduced. Postmarketing reports suggest a link between montelukast and neuropsychiatric effects, especially mood changes and suicidality. Fortunately, these effects are rare.

Montelukast appears devoid of serious drug interactions. Unlike zileuton and zafirlukast, it does not increase levels of theophylline or warfarin. Concurrent use of phenytoin (an anticonvulsant that induces P450 isoenzymes) can decrease levels of montelukast.

Preparations, Dosage, and Administration

Montelukast is available in three formulations: standard tablets (10 mg), chewable tablets (4 and 5 mg), and oral granules (4 mg/packet). The oral granules may be put directly in the mouth or may be mixed with one spoonful of either applesauce, carrots, rice, or ice cream. For prophylaxis or chronic treatment of asthma, dosing is done once a day in the evening, with or without food. Dosage is based on patient age as follows:

- Age 15 years and older—one 10-mg tablet daily
- Age 6 to 14 years—one 5-mg chewable tablet daily
- Age 2 to 5 years—one 4-mg chewable tablet *or* 4 mg of oral granules daily
- Age 12 to 23 months—4 mg of oral granules daily

To prevent EIB, patients should take one 10-mg tablet at least 2 hours before exercising. No additional dose should be taken for at least 24 hours. Patients already taking montelukast daily should not take any more to prevent EIB.

Cromolyn

Cromolyn is an inhalational agent that suppresses bronchial inflammation. The drug is used for prophylaxis—not quick relief—in patients with mild to moderate asthma. Antiinflammatory effects are less than with glucocorticoids; therefore, cromolyn is not a preferred drug for asthma therapy. When glucocorticoids create problems, however, cromolyn may be prescribed as alternative therapy.

Mechanism of Action

Cromolyn suppresses inflammation; it does not cause bronchodilation. The drug acts in part by stabilizing the cytoplasmic membrane of mast cells, preventing release of histamine and other mediators. In addition, cromolyn inhibits eosinophils, macrophages, and other inflammatory cells.

Pharmacokinetics

Cromolyn is administered by nebulizer. The fraction absorbed from the lungs is small and rarely produces significant systemic effects. Absorbed cromolyn is excreted unchanged in the urine.

Therapeutic Uses

Chronic Asthma

Cromolyn is an alternative to inhaled glucocorticoids for prophylactic therapy of mild persistent asthma. When administered on a fixed schedule, cromolyn reduces both the frequency and intensity of asthma attacks. Maximal effects may take several weeks to develop. No tolerance to effects is seen with long-term use. Cromolyn is especially effective for prophylaxis of seasonal allergic attacks and for acute allergy prophylaxis immediately before allergen exposure (e.g., before mowing the lawn).

Exercise-Induced Bronchospasm

Cromolyn can prevent bronchospasm in patients at risk for EIB. For best results, cromolyn should be administered 10 to 15 minutes before anticipated exertion but no longer than 1 hour before exercise.

> **Patient Education**
>
> **CROMOLYN**
>
> Instruct patients on the proper use and care of nebulizers.
>
> For acute prophylaxis, instruct patients to administer cromolyn 15 minutes before exercise and exposure to other precipitating factors (e.g., cold, environmental agents).
>
> For long term use, instruct patients to administer cromolyn on a regular schedule. Be sure to inform them that full therapeutic effects may take several weeks to develop.
>
> Teach patients with chronic asthma to monitor and record PEF, symptom frequency and symptom intensity, nighttime awakenings, effect on normal activity, and SABA use.

Allergic Rhinitis

Intranasal cromolyn [NasalCrom] can relieve symptoms of allergic rhinitis (see Chapter 61).

Adverse Effects

Cromolyn is the safest of all antiasthma medications. Significant adverse effects occur in fewer than 1 of every 10,000 patients. Occasionally, cough or bronchospasm occurs in response to cromolyn inhalation.

Preparations, Dosage, and Administration

Cromolyn is administered using a power-driven nebulizer. The initial dosage for adults and children is 20 mg 4 times a day. For maintenance therapy, the lowest effective dosage should be established.

Omalizumab

Omalizumab [Xolair] is a monoclonal antibody with a unique mechanism of action: antagonism of IgE, a type of antibody. The drug is a second-line agent indicated only for allergy-related asthma and only when preferred options have failed. Omalizumab offers modest benefits and has significant drawbacks: the drug poses a risk for anaphylaxis and cancer, must be given subcutaneously, and costs more than $10,000 a year. Furthermore, its long-term safety is unknown.

Mechanism of Action

Omalizumab forms complexes with free IgE in the blood and thereby reduces the amount of IgE available to bind with its receptors on mast cells. This greatly reduces the number of IgE molecules on the mast cell surface and thus limits the ability of allergens to trigger release of histamine, leukotrienes, and other mediators that promote bronchospasm and airway inflammation. At recommended doses, omalizumab decreases free IgE in serum by 96%. When treatment stops, about 1 year is required for free IgE to return to its pretreatment level.

Therapeutic Use

Omalizumab is approved only for patients age 12 years and older with moderate to severe asthma that (1) is allergy related and that (2) cannot be controlled with an inhaled glucocorticoid. In clinical trials, the drug produced a modest decrease in the number of exacerbations and often permitted a reduction in glucocorticoid use. Because of its mechanism of action, omalizumab can only help patients whose asthma is caused by a specific allergen (e.g., pet dander, dust mite feces). Accordingly, a skin test or blood test proving allergen reactivity is required. Unless instructed otherwise, patients should continue all asthma medications they were using before starting omalizumab.

Pharmacokinetics

Omalizumab is administered by subcutaneous (subQ) injection, and absorption is slow, producing peak plasma levels in 7 to 8 days. Degradation occurs in the liver. The drug's half-life is prolonged, about 26 days.

Adverse Effects

Omalizumab can cause a variety of adverse effects. The most common are injection-site reactions, viral infection, upper respiratory infection, sinusitis, headache, and pharyngitis. Early clinical trials suggested a very small risk for cardiovascular problems and malignancy. A meta-analysis of postmarketing studies revealed no significant increase in cardiovascular events between subjects taking omalizumab and a placebo. There was a small increase in rare malignancy occurrence in subjects taking omalizumab; however, a clear relationship to the drug has not been established. Possible adverse consequences of long-term IgE suppression are unknown.

Life-threatening anaphylaxis—characterized by urticaria and edema of the throat and/or tongue—has occurred rarely (in less than 0.1% of patients). Anaphylaxis is most likely with the first dose but can also occur after receiving repeated doses with no apparent sensitivity. To minimize injury from anaphylaxis, patients should be observed for 2 hours after the first three doses and for 30 minutes after all subsequent doses. Facilities for managing anaphylaxis should be immediately available. Patients who experience a severe reaction should not be given omalizumab again.

> **BLACK BOX WARNING: OMALIZUMAB (XOLAIR)**
>
> Omalizumab carries a risk for anaphylaxis that may occur at any time during the course of treatment. Patients should be notified of signs or symptoms that necessitate seeking medical care. Patients should be routinely monitored after administration in health care settings.

Preparations, Dosage, and Administration

Omalizumab [Xolair] is available as a powder (202.5 mg) in single-use vials for reconstitution with 1.4 mL of sterile water. Dissolving the powder, which can take 20 minutes or longer, yields a final solution of 150 mg/1.2 mL. Administration is by subQ injection, which may take 5 to 10 seconds because the solution is somewhat viscous. The reconstituted solution should be used within 4 hours (if stored at room temperature) or within 8 hours (if stored cold). Omalizumab powder should be kept refrigerated.

The size of each dose and the dosing interval are determined by body weight and total serum IgE, measured at baseline. Dosages range from 150 to 300 mg every 4 weeks, to 225 to 375 mg every 2 weeks. No more than 150 mg should be injected at any site. If a dose exceeds 150 mg, it should be divided among two or more sites.

BRONCHODILATORS

Bronchodilators provide symptomatic relief in patients with asthma and COPD, but do not alter the underlying inflammation that is part of the disease process. This is why most patients who require a bronchodilator also use an inhaled glucocorticoid for long-term suppression of inflammation. Monotherapy with a bronchodilator is appropriate only when asthma is very mild and attacks are infrequent.

Beta$_2$-Adrenergic Agonists

Inhaled beta$_2$ agonists are the most effective drugs available for relieving acute bronchospasm and preventing EIB. Virtually all patients with asthma use these first-line drugs as a component of an asthma management regimen. The basic pharmacology of the beta$_2$ agonists is presented in Chapter 13. Discussion here is limited to their use in asthma.

Mechanism of Action

The beta$_2$ agonists are sympathomimetic drugs that activate beta$_2$-adrenergic receptors. By activating beta$_2$ receptors in smooth muscle of the lung, these drugs promote *bronchodilation* and thus relieve bronchospasm. In addition, beta$_2$ agonists

PATIENT-CENTERED CARE ACROSS THE LIFE SPAN

Bronchodilators

Life Stage	Patient Care Concerns
Children	Although they may be used for younger children, SABAs are approved for children 2 years and older. Special delivery devices such as nebulizers may be used for very young children. Safety and efficacy of anticholinergics has not been established for children younger than 11 years. Methylxanthines are approved for children of all ages, including neonates. It is important to consider variable drug clearance across age ranges when dosing.
Pregnant women	$Beta_2$ agonists are classified in FDA Pregnancy Risk Category C owing to uterine relaxation; however, NAEPP guidelines note that benefits are greater than risks. Pregnant women must have adequate respiratory exchange to ensure adequate oxygenation of the developing fetus. Anticholinergics are classified in FDA Pregnancy Risk Category B. Methylxanthines are Pregnancy Risk Category C.
Breastfeeding women	Breastfeeding is not contraindicated with $beta_2$ agonists or anticholinergics; however, manufacturers of both drugs recommend caution. Labeling for methylxanthines warns against breastfeeding only if the mother may have toxic levels.
Older adults	Benefits exceed risks for beta agonists and anticholinergics. Systemic anticholinergics are included in Beers Criteria for Potentially Inappropriate Use in Older Adults; they should not be substituted for inhaled anticholinergics. Older patients are at much higher risk for toxicity when taking methylxanthines.

have a limited role in suppressing histamine release in the lung and increasing ciliary motility.

Classification by Route and Time Course

$Beta_2$ agonists may be administered orally or by inhalation, and their effects may be brief or prolonged. All of the oral agents are long acting. Among the inhaled agents, some are short acting and some are long acting. With the short-acting inhaled preparations, effects begin almost immediately, peak in 30 to 60 minutes, and persist for 3 to 5 hours. Because of this time course, the short-acting $beta_2$ agonists (SABAs) can be used to abort an ongoing attack, but cannot be used for prolonged prophylaxis. With the inhaled long-acting $beta_2$ agonists (LABAs), onset depends on the drug: with formoterol and arformoterol, onset is relatively rapid; whereas with salmeterol, onset is delayed. However, because these drugs are used on a fixed schedule for long-term control, the difference in onset is not very important.

Use in Asthma and Chronic Obstructive Pulmonary Disease

$Beta_2$ agonists are employed for quick relief and long-term control. Drug selection depends on the goal.

Inhaled Short-Acting $Beta_2$ Agonists

SABAs are taken PRN to abort an ongoing attack. In patients with EIB, they are taken before exercise to prevent an attack from occurring. For hospitalized patients undergoing a severe acute attack, a nebulized SABA is the traditional treatment of choice. However, delivery with an MDI in the outpatient setting may be equally effective.

Long-Acting Inhaled $Beta_2$ Agonists

Patients who experience frequent attacks may be prescribed a LABA for long-term control. Dosing is done on a fixed schedule, not PRN. LABAs are preferred over SABAs for patients with stable COPD. In patients with asthma, however, LABAs are not first-line therapy, and they must always be *combined with a glucocorticoid.* In fact, their use *alone* in asthma is *contraindicated* because LABA monotherapy has been associated with increased incidence of asthma-associated death.[a] For combined LABA-glucocorticoid therapy, the U.S. Food and Drug Administration (FDA) recommends using a product that contains both drugs in the same inhaler.

BLACK BOX WARNING: LONG-ACTING $BETA_2$-ADRENERGIC AGONISTS

All LABAs carry a risk for asthma-related deaths. To attenuate this risk, the use of LABAs as monotherapy is contraindicated. LABAs should only be prescribed as a component of long-term therapy with medications such as inhaled glucocorticoids.

Oral $Beta_2$ Agonists

These drugs are used only for long-term control. Onset is too slow to abort an ongoing attack. Like the long-acting inhaled $beta_2$ agonists, the oral agents are not first-line therapy.

Adverse Effects

Inhaled Preparations: Short Acting

Inhaled SABAs are well tolerated. Systemic effects—tachycardia, angina, and tremor—can occur, but are usually minimal.

Inhaled Preparations: Long Acting

Inhaled LABAs may increase the risk for severe asthma and asthma-related death when used as monotherapy for long-term control. To minimize risk, LABAs should be used only in patients taking a recommended medication for long-term control, and only if that medication has been inadequate by itself. LABAs should never be used as first-line therapy for prolonged control and should never be used alone.

[a]Although using a LABA alone is contraindicated for patients with asthma, LABAs can still be used alone in patients with COPD.

Oral Preparations

The selectivity of the $beta_2$-adrenergic agonists is only relative, not absolute. Accordingly, when these drugs are administered orally, they are likely to produce some activation of $beta_1$ receptors in the heart. If dosage is excessive, stimulation of cardiac $beta_1$ receptors can cause *angina pectoris* and *tachydysrhythmias*. Patients should be instructed to report chest pain or changes in heart rate or rhythm.

Oral $beta_2$ agonists often cause *tremor* by activating $beta_2$ receptors in skeletal muscle. Tremor can be reduced by lowering the dosage. With continued drug use, tremor declines spontaneously.

Patient Education

$BETA_2$ ADRENERGIC AGONISTS

Instruct patients on the proper use of this inhalers. Have patients demonstrate proper technique.

For patients who have difficulty with hand-breath coordination, using a spacer with a one-way valve may improve results.

Advise patients with asthma to assess PEF daily and compare with personal best. Counsel patients to keep a record of these assessments along with symptom frequency and symptom intensity, nighttime awakenings, effect on normal activity, and SABA use.

Inform patients who are using MDIs or DPIs that, when 2 inhalations are needed, an interval of at least 1 minute should elapse between inhalations.

Instruct patients to report chest pain associated with changes in heart rate or rhythm. This could indicate cardiac stress secondary to adrenergic effects.

Warn patients against exceeding recommended dosages. If worsening symptoms require more frequent use of an SABA, the provider should be notified.

Inform patients that inhaled LABAs (formoterol, arformoterol, and salmeterol) should be taken on a fixed schedule—not PRN—and always in combination with an inhaled glucocorticoid.

Instruct patients to take oral $beta_2$ agonists on a fixed schedule—not PRN. Sustained-release preparations should be swallowed intact, without crushing or chewing.

Preparations, Dosage, and Administration

Nine selective $beta_2$ agonists are available (Table 60.3). Some are used for quick relief and some for long-term control.

Inhaled Preparations for Quick Relief

To provide quick relief, $beta_2$ agonists must be administered by inhalation. Three types of devices may be used: MDIs, DPIs, and nebulizers.

For drugs administered with an MDI or DPI, the initial dosing schedule is 1 or 2 inhalations 3 or 4 times a day. Additional drugs are added to the asthma management regimen (Table 60.4) with a goal of decreasing reliance on a SABA to no more than twice a week.

When 2 inhalations are needed, an interval of 1 minute or longer should separate them. During this interval, some bronchodilation develops, facilitating penetration of the second inhalation.

For certain patients, nebulizers may be superior to inhalers. Some patients who have become unresponsive to a $beta_2$ agonist delivered with an inhaler may respond to the same drug when it is given with a nebulizer. The nebulizer delivers the dose slowly (over several minutes); as the bronchi gradually dilate, the drug gains deeper and deeper access to the lungs.

Inhaled Preparations for Long-Term Control

Three single-agent inhaled LABAs are approved for treatment of asthma: salmeterol [Serevent Diskus], formoterol [Foradil Aerolizer], and arformoterol [Brovana], the *(R,R)*-enantiomer of formoterol. Vilanterol, another LABA, is available only in combination with a glucocorticoid (fluticasone/vilanterol [Breo Ellipta] and umeclidinium/vilanterol [Anoro Ellipta]). LABAs have a long duration of action and thus are suited for long-term control. Dosing is every 12 hours. If supplemental bronchodilation is needed between doses, a SABA should be used. As discussed previously, LABAs are not first-choice agents for long-term control, and they should not be used alone. Rather, they should always be combined with an inhaled glucocorticoid, preferably in the same inhaler device.

Although salmeterol is usually inhaled twice daily (every 12 hours), with continuous use, more frequent dosing may be needed because benefits seem to persist for a shorter time as the duration of treatment increases.

Oral Preparations for Long-Term Control

Two oral $beta_2$ agonists—albuterol and terbutaline—are approved for long-term control of asthma. Dosing is 3 or 4 times a day. (In Canada, terbutaline is also available in an inhaled form as Bricanyl Turbuhaler offering 500 mcg/actuation for PRN dosing.)

Methylxanthines

We first encountered the methylxanthines (theophylline, caffeine, others) in Chapter 29. As discussed there, the most prominent actions of these drugs are (1) central nervous system (CNS) excitation and (2) bronchodilation. Other actions include cardiac stimulation, vasodilation, and diuresis.

Theophylline

Theophylline [Theo-24, Theochron, Elixophyllin, Theolair ♣, Uniphyl ♣] is the principal methylxanthine employed in asthma. Benefits derive primarily from bronchodilation. Theophylline has a narrow therapeutic range, so dosage must be carefully controlled. The drug is usually administered by mouth but may also be administered intravenously.

Mechanism of Action

Theophylline produces bronchodilation by relaxing smooth muscle of the bronchi. Although the mechanism of bronchodilation has not been firmly established, the most probable is blockade of receptors for adenosine.

Use in Asthma and Chronic Obstructive Pulmonary Disease

Oral theophylline is used for maintenance therapy of chronic stable asthma. Although less effective than $beta_2$ agonists, theophylline has a longer duration of action (when administered in a sustained-release formulation). With regular use, theophylline can decrease the frequency and severity of asthma attacks. Because its effects are prolonged, theophylline may be most appropriate for patients who experience nocturnal attacks.

Once standard therapy in management of COPD, theophylline is no longer recommended. Evidence-based guidelines recommend its use only if $beta_2$ agonists and anticholinergics are not available or if the patient cannot afford long-term therapy with other drugs.

Intravenous theophylline has been employed in emergencies. However, the drug is no more effective than $beta_2$ agonists and glucocorticoids and is clearly more dangerous.

TABLE 60.3 ▪ Beta$_2$-Adrenergic Agonists

Drug [Trade Name]	Formulation	Initial Dosage: Adults	Initial Dosage: Children
INHALED AGENTS: SHORT ACTING			
Albuterol			
[ProAir HFA, ProAir RespiClick, Proventil HFA, Ventolin HFA]	MDI (90 mcg/inhalation)	2 inhalations every 4–6 hours PRN	2 inhalations every 4–6 hours PRN
[Proventil]	Solution for nebulization	1.25–5 mg every 4–8 hours PRN	0.63–2.5 mg/kg every 4–6 hours PRN
Levalbuterol			
[Xopenex HFA]	MDI (45 mcg/inhalation)	2 inhalations every 4–6 hours PRN	2 inhalations every 4–6 hours PRN
[Xopenex]	Solution for nebulization	0.63 mg every 6–8 hours PRN	0.31–1.25 mg every 4–6 hours PRN
INHALED AGENTS: LONG ACTING†			
Aclidinium bromide‡ [Tudorza Pressair]	DPI (400 mcg/inhalation)	1 inhalation every 12 hours	Safety and efficacy not established
Arformoterol‡ [Brovana]	Solution for nebulization	15 mcg every 12 hours	Safety and efficacy not established
Formoterol			
[Foradil Aerolizer]†	DPI (12 mcg/inhalation)	1 inhalation every 12 hours	1 inhalation every 12 hours
[Perforomist]‡	Solution for nebulization	20 mcg every 12 hours	Safety and efficacy not established
Indacaterol‡ [Arcapta Neohaler]	DPI (75 mcg/inhalation)	1 inhalation every 24 hours	N/A
Olodaterol [Striverdi Respimat]‡	Respimat: 2.5 mcg/ inhalation	2 inhalations once daily	Safety and efficacy not established
Salmeterol† [Serevent Diskus]	DPI (50 mcg/inhalation)	1 inhalation every 12 hours	1 inhalation every 12 hours
ORAL AGENTS			
Albuterol			
Generic	Tablets, syrup	2 or 4 mg 3–4 times/day	2 mg 3–4 times/day
[VoSpire ER]	Tablets (extended release)	8 mg every 12 hours	4 mg every 12 hours
Terbutaline (generic only)	Tablets	5 mg 3 times/day	2.5 mg 3 times/day

†When used to treat asthma, must always be combined with an inhaled glucocorticoid.
‡Approved only for chronic obstructive pulmonary disease, not asthma.
DPI, dry-powder inhaler; HFA, hydrofluoroalkane propellant; MDI, metered-dose inhaler.

TABLE 60.4 ▪ Classification of Asthma Severity and Recommended Step for Initial Treatment

	Intermittent Asthma	Persistent Asthma: Mild	Persistent Asthma: Moderate	Persistent Asthma: Severe
CURRENT IMPAIRMENT				
Symptoms	≤2 days/week	>2 days/week, but not daily	Daily	Throughout the day
Nighttime awakenings	≤2 times/month	3–4 times/month	>Once a week, but not nightly	Often 7 times/week
SABA used to control symptoms (but not to prevent EIB)	≤2 days/week	>2 days/week, but not daily, and not more than once on any day	Daily	Several times a day
Effect on normal activity	None	Minor limitation	Some limitation	Severe limitation
Lung function tests	• Normal FEV_1 between exacerbations • FEV_1 >80% of predicted • FEV_1/FVC normal*	• FEV_1 >80% of predicted • FEV_1/FVC normal*	• FEV_1 >60% but <80% of predicted • FEV_1/FVC reduced 5%*	• FEV_1 <60% of predicted • FEV_1/FVC reduced >5%*
FUTURE RISK				
Exacerbations requiring oral glucocorticoids	0–1/year	≥2/year	≥2/year	≥2/year
Recommended step for initial treatment†	Step 1	Step 2	Step 3	Step 4 or 5

*Normal values for FEV_1/FVC by age group: 8–19 years, 85%; 20–39 years, 80%; 40–59 years, 75%; 60–80 years, 70%.
†See Table 60.6 and text for drugs used at each step.
EIB, exercise-induced bronchospasm; FEV_1, forced expiratory volume in 1 second; FVC, forced vital capacity; SABA, short-acting beta$_2$ agonist.

Pharmacokinetics

Absorption. Oral theophylline is available in sustained-release formulations and as an elixir. Absorption from sustained-release preparations is slow, but the resulting plasma levels are stable, being free of the wide fluctuations associated with the immediate-release products. Absorption from some sustained-release preparations can be affected by food.

Metabolism. Theophylline is metabolized in the liver. Rates of metabolism are affected by multiple factors—age, disease, drugs—and show wide individual variation. As a result, the plasma half-life of theophylline varies considerably among patients. For example, although the average half-life in nonsmoking adults is about 8 hours, the half-life can be as short as 2 hours in some adults and as long as 15 hours in others. Smoking either tobacco or marijuana accelerates metabolism and decreases the half-life. The average half-life in children is 4 hours. Metabolism is slowed in patients with certain pathologies (e.g., heart disease, liver disease, prolonged fever). Some drugs (e.g., cimetidine, fluoroquinolone antibiotics) decrease theophylline metabolism. Other drugs (e.g., phenobarbital) accelerate metabolism. Because of these variations in metabolism, dosage must be individualized.

Drug Levels. Safe and effective therapy requires periodic measurement of theophylline blood levels. Traditionally, dosage has been adjusted to produce theophylline levels between 10 and 20 mcg/mL. However, many patients respond well at 5 mcg/mL, and, as a rule, there is little benefit to increasing levels above 15 mcg/mL. Therefore levels between 5 and 15 mcg/mL are appropriate for most patients. At levels above 20 mcg/mL, the risk for significant adverse effects is high.

Patient Education

THEOPHYLLINE

Warn patients that, if a dose is missed, the following dose should not be doubled.

Instruct patients to swallow enteric-coated and sustained-release formulations intact, without crushing or chewing.

Warn patients against consuming caffeine-containing beverages (e.g., coffee, many soft drinks) and other sources of caffeine. Explain that caffeine can intensify adverse effects while decreasing theophylline breakdown.

Instruct patients to call the clinic if they start to develop symptoms of nausea, vomiting, abdominal discomfort, diarrhea, insomnia, restlessness, or palpitations as these may signify theophylline toxicity.

Warn patients that smoking tobacco or marijuana can increase theophylline clearance resulting in ineffective dosing.

Toxicity

Symptoms. Toxicity is related to theophylline levels. Adverse effects are uncommon at plasma levels below 20 mcg/mL. At 20 to 25 mcg/mL, relatively mild reactions occur (e.g., nausea, vomiting, diarrhea, insomnia, restlessness). Serious adverse effects are most likely at levels above 30 mcg/mL. These reactions include severe dysrhythmias (e.g., ventricular fibrillation) and convulsions that can be highly resistant to treatment. Death may result from cardiorespiratory collapse.

Treatment. At the first indication of toxicity, dosing with theophylline should stop. Absorption can be decreased by administering activated charcoal together with a cathartic. Ventricular dysrhythmias respond to lidocaine. Intravenous diazepam may help control seizures.

Drug Interactions

Caffeine. Caffeine is a methylxanthine with pharmacologic properties like those of theophylline (see Chapter 29). Accordingly, caffeine can intensify the adverse effects of theophylline on the CNS and heart. In addition, caffeine can compete with theophylline for drug-metabolizing enzymes, causing theophylline levels to rise. Because of these interactions, individuals taking theophylline should avoid caffeine-containing beverages (e.g., coffee, many soft drinks) and other sources of caffeine.

Tobacco and Marijuana Smoke. Smoking tobacco or marijuana can induce theophylline metabolism, resulting in increased drug clearance of up to 50% in adults and 80% in older adults. (Secondhand smoke can result in similarly decreased drug levels.) Consequently, if a smoking patient stops smoking but the dose of theophylline is not decreased, the patient is at risk for theophylline toxicity over time.

Drugs That Reduce Theophylline Levels. Several agents—including phenobarbital, phenytoin, and rifampin—can lower theophylline levels by inducing hepatic drug-metabolizing enzymes. Concurrent use of these agents may necessitate an increase in theophylline dosage.

Drugs That Increase Theophylline Levels. Several drugs—including cimetidine and the fluoroquinolone antibiotics (e.g., ciprofloxacin)—can elevate plasma levels of theophylline, primarily by inhibiting hepatic metabolism. To avoid theophylline toxicity, the dosage of theophylline should be reduced when the drug is combined with these agents.

Formulations

Theophylline is available for IV and oral use. For IV use, generic solutions are available in concentrations of 400 mg/250 mL, 400 mg/500 mL, or 800 mg/500 mL of solution.

For oral use, the following concentrations are available:

- Elixophyllin oral elixir: 80 mg/15 mL
- Generic oral solution: 80 mg/15 mL
- Theochron 12-hour extended-release tablets: 100 mg, 200 mg, and 300 mg
- Generic 12-hour extended-release tablets: 100 mg, 200 mg, 300 mg, and 450 mg
- Theo-24 24-hour extended-release capsule: 100 mg, 200 mg, 300 mg, and 400 mg
- Generic 24-hour extended release tablets: 400 mg and 600 mg

Unlike the elixir and oral solution, the sustained-release tablets and capsules produce drug levels that are relatively stable. Accordingly, the sustained-release formulations are preferred for routine therapy.

Dosage and Administration

Oral. Dosage must be individualized. To minimize chances of toxicity, doses should be low initially and then gradually increased. If a dose is missed, the following dose should not be doubled because doing so could produce toxicity. Smokers require higher than average doses. Conversely, patients with heart disease, liver dysfunction, or prolonged fever are likely to require lower doses. Patients should be instructed not to chew the sustained-release tablets or capsules. Product information should be consulted for compatibility with food.

The initial dosage is based on the age and weight of the patient and on the presence or absence of factors that can impair theophylline elimination. Specific initial dosages are described in the prescribing information in the package insert. As noted previously, maintenance doses should be adjusted to produce drug levels in the therapeutic range—typically 5 to 15 mcg/mL.

Intravenous. Intravenous theophylline is reserved for emergencies. Administration must be done slowly because rapid injection can cause fatal cardiovascular reactions. Intravenous theophylline is incompatible with many other drugs. Accordingly, compatibility should be verified before mixing theophylline with other IV agents. For specific IV dosages, refer to the discussion of aminophylline below.

Other Methylxanthines

Aminophylline

Aminophylline is a theophylline salt that is considerably more soluble than theophylline itself. In solution, each molecule of aminophylline dissociates to yield two molecules of theophylline. Hence, the pharmacologic properties of aminophylline and theophylline are identical. Aminophylline is available in formulations for oral and IV dosing. Intravenous administration is employed most often.

Administration and Dosage

Intravenous. Because of its relatively high solubility, aminophylline is the preferred form of theophylline for IV use. Infusions should be done slowly (no faster than 25 mg/min) because rapid injection can produce severe hypotension and death. The usual loading dose is 5.7 mg/kg. The maintenance infusion rate should be adjusted to provide plasma levels of theophylline that are within the therapeutic range (10–20 mcg/mL). Aminophylline solutions are incompatible with a number of other drugs. Therefore compatibility must be verified before mixing aminophylline with other IV agents.

Oral. Aminophylline is available in 100- and 200-mg tablets. Dosing guidelines are the same as for theophylline.

Anticholinergic Drugs

Anticholinergic drugs improve lung function by blocking muscarinic receptors in the bronchi, reducing bronchoconstriction. Two agents are available:

ipratropium and tiotropium. These drugs are approved only for COPD but are used off-label for asthma. Both drugs are administered by inhalation. The principal difference between the two is pharmacokinetic: tiotropium has a much longer duration of action and thus can be dosed less often. With both drugs, systemic effects are minimal.

Ipratropium

Actions and Therapeutic Use

Ipratropium [Atrovent HFA] is an atropine derivative administered by inhalation to relieve bronchospasm. The drug has FDA approval only for bronchospasm associated with COPD but is often used off-label for asthma and is included in current evidence-based guidelines from the NAEPP for asthma management. Like atropine, ipratropium is a muscarinic antagonist. By blocking muscarinic cholinergic receptors in the bronchi, ipratropium prevents bronchoconstriction. Therapeutic effects begin within 30 seconds, reach 50% of their maximum in 3 minutes, and persist about 6 hours. Ipratropium is effective against allergen-induced asthma and EIB, but is less effective than the beta$_2$ agonists. However, because ipratropium and the beta$_2$-adrenergic agonists promote bronchodilation by different mechanisms, their beneficial effects are additive.

Adverse Effects

Systemic effects are minimal because ipratropium is a quaternary ammonium compound and therefore always carries a positive charge. As a result, the drug is not readily absorbed from the lungs or from the digestive tract. The most common adverse reactions are dry mouth and irritation of the pharynx. If systemic absorption is sufficient, the drug may raise intraocular pressure in patients with glaucoma. Adverse cardiovascular events (heart attack, stroke, death) have occurred in people taking ipratropium; however, because absorption is minimal, it seems unlikely that ipratropium is the cause.

Preparations, Dosage, and Administration

Ipratropium [Atrovent HFA] is supplied (1) in solution (500 mcg/vial) and (2) in MDIs that deliver 17 mcg per actuation. For patients using an MDI, the usual dosage is 2 inhalations 4 times a day, and the maximal dosage is 12 inhalations in 24 hours. For patients using the solution, the usual dosage is 500 mcg 3 or 4 times a day, administered by a nebulizer.

Tiotropium

Actions and Therapeutic Use

Tiotropium [Spiriva] is a long-acting, inhaled anticholinergic agent approved for maintenance therapy of bronchospasm associated with COPD. The drug is not approved for asthma but has been used off-label for patients who have not responded to other medications. Like ipratropium, tiotropium relieves bronchospasm by blocking muscarinic receptors in the lungs. Therapeutic effects begin about 30 minutes after inhalation, peak in 3 hours, and persist about 24 hours. With subsequent doses, bronchodilation gets better and better, reaching a plateau after eight consecutive doses (8 days). Compared with ipratropium, tiotropium is more effective, and its dosing schedule is more convenient (once daily vs. 4 times daily). Tiotropium is indicated only for long-term maintenance. For rapid relief of ongoing bronchospasm, patients should inhale a SABA.

Adverse Effects

The most common adverse effect is dry mouth, which develops in 16% of patients. Fortunately, this response is generally mild and diminishes over time. Patients can suck on sugarless candy for relief.

Systemic anticholinergic effects (e.g., constipation, urinary retention, tachycardia, blurred vision) are minimal. Like ipratropium, tiotropium is a quaternary ammonium compound, and thus absorption into the systemic circulation is very limited. Like ipratropium, tiotropium has been associated with adverse cardiovascular events; however, because absorption is low, tiotropium is unlikely to be the cause.

Preparations, Dosage, and Administration

Tiotropium [Spiriva] is supplied both as a Respimat inhaler and in 18-mcg capsules along with a HandiHaler DPI device. Dosage for the Respimat inhaler is two inhalations one daily. Dosage for the HandiHaler DPI is 18 mcg once daily. Administration is by inhalation only. The capsules should not be swallowed.

Aclidinium

Actions and Therapeutic Use

Aclidinium [Tudorza Pressair], which received FDA approval in 2012, is indicated for management of bronchospasm associated with COPD. It relieves bronchospasm by blocking muscarinic receptors in the lung. Peak levels have occurred within 10 minutes of drug delivery; however, it is intended only for maintenance therapy and not for acute symptom relief.

Adverse Effects

The most common adverse reactions reported in clinical trials were headache, nasopharyngitis, and cough. As with any anticholinergic, there is a theoretical risk for worsening narrow-angle glaucoma, urinary retention, and other systemic anticholinergic effects; however, these have not been reported.

Preparations, Dosage, and Administration

Aclidinium is available as a breath-activated multidose DPI. Each metered dose contains 400 mcg of aclidinium bromide. Recommended use is twice a day.

Umeclidinium

Actions and Therapeutic Use

Umeclidinium [Incruse Ellipta] which received FDA approval in 2013, is the newest long-acting anticholinergic indicated for management of bronchospasm associated with COPD. In addition to its availability as a single agent, it is also available in combination with the LABA vilanterol as the Anoro Ellipta. Both the single and combination drugs are indicated for COPD maintenance therapy only; they are not approved for asthma treatment.

Adverse Effects

Umeclidinium contains lactose as a component of the powder mix. Theoretically, it may cause severe hypersensitivity reactions when taken by people who have milk protein allergies. In clinical trials, adverse effects were negligible: nasopharyngitis was reported by 8% of subjects; however, this was reported by 7% of those taking a placebo. Similarly, 5% reported upper respiratory tract infections; yet this was reported by 4% of those taking a placebo. Although it is possible for this anticholinergic drug to cause typical anticholinergic adverse effects because it is inhaled, the likelihood of this occurrence is markedly decreased.

Preparations, Dosage, and Administration

Umeclidinium is available for inhalation. Each metered dose contains 62.5 mcg of umeclidinium. It should be used once every 24 hours.

GLUCOCORTICOID/LONG-ACTING BETA$_2$ AGONIST COMBINATIONS

Fluticasone/salmeterol [Advair Diskus, Advair HFA], fluticasone/vilanterol [Breo Ellipta], *budesonide/formoterol* [Symbicort], and *mometasone/formoterol* [Dulera] are available in fixed-dose combinations for inhalational therapy of asthma and COPD. The glucocorticoids (fluticasone, budesonide, and mometasone) provide antiinflammatory benefits, and the LABAs (salmeterol and formoterol) provide bronchodilation. All four products are indicated for long-term maintenance in adults and children. These combinations are more convenient than taking a glucocorticoid and LABA separately but have the disadvantage of restricting dosage flexibility. These products carry a black box warning about possible increased risk for asthma severity or asthma-related death (from the LABA in the combination). However, because the LABA is combined with a glucocorticoid, risk should be minimal. The four combination products have not been directly compared. Nonetheless, when used in equivalent dosages, they are likely to be equally effective.

Fluticasone/Salmeterol

Fluticasone and salmeterol are available in a DPI sold as Advair Diskus and an MDI sold as Advair HFA. Advair Diskus is approved for patients 4 years and older, whereas Advair HFA is approved for patients 12 years and older.

Advair Diskus is available in three strengths that deliver the following doses of salmeterol/fluticasone per inhalation: 50/100 mcg, 50/250 mcg, and 50/500 mcg. Dosing consists of 1 inhalation every morning and evening. The dose of fluticasone selected should be equivalent to the dose of the glucocorticoid already in use.

Advair HFA is available in three strengths that deliver the following doses of salmeterol/fluticasone per inhalation: 21/45 mcg, 21/115 mcg, and 21/230 mcg. Dosing consists of 2 inhalations every morning and evening. As with Advair Diskus, the fluticasone dosage should be equivalent to the dosage of glucocorticoid in current use.

Fluticasone/Vilanterol [Breo Ellipta]

Fluticasone/vilanterol [Breo Ellipta] is approved only for adults and is indicated for treatment of both asthma and COPD. Breo Ellipta is available in two strengths: 100 mcg/25 mcg and 200 mcg/25 mcg per actuation of the dry-powder delivery device. Dosing for both conditions is 1 inhalation of the 100 mcg/25 mcg strength once daily. This is the maximal recommended dose for COPD. For asthma, if there is inadequate improvement, patients may use the 200 mcg/25 mcg strength once daily.

Budesonide/Formoterol

Budesonide/formoterol [Symbicort] is supplied in an MDI for use by patients 12 years and older. Symbicort is available in two strengths that deliver either 80/4.5 mcg or 160/4.5 mcg of budesonide/formoterol per inhalation. Dosing consists of 2 inhalations every morning and evening. Patients currently taking low to medium glucocorticoid doses should start with the 80/4.5-mcg formulation. Patients taking medium to high glucocorticoid doses should start with the 160/4.5-mcg formulation.

Mometasone/Formoterol

Mometasone/formoterol [Dulera] is supplied in an MDI for use by patients 12 years and older. Dulera is available in two strengths that deliver either 100/5 mcg or 200/5 mcg of mometasone/formoterol per inhalation. Dosing consists of 2 inhalations every morning and evening. Patients currently taking low to medium glucocorticoid doses should start with the 100/5-mcg formulation. Patients taking medium to high glucocorticoid doses should start with the 160/5-mcg formulation.

BETA$_2$-ADRENERGIC AGONIST/ ANTICHOLINERGIC COMBINATIONS

The combination of a beta$_2$ agonist with a cholinergic antagonist optimizes bronchodilation by capitalizing on the unique action of the individual agents. As mentioned previously, beta$_2$ agonists promote bronchodilation by stimulating adrenergic receptors. In the lung, this relaxes smooth muscle in the airways. Cholinergic antagonists (anticholinergics) promote bronchodilation by blocking cholinergic receptors. This relaxes smooth muscle tone by preventing stimulation of cholinergic receptors. Additionally, beta$_2$ agonists primarily affect the bronchioles, whereas anticholinergics primarily affect the bronchi. This action on different areas of the airways further enhances bronchodilation.

All beta agonist/anticholinergic combinations are inhaled. Four combinations are available: Albuterol/ipratropium [Combivent Respimat, Combivent UDV], indacaterol/glycopyrronium [Utibron Neohaler, Ultibro Breezhaler ♣], olodaterol/tiotropium [Stiolto Respimat], and vilanterol/umeclidinium, inhaled [Anoro Ellipta]. These are only approved for management of COPD; however, Combivent (the only combination with a SABA), has been used off-label for management of asthma.

Ipratropium/Albuterol [Combivent Respimat, Duoneb]

Ipratropium plus albuterol is available in two formulations: solution for nebulization [DuoNeb] and an inhaler [Combivent Respimat]. DuoNeb solution contains 500 mcg of ipratropium, an anticholinergic, and 2500 mcg of albuterol, a SABA, in 3-mL, single-use vials. The recommended dosage is 3 mL administered 4 times a day by oral inhalation using a nebulizer. The Combivent Respimat inhaler delivers 20 mcg of ipratropium and 100 mcg of albuterol with each actuation. The recommended dosage is 1 inhalation 4 times a day with a maximum of 6 inhalations in 24 hours.

Indacaterol/Glycopyrronium [Utibron Neohaler]

The Utibron Neohaler contains 27.5 mcg of the LABA indacaterol and 15 mcg of the anticholinergic glycopyrronium (glycopyrrolate) per inhalation. Dosing is twice daily on a scheduled regimen.

Olodaterol/Tiotropium [Stiolto Respimat]

Olodaterol, a LABA, is combined with tiotropium, an anticholinergic, in Stiolto Respimat. There are 2.5 mcg of olodaterol and 2.5 mcg of tiotropium per actuation. Dosing is two inhalations once a day.

Umeclidinium/Vilanterol [Anoro Ellipta]

The combination product Anoro Ellipta contains umeclidinium 62.5 mcg and vilanterol 25 mcg per inhalation. One inhalation should be taken once a day.

MANAGEMENT OF ASTHMA

In 2007, the National Asthma Education and Prevention Program (NAEPP) of the National Heart, Lung, and Blood Institute issued *Expert Panel Report 3 (EPR-3): Guidelines for the Diagnosis and Management of Asthma.* These are still the most current U.S. recommendations for asthma management. The following discussion reflects EPR-3 recommendations, which are available online at http://www.nhlbi.nih.gov/health-pro/guidelines/current/asthma-guidelines. These are currently undergoing a process of revision and update with a proposal to have new guidelines available in 2018. To follow updates and draft summary reports go to http://www.nhlbi.nih.gov/about/org/naepp.

In EPR-3, management recommendations are made for three age groups: 0 to 4 years, 5 to 11 years, and 12 years and older. Recommendations for all three groups are similar, although there are some important differences. *Discussion here is limited to adults and older children.* For recommendations that apply to younger patients, please consult EPR-3.

Measuring Lung Function

Before considering asthma therapy, we need to address tests of lung function. Three tests are described here.

Forced expiratory volume in 1 second (FEV_1) is the single most useful test of lung function. To determine FEV_1, the patient inhales completely and then exhales as completely and forcefully as possible into the spirometer. The spirometer measures how much air was expelled during the first second of exhalation. Results are then compared with a "predicted normal value" for a healthy person of similar age, sex, height, and weight. For a patient with asthma, the FEV_1 might be 75% of the predicted value.

Forced vital capacity (FVC), also measured with a spirometer, is defined as the total volume of air the patient can exhale after a full inhalation.

FEV_1/FVC (i.e., FEV_1 divided by FVC) is the fraction (percentage) of vital capacity exhaled during the first second of forced expiration. Normal values for FEV_1/FVC range from 85% (for people 8–19 years old) down to 70% (for people 60–80 years old). In patients with asthma, the value

for FEV_1/FVC may be in the normal range, or it may be reduced by 5% or more, depending on asthma severity.

Peak expiratory flow (PEF) is defined as the maximal rate of airflow during expiration. To determine PEF, the patient exhales as forcefully as possible into a *peak flowmeter,* a relatively inexpensive, hand-held device. Patients should measure their peak flow every morning. If the value is less than 80% of their personal best, more frequent monitoring should be done.

Classification of Asthma Severity

As described in the EPR-3, chronic asthma has four classes of increasing severity: (1) intermittent, (2) mild persistent, (3) moderate persistent, and (4) severe persistent. Diagnostic criteria for these classes are shown in Table 60.4. Note that severity classification is based on two separate domains: *impairment* and *risk.* Impairment refers to the effect of asthma on quality of life and functional capacity *in the present.* Risk refers to possible adverse events *in the future,* such as exacerbations and progressive loss of lung function. As we progress from intermittent asthma to severe persistent asthma, both impairment and risk increase: asthma symptoms occur more often and last longer, use of SABAs for symptomatic control increases, limitations on physical activity become more substantial, FEV_1 decreases to less than 60% of predicted, FEV_1/FVC drops to 5% or more below normal, and the number of exacerbations that require oral glucocorticoids gets larger. It is important to note that the two domains of asthma—impairment and risk—may respond differently to drugs. Furthermore, patients can be at high risk for future events, even if their current level of impairment is low.

Treatment Goals

Treatment of chronic asthma is directed at two basic goals: reducing impairment and reducing risk. Components of each goal are listed here.

Reducing Impairment

- Preventing chronic and troublesome symptoms (e.g., coughing or breathlessness after exertion and at all other times)
- Reducing use of SABAs for symptom relief to 2 days a week or less
- Maintaining normal (or near-normal) pulmonary function
- Maintaining normal activity levels, including exercise and attendance at school or work
- Meeting patient and family expectations regarding asthma care

Reducing Risk

- Preventing recurrent exacerbations
- Minimizing the need for emergency department visits or hospitalizations
- Preventing progressive loss of lung function (for children, preventing reduced lung growth)
- Providing maximal benefits with minimal adverse effects

Chronic Drug Therapy

In patients with chronic asthma, drugs are employed in two ways: some agents are taken to establish *long-term control,* and some are taken for *quick relief* of an ongoing attack (Table 60.5). The long-term control drugs are taken every day, whereas the quick-relief drugs are taken PRN. Of the long-term control agents in current use, inhaled glucocorticoids are by far the most important. With regular dosing, these drugs reduce the frequency and severity of attacks, as well as the need for quick-relief medications. Of the quick-relief drugs in current use, inhaled SABAs are the most important. These drugs act promptly to reverse bronchoconstriction and provide rapid relief from cough, chest tightness, and wheezing.

For chronic drug therapy, EPR-3 recommends a *stepwise* approach, in which drug dosages and drug classes are stepped up as needed and stepped down when possible. Six steps are described (Table 60.6). The basic concept is simple. First, all patients, starting with step 1, should use an inhaled SABA as

TABLE 60.5 ▪ Drugs for Asthma: Agents for Long-Term Control Versus Quick Relief

LONG-TERM CONTROL MEDICATIONS	
Antiinflammatory drugs	Glucocorticoids (inhaled or oral)
	Leukotriene modifiers
	Cromolyn
	Omalizumab
Bronchodilators	Long-acting inhaled $beta_2$ agonists*
	Long-acting oral $beta_2$ agonists
	Theophylline
QUICK-RELIEF MEDICATIONS	
Bronchodilators	Short-acting inhaled $beta_2$ agonists
	Anticholinergics
Antiinflammatory drugs	Glucocorticoids, systemic†

*For treatment of asthma, should always be combined with an inhaled glucocorticoid.

†Considered quick-relief drugs when used in a short burst (3–10 days) at the start of therapy or during a period of gradual deterioration. Glucocorticoids are not used for immediate relief of an ongoing attack.

TABLE 60.6 ▪ Stepwise Approach to Managing Asthma in Patients 12 Years and Older

	Long-Term Control Drugs (Taken Daily): Preferred	Long-Term Control Drugs (Taken Daily): Alternative	Quick-Relief Drugs (Taken PRN)
Step 1	No daily medication needed		SABA
Step 2	Low-dose IGC	Cromolyn, LTRA, or theophylline	SABA
Step 3	Low-dose IGC + LABA *or* Medium-dose IGC	Low-dose IGC + either LTRA, theophylline, or zileuton	SABA
Step 4	Medium dose IGC + LABA	Medium-dose IGC + either LTRA, theophylline, or zileuton	SABA
Step 5	High-dose IGC + LABA		SABA
Step 6	High-dose IGC + LABA + oral glucocorticoid		SABA

IGC, inhaled glucocorticoid; LABA, long-acting $beta_2$ agonist; LTRA, leukotriene receptor antagonist; SABA, short-acting $beta_2$ agonist.

needed for quick relief. Second, all patients—except those on step 1—should use a long-term control medication (preferably an inhaled glucocorticoid) to provide baseline control. Third, when patients move up a step, owing to increased impairment and risk, dosage of the control medication is increased or another control medication is added (typically a LABA), or both. And fourth, after a period of sustained control, moving down a step should be tried.

For patients just beginning drug therapy, the step they start on is determined by the pretreatment classification of asthma severity. For example, a patient diagnosed with intermittent asthma would begin at step 1 (PRN use of an inhaled SABA), whereas a patient diagnosed with moderate persistent asthma would begin at step 3 (daily inhalation of a low-dose glucocorticoid plus daily inhalation of a LABA, supplemented with an inhaled SABA as needed).

After treatment has been ongoing, stepping up or down is based on *assessment of asthma control*. Like the diagnosis of pretreatment severity, assessment of control is based on two domains: current impairment and future risk. In EPR-3, three classes of control are defined: well controlled, not well controlled, and very poorly controlled. Diagnostic criteria for each class are shown in Table 60.7 along with recommended actions for treatment.

Drugs for Acute Severe Exacerbations

Acute severe exacerbations of asthma require immediate attention. The goals are to relieve airway obstruction and hypoxemia and normalize lung function as quickly as possible. Initial therapy consists of the following:

- Giving oxygen to relieve hypoxemia
- Giving a systemic glucocorticoid to reduce airway inflammation
- Giving a nebulized high-dose SABA to relieve airflow obstruction
- Giving nebulized ipratropium to further reduce airflow obstruction

TABLE 60.7 ■ Assessment of Asthma Control in Patients 12 Years and Older and Recommended Action for Treatment

	Classification of Control*		
Components of Control	**Well Controlled**	**Not Well Controlled**	**Very Poorly Controlled**
CURRENT IMPAIRMENT			
Symptoms	≤2 days/week	>2 days/week	Throughout the day
Nighttime awakenings	≤2 times/month	1–3 times/week	≥4 times/week
SABA used to control symptoms (not to prevent EIB)	≤2 days/week	>2 days/week	Several times a day
Effect on normal activity	None	Some limitation	Severe limitation
Lung function tests:			
FEV_1 (% of predicted)	FEV_1 >80% *or*	FEV_1 60%–80% *or*	FEV_1 <60% *or*
PEF (% of personal best)	PEF >80%	PEF 60%–80%	PEF <60%
Questionnaire scores			
ATAQ	0	1–2	3–4
ACQ	≤0.75	≥1.5	N/A
ACT	≥20	16–19	≤15
FUTURE RISK			
Exacerbations requiring oral glucocorticoids	0–1/year	≥2/year†	≥2/year†
Progressive loss of lung function	Evaluation requires long-term follow-up care.		
Treatment-related adverse effects	Medication side effects can vary in intensity from none to very troublesome and worrisome. The level of intensity does not correlate to specific levels of control but should be considered in the overall assessment of risk.		
RECOMMENDED ACTION FOR TREATMENT‡	Maintain current treatment step. Follow up every 1–6 months to maintain control. Consider step down if well controlled for 3 months or longer.	Move up 1 step and reassess in 2–6 weeks. To reduce side effects, consider changing drugs.	Consider short course of oral glucocorticoids. Move up 1 or 2 steps and reassess in 2 weeks. To reduce side effects, consider changing drugs.

*The level of control is based on the most severe impairment or risk category. Assess impairment domain by patient's recall of previous 2 to 4 weeks and by FEV_1 or PEF. Symptom assessment for longer periods should reflect a global assessment, such as inquiring whether the patient's asthma is better or worse since the last visit.

†At present, there are inadequate data to correspond frequencies of exacerbations with different levels of asthma control. In general, more frequent and intense exacerbations (e.g., requiring urgent, unscheduled care, hospitalization, or intensive care unit admission) indicate poorer disease control. For treatment purposes, patients who had two or more exacerbations requiring oral glucocorticoids in the past year may be considered the same as patients who have not-well-controlled asthma, even in the absence of impairment levels consistent with not-well-controlled asthma.

‡Treatment steps are shown in Table 60.6.

ACQ, Asthma Control Questionnaire; ACT, Asthma Control Test; ATAQ, Asthma Therapy Assessment Questionnaire; EIB, exercise-induced bronchospasm; FEV_1, forced expiratory volume in 1 second; N/A, not applicable; PEF, peak expiratory flow rate.

Severe cases may benefit from IV magnesium sulfate or inhalation of heliox (79% helium/21% oxygen). After resolution of the crisis and hospital discharge, an oral glucocorticoid is taken for 5 to 10 days. All patients should also take a medium-dose inhaled glucocorticoid. Full recovery of lung function may take weeks.

Drugs for Exercise-Induced Bronchospasm

Exercise increases airway obstruction in practically all people with chronic asthma. The cause is bronchospasm secondary to loss of heat or water from the lung. EIB usually starts either during or immediately after exercise, peaks in 5 to 10 minutes, and resolves 20 to 30 minutes later.

With proper medication, most people with asthma can be as active as they wish. Indeed, many world-class athletes have had asthma. To prevent EIB, patients can inhale a SABA or cromolyn prophylactically. Inhaled SABAs, which prevent EIB in more than 80% of patients, are generally preferred over cromolyn, which is less effective. Beta$_2$ agonists should be inhaled immediately before exercise; cromolyn should be inhaled 15 minutes before exercise.

Reducing Exposure to Allergens and Triggers

For patients with chronic asthma, the treatment plan should include measures to control allergens and other factors that can cause airway inflammation and exacerbate symptoms. Important sources of asthma-associated allergens include the house dust mite, warm-blooded pets, cockroaches, and molds. Factors that can exacerbate asthma include tobacco smoke, wood smoke, and household sprays. To the extent possible, exposure to these factors should be reduced or eliminated.

MANAGEMENT OF CHRONIC OBSTRUCTIVE PULMONARY DISEASE

Diagnosis and treatment of COPD are addressed in the *Global Strategy for the Diagnosis, Management, and Prevention of Chronic Obstructive Pulmonary Disease.* These evidence-based practice guidelines, developed by the Global Initiative for Chronic Obstructive Lung Disease (GOLD), were updated in 2016. These guidelines are available at http://goldcopd.org/gold-reports/.

Measuring Lung Function

Patients who have signs and symptoms of COPD, such as dyspnea that has worsened over time, chronic cough, sputum production, and a history of smoking tobacco or other risk factors, should be tested with a spirometer to measure the degree of airway obstruction. A postbronchodilator FEV$_1$/FVC of less than 0.70 is needed to confirm the COPD diagnosis.

Classification of Airflow Limitation Severity

Severity of airflow limitation is based on spirometry. The four classes of increasing severity are (1) mild, (2) moderate, (3) severe, and (4) very severe. Remember that, for all patients, a diagnosis of COPD requires an FEV$_1$/FVC of less than 0.70.

- Mild: FEV$_1$ greater than 80% predicted
- Moderate: FEV$_1$ is 50% or greater than predicted but less than 80% predicted
- Severe: FEV$_1$ is 30% or greater than predicted but less than 50% predicted
- Very severe: FEV$_1$ less than 30% predicted

Treatment Goals

There are two primary goals of COPD management. The first is to reduce symptoms, improve the patient's health status, and increase exercise tolerance. The second goal is to reduce risks and mortality. The latter is accomplished by preventing COPD progression and by preventing and managing exacerbations.

Treatment goals are based on the overall level of COPD severity. The GOLD guidelines classify COPD severity from A to D based on consideration of the patient's symptoms, their airflow limitation severity (see earlier discussion), their risk level for COPD exacerbations, and any comorbid conditions they may have. Symptoms are quantified using instruments such as the COPD Assessment Test (available at http://www.catestonline.org) and the COPD Control Questionnaire (available at http://www.ccq.nl). For full instructions determining severity, please see the Global Strategy for Diagnosis, Management, and Prevention of COPD – 2016 report available at http://goldcopd.org/gold-reports.

- Group A (few symptoms; low risk): mild/moderate airflow limitation + low symptom scores + 1 or fewer exacerbations per year
- Group B (increased symptoms; low risk): mild/moderate airflow limitation + low symptom scores + 1 or fewer exacerbations per year
- Group C (few symptoms; high risk): severe/very severe airflow limitation + high symptom scores + 2 or more exacerbations per year
- Group D (increased symptoms; high risk): severe/very severe airflow limitation + high symptom scores + 2 or more exacerbations per year

Management is often challenging because patients with COPD commonly have comorbidities that complicate management choices, so COPD management must be individualized.

Management of Stable Chronic Obstructive Pulmonary Disease

Pharmacologic management of stable COPD relies primarily on bronchodilators, glucocorticoids, and phosphodiesterase type 4 (PDE-4) inhibitors. The GOLD guidelines offer recommendations for each.

Bronchodilators

Inhaled long-acting formulations of either beta$_2$ agonists or anticholinergics are preferred for bronchodilation. Theophylline is reserved for use only when other bronchodilators are not available.

Glucocorticoids

Long-term inhaled glucocorticoids are recommended when symptoms are severe or when long-acting bronchodilators are inadequate for management of exacerbations. When given for

COPD, glucocorticoids should be given in combination with a LABA; glucocorticoid monotherapy is no longer recommended for long-term therapy because of decreased efficacy when used alone.

Phosphodiesterase Type 4 Inhibitors

In patients with severe, chronic COPD, the risk for exacerbations may be reduced with roflumilast [Daliresp]. Roflumilast is a selective inhibitor of PDE, an enzyme that inactivates cyclic adenosine monophosphate (cAMP). The drug reduces inflammation, cough, and excessive mucus production by raising levels of cAMP in lung cells. Adverse effects include diarrhea, reduced appetite, weight loss, nausea, headache, back pain, insomnia, and depression. Safety in pregnancy has not been established. The dosage is 500 mcg once a day, taken with or without food. Roflumilast should be used in combination with tiotropium, a LABA, or an inhaled glucocorticoid.

Management of Chronic Obstructive Pulmonary Disease Exacerbations

Although some of the same drugs used for management of stable COPD are also used for management of COPD exacerbations, the drug formulations used differ. For example, although LABAs are preferred for stable COPD management, SABAs (specifically inhaled either alone or in combination with inhaled anticholinergics) are preferred for bronchodilation during COPD exacerbations. Further, systemic glucocorticoids greatly improve outcomes when used in management of COPD exacerbations. Other agents that may be used to control and shorten exacerbations include antibiotics for patients who have signs and symptoms of infection and supplemental oxygen to maintain an oxygen saturation of 88% to 92%.

PRESCRIBING AND MONITORING CONSIDERATIONS

Glucocorticoids

Inhaled

Beclomethasone
Budesonide
Ciclesonide
Flunisolide
Fluticasone
Mometasone

Oral

Methylprednisolone
Prednisolone
Prednisone

The nursing implications summarized in the following discussion refer specifically to the use of glucocorticoids in asthma. A full summary of nursing implications for glucocorticoids is presented in Chapter 56.

Preadministration Assessment

Therapeutic Goal. Glucocorticoids are used on a fixed schedule to suppress inflammation. They are not used to abort an ongoing attack.

Baseline Data. Determine FEV_1 and the frequency and severity of attacks, and attempt to identify trigger factors.

Identifying High-Risk Patients

INHALED GLUCOCORTICOIDS. These preparations are *contraindicated* for patients with persistently positive sputum cultures for *Candida albicans. (They are not contraindicated for oral candidiasis; however, they create an environment that supports growth of C. albicans.)*

ORAL GLUCOCORTICOIDS. These preparations are *contraindicated* for patients with systemic fungal infections and for individuals receiving live virus vaccines.

Use with *caution* in pediatric patients and in women who are pregnant or breastfeeding. Also, exercise *caution* in patients with hypertension, heart failure, renal impairment, esophagitis, gastritis, peptic ulcer disease, myasthenia gravis, diabetes mellitus, osteoporosis, or infections that are resistant to treatment and in patients receiving potassium-depleting diuretics, digitalis glycosides, insulin, oral hypoglycemics, or nonsteroidal antiinflammatory drugs.

Administration Considerations

Routes

INHALATION. Inhaled glucocorticoids are administered with an MDI, DPI, or nebulizer.

ORAL. Alternate-day therapy is recommended to minimize adrenal suppression. During long-term treatment, supplemental doses must be given at times of severe stress.

Ongoing Monitoring and Interventions

Evaluating Therapeutic Effects. Providers should monitor status of patients with asthma at each appointment. Monitoring includes tracking PEF, symptom frequency and symptom intensity, nighttime awakenings, effect on normal activity, and SABA use.

Minimizing Adverse Effects

INHALED GLUCOCORTICOIDS. If candidiasis develops, it can be treated with antifungal medication. Also, using a spacer will decrease deposits onto the oropharynx, thereby decreasing the risk of developing this condition.

ORAL GLUCOCORTICOIDS. Prolonged therapy can cause serious adverse effects, including *osteoporosis, hyperglycemia, peptic ulcer disease,* and *growth suppression.* These effects can be reduced with alternate-day dosing. Additional interventions that apply to adverse effects of long-term glucocorticoid therapy are summarized in Chapter 56.

Adrenal suppression is a potentially life-threatening adverse effect of long-term glucocorticoid use. When discontinuing a systemic glucocorticoid, you must be sure it is done gradually to allow the body to resume producing the endogenous hormone. During times of severe physical stress when the body would normally produce high levels of glucocorticoids, it is essential to increase the dose of systemic glucocorticoids.

$Beta_2$-Adrenergic Agonists

Inhaled, Short Acting

Albuterol
Levalbuterol

Inhaled, Long Acting

Arformoterol
Formoterol

Indacaterol
Olodaterol
Salmeterol

Oral

Albuterol
Terbutaline

Preadministration Assessment

Therapeutic Goal. Short-acting inhaled $beta_2$ agonists are used PRN for prophylaxis of EIB and to relieve ongoing asthma attacks and COPD exacerbations. Oral and inhaled LABAs are used for maintenance therapy.

Baseline Data. Determine FEV_1 and the frequency and severity of attacks, and attempt to identify trigger factors. Monitor home assessments of PEF at each clinic encounter.

Identifying High-Risk Patients. Systemic (oral, parenteral) $beta_2$ agonists are *contraindicated* for patients with tachydysrhythmias or tachycardia associated with digitalis toxicity.

Use systemic $beta_2$ agonists with *caution* in patients with diabetes, hyperthyroidism, organic heart disease, hypertension, or angina pectoris.

Administration Considerations

Inhaled $beta_2$ agonists are administered with an MDI, DPI, or nebulizer. Some pharmaceutical companies also have developed specialized inhaler devices for their products. Instructions for use, with return demonstration by patients, should be undertaken when prescribed and periodically to verify that proper technique is used.

Ongoing Monitoring and Interventions

Evaluating Therapeutic Effects. Asthma control should be assessed at each clinic encounter. (See Table 60.4.) Monitor PEF, symptom frequency and symptom intensity, nighttime awakenings, effect on normal activity, and SABA use. It is also important to discuss medication adherence or deviation from the management plan. Because patients may forget some of the finer points of inhaled medication administration, this is a good time to have the patient demonstrate their technique for using inhalers.

Minimizing Adverse Effects

INHALED SHORT-ACTING $BETA_2$ AGONISTS. When used at recommended doses, SABAs are generally devoid of significant adverse effects. Cardiac stimulation and tremors are most likely with systemic therapy.

INHALED LONG-ACTING $BETA_2$ AGONISTS. When used correctly, LABAs are safe; however, when used *alone* for prophylaxis, they may increase the risk for severe asthma attacks and asthma-related death. To minimize risk, these drugs should always be combined with an inhaled glucocorticoid, preferably in the same inhalation device.

ORAL $BETA_2$ AGONISTS. Excessive dosing can activate $beta_1$ receptors on the heart, resulting in anginal pain and tachydysrhythmias. For this reason, selective beta-2 adrenergic agonists should be prescribed (see Table 60.3) rather than nonselective beta adrenergic drugs (e.g. isoproterenol).

Tremor is common with systemic $beta_2$ agonists and usually subsides with continued drug use. If necessary, tremor can be reduced by lowering the dosage.

Cromolyn

Preadministration Assessment

Therapeutic Goal

Cromolyn is used for acute and long-term prophylaxis of asthma. The drug will not abort an ongoing asthma attack.

Baseline Data

Determine FEV_1 and the frequency and severity of attacks and attempt to identify trigger factors.

Identifying High-Risk Patients

Cromolyn is *contraindicated* for the rare patient who has experienced an allergic response to cromolyn in the past.

Administration Considerations

Cromolyn is administered with a nebulizer.

Acute Prophylaxis

When administered 15 minutes before exercise or prior to exposure to other precipitating factors (eg, cold, environmental agents), cromolyn can prevent an asthma attack.

Long-Term Prophylaxis

When taken on a regular schedule, cromolyn provides long-term prophylaxis for asthma. Full therapeutic effects may take several weeks to develop.

Ongoing Monitoring and Interventions

Evaluating Therapeutic Effects

Monitor and PEF, symptom frequency and symptom intensity, nighttime awakenings, effect on normal activity, and SABA use at each clinic encounter.

Minimizing Adverse Effects and Interactions

Cromolyn is devoid of significant adverse effects and drug interactions.

Theophylline

Preadministration Assessment

Therapeutic Goal

Theophylline is a bronchodilator taken on a regular schedule to decrease the intensity and frequency of moderate to severe asthma attacks.

Baseline Data

Determine FEV_1 and the frequency and severity of attacks.

Identifying High-Risk Patients

Theophylline is *contraindicated* for patients with untreated seizure disorders or peptic ulcer disease.

Use with *caution* in patients with heart disease, liver or kidney dysfunction, or severe hypertension.

Administration Considerations

Routes

Oral, intravenous.

Oral

Dosage must be individualized. Doses are low initially and then increased gradually. The dosing objective is to produce plasma theophylline levels in the therapeutic range, which for most patients is 5 to 15 mcg/mL.

Intravenous

Dosage is individualized. Administer slowly. Verify compatibility with other IV drugs before mixing.

Ongoing Monitoring and Interventions

Evaluating Therapeutic Effects

Monitor theophylline levels to ensure that they are in the therapeutic range (5–15 mcg/mL for most patients).

Minimizing Adverse Effects

Adverse effects (e.g., nausea, vomiting, diarrhea, insomnia, restlessness) develop as plasma drug levels rise above 20 mcg/mL. Severe effects (convulsions, ventricular fibrillation) can occur at drug levels above 30 mcg/mL. Dosage should be adjusted to keep theophylline levels below 20 mcg/mL.

Minimizing Adverse Interactions

Caffeine. Caffeine can intensify the adverse effects of theophylline on the heart and CNS and can decrease theophylline metabolism.

Smoking Tobacco or Marijuana. Tobacco and marijuana smoking can increase clearance to 50% in adults and 80% in older adults. Secondhand smoke also increases theophylline clearance. Accordingly, it is important to inquire regarding smoking habits in order to optimize dosing.

Drugs That Reduce Theophylline Levels. Phenobarbital, phenytoin, rifampin, and other drugs can lower theophylline levels. In the presence of these drugs, the dosage of theophylline may need to be increased.

Drugs That Increase Theophylline Levels. Cimetidine, fluoroquinolone antibiotics, and other drugs can elevate theophylline levels. When combined with these drugs, theophylline should be used in reduced dosage.

Management of Toxicity. Theophylline overdose can cause severe dysrhythmias and convulsions. Death from cardiorespiratory collapse may occur. Manage toxicity by (1) discontinuing theophylline and (2) administering activated charcoal (to decrease theophylline absorption) plus a cathartic (to accelerate fecal excretion). Give lidocaine to control ventricular dysrhythmias and IV diazepam to control seizures.

CHAPTER

61

Drugs for Allergic Rhinitis, Cough, and Colds

Jacqueline Rosenjack Burchum, DNSc, FNP-BC, CNE

The drugs addressed in this chapter are given to alleviate symptoms of common upper respiratory disorders. Our principal focus is on the symptoms of allergic rhinitis and the common cold.

DRUGS FOR ALLERGIC RHINITIS

Allergic rhinitis is an inflammatory disorder that affects the upper airway. Major symptoms are sneezing, rhinorrhea, pruritus, and nasal congestion caused by dilation and increased permeability of nasal blood vessels. In addition, some patients experience associated conjunctivitis, sinusitis, and even asthma. Symptoms are triggered by airborne allergens, which bind to immunoglobulin E (IgE) antibodies on mast cells, and thereby cause release of inflammatory mediators, including histamine, leukotrienes, and prostaglandins. Allergic rhinitis is the most common allergic disorder, affecting almost one out of every six people living in the United States.

Allergic rhinitis has two major forms: seasonal and perennial. Seasonal rhinitis, also known as *hay fever,* occurs in the spring and fall in reaction to outdoor allergens such as fungi and pollens from weeds, grasses, and trees. Perennial (nonseasonal) rhinitis is triggered by indoor allergens, especially the house dust mite and pet dander.

Several classes of drugs are used for allergic rhinitis (Table 61.1). Principal among these are (1) glucocorticoids (intranasal), (2) antihistamines (oral and intranasal), and (3) sympathomimetics (oral and intranasal).

Approaches to rhinitis management are based in large part on *The Diagnosis and Management of Rhinitis: An Updated Practice Parameter* (2008), an evidence-based guideline developed by the Joint Task Force on Practice Parameters, representing the American Academy of Allergy, Asthma & Immunology; the American College of Allergy, Asthma and Immunology; and the Joint Council of Allergy, Asthma and Immunology. The American Academy of Otolaryngology's (AAO) *Clinical Practice Guideline: Allergic Rhinitis* (2015) provides further guidance by individualizing drug choice for symptom control. An algorithm for management of allergic rhinitis, developed by the AAO, is shown in Fig. 61.1.

Intranasal Glucocorticoids

The basic pharmacology of the glucocorticoids is discussed in Chapter 56. Consideration here is limited to their use in allergic rhinitis.

Actions and Uses

Intranasal glucocorticoids are the most effective drugs for prevention and treatment of seasonal and perennial rhinitis. Because of their antiinflammatory actions, these drugs can prevent or suppress the major symptoms of allergic rhinitis: congestion, rhinorrhea, sneezing, nasal itching, and erythema in 90% of patients who use them properly. Seven intranasal glucocorticoids are available (Table 61.2). Three of these—budesonide [Rhinocort Aqua], fluticasone propionate [Flonase], and triamcinolone [Nasacort Allergy 24 hours]–are available in the United States without a prescription. All appear equally effective.

Adverse Effects

Adverse effects of intranasal glucocorticoids are generally mild. The most common are *drying of the nasal mucosa* and a *burning or itching sensation. Sore throat, epistaxis*, and *headache* may also occur.

Systemic effects are possible but are rare at recommended doses. Of greatest concern are adrenal suppression and slowing of linear growth in children (whether final adult height is reduced is unknown). Systemic effects are least likely with ciclesonide, fluticasone, and mometasone, which have very low bioavailability (see Table 61.2).

Preparations, Dosage, and Administration

Intranasal glucocorticoids are administered using a metered-dose spray device. Benefits are greatest when dosing is done daily, rather than irregularly. Full doses are given initially (see Table 61.2). After symptoms are under control, the dosage should be reduced to the lowest effective amount. For patients with seasonal allergic rhinitis, maximal effects may require a week or more to develop. However, an initial response can be seen within hours. For patients with perennial rhinitis, maximal responses may take 2 to 3 weeks to develop. If nasal passages are blocked because of nasal congestion, they should be cleared with a topical decongestant before glucocorticoid administration.

Antihistamines

The antihistamines are discussed in Chapter 54. Consideration here is limited to their use in allergic rhinitis.

Oral Antihistamines

Oral antihistamines (histamine-1 [H_1] receptor antagonists) are first-line drugs for mild to moderate allergic rhinitis. For therapy of allergic rhinitis, antihistamines are most effective

TABLE 61.1 ■ Overview of Drugs for Allergic Rhinitis

Drug or Class	Route	Actions	Adverse Effects
Glucocorticoids	Nasal	Prevent inflammatory response to allergens and thereby reduce all symptoms.	Nasal irritation; possible slowing of linear growth in children
Antihistamines	Oral/nasal	Block histamine-1 receptors and thereby decrease itching, sneezing, and rhinorrhea; do *not* reduce congestion.	*Oral:* Sedation and anticholinergic effects (mostly with first-generation agents) *Nasal:* Bitter taste
Cromolyn	Nasal	Prevents release of inflammatory mediators from mast cells and thereby can decrease all symptoms. However, benefits are modest.	None
Sympathomimetics	Oral/nasal	Activate vascular alpha$_1$ receptors and thereby cause vasoconstriction, which reduces nasal congestion; do *not* decrease sneezing, itching, or rhinorrhea.	*Oral:* Restlessness, insomnia, increased blood pressure *Nasal:* Rebound nasal congestion
Anticholinergics	Nasal	Block nasal cholinergic receptors and thereby reduce secretions; do *not* decrease sneezing, nasal congestion, or postnasal drip.	Nasal drying and irritation
Antileukotrienes	Oral	Block leukotriene receptors and thereby reduce nasal congestion.	Rare neuropsychiatric effects

TABLE 61.2 ■ Some Glucocorticoid Nasal Sprays for Allergic Rhinitis

Drug	Trade Name	Intranasal Bioavailability (%)	Dose/Spray (mcg)	Patient Age (yr)	Initial Dosage (Sprays/Nostril)
FIRST GENERATION: INCREASED SYSTEMIC ABSORPTION					
Beclomethasone	Beconase AQ	44	42	6–11	1 twice daily
				12 and older	1 or 2 twice daily
	Qnasl	—	80	12 and older	2 once daily
Budesonide	Rhinocort Aqua	34	32	6–11	1 or 2 once daily
				12 and older	1–4 once daily
Triamcinolone	Nasacort AQ	46	55	6 and older	1 or 2 once daily
Flunisolide	Generic only	49	25	6–13	2 twice daily or 1 thrice daily
				14 and older	2 twice or thrice daily
SECOND GENERATION: DECREASED SYSTEMIC ABSORPTION					
Ciclesonide	Omnaris	—	50	6 and older	2 once daily
Fluticasone propionate	Flonase	0.5–2	50	4–11	1 once daily
				12 and older	2 once daily
Fluticasone furoate	Veramyst	—	27.5	2–11	1 once daily
				12 and older	2 once daily
Mometasone	Nasonex	0.1	50	2–11	1 once daily
				12 and older	2 once daily

when taken *prophylactically* and less helpful when taken after symptoms appear.

Actions and Uses

These drugs can relieve sneezing, rhinorrhea, and nasal itching; however, they do not reduce nasal congestion. Because histamine is only one of several mediators of allergic rhinitis, antihistamines are less effective than glucocorticoids. Antihistamines should be administered on a regular basis throughout the allergy season, even when symptoms are absent, to prevent an initial histamine receptor activation.

Because histamine does not contribute to symptoms of infectious rhinitis, antihistamines are of no value against the common cold. Some patients take first-generation antihistamines for their drying effect; however, this may complicate treatment of colds by increasing the viscosity of secretions.

Adverse Effects

Adverse effects are usually mild. The most common complaint is *sedation,* which occurs frequently with the first-generation antihistamines (e.g., diphenhydramine) and much less often with the second-generation agents (e.g., fexofenadine). Accordingly, second-generation agents are clearly preferred for students who need to remain alert in class and for patients who do work that requires alertness. *Anticholinergic effects* (e.g., drying of nasal secretions, dry mouth, constipation, urinary hesitancy) are common with first-generation agents and relatively rare with the second-generation agents.

Preparations, Dosage, and Administration

Dosages for some popular H_1 antagonists are presented in Table 61.3. A more complete list appears in Chapter 54.

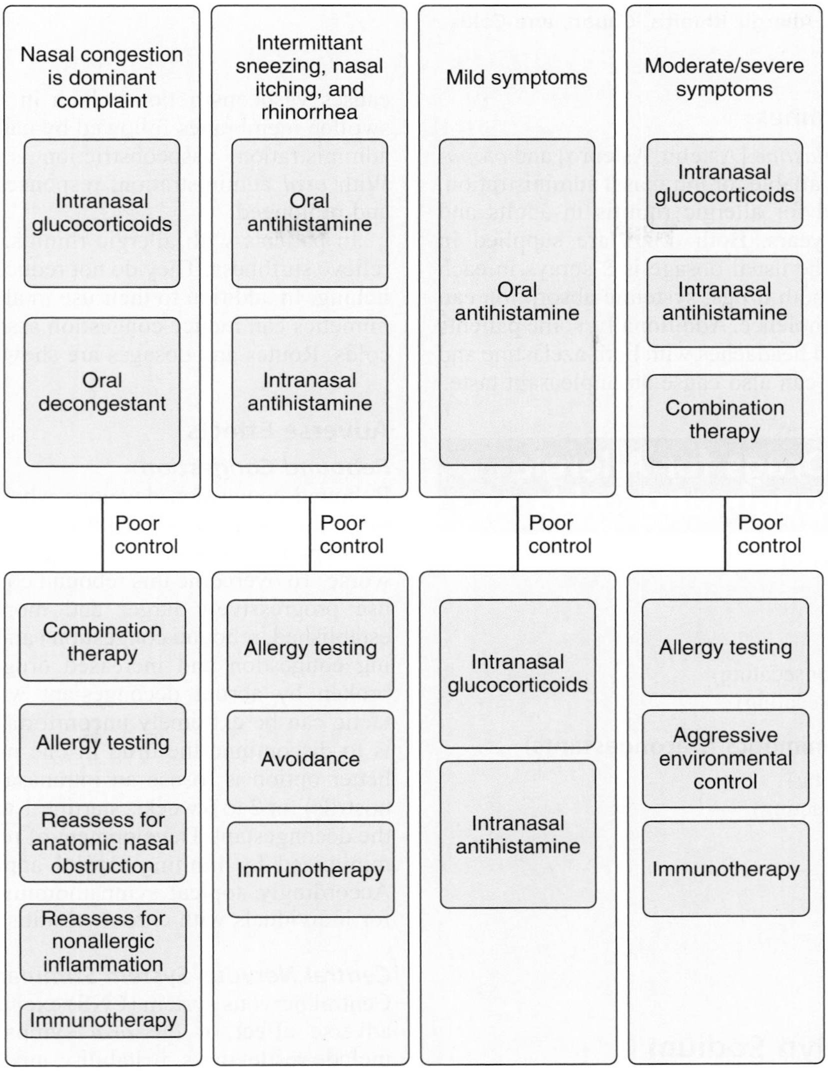

Figure 61.1 ■ Pharmacologic management of allergic rhinitis.
INS, intranasal steroids. (From American Academy of Otolaryngology. Clinical practice guideline: allergic rhinitis. 2015. http://www.entnet.org/content/clinical-practice-guideline-allergic-rhinitis.)

TABLE 61.3 ■ Some Antihistamines for Allergic Rhinitis

Generic Name	Trade Name	Dosage
ORAL ANTIHISTAMINES		
First Generation (Sedating)		
Chlorpheniramine	Chlor-Trimeton Allergy, Chlor-Tripolon ♣, others	*Adults and children 12 yr and older:* 4 mg every 4–6 hr *Children 6–11 yr:* 2 mg every 4–6 hr
Diphenhydramine	Benadryl, others	*Adults:* 25–50 mg every 4–6 hr *Children under 10 kg:* 12.5–25 mg 3 or 4 times/day
Second Generation (Nonsedating)		
Cetirizine*	Zyrtec, Reactine ♣	*Adults and children 6 yr and older:* 5 or 10 mg once daily
Levocetirizine	Xyzal	*Adults and children 12 yr and older:* 5 mg once daily *Children 6–11 yr:* 2.5 mg once daily
Fexofenadine	Allegra	*Adults and children 12 yr and older:* 60 mg twice daily or 180 mg once daily
Loratadine	Claritin, Alavert	*Adults and children 6 yr and older:* 10 mg once daily
Desloratadine	Clarinex, Aerius ♣	*Adults and children 12 yr and older:* 5 mg once daily
INTRANASAL ANTIHISTAMINES		
Second Generation (Nonsedating)		
Azelastine*	Astelin, Astepro	*Adults and children 12 yr and older:* 2 sprays/nostril twice daily *Children 5–11 yr:* 1 spray/nostril twice daily†
Olopatadine	Patanase	*Adults and children 12 yr and older:* 2 sprays/nostril twice daily (665 mcg/spray)

*May cause some sedation at recommended doses.
†Astelin only. Astepro is not approved for children younger than 12 years.

Intranasal Antihistamines

Two antihistamines—*azelastine* [Astelin, Astepro] and *olopatadine* [Patanase]—are available for intranasal administration. Both drugs are indicated for allergic rhinitis in adults and children older than 12 years. Both drugs are supplied in metered-spray devices. The usual dosage is 2 sprays in each nostril twice daily. With both drugs, systemic absorption can be sufficient to cause somnolence. Additionally, some patients experience nosebleeds and headaches with both azelastine and olopatadine. These drugs can also cause an unpleasant taste.

Prototype Drugs for Allergic Rhinitis, Cough, and Colds

Intranasal Glucocorticoid

Beclomethasone

Antihistamines

Azelastine (intranasal, nonsedating)
Loratadine (oral, nonsedating)

Intranasal Sympathomimetics (Decongestants)

Phenylephrine (short acting)
Oxymetazoline (long acting)

Opioid

Hydrocodone

Nonopioid

Dextromethorphan

Intranasal Cromolyn Sodium

The basic pharmacology of cromolyn sodium is discussed in Chapter 60. Consideration here is limited to its use in allergic rhinitis.

Actions and Uses

For treatment of allergic rhinitis, intranasal cromolyn [NasalCrom] is extremely safe but only moderately effective. Benefits are much less than those of intranasal glucocorticoids. Cromolyn reduces symptoms by suppressing release of histamine and other inflammatory mediators from mast cells. Accordingly, the drug is best suited for prophylaxis and hence should be given before symptoms start. Responses may take a week or two to develop; patients should be informed of this delay. Adverse reactions are minimum—less than with any other drug for allergic rhinitis.

Preparations, Dosage, and Administration

For treatment of allergic rhinitis, cromolyn sodium is available in a metered-dose spray device that delivers 5.2 mg/actuation. The usual dosage for adults and children over 2 years is 1 spray (5.2 mg) per nostril 4 to 6 times a day. If nasal congestion is present, a topical decongestant should be used before cromolyn. Like the antihistamines and glucocorticoids, cromolyn should be dosed on a regular schedule throughout the allergy season.

Sympathomimetics (Decongestants)

Actions and Uses

Sympathomimetics reduce nasal congestion by activating alpha$_1$-adrenergic receptors on nasal blood vessels. This causes vasoconstriction, which in turn causes shrinkage of swollen membranes followed by nasal drainage. With *topical* administration, vasoconstriction is both rapid and intense. With *oral* administration, responses are delayed, moderate, and prolonged.

In patients with allergic rhinitis, sympathomimetics only relieve stuffiness. They do not reduce rhinorrhea, sneezing, or itching. In addition to their use in allergic rhinitis, sympathomimetics can reduce congestion associated with sinusitis and colds. Routes and dosages are shown in Table 61.4.

Adverse Effects

Rebound Congestion

Rebound congestion develops when *topical* agents are used more than a few days. With prolonged use, as the effects of each application wear off, congestion becomes progressively worse. To overcome this rebound congestion, the patient must use progressively larger and more frequent doses. Once established, rebound congestion can lead to a cycle of escalating congestion and increased drug use. The cycle can be broken by abrupt decongestant withdrawal; however, this tactic can be extremely uncomfortable. A less drastic option is to discontinue the drug in one nostril at a time. An even better option is to use an intranasal glucocorticoid (in both nostrils) for 2 to 6 weeks, starting 1 week before discontinuing the decongestant. Development of rebound congestion can be minimized by limiting topical application to 3 to 5 days. Accordingly, topical sympathomimetics are not appropriate for individuals with chronic rhinitis.

Central Nervous System Stimulation

Central nervous system (CNS) excitation is the most common adverse effect of the *oral* sympathomimetics. Symptoms include restlessness, irritability, anxiety, and insomnia. These responses are uncommon with topical agents when used as recommended.

Cardiovascular Effects

By activating alpha$_1$-adrenergic receptors on systemic blood vessels, sympathomimetics can cause widespread vasoconstriction. Generalized vasoconstriction is most likely with *oral* agents. However, if used in excess, even the topical agents can cause significant systemic vasoconstriction. For most patients, effects on systemic vessels are inconsequential. However, for individuals with cardiovascular disorders—hypertension, coronary artery disease, cardiac arrhythmias, cerebrovascular disease—widespread vasoconstriction can be hazardous.

Abuse

Pseudoephedrine is associated with abuse. By causing CNS stimulation, this sympathomimetic can produce subjective effects similar to those of amphetamine. Also, it can be readily converted to methamphetamine, a widely used drug of abuse. To reduce the availability of pseudoephedrine for methamphetamine production, Congress passed the *Combat Methamphetamine Epidemic Act of 2005,* which requires that all products containing pseudoephedrine be placed behind the counter (even though it can still be purchased without a prescription in some states). Furthermore, purchasers must present identification and sign a log. Also, individuals can

TABLE 61.4 ▪ Sympathomimetics Used for Nasal Decongestion

Decongestant	Mode of Use	Dosing Interval	Dosage Size*
Phenylephrine [Neo-Synephrine, others]	Drops	Every 4 or more hr	*6 yr and older:* 2–3 drops (0.25%–1%) *2–6 yr:* 2–3 drops (0.125%)
	Spray	Every 4 or more hr	*12 yr and older:* 2–3 sprays (0.25%–1%) *6–12 yr:* 2–3 sprays (0.25%) *2–6 yr:* Not recommended
	Oral	Every 4 hr	*12 yr and older:* 10 mg *6–11 yr:* 5 mg *4–5 yr:* 2.5 mg *Younger than 4 yr:* Not recommended
Pseudoephedrine [Sudafed, others]	Oral	Every 4–6 hr	*12 yr and older:* 60 mg *6–12 yr:* 30 mg *Younger than 6 yr:* 15 mg
	Oral SR	Every 12 hr	*12 yr and older:* 120 mg *Younger than 12 yr:* Not recommended
	Oral CR	Every 24 hr	*12 yr and older:* 240 mg *Younger than 12 yr:* Not recommended
Naphazoline [Privine]	Drops	Every 6 or more hr	*12 yr and older:* 1 or 2 drops (0.05%) *Younger than 12 yr:* Not recommended
	Spray	Every 6 or more hr	*12 yr and older:* 1 or 2 sprays (0.05%) *Younger than 12 yr:* Not recommended
Oxymetazoline [Afrin 12-Hour, Neo-Synephrine 12-Hour, Dristan 12-Hour, others]	Spray	Every 10–12 hr	*6 yr and older:* 2–3 sprays (0.05%) *Younger than 6 yr:* Not recommended
Tetrahydrozoline [Tyzine]	Drops	Every 3 or more hr	*6 yr and older:* 2–4 drops (0.1%) *2–6 yr:* 2–3 drops (0.05%)
	Spray	Every 3 or more hr	*6 yr and older:* 3–4 sprays (0.1%) *Younger than 6 yr:* Not recommended
Xylometazoline [Otrivin]	Drops	Every 8–10 hr	*12 yr and older:* 2–3 drops (0.1%) *2–12 yr:* 2–3 drops (0.05%)
	Spray	Every 8–10 hr	*12 yr and older:* 1–3 sprays (0.1%) *2–12 yr:* 1 spray (0.05%)

*For drops and sprays, dosage listed is applied to *each* nostril; numbers in parentheses indicate concentration of solution employed.
CR, controlled release; SR, sustained release.

purchase no more than 9 g per month or 3.6 g on any day. Because of these constraints, many products are being reformulated to contain phenylephrine rather than ephedrine and pseudoephedrine. Unfortunately, when taken orally, phenylephrine is not very effective.

Factors in Topical Administration

General Considerations

Because of the risk for rebound congestion, topical sympathomimetics should be used for no more than 3 to 5 consecutive days. To avoid systemic effects, doses should not exceed those recommended by the manufacturer. The applicator should be cleansed after each use to prevent contamination.

Drops

Drops should be administered with the patient in a lateral, head-low position. This causes the drops to spread slowly over the nasal mucosa, thereby promoting beneficial effects while reducing the amount that is swallowed. Because the number of drops can be precisely controlled, drops allow better control of dosage than do sprays. Accordingly, because young children are particularly susceptible to toxicity, drops are preferred for these patients.

Sprays

Sprays deliver the decongestant in a fine mist. Although convenient, sprays are less effective than an equal volume of properly instilled drops.

Contrasts Between Oral and Topical Agents

Oral and topical sympathomimetics differ in several important respects. First, topical agents act faster than the oral agents and are usually more effective. Second, oral agents act longer than topical preparations. Third, systemic effects (vasoconstriction, CNS stimulation) occur primarily with oral agents; topical agents usually elicit these responses only when dosage is higher than recommended. And fourth, rebound congestion is common with prolonged use of topical agents but is rare with oral agents.

Comparison of Phenylephrine and Pseudoephedrine

Phenylephrine is one of the most widely used nasal decongestants. The drug is administered topically as a single agent and orally as a component of combination preparations. When administered topically, phenylephrine is both fast and effective. When taken orally, the drug effect is insignificant, in large part because of extensive first-pass metabolism. Although it might seem logical to simply increase the dosage, this is not advisable because, even though absorption is poor, phenylephrine can still cause adverse cardiovascular and CNS effects.

Pseudoephedrine is available for oral administration. Compared with oral phenylephrine, pseudoephedrine is better absorbed, has a longer half-life, and is much more effective.

Antihistamine/Sympathomimetic and Antihistamine/Glucocorticoid Combinations

Some patients require combined therapy with a sympathomimetic or glucocorticoid in addition to an antihistamine. Although antihistamines alone are a first-line treatment, they do not relieve nasal congestion and may be inadequate for some patients. For these patients, addition of a sympathomimetic or glucocorticoid may be indicated. This can be accomplished in one of two ways: by giving the drugs separately or by using a combination product. Some popular combination products are listed in Table 61.5.

Ipratropium, an Anticholinergic Agent

Ipratropium bromide [Atrovent] is an anticholinergic agent. The drug is indicated for allergic rhinitis, asthma, and the common cold. To treat allergic rhinitis, ipratropium is administered as a nasal spray (0.03% and 0.06%). Blockade of cholinergic receptors inhibits secretions from the serous and seromucous glands lining the nasal mucosa and thereby decreases rhinorrhea. The drug does not decrease sneezing, nasal congestion, or postnasal drip. At the doses used for allergic rhinitis, side effects are minimal. The most common side effects are nasal drying and irritation. Ipratropium does not readily cross membranes because it is a quaternary ammonium compound, and hence systemic effects are absent. Dosages for allergic rhinitis in patients 12 years and older range from 2 sprays of 0.03% ipratropium (42 mcg total) per nostril 2 to 3 times a day to 2 sprays of 0.06% ipratropium (84 mcg total) per nostril 4 times a day. Use of ipratropium for asthma is discussed in Chapter 60.

Montelukast, a Leukotriene Antagonist

Montelukast [Singulair], originally approved for asthma, is now approved for seasonal and perennial allergic rhinitis as well. Benefits derive from blocking binding of leukotrienes to their receptors. In people with allergic rhinitis, leukotrienes act primarily to cause nasal congestion (by promoting vasodilation and by increasing vascular permeability). Hence, by blocking leukotriene receptors, montelukast relieves nasal congestion, although it has little effect on sneezing or itching. When used alone or in combination with an antihistamine, montelukast is less effective than intranasal glucocorticoids. Although montelukast is generally well tolerated, it can cause rare but serious neuropsychiatric effects, including agitation, aggression, hallucinations, depression, insomnia, restlessness, and suicidal thinking and behavior. Because of these adverse effects, and because beneficial effects are limited, it is probably best to reserve montelukast for patients who do not respond to or cannot tolerate intranasal glucocorticoids, antihistamines, or both. Administration is oral. Dosage, which varies with age, is the same as that used for asthma.

TABLE 61.5 ■ Some Antihistamine Combination Products

	Trade Name	Dosage
ANTIHISTAMINE/SYMPATHOMIMETIC		
Acrivastine/ pseudoephedrine	Semprex-D Capsules	8 mg/60 mg 4 times daily
Chlorpheniramine/ pseudoephedrine	Allerest Maximum Strength Tablets	4 mg/60 mg every 4–6 hr
Fexofenadine/ pseudoephedrine	Allegra-D 12-Hour Tablets	60 mg/120 mg twice daily
Loratadine/ pseudoephedrine	Claritin-D 12-Hour Tablets	5 mg/120 mg every 12 hr
Desloratadine/ pseudoephedrine	Clarinex-D 12-Hour Tablets	2.5 mg/120 mg every 12 hr
Triprolidine/ pseudoephedrine	Actifed Cold & Allergy Tablets	2.5 mg/60 mg every 4–6 hr
ANTIHISTAMINE/GLUCOCORTICOID		
Azelastine/ fluticasone propionate	Dymista	*Adults and children 12 yr and older:* 1 spray/nostril twice daily

Omalizumab

Omalizumab [Xolair] is a monoclonal antibody directed against IgE, an immunoglobulin (antibody) that plays a central role in the allergic release of inflammatory mediators from mast cells and basophils. Omalizumab is approved only for allergy-mediated asthma; however, several studies have demonstrated significant improvement of allergic symptoms. Because patients with ragweed-induced seasonal allergic rhinitis have achieved symptom relief with omalizumab when other drugs have been ineffective, this drug is sometimes prescribed off-label for management while clinical trials continue.

DRUGS FOR COUGH

Cough is a complex reflex involving the CNS, the peripheral nervous system, and the muscles of respiration. The cough reflex can be initiated by irritation of the bronchial mucosa as well as by stimuli arising at sites distant from the respiratory tract. Cough is often beneficial, serving to remove foreign matter and excess secretions from the bronchial tree. The productive cough that is characteristic of chronic lung disease (e.g., emphysema, asthma, bronchitis) should not be suppressed, for example. Not all cough, however, is useful. When cough is nonproductive, creates discomfort, or deprives patients of comfort or sleep, cough suppressant medication is appropriate. The most common use of cough medicines is suppression of nonproductive cough associated with the common cold and other upper respiratory infections.

Antitussives

Antitussives are drugs that suppress cough. Some agents act within the CNS; others act peripherally. The antitussives fall into two major groups: (1) opioid antitussives and (2) nonopioid antitussives. Interestingly, although the major antitussives—codeine, dextromethorphan, and diphenhydramine—are clearly effective against chronic nonproductive cough and experimentally induced cough, there is no good evidence that these drugs can suppress cough associated with the common cold.

Opioid Antitussives

All of the opioid analgesics have the ability to suppress cough. The two opioids used most often for cough suppression are *codeine* and *hydrocodone.* Both drugs act in the CNS to elevate cough threshold. Hydrocodone is somewhat more potent than codeine and carries a greater liability for abuse. The basic pharmacology of the opioids is discussed in Chapter 22.

Codeine

Codeine is the most effective cough suppressant available. The drug is active orally and can decrease both the frequency and intensity of cough. Doses are low, about $\frac{1}{10}$ those needed to relieve pain. At these doses, the risk for physical dependence is small.

Like all other opioids, codeine can suppress respiration. Accordingly, the drug should be employed with caution in patients with reduced respiratory reserve. In the event of overdose, respiratory depression may prove fatal. An opioid antagonist (e.g., naloxone) should be used to reverse toxicity.

When dispensed by itself, codeine has a significant potential for abuse and therefore is classified under Schedule II of the Controlled Substances Act. However, the abuse potential of the antitussive mixtures that contain codeine is low. Accordingly, these mixtures are classified under Schedule V.

For treatment of cough, the adult dosage is 10 to 20 mg orally, 4 to 6 times a day. Codeine is rarely recommended for children.

Nonopioid Antitussives

Dextromethorphan

Dextromethorphan is the most effective over-the-counter (OTC) nonopioid cough medicine and the most widely used of all cough medicines. Like the opioids, dextromethorphan acts in the CNS. Dextromethorphan is a derivative of the opioids; however, it does not produce typical opioid-like euphoria or physical dependence. Nonetheless, when taken in high doses, dextromethorphan can cause euphoria and is sometimes abused for this effect (see Chapter 33). Depending on the dose, subjective effects can range from mild inebriation to a state of mind-body dissociation, much like that caused by phencyclidine (PCP). At therapeutic doses, dextromethorphan does not depress respiration. Adverse effects are mild and rare. Dextromethorphan is the active ingredient in more than 140 nonprescription cough medicines. The usual adult dosage is 10 to 30 mg every 4 to 8 hours.

In the past, dextromethorphan was considered devoid of analgesic actions; however, it now appears the drug *can* reduce pain. The mechanism is blockade of receptors for *N*-methyl-D-aspartate (NMDA) in the brain and spinal cord. In contrast, opioids relieve pain primarily through activation of mu receptors. Although dextromethorphan has minimal analgesic effects when used alone, it can enhance analgesic effects of the opioids. For example, we can double the analgesic response to 30 mg of morphine by combining the morphine with 30 mg of dextromethorphan.

Other Nonopioid Antitussives

Diphenhydramine is an antihistamine with the ability to suppress cough. The mechanism is unclear. Like other antihistamines, diphenhydramine has sedative and anticholinergic properties. Cough suppression is achieved only at doses that produce prominent sedation. The usual adult dosage is 25 mg every 4 hours.

Benzonatate [Tessalon, Zonatuss] is a structural analog of two local anesthetics: tetracaine and procaine. The drug suppresses cough by decreasing the sensitivity of respiratory tract stretch receptors (components of the cough-reflex pathway). Adverse effects are usually mild (e.g., sedation, dizziness, constipation). Nonetheless, severe effects can occur in children and adults. In children younger than 2 years, accidental ingestion of just one or two capsules has been fatal. In older children and adults, overdose can cause seizures, dysrhythmia, and death. Smaller doses can cause confusion, chest numbness, visual hallucinations, and a burning sensation in the eyes. If the capsules are sucked or chewed, rather than swallowed, the drug can cause laryngospasm, bronchospasm, and circulatory collapse. Accordingly, benzonatate capsules should be swallowed intact. The usual adult dosage is 100 mg 3 times a day. Safety and efficacy have not been established in children younger than 10 years.

Expectorants and Mucolytics

Expectorants

An expectorant is a drug that renders cough more productive by stimulating the flow of respiratory tract secretions. A variety of compounds (e.g., ammonium chloride, iodide products) have been promoted for their supposed expectorant actions. However, in almost all cases, efficacy is questionable. One agent—guaifenesin [Mucinex, Humibid, others]—may be an exception. However, for this drug to be effective, doses higher than those normally employed may be needed.

Mucolytics

A mucolytic is a drug that reacts directly with mucus to make it more watery. This action should help make cough more productive. Two preparations—hypertonic saline and acetylcysteine—are employed for their mucolytic actions. Both are administered by inhalation. Unfortunately, both can trigger bronchospasm. Because of its sulfur content, acetylcysteine has the additional drawback of smelling like rotten eggs.

COLD REMEDIES: COMBINATION PREPARATIONS

Basic Considerations

The common cold is an acute *upper* respiratory infection of viral origin. Between 50% and 80% of colds are caused by the human rhinovirus, which can also cause serious infection of the *lower* respiratory tract. Characteristic symptoms of the common cold are rhinorrhea, nasal congestion, cough, sneezing, sore throat, hoarseness, headache, malaise, and myalgia; fever is common in children but rare in adults. Colds are self-limited and usually benign. Persistence or worsening of symptoms suggests development of a secondary bacterial infection. In the United States the economic burden of the cold is estimated at more than $60 billion a year.

There is no cure for the cold, so treatment is purely symptomatic. Because colds are caused by viruses, there is no justification for the routine use of antibiotics. These agents are appropriate only if a bacterial coinfection arises. There is no evidence that vitamin C or zinc can prevent or cure colds.

Because no single drug can relieve all symptoms of a cold, the pharmaceutical industry has formulated a vast number of cold remedies that contain a mixture of ingredients. These combination cold remedies should be reserved for patients with multiple symptoms. In addition, the combination chosen should contain only those agents that are appropriate for the symptoms at hand. Patients who require relief from just a single symptom (e.g., rhinitis, cough, or headache) are best treated with single-drug preparations.

Combination cold remedies frequently contain two or more of the following: (1) a nasal decongestant, (2) an antitussive, (3) an analgesic, (4) an antihistamine, and (5) caffeine. The purpose of the first three agents is self-evident. In contrast, the roles of antihistamines and caffeine require explanation. Because histamine has nothing to do with the symptoms of a cold, the purpose of including antihistamines is not to block histamine receptors. Rather, because of their anticholinergic actions, antihistamines are included to suppress mucus secretion. (This action can potentially worsen upper respiratory infections by thickening secretions, making them more difficult to drain. This may create an environment conducive to bacterial proliferation, which may lead to secondary bacterial infections such as sinusitis.) Caffeine is added to offset the sedative effects of the antihistamine.

Although they can be convenient, combination cold remedies do have disadvantages. As with all fixed-dose combinations, there is the chance that a dosage (e.g., 1 capsule or 1 tablet) that produces therapeutic levels of one ingredient may produce levels of other ingredients that are either excessive or subtherapeutic. In addition, the combination may contain ingredients that the patient does not need. Furthermore, under U.S. Food and Drug Administration (FDA) regulations, a brand-name product can be reformulated and then sold under the same name. Hence, without carefully reading the label, the consumer has no assurance that the brand-name product purchased contains the same amounts of the same drugs that were present in a previous version of that combination product.

Use in Young Children

Many experts believe that OTC cold remedies should not be used by young children. There is no proof of efficacy or safety in pediatric patients—and there *is* proof of the potential for serious harm. According to the Centers for Disease Control and Prevention, thousands of children have been taken to emergency departments for management of adverse effects related to cough or cold products. Presenting symptoms have included convulsions, tachycardia, hallucinations, and impaired consciousness. Some children died. In early 2008, the FDA recommended that OTC cold remedies no longer be given to children younger than 2 years, owing to the risk for potentially life-threatening events. The FDA is still reviewing the safety of these drugs in children 2 to 11 years old. In the meantime, citing inadequate effectiveness, significant adverse effects, and common misuse, the American Academy of Pediatrics recommended restricting use of cough and cold medicines to children older than 6 years. Manufacturers voluntarily revised the labels of children's cold and cough preparations to indicate they should not be used in children younger than 4 years. In addition, for products that contain an antihistamine, manufacturers added a warning against using these drugs to sedate children.

After these interventions, emergency visits related to cold and cough medications decreased significantly for children younger than 4 years. To minimize harm to pediatric patients, parents should do the following:

- Avoid OTC cold remedies in children younger than 4 to 6 years.
- Only use products labeled for pediatric use.
- Consult a health care professional before giving these drugs to a child.
- Read all product safety information before dosing.
- Use the measuring device provided with the product.
- Discontinue the medicine and seek professional care if the child's condition worsens or fails to improve.
- Avoid using antihistamine-containing products to sedate children.

UNIT XVI
Gastrointestinal Drugs

CHAPTER 62
Drugs for Peptic Ulcer Disease

Laura D. Rosenthal, DNP, ACNP, FAANP

Peptic ulcer disease (PUD) refers to a group of upper gastrointestinal (GI) disorders characterized by varying degrees of erosion of the gut wall. Severe ulcers can be complicated by hemorrhage and perforation. Although peptic ulcers can develop in any region exposed to acid and pepsin, ulceration is most common in the lesser curvature of the stomach and the duodenum. PUD is a common disorder that affects about 10% of Americans at some time in their lives. About 4 million Americans get ulcers each year. Before the mid-1990s, PUD was considered a chronic, relapsing disorder of unknown cause and with no known cure; therapy promoted healing but did not prevent ulcer recurrence. Today, thanks to the pioneering work of two Australians—Barry J. Marshall and J. Robin Warren—we know that most cases of PUD are caused by infection with *Helicobacter pylori* and that eradication of this bacterium not only promotes healing but also greatly reduces the chance of recurrence.

PATHOGENESIS OF PEPTIC ULCERS

Peptic ulcers develop when there is an imbalance between mucosal defensive factors and aggressive factors (Fig. 62.1). The major defensive factors are mucus and bicarbonate. The major aggressive factors are *H. pylori,* nonsteroidal antiinflammatory drugs (NSAIDs), gastric acid, and pepsin.

Defensive Factors

Defensive factors serve the physiologic role of protecting the stomach and duodenum from self-digestion. When defenses are intact, ulcers are unlikely. Conversely, when defenses are compromised, aggressive factors are able to cause injury. Two important agents that can weaken defenses are *H. pylori* and NSAIDs.

Mucus

Mucus is secreted continuously by cells of the GI mucosa, forming a barrier that protects underlying cells from attack by acid and pepsin.

Bicarbonate

Bicarbonate is secreted by epithelial cells of the stomach and duodenum. Most bicarbonate remains trapped in the mucus layer, where it serves to neutralize any hydrogen ions that penetrate the mucus. Bicarbonate produced by the pancreas is secreted into the lumen of the duodenum, where it neutralizes acid delivered from the stomach.

Blood Flow

Sufficient blood flow to cells of the GI mucosa is essential for maintaining mucosal integrity. If submucosal blood flow is reduced, the resultant local ischemia can lead to cell injury, thereby increasing vulnerability to attack by acid and pepsin.

Prostaglandins

Prostaglandins play an important role in maintaining defenses. These compounds stimulate secretion of mucus and bicarbonate, and they promote vasodilation, which helps maintain submucosal blood flow. They provide additional protection by suppressing secretion of gastric acid.

Aggressive Factors

Helicobacter pylori

H. pylori is a gram-negative bacillus that can colonize the stomach and duodenum. By taking up residence in the space between epithelial cells and the mucus barrier that protects these cells, the bacterium manages to escape destruction by acid and pepsin. When established, *H. pylori* can remain in the GI tract for decades. Although about half of the world's population is infected with *H. pylori,* most infected people never develop symptomatic PUD.

Why do we think *H. pylori* causes PUD? First, between 60% and 75% of patients with PUD have *H. pylori* infection. Second, duodenal ulcers are much more common among people with *H. pylori* infection than among people who are not infected. Third, eradication of the bacterium promotes ulcer healing. And fourth, eradication of the bacterium minimizes ulcer recurrence. (One-year recurrence rates approach 80% when *H. pylori* remains present, compared with only 10% when the organism is gone.)

Although the mechanism by which *H. pylori* promotes ulcers has not been firmly established, likely possibilities are enzymatic degradation of the protective mucus layer, elaboration of a cytotoxin that injures mucosal cells, and infiltration of neutrophils and other inflammatory cells in response to the bacterium's presence. Also, *H. pylori* produces *urease,* an

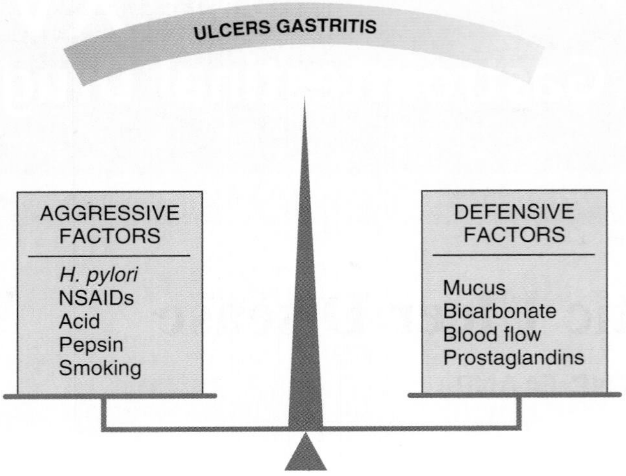

Figure 62.1 ▪ The relationship of mucosal defenses and aggressive factors to health and peptic ulcer disease. When aggressive factors outweigh mucosal defenses, gastritis and peptic ulcers result. NSAIDs, nonsteroidal antiinflammatory drugs.

enzyme that forms carbon dioxide and ammonia (from urea in gastric juice); both compounds are potentially toxic to the gastric mucosa.

In addition to its role in PUD, *H. pylori* appears to promote gastric cancer. In fact, the bacterium has been declared a type 1 carcinogen by the International Agency for Research on Cancer. There is a strong association between *H. pylori* infection and the presence of gastric mucosa-associated lymphoid tissue (MALT) lymphomas. Furthermore, among patients with localized MALT lymphoma, eradicating *H. pylori* produces tumor regression in 60% to 90% of cases. In one long-term study, treatment of *H. pylori* reduced the risk for gastric adenocarcinoma by 40% after 15 years.

Nonsteroidal Antiinflammatory Drugs

NSAIDs are the underlying cause of many gastric ulcers and some duodenal ulcers. As discussed in Chapter 55, aspirin and other NSAIDs inhibit the biosynthesis of prostaglandins. By doing so, they can decrease submucosal blood flow, suppress secretion of mucus and bicarbonate, and promote secretion of gastric acid. Furthermore, NSAIDs can irritate the mucosa directly. NSAID-induced ulcers are most likely with long-term, high-dose therapy.

Gastric Acid

Gastric acid is an absolute requirement for peptic ulcer generation: in the absence of acid, no ulcer will form. Acid causes ulcers directly by injuring cells of the GI mucosa and indirectly by activating pepsin, a proteolytic enzyme. In most cases, acid hypersecretion, by itself, is insufficient to cause ulcers. In fact, in most patients with gastric ulcers, acid secretion is normal or reduced, and among patients with duodenal ulcers, only one third produce excessive amounts of acid. From these observations, we can conclude that, in most patients with peptic ulcers, factors in addition to acid must be involved.

Zollinger-Ellison syndrome is the primary disorder in which hypersecretion of acid alone causes ulcers. The syndrome is caused by a tumor that secretes gastrin, a hormone that stimulates gastric acid production. The amount of acid produced is so large that it overwhelms mucosal defenses. Zollinger-Ellison syndrome is a rare disorder that accounts for only 0.1% of duodenal ulcers.

Pepsin

Pepsin is a proteolytic enzyme present in gastric juice. Like gastric acid, pepsin can injure unprotected cells of the gastric and duodenal mucosa.

Smoking

Smoking delays ulcer healing and increases the risk for recurrence. Possible mechanisms include reduction of the beneficial effects of antiulcer medications, reduced secretion of bicarbonate, and accelerated gastric emptying, which would deliver more acid to the duodenum.

Summary

Infection with *H. pylori* is the most common cause of gastric and duodenal ulcers. However, among people whose PUD can be ascribed to *H. pylori,* additional factors must be involved because more than 50% of the population harbors *H. pylori* but only 10% develop ulcers. Factors that may increase the risk for PUD in people infected with *H. pylori* include smoking, increased acid secretion, and reduced bicarbonate production. The second most common cause of gastric ulcers is NSAIDs. Hypersecretion of acid underlies a few cases of PUD that are not caused by *H. pylori* or NSAIDs.

OVERVIEW OF TREATMENT

Drug Therapy

The goals of drug therapy are to (1) alleviate symptoms, (2) promote healing, (3) prevent complications (hemorrhage, perforation, obstruction), and (4) prevent recurrence. With the exception of antibiotics, the drugs employed do not alter the disease process. Rather, they simply create conditions conducive to healing. Because nonantibiotic therapies do not cure ulcers, the relapse rate after their discontinuation is high. In contrast, the relapse rate after antibiotic therapy is low.

Classes of Antiulcer Drugs

As shown in Table 62.1, the antiulcer drugs fall into five major groups:

- Antibiotics
- Antisecretory agents (proton pump inhibitors [PPIs], histamine-2 [H_2] receptor antagonists)
- Mucosal protectants
- Antisecretory agents that enhance mucosal defenses
- Antacids

From this classification, we can see that drugs act in three basic ways to promote ulcer healing. Specifically, they can (1) eradicate *H. pylori* (antibiotics do this), (2) reduce gastric acidity (antisecretory agents, misoprostol, and antacids do this), and (3) enhance mucosal defenses (sucralfate and misoprostol do this).

TABLE 62.1 ■ Classification of Antiulcer Drugs

Class	Drugs	Availability	Usual Daily Adult Dosing	Mechanism of Action
ANTIBIOTICS	Amoxicillin [Amoxil]	500-mg capsules	2000 mg	Eradicate *Helicobacter pylori*
	Bismuth [Pepto-Bismol]	262.4-mg tablets	3000 mg	
	Clarithromycin [Biaxin]	500-mg tablets	1000 mg	
	Metronidazole [Flagyl]	125-mg tablets	1000 mg	
	Tetracycline (generic only)	125-mg tablets	1500 mg	
	Tinidazole [Tindamax]	500-mg tablets	1000 mg	
ANTISECRETORY AGENTS				
H_2 receptor antagonists	Cimetidine [Tagamet]	200-, 300-, 400-, 800-mg tablets 300-mg/mL solution	800 mg Lower dose with renal impairment	Suppress acid secretion by blocking H_2 receptors on parietal cells
	Famotidine [Pepcid]	20-, 40-mg tablets 20-, 40-mg orally disintegrating tablets	Ulcer treatment 40 mg GERD 20–40 mg	
	Nizatidine [Axid]	75-, 150-, 300-mg capsules 15-mg/mL solution	300 mg	
	Ranitidine [Zantac]	75-, 150-, 300-mg tablets 150-, 300-mg capsules 15-mg/mL syrup	300 mg	
Proton pump inhibitors	Dexlansoprazole [Dexilant]	30-, 60-mg capsules	Initial erosive esophagitis: 60 mg Maintenance: 30 mg	Suppress acid secretion by inhibiting H^+,K^+-ATPase, the enzyme that makes gastric acid
	Esomeprazole [Nexium]	20-, 40-mg delayed-release capsules 2.5-, 5-, 10-, 20-, 40-mg enteric-coated granules	20 mg	
	Lansoprazole [Prevacid]	15-, 30-mg delayed-release capsules 15-, 30-mg orally disintegrating delayed-release tablets	30 mg	
	Omeprazole [Prilosec, Zegerid, Losec ♣]	10-, 20-, 40-mg delayed-release capsules 20-, 40-mg delayed-release tablets 2.5-, 10-mg suspension 20-, 40-mg powder for reconstitution	20 mg	
	Pantoprazole [Protonix, Pantoloc ♣]	20-, 40-mg delayed-release tablets 40-mg enteric-coated granules	40 mg	
	Rabeprazole [Aciphex, Pariet ♣]	20-mg delayed-release tablets 5-, 10-mg delayed-release capsules	20 mg	
MUCOSAL PROTECTANT	Sucralfate [Carafate, Sulcrate ♣]	1-mg tablets 1-g/10 mL oral suspension	4 g	Forms a barrier over the ulcer crater that protects against acid and pepsin
ANTISECRETORY AGENT THAT ENHANCES MUCOSAL DEFENSES	Misoprostol [Cytotec]	100-, 200-mcg tablets	800 mcg	Protects against NSAID-induced ulcers by stimulating secretion of mucus and bicarbonate, maintaining submucosal blood flow, and suppressing secretion of gastric acid
ANTACIDS	Aluminum hydroxide	Many forms	—	React with gastric acid to form neutral salts
	Calcium carbonate	Many forms	—	
	Magnesium hydroxide	Many forms	—	

GERD, gastroesophageal reflux disease; NSAID, nonsteroidal antiinflammatory drug.

Drug Selection

Helicobacter pylori–Associated Ulcers

In 1997, a National Institutes of Health Consensus Development Conference recommended that all patients with gastric or duodenal ulcers and documented *H. pylori* infection be treated with antibiotics. This recommendation applies to patients with newly diagnosed PUD, recurrent PUD, and PUD in which use of NSAIDs is a contributing factor. To hasten healing and relieve symptoms, an antisecretory agent should be given along with the antibiotics. By eliminating *H. pylori,* antibiotics can cure PUD and can thereby prevent recurrence. Diagnosis of *H. pylori* infection and specific antibiotic regimens are discussed later under "Antibacterial Drugs."

NSAID-Induced Ulcers

Prophylaxis. For patients with risk factors for ulcer development (e.g., older than 60 years, history of ulcers, high-dose NSAID therapy), prophylactic therapy is indicated. PPIs (e.g., omeprazole) are preferred. Misoprostol is also effective but can cause diarrhea. Antacids, sucralfate, and H_2 receptor blockers are not recommended.

Treatment. NSAID-induced ulcers can be treated with any ulcer medication. However, H_2 receptor blockers and PPIs are preferred. If possible, the offending NSAID should be discontinued, so as to accelerate healing. If the NSAID cannot be discontinued, a PPI is the best choice to promote healing.

Evaluation

We can evaluate ulcer healing by monitoring for relief of pain and by radiologic or endoscopic examination of the ulcer site. Unfortunately, evaluation is seldom straightforward because cessation of pain and disappearance of the ulcer rarely coincide: in most cases, pain subsides before complete healing. However, the converse may also be true: pain may persist even though endoscopic or radiologic examination reveals healing is complete.

Eradication of *H. pylori* can be determined with several methods, including breath tests, serologic tests, stool tests, and microscopic observation of a stained biopsy sample.

A Note About the Effects of Drugs on Pepsin

Pepsin is a proteolytic enzyme that can contribute to ulcer formation. The enzyme promotes ulcers by breaking down protein in the gut wall.

Like most enzymes, pepsin is sensitive to pH. As pH rises from 1.3 (the usual pH of the stomach) to 2, peptic activity increases by a factor of 4. As pH goes even higher, peptic activity begins to decline. At a pH of 5, peptic activity drops below baseline rates. When pH exceeds 6 to 7, pepsin undergoes irreversible inactivation.

Because the activity of pepsin is pH dependent, drugs that elevate gastric pH (e.g., antacids, H_2 antagonists, PPIs) can cause peptic activity to increase, thereby enhancing pepsin's destructive effects. For example, treatment that produces a 99% reduction in gastric acidity will cause pH to rise from a base level of 1.3 up to 3.3. At pH 3.3, peptic activity will be significantly increased. To avoid activation of pepsin, drugs that reduce acidity should be administered in doses sufficient to raise gastric pH above 5.

Nondrug Therapy

Optimal antiulcer therapy requires implementation of nondrug measures in addition to drug therapy.

Diet

Despite commonly held beliefs, diet plays a minor role in ulcer management. The traditional "ulcer diet," consisting of bland foods together with milk or cream, does not accelerate healing. Furthermore, there is no convincing evidence that caffeine-containing beverages (coffee, tea, colas) promote ulcer formation or interfere with recovery. A change in *eating pattern* may be beneficial: consumption of five or six small meals a day, rather than three larger ones, can reduce fluctuations in intragastric pH and may thereby facilitate recovery.

Other Nondrug Measures

Smoking is associated with an increased incidence of ulcers and also delays recovery. Accordingly, cigarettes should be avoided. Because of their ulcerogenic actions, *aspirin and other NSAIDs* should be avoided by patients with PUD. The exception to this rule is use of aspirin to prevent cardiovascular disease; in the low doses employed, aspirin is only a small factor in PUD. There are no hard data indicating that *alcohol* contributes to PUD. However, if the patient notes a temporal relationship between alcohol consumption and exacerbation of symptoms, then alcohol use should stop. Many people feel that reduction of *stress and anxiety* may encourage ulcer healing; however, there is no good evidence that this is true.

ANTIBACTERIAL DRUGS

Antibacterial drugs should be given to all patients with gastric or duodenal ulcers and confirmed infection with *H. pylori.* Antibiotics are not recommended for asymptomatic individuals who test positive for *H. pylori.*

Antibiotics Employed

The antibiotics employed most often are clarithromycin, amoxicillin, bismuth, metronidazole, and tetracycline. None is effective alone. Furthermore, if these drugs *are* used alone, the risk for developing resistance is increased.

Clarithromycin

Clarithromycin [Biaxin] suppresses growth of *H. pylori* by inhibiting protein synthesis. In the absence of resistance, treatment is highly effective. Unfortunately, the rate of resistance is rising, exceeding 20% in some areas. The most common side effects are nausea, diarrhea, and distortion of taste. The basic pharmacology of clarithromycin is presented in Chapter 71.

Amoxicillin

H. pylori is highly sensitive to amoxicillin. The rate of resistance is low, only about 3%. Amoxicillin kills bacteria by disrupting the cell wall. Antibacterial activity is highest at neutral pH and hence can be enhanced by reducing gastric acidity with an antisecretory agent (e.g., omeprazole). The most common side effect is diarrhea. The basic pharmacology of amoxicillin is discussed in Chapter 69.

Bismuth

Bismuth compounds—bismuth subsalicylate and bismuth subcitrate—act topically to disrupt the cell wall of *H. pylori,* thereby causing lysis and death. Bismuth may also inhibit urease activity and may prevent *H. pylori* from adhering to the gastric surface.

Bismuth can impart a harmless black coloration to the tongue and stool. Patients should be forewarned. Stool discoloration may confound interpretation of gastric bleeding. Long-term therapy may carry a risk for neurologic injury.

Tetracycline

Tetracycline, an inhibitor of bacterial protein synthesis, is highly active against *H. pylori.* Resistance is rare (less than 1%). Because tetracycline can stain developing teeth, it should not be used by pregnant women or young children. The pharmacology of tetracycline is discussed in Chapter 71.

Metronidazole

Metronidazole [Flagyl] is very effective against sensitive strains of *H. pylori.* Unfortunately, more than 40% of strains are now resistant. The most common side effects are nausea and headache. A disulfiram-like reaction can occur if metronidazole is used with alcohol, and hence alcohol must be avoided. Metronidazole should not be taken during pregnancy. The basic pharmacology of metronidazole is discussed in Chapter 81.

Tinidazole

Tinidazole [Tindamax] is very similar to metronidazole and shares that drug's adverse effects and interactions. Like metronidazole, tinidazole can cause a disulfiram-like reaction and hence must not be combined with alcohol. The basic pharmacology of tinidazole is discussed in Chapter 81.

Antibiotic Regimens

In 2007, the American College of Gastroenterology (ACG) issued updated guidelines for managing *H. pylori* infection. To minimize emergence of resistance, the guidelines recommend using at least two antibiotics, and preferably three. An antisecretory agent—PPI or histamine-2 receptor antagonist (H_2RA)—should be included as well. Eradication rates are good with a 10-day course and slightly better with a 14-day course.

Table 62.2 presents four ACG-recommended regimens. In regions where resistance to clarithromycin is low (below 20%), the preferred treatment is *clarithromycin-based triple therapy,* consisting of clarithromycin plus amoxicillin plus a PPI. For patients with penicillin allergy, metronidazole can be substituted for amoxicillin. In regions where resistance to clarithromycin is high (above 20%), the preferred regimen is *bismuth-based quadruple therapy,* consisting of bismuth subsalicylate plus metronidazole plus tetracycline, all three combined with a PPI or an H_2RA. For patients who can't use triple therapy or quadruple therapy, *sequential therapy* is an option. This regimen consists of taking a PPI plus amoxicillin for 5 days, followed by a PPI plus clarithromycin plus tinidazole for 5 days. At this time, the efficacy of sequential therapy in North America has not been established.

For several reasons, compliance with antibiotic therapy can be difficult. First, antibiotic regimens are complex, requiring the patient to ingest as many as 12 pills a day. Second, side effects—especially nausea and diarrhea—are common. Third, a course of treatment is somewhat expensive. However, it costs much less to eradicate *H. pylori* with antibiotics than it does to treat ulcers over and over again with traditional antiulcer drugs, which merely promote healing without eliminating the cause.

HISTAMINE-2 RECEPTOR ANTAGONISTS

The H_2RAs are effective drugs for treating gastric and duodenal ulcers. These agents promote ulcer healing by suppressing secretion of gastric acid. Four H_2RAs are available: cimetidine, ranitidine, famotidine, and nizatidine. All four are equally effective. Serious side effects are uncommon.

TABLE 62.2 ▪ First-Line Regimens for Eradicating *Helicobacter pylori*

Drugs	Duration (days)	Eradication Rate (%)	Comments
CLARITHROMYCIN-BASED TRIPLE THERAPY 1 Standard-dose PPI* Clarithromycin (500 mg twice daily) Amoxicillin (1 g twice daily)	10–14	70–85	Consider in non–penicillin-allergic patients who have not previously received clarithromycin or another macrolide
CLARITHROMYCIN-BASED TRIPLE THERAPY 2 Standard-dose PPI* Clarithromycin (500 mg twice daily) Metronidazole (500 mg twice daily)	10–14	70–85	Consider in penicillin-allergic patients who have not previously received a macrolide or are unable to tolerate bismuth quadruple therapy
BISMUTH-BASED QUADRUPLE THERAPY Bismuth subsalicylate (525 mg 4 times daily) Metronidazole (250 mg 4 times daily) Tetracycline (500 mg 4 times daily) Standard-dose PPI* or ranitidine (150 mg twice daily)	10–14	75–90	Consider in penicillin-allergic patients and in patients with clarithromycin-resistant *H. pylori*
SEQUENTIAL THERAPY Standard-dose PPI* + amoxicillin (1 g twice daily) for 5 days, followed by: Standard-dose PPI* + clarithromycin (500 mg once daily) + tinidazole (500 mg twice daily) for 5 days	10	More than 90	Efficacy in North America requires validation

*Standard doses for PPIs are as follows: dexlansoprazole, 30 to 60 mg once daily; esomeprazole, 40 mg once daily; lansoprazole, 30 mg twice daily; omeprazole, 40 mg twice daily; pantoprazole, 40 mg twice daily; and rabeprazole, 20 mg twice daily.

Adapted from Chey WD, Wong BCY, and Practice Parameters Committee of the American College of Gastroenterology. American College of Gastroenterology guideline on the management of *Helicobacter pylori* infection. Am J Gastroenterol 2007;102:1808-1825.

Cimetidine

Cimetidine [Tagamet] was the first H_2RA available and will serve as our prototype for the group. At one time, cimetidine was the most frequently prescribed drug in the United States.

Prototype Drugs

DRUGS FOR PEPTIC ULCER DISEASE

Antibiotic (for *Helicobacter pylori*)
Amoxicillin/clarithromycin/omeprazole

Histamine-2 Receptor Antagonist
Cimetidine

Proton Pump Inhibitor
Omeprazole

Mucosal Protectant
Sucralfate

Antacid
Aluminum hydroxide/magnesium hydroxide

Mechanism of Action

Histamine acts through two types of receptors, named H_1 and H_2. Activation of H_1 receptors produces symptoms of allergy. Activation of H_2 receptors, which are located on parietal cells of the stomach (Fig. 62.2), promotes secretion of gastric acid. By blocking H_2 receptors, cimetidine reduces both the volume of gastric juice and its hydrogen ion concentration. Cimetidine suppresses basal acid secretion and secretion stimulated by gastrin and acetylcholine. Because cimetidine produces selective blockade of H_2 receptors, the drug cannot suppress symptoms of allergy.

Pharmacokinetics

Cimetidine may be administered by the oral, intramuscular (IM), or intravenous (IV) route. Comparable blood levels are achieved with all three routes. When the drug is taken orally, food decreases the rate of absorption but not the extent. Hence, if cimetidine is taken with meals, absorption will be slowed and beneficial effects prolonged. Cimetidine crosses the blood-brain barrier—albeit with difficulty—and central nervous system (CNS) side effects can occur. Although some hepatic metabolism takes place, most of each dose is eliminated intact in the urine. The half-life is relatively short (about 2 hours) but increases in patients with renal impairment. Accordingly, dosage should be reduced in these patients.

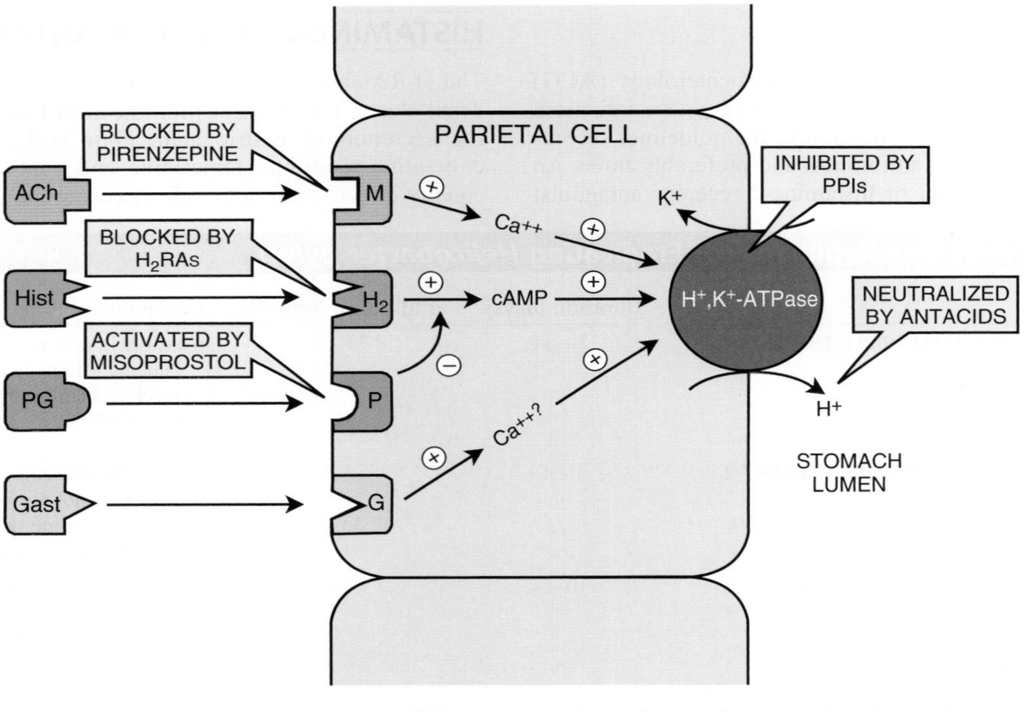

Figure 62.2 ■ A model of the regulation of gastric acid secretion showing the actions of antisecretory drugs and antacids.
Production of gastric acid is stimulated by three endogenous compounds: (1) acetylcholine (ACh) acting at muscarinic (M) receptors; (2) histamine (Hist) acting at histamine-2 (H_2) receptors; and (3) gastrin (Gast) acting at gastrin (G) receptors. As indicated, all three compounds act through intracellular messengers—either calcium (Ca^{++}) or cyclic adenosine monophosphate (cAMP)—to increase the activity of H^+,K^+-ATPase, the enzyme that actually produces gastric acid. Prostaglandins (PG) decrease acid production, perhaps by suppressing production of intracellular cAMP. The actions of H_2 receptor antagonists (H_2RAs), proton pump inhibitors (PPIs), and other drugs are indicated. (P, prostaglandin receptor.)

Therapeutic Uses

Gastric and Duodenal Ulcers

Cimetidine promotes healing of gastric and duodenal ulcers. To heal duodenal ulcers, 4 to 6 weeks of therapy are generally required. To heal gastric ulcers, 8 to 12 weeks may be needed. Long-term therapy with low doses may be given as prophylaxis against recurrence of gastric and duodenal ulcers.

Gastroesophageal Reflux Disease (GERD)

Reflux esophagitis is an inflammatory condition caused by reflux of gastric contents back into the esophagus. Cimetidine is a drug of choice for relieving symptoms. However, cimetidine does little to hasten healing.

Zollinger-Ellison Syndrome

This syndrome is characterized by hypersecretion of gastric acid and development of peptic ulcers. The underlying cause is secretion of gastrin from a gastrin-producing tumor. Cimetidine can promote healing of ulcers in patients with Zollinger-Ellison syndrome, but only if high doses are employed. At these doses, significant adverse effects can occur.

Heartburn, Acid Indigestion, and Sour Stomach

Cimetidine is available over the counter to treat these common acid-related symptoms.

Adverse Effects

The incidence of side effects is low, and those that do occur are usually benign.

Antiandrogenic Effects

Cimetidine binds to androgen receptors, producing receptor blockade. As a result, the drug can cause gynecomastia, reduced libido, and impotence—all of which reverse when dosing stops.

CNS Effects

Effects on the CNS are most likely in older adults who have renal or hepatic impairment. Possible reactions include confusion, hallucinations, CNS depression, and CNS excitation.

Pneumonia

Elevation of gastric pH with an antisecretory agent increases the risk for pneumonia because, when gastric acidity is reduced, bacterial colonization of the stomach increases, resulting in a secondary increase in colonization of the respiratory tract. Among people using an H_2RA, the *relative* risk for acquiring pneumonia is doubled. However, the *absolute* risk is still low (about 1 extra case for every 500 people using the drug).

Other Adverse Effects

When administered by IV bolus, cimetidine can cause hypotension and dysrhythmias. These reactions are rare and do not occur with oral therapy. By reducing gastric acidity, cimetidine may permit growth of Candida in the stomach. Hematologic effects (neutropenia, leukopenia, thrombocytopenia) occur rarely. Minor side effects include headache, dizziness, myalgia, nausea, diarrhea, constipation, rash, and pruritus.

Drug Interactions

Interactions Related to Inhibition of Drug Metabolism

Cimetidine inhibits hepatic drug-metabolizing enzymes and hence can cause levels of many other drugs to rise. Drugs of particular concern are *warfarin, phenytoin, theophylline,* and *lidocaine,* all of which have a narrow margin of safety. If these drugs are used with cimetidine, their dosages should be reduced.

Antacids

Antacids can decrease absorption of cimetidine. Accordingly, cimetidine and antacids should be administered at least 1 hour apart.

Ranitidine

Ranitidine [Zantac] shares many of the properties of cimetidine. However, although similar to cimetidine, the drug differs in three important respects: ranitidine is more potent, produces fewer adverse effects, and causes fewer drug interactions.

Actions

Like cimetidine, ranitidine suppresses secretion of gastric acid by blocking H_2 receptors on gastric parietal cells. It does not block H_1 receptors and hence does not reduce symptoms of allergy.

Pharmacokinetics

Ranitidine can be administered by the oral, IM, or IV route. Oral bioavailability is about 50%. In contrast to cimetidine, ranitidine is absorbed at the same rate in the presence or absence of food. Ranitidine's ability to enter the CNS is even less than that of cimetidine. Elimination is by hepatic metabolism and renal excretion. Accumulation will occur in patients with renal impairment unless the dosage is reduced. The half-life is 2 to 3 hours.

Adverse Effects

Significant side effects are uncommon. Because ranitidine penetrates the blood-brain barrier poorly, CNS effects are rare. In contrast to cimetidine, ranitidine does not bind to androgen receptors and hence does not cause antiandrogenic effects (e.g., gynecomastia, impotence). Elevation of gastric pH may increase the risk for pneumonia.

Drug Interactions

Ranitidine has few drug interactions. In contrast to cimetidine, ranitidine is a weak inhibitor of hepatic drug-metabolizing enzymes and therefore does not greatly depress metabolism of other drugs. Antacids have a small effect on ranitidine absorption.

Therapeutic Uses

Ranitidine has the same indications as cimetidine: (1) short-term treatment of gastric and duodenal ulcers, (2) prophylaxis of recurrent duodenal ulcers, (3) treatment of Zollinger-Ellison syndrome and other hypersecretory states, and (4) treatment of GERD. Because it produces fewer side effects than cimetidine, and because of its greater potency, ranitidine is preferred to cimetidine for treating hypersecretory states (e.g., Zollinger-Ellison syndrome).

Famotidine

Basic and Clinical Pharmacology

Famotidine [Pepcid, Pepcid AC] is much like ranitidine. The drug is approved for treatment and prevention of duodenal ulcers and for treatment of gastric ulcers, GERD, and hypersecretory states (e.g., Zollinger-Ellison syndrome). An over-the-counter formulation is approved for heartburn, acid indigestion, and sour stomach. Like ranitidine, famotidine does not bind to androgen receptors and hence does not have antiandrogenic effects. Elevation of gastric pH may increase the risk for pneumonia. Famotidine does not inhibit hepatic drug-metabolizing enzymes and hence does not suppress the metabolism of other drugs.

Nizatidine

Basic and Clinical Pharmacology

Nizatidine [Axid] is much like ranitidine and famotidine. The drug is used to treat and prevent duodenal ulcers and to treat gastric ulcers, GERD, heartburn, acid indigestion, and sour stomach. Like ranitidine and famotidine, nizatidine does not have antiandrogenic effects and does not inhibit the metabolism of other drugs. Elevation of gastric pH may increase the risk for pneumonia.

PROTON PUMP INHIBITORS

The PPIs are the most effective drugs we have for suppressing gastric acid secretion. Indications include gastric and duodenal ulcers and GERD. Similarities among the PPIs are more profound than the differences. Therefore selecting among them is based largely on cost and prescriber preference.

Although PPIs are generally well tolerated, they *can* increase the risk for serious adverse events, including fractures, pneumonia, acid rebound, and, possibly, intestinal infection with *Clostridium difficile.* To ensure that the benefits of treatment outweigh the risks, treatment should be limited to appropriate candidates, who should take the lowest dose needed for the shortest time possible.

Omeprazole

Omeprazole [Prilosec, Prilosec OTC, Zegerid, Zegerid OTC, Losec ♣] was the first PPI available and will serve as our prototype for the group. Acid suppression is greater than with the H_2RAs. Side effects from short-term therapy are minimal.

Mechanism of Action

Omeprazole is a prodrug that undergoes conversion to its active form within parietal cells of the stomach. The active form then causes irreversible inhibition of H^+,K^+-ATPase (proton pump), the enzyme that generates gastric acid (see Fig. 62.2). Because it blocks the final common pathway of gastric acid production, omeprazole can inhibit basal and stimulated acid release. A single 30-mg oral dose reduces acid production by 97% within 2 hours. Because inhibition of the ATPase is not reversible, effects persist until new enzyme is synthesized. Partial recovery occurs 3 to 5 days after stopping treatment. Full recovery may take weeks.

Pharmacokinetics

After oral dosing, about 50% of the drug reaches the systemic circulation. Omeprazole undergoes hepatic metabolism followed by renal excretion. The plasma half-life is short—about 1 hour. However, because omeprazole acts by irreversible enzyme inhibition, effects persist long after the drug has left the body.

Omeprazole is acid labile and hence must be protected from stomach acid. To accomplish this, the drug is formulated in a capsule that contains protective enteric-coated granules. The capsule dissolves in the stomach, but the granules remain intact until they reach the relatively alkaline environment of the duodenum.

Therapeutic Use

Omeprazole is approved for short-term therapy of duodenal ulcers, gastric ulcers, erosive esophagitis, and GERD and for long-term therapy of hypersecretory conditions (e.g., Zollinger-Ellison syndrome). Except for therapy of hypersecretory states, treatment should be limited to 4 to 8 weeks.

In hospitals, omeprazole and other PPIs are widely used to prevent stress ulcers. However, about two thirds of patients who receive PPIs don't really need them. Ulcer prophylaxis is indicated only for patients in intensive care units, and then only if they have an additional risk factor, such as multiple trauma, spinal cord injury, or prolonged mechanical ventilation (more than 48 hours). General medical and surgical patients are at low risk for stress ulcers and should not receive PPIs for prophylaxis.

How does omeprazole compare with H_2RAs? Omeprazole and other PPIs reduce 24-hour acid secretion by 90%, compared with 65% for H_2RAs. Also, PPIs act faster than H_2RAs to reduce gastric acidity and relieve ulcer symptoms. Patients who fail to respond to H_2RAs can often benefit from a PPI.

GERD is a common disorder characterized by heartburn and acid regurgitation. The disease is formally defined by the presence of troublesome symptoms or complications caused by passage of gastric contents into the esophagus. Among American adults, heartburn develops in 44% at least once a month, in 14% at least once a week, and in up to 7% every day. GERD is also common among children.

GERD is associated with a wide range of symptoms and complications. On the basis of endoscopic examination, patients fall into two major groups: those with *erosive esophagitis* and those with *nonerosive reflux disease* (NERD). Erosive esophagitis is characterized by breaks in the esophageal mucosa. In contrast, mucosal breaks are absent in people with NERD. Less than 50% of patients with GERD have the erosive form. Complications of erosive GERD include difficulty swallowing, painful swallowing, esophageal stricture, ulcers, GI bleeding, anemia, and persistent vomiting. Erosive GERD can also lead to esophageal adenocarcinoma and Barrett esophagus, a premalignant condition that can evolve into adenocarcinoma.

The primary problem is inappropriate relaxation of the lower esophageal sphincter (LES), a ring of smooth muscle that normally prevents reflux of gastric acid. In people with GERD, the LES undergoes frequent, transient relaxation, thereby allowing pressure in the stomach to force gastric contents up into the esophagus. Other factors that can contribute to GERD include obesity, hiatal hernia, delayed gastric emptying, and impaired clearance of acid from the esophagus. Of note, *Helicobacter pylori,* the bacterium that causes most gastric and duodenal ulcers, appears to play little or no role in GERD.

We can treat GERD with drugs or with surgery. For most patients, drugs are preferred. As a rule, surgery should be reserved for young, healthy patients who either cannot or will not take drugs chronically. With either drug therapy or surgery, treatment has three goals: relief of symptoms, promotion of healing, and prevention of complications.

For drug therapy, the principal options are PPIs and H_2RAs. However, because PPIs are much better than H_2RAs at healing esophagitis and maintaining remission, PPIs are considered the clear drugs of choice. For patients with NERD, PPIs may be taken PRN. For patients with erosive GERD, PPIs should be taken continuously until symptoms resolve (typically 4–8 weeks). Unfortunately, when PPIs are discontinued, the relapse rate is high, occurring in 80% to 90% of patients within 6 to 12 months. Accordingly, for patients with severe GERD, long-term maintenance therapy is recommended.

Lifestyle changes can complement drug therapy—but should not be substituted for drugs. Measures that may help include smoking cessation, weight loss, avoidance of alcohol and late-night meals, and sleeping with the head elevated. Certain foods—citrus fruits, tomatoes, onions, spicy foods, and carbonated beverages—aggravate symptoms for some patients and in these cases should be avoided.

Adverse Effects

Minor Effects

Effects seen with short-term therapy are generally inconsequential. Like the H_2RAs, omeprazole can cause headache, diarrhea, nausea, and vomiting. The incidence of these effects is less than 1%.

Pneumonia

Omeprazole and other PPIs increase the risk for community-acquired and hospital-acquired pneumonia. Possible causes include alteration of upper GI flora (owing to reduced gastric acidity) and impairment of white blood cell function. Of note, the time frame for increased risk is limited to the first few days of PPI use. After that, risk is no higher than in nonusers.

Fractures

Long-term therapy, especially in high doses, increases the risk for osteoporosis and fractures by reducing acid secretion, which may decrease absorption of calcium. However, the risk appears to be low. For example, only 1 extra hip fracture would be expected for each 1200 patients. To minimize fracture risk, treatment should use the lowest dose needed for the shortest duration possible. Also, patients should be encouraged to maintain adequate intake of calcium and vitamin D.

Rebound Acid Hypersecretion

When patients stop taking PPIs, they often experience dyspepsia brought on by rebound hypersecretion of gastric acid. Acid rebound can be minimized by using PPIs in the lowest effective dose for the shortest time needed and by tapering the dose when stopping treatment. Dyspepsia can be managed with an antacid and perhaps with an H_2RA. Acid rebound can persist for several months after the PPI is discontinued.

Hypomagnesemia

With long-term use, PPIs can lower magnesium levels, perhaps by reducing intestinal magnesium absorption. In severe cases, serum magnesium may drop below 1 mg/dL. Symptoms include tremors, muscle cramps, seizures, and dysrhythmias. The risk for hypomagnesemia is increased by other drugs that lower magnesium, especially thiazide and loop diuretics. Low magnesium can be treated with oral magnesium (e.g., Slow-Mag, MagOx). Severe cases may require IV magnesium. If magnesium levels remain low, the patient can be switched to an H_2 blocker. After PPI withdrawal, magnesium levels usually normalize within 2 weeks. For long-term PPI therapy, consider measuring magnesium at baseline and periodically thereafter.

Diarrhea

In retrospective, observational studies, omeprazole and other PPIs have been associated with a dose-related increase in the risk for infection with *C. difficile,* a bacterium that can cause severe diarrhea. Patients experiencing diarrhea while taking omeprazole or other PPIs should report immediately to their health care provider for testing.

Drug Interactions

By elevating gastric pH, omeprazole and other PPIs can significantly reduce absorption of *atazanavir* [Reyataz], *delavirdine* [Rescriptor], and *nelfinavir* [Viracept], all used to treat HIV/AIDS. These drugs should not be combined with a PPI. Reducing gastric pH can also decrease the absorption of two antifungal drugs: *ketoconazole* and *itraconazole.*

Clopidogrel

Omeprazole and other PPIs can reduce the *adverse* effects of clopidogrel [Plavix] but may also reduce its *beneficial* effects. Clopidogrel is an antiplatelet drug used to decrease thrombotic events. Unfortunately, by suppressing platelet aggregation, the drug can promote gastric bleeding. To reduce the risk for GI bleeding, clopidogrel is often combined with a PPI. Unfortunately, in addition to protecting against GI bleeding, the PPI may reduce the beneficial effects of clopidogrel because PPIs inhibit CYP2C19, the isoenzyme of cytochrome P450 that converts clopidogrel to its active form. Hence the dilemma: if clopidogrel is used alone, there is a significant risk for GI bleeding; however, if clopidogrel is combined with a PPI, the risk for GI bleeding will be reduced, but antiplatelet effects may be reduced as well. After considering the available evidence, three organizations—the American College of Cardiology, the American Heart Association, and the American College of Gastroenterology—issued a consensus document on the problem. This document concludes that, although PPIs may reduce the antiplatelet effects of clopidogrel, there is no evidence that the reduction is large enough to be clinically relevant. Accordingly, *for patients with risk factors for GI bleeding* (e.g., advanced age, use of NSAIDs or anticoagulants), the benefits of combining a PPI with clopidogrel probably outweigh any risk from reduced antiplatelet effects, and hence combining a PPI with clopidogrel is probably okay. Conversely, *for patients who lack risk factors for GI bleeding,* combined use of clopidogrel with a PPI may reduce the antiplatelet effects of clopidogrel without offering any real benefit, so combining a PPI with clopidogrel in these patients should generally be avoided.

Esomeprazole

Esomeprazole [Nexium] is nearly identical to omeprazole [Prilosec]. Esomeprazole is metabolized more slowly than omeprazole, and hence esomeprazole achieves higher blood levels, and its effects last somewhat longer. Otherwise the two drugs are essentially the same. The most common adverse effects are headache and diarrhea. In addition, esomeprazole may cause nausea, flatulence, abdominal pain, and dry mouth. Elevation of gastric pH may increase the risk for pneumonia. As with omeprazole, long-term therapy may pose a risk for hypomagnesemia as well as osteoporosis and fractures. Approved indications are erosive esophagitis, GERD, and duodenal ulcers associated with *H. pylori* infection. In addition, the drug may be used for prophylaxis of NSAID-induced ulcers.

Lansoprazole

Lansoprazole [Prevacid, Prevacid 24 HR] is very similar to omeprazole. Both drugs cause prolonged inhibition of H^+,K^+-ATPase. Hence, suppression of acid secretion is sustained. Like omeprazole, lansoprazole is well tolerated. The most common adverse effects are diarrhea, abdominal pain, and nausea. Elevation of gastric pH may increase the risk for pneumonia. Prolonged, high-dose therapy may pose a risk for hypomagnesemia, as well as osteoporosis and fracture.

Dexlansoprazole

Dexlansoprazole [Dexilant] is similar to lansoprazole but has a longer duration. Like lansoprazole and all other PPIs, dexlansoprazole reduces gastric acidity by inhibiting gastric H^+,K^+-ATPase. To prolong effects, dexlansoprazole is formulated in dual delayed-release capsules that contain two types of pH-sensitive granules. After ingestion, some of these granules release lansoprazole when they reach the proximal small intestine, and the remainder release lansoprazole when they reach the distal small intestine. As a result, drug levels first peak 1 to 2 hours after dosing and then peak again 4 to 5 hours after dosing. In clinical trials, the most common adverse effects were diarrhea, abdominal pain, nausea, vomiting, flatulence, and upper respiratory infection. Long-term therapy may pose a risk for hypomagnesemia, as well as osteoporosis and fractures. Dexlansoprazole is approved for treatment and maintenance of erosive esophagitis and for treatment of symptomatic GERD (heartburn).

Rabeprazole

Rabeprazole [Aciphex, Pariet ♣] is much like omeprazole and lansoprazole in actions, uses, and adverse effects. The drug is approved for *H. pylori* eradication, duodenal ulcers, GERD, and hypersecretory states, such as Zollinger-Ellison syndrome. Like other PPIs, rabeprazole suppresses acid secretion by inhibiting H^+,K^+-ATPase in parietal cells. However, in contrast to omeprazole, the drug causes reversible inhibition of H^+,K^+-ATPase, and hence its effects are less durable. In addition to suppressing acid secretion, rabeprazole has antibacterial activity. As a result, it may help other antibacterial drugs eradicate *H. pylori*. The most common adverse effects are diarrhea, headache, dizziness, malaise, nausea, and rash. Elevation of gastric pH may increase the risk for pneumonia. Long-term therapy may pose a risk for hypomagnesemia, as well as osteoporosis and fractures. Although rabeprazole is metabolized by cytochrome P450 enzymes, it does not appear to influence the metabolism of other drugs. However, it can increase digoxin levels by 20%. Accordingly, levels of digoxin should be monitored.

Pantoprazole

Pantoprazole [Protonix, Pantoloc ♣] is similar to omeprazole and the other PPIs. The drug is approved for treating GERD and hypersecretory states. Like other PPIs, pantoprazole is well tolerated. With oral therapy, the most common adverse effects are diarrhea, headache, and dizziness. Elevation of gastric pH may increase the risk for pneumonia. Long-term therapy may pose a risk for hypomagnesemia, as well as osteoporosis and fractures. Pantoprazole does not affect cytochrome P450 enzymes and hence does not affect the metabolism of other drugs.

OTHER ANTIULCER DRUGS

Sucralfate

Sucralfate [Carafate, Sulcrate ♣] is an effective antiulcer medication notable for minimal side effects and lack of significant drug interactions. The drug promotes ulcer healing by creating a protective barrier against acid and pepsin. Sucralfate has no acid-neutralizing capacity and does not decrease acid secretion.

Mechanism of Antiulcer Action

Sucralfate is a complex substance composed of sulfated sucrose and aluminum hydroxide. Under mildly acidic conditions (pH less than 4), sucralfate undergoes polymerization and cross-linking reactions. The resultant product is a viscid and very sticky gel that adheres to the ulcer crater, creating a barrier to back-diffusion of hydrogen ions, pepsin, and bile salts. Attachment to the ulcer appears to last up to 6 hours.

Pharmacokinetics

Sucralfate is administered orally, and systemic absorption is minimal (3%–5%). About 90% of each dose is eliminated in the feces.

Therapeutic Uses

Sucralfate is approved for acute therapy and maintenance therapy of duodenal ulcers. Rates of healing are comparable to those achieved with cimetidine. Controlled trials indicate that sucralfate can also promote healing of gastric ulcers.

Adverse Effects

Sucralfate has no known serious adverse effects. The most significant side effect is constipation, which occurs in 2% of patients. Because sucralfate is not absorbed, systemic effects are absent.

Drug Interactions

Interactions with other drugs are minimal. By raising gastric pH above 4, antacids may interfere with sucralfate's effects. This interaction can be minimized by administering these drugs at least 30 minutes apart.

Sucralfate may impede the absorption of some drugs, including phenytoin, theophylline, digoxin, warfarin, and fluoroquinolone antibiotics (e.g., ciprofloxacin, norfloxacin). These interactions can be minimized by administering sucralfate at least 2 hours apart from these other drugs.

Misoprostol

Therapeutic Use

Misoprostol [Cytotec] is an analog of prostaglandin E_1. In the United States the drug's only approved GI indication is prevention of gastric ulcers caused by long-term therapy with NSAIDs. In other countries, misoprostol is also used to treat peptic ulcers unrelated to NSAIDs. In addition to its use in PUD, misoprostol is used to promote cervical ripening.

Mechanism of Action

In normal individuals, prostaglandins help protect the stomach by suppressing secretion of gastric acid, promoting secretion of bicarbonate and cytoprotective mucus, and maintaining submucosal blood flow (by promoting vasodilation). As discussed in Chapter 55, aspirin and other NSAIDs cause gastric ulcers in part by inhibiting prostaglandin biosynthesis. Misoprostol prevents NSAID-induced ulcers by serving as a replacement for endogenous prostaglandins.

Adverse Effects

The most common reactions are dose-related diarrhea (13%–40%) and abdominal pain (7%–20%). Some women experience spotting and dysmenorrhea.

PATIENT-CENTERED CARE ACROSS THE LIFE SPAN

Peptic Ulcer Disease

Life Stage	Patient Care Concerns
Infants	Both PPIs and H_2 receptor antagonists are used safely in infants as young as 1 month to treat GERD and duodenal ulcers.
Children/adolescents	PPIs and H_2 receptor antagonists can be used safely in children, just in smaller doses. Side-effect profiles are similar to those of adults.
Pregnant women	Misoprostol is classified in FDA Pregnancy Risk Category X. This drug must be avoided at all costs. Some PPIs (esomeprazole) and H_2 receptor antagonists (ranitidine) are safe for use in pregnancy.
Breastfeeding women	Use of drugs such as omeprazole, esomeprazole, and ranitidine is not predicted to cause any adverse effects in breastfed infants.
Older adults	PPIs are associated with increased risk for fractures from osteoporosis. PPIs can also cause medication interactions and vitamin or mineral deficiencies. There should be a clear indication for prescribing these medications in this older population.

Misoprostol is classified in U.S. Food and Drug Administration (FDA) Pregnancy Risk Category X. If women of childbearing age are to use misoprostol, they must (1) be able to comply with birth control measures, (2) be given oral and written warnings about the dangers of misoprostol, (3) have a negative serum pregnancy test result within 2 weeks before beginning therapy, and (4) begin therapy only on the second or third day of the next normal menstrual cycle.

BLACK BOX WARNING: MISOPROSTOL IN PREGNANCY

Misoprostol is contraindicated during pregnancy. The drug is classified in *FDA Pregnancy Risk Category X: the risk of use by pregnant women clearly outweighs any possible benefits.* Because prostaglandins stimulate uterine contractions, use of misoprostol during pregnancy has caused partial or complete expulsion of the developing fetus.

Antacids

Antacids are alkaline compounds that neutralize stomach acid. Their principal indications are PUD and GERD.

Beneficial Actions

Antacids react with gastric acid to produce neutral salts or salts of low acidity. By neutralizing acid, these drugs decrease destruction of the gut wall. In addition, if treatment raises gastric pH above 5, these drugs will reduce pepsin activity as well. Antacids may also enhance mucosal protection by stimulating production of prostaglandins. These drugs do not coat the ulcer crater to protect it from acid and pepsin. With the exception of sodium bicarbonate, antacids are poorly absorbed and therefore do not alter systemic pH.

Therapeutic Uses

Peptic Ulcer Disease

The primary indication for antacids is PUD. Rates of healing are equivalent to those achieved with H_2RAs. In the past, antacids were the mainstay of antiulcer therapy. However, these drugs have been largely replaced by newer options (H_2RAs, PPIs, sucralfate) that are equally effective and more convenient to administer and cause fewer side effects.

Other Uses

Antacids are administered before anesthesia to prevent aspiration pneumonitis. In addition, they can provide prophylaxis against stress-induced ulcers. For patients with GERD, antacids can produce symptomatic relief, but they do not accelerate healing. Although antacids are used widely by the general public to relieve functional symptoms (dyspepsia, heartburn, acid indigestion), there are no controlled studies that demonstrate efficacy in these conditions.

Dosage and Formulations

Dosage

The objective of peptic ulcer therapy is to promote healing and not simply to relieve pain. Consequently, antacids should be taken on a regular schedule, not just in response to discomfort. In the usual dosing schedule, antacids are administered 7 times a day: 1 and 3 hours after each meal and at bedtime.

To provide maximal benefits, treatment should elevate gastric pH above 5. At this pH there is inhibition of pepsin activity in addition to nearly complete (greater than 99.9%) neutralization of acid.

Antacids are inconvenient and unpleasant to ingest, making adherence difficult—especially in the absence of pain. Patients should be encouraged to take their medication as prescribed, even after symptoms are gone.

Formulations

Antacids are available in tablet and liquid formulations. Antacid tablets should be chewed thoroughly and followed with a glass of water or milk. Liquid preparations should be shaken before dispensing. As a rule, liquids (suspensions) are more effective than tablets.

Adverse Effects

Constipation and Diarrhea

Most antacids affect the bowel. Some (e.g., aluminum hydroxide) promote constipation, whereas others (e.g., magnesium hydroxide) promote diarrhea. Effects on the bowel can be minimized by combining an antacid that promotes constipation with one that promotes diarrhea. Patients should be taught to adjust the dosage of one agent or the other to normalize bowel function.

Sodium Loading

Some antacid preparations contain substantial amounts of sodium. Because sodium excess can exacerbate hypertension and heart failure, patients with these disorders should avoid preparations that have a high sodium content.

Drug Interactions

By raising gastric pH, antacids can influence the dissolution and absorption of many other drugs, including cimetidine and ranitidine. These interactions can be minimized by allowing 1 hour between taking antacids and these other drugs.

Antacids can interfere with the actions of sucralfate. To minimize this interaction, administer these drugs at least 1 hour apart.

If absorbed in substantial amounts, antacids can alkalinize the urine. Elevation of urinary pH can accelerate excretion of acidic drugs and delay excretion of basic drugs.

Antacid Families

There are four major groups of antacids: (1) aluminum compounds, (2) magnesium compounds, (3) calcium compounds, and (4) sodium compounds. Individual agents that belong to each group are shown in Table 62.3. Representative members of these groups are discussed next.

Representative Antacids

Antacids differ from one another with respect to onset and duration of action, effects on the bowel, systemic effects, and special applications. In this section, we discuss the two most commonly used antacids—magnesium hydroxide and aluminum hydroxide—and two less commonly used drugs—calcium carbonate and sodium bicarbonate. The distinguishing properties of these agents are shown in Table 62.4.

Magnesium Hydroxide

This antacid is rapid acting and produces long-lasting effects. These properties make magnesium hydroxide an antacid of choice. The liquid formulation of magnesium hydroxide is often referred to as milk of magnesia.

The most prominent adverse effect is diarrhea, which results from retention of water in the intestinal lumen. To compensate for this effect, magnesium hydroxide is usually administered in combination with aluminum hydroxide, an antacid that promotes constipation. However, if the dose of magnesium hydroxide is sufficiently high, no amount of aluminum hydroxide will prevent diarrhea. Because stimulation of the bowel can be hazardous for patients with intestinal obstruction or appendicitis, magnesium hydroxide should be avoided in those with undiagnosed abdominal pain. Because of its effect on the bowel, magnesium hydroxide is frequently employed as a laxative (see Chapter 63). In patients with renal impairment, magnesium may accumulate to high levels, causing signs of toxicity (e.g., CNS depression).

Aluminum Hydroxide

This drug is slow acting but produces effects of long duration. Although rarely used alone, this compound is widely used in combination with magnesium hydroxide (see Table 62.3). Aluminum hydroxide preparations contain significant amounts of sodium; appropriate caution should be exercised. The most common adverse effect is constipation.

TABLE 62.3 ▪ Classification of Antacids

Aluminum compounds	Aluminum hydroxide
Magnesium compounds	Magnesium hydroxide (milk of magnesia) Magnesium oxide
Calcium compounds	Calcium carbonate
Sodium compounds	Sodium bicarbonate
Other	Magaldrate (a complex of magnesium and aluminum compounds)

Aluminum hydroxide adsorbs a variety of compounds. Binding of certain drugs (e.g., tetracyclines, warfarin, digoxin) may reduce their effects. Aluminum hydroxide has a high affinity for phosphate. By binding with phosphate, the drug can reduce phosphate absorption and can thereby cause hypophosphatemia. Aluminum hydroxide can also bind to pepsin, which may facilitate ulcer healing.

Calcium Carbonate

Calcium carbonate, like magnesium hydroxide, is rapid acting and produces effects of long duration. Because of these properties, calcium carbonate was once considered the ideal antacid. However, because of concerns about acid rebound (stimulation of acid secretion), use of calcium carbonate has declined. The principal adverse effect is constipation, which can be overcome by combining calcium carbonate with a magnesium-containing antacid (e.g., magnesium hydroxide). Calcium carbonate releases carbon dioxide in the stomach and can thereby cause eructation (belching) and flatulence. Rarely, systemic absorption is sufficient to produce the milk-alkali syndrome, a condition characterized by hypercalcemia, metabolic alkalosis, soft tissue calcification, and impaired renal function. The palatability of calcium carbonate is low and can detract from adherence.

Combination Packs

Three combination packs—Omeclamox-Pak, Pylera, and Prevpac—are available for treating *H. pylori*–associated ulcers. The purpose of these packs is to simplify the purchase and administration of drugs for triple and quadruple therapy of PUD.

Omeclamox-Pak

The Omeclamox-Pak contains omeprazole delayed-release capsules (20 mg), clarithromycin tablets (500 mg), and amoxicillin (500 mg). One dose consists of 1 omeprazole capsule, 1 clarithromycin tablet, and 2 amoxicillin capsules. Patients should take the Omeclamox-Pak before meals.

Pylera

The Pylera pack consists of capsules that contain three drugs each: bismuth subcitrate potassium (140 mg), metronidazole (125 mg), and tetracycline (125 mg). One dose consists of 3 capsules. Patients take four such doses a day, along with omeprazole.

Prevpac

The Prevpac pack contains lansoprazole [Prevacid] capsules (30 mg), amoxicillin capsules (500 mg), and clarithromycin tablets (500 mg). One dose consists of 1 lansoprazole capsule, 2 amoxicillin capsules, and 1 clarithromycin tablet. Patients take two of these doses a day.

TABLE 62.4 ▪ Representative Antacids: Distinguishing Properties

	Effect on the Bowel			
Antacid	**Constipation**	**Diarrhea**	**Effect on Systemic pH**	**Comments**
Aluminum hydroxide	Yes	No	None	Can cause hypophosphatemia; can treat hyperphosphatemia
Magnesium hydroxide	No	Yes	None	Can cause magnesium toxicity (CNS depression) in patients with renal impairment
Calcium carbonate	Yes	No	None	May cause acid rebound or milk-alkali syndrome; releases CO_2
Sodium bicarbonate	No	No	Increase	Not used routinely for ulcers; used to treat acidosis and to alkalinize urine; high risk for sodium loading; releases CO_2

CNS, central nervous system.

CHAPTER

63 Laxatives

Laura D. Rosenthal, DNP, ACNP, FAANP

Laxatives are used to ease or stimulate defecation. These agents can soften the stool, increase stool volume, hasten fecal passage through the intestine, and facilitate evacuation from the rectum. When properly employed, laxatives are valuable medications. However, these agents are also subject to abuse. Misuse of laxatives is largely the result of misconceptions about what constitutes normal bowel function.

Before we talk about laxatives, we need to distinguish between two terms: *laxative effect* and *catharsis*. The term *laxative effect* refers to production of a soft, formed stool over a period of 1 or more days. In contrast, the term *catharsis* refers to a prompt, fluid evacuation of the bowel. Hence a laxative effect is slower and relatively mild, whereas catharsis is relatively fast and intense.

GENERAL CONSIDERATIONS

Function of the Colon

The principal function of the colon is to absorb water and electrolytes. Absorption of nutrients is minimal. Normally, about 1500 mL of fluid enters the colon each day, and approximately 90% gets absorbed. When the colon is working correctly, the extent of fluid absorption is such that the resulting stool is soft (but formed) and capable of elimination without strain. However, when fluid absorption is excessive, as can happen when transport through the intestine is delayed, the resultant stool is dehydrated and hard. Conversely, if insufficient fluid is absorbed, watery stools result.

Frequency of bowel evacuation varies widely among individuals. For some people, bowel movements occur 2 or 3 times a day. For others, elimination may occur only 2 times a week. Because of this wide individual variation, we can't define a normal frequency for bowel movements. Put another way, although a daily bowel movement may be normal for many people, it may be abnormal for many others.

Dietary Fiber

Proper function of the bowel is highly dependent on dietary fiber—the component of vegetable matter that escapes digestion in the stomach and small intestine. Fiber facilitates colonic function in two ways. First, fiber absorbs water, thereby softening the feces and increasing their mass. Second, fiber can be digested by colonic bacteria, whose subsequent growth increases fecal mass. The best source of fiber is bran. Fiber can also be obtained from fruits and vegetables. Ingestion of 20 to 60 g of fiber a day should optimize intestinal function.

Constipation

Constipation is one of the most common gastrointestinal (GI) disorders. In the United States people seek medical help for constipation at least 2.5 million times a year and spend hundreds of millions of dollars on laxatives.

Constipation is defined in terms of symptoms, which include hard stools, infrequent stools, excessive straining, prolonged effort, a sense of incomplete evacuation, and unsuccessful defecation. Scientists who do research on constipation usually define it using the Rome III criteria (Table 63.1). Constipation is determined more by stool *consistency* (degree of hardness) than by *how often* bowel movements occur. Hence, if the interval between bowel movements becomes prolonged, but the stool remains soft and hydrated, a diagnosis of constipation would be improper. Conversely, if bowel movements occur with regularity, but the feces are hard and dry, constipation can be diagnosed—despite the regular and frequent passage of stool.

A common cause of constipation is poor diet—specifically, a diet deficient in fiber and fluid. Other causes include dysfunction of the pelvic floor and anal sphincter, slow intestinal transit, and use of certain drugs (e.g., opioids, anticholinergics, some antacids).

In most cases, constipation can be readily corrected. Stools will become softer and more easily passed within days of increasing fiber and fluid in the diet. Mild exercise, especially after meals, also helps improve bowel function. If necessary, a laxative may be employed—but only briefly and only as an adjunct to improved diet and exercise.

Indications for Laxative Use

Laxatives can be highly beneficial when employed for valid indications. By softening the stool, laxatives can reduce the painful elimination that can be associated with episiotomy and with hemorrhoids and other anorectal lesions. In patients with cardiovascular diseases (e.g., aneurysm, myocardial infarction, disease of the cerebral or cardiac vasculature), softening the stool decreases the amount of strain needed to defecate, avoiding dangerous elevation of blood pressure. In older-adult patients, laxatives can help compensate for loss of tone in abdominal and perineal muscles. As an adjunct to anthelmintic therapy, laxatives can be used for (1) obtaining a fresh stool sample for diagnosis; (2) emptying the bowel before treatment (so as to increase parasitic exposure to anthelmintic medication); and (3) facilitating export of dead parasites after anthelmintic use. Additional applications include (1) emptying of the bowel before surgery and diagnostic procedures

PATIENT-CENTERED CARE ACROSS THE LIFE SPAN

Laxatives

Life Stage	Patient Care Concerns
Infants	Docusate, lactulose, and glycerin suppositories have been used to treat constipation safely in infants.
Children/adolescents	Milk of magnesia, mineral oil, senna, docusate, and bisacodyl can be used to treat constipation in children and adolescents.
Pregnant women	Laxatives should be used cautiously in pregnancy because GI stimulation can induce labor.
Breastfeeding women	Senna is safe for use in breastfeeding. Data are lacking regarding the use of PEG and Dulcolax; caution is advised.
Older adults	All laxatives discussed in this chapter can be used in the older-adult population. Monitor closely for dehydration in the older adult.

TABLE 63.1 ▪ Rome III Criteria for Constipation

ADULTS

Two or more of the following for the past 3 months with symptom onset at least 6 months before diagnosis:

- Straining during at least 25% of bowel movements
- Lumpy or hard stools in at least 25% of bowel movements
- Sensation of incomplete evacuation for at least 25% of bowel movements
- Sensation of anorectal blockage for at least 25% of bowel movements
- Manual maneuvers (e.g., digital evacuation; support of the pelvic floor) to facilitate at least 25% of bowel movements
- Fewer than three bowel movements per week
- Loose stools rarely present without the use of laxatives, and insufficient criteria to permit diagnosis of irritable bowel syndrome

INFANTS AND CHILDREN

Must include 1 month of at least two of the following in infants and children up to age 4 years:

- Two or fewer defecations per week
- History of excessive stool retention
- History of painful or hard bowel movements
- History of large-diameter stools that may obstruct the toilet
- At least one episode per week of incontinence after the acquisition of toileting skills

(e.g., radiologic examination, colonoscopy); (2) modifying the effluent from an ileostomy or colostomy; (3) preventing fecal impaction in bedridden patients; (4) removing ingested poisons; and (5) correcting constipation associated with pregnancy and certain drugs, especially opioid analgesics.

Precautions and Contraindications to Laxative Use

Laxatives are contraindicated for individuals with certain disorders of the bowel. Specifically, laxatives must be avoided by individuals experiencing abdominal pain, nausea, cramps, or other symptoms of appendicitis, regional enteritis, diverticulitis, and ulcerative colitis. Laxatives are also contraindicated for patients with acute surgical abdomen. In addition, laxatives should not be used in patients with fecal impaction or obstruction of the bowel because increased peristalsis could cause bowel perforation. Lastly, laxatives should not be employed habitually to manage constipation. Reasons for this are discussed under "Laxative Abuse."

Laxatives should be used with caution during pregnancy (because GI stimulation might induce labor) and during lactation (because the laxative may be excreted in breast milk).

Laxative Classification Schemes

Traditionally, laxatives have been classified according to general *mechanism of action.* This scheme has four major categories: (1) bulk-forming laxatives, (2) surfactant laxatives, (3) stimulant laxatives, and (4) osmotic laxatives. Representative drugs are shown in Table 63.2.

From a clinical perspective, it can be useful to classify laxatives according to *therapeutic effect* (time of onset and effect on stool consistency). When these properties are considered, most laxatives fall into one of three groups, labeled I, II, and III in this chapter. Group I agents act rapidly (within 2–6 hours) and give a watery consistency to the stool. Laxatives in group I are especially useful when preparing the bowel for diagnostic procedures or surgery. Group II agents have an intermediate latency (6–12 hours) and produce a stool that is semifluid. Group II agents are the ones most frequently abused by the general public. Group III laxatives act slowly (in 1–3 days) to produce a soft but formed stool. Uses for this group include treating chronic constipation and preventing straining at stool. Representative members of groups I, II, and III are shown in Table 63.3.

BASIC PHARMACOLOGY OF LAXATIVES

Bulk-Forming Laxatives

The bulk-forming laxatives (e.g., methylcellulose, psyllium, polycarbophil) have actions and effects much like those of dietary fiber. These agents consist of natural or semisynthetic polysaccharides and celluloses derived from grains and other plant material. The bulk-forming agents belong to our therapeutic group III, producing a soft, formed stool after 1 to 3 days of use.

Mechanism of Action

Bulk-forming agents have the same effect on bowel function as dietary fiber. After ingestion, these agents, which are nondigestible and nonabsorbable, swell in water to form a viscous solution or gel, thereby softening the fecal mass and

TABLE 63.2 ▪ Classification of Laxatives by Pharmacologic Category

Class and Agent	Site of Action	Mechanism of Action
BULK-FORMING LAXATIVES		
Methylcellulose Psyllium Polycarbophil	Small intestine and colon	Absorb water, thereby softening and enlarging the fecal mass; fecal swelling promotes peristalsis
SURFACTANT LAXATIVES		
Docusate sodium Docusate calcium	Small intestine and colon	Surfactant action softens stool by facilitating penetration of water; also cause secretion of water and electrolytes into intestine
STIMULANT LAXATIVES		
Bisacodyl Senna Castor oil	Colon Colon Small intestine	(1) Stimulate peristalsis and (2) soften feces by increasing secretion of water and electrolytes into the intestine and decreasing water and electrolyte absorption
OSMOTIC LAXATIVES		
Magnesium hydroxide Magnesium sulfate Magnesium citrate Sodium phosphate Polyethylene glycol Lactulose	Small intestine and colon	Osmotic action retains water and thereby softens the feces; fecal swelling promotes peristalsis
MISCELLANEOUS LAXATIVES		
Lubiprostone	Small intestine and colon	Opens chloride channels in the intestinal epithelium and thereby increases intestinal motility and secretion of fluid into the lumen
Mineral oil	Colon	Lubricates and reduces water absorption
Glycerin suppository	Colon	Lubricates and causes reflex rectal contraction
Polyethylene glycol–electrolyte solution	Small intestine and colon	Similar to osmotic laxatives
Sodium picosulfate/magnesium oxide/anhydrous citric acid	Colon	Stimulates colonic peristalsis and draws water into the GI tract

TABLE 63.3 ▪ Classification of Laxatives by Therapeutic Response

Group I: Produce Watery Stool in 2–6 Hours	Group II: Produce Semifluid Stool in 6–12 Hours	Group III: Produce Soft Stool in 1–3 Days
OSMOTIC LAXATIVES (IN HIGH DOSES)	**OSMOTIC LAXATIVES (IN LOW DOSES)**	**BULK-FORMING LAXATIVES**
Magnesium salts Sodium salts Polyethylene glycol	Magnesium salts Sodium salts Polyethylene glycol	Methylcellulose Psyllium Polycarbophil
OTHERS	**STIMULANT LAXATIVES (EXCEPT CASTOR OIL)**	**SURFACTANT LAXATIVES**
Castor oil Polyethylene glycol–electrolyte solution	Bisacodyl, oral* Senna	Docusate sodium Docusate calcium
		OTHERS
		Lactulose Lubiprostone

*Bisacodyl *suppositories* act in 15 minutes.

increasing its bulk. Fecal volume may be further enlarged by growth of colonic bacteria, which can utilize these materials as nutrients. Transit through the intestine is hastened because swelling of the fecal mass stretches the intestinal wall and thereby stimulates peristalsis.

Indications

Bulk-forming laxatives are preferred agents for temporary treatment of constipation. Also, they are widely used in patients with diverticulosis and irritable bowel syndrome. In addition, by altering fecal consistency, they can provide symptomatic relief of diarrhea and can reduce discomfort and inconvenience for patients with an ileostomy or colostomy.

Adverse Effects

Untoward effects are minimal. Because the bulk-forming agents are not absorbed, systemic reactions are rare. *Esophageal obstruction* can occur if they are swallowed in the absence of sufficient fluid. Accordingly, bulk-forming laxatives should be administered with a full glass of water or juice. If their passage through the intestine is impeded, they may produce *intestinal obstruction* or *impaction.* Accordingly, they should be avoided if there is narrowing of the intestinal lumen.

Preparations, Dosage, and Administration

Psyllium (prepared from *Plantago* seed), *methylcellulose,* and *polycarbophil* are the principal bulk-forming laxatives. All three preparations should be administered with a full glass of water or juice. Dosages and trade names are shown in Table 63.4.

Surfactant Laxatives

Actions

The surfactants (e.g., docusate sodium) are group III laxatives: they produce a soft stool several days after the onset of treatment. Surfactants alter stool consistency by lowering surface tension, which facilitates penetration of water into the feces. The surfactants may also act on the intestinal wall to (1) inhibit fluid absorption and (2) stimulate secretion of water and electrolytes into the intestinal lumen. In this respect, surfactants resemble the stimulant laxatives (see later).

Preparations, Dosage, and Administration

The surfactant family consists of two *docusate salts:* docusate sodium and docusate calcium. The dosage for docusate sodium [Colace], the prototype surfactant, is shown in Table 63.4. Administration should be accompanied by a full glass of water.

Prototype Drugs

LAXATIVES

Bulk-Forming Agent
Methylcellulose

Surfactant
Docusate sodium

Stimulant Laxative
Bisacodyl

Osmotic Laxative
Magnesium hydroxide

Chloride Channel Activator
Lubiprostone

TABLE 63.4 ▪ Representative Laxatives: Trade Names, Dosage Forms, and Dosages

Drug Class and Generic Name	Trade Names	Dosage Forms	Dosage and Administration
BULK-FORMING			
Methylcellulose	Citrucel	Powder	*Powder:* 1 heaping tbsp in 8 ounces cold water 1–3 times a day
Psyllium	Metamucil, others	Powder, wafer	*Adults:* 1 rounded tsp (or 1 packet) mixed with water or other fluid, taken 1–3 times daily *Children older than 6 yr:* ⅓ to ½ adult dose
Polycarbophil	FiberCon, others	Tablets	*Adults:* 1250 mg 1–4 times a day *Children 6–12 yr:* 625 mg 1–4 times a day
SURFACTANT			
Docusate sodium	Colace, others	Capsules, tablets, syrup, liquid	*Adults and children older than 12 yr:* 50–500 mg/day *Children 6–12 yr:* 40–120 mg/day (All doses taken with a full glass of water)
STIMULANT			
Bisacodyl	Correctol, Dulcolax, Fleet Laxative, others	Tablets, suppositories	*Adults:* 10–15 mg (tablets) or 10-mg suppository once daily *Children:* 5-mg tablet or 5-mg suppository once daily
Senna	Senokot, Ex-Lax, others	Tablets	*Adults:* 2 tablets once or twice a day *Children 6–12 yr:* 1 tablet once or twice a day
OSMOTIC			
Polyethylene glycol	GlycoLax, MiraLax, Peglax ♣	Powder	*Adults:* 17 g (dissolved in 8 ounces of water) once a day
Lactulose	Cephulac, Cholac, others	Liquid	*Children:* 1 mL/kg PO once or twice daily
Magnesium hydroxide (milk of magnesia)	Phillips' Milk of Magnesia, others	Liquid	*Adults:* 15–30 mL daily, increased to 60 mL if needed *Children 6 mo–1 yr:* 40 mg/kg PO daily *Children 2–5 yr:* 400–1200 mg PO daily *Children 6–11 yr:* 1200–2400 mg PO daily *Children >12 yr:* 2400–4800 mg PO daily
OTHER			
Lubiprostone	Amitiza	Capsule	*Adults:* 24 mcg twice a day with food
Mineral oil	Generic only	Liquid	*Adults:* 15–45 mL daily; may take in divided doses *Children:* 5–45 mL daily; may take in divided doses

Stimulant Laxatives

The stimulant laxatives (e.g., bisacodyl, senna, castor oil) have two effects on the bowel. First, they stimulate intestinal motility—hence their name. Second, they increase the amount of water and electrolytes within the intestinal lumen by increasing secretion of water and ions into the intestine and by reducing water and electrolyte absorption. Most stimulant laxatives are group II agents: they act on the colon to produce a semifluid stool within 6 to 12 hours.

Stimulant laxatives are widely used—and abused—by the general public and are of concern for this reason. They have few legitimate applications. Two applications that *are* legitimate are (1) treatment of opioid-induced constipation and (2) treatment of constipation resulting from slow intestinal transit. Properties of individual agents are discussed next.

Bisacodyl

Bisacodyl [Correctol, Dulcolax] is unique among the stimulant laxatives in that it can be administered by rectal suppository as well as by mouth. *Oral* bisacodyl acts within 6 to 12 hours. Hence tablets may be given at bedtime to produce a response the following morning. Bisacodyl *suppositories* act rapidly (in 15–60 minutes). Dosages for bisacodyl are shown in Table 63.4.

Bisacodyl tablets are enteric coated to prevent gastric irritation. Accordingly, patients should be advised to swallow them intact, without chewing or crushing. Because milk and antacids accelerate dissolution of the enteric coating, the tablets should be administered no sooner than 1 hour after ingesting these substances.

Bisacodyl suppositories may cause a burning sensation and, with continued use, proctitis may develop. Accordingly, long-term use should be discouraged.

Senna

Senna [Senokot, Ex-Lax] is a plant-derived laxative that contains *anthraquinones* as active ingredients. The actions and applications of senna are similar to those of bisacodyl. Anthraquinones act on the colon to produce a soft or semifluid stool in 6 to 12 hours. Systemic absorption followed by renal secretion may impart a harmless yellow-brown or pink color to the urine. Dosages are presented in Table 63.4.

Castor Oil

Castor oil is the only stimulant laxative that acts on the *small intestine.* As a result, the drug acts quickly (in 2–6 hours) to produce a watery stool. Hence, unlike other stimulant laxatives, which are all group II agents, castor oil belongs to group I. Use of castor oil is limited to situations in which rapid and thorough evacuation of the bowel is desired (e.g., preparation for radiologic procedures). The drug is far too powerful for routine treatment of constipation. Because of its relatively prompt action, castor oil should not be administered at bedtime. The drug has an unpleasant taste that can be improved by chilling and mixing with fruit juice.

Osmotic Laxatives

Laxative Salts

Actions and Uses

The laxative salts (e.g., sodium phosphate, magnesium hydroxide) are poorly absorbed salts whose osmotic action draws water into the intestinal lumen. Accumulation of water causes the fecal mass to soften and swell, thereby stretching the intestinal wall, which stimulates peristalsis. When administered in low doses, the osmotic laxatives produce a soft or semifluid stool in 6 to 12 hours. In high doses, these agents act rapidly (in 2–6 hours) to cause a fluid evacuation of the bowel. High-dose therapy is employed to empty the bowel in preparation for diagnostic and surgical procedures. High doses are also employed to purge the bowel of ingested poisons and to evacuate dead parasites after anthelmintic therapy.

Preparations

We have two groups of laxative salts: (1) *magnesium salts* (magnesium hydroxide, magnesium citrate, and magnesium sulfate) and (2) one *sodium salt* (sodium phosphate). Dosages for magnesium hydroxide solution (also known as milk of magnesia) and sodium phosphate are shown in Table 63.4.

Adverse Effects

Osmotic laxatives can cause substantial *loss of water.* To avoid dehydration, patients should increase fluid intake. Although the osmotic laxatives are poorly and slowly absorbed, some absorption does take place. In patients with renal impairment, *magnesium can accumulate to toxic levels.* Accordingly, magnesium salts are contraindicated in patients with kidney disease. Sodium absorption (from sodium phosphate) can cause *fluid retention,* which in turn can exacerbate heart failure, hypertension, and edema. Accordingly, sodium phosphate is contraindicated for patients with these disorders. Sodium phosphate can also cause *acute renal failure* in vulnerable patients, especially those with kidney disease and those taking drugs that alter renal function (e.g., diuretics, angiotensin-converting enzyme [ACE] inhibitors, angiotensin receptor blockers [ARBs]). The mechanism involves dehydration and precipitation of calcium and phosphate in renal tubules. Accordingly, sodium phosphate should be avoided in this vulnerable group.

Polyethylene Glycol

Polyethylene glycol (PEG) [MiraLax, GlycoLax, Peglax ♣] is an osmotic laxative used widely for chronic constipation. Like the laxative salts, PEG is a nonabsorbable compound that retains water in the intestinal lumen, causing the fecal mass to soften and swell. The most common adverse effects are nausea, abdominal bloating, cramping, and flatulence. High doses may cause diarrhea. For management of chronic constipation, PEG is superior to lactulose with regard to relief of abdominal pain and improvements in stool consistency and frequency per week, although side effects are similar. The recommended dosage is 17 g once a day, dissolved in 4 to 8 ounces of water, juice, soda, coffee, or tea. Bowel movement may not occur for another 2 to 4 days. As discussed later, products that contain PEG plus electrolytes can be used to cleanse the bowel before colonoscopy and other procedures.

Lactulose

Lactulose [Constulose, Enulose] is a semisynthetic disaccharide composed of galactose and fructose. Lactulose is poorly absorbed and cannot be digested by intestinal enzymes. In the colon, resident bacteria metabolize lactulose to lactic acid, formic acid, and acetic acid. These acids exert a mild osmotic action, producing a soft, formed stool in 1 to 3 days. Although lactulose can relieve constipation, this agent is more expensive than equivalent drugs (bulk-forming laxatives) and causes more unpleasant side effects (flatulence and cramping are common). Accordingly, lactulose should be reserved for patients who do not respond adequately to a bulk-forming agent.

In addition to its laxative action, lactulose can enhance intestinal excretion of ammonia. This property has been exploited to lower blood ammonia content in patients with portal hypertension and hepatic encephalopathy secondary to chronic liver disease.

Other Laxatives

Lubiprostone

Lubiprostone [Amitiza] is the first representative of a new class of drugs: the selective *chloride channel activators*. By activating (opening) chloride channels in epithelial cells lining the intestine, lubiprostone (1) promotes secretion of chloride-rich fluid into the intestine and (2) enhances motility in the small intestine and colon. The result is spontaneous evacuation of a semisoft stool, usually within 24 hours. Lubiprostone has three indications: (1) chronic idiopathic constipation in adults, (2) irritable bowel syndrome with constipation (IBS-C) in women at least 18 years old, and (3) treatment of opioid-induced constipation in chronic noncancer pain. In clinical trials, the drug reduced constipation severity, abdominal bloating, and discomfort.

Lubiprostone is taken orally, and very little is absorbed. Nausea is the most common side effect and can be reduced by taking lubiprostone with food and water. Other GI effects include diarrhea, abdominal distention, abdominal pain, gas, vomiting, and loose stools. Headache is the major non-GI effect. A small percentage of patients experience difficulty breathing in association with a sense of tightness in the chest, starting 30 to 60 minutes after the first dose and resolving in a few hours. Lubiprostone is categorized in U.S. Food and Drug Administration (FDA) Pregnancy Risk Category C and hence should be used only if benefits are deemed to outweigh potential risks to the fetus. (In animal studies, lubiprostone was not teratogenic. However, when given to guinea pigs in doses more than 100 times the human dose, lubiprostone did cause fetal loss.) Interactions with other drugs have not been studied but seem unlikely because lubiprostone is poorly absorbed and does not alter the activity of cytochrome P450 drug-metabolizing enzymes.

Lubiprostone is available in 8- and 24-mcg soft-gelatin capsules that should be taken with food and water. The recommended dosage is 24 mcg twice daily for constipation and 8 mcg twice daily for IBS-C. The role of lubiprostone in IBS-C is discussed in Chapter 64.

Mineral Oil

Mineral oil is a mixture of indigestible and poorly absorbed hydrocarbons. Laxative action is produced by lubrication. Mineral oil is especially useful when administered by enema to treat fecal impaction.

Mineral oil can produce a variety of adverse effects. Aspiration of oil droplets can cause lipid pneumonia. Anal leakage can cause pruritus and soiling. Systemic absorption can produce deposition of mineral oil in the liver. Excessive dosing can decrease absorption of fat-soluble vitamins. Dosages for adults and children are shown in Table 63.4.

Glycerin Suppository

Glycerin is an osmotic agent that softens and lubricates inspissated (hardened, impacted) feces. The drug may also stimulate rectal contraction. Evacuation occurs about 30 minutes after suppository insertion. Glycerin suppositories have been useful for reestablishing normal bowel function after termination of chronic laxative use.

Bowel Cleansing Products for Colonoscopy

Colonoscopy is the most effective method for early detection of colorectal cancer, the second leading cause of cancer deaths in the United States. Before the procedure, the bowel must be cleansed to permit good visualization. Three kinds of bowel cleansers are used: (1) sodium phosphate; (2) a combination of sodium picosulfate, magnesium oxide, and citric acid; and (3) PEG plus electrolytes (ELS). The PEG-ELS products are isotonic with body fluids and hence do not alter water or electrolyte status. In contrast, the sodium phosphate and combination products are hypertonic and can cause dehydration and electrolyte disturbances. In addition, the sodium phosphate products can cause kidney damage. However, despite their greater potential for harm, the sodium phosphate products have better patient acceptance because the PEG-ELS products require ingestion of a large volume of liquid, whereas the sodium phosphate products do not. Nonetheless, sodium phosphate products should be avoided by patients at risk, including those with electrolyte abnormalities, renal impairment, and hypovolemia. Representative bowel cleansers are shown in Table 63.5.

Polyethylene Glycol–Electrolyte Solutions

These bowel-cleansing solutions [CoLyte, GoLYTELY, others] contain PEG, a nonabsorbable osmotic agent, together with ELS (usually potassium chloride, sodium chloride, sodium sulfate, and sodium bicarbonate). The mixture is isosmotic with body fluids, and hence water and electrolytes are neither absorbed from nor secreted into the intestinal lumen. As a result, dehydration does not occur and electrolyte balance is preserved. Because effects on water and electrolytes are minimal, PEG-ELS solutions can be used safely by patients who are dehydrated and by those who are especially sensitive to alteration of electrolyte levels (e.g., patients with renal impairment or cardiovascular disease).

With traditional PEG-ELS products (e.g., CoLyte, GoLYTELY), the volume administered is huge, typically 4 L. Patients must ingest 250 to 300 mL every 10 minutes for 2 to 3 hours. With two newer products—HalfLytely and MoviPrep—the volume is cut in half. Patients using HalfLytely take a stimulant laxative—bisacodyl—along with the PEG-ELS solution and hence don't need the full 4-L dose. Volume reduction with MoviPrep is possible owing to addition of ascorbic acid and sodium ascorbate to the PEG-ELS solution. With all PEG products, bowel movements commence about 1 hour after the first dose.

PEG-ELS products are generally well tolerated. The most common adverse effects are nausea, bloating, and abdominal discomfort. These effects are less intense with the reduced-volume formulations. Because PEG-ELS products don't alter water and electrolyte status, they are safer than sodium phosphate products for patients with electrolyte imbalances, heart failure, kidney disease, or advanced liver disease.

Sodium Phosphate Products

As discussed previously, sodium phosphate is an osmotic laxative that draws water into the intestinal lumen, which then softens and swells the fecal mass, which then stretches the intestinal wall to stimulate peristalsis. Dosing consists of swallowing tablets along with a large volume of water or

TABLE 63.5 ■ Oral Bowel Cleansing Products for Colonoscopy

		Total Volume to Swallow	
Product Type and Brand Name	**Adult Dosage**	**Bowel Cleanser**	**Clear Liquid**
SODIUM PHOSPHATE TABLETS			
Visicol	20 tablets with clear liquid in the evening *plus* 12 tablets with clear liquid the next day		3.4 L
OsmoPrep	20 tablets with clear liquid in the evening *plus* 20 tablets with clear liquid the next day		1.9 L
POLYETHYLENE GLYCOL PLUS ELECTROLYTES			
GoLYTELY, NuLytely, CoLyte, TriLyte	240 mL every 10 min until 4 L is ingested or until rectal effluent is clear	4 L	
HalfLytely and bisacodyl	240 mL every 10 min until 2 L is ingested*	2 L	
MoviPrep†	240 mL every 15 min until 1 L is ingested, then repeat 1.5 hr later, then drink 1 more L of clear liquid‡	2 L	1 L
COMBINATION PRODUCT			
Prepopik	1 package (16.1 g) mixed in 5 ounces of water the evening before the colonoscopy and 1 package mixed in 5 ounces of water the morning of the colonoscopy.§		2.5 L

*Before drinking the solution, patients should take 4 bisacodyl delayed-release tablets and wait for a bowel movement or for 6 hours, whichever comes first.

†Formulated with ascorbic acid, which allows use of a smaller volume than traditional PEG-electrolyte products.

‡Dosage can be split by ingesting 1 L of the prep plus 0.5 L clear liquid in the evening, followed by 1 L of the prep plus 0.5 L clear liquid the next day.

§Dose should be followed by 40 ounces of clear liquid the evening before the colonoscopy and 32 ounces of clear liquid in the morning of the procedure.

some other clear liquid. Because the clear liquid is more palatable than the PEG-ELS solutions, patients find the sodium phosphate regimens more appealing.

Like the PEG-ELS products, the sodium phosphate products can cause nausea, bloating, and abdominal discomfort. In addition, the sodium phosphate products can cause adverse effects not seen with the PEG-ELS products, especially dehydration, electrolyte disturbances, and kidney damage. By drawing a large volume of fluid into the intestinal lumen, sodium phosphate can cause dehydration. To prevent dehydration, patients must drink a large volume of clear fluid before, during, and after dosing.

Rarely, phosphate is absorbed in amounts sufficient to cause hyperphosphatemia, which can cause *acute, reversible renal damage, and possibly chronic, irreversible renal damage.* Risk factors for hyperphosphatemia and kidney damage include hypovolemia, advanced age, delayed bowel transit, active colitis, preexisting kidney disease, and use of drugs that can alter kidney function, including diuretics, ACE inhibitors, ARBs, and nonsteroidal antiinflammatory drugs. Patients who have these risk factors should probably use a PEG-ELS product rather than sodium phosphate.

Combination Products

One combination product—magnesium oxide/anhydrous citric acid/sodium picosulfate [Prepopik]—is approved for preparation for colonoscopy in adults. Sodium picosulfate is a stimulant laxative, and magnesium oxide and citric acid combine to form magnesium citrate, an osmotic laxative. When given in a split-dose regimen, results were superior to colon preparation with PEG-ELS.

Prepopik is given in a split-dose regimen. It is supplied in 2 packets containing 16.1 g each of powder that must be mixed with water for consumption. The first dose is taken the evening before the colonoscopy and the second dose the next morning before the procedure.

As with sodium phosphate products, Prepopik can cause electrolyte and fluid imbalances, renal impairment, seizures, and dysrhythmia secondary to electrolyte abnormalities. Caution must be employed in patients with reduced renal function. The most common adverse reactions are nausea, headache, and vomiting.

LAXATIVE ABUSE

Causes

Many people believe that a daily bowel movement is a requisite of good health and that any deviation from this pattern merits correction. Such misconceptions are reinforced by aggressive marketing of over-the-counter laxative preparations. Not infrequently, the combination of tradition supported by advertising has led to habitual self-prescribing of laxatives by people who don't need them.

Laxatives can help perpetuate their own use. Strong laxatives can purge the entire bowel. When this occurs, spontaneous evacuation is impossible until bowel content has been replenished, which can take 2 to 5 days. During this time, the laxative user, having experienced no movement of the bowel, often becomes convinced that constipation has returned. In response, he or she takes yet another dose, which purges the bowel once more, and thereby sets the stage for a repeating cycle of laxative use and purging.

Consequences

Chronic exposure to laxatives can diminish defecatory reflexes, leading to further reliance on laxatives. Laxative abuse may also cause more serious pathologic changes, including electrolyte imbalance, dehydration, and colitis.

Treatment

The first step in breaking the laxative habit is abrupt cessation of laxative use. After drug withdrawal, bowel movements will be absent for several days; the patient should be informed of this fact. Any misconceptions that the patient has regarding bowel function should be corrected: the patient should be taught that a once-daily bowel movement may not be normal for him or her and that stool *quality* is more important than frequency or quantity. Instruction on bowel training (heeding the defecatory reflex, establishing a consistent time for bowel movements) should be provided. Increased consumption of fiber (bran, fruits, vegetables) and fluid should be stressed. The patient should be encouraged to exercise daily, especially after meals. Finally, the patient should be advised that, if a laxative must be used, it should be used briefly and in the smallest effective dose. Agents that produce catharsis must be avoided.

CHAPTER

64

Other Gastrointestinal Drugs

Laura D. Rosenthal, DNP, ACNP, FAANP

In this chapter we discuss an assortment of gastrointestinal (GI) drugs with indications ranging from emesis to colitis to hemorrhoids. Four groups are emphasized: (1) antiemetics, (2) antidiarrheals, (3) drugs for irritable bowel syndrome, and (4) drugs for inflammatory bowel disease.

ANTIEMETICS

Antiemetics are given to suppress nausea and vomiting. We begin our discussion by reviewing the emetic response. Next we discuss the major antiemetic classes. We finish by considering the most important application of these drugs: management of chemotherapy-induced nausea and vomiting (CINV).

The Emetic Response

Emesis is a complex reflex brought about by activating the vomiting center, a nucleus of neurons located in the medulla oblongata. Some stimuli activate the vomiting center directly; others act indirectly (Fig. 64.1). Direct-acting stimuli include signals from the cerebral cortex (anticipation or fear), signals from sensory organs (upsetting sights, noxious odors, or pain), and signals from the vestibular apparatus of the inner ear. Indirect-acting stimuli first activate the chemoreceptor trigger zone (CTZ), which in turn activates the vomiting center. Activation of the CTZ occurs in two ways: (1) by signals from the stomach and small intestine (traveling along vagal afferents) and (2) by the direct action of emetogenic compounds (e.g., anticancer drugs, opioids, ipecac) that are carried to the CTZ in the blood. When activated, the vomiting center signals the stomach, diaphragm, and abdominal muscles; the resulting coordinated response expels gastric contents.

Several types of receptors are involved in the emetic response. Important among these are receptors for serotonin, glucocorticoids, substance P, neurokinin-1, dopamine, acetylcholine, and histamine. Many antiemetics, including ondansetron [Zofran], dexamethasone, aprepitant [Emend], prochlorperazine, and dimenhydrinate, act by blocking (or activating) one or more of these receptors.

Antiemetic Drugs

Several types of antiemetics are available. Their classes, trade names, and dosages are shown in Table 64.1. Uses and mechanisms are shown in Table 64.2. Properties of the principal classes are discussed next.

Prototype Drugs

GASTROINTESTINAL DRUGS

Serotonin Antagonist
Ondansetron

Glucocorticoids
Dexamethasone

Substance P/Neurokinin-1 Antagonist
Aprepitant

Dopamine Antagonist
Prochlorperazine

Cannabinoid
Dronabinol

Benzodiazepine
Lorazepam

Drug for Constipation-Predominant IBS
Lubiprostone

Drug for Diarrhea-Predominant IBS
Alosetron

5-Aminosalicylate
Sulfasalazine

Glucocorticoid
Budesonide

Immunomodulators/Immunosuppressants
Mercaptopurine
Infliximab

Serotonin Receptor Antagonists

Serotonin receptor antagonists are the most effective drugs available for suppressing nausea and vomiting caused by

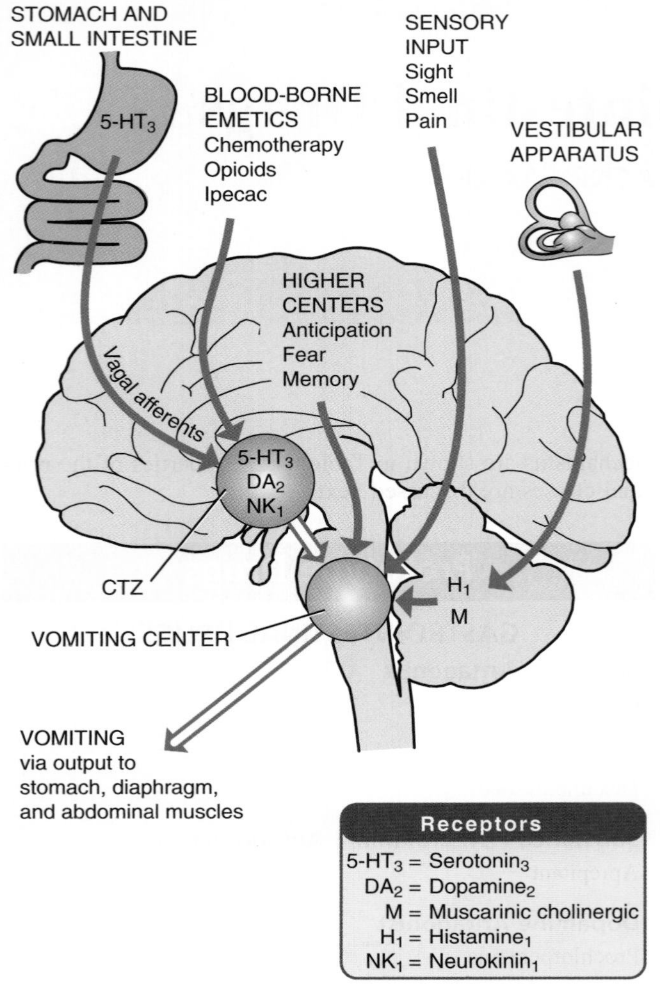

Figure 64.1 ■ The emetic response: stimuli, pathways, and receptors.
CTZ, chemoreceptor trigger zone.

cisplatin and other highly emetogenic anticancer drugs. These drugs are also highly effective against nausea and vomiting associated with radiation therapy, anesthesia, viral gastritis, and pregnancy. Four serotonin antagonists are available for treating emesis: ondansetron, granisetron, dolasetron, and palonosetron.

Ondansetron

Ondansetron [Zofran, Zofran ODT, Zuplenz] was the first serotonin receptor antagonist approved for CINV. The drug is also used to prevent nausea and vomiting associated with radiotherapy and anesthesia. In addition, the drug is used off-label to treat nausea and vomiting from other causes, including childhood viral gastritis and morning sickness of pregnancy. In all cases, benefits derive from blocking type 3 serotonin receptors ($5\text{-}HT_3$ receptors[1]) located in the CTZ and on afferent vagal neurons in the upper GI tract. The drug is very effective by itself, and even more effective when combined with dexamethasone. Administration may be oral or parenteral. The most common side effects are headache, diarrhea, and dizziness. Of much greater concern, ondansetron prolongs the QT interval and hence poses a risk for torsades de pointes, a potentially life-threatening dysrhythmia. Accordingly, the drug should not be given to patients with long QT syndrome and should be used with caution in patients with electrolyte abnormalities, heart failure, or bradydysrhythmias and in those taking other QT drugs. Because ondansetron does not block dopamine receptors, it does not cause the extrapyramidal effects (e.g., akathisia, acute dystonia) seen with antiemetic phenothiazines.

Administration is by the oral (PO), intramuscular (IM), or intravenous (IV) route. For oral dosing, ondansetron is available in solution (sold as Zofran), standard tablets (sold as Zofran), orally disintegrating tablets (sold as Zofran ODT), and a soluble film (sold as Zuplenz). To prevent CINV, the recommended IV dose is 0.15 mg/kg infused slowly (over 15 minutes) beginning 30 minutes before chemotherapy; this dose is repeated 4 and 8 hours later. The dosage for patients undergoing radiation therapy is 8 mg PO (tablets, solution, or soluble film) 3 times a day. The dosage for postoperative nausea and vomiting is 16 mg PO (tablets, solution, or soluble film) 1 hour before induction of anesthesia.

Granisetron

Like ondansetron, granisetron [Granisol, Kytril ♣, Sancuso] suppresses emesis by blocking $5\text{-}HT_3$ receptors on afferent vagal neurons and in the CTZ. The drug is approved for preventing nausea and vomiting associated with cancer chemotherapy, radiation therapy, and surgery. Principal adverse effects are headache (responsive to acetaminophen), weakness, tiredness, and either diarrhea or constipation. Administration is PO, IV, or transdermal. The recommended dosage for CINV is either (1) 10 mcg/kg IV infused over 5 minutes, starting 30 minutes before chemotherapy or (2) a single transdermal patch [Sancuso] applied 24 to 48 hours before chemotherapy and removed 24 hours after chemotherapy is completed (but no more than 7 days after application). The dosage for patients undergoing radiation therapy is 2 mg (tablets or oral solution) once daily given within 1 hour of radiation treatment. The dosage for preventing postoperative nausea and vomiting is 1 mg IV injected slowly (over 30 seconds) either before induction of anesthesia or just before reversing anesthesia.

Dolasetron

Dolasetron [Anzemet] is approved for CINV and postoperative nausea and vomiting. Administration is PO or IV. Side effects are like those of other serotonin antagonists, with one important exception: when given by IV injection in high doses, dolasetron poses a significant risk for fatal dysrhythmias. Accordingly, high-dose IV therapy should not be used. Oral therapy and low-dose IV therapy are considered safe. The recommended dosage for CINV in adults is 100 mg PO 1 hour before chemotherapy. The dosage to prevent postoperative nausea and vomiting is 100 mg PO 2 hours before anesthesia or 12.5 mg IV 15 minutes before anesthesia is stopped.

Palonosetron

Palonosetron [Aloxi], indicated for CINV and postoperative nausea and vomiting, has the same mechanism, efficacy, and side effects as other serotonin antagonists, but differs from the others in two clinically significant ways. First, palonosetron has a much longer half-life (40 hours vs. about 8 hours). Second, because of its long half-life, palonosetron is effective against delayed emesis (as well as acute emesis), whereas the others are most effective against acute emesis. Palonosetron also has much greater affinity for $5\text{-}HT_3$ receptors than the other serotonin antagonists, but this difference does not appear to have clinical significance. Palonosetron is available only in an IV formulation. The recommended dosage for CINV in adults is 250 mcg IV delivered over 30 seconds starting 30 minutes before chemotherapy. To prevent postoperative nausea and vomiting, the dosage is 75 mcg IV delivered over 10 seconds immediately before induction of anesthesia.

Glucocorticoids

Two glucocorticoids—*methylprednisolone* [Solu-Medrol] and *dexamethasone*—are commonly used to suppress CINV, even though they are not approved by the U.S. Food and Drug Administration (FDA) for this application. Glucocorticoids are effective alone and in combination with other antiemetics. The mechanism by which glucocorticoids suppress emesis is unknown. Both dexamethasone and methylprednisolone are administered by IV route. Because antiemetic use is intermittent and short term, serious side effects are absent. The pharmacology of the glucocorticoids is discussed in Chapter 56.

---

[1]Serotonin is also known as 5-hydroxytryptamine (5-HT), so type 3 serotonin receptors are abbreviated as *$5\text{-}HT_3$*.

TABLE 64.1 ■ Antiemetic Drugs: Classes, Trade Names, and Dosages

Class and Generic Name	Trade Name	Adult Dosage
SEROTONIN ANTAGONISTS		
Ondansetron	Zofran, Zuplenz	See text
Granisetron	Granisol, Kytril ♣, Sancuso	See text
Dolasetron	Anzemet	See text
Palonosetron	Aloxi	See text
GLUCOCORTICOIDS		
Dexamethasone	Generic only	10–20 mg IV before chemotherapy, then 4–8 mg
Methylprednisolone	Solu-Medrol	2 doses of 125–500 mg IV 6 hr apart before chemotherapy
SUBSTANCE P/NEUROKININ-1 ANTAGONISTS		
Aprepitant	Emend	125 mg PO on day 1, then 80 mg PO on days 2 and 3
Netupitant/Palonosetron	Akynzeo	300/0.5 mg PO 1 hr before chemotherapy
Fosaprepitant	Emend	115 mg IV, used in place of the first (125-mg) dose of aprepitant in the regimen above
Rolapitant	Varubi	180 mg PO 1–2 hours before the start of chemotherapy
BENZODIAZEPINE		
Lorazepam	Ativan	1–1.5 mg IV before chemotherapy
DOPAMINE ANTAGONISTS		
Phenothiazines		
Chlorpromazine	Generic only	10–25 mg (PO, IM, IV) every 4–6 hr PRN
Perphenazine	Generic only	8–16 mg/day in divided doses (PO, IM, IV)
Prochlorperazine	Generic only	5–10 mg (PO, IM, IV) 3–4 times a day PRN
Promethazine*	Phenergan	12.5–25 mg (PO, IM, IV) every 4–6 hr
Butyrophenones		
Haloperidol†	Haldol	1–5 mg (PO, IM, IV) every 12 hr PRN
Droperidol	Inapsine	0.625–2.5 mg (IM, IV) every 4–6 hr PRN
Others		
Metoclopramide‡	Reglan	See Table 64.3
CANNABINOIDS		
Dronabinol	Marinol	5 mg/m^2 PO every 2–4 hr PRN
Nabilone	Cesamet	1–2 mg PO twice daily
ANTICHOLINERGICS		
Antihistamines		
Cyclizine	Cyclivert	50 mg PO every 4–6 hr PRN
Dimenhydrinate	Dramamine	50–100 mg (PO, IM, IV) every 4–6 hr PRN
Diphenhydramine	Benadryl	10–50 mg (PO, IM, IV) every 4–6 hr PRN
Hydroxyzine	Vistaril	25–100 mg IM every 6 hr PRN
Meclizine	Bonine, Antivert	25–50 mg PO every 24 hr PRN
Others		
Scopolamine	Transderm Scōp	0.5 mg transdermal every 72 hr PRN

*Promethazine is contraindicated for children younger than 2 years owing to a risk for fatal respiratory depression.
†Off-label use.
‡Also blocks serotonin receptors.

Substance P/Neurokinin-1 Antagonists

Four substance P/neurokinin-1 antagonists are currently available: aprepitant, rolapitant, netupitant, and fosaprepitant, a prodrug that undergoes conversion to aprepitant in the body. Their principal application is prevention of CINV.

Aprepitant

Actions and Use. Aprepitant [Emend] is an important antiemetic. The drug is approved for preventing postoperative nausea and vomiting and CINV. Owing to its unique mechanism of action—blockade of neurokinin-1–type receptors (for substance P) in the CTZ—aprepitant can enhance responses when combined with other antiemetic drugs. Aprepitant has a prolonged duration of action and hence can prevent *delayed* CINV as well as *acute* CINV. Aprepitant can be used *alone* for managing postoperative nausea and vomiting. However, because the drug is only moderately effective, it must be combined with other antiemetic drugs—specifically, a glucocorticoid (e.g., dexamethasone) and a serotonin antagonist (e.g., ondansetron)—for managing CINV.

Pharmacokinetics. Oral aprepitant is well absorbed, both in the presence and absence of food. Plasma levels peak 4 hours after dosing. The drug undergoes extensive hepatic

TABLE 64.2 ▪ Antiemetic Drugs: Uses and Mechanism of Action

Class	Prototype	Antiemetic Use	Mechanism of Antiemetic Action
Serotonin antagonists	Ondansetron [Zofran, Zuplenz]	Chemotherapy, radiation, postoperative	Block serotonin receptors on vagal afferents and in the CTZ
Glucocorticoids	Dexamethasone (generic only)	Chemotherapy	Unknown
Substance P/neurokinin-1 antagonists	Aprepitant [Emend]	Chemotherapy	Block receptors for substance P/neurokinin-1 in the brain
Dopamine antagonists	Prochlorperazine (generic only)	Chemotherapy, postoperative, general	Block dopamine receptors in the CTZ
Cannabinoids	Dronabinol [Marinol]	Chemotherapy	Unknown, but probably activate cannabinoid receptors associated with the vomiting center
Anticholinergics	Scopolamine [Transderm Scōp]	Motion sickness	Block muscarinic receptors in the pathway from the inner ear to the vomiting center
Antihistamines	Dimenhydrinate (generic only)	Motion sickness	Block histamine-1 receptors and muscarinic receptors in the pathway from the inner ear to the vomiting center

CTZ, chemoreceptor trigger zone.

metabolism—primarily by CYP3A4 (the 3A4 isoenzyme of cytochrome P450)—followed by excretion in the urine and feces. The plasma half-life is 9 to 13 hours.

Adverse Effects. Aprepitant is generally well tolerated. Compared with patients receiving ondansetron and dexamethasone, those receiving aprepitant plus ondansetron and dexamethasone experience more fatigue and asthenia (17.8% vs. 11.8%), hiccups (10.8% vs. 5.6%), dizziness (6.6% vs. 4.4%), and diarrhea (10.3% vs. 7.5%). Aprepitant may also cause a mild, transient elevation of circulating aminotransferases, indicating possible liver injury.

Drug Interactions. The potential for drug interactions is complex because aprepitant is a substrate for, inhibitor of, and inducer of CYP3A4, a major drug-metabolizing enzyme. Inhibitors of CYP3A4 (e.g., itraconazole, ritonavir) can raise levels of aprepitant. Conversely, inducers of CYP3A4 (e.g., rifampin, phenytoin) can decrease levels of aprepitant. By inhibiting CYP3A4, aprepitant can raise levels of CYP3A4 substrates, including many drugs used for cancer chemotherapy. Among these are docetaxel, paclitaxel, etoposide, irinotecan, ifosfamide, imatinib, vinorelbine, vinblastine, and vincristine. Also, aprepitant can raise levels of glucocorticoids used to prevent CINV. Accordingly, doses of these drugs (dexamethasone and methylprednisolone) should be reduced.

In addition to affecting CYP3A4, aprepitant can induce CYP2D6, another drug-metabolizing enzyme. As a result, aprepitant can decrease levels of CYP2D6 substrates, including warfarin (an anticoagulant) and ethinyl estradiol (found in oral contraceptives). Patients receiving warfarin should be monitored closely. Patients using oral contraceptives may need an alternative form of birth control.

Preparations, Dosage, and Administration. Aprepitant [Emend] is available in 40-, 80- and 125-mg capsules. Dosing may be done with or without food.

For CINV, dosing is done once a day for 3 days. The first dose (125 mg) is given 1 hour before chemotherapy. The second and third doses (80 mg each) are given early on the following 2 days. As noted, aprepitant should be used in combination with dexamethasone and ondansetron.

For postoperative nausea and vomiting, treatment consists of a single 40-mg dose given within 3 hours of anesthesia induction.

Fosaprepitant

Fosaprepitant [Emend] is an intravenous prodrug that undergoes rapid conversion to aprepitant in the body. Accordingly, the pharmacology of fosaprepitant is nearly identical to that of aprepitant. Fosaprepitant is indicated only for preventing CINV. In contrast, aprepitant is approved for CINV and postoperative nausea and vomiting. For prevention of CINV, fosaprepitant is used as a substitute for aprepitant—but only for the first dose in the three-dose regimen (see earlier). Because IV fosaprepitant has greater bioavailability than PO aprepitant, the dosage for fosaprepitant is only 115 mg, compared with 125 mg for aprepitant. In addition to causing the same adverse effects as aprepitant, fosaprepitant can cause pain and induration at the infusion site.

Rolapitant

Actions and Use. Rolapitant [Varubi] is approved for the prevention of delayed nausea and vomiting associated with chemotherapy. Like aprepitant, rolapitant works well when combined with other antiemetic agents, including dexamethasone and 5-HT_3 receptor antagonists.

Pharmacokinetics. Oral rolapitant is well absorbed, in both the presence and absence of food. Plasma levels peak 4 hours after dosing. The drug undergoes extensive hepatic metabolism—primarily by CYP3A4—followed by excretion in the urine and feces. The plasma half-life is very long—approximately 7 days.

Adverse Effects. Rolapitant is generally well tolerated. Common adverse reactions include decreased appetite, neutropenia, dizziness, and dyspepsia. Compared with the combination of dexamethasone and a 5-HT_3 receptor antagonist alone, there are no significant differences in side effects.

Drug Interactions. Like aprepitant, concomitant use with inhibitors of CYP3A4 (e.g., itraconazole, ritonavir) can raise levels of rolapitant. Conversely, inducers of CYP3A4 (e.g., rifampin, phenytoin) can decrease levels of rolapitant.

Preparations, Dosage, and Administration. Rolapitant [Varubi] is available in 90-mg tablets. The recommended dose is 180 mg administered 1 to 2 hours before the start of chemotherapy. Dosing should be in conjunction with prescribed dexamethasone and a 5-HT_3 receptor antagonist.

Netupitant/Palonosetron

Netupitant/palonosetron [Akynzeo] is a combination drug that contains both a substance P antagonist (netupitant) and a 5-HT_3 receptor antagonist (Palonosetron). The drug is approved for preventing acute and delayed nausea and vomiting associated with chemotherapy. Pharmacokinetics, adverse effects, and drug interactions are similar to the other agents that block substance P and 5-HT_3 receptors. Netupitant/palonosetron [Akynzeo] is available in 300/0.5-mg capsules. Dosing can be with or without food. Patients should take one capsule approximately 1 hour before chemotherapy.

Benzodiazepines

Lorazepam [Ativan] is used in combination regimens to suppress CINV. The drug has three principal benefits: sedation, suppression of anticipatory emesis, and production of anterograde amnesia. In addition, lorazepam may help control extrapyramidal reactions caused by phenothiazine antiemetics. The basic pharmacology of lorazepam and other benzodiazepines is discussed in Chapter 27.

Dopamine Antagonists

Phenothiazines

The phenothiazines (e.g., prochlorperazine) suppress emesis by blocking dopamine-2 receptors in the CTZ. These drugs can reduce emesis associated with surgery, cancer chemotherapy, and toxins. Side effects include extrapyramidal reactions, anticholinergic effects, hypotension, and sedation. The basic pharmacology of the phenothiazines is discussed in Chapter 24.

One phenothiazine—*promethazine* [Phenergan]—requires comment. Promethazine is the most widely used antiemetic in young children, despite its adverse side effects (respiratory depression and local tissue injury) and despite the availability of potentially safer alternatives (e.g., ondansetron).

BLACK BOX WARNING: PROMETHAZINE

Respiratory depression from promethazine can be severe. Deaths have occurred. Because of this risk, promethazine is contraindicated in children younger than 2 years and should be used with caution in children older than 2 years.

Tissue injury can result in several ways. For example, extravasation of IV promethazine can cause abscess formation, tissue necrosis, and gangrene that requires amputation. Severe injury can also occur with inadvertent perivascular or intraarterial administration, or with administration into or near a nerve. Risk for local injury is lower with IM dosing than with IV dosing. Accordingly, when parenteral administration is needed, the IM route is preferred. Subcutaneous (subQ) promethazine is contraindicated. If IV administration *must* be done, promethazine should be given through a large-bore, freely flowing line, in a concentration of 25 mg/mL or less at a rate of 25 mg/min or less. Patients should be advised to report local burning or pain immediately.

Butyrophenones

Two butyrophenones—*haloperidol* [Haldol] and *droperidol* [Inapsine]—are used as antiemetics. Like the phenothiazines, the butyrophenones suppress emesis by blocking dopamine-2 receptors in the CTZ. Butyrophenones are effective against postoperative nausea and vomiting and against emesis caused by cancer chemotherapy, radiation therapy, and toxins. Potential side effects are similar to those of the phenothiazines: extrapyramidal reactions, sedation, and hypotension. The pharmacology of the butyrophenones is discussed in Chapter 24.

BLACK BOX WARNING: DROPERIDOL

Droperidol may pose a risk for fatal dysrhythmias owing to prolongation of the QT interval. Accordingly, patients receiving the drug should undergo an electrocardiographic evaluation before administration.

Metoclopramide

Metoclopramide [Reglan] suppresses emesis through blockade of dopamine receptors in the CTZ. The drug can suppress postoperative nausea and vomiting as well as emesis caused by anticancer drugs, opioids, toxins, and radiation therapy. The pharmacology of metoclopramide is discussed later under "Prokinetic Agents."

Cannabinoids

Two cannabinoids—*dronabinol* [Marinol] and *nabilone* [Cesamet]—are approved for medical use in the United States. Both drugs are related to marijuana (*Cannabis sativa*). Dronabinol (delta-9-tetrahydrocannabinol; THC) is the principal psychoactive agent in *C. sativa.* Nabilone is a synthetic derivative of dronabinol. A third cannabinoid preparation, sold as *Sativex* ♣ (a combination of THC and cannabidiol), is available in Canada (for treating neuropathic pain) but is not FDA approved in the United States. The basic pharmacology of THC and other cannabinoids is discussed in Chapter 33.

Therapeutic Uses

Both dronabinol and nabilone are approved for suppressing CINV. The mechanism underlying benefits is unknown but most likely results from activating cannabinoid receptors in and around the vomiting center. Because of their psychotomimetic effects and abuse potential (see later), the cannabinoids are considered second-line drugs for CINV and hence should be reserved for patients who are unresponsive to or intolerant of preferred agents.

In addition to its use in CINV, dronabinol (but not nabilone) is approved for stimulating appetite in patients with AIDS. The goal is to reduce AIDS-induced anorexia and prevent or reverse weight loss.

Adverse Effects and Drug Interactions

In theory, the cannabinoids used medically can produce subjective effects identical to those caused by smoking marijuana. Potential unpleasant effects include temporal disintegration, dissociation, depersonalization, and dysphoria. Because of these effects, cannabinoids are contraindicated for patients with psychiatric disorders. In addition to their subjective effects, cannabinoids can cause tachycardia and hypotension and therefore must be used with caution in patients with cardiovascular diseases. The cannabinoids can cause drowsiness and hence should not be combined with alcohol, sedatives, and central nervous system (CNS) depressants.

Abuse Potential

Because they can mimic the subjective effects of marijuana, cannabinoids have some potential for abuse. When first approved for medical use, both drugs were classified under Schedule II of the Controlled Substances Act (CSA)—a classification reserved for drugs with a high abuse potential. However, in 1998, the manufacturer of dronabinol petitioned the Drug Enforcement Agency (DEA) to reclassify the drug under Schedule III. Two arguments for the reduced classification were offered: (1) because of its slow onset, dronabinol does not produce the same "high" produced by smoking marijuana and (2) there is little or no interest in dronabinol on the street. Apparently, the DEA agreed: dronabinol is now classified under Schedule III. Nabilone remains under Schedule II, although its abuse potential seems no greater than that of dronabinol.

Preparations, Dosage, and Administration

Dronabinol. Dronabinol [Marinol] is supplied in capsules (2.5, 5, and 10 mg) for oral use. To prevent emesis, the usual dosage is 5 mg/m^2 every 4 to 6 hours as needed. To stimulate appetite in patients with AIDS, the recommended initial dosage is 2.5 mg before lunch and supper. If this dosage is intolerable, 2.5 mg once daily may be tried.

Nabilone. Nabilone [Cesamet] is supplied in 1-mg capsules for oral use. The usual dosage is 1 to 2 mg twice daily.

Chemotherapy-Induced Nausea and Vomiting

Many anticancer drugs cause severe nausea and vomiting, leading to dehydration, electrolyte imbalances, nutrient depletion, and esophageal tears. Worse yet, these reactions can be so intense that patients may discontinue chemotherapy rather than endure further discomfort. Fortunately, CINV can be minimized with the antiemetics.

Chemotherapy is associated with three types of emesis: (1) anticipatory, (2) acute, and (3) delayed. *Anticipatory emesis* occurs before anticancer drugs are actually given; it is triggered by the memory of severe nausea and vomiting from a previous round of chemotherapy. *Acute emesis* begins within minutes to a few hours after receiving chemotherapy and often resolves within 24 hours. In contrast, *delayed emesis* develops a day or more after drug administration. For example, with cisplatin, emesis is maximum 48 to 72 hours after dosing and can persist for 6 to 7 days.

Antiemetics are more effective at *preventing* CINV than at *suppressing* CINV that has already begun. Accordingly, antiemetics should be administered *before* chemotherapy. For prevention, antiemetics may be given orally or parenterally. Both routes are equally effective (although dosage may differ). In general, oral therapy is preferred. However, if emesis is ongoing, oral therapy won't work, and hence parenteral therapy is required.

The antiemetic regimen for a particular patient is based on the emetogenic potential of the chemotherapy drugs being used. For drugs with a low risk for causing emesis, a single antiemetic (dexamethasone) may be adequate. For drugs with a moderate or high risk for causing emesis, a combination of antiemetics is needed. The current regimen of choice for patients taking highly emetogenic drugs consists of three agents: aprepitant plus dexamethasone plus a 5-HT_3 antagonist (e.g., ondansetron, palonosetron). Lorazepam may be added to reduce anxiety and anticipatory emesis and to provide amnesia. The superior efficacy of combination therapy suggests that anticancer drugs may induce emesis by multiple mechanisms. Table 64.3 shows representative regimens for preventing CINV in patients receiving anticancer drugs with low, moderate, and high emetogenic risk.

TABLE 64.3 ▪ Representative Regimens for Preventing Chemotherapy-Induced Nausea and Vomiting

CHEMOTHERAPY WITH HIGH EMETOGENIC RISK	
Aprepitant	125 mg PO on day 1, 80 mg PO on days 2 and 3, *plus*
Dexamethasone	12 mg PO or IV on day 1, 8 mg PO or IV on days 2–4, *plus*
Ondansetron	8 mg PO twice on day 1 *or* 8 mg or 1.5 mg/kg IV on day 1
CHEMOTHERAPY WITH MODERATE EMETOGENIC RISK	
Dexamethasone	8 mg PO or IV, *plus*
Palonosetron	0.25 mg IV or 0.5 mg PO
CHEMOTHERAPY WITH LOW EMETOGENIC RISK	
Dexamethasone	8 mg PO or IV

Data from Basch E, Prestrud AA, et al. Antiemetics: American Society of Clinical Oncology. Clinical Practice Guideline Update *J Clin Oncol* 2011;29:4189–4198.

Nausea and Vomiting of Pregnancy

Nausea and vomiting of pregnancy (NVP) is extremely common, especially during the first trimester. About 50% of women experience nausea *plus* vomiting, and another 25% experience nausea alone. A few women experience *hyperemesis gravidarum,* a severe form of NVP characterized by dehydration, ketonuria, hypokalemia, and loss of 5% or more of body weight. Fortunately, most cases of NVP abate early in pregnancy: about 60% resolve within 13 weeks, and 90% resolve by the end of 20 weeks. Although NVP is commonly called *morning sickness,* it can occur any time of the day.

NVP can be managed with drugs and with nondrug measures. Nondrug measures include (1) eating small portions of food throughout the day; (2) avoiding odors, foods, and supplements that can trigger NVP (e.g., fatty foods, spicy foods, iron tablets); and (3) use of alternative treatments, such as acupuncture and ginger. Despite use of these nondrug measures, about 10% of women require drug therapy.

First-line therapy consists of a two-drug combination: *doxylamine* plus *vitamin B_6 (pyridoxine).* In randomized, controlled trials, the combination reduced NVP by 70% and showed no evidence of adverse fetal outcomes. Doxylamine and vitamin B_6 are available in a fixed-dose combination sold as *Diclectin* ♣ and *Diclegis.* Diclegis is sold in delayed-release tablets containing 10 mg each of doxylamine and pyridoxine. Dosing starts with 2 tablets at bedtime. If doxylamine and vitamin B_6 fail to suppress NVP, alternatives include prochlorperazine, metoclopramide, and ondansetron. Methylprednisolone may be tried as a last resort, but only after 10 weeks of gestation (earlier use greatly increases the risk for cleft lip, with or without cleft palate).

DRUGS FOR MOTION SICKNESS

Motion sickness can be caused by sea, air, automobile, and space travel. Symptoms are nausea, vomiting, pallor, and cold sweats. Drug therapy is most effective when given prophylactically, rather than after symptoms begin.

Scopolamine

Scopolamine, a muscarinic antagonist, is our most effective drug for prevention and treatment of motion sickness. Benefits derive from suppressing nerve traffic in the neuronal pathway that connects the vestibular apparatus of the inner ear to the vomiting center (see Fig. 64.1). The most common side effects are dry mouth, blurred vision, and drowsiness. More severe but less common effects are urinary retention, constipation, and disorientation.

PATIENT-CENTERED CARE ACROSS THE LIFE SPAN

Other Gastrointestinal Drugs

Life Stage	Patient Care Concerns
Infants	See later entry "Breastfeeding Women"
Children/adolescents	Promethazine is a commonly used antiemetic in children, but it is contraindicated in children younger than 2 years. Other antiemetics, including dronabinol, are approved for nausea and vomiting in children. Side effects are similar to those that occur in adults.
Pregnant women	First-line therapy in NVP includes doxylamine and vitamin B_6 in addition to diet changes. Other alternatives include prochlorperazine, metoclopramide, and ondansetron. The use of chenodiol is contraindicated during pregnancy.
Breastfeeding women	Prochlorperazine and promethazine appear safe for short-term use while breastfeeding. Observe infant for sedation. Metoclopramide, dronabinol, and droperidol should be avoided while breastfeeding.
Older adults	Benzodiazepines, scopolamine, and metoclopramide should be avoided in older adults.

Scopolamine is available for oral, subcutaneous, and transdermal dosing. The transdermal system [Transderm Scōp], an adhesive patch that contains scopolamine, is applied behind the ear. Anticholinergic side effects with transdermal administration may be less intense than with oral or subcutaneous dosing.

Antihistamines

The antihistamines used most often for motion sickness are *dimenhydrinate, meclizine* [Antivert, others], and *cyclizine* [Cyclivert]. Because these drugs block receptors for acetylcholine in addition to receptors for histamine, they appear in Table 64.1 as a subclass under "Anticholinergics." Suppression of motion sickness appears to result from blocking histaminergic (histamine-1, or H_1) and muscarinic cholinergic receptors in the neuronal pathway that connects the inner ear to the vomiting center (see Fig. 64.1). The most prominent side effect—sedation—results from blocking H_1 receptors. Other side effects—dry mouth, blurred vision, urinary retention, and constipation—result from blocking muscarinic receptors. Antihistamines are less effective than scopolamine for treating motion sickness, and sedation further limits their utility.

ANTIDIARRHEAL AGENTS

Diarrhea is characterized by stools of excessive volume and fluidity and by increased frequency of defecation. Diarrhea is a symptom of GI disease and not a disease per se. Causes include infection, maldigestion, inflammation, and functional disorders of the bowel (e.g., irritable bowel syndrome). The most serious complications of diarrhea are dehydration and electrolyte depletion. Management is directed at (1) diagnosis and treatment of the underlying disease, (2) replacement of lost water and salts, (3) relief of cramping, and (4) reducing passage of unformed stools.

Antidiarrheal drugs fall into two major groups: (1) specific antidiarrheal drugs and (2) nonspecific antidiarrheal drugs. The specific agents are drugs that treat the underlying cause of diarrhea. Included in this group are antiinfective drugs and drugs used to correct malabsorption syndromes. Nonspecific antidiarrheals are agents that act on or within the bowel to provide symptomatic relief; these drugs do not influence the underlying cause.

Nonspecific Antidiarrheal Agents

Opioids

Opioids are our most effective antidiarrheal agents. By activating opioid receptors in the GI tract, these drugs decrease intestinal motility and thereby slow intestinal transit, which allows more time for absorption of fluid and electrolytes. In addition, activation of opioid receptors decreases secretion of fluid into the small intestine and increases absorption of fluid and salt. The net effect is to present the large intestine with less water. As a result, the fluidity and volume of stools are reduced, as is the frequency of defecation.

At the doses employed to relieve diarrhea, subjective effects and dependence do not occur. However, excessive doses *can* elicit typical morphine-like subjective effects. If severe overdose occurs, it should be treated with an opioid antagonist (e.g., naloxone). In patients with inflammatory bowel disease, opioids may cause toxic megacolon.

Several opioid preparations—diphenoxylate, difenoxin, loperamide, paregoric, and opium tincture—are approved for diarrhea. Of these, diphenoxylate [Lomotil, others] and loperamide [Imodium, others] are the most frequently employed. Pharmacologic properties of these agents are discussed later. Dosages for diarrhea are shown in Table 64.4.

Diphenoxylate

Diphenoxylate is an opioid used only for diarrhea. The drug is insoluble in water and hence cannot be abused by parenteral routes. When taken orally in antidiarrheal doses, diphenoxylate has no significant effect on the CNS. However, if taken in high doses, the drug can elicit typical morphine-like subjective effects.

Diphenoxylate is formulated in combination with atropine. The combination, best known as *Lomotil,* is available in tablets and an oral liquid. Each tablet or 5 mL of liquid contains 2.5 mg of diphenoxylate and 0.025 mg of atropine sulfate. The atropine is present to discourage diphenoxylate abuse: doses of the combination that are sufficiently high to produce euphoria from the diphenoxylate would produce unpleasant side effects from the correspondingly high dose of atropine. Accordingly, the combination has a very low potential for abuse and is classified under Schedule V of the CSA.

TABLE 64.4 ▪ Opioids Used to Treat Diarrhea

Generic Name	Trade Name	CSA Schedule	Antidiarrheal Dosage
Diphenoxylate (plus atropine)*	Lomotil	V	*Adults:* 5 mg, 4 times/day *Children (initial dosage):* Ages 2–5 yr: 1 mg, 4 times/day Ages 5–12 yr: 1–2 mg, 4 times/day
Difenoxin (plus atropine)*	Motofen	IV	*Adults:* 2 mg initially, then 1 mg after each loose stool
Loperamide	Imodium, Pepto Diarrhea Control, others	NR	*Adults* (initial dose): 4 mg *Children (initial dosage):* Ages 2–5 yr: 1 mg, 3 times/day Ages 5–8 yr: 2 mg, 2 times/day Ages 8–12 yr: 2 mg, 3 times/day
Paregoric (camphorated tincture of opium; contains 0.4 mg morphine/mL)		III	*Adults:* 5–10 mL, 1–4 times/day *Children:* 0.25–0.5 mL/kg, 1–4 times/day
Opium tincture (opioid content equivalent to 10 mg morphine/mL)		II	0.6 mL, 4 times/day

*Diphenoxylate and difenoxin are available only in combination with atropine. The atropine dose is subtherapeutic and is present to discourage abuse.
CSA, Controlled Substances Act; NR, not regulated under the CSA.

Loperamide

Loperamide [Imodium, others] is a structural analog of meperidine. The drug is employed to treat diarrhea and to reduce the volume of discharge from ileostomies. Benefits derive from suppressing bowel motility and from suppressing fluid secretion into the intestinal lumen. The drug is poorly absorbed and does not readily cross the blood-brain barrier. Very large oral doses do not elicit morphine-like subjective effects. Loperamide has little or no potential for abuse and is not regulated under the CSA. The drug is supplied in 2-mg capsules, in 2-mg tablets, and in two liquid formulations (1 mg/5 mL and 1 mg/7.5 mL).

Difenoxin

Difenoxin is the major active metabolite of diphenoxylate. Like diphenoxylate, difenoxin can elicit morphine-like subjective effects at high doses. To discourage excessive dosing, difenoxin, like diphenoxylate, is formulated in combination with atropine. The combination is marketed as Motofen. Because its abuse potential is somewhat greater than that of diphenoxylate plus atropine, Motofen is classified as a Schedule IV product.

Paregoric

Paregoric (camphorated tincture of opium) is a dilute solution of opium, containing morphine (0.4 mg/mL) as its main active ingredient. The primary use is diarrhea, although paregoric has the same approved uses as morphine. Antidiarrheal doses cause neither euphoria nor analgesia. Very high doses can cause typical morphine-like responses. Paregoric has a moderate potential for abuse and is classified under Schedule III of the CSA.

Opium Tincture

Opium tincture is an alcohol-based solution that contains 10% opium by weight. The principal active ingredient—morphine—is present at 10 mg/mL. The primary indication is diarrhea. In addition, opium tincture (after dilution) may be given to suppress symptoms of withdrawal in opioid-dependent neonates. When administered in antidiarrheal doses, opium tincture does not produce analgesia or euphoria. However, high doses can cause typical opioid agonist effects. Opium tincture has a high potential for abuse and is classified as a Schedule II agent.

Other Nonspecific Antidiarrheals

Bismuth Subsalicylate

Bismuth subsalicylate [Pepto-Bismol, others] is effective for the prevention and treatment of mild diarrhea. For prevention, the dosage is two 262-mg tablets 4 times a day for up to 3 weeks. For treatment, the dosage is 2 tablets every 30 minutes for up to eight doses. Users should be aware that the drug may blacken stools and the tongue.

Bulk-Forming Agents

Paradoxically, methylcellulose, polycarbophil, and other bulk-forming laxatives can help manage diarrhea. Benefits derive from making stools more firm and less watery. Stool volume is not decreased. The bulk-forming laxatives are discussed in Chapter 63.

Anticholinergic Antispasmodics

Muscarinic antagonists (e.g., atropine) can relieve cramping associated with diarrhea, but do not alter fecal consistency or volume. However, owing to undesirable side effects (e.g., blurred vision, photophobia, dry mouth, urinary retention, tachycardia), anticholinergic drugs are of limited use. The pharmacology of the muscarinic blockers is discussed in Chapter 12.

Management of Infectious Diarrhea

General Considerations

Infectious diarrhea may be produced by enteric infection with a variety of bacteria and protozoa. These infections are usually self-limited. Mild diarrhea can be managed with nonspecific antidiarrheals. In many cases, no treatment is required at all. Antibiotics should be administered only when clearly indicated. Indiscriminate use of antibiotics is undesirable in that it (1) can promote emergence of antibiotic resistance and (2) can produce an asymptomatic carrier state by killing most of the infectious agents. Conditions that *do* merit antibiotic treatment include severe infections with *Salmonella, Shigella, Campylobacter,* or *Clostridium* species.

Traveler's Diarrhea

Tourists are often plagued by infectious diarrhea. In most cases, the causative organism is *Escherichia coli.* As a rule, treatment is unnecessary: infection with *E. coli* is self-limited and will run its course in a few days. However, if symptoms are especially severe, treatment with one of the fluoroquinolone antibiotics—*ciprofloxacin* (500 mg twice daily) or *norfloxacin* (400 mg twice daily)—is indicated. *Azithromycin* [Zithromax] is preferred for children (10 mg/kg on day 1 and 5 mg/kg on days 2 and 3) and for pregnant women (1000 mg once or 500 mg once daily for 3 days). *Rifaximin* [Xifaxan] (200 mg 3 times a day for 3 days) may also be used, provided the patient is not pregnant or febrile and that stools are not bloody. For patients with mild symptoms, relief can be achieved with *loperamide,* a nonspecific antidiarrheal. However, by slowing peristalsis, loperamide may delay export of the offending organism and may thereby prolong the infection.

Several measures can reduce acquisition of traveler's diarrhea. Two measures—avoiding local drinking water and carefully washing foods—are highly effective. Certain drugs—*ciprofloxacin* and *norfloxacin*—can be taken for prophylaxis. However, because these drugs can cause serious side effects, prophylaxis is not generally recommended. Lastly, travelers can be vaccinated against some pathogens. Oral vaccination with *Dukoral* ♣ protects against diarrhea caused by *E. coli* and *Vibrio cholera.*

Clostridium difficile–Associated Diarrhea

Clostridium difficile is a gram-positive, anaerobic bacillus that infects the bowel. Injury results from release of bacterial toxins. Symptoms range from relatively mild (abdominal discomfort, nausea, fever, diarrhea) to very severe (toxic megacolon, pseudomembranous colitis, colon perforation, sepsis, and death). *C. difficile* infection and its treatment are discussed in Chapter 70.

DRUGS FOR IRRITABLE BOWEL SYNDROME

Irritable bowel syndrome (IBS) is the most common disorder of the GI tract, affecting an estimated 20% of Americans—about 54 million people. The incidence in women is 3 times the incidence in men. IBS is responsible for 12% of all visits to primary care physicians and 28% of all visits to gastroenterologists. The direct medical costs are estimated at $8 billion a year; the indirect costs are much higher—about $25 billion a year. IBS is second only to the common cold as the leading cause of days missed from work.

IBS is a GI disorder characterized by crampy abdominal pain—sometimes severe—occurring in association with diarrhea, constipation, or both. Formally, IBS is defined by the presence, for at least 12 weeks in the past year, of abdominal pain or discomfort that cannot be explained by structural or chemical abnormalities and that has at least two of the following features:

- Pain is relieved by defecation.
- Onset was associated with a change in frequency of stool.
- Onset of pain occurred in association with a change in stool consistency (from normal to loose, watery, or pellet-like).

IBS has four major forms, characterized as follows:

- Abdominal pain in association with diarrhea (diarrhea-predominant IBS; IBS-D)
- Abdominal pain in association with constipation (constipation-predominant IBS; IBS-C)
- Abdominal pain in association with alternating episodes of diarrhea and constipation (mixed IBS; IBS-M)
- Abdominal pain in association with alternating episodes of diarrhea and constipation less than 25% of the time (unsubtyped IBS; IBS-U)

No one knows what causes IBS. Despite extensive research, no underlying pathophysiologic mechanism has been identified. What we do know is that the bowel appears hypersensitive and hyperresponsive. As a result, mild stimuli that would have no effect on most people can trigger an intense response. In addition, we know that symptoms can be triggered by stress, depression, and dietary factors, including caffeine, alcohol, fried foods, high-fat foods, gas-generating vegetables (beans, broccoli, cabbage), and too much sorbitol, a sweetener found in chewing gum and some diet products. Overproduction of gastric acid and excessive bacterial colonization of the small intestine have also been implicated.

Fortunately, many people achieve significant relief with treatment. Nondrug measures and drug therapy are employed. Patients should keep a log to identify foods and stressors that trigger symptoms. Because large meals stretch and stimulate the bowel, switching to smaller, more frequent meals may help. Increasing dietary fluid and fiber may reduce constipation.

Two groups of drugs are used for treatment: nonspecific drugs and drugs specific for IBS. Both groups are discussed next.

Nonspecific Drugs

Four groups of drugs—*antispasmodics* (e.g., hyoscyamine, dicyclomine), *bulk-forming agents* (e.g., psyllium, polycarbophil), *antidiarrheals* (e.g., loperamide), and *tricyclic antidepressants* (TCAs)—have been employed for years to provide symptomatic relief. However, a report from the American College of Gastroenterology (ACG) concluded that, for most of these agents, there is no good proof of clinical benefits. Specifically, after reviewing available data, the authors concluded that loperamide and the bulk-forming agents are no better than placebo at relieving global symptoms of IBS. In contrast, they concluded there is good evidence that TCAs can reduce abdominal pain and that this benefit is unrelated to relief of depression. Regarding antispasmodic agents, they concluded that the available data are insufficient to make a recommendation for or against use.

Studies suggest that, for some patients, symptoms can be relieved with *antibiotics* or an *acid suppressant.* For example, in one study, researchers observed that many patients with IBS have excessive bacteria in the small intestine. When these people were treated with antibiotics, bacterial colonization was reduced—and so were symptoms of IBS. In a more recent study, treatment with oral rifaximin (a poorly absorbed, broad-spectrum antibiotic) reduced symptoms in some patients with IBS. Another study evaluated the effects of drugs that suppress production of stomach acid in patients who routinely experienced exacerbation of symptoms after eating. Two kinds of acid suppressants were used: proton pump inhibitors (lansoprazole or omeprazole) and histamine-2 receptor blockers (famotidine or ranitidine). In all cases, patients experienced a significant reduction of postprandial urgency and other symptoms. Benefits developed quickly (within days) and reversed when the drugs were stopped.

Inflammatory Bowel Syndrome–Specific Drugs

In this section we discuss three drugs approved for IBS. These are alosetron and eluxadoline (approved for IBS-D) and lubiprostone (approved for IBS-C). Although a fourth drug, tegaserod, exists, it is used only in emergency situations owing to a risk for serious cardiovascular events.

Alosetron

Alosetron [Lotronex] is a potentially hazardous drug approved for IBS-D in women. (Safety and efficacy in men have not been demonstrated.) Alosetron was first approved on February 9, 2000, and then, in response to reports of severe GI toxicity and several deaths, approval was withdrawn on November 28, 2000, less than 10 months after being introduced. However, in 2002, alosetron was *reapproved* by the FDA, marking the first time the agency has allowed a drug back on the market after it had been pulled for safety reasons. To reduce risk, prescribers, patients, and pharmacists must adhere to a strict risk management program (see later).

Indications

Alosetron is approved only for treating women with severe IBS-D that has lasted for 6 months or more and has not responded to conventional treatment. IBS-D is considered severe if the patient experiences one or more of the following: (1) frequent and severe abdominal pain or discomfort, (2) frequent bowel urgency or fecal incontinence, and (3) disability or restriction of daily activities because of IBS. Less than 5% of IBS cases qualify as severe.

Mechanism of Action and Clinical Effects

Alosetron causes selective blockade of 5-HT_3 receptors, which are found primarily on neurons that innervate the viscera. In patients with IBS-D, alosetron can decrease abdominal pain, increase colonic transit time, reduce intestinal secretions, and increase absorption of water and sodium. As a result, the drug can increase stool firmness and decrease both fecal urgency and frequency. Presumably, all of these effects result from 5-HT_3 blockade. Symptoms decline 1 to 4 weeks after starting the drug and resume 1 week after stopping the drug.

Pharmacokinetics

Administration is oral, and absorption is rapid but incomplete (50%–60%). Bioavailability is decreased by food. Plasma levels peak about 1 hour after dosing. Alosetron undergoes extensive metabolism by hepatic cytochrome P450 enzymes, followed by excretion primarily in the urine. The half-life is 1.5 hours.

Drug Interactions

Alosetron does not interact with theophylline, oral contraceptives, cisapride, ibuprofen, alprazolam, amitriptyline, fluoxetine, or hydrocodone combined with acetaminophen. Because alosetron is metabolized by cytochrome P450 enzymes, drugs that interfere with these enzymes (e.g., carbamazepine, phenobarbital, cimetidine, quinolone antibiotics, ketoconazole, clarithromycin, voriconazole, and protease inhibitors) may alter alosetron levels.

Adverse Effects and Contraindications

Although alosetron is generally well tolerated, it *can* cause severe adverse effects. Deaths have occurred. The most common problem is constipation (29%), which can be complicated by impaction, bowel obstruction, and perforation.

BLACK BOX WARNING: ALOSETRON

Alosetron can cause *ischemic colitis* (intestinal damage secondary to reduced blood flow). Ischemic colitis and complications of constipation have led to hospitalization, blood transfusion, surgery, and death. Owing to its potential for GI toxicity, alosetron is *contraindicated* for patients with ongoing constipation or a history of any of the following:

- Chronic constipation, severe constipation, or sequelae from constipation
- Intestinal obstruction or stricture, toxic megacolon, or GI perforation or adhesions
- Ischemic colitis, impaired intestinal circulation, thrombophlebitis, or hypercoagulable state
- Crohn disease or ulcerative colitis
- Diverticulitis

Risk Management Program

To ensure the best possible benefit-to-risk ratio, the manufacturer and the FDA have established a risk management program that involves active participation of the patient, prescriber, and pharmacist. Details of this program can be found at lotronexppl.com.

Preparations, Dosage, and Administration

Alosetron [Lotronex] is supplied in 0.5- and 1-mg tablets. The recommended initial dosage is currently 0.5 mg twice daily. If, after 4 weeks, the dosage is well tolerated but inadequate, it can be increased to 1 mg twice a day. If, after 4 weeks at the higher dosage, treatment is still inadequate, the drug is not likely to help and should be stopped.

Patients who develop constipation or signs of ischemic colitis (rectal bleeding, bloody diarrhea, new or worsening abdominal pain) should immediately inform the prescriber and discontinue the drug. Those with ischemic colitis should never use alosetron again. Those with constipation may resume treatment, but only after constipation has resolved and only on the advice of the prescriber. If constipation does not resolve, the prescriber should be seen for evaluation.

Eluxadoline

Eluxadoline [Viberzi] is approved for IBS-D in both men and women. Eluxadoline is a mu- and kappa-opioid receptor agonist. By triggering these receptors, motility in the bowel is slowed. The dosage is 100 mg twice daily taken with food. A decreased dose of 75 mg twice daily is recommended for patients without a gallbladder, those who are unable to tolerate the higher dose, and those who have mild or moderate hepatic impairment. The most common adverse reactions include constipation, nausea, and abdominal pain.

Lubiprostone

Lubiprostone [Amitiza] is approved for IBS-C in women 18 years and older. Unfortunately, benefits are modest: the drug can reduce abdominal pain and discomfort, but only in a small percentage of patients. Efficacy against IBS-C in men has not been established. In addition to its use in IBS-C, lubiprostone is used for chronic idiopathic constipation (CIC) in women and men. As discussed in Chapter 63, lubiprostone causes selective activation of chloride channels in epithelial cells of the intestine and thereby (1) promotes secretion of chloride-rich fluid into the intestinal lumen and (2) enhances motility of the small intestine and colon. The dosage for IBS-C is lower than for CIC: 8 mcg twice daily versus 24 mcg twice daily. As a result, compared with patients treated for CIC, patients treated for IBS-C experience less nausea (8% vs. 30%), diarrhea (7% vs. 13%), and chest discomfort (0.4% vs. 2.5%). To reduce the incidence of nausea, all doses should be taken with food and water.

DRUGS FOR INFLAMMATORY BOWEL DISEASE

Inflammatory bowel disease (IBD) has two forms: *Crohn disease* and *ulcerative colitis.* Crohn disease is characterized by transmural inflammation and usually affects the terminal ileum but can also affect all other parts of the GI tract. Ulcerative colitis is characterized by inflammation of the mucosa and submucosa of the colon and rectum. Both diseases produce abdominal cramps and diarrhea. Ulcerative colitis may cause rectal bleeding as well. About 15% of patients with ulcerative colitis eventually have an attack severe enough to require hospitalization for IV glucocorticoid therapy, which produces remission in 60% of patients; the remaining 40% usually require total colectomy. In the United States IBD afflicts about 1.4 million people.

There is general agreement that IBD results from an exaggerated immune response directed against normal bowel flora—but only in genetically predisposed people.

Drug therapy of IBD is shown in Table 64.5. Five types of drugs are employed: *5-aminosalicylates* (e.g., sulfasalazine), *glucocorticoids* (e.g., hydrocortisone), *immunosuppressants* (e.g., azathioprine), *immunomodulators* (e.g., infliximab), and *antibiotics* (e.g., metronidazole). None of these drugs is curative; at best, drugs may control the disease process. Patients frequently require therapy with more than one agent.

5-Aminosalicylates

The 5-aminosalicylates are used to treat mild or moderate ulcerative colitis and Crohn disease and to maintain remission after symptoms have subsided. Four aminosalicylates are available: sulfasalazine, mesalamine, olsalazine, and balsalazide.

Sulfasalazine

Sulfasalazine [Azulfidine] belongs to the same chemical family as the sulfonamide antibiotics. However, although similar to the sulfonamides, sulfasalazine is not employed to treat infections. Its only approved indications are IBD and rheumatoid arthritis (see Chapter 57).

Actions

Sulfasalazine is metabolized by intestinal bacteria into two compounds: 5-aminosalicylic acid (5-ASA) and sulfapyridine. 5-ASA is the component responsible for reducing inflammation; sulfapyridine is responsible for adverse effects. Possible mechanisms by which 5-ASA reduces inflammation include suppression of prostaglandin synthesis and suppression of the migration of inflammatory cells into the affected region.

Therapeutic Uses

Sulfasalazine is most effective against acute episodes of mild to moderate ulcerative colitis. Responses are less satisfactory when symptoms are severe. Sulfasalazine can also benefit patients with Crohn disease.

Adverse Effects

Nausea, fever, rash, and arthralgia are common. Hematologic disorders (e.g., agranulocytosis, hemolytic anemia, macrocytic anemia) may also occur. Accordingly, complete blood counts should be obtained periodically. Sulfasalazine appears safe during pregnancy and lactation.

Preparations, Dosage, and Administration

Sulfasalazine [Azulfidine] is available in 500-mg immediate- and delayed-release oral tablets. The initial adult dosage is 500 mg/day. Maintenance dosages range from 2 to 4 g/day, given in divided doses.

Mesalamine

Mesalamine [Apriso, Asacol HD, Canasa, Delzicol, Lialda, Pentasa, Rowasa] is the generic name for 5-ASA, the active component in sulfasalazine. The drug is used for acute treatment of mild to moderate IBD and for maintenance therapy of IBD. Mesalamine can be administered by retention enema, by rectal suppository, or by mouth (in tablets and capsules that dissolve when they reach the terminal ileum). Adverse effects are milder than with sulfasalazine. The most common side effects of oral therapy are headache and GI upset. The adult oral dosage is 800 mg 3 times a day (for Asacol HD tablets or Delzicol capsules) or 1 g 4 times a day (for Pentasa capsules) or 1.5 g once a day (for Apriso capsules) or 2.4 to 4.8 g once a day (for Lialda tablets). The 1000-mg rectal suppositories [Canasa] are administered once daily at bedtime. The retention enema [Rowasa] is administered once daily (4 g in 60 mL).

Olsalazine

Olsalazine [Dipentum] is a dimer composed of two molecules of 5-ASA, the active component of sulfasalazine. Olsalazine is approved for maintenance therapy of ulcerative colitis in patients who can't tolerate sulfasalazine. The most common adverse effect is watery diarrhea, which occurs in 17% of patients. Other adverse effects include abdominal pain, cramps, acne, rash, and joint pain. Olsalazine is supplied in 250-mg oral capsules. The adult dosage is 500 mg twice daily with food.

Balsalazide

Balsalazide [Colazal] is an aminosalicylate indicated for mildly to moderately active ulcerative colitis. As with sulfasalazine, colonic bacteria act on balsalazide to release 5-ASA, the active portion of the molecule. Nearly all of the drug remains in the intestine; less than 1% is absorbed. As a result, balsalazide is well tolerated. The most common adverse effects are headache, abdominal pain, diarrhea, and nausea. Balsalazide is available in 750-mg oral capsules. The recommended dosage is 3 capsules 3 times a day for 8 to 12 weeks. This dosage delivers 2.4 g of free 5-ASA to the colon daily.

Glucocorticoids

The basic pharmacology of the glucocorticoids is presented in Chapter 56; discussion here is limited to their use in IBD. Glucocorticoids (e.g., dexamethasone, budesonide) can

TABLE 64.5 ■ Therapeutic Options for Inflammatory Bowel Disease

Disease Intensity	Disease Form: Ulcerative Colitis	Crohn Disease
Mild	5-Aminosalicylate: PO or rectal	Mesalamine: PO Metronidazole: PO Budesonide: PO Ciprofloxacin: PO
Moderate	5-Aminosalicylate: PO or rectal Infliximab: IV	Glucocorticoid: PO Azathioprine: PO Mercaptopurine: PO Infliximab: IV
Severe	Glucocorticoid: PO or IV Cyclosporine: IV Infliximab: IV	Glucocorticoid: PO or IV Methotrexate: IV or subQ Infliximab: IV
Refractory	Glucocorticoid: PO or IV Azathioprine: PO Mercaptopurine: PO	Infliximab: IV
Remission	5-Aminosalicylate: PO Azathioprine: PO Mercaptopurine: PO	Mesalamine: PO Azathioprine: PO Metronidazole: PO Mercaptopurine: PO Infliximab: IV

IV, intravenous; PO, oral; subQ, subcutaneous.

relieve symptoms of ulcerative colitis and Crohn disease. Benefits derive from antiinflammatory actions. Prolonged use of glucocorticoids can cause severe adverse effects, including adrenal suppression, osteoporosis, increased susceptibility to infection, and a cushingoid syndrome.

Glucocorticoids are indicated primarily for induction of remission—not for long-term maintenance. Administration is IV or PO.

Oral *budesonide* [Entocort EC] is approved for mild to moderate Crohn disease that involves the ileum and ascending colon. Entocort EC capsules are formulated to release budesonide when it reaches the ileum and ascending colon. As a result, high local concentrations are produced. Systemic effects are lower than with other glucocorticoids because absorbed budesonide undergoes extensive first-pass metabolism.

Immunosuppressants

Immunosuppressants are used for long-term therapy of selected patients with ulcerative colitis and Crohn disease. Clinical experience is greatest with azathioprine and mercaptopurine.

Thiopurines: Azathioprine and Mercaptopurine

These drugs are discussed together because one is the active form of the other. (Mercaptopurine is the active drug; azathioprine is a prodrug that undergoes conversion to mercaptopurine in the body.)

Although not approved for IBD, azathioprine [Imuran] and mercaptopurine [Purinethol] have been employed with success to induce and maintain remission in both ulcerative colitis and Crohn disease. Because onset of effects may be delayed for up to 6 months, these agents cannot be used for acute monotherapy. Furthermore, because these drugs are potentially more toxic than aminosalicylates or glucocorticoids, they are generally reserved for patients who have not responded to traditional therapy. Major adverse effects are pancreatitis and neutropenia (secondary to bone marrow suppression). At the doses used for IBD, these drugs are neither carcinogenic nor teratogenic.

Cyclosporine

Cyclosporine [Sandimmune, Neoral, Gengraf] is a stronger immunosuppressant than azathioprine or mercaptopurine—and acts faster, too. When used for IBD, the drug is generally reserved for patients with acute, severe ulcerative colitis or Crohn disease that has not responded to glucocorticoids. For these patients, continuous IV infusion can rapidly induce remission. In addition to IV administration, the drug has been administered orally in low doses to maintain remission, but results have been inconsistent. Cyclosporine is a potentially toxic compound that can cause renal impairment, neurotoxicity, and generalized suppression of the immune system.

Methotrexate

In patients with Crohn disease, methotrexate can promote short-term remission and thereby reduce the need for glucocorticoids. Because the doses employed are low (25 mg once a week), the toxicity associated with high-dose therapy in cancer patients is avoided.

Immunomodulators

The drugs discussed in this section are monoclonal antibody products that modulate immune responses. Three of these drugs—infliximab, certolizumab, and adalimumab—are inhibitors of *tumor necrosis factor-alpha* (TNF-alpha). The fourth drug—natalizumab—interferes with $alpha_4$ integrin. These drugs are generally considered second-line agents. However, some authorities now recommend their use early in treatment, with the hope of inducing remission quickly and maintaining remission longer.

Infliximab

Infliximab [Remicade] is a monoclonal antibody designed to neutralize TNF-alpha, a key immunoinflammatory modulator. The drug is indicated for moderate to severe Crohn disease and ulcerative colitis. In clinical trials, infliximab reduced symptoms in 65% of patients with moderate to severe Crohn disease and produced clinical remission in 33%. Good responses are also seen in ulcerative colitis. As discussed in Chapter 57, infliximab is also used for rheumatoid arthritis.

During clinical trials, 5% of patients dropped out because of serious adverse effects. Infections and infusion reactions are most common. Tuberculosis and opportunistic infections are of particular concern. Infusion reactions include fever, chills, pruritus, urticaria, and cardiopulmonary reactions (chest pain, hypotension, hypertension, dyspnea). Infliximab may also increase the risk for lymphoma, especially among patients with highly active disease or those on long-term immunosuppressive therapy.

For patients with Crohn disease or ulcerative colitis, treatment consists of an induction regimen (5 mg/kg infused at 0, 2, and 6 weeks) followed by maintenance infusions of 5 mg/kg every 8 weeks thereafter.

The basic pharmacology of infliximab is discussed in Chapter 57.

Antibiotics

Antibiotics, such as metronidazole and ciprofloxacin, can help control symptoms in patients with mild or moderate Crohn disease. In contrast, antibiotics are largely ineffective against ulcerative colitis.

Metronidazole

In patients with mild or moderate Crohn disease, metronidazole [Flagyl] is as effective as sulfasalazine. The dosages employed—up to 750 mg 3 times a day—are high. Furthermore, because relapse is likely if metronidazole is discontinued, long-term therapy is required. Unfortunately, prolonged use of high-dose metronidazole poses a risk of peripheral neuropathy. Although metronidazole can help patients with Crohn disease, benefits are minimal in those with ulcerative colitis. The pharmacology of metronidazole is discussed in Chapter 76.

Ciprofloxacin

Like metronidazole, ciprofloxacin [Cipro] is highly effective in patients with mild or moderate Crohn disease. A typical dosage is 500 mg twice daily. In one study, ciprofloxacin produced complete or partial remission in 72% of those treated. Combining ciprofloxacin with infliximab is superior to either drug used alone. Like metronidazole, ciprofloxacin is of little benefit in ulcerative colitis. The pharmacology of ciprofloxacin is presented in Chapter 76.

PROKINETIC AGENTS

Prokinetic drugs increase the tone and motility of the GI tract. Indications include gastroesophageal reflux disease (GERD), CINV, and diabetic gastroparesis.

Metoclopramide

Actions

Metoclopramide [Reglan, Metozolv ODT] has two beneficial actions: it (1) suppresses emesis (by blocking receptors for dopamine and serotonin in the CTZ) and (2) increases upper GI motility (by enhancing the actions of acetylcholine).

Therapeutic Uses

Indications depend on the route (oral or IV). *Oral* metoclopramide has two approved uses: diabetic gastroparesis and suppression of gastroesophageal reflux. *Intravenous* metoclopramide has four approved uses: suppression of postoperative nausea and vomiting, suppression of CINV, facilitation of small bowel intubation, and facilitation of radiologic examination of the GI tract. Off-label uses include for hiccups and for nausea and vomiting of early pregnancy.

Adverse Effects

With high-dose therapy, sedation and diarrhea are common. Long-term high-dose therapy can cause irreversible *tardive dyskinesia,* characterized by repetitive, involuntary movements of the arms, legs, and facial muscles. Older adults are especially vulnerable. To reduce the risk for tardive dyskinesia, treatment should be as brief as possible using the lowest effective dose. Owing to its ability to increase gastric and intestinal motility, metoclopramide is contraindicated in patients with GI obstruction, perforation, or hemorrhage. Of note, exposure to metoclopramide during the first trimester of pregnancy is not associated with an excess risk for congenital malformations.

Preparations, Dosage, and Administration

Metoclopramide is available in four formulations: standard tablets (5 and 10 mg) sold as Reglan, orally disintegrating tablets (5 and 10 mg) sold as Metozolv ODT, an oral syrup (1 mg/mL) sold generically, and a solution for injection (5 mg/mL) sold as Reglan. Dosages are as follows.

Diabetic Gastroparesis

The adult dosage is 10 mg PO 30 minutes before each meal and at bedtime for 2 to 8 weeks. The maximal duration is 12 weeks.

Symptomatic Gastroesophageal Reflux

The usual adult dosage is 10 to 15 mg PO 30 minutes before each meal and at bedtime, for a maximum of 12 weeks. If symptoms are sporadic, a single dose can be taken as needed (up to 20 mg PO 30 minutes before the precipitating situation).

PANCREATIC ENZYMES

The pancreas produces three types of digestive enzymes: lipases, amylases, and proteases. These enzymes are secreted into the duodenum, where they help digest fats, carbohydrates, and proteins. To protect the enzymes from stomach acid and pepsin, the pancreas secretes bicarbonate. The bicarbonate neutralizes acid in the duodenum, and the resulting elevation in pH inactivates pepsin.

Deficiency of pancreatic enzymes can compromise digestion, especially digestion of fats. Fatty stools are characteristic of the deficiency. When secretion of pancreatic enzymes is reduced, replacement therapy is needed. Causes of deficiency include cystic fibrosis, pancreatectomy, pancreatitis, and obstruction of the pancreatic duct.

Pancreatic enzymes for clinical use are available as pancrelipase, a mixture of lipases, amylases, and proteases prepared from hog pancreas. Trade names are Creon, Pancreaze, Pertzye, Ultresa, Viokace, and Zenpep. All drugs, with the exception of Viokace, are supplied in delayed-release capsules designed to dissolve in the duodenum and upper jejunum. Viokace is supplied in tablets. The capsules should not be crushed, chewed, or retained in the mouth, owing to a risk for irritating the oral mucosa.

Pancrelipase is generally well tolerated. The most common adverse effects are abdominal discomfort, flatulence, headache, and cough. Large doses can cause diarrhea, nausea, and cramping. The most serious concern is fibrosing colonopathy, seen rarely during high-dose therapy in patients with cystic fibrosis. Porcine pancrelipase contains high levels of purines and hence may pose a risk to patients with gout or hyperuricemia. Allergic reactions occur occasionally.

Acid suppressants (e.g., histamine-2 receptor blockers, proton pump inhibitors) may be employed as adjuvants to pancreatic enzyme therapy. The objective is to raise gastric pH, protecting the enzymes from inactivation. However, acid suppressants are beneficial only when acid secretion is excessive.

Dosage is adjusted on an individual basis. Determining factors include the extent of enzyme deficiency, dietary fat content, and enzyme activity of the preparation selected. The efficacy of therapy can be evaluated by measuring the reduction in 24-hour fat excretion. Pancreatic enzymes should be taken with every meal and snack.

ANORECTAL PREPARATIONS

Nitroglycerin for Anal Fissures

Rectogesic is a 0.4% nitroglycerin ointment used for relief of moderate to severe pain caused by chronic anal fissures (small tears in the skin that lines the anus). These fissures afflict about 700,000 Americans every year, often causing unrelenting and debilitating pain. Topical nitroglycerin relieves pain and promotes healing by relaxing the internal anal sphincter. Nitroglycerin ointment has been used in other countries for years and is considered by many experts to be a first-line therapy. The principal adverse effect is headache.

Other Anorectal Preparations

Various preparations can help relieve discomfort from hemorrhoids and other anorectal disorders. Local anesthetics (e.g., benzocaine, dibucaine) and hydrocortisone (a glucocorticoid) are common ingredients. Hydrocortisone suppresses inflammation, itching, and swelling. Local anesthetics reduce itching and pain. Anorectal preparations may also contain emollients (e.g., mineral oil, lanolin), whose lubricant properties reduce irritation, and astringents (e.g., bismuth subgallate, witch hazel, zinc oxide), which reduce irritation and inflammation. Anorectal preparations are available in multiple formulations: suppositories, creams, ointments, lotions, foams, tissues, and pads. Trade names include Preparation H, Rectagene, and Anusol.

UNIT XVII

Nutrition and Complementary Therapies

CHAPTER 65

Vitamins

Jacqueline Rosenjack Burchum, DNSc, FNP-BC, CNE

Vitamins have the following defining characteristics: (1) they are *organic compounds,* (2) they are required in *minute amounts* for growth and maintenance of health, and (3) they do not serve as a source of energy (in contrast to fats, carbohydrates, and proteins), but rather are *essential for energy transformation and regulation of metabolic processes.* Several vitamins are inactive in their native form and must be converted to active compounds in the body.

BASIC CONSIDERATIONS

Dietary Reference Intakes

Reference values on dietary vitamin intake, as set by the Food and Nutrition Board of the Institute of Medicine of the National Academy of Sciences, were established to provide a standard for good nutrition. In a 2006 report—*Dietary Reference Intakes: The Essential Guide to Nutrient Requirements*—the Food and Nutrition Board defined five reference values: *Recommended Dietary Allowance* (RDA), *Adequate Intake* (AI), *Tolerable Upper Intake Level* (UL), *Estimated Average Requirement* (EAR), and *Acceptable Macronutrient Distribution Range* (AMDR). Collectively, these five values are referred to as *Dietary Reference Intakes* (DRIs). Of these, the RDA, AI, UL, and EAR apply to vitamins. (The AMDR is used for macronutrients such as fats and carbohydrates.)

Recommended Dietary Allowance

The RDA is the average daily dietary intake sufficient to meet the nutrient requirements of nearly all (97%–98%) healthy individuals. These figures are not absolutes. RDAs change as we grow older. In addition, they often differ for males and females and typically increase for women who are pregnant or breastfeeding. Furthermore, RDAs apply only to individuals in good health. Vitamin requirements can be increased by illness, and therefore published RDA values may not be appropriate for sick people. RDAs, which are based on extensive experimental data, are revised periodically as new information becomes available. Current values are available at http://fnic.nal.usda.gov/dietary-guidance/dietary-reference-intakes/dri-reports.

Adequate Intake

The AI is an *estimate* of the average daily intake required to meet nutritional needs. AIs are employed when experimental evidence is not strong enough to establish an RDA. AIs are set with the expectation that they will meet the needs of all individuals. However, because AIs are only estimates, there is no guarantee they are adequate.

Tolerable Upper Intake Level

The UL is the highest average daily intake that can be consumed by nearly everyone without a significant risk for adverse effects. Please note that the UL is not a *recommended* upper limit for intake. It is simply an index of safety.

Estimated Average Requirement

The EAR is the level of intake that will meet nutrition requirements for 50% of the healthy individuals in any life-stage or gender group. By definition, the EAR may be insufficient for the other 50%. The EAR for a vitamin is based on extensive experimental data and serves as the basis for establishing an RDA. If there is not enough information to establish an EAR, no RDA can be set. Instead, an AI is assigned, using the limited data on hand.

Acceptable Macronutrient Distribution Range

The AMDR is a range for macronutrients (e.g., proteins, carbohydrates, fats) associated with optimal health. Intake of a nutrient below the established range for that nutrient increases the risk for malnourishment. Intake of a nutrient above the established range for that nutrient increases the risk for chronic diseases.

Classification of Vitamins

The vitamins are divided into two major groups: *fat-soluble vitamins* and *water-soluble vitamins.* In the fat-soluble group are vitamins A, D, E, and K. The water-soluble group consists of vitamin C and members of the vitamin B complex (thiamine, riboflavin, niacin, pyridoxine, pantothenic acid, biotin, folic acid, and cyanocobalamin). Except for vitamin B_{12}, water-soluble vitamins undergo minimal storage in the body, and hence frequent ingestion is needed to replenish supplies. In contrast, fat-soluble vitamins can be stored in massive amounts, which is good news and bad news. The good news is that extensive storage minimizes the risk for deficiency. The bad news is that extensive storage greatly increases the potential for toxicity if intake is excessive.

Should We Take Multivitamin Supplements?

In the United States we spend billions each year on multivitamin and multimineral supplements. Is the money well spent? Maybe. Maybe not. An expert panel—convened by the Office of Dietary Supplements at the National Institutes of Health—has spoken out on this issue. They report that there is insufficient evidence to recommend either for or against the use of multivitamins by Americans to prevent chronic disease.

For people who *do* take a multivitamin supplement, the dosage should be moderate because excessive doses can cause harm. For example, too much vitamin A increases the risk for osteoporosis in postmenopausal women and can cause birth defects when taken early in pregnancy. In older people with chronic health problems, too much vitamin E increases the risk for death. Because of these and other concerns, high-dose multivitamin supplements should be avoided. Instead, supplements that supply 100% or *less* of the RDA should be used.

Although research supporting the use of *multi*vitamin supplements is inconclusive, we do have solid data supporting the use of three *individual* vitamins—vitamin B_{12}, folic acid, and vitamin D. Who should take these vitamins? Nutrition experts recommend vitamin B_{12} for all people over age 50, folic acid for all women of childbearing age, and vitamin D (plus calcium) for postmenopausal women and other people at risk for fractures.

What About Protective Antioxidant Effects?

Dietary antioxidants are defined as substances present in food that can significantly decrease cellular and tissue injury caused by highly reactive forms of oxygen and nitrogen, known as *free radicals.* These free radicals, which are normal byproducts of metabolism, readily react with other molecules. The result is tissue injury known as *oxidative stress.* Antioxidants help reduce oxidative stress by neutralizing free radicals before they can cause harm.

Although high doses of antioxidant supplements have been touted for their ability to prevent chronic diseases such as cardiovascular disease and cancer, much of this is information carried over from assumptions made a quarter century ago. Despite plausible theories and observational studies that provided support for protective effects of antioxidant supplements, more recent and more rigorous trials have failed to show protection against heart disease, cancer, or any other long-term illness. The National Center for Complementary and Alternative Medicine examined well-designed experimental studies that included more than 100,000 subjects and concluded that most studies failed to demonstrate a role for antioxidant-related reduction in disease development. Further, they identified that high doses of certain antioxidants might actually increase the risk for disease. For example, high doses of beta-carotene were associated with an increase of lung cancer in people who smoked, and high doses of vitamin E were associated with an increase of prostate cancer and stroke. Additionally, some antioxidant supplements were responsible for significant drug interactions.

What's the bottom line? The National Academy of Sciences recommends limiting intake of antioxidant supplements to amounts that will prevent nutritional deficiency and avoiding doses that are potentially harmful. Of course, people should continue to obtain antioxidants as part of a healthy diet.

FAT-SOLUBLE VITAMINS

Vitamin A (Retinol)

Actions

Vitamin A, also known as retinol, has multiple functions. In the eye, vitamin A plays an important role in adaptation to dim light. The vitamin also has a role in embryogenesis, spermatogenesis, immunity, growth, and maintaining the structural and functional integrity of the skin and mucous membranes.

Sources

Requirements for vitamin A can be met by (1) consuming foods that contain preformed vitamin A (retinol) and (2) consuming foods that contain provitamin A carotenoids (beta-carotene, alpha-carotene, beta-cryptoxanthin), which are converted to retinol by cells of the intestinal mucosa. Preformed vitamin A is present only in foods of animal origin. Good sources are dairy products, meat, fish oil, and fish. Provitamin A carotenoids are found in darkly colored, carotene-rich fruits and vegetables. Especially rich sources are carrots, cantaloupe, mangoes, spinach, tomatoes, pumpkins, and sweet potatoes.

Units

The unit employed to measure vitamin A activity is called the retinol activity equivalent (RAE). By definition, 1 RAE equals 1 mcg of retinol, 12 mcg of beta-carotene, 24 mcg of alpha-carotene, or 24 mcg of beta-cryptoxanthin. Why are the RAEs for the provitamin A carotenoids 12 to 24 times higher than the RAE for retinol? Because dietary carotenoids are poorly absorbed and incompletely converted into retinol. Hence, to produce the nutritional equivalent of retinol, we need to ingest much higher amounts of the carotenoids. In the past, vitamin A activity was measured in international units (IU). This IU designation is still commonly used on product labels.

Requirements

The current RDA for vitamin A for adult males is 900 RAEs, and the RDA for adult females is 700 RAEs. RDAs for individuals in other life-stage groups are shown in Table 65.1.

Pharmacokinetics

Under normal conditions, dietary vitamin A is readily absorbed and then stored in the liver. As a rule, liver reserves of vitamin A are large and will last for months if intake of retinol ceases. Normal plasma levels for retinol range between 30 and 70 mcg/dL. In the absence of vitamin A intake, levels are maintained through mobilization of liver reserves. As liver stores approach depletion, plasma levels begin to decline. Signs and symptoms of deficiency appear when plasma levels fall below 20 mcg/dL.

Deficiency

Because vitamin A is needed for dark adaptation, night blindness is often the first indication of deficiency. With time, vitamin A deficiency may lead to *xerophthalmia* (a dry, thickened condition of the conjunctiva) and *keratomalacia* (degeneration of the cornea with keratinization of the

TABLE 65.1 ▪ Recommended Vitamin Intakes for Individuals

Life-Stage Group	Recommended Vitamin Intake Per Day												
	Vitamin A (mcg)[a]	Vitamin C (mg)	Vitamin D (IU)[b,c]	Vitamin E (mg)[d]	Vitamin K (mcg)	Thiamine (mg)	Riboflavin (mg)	Niacin (mg)[e]	Vitamin B_6 (mg)	Folate (mcg)[f]	Vitamin B_{12} (mcg)	Pantothenic Acid (mg)	Biotin (mcg)
INFANTS													
0–6 mo	400*	40*	400*	4*	2*	0.2*	0.3*	2*	0.1*	65*	0.4*	1.7*	5*
7–12 mo	500*	50*	400*	5*	2.5*	0.3*	0.4*	4*	0.3*	80*	0.5*	1.8*	6*
CHILDREN													
1–3 yr	300	15	600	6	30*	0.5	0.5	6	0.5	150	0.9	2*	8*
4–8 yr	400	25	600	7	55*	0.6	0.6	8	0.6	200	1.2	3*	12*
MALES													
9–13 yr	600	45	600	11	60*	0.9	0.9	12	1	300	1.8	4*	20*
14–18 yr	900	75	600	15	75*	1.2	1.3	16	1.3	400	2.4	5*	25*
19–30 yr	900	90	600	15	120*	1.2	1.3	16	1.3	400	2.4	5*	30*
31–50 yr	900	90	600	15	120*	1.2	1.3	16	1.3	400	2.4	5*	30*
51–70 yr	900	90	600	15	120*	1.2	1.3	16	1.7	400	2.4[g]	5*	30*
>70 yr	900	90	800	15	120*	1.2	1.3	16	1.7	400	2.4[g]	5*	30*
FEMALES													
9–13 yr	600	45	600	11	60*	0.9	0.9	12	1	300	1.8	4*	20*
14–18 yr	700	65	600	15	75*	1	1	14	1.2	400[h]	2.4	5*	25*
19–30 yr	700	75	600	15	90*	1.1	1.1	14	1.3	400[h]	2.4	5*	30*
31–50 yr	700	75	600	15	90*	1.1	1.1	14	1.3	400[h]	2.4	5*	30*
51–70 yr	700	75	600	15	90*	1.1	1.1	14	1.5	400	2.4[g]	5*	30*
>70 yr	700	75	800	15	90*	1.1	1.1	14	1.5	400	2.4[g]	5*	30*
DURING PREGNANCY													
≤18 yr	750	80	600	15	75*	1.4	1.4	18	1.9	600[i]	2.6	6*	30*
19–30 yr	770	85	600	15	90*	1.4	1.4	18	1.9	600[i]	2.6	6*	30*
31–50 yr	770	85	600	15	90*	1.4	1.4	18	1.9	600[i]	2.6	6*	30*
DURING LACTATION													
≤18 yr	1200	115	600	19	75*	1.4	1.6	17	2	500	2.8	7*	35*
19–30 yr	1300	120	600	19	90*	1.4	1.6	17	2	500	2.8	7*	35*
31–50 yr	1300	120	600	19	90*	1.4	1.6	17	2	500	2.8	7*	35*

NOTE: This table presents recommended dietary allowances (RDAs) in **bold type** and Adequate Intakes (AIs) in ordinary type followed by an asterisk (*). RDAs and AIs may both be used as goals for individual intake. RDAs are set to meet the needs of almost all (97%–98%) individuals in a group. For healthy breastfed infants, the AI is the mean intake. The AI for other life-stage and gender groups is believed to cover needs of all individuals in the group, but lack of data or uncertainty in the data prevents being able to specify with confidence the percentage of individuals covered by this intake.

[a] As retinol activity equivalents (RAEs): 1 RAE = 1 mcg retinol, 12 mcg beta-carotene, 24 mcg alpha-carotene, or 24 mcg beta-cryptoxanthin. To calculate RAEs from retinol equivalents (REs) of provitamin A carotenoids in foods, divide the REs by 2. For preformed vitamin A in foods or supplements and for provitamin A carotenoids in supplements, 1 RE = 1 RAE.

[b] These new RDAs and AIs were issued by the Institute of Medicine on November 30, 2010.

[c] In the absence of adequate exposure to sunlight.

[d] As alpha-tocopherol. Alpha-tocopherol includes *RRR*-alpha-tocopherol, the only form of alpha-tocopherol that occurs naturally in foods, and the 2R-stereoisomeric forms of alpha-tocopherol (*RRR*-, *RSR*-, *RRS*-, and *RSS*-alpha-tocopherol) that occur in fortified foods and supplements. It does not include the 2S-stereoisomeric forms of alpha-tocopherol (*SRR*-, *SSR*-, *SRS*-, and *SSS*-alpha-tocopherol), also found in fortified foods and supplements.

[e] As niacin equivalents (NE): 1 mg of niacin = 60 mg of tryptophan; 0 to 6 months = preformed niacin (not NE).

[f] As dietary folate equivalents (DFEs): 1 DFE = 1 mcg food folate = 0.6 mcg of folic acid from fortified food or as a supplement consumed with food = 0.5 mcg of a supplement taken on an empty stomach.

[g] Because 10% to 30% of older people may absorb food-bound B_{12} poorly, it is advisable for those older than 50 years to meet their RDA mainly by consuming foods fortified with B_{12} or by consuming a supplement containing B_{12}.

[h] In view of evidence linking folate deficiency with neural tube defects in the fetus, the USPSTF recommends that all women capable of becoming pregnant consume 400 to 800 mcg from supplements in addition to intake of food folate from a varied diet.

[i] It is assumed that women will continue consuming 400 mcg from supplements or fortified food until their pregnancy is confirmed and they enter prenatal care, which ordinarily occurs after the end of the periconceptional period—the critical time for formation of the neural tube.

corneal epithelium). When vitamin A deficiency is severe, blindness may occur. In addition to effects on the eye, deficiency can produce skin lesions and dysfunction of mucous membranes.

Toxicity

In high doses, vitamin A can cause birth defects, liver injury, and bone-related disorders. To reduce risk, the Food and Nutrition Board has set the UL for vitamin A at 3000 mcg/day.

Vitamin A is highly teratogenic. Excessive intake during pregnancy can cause malformation of the fetal heart, skull, and other structures of cranial–neural crest origin. Pregnant women should definitely not exceed the UL for vitamin A and should probably not exceed the RDA.

Excessive doses can cause a toxic state referred to as *hypervitaminosis A*. Chronic intoxication affects multiple organ systems, especially the liver. Symptoms are diverse and may include vomiting, jaundice, hepatosplenomegaly, skin changes, hypomenorrhea, and elevation of intracranial pressure. Most symptoms disappear after vitamin A withdrawal.

Vitamin A excess can damage bone. In infants and young children, vitamin A can cause bulging of the skull at sites where bone has not yet formed. In adult females, too much vitamin A can increase the risk for hip fracture—apparently by blocking the ability of vitamin D to enhance calcium absorption.

Therapeutic Uses

The only indication for vitamin A is prevention or correction of vitamin A deficiency. Contrary to earlier hopes, it is now clear that vitamin A, in the form of beta-carotene supplements, does not decrease the risk for cancer or cardiovascular disease. In fact, in a study comparing placebo with dietary supplements (beta-carotene plus vitamin A), subjects taking the supplements had a significantly *increased* risk for lung cancer and overall mortality. As discussed in Chapter 85, certain derivatives of vitamin A (e.g., isotretinoin, etretinate) are used to treat acne and other dermatologic disorders.

Preparations and Routes of Administration

Vitamin A (retinol) is available in drops, tablets, and capsules for oral dosing and in solution for intramuscular (IM) injection. Oral dosing is generally preferred. To prevent deficiency, dietary plus supplemental vitamin A should add up to the RDA. To treat deficiency, doses up to 100 times the RDA may be required.

Vitamin D

Vitamin D plays a critical role in calcium metabolism and maintenance of bone health. The classic effects of deficiency are *rickets* (in children) and *osteomalacia* (in adults). Does vitamin D offer health benefits beyond bone health? Possibly. Studies suggest that vitamin D may protect against arthritis, diabetes, heart disease, autoimmune disorders, and cancers of the colon, breast, and prostate. However, in a 2011 report—*Dietary Reference Intakes for Calcium and Vitamin D*—an expert panel concluded that, although such claims might eventually prove true, the current evidence does not prove any benefits beyond bone health. The pharmacology and physiology of vitamin D are discussed in Chapter 59. Values for RDAs and adequate intake are shown in Table 65.1.

Vitamin E (Alpha-Tocopherol)

Vitamin E (alpha-tocopherol) is essential to the health of many animal species but has no clearly established role in human nutrition. Unlike other vitamins, vitamin E has no known role in metabolism. Deficiency, which is rare, can result in neurologic deficits.

Vitamin E helps maintain health primarily through antioxidant actions. Specifically, the vitamin helps protect against peroxidation of lipids. It also inhibits oxidation of vitamins A and C. Observational studies of the past suggested that vitamin E protected against cardiovascular disease, Alzheimer disease, and cancer. However, more rigorous studies have failed to show any such benefits. Moreover, there *is* evidence that high-dose vitamin E may actually increase the risk for heart failure, cancer progression, and all-cause mortality.

Forms of Vitamin E

Vitamin E exists in a variety of forms (e.g., alpha-tocopherol, beta-tocopherol, alpha-tocotrienol), each of which has multiple stereoisomers. However, only four stereoisomers are found in our blood, all of them variants of alpha-tocopherol. These isomers are designated RRR-, RRS-, RSR-, and RSS-alpha-tocopherol. Of the four, only RRR-alpha-tocopherol occurs naturally in foods. However, all four can be found in fortified foods and dietary supplements. Why are other forms of vitamin E absent from blood? Because they are unable to bind to alpha-tocopherol transfer protein (alpha-TTP), the hepatic protein required for secretion of vitamin E from the liver and subsequent transport throughout the body.

Sources

Most dietary vitamin E comes from vegetable oils (e.g., corn oil, olive oil, cottonseed oil, safflower oil, canola oil). The vitamin is also found in nuts, wheat germ, whole-grain products, and mustard greens.

Requirements

The RDA for vitamin E, for men and women, is 15 mg/day (22.5 IU). RDAs increase for women who are breastfeeding, but not for those who are pregnant. Taking more than 200 mg/day increases the risk for hemorrhagic stroke. Accordingly, this limit should be exceeded only when there is a need to manage a specific disorder (e.g., advanced macular degeneration) and only when advised by a health care professional.

Deficiency

Vitamin E deficiency is rare. In the United States deficiency is limited primarily to people with an inborn deficiency of alpha-TTP and to those who have fat malabsorption syndromes and hence cannot absorb fat-soluble vitamins. Symptoms of deficiency include ataxia, sensory neuropathy, areflexia, and muscle hypertrophy.

Potential Benefits

Vitamin E has a role in protecting red blood cells from hemolysis. There is evidence that 200 IU of vitamin E daily may reduce the risk for colds in older adults, and 400 IU daily (in combination with vitamin C, beta-carotene, zinc, and copper) may delay progression of age-related macular degeneration. The higher dose associated with halting macular degeneration carries substantial risk, as detailed in the discussion that follows.

Potential Risks

High-dose vitamin E appears to increase the risk for hemorrhagic stroke by inhibiting platelet aggregation. According to a 2010 report, for every 10,000 people taking more than 200 IU of vitamin E daily for 1 year, there would be 8 additional cases of hemorrhagic stroke. Accordingly, doses higher than 200 IU/day should generally be avoided.

Some studies have demonstrated a relationship between high doses of vitamin E (400 IU daily) and increased cancer risk or poor cancer outcomes. These results are consistent with the theory that high doses of antioxidants may cause cancer or accelerate cancer progression.

Studies have also linked *high-dose* vitamin E therapy with an increased risk for death, especially in older people. Others have demonstrated higher mortality with *long-term* vitamin E therapy at doses above 400 IU (266 mg). Accordingly, recommendations have been put forward to decrease the current UL of 1500 IU daily to 200 IU daily.

Finally, high-dose vitamin E (in combination with vitamin C) can blunt the beneficial effects of exercise on insulin sensitivity. Under normal conditions, exercising enhances cellular responses to insulin. However, among subjects who took vitamin E (400 IU/day) plus vitamin C (500 mg twice daily), exercising failed to yield this benefit.

Vitamin K

Action

Vitamin K is required for synthesis of prothrombin and clotting factors VII, IX, and X. All of these vitamin K–dependent factors are needed for coagulation of blood.

Forms and Sources of Vitamin K

Vitamin K occurs in nature in two forms: (1) vitamin K_1, or phytonadione (phylloquinone), and (2) vitamin K_2. Phytonadione is present in a wide variety of foods. Vitamin K_2 is synthesized by the normal flora of the gut. Two other forms—vitamin K_4 (menadiol) and vitamin K_3 (menadione)—are produced synthetically. At this time, phytonadione is the only form of vitamin K available for therapeutic use.

Requirements

Human requirements for vitamin K have not been precisely defined. In 2002 the Food and Nutrition Board set the AI for adult males at 120 mcg and the AI for adult females at 90 mcg. AIs for other life-stage groups are shown in Table 65.1. For most individuals, vitamin K requirements are readily met through dietary sources and through vitamin K synthesized by intestinal bacteria. Because bacterial colonization of the gut is not complete until several days after birth, levels of vitamin K may be low in newborns.

Pharmacokinetics

Intestinal absorption of the natural forms of vitamin K (phytonadione and vitamin K_2) is adequate only in the presence of bile salts. Menadione and menadiol do not require bile salts for absorption. After absorption, vitamin K is concentrated in the liver. Metabolism and secretion occur rapidly. Very little is stored.

Deficiency

Vitamin K deficiency produces bleeding tendencies. If the deficiency is severe, spontaneous hemorrhage may occur. In newborns, intracranial hemorrhage is of particular concern.

An important cause of deficiency is reduced absorption. Because the natural forms of vitamin K require bile salts for their uptake, any condition that decreases availability of these salts (e.g., obstructive jaundice) can lead to deficiency. Malabsorption syndromes (sprue, celiac disease, cystic fibrosis of the pancreas) can also decrease vitamin K uptake. Other potential causes of impaired absorption are ulcerative colitis, regional enteritis, and surgical resection of the intestine.

Disruption of intestinal flora may result in deficiency by eliminating vitamin K–synthesizing bacteria. Hence deficiency may occur secondary to use of antibiotics. In infants, diarrhea may cause bacterial losses sufficient to result in deficiency.

The normal infant is born vitamin K deficient. Consequently, to rapidly elevate prothrombin levels and reduce the risk for neonatal hemorrhage, the American Academy of Pediatrics and the Centers for Disease Control and Prevention recommend that all infants receive a single injection of phytonadione (vitamin K_1) immediately after delivery. This previously routine prophylactic intervention has recently been challenged by parents who believe that the risks outweigh benefits. Subsequent to increases in parents declining prophylaxis, there has been an increase in life-threatening vitamin K deficiency bleeding in recent years.

As discussed in Chapter 44, the anticoagulant warfarin acts as an antagonist of vitamin K and thereby decreases synthesis of vitamin K–dependent clotting factors. As a result, warfarin produces a state that is functionally equivalent to vitamin K deficiency. If the dosage of warfarin is excessive, hemorrhage can occur secondary to lack of prothrombin.

Adverse Effects

Severe Hypersensitivity Reactions

Intravenous (IV) phytonadione can cause serious reactions (shock, respiratory arrest, cardiac arrest) that resemble anaphylaxis or hypersensitivity reactions. Death has occurred. Consequently, phytonadione should not be administered by the IV route unless other routes are not feasible, and then only if the potential benefits clearly outweigh the risks.

Hyperbilirubinemia

When administered *parenterally* to newborns, vitamin K derivatives can elevate plasma levels of bilirubin, thereby posing a risk for *kernicterus*. The incidence of hyperbilirubinemia is greater in premature infants than in full-term infants. Although all forms of vitamin K can raise bilirubin levels, the risk is higher with menadione and menadiol than with phytonadione.

Therapeutic Uses and Dosage

Vitamin K has two major applications: (1) correction or prevention of hypoprothrombinemia and bleeding caused by vitamin K deficiency and (2) control of hemorrhage caused by warfarin.

Vitamin K Replacement

As discussed, vitamin K deficiency can result from impaired absorption and from insufficient synthesis of vitamin K by intestinal flora. Rarely, deficiency results from inadequate diet. For children and adults, the usual dosage for correction of vitamin K deficiency ranges between 5 and 15 mg/day.

As noted, infants are born vitamin K deficient. To prevent hemorrhagic disease in neonates, it is recommended that all newborns be given an injection of phytonadione (0.5–1 mg) immediately after delivery.

Warfarin Antidote

Vitamin K reverses hypoprothrombinemia and bleeding caused by excessive dosing with warfarin, an oral anticoagulant. Bleeding is controlled within hours of vitamin K administration.

Preparations and Routes of Administration

Phytonadione (vitamin K_1) is available in 5-mg tablets, marketed as Mephyton, and in parenteral formulations (2 and 10 mg/mL) sold generically. Parenteral phytonadione may be administered by IM, subcutaneous (subQ), and IV route. However, because IV administration is dangerous, this route should be used only when other routes are not feasible and only if the perceived benefits outweigh the substantial risks. For example, this might be indicated in management of life-threatening bleeding due to vitamin K antagonists (e.g., poisoning by coumarins in rodenticides).

WATER-SOLUBLE VITAMINS

The group of water-soluble vitamins consists of vitamin C and members of the vitamin B complex: thiamine, riboflavin, niacin, pyridoxine, pantothenic acid, biotin, folic acid, and cyanocobalamin. The B vitamins differ widely from one another in structure and function. They are grouped together because they were first isolated from the same sources (yeast and liver). Vitamin C is not found in the same foods as the B vitamins and hence is classified by itself.

Two compounds—*pangamic acid* and *laetrile*—have been falsely promoted as B vitamins. Pangamic acid has been marketed as "vitamin B_{15}" and laetrile as "vitamin B_{17}." There is no proof these compounds act as vitamins or have any other role in human nutrition.

Vitamin C (Ascorbic Acid)

Actions

Vitamin C participates in multiple biochemical reactions. Among these are synthesis of adrenal steroids, conversion of folic acid to folinic acid, and regulation of the respiratory cycle in mitochondria. At the tissue level, vitamin C is required for production of collagen and other compounds that comprise the intercellular matrix that binds cells together. In addition, vitamin C has antioxidant activity and facilitates absorption of dietary iron.

Sources

The main dietary sources of ascorbic acid are citrus fruits and juices, tomatoes, potatoes, strawberries, melons, spinach, and broccoli. Orange juice and lemon juice are especially rich sources.

Requirements

Current RDAs for vitamin C are shown in Table 65.1. As in the past, RDAs increase for women who are pregnant or breastfeeding. For smokers, the RDA is increased by 35 mg/day.

Deficiency

Deficiency of vitamin C can lead to *scurvy,* a disease rarely seen in the United States. Symptoms include faulty bone and tooth development, loosening of the teeth, gingivitis, bleeding gums, poor wound healing, hemorrhage into muscles and joints, and ecchymoses (skin discoloration caused by leakage of blood into subcutaneous tissues). Many of these symptoms result from disruption of the intercellular matrix of capillaries and other tissues.

Adverse Effects

Excessive doses can cause *nausea, abdominal cramps,* and *diarrhea.* The mechanism is direct irritation of the intestinal mucosa. To protect against gastrointestinal (GI) disturbances, the Food and Nutrition Board has set 2 g/day as the adult UL for vitamin C.

Therapeutic Use

The only *established* indication for vitamin C is prevention and treatment of scurvy. For severe, acute deficiency, parenteral administration is recommended.

Vitamin C has been advocated for therapy of many conditions unrelated to deficiency, including cancers, asthma, osteoporosis, and the common cold. Claims of efficacy for several of these conditions have been definitively disproved. Other claims remain unproved. Studies have shown that large doses of vitamin C do not reduce the incidence of colds, although the intensity or duration of illness may be decreased slightly. Research has failed to show any benefit of vitamin C therapy for patients with advanced cancer, atherosclerosis, or schizophrenia. Vitamin C does not promote healing of wounds.

Preparations and Routes of Administration

Vitamin C is available in formulations for oral and parenteral administration. Oral products include tablets (ranging from 25–1000 mg), timed-release capsules (500–1500 mg), and syrups (20 and 100 mg/mL), as well as granules, crystals, powders, effervescent powders, and wafers. Parenteral administration may be subQ, IM, or IV.

Niacin (Nicotinic Acid)

Niacin has a role as both a vitamin and a medicine. In its medicinal role, niacin is used to reduce cholesterol levels; the doses required are much higher than those used to correct or prevent nutritional deficiency. Discussion in this chapter focuses on niacin as a vitamin. Use of nicotinic acid to reduce cholesterol levels is discussed in Chapter 42.

Physiologic Actions

Before it can exert physiologic effects, niacin must first be converted into nicotinamide adenine dinucleotide (NAD) or nicotinamide adenine dinucleotide phosphate (NADP). NAD and NADP then act as coenzymes in oxidation-reduction reactions essential for cellular respiration.

Sources

Nicotinic acid (or its nutritional equivalent, nicotinamide) is present in many foods of plant and animal origin. Particularly rich sources are liver, poultry, fish, potatoes, peanuts, cereal bran, and cereal germ.

In humans, the amino acid tryptophan can be converted to nicotinic acid. Hence proteins can be a source of the vitamin. About 60 mg of dietary tryptophan is required to produce 1 mg of nicotinic acid.

Requirements

RDAs for nicotinic acid are stated as niacin equivalents (NEs). By definition, 1 NE is equal to 1 mg of niacin (nicotinic acid) or 60 mg of tryptophan. Current RDAs for niacin are provided in Table 65.1.

Deficiency

The syndrome caused by niacin deficiency is called *pellagra,* a term that is a condensation of the Italian words *pelle agra,* meaning "rough skin." As suggested by this name, a prominent symptom of pellagra is dermatitis, characterized by scaling and cracking of the skin in areas exposed to the sun.

Other symptoms involve the GI tract (abdominal pain, diarrhea, soreness of the tongue and mouth) and central nervous system (irritability, insomnia, memory loss, anxiety, dementia). All symptoms reverse with niacin replacement therapy.

Adverse Effects

Nicotinic acid has very low toxicity. Small doses are completely devoid of adverse effects. When taken in large doses, nicotinic acid can cause vasodilation with resultant *flushing, dizziness,* and *nausea.* Using flushing as an index of excess niacin consumption, the Food and Nutrition Board has set 50 mg as the adult UL. Toxicity associated with high-dose therapy is discussed in Chapter 42.

Nicotinamide, a compound that can substitute for nicotinic acid in the treatment of pellagra, is not a vasodilator, and this does not produce the adverse effects associated with large doses of nicotinic acid. Accordingly, nicotinamide is often preferred to nicotinic acid for treating pellagra.

Therapeutic Uses

In its capacity as a vitamin, nicotinic acid is indicated only for the prevention or treatment of niacin deficiency. It is used off-label for treatment of pellagra.

Preparations, Dosage, and Administration

Nicotinic acid (niacin) is available in immediate-release tablets (50–500 mg), extended-release tablets (250–1000 mg), and extended-release capsules (250–500 mg). Dosages for mild deficiency range from 10 to 20 mg/day. For treatment of pellagra, daily doses may be as high as 500 mg/day; however, the usual dose is 50-100 mg every 6-8 hours. Dosages for hyperlipidemia are given in Chapter 42.

Nicotinamide (niacinamide) is available in 100- and 500-mg tablets. The usual dosage for treatment of pellagra is 100 mg every 6 hours initially. Once major signs and symptoms have resolved, dosing can be decreased to 10 mg every 8-12 hours until resolution of skin lesions. Unlike nicotinic acid, nicotinamide has no effect on plasma lipoproteins and hence is not used to treat hyperlipidemias.

Riboflavin (Vitamin B_2)

Actions

Riboflavin participates in numerous enzymatic reactions. However, to do so, the vitamin must first be converted into one of two active forms: flavin adenine dinucleotide (FAD) or flavin mononucleotide (FMN). In the form of FAD or FMN, riboflavin acts as a coenzyme for multiple oxidative reactions.

Sources and Requirements

In the United States most dietary riboflavin comes from milk, yogurt, cheese, bread products, and fortified cereals. Organ meats are also rich sources. RDAs for riboflavin are listed in Table 65.1.

Toxicity

Riboflavin appears devoid of toxicity to humans. When large doses are administered, the excess is rapidly excreted in the urine. Because large doses are harmless, no UL has been set.

Use in Riboflavin Deficiency

Riboflavin is indicated only for prevention and correction of riboflavin deficiency, which usually occurs in conjunction with deficiency of other B vitamins. In its early state, riboflavin deficiency manifests as sore throat and angular stomatitis (cracks in the skin at the corners of the mouth). Later symptoms include cheilosis (painful cracks in the lips), glossitis (inflammation of the tongue), vascularization of the cornea, and itchy dermatitis of the scrotum or vulva. Oral riboflavin is used for treatment. The dosage is 10 to 15 mg/day.

Use in Migraine Headache

As discussed in Chapter 23, riboflavin can help prevent migraine headaches; however, prophylactic effects do not develop until after 3 months of treatment. The daily dosage is 400 mg—much higher than the dosage for riboflavin deficiency.

Thiamine (Vitamin B_1)

Actions and Requirements

The active form of thiamine (thiamine pyrophosphate) is an essential coenzyme for carbohydrate metabolism. Thiamine requirements are related to caloric intake and are greatest when carbohydrates are the primary source of calories. For maintenance of good health, thiamine consumption should be at least 0.3 mg/1000 kcal in the diet. Current RDAs for thiamine appear in Table 65.1. As indicated, thiamine requirements increase significantly during pregnancy and lactation.

Sources

In the United States the principal dietary sources of thiamine are enriched, fortified, or whole-grain products, especially breads and ready-to-eat cereals. The richest source of the natural vitamin is pork.

Deficiency

Severe thiamine deficiency produces *beriberi,* a disorder having two distinct forms: *wet beriberi* and *dry beriberi. Wet beriberi* is so named because its primary symptom is fluid accumulation in the legs. Cardiovascular complications (palpitations, electrocardiogram abnormalities, high-output heart failure) are common and may progress rapidly to circulatory collapse and death. *Dry beriberi* is characterized by neurologic and motor deficits (e.g., anesthesia of the feet, ataxic gait, footdrop, wristdrop); edema and cardiovascular symptoms are absent. Wet beriberi responds rapidly and dramatically to replacement therapy. In contrast, recovery from dry beriberi can be very slow.

In the United States thiamine deficiency occurs most commonly among people with chronic alcohol consumption. In this population, deficiency manifests as *Wernicke-Korsakoff syndrome* rather than frank beriberi. This syndrome is a serious disorder of the central nervous system, having neurologic and psychological manifestations. Symptoms include nystagmus, diplopia, ataxia, and an inability to remember the recent past. Failure to correct the deficit may result in irreversible brain damage. Accordingly, if Wernicke-Korsakoff syndrome is suspected, parenteral thiamine should be administered immediately.

Adverse Effects

When taken orally, thiamine is devoid of adverse effects. Accordingly, no UL for the vitamin has been established.

Therapeutic Use

The only indication for thiamine is treatment and prevention of thiamine deficiency.

Preparations, Dosage, and Administration

Thiamine is available in standard tablets (50, 100, and 250 mg) and in solution (100 mg/mL) for IM or IV administration. For mild deficiency, oral thiamine is preferred. Parenteral administration is reserved for severe deficiency states (wet or dry beriberi, Wernicke-Korsakoff syndrome). The dosage for beriberi is 5 to 30 mg/day orally in single or divided doses 3 times/day for 1 month. For critically ill patients, therapy is initiated at the same dosage but via the IM or IV route 3 times/day. For Wernicke's encephalopathy, typical dosage is 100 mg IV initially followed by 50 to 100 mg/day IM or IV until the patient begins eating a balanced diet. In some instances, dosage may need to be increased.

Pyridoxine (Vitamin B_6)

Actions

Pyridoxine functions as a coenzyme in the metabolism of amino acids and proteins. However, before it can do so, pyridoxine must first be converted to its active form: pyridoxal phosphate.

Requirements

Current RDAs for pyridoxine are listed in Table 65.1. RDAs increase significantly for women who are pregnant or breastfeeding.

Sources

In the United States the principal dietary sources of pyridoxine are fortified, ready-to-eat cereals; meat, fish, and poultry; white potatoes and other starchy vegetables; and noncitrus fruits. Especially rich sources are organ meats (e.g., beef liver) and cereals or soy-based products that have been highly fortified.

Deficiency

Pyridoxine deficiency may result from poor diet, isoniazid therapy for tuberculosis, and inborn errors of metabolism. Symptoms include seborrheic dermatitis, anemia, peripheral neuritis, convulsions, depression, and confusion.

In the United States dietary deficiency of vitamin B_6 is rare, except among people who abuse alcohol on a long-term basis. Within this population, vitamin B_6 deficiency is estimated at 20% to 30% and occurs in combination with deficiency of other B vitamins.

Isoniazid (a drug for tuberculosis) prevents conversion of vitamin B_6 to its active form and may thereby induce symptoms of deficiency (peripheral neuritis). Patients who are predisposed to this neuropathy (e.g., people with diabetes or alcoholism) should receive daily pyridoxine supplements.

Inborn errors of metabolism can prevent efficient utilization of vitamin B_6, resulting in greatly increased pyridoxine requirements. Among infants, symptoms include irritability, convulsions, and anemia. Unless treatment with vitamin B_6 is initiated early, permanent cognitive deficits may result.

Adverse Effects

At low doses, pyridoxine is devoid of adverse effects. However, if extremely large doses are taken, neurologic injury may result. Symptoms include ataxia and numbness of the feet and hands. To minimize risk, adults should not consume more than 100 mg/day, the UL for this vitamin.

Drug Interactions

Vitamin B_6 interferes with the utilization of levodopa, a drug for Parkinson disease. Accordingly, patients receiving levodopa should be advised against taking the vitamin.

Therapeutic Uses

Pyridoxine is indicated for prevention and treatment of all vitamin B_6 deficiency states (dietary deficiency, isoniazid-induced deficiency, pyridoxine dependency syndrome).

Preparations, Dosage, and Administration

Pyridoxine is available in solution (200 mg/5 mL), standard tablets (25, 50, 100, 250, and 500 mg), extended-release tablets (200 mg), and capsules (150 mg) for oral use. It is available in solution (100 mg/mL) for IM or IV administration. To correct dietary deficiency, the dosage is 10 to 20 mg/day for 3 weeks followed by 1.5 to 2.5 mg/day thereafter for maintenance. To treat deficiency induced by isoniazid, the dosage is typically 100 mg/day IM or IV for 3 weeks and then 30 mg/day as a maintenance dose. To protect against developing isoniazid-induced deficiency, the dosage is 25 to 50 mg/day. Pyridoxine dependency syndrome may require initial doses up to 600 mg/day followed by 25 to 50 mg/day for life.

Cyanocobalamin (Vitamin B_{12}) and Folic Acid

Cyanocobalamin (vitamin B_{12}) and folic acid (folacin) are essential factors in the synthesis of DNA. Deficiency of either vitamin manifests as megaloblastic anemia. Cyanocobalamin deficiency produces neurologic damage as well. Because deficiency presents as anemia, folic acid and cyanocobalamin are discussed in Chapter 45.

Recommended Dietary Allowances and Tolerable Upper Intake Levels

RDAs for vitamin B_{12} and folate are provided in Table 65.1. Because adults older than 50 years often have difficulty absorbing dietary vitamin B_{12}, they should ingest at least 2.4 mcg/day in the form of a supplement. A UL of 1000 mcg/day has been set for folic acid. Owing to insufficient data, no UL has been set for B_{12}.

Food Folate Versus Synthetic Folate

The form of folate that occurs naturally (food folate) has a different chemical structure than synthetic folate (pteroylglutamic acid). Synthetic folate is more stable than food folate and has greater bioavailability. In the presence of food, the bioavailability of synthetic folate is at least 85%. In contrast, bioavailability of food folate is less than 50%.

To increase folate in the American diet, the U.S. Food and Drug Administration requires that all enriched grain products (e.g., enriched bread, pasta, flour, breakfast cereal, grits, rice) must be fortified with synthetic folate—specifically, 140 mcg/100 g of grain. As a result of grain fortification, the incidence of folic acid deficiency in the United States has declined dramatically. Unfortunately, the incidence of birth defects from folate deficiency (see later) has only dropped by 32%.

Folic Acid Deficiency and Fetal Development

Deficiency of folic acid during pregnancy can impair development of the central nervous system, resulting in *neural tube defects* (NTDs), manifesting as *anencephaly* or *spina bifida.* Anencephaly (failure of the brain to develop) is uniformly fatal. Spina bifida, a condition characterized by defective development of the bony encasement of the spinal cord, can result in nerve damage, paralysis, and other complications. The time of vulnerability for NTDs is days 21 through 28 after conception. As a result, damage can occur before a woman recognizes that she is pregnant. Because NTDs occur very early in pregnancy, it is essential that adequate levels of folic acid be present *when pregnancy begins;* women cannot wait until pregnancy is confirmed before establishing adequate intake. To ensure sufficient folate at the onset of pregnancy, the U.S. Preventive Services Task Force (USPSTF) now recommends that *all women who are capable of becoming pregnant consume 400 to 800 mcg of supplemental folic acid each day—in addition to the folate they get from food.*

Folic Acid and Cancer Risk

There is evidence that folic acid in *low* doses may *reduce* cancer risk, whereas folic acid in *higher* doses may *increase* cancer risk—suggesting that cancer risk is increased by having either *too little* folic acid (folic acid deficiency) or by having *too much* folic acid (folic acid excess). The bottom line? Taking high-dose folic acid to reduce cancer risk is ineffective and should be discouraged. Women who might become pregnant should continue taking at least 400 mcg of folic acid every day to prevent NTDs.

Pantothenic Acid

Pantothenic acid is an essential component of two biologically important molecules: coenzyme A and acyl carrier protein. Coenzyme A is an essential factor in multiple biochemical processes, including gluconeogenesis, intermediary metabolism of carbohydrates, and biosynthesis of steroid hormones, porphyrins, and acetylcholine. Acyl carrier protein is required for synthesis of fatty acids. Pantothenic acid is present in virtually all foods. As a result, spontaneous deficiency has not been reported. There are insufficient data to establish RDAs for pantothenic acid. However, the Food and Nutrition Board has assigned AIs (see Table 65.1). There are no reports of toxicity from pantothenic acid. Accordingly, no UL has been set. Pantothenic acid is available in single-ingredient tablets and in multivitamin preparations. However, because deficiency does not occur, there is no reason to take supplements.

Biotin

Biotin is an essential cofactor for several reactions involved in the metabolism of carbohydrates and fats. The vitamin is found in a wide variety of foods, although the exact amount in most foods has not been determined. In addition to being available in foods, biotin is synthesized by intestinal bacteria. Biotin deficiency is extremely rare. In fact, to determine the effects of deficiency, scientists had to induce it experimentally. When this was done, subjects experienced dermatitis, conjunctivitis, hair loss, muscle pain, peripheral paresthesias, and psychological effects (lethargy, hallucinations, depression). At this time, the data are insufficient to establish RDAs for biotin. However, as with pantothenic acid, the Food and Nutrition Board has assigned AIs (see Table 65.1). Biotin appears devoid of toxicity: subjects given large doses experienced no adverse effects. Accordingly, no UL has been set.

CHAPTER

66 Drugs for Weight Loss

Jacqueline Rosenjack Burchum, DNSc, FNP-BC, CNE

In the United States 69.2% of adults are overweight. Of these, 35.9% are obese. Excessive body fat may be associated with increased risk for morbidity from hypertension, coronary heart disease, ischemic stroke, type 2 diabetes, gallbladder disease, liver disease, kidney stones, osteoarthritis, sleep apnea, dementia, and certain cancers. Among women, obesity may increase the risk for menstrual irregularities, amenorrhea, and polycystic ovary syndrome. During pregnancy, obesity may increase the risk for morbidity and mortality for both mother and child. In young men, obesity may reduce the quality and quantity of sperm. The Centers for Disease Control and Prevention (CDC) estimate that 112,000 Americans die per year from obesity-associated illnesses.

Pediatric obesity is a special concern. Despite recent declines in obesity prevalence, almost one third of American children and adolescents are overweight or obese. This increases the risk for hypertension, heart disease, and asthma. In addition, type 2 diabetes, formerly seen almost exclusively in adults, has increased 10-fold among children and teens, and gallbladder disease has tripled.

Obesity is now viewed as a chronic disease, much like hypertension and diabetes. Despite intensive research, the underlying cause remains incompletely understood. Contributing factors include genetics, metabolism, and appetite regulation, along with environmental, psychosocial, and cultural factors. Although obese people can lose weight, the tendency to regain weight cannot be eliminated. Put another way, obesity cannot yet be cured. Accordingly, for most patients, lifelong management is indicated.

ASSESSMENT OF WEIGHT-RELATED HEALTH RISK

Health risk is determined by (1) the degree of obesity (as reflected in the body mass index), (2) the pattern of fat distribution (as reflected in the waist circumference measurement), and (3) the presence of obesity-related diseases or cardiovascular risk factors. Accordingly, all three factors must be assessed when establishing a treatment plan.

Body Mass Index

The body mass index (BMI), which is derived from the patient's weight and height, is a simple way to estimate body fat content. Studies indicate a close correlation between BMI and total body fat. These can be calculated manually (Fig. 66.1) or by using an application such as the online CDC resource at http://www.cdc.gov/healthyweight/assessing/bmi/adult_bmi/english_bmi_calculator/bmi_calculator.html. Tables that assign BMI according to height and weight are also available (Fig. 66.2).

According to the federal guidelines, a BMI of 30 or higher indicates obesity. Individuals with a BMI of 25 to 29.9 are considered overweight, but not obese. There is evidence that the risk for cardiovascular disease and other disorders rises when the BMI exceeds 25. These associations between BMI and health risk do not apply to older adults, growing children, or women who are pregnant or lactating. Nor do they apply to competitive athletes or bodybuilders, who are heavy because of muscle mass rather than excess fat.

Waist Circumference

Waist circumference (WC) is an indicator of *abdominal* fat content, an independent risk factor for obesity-related diseases. Accumulation of fat in the upper body, and especially within the abdominal cavity, poses a greater risk to health than does accumulation of fat in the lower body (hips and thighs). People with too much abdominal fat are at increased risk for insulin resistance, diabetes, hypertension, coronary atherosclerosis, ischemic stroke, and dementia. Fat distribution can be estimated simply by looking in the mirror: an apple shape indicates too much abdominal fat, whereas a pear shape indicates fat on the hips and thighs. Measurement of WC provides a quantitative estimate of abdominal fat. A WC exceeding 40 inches (102 cm) in men or 35 inches (88 cm) in women signifies an increased health risk—but only for people with a BMI between 25 and 34.9.

Risk Status

Overall weight-related health risk is determined by BMI, WC, and the presence of weight-related diseases and cardiovascular risk factors. Certain weight-related diseases—established coronary heart disease, other atherosclerotic diseases, type 2 diabetes, and sleep apnea—confer a risk for complications and mortality. Other weight-related diseases—gynecologic abnormalities, osteoarthritis, gallstones, and stress incontinence—confer less risk. Cardiovascular risk factors—smoking, hypertension, high levels of low-density lipoprotein (LDL) cholesterol, low levels of high-density lipoprotein (HDL) cholesterol, high fasting glucose, family history of premature coronary heart disease, physical inactivity, and advancing age—confer a high risk when three or more of these factors are present.

$$\text{BMI} = \frac{\text{weight in pounds} \times 703}{(\text{height in inches})^2}$$

OR

$$\text{BMI} = \frac{\text{weight in kilograms}}{(\text{height in metres})^2}$$

BMI	Weight status
Less than 18.5	Underweight
18.5–24.9	Normal weight
25–29.9	Overweight
30–39.9	Obese
40 and greater	Morbidly obese

Figure 66.1 ■ Body mass index calculation.

BMI	19	20	21	22	23	24	25	26	27	28	29	30	31	32	33	34	35	36	37	38	39	40	41	42	43	44	45	46	47	48
Height	**Weight in Pounds**																													
4'10"	91	96	100	105	110	115	119	124	129	134	138	143	148	153	158	162	167	172	177	181	186	191	196	201	205	210	215	220	224	229
4'11"	94	99	104	109	114	119	124	128	133	138	143	148	153	158	163	168	173	178	183	188	193	198	203	208	212	217	222	227	232	237
5'	97	102	107	112	118	123	128	133	138	143	148	153	158	163	168	174	179	184	189	194	199	204	209	215	220	225	230	235	240	245
5'1"	100	106	111	116	122	127	132	137	143	148	153	158	164	169	174	180	185	190	195	201	206	211	217	222	227	232	238	243	248	254
5'2"	104	109	115	120	126	131	136	142	147	153	158	164	169	175	180	186	191	196	202	207	213	218	224	229	235	240	246	251	256	262
5'3"	107	113	118	124	130	135	141	146	152	158	163	169	175	180	186	191	197	203	208	214	220	225	231	237	242	248	254	259	265	270
5'4"	110	116	122	128	134	140	145	151	157	163	169	174	180	186	192	197	204	209	215	221	227	232	238	244	250	256	262	267	273	279
5'5"	114	120	126	132	138	144	150	156	162	168	174	180	186	192	198	204	210	216	222	228	234	240	246	252	258	264	270	276	282	288
5'6"	118	124	130	136	142	148	155	161	167	173	179	186	192	198	204	210	216	223	229	235	241	247	253	260	266	272	278	284	291	297
5'7"	121	127	134	140	146	153	159	166	172	178	185	191	198	204	211	217	223	230	236	242	249	255	261	268	274	280	287	293	299	306
5'8"	125	131	138	144	151	158	164	171	177	184	190	197	203	210	216	223	230	236	243	249	256	262	269	276	282	289	295	302	308	315
5'9"	128	135	142	149	155	162	169	176	182	189	196	203	209	216	223	230	236	243	250	257	263	270	277	284	291	297	304	311	318	324
5'10"	132	139	146	153	160	167	174	181	188	195	202	209	216	222	229	236	243	250	257	264	271	278	285	292	299	306	313	320	327	334
5'11"	136	143	150	157	165	172	179	186	193	200	208	215	222	229	236	243	250	257	265	272	279	286	293	301	308	315	322	329	338	343
6'	140	147	154	162	169	177	184	191	199	206	213	221	228	235	242	250	258	265	272	279	287	294	302	309	316	324	331	338	346	353
6'1"	144	151	159	166	174	182	189	197	204	212	219	227	235	242	250	257	265	272	280	288	295	302	310	318	325	333	340	348	355	363
6'2"	148	155	163	171	179	186	194	202	210	218	225	233	241	249	256	264	272	280	287	295	303	311	319	326	334	342	350	358	365	373
6'3"	152	160	168	176	184	192	200	208	216	224	232	240	248	256	264	272	279	287	295	303	311	319	327	335	343	351	359	367	375	383
6'4"	156	164	172	180	189	197	205	213	221	230	238	246	254	263	271	279	287	295	304	312	320	328	336	344	353	361	369	377	385	394

□ = Healthy weight: BMI 18.5 to 24.9
□ = Overweight: BMI 25 to 29.9
□ = Obese: BMI 30 to 39.9
□ = Severely obese: BMI 40 and higher

Figure 66.2 ■ Adult weight classification based on body mass index (BMI). (Adapted from National Heart, Lung, and Blood Institute Body Mass Index Table, 2012. Complete table available online at http://www.nhlbi.nih.gov/health/educational/lose_wt/BMI/bmi_tbl.pdf.)

Health risk rises as BMI gets larger. In addition, the risk is increased by the presence of an excessive WC. The risk is further increased by weight-related diseases and cardiovascular risk factors. In the absence of an excessive WC and other risk factors, health risk is minimal with a BMI below 25 and relatively low with a BMI below 30. Conversely, a BMI of 30 or more indicates significant risk. In the presence of an excessive WC, health risk is high for all individuals with a BMI above 25.

OVERVIEW OF OBESITY TREATMENT

The strategy for losing weight is simple: take in fewer calories per day than are burned. Of course, implementation is much more challenging. The key components of a weight-loss program are diet and exercise. Drugs and other measures are employed only as adjuncts.

Who Should Be Treated?

According to the federal guidelines, weight-loss therapy is indicated for people with any the following:

- A BMI of 30 or more
- A BMI of 25 to 29.9 *plus* two risk factors
- A WC greater than 40 inches (in men) or greater than 35 inches (in women) *plus* two risk factors

Benefits of Treatment

In overweight and obese people, weight reduction may confer these benefits:

- Reduction of high blood pressure in patients with hypertension
- Improvement of blood lipid status (elevation of HDL cholesterol and reduction of LDL cholesterol, total cholesterol, and triglycerides)

- Reduction in development of type 2 diabetes mellitus (DM) and, in patients with type 2 DM, reduction of elevated blood glucose
- Reduced mortality

Treatment Goal

The goal of treatment is to promote and maintain weight loss. The initial objective is to reduce weight by 10% over 6 months. For patients with a BMI of 27 to 35, this can usually be achieved by reducing energy intake by 300 to 500 kcal/day, which should allow a loss of 0.5 to 1 pound a week—or 13 to 26 pounds in 6 months. People with a BMI above 35 require greater caloric restriction (500–1000 kcal/day) to lose 10% of their weight in 6 months. After 6 months, the goal for all patients is to prevent lost weight from returning. This may be accomplished by a combination of diet, physical activity, and behavioral therapy. If appropriate, additional weight reduction can be attempted.

Although these goals are laudable and a return to a normal BMI is desirable, this is rarely achieved in obese individuals, even with drug therapy. A more realistic goal is to target a percentage of body weight at which risk is decreased and comorbidities prevented. A weight loss of 10% to 15% is typical for those who diligently adhere to medication and lifestyle regimen, whereas a loss greater than 15% is exceptional.

Treatment Modalities

Weight loss can be accomplished with five treatment modalities: caloric restriction, physical activity, behavioral therapy, drug therapy, and surgery. For any individual, the treatment mode is determined by the degree of obesity and personal preference.

Caloric Restriction

A reduced-calorie diet is central to any weight-loss program. As noted, the only way to lose weight is to take in fewer calories than are burned. Depending on the individual, the caloric deficit should range from 300 to 1000 kcal/day. Because fats contain more calories than either carbohydrates or proteins (on an ounce-for-ounce basis), reducing dietary fat is the easiest way to reduce calorie intake.

To succeed at losing weight, it helps to know just how many calories are taken in each day and how many you burn. The following websites, which are free, have databases on foods and physical activities, along with tools to calculate and log calories taken in and calories burned:

- Choose My Plate: www.choosemyplate.gov
- Super Tracker: www.supertracker.usda.gov

Exercise

Physical activity should be a component of all weight-loss and weight-maintenance programs. Exercise makes a modest contribution to weight loss by increasing energy expenditure. In addition, exercise can help reduce abdominal fat, increase cardiorespiratory fitness, and maintain weight once loss has occurred. According to the American College of Sports Medicine, people trying to *lose* weight should exercise at least 150 minutes per week (and preferably more), and those trying to *maintain* weight loss should exercise 200 to 300 minutes per week.

Behavior Modification

Behavioral therapy is directed at modifying eating and exercise habits. As such, behavioral therapy can strengthen a program of diet and exercise. Techniques of behavioral therapy include self-monitoring of eating and exercise habits, stress management (because stress can trigger eating), and stimulus control (limiting exposure to stimuli that promote eating). There is no evidence that any one of these techniques is superior to others.

Drug Therapy

In theory, drugs can promote weight loss in three ways: they can suppress appetite, reduce absorption of nutrients, or increase metabolic rate. Drugs can be used as an adjunct to diet and exercise—but only for people at increased health risk, and only after a 6-month program of diet and exercise has failed. Drugs should never be used alone; rather, they should be part of a comprehensive weight-reduction program—one that includes exercise, behavior modification, and a reduced-calorie diet.

Drugs should be reserved for patients whose BMI is 30 or greater or 27 or greater in the presence of additional risk factors. Drugs are not appropriate for patients whose BMI is relatively low. Drugs are also not appropriate for women who are pregnant. The American College of Obstetricians and Gynecologists recommends weight gain, not loss, for obese women who are pregnant, although the total amount of gain is less than that of women who are within normal limits for weight.

Benefits of drugs are usually modest. Weight loss attributable to drugs generally ranges between 4.4 and 22 pounds, although some people lose significantly more. As a rule, most weight loss occurs during the first 6 months of treatment.

Duration of therapy varies depending on the drug selected. Today, long-term treatment is recommended more often than in the past because we now know that, when drugs are discontinued, most patients regain lost weight. Accordingly, when treatment has been effective and well tolerated, it may need to continue indefinitely. Unfortunately, not all drugs are approved for long-term use.

Not everyone responds to drugs, so regular assessment is required. Patients should lose at least 4 pounds during the first 4 weeks of drug treatment. If this initial response is absent, further drug use should be questioned. For patients who *do* respond, ongoing assessment must show that (1) the drug is effective at *maintaining* weight loss and (2) serious adverse effects are absent. Otherwise, drug therapy should cease.

Bariatric Surgery

Surgical procedures can produce significant weight loss by reducing food intake. However, they are indicated only for patients with a BMI of 40 or more (in the absence of severe comorbidity). The two most widely used procedures are *gastric bypass surgery* (Roux-en-Y procedure) and laparoscopic implantation of an adjustable gastric band, which reduces the effective volume of the upper part of the stomach. Surgery is effective: in 6 months to a year, patients can lose between 110 and 220 pounds. Unfortunately, the surgery can carry significant risk: in one study, mortality rates at 30 days, 90 days, and 1 year after gastric surgery were 2%, 2.8%, and 4.6%, respectively.

WEIGHT-LOSS DRUGS

As previously mentioned, weight loss drugs vary in their ability to promote weight loss. The combination drug topiramate/phentermine is associated with the greatest amount of weight loss (greater than 5% of body weight). This is followed by phentermine as monotherapy and another combination drug naltrexone/bupropion, which generally achieve a weight loss of greater than 3% to 5%. Orlistat provides the least weight loss (2%–3%). The individual classes of weight loss drugs are discussed next. Dosages and administration guidelines are summarized in Table 66.1.

Lipase Inhibitor: Orlistat

Actions and Use

Orlistat [Alli, Xenical] is a novel drug approved for promoting and maintaining weight loss in obese patients 12 years and older. Unlike most other weight-loss drugs, which act in the brain to curb appetite, orlistat acts in the GI tract to reduce absorption of fat. Specifically, the drug acts in the stomach and small intestine to cause irreversible inhibition of gastric and pancreatic lipases, enzymes that break down triglycerides into monoglycerides and free fatty acids. If triglycerides are not broken down, they can't be absorbed. In patients taking orlistat, absorption of dietary fat is reduced about 30%. Patients must adopt a reduced-calorie diet in which 30% of calories come from fat.

In clinical trials, orlistat produced modest benefits. Patients treated for 2 years lost an average of 19 pounds, compared with 12 pounds for those taking placebo. In addition, treatment reduced total and LDL cholesterol, raised HDL cholesterol, reduced fasting blood glucose, and lowered systolic and diastolic blood pressure.

Adverse Effects

Gastrointestinal Effects

Orlistat undergoes less than 1% absorption, and hence systemic effects are absent. In contrast, GI effects are common. Approximately 20% to 30% of patients experience oily rectal leakage, flatulence with discharge, fecal urgency, and fatty or oily stools. Another 10% experience increased defecation and fecal incontinence. All of these are the result of reduced fat absorption, and all can be minimized by reducing fat intake. Dosing with psyllium [Metamucil, others], a bulk-forming laxative, can greatly reduce GI effects. The underlying mechanism is adsorption of dietary fat by psyllium.

Possible Liver Damage

Orlistat has been associated with rare cases of *severe liver damage.* Signs and symptoms include itching, vomiting, jaundice, anorexia, fatigue, dark urine, and light-colored stools. *Patients who experience these signs and symptoms should report them immediately.* Orlistat should be discontinued until liver injury has been ruled out.

Other Adverse Effects

Rarely, orlistat has been associated with *acute pancreatitis* and *kidney stones,* although a causal relationship has not been established. Cholelithiasis may occur if weight loss is substantial.

Contraindications

Orlistat is contraindicated for patients with malabsorption syndrome or cholestasis.

Drug and Nutrient Interactions

Reduced Absorption of Vitamins

By reducing fat absorption, orlistat can reduce absorption of fat-soluble vitamins (vitamins A, D, E, and K). Vitamin K deficiency can intensify the effects of *warfarin,* an anticoagulant. In patients taking warfarin, anticoagulant effects should be monitored closely. To avoid deficiency, patients should take a daily multivitamin supplement. Administration should be done 2 hours before or 2 hours after taking orlistat

Drug Interactions

Orlistat may cause hypothyroidism in patients taking levothyroxine by decreasing the absorption of thyroid hormone. To minimize this effect, levothyroxine and orlistat should be administered at least 4 hours apart. Orlistat also can reduce absorption of cyclosporine. At least 3 hours is recommended between doses of these two drugs.

Serotonin Receptor Agonist: Lorcaserin

Actions and Use

Lorcaserin [Belviq] is a selective type 2C serotonin ($5\text{-}HT_{2C}$) agonist with indications for chronic weight loss. It suppresses appetite and creates a sense of satiety by activating hypothalamic and mesolimbic pathways that control appetite. Studies have demonstrated an average loss of 5.8% of baseline weight after 1 year, compared with 2.2% in patients taking placebo. In addition, lorcaserin reduces waist circumference, fasting glucose, insulin, total cholesterol, LDL cholesterol, and triglycerides.

Adverse Effects

Ten percent or more of patients will experience headaches, back pain, a decrease in lymphocytes, and upper respiratory infections. About 30% of patients with diabetes will experience an increase in hypoglycemic episodes.

Less common but serious adverse effects include blood dyscrasias, cognitive impairment, psychiatric disorders, priapism (prolonged penile erection), pulmonary hypertension, and valvular heart disease. Accordingly, this drug should not be given to patients at risk for these conditions.

Lorcaserin has potential for abuse. It is classified as a Schedule IV drug under the Controlled Substances Act (CSA).

Contraindications

There are life span–associated contraindications with this drug.

Drug Interactions

Lorcaserin is an inhibitor of the CYP2D6 isoenzyme of cytochrome P450. When given with CYP2D6 substrates (i.e., drugs metabolized by CYP2D6 isoenzymes), the serum levels of the substrates can be increased. To decrease the risk for toxicity, when both drugs are prescribed, the substrate may need to be prescribed at a lower dose.

Risk for serotonin syndrome is associated with serotonergic drugs. When serotonergic drugs such as lorcaserin are given with other serotonergic drugs, this risk increases. We do not yet have sufficient studies to evaluate the effects of prescribing lorcaserin with specific serotonergic drugs; therefore, caution and close monitoring are advised when administering this drug along with bupropion, dextromethorphan, monoamine oxidase (MAO) inhibitors, serotonin-norepinephrine reuptake inhibitors, selective serotonin reuptake inhibitors, St. John's wort, and triptans.

Sympathomimetic Amines: Diethylpropion and Phentermine

The sympathomimetics fall into two groups: amphetamines and nonamphetamines. The amphetamines are not FDA approved for weight loss because they have a high abuse potential, so they are not addressed here.

Four noradrenergic drugs are approved for weight loss. However, only two—diethylpropion (generic) and phentermine (Adipex-P, Suprenza)—should be used. The other two—benzphetamine and phendimetrazine—have a higher potential for abuse.

TABLE 66.1 ▪ Dosages and Administration

Drug Class and Drug	Preparation	Dosage	Administration
LIPASE INHIBITOR			
Orlistat (Alli, Xenical)	Alli: 60-mg tablet (over the counter) Xenical: 120-mg tablet	Alli: 60-mg 3 times daily with meals Xenical: 120-mg 3 times daily with meals	Take with, or 1 hour after, meals that contain fat. Omit dose if a meal is missed or if a meal does not contain fat. Fat-soluble vitamins (A, D, E, K) should be taken at least 2 hours before or after orlistat.
SEROTONIN 5-HT_{2C} RECEPTOR AGONIST			
Lorcaserin (Belviq)	10-mg tablet	10 mg twice daily	Oral administration. May be taken with or without food.
SYMPATHOMIMETIC AMINES			
Diethylpropion (generic)	25-mg immediate-release tablet 75-mg extended-release tablet	Immediate release: 25 mg 3 times daily Extended release: 75 mg daily	Oral administration. Administer immediate release tablets 1 hour before meals. Administer extended-release tablets at midmorning. Avoid evening or nighttime administration to prevent insomnia.
Phentermine (Adipex-P, Suprenza)	Adipex-P: 37.5-mg tablet; 37.5-mg capsule Suprenza: 15-, 30-, or 37.5-mg disintegrating tablet	Adipex-P: Usual dosage is 37.5 mg daily. Alternate dosing schedules are ½ tablet (18.75 mg) daily or ½ tablet twice daily. Lowest effective dose is recommended. Suprenza: Individualize dosage to the lowest effective dose.	Oral administration. May be taken with or without food. Administer before breakfast or 1–2 hours after breakfast. Avoid evening or night time administration to prevent insomnia.
GLUCAGON-LIKE PEPTIDE-1 AGONIST			
Liraglutide (Saxenda)	Prefilled multidose pens hold 3 mL of a 6-mg/mL solution. Pen contains a dose selector that allows delivery of specific doses at 0.6-, 1.2-, 1.8-, 2.4-, and 3-mg doses	Week 1: 0.6 mg daily Week 2: 1.2 mg daily Week 3: 1.8 mg daily Week 4: 2.4 mg daily Week 5 and thereafter: 3 mg daily	Injected subcutaneously in upper arm, abdomen, or thigh. Does not need to be coordinated with intake.
COMBINATION PRODUCTS			
Phentermine/topiramate (Qsymia)	24-hour extended-release tablet in four strengths 3.75/23 (Phentermine 3.75 mg/topiramate 23 mg) 7.5/46 (Phentermine 7.5 mg/topiramate 46 mg) 11.25/69 (Phentermine 11.25 mg/topiramate 69 mg) 15/92 (Phentermine 15 mg/topiramate 92 mg)	Weeks 1 and 2: One 3.75/23 tablet daily, followed by one 75/46 tablet daily for 12 weeks Evaluate weight loss. If 3% of baseline body weight has not occurred, discontinue or increase to one 11.25/69 tablet once daily for 2 weeks followed by one 15/92 tablet for 12 weeks. Evaluate weight loss. If 5% of baseline weight has not been lost, taper off therapy.	Administer in the morning. May be taken with or without food. Avoid evening or nighttime administration to prevent insomnia.
Naltrexone/bupropion (Contrave)	12-hour extended-release tablet containing naltrexone 8 mg/bupropion 90 mg	Week 1: one tablet in the morning Week 2: one tablet in the morning; one tablet in the evening Week 3: two tablets in the morning; one tablet in the evening Week 4 and thereafter: two tablets in the morning; two tablets in the evening	Substantial increases in bupropion and naltrexone occur when taken with high-fat meals, so this should be avoided. If a dose is skipped, wait until the next scheduled dose to resume schedule.

PATIENT-CENTERED CARE ACROSS THE LIFE SPAN

Weight Loss

Life Stage	Considerations or Concerns
Children	Liraglutide, lorcaserin, and the combination drugs phentermine/topiramate and naltrexone/bupropion are not approved for children. Orlistat is not approved for children younger than 12 years. Diethylpropion and phentermine are not recommended for children younger than 16 years.
Pregnant women	Weight loss is not advisable for pregnant women. All drugs mentioned in this chapter are Pregnancy Risk Category X with the exception of diethylpropion. Although labeled as Pregnancy Risk Category B, neonates born to women who take diethylpropion may experience withdrawal symptoms.
Breastfeeding women	For all drugs listed, breastfeeding is not recommended.
Older adults	For patients with moderate renal impairment, naltrexone/bupropion should be limited to one tablet daily. If the creatinine clearance is <50, phentermine/topiramate should be limited to one 7.5/46 capsule daily. If the creatinine clearance is <30, lorcaserin should not be given. For patients with hepatic impairment, both naltrexone/bupropion and phentermine/topiramate should be limited to one tablet daily. Phentermine/topiramate should not be prescribed for patients with severe hepatic impairment. The manufacturer of liraglutide recommends caution when prescribing for patients with renal or hepatic impairment. Dosage adjustments are not indicated for orlistat, diethylpropion, and phentermine.

Actions and Use

Diethylpropion and phentermine promote weight loss by decreasing appetite. They are central nervous system (CNS) stimulants that suppress appetite by increasing the availability of norepinephrine at receptors in the brain. This same mechanism underlies their stimulant effects and potential for abuse. Weight loss is usually modest: about 7 to 8 pounds. These drugs should be used only in the short term (for 3 months or less).

Adverse Effects

Like the amphetamines, diethylpropion and phentermine can increase alertness, decrease fatigue, and induce nervousness and insomnia. Because they can interfere with sleep, these drugs should be administered no later than 4:00 PM. After drug withdrawal, fatigue and depression may replace CNS stimulation.

Diethylpropion and phentermine have effects in the periphery as well as in the CNS. Peripheral effects of greatest concern are tachycardia, anginal pain, and hypertension. Accordingly, these drugs should be used with caution in patients with cardiovascular disease.

Although the risk for abuse is lower than with the amphetamines, abuse can still occur. Both diethylpropion and phentermine are regulated under Schedule IV of the CSA (benzphetamine and phendimetrazine are regulated under Schedule III). Tolerance is common and may be seen in 6 to 12 weeks. If tolerance develops, the appropriate response is to discontinue the drug rather than to increase the dosage.

Contraindications

Contraindications are associated with development across the life span (see the box for Patient-Centered Care across the Life Span: Weight Loss)

Glucagon-Like Peptide-1 Agonist: Liraglutide

Actions and Use

Liraglutide (Saxenda) is a glucagon-like peptide-1 (GLP-1) agonist that is approved for chronic weight management in adults. It acts by slowing gastric emptying, which increases a feeling of fullness, which leads to decreased food intake. GLP-1 agonists are also used in management of type 2 diabetes (see Chapter 46) to enhance glycemic control. In this regard, it also increases insulin secretion and decreases glucagon secretion.

Adverse Effects

More than one third of patients taking liraglutide experience an increase in heart rate 10 to 20 beats/min from baseline. Approximately 1 in 20 will develop tachycardia. Other common adverse effects include nausea, vomiting, and either constipation or diarrhea. Hypoglycemia is a concern if taken by patients with diabetes who are taking other antidiabetic drugs; however, this is a rare occurrence in patients who do not have diabetes. Headache may occur, as may generalized fatigue and weakness, although these symptoms are less common. Because of the effects on gastric emptying, dyspepsia and abdominal discomfort may occur. Liraglutide is administered subcutaneously; as with any injection, local site reactions such as redness or pruritus may occur.

Several uncommon effects warranting special precautions occur in less than 1% of patients taking liraglutide. These include acute pancreatitis, renal impairment (likely associated with dehydration secondary to nausea, vomiting, and diarrhea) and acute gallbladder disease (typically associated with significant or rapid weight loss regardless of medication).

Contraindications

Liraglutide is known to cause thyroid cancer development in rodents, so cautious use is warranted until the effects on humans are known. Liraglutide is contraindicated in patients who have multiple endocrine neoplasia syndrome type 2 (MEN 2) or who have a personal or family history of medullary thyroid carcinoma (MTC).

BLACK BOX WARNING: LIRAGLUTIDE (SAXENDA)

Liraglutide is associated with a risk for thyroid C-cell tumors based on studies in rodents. It is contraindicated in patients who have multiple neoplasia syndrome type 2 (MEN 2) or a personal or family history of medullary thyroid carcinoma (MTC).

Life span–associated contraindications are provided the box for Patient-Centered Care across the Life Span: Weight Loss.

Drug Interactions

Liraglutide may potentiate the hypoglycemic effect of drugs given for glycemic control in diabetes mellitus. Additionally, it will enhance the glucose-lowering side effects of other drugs with this feature, including androgens, fluoroquinolone antibiotics, MAO inhibitors, and selective serotonin reuptake inhibitors (SSRIs).

Combination Products

There are currently two combination products approved for weight loss. Each combination is unique with different mechanisms of action and different side effect profiles.

Phentermine/Topiramate

Actions and Use

A combination product phentermine and topiramate [Qsymia] is a Schedule IV drug indicated for chronic weight-loss therapy. Phentermine, as mentioned previously, is a sympathomimetic amine already approved for short-term management of obesity. Topiramate is currently approved for seizure disorders (see Chapter 19) and prophylaxis of migraine (see Chapter 23). Phentermine suppresses appetite, and topiramate induces a sense of satiety. Possible mechanisms for topiramate include antagonism of glutamate (an excitatory neurotransmitter), modulation of receptors for gamma-aminobutyric acid, and inhibition of carbonic anhydrase. In a 56-week trial, phentermine/topiramate produced a 10% reduction in weight and a significant decrease in systolic blood pressure. Long-term results are not available.

Adverse Effects

The most common adverse effects are dry mouth, constipation, altered taste, nausea, blurred vision, dizziness, insomnia, and numbness and tingling in the limbs. The most serious effects are memory impairment, difficulty concentrating, hypertension and tachycardia, birth defects, acute myopia with angle-closure glaucoma, acidosis, and, for patients who take insulin secretagogues or insulin, an increased risk for hypoglycemia beyond that of antidiabetic drugs alone.

Contraindications

There are life span–associated contraindications with phentermine/topiramate (see the box for Patient-Centered Care across the Life Span: Weight Loss). Its use is also contraindicated for patients with glaucoma or hyperthyroidism.

Drug Interactions

Phentermine/topiramate should not be given with MAO inhibitors. In fact, at least 2 weeks should pass after taking an MAO inhibitor before phentermine/topiramate is begun. Similarly, at least 2 weeks should pass after ending phentermine/topiramate before an MAO inhibitor is begun. Phentermine/topiramate can potentiate CNS depressants. When given with the antiepileptic drugs carbamazepine or phenytoin, levels of topiramate (which is also an antiepileptic drug) may be increased. Administration with carbonic anhydrase inhibitors increases the risk for metabolic acidosis, whereas administration with diuretics that are not potassium sparing increases the risk for hypokalemia. Finally, studies show that concomitant administration with oral contraceptives increases the estrogen level while decreasing the progestin level.

Naltrexone/Bupropion

Actions and Use

The anorexiant naltrexone/bupropion (Contrave) combines the effects of a dopamine and norepinephrine-reuptake inhibitor with an opioid antagonist. The mechanism of action by which this drug combination promotes weight loss is unknown, but it has been hypothesized that it acts on the regulation of appetite in the hypothalamus and on the mesolimbic dopamine system, which is the key reward pathway in the brain. The individual drugs are discussed separately. (See Chapter 22 for naltrexone and Chapter 25 for bupropion.)

Adverse Effects

The most common adverse reactions (experienced by more than 10% of those taking naltrexone with bupropion) are nausea, vomiting, constipation, headache, dizziness, and insomnia. Approximately 5% of patients experience an increase in blood pressure, dry mouth, diarrhea, abdominal discomfort, anxiety, and fatigue. There is also a suicide risk associated with this drug.

BLACK BOX WARNING: NALTREXONE AND BUPROPION (CONTRAVE)

The naltrexone/bupropion combination is associated with an increased risk for suicidal ideation and suicide attempts in children, adolescents, and young adults.

Contraindications

This product is contraindicated for patients taking other products containing bupropion. Because naltrexone is an opioid antagonist, it will decrease the ability of opioid analgesics to relieve pain. It should not be taken within 2 weeks of MAO inhibitors.

BLACK BOX WARNING: NALTREXONE AND BUPROPION (CONTRAVE)

When the naltrexone/bupropion combination is given to patients who are taking or discontinuing bupropion (Aplenzin, Budeprion, Bupropion, Wellbutrin, Zyban), severe neuropsychiatric reactions, including depression, mania, psychosis, and homicidal ideation, have occurred.

Naltrexone-bupropion is also contraindicated for people with selected conditions. It should not be used for weight loss in patients with uncontrolled hypertension, seizure disorders, or eating disorders such as anorexia or bulimia. Patients who are undergoing alcohol, barbiturate, or benzodiazepine withdrawal should not take this drug. Life span–associated contraindications are listed in the box for Patient-Centered Care across the Life Span: Weight Loss.

Drug Interactions

Drug interactions are numerous and reflect interactions of the individual agents. (See Chapter 22 for naltrexone and Chapter 25 for bupropion). Dangerous interactions occur with MAO inhibitors and opioid antagonists. The bupropion component of naltrexone/bupropion is a minor substrate of numerous hepatic enzyme families and a major substrate of CYP2B6 enzymes. Inhibitors of these enzymes can increase naltrexone/bupropion levels, requiring a lowered dosage. When CYP2B6 inducers are given with this drug, it may result in subtherapeutic doses. Naltrexone/bupropion is also a strong inhibitor of CYP2D6 enzymes. Accordingly, when given with CYP2D6 substrates, naltrexone/bupropion can increase their drug levels.

A NOTE REGARDING DRUGS FOR WEIGHT LOSS

Weight-loss drugs share a disturbing history: they receive regulatory approval, undergo widespread use, and then are withdrawn owing to discovery of serious adverse effects. It is quite likely that new drugs may be approved by the time you read this chapter. It is also possible that drugs in this chapter, especially those most recently approved, will have been taken off the market.

CHAPTER

67 Complementary and Alternative Therapy

Jacqueline Rosenjack Burchum, DNSc, FNP-BC, CNE

The National Center for Complementary and Integrative Health (NCCIH) defines *complementary* health approaches as "a nonmainstream practice used together with conventional medicine" and *alternative* health approaches as "a nonmainstream practice that is used in place of conventional medicine." Examples include both products (e.g., herbs, probiotics, and vitamins) and practices (e.g., meditation, acupuncture, and therapeutic touch). According to the National Health Statistics Reports published in 2015, 32.3% of adults in the United States used some form of complementary and alternative medicine (CAM) in 2012 (the year of the most recent national study).

Dietary supplements are the most common form of CAM. Dietary supplements are defined by the U.S. Food and Drug Administration (FDA) as "a product intended for ingestion that contains a 'dietary ingredient' intended to add further nutritional value to (supplement) the diet. A 'dietary ingredient' may be one, or any combination, of the following substances: a vitamin, a mineral, an herb or other botanical, an amino acid, a dietary substance for use by people to supplement the diet by increasing the total dietary intake, a concentrate, metabolite, constituent, or extract."

The popularity of supplements may be explained by several factors (Box 67.1). Some people like the sense of empowerment that comes from self-diagnosis and self-prescribing. Others may turn to supplements out of anger or frustration with their health care providers. Still others may distrust conventional medicine or may feel it has failed them. In addition, supplements may be a way to save money: because these products are available without prescription, they can be purchased without the cost of visiting a prescriber. In fact, according to the National Health Interview Survey (NHIS), there is a clear relationship between concern about the costs of conventional care and the likelihood of turning to CAM. However, perhaps the strongest force driving the demand for nutritional supplements is aggressive marketing.

Our understanding of CAM is far from adequate. To advance our knowledge, the National Institutes of Health (NIH) created the National Center for Complementary and Alternative Medicine (NCCAM) in the late 1990s. This organization (renamed the National Center for Complementary and Integrative Health [NCCIH] in 2014) is charged with promoting and funding basic research and clinical trials designed to address open questions on the safety and efficacy of CAM. The NCCIH website, which provides a wealth of information on CAM, is available at https://nccih.nih.gov.

REGULATION OF DIETARY SUPPLEMENTS

Dietary Supplement Health and Education Act of 1994

Core Provisions

In 1994, after intensive lobbying efforts from the multibillion-dollar dietary supplement industry aimed at minimizing FDA oversight, Congress passed the Dietary Supplement Health and Education Act of 1994 (DSHEA). The Food, Drug, and Cosmetic Act requires that conventional drugs—both prescription and over-the-counter agents—undergo rigorous evaluation of safety and efficacy before receiving FDA approval for marketing. The DSHEA categorizes botanical products (herbal supplements), vitamins, and minerals as dietary (food) supplements rather than as drugs. By classifying products as dietary supplements, the DSHEA exempts them from undergoing FDA scrutiny and approval before marketing. In fact, dietary supplements can be manufactured and marketed without giving the FDA any proof they are safe or effective. All the manufacturer must do is notify the FDA of efficacy claims. If a product eventually proves harmful or makes false claims, the FDA does have the authority to intervene—but only *after* the product had been released for marketing. Furthermore, to challenge a claim of efficacy, the FDA must file suit in court; the challenge cannot be made through a simple administrative procedure.

Package Labeling

The DSHEA does impose some restrictions on labeling. All herbal products must be labeled as dietary supplements. In addition, the label must not claim that the product can be used to diagnose, prevent, treat, or cure a disease. In fact, it must state the opposite: *this product is not intended to diagnose, treat, cure, or prevent any disease.* However, the label *is* allowed to make claims about the product's ability to favorably influence *body structure or function.* Put another way, the label can insinuate specific benefits but can't make overt claims. By way of illustration, labels *can* bear statements such as these:

- Helps promote urinary tract health
- Helps maintain cardiovascular function
- Energizes and rejuvenates
- Reduces stress and frustration
- Improves absentmindedness
- Supports the immune system

BOX 67.1 ▪ WHY PEOPLE USE DIETARY SUPPLEMENTS

- Perception that supplements are safer and "healthier" than conventional drugs
- Sense of control over one's care
- Emotional comfort from taking action
- Cultural influence
- Limited access to professional care
- Lack of health insurance
- Convenience
- Media hype and aggressive marketing
- Recommendation from family and friends

But labels *can't* bear statements or terms such as these:

- Protects against cancer
- Reduces pain and stiffness of arthritis
- Lowers cholesterol
- Supports the body's antiviral capabilities
- Improves symptoms of Alzheimer disease
- Relieves menopausal hot flashes
- "Antibiotic," "antiseptic," "antidepressant," "laxative," or "diuretic"

If all of this sounds like semantic hair splitting—it largely is. Furthermore, regardless of what the label says, common sense assumes that people *will* take herbal products with the intent to prevent or treat disease.

Under the provisions of the DSHEA, there is no assurance that a product actually contains what the label proclaims: the package may contain ingredients that are *not* listed, or it may *lack* ingredients that *are* listed. These shortcomings and others have been addressed by the Current Good Manufacturing Practices (CGMPs) ruling, issued by the FDA in 2007.

Adverse Effects

With dietary supplements, as with conventional drugs, the manufacturer is responsible for safety. However, the similarity ends there. Under the DSHEA, a product is presumed safe until proved hazardous. Furthermore, the burden for proving danger lies with the consumer and the FDA. With conventional drugs, opposite logic and regulations apply: drugs are presumed dangerous until rigorous testing by the manufacturer reveals an absence of serious adverse effects. Because of this system, the number of dangerous drugs that reach the market is kept to a minimum. Ask yourself, "Which product would I be more comfortable using—one that has been tested for adverse effects *before* I take it, or one that is evaluated for adverse effects only *after* it caused me harm?"

Impurities, Adulterants, and Variability

The DSHEA does not address the issues of impurities, adulterants, or variability. As a result, dangerous products have been allowed to reach consumers. A few examples illustrate the problem:

- A combination product used to "cleanse the bowel" caused life-threatening heart block. Analysis revealed contamination with *Digitalis lanata,* a plant with powerful effects on the heart.
- Among 125 ephedra products analyzed by the FDA, ephedrine content per dose ranged from undetectable to 110 mg. Also, some products had 6 to 20 additional ingredients.
- Testing of 10 brands of ginseng products revealed a 20-fold variation in ginsenoside content.
- When the California Department of Health Sciences analyzed 243 Asian patent medicines, they found 24 containing lead, 35 containing mercury, and 36 containing arsenic—all in levels above those permitted in drugs. Of these products, 7% were adulterated with undeclared pharmaceuticals, including ephedrine, chlorpheniramine, methyltestosterone, and phenacetin.

As discussed later, the CGMPs ruling, issued by the FDA in 2007, should prevent the sale of such products in the future.

Current Good Manufacturing Practices Ruling

In June 2007, the FDA issued a set of standards to regulate manufacturing and labeling of dietary supplements. These standards, referred to as Current Good Manufacturing Practices, are designed to ensure that dietary supplements be devoid of adulterants, contaminants, and impurities, and that package labels accurately reflect the identity, purity, quality, and strength of what's inside. In addition, the label should indicate not only active ingredients but also inactive ingredients. The CGMPs also mandate that manufacturers establish quality-control procedures, with the objective of preventing mislabeled, underfilled, or overfilled formulations; variations in tablet size, color, or potency; and contamination with drugs, bacteria, pesticides, glass, lead, and other potential contaminants. Unfortunately, even with the new standards and rules, there is still no assurance that dietary supplements will be either safe or effective—but at least we will have improved confidence regarding package contents.

Dietary Supplement and Nonprescription Drug Consumer Protection Act

The Dietary Supplement and Nonprescription Drug Consumer Protection Act, passed in 2006, mandates reporting of serious adverse events for nonprescription drugs and dietary supplements. The following events should be reported: deaths, hospitalizations, life-threatening experiences, persistent or significant disabilities, and birth defects. Manufacturers and distributors must report these to the FDA within 15 days. Reports can be filed by telephone or by mail, or through the MEDWATCH program at http://www.fda.gov/Safety/MedWatch.

A Comment on the Regulatory Status of Dietary Supplements

Although herbal products and other dietary supplements are not regulated for either safety or efficacy, many of these products have components that can produce profound beneficial and adverse pharmacologic effects. Nonetheless, reliable information on clinical effects is largely lacking. Many of those working in the fields of pharmacy, medicine, and nursing are concerned that the exceptions made for dietary supplements are both irrational and dangerous.

PRIVATE QUALITY CERTIFICATION PROGRAMS

Four *private* organizations—the U.S. Pharmacopeia (USP), ConsumerLab, the Natural Products Association, and NSF International (formerly known as the National Sanitation Foundation)—test dietary supplements for quality. A "seal of approval" is given to products that meet their standards, which are very similar to the CGMPs described previously. The USP standards are enforceable by the FDA. All four organizations require manufacturers to pay for the tests, and all four report on the following:

- Current Good Manufacturing Practices
- Purity
- Identity
- Potency
- Dissolution
- Accuracy of labeling

In addition, two organizations—the USP and ConsumerLab—report on postapproval surveillance.

STANDARDIZATION OF HERBAL PRODUCTS

With herbal products, there is often uncertainty about the amounts of active ingredients. The concentration of active ingredients in herbal crops can vary from year to year and from place to place. Reasons include differences in sunshine, rainfall, temperature, and soil nutrients. As a result, the potency of herbal products can vary widely.

Variability can be reduced through standardization, a three-step process in which the manufacturer (1) prepares an *extract* of plant parts, (2) analyzes the extract for one or two known active ingredients, and (3) dilutes or concentrates the extract such that the final product contains a predetermined amount of the active ingredients. The objective is to achieve therapeutic equivalence from batch to batch made by the same manufacturer, and among batches made by different manufacturers. Table 67.1 lists the concentrations of active ingredients in some standardized preparations.

Standardization has two important benefits. First, it permits accurate dosing. Second, it permits extrapolation of data obtained in clinical trials to the public in general.

Unfortunately, standardization also has drawbacks. The extraction process might destroy active compounds. Furthermore, the process may fail to extract as-yet unidentified active agents, and hence the extract may have a different spectrum of effects than the intact plant. To the extent this is true, historical data obtained with whole plants will lose some value as a basis for helping us understand clinical responses to the standardized extract.

TABLE 67.1 ■ Concentrations of Active Agents in Some Standardized Herbal Preparations

Herb	Amount of Active Agent
Black cohosh	2.5% Triterpene glycosides
Echinacea	4% Phenolic compounds
Feverfew	0.2% Parthenolide
Ginkgo biloba	24% Ginkgo flavonoids, 6% terpenoids
St. John's wort	0.3% Hypericin
Valerian root	1% Valerianic acid

ADVERSE INTERACTIONS WITH CONVENTIONAL DRUGS

Herbal products and other dietary supplements can interact with conventional drugs, sometimes with significant harmful results. The principal concerns are increased toxicity and decreased therapeutic effects. Clinicians and consumers should be alert to these possibilities. Unfortunately, with many supplements, reliable information on adverse interactions is lacking—in large part because potential interactions have not been systematically studied. Hence, if a patient is taking a conventional medication and a dietary supplement, and therapeutic effects are lost or toxicity appears, it may be impossible to say for sure that the supplement was (or was not) responsible.

A few important interactions *have* been identified, including the following:

- St. John's wort can induce CYP3A4 (the 3A4 isoenzyme of cytochrome P450) and can thereby accelerate the metabolism of many drugs, causing a loss of therapeutic effects.
- Several herbal products, including *Ginkgo biloba,* feverfew, and garlic, suppress platelet aggregation and hence can increase the risk for bleeding in patients receiving antiplatelet drugs (e.g., aspirin) or anticoagulants (e.g., warfarin, heparin).
- Ma huang (ephedra) contains ephedrine, a compound that can elevate blood pressure and stimulate the heart and central nervous system (CNS). Accordingly, ephedra can intensify the effects of pressor agents, cardiac stimulants, and CNS stimulants, and counteract the beneficial effects of antihypertensive drugs and CNS depressants.

These interactions, at least, can be avoided—provided the prescriber is aware of them, and provided the patient informs the prescriber about supplement use. Unfortunately, up to 70% of patients neglect to do so.

SOME COMMONLY USED DIETARY SUPPLEMENTS

Black Cohosh

Uses

Black cohosh has a long history in America. The herb was used by Native Americans and later by American colonists. Between 1820 and 1926, it was listed as an official drug in the USP.

Black cohosh (*Cimicifuga racemosa*) is used for treating symptoms of menopause, including hot flashes, vaginal dryness, palpitations, depression, irritability, and sleep disturbance. The preparation should *not* be used to reduce hot flashes caused by tamoxifen and other selective estrogen receptor modulators (SERMs).

Actions

How black cohosh works is unknown. At one time, we believed it suppressed release of luteinizing hormone (LH). However, clinical studies have failed so show an effect on female hormones, including LH, estradiol, prolactin, and follicle-stimulating hormone. In laboratory studies, black cohosh does not interact with estrogen receptors: it doesn't bind to these receptors, upregulate estrogen-dependent genes, or promote growth of estrogen-dependent tumors (at least in animals).

Effectiveness

Early studies carried out in Germany supported the ability of black cohosh to effectively relieve menopausal symptoms. In 2012, however, a Cochrane meta-analysis of 16 randomized controlled trials involving more than 2000 women concluded that there was insufficient evidence to support black cohosh for management of menopausal symptoms. After a review of the evidence, the NCCIH concluded, "[T]here is overall insufficient evidence to support the use of black cohosh for menopausal symptoms." These conclusions were echoed by the American College of Obstetricians and Gynecologists (ACOG) when they updated their clinical guidelines for management of menopausal symptoms in 2014. Conversely, at the time of this writing, the North American Menopause Society continues to include black cohosh among the natural remedies for hot flashes listed on its website.

Adverse Effects

Some women taking black cohosh have developed liver inflammation. In some instances, this has led to liver failure. The association is tenuous, however, because the occurrence has been rare, and a distinction from other possible causes of liver injury has not been ruled out.

Less serious and more common adverse effects include rash, headache, dizziness, and abdominal discomfort. Safety in pregnancy and breastfeeding has not been established; however, for those taking black cohosh for menopausal benefit, this would only be a concern in rare circumstances. One caveat acknowledged almost universally is the need to limit the use of black cohosh to 6 months because long-term studies have not been conducted.

Interactions With Conventional Drugs

Black cohosh may potentiate the hypotensive effects of antihypertensive drugs as well as the hypoglycemic effects of insulin and other drugs for diabetes. Black cohosh may potentiate the effects of estrogens used for hormone therapy. Black cohosh should be used with caution in patients taking other drugs that may harm the liver.

Comments

Users must not confuse black cohosh with blue cohosh (Caulophyllum thalictroides). Although blue cohosh has legitimate uses, including promotion of menstruation and labor, it is very different from black cohosh and potentially more dangerous. Blue cohosh can elevate blood pressure, increase intestinal motility, and accelerate respiration. It can also induce uterine contractions and hence should be avoided during pregnancy. Some commercial products contain both black cohosh and blue cohosh. Women who want only black cohosh should avoid these products.

Butterbur

Butterbur (*Petasites hybridus*) is a bush that grows in marshy areas across North America. Products are made from the rhizomes and roots as well as the stems of this plant.

Uses

Butterbur is most commonly taken for migraine headaches, allergies, and asthma. It is one of the few botanicals recommended as a drug of first choice based on outcomes of randomized controlled trials.

Actions

Butterbur has antiinflammatory, antispasmodic, and vasodilatory effects. As with many herbal products, the exact mechanism of action is unknown. Some believe that butterbur works as a calcium channel blocker. Laboratory studies point to inhibition of lipoxygenase, an enzyme which contributes to the synthesis of leukotrienes and other proinflammatory substances.

Effectiveness

Although evidence remains lacking for the efficacy of butterbur in the treatment of skin allergies and asthma, substantial evidence supports other uses. According to the NCCIH:

- A sponsored literature review found that butterbur is just as effective as an antihistamine for allergy symptoms.
- Butterbur appears to relieve nasal allergy symptoms.
- Research findings indicate that butterbur can be effective in treating migraine headache.

The American Academy of Neurology (AAN) and the American Headache Society (AHA) also noted the effects of butterbur on preventing migraine headache. In 2012 they published a joint report in which they not only pronounced that butterbur was effective in decreasing migraine headache frequency, but also gave it the highest (Level A) rating. Their conclusion? "Petasites (butterbur) is effective for migraine prevention and should be offered to patients with migraine to reduce the frequency and severity of migraine attacks." For this purpose, the AAN recommends 50 to 75 mg twice a day. (See the AAN 2014 report *Headache: Quality Measurement Set* available through http://www.aan.com.)

Adverse Effects

Long-term safety has not been established; however, butterbur appears to be safe for short-term use of less than 4 months' duration when taken at recommended doses. The most common adverse effects are eructation (belching), headache, and fatigue. Those who have allergies to ragweed, daisies, marigolds, and chrysanthemums may have allergic reactions to butterbur.

With the increased use of butterbur, the concern has arisen regarding new reports of liver injury. According to the NCCIH, this can be the result of pyrrolizidine alkaloids (PAs) found in butterbur. The NCCIH recommends using only butterbur products where these have been removed and are certified as PA-free. Whether this type of product was taken by those who developed liver injury is unknown.

Interactions With Conventional Drugs

Interactions can occur if butterbur is given with drugs that induce CYP3A4 isoenzymes. Examples include not only drugs such as carbamazepine, phenobarbital, and phenytoin but also dietary supplements such as echinacea, garlic, and St. John's wort. The greatest concern comes when a non-PA-free form of butterbur is used because PAs are substrates of CYP3A4 isoenzymes; metabolism converts these to their toxic metabolites.

Coenzyme Q-10

Coenzyme Q-10 (ubiquinone, CoQ-10) is an antioxidant that serves a vital role in cellular energy production. As we age, CoQ-10 levels decrease. This has led to increased interest in the use of CoQ-10 in treatment of conditions associated with aging and with cellular energy production.

Uses

CoQ-10 is used to treat heart failure, muscle injury caused by HMG-CoA reductase inhibitors (statins), and mitochondrial encephalomyopathies (i.e., muscle and nervous system injury caused by deranged mitochondrial metabolism).

Actions

CoQ-10 is a potent antioxidant. It participates in many metabolic pathways, most notably production of adenosine triphosphate (ATP).

Effectiveness

In patients with documented CoQ-10 deficiency, replacement therapy with CoQ-10 offers clear benefits. Although some study findings have been mixed, the NCCIH reports a number of positive outcomes associated with the use of CoQ-10.

- Patients with heart failure who took CoQ-10 had improved cardiac function.
- Patients who took CoQ-10 after cardiac surgery had faster recovery.
- CoQ-10 may improve sperm count and semen quality; however, further studies are needed to identify an improvement in conception.

Research studies that examined the effect of CoQ-10 on statin-associated muscle injury, cancer prevention and treatment, and hypertension were inconclusive.

Adverse Effects

CoQ-10 is well tolerated. High doses may produce gastrointestinal (GI) disturbances, including gastritis, reduced appetite, nausea, and diarrhea. Liver enzymes may increase, although no reports of actual liver injury have been made. Women who are pregnant or breastfeeding should not take CoQ-10 because safety has not been established.

Interactions With Conventional Drugs

CoQ-10 is structurally similar to vitamin K_2 and hence may antagonize the effects of warfarin.

Biosynthesis of CoQ-10 shares a common pathway with cholesterol. As a result, drugs such as the statins, which inhibit synthesis of cholesterol, can also inhibit synthesis of CoQ-10, causing levels of endogenous CoQ-10 to decline. (Statin-induced reductions in CoQ-10 may explain why statins cause muscle injury.)

Cranberry Juice

Uses

Cranberry juice is used to prevent urinary tract infections (UTIs) and to decrease urine odor in patients with urinary incontinence.

Actions

Benefits derive from the presence of proanthocyanidins, a group of compounds that prevent bacteria from adhering to the urinary tract wall. Bacteria that have already attached themselves are not affected. Cranberry juice does not acidify the urine as previously thought.

Effectiveness

Daily consumption of cranberry juice can *prevent* recurrent UTIs, but this has been demonstrated only in certain age groups. Specifically, it appears to benefit older-adult women and women in their teens or 20s, but not middle-aged adults or young girls. Furthermore, although cranberry juice can prevent UTIs, it is not effective as treatment for an established infection. In patients with urinary incontinence, cranberry juice can reduce unpleasant odor. Little is known about the efficacy of cranberry-extract capsules. Accordingly, cranberry juice itself is the preferred formulation.

Adverse Effects

Drinking more than 1 L/day may increase the risk for GI upset and formation of kidney stones.

Interactions With Conventional Drugs

There is some evidence that cranberry juice may increase the risk for bleeding in patients taking warfarin. Accordingly, these patients should be monitored closely.

Echinacea

Echinacea is the scientific name of the coneflower plant which is native to the United States and parts of Canada. Echinacea was listed in the National Formulary from 1916 to 1950, but fell from favor owing to development of antibiotics and a lack of scientific data to support its use.

Uses

Echinacea (*Echinacea angustifolia, E. purpurea, E. pallida*) is administered orally and topically. Oral echinacea is taken to stimulate immune function, suppress inflammation, and treat viral infections, including influenza and the common cold. Topical echinacea is used to treat wounds, burns, eczema, psoriasis, and herpes simplex infections.

Actions

Active ingredients in echinacea preparations include cichoric acid, polysaccharides, flavonoids, and essential oils. These ingredients have been thought to produce antiviral, antiinflammatory, and immunostimulant effects through a combination of actions, including mobilization of phagocytes, stimulation of T-lymphocyte proliferation, stimulation of interferon and tumor necrosis factor production, and inhibition of hyaluronidase, a proinflammatory enzyme.

Effectiveness

Although echinacea is taken widely to prevent and treat colds, its efficacy is highly questionable. Recent randomized, placebo-controlled trials designed to evaluate the ability of echinacea to *prevent* colds found no effect on (1) the time to developing an upper respiratory tract infection (URI); (2) the incidence, duration, or severity of URIs that did develop; or (3) development of experimentally induced URIs. Other recent trials conducted on adults and children who already had a URI found echinacea no better than placebo at reducing either the duration or severity of symptoms. The NCCIH continues to support research for its effects on the immune system.

Adverse Effects

Very few adverse effects have been reported. The most common complaint is unpleasant taste. Fever, nausea, and vomiting occur infrequently.

Rarely, echinacea causes allergic reactions, including acute asthma, urticaria, angioedema, and anaphylaxis. Echinacea belongs to the daisy family of plants, whose members include ragweed, asters, chamomile, and chrysanthemums. People allergic to any of these plants are at increased risk for reacting to echinacea. Individuals with atopy (a genetic tendency toward allergic conditions) appear at increased risk for reacting to echinacea.

Until echinacea's effects on the immune system are fully known, it would be prudent to avoid the drug in patients with autoimmune diseases, such as lupus erythematosus or rheumatoid arthritis. Although short-term exposure to echinacea *may* stimulate immune function, there is concern that long-term exposure can *suppress* immune function. Accordingly, long-term therapy should be avoided in immunocompromised patients, including those with HIV infection. In addition, prolonged therapy should be avoided in people with tuberculosis and other chronic infections that require optimal immune function for cure.

Interactions With Conventional Drugs

By stimulating the immune system, echinacea can oppose the effects of immunosuppressant drugs. Conversely, by suppressing immune function (in response to long-term use), echinacea can compromise drug therapy of tuberculosis, cancer, and HIV infection.

Feverfew

Feverfew *(Tanacetum parthenium)* is a bushy plaint with small daisy-like flowers that grows throughout North and South America and Europe. Supplements are made from the dried leaves, although sometimes the flowers and stems are included.

Uses

Feverfew is used primarily for prophylaxis of migraine. It is also taken for a number of conditions associated with hypersensitivity and altered immune responses such as allergies, asthma, rheumatoid arthritis, and psoriasis.

Actions

The principal active agent in feverfew is *parthenolide,* a compound found in feverfew leaves. How parthenolide suppresses migraine is poorly understood. Possibilities include inhibition of vasoconstriction in the brain, suppression of serotonin release from platelets and leukocytes, and suppression of inflammation secondary to inhibition of arachidonic acid release.

Effectiveness

Clinical studies on feverfew's effect on migraine headaches have had mixed results. Some findings suggest that, when taken prophylactically, the herb can reduce the frequency of attacks and the severity of symptoms (nausea, photophobia, phonophobia, and pain). Feverfew was found less effective when taken to abort an ongoing attack, however. Furthermore, the doses required are much higher than those for prophylaxis.

In 2012, the AAN and the AHS published a joint report on the evidence for CAM on episodic migraine prophylaxis. Their conclusion was that feverfew was probably effective for this purpose. (See earlier section "Butterbur.") The AAN recommends dosing at 50 to 300 mg to be taken twice a day for migraine prophylaxis.

What about the other purposes for which people use feverfew? Unfortunately, there is no reliable evidence that feverfew can benefit patients with rheumatoid arthritis or other inflammatory conditions.

Adverse Effects

Feverfew is very well tolerated. No serious adverse effects have been reported, although long-term studies of safety are lacking. Mild reactions include abdominal pain, indigestion, diarrhea, flatulence, nausea, and vomiting. Chewing feverfew leaves, a rare practice today, can cause oral ulceration, tongue irritation, and swollen lips. Some patients develop *postfeverfew syndrome,* characterized by nervousness, fatigue, insomnia, tension headache, and joint pain or stiffness.

Feverfew belongs to the same plant family as echinacea. Accordingly, individuals allergic to ragweed, chrysanthemums, daisies, and marigolds may also be allergic to feverfew. By suppressing release of arachidonic acid in platelets, feverfew can decrease platelet aggregation and may thereby pose a risk for bleeding. Accordingly, the product should be discontinued 2 weeks before elective surgery.

Some reports suggest that feverfew may cause uterine contractions. For this reason, women who are pregnant should not take this drug. Safety regarding breastfeeding has not been established.

Interactions With Conventional Drugs

By suppressing platelet aggregation, feverfew can increase the risk for bleeding in patients taking antiplatelet drugs (e.g., aspirin) or anticoagulants (e.g., warfarin, heparin).

Comments

There is great variability in feverfew products. Some contain little or no active ingredient.

Flaxseed

Flaxseeds are small seeds of the flax plant that grows in the Northwest United States and Canada. They may be processed in various products or added whole to cereals and other food products.

Uses

Flaxseed powders are used to treat constipation and dyslipidemias. Because it is a phytoestrogen, some women take it to combat hot flashes associated with menopause. Flaxseed also represents a vegetarian source of omega-3 fatty acids.

Actions

Ground flaxseed provides soluble plant fiber and alpha-linolenic acid. Like other high-fiber products, flaxseed can reduce serum cholesterol.

Flaxseed is an important food source of phytoestrogens called lignans. In the colon, bacteria convert these lignans into enterolactone and enterodial, compounds that have both mild estrogenic and antiestrogenic actions. The antiestrogenic actions can decrease cellular proliferation in breast tissue.

Effectiveness

Like other fiber products, flaxseed has the potential to decrease plasma levels of total cholesterol and low-density lipoprotein (LDL) cholesterol but does not affect high-density lipoprotein (HDL) cholesterol or triglycerides. These effects occur predominantly among people with high cholesterol levels and in women who are postmenopausal. In contrast, *defatted* flaxseed may *increase* triglyceride levels, so it should be avoided by patients with hypertriglyceridemia.

Owing to its soluble fiber content, flaxseed acts like a bulk-forming laxative to relieve constipation. As with any bulk-forming laxative, adequate fluid intake is an important component of therapy.

Other than for management of hypercholesterolemia, current studies do not support the use of flaxseed for cardiovascular disease. They also do not support its use for relief of menopausal symptoms or cancer prevention. However, NCCIH funding of flaxseed research is ongoing.

Adverse Effects

Like other sources of dietary fiber, flaxseed can cause GI effects, including bloating, flatulence, and abdominal discomfort.

Interactions With Conventional Drugs

Flaxseed may reduce the absorption of conventional medications. Hence, it should be taken 1 hour before or 2 hours after these drugs.

Garlic

Garlic *(Allium sativum)* is a common plant known for its edible bulb. It has been used throughout history for a myriad of uses and remains one of the most popular dietary supplements in use today.

Uses

Garlic is used primarily for effects on the cardiovascular system. The herb is taken to reduce levels of triglycerides and LDL cholesterol and to raise levels of HDL cholesterol. Garlic is also employed to reduce blood pressure, suppress platelet aggregation, increase arterial elasticity, and decrease formation of atherosclerotic plaque. In addition, garlic has been used for antimicrobial and anticancer effects.

Actions

Beneficial effects are presumed to result from the actions of sulfides in garlic oil. Intact garlic cells contain *alliin,* an odorless amino acid. When garlic cells are crushed, they release allinase, an enzyme that converts alliin into *allicin.* Allicin is the major active agent in garlic oil and the compound that gives garlic its distinctive aroma. In addition to allicin, garlic oil contains *ajoenes* (pronounced AH-ho-weens), biologically active compounds that contribute to beneficial effects.

Garlic is thought to reduce cholesterol levels by interfering with cholesterol synthesis in the liver. There is conflicting evidence regarding inhibition of HMG-CoA reductase, the rate-limiting enzyme in cholesterol synthesis and the enzyme that "statin" drugs inhibit.

Antiplatelet effects, which are well documented, result in part from inhibiting thromboxane synthesis. Methylallyltrisulfide is the chemical in garlic believed responsible. In addition, garlic may suppress platelet aggregation by disrupting calcium-dependent processes. Coagulation is also affected by the ajoenes, which have antithrombotic actions and may also stimulate fibrinolysis.

Lowering of blood pressure may be explained by garlic's ability to increase the activity of nitric oxide synthase, the enzyme in blood vessels that makes nitric oxide. Nitric oxide, also known as endothelium-derived relaxant factor, is a powerful vasodilator.

Effectiveness

As with many dietary supplements, research findings regarding garlic have been mixed. Outcomes of small trials in the 1990s demonstrated that garlic can produce favorable effects on plasma lipids. More recent and larger studies, however, have cast doubt on those findings.

After reviewing the scientific research, the NCCIH has concluded the following, for now:

- Garlic does not appear to lower LDL cholesterol.
- Garlic *may* lower blood pressure, but any benefit appears modest, at best.
- Garlic *may* decrease the rate of atherosclerosis development.

Regarding the effect of garlic on cancer prevention, at this time, the National Cancer Institute recognizes that garlic *may* have a role in cancer prevention but, in the absence of adequate reliable data, does not recommend it.

Adverse Effects

Garlic is generally well tolerated. The most common side effects are bad breath and body odor. (This occurs because a product of garlic metabolism is allyl methyl sulfide, a sulfur compound that is excreted through respiration and skin pores.) Rarely, garlic causes heartburn, flatulence, nausea, vomiting, diarrhea, and a burning sensation in the mouth. These effects are most pronounced with raw garlic and in people who don't eat garlic often. Patients suffering from infectious or inflammatory GI disorders should avoid garlic owing to its potential for GI irritation.

Interactions With Conventional Drugs

Garlic has significant antiplatelet effects. Accordingly, it can increase the risk for bleeding in patients taking antiplatelet drugs (e.g., aspirin) or anticoagulants (e.g., warfarin, heparin).

Garlic can reduce levels of at least two drugs: cyclosporine (an immunosuppressant) and saquinavir (a protease inhibitor used to treat HIV infection).

Ginger Root

Ginger grows primarily in the tropics. Its root, actually a rhizome, is the source of the ginger root used in CAM.

Uses

Ginger root (*Zingiber officinale*) is used primarily to treat vertigo and to suppress nausea and vomiting associated with motion sickness, morning sickness, seasickness, and general anesthesia. In addition, ginger has antiinflammatory and analgesic properties that may help people with arthritis and other chronic inflammatory conditions. Some practitioners use ginger for URIs, although proof of efficacy is lacking.

Actions

The mechanism by which ginger suppresses nausea and vomiting is unclear. A good possibility is blockade of serotonin (5-hydroxytryptamine$_3$, or 5-HT$_3$) receptors located in the chemoreceptor trigger zone of the medulla and on afferent vagal neurons in the GI tract. Activation of these receptors triggers emesis. Conversely, blockade of these receptors suppresses emesis. In fact, drugs that block 5-HT$_3$ receptors (e.g., ondansetron [Zofran]) are the most effective antiemetics available. Galanolactone, a major constituent of ginger, can block 5-HT$_3$ receptors in vitro, suggesting that receptor blockade may underlie antiemetic effects. Other actions that may contribute to beneficial effects include stimulation of intestinal motility, salivation, and gastric mucus production and suppression of GI spasm secondary to anticholinergic and antihistaminic actions.

The antiinflammatory effects of ginger have been attributed to inhibiting synthesis of prostaglandins and leukotrienes, which are powerful inflammatory mediators.

How ginger may reduce vertigo is unknown.

Effectiveness

There is good evidence supporting the benefits of ginger root for prevention and treatment of morning sickness. A 2014 meta-analysis of the evidence demonstrated a decrease in nausea but not in episodes of vomiting. Unfortunately, studies focused on nausea due to motion sickness and postoperative nausea and vomiting (in the absence of opioids) have had conflicting results.

In patients with rheumatoid arthritis, ginger root *appears* to reduce pain, improve joint mobility, and decrease swelling and morning stiffness. These studies are inconclusive, however, and further research is ongoing.

Adverse Effects

Ginger is very well tolerated. Severe toxicity has not been reported—although excessive doses (above 5 g/day) have the potential to cause CNS depression and cardiac dysrhythmias. Huge doses may also cause GI disturbances.

Although ginger has effectiveness in relieving morning sickness, it should be used with caution during pregnancy because safety in pregnancy has not been proved. High-dose ginger is believed to stimulate the uterus and thus may theoretically cause spontaneous abortion, although there are no reports of this ever happening. A 2012 population study of women in Norway included data on 1020 women who used ginger during pregnancy. Research findings showed no increased risk for malformations, spontaneous abortion, or other complications compared with women who did not take ginger.

Interactions With Conventional Drugs

Ginger can inhibit production of thromboxane by platelets and can thereby suppress platelet aggregation. Accordingly, ginger can increase the risk for bleeding in patients receiving antiplatelet drugs (e.g., aspirin) or anticoagulants (e.g., warfarin, heparin). Ginger can lower blood sugar and hence may potentiate the hypoglycemic effects of insulin and other drugs for diabetes.

Ginkgo biloba

Medicinal ginkgo is prepared by acetone extraction of leaves from the *Ginkgo biloba* tree. These leaves contain two classes of active compounds: *flavonoids* (ginkgoflavone glycosides) and *terpenoids* (ginkgolides, bilobalide). *Ginkgo biloba extracts* (GBEs) are standardized to contain 24% flavonoids and 6% terpenoids. Daily oral doses of standardized GBE range from 60 to 240 mg.

Uses

Ginkgo (*Ginkgo biloba*) is used primarily to improve memory, to halt progression of dementia, and to decrease intermittent claudication. Less common uses include treatment of erectile dysfunction and other conditions associated with decreased perfusion.

Actions

Any benefits are believed to derive from improved blood flow secondary to ginkgo-induced vasodilation. GBEs also suppress production of platelet-activating factor (PAF), a mediator of platelet aggregation, bronchospasm, and other processes. Reduced PAF production may help protect against thrombosis as well as bronchospasm and other allergic disorders.

Effectiveness

Gingko is one of the most studied of the herbal products. As with many of these, early studies showed promising findings that conflicted with more recent and rigorous clinical trials.

Studies that examine the effects of gingko on intermittent claudication have had mixed results. Most have not demonstrated a significant benefit. In those in which improvement was noted, the degree of improvement was small.

What about benefits in dementia? In a large placebo-controlled trial—the Ginkgo Evaluation of Memory (GEM) study, sponsored by the NIH—GBE failed to prevent dementia of any sort, including Alzheimer disease. This study enrolled more than 3000 participants 75 years or older. Half received a GBE formulation (120 mg twice daily), and the other half received a placebo. The result? After 6 years of treatment, the incidence of dementia was nearly identical in both groups.

The NCCIH is currently studying ginkgo effects in multiple sclerosis, sexual dysfunction caused by antidepressants, insulin resistance, and memory loss due to electroconvulsive therapy. Additional studies continue for intermittent claudication and dementia.

Adverse Effects

Ginkgo is generally well tolerated. In some patients, it causes stomach upset, headache, dizziness, or vertigo, all of which can be minimized by avoiding rapid increases in dosage. There have been case reports of spontaneous bleeding, although no bleeding was observed in the GEM study.

There have been reports of people eating raw or roasted ginkgo seeds. Unlike ginkgo leaves, the seeds contain significant amounts of toxins. Seizures and fatalities have occurred after ingestion.

Interactions With Conventional Drugs

Ginkgo may suppress coagulation. Accordingly, it should be used with caution in patients taking antiplatelet drugs (e.g., aspirin) or anticoagulants (e.g., warfarin, heparin).

There is concern that ginkgo may promote seizures. Accordingly, the herb should be avoided by patients at risk for seizures, including those taking drugs that can lower the seizure threshold, including some antipsychotics, antidepressants, cholinesterase inhibitors, decongestants, first-generation antihistamines, and systemic glucocorticoids.

Glucosamine and Chondroitin

Glucosamine and chondroitin are individual products that are usually administered together. Both are innate substances in the body that serve as essential components of cartilage. Products containing these substances can come from natural sources (e.g., animal cartilage) or may be manufactured in a laboratory.

Uses

These agents are used widely to treat osteoarthritis. Osteoarthritis primarily affects the knee, hip, and wrist joints.

Actions

Glucosamine is employed by the body in the synthesis of cartilage and synovial fluid. Chondroitin helps to keep cartilage hydrated. When given to people with osteoarthritis, glucosamine may help in several ways. First, it can act as a substrate for making cartilage and synovial fluid. Second, it can stimulate the activity of chondrocytes, the cells in joints that make cartilage and synovial fluid. And third, it can suppress production of cytokines that mediate joint inflammation and cartilage degradation. Chondroitin has a role in maintaining cartilage integrity.

Effectiveness

Studies on the efficacy of glucosamine and chondroitin in osteoarthritis have yielded mixed results. Most studies do not show improvement in pain relief; however, some studies have demonstrated a modest improvement in joint structure.

In 2012, the American College of Rheumatology updated their recommendations for the management for osteoarthritis. After an examination of the evidence, the expert panel advised providers *not* to use glucosamine and chondroitin for osteoarthritis management.

Adverse Effects

The most common side effects are GI disturbances, such as nausea and heartburn. Because commercial glucosamine is produced from the exoskeletons of shellfish (shrimp), glucosamine should be used with caution in patients with shellfish allergy. In theory, glucosamine can raise blood levels of glucose, but this has not been observed in clinical trials.

Interactions With Conventional Drugs

Several case reports suggest glucosamine may increase the risk for bleeding. Accordingly, patients taking antiplatelet drugs (e.g., aspirin) or anticoagulants (e.g., warfarin, heparin) should probably avoid this product.

Green Tea

Green tea is produced from the *Camellia sinensis* plant. This is the same plant used to produce black tea and oolong tea. The differences lie in the method of production.

Uses

Green tea and green tea extracts have been used to lose weight, improve mental clarity, and prevent and treat cancers of the stomach, skin, bladder, and breast.

Actions

The mechanism underlying beneficial effects is poorly understood and probably multifactorial. Polyphenols in green tea may underlie antiinflammatory, chemoprotective, and antioxidant effects. Chemoprotection may also stem from epigallocatechin-3-gallate (EGCG), a compound in green tea extracts. The caffeine in green tea may be responsible for weight loss and improved mental clarity.

Effectiveness

Data on green tea efficacy are limited. There is evidence that drinking green tea throughout the day can improve mental clarity and may help with weight loss. In both cases, any benefits are probably due to caffeine and not a substance unique to green tea.

Studies done in animals and cultured cancer cells have shown that green tea and EGCG may prevent or slow the growth of certain cancers. Also, there is a small body of evidence indicating that drinking green tea may help prevent recurrence after treatment of early-stage breast cancer. These studies have shown mixed results; however, research is ongoing.

Adverse Effects

Moderate consumption appears to be safe. As with other caffeine-containing products, overconsumption may result in headache, nausea, anxiety, insomnia, increased heart rate, and increased urination. Hepatotoxicity has been reported, primarily in people using concentrated green tea extracts. The mechanism of the hepatotoxicity remains unknown.

Interactions With Conventional Drugs

There is a long list of potential drug interactions. Green tea should be consumed with caution by patients taking vasodilators, stimulants and other psychoactive medications, and medications with a known risk for liver damage. Green tea contains a small amount of vitamin K, which may decrease the anticoagulant effects of warfarin.

Peppermint

Peppermint (*Mentha piperita*) is a common herb in North America as well as Europe and the Middle East. It is often found in near streams, especially in partially shaded areas.

Uses

Peppermint is best known as a culinary flavoring. Peppermint tea is a popular drink in some regions. When used as a medicinal preparation, peppermint oil is the form most commonly used. It is available over the counter in gel tablets or capsules.

Randomized controlled trials (RCTs) have demonstrated a beneficial effect of peppermint oil for management of irritable bowel syndrome (IBS). In their 2014 Monograph on the Management of Irritable Bowel Syndrome and Chronic Idiopathic Constipation (available at http://gi.org/wp-content/uploads/2014/08/IBS_CIC_Monograph_AJG_Aug_2014.pdf), the American College of Gastroenterology included peppermint oil among their recommendations for IBS management.

Peppermint oil is also gaining recognition as therapy for small intestine bacterial overgrowth (SIBO). SIBO is a condition that has become increasingly common as a result of increases in over-the-counter proton pump inhibitor use as well as following certain bariatric surgeries such as the Roux-en-Y gastric bypass. As bacteria break down carbohydrates and other substances, excessive gas forms. This results in severe abdominal cramps and low volume diarrhea. SIBO is typically treated with antibiotics; therefore, the antibiotic properties of peppermint oil are beneficial in this regard.

Small studies have also supported the use of peppermint oil to manage esophageal spasms in adults and functional abdominal pain in children. Numerous anecdotal reports suggest topical use of peppermint oil applied to the temples may help ease tension headaches. This is supported by two small trials comparing peppermint oil to a placebo and peppermint oil to acetaminophen. In these, peppermint oil was significantly more effective than the placebo and equal in effectiveness compared to acetaminophen.

Actions

Peppermint oil inhibits smooth muscle activity in the gastrointestinal tract. The exact mechanism is unclear; however, animal studies have indicated a possible relationship to blocking of calcium channels in the GI system.

Antibacterial properties of peppermint may come, in part, from menthol and other volatile oils. Research has demonstrated that peppermint oil has a bacteriostatic effect against 22 strains of both gram positive and gram negative bacteria and bactericidal activity against *Escherichia coli, Helicobacter pylori,* and *Salmonella enteritidis*.

It has been theorized that peppermint activates opioid receptors. Recent studies point to a different mechanism for pain relief: stimulation of transient receptor potential ion channel melastatin subtype 8 (TRPM8) in gastrointestinal pathways. TRPM8 receptors are activated by cold temperatures and by cooling agents such as menthol, which is a component of peppermint,

Effectiveness

Numerous studies demonstrate that peppermint oil is significantly superior to a placebo for management of IBS. Smaller studies support its use for SIBO, functional abdominal pain, and tension headache.

Adverse Effects

Peppermint can lower esophageal sphincter pressure leading to gastroesophageal reflux. This is more likely to occur with peppermint teas. Peppermint gels do not usually cause such problems because their enteric coating allows them to pass through the stomach intact.

Allergic reactions have been reported. Perianal burning has been reported following high doses. Excessive doses have also been tied to renal problems. At standard doses, peppermint oil appears to be devoid of serious adverse effects.

Interactions With Conventional Drugs

Over a decade ago, questions were raised regarding CYP1A2 inhibition by peppermint oil; however, this has not been demonstrated in humans. Peppermint oil may have an additive effect when administered with antispasmodics.

Probiotics

Probiotics are dietary supplements composed of potentially beneficial bacteria or yeasts. These preparations typically contain two types of bacteria—lactobacilli and bifidobacteria—as well as *Saccharomyces boulardii,* a specific strain of yeast. All of these microorganisms are normal components of our gut flora.

Uses

The *bacteria* in probiotics may help treat irritable bowel syndrome (IBS), ulcerative colitis, *Clostridium difficile*–associated diarrhea (CDAD), and, in children, rotavirus diarrhea. Products containing *S. boulardii* are used for CDAD.

Actions

Normal intestinal and colonic bacteria play several important roles: they help metabolize foods and some drugs; they promote nutrient absorption; and they reduce colonization of the gut by pathogenic bacteria. *Lactobacillus* and *Bifidobacterium* species adhere to the intestinal wall and thereby prevent attachment of bacterial pathogens. They also control bacterial overgrowth by producing lactic acid and to some degree by producing hydrogen peroxide. Benefits may also derive from increasing nonspecific cellular and humeral immunity. The yeast *S. boulardii* produces proteases that can degrade toxins produced by *C. difficile.* Benefits of *S. boulardii* in Crohn disease derive in part from increasing intestinal secretion of immunoglobulin A.

Effectiveness

According to information available at NCCIH (https://nccih.nih.gov/health/probiotics), studies on probiotics have yielded conflicting results. Larger and more rigorous research studies are needed. There is some evidence that *Lactobacillus* species may reduce the duration of diarrhea in patients with rotavirus infection and other GI conditions. Effectiveness appears to vary among *Lactobacillus* species. VSL#3, a product composed of lactobacilli, bifidobacteria, *Streptococcus thermophilus,* and other bacteria, appears to have a role in inducing remission of ulcerative colitis, perhaps in as many as 50% of patients. In patients with IBS, VSL#3 may reduce bloating and abdominal pain. However, the product does not improve bowel movement frequency or consistency. Additional testing is needed.

Adverse Effects

Probiotics are generally well tolerated. Flatulence and bloating are the most common adverse effects. Infection of the blood with lactobacilli and fungi has been reported after ingestion of yogurt, but only in severely ill, immunocompromised patients taking broad-spectrum antibiotics long term. Fungemia has occurred most often when packets of *S. boulardii* [Florastor] have been opened at the bedside in the intensive care unit. Florastor is contraindicated in patients who have central lines.

Interactions With Conventional Drugs

Antibacterial and antifungal drugs can kill the bacteria and yeasts in probiotic products. Accordingly, to help preserve probiotic activity, these preparations should be administered no sooner than 2 hours after dosing with antibacterial or antifungal drugs.

Resveratrol

Resveratrol is a chemical found in grapes (mainly the skin), red wine, purple grape juice, blueberries, cranberries, and peanuts. Resveratrol content of dietary supplements ranges from 16 to 600 mg per tablet or capsule. The amount in red wine is quite low, only 0.3 to 1.9 mg per 150-mL serving.

Uses

Resveratrol is an antioxidant promoted for antiaging effects and for protection against chronic diseases. Owing to the presence of resveratrol in red wine, researchers thought it might explain the *French paradox:* how can it be that French people have a relatively low incidence of coronary heart disease, despite having a diet relatively high in saturated fats? However, the amount of resveratrol in red wine seems much too low for significant cardioprotectant effects.

Recent research findings have opened the door to the potential for resveratrol to improve outcomes in a number of conditions. Research is ongoing to determine resveratrol's role in management of heart disease, diabetes, obesity, and Alzheimer disease.

Actions

In 2012, a breakthough NIH study of resveratrol identified the mechanism of action, heretofore believed to be due to direct interaction with sirtuin enzymes. Resveratrol inhibits phosphodiesterases (PDEs). This, in turn, increases levels of cyclic adenosine monophosphate (AMP) and activation of AMP-dependent kinase. This is important because PDEs play a role in many chronic conditions (e.g., heart disease, diabetes, chronic obstructive pulmonary disease), and PDE inhibitors are proving to be important drugs in managing these.

Effectiveness

Resveratrol has produced clear benefits in animal studies. In middle-aged mice on a high-calorie diet, resveratrol increased insulin sensitivity and reduced mortality. In normal-weight mice, resveratrol failed to reduce mortality, but did improve cardiovascular function, bone density, and motor coordination, and delayed formation of cataracts. In rodent models of human cancers, resveratrol suppressed tumor growth, including tumors of the lung, skin, breast, and prostate. In diabetic rats, resveratrol lowered blood glucose, and in human cells grown in culture, resveratrol increased glucose uptake. In one human study, resveratrol suppressed production of tumor necrosis factor and free radicals; both actions could reduce blood vessel inflammation and subsequent atherosclerosis.

Although studies done in cell cultures and animals have been encouraging, very little is known about the long-term benefits of resveratrol in humans. In fact, we have no data at all showing that resveratrol either slows aging or reduces the incidence or severity of any disease.

Adverse Effects and Interactions With Conventional Drugs

Information on adverse effects is limited. We do know that resveratrol has antiplatelet actions, which might intensify the effects of anticoagulants and antiplatelet drugs. Also, resveratrol can mimic the effects of estrogen and hence is not recommended for women with estrogen-dependent breast cancer. In addition, resveratrol may increase insulin sensitivity and hence should be used with caution by patients taking antidiabetic agents.

Saw Palmetto

The American saw palmetto (*Serenoa repens, Sabal serrulata*) is a small palm tree that grows in the eastern United States. The product employed clinically is an extract made from its berries.

Uses

Saw palmetto is taken to relieve urinary symptoms associated with benign prostatic hyperplasia (BPH). No other use has been identified.

Actions

How does saw palmetto affect prostate function? Some have postulated that it causes blockade of testosterone receptors, blockade of alpha-adrenergic receptors, and suppression of inflammation. Contrary to prior belief, the preparation does not seem to inhibit 5-alpha-reductase, the enzyme that converts testosterone into dihydrotestosterone (DHT), the active form of testosterone in the prostate. Saw palmetto does not reduce prostate size or serum levels of testosterone, DHT, or prostate-specific antigen (PSA).

Effectiveness

At this time, there is insufficient evidence to support using saw palmetto for BPH or any other condition. Although early studies suggested that saw palmetto might reduce symptoms of BPH, these results have not been confirmed by more rigorous studies. Two clinical trials funded by the NIH showed that saw palmetto extract is no more effective than placebo at reducing symptoms of BPH. A 2012 Cochrane review of 32 RCTs involving 5666 men found no significant difference between saw palmetto and a placebo. It continues to be widely used, however, and promoted in nonprofessional magazines and other resources.

Adverse Effects

Saw palmetto is very well tolerated. Significant adverse effects have not been reported. Rarely, saw palmetto causes nausea or headache. Although antiandrogenic effects (e.g., gynecomastia) have not been reported, it may be wise to monitor for them. Saw palmetto may have antiplatelet actions, but increased bleeding has not been reported.

Because of its antiandrogenic effects, saw palmetto represents a danger to the developing fetus. Pregnant women should not ingest this herb, but then we would hope that women would not anticipate needing a preparation whose only indication is treatment of BPH.

Interactions with Conventional Drugs

Because of its antiplatelet effects, saw palmetto should be used with caution in patients taking antiplatelet drugs (e.g., aspirin) or anticoagulants (e.g., warfarin, heparin).

Soy

Soy is a member of the pea (legume) family. Although it is processed in tablets and capsules for CAM, it has become a common staple in American diets both in its original form (edamame) and in processed foods such as soy sauce and tofu.

Uses

Soy protein and soy isoflavones have several uses, including prevention of breast cancer and, in postmenopausal women, treatment of vasomotor symptoms (hot flashes) and prevention of osteoporosis.

Actions

Soy's major active components are phytoestrogens (isoflavones and lignans) and phytosterols (betasitosterol). Two isoflavones—genistein and daidzein—undergo enzymatic conversion to equol, a compound with estrogenic actions. Soy isoflavones are structurally similar to estradiol (the major endogenous estrogen) and can bind with estrogen receptors. However, like the SERMs, isoflavones exert mixed estrogenic and antiestrogenic actions. In women with normal estrogen levels, soy isoflavones appear to *antagonize* endogenous estrogen. By contrast, in postmenopausal women, soy isoflavones act as estrogen agonists.

Effectiveness

Clinical trials using soy-derived phytoestrogens to relieve menopausal hot flashes have yielded mixed results. Overall, the studies lean toward a reduction in hot flashes.

Several epidemiologic studies infer that soy consumption may reduce the risk for developing breast cancer. In particular, population studies have documented that Asian women who eat a diet high in soy are at reduced risk. However, clinical trials confirming this benefit are lacking.

Several early studies suggested that isoflavones either increase bone mineral density or slow the progression of osteoporosis in perimenopausal and postmenopausal women. However, with one exception, several meta-analyses of studies published between 2010 and 2015 do not demonstrate significant improvement in bone mineral density. The exception? A meta-analysis on the effects of phytoestrogens on osteoporosis in ovariectomized rats.

Adverse Effects

Soy and soy extracts are very well tolerated. Gastrointestinal effects—bloating, nausea, constipation or diarrhea—are most common. Rarely, soy can cause migraine, probably because of its estrogenic effects. Large amounts of soy products may increase the risk for oxalate kidney stones. There have been several cases of goiter and hypothyroidism in infants who drank soy-based formula. Concerns that soy formulas might cause feminization of male infants were dispelled by a 2008 review from the American Academy of Pediatrics.

Interactions With Conventional Drugs

Soy should not be combined with tamoxifen and other drugs that can block estrogen receptors. By killing intestinal flora, antibiotics may reduce conversion of isoflavones to their active form, thus decreasing any potential positive effects of soy.

St. John's Wort

St. John's wort (*Hypericum perforatum*) is a plant that grows wild in the western United States and parts of Canada. Its yellow flowers are used in the preparation of extracts and other preparations.

Uses

St. John's wort is used primarily for oral therapy of mild to moderate depression. The herb has also been used topically to manage local infection and orally to relieve pain and inflammation.

Actions

Benefits of St. John's wort appear to derive from two compounds—hyperforin and hypericin—that are extracted from flowers of the plant. These compounds can decrease reuptake of three neurotransmitters: serotonin, norepinephrine (NE), and dopamine. Blockade of serotonin and NE uptake mimics the actions of some conventional antidepressants. Early research attributed antidepressant effects to inhibition of monoamine oxidase (MAO). However, we now know that the degree of MAO inhibition is too small to explain clinical effects.

Effectiveness

How effective is St. John's wort? At this time, it's hard to say. Although numerous studies have been conducted, evidence for efficacy is mixed, owing to poor study design, heterogeneous study populations, and variable hypericin content of the preparations used, as well as other confounding factors. The bottom line? For patients with *mild to moderate* major depression, St. John's wort appears superior to placebo and equal to tricyclic antidepressants. For patients with *severe* depression, there is no convincing proof of efficacy.

Adverse Effects

St. John's wort is generally well tolerated. Allergic skin reactions may occur, especially in people allergic to ragweed and daisies. In addition, the herb may cause CNS effects (e.g., insomnia, vivid dreams, restlessness, anxiety, agitation, and irritability) as well as GI discomfort, fatigue, dry mouth, and headache. High-dose therapy may pose a risk for phototoxicity. To reduce this risk, patients should minimize exposure to sunlight, wear protective clothing, and apply a sunscreen to exposed skin.

Interactions With Conventional Drugs

St. John's wort is known to interact adversely with many drugs—and the list continues to grow. Three mechanisms are involved: induction of cytochrome P450 enzymes, induction of P-glycoprotein, and intensification of serotonin effects. Let's consider these one by one:

- *Induction of 3A4 isoenzymes of cytochrome P450* can accelerate the metabolism of many drugs, thereby decreasing their effects. This mechanism appears responsible for breakthrough bleeding and unintended pregnancy in women taking oral contraceptives, transplant rejection in patients taking cyclosporine (an immunosuppressant), reduced anticoagulation in patients taking warfarin, and reduced antiretroviral effects in patients taking protease inhibitors or nonnucleoside reverse transcriptase inhibitors.
- *P-glycoprotein* is a transport protein found in cells that line the intestine and renal tubules. In the intestine, P-glycoprotein transports drugs *out* of cells into the intestinal lumen; in renal tubules, P-glycoprotein transports drugs *out* of tubular cells into the urine. Hence, by increasing P-glycoprotein synthesis, St. John's wort can accelerate elimination of drugs and can thereby reduce their effects. This is the mechanism by which St. John's wort greatly reduces levels of *digoxin,* a drug for heart failure. Other drugs whose levels can probably be reduced by this mechanism include calcium channel blockers, steroid hormones, protease inhibitors, and certain anticancer drugs (e.g., etoposide, paclitaxel, vinblastine, vincristine).
- Combining St. John's wort with certain drugs can intensify serotonergic transmission to a degree sufficient to cause potentially fatal *serotonin syndrome.* Although St. John's wort can enhance serotonergic transmission by itself, its effect is relatively weak. Hence, when used alone, the herb poses little risk. However, if St. John's wort is combined with other serotonin-enhancing agents, the risk is greatly increased, and hence St. John's wort should not be combined with such drugs. Among these are amphetamine, cocaine, and many antidepressants, including MAO inhibitors, selective serotonin reuptake inhibitors, certain tricyclic agents (e.g., amitriptyline, clomipramine), and duloxetine, nefazodone, and venlafaxine.

Because St. John's wort has a variety of known adverse interactions—and is likely to have more that are as yet unknown—caution is clearly advised. St. John's wort is not recommended for treating depression in patients taking other medications.

Valerian

Valerian (*Valeriana officinalis*), also known as garden heliotrope, is a common plant in Europe and Asia, although it is grown in some areas of North America. The plant's rhizomes and roots are used in the preparation of medicinal products.

Uses

Valerian root is a sedative preparation used primarily to promote sleep. In addition, some people take it to reduce anxiety-associated restlessness.

Actions

Valerian may work by increasing the availability of gamma-aminobutyric acid (GABA, an inhibitory neurotransmitter) at synapses in the CNS. (Benzodiazepines and benzodiazepine-like drugs, which are the major conventional hypnotics, act by potentiating the actions of GABA.) In addition, valerian may act as a direct GABA agonist. The active ingredients in valerian have not been identified.

Effectiveness

Although valerian has been used for centuries in Europe, China, and other countries, objective evidence of efficacy is lacking. According to the NCCIH at https://nccih.nih.gov/health/providers/digest/sleep-disorders-science, "Various herbs such as valerian, chamomile, and kava, and homeopathic medicines sometimes used as sleep aids have not been shown to be effective for insomnia." Even so, some suggest it may still have mild sedative effects that may be useful for anxiety.

Adverse Effects

Valerian is generally very well tolerated. The FDA has given valerian a Generally Recognized as Safe (GRAS) rating when the product is consumed in amounts commonly used in food. Possible side effects include daytime drowsiness, dizziness, depression, dyspepsia, and pruritus. Prolonged use may cause headache, nervousness, or cardiac abnormalities. Because valerian can reduce alertness, users should exercise caution when performing dangerous activities, such as driving or operating dangerous machinery. In addition, valerian should be used with caution by people with psychiatric illnesses (e.g., depression, dementia). As with benzodiazepines, there may be a risk for paradoxical excitation and physical dependence. We do not know if valerian enters breast milk or harms the developing fetus. Until more is known, valerian should be avoided by women who are pregnant or breastfeeding.

Interactions With Conventional Drugs

In theory, valerian can potentiate the actions of other drugs with CNS-depressant actions. Among these are alcohol, benzodiazepines, barbiturates, opioids, antihistamines, and centrally acting skeletal muscle relaxants. These combinations should be used with caution.

HARMFUL SUPPLEMENTS TO AVOID

To help protect the public from dangerous botanical products, the FDA and the Federal Trade Commission are monitoring adverse event data and issuing warnings to consumers and manufacturers. Three potentially harmful products—comfrey, kava, and Ma huang—are discussed here.

Comfrey

Comfrey (*Symphytum officinale*) is an herbal supplement used topically and orally. Topical use appears safe. Oral use is not. Why? Because comfrey contains pyrrolizidine alkaloids, which can cause venoocclusive disease (VOD) in animals and hepatic VOD in humans. Hepatic VOD can result in severe liver damage. In addition to causing VOD, pyrrolizidine alkaloids may also be carcinogenic. Accordingly, in July of 2001, the FDA issued a letter to dietary supplement manufacturers advising them to remove comfrey from the market. They urged manufacturers to discontinue production, pull existing product off the shelves, and to warn consumers of the possible dangers; however, comfrey remains widely available for sale on the Internet and elsewhere.

Kava

Kava (*Piper methysticum*), also known as *kava-kava* or *awa,* is used to relieve anxiety, promote sleep, and relax muscles. In the United States the herb has been promoted as a natural alternative to benzodiazepines (e.g., diazepam [Valium]) for treating anxiety and stress. Unfortunately, kava can cause severe liver injury, leading the FDA to issue a public warning in March 2002. Later that year, the Centers for Disease Control and Prevention issued a report on kava-related hepatotoxicity. In the report, they discussed 11 cases of hepatotoxicity from the United States and Europe in which the victims required a liver transplant owing to severe liver failure. Because of concerns over hepatotoxicity, kava sales have been restricted in Germany, Canada, Switzerland, France, and Australia—but not yet in the United States.

Ma Huang (Ephedra)

Ma huang (ephedra) contains ephedrine, a compound that can elevate blood pressure and stimulate the heart and CNS. High-dose ephedra has been associated with stroke, myocardial infarction, and death. To date, more than 17,000 adverse events have been reported, and at least 155 users have died. In 2004 the FDA banned U.S. sales of all ephedra products, marking the first time that a dietary supplement has been ordered off the market. The ban was challenged by an ephedra producer and, in 2005, was partially reversed: a federal court upheld the ban for ephedra products that contain more than 10 mg/dose, but reversed the ban for products that contain 10 mg or less, arguing that there are insufficient data to prove that low doses pose a "significant or unreasonable risk." In 2006, a federal appeals court upheld the FDA ban of ephedra. This ban was challenged again in 2007, but the U.S. Court of Appeals denied the petition for rehearing. At this time, the FDA ban does not apply to ephedra in traditional Asian medicines or in herbal teas, which are not marketed as dietary supplements.

UNIT XVIII

Therapy of Infectious and Parasitic Diseases

CHAPTER 68

Basic Principles of Antimicrobial Therapy

Laura D. Rosenthal, DNP, ACNP, FAANP

With this chapter we begin our study of drugs used to treat infectious diseases. Each day, 190 million doses of antibiotics are given in hospitals, making these drugs one of our most widely used groups of medicines.

Modern antimicrobial agents had their debut in the 1930s and 1940s and have greatly reduced morbidity and mortality from infection. As newer drugs are introduced, our ability to fight infections increases even more. However, despite impressive advances, continued progress is needed. There remain organisms that respond poorly to available drugs; there are effective drugs whose use is limited by toxicity; and there is, because of evolving microbial resistance, the constant threat that currently effective antibiotics will be rendered useless.

Here we focus on two principal themes. The first is microbial susceptibility to drugs, with special emphasis on resistance. The second is clinical use of antimicrobials. Topics addressed include criteria for drug selection, host factors that modify drug use, use of antimicrobial combinations, and use of antimicrobial agents for prophylaxis.

Before going further, we need to consider two terms: *antibiotic* and *antimicrobial drug*. In common practice, the terms *antibiotic* and *antimicrobial drug* are used interchangeably, as they are in this book. However, be aware that the formal definitions of these words are not identical. Strictly speaking, an *antibiotic* is a chemical that is produced by one microbe and has the ability to harm other microbes. Under this definition, only those compounds that are actually made by microorganisms qualify as antibiotics. Drugs such as the sulfonamides, which are produced in the laboratory, would not be considered antibiotics under the strict definition. In contrast, an *antimicrobial drug* is defined as any agent, natural or synthetic, that has the ability to kill or suppress microorganisms. Under this definition, no distinction is made between compounds produced by microbes and those made by chemists. From the perspective of therapeutics, there is no benefit to distinguishing between drugs made by microorganisms and drugs made by chemists. Hence, the current practice is to use the terms *antibiotic* and *antimicrobial drug* interchangeably.

SELECTIVE TOXICITY

Selective toxicity is defined as the ability of a drug to injure a target cell or target organism without injuring other cells or organisms that are in intimate contact with the target. As applied to antimicrobial drugs, selective toxicity indicates the ability of an antibiotic to kill or suppress microbial pathogens without causing injury to the host. Selective toxicity is the property that makes antibiotics valuable. If it weren't for selective toxicity—that is, if antibiotics were as harmful to the host as they are to infecting organisms—these drugs would have no therapeutic utility.

Achieving Selective Toxicity

How can a drug be highly toxic to microbes but harmless to the host? The answer lies with differences in the cellular chemistry of mammals and microbes. There are biochemical processes critical to microbial well-being that do not take place in mammalian cells. Hence, drugs that selectively interfere with these unique microbial processes can cause serious injury to microorganisms while leaving mammalian cells intact. Three examples of how we achieve selective toxicity are discussed here.

Disruption of the Bacterial Cell Wall

Unlike mammalian cells, bacteria are encased in a rigid cell wall. The protoplasm within this wall has a high concentration of solutes, making osmotic pressure within the bacterium high. If it were not for the cell wall, bacteria would absorb water, swell, and then burst. Several families of drugs (e.g., penicillins, cephalosporins) weaken the cell wall and thereby promote bacterial lysis. Because mammalian cells have no cell wall, drugs directed at this structure do not affect us.

Inhibition of an Enzyme Unique to Bacteria

The sulfonamides represent antibiotics that are selectively toxic because they inhibit an enzyme critical to bacterial survival but not to our survival. Specifically, sulfonamides inhibit an enzyme needed to make folic acid, a compound required by all cells, both mammalian and bacterial. Because we can use folic acid from dietary sources, sulfonamides are safe for human consumption. In contrast, bacteria must synthesize folic acid themselves (because, unlike us, they can't take up folic acid from the environment). Hence, to meet their needs, bacteria first take up *para*-aminobenzoic acid (PABA), a precursor of folic acid, and then convert the PABA into folic acid. Sulfonamides block this conversion. Because mammalian cells do not make their own folic acid, sulfonamide toxicity is limited to microbes.

Disruption of Bacterial Protein Synthesis

In bacteria, as in mammalian cells, protein synthesis is done by ribosomes. However, bacterial and mammalian ribosomes are not identical, and hence we can make drugs that disrupt function of one but not the other. As a result, we can impair protein synthesis in bacteria while leaving mammalian protein synthesis untouched.

CLASSIFICATION OF ANTIMICROBIAL DRUGS

Various schemes are employed to classify antimicrobial drugs. The two schemes most suited to our objectives are considered here.

Classification by Susceptible Organism

Antibiotics differ widely in their antimicrobial activity. Some agents, called *narrow-spectrum antibiotics,* are active against only a few species of microorganisms. In contrast, *broad-spectrum antibiotics* are active against a wide variety of microbes. As discussed later, *narrow-spectrum drugs are generally preferred to broad-spectrum drugs.*

Table 68.1 classifies the major antimicrobial drugs according to susceptible organisms. The table shows three major groups: *antibacterial drugs, antifungal drugs,* and *antiviral drugs.* In addition, the table subdivides the antibacterial drugs into narrow-spectrum and broad-spectrum agents and indicates the principal classes of bacteria against which they are active.

TABLE 68.1 ■ Classification of Antimicrobial Drugs by Susceptible Organisms

ANTIBACTERIAL DRUGS	
Narrow Spectrum	
Gram-positive cocci and gram-positive bacilli	Penicillin G and V Penicillinase-resistant penicillins: oxacillin, nafcillin Vancomycin Erythromycin Clindamycin
Gram-negative aerobes	Aminoglycosides: gentamicin, others Cephalosporins (first and second generations)
Mycobacterium tuberculosis	Isoniazid Rifampin Ethambutol Pyrazinamide
Broad Spectrum	
Gram-positive cocci and gram-negative bacilli	Broad-spectrum penicillins: ampicillin, others Extended-spectrum penicillins: piperacillin, others Cephalosporins (third generation) Tetracyclines: tetracycline, others Carbapenems: imipenem, others Trimethoprim Sulfonamides: sulfisoxazole, others Fluoroquinolones: ciprofloxacin, others
ANTIVIRAL DRUGS	
Drugs for HIV infection	Reverse transcriptase inhibitors: zidovudine, others Protease inhibitors: ritonavir, others Fusion inhibitors: enfuvirtide Integrase inhibitors: raltegravir CCR5 antagonists: maraviroc
Drugs for influenza	Adamantanes: amantadine, others Neuraminidase inhibitors: oseltamivir, others
Other antiviral drugs	Acyclovir Ribavirin Interferon alfa
ANTIFUNGAL DRUGS	Polyene antibiotics: amphotericin B, others Azoles: itraconazole, others Echinocandins: caspofungin, others

Classification by Mechanism of Action

The antimicrobial drugs fall into seven major groups based on mechanism of action. This classification is shown in Table 68.2. Properties of the seven major classes are discussed briefly here.

- *Drugs that inhibit bacterial cell wall synthesis or activate enzymes that disrupt the cell wall.* These drugs (e.g., penicillins, cephalosporins) weaken the cell wall and thereby promote bacterial lysis and death.
- *Drugs that increase cell membrane permeability.* Drugs in this group (e.g., amphotericin B) increase the permeability of cell membranes, causing leakage of intracellular material.
- *Drugs that cause lethal inhibition of bacterial protein synthesis.* The aminoglycosides (e.g., gentamicin) are the only drugs in this group. We do not know why inhibition of protein synthesis by these agents results in cell death.
- *Drugs that cause nonlethal inhibition of protein synthesis.* Like the aminoglycosides, these drugs (e.g., tetracyclines) inhibit bacterial protein synthesis. However, in contrast to the aminoglycosides, these agents only slow microbial growth—they do not kill bacteria at clinically achievable concentrations.
- *Drugs that inhibit bacterial synthesis of DNA and RNA or disrupt DNA function.* These drugs inhibit synthesis of DNA or RNA by binding directly to nucleic acids or by interacting with enzymes required for nucleic acid synthesis. They may also bind with DNA and disrupt its function. Members of this group include rifampin, metronidazole, and the fluoroquinolones (e.g., ciprofloxacin).
- *Antimetabolites.* These drugs disrupt specific biochemical reactions. The result is either a decrease in the synthesis of essential cell constituents or synthesis of nonfunctional

TABLE 68.2 ▪ Classification of Antimicrobial Drugs by Mechanism of Action

Drug Class	Representative Antibiotics
Inhibitors of cell wall synthesis	Penicillins
	Cephalosporins
	Imipenem
	Vancomycin
	Caspofungin
Drugs that disrupt the cell membrane	Amphotericin B
	Daptomycin
	Itraconazole
Bactericidal inhibitors of protein synthesis	Aminoglycosides
Bacteriostatic inhibitors of protein synthesis	Clindamycin
	Erythromycin
	Linezolid
	Tetracyclines
Drugs that interfere with synthesis or integrity of bacterial DNA and RNA	Fluoroquinolones
	Metronidazole
	Rifampin
Antimetabolites	Flucytosine
	Sulfonamides
	Trimethoprim
Drugs that suppress viral replication	
Viral DNA polymerase inhibitors	Acyclovir
	Ganciclovir
HIV reverse transcriptase inhibitors	Zidovudine
	Lamivudine
HIV protease inhibitors	Ritonavir
	Saquinavir
HIV fusion inhibitors	Enfuvirtide
HIV integrase inhibitors	Raltegravir
HIV CCR5 antagonists	Maraviroc
Influenza neuraminidase inhibitors	Oseltamivir
	Zanamivir

analogs of normal metabolites. Examples of antimetabolites include trimethoprim and the sulfonamides.

- *Drugs that suppress viral replication.* Most of these drugs inhibit specific enzymes—DNA polymerase, reverse transcriptase, protease, integrase, or neuraminidase—required for viral replication and infectivity.

When considering the *antibacterial* drugs, it is useful to distinguish between agents that are *bactericidal* and agents that are *bacteriostatic. Bactericidal* drugs are directly lethal to bacteria at clinically achievable concentrations. In contrast, *bacteriostatic* drugs can slow bacterial growth but do not cause cell death. When a bacteriostatic drug is used, elimination of bacteria must ultimately be accomplished by host defenses (i.e., the immune system working in concert with phagocytic cells).

ACQUIRED RESISTANCE TO ANTIMICROBIAL DRUGS

In this section, we discuss bacterial resistance to antibiotics, which may be *innate* (natural, inborn) or *acquired* over time. Discussion here is limited to acquired resistance, which is a much greater clinical concern than innate resistance.

Over time, an organism that had once been highly sensitive to an antibiotic may become less susceptible, or it may lose drug sensitivity entirely. In some cases, resistance develops to several drugs. Acquired resistance is of great concern in that it can render currently effective drugs useless, thereby creating a clinical crisis and a constant need for new antimicrobial agents. As a rule, antibiotic resistance is associated with extended hospitalization, significant morbidity, and excess mortality. Organisms for which drug resistance is now a serious problem include *Enterococcus faecium, Staphylococcus aureus, Enterobacter* species, *Pseudomonas aeruginosa, Acinetobacter baumannii, Klebsiella* species, and *Clostridium difficile* (Table 68.3). Two of these resistant bacteria—methicillin-resistant *S. aureus* and *C. difficile*—are discussed in Chapters 69 and 70 respectively.

In the discussion that follows, we examine the mechanisms by which microbial drug resistance is acquired and the measures by which emergence of resistance can be delayed. As you read this section, keep in mind that it is the *microbe* that becomes drug resistant, *not the patient.*

Microbial Mechanisms of Drug Resistance

Microbes have four basic mechanisms for resisting drugs. They can (1) decrease the concentration of a drug at its site of action, (2) alter the structure of drug target molecules, (3) produce a drug antagonist, and (4) cause drug inactivation.

Reduction of Drug Concentration at Its Site of Action

For most antimicrobial drugs, the site of action is intracellular. Accordingly, if a bug can reduce the intracellular concentration of a drug, it can resist harm. Two basic mechanisms are involved. First, microbes can *cease active uptake* of certain drugs—tetracyclines and gentamicin, for example. Second, microbes can *increase active export* of certain drugs—tetracyclines, fluoroquinolones, and macrolides, for example.

Alteration of Drug Target Molecules

Most antibiotics, like most other drugs, must interact with target molecules (receptors) to produce their effects. Hence, if the structure of the target molecule is altered, resistance can result. For example, some bacteria are now resistant to streptomycin because of structural changes in bacterial ribosomes, the sites at which streptomycin acts to inhibit protein synthesis.

Antagonist Production

In rare cases, a microbe can synthesize a compound that antagonizes drug actions. For example, by acquiring the ability to synthesize increased quantities of PABA, some bacteria have developed resistance to sulfonamides.

Drug Inactivation

Microbes can resist harm by producing drug-metabolizing enzymes. For example, many bacteria are resistant to penicillin G because of increased production of penicillinase, an enzyme that inactivates penicillin. In addition to penicillins, bacterial enzymes can inactivate other antibiotics, including cephalosporins, carbapenems, and fluoroquinolones.

TABLE 68.3 ■ Drugs for Some Highly Resistant Bacteria

Bacterium	Resistance	Resistance Mechanism	Alternative Treatments
Enterococcus faecium	Ampicillin	Mutation and overexpression of PBP5	Quinupristin/dalfopristin, daptomycin, tigecycline, linezolid
	Linezolid	Production of altered 23S ribosomes	Quinupristin/dalfopristin, daptomycin, tigecycline
	Daptomycin	Unknown	Quinupristin/dalfopristin
	Quinupristin/dalfopristin	Production of enzymes that inactivate quinupristin/dalfopristin, altered drug target	Daptomycin, tigecycline, linezolid
	Aminoglycosides	Production of aminoglycoside-modifying enzymes, ribosomal mutations	May attempt to test for streptomycin sensitivity
*Staphylococcus aureus**	Vancomycin	Thickening of cell wall and altered structure of cell wall precursor molecules	Quinupristin/dalfopristin, daptomycin, tigecycline, linezolid, telavancin
	Daptomycin	Altered structure of cell wall and cell membrane	Quinupristin/dalfopristin, tigecycline, linezolid, telavancin
	Linezolid	Production of altered 23S ribosomes	Quinupristin/dalfopristin, daptomycin, tigecycline, telavancin, ceftobiprole, ceftaroline
Enterobacter species	Ceftriaxone, cefotaxime, ceftazidime, cefepime	Production of extended-spectrum beta-lactamases	Carbapenems, tigecycline
	Carbapenems	Production of carbapenemases, decreased permeability	Polymyxins, tigecycline
Klebsiella species	Ceftriaxone, cefotaxime, ceftazidime, cefepime	Production of extended-spectrum beta-lactamases	Carbapenems, tigecycline
	Carbapenems	Production of carbapenemases, decreased permeability	Polymyxins, tigecycline
Pseudomonas aeruginosa	Carbapenems	Decreased permeability, increased drug efflux, production of carbapenemases	Polymyxins
Acinetobacter baumannii	Carbapenems	Decreased permeability, increased drug efflux, production of carbapenemases	Polymyxins
Clostridium difficile†	Metronidazole	Reduced drug activation, increased drug efflux, increased repair of drug-induced DNA damage	Vancomycin, rifaximin

*Methicillin-resistant *Staphylococcus aureus* is discussed in Chapter 69.
†*Clostridium difficile* infection is discussed in Chapter 70.
PBP5, penicillin-binding protein 5.

New Delhi Metallo-Beta-Lactamase 1 (NDM-1) Gene

Extensive drug resistance is conferred by the *NDM-1* gene, which codes for a powerful form of beta-lactamase. As discussed in Chapters 69 and 70, beta-lactamases are enzymes that can inactivate drugs that have a beta-lactam ring. The form of beta-lactamase encoded by *NDM-1* is both unusual and troubling in that it can inactivate essentially all beta-lactam antibiotics, a group that includes penicillins, cephalosporins, and carbapenems. Because the *NDM-1* gene is resistant to carbapenems, it is also classified as a type of carbapenem-resistant Enterobacteriaceae (CRE). Worse yet, the DNA segment that contains the *NDM-1* gene also contains genes that code for additional resistance determinants, including drug efflux pumps, and enzymes that can inactivate other important antibiotics, including erythromycin, rifampin, chloramphenicol, and fluoroquinolones. Furthermore, all of these genes are present on a plasmid, a piece of DNA that can be easily transferred from one bacterium to another (see later). Of note, bacteria that have the *NDM-1* gene are resistant to nearly all antibiotics, except for tigecycline and colistin. Since its discovery in *Klebsiella pneumoniae* in 2008, *NDM-1* has been found in other common enteric bacteria, including *Escherichia coli, Enterobacter* and *Salmonella* species, *Citrobacter freundii, Providencia rettgeri,* and *Morganella morganii.* Before 2012, only a few cases of *NDM-1* infection were reported in the United States and Canada, but that number is increasing. Between July 2012 and February 2013, 15 additional cases were reported in the United States alone.

Mechanisms by Which Resistance Is Acquired

How do microbes acquire mechanisms of resistance? Ultimately, all of the alterations in structure and function discussed previously result from changes in the microbial genome. These genetic changes may result either from spontaneous mutation or from acquisition of DNA from an external source. One important mechanism of DNA acquisition is conjugation with other bacteria.

Spontaneous Mutation

Spontaneous mutations produce random changes in a microbe's DNA. The result is a gradual increase in resistance. Low-level resistance develops first. With additional mutations, resistance becomes greater. As a rule, spontaneous mutations confer resistance *to only one drug.*

Conjugation

Conjugation is a process by which extrachromosomal DNA is transferred from one bacterium to another. To transfer resistance by conjugation, the donor organism must possess two unique DNA segments, one that codes for the mechanisms of drug resistance and one that codes for the "sexual" apparatus required for DNA transfer. Together, these two DNA segments constitute an *R factor* (resistance factor).

Conjugation takes place primarily among *gram-negative* bacteria. Genetic material may be transferred between members of the same species or between members of different species. Because transfer of R factors is not species specific, it is possible for pathogenic bacteria to acquire R factors from the normal flora of the body. Because R factors are becoming common in normal flora, the possibility of transferring resistance from normal flora to pathogens is a significant clinical concern.

In contrast to spontaneous mutation, conjugation frequently confers *multiple-drug resistance.* This can be achieved, for example, by transferring DNA that codes for several different drug-metabolizing enzymes. Hence, in a single event, a drug-sensitive bacterium can become highly drug resistant.

Relationships Between Antibiotic Use and Emergence of Drug-Resistant Microbes

Use of antibiotics promotes the emergence of drug-resistant microbes. Please note, however, that although antibiotics promote drug resistance, they are not mutagenic and do not directly cause the genetic changes that underlie reduced drug sensitivity. Spontaneous mutation and conjugation are random events whose incidence is independent of drug use. Drugs simply make conditions favorable for overgrowth of microbes that have acquired mechanisms for resistance.

How Do Antibiotics Promote Resistance?

To answer this question, we need to recall two aspects of microbial ecology: (1) microbes secrete compounds that are toxic to other microbes and (2) microbes within a given ecologic niche (e.g., large intestine, urogenital tract, skin) compete with each other for available nutrients. Under drug-free conditions, the various microbes in a given niche keep each other in check. Furthermore, if none of these organisms is drug resistant, introduction of antibiotics will be equally detrimental to all members of the population and therefore will not promote the growth of any individual microbe. However, *if a drug-resistant organism is present, antibiotics will create selection pressure favoring its growth* by killing off sensitive organisms. In doing so, the drug will eliminate the toxins they produce and will thereby facilitate survival of the microbe that is drug resistant. Also, elimination of sensitive organisms will remove competition for available nutrients, thereby making conditions even more favorable for the resistant microbe to flourish. Hence, although drug resistance is of no benefit to an organism when there are no antibiotics present, when antibiotics are introduced, they create selection pressure favoring overgrowth of microbes that are resistant.

Which Antibiotics Promote Resistance?

All antimicrobial drugs promote the emergence of drug-resistant organisms. However, some agents are more likely to promote resistance than others. Because broad-spectrum antibiotics kill more competing organisms than do narrow-spectrum drugs, broad-spectrum agents do the most to facilitate emergence of resistance.

Influence of Increased Antibiotic Use on the Emergence of Resistance

The more that antibiotics are used, the faster drug-resistant organisms will emerge. Not only do antibiotics promote emergence of resistant pathogens, they also promote overgrowth of normal flora that possess mechanisms for resistance. Because drug use can increase resistance in normal flora, and because normal flora can transfer resistance to pathogens, every effort should be made to avoid use of antibiotics by individuals who don't actually need them (i.e., individuals who don't have a bacterial infection). Because all antibiotic use will further the emergence of resistance, there can be no excuse for casual or indiscriminate dispensing of these drugs.

Health Care–Associated Infections

Because hospitals are sites of intensive antibiotic use, resident organisms can be extremely drug resistant. As a result, *health care–associated infections (HAIs)* are among the most difficult to treat. According to the Centers for Disease Control and Prevention (CDC), 1 of every 20 patients will fall victim to an HAI. Measures to delay emergence of resistant organisms in hospitals are discussed later.

Superinfection

Superinfection is a special example of the emergence of drug resistance. A superinfection is defined as a *new* infection that appears during the course of treatment for a primary infection.

New infections develop when antibiotics eliminate the inhibitory influence of normal flora, thereby allowing a second infectious agent to flourish.

When there is normal flora that contains a resistant organism, the antibiotic will selectively promote the growth of that specific resistant flora. Although the antibiotic promotes the overgrowth of resistant flora, it kills off sensitive strains, thus facilitating the survival of the resistant flora. Although there is selective overgrowth of the normal flora with resistance, there is still a decrease in the inhibitory effects of the sensitive flora.

Because broad-spectrum antibiotics kill off more normal flora than do narrow-spectrum drugs, superinfections are more likely in patients receiving broad-spectrum agents. Because superinfections are caused by drug-resistant microbes, these infections are often difficult to treat.

Antimicrobial Stewardship

Many organizations have begun to address the issue of antibiotic resistance in health care. In 2012 the Infectious Diseases Society of America (IDSA), in conjunction with the Society for Healthcare Epidemiology of America (SHEA) and the Pediatric Infectious Diseases Society (PIDS), released its first *Statement on Antimicrobial Stewardship.* The statement included five recommendations, with suggestions for monitoring, education, and research to assist in the prevention of antibiotic resistance. The statement can be found online at http://www.jstor.org/stable/10.1086/665010.

The American Board of Internal Medicine (ABIM) Foundation also created the *Choosing Wisely* Campaign in 2012 to decrease the amount of wasteful practice in health care. More than 70 specialty organizations have contributed guidelines to promote evidence based practice. Many of these guidelines address the appropriate use of antimicrobial therapy. *Choosing Wisely* can be located at http://www.choosingwisely.org. The *Get Smart for Healthcare* Campaign initiated by the CDC provides information on proper use of antibiotics in humans and animals. The campaign has three objectives: to promote adherence to appropriate prescribing guidelines, to decrease demand for antibiotics among healthy adults and parents of young children, and to increase adherence to prescribed antibiotics. Target audiences include patient and providers. More information is available at www.cdc.gov/drugresistance.

In addition to the CDC Campaign, in 2014 the Interagency Task Force on Antimicrobial Resistance published an update to its original 2012 publication, *A Public Health Action Plan to Combat Antimicrobial Resistance*. This updated action plan discusses three focus areas developed to decrease resistance to antibiotics:

- *Focus Area I: Surveillance, Prevention and Control of Antimicrobial Resistant Infections.* Goals include improving the detection, monitoring, and characterization of drug-resistant infections in humans and animals as well as improving the definition, characterization, and measurement of the impact of antimicrobial drug use.
- *Focus Area II: Research.* Goals include facilitation of basic research on antimicrobial resistance as well as translation of basic research into practice. Support for epidemiologic studies to identify key drivers of the emergence and spread of antimicrobial resistance is of great importance.
- *Focus Area III: Regulatory Pathways for New Products.* Aims for product development include provision of information on the status of antibacterial drug product development and encouraging development of rapid diagnostic tests and vaccines.

SELECTION OF ANTIBIOTICS

When treating infection, the therapeutic objective is to produce maximal antimicrobial effects while causing minimal harm to the host. To achieve this goal, we must select the most appropriate antibiotic for the individual patient. When choosing an antibiotic, three principal factors must be considered: (1) the identity of the infecting organism (Table 68.4), (2) drug sensitivity of the infecting organism, and (3) host factors, such as the site of infection and the status of host defenses.

For any given infection, several drugs may be effective. However, for most infections, there is usually one drug that is superior to the alternatives (Table 68.5). This drug of first choice may be preferred for several reasons, such as greater efficacy, lower toxicity, or more narrow spectrum. Whenever possible, the drug of first choice should be employed.

TABLE 68.4 ■ Common Infections Caused by Common "Bugs"

Infection	Bacteria
Bacterial meningitis	*Streptococcus pneumoniae, Neisseria meningitides*
Acute sinusitis	*Streptococcus pneumoniae, Haemophilus influenzae*
Pharyngitis	*Streptococcus pyogenes*
Community-acquired pneumonia	*S. pneumoniae, Mycoplasma* spp., *Haemophilus influenzae, Staphylococcus aureus*
Hospital-acquired pneumonia	*Pseudomonas* spp., *Klebsiella* spp., *S. aureus*
Endocarditis	*Streptococcus viridans,* coagulase-negative *Staphylococcus* spp., *S. aureus*
Cholangitis	Enterobacteriaceae, anaerobes
Urinary tract infection, pyelonephritis	*Escherichia coli,* Enterobacteriaceae
Osteomyelitis	*S. aureus*
Cellulitis	*S. aureus, Streptococcus* spp.

Alternative agents should be used only when the first-choice drug is inappropriate. Conditions that might rule out a first-choice agent include (1) allergy to the drug of choice, (2) inability of the drug of choice to penetrate to the site of infection, and (3) heightened susceptibility of the patient to toxicity of the first-choice drug.

Empiric Therapy Before Completion of Laboratory Tests

Optimal antimicrobial therapy requires identification of the infecting organism and determination of its drug sensitivity. However, when the patient has a severe infection, we may have to initiate treatment before test results are available. Under these conditions, drug selection must be based on clinical evaluation and knowledge of which microbes are most likely to cause infection at a particular site. If necessary, a broad-spectrum agent can be used for initial treatment. After the identity and drug sensitivity of the infecting organism have been determined, we can switch to a more selective antibiotic. When conditions demand that we start therapy in the absence of laboratory data, it is essential that samples of exudates and body fluids be obtained for culture *before initiation of treatment;* if antibiotics are present at the time of sampling, they can suppress microbial growth in culture and can thereby confound identification.

Identifying the Infecting Organism

The first rule of antimicrobial therapy is to *match the drug with the bug.* Hence, whenever possible, the infecting organism should be identified before starting treatment. If treatment is begun in the absence of a definitive diagnosis, positive identification should be established as soon as possible so as to permit adjustment of the regimen to better conform with the drug sensitivity of the infecting organism.

The quickest, simplest, and most versatile technique for identifying microorganisms is microscopic examination of a

TABLE 68.5 ■ Antibacterial Drugs of Choice

Organism	Drug of First Choice	Some Alternative Drugs
GRAM-POSITIVE COCCI		
*Enterococcus**		
Endocarditis and other severe infections	Penicillin G *or* ampicillin *with either* gentamicin or streptomycin	Vancomycin *with either* gentamicin or streptomycin, quinupristin/dalfopristin, linezolid, daptomycin
Uncomplicated urinary tract infection	Ampicillin, amoxicillin	Nitrofurantoin, a fluoroquinolone; fosfomycin
Staphylococcus aureus or *epidermidis**		
Penicillinase producing	A penicillinase-resistant penicillin	A cephalosporin, vancomycin, imipenem, linezolid, clindamycin, daptomycin, a fluoroquinolone
Methicillin resistant	Vancomycin *with or without* gentamicin *with or without* rifampin	Linezolid, quinupristin/dalfopristin, daptomycin, tigecycline, doxycycline, ceftaroline, trimethoprim/sulfamethoxazole, a fluoroquinolone
Streptococcus pyogenes (group A) and groups C and G	Penicillin G, penicillin V	Clindamycin, vancomycin, erythromycin, clarithromycin, azithromycin, daptomycin, linezolid, a cephalosporin
Streptococcus, group B	Penicillin G or ampicillin	A cephalosporin, vancomycin, erythromycin, daptomycin
Streptococcus viridans group	Penicillin G *with or without* gentamicin	A cephalosporin, vancomycin
Streptococcus bovis	Penicillin G	A cephalosporin, vancomycin
Streptococcus, anaerobic	Penicillin G	Clindamycin, a cephalosporin, vancomycin
Streptococcus pneumoniae (pneumococcus)	Penicillin G, penicillin V, amoxicillin	A cephalosporin, erythromycin, azithromycin, clarithromycin, levofloxacin, gemifloxacin, moxifloxacin, meropenem, imipenem, ertapenem, trimethoprim/sulfamethoxazole, clindamycin, a tetracycline, vancomycin
GRAM-NEGATIVE COCCI		
Neisseria gonorrhoeae (gonococcus)	See Chapter 80	
Neisseria meningitides (meningococcus)	Penicillin G	Cefotaxime, ceftriaxone, chloramphenicol, a sulfonamide, a fluoroquinolone
GRAM-POSITIVE BACILLI		
Bacillus anthracis (anthrax)	Ciprofloxacin	Doxycycline, Amoxicillin
Clostridium difficile	See Chapter 70	
Clostridium perfringens	Penicillin G, clindamycin	Metronidazole, chloramphenicol, imipenem, meropenem, ertapenem
Clostridium tetani	Metronidazole	Penicillin G, doxycycline
Corynebacterium diphtheriae	Erythromycin	Penicillin G
Listeria monocytogenes	Ampicillin *with or without* gentamicin	Trimethoprim/sulfamethoxazole
ENTERIC GRAM-NEGATIVE BACILLI		
Campylobacter jejuni	Erythromycin, azithromycin	A fluoroquinolone, gentamicin, a tetracycline
Escherichia coli	Cefotaxime, ceftazidime, cefepime, ceftriaxone	Ampicillin *with or without* gentamicin, ticarcillin/clavulanic acid, trimethoprim/sulfamethoxazole, imipenem, meropenem, others
*Enterobacter**	Imipenem, meropenem, cefepime	Trimethoprim/sulfamethoxazole, gentamicin, tobramycin, amikacin, ciprofloxacin, cefotaxime, ticarcillin/clavulanic acid, piperacillin/tazobactam, aztreonam, ceftazidime, tigecycline
*Klebsiella pneumoniae**	Cefotaxime, ceftriaxone, cefepime, ceftazidime	Imipenem, meropenem, ertapenem, gentamicin, tobramycin, amikacin, others
Proteus, indole positive (including *Providencia rettgeri* and *Morganella morganii*)	Cefotaxime, ceftriaxone, cefepime, ceftazidime	Imipenem, meropenem, ertapenem, gentamicin, a fluoroquinolone, trimethoprim/sulfamethoxazole, others
Proteus mirabilis	Ampicillin	A cephalosporin, ticarcillin, trimethoprim/sulfamethoxazole, imipenem, meropenem, ertapenem, gentamicin, others
Salmonella typhi	Ceftriaxone, a fluoroquinolone	Trimethoprim/sulfamethoxazole, ampicillin, amoxicillin, chloramphenicol, azithromycin
Other *Salmonella*	Ceftriaxone, cefotaxime, a fluoroquinolone	Trimethoprim/sulfamethoxazole, chloramphenicol, ampicillin, amoxicillin
Serratia	Imipenem, meropenem	Gentamicin, amikacin, cefotaxime, a fluoroquinolone, trimethoprim/sulfamethoxazole, aztreonam, others

Continued

TABLE 68.5 ▪ Antibacterial Drugs of Choice—cont'd

Organism	Drug of First Choice	Some Alternative Drugs
Shigella	A fluoroquinolone	Trimethoprim/sulfamethoxazole, ampicillin, ceftriaxone, azithromycin
Yersinia enterocolitica	Trimethoprim/sulfamethoxazole	A fluoroquinolone, gentamicin, tobramycin, amikacin, cefotaxime
OTHER GRAM-NEGATIVE BACILLI		
*Acinetobacter**	Imipenem, meropenem	An aminoglycoside, trimethoprim/sulfamethoxazole, doxycycline, ciprofloxacin, ceftazidime, ticarcillin/clavulanic acid, piperacillin/tazobactam
Bacteroides	Metronidazole	Imipenem, ertapenem, meropenem, amoxicillin/clavulanic acid, ticarcillin/clavulanic acid, piperacillin/tazobactam, ampicillin/sulbactam, chloramphenicol
Bordetella pertussis (whooping cough)	Azithromycin, clarithromycin, erythromycin	Trimethoprim/sulfamethoxazole
Brucella (brucellosis)	A tetracycline *plus* rifampin	A tetracycline *plus either* gentamicin or streptomycin, trimethoprim/sulfamethoxazole *with or without* gentamicin, chloramphenicol *with or without* streptomycin, ciprofloxacin *plus* rifampin
Klebsiella (formerly *Calymmatobacterium*) *granulomatis*	Trimethoprim/sulfamethoxazole	Doxycycline or ciprofloxacin
Francisella tularensis (tularemia)	Streptomycin	Gentamycin, doxycycline, ciprofloxacin
Gardnerella vaginalis	Metronidazole (PO)	Topical clindamycin or metronidazole, clindamycin (PO)
Haemophilus ducreyi (chancroid)	Azithromycin, ceftriaxone	Ciprofloxacin, erythromycin
Haemophilus influenzae		
Meningitis, epiglottitis, arthritis, and other serious infections	Cefotaxime, ceftriaxone	Cefuroxime, chloramphenicol, meropenem
Upper respiratory infection and bronchitis	Trimethoprim/sulfamethoxazole	Cefuroxime, amoxicillin/clavulanic acid, a fluoroquinolone, others
Helicobacter pylori	Clarithromycin *plus* amoxicillin *plus* esomeprazole (a proton pump inhibitor)	Tetracycline *plus* metronidazole *plus* bismuth subsalicylate *plus* esomeprazole (a proton pump inhibitor)
Legionella spp.	Azithromycin, a fluoroquinolone *with or without* rifampin	Doxycycline *with or without* rifampin, trimethoprim/sulfamethoxazole, erythromycin
Pasteurella multocida	Penicillin G	Doxycycline, a second- or third-generation cephalosporin, amoxicillin/clavulanic acid, ampicillin/sulbactam
*Pseudomonas aeruginosa**		
Urinary tract infection	Ciprofloxacin	Levofloxacin, piperacillin/tazobactam, ceftazidime, cefepime, imipenem, meropenem, gentamicin, tobramycin, amikacin, aztreonam
Other infections	Piperacillin/tazobactam (or ticarcillin/clavulanic acid) *with or without* tobramycin, gentamicin, or amikacin	Ceftazidime, ciprofloxacin, imipenem, meropenem, aztreonam, or cefepime, *any one with or without* tobramycin, gentamicin, or amikacin
Spirillum minus (rat-bite fever)	Penicillin G	Doxycycline, streptomycin
Streptobacillus moniliformis (rat-bite fever)	Penicillin G	Doxycycline, streptomycin
Vibrio cholerae (cholera)	A tetracycline	Trimethoprim/sulfamethoxazole, a fluoroquinolone
Yersinia pestis (plague)	Streptomycin *with* Gentamycin	Doxycycline, ciprofloxacin, chloramphenicol
MYCOBACTERIA		
Mycobacterium tuberculosis	See Chapter 75	
Mycobacterium leprae (leprosy)	See Chapter 75	
Mycobacterium avium complex	See Chapter 75	
ACTINOMYCETES		
Actinomycetes israelii	Penicillin G	Doxycycline, erythromycin, clindamycin
Nocardia	Trimethoprim/sulfamethoxazole	Sulfisoxazole, imipenem, meropenem, amikacin, a tetracycline, linezolid, ceftriaxone, cycloserine

TABLE 68.5 ▪ Antibacterial Drugs of Choice—cont'd

Organism	Drug of First Choice	Some Alternative Drugs
CHLAMYDIAE		
Chlamydia psittaci	Doxycycline	Chloramphenicol
Chlamydia trachomatis	See Chapter80	
MYCOPLASMA		
Mycoplasma pneumoniae	Erythromycin, clarithromycin, azithromycin, a tetracycline	A fluoroquinolone
Ureaplasma urealyticum	Azithromycin	A tetracycline, clarithromycin, erythromycin, ofloxacin
RICKETTSIA		
Rocky Mountain spotted fever, endemic typhus (murine), trench fever, typhus, scrub typhus, Q fever	Doxycycline	Chloramphenicol, a fluoroquinolone
SPIROCHETES		
Borrelia burgdorferi (Lyme disease)	Doxycycline, amoxicillin, cefuroxime	Ceftriaxone, cefotaxime, penicillin G, azithromycin, clarithromycin
Borrelia recurrentis (relapsing fever)	A tetracycline	Penicillin G, erythromycin
Leptospira	Penicillin G	Doxycycline, ceftriaxone
Treponema pallidum (syphilis)	Penicillin G	Doxycycline, ceftriaxone
Treponema pertenue (yaws)	Penicillin G	Doxycycline

*Many of these drugs have resistant strains that must be treated with alternative antibiotics.

Gram-stained preparation. Samples for examination can be obtained from exudate, sputum, urine, blood, and other body fluids. The most useful samples are direct aspirates from the site of infection.

In some cases, only a small number of infecting organisms will be present. Under these conditions, positive identification may require that the microbes be grown out in culture. As stressed previously, material for culture should be obtained before initiating treatment. Furthermore, the samples should be taken in a fashion that minimizes contamination with normal body flora. Also, the samples should not be exposed to low temperature, antiseptics, or oxygen.

A relatively new method, known as the *polymerase chain reaction (PCR) test* or *nucleic acid amplification test,* can detect very low titers of bacteria and viruses. Testing is done by using an enzyme—either DNA polymerase or RNA polymerase—to generate thousands of copies of DNA or RNA unique to the infecting microbe. As a result of this nucleic acid amplification, there is enough material for detection. Microbes that we can identify with a PCR test include important bacterial pathogens (e.g., *C. difficile, S. aureus, Mycobacterium tuberculosis, Neisseria gonorrhoeae, Chlamydia trachomatis, Helicobacter pylori*) and important viral pathogens (e.g., HIV, influenza virus). Compared with Gram staining, PCR tests are both more specific and more sensitive.

Determining Drug Susceptibility

Owing to the emergence of drug-resistant microbes, testing for drug sensitivity is common. However, sensitivity testing is not always needed. Rather, testing is indicated only when the infecting organism is one in which resistance is likely. Hence, for microbes such as the group A streptococci, which have remained highly susceptible to penicillin G, sensitivity testing is unnecessary. In contrast, when resistance *is* common, as it is with *S. aureus* and the gram-negative bacilli, tests for drug sensitivity should be performed. Most tests used today are based on one of three methods: disk diffusion, serial dilution, or gradient diffusion.

Before sensitivity testing can be done, we must first identify the microbe so that we can test for sensitivity to the appropriate drugs. For example, if the infection is caused by *C. difficile,* we might test for sensitivity to metronidazole or vancomycin. We would not test for sensitivity to aminoglycosides or cephalosporins—because we already know these drugs won't work.

HOST FACTORS THAT MODIFY DRUG CHOICE, ROUTE OF ADMINISTRATION, OR DOSAGE

In addition to matching the drug with the bug and determining the drug sensitivity of an infecting organism, we must consider host factors when prescribing an antimicrobial drug. Two host factors—host defenses and infection site—are unique to the selection of antibiotics. Other host factors, such as age, pregnancy, and previous drug reactions, are the same factors that must be considered when choosing any other drug.

Host Defenses

Host defenses consist primarily of the immune system and phagocytic cells (macrophages, neutrophils). Without the contribution of these defenses, successful antimicrobial therapy would be rare. In most cases, the drugs we use don't cure infection on their own. Rather, they work in concert with host defense systems to subdue infection. Accordingly, the usual objective of antibiotic treatment is not outright kill of infecting organisms. Rather, the goal is to suppress microbial growth to the point at which the balance is tipped in favor of the host. Underscoring the critical role of host defenses is the grim fact that people whose defenses are impaired, such as those with AIDS and those undergoing cancer chemotherapy, frequently die of infections that drugs alone are unable to control. When treating the immunocompromised host, our only hope lies with drugs that are rapidly bactericidal, and even these may prove inadequate.

Site of Infection

To be effective, an antibiotic must be present at the site of infection in a concentration greater than the minimal inhibitory concentration (MIC). At some sites, drug penetration may be hampered, making it difficult to achieve the MIC. For example, drug access can be impeded in meningitis (because of the blood-brain barrier), endocarditis (because bacterial vegetations in the heart are difficult to penetrate), and infected abscesses (because of poor vascularity and the presence of purulent material). When treating meningitis, two approaches may be used: (1) we can select a drug that readily crosses the blood-brain barrier, and (2) we can inject an antibiotic directly into the subarachnoid space. When exudate and other fluids hinder drug access, surgical drainage is indicated.

Foreign materials (e.g., cardiac pacemakers, prosthetic joints and heart valves, synthetic vascular shunts) present a special local problem. Phagocytes react to these objects and attempt to destroy them. Because of this behavior, the phagocytes are less able to attack bacteria, thereby allowing microbes to flourish. Treatment of these infections often results in failure or relapse. In many cases, the infection can be eliminated only by removing the foreign material.

Other Host Factors

Previous Allergic Reaction

Severe allergic reactions are more common with the penicillins than with any other family of drugs. As a rule, patients with a history of severe allergy to the penicillins should not receive them again. The exception is treatment of a life-threatening infection for which no suitable alternative is available. In addition to the penicillins, other antibiotics (sulfonamides, trimethoprim, erythromycin) are associated with a high incidence of allergic responses. However, severe reactions to these agents are rare.

Genetic Factors

As with other drugs, responses to antibiotics can be influenced by the patient's genetic heritage. For example, some antibiotics (e.g., sulfonamides) can cause hemolysis in patients who, because of their genetic makeup, have red blood cells that are deficient in glucose-6-phosphate dehydrogenase. Clearly, people with this deficiency should not be given antibiotics that are likely to induce red cell lysis.

Genetic factors can also affect rates of metabolism. For example, hepatic inactivation of isoniazid is rapid in some people and slow in others. If the dosage is not adjusted accordingly, isoniazid may accumulate to toxic levels in the slow metabolizers and may fail to achieve therapeutic levels in the rapid metabolizers.

DOSAGE AND DURATION OF TREATMENT

Success requires that the antibiotic be present at the site of infection in an effective concentration for a sufficient time. Dosages should be adjusted to produce drug concentrations that are equal to or greater than the MIC for the infection being treated. Drug levels 4 to 8 times the MIC are often desirable.

Duration of therapy depends on a number of variables, including the status of host defenses, the site of the infection, and the identity of the infecting organism.

THERAPY WITH ANTIBIOTIC COMBINATIONS

Therapy with a combination of antimicrobial agents is indicated only in specific situations. Under these well-defined conditions, use of multiple drugs may be lifesaving. However, it should be stressed that, although antibiotic combinations do have a valuable therapeutic role, routine use of two or more antibiotics should be discouraged. When an infection is

PATIENT-CENTERED CARE ACROSS THE LIFE SPAN

Antimicrobials

Life Stage	Patient Care Concerns
Infants	Infants are highly vulnerable to drug toxicity. Because of poorly developed kidney and liver function, neonates eliminate drugs slowly. Use of sulfonamides in newborns can produce kernicterus, a severe neurologic disorder caused by displacement of bilirubin from plasma proteins (see Chapter 73).
Children/adolescents	The tetracyclines provide another example of toxicity unique to the young: these antibiotics bind to developing teeth, causing discoloration.
Pregnant women	Antimicrobial drugs can cross the placenta, posing a risk to the developing fetus. For example, when gentamicin is used during pregnancy, irreversible hearing loss in the infant may result. Antibiotic use during pregnancy may also pose a risk to the expectant mother.
Breastfeeding women	Antibiotics can enter breast milk, possibly affecting the nursing infant. Sulfonamides, for example, can reach levels in milk that are sufficient to cause kernicterus in nursing newborns. As a general guideline, antibiotics and all other drugs should be avoided by women who are breastfeeding.
Older adults	In the older adult, heightened drug sensitivity is due in large part to reduced rates of drug metabolism and drug excretion, which can result in accumulation of antibiotics to toxic levels.

Patient Education

FINISHING THE PRESCRIBED COURSE

It is imperative that antibiotics not be discontinued prematurely. Accordingly, *patients should be instructed to take their medication for the entire prescribed course, even though symptoms may subside before the full course has been completed.* Early discontinuation is a common cause of recurrent infection, and the organisms responsible for relapse are likely to be more drug resistant than those present when treatment began.

caused by a single, identified microbe, treatment with just one drug is usually most appropriate.

Antimicrobial Effects of Antibiotic Combinations

When two antibiotics are used together, the result may be *additive, potentiative,* or, in certain cases, *antagonistic.* An *additive* response is one in which the antimicrobial effect of the combination is equal to the sum of the effects of the two drugs alone. A *potentiative* interaction (also called a *synergistic* interaction) is one in which the effect of the combination is greater than the sum of the effects of the individual agents. A classic example of potentiation is produced by trimethoprim plus sulfamethoxazole, drugs that inhibit sequential steps in the synthesis of tetrahydrofolic acid (see Chapter 73).

In certain cases, a combination of two antibiotics may be *less* effective than one of the agents by itself, indicating *antagonism* between the drugs. Antagonism is most likely when a *bacteriostatic* agent (e.g., tetracycline) is combined with a *bactericidal* drug (e.g., penicillin). Antagonism occurs because bactericidal drugs are usually effective only against organisms that are actively growing. Hence, when bacterial growth has been suppressed by a bacteriostatic drug, the effects of a bactericidal agent can be reduced. If host defenses are intact, antagonism between two antibiotics may have little significance. However, if host defenses are compromised, the consequences can be dire.

Indications for Antibiotic Combinations

Initial Therapy of Severe Infection

The most common indication for using multiple antibiotics is initial therapy of severe infection of unknown etiology, especially in the neutropenic host. Until the infecting organism has been identified, wide antimicrobial coverage is appropriate. Just how broad the coverage should be depends on the clinician's skill in narrowing the field of potential pathogens. After the identity of the infecting microbe is known, drug selection can be adjusted accordingly. As discussed earlier, samples for culture should be obtained before drug therapy starts.

Mixed Infections

An infection may be caused by more than one microbe. Multiple infectious organisms are common in brain abscesses, pelvic infections, and infections resulting from perforation of abdominal organs. When the infectious microbes differ from one another in drug susceptibility, treatment with more than one antibiotic is required.

Preventing Resistance

Although use of multiple antibiotics is usually associated with *promoting* drug resistance, there is one infectious disease—tuberculosis—in which drug combinations are employed for the specific purpose of *suppressing* the emergence of resistant bacteria. Why tuberculosis differs from other infections in this regard is discussed in Chapter 75.

Decreased Toxicity

In some situations, an antibiotic combination can reduce toxicity to the host. For example, by combining flucytosine with amphotericin B in the treatment of fungal meningitis, the dosage of amphotericin B can be reduced, thereby decreasing the risk for amphotericin-induced damage to the kidneys.

Enhanced Antibacterial Action

In specific infections, a combination of antibiotics can have greater antibacterial action than a single agent. This is true of the combined use of penicillin plus an aminoglycoside in the treatment of enterococcal endocarditis. Penicillin acts to weaken the bacterial cell wall; the aminoglycoside acts to suppress protein synthesis. The combination has enhanced antibacterial action because, by weakening the cell wall, penicillin facilitates penetration of the aminoglycoside to its intracellular site of action.

Disadvantages of Antibiotic Combinations

Use of multiple antibiotics has several drawbacks, including (1) increased risk for toxic and allergic reactions, (2) possible antagonism of antimicrobial effects, (3) increased risk for superinfection, (4) selection of drug-resistant bacteria, and (5) increased cost. Accordingly, antimicrobial combinations should be employed only when clearly indicated.

PROPHYLACTIC USE OF ANTIMICROBIAL DRUGS

Estimates indicate that between 30% and 50% of the antibiotics used in the United States are administered for prophylaxis. That is, these agents are given to prevent an infection rather than to treat an established infection. Much of this prophylactic use is uncalled for. However, in certain situations, antimicrobial prophylaxis is both appropriate and effective. Whenever prophylaxis is proposed, the benefits must be weighed against the risks for toxicity, allergic reactions, superinfection, and selection of drug-resistant organisms. Generally approved indications for prophylaxis are discussed next.

Surgery

Prophylactic use of antibiotics can decrease the incidence of infection in certain kinds of surgery. Procedures in which prophylactic efficacy has been documented include cardiac surgery, peripheral vascular surgery, orthopedic surgery, and surgery on the gastrointestinal (GI) tract (stomach, duodenum, colon, rectum, and appendix). Prophylaxis is also beneficial for women undergoing a hysterectomy or an emergency cesarean section. In contaminated surgery (operations performed on perforated abdominal organs, compound fractures, or lacerations from animal bites), the risk for infection is nearly 100%. Hence, for these operations, use of antibiotics is considered *treatment,* not prophylaxis. When antibiotics are given for prophylaxis, they should be given before the surgery. If the procedure is unusually long, dosing again during surgery may be indicated. As a rule, postoperative antibiotics are unnecessary. For most operations, a first-generation cephalosporin (e.g., cefazolin) will suffice.

Bacterial Endocarditis

Individuals with congenital or valvular heart disease and those with prosthetic heart valves are unusually susceptible to bacterial endocarditis. For these people, endocarditis can develop after certain dental and medical procedures that dislodge bacteria into the bloodstream. Thus before undergoing such procedures, these patients may need prophylactic antimicrobial medication. However, according to guidelines released by the American Heart Association, antibiotic prophylaxis is less necessary than previously believed and hence should be done much less often than in the past.

Neutropenia

Severe neutropenia puts individuals at high risk for infection. There is some evidence that the incidence of bacterial infection may be reduced through antibiotic prophylaxis. However, prophylaxis may increase the risk for infection with fungi: by killing normal flora, whose presence helps suppress fungal growth, antibiotics can encourage fungal invasion.

Other Indications for Antimicrobial Prophylaxis

For young women with recurrent urinary tract infection, prophylaxis with trimethoprim/sulfamethoxazole may be helpful. Oseltamivir (an antiviral agent) may be employed for prophylaxis against influenza. For individuals who have had severe rheumatic endocarditis, lifelong prophylaxis may be needed. Antimicrobial prophylaxis is indicated after exposure to organisms responsible for sexually transmitted diseases (e.g., syphilis, gonorrhea).

MISUSES OF ANTIMICROBIAL DRUGS

Misuse of antibiotics is common. According to the CDC, about 50% of antibiotic prescriptions are either inappropriate or entirely unnecessary. Ways that we misuse antibiotics are discussed next.

Attempted Treatment of Viral Infection

Most viral infections—including mumps, chickenpox, and the common cold—do not respond to currently available drugs. Hence, when drug therapy of these disorders is attempted, patients are exposed to all the risks of drugs but have no chance of receiving benefits.

Acute upper respiratory tract infections, including the common cold, are a particular concern. When these infections are treated with antibiotics, only 1 patient out of 4000 is likely to benefit. However, the risks remain high: 1 in 4 patients will get diarrhea, 1 in 50 will get a rash, and 1 in 1000 will need to visit an emergency department, usually because of a severe allergic reaction.

Treatment of Fever of Unknown Origin

Although fever can be a sign of infection, it can also signify other diseases, including hepatitis, arthritis, and cancer. Unless the cause of a fever is a proven infection, antibiotics should not be employed. If the fever is *not* due to an infection, antibiotics would not only be inappropriate, they would also expose the patient to unnecessary toxicity and delay correct diagnosis of the fever's cause. If the fever *is* caused by infection, antibiotics could hamper later attempts to identify the infecting organism.

The only situation in which fever, by itself, constitutes a legitimate indication for antibiotic use is when fever occurs in the severely immunocompromised host. Because fever may indicate infection, and because infection can be lethal to the immunocompromised patient, these patients should be given antibiotics when fever occurs—even if fever is the only indication that an infection may be present.

Improper Dosage

Like all other medications, antibiotics must be used in the right dosage. If the dosage is too low, the patient will be exposed to a risk for adverse effects without benefit of antibacterial effects. If the dosage is too high, the risks for superinfection and adverse effects become unnecessarily high.

Treatment in the Absence of Adequate Bacteriologic Information

As stressed earlier, proper antimicrobial therapy requires information on the identity and drug sensitivity of the infecting organism. Except in life-threatening situations, therapy should not be undertaken in the absence of bacteriologic information. This important guideline is often ignored.

Omission of Surgical Drainage

Antibiotics may have limited efficacy in the presence of foreign material, necrotic tissue, or exudate. Hence, when appropriate, surgical drainage and cleansing should be performed to promote antimicrobial effects.

MONITORING ANTIMICROBIAL THERAPY

Antimicrobial therapy is assessed by monitoring clinical responses and laboratory results. The frequency of monitoring is directly proportional to the severity of infection. Important clinical indicators of success are reduction of fever and resolution of signs and symptoms related to the affected organ system (e.g., improvement of breath sounds in patients with pneumonia).

Various laboratory tests are used to monitor treatment. Serum drug levels may be monitored for two reasons: to ensure that levels are sufficient for antimicrobial effects and to avoid toxicity from excessive levels. Success of therapy is indicated by the disappearance of infectious organisms from posttreatment cultures. Cultures may become sterile within hours of the onset of treatment (as may happen with urinary tract infections), or they may not become sterile for weeks (as may happen with tuberculosis).

CHAPTER 69

Drugs That Weaken the Bacterial Cell Wall I: Penicillins

Laura D. Rosenthal, DNP, ACNP, FAANP

INTRODUCTION TO THE PENICILLINS

The penicillins are practically ideal antibiotics because they are active against a variety of bacteria and their direct toxicity is low. Allergic reactions are the principal adverse effects. Owing to their safety and efficacy, the penicillins are widely prescribed.

Because they have a beta-lactam ring in their structure, the penicillins are known as *beta-lactam antibiotics.* The beta-lactam family also includes the cephalosporins, carbapenems, and aztreonam (see Chapter 70). All of the beta-lactam antibiotics share the same mechanism of action: disruption of the bacterial cell wall.

Mechanism of Action

To understand the actions of the penicillins, we must first understand the structure and function of the bacterial cell wall—a rigid, permeable, mesh-like structure that lies outside the cytoplasmic membrane. Inside the cytoplasmic membrane, osmotic pressure is very high. Hence, were it not for the rigid cell wall, which prevents expansion, bacteria would take up water, swell, and then burst.

Penicillins weaken the cell wall, causing bacteria to take up excessive amounts of water and rupture. As a result, penicillins are generally *bactericidal.* However, it is important to note that penicillins are active only against bacteria that are undergoing growth and division (see later).

Penicillins weaken the cell wall by two actions: (1) *inhibition of transpeptidases* and (2) *disinhibition (activation) of autolysins.* Transpeptidases are enzymes critical to cell wall synthesis. Specifically, they catalyze the formation of cross-bridges between the peptidoglycan polymer strands that form the cell wall and thus give the cell wall its strength (Fig. 69.1). Autolysins are bacterial enzymes that cleave bonds in the cell wall. Bacteria employ these enzymes to break down segments of the cell wall to permit growth and division. By simultaneously inhibiting transpeptidases and activating autolysins, the penicillins (1) disrupt synthesis of the cell wall and (2) promote its active destruction. These combined actions result in cell lysis and death.

The molecular targets of the penicillins (transpeptidases, autolysins, other bacterial enzymes) are known collectively as *penicillin-binding proteins* (PBPs). These molecules are so named because penicillins must bind to them to produce antibacterial effects. As indicated in Fig. 69.2, PBPs are located on the outer surface of the cytoplasmic membrane. More than eight different PBPs have been identified. Of these, PBP1 and PBP3 are most critical to penicillin's antibacterial effects. Bacteria express PBPs only during growth and division. Accordingly, because PBPs must be present for penicillins to work, these drugs work only when bacteria are growing.

Because mammalian cells lack a cell wall, and because penicillins act specifically on enzymes that affect cell wall integrity, the penicillins have virtually no *direct* effects on cells of the host. As a result, the penicillins are among our safest antibiotics.

Mechanisms of Bacterial Resistance

Bacterial resistance to penicillins is determined primarily by three factors: (1) inability of penicillins to reach their targets (PBPs), (2) inactivation of penicillins by bacterial enzymes, and (3) production of PBPs that have a low affinity for penicillins.

The Gram-Negative Cell Envelope

All bacteria are surrounded by a cell envelope. However, the cell envelope of gram-negative organisms differs from that of gram-positive organisms. Because of this difference, some penicillins are ineffective against gram-negative bacteria.

The cell envelope of *gram-positive* bacteria has only two layers: the cytoplasmic membrane and a relatively thick cell wall. Despite its thickness, the cell wall can be readily penetrated by penicillins, giving them easy access to PBPs on the cytoplasmic membrane. As a result, penicillins are generally very active against gram-positive organisms.

The *gram-negative* cell envelope has three layers: the cytoplasmic membrane, a relatively thin cell wall, and an additional *outer membrane* (see Fig. 69.2). Like the gram-positive cell wall, the gram-negative cell wall can be easily penetrated by penicillins. The outer membrane, however, is difficult to penetrate. As a result, only certain penicillins (e.g., ampicillin) are able to cross it and thereby reach PBPs on the cytoplasmic membrane.

Penicillinases (Beta-Lactamases)

Beta-lactamases are enzymes that cleave the beta-lactam ring and thereby render penicillins and other beta-lactam antibiotics inactive. Bacteria produce a large variety of beta-lactamases; some are specific for penicillins, some are specific for other beta-lactam antibiotics (e.g., cephalosporins), and some act on several kinds of beta-lactam antibiotics. Beta-lactamases that act selectively on penicillins are known as *penicillinases.*

Penicillinases are synthesized by gram-positive and gram-negative bacteria. Gram-positive organisms produce large amounts of these enzymes and then export them into the surrounding medium. In contrast, gram-negative bacteria produce penicillinases in relatively small amounts and, rather than exporting them to the environment, secrete them into the periplasmic space (see Fig. 69.2).

The genes that code for beta-lactamases are located on chromosomes and on plasmids (extrachromosomal DNA). The genes on plasmids may be transferred from one bacterium to another, thereby promoting the spread of penicillin resistance.

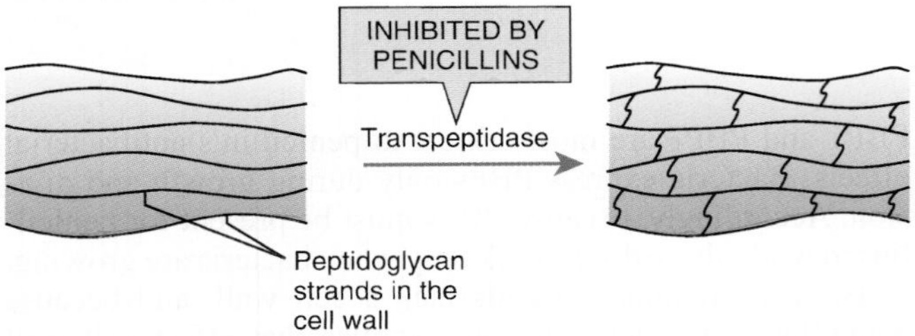

Figure 69.1 ■ Inhibition of transpeptidase by penicillins. The bacterial cell wall is composed of long strands of a peptidoglycan polymer. As depicted, transpeptidase enzymes create cross-bridges between the peptidoglycan strands, giving the cell wall added strength. By inhibiting transpeptidases, penicillins prevent cross-bridge synthesis and thereby weaken the cell wall.

Transfer of resistance is of special importance with *Staphylococcus aureus*. When penicillin was first introduced in the early 1940s, all strains of *S. aureus* were sensitive. However, by 1960, as many as 80% of *S. aureus* isolates in hospitals displayed penicillin resistance. Fortunately, a penicillin derivative (methicillin) that has resistance to the actions of beta-lactamases was introduced at this time. To date, no known strains of *S. aureus* produce beta-lactamases capable of inactivating methicillin or related penicillinase-resistant penicillins (although some strains are resistant to these drugs for other reasons).

Altered Penicillin-Binding Proteins

Certain bacterial strains, known collectively as methicillin-resistant *Staphylococcus aureus* (MRSA), have a unique mechanism of resistance: production of PBPs with a low affinity for penicillins and all other beta-lactam antibiotics. MRSA developed this ability by acquiring genes that code for low-affinity PBPs from other bacteria.

Methicillin-Resistant *Staphylococcus aureus*

S. aureus is a gram-positive bacterium that often colonizes the skin and nostrils of healthy people. Infection usually involves the skin and soft tissues, causing abscesses, boils, cellulitis, and impetigo. However, more serious infections can also

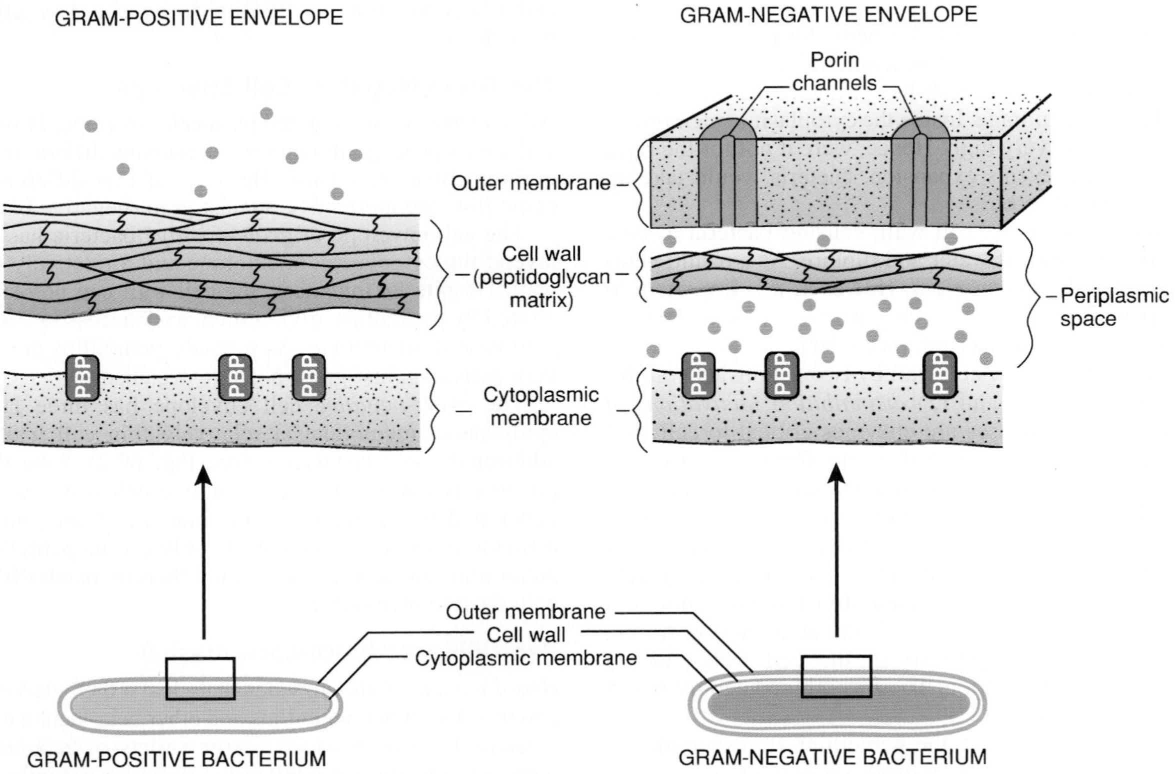

Figure 69.2 ■ The bacterial cell envelope.
Note that the gram-negative cell envelope has an outer membrane, whereas the gram-positive envelope does not. The outer membrane of the gram-negative cell envelope prevents certain penicillins from reaching their target molecules. (PBP, penicillin-binding protein.)

develop, including infections of the lungs and bloodstream, which can be fatal.

Like other pathogens, *S. aureus* has developed resistance over the years. When penicillins were introduced in the 1940s, all strains of *S. aureus* were susceptible. However, penicillin-resistant strains quickly emerged, owing to bacterial production of penicillinases. In 1959 this resistance was overcome with methicillin, the first penicillinase-resistant penicillin. Unfortunately, by 1968, strains resistant to methicillin had emerged. These highly resistant bacteria, known as *MRSA,* are resistant not only to methicillin (now obsolete) but also to all penicillins and all cephalosporins as well. The basis of MRSA resistance is acquisition of genes that code for penicillin-binding proteins that have very low affinity for penicillins and cephalosporins. Resistant strains were initially limited to health care facilities but are now found in the community as well.

In the United States MRSA is a serious public health problem. In 2014 it was estimated that 75,309 infections were caused by MRSA. Not only does MRSA increase mortality, it also increases costs: treating hospitalized MRSA patients costs about $35,000, compared with $14,000 for patients with methicillin-sensitive infections. Fortunately, the MRSA news isn't all bad. For one thing, although MRSA infections are now common, most patients can be cured. Also, rates of MRSA infection among hospitalized patients are now falling, after rising steadily for many years. MRSA infections that began in hospitals declined 54% between 2005 and 2011, with 30,800 fewer severe infections.

There are two distinct types of MRSA, referred to as *health care–associated MRSA* (HCA-MRSA) and *community-associated MRSA* (CA-MRSA). Of the two, HCA-MRSA is more prevalent (80% vs. 20%) and emerged earlier (1968 vs. 1981). Also, HCA-MRSA infection is generally more serious and harder to treat. Molecular typing indicates that HCA-MRSA and CA-MRSA are genetically distinct strains, known as USA100 and USA300, respectively.

Health Care–Associated MRSA

Methicillin resistance in *S. aureus* was first reported in isolates from hospitalized patients in 1968. For most of the next four decades, the prevalence of HCA-MRSA among hospitalized patients climbed steadily, reaching 85% of all invasive *S. aureus* infections by 2004.

Although many infections with HCA-MRSA *surface* in the community, nearly all occur in people who had been exposed to a health care facility within the prior year, indicating that acquisition of the infection probably occurred in a health care setting—not out in the community. Transmission of HCA-MRSA is usually through person-to-person contact, very often between health care workers and patients. Risk factors for acquiring HCA-MRSA include advanced age, recent surgery or hospitalization, dialysis, treatment in an intensive care unit, prolonged antibiotic therapy, an indwelling catheter, and residence in a long-term care facility.

The treatment of HCA-MRSA infection is addressed at length in a guideline—Clinical Practice Guidelines by the Infectious Diseases Society of America for the Treatment of Methicillin-Resistant *Staphylococcus aureus* Infections in Adults and Children. The guideline stresses the importance of selecting drugs based on the site of the infection, age of the patient, and drug sensitivity of the pathogen. For complicated skin and soft tissue infections in adults, the preferred drugs are intravenous (IV) vancomycin, linezolid [Zyvox], daptomycin [Cubicin], telavancin [Vibativ], clindamycin, and ceftaroline [Teflaro]. IV vancomycin is the preferred drug for children. For bacteremia or endocarditis in adults or children, IV vancomycin and daptomycin are drugs of choice. Preferred drugs for pneumonia in adults and children are IV vancomycin, linezolid, and clindamycin. Because most strains of MRSA are multidrug resistant, many other antibiotics are ineffective, including tetracyclines, clindamycin, trimethoprim/sulfamethoxazole, and beta-lactam agents (except ceftaroline).

Community-Associated MRSA

Infection with CA-MRSA, first reported in 1981, is caused by staphylococcal strains that are genetically distinct from HCA-MRSA. For example, most strains of CA-MRSA carry a gene for Panton-Valentine leukocidin (a cytotoxin that causes necrosis), whereas HCA-MRSA strains do not. Many people are now asymptomatic carriers of CA-MRSA. In fact, between 20% and 30% of the population is colonized, typically on the skin and in the nostrils.

Infection with CA-MRSA is generally less dangerous than with HCA-MRSA but is more dangerous than with methicillin-sensitive *S. aureus.* In most cases, CA-MRSA causes mild infections of the skin and soft tissues, manifesting as boils, impetigo, and so forth. However, CA-MRSA can also cause more serious infections, including necrotizing fasciitis, severe necrotizing pneumonia, and severe sepsis. Fortunately, these invasive infections are relatively rare. On the other hand, infections of the skin and soft tissues are now common, with CA-MRSA accounting for more than 50% of the *S. aureus* isolates from these sites.

CA-MRSA transmission is by skin-to-skin contact and by contact with contaminated objects, including frequently touched surfaces, sports equipment, and personal items (e.g., razors). In contrast to HCA-MRSA infection, CA-MRSA infection is seen primarily in young, healthy people with no recent exposure to health care facilities. Individuals at risk include athletes in contact sports (e.g., wrestling), men who have sex with men, and people who live in close quarters, such as family members, child care clients, prison inmates, military personnel, and college students.

Several measures can reduce the risk for CA-MRSA transmission. Topping the list is good hand hygiene—washing with soap and water or applying an alcohol-based sanitizer. Other measures include showering after contact sports, cleaning frequently touched surfaces, keeping infected sites covered, and not sharing towels and personal items.

Treatment depends on infection severity. For boils, small abscesses, and other superficial infections, surgical drainage may be all that is needed. For more serious infections, drugs may be indicated. Preferred agents are trimethoprim/sulfamethoxazole, minocycline, doxycycline, and clindamycin. Alternative drugs—vancomycin, daptomycin, and linezolid—should be reserved for severe infections and treatment failures. To eradicate the carrier state, intranasal application of a topical antibiotic—mupirocin or retapamulin—can be effective. Like HCA-MRSA, CA-MRSA does not respond to beta-lactam antibiotics, except ceftaroline.

Chemistry

All of the penicillins are derived from a common nucleus: 6-aminopenicillanic acid. This nucleus contains a beta-lactam ring joined to a second ring. The beta-lactam ring is essential for antibacterial actions. Properties of individual penicillins are determined by additions made to the basic nucleus. These modifications determine (1) affinity for PBPs, (2) resistance to penicillinases, (3) ability to penetrate the gram-negative cell envelope, (4) resistance to stomach acid, and (5) pharmacokinetic properties.

Classification

The most useful classification of penicillins is based on antimicrobial spectrum. When classified this way, the penicillins fall into four major groups: (1) narrow-spectrum penicillins that are penicillinase sensitive, (2) narrow-spectrum penicillins that are penicillinase resistant (antistaphylococcal penicillins), (3) broad-spectrum penicillins (aminopenicillins), and (4) extended-spectrum penicillins (antipseudomonal penicillins). Table 69.1 lists the members of each group and their principal target organisms.

TABLE 69.1 ▪ Classification of the Penicillins

Penicillin Class	Drug	Clinically Useful Antimicrobial Spectrum
Narrow-spectrum penicillins: penicillinase sensitive	Penicillin G Penicillin V	*Streptococcus* spp., *Neisseria* spp., many anaerobes, spirochetes, others
Narrow-spectrum penicillins: penicillinase resistant (antistaphylococcal penicillins)	Nafcillin Oxacillin Dicloxacillin	*Staphylococcus aureus*
Broad-spectrum penicillins (aminopenicillins)	Ampicillin Amoxicillin	*Haemophilus influenzae, Escherichia coli, Proteus mirabilis,* enterococci, *Neisseria gonorrhoeae*
Extended-spectrum penicillin (antipseudomonal penicillin)	Piperacillin	Same as broad-spectrum penicillins plus *Pseudomonas aeruginosa, Enterobacter* spp., *Proteus* (indole positive), *Bacteroides fragilis,* many *Klebsiella* spp.

PROPERTIES OF INDIVIDUAL PENICILLINS

Penicillin G

Penicillin G (benzylpenicillin) was the first penicillin available and will serve as our prototype for the penicillin family. This drug is often referred to simply as *penicillin.* Penicillin G is bactericidal to a number of gram-positive bacteria as well as to some gram-negative bacteria. Despite the introduction of newer antibiotics, penicillin G remains a drug of choice for many infections.

Antimicrobial Spectrum

Penicillin G is active against most *gram-positive bacteria* (except penicillinase-producing staphylococci), gram-negative cocci (*Neisseria meningitidis* and non–penicillinase-producing strains of *Neisseria gonorrhoeae*), anaerobic bacteria, and spirochetes (including *Treponema pallidum*). With few exceptions, gram-negative bacilli are resistant. Although many organisms respond to penicillin G, the drug is considered a narrow-spectrum agent compared with other members of the penicillin family.

Therapeutic Uses

Penicillin G is a drug of first choice for infections caused by sensitive gram-positive cocci. Important among these are pneumonia and meningitis caused by *Streptococcus pneumoniae* (pneumococcus), pharyngitis caused by *Streptococcus pyogenes,* and infectious endocarditis caused by *Streptococcus viridans.* Penicillin is also the preferred drug for those few strains of *S. aureus* that do not produce penicillinase.

Penicillin is a preferred agent for infections caused by several gram-positive bacilli, specifically, gas gangrene (caused by *Clostridium perfringens*), tetanus (caused by *Clostridium tetani*), and anthrax (caused by *Bacillus anthracis*).

Penicillin is also the drug of first choice for meningitis caused by *N. meningitidis* (meningococcus). Although once the drug of choice for gonorrhea (caused by *N. gonorrhoeae*), penicillin has been replaced by ceftriaxone as the primary treatment. Penicillin is now limited to infections caused by non–penicillinase-producing strains of *N. gonorrhoeae.* Penicillin is the drug of choice for syphilis, an infection caused by the spirochete *T. pallidum.*

In addition to treating active infections, penicillin G has important prophylactic applications. The drug is used to prevent syphilis in sexual partners of individuals who have this infection. Benzathine penicillin G is employed for prophylaxis against recurrent attacks of rheumatic fever; treatment is recommended for patients with a history of recurrent rheumatic fever and for those with clear evidence of rheumatic heart disease. Penicillin is also employed for prophylaxis of bacterial endocarditis; candidates include individuals with (1) prosthetic heart valves, (2) most congenital heart diseases, (3) acquired valvular heart disease, (4) mitral valve prolapse, and (5) previous history of bacterial endocarditis. For prevention of endocarditis, penicillin is administered before dental procedures and other procedures that are likely to produce temporary bacteremia.

Pharmacokinetics

Absorption

Penicillin G is available as four salts: (1) *potassium* penicillin G, (2) *procaine* penicillin G, (3) *benzathine* penicillin G, and (4) *sodium* penicillin G. These salts differ with respect to route of administration and time course of action. With all forms, the salt dissociates to release penicillin G, the active component.

Intramuscular. All forms of penicillin may be administered by the intramuscular (IM) route. However, it is important to note that the different salts are absorbed at very different rates. As indicated in Fig. 69.3, absorption of *potassium* and *sodium* penicillin G is rapid; blood levels peak about 15 minutes after injection. In contrast, the *procaine* and *benzathine* salts are absorbed slowly and hence are considered *repository* preparations. When benzathine penicillin is administered by IM injection, penicillin G is absorbed for weeks, producing blood levels that are persistent but very low. Consequently, this preparation is useful only against highly sensitive organisms (e.g., *T. pallidum,* the bacterium that causes syphilis).

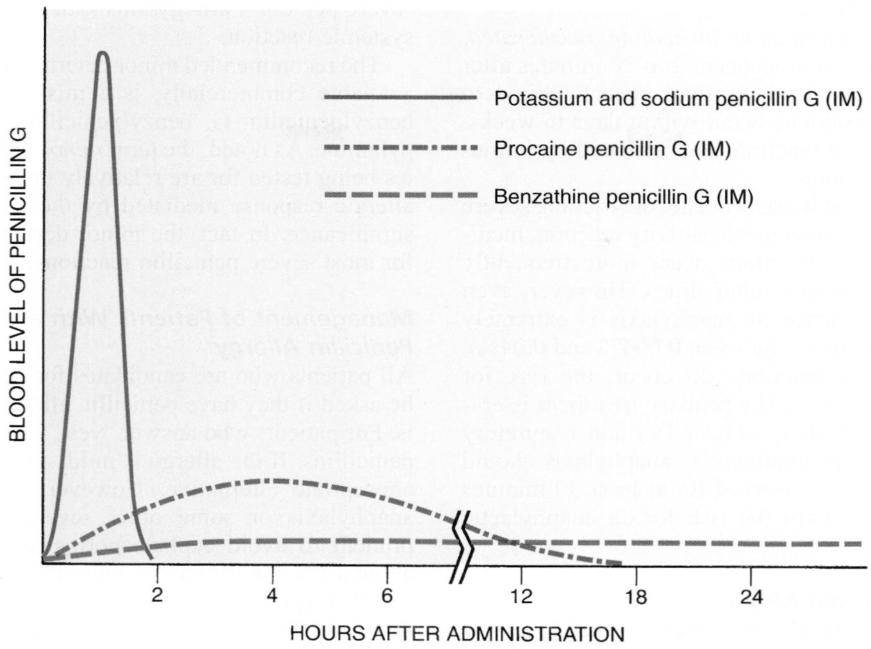

Figure 69.3 ▪ Blood levels of penicillin G following intramuscular injection of four different penicillin G salts.

Distribution

Penicillin distributes well to most tissues and body fluids. In the absence of inflammation, penetration of the meninges and into fluids of joints and the eyes is poor. By contrast, in the presence of inflammation, entry into cerebrospinal fluid, joints, and the eyes is enhanced, permitting treatment of infections caused by susceptible organisms.

Metabolism and Excretion

Penicillin undergoes minimal metabolism and is eliminated by the kidneys, primarily as the unchanged drug. Renal excretion is accomplished mainly (90%) by active tubular secretion; the remaining 10% results from glomerular filtration. In older children and adults, the half-life is very short (about 30 minutes). Renal impairment causes the half-life to increase dramatically and may necessitate a reduction in dosage. In patients at high risk for toxicity (those with renal impairment, the acutely ill, the very young, older adults), kidney function should be monitored.

Side Effects and Toxicities

Penicillin G is the least toxic of all antibiotics and is among the safest of all medications. Allergic reactions, the principal concern with penicillin, are discussed separately later. Other reactions include *pain at sites of IM injection,* prolonged (but reversible) *sensory and motor dysfunction* after accidental injection into a peripheral nerve, and *neurotoxicity* (seizures, confusion, hallucinations) if blood levels are too high. Inadvertent *intraarterial* injection can produce severe reactions—gangrene, necrosis, sloughing of tissue—and must be avoided.

Certain adverse effects may be caused by compounds coadministered with penicillin. For example, the procaine component of procaine penicillin G may cause bizarre behavioral effects when procaine penicillin is given in large doses. When large IV doses of potassium penicillin G are administered rapidly, hyperkalemia can result, possibly causing dysrhythmias and even cardiac arrest. Similarly, use of IV sodium penicillin G may lead to electrolyte imbalance. Sodium penicillin G should be used with caution in patients on sodium-restricted diets.

Penicillin Allergy

General Considerations

Penicillins are the most common cause of drug allergy. Between 0.4% and 7% of patients who receive penicillins experience an allergic reaction. Severity can range from a minor rash to life-threatening anaphylaxis.
As with most allergic reactions, there is no direct relationship between the size of the dose and the intensity of the response. Although prior exposure to penicillins is required for an allergic reaction, responses may occur in the absence of prior penicillin use because patients may have been exposed to penicillins produced by fungi or to penicillins present in foods of animal origin.

Because of cross sensitivity, patients allergic to one penicillin should be considered allergic to all other penicillins. In addition, a few patients (about 1%) display cross sensitivity to *cephalosporins.* If at all possible, patients with penicillin allergy should not be treated with any member of the penicillin family. Use of cephalosporins depends on the intensity of allergic response: if the penicillin allergy is mild, use of cephalosporins is probably safe; however, if the allergy is severe, cephalosporins should be avoided.

Individuals allergic to penicillin should be encouraged to wear a medical identification bracelet to alert health care personnel to their condition.

Types of Allergic Reactions

Penicillin reactions are classified as *immediate, accelerated,* and *delayed.* Immediate reactions occur 2 to 30 minutes after drug administration; accelerated reactions occur within 1 to 72 hours; and delayed reactions occur within days to weeks. Immediate and accelerated reactions are mediated by immunoglobulin E (IgE) antibodies.

Anaphylaxis (laryngeal edema, bronchoconstriction, severe hypotension) is an immediate hypersensitivity reaction, mediated by IgE. Anaphylactic reactions occur more frequently with penicillins than with any other drugs. However, even with penicillins, the incidence of anaphylaxis is extremely low (the estimated incidence is between 0.004% and 0.04%). Nonetheless, when these reactions do occur, the risk for mortality is high (about 10%). The primary treatment is *epinephrine* (subcutaneous [subQ], IM, or IV) and respiratory support. To ensure prompt treatment if anaphylaxis should develop, patients should be observed for at least 30 minutes after drug injection (i.e., until the risk for an anaphylactic reaction has passed).

Development of Penicillin Allergy

Before discussing penicillin allergy further, we need to review development of allergy to small molecules as a class. Small molecules, such as penicillin and most other drugs, are unable to induce antibody formation directly. Therefore, to promote antibody formation, the small molecule must first bond covalently to a larger molecule, usually a protein. In these combinations, the small molecule is referred to as a *hapten.* The hapten-protein combination constitutes the complete *antigen* that stimulates antibody formation.

The hapten that stimulates production of penicillin antibodies is rarely intact penicillin itself. Rather, compounds formed from the degradation of penicillin are the actual cause. As a result, most "penicillin antibodies" are not directed at penicillin itself. Rather, they are directed at various penicillin degradation products.

Skin Tests for Penicillin Allergy

Allergy to penicillin can decrease over time. Hence, an intense allergic reaction in the past does not necessarily mean that an intense reaction will occur again. In patients with a history of penicillin allergy, skin tests can be employed to assess current risk. These tests are performed by injecting a tiny amount of allergen intradermally and observing for a local allergic response. A positive test indicates the presence of IgE antibodies, which can mediate severe penicillin allergy. Accordingly, if skin testing is negative, a severe allergic reaction (anaphylaxis) is unlikely.

It is important to note that skin testing can be dangerous: in patients with severe penicillin allergy, the skin test itself can precipitate an anaphylactic reaction. Accordingly, the test should be performed only if epinephrine and facilities for respiratory support are immediately available.

Current guidelines recommend skin testing with two reagents, which test for the major and minor determinants of penicillin allergy. The minor determinants, although less common, mediate most severe penicillin reactions.

The major determinant reagent, available commercially as Pre-Pen, contains a single component: *benzylpenicilloyl-polylysine.* Benzylpenicilloyl-polylysine is a large polymeric molecule that is poorly absorbed. Hence, even in patients with severe penicillin allergy, this skin test carries a low risk for a systemic reaction.

The recommended minor determinant reagent, which is not available commercially, is a mixture of three compounds: benzylpenicillin G, benzylpenicilloate, and penicilloyl propylamine. As noted, the term *minor* indicates that the antibodies being tested for are relatively uncommon and not that the allergic response mediated by these antibodies is of minor significance. In fact, the minor determinants are responsible for most severe penicillin reactions.

Management of Patients With a History of Penicillin Allergy

All patients who are candidates for penicillin therapy should be asked if they have penicillin allergy and what the reaction is. For patients who answer "yes," the general rule is to avoid penicillins. If the allergy is mild, a *cephalosporin* is often an appropriate alternative. However, if there is a history of anaphylaxis or some other severe allergic reaction, it is prudent to avoid cephalosporins as well (because there is about a 1% risk for cross sensitivity to cephalosporins). When a cephalosporin is indicated, an oral cephalosporin is preferred (because the risk for a severe reaction is lower than with parenteral therapy). For many infections, *vancomycin, erythromycin,* and *clindamycin* are effective and safe alternatives for patients with penicillin allergy.

Rarely, a patient with a history of anaphylaxis may have a life-threatening infection (e.g., enterococcal endocarditis) for which alternatives to penicillins are ineffective. In these cases, the potential benefits of penicillin therapy outweigh the risks, and treatment should be instituted. To minimize the chances of an anaphylactic reaction, penicillin should be administered according to a desensitization schedule. In this procedure, an initial small dose is followed at 60-minute intervals by progressively larger doses until the full therapeutic dose has been achieved. It should be noted that the desensitization procedure is not without risk. Accordingly, epinephrine and facilities for respiratory support should be immediately available.

Drug Interactions

Bacteriostatic Antibiotics

Because penicillins are most effective against actively growing bacteria, concurrent use of a bacteriostatic antibiotic (e.g., tetracycline) could, in theory, reduce the bactericidal effects of the penicillin. However, the clinical significance of such interactions is not known. Nonetheless, combined use of penicillin and bacteriostatic agents is generally avoided.

Penicillin V

Penicillin V, also known as penicillin VK, is similar to penicillin G in most respects. The principal difference is acid stability: Penicillin V is stable in stomach acid, whereas penicillin G is not. Because of its acid stability, penicillin V has replaced penicillin G for oral therapy. Penicillin V may be taken with meals.

Penicillinase-Resistant Penicillins (Antistaphylococcal Penicillins)

By altering the penicillin side chain, pharmaceutical chemists have created a group of penicillins that are highly resistant to inactivation by beta-lactamases. In the United States three such drugs are available: *nafcillin, oxacillin,* and *dicloxacillin.* These agents have a very narrow antimicrobial spectrum and are used only against penicillinase-producing strains of staphylococci (*S. aureus* and *S. epidermidis*). Because most

PATIENT-CENTERED CARE ACROSS THE LIFE SPAN

Penicillins

Life Stage	Patient Care Concerns
Infants	Penicillins are used safely in infants with bacterial infections, including syphilis, meningitis, and group A streptococcus.
Children/adolescents	Penicillins are a common drug used to treat bacterial infections in children.
Pregnant women	Penicillins are classified in U.S. Food and Drug Administration Pregnancy Risk Category B. There is no evidence of second- or third-trimester fetal risk.
Breastfeeding women	Amoxicillin is safe for use in breastfeeding mothers. Data are lacking regarding transmission of some other penicillins from mother to infant through breast milk.
Older adults	Doses should be adjusted in older adults with renal dysfunction.

strains of staphylococci produce penicillinase, the penicillinase-resistant penicillins are drugs of choice for most staphylococcal infections. It should be noted that these agents should not be used against infections caused by non–penicillinase-producing staphylococci because they are less active than penicillin G against these bacteria.

An increasing clinical problem is the emergence of staphylococcal strains referred to as *MRSA*, a term used to indicate lack of susceptibility to methicillin (an obsolete penicillinase-resistant penicillin) and all other penicillinase-resistant penicillins. Resistance appears to result from production of PBPs to which the penicillinase-resistant penicillins cannot bind. Vancomycin is the treatment of choice.

Nafcillin

Nafcillin is usually administered by the IV route. IM use is rare. Absorption from the gastrointestinal (GI) tract is erratic and incomplete, and hence oral formulations have been discontinued.

Oxacillin and Dicloxacillin

Oxacillin and dicloxacillin are similar in structure and pharmacokinetic properties. Both are acid stable, but only dicloxacillin is formulated for oral dosing. Oxacillin is administered by the IV route.

Broad-Spectrum Penicillins (Aminopenicillins)

Only two broad-spectrum penicillins are available: *ampicillin* and *amoxicillin.* Both have the same antimicrobial spectrum as penicillin G, *plus* increased activity against certain gram-negative bacilli, including *Haemophilus influenzae, Escherichia coli,* and *Salmonella* and *Shigella* species. This broadened spectrum is due in large part to an increased ability to penetrate the gram-negative cell envelope. Both drugs are readily inactivated by beta-lactamases and hence are ineffective against most infections caused by *S. aureus.*

Ampicillin

Ampicillin was the first broad-spectrum penicillin in clinical use. The drug is useful against infections caused by *Enterococcus fecalis, Proteus mirabilis, E. coli, Salmonella* and *Shigella* species, and *H. influenzae.* The most common side effects are rash and diarrhea, both of which occur more frequently with ampicillin than with any other penicillin. Administration may be oral or IV. It should be noted that for oral therapy, amoxicillin is preferred (see later). Dosages for patients with normal kidney function are shown in Table 69.2. For patients with renal impairment, dosage should be reduced.

As discussed later, ampicillin is also available in a fixed-dose combination with sulbactam, an inhibitor of bacterial beta-lactamase. The combination is sold as *Unasyn.*

Amoxicillin

Amoxicillin [Moxatag] is similar to ampicillin in structure and actions. The drugs differ primarily in acid stability, amoxicillin being the more acid stable. Hence, when the two are administered orally in equivalent doses, blood levels of amoxicillin are greater. Accordingly, when oral therapy is indicated, amoxicillin is preferred. Amoxicillin produces less diarrhea than ampicillin, perhaps because less amoxicillin remains unabsorbed in the intestine.

As discussed later, amoxicillin is also available in a fixed-dose combination with clavulanic acid, an inhibitor of bacterial beta-lactamases. The combination is marketed as *Augmentin.* Amoxicillin, by itself, is one of our most frequently prescribed antibiotics.

Extended-Spectrum Penicillins (Antipseudomonal Penicillins)

Only one extended-spectrum penicillin is available: *piperacillin.* The antimicrobial spectrum of piperacillin includes organisms that are susceptible to the aminopenicillins plus *Pseudomonas aeruginosa, Enterobacter* species, *Proteus* species (indole positive), *Bacteroides fragilis,* and many *Klebsiella* species. This extended-spectrum penicillin is susceptible to beta-lactamases and hence is ineffective against most strains of *S. aureus.*

Piperacillin is used primarily for infections with *P. aeruginosa.* These infections often occur in the immunocompromised host and can be very difficult to eradicate. To increase killing of *Pseudomonas,* an antipseudomonal aminoglycoside (gentamicin, tobramycin, amikacin, netilmicin) may be added to the regimen. When these combinations are employed, the penicillin and the aminoglycoside should not be mixed in the same IV solution because high concentrations of penicillins can inactivate aminoglycosides.

TABLE 69.2 ▪ Dosages for Penicillins

Generic Name	Trade Name	Usual Routes	Dosing Interval (hr)	Total Daily Dosage[a] Adults	Total Daily Dosage[a] Children
NARROW-SPECTRUM PENICILLINS: PENICILLINASE SENSITIVE					
Penicillin G	Bicillin C-R, Bicillin LA, Pfizerpen	IM, IV	4	1.2–24 million units[b]	100,000–400,000 units/kg[b]
Penicillin V	Generic only	PO	4–6	0.5–2 g	25–50 mg/kg
NARROW-SPECTRUM PENICILLINS: PENICILLINASE-RESISTANT (ANTISTAPHYLOCOCCAL PENICILLINS)					
Nafcillin		IV	4–6	2–12 g	100–200 mg/kg
Oxacillin		IV	4–6	1–12 g	100–200 mg/kg
Dicloxacillin		PO	6	0.5–4 g	12.5–25 mg/kg
BROAD-SPECTRUM PENICILLINS (AMINOPENICILLINS)					
Ampicillin	Generic only	PO	6–8	2–4 g	50–100 mg/kg
		IV	6–8	4–12 g	50–400 mg/kg
Ampicillin/sulbactam	Unasyn	IV	6	4–8 g[c]	150–600 mg/kg[c]
Amoxicillin	Generic only	PO	8	750–1750 mg	20–90 mg/kg
Amoxicillin, ER	Moxatag	PO	24	775 mg	775 mg
Amoxicillin/clavulanate	Augmentin, Clavulin ♣	PO	8–12	250–1750 mg[d]	20–90 mg/kg[d]
	Augmentin ES-600	PO	12	—	90 mg/kg
	Augmentin XR	PO	12	4000 mg	—
EXTENDED-SPECTRUM PENICILLIN (ANTIPSEUDOMONAL PENICILLIN)					
Piperacillin/tazobactam	Zosyn, Tazocin ♣	IV	4–6	12–18 g[e]	80–100 mg/kg[e]

[a]Doses vary widely, depending on the type and severity of infection; doses and dosing intervals presented here may not be appropriate for all patients.
[b]10,000 units = 6 mg.
[c]Dose based on ampicillin content.
[d]Dose based on amoxicillin content.
[e]Dose based on piperacillin content.
ER, extended release; IM, intramuscular; IV, intravenous; PO, oral.

Piperacillin

Piperacillin has a broad antimicrobial spectrum; however, the drug is penicillinase sensitive. Piperacillin is highly active against *P. aeruginosa,* its principal target. Piperacillin can cause bleeding secondary to disrupting platelet function. The drug is acid labile and hence must be administered parenterally, usually by the IV route. Dosages for patients with normal kidney function are shown in Table 69.2. Dosage should be reduced in patients with renal impairment. As discussed later, piperacillin is also available in a fixed-dose combination with tazobactam, a beta-lactamase inhibitor. The combination is marketed as Zosyn.

Penicillins Combined With a Beta-Lactamase Inhibitor

As their name indicates, beta-lactamase inhibitors are drugs that inhibit bacterial beta-lactamases. By combining a beta-lactamase inhibitor with a penicillinase-sensitive penicillin, we can extend the antimicrobial spectrum of the penicillin. In the United States three beta-lactamase inhibitors are used: *sulbactam, tazobactam,* and *clavulanic acid* (clavulanate). These drugs are not available alone. Rather, they are available only in fixed-dose combinations with a penicillin. Four such combination products are available:

- Ampicillin/sulbactam [Unasyn]
- Amoxicillin/clavulanate [Augmentin, Clavulin ♣]
- Piperacillin/tazobactam [Zosyn, Tazocin ♣]

Because beta-lactamase inhibitors have minimal toxicity, any adverse effects that occur with the combination products are due to the penicillin.

CHAPTER

70 Drugs That Weaken the Bacterial Cell Wall II: Other Drugs

Laura D. Rosenthal, DNP, ACNP, FAANP

Like the penicillins, the drugs discussed here are inhibitors of cell wall synthesis. By disrupting the cell wall, these drugs produce bacterial lysis and death. Much of the chapter focuses on the cephalosporins, our most widely used antibacterial drugs. With only three exceptions—vancomycin, telavancin, and fosfomycin—the agents addressed here are beta-lactam drugs.

CEPHALOSPORINS

The cephalosporins are beta-lactam antibiotics similar in structure and actions to the penicillins. These drugs are bactericidal, often resistant to beta-lactamases, and active against a broad spectrum of pathogens. Their toxicity is low. Because of these attributes, the cephalosporins are popular therapeutic agents and constitute our most widely used group of antibiotics.

Chemistry

All cephalosporins are derived from the same nucleus. This nucleus contains a *beta-lactam ring* fused to a second ring. The beta-lactam ring is required for antibacterial activity.

Mechanism of Action

The cephalosporins are bactericidal drugs with a mechanism like that of the penicillins. These agents bind to penicillin-binding proteins (PBPs) and thereby (1) disrupt cell wall synthesis and (2) activate autolysins (enzymes that cleave bonds in the cell wall). The resultant damage to the cell wall causes death by lysis. Like the penicillins, cephalosporins are most effective against cells undergoing active growth and division.

Resistance

The principal cause of cephalosporin resistance is production of beta-lactamases, enzymes that cleave the beta-lactam ring and thereby render these drugs inactive. Beta-lactamases that act on cephalosporins are sometimes referred to as *cephalosporinases*. Some of the beta-lactamases that act on cephalosporins can also cleave the beta-lactam ring of penicillins.

Not all cephalosporins are equally susceptible to beta-lactamases. Most *first-generation* cephalosporins are destroyed by beta-lactamases; *second-generation* cephalosporins are less sensitive to destruction; and *third-, fourth-, and fifth-generation* cephalosporins are highly resistant.

In some cases, bacterial resistance results from producing altered PBPs that have a low affinity for cephalosporins. Methicillin-resistant staphylococci produce these unusual PBPs and are resistant to most cephalosporins as a result. Ceftaroline, a fifth-generation cephalosporin, has demonstrated activity against methicillin-resistant *Staphylococcus aureus* (MRSA).

Classification and Antimicrobial Spectra

The cephalosporins can be grouped into five "generations" based on the order of their introduction to clinical use. The generations differ significantly with respect to antimicrobial spectrum and susceptibility to beta-lactamases (Table 70.1). In general, *as we progress from first-generation agents to fifth-generation agents, there is (1) increasing activity against gram-negative bacteria and anaerobes, (2) increasing resistance to destruction by beta-lactamases, and (3) increasing ability to reach the cerebrospinal fluid (CSF).*

First Generation

First-generation cephalosporins, represented by cephalexin, are highly active against gram-positive bacteria. These drugs are the most active of all cephalosporins against staphylococci and nonenterococcal streptococci. However, staphylococci that are resistant to methicillin-like drugs are also resistant to first-generation cephalosporins (and to most other cephalosporins as well). The first-generation agents have only modest activity against gram-negative bacteria and do not reach effective concentrations in the CSF.

Second Generation

Second-generation cephalosporins (e.g., cefoxitin) have enhanced activity against gram-negative bacteria. The increase is due to a combination of factors: (1) increased affinity for PBPs of gram-negative bacteria, (2) increased ability to penetrate the gram-negative cell envelope, and (3) increased resistance to beta-lactamases produced by gram-negative organisms. However, none of the second-generation agents is active against *Pseudomonas aeruginosa.* These drugs do not reach effective concentrations in the CSF.

Third Generation

Third-generation cephalosporins (e.g., cefotaxime) have a broad spectrum of antimicrobial activity. Because of increased resistance to beta-lactamases, these drugs are considerably more active against gram-negative aerobes than are the first- and second-generation agents. Some third-generation cephalosporins (e.g., ceftazidime) have important activity against *P. aeruginosa.* Others (e.g., cefixime) lack such activity. In contrast to first- and second-generation cephalosporins, the third-generation agents reach clinically effective concentrations in the CSF.

Fourth Generation

Cefepime and ceftolozane have a very broad antibacterial spectrum. Although cefepime itself is highly resistant to beta-lactamases, ceftolozane must be paired with tazobactam to prevent breakdown of the drug. This pairing is marketed as Zerbaxa.

Fifth Generation

Ceftaroline [Teflaro]—has a spectrum like that of the third-generation agents, but with one important exception: ceftaroline is the only cephalosporin with activity against MRSA.

Pharmacokinetics

Absorption

Because of poor absorption from the gastrointestinal (GI) tract, *many cephalosporins must be administered parenterally* (by intramuscular [IM] or intravenous [IV] route). Of the cephalosporins used in the United States, only 10 can be administered by mouth (Table 70.2). Of these, only one—*cefuroxime*—can be administered orally *and* by injection.

Distribution

Cephalosporins distribute well to most body fluids and tissues. Therapeutic concentrations are achieved in pleural, pericardial, and peritoneal fluids. However, concentrations in ocular fluids are generally low. Penetration to the CSF by first- and second-generation drugs is unreliable, and hence these drugs should not be used for bacterial meningitis. In contrast, CSF levels achieved with third-, and fourth-, and fifth-generation drugs are generally sufficient for bactericidal effects.

Elimination

Practically all cephalosporins are eliminated by the *kidneys;* excretion is by a combination of glomerular filtration and active tubular secretion. Probenecid can decrease tubular secretion of some cephalosporins, thereby prolonging their effects. In patients with renal insufficiency, dosages of most cephalosporins must be reduced (to prevent accumulation to toxic levels).

One cephalosporin—*ceftriaxone*—is eliminated largely by the liver. Consequently, dosage reduction is unnecessary in patients with renal impairment.

TABLE 70.1 ▪ Major Differences Between Cephalosporin Generations

Class	Activity Against Gram-Negative Bacteria	Resistance to Beta-Lactamases	Distribution to Cerebrospinal Fluid
First generation (e.g., cephalexin)	Low	Low	Poor
Second generation (e.g., cefoxitin)	Higher	Higher	Poor
Third generation (e.g., cefotaxime)	Higher	Higher	Good
Fourth generation (cefepime)	Highest	Highest	Good
Fifth generation (ceftaroline)	High	Highest	Good

TABLE 70.2 ▪ Pharmacokinetic Properties of the Cephalosporins

				Half-Life (hr)	
Class	Drug	Routes of Administration	Major Route of Elimination	Normal Renal Function	Severe Renal Impairment
First generation	Cefadroxil	PO	Renal	1.2–1.3	20–25
	Cefazolin	IM, IV	Renal	1.5–2.2	24–50
	Cephalexin	PO	Renal	0.4–1	10–20
Second generation	Cefaclor	PO	Renal	0.6–0.9	2–3
	Cefotetan	IM, IV	Renal	3–4.5	13–35
	Cefoxitin	IM, IV	Renal	0.7–1	13–22
	Cefprozil	PO	Renal	1.3	5–6
	Cefuroxime	PO, IM, IV	Renal	1–1.9	15–22
Third generation	Cefdinir	PO	Renal	1.7	16
	Cefditoren	PO	Renal	1.6	—
	Cefixime	PO	Renal	3–4	11.5
	Cefotaxime	IM, IV	Renal	0.9–1.4	3–11
	Cefpodoxime	PO	Renal	2–3	9.8
	Ceftazidime	IM, IV	Renal	1.9–2	—
	Ceftibuten	PO	Renal	2	Increased
	Ceftriaxone	IM, IV	Hepatic	5.8–8.7	15.7
Fourth generation	Cefepime	IM, IV	Renal	2	Increased
				2.8–3.1	Increased
			Renal		
	Ceftolozane	IV			
Fifth generation	Ceftaroline	IV	Renal	2.6	Increased

Adverse Effects

Cephalosporins are generally well tolerated and constitute one of our safest groups of antimicrobial drugs. Serious adverse effects are rare.

Allergic Reactions

Hypersensitivity reactions are the most frequent adverse events. Maculopapular rash that develops several days after the onset of treatment is most common. Severe, immediate reactions (e.g., bronchospasm, anaphylaxis) are rare. If, during the course of treatment, signs of allergy appear (e.g., urticaria, rash, hypotension, difficulty in breathing), the cephalosporin should be discontinued immediately. Anaphylaxis is treated with respiratory support and parenteral epinephrine. Patients with a history of cephalosporin allergy should not be given these drugs.

Because of structural similarities between penicillins and cephalosporins, a few patients allergic to one type of drug may experience cross-reactivity with the other. In clinical practice, the incidence of cross-reactivity has been low: only 1% of penicillin-allergic patients experience an allergic reaction if given a cephalosporin. For patients with mild penicillin allergy, cephalosporins can be used with minimal concern. However, because of the potential for fatal anaphylaxis, *cephalosporins should not be given to patients with a history of severe reactions to penicillins.*

Bleeding

Two cephalosporins—*cefotetan* and *ceftriaxone*—can cause bleeding tendencies. The mechanism is reduction of prothrombin levels through interference with vitamin K metabolism.

Several measures can reduce the risk for hemorrhage. During prolonged treatment, patients should be monitored for prothrombin time, bleeding time, or both. Parenteral vitamin K can correct an abnormal prothrombin time. Patients should be observed for signs of bleeding, and, if bleeding develops, the cephalosporin should be withdrawn. Caution should be exercised during concurrent use of anticoagulants or thrombolytic agents. Because of their antiplatelet effects, aspirin and other nonsteroidal antiinflammatory drugs (NSAIDs) should be used with care. Caution is needed in patients with a history of bleeding disorders.

Thrombophlebitis

Thrombophlebitis may develop during IV infusion. This reaction can be minimized by rotating the infusion site and by administering cephalosporins slowly and in dilute solution. Patients should be observed for phlebitis. If it develops, the infusion site should be changed.

Hemolytic Anemia

Rarely, cephalosporins have induced immune-mediated hemolytic anemia, a condition in which antibodies mediate destruction of red blood cells. If hemolytic anemia develops, the cephalosporin should be discontinued. Blood transfusions may be given as needed.

Other Adverse Effects

Cephalosporins may cause pain at sites of IM injection; patients should be forewarned. Rarely, cephalosporins may be the cause of pseudomembranous colitis due to colonic overgrowth with *Clostridium difficile.* If this superinfection develops, the cephalosporin should be discontinued and, if necessary, oral vancomycin should be given.

With one cephalosporin—cefditoren—there are two unique concerns. First, the drug contains a milk protein (sodium caseinate) and hence should be avoided by patients with milk-protein hypersensitivity (as opposed to lactose intolerance). Second, cefditoren is excreted in combination with carnitine and can cause carnitine loss. Therefore the drug is contraindicated for patients with existing carnitine deficiency or with conditions that predispose to carnitine deficiency.

Drug Interactions

Alcohol

Two cephalosporins—*cefazolin* and *cefotetan*—can induce a state of alcohol intolerance. If a patient taking these drugs were to ingest alcohol, a disulfiram-like reaction could occur. (As discussed in Chapter 31 the disulfiram effect, which can be very dangerous, is brought on by accumulation of acetaldehyde secondary to inhibition of aldehyde dehydrogenase.) Patients using these cephalosporins must not consume alcohol in any form.

Drugs That Promote Bleeding

As noted, *cefotetan* and *ceftriaxone* can promote bleeding. Caution is needed if these drugs are combined with other agents that promote bleeding (anticoagulants, thrombolytics, NSAIDs, and other antiplatelet agents).

Therapeutic Uses

The therapeutic role of the cephalosporins is continually evolving as new agents are introduced and more experience is gained with older ones. Only general recommendations are considered here.

The cephalosporins are broad-spectrum, bactericidal drugs with a high therapeutic index. They have been employed widely and successfully against a variety of infections. Cephalosporins can be useful alternatives for patients with mild penicillin allergy.

The five generations of cephalosporins differ significantly in their applications. With one important exception—the use of first-generation agents for infections caused by sensitive staphylococci—the *first- and second-generation cephalosporins* are rarely drugs of choice for active infections. In most cases, equally effective and less expensive alternatives are available. In contrast, the *third-generation agents* have qualities that make them the preferred therapy for several infections. The *fourth- and fifth-generation agents* are effective against resistant organisms. The *fifth-generation* agent is used to treat skin infections, including MRSA, and health care–associated pneumonias.

First-Generation Cephalosporins

When a cephalosporin is indicated for a gram-positive infection, a first-generation drug should be used; these agents are the most active of the cephalosporins against gram-positive organisms and are less expensive than other cephalosporins. First-generation agents are frequently employed as alternatives to penicillins to treat infections caused by staphylococci or streptococci (except enterococci) in patients with penicillin allergy. However, it is important to note that cephalosporins should be given only to patients with a history of mild penicillin allergy—not to those who have experienced a severe, immediate hypersensitivity reaction.

The first-generation agents have been employed widely for prophylaxis against infection in surgical patients. First-generation agents are preferred to second- or third-generation cephalosporins for surgical prophylaxis because they are as effective as the newer drugs, are less expensive, and have a more narrow antimicrobial spectrum.

Second-Generation Cephalosporins

Specific indications for second-generation cephalosporins are limited. Cefuroxime has been used with success against pneumonia caused by *Haemophilus influenzae,* Klebsiella species, pneumococci, and staphylococci. Oral cefuroxime is useful for otitis, sinusitis, and respiratory tract infections. Cefoxitin is useful for abdominal and pelvic infections.

Prototype Drugs

DRUGS THAT INHIBIT CELL WALL SYNTHESIS

Cephalosporin
Cephalexin

Carbapenem
Imipenem

Other
Vancomycin

Third-Generation Cephalosporins

Because they are highly active against gram-negative organisms, and because they penetrate to the CSF, third-generation cephalosporins are drugs of choice for meningitis caused by enteric, gram-negative bacilli. Ceftazidime is of special utility for treating meningitis caused by *P. aeruginosa.* Nosocomial infections caused by gram-negative bacilli, which are often resistant to first- and second-generation cephalosporins (and most other commonly used antibiotics), are appropriate indications for the third-generation drugs. Two third-generation agents—ceftriaxone and cefotaxime—are drugs of choice for infections caused by *Neisseria gonorrhoeae* (gonorrhea), *H. influenzae,* and Proteus, Salmonella, Klebsiella, and Serratia species; these drugs are also effective against meningitis caused by *Streptococcus pneumoniae,* a gram-positive bacterium.

The third-generation cephalosporins should not be used routinely. Rather, they should be given only when conditions demand so as to delay emergence of resistance.

Fourth-Generation Cephalosporins

There are only two drugs in this category: cefepime [Maxipime] and ceftolozane/tazobactam [Zerbaxa]. Cefepime is commonly used to treat health care– and hospital-associated pneumonias, including those caused by the resistant organism Pseudomonas. Zerbaxa was approved in 2014 for the treatment of complicated intraabdominal and urinary tract infections.

Fifth-Generation Cephalosporins

Ceftaroline [Teflaro] is the only cephalosporin adequate for the treatment of MRSA-associated infections.

Drug Selection

Nineteen cephalosporins are currently employed in the United States, and selection among them can be a challenge. Within each generation, the similarities among cephalosporins are more pronounced than the differences. Hence, aside from cost, there is frequently no rational basis for choosing one drug over another in the outpatient setting. However, there *are* some differences between cephalosporins, and these differences may render one agent preferable to another for treating a specific infection in a specific host. The differences that do exist can be grouped into three main categories: (1) antimicrobial spectrum, (2) adverse effects, and (3) pharmacokinetics (e.g., route of administration, penetration to the CSF, time course, mode of elimination). Drug selection based on these differences is discussed here.

Antimicrobial Spectrum

A prime rule of antimicrobial therapy is to match the drug with the bug: the drug should be active against known or suspected pathogens, but its spectrum should be no broader than required. When a cephalosporin is appropriate, we should select from among those drugs known to have good activity against the causative pathogen. The third- and fourth-generation agents, with their very broad antimicrobial spectra, should be avoided in situations in which a narrower spectrum, first- or second-generation drug would suffice.

For some infections, one cephalosporin may be decidedly more effective than all others and should be selected on this basis. For example, ceftazidime (a third-generation drug) is the most effective of all cephalosporins against *P. aeruginosa* and is clearly the preferred cephalosporin for treating infections caused by this microbe. Similarly, ceftaroline is the only cephalosporin with activity against MRSA and hence is preferred to all other cephalosporins for treating these infections.

Adverse Effects

Although most cephalosporins produce the same spectrum of adverse effects, a few can cause unique reactions. For example, cefotetan and ceftriaxone can cause bleeding tendencies. When an equally effective alternative is available, it would be prudent to avoid these drugs.

Pharmacokinetics

Four pharmacokinetic properties are of interest: (1) route of administration, (2) duration of action, (3) distribution to the CSF, and (4) route of elimination. The relationship of these properties to drug selection is discussed next.

Route of Administration

Ten cephalosporins can be administered orally. These drugs may be preferred for mild to moderate infections in patients who can't tolerate parenteral agents.

Duration of Action

In patients with normal renal function, the half-lives of the cephalosporins range from about 30 minutes to 9 hours (see Table 70.2). Because they require fewer doses per day, drugs with a long half-life are frequently preferred. Cephalosporins with the longest half-lives in each generation are as follows: first generation, cefazolin (1.5–2 hours); second generation, cefotetan (3–4.5 hours); and third generation, ceftriaxone (6–9 hours).

Distribution to Cerebrospinal Fluid

Only the third- and fourth-generation agents achieve CSF concentrations sufficient for bactericidal effects. Hence, for meningitis caused by susceptible organisms, these drugs are preferred over first- and second-generation agents.

Route of Elimination

Most cephalosporins are eliminated by the kidneys and, if dosage is not carefully adjusted, they may accumulate to toxic levels in patients with renal impairment. Only one agent—ceftriaxone—is eliminated primarily by nonrenal routes and hence can be used with relative safety in patients with kidney dysfunction.

Dosage and Administration

Routes

Many cephalosporins cannot be absorbed from the GI tract and must therefore be administered parenterally (IM or IV). Only 10 cephalosporins can be given orally. One drug—cefuroxime—can be administered both orally and by injection.

Dosage

Dosages are shown in Table 70.3. For most cephalosporins (ceftriaxone excepted), dosage should be reduced in patients with significant renal impairment.

Administration

Oral

If oral cephalosporins produce nausea, administration with food can reduce the response. Oral suspensions should be stored cold.

Intramuscular

Intramuscular injections should be made deep into a large muscle. Intramuscular injection of cephalosporins is frequently painful; the patient should be forewarned. The injection site should be checked for induration, tenderness, and redness, and the prescriber informed if these occur.

TABLE 70.3 ▪ Cephalosporin Dosages

				Total Daily Dosage*	
Drug	**Trade Name**	**Route**	**Dosing Interval (hr)**	**Adults (g)**	**Children (mg/kg)**
FIRST GENERATION					
Cefadroxil	Generic only	PO	12, 24	1–2	30
Cefazolin	Generic only	IM, IV	6, 8	2–12	80–160
Cephalexin	Keflex	PO	6	1–4	25–100
SECOND GENERATION					
Cefaclor	Raniclor ♣	PO	8	0.75–1.5	20–40
Cefotetan	Generic only	IM, IV	12	1–6	—
Cefoxitin	Mefoxin	IM, IV	4, 8	3–12	80–160
Cefprozil	Generic only	PO	12, 24	0.5–1	15–30
Cefuroxime	Ceftin	PO	12	0.5–1	250–500
	Zinacef	IM, IV	8	1.5–6	50–100
THIRD GENERATION					
Cefdinir	Omnicef	PO	12, 24	0.6	14
Cefditoren	Spectracef	PO	12	0.4–0.8	—
Cefixime	Suprax	PO	24	0.4	8
Cefotaxime	Claforan	IM, IV	4, 8	2–12	100–200
Cefpodoxime	Vantin	PO	12	0.2–0.4	10
Ceftazidime	Fortaz, Tazicef	IM, IV	8, 12	0.5–6	60–150
Ceftibuten	Cedax	PO	24	0.4	9
Ceftriaxone	Rocephin	IM, IV	12, 24	1–4	50–100
FOURTH GENERATION					
Cefepime	Maxipime	IM, IV	12	1–6	100–150
Ceftolozane/tazobactam	Zerbaxa	IV	8	4.5	—
FIFTH GENERATION					
Ceftaroline	Teflaro	IV	12	1.2	—

*With the exception of ceftriaxone, cephalosporins require a dosage reduction in patients with severe renal impairment.

Intravenous

For IV therapy, cephalosporins may be administered by three techniques: (1) bolus injection, (2) slow injection (over 3–5 minutes), and (3) continuous infusion over 30 to 60 minutes. Your prescriber order should state which method to use.

CARBAPENEMS

Carbapenems are beta-lactam antibiotics that have very broad antimicrobial spectra—although none is active against MRSA. Four carbapenems are available: imipenem, meropenem, ertapenem, and doripenem. With all four, administration is parenteral. To delay emergence of resistance, these drugs should be reserved for patients who cannot be treated with a more narrow-spectrum agent.

Imipenem

Imipenem [Primaxin], a beta-lactam antibiotic, has an extremely broad antimicrobial spectrum—broader, in fact, than nearly all other antimicrobial drugs. As a result, imipenem may be of special use for treating mixed infections in which anaerobes, *S. aureus,* and gram-negative bacilli may all be involved. Imipenem is supplied in fixed-dose combinations with cilastatin, a compound that inhibits destruction of imipenem by renal enzymes.

Mechanism of Action

Imipenem binds to two PBPs (PBP1 and PBP2), causing weakening of the bacterial cell wall with subsequent cell lysis and death. Antimicrobial effects are enhanced by the drug's resistance to practically all beta-lactamases and by its ability to penetrate the gram-negative cell envelope.

Antimicrobial Spectrum

Imipenem is active against most bacterial pathogens, including organisms resistant to other antibiotics. The drug is highly active against gram-positive cocci and most gram-negative cocci and bacilli. In addition, imipenem is the most effective beta-lactam antibiotic for use against anaerobic bacteria.

Pharmacokinetics

Imipenem is not absorbed from the GI tract and hence must be given intravenously. The drug is well distributed to body fluids and tissues. Imipenem penetrates the meninges to produce therapeutic concentrations in the CSF.

Elimination is primarily renal. When employed alone, imipenem is inactivated by dipeptidase, an enzyme present in the kidneys. As a result, drug levels in urine are low. To increase urinary concentrations, imipenem is administered in combination with *cilastatin,* a dipeptidase inhibitor. When the combination is used, about 70% of imipenem is excreted unchanged in the urine. The elimination half-life is about 1 hour.

Adverse Effects

Imipenem is generally well tolerated. Gastrointestinal effects (nausea, vomiting, diarrhea) are most common. Superinfections with bacteria or fungi develop in about 4% of patients. Rarely, seizures have occurred.

Hypersensitivity reactions (rashes, pruritus, drug fever) have occurred, and patients allergic to other beta-lactam antibiotics may be cross-allergic with imipenem. Fortunately, the incidence of cross sensitivity with penicillins is low—only about 1%.

Interaction With Valproate

Imipenem can reduce blood levels of valproate, a drug used to control seizures (see Chapter 19). Breakthrough seizures have occurred. If possible, combined use of imipenem and valproate should be avoided. If no other antibiotic will suffice, supplemental antiseizure therapy should be considered.

Therapeutic Use

Because of its broad spectrum and low toxicity, imipenem is used widely. The drug is effective for serious infections caused by gram-positive cocci, gram-negative cocci, gram-negative bacilli, and anaerobic bacteria. This broad antimicrobial spectrum gives imipenem special utility for antimicrobial therapy of mixed infections (e.g., simultaneous infection with aerobic and anaerobic bacteria). When imipenem has been given alone to treat infection with *P. aeruginosa,* resistant organisms have emerged. Consequently, imipenem should be combined with another antipseudomonal drug when used against this microbe. Dosing for the carbapenems is provided in Table 70.4.

Other Carbapenems

Meropenem

Actions and Uses

Meropenem [Merrem] is a beta-lactam antibiotic similar in structure and actions to imipenem. Meropenem is active against most clinically important gram-positive and gram-negative aerobes and anaerobes. Approved indications are (1) bacterial meningitis in children age 3 months or older, (2) intraabdominal infections in children and adults, and (3) complicated skin and skin structure infections in children and adults. Meropenem may prove especially useful for health care– or community-associated infections caused by organisms resistant to other antibiotics.

Pharmacokinetics

Meropenem is given by IV route and distributes to all body fluids and tissues. The drug has a plasma half-life of 1 hour and is eliminated primarily unchanged in the urine. In contrast to imipenem, meropenem is not degraded by renal dipeptidases and hence is not combined with cilastatin.

Adverse Effect and Interactions

Like other beta-lactam antibiotics, meropenem is generally well tolerated. Principal adverse effects are rashes, diarrhea, nausea, and vomiting. The risk for cross sensitivity in patients allergic to penicillins is about 1%. As with imipenem, seizures occur rarely. The risk for seizures is highest in patients with central nervous system (CNS) disorders (e.g., brain lesions, history of seizures) and bacterial meningitis. Like imipenem, meropenem can reduce levels of valproate and may permit breakthrough seizures in patients taking the drug.

Ertapenem

Actions and Uses

Like other carbapenems, ertapenem [Invanz] weakens the bacterial cell wall and thereby causes cell lysis and death. Also like other carbapenems, ertapenem is highly resistant to beta-lactamases and thus has a very broad antimicrobial spectrum—but less broad than that of imipenem or meropenem. Ertapenem is active against most gram-positive bacteria and most anaerobes. However, in contrast to imipenem and meropenem, the drug has little or no activity against *P. aeruginosa* or Acinetobacter species. In addition, ertapenem

PATIENT-CENTERED CARE ACROSS THE LIFE SPAN

Cephalosporins, Carbapenems, and Others

Life Stage	Patient Care Concerns
Infants	Third-generation cephalosporins are used to treat bacterial infections in neonates as well as infants.
Children/adolescents	Cephalosporins are commonly used to treat bacterial infections in children, including otitis media and gonococcal and pneumococcal infections.
Pregnant women	Administration of telavancin during pregnancy should be avoided because of risk for adverse developmental outcomes. All cephalosporins appear safe for use in pregnancy and are classified in FDA Pregnancy Risk Category B.
Breastfeeding women	Cephalosporins are generally not expected to cause adverse effects in breastfed infants.
Older adults	Doses should be adjusted in older adults with decreased renal function.

TABLE 70.4 ▪ Carbapenem Dosages

				Total Daily Dosage in Normal Renal Function	
Drug	**Trade Name**	**Route**	**Dosing Interval (hr)**	**Adults (g)**	**Children (mg/kg)**
Doripenem	Doribax	IV	8	1.5	—
Ertapenem	Invanz	IM, IV	24	1	30
Imipenem/cilastatin	Primaxin	IV	6	1–2	50–100
Meropenem	Merrem	IV	8	3	60–120

has minimal activity against pneumococci that are highly resistant to penicillin and has no activity against methicillin-resistant staphylococci, *Enterococcus faecium, Enterococcus fecalis,* or atypical respiratory tract pathogens, including Chlamydia species, Legionella species, and *Mycoplasma pneumoniae.* Ertapenem is indicated for parenteral therapy of acute pelvic infections, community-acquired pneumonia, prophylaxis after elective colorectal surgery, and complicated infections of the urinary tract, abdomen, skin, and skin structures.

Pharmacokinetics

Ertapenem may be administered by IM injection or IV infusion. Absorption after IM injection is complete. In the blood, ertapenem is highly bound to plasma proteins. The drug undergoes some hydrolysis of the beta-lactam ring before excretion in the urine and feces. Its half-life is approximately 4 hours (compared with only 1 hour for imipenem or meropenem).

Adverse Effects and Interactions

Like other carbapenems, ertapenem is generally well tolerated. In clinical trials, the most common adverse effects were diarrhea, nausea, infused-vein complications, headache, vomiting, and edema. In addition, CNS effects (agitation, confusion, disorientation, decreased mental acuity, somnolence, stupor) were reported in 5.1% of patients. Like most other antibiotics, ertapenem can promote *C. difficile* infection. Like imipenem and meropenem, ertapenem can cause seizures, but the incidence is relatively low (0.5%). Like other carbapenems, ertapenem can reduce levels of valproate and may thereby cause loss of seizure control.

Doripenem

Actions and Uses

Doripenem [Doribax] is active against a broad spectrum of gram-positive, gram-negative, and anaerobic bacteria. Activity against *P. aeruginosa* is greater than with other carbapenems. Cell kill results from disrupting cell wall synthesis. Doripenem has two approved indications: complicated intraabdominal infections and complicated urinary tract infections. To delay emergence of resistance, the drug should be reserved for seriously ill patients with mixed infections or infection with multidrug-resistant, gram-negative bacteria or Pseudomonas species.

Pharmacokinetics

Doripenem is administered by IV infusion. Binding to plasma proteins is low, and hepatic metabolism is minimal. Elimination is renal, primarily as unchanged drug. In patients with normal kidney function, the half-life is about 1 hour. In patients with renal impairment, the half-life is longer, and hence these people require a reduced dosage to prevent doripenem from accumulating to dangerous levels.

Adverse Effects and Interactions

Like other carbapenems, doripenem is generally well tolerated. The most common side effects are headache, nausea, diarrhea, rash, and injection-site phlebitis. In contrast to other carbapenems, doripenem does not cause seizures. However, like other carbapenems, doripenem can reduce levels of valproic acid and may cause loss of seizure control.

OTHER INHIBITORS OF CELL WALL SYNTHESIS

Vancomycin

Vancomycin [Vancocin] is the most widely used antibiotic in U.S. hospitals. Principal indications are *C. difficile* infection (CDI), MRSA infection, and treatment of serious infections with susceptible organisms in patients allergic to penicillins. The major toxicity is renal failure. Unlike most other drugs discussed here, vancomycin does not contain a beta-lactam ring.

Mechanism of Action

Like the beta-lactam antibiotics, vancomycin inhibits cell wall synthesis and thereby promotes bacterial lysis and death. However, in contrast to the beta-lactams, vancomycin does not interact with PBPs. Instead, it disrupts the cell wall by binding to molecules that serve as precursors for cell wall biosynthesis.

Antimicrobial Spectrum

Vancomycin is active only against gram-positive bacteria. The drug is especially active against *S. aureus* and *Staphylococcus epidermidis,* including strains of both species that are methicillin resistant. Other susceptible organisms include streptococci, penicillin-resistant pneumococci, and *C. difficile.*

Pharmacokinetics

Absorption from the GI tract is poor. Hence, for most infections, vancomycin is given parenterally. Oral administration is employed only for infections of the intestine, mainly CDI.

Vancomycin is well distributed to most body fluids and tissues. Although it enters the CSF, levels may be insufficient to treat meningitis. Hence, if meningeal infection fails to respond to IV therapy, concurrent intrathecal dosing may be required.

Vancomycin is eliminated unchanged by the kidneys. In patients with renal impairment, dosage must be reduced.

Therapeutic Use

Vancomycin should be reserved for serious infections. This agent is the drug of choice for infections caused by MRSA or *S. epidermidis;* most strains of these bacteria are still sensitive to vancomycin. Vancomycin is also the drug of choice for severe CDI, but not for mild CDI. The drug is also employed as an alternative to penicillins and cephalosporins to treat severe infections (e.g., staphylococcal and streptococcal endocarditis) in patients allergic to beta-lactam antibiotics.

Adverse Effects

The major toxicity is *renal failure.* Risk is dose related and increased by concurrent use of other nephrotoxic drugs (e.g., aminoglycosides, cyclosporine, NSAIDs). To minimize risk, trough serum levels of vancomycin should be no greater than needed (see later). If significant kidney damage develops, as indicated by a 50% increase in serum creatinine level, vancomycin dosage should be reduced.

Ototoxicity develops rarely and is usually reversible. Risk is increased by prolonged treatment, renal impairment, and concurrent use of other ototoxic drugs (e.g., aminoglycosides, ethacrynic acid).

Rapid infusion of vancomycin can cause a constellation of disturbing effects—flushing, rash, pruritus, urticaria, tachycardia, and hypotension—known collectively as red man syndrome. These effects, which may result from release of histamine, can usually be avoided by infusing vancomycin slowly (over 60 minutes or more).

Thrombophlebitis is common. The reaction can be minimized by administering vancomycin in dilute solution and by changing the infusion site frequently.

Rarely, vancomycin causes immune-mediated thrombocytopenia, a condition in which platelets are lost and spontaneous bleeding results. The underlying mechanism is development of unusual antibodies that bind to platelets—but only if the platelets first bind with vancomycin (forming a vancomycin-platelet complex). The resulting antibody-vancomycin-platelet complexes are then removed from the circulation by macrophages.

Patients allergic to penicillins do not show cross-reactivity with vancomycin. Accordingly, vancomycin is an alternative to penicillins in patients with penicillin allergy.

Preparations, Dosage, and Administration

Intravenous Dosing

For systemic infection, vancomycin is administered by intermittent infusion over 60 minutes or longer. The traditional dosage is 15 mg/kg every 12 hours. However, a higher dosage (15–20 mg/kg every 8–12 hours) is now recommended. For patients with severe infection, a loading dose (25–30 mg/kg) may be used. In patients with renal impairment, dosages must be reduced.

Dosage should be adjusted to achieve effective trough serum levels of vancomycin. For serious infections (e.g., bacteremia, osteomyelitis, meningitis, health care–acquired pneumonia), trough levels should be 15 to 20 mcg/mL. For less serious infections, trough levels should be at least 10 mcg/mL.

Oral Dosing

Vancomycin is given orally for CDI and other intestinal infections. (Dosages for CDI are shown in Table 70.5) Because vancomycin is not absorbed from the GI tract, there is no need to decrease oral doses in patients with renal impairment.

Rectal Dosing

Rectal dosing may be used for patients with complicated CDI. One recommended regimen consists of giving 500 mg in 100 mL of normal saline every 6 hours, using a retention enema.

Clostridium difficile Infection

C. difficile (sometimes called *C. diff*) is a gram-positive, spore-forming, anaerobic bacillus that infects the bowel. Injury results from release of two toxins: toxin A and toxin B. Symptoms range from mild (abdominal discomfort, nausea, fever, diarrhea) to very severe (toxic megacolon, pseudomembranous colitis, colon perforation, sepsis, death). CDI has become more common and more severe owing to the spread of a more virulent strain—known as NAP1/BI/027—that releases more toxin than older strains. In many hospitals, rates of infection caused by *C. diff* exceed those caused by MRSA. Fortunately, most cases of CDI can be managed well with antibiotics, usually metronidazole [Flagyl] or vancomycin [Vancocin].

CDI is almost always preceded by use of antibiotics, which kill off normal gut flora and allow *C. diff* to flourish. Antibiotics most likely to promote CDI are clindamycin, second- and third-generation cephalosporins, and fluoroquinolones. In fact, intensive use of fluoroquinolones, such as ciprofloxacin [Cipro] and levofloxacin [Levaquin], is believed responsible for the rapid spread of the NAP1/BI/027 strain.

CDI is acquired by ingesting *C. difficile* spores, which are shed in the feces. Any object that feces contact—including toilets, bathtubs, and rectal thermometers—can be a source of infection. Within hospitals, spores are transferred to patients primarily on the hands of health care workers who have touched a contaminated person or object. Spores of *C. diff* are resistant to drying, temperature changes, and alcohol, so viable spores can remain in the environment for weeks.

CDI is defined by (1) the passage of three or more unformed stools in 24 hours or less plus (2) a positive stool test for *C. difficile* or its toxins. Intestinal damage is caused by toxins A and B, which attack the lining of the colon. Symptoms range from watery diarrhea to life-threatening pseudomembranous colitis, characterized by patches of severe inflammation and pus. Complications of severe *C. difficile* colitis include dehydration, electrolyte disturbances, toxic megacolon, bowel perforation, renal failure, sepsis, and death. Among patients successfully treated for CDI, the recurrence rate is 15% to 30%.

The principal risk factor for CDI is treatment with antibiotics. Risk is especially high among older adults who take antibiotics. Other risk factors include GI surgery, serious illness, prolonged hospitalization, and immunosuppression, which may result from cancer chemotherapy, immunosuppressive therapy, or HIV.

Treatment of CDI consists of stopping one antibiotic and starting another, as recommended in a clinical guideline issued by the Infectious Disease Society of America (IDSA) and the Society for Healthcare Epidemiology of America (SHEA). As soon as possible after CDI has been diagnosed, we should stop the antibiotic that facilitated *C. diff* overgrowth because doing so (1) will reduce the risk for reinfection after CDI has cleared, and (2) in 25% of patients with mild CDI, will cause the infection to resolve. At the same time, we should start an antibiotic to eradicate *C. diff.* Drug selection is based on infection severity, as judged by two laboratory values: white blood cell (WBC) counts and serum creatinine (SCr) values. Higher WBC counts indicate more severe colonic inflammation. Higher SCr values indicate more severe dehydration (from diarrhea) and worsening renal perfusion (from dehydration). As shown later, oral *metronidazole* is recommended for a mild or moderate initial episode, and oral *vancomycin* is recommended for a severe initial episode. For a complicated severe initial episode, the guidelines recommend IV metronidazole *plus* vancomycin given either PO or through a nasogastric tube. If the patient has complete ileus (absence of intestinal motility), rectal instillation of

TABLE 70.5 ▪ Recommended Treatments for *Clostridium difficile* Infection

Clinical Definition	Supportive Clinical Data	Drug Therapy
Initial episode: mild or moderate	Leukocytosis with a WBC count of 15,000 cells/mcL or lower *and* SCr less than 1.5 times baseline	Metronidazole, 500 mg PO 3 times daily for 10–14 days
Initial episode: severe	Leukocytosis with a WBC count of 15,000 cells/mcL or higher *or* SCr 1.5 times baseline or higher	Vancomycin, 125 mg PO 4 times daily for 10–14 days
Initial episode: severe, complicated	Leukocytosis with a WBC count of 15,000 cells/mcL or higher *or* SCr 1.5 times baseline or higher, *either one, plus* hypotension/shock, ileus, megacolon	Metronidazole 500 mg IV every 8 hr *plus* vancomycin, 500 mg PO/NG 4 times daily for 10–14 days If complete ileus is present, consider adding vancomycin retention enema
First recurrence		Same as initial episode
Second recurrence		Vancomycin PO in a tapered regimen, for example: 125 mg 4 times daily for 10–14 days, then 125 mg twice daily for 7 days, then 125 mg once daily for 7 days, then 125 mg every 2 or 3 days for 2–8 weeks

mcL, microliter; NG, by nasogastric tube; PO, by mouth; SCr, serum creatinine; WBC, white blood cell.
Recommendation data are from Cohen SH, Gerding DN, Johnson S, et al. Clinical practice guidelines for *Clostridium difficile* infection in adults: 2010 update by the Society for Healthcare Epidemiology of America (SHEA) and the Infectious Disease Society of America (IDSA). Infect Control Hosp Epidemiol 2010;31:431-455.

vancomycin may be added. If CDI recurs after being cleared, the regimen used for initial therapy should be tried again. If there is a second recurrence, the guidelines recommend a prolonged course of oral vancomycin in which the number of daily doses is gradually decreased.

Alternatives and supplements to metronidazole and vancomycin are being studied. Promising options include the following:

- *Fidaxomicin* [Dificid]—a narrow-spectrum macrolide antibiotic with high selectivity for *C. difficile*—was approved for treating *C. difficile*–associated diarrhea in 2011. In a phase 3 trial, the cure rate with fidaxomicin was higher than with vancomycin, and the recurrence rate was lower. Parameters for use of fidaxomicin are still being defined.
- *Nitazoxanide,* approved for diarrhea caused by *Giardia* species and *Cryptosporidium* species, appears equal to metronidazole or vancomycin for treating CDI. Prospective trials are still needed.
- *Rifaximin,* approved for diarrhea caused by *Escherichia coli,* can reduce CDI recurrence following treatment with vancomycin.
- *Monoclonal antibodies* directed against *C. difficile* toxins A and B can reduce CDI recurrence when given concurrently with metronidazole or vancomycin. These antibodies are not yet available for routine clinical use, yet there is one drug in phase 3 trials at this time.
- Inoculating the bowel with a *benign strain* of *C. difficile* can protect against developing CDI. Presumably, when the benign strain colonizes the bowel, it occupies the same niche that a virulent strain would occupy and thereby prevents the virulent strain from becoming established.

How can we control the spread of CDI? The IDSA/SHEA guidelines offer the following recommendations:

- Use antibiotics judiciously, especially those associated with a high risk for CDI (clindamycin, cephalosporins, and fluoroquinolones).
- If possible, isolate patients with CDI in a private room or have them share a room with another patient with CDI.
- Wear gloves and a gown when entering the room of a patient with CDI.
- After contact with a patient with CDI, wash hands with soap and running water. Soap and water won't kill *C. diff* spores, but it will flush them off the hands. Alcohol-based hand rubs will not kill spores and will not remove them from the hands.
- Use disposable rectal thermometers.
- In areas associated with increased rates of CDI, decontaminate surfaces with a chlorine-containing cleaning agent (or any other agent that can kill *C. diff* spores).

Telavancin

Actions and Uses

Telavancin [Vibativ] is the first representative of a new class of agents, the lipoglycoproteins, synthetic derivatives of vancomycin. Like vancomycin, telavancin is active only against gram-positive bacteria. Cell kill results from two mechanisms. First, like vancomycin, telavancin inhibits bacterial cell wall synthesis. Second, telavancin binds to the bacterial cell membrane and thereby disrupts membrane function. Telavancin is approved only for IV therapy of complicated skin and skin structure infections caused by susceptible strains of the following gram-positive organisms: *S. aureus* (including methicillin-sensitive and methicillin-resistant strains), *Streptococcus pyogenes, Streptococcus agalactiae, Streptococcus anginosus* group, and *Enterococcus fecalis* (but only vancomycin-sensitive strains). To delay development of resistance, telavancin should be reserved for treating vancomycin-resistant infections or for use as an alternative to linezolid [Zyvox], daptomycin [Cubicin], or tigecycline [Tygacil] in patients who cannot take these drugs.

Pharmacokinetics

After IV infusion, telavancin undergoes 90% binding to plasma proteins. Elimination is primarily renal. In healthy volunteers, the plasma half-life was approximately 8 hours. In patients with renal impairment, the half-life is prolonged and blood levels increase. In patients with moderate hepatic impairment, the kinetics of telavancin remain unchanged.

Adverse Effects

Telavancin can cause multiple adverse effects. The most common are taste disturbance, nausea, vomiting, and foamy urine. As with vancomycin, rapid infusion can cause red man syndrome, characterized by flushing, rash, pruritus, urticaria, tachycardia, and hypotension.

Kidney damage develops in 3% of patients, as indicated by increased serum creatinine, renal insufficiency, or even renal failure. To reduce risk, kidney function should be measured at baseline, every 72 hours during treatment, and at the end of treatment. If these tests indicate nephrotoxicity, switching to a different antibiotic should be considered. In most cases, kidney function normalizes after telavancin is withdrawn. The risk for kidney damage is increased by using other nephrotoxic drugs.

BLACK BOX WARNING: TELAVANCIN

Telavancin, when used to treat hospital-acquired or ventilator-associated bacterial pneumonia in patients with a creatinine clearance of <50 mL/min, has been associated with increased mortality compared with vancomycin.

Telavancin can prolong the QT interval. However, serious dysrhythmias have not been reported. Nonetheless, telavancin should not be given to patients at high risk, including those with congenital long QT syndrome, uncompensated heart failure, or severe left ventricular hypertrophy and those using other QT drugs.

Avoid telavancin during pregnancy. When given to pregnant animals, telavancin reduced fetal weight and increased the risk for digit and limb deformities. The drug has not been studied in pregnant women. Nonetheless, because telavancin is fetotoxic in animals, it is classified in U.S. Food and Drug Administration (FDA) Pregnancy Risk Category C (risk cannot be ruled out). Accordingly, telavancin should not be used during pregnancy unless the benefits to the patient are deemed to outweigh the risks to the fetus. Before telavancin is used, pregnancy should be ruled out with a serum pregnancy test.

Drug Interactions

Telavancin should be used with caution in patients taking other drugs that can damage the kidneys (e.g., NSAIDs, angiotensin-converting enzyme inhibitors, aminoglycosides) and in patients taking drugs that prolong the QT interval (e.g., clarithromycin, ketoconazole). Clinically significant interactions involving cytochrome P450 enzymes have not been observed.

Preparations, Dosage, and Administration

The usual dosage of telavancin [Vibativ] is 10 mg/kg once daily, infused over 60 minutes to reduce the risk for red man syndrome. Treatment duration is 7 to 14 days. Monitoring telavancin blood levels is unnecessary. In patients with renal impairment, as indicated by reduced creatinine clearance, dosage should be decreased. In patients with moderate hepatic impairment, no dosage adjustment is needed.

Aztreonam

Chemistry

Aztreonam [Azactam, Cayston] belongs to a class of beta-lactam antibiotics known as monobactams. These agents contain a beta-lactam ring, but the ring is not fused with a second ring.

Mechanism of Action

Aztreonam binds to PBP3. Therefore, like most beta-lactam antibiotics, the drug inhibits bacterial cell wall synthesis and thereby promotes cell lysis and death. The drug does not bind to PBPs produced by anaerobes or gram-positive bacteria.

Antimicrobial Spectrum and Therapeutic Use

Aztreonam has a narrow antimicrobial spectrum, being active only against gram-negative aerobic bacteria. Susceptible organisms include Neisseria species, *H. influenzae, P. aeruginosa,* and Enterobacteriaceae (e.g., *E. coli,* Klebsiella, Proteus, Serratia, Salmonella, Shigella). Aztreonam is highly resistant to beta-lactamases and therefore is active against many gram-negative aerobes that produce them. The drug is not active against gram-positive bacteria and anaerobes.

Pharmacokinetics

Aztreonam is not absorbed from the GI tract and hence must be administered parenterally (IM or IV) for systemic therapy. When in the blood, the drug distributes widely to most body fluids and tissues. Therapeutic concentrations can be achieved in the CSF. Aztreonam is eliminated by the kidneys, primarily unchanged.

In addition to being administered IM and IV, aztreonam can be inhaled for delivery directly to the lungs. This route is used to treat *P. aeruginosa* lung infection in patients with cystic fibrosis.

Adverse Effects

Aztreonam is generally well tolerated. Adverse effects are like those of other beta-lactam antibiotics. The most common effects are pain and thrombophlebitis at the site of injection. Because aztreonam differs greatly in structure from penicillins and cephalosporins, there is little cross-allergenicity with them. Hence aztreonam appears safe for patients with allergies to other beta-lactam antibiotics.

Preparations, Dosage, and Administration

Parenteral

Aztreonam, sold as Azactam, is available for IM or IV administration. The usual adult dosage is 1 to 2 g every 8 to 12 hours. Dosage should be reduced in patients with renal impairment.

Inhalational

Aztreonam, sold as Cayston, should be inhaled using the Altera Nebulizer System. Dosing is done as a repeating cycle of 75 mg 3 times a day for 28 days, followed by 28 days off.

Fosfomycin

Fosfomycin [Monurol] is a unique antibiotic approved for single-dose therapy in women with uncomplicated urinary tract infections (i.e., acute cystitis) caused by *E. coli* or *Enterococcus faecalis.* The drug kills bacteria by disrupting synthesis of the peptidoglycan polymer strands that compose the cell wall. (As discussed in Chapter 69, penicillins kill bacteria in part by preventing cross-linking of peptidoglycan strands.)

The most common adverse effects are diarrhea, headache, vaginitis, and nausea. Fosfomycin may also cause abdominal pain, rhinitis, drowsiness, dizziness, and rash.

Fosfomycin dosing may be done with or without food. Symptoms of cystitis should improve in 2 to 3 days. If symptoms fail to improve, additional doses will not help—but will increase the risk for side effects.

CHAPTER

71 Bacteriostatic Inhibitors of Protein Synthesis

Laura D. Rosenthal, DNP, ACNP, FAANP

All the drugs discussed in this chapter inhibit bacterial protein synthesis. However, unlike the aminoglycosides, which are bactericidal, the drugs considered here are largely bacteriostatic. That is, they suppress bacterial growth and replication but do not produce outright kill. In general, the drugs presented here are second-line agents, used primarily for infections resistant to first-line agents.

TETRACYCLINES

The tetracyclines are *broad-spectrum* antibiotics. In the United States four tetracyclines are available for systemic therapy. All four—tetracycline, demeclocycline, doxycycline, and minocycline—are similar in structure, antimicrobial actions, and adverse effects. Principal differences among them are pharmacokinetic. Because the similarities among these drugs are more pronounced than their differences, we will discuss the tetracyclines as a group, rather than focusing on a prototype. Unique properties of individual tetracyclines are indicated as appropriate.

Mechanism of Action

The tetracyclines suppress bacterial growth by inhibiting protein synthesis. These drugs bind to the 30S ribosomal subunit and thereby inhibit binding of transfer RNA to the messenger RNA–ribosome complex. As a result, addition of amino acids to the growing peptide chain is prevented. At the concentrations achieved clinically, the tetracyclines are bacteriostatic.

Selective toxicity of the tetracyclines results from their poor ability to cross mammalian cell membranes. To influence protein synthesis, tetracyclines must first gain access to the cell interior. These drugs enter bacteria by way of an energy-dependent transport system. Mammalian cells lack this transport system and hence do not actively accumulate the drug. Consequently, although tetracyclines are inherently capable of inhibiting protein synthesis in mammalian cells, their levels within host cells remain too low to be harmful.

Microbial Resistance

Bacterial resistance results from increased drug inactivation, decreased access to ribosomes (owing to the presence of ribosome protection proteins), and reduced intracellular accumulation (owing to decreased uptake and increased export).

Antimicrobial Spectrum

The tetracyclines are broad-spectrum antibiotics, active against a wide variety of gram-positive and gram-negative bacteria. Sensitive organisms include *Rickettsia,* spirochetes, *Brucella, Chlamydia, Mycoplasma, Helicobacter pylori, Borrelia burgdorferi, Bacillus anthracis*, and *Vibrio cholerae*.

Therapeutic Uses

Treatment of Infectious Diseases

Extensive use of tetracyclines has resulted in increasing bacterial resistance. Because of resistance, and because antibiotics with greater selectivity and less toxicity are now available, use of tetracyclines has declined. Today, tetracyclines are rarely drugs of first choice. Disorders for which they *are* first-line drugs include (1) rickettsial diseases (e.g., Rocky Mountain spotted fever, typhus fever, Q fever); (2) infections caused by *Chlamydia trachomatis* (trachoma, lymphogranuloma venereum, urethritis, cervicitis); (3) brucellosis; (4) cholera; (5) pneumonia caused by *Mycoplasma pneumoniae;* (6) Lyme disease; (7) anthrax; and (8) gastric infection with *H. pylori.*

Treatment of Acne

Tetracyclines are used topically and orally for severe acne vulgaris. Beneficial effects derive from suppressing the growth and metabolic activity of *Propionibacterium acnes,* an organism that secretes inflammatory chemicals. Oral doses for acne are relatively low. As a result, adverse effects are minimal. Acne is discussed in Chapter 85.

Peptic Ulcer Disease

H. pylori, a bacterium that lives in the stomach, is a major contributing factor to peptic ulcer disease. Tetracyclines, in combination with metronidazole and bismuth subsalicylate, are a treatment of choice for eradicating this bug. The role of *H. pylori* in ulcer formation is discussed in Chapter 62.

Periodontal Disease

Two tetracyclines—*doxycycline* and *minocycline*—are used for periodontal disease. Doxycycline is used orally *and* topically, whereas minocycline is used only topically.

Oral Therapy

Benefits of oral doxycycline [Periostat] result from inhibiting collagenase, an enzyme that destroys connective tissue in the gums. The small doses employed—20 mg twice daily—are too low to harm bacteria.

Topical Therapy

Topical minocycline [Arestin] and doxycycline [Atridox] are employed as adjuncts to scaling and root planing. The objective is to reduce pocket depth and bleeding in adults with periodontitis. Benefits derive from suppressing bacterial growth. Both products are applied directly to the site of periodontal disease.

Rheumatoid Arthritis

Minocycline can reduce symptoms in patients with rheumatoid arthritis, suggesting a possible infectious component to the disease.

Pharmacokinetics

Individual tetracyclines differ significantly in their pharmacokinetic properties. Of particular significance are differences in half-life and route of elimination. Also important is the degree to which food decreases absorption. The pharmacokinetic properties of individual tetracyclines are shown in Table 71.1.

Duration of Action

The tetracyclines can be divided into three groups: short acting, intermediate acting, and long acting. These differences are related to differences in lipid solubility: the only short-acting agent (tetracycline) has relatively low lipid solubility, whereas the long-acting agents (doxycycline, minocycline) have relatively high lipid solubility.

Absorption

All of the tetracyclines are orally effective, although the extent of absorption differs among individual agents. Absorption of three agents—tetracycline, demeclocycline, and doxycycline—is reduced by food, whereas absorption of minocycline is not.

The tetracyclines form insoluble chelates with calcium, iron, magnesium, aluminum, and zinc. The result is decreased absorption.

Patient Education

DRUG INTERACTIONS WITH TETRACYCLINES

Tetracyclines should not be administered together with (1) *calcium supplements,* (2) *milk products* (because they contain calcium), (3) *iron supplements,* (4) *magnesium-containing laxatives,* and (5) *most antacids* (because they contain magnesium, aluminum, or both).

Distribution

Tetracyclines are widely distributed to most tissues and body fluids. However, penetration to the cerebrospinal fluid (CSF) is poor, and hence levels in the CSF are too low to treat meningeal infections. Tetracyclines readily cross the placenta and enter the fetal circulation.

Elimination

Tetracyclines are eliminated by the kidneys and liver. All tetracyclines are excreted by the liver into the bile. After the bile enters the intestine, most tetracyclines are reabsorbed.

Ultimate elimination of short- and intermediate-acting tetracyclines—tetracycline and demeclocycline—is in the urine, largely as the unchanged drug. Because these agents undergo renal elimination, they can accumulate to toxic levels if the kidneys fail. Consequently, *tetracycline and demeclocycline should not be given to patients with significant renal impairment.*

Long-acting tetracyclines are eliminated by the liver, primarily as metabolites. Because these agents are excreted by the liver, their half-lives are unaffected by kidney dysfunction. Accordingly, *the long-acting agents (doxycycline and minocycline) are drugs of choice for tetracycline-responsive infections in patients with renal impairment.*

Adverse Effects

Gastrointestinal Irritation

Tetracyclines irritate the gastrointestinal (GI) tract. As a result, oral therapy is frequently associated with epigastric burning, cramps, nausea, vomiting, and diarrhea. These reactions can be reduced by giving tetracyclines with meals—although food may decrease absorption. Occasionally, tetracyclines cause esophageal ulceration. Risk can be minimized by avoiding dosing at bedtime. Because diarrhea may result from superinfection of the bowel (in addition to nonspecific irritation), it is important that the cause of diarrhea be determined.

Effects on Bones and Teeth

Tetracyclines bind to calcium in developing teeth, resulting in yellow or brown discoloration; hypoplasia of the enamel may also occur. The intensity of tooth discoloration is related to the total cumulative dose: staining is darker with prolonged and repeated treatment. When taken after the fourth month of gestation, tetracyclines can cause staining of *deciduous* teeth of the infant. However, use during pregnancy will not affect *permanent* teeth. Discoloration of permanent teeth occurs when tetracyclines are taken by patients aged 4 months to 8 years, the interval during which tooth enamel is being formed. Accordingly, these drugs should be avoided by children younger than 8 years. The risk for tooth discoloration with *doxycycline* may be less than with other tetracyclines.

TABLE 71.1 ■ Pharmacokinetic Properties of the Tetracyclines

Class	Drug	Lipid Solubility	Oral Dose Absorbed (%)*	Effect of Food on Absorption	Route of Elimination	Half-Life	
						Normal (hr)	Anuric (hr)
Short acting	Tetracycline	Low	60–80	Large decrease	Renal	8	57–108†
Intermediate acting	Demeclocycline	Moderate	60–80	Large decrease	Renal	12	40–60†
Long acting	Doxycycline	High	90–100	Small decrease	Hepatic	18	17–30
	Minocycline	High	90–100	No change	Hepatic	16	11–23

*Percentage absorbed when taken on an empty stomach.

†Do not use in patients with renal impairment because the drug could accumulate to toxic levels.

Tetracyclines can suppress long-bone growth in premature infants. This effect is reversible on discontinuation of treatment.

Superinfection

A superinfection is an overgrowth with drug-resistant microbes, which occurs secondary to suppression of drug-sensitive organisms. Because the tetracyclines are broad-spectrum agents and therefore can decrease viability of a wide variety of microbes, the risk for superinfection is greater than with antibiotics that have a more narrow spectrum.

Superinfection of the bowel with staphylococci or with *Clostridium difficile* produces severe diarrhea and can be life-threatening. The infection caused by *C. difficile* is known as *C. difficile*–associated diarrhea (CDAD), also known as *antibiotic-associated pseudomembranous colitis.* Patients should notify the prescriber if significant diarrhea occurs so that the possibility of bacterial superinfection can be evaluated. If a diagnosis of superinfection with staphylococci or *C. difficile* is made, tetracyclines should be discontinued immediately. Treatment of CDAD consists of oral *vancomycin* or *metronidazole* plus vigorous fluid and electrolyte replacement (see Chapter 64).

Overgrowth with fungi (commonly *Candida albicans*) may occur in the mouth, pharynx, vagina, and bowel. Symptoms include vaginal or anal itching; inflammatory lesions of the anogenital region; and a black, furry appearance of the tongue. Superinfection with *Candida* can be managed by discontinuing tetracyclines. When this is not possible, antifungal therapy is indicated.

Hepatotoxicity

Tetracyclines can cause fatty infiltration of the liver. Hepatotoxicity manifests clinically as lethargy and jaundice. Rarely, the condition progresses to massive liver failure. Liver damage is most likely when tetracyclines are administered intravenously in high doses (greater than 2 g/day). Pregnant and postpartum women with kidney disease are at especially high risk.

Renal Toxicity

Tetracyclines may exacerbate renal impairment in patients with preexisting kidney disease. Because *tetracycline* and *demeclocycline* are eliminated by the kidneys, these agents should not be given to patients with renal impairment. If a patient with renal impairment requires a tetracycline, either *doxycycline* or *minocycline* should be used because these drugs are eliminated primarily by the liver.

Patient Education

SUN EXPOSURE RISK WITH TETRACYCLINES

All tetracyclines can increase the sensitivity of the skin to ultraviolet light. The most common result is exaggerated sunburn. Advise patients to avoid prolonged exposure to sunlight, wear protective clothing, and apply a sunscreen to exposed skin.

Other Adverse Effects

Vestibular toxicity—manifesting as dizziness, lightheadedness, and unsteadiness—has occurred with minocycline. Rarely, tetracyclines have produced pseudotumor cerebri (a benign elevation in intracranial pressure). In a few patients, demeclocycline has produced nephrogenic diabetes insipidus, a syndrome characterized by thirst, increased frequency of urination, and unusual weakness or tiredness. Because of their irritant properties, tetracyclines can cause pain at sites of intramuscular (IM) injection and thrombophlebitis when administered intravenously.

Drug and Food Interactions

As noted, tetracyclines can form nonabsorbable chelates with certain metal ions (calcium, iron, magnesium, aluminum, zinc). Substances that contain these ions include *milk products, calcium supplements, iron supplements, magnesium-containing laxatives,* and *most antacids.* If a tetracycline is administered with these agents, its absorption will be decreased. To minimize interference with absorption, tetracyclines should be *administered at least 1 hour before or 2 hours after ingestion of chelating agents.*

Tetracyclines can also increase digoxin levels through increasing absorption in the GI tract and increase international normalized ratio (INR) levels by altering the vitamin K–producing flora in the gut. Patients on digoxin or warfarin should undergo careful drug level monitoring.

Dosage and Administration

Administration

For systemic therapy, tetracyclines may be administered orally or intravenously. Oral administration is preferred, and

PATIENT-CENTERED CARE ACROSS THE LIFE SPAN

Tetracyclines

Life Stage	Patient Care Concerns
Infants	Tetracyclines should not be used in children younger than 8 years because they may cause permanent discoloration of the teeth.
Children/adolescents	Tetracyclines should not be used in children younger than 8 years.
Pregnant women	Animal studies reveal that tetracyclines can cause fetal harm in pregnancy. Thus this class of drugs should be avoided in pregnant women.
Breastfeeding women	Use of tetracyclines during tooth development can cause permanent staining. Tetracyclines should be avoided by breastfeeding women.
Older adults	Tetracyclines can interact with drugs, including digoxin. In the older adult who takes many medications, check for interactions.

all tetracyclines are available in oral formulations. As a rule, oral tetracyclines should be taken on an empty stomach (1 hour before meals or 2 hours after) and with a full glass of water. An interval of at least 2 hours should separate tetracycline ingestion and ingestion of products that can chelate these drugs (e.g., milk, calcium or iron supplements, antacids). Two tetracyclines can be given intravenously (Table 71.2), but this route should be employed only when oral therapy cannot be tolerated or has proved inadequate.

In addition to their systemic use, two agents—doxycycline and minocycline—are available in formulations for topical therapy of periodontal disease.

Dosage

Dosage is determined by the nature and intensity of the infection. Typical systemic doses for adults and children are shown in Table 71.2.

Major Precautions

Two tetracyclines—*tetracycline* and *demeclocycline*—are eliminated primarily in the urine and hence will accumulate to toxic levels in patients with kidney disease. Accordingly, patients with kidney disease should not use these drugs.

Tetracyclines can cause discoloration of deciduous and permanent teeth. Tooth discoloration can be avoided by withholding these drugs from pregnant women and from children younger than 8 years.

Diarrhea may indicate a potentially life-threatening superinfection of the bowel. Advise patients to notify the prescriber if diarrhea occurs.

High-dose intravenous (IV) therapy has been associated with severe liver damage, particularly in pregnant and postpartum women with kidney disease. As a rule, these women should not receive tetracyclines.

Unique Properties of Individual Tetracyclines

Tetracycline

Tetracycline hydrochloride is the least expensive and most widely used member of the family. When employed systemically, the drug has the indications, pharmacokinetics, adverse effects, and drug interactions described for the tetracyclines as a group. Like most tetracyclines, tetracycline hydrochloride should not be administered with food and is contraindicated for patients with renal impairment.

Demeclocycline

Demeclocycline [Declomycin] shares the actions, indications, and adverse effects described previously for the tetracyclines as a group. Because of its intermediate duration of action, demeclocycline can be administered at dosing intervals that are longer than those used for tetracycline. Like tetracycline, demeclocycline should not be administered with food.

Demeclocycline is unique among the tetracyclines in that it stimulates urine flow. This side effect can lead to excessive urination, thirst, and tiredness. Interestingly, because of its effect on renal function, demeclocycline has been employed therapeutically to promote urine production in patients suffering from the syndrome of inappropriate secretion of antidiuretic hormone (SIADH).

Doxycycline

Doxycycline [Vibramycin, others] is a long-acting agent that shares the actions and adverse effects described for the tetracyclines as a group. Because of its extended half-life, doxycycline can be administered once daily in some situations. Absorption of oral doxycycline is greater than that of tetracycline. However, food can still reduce the absorption of doxycycline somewhat, and hence it is best to give this drug on an empty stomach. Doxycycline is eliminated primarily by nonrenal mechanisms. As a result, it is safe for patients with renal failure. Doxycycline is a first-line drug for Lyme disease, anthrax, chlamydial infections (urethritis, cervicitis, and lymphogranuloma venereum), and sexually acquired proctitis (in combination with ceftriaxone). A topical formulation [Atridox] is used for periodontal disease, as is a low-dose oral formulation [Periostat]. Another low-dose oral formulation [Oracea] is used for acne.

Minocycline

Minocycline [Minocin, others] is a long-acting agent similar to doxycycline. Unlike other tetracyclines, minocycline can be taken with food. Like doxycycline, and unlike tetracycline and demeclocycline, minocycline is safe for patients with kidney disease. Minocycline is unique among the tetracyclines in that it can damage the vestibular system, causing unsteadiness, lightheadedness, and dizziness. This toxicity limits its use. Minocycline is expensive, costing significantly more than tetracycline. In addition to fighting systemic infection, minocycline can reduce symptoms of arthritis (see Chapter 57) and is available in an extended-release formulation [Solodyn] for acne and a topical formulation [Arestin] for periodontal disease.

MACROLIDES

The macrolides are broad-spectrum antibiotics that inhibit bacterial protein synthesis. They are called macrolides because they are big. Erythromycin is the oldest member of the family. The newer macrolides—azithromycin and clarithromycin—are derivatives of erythromycin.

TABLE 71.2 ■ Tetracyclines: Routes of Administration, Dosing Interval, and Dosage

Class	Drug	Trade Names	Route	Usual Dosing Interval (hr)	Total Daily Dose	
					Adult (mg)	Pediatric (mg/kg)[a]
Short acting	Tetracycline	Generic only	PO	6	1000–2000	25–50
Intermediate acting	Demeclocycline	Declomycin	PO	12	600	7–13
Long acting	Doxycycline	Vibramycin,	PO	24	100–200	2.2[b]
		others	IV	24	100–200[c]	2.2–4.4[d]
	Minocycline	Minocin,	PO	12	200[e]	4[f]
		others	IV	12	200[e]	4[f]

[a]Doses presented are for children older than 8 years. Use in children younger than this age may cause permanent staining of teeth.
[b]First-day regimen is 2.2 mg/kg initially, followed by 2.2 mg/kg 12 hours later.
[c]First-day regimen is 200 mg in one or two slow infusions (1–4 hours).
[d]First-day regimen is 4.4 mg/kg in one or two slow infusions (1–4 hours).
[e]First-day regimen is 200 mg initially, followed by 100 mg 12 hours later.
[f]First-day regimen is 4 mg/kg initially, followed by 2 mg/kg 12 hours later.

Erythromycin

Erythromycin has a relatively broad antimicrobial spectrum and is a preferred or alternative treatment for a number of infections. The drug is one of our safer antibiotics and will serve as our prototype for the macrolide family.

Prototype Drugs

BACTERIOSTATIC INHIBITORS OF PROTEIN SYNTHESIS

Tetracycline
Tetracycline

Macrolide
Erythromycin

Oxazolidinone
Linezolid

Glycylcycline
Tigecycline

Other
Clindamycin

Mechanism of Action

Antibacterial effects result from inhibition of protein synthesis: erythromycin binds to the 50S ribosomal subunit and thereby blocks addition of new amino acids to the growing peptide chain. The drug is usually bacteriostatic but can be bactericidal against highly susceptible organisms or when present in high concentration. Erythromycin is selectively toxic to bacteria because ribosomes in the cytoplasm of mammalian cells do not bind the drug. Also, in contrast to chloramphenicol (see later), erythromycin cannot cross the mitochondrial membrane and therefore does not inhibit protein synthesis in host mitochondria.

Acquired Resistance

Bacteria can become resistant by two mechanisms: (1) production of a pump that exports the drug and (2) modification (by methylation) of target ribosomes so that binding of erythromycin is impaired.

Antimicrobial Spectrum

Erythromycin has an antibacterial spectrum similar to that of penicillin. The drug is active against most gram-positive bacteria as well as some gram-negative bacteria. Bacterial sensitivity is determined in large part by the ability of erythromycin to gain access to the cell interior.

Therapeutic Uses

Erythromycin is a commonly used antibiotic. *The drug is a treatment of first choice for several infections and may be used as an alternative to penicillin G in patients with penicillin allergy.*

Erythromycin is considered the drug of first choice for individuals infected with *Bordetella pertussis,* the causative agent of *whooping cough.* Because symptoms are caused by a toxin produced by *B. pertussis,* erythromycin does little to alter the course of the disease. However, by eliminating *B. pertussis* from the nasopharynx, treatment does lower infectivity.

Corynebacterium diphtheriae is highly sensitive to erythromycin. Accordingly, erythromycin is the treatment of choice for *acute diphtheria* and eliminating the diphtheria carrier state.

Several infections respond equally well to macrolides and tetracyclines. Both are drugs of first choice for certain chlamydial infections (urethritis, cervicitis) and for pneumonia caused by *M. pneumoniae.*

Pharmacokinetics

Absorption and Bioavailability

Erythromycin for oral administration is available in three forms: *erythromycin base* and two derivatives of the base: *erythromycin stearate* and *erythromycin ethylsuccinate.* The base is unstable in stomach acid, and its absorption can be variable; the derivatives were synthesized to improve bioavailability. Bioavailability has also been enhanced by formulating tablets with an acid-resistant coating, which protects erythromycin while in the stomach and then dissolves in the duodenum, permitting absorption from the small intestine. As a rule, *food decreases the absorption of erythromycin base and erythromycin stearate,* whereas absorption of erythromycin ethylsuccinate is not affected. Only erythromycin base is biologically active; the derivatives must be converted to the base (either in the intestine or after absorption) in order to work. When used properly (i.e., when dosage is correct and the effects of food are accounted for), all of the oral erythromycins produce equivalent responses.

In addition to its oral forms, erythromycin is available as *erythromycin lactobionate* for IV use. IV dosing produces drug levels that are higher than those achieved with oral dosing (Table 71.3).

Distribution

Erythromycin readily distributes to most tissues and body fluids. Penetration to the CSF, however, is poor. Erythromycin crosses the placenta, but adverse effects on the fetus have not been observed.

Elimination

Erythromycin is eliminated primarily by hepatic mechanisms, including metabolism by CYP3A4 (the 3A4 isoenzyme of cytochrome P450). Erythromycin is concentrated in the liver and then excreted in the bile. A small amount (10%–15%) is excreted unchanged in the urine.

Adverse Effects

Erythromycin is generally free of serious toxicity and is considered one of our safest antibiotics. However, the drug does carry a very small risk for sudden cardiac death from QT prolongation.

Gastrointestinal Effects

Gastrointestinal disturbances (epigastric pain, nausea, vomiting, diarrhea) are the most common side effects. These can be reduced by administering erythromycin with meals. However, this should be done only when using erythromycin

TABLE 71.3 ■ Macrolides: Routes of Administration, Dosing Interval, and Dosage

				Total Daily Dose	
Drug	Trade Names	Route	Usual Dosing Interval (hr)	Adult (mg)	Pediatric (mg/kg)
Azithromycin	Zithromax	PO	24	250–500*	5–12†
		IV	24	500	5–10†
Clarithromycin	Biaxin Biaxin XL	PO	12–24	500–1000	
Erythromycin	Ery-Tab	PO	6	1000–2000	30–50
	Erythromycin Filmtabs	IV	24	1000–4000	60–200

*500 mg on day 1 and 250 mg on days 2–4.
†10 mg/kg on days 1–2 and 5 mg/kg on days 3–5.

products whose absorption is unaffected by food (erythromycin ethylsuccinate, certain enteric-coated formulations of erythromycin base). Patients who experience persistent or severe GI reactions should notify the prescriber.

QT Prolongation and Sudden Cardiac Death

A study published in 2004 raised concerns about cardiotoxicity, especially when erythromycin is combined with drugs that can raise its plasma level. When present in high concentrations, erythromycin can prolong the QT interval, thereby posing a risk for torsades de pointes, a potentially fatal ventricular dysrhythmia. Sudden death can result. The study revealed that, when erythromycin is combined with a CYP3A4 inhibitor, there is a fivefold increase in the risk for sudden cardiac death—or 6 extra deaths for every 100,000 patients using the drug. To minimize risk, erythromycin should be avoided by patients with congenital QT prolongation and by those taking class IA or class III antidysrhythmic drugs. Also, the drug should be avoided by patients taking CYP3A4 inhibitors, including certain calcium channel blockers (verapamil and diltiazem), azole antifungal drugs (e.g., ketoconazole, itraconazole), HIV protease inhibitors (e.g., ritonavir, saquinavir), and nefazodone (an antidepressant).

Other Adverse Effects

By killing off sensitive gut flora, erythromycin can promote superinfection of the bowel. Thrombophlebitis can occur with IV administration; this reaction can be minimized by infusing the drug slowly in dilute solution. Transient hearing loss occurs rarely with high-dose therapy. There is evidence that erythromycin may cause hypertrophic pyloric stenosis in infants, especially those younger than 2 weeks.

Drug Interactions

Erythromycin can increase the plasma levels and half-lives of several drugs, thereby posing a risk for toxicity. The mechanism is inhibition of hepatic cytochrome P450 drug-metabolizing enzymes. Elevated levels are a concern with *theophylline* (used for asthma), *carbamazepine* (used for seizures and bipolar disorder), and *warfarin* (an anticoagulant). Accordingly, when these agents are combined with erythromycin, the patient should be monitored closely for signs of toxicity.

Erythromycin prevents binding of *chloramphenicol* and *clindamycin* to bacterial ribosomes, thereby antagonizing their antibacterial effects. Accordingly, concurrent use of erythromycin with these two drugs is not recommended.

As noted, erythromycin should not be combined with drugs that can inhibit erythromycin metabolism. Among these are verapamil, diltiazem, HIV protease inhibitors, and azole antifungal drugs.

Clarithromycin

Actions and Therapeutic Uses

Like erythromycin, clarithromycin [Biaxin, Biaxin XL] binds the 50S subunit of bacterial ribosomes, causing inhibition of protein synthesis. The drug is approved for respiratory tract infections, uncomplicated infections of the skin and skin structures, and prevention of disseminated Mycobacterium avium complex infections in patients with advanced HIV infection. It is also used for *H. pylori* infection and as a substitute for penicillin G in penicillin-allergic patients.

Pharmacokinetics

Clarithromycin is available in three oral formulations: immediate-release (IR) tablets, extended-release (ER) tablets, and granules for solution. The IR tablets and granules are well absorbed, in the presence and absence of food. In contrast, the ER tablets are absorbed poorly if food is absent. After absorption, clarithromycin is widely distributed and readily penetrates cells. Elimination is by hepatic metabolism and renal excretion. A reduction in dosage may be needed for patients with severe renal impairment.

Adverse Effects and Interactions

Clarithromycin is well tolerated and does not produce the intense nausea seen with erythromycin. The most common reactions (3%) have been diarrhea, nausea, and distorted taste—all described as mild to moderate. In clinical trials, only 3% of patients withdrew because of side effects, compared with 20% of those taking erythromycin. High doses of clarithromycin have caused fetal abnormalities in laboratory animals; possible effects on the human fetus are unknown. Like erythromycin, clarithromycin may prolong the QT interval and hence may pose a risk for serious dysrhythmias.

Like erythromycin, clarithromycin can inhibit hepatic metabolism of other drugs and can thereby elevate their levels. Affected drugs include warfarin, carbamazepine, and theophylline. Dosages of these drugs may need to be reduced.

Azithromycin

Actions and Therapeutic Uses

Like erythromycin, azithromycin [Zithromax, Zmax] binds the 50S subunit of bacterial ribosomes, causing inhibition of protein synthesis. The drug is used for respiratory tract infections, cholera, chancroid, otitis media, uncomplicated infections of the skin and skin structures, disseminated M. avium complex disease, and infections caused by *C. trachomatis*, for which it is a drug of choice. It may also be used as a substitute for penicillin G in penicillin-allergic patients.

Pharmacokinetics

Absorption of azithromycin is decreased by food, and hence dosing should occur on an empty stomach. After absorption, azithromycin is widely distributed to tissues and becomes concentrated in cells. Elimination is through the bile as metabolites and parent drug.

Adverse Effects and Interactions

Like clarithromycin, azithromycin is well tolerated and does not produce the intense nausea seen with erythromycin. The most common reactions are diarrhea, mild nausea, and abdominal pain. In one trial, only 0.7% of patients withdrew because of side effects. Aluminum- and magnesium-containing antacids reduce the rate (but not the extent) of absorption. In contrast to erythromycin and clarithromycin, azithromycin does not inhibit the metabolism of other drugs. However, there is concern that azithromycin may enhance the effects of warfarin (an anticoagulant) and may thereby pose a risk for bleeding. In patients taking both drugs, prothrombin time should be closely monitored to ensure that anticoagulation remains at a safe level.

QT Prolongation

Like erythromycin, azithromycin has the potential to cause fatal heart dysrhythmias secondary to prolonging the QT interval. Patients at highest risk include those with existing QT interval prolongation, low blood levels of potassium or magnesium, or a slower-than-normal heart rate, and those who use drugs to treat abnormal heart rhythms.

OTHER BACTERIOSTATIC INHIBITORS OF PROTEIN SYNTHESIS

Clindamycin

Clindamycin [Cleocin, Dalacin C ♣] can promote severe CDAD, a condition that can be fatal. Because of the risk for CDAD, indications for clindamycin are limited. Currently, systemic use is indicated only for certain anaerobic infections located outside the central nervous system (CNS).

Mechanism of Action

Clindamycin binds to the 50S subunit of bacterial ribosomes and thereby inhibits protein synthesis. The site at which clindamycin binds overlaps the binding sites for erythromycin and chloramphenicol. As a result, these agents may antagonize each other's effects. Accordingly, there are no indications for concurrent use of clindamycin with these other antibiotics.

Antimicrobial Spectrum

Clindamycin is active against most anaerobic bacteria (gram positive and gram negative) and most gram-positive aerobes. Gram-negative aerobes are generally resistant. Susceptible anaerobes include *Bacteroides fragilis, Fusobacterium* species, *Clostridium perfringens,* and anaerobic streptococci. Clindamycin is usually bacteriostatic. However, it can be bactericidal if the target organism is especially sensitive. Resistance can be a significant problem with *B. fragilis.*

Therapeutic Use

Because of its efficacy against gram-positive cocci, clindamycin has been used widely as an alternative to penicillin. The drug is employed primarily for anaerobic infections outside the CNS (it doesn't cross the blood-brain barrier). Clindamycin is the drug of choice for severe group A streptococcal infection and for gas gangrene (an infection caused by *C. perfringens*), owing to its ability to rapidly suppress synthesis of bacterial toxins. In addition, clindamycin is a preferred drug for abdominal and pelvic infections caused by *B. fragilis.*

Pharmacokinetics

Absorption and Distribution

Clindamycin may be administered by the oral, IM, or IV route. Absorption from the GI tract is nearly complete and not affected by food. The drug is widely distributed to most body fluids and tissues, including synovial fluid and bone. However, penetration to the CSF is poor.

Elimination

Clindamycin undergoes hepatic metabolism to active and inactive products, which are later excreted in the urine and bile. Only 10% of the drug is eliminated unchanged by the kidneys. The half-life is approximately 3 hours. In patients with substantial reductions in liver function or kidney function, the half-life increases slightly, but adjustments in dosage are not needed. However, in patients with combined hepatic and renal disease, the half-life increases significantly, and hence the drug may accumulate to toxic levels if dosage is not reduced.

Adverse Effects

Clostridium Difficile–*Associated Diarrhea*

CDAD, formerly known as *antibiotic-associated pseudomembranous colitis,* is the most severe toxicity of clindamycin. The cause is superinfection of the bowel with *C. difficile,* an anaerobic gram-positive bacillus. CDAD is characterized by profuse, watery diarrhea (10–20 watery stools per day), abdominal pain, fever, and leukocytosis. Stools often contain mucus and blood. Symptoms usually begin during the first week of treatment but may develop as long as 4 to 6 weeks after clindamycin withdrawal. Left untreated, the condition can be fatal. CDAD occurs with parenteral and oral therapy. Because of the risk for CDAD, patients should be instructed to report significant diarrhea (more than five watery stools per day). If superinfection with *C. difficile* is diagnosed, clindamycin should be discontinued and the patient given oral vancomycin or metronidazole, which are drugs of choice for eliminating *C. difficile* from the bowel. Diarrhea usually ceases 3 to 5 days after starting vancomycin. Vigorous replacement therapy with fluids and electrolytes is usually indicated. Drugs that decrease bowel motility (e.g., opioids, anticholinergics) may worsen symptoms and should not be used. CDAD is discussed further in Chapter 64.

BLACK BOX WARNING: CLINDAMYCIN

Clindamycin can cause potentially fatal *Clostridium difficile* diarrhea. Patients should promptly report any diarrhea to their health care provider.

Other Adverse Effects

Diarrhea (unrelated to CDAD) is relatively common. Hypersensitivity reactions (especially rashes) occur frequently. Hepatotoxicity and blood dyscrasias (agranulocytosis, leukopenia, thrombocytopenia) develop rarely. Rapid IV administration can cause electrocardiographic changes, hypotension, and cardiac arrest.

Preparations, Dosage, and Administration

Preparations

Clindamycin is available as clindamycin hydrochloride and clindamycin palmitate for oral dosing and as clindamycin phosphate for IM, IV, or topical (vaginal) dosing. Clindamycin hydrochloride [Cleocin] is supplied in capsules (75, 150, and 300 mg). Clindamycin palmitate [Cleocin Pediatric] is supplied in flavored granules, which are reconstituted with fluid to make an oral solution containing 15 mg of clindamycin per milliliter. Clindamycin phosphate is supplied in concentrated solution (150 mg/mL) and dilute solution (6, 12, and 18 mg/mL) sold as Cleocin Phosphate for parenteral therapy and in a 2% cream [Cleocin, Clindesse] and 100-mg suppositories [Cleocin] for intravaginal dosing.

Oral Dosage and Administration

For clindamycin hydrochloride, the adult dosage range is 150 to 450 mg every 6 hours; the pediatric dosage range is 8 to 20 mg/kg daily in three or four divided doses. For clindamycin palmitate, adult and pediatric dosages range from 8 to 25 mg/kg/day administered in three or four divided doses. Oral clindamycin should be taken with a full glass of water. The drug may be administered with meals.

Parenteral Dosage and Administration

For parenteral (IM or IV) therapy, clindamycin phosphate is employed. IM and IV dosages are the same. The usual adult dosage is 1.2 to 2.7 g/day administered in three or four divided doses. The usual pediatric dosage is 15 to 40 mg/kg/day in three or four divided doses.

Intravaginal Administration

Intravaginal clindamycin (suppositories or cream) is indicated for bacterial vaginosis. The suppositories are approved only for nonpregnant women; the cream can be used by pregnant women, but only during the second and third trimesters. Women using clindamycin cream should insert 1 applicatorful (5 g containing 100 mg clindamycin) nightly for 7 days (if pregnant) or for 3 to 7 days (if nonpregnant). Women using clindamycin suppositories should insert 1 suppository (100 mg) on three consecutive evenings.

Linezolid

Linezolid [Zyvox] is a first-in-class *oxazolidinone* antibiotic. The drug is important because it has activity against multidrug-resistant gram-positive pathogens, including vancomycin-resistant enterococci (VRE) and methicillin-resistant *Staphylococcus aureus* (MRSA). For treatment of MRSA, the drug is at least as effective as vancomycin. To delay the emergence of resistance, linezolid should generally be reserved for infections caused by VRE or MRSA, even though it has additional approved uses.

Mechanism, Resistance, and Antimicrobial Spectrum

Linezolid is a bacteriostatic inhibitor of protein synthesis. The drug binds to the 23S portion of the 50S ribosomal subunit and thereby blocks formation of the initiation complex. As a result, cross-resistance with other agents is unlikely. In clinical trials, development of resistance to linezolid was rare and occurred only in association with prolonged treatment of VRE infections and the presence of a prosthetic implant or undrained abscess. In real practice, resistance has been reported in association with extensive linezolid use.

Linezolid is active primarily against aerobic and facultative gram-positive bacteria. Susceptible pathogens include *Enterococcus faecium* (vancomycin-sensitive and vancomycin-resistant strains), *Enterococcus fecalis* (vancomycin-resistant strains), *S. aureus* (methicillin-sensitive and methicillin-resistant strains), *Staphylococcus epidermidis* (including methicillin-resistant strains), and *Streptococcus pneumoniae* (penicillin-sensitive and penicillin-resistant strains). Linezolid is not active against gram-negative bacteria, which readily export the drug.

Therapeutic Use

Linezolid has five approved indications:

- Infections caused by VRE
- Health care–associated pneumonia caused by *S. aureus* (methicillin-susceptible and methicillin-resistant strains) or *S. pneumoniae* (penicillin-susceptible strains only)
- Community-associated pneumonia (CAP) caused by *S. pneumoniae* (penicillin-susceptible strains only)
- Complicated skin and skin structure infections caused by *S. aureus* (methicillin-susceptible and methicillin-resistant strains), *Streptococcus pyogenes,* or *Streptococcus agalactiae*
- Uncomplicated skin and skin structure infections caused by *S. aureus* (methicillin-susceptible strains only) or *S. pyogenes*

As noted previously, to delay the emergence of resistance, linezolid should generally be reserved for infections caused by VRE or MRSA, even though it has other approved uses.

Pharmacokinetics

Oral linezolid is rapidly and completely absorbed. Food decreases the rate of absorption but not the extent. Linezolid is eliminated by hepatic metabolism and renal excretion. Its half-life is about 5 hours.

Adverse Effects

Linezolid is generally well tolerated. The most common side effects are diarrhea, nausea, and headache. Linezolid oral suspension contains phenylalanine and hence must not be used by patients with phenylketonuria.

Linezolid can cause reversible *myelosuppression,* manifesting as anemia, leukopenia, thrombocytopenia, or even pancytopenia. Risk is related to duration of use. Complete blood counts should be done weekly. Special caution is needed in patients with preexisting myelosuppression, those taking other myelosuppressive drugs, and those receiving linezolid for more than 2 weeks. If existing myelosuppression worsens or new myelosuppression develops, discontinuing linezolid should be considered.

Rarely, prolonged therapy has been associated with *neuropathy.* Patients taking the drug for more than 5 months have developed reversible optic neuropathy and irreversible peripheral neuropathy.

Drug Interactions

Linezolid is a weak inhibitor of monoamine oxidase (MAO) and hence poses a risk for hypertensive crisis. As discussed in Chapter 25, MAO inhibitors can cause severe hypertension if combined with *indirect-acting sympathomimetics* (e.g., ephedrine, pseudoephedrine, methylphenidate, cocaine) or with foods that contain large amounts of *tyramine.* Accordingly, patients using linezolid should be warned to avoid these agents.

Combining linezolid with a *selective serotonin reuptake inhibitor* (SSRI) can increase the risk for serotonin syndrome (because inhibition of MAO increases the serotonin content of CNS neurons). Deaths have been reported. Patients using SSRIs (e.g., paroxetine [Paxil, Pexeva], duloxetine [Cymbalta]) should not take linezolid.

Preparations, Dosage, and Administration

Linezolid is available in three formulations: (1) 600-mg tablets, (2) a powder for reconstitution to a 20-mg/mL oral suspension, and (3) a 2-mg/mL intravenous solution. Oral linezolid can be taken with or without food. Intravenous linezolid is infused over 30 to 120 minutes and should not be combined with additives or other drugs. Adult dosages for specific infections are as follows:

- *VRE infections*—600 mg oral (PO) or IV every 12 hours for 14 to 28 days
- *Pneumonia (healthcare or community associated)*—600 mg PO or IV every 12 hours for 10 to 14 days
- *Complicated skin and skin structure infections (including MRSA infections)*—same as pneumonia
- *Uncomplicated skin and skin structure infections*—400 mg PO every 12 hours for 10 to 14 days

Tedizolid

Tedizolid [Sivextro] was the second *oxazolidinone* antibiotic approved after linezolid. Like linezolid, tedizolid is effective in the treatment of MRSA as well as other bacterial skin and soft tissue infections caused by sensitive *Staphylococcus* and *Streptococcus* species.

Therapeutic Use

Tedizolid is used in the treatment of skin and soft tissue infections caused by MRSA, methicillin-sensitive *S. aureus* (MSSA), *S. pyogenes, S. agalactiae, Streptococcus anginosus* group (including *Streptococcus anginosus, Streptococcus intermedius,* and *Streptococcus constellatus),* and *E. fecalis.*

Pharmacokinetics

Peak plasma concentrations of oral tedizolid are reached within 3 hours of administration. After intravenous administration, peak concentrations are reached within 1 hour. Tedizolid is eliminated largely in the feces (82%).

Adverse Effects

The most common side effects associated with tedizolid are diarrhea, nausea, vomiting, dizziness, and headache. More serious adverse effects such as neuropathy and myelosuppression were seen with tedizolid as with linezolid.

Drug Interactions

Tedizolid interacts with few drugs. Of note, tedizolid, like linezolid, is a weak inhibitor of MAO and hence poses a risk for hypertensive crisis. Accordingly, patients using tedizolid should be warned to avoid these agents. The same principle applies to the SSRIs as well.

Preparations, Dosage, and Administration

Tedizolid is available in two formulations: 200-mg tablets and an intravenous solution. Oral tedizolid can be taken with or without food. The dose, whether intravenous or oral, is 200 mg once daily for 6 days.

Telithromycin

Therapeutic Use

Telithromycin [Ketek], a close relative of erythromycin and other macrolides, is a first-in-class ketolide antibiotic. Antibacterial activity is similar to that of the macrolides, with one important exception: telithromycin has significant activity against strains of *S. pneumoniae* that are penicillin and macrolide resistant. Currently, the only approved indication is CAP caused by *S. pneumoniae* (including multidrug-resistant isolates), *Haemophilus influenzae, Moraxella catarrhalis, Chlamydia pneumoniae,* or *M. pneumoniae*.

Unfortunately, although telithromycin is an effective antibiotic, it carries a significant risk for adverse effects (especially severe liver injury) and drug interactions. As a result, it should be reserved for infections caused by multidrug-resistant *S. pneumoniae* (MDRSP) that cannot be treated with other agents.

Mechanism of Action

Like the macrolides, telithromycin binds to the 50S ribosomal subunit and thereby inhibits bacterial protein synthesis. However, in contrast to the macrolides, telithromycin has properties that give it activity against bacteria that are macrolide resistant. Among respiratory tract pathogens, macrolide resistance occurs by two mechanisms: (1) removal of the macrolide with export pumps and (2) modification (by methylation) of the bacterial ribosome in a way that decreases macrolide binding. Because telithromycin differs in structure from the macrolides, the drug is less subject to removal by bacterial export pumps and can bind strongly to bacterial ribosomes even if they are methylated.

Pharmacokinetics

Telithromycin undergoes rapid but incomplete absorption after oral administration. Bioavailability is about 57%, both in the presence and absence of food. When in the blood, telithromycin becomes concentrated in white cells. About 70% of absorbed drug is metabolized in the liver—half by CYP3A4 and half by P450-independent pathways. Excretion of parent drug and metabolites occurs in the urine and feces. The half-life is 10 hours.

Adverse Effects

Although telithromycin is generally well tolerated, the drug can cause serious adverse effects, especially injury to the liver (see later). As a result, telithromycin should be used only when absolutely necessary.

In clinical trials, most adverse effects were mild to moderate. Furthermore, the rate of discontinuation because of adverse effects was nearly the same as with a comparator antibiotic. The most common adverse effects are gastrointestinal disturbances, including diarrhea, nausea, vomiting, and loose stools.

Telithromycin can cause severe liver injury (fulminant hepatitis, hepatic necrosis) and acute hepatic failure. Liver transplantation has been required, and deaths have occurred. Liver damage can develop early in telithromycin treatment and can progress rapidly. Patients should be monitored for signs of hepatitis (e.g., jaundice, fatigue, abdominal pain, dark urine). If liver injury is diagnosed, telithromycin should be discontinued and never used again.

BLACK BOX WARNING: TELITHROMYCIN

In patients with myasthenia gravis, telithromycin can make muscle weakness much worse, sometimes within hours of taking the first dose. Some patients have died from respiratory failure. Accordingly, telithromycin is contraindicated for patients with this disorder.

About 1% of patients experience visual disturbances, including blurred vision, double vision, and difficulty focusing. Females and patients younger than 40 years are at highest risk. These disturbances usually develop after the first or second dose and can persist for several hours. Symptoms may or may not recur with subsequent doses.

Like erythromycin and clarithromycin, telithromycin can prolong the QT interval and hence may pose a risk for adverse cardiac events. Telithromycin should be avoided by patients with congenital QT prolongation and by those taking class IA or class III antidysrhythmics.

Drug Interactions

Telithromycin is both a substrate for and inhibitor of CYP3A4 and hence has the potential for numerous drug interactions.

Because telithromycin is a substrate for CYP3A4, agents that inhibit the enzyme (e.g., itraconazole, ketoconazole) can elevate telithromycin levels. Conversely, agents that induce CYP3A4 (e.g., rifampin, phenytoin, carbamazepine, phenobarbital) can decrease telithromycin levels, possibly resulting in therapeutic failure.

By inhibiting CYP3A4, telithromycin can increase levels of many drugs that are substrates for the enzyme, thereby posing a risk for toxicity. Two such substrates—cisapride and pimozide—are contraindicated for use with telithromycin. Similarly, use of three statin-type cholesterol-lowering agents—simvastatin, lovastatin, and atorvastatin—should be interrupted during telithromycin therapy. However, use of two other statins—pravastatin and fluvastatin—may continue. Telithromycin is likely to increase levels of ergotamine and dihydroergotamine (ergot alkaloids used for migraine) and may thereby cause severe peripheral vasospasm. Accordingly, use of these alkaloids must be avoided. Telithromycin increases peak levels of digoxin by 73%. Accordingly, digoxin levels and side effects should be monitored closely. Other CYP3A4 substrates whose levels can be increased include midazolam [Versed], ritonavir, sirolimus, and tacrolimus. Finally, telithromycin can increase levels of metoprolol, a substrate for CYP2D6. Patients with heart failure who are using metoprolol should be monitored closely.

Preparations, Dosage, and Administration

Telithromycin [Ketek] is available in 300- and 400-mg tablets for oral dosing, with or without food. The dosage for CAP is 800 mg once a day for 7 to 10 days. Dosage reduction may be needed for patients with severe renal impairment, but not for patients with mild to moderate renal impairment or those with hepatic impairment.

Dalfopristin/Quinupristin

Dalfopristin and quinupristin are first-in-class streptogramin antibiotics. The two drugs are available in a fixed-dose combination (70 parts dalfopristin/30 parts quinupristin) under the trade name Synercid.

Mechanism of Action

Dalfopristin and quinupristin inhibit bacterial protein synthesis. When used separately, dalfopristin and quinupristin are bacteriostatic. However, in combination they are bactericidal.

Therapeutic Use

The principal indication for dalfopristin/quinupristin is vancomycin-resistant *E. faecium*. (The drugs are not active against *E. fecalis*.) Other indications include MRSA, methicillin-resistant *S. epidermidis*, and drug-resistant *S. pneumoniae*. Dalfopristin/quinupristin is safe for patients who are allergic to penicillins and cephalosporins.

BLACK BOX WARNING: DALFOPRISTIN/QUINUPRISTIN

To delay emergence of resistance, dalfopristin/quinupristin should be reserved for infections that have not responded to vancomycin.

Adverse Effects

Hepatotoxicity is the major concern. Blood should be tested for liver enzymes and bilirubin at least twice during the first week of therapy and weekly thereafter. About 50% of patients develop infusion-related thrombophlebitis. When this occurs, administration must be switched to a central venous line, or the solution should be further diluted. Other adverse effects include joint and muscle pain, rash, pruritus, vomiting, and diarrhea.

Drug Interactions

Dalfopristin and quinupristin inhibit hepatic drug-metabolizing enzymes, specifically CYP3A4. Accordingly, the combination is likely to inhibit the metabolism of many other drugs, including cyclosporine, tacrolimus, and cisapride.

Preparations, Dosage, and Administration

Dalfopristin/quinupristin [Synercid] is supplied as a powder in 500-mg vials to be reconstituted for IV administration. The usual dosage is 7.5 mg/kg infused slowly (over 1 hour) 2 or 3 times a day. Because dalfopristin and quinupristin are eliminated by hepatic metabolism, dosage should be reduced in patients with liver impairment.

Chloramphenicol

Chloramphenicol is a broad-spectrum antibiotic with the potential for causing fatal aplastic anemia and other blood dyscrasias. Because of the risk for severe blood disorders, use of chloramphenicol is limited to serious infections for which less toxic drugs are not effective.

Mechanism of Action

Chloramphenicol inhibits bacterial protein synthesis. The drug binds reversibly to the 50S subunit of bacterial ribosomes and thereby prevents addition of new amino acids to the growing peptide chain. Chloramphenicol is usually bacteriostatic but can be bactericidal against highly susceptible organisms or when its concentration is high.

Because most protein synthesis in mammalian cells is carried out in the cytoplasm employing ribosomes that are insensitive to chloramphenicol, toxic effects are restricted largely to bacteria. However, the ribosomes of mammalian mitochondria are very similar to those of bacteria, so chloramphenicol can decrease mitochondrial protein synthesis in the host. This action may underlie certain adverse effects (e.g., dose-dependent bone marrow suppression, gray syndrome in infants).

Antimicrobial Spectrum

Chloramphenicol is active against a broad spectrum of bacteria. A large number of gram-positive and gram-negative aerobic organisms are sensitive. Among these are *Salmonella typhi, H. influenzae, Neisseria meningitidis,* and *S. pneumoniae.* Most anaerobic bacteria (e.g., *B. fragilis*) are also susceptible. In addition, chloramphenicol is active against rickettsiae, chlamydiae, mycoplasmas, and treponemes.

Resistance

Resistance among gram-negative bacteria results from acquisition of an R factor that codes for acetyltransferase, an enzyme that inactivates chloramphenicol. This same R factor also codes for resistance to tetracyclines and frequently confers resistance to penicillins, too.

Pharmacokinetics

Chloramphenicol is available as an inactive prodrug—chloramphenicol sodium succinate—for IV dosing. Conversion to the active form (free chloramphenicol) is variable and incomplete. Production of active drug is especially erratic in newborns, infants, and young children.

Chloramphenicol is highly lipid soluble and widely distributed to body tissues and fluids. Therapeutic concentrations are readily achieved in the CSF, and drug levels in the brain may be as much as 9 times those in plasma. As a result, chloramphenicol is of special value for treating meningitis and brain abscesses caused by susceptible bacteria. The drug crosses the placenta and is secreted in breast milk.

Chloramphenicol is eliminated primarily by hepatic metabolism. Inactive metabolites are excreted in the urine. In patients with liver impairment, the half-life is prolonged and accumulation can occur. Accordingly, dosage should be reduced. Because the kidneys serve only to excrete inactive metabolites, there is no need for dosage reduction in patients with renal impairment. In neonates, hepatic metabolism is not fully developed, and hence the half-life of chloramphenicol is prolonged.

Because chloramphenicol has a low therapeutic index, and because serum levels of the drug can vary substantially among patients, monitoring drug levels is frequently indicated. Monitoring is especially important for neonates, infants, and young children because chloramphenicol levels in these patients can be especially variable. For most infections, effective therapy is achieved with peak serum drug levels of 10 to 20 mcg/mL and trough levels of 5 to 10 mcg/mL. The risk for dose-dependent bone marrow suppression is significantly increased when peak levels rise above 25 mcg/mL.

Therapeutic Use

When first introduced, chloramphenicol was employed widely. However, use dropped sharply when its ability to cause fatal aplastic anemia became evident. Today, chloramphenicol is indicated only for life-threatening infections for which safer drugs are ineffective or contraindicated.

Adverse Effects

The most important adverse effects are gray syndrome and toxicities related to the blood. Because of these toxicities, indications for chloramphenicol are limited.

Gray Syndrome

Gray syndrome, originally known as gray baby syndrome, is a potentially fatal toxicity observed most commonly in newborns. Initial symptoms are vomiting, abdominal distention, cyanosis, and gray discoloration of the skin. These may be followed by vasomotor collapse and death. The syndrome results from accumulation of chloramphenicol to high levels. Newborns are especially vulnerable to gray syndrome because (1) hepatic function is insufficient to detoxify chloramphenicol and (2) renal function is insufficient to excrete active drug. Although gray syndrome is usually observed in neonates, it can occur in older children and adults if dosage is excessive. If drug use is discontinued immediately when early symptoms appear, the syndrome is usually reversible. The risk for gray syndrome in infants can be reduced by using low doses and by monitoring chloramphenicol levels in serum.

Reversible Bone Marrow Suppression

Chloramphenicol can produce dose-related suppression of the bone marrow, resulting in anemia, and sometimes leukopenia and thrombocytopenia. Marrow suppression occurs most commonly when plasma drug levels exceed 25 mcg/mL. The cause of bone marrow suppression appears to be inhibition of protein synthesis in host mitochondria. To promote early detection of bone marrow suppression, complete blood counts should be performed before therapy and every 2 days thereafter. Advise patients to notify the prescriber if signs of blood disorders develop (e.g., sore throat, fever, unusual bleeding or bruising). Chloramphenicol should be withdrawn if evidence of bone marrow suppression is detected. Suppression of bone marrow usually reverses within 1 to 3 weeks after drug withdrawal. The anemia associated with toxic bone marrow suppression is not related to aplastic anemia (discussed next).

BLACK BOX WARNING: CHLORAMPHENICOL

Rarely, chloramphenicol produces aplastic anemia, a condition characterized by pancytopenia and bone marrow aplasia. The reaction is usually fatal.

Aplastic Anemia

Aplastic anemia develops in 1 of 35,000 patients and is not related to dosage. As a rule, the reaction develops weeks or months after termination of treatment. Aplastic anemia can occur with oral, IV, or even topical (ophthalmic) use of the drug. The mechanism underlying aplastic anemia has not been determined, but toxicity may result from a genetic predisposition. Unfortunately, aplastic anemia cannot be predicted by monitoring the blood.

Other Adverse Effects

Gastrointestinal effects (vomiting, diarrhea, glossitis) occur occasionally. Neurologic effects (peripheral neuropathy, optic neuritis, confusion, delirium) develop rarely, usually in association with prolonged treatment. Other rare toxicities include superinfection of the bowel, allergic reactions, and fever.

Drug Interactions

Chloramphenicol can inhibit hepatic drug-metabolizing enzymes, thereby prolonging the half-lives of other drugs. Agents that may be affected include phenytoin (an anticonvulsant), warfarin (an anticoagulant), and two oral hypoglycemics: tolbutamide and chlorpropamide. If any of these drugs are taken concurrently with chloramphenicol, their dosages should be reduced.

Preparations, Dosage, and Administration

Chloramphenicol sodium succinate is available as a powder for reconstitution to a 100-mg/mL solution. Administration is by slow IV injection. As a rule, the dosing objective is to produce peak chloramphenicol plasma levels that range between 10 and 20 mcg/mL. The usual IV dosage for adults and children is 12.5 to 25 mg/kg every 6 hours. For infants 7 days old or younger, the usual dosage is 25 mg/kg once a day. For infants more than 7 days old, the recommended dosage is 25 mg/kg every 12 hours. Dosage should be reduced for patients with liver dysfunction.

Tigecycline

Tigecycline [Tygacil] is a first-in-class glycylcycline antibiotic. The drug is a tetracycline derivative designed to overcome drug resistance. Tigecycline is active against a broad spectrum of bacteria, including many drug-resistant strains. Unfortunately, tigecycline is associated with an increased mortality (see later), and hence using another antibiotic drug should be considered.

Mechanism of Action and Resistance

Tigecycline is a bacteriostatic inhibitor of protein synthesis. Like the tetracyclines, tigecycline binds to the 30S ribosomal subunit and thereby inhibits binding of transfer RNA to the messenger RNA–ribosome complex. As a result, addition of amino acids to the growing peptide chain is stopped.

Bacterial resistance to tigecycline is much less than with the tetracyclines. First, bacteria are unable to extrude tigecycline. Second, bacteria cannot block binding of tigecycline to ribosomes.

Antimicrobial Spectrum

Tigecycline is a broad-spectrum antibiotic with activity against gram-positive and gram-negative bacteria, including many strains that are drug resistant. Susceptible gram-positive organisms include *S. aureus* (vancomycin sensitive, methicillin sensitive, and methicillin resistant), vancomycin-resistant enterococci, penicillin-resistant *S. pneumoniae, C. perfringens, and C. difficile*. Susceptible gram-negative organisms include *Acinetobacter baumannii, Stenotrophomonas maltophilia, B. fragilis, Escherichia coli,* and *Enterobacter* species. Of note, tigecycline is not active against *Pseudomonas aeruginosa* or *Proteus* species.

Therapeutic Use

Tigecycline was originally approved only for complicated intraabdominal infections and complicated skin infections that need broad empiric coverage and was later approved for CAP caused by *S. pneumoniae* (penicillin-susceptible isolates). To delay emergence of resistance, tigecycline should be used only when other drugs are considered likely to fail.

Pharmacokinetics

Tigecycline is administered intravenously and undergoes moderate binding to plasma proteins (about 80%). Very little of the drug is metabolized. Excretion occurs in the bile (59%) and urine (33%), mainly as unchanged drug. The plasma half-life is 42 hours.

Adverse Effects

Tigecycline is a tetracycline analog and hence may have adverse effects like those of the tetracyclines. In clinical trials, the most common reactions were nausea and vomiting. Like the tetracyclines, tigecycline may pose a risk for pseudotumor cerebri (a benign elevation of intracranial pressure) and may increase sensitivity to ultraviolet light, thereby increasing the risk for sunburn. Being a broad-spectrum antibiotic, tigecycline may pose a risk for superinfection, including CDAD. Acute pancreatitis, including fatal cases, has occurred during tigecycline treatment. If pancreatitis is suspected, withdrawal of the drug should be considered. Tigecycline is in U.S. Food and Drug Administration (FDA) Pregnancy Risk Category D and hence should be avoided by pregnant women.

BLACK BOX WARNING: TIGECYCLINE

Among patients treated for severe infections, mortality is higher for those receiving tigecycline than for those receiving other antibiotics. Accordingly, the FDA recommends considering an alternative to tigecycline for patients with severe infections.

Drug Interactions

Drug interactions appear minimal. Tigecycline does not affect the cytochrome P450 system and hence will not alter the kinetics of drugs metabolized by P450. Similarly, because tigecycline undergoes very little metabolism, drugs that alter P450 activity should not alter the kinetics of tigecycline. Tigecycline can delay the clearance of warfarin (an anticoagulant). Accordingly, if the drugs are used concurrently, coagulation status should be monitored.

Preparations, Dosage, and Administration

Tigecycline [Tygacil] is supplied as a lyophilized powder in single-dose 50-mg vials, to be reconstituted for IV infusion. Treatment consists of a 100-mg initial dose followed by 50 mg every 12 hours for 5 to 14 days. No adjustment in dosage is needed for patients with renal impairment or with mild to moderate hepatic impairment. For patients with severe hepatic impairment, the initial dose is unchanged, but maintenance dosing should be reduced to 25 mg every 12 hours.

Retapamulin and Mupirocin

Retapamulin and mupirocin are topical antibiotics. Both drugs are indicated for impetigo; mupirocin is also indicated for clearing the nostrils of MRSA. For impetigo therapy, retapamulin is more convenient than mupirocin, but generic mupirocin is cheaper.

Retapamulin

Retapamulin [Altabax] is a first-in-class pleuromutilin antibiotic. The drug binds to the 50S bacterial ribosomal subunit and thereby inhibits protein synthesis. However, the 50S binding site is different from that of other antibiotics, and hence cross-resistance with other antibiotics is not expected. Retapamulin is bacteriostatic at therapeutic concentrations. At this time, the drug is approved only for topical therapy of impetigo caused by *S. pyogenes* or MRSA. However, in vitro data indicate that the drug may be effective against MRSA and mupirocin-resistant *S. aureus.* Significant resistance among *S. aureus* has not been observed and is considered unlikely. The principal adverse effect is local irritation, which only 2% of users experience. Systemic toxicity does not occur, owing to minimal absorption from topical sites. Retapamulin is available as a 1% ointment in 15- and 30-g tubes. Application is done twice daily for 5 days.

Mupirocin

Mupirocin [Bactroban, Bactroban Nasal] is a topical antibiotic with two indications: (1) impetigo caused by *S. aureus, S. pyogenes,* or beta-hemolytic streptococci and (2) elimination of nasal colonization by MRSA. Mupirocin has a unique mechanism: the drug binds with bacterial isoleucyl transfer RNA synthetase and thereby blocks protein synthesis. The drug is bactericidal at therapeutic concentrations. Resistance has developed owing to production of a modified form of isoleucyl transfer RNA synthetase, but cross-resistance with other antibiotics has not been reported.

Adverse effects depend on the application site. With application to the skin, local irritation can occur, but systemic effects occur rarely, if at all. (Absorption from intact skin is minimum, and any absorbed drug undergoes rapid conversion to inactive products.) With intranasal application, the most common side effects are headache, rhinitis, upper respiratory congestion, and pharyngitis.

Mupirocin is available as a 2% cream and a 2% ointment. For impetigo, the cream or ointment is applied 3 times a day for 7 to 14 days. To eradicate MRSA nasal colonization, the ointment is applied twice daily for 5 days.

CHAPTER 72

Aminoglycosides: Bactericidal Inhibitors of Protein Synthesis

Laura D. Rosenthal, DNP, ACNP, FAANP

The aminoglycosides are narrow-spectrum antibiotics used primarily against aerobic gram-negative bacilli. These drugs disrupt protein synthesis, resulting in rapid bacterial death. The aminoglycosides can cause serious injury to the inner ears and kidneys. Because of these toxicities, indications for these drugs are limited. All of the aminoglycosides carry multiple positive charges. As a result, they are not absorbed from the gastrointestinal (GI) tract and must be administered parenterally to treat systemic infections. In the United States seven aminoglycosides are approved for clinical use. The agents employed most commonly are gentamicin, tobramycin, and amikacin.

BASIC PHARMACOLOGY OF THE AMINOGLYCOSIDES

Chemistry

The aminoglycosides are composed of two or more amino sugars connected by a glycoside linkage. At physiologic pH, these drugs are highly polar polycations (i.e., they carry several positive charges) and therefore cannot readily cross membranes. As a result, aminoglycosides are not absorbed from the GI tract, do not enter the cerebrospinal fluid, and are rapidly excreted by the kidneys.

Mechanism of Action

The aminoglycosides disrupt bacterial protein synthesis. As indicated in Fig. 72.1, these drugs bind to the 30S ribosomal subunit, causing (1) inhibition of protein synthesis, (2) premature termination of protein synthesis, and (3) production of abnormal proteins (secondary to misreading of the genetic code).

The aminoglycosides are *bactericidal.* Cell kill is *concentration dependent.* Hence the higher the concentration, the more rapidly the infection will clear. Of note, bactericidal activity persists for several hours *after* serum levels have dropped below the minimal bactericidal concentration, a phenomenon known as the *postantibiotic effect.*

Bacterial kill appears to result from production of abnormal proteins rather than from simple inhibition of protein synthesis. Studies suggest that abnormal proteins become inserted in the bacterial cell membrane, causing it to leak. The resultant loss of cell contents causes death. Inhibition of protein synthesis per se does not seem the likely cause of bacterial death because complete blockade of protein synthesis by other antibiotics (e.g., tetracyclines, chloramphenicol) is usually bacteriostatic—not bactericidal.

Microbial Resistance

The principal cause for bacterial resistance is production of enzymes that can inactivate aminoglycosides. Among gram-negative bacteria, the genetic information needed to synthesize these enzymes is acquired through transfer of R factors. To date, more than 20 different aminoglycoside-inactivating enzymes have been identified. Because each of the aminoglycosides can be modified by more than one of these enzymes, and because each enzyme can act on more than one aminoglycoside, patterns of bacterial resistance can be complex.

Of all the aminoglycosides, *amikacin* is least susceptible to inactivation by bacterial enzymes. As a result, resistance to amikacin is uncommon. To minimize emergence of resistant bacteria, amikacin should be reserved for infections that are unresponsive to other aminoglycosides.

Antimicrobial Spectrum

Bactericidal effects of the aminoglycosides are limited almost exclusively to *aerobic gram-negative bacilli.* Sensitive organisms include *Escherichia coli, Klebsiella pneumoniae, Serratia marcescens, Proteus mirabilis,* and *Pseudomonas aeruginosa.* Aminoglycosides are inactive against most gram-positive bacteria.

Aminoglycosides *cannot kill anaerobes.* To produce antibacterial effects, aminoglycosides must be transported across the bacterial cell membrane, a process that is oxygen dependent. Because, by definition, anaerobic organisms live in the absence of oxygen, these microbes cannot take up aminoglycosides and hence are resistant. For the same reason, aminoglycosides are inactive against facultative bacteria when these organisms are living under anaerobic conditions.

Therapeutic Use

Parenteral Therapy

The principal use for parenteral aminoglycosides is treatment of *serious infections due to aerobic gram-negative bacilli.* Primary target organisms are *P. aeruginosa* and the Enterobacteriaceae (e.g., *E. coli, Klebsiella* and *Serratia* species, *P. mirabilis*).

One aminoglycoside—gentamicin—is now commonly used in combination with either vancomycin or a beta-lactam antibiotic to treat *serious infections with certain gram-positive cocci,* specifically *Enterococcus* species, some streptococci, and *Staphylococcus aureus.*

The aminoglycosides used most commonly for parenteral therapy are gentamicin, tobramycin, and amikacin. Selection among the three depends in large part on patterns of resistance in a given community or hospital. In

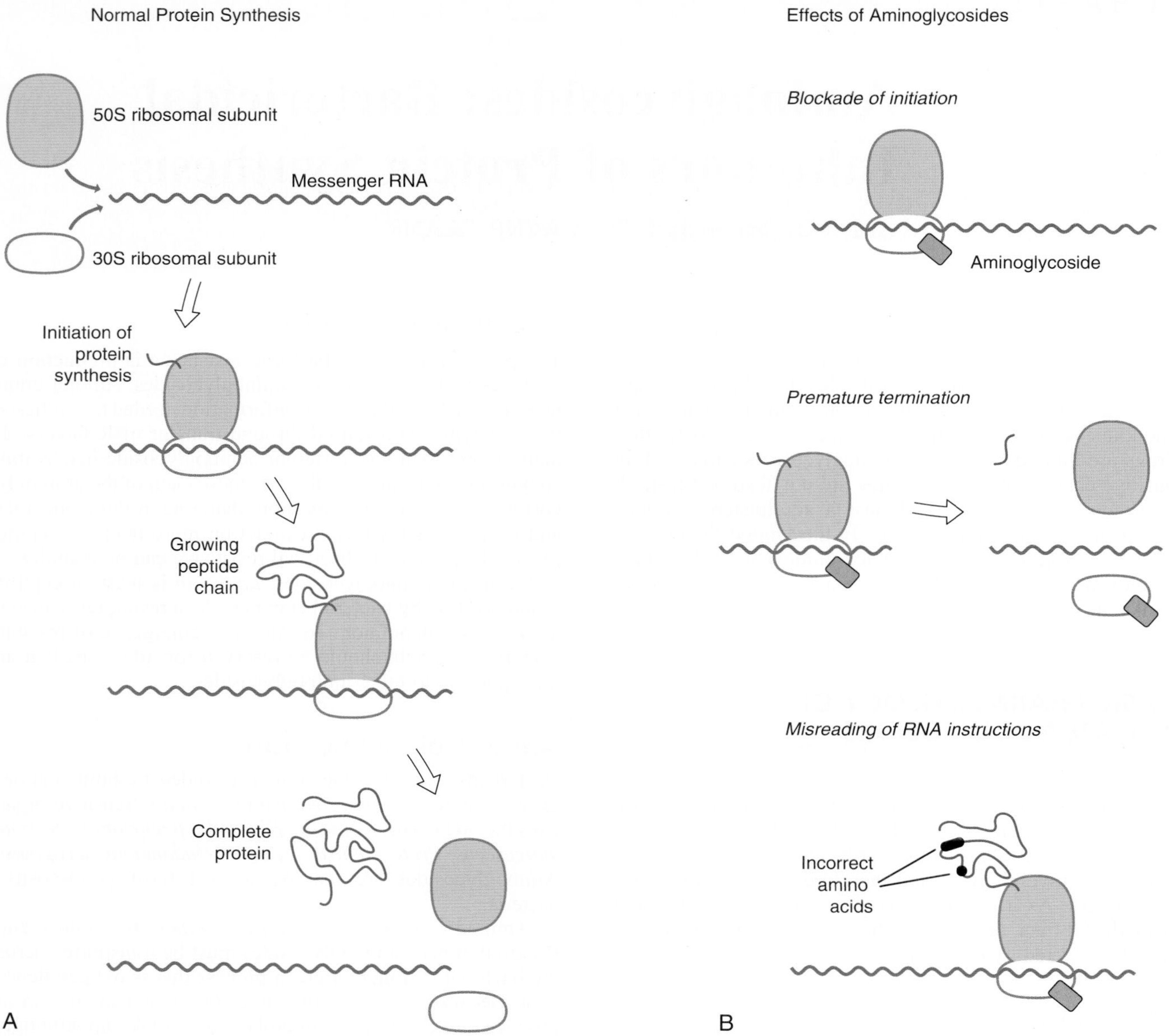

Figure 72.1 ▪ Mechanism of action of aminoglycosides.
A, Protein synthesis begins with binding of the 50S and 30S ribosomal subunits to messenger RNA (mRNA), followed by attachment of the first amino acid of the new protein to the 50S subunit. As the ribosome moves down the mRNA strand, additional amino acids are added to the growing peptide chain. When the new protein is complete, it separates from the ribosome, and the ribosomal subunits separate from the mRNA. **B,** Aminoglycosides bind to the 30S ribosomal subunit and can (1) block initiation, (2) terminate synthesis before the new protein is complete, and (3) cause misreading of the genetic code, which causes synthesis of faulty proteins.

settings where resistance to aminoglycosides is uncommon, either gentamicin or tobramycin is usually preferred. Of the two, gentamicin is less expensive and may be selected on this basis. Organisms resistant to both gentamicin and tobramycin are usually sensitive to amikacin. Accordingly, in settings where resistance to gentamicin and tobramycin is common, amikacin may be preferred for initial therapy.

Oral Therapy

Aminoglycosides are not absorbed from the GI tract, and hence oral therapy is used only for local effects within the intestine. In patients anticipating elective colorectal surgery, oral aminoglycosides have been given prophylactically to suppress bacterial growth in the bowel. One aminoglycoside—paromomycin—is used to treat intestinal amebiasis.

Topical Therapy

Neomycin is available in formulations for application to the eyes, ears, and skin. Topical preparations of gentamicin and tobramycin are used to treat conjunctivitis caused by susceptible gram-negative bacilli.

Pharmacokinetics

All of the aminoglycosides have similar pharmacokinetic profiles. Pharmacokinetic properties of the principal aminoglycosides are shown in Table 72.1.

Absorption

Because they are polycations, the aminoglycosides cross membranes poorly. As a result, very little (about 1%) of an oral dose is absorbed. Hence, for treatment of systemic infections, aminoglycosides must be given parenterally (by intramuscular [IM] or intravenous [IV] route). Absorption after application to the intact skin is minimal. However, when used for wound irrigation, aminoglycosides may be absorbed in amounts sufficient to produce systemic toxicity.

Distribution

Distribution of aminoglycosides is limited largely to extracellular fluid. Entry into the cerebrospinal fluid is insufficient to treat meningitis in adults. Aminoglycosides bind tightly to renal tissue, achieving levels in the kidneys up to 50 times higher than levels in serum. These high levels are responsible for nephrotoxicity (see later). Aminoglycosides penetrate readily to the perilymph and endolymph of the inner ears and can thereby cause ototoxicity (see later). Aminoglycosides can cross the placenta and may be toxic to the fetus.

Elimination

The aminoglycosides are eliminated primarily by the kidneys. These drugs are not metabolized. In patients with normal renal function, half-lives of the aminoglycosides range from 2 to 3 hours. However, because elimination is almost exclusively renal, half-lives increase dramatically in patients with renal impairment. *Accordingly, to avoid serious toxicity, we must reduce dosage size or increase the dosing interval in patients with kidney disease.*

Interpatient Variation

Different patients receiving the same aminoglycoside dosage (in milligrams per kilogram of body weight) can achieve widely different serum levels of drug. This interpatient variation is caused by several factors, including age, percent body fat, and pathophysiology (e.g., renal impairment, fever, edema, dehydration). Because of variability among patients, aminoglycoside dosage must be individualized. As dramatic evidence of this need, in one clinical study it was observed that, to produce equivalent serum drug levels, the doses required ranged from as little as 0.5 mg/kg in one patient to

PATIENT-CENTERED CARE ACROSS THE LIFE SPAN

Aminoglycosides

Life Stage	Patient Care Concerns
Infants	Aminoglycosides are approved to treat bacterial infections in infants younger than 8 days. Dosing is based on weight and length of gestation.
Children/adolescents	Aminoglycosides are safe for use against bacterial infections in children and adolescents.
Pregnant women	There is evidence that use of aminoglycosides in pregnancy can harm the fetus. They are classified in U.S. Food and Drug Administration Pregnancy Risk Category D.
Breastfeeding women	Gentamycin is probably safe to use in lactation. There is limited information regarding its use.
Older adults	Caution must be used regarding decreased renal function in the older adult.

TABLE 72.1 ▪ Dosages and Pharmacokinetics of Systemic Aminoglycosides

Generic Name	Trade Name	Total Daily Dose (mg/kg)[a,b] Adults	Children	Half-Life in Adults (hr) Normal	Anuric	Therapeutic (Peak) Level[c,d] (mcg/mL)	Recommended Trough Level[e,f] (mcg/mL)
Amikacin	Amikin	15	15	2–3	24–60	15–30	Less than 5–10
Gentamicin	Generic only	3–5[g]	6–7.5[g]	2	24–60	4–10[h]	Less than 1–2[i]
Tobramycin	Generic only	3–6	6–7.5	2–2.5	24–60	4–10	Less than 1–2[i]

[a]The total daily dose may be administered as one large dose each day or as two or three divided doses given at equally spaced intervals around-the-clock.
[b]Because of interpatient variability, standard doses cannot be relied on to produce appropriate serum drug levels, and hence dosage should be adjusted on the basis of serum drug measurements.
[c]Measured 30 minutes after IM injection or after completing a 30-minute IV infusion.
[d]The peak values presented refer to levels obtained when the total daily dosage is given in *divided* doses, rather than as a single large daily dose.
[e]Measured just before the next dose.
[f]To minimize ototoxicity and nephrotoxicity, drug levels should drop *below* the listed values between doses.
[g]When gentamicin is combined with either vancomycin or a beta-lactam antibiotic to treat certain gram-positive infections, the total daily dose is much lower (e.g., about 1 mg/kg for adults).
[h]These peak values apply when gentamicin is used to treat gram-negative infections, not when gentamicin is combined with vancomycin or a beta-lactam antibiotic to treat gram-positive infections.
[i]For severe infections, the trough may be higher (e.g., less than 2–4 mcg/mL).

a high of 25.8 mg/kg in another—a difference of more than 50-fold.

Adverse Effects

The aminoglycosides can produce serious toxicity, especially to the inner ears and kidneys. The inner ears and kidneys are vulnerable because aminoglycosides become concentrated within cells of these structures.

Ototoxicity

All aminoglycosides can accumulate within the inner ears, causing cellular injury that can impair both hearing and balance. *Hearing impairment* is caused by damage to sensory hair cells in the *cochlea. Disruption of balance* is caused by damage to sensory hair cells of the *vestibular apparatus.*

The risk for ototoxicity is related primarily to excessive *trough levels*[a] of drug—rather than to excessive *peak* levels. When trough levels remain persistently elevated, aminoglycosides are unable to diffuse out of inner ear cells, and hence the cells are exposed to the drug continuously for an extended time. It is this prolonged exposure, rather than brief exposure to high levels, that underlies cellular injury. In addition to high trough levels, the risk for ototoxicity is increased by (1) renal impairment (which can cause accumulation of aminoglycosides); (2) concurrent use of ethacrynic acid (a drug that has ototoxic properties of its own); and (3) administering aminoglycosides in excessive doses or for more than 10 days.

BLACK BOX WARNING: AMINOGLYCOSIDE NEUROTOXICITY/ OTOTOXICITY

Use of aminoglycosides is associated with irreversible ototoxicity. Neurotoxic symptoms may also include numbness, tingling, muscle twitching, and seizures. This risk increases in patients with use of high doses or prolonged use and in patients with preexisting renal impairment.

Patients on aminoglycoside therapy should be monitored for ototoxicity. The first sign of impending *cochlear* damage is high-pitched tinnitus. Ototoxicity is largely *irreversible.* Accordingly, if permanent injury is to be avoided, aminoglycosides should be withdrawn at the first sign of damage (i.e., tinnitus, persistent headache, or both).

As injury to cochlear hair cells proceeds, hearing in the high-frequency range begins to decline. Loss of low-frequency hearing develops with continued drug use. Because the initial decline in high-frequency hearing is subtle, audiometric testing is needed to detect it. The first sign of impending *vestibular* damage is headache, which may last for 1 or 2 days. After that, nausea, unsteadiness, dizziness, and vertigo begin to appear. Patients should be informed about the symptoms of vestibular and cochlear damage and instructed to report them.

BLACK BOX WARNING: NEPHROTOXICITY

Use of aminoglycosides is associated with nephrotoxicity. This risk increases in patients with use of high doses or prolonged use and in patients with preexisting renal impairment.

[a]The trough serum level is the lowest level between doses. It occurs just before administration of the next dose.

Nephrotoxicity

Aminoglycosides can injure cells of the proximal renal tubules. These drugs are taken up by tubular cells and achieve high intracellular concentrations. Nephrotoxicity correlates with (1) the *total cumulative dose* of aminoglycosides and (2) *high trough levels.* High *peak levels* do not seem to increase toxicity. Aminoglycoside-induced nephrotoxicity usually manifests as acute tubular necrosis. Prominent symptoms are proteinuria, casts in the urine, production of dilute urine, and elevations in serum creatinine and blood urea nitrogen (BUN). Serum creatinine and BUN should be monitored. The risk for nephrotoxicity is especially high in older adults, in patients with preexisting kidney disease, and in patients receiving other nephrotoxic drugs (e.g., amphotericin B, cyclosporine). Fortunately, cells of the proximal tubule readily regenerate. As a result, injury to the kidneys usually reverses after aminoglycoside use.[b] The most significant consequence of renal damage is accumulation of aminoglycosides themselves, which can lead to ototoxicity and even more kidney damage.

BLACK BOX WARNING: AMINOGLYCOSIDE-INDUCED NEUROMUSCULAR BLOCKADE

Aminoglycosides can inhibit neuromuscular transmission, causing flaccid paralysis and potentially fatal respiratory depression. Most episodes of neuromuscular blockade have occurred after intraperitoneal or intrapleural instillation of aminoglycosides.

Neuromuscular Blockade

The risk for paralysis is increased by concurrent use of neuromuscular blocking agents and general anesthetics. Myasthenia gravis is an additional risk. Neuromuscular blockade can be reversed with calcium; IV infusion of a calcium salt (e.g., calcium gluconate) is the treatment of choice. Because of increased prescriber awareness, aminoglycoside-induced neuromuscular blockade is now rare.

Other Adverse Effects

Hypersensitivity reactions (e.g., rash, pruritus, urticaria) occur occasionally. Blood dyscrasias (neutropenia, agranulocytosis, aplastic anemia) are rare. Streptomycin has been associated with neurologic disorders (optic nerve dysfunction, peripheral neuritis, paresthesias of the face and hands). Oral neomycin has caused superinfection of the bowel and intestinal malabsorption. Tobramycin has caused *Clostridium difficile*–associated diarrhea. Topical neomycin can cause contact dermatitis.

Beneficial Drug Interactions

Penicillins

Penicillins and aminoglycosides are frequently employed in combination to enhance bacterial kill. The combination is effective because penicillins disrupt the cell wall and thereby facilitate access of aminoglycosides to their site of action. Unfortunately, when present in high concentrations, penicillins can inactivate aminoglycosides. Therefore *penicillins and aminoglycosides should not be mixed together in the same IV solution.* (Inactivation is not likely to occur after the drugs are in the body because drug concentrations are usually too low for significant chemical interaction.)

[b]If interstitial fibrosis or renal tubular necrosis develops, damage to the kidneys may be permanent.

Cephalosporins and Vancomycin

Like the penicillins, cephalosporins and vancomycin weaken the bacterial cell wall and can thereby act in concert with aminoglycosides to enhance bacterial kill.

Adverse Drug Interactions

Ototoxic Drugs

The risk for injury to the inner ears is significantly increased by concurrent use of *ethacrynic acid,* a loop diuretic that has ototoxic actions of its own. Combining aminoglycosides with two other loop diuretics—furosemide and bumetanide—appears to cause no more ototoxicity than aminoglycosides alone.

Nephrotoxic Drugs

The risk for renal damage is increased by concurrent therapy with other nephrotoxic agents. Additive or potentiative nephrotoxicity can occur with *amphotericin B, cephalosporins, polymyxins, vancomycin,* and *cyclosporine,* as well as with *aspirin* and *other nonsteroidal antiinflammatory drugs (NSAIDs).*

Skeletal Muscle Relaxants

Aminoglycosides can intensify neuromuscular blockade induced by pancuronium and other skeletal muscle relaxants. If aminoglycosides are used with these agents, caution must be exercised to avoid respiratory arrest.

Dosing Schedules

Systemic aminoglycosides may be administered as a single large dose each day or as two or three smaller doses. Traditionally, these drugs have been administered in divided doses, given at equally spaced intervals around-the-clock (e.g., every 8 hours). Today, however, it is common to administer the total daily dose all at once, rather than dividing it up. Several studies have shown that once-daily doses are just as effective as divided doses, and probably safer. Because once-daily dosing is both safe and effective, and because it's easier and cheaper than giving divided doses, once-daily dosing has become the preferred schedule. Keep in mind, however, that this schedule is not appropriate for some patients, including neonates, patients who are pregnant, patients undergoing dialysis, and patients with ascites.

Monitoring Serum Drug Levels

Monitoring serum drug levels provides the best basis for adjusting aminoglycoside dosage. To produce bacterial kill, peak levels must be sufficiently high. To minimize ototoxicity and nephrotoxicity, trough levels must be sufficiently low.

How monitoring is done depends on the dosing schedule employed (i.e., once-daily dosing or use of divided doses). When once-daily dosing is employed, we only need to measure trough levels. As a rule, there is no need to measure peak levels because, when the entire daily dose is given at once, high peak levels are guaranteed. (They're typically 3–4 times those achieved with divided doses.) In contrast, when divided doses are employed, we need to measure both the peak and the trough.

When drawing blood samples for aminoglycoside levels, timing is important. Samples for *peak* levels should be taken 30 minutes after giving an IM injection or after completing a 30-minute IV infusion. Sampling for *trough* levels depends on the dosing schedule. For patients receiving *divided doses,* trough samples should be taken just before the next dose. For patients receiving *once-daily doses,* a single sample can be drawn 1 hour before the next dose. The value should be very low, preferably close to zero.

PROPERTIES OF INDIVIDUAL AMINOGLYCOSIDES

Gentamicin

Therapeutic Use

Gentamicin is used primarily to treat serious infections caused by aerobic gram-negative bacilli. Primary targets are *P. aeruginosa* and the Enterobacteriaceae (e.g., *E. coli, Klebsiella* and *Serratia* species, *P. mirabilis*). In hospitals where resistance is not a problem, gentamicin is often the preferred aminoglycoside for use against these bacteria because gentamicin is cheaper than the alternatives (tobramycin and amikacin). Unfortunately, resistance to gentamicin is increasing, and cross-resistance to tobramycin is common. For infections that are resistant to gentamicin and tobramycin, amikacin is usually effective.

In addition to its use against gram-negative bacilli, gentamicin can be combined with vancomycin, a cephalosporin, or a penicillin to treat serious infections caused by certain gram-positive cocci, namely, *Enterococcus* species, some streptococci, and *S. aureus.*

Adverse Effects and Interactions

Like all other aminoglycosides, gentamicin is toxic to the kidneys and inner ears. Caution must be exercised when combining gentamicin with other nephrotoxic or ototoxic drugs. Gentamicin is inactivated by direct chemical interaction with penicillins, and hence these drugs should not be mixed in the same IV solution.

Preparations, Dosage, and Administration

Treatment of Gram-Negative Infections

Intravenous and Intramuscular. Gentamicin sulfate is supplied in solution (0.8, 0.9, 1, 1.2, 1.4, 1.6, 10, and 40 mg/mL) and as a powder (60, 80, and 100 mg for reconstitution) for IM and IV administration. The dosage for both routes is the same. For adults, the traditional dosing scheme consists of a loading dose (2 mg/kg) followed by doses of 1 to 1.7 mg/kg every 8 hours—for a total of 3 to approximately 5 mg/kg/day. When once-daily dosing is employed, the dosage is 5 mg/kg every 24 hours; no loading dose is needed. For children, the traditional maintenance dosage is 2 to 2.5 mg/kg every 8 hours. In adults and children with renal impairment, the total daily dosage should be reduced. Duration of treatment is usually 7 to 10 days.

Because of substantial interpatient variation, it is desirable to monitor serum drug levels and to adjust dosage accordingly. Peak levels should range between 4 and 10 mcg/mL (for traditional dosing) or between 16 and 24 mcg/mL (for once-daily dosing). As a rule, the trough should not exceed 2 mcg/mL.

Intrathecal. Intrathecal therapy is done with a 2-mg/mL solution devoid of preservatives. The usual dosage for children is 1 to 2 mg once daily. The usual dosage for adults is 4 to 8 mg once daily. For all patients, treatment should continue for 1 day after samples of cerebrospinal fluid become negative for the infecting organism.

Treatment of Gram-Positive Infections

As noted, gentamicin may be combined with vancomycin, a penicillin, or a cephalosporin to treat serious infections caused by *Enterococcus* species, certain streptococci, and *S. aureus*. When gentamicin is used in this way, dosages are much lower than when the drug is used against gram-negative infections. For combination therapy, a typical dosage for adults is 1 mg/kg/day, compared with 3 to 5 mg/kg/day when the drug is used by itself.

Tobramycin

Uses, Adverse Effects, and Interactions

Tobramycin is similar to gentamicin with respect to uses, adverse effects, and interactions. The drug is more active than gentamicin against *P. aeruginosa,* but less active against enterococci and *Serratia* species. Tobramycin is used for patients with cystic fibrosis. Like all other aminoglycosides, tobramycin can injure the inner ears and kidneys. If possible, concurrent therapy with other ototoxic or nephrotoxic drugs should be avoided. Tobramycin may also cause *C. difficile*–associated diarrhea.

Preparations, Dosage, and Administration

Intravenous and Intramuscular

Tobramycin sulfate is supplied in solution (0.8, 1.2, 10, and 40 mg/mL) and as a 1.2-g powder (40 mg/mL after reconstitution) for IM and IV administration. Dosages and serum levels are the same as those given for gentamicin. Ideally, dosages should be individualized to produce peak and trough levels within the ranges shown in Table 72.1. In patients with renal impairment, the total daily dosage should be reduced. Duration of treatment is usually 7 to 10 days.

Nebulization

For patients with cystic fibrosis, tobramycin [TOBI] is available in solution (300 mg/5 mL) for use in a nebulizer. The dosage is 300 mg twice daily administered in a repeating cycle consisting of 28 days of drug use followed by 28 days off.

Amikacin

Uses, Adverse Effects, and Interactions

Amikacin has two outstanding features: (1) of all the aminoglycosides, amikacin is active against the broadest spectrum of gram-negative bacilli and (2) of all the aminoglycosides, amikacin is the least vulnerable to inactivation by bacterial enzymes. Because most aminoglycoside-inactivating enzymes do not affect amikacin, the incidence of bacterial resistance to this agent is lower than with other major aminoglycosides (gentamicin and tobramycin). In hospitals where resistance to gentamicin and tobramycin is common, amikacin is the preferred agent for initial treatment of infections caused by aerobic gram-negative bacilli. However, in settings where resistance to the other aminoglycosides is infrequent, amikacin should be reserved for infections of proven aminoglycoside resistance because this practice will delay emergence of organisms resistant to amikacin. Like all other aminoglycosides, amikacin is toxic to the kidneys and inner ears. Caution should be exercised if amikacin is used in combination with other ototoxic or nephrotoxic drugs.

Preparations, Dosage, and Administration

Amikacin sulfate is available in solution (500 mg/2 mL and 1 g/4 mL) for IM and IV administration. The recommended dosage for adults and children is 15 mg/kg/day administered either (1) as a single daily dose or (2) in equally divided doses given 8 or 12 hours apart. In patients with renal impairment, dosage should be reduced or the dosing interval increased. Dosage adjustments should be based on measurements of serum drug levels. As a rule, duration of treatment should not exceed 10 days.

Other Aminoglycosides

Neomycin

Neomycin is more ototoxic and nephrotoxic than any other aminoglycoside. As a result, neomycin is not used parenterally. Instead, the drug is employed for topical treatment of infections of the eyes, ears, and skin. Neomycin is also administered orally to suppress bowel flora before surgery of the intestine. Because aminoglycosides are not absorbed from the GI tract, oral administration constitutes a local (nonsystemic) use of the drug. Oral neomycin can cause superinfection of the bowel as well as an intestinal malabsorption syndrome.

Kanamycin

Kanamycin is an older aminoglycoside to which bacterial resistance is common. The drug is still active against some gram-negative bacilli, but *Serratia* species and *P. aeruginosa* are resistant. Because of resistance, systemic use of the drug has sharply declined; gentamicin, tobramycin, and amikacin are preferred. Like neomycin, kanamycin is employed to suppress bacterial flora of the bowel before elective colorectal surgery. Kanamycin is supplied in solution for IM and IV use.

Streptomycin

Streptomycin, discovered in 1943, was the first aminoglycoside drug. Although once employed widely, streptomycin has been largely replaced by safer or more effective medications. Streptomycin can be used in combination with other drugs to treat tuberculosis, but newer and safer agents (rifampin, isoniazid, ethambutol) are generally preferred. Streptomycin is also indicated for several uncommon infections (plague, tularemia, brucellosis). When combined with ampicillin or penicillin G, streptomycin may be used for enterococcal endocarditis.

Paromomycin

Paromomycin is an aminoglycoside employed only for local effects within the intestine. The drug is approved for oral therapy of intestinal amebiasis and has been used investigationally against other intestinal parasites. The dosage for amebiasis in adults and children is 8 to 12 mg/kg 3 times daily for 7 days. Principal adverse effects are nausea, cramps, and diarrhea. Paromomycin is supplied in 250-mg capsules.

CHAPTER

73 Sulfonamides and Trimethoprim

Jacqueline Rosenjack Burchum, DNSc, FNP-BC, CNE

The sulfonamides and trimethoprim are broad-spectrum antimicrobials that have closely related mechanisms: they all disrupt the synthesis of tetrahydrofolic acid, a derivative of folic acid or folate. In approaching these drugs, we begin with the sulfonamides, followed by trimethoprim, and then conclude with trimethoprim/sulfamethoxazole, an important fixed-dose combination.

SULFONAMIDES

Sulfonamides were the first drugs available for systemic treatment of bacterial infections. After their introduction in the 1930s, their use produced a sharp decline in morbidity and mortality from susceptible infections. With the advent of penicillin and newer antimicrobial drugs, use of sulfonamides has greatly declined. Nonetheless, the sulfonamides still have important uses, primarily against urinary tract infections (UTIs). With the introduction of trimethoprim/sulfamethoxazole in the 1970s, indications for the sulfonamides expanded.

Basic Pharmacology

Similarities among the sulfonamides are more striking than the differences. Accordingly, rather than focusing on a representative prototype, we will discuss the sulfonamides as a group.

Chemistry

The general structural formula for the sulfonamides is shown in Fig. 73.1. Sulfonamides are structural analogs of *para*-aminobenzoic acid (PABA). The antimicrobial actions of sulfonamides are based on this similarity.

Individual sulfonamides vary greatly with respect to solubility in water. Older sulfonamides had low solubility; therefore they often crystallized out in the urine, causing injury to the kidneys. The sulfonamides in current use are much more water soluble, and hence the risk for renal damage is low.

Mechanism of Action

Sulfonamides are usually bacteriostatic. Accordingly, adequate host defenses are essential for elimination of infection.

Sulfonamides suppress bacterial growth by inhibiting synthesis of tetrahydrofolate, a derivative of *folic acid* (folate). Folate is required by all cells to make DNA, RNA, and proteins. The steps in folate synthesis are shown in Fig. 73.2. Sulfonamides block the step in which PABA is combined with pteridine to form dihydropteroic acid. Because of their structural similarity to PABA, sulfonamides act as competitive inhibitors of this reaction.

If all cells require folate, why don't sulfonamides harm us? The answer lies in how bacteria and mammalian cells acquire folic acid. Bacteria are unable to take up folate from their environment, so they must synthesize folic acid from precursors. In contrast to bacteria, mammalian cells do not manufacture their own folate. Rather, they simply take up folic acid obtained from the diet, using a specialized transport system for uptake. Because mammalian cells use preformed folic acid rather than synthesizing it, sulfonamides are harmless to us.

Microbial Resistance

Many bacterial species have developed resistance to sulfonamides. Resistance is especially high among gonococci, meningococci, streptococci, and shigellae. Resistance may be acquired by spontaneous mutation or by transfer of plasmids that code for antibiotic resistance (R factors). Principal resistance mechanisms are (1) reduced sulfonamide uptake, (2) synthesis of PABA in amounts sufficient to overcome sulfonamide-mediated inhibition of dihydropteroate synthetase, and (3) alteration in the structure of dihydropteroate synthetase such that binding and inhibition by sulfonamides is reduced.

Antimicrobial Spectrum

The sulfonamides are active against a broad spectrum of microbes. Susceptible organisms include gram-positive cocci (including methicillin-resistant *Staphylococcus aureus*), gram-negative bacilli, *Listeria monocytogenes*, actinomycetes (e.g., *Nocardia*), chlamydiae (e.g., *Chlamydia trachomatis*), some protozoa (e.g., *Toxoplasma* species, plasmodia, *Isospora belli*), and two fungi: *Pneumocystis jiroveci* (formerly thought to be *Pneumocystis carinii*) and *Paracoccidioides brasiliensis*.

Therapeutic Uses

Although the sulfonamides were once employed widely, their applications are now limited. Two factors explain why: (1) introduction of bactericidal antibiotics that are less toxic than the sulfonamides and (2) development of sulfonamide resistance. Today, UTI is the principal indication for these drugs.

Urinary Tract Infections

Sulfonamides are often preferred drugs for acute UTIs. About 90% of these infections are due to *Escherichia coli,* a bacterium that is usually sulfonamide sensitive. Of the sulfonamides available, *sulfamethoxazole* (in combination with trimethoprim) is generally favored. Sulfamethoxazole has good solubility in urine and achieves effective concentrations within the urinary tract. UTIs are discussed in Chapter 74.

Other Uses

Sulfonamides are useful drugs for nocardiosis (infection with *Nocardia asteroides*), *Listeria* species infection, and infection with *P. jiroveci.* In addition, sulfonamides are alternatives to doxycycline and erythromycin for infections caused by *C. trachomatis* (trachoma, inclusion conjunctivitis, urethritis, lymphogranuloma venereum). Sulfonamides are used in conjunction with pyrimethamine to treat two protozoal infections: toxoplasmosis and malaria caused by chloroquine-resistant *Plasmodium falciparum*. Topical sulfonamides are used to treat superficial infections of the eyes and to suppress bacterial colonization in burn patients.

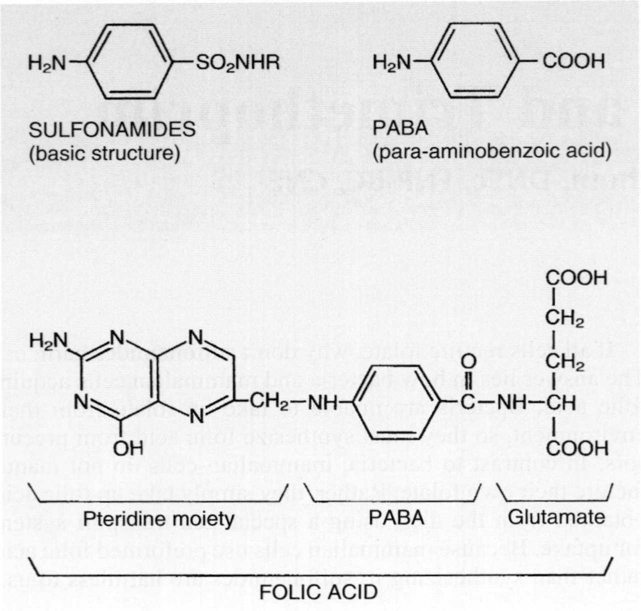

Figure 73.1 ■ Structural relationships among sulfonamides, *para*-aminobenzoic acid (PABA), and folic acid.

One sulfonamide—sulfasalazine—is used to treat ulcerative colitis. However, benefits in this disorder do not result from inhibiting microbial growth. Ulcerative colitis is discussed in Chapter 64.

Pharmacokinetics

Absorption

Sulfonamides are well absorbed after oral administration. When applied topically to the skin or mucous membranes, these drugs may be absorbed in amounts sufficient to cause systemic effects.

Distribution

Sulfonamides are well distributed to all tissues. Concentrations in pleural, peritoneal, ocular, and similar body fluids may be as much as 80% of the concentration in blood. Sulfonamides readily cross the placenta, and levels achieved in the fetus are sufficient to produce antimicrobial effects and toxicity.

Metabolism

Sulfonamides are metabolized in the liver, principally by acetylation. Acetylated derivatives lack antimicrobial activity but are just as toxic as the parent compounds. Acetylation may decrease sulfonamide solubility, thereby increasing the risk for renal damage from crystal formation.

Excretion

Sulfonamides are excreted primarily by the kidneys. Thus the rate of renal excretion is the principal determinant of their half-lives.

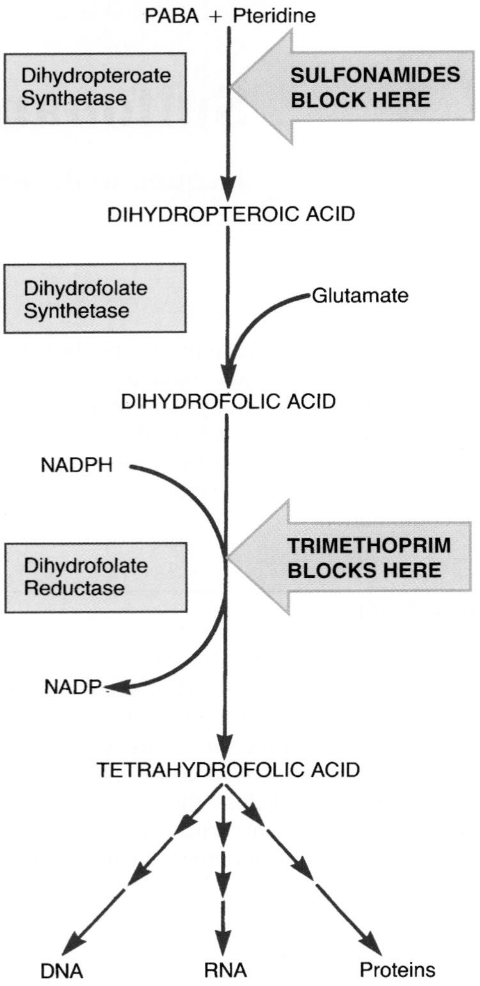

Figure 73.2 ■ Sites of action of sulfonamides and trimethoprim.
Sulfonamides and trimethoprim inhibit sequential steps in the synthesis of tetrahydrofolic acid (FAH_4). In the absence of FAH_4, bacteria are unable to synthesize DNA, RNA, and proteins.

Adverse Effects

Sulfonamides can cause multiple adverse effects. Prominent among these are hypersensitivity reactions, blood dyscrasias, and kernicterus, which occurs in newborns. Renal damage from crystalluria was a problem with older sulfonamides but is less common with the sulfonamides used today.

Hypersensitivity Reactions

Sulfonamides can induce a variety of hypersensitivity reactions, which are seen in about 3% of patients. Mild reactions—rash, drug fever, photosensitivity—are relatively common. To minimize photosensitivity reactions, patients should avoid prolonged exposure to sunlight, wear protective clothing, and apply a sunscreen to exposed skin.

Hypersensitivity reactions are especially frequent with *topical* sulfonamides. As a result, these preparations are no longer employed routinely. Rather, they are usually reserved for ophthalmic infections, burns, and bacterial vaginosis caused by *Gardnerella vaginalis* and a mixed population of anaerobic bacteria.

The most severe hypersensitivity response to sulfonamides is *Stevens-Johnson syndrome,* a rare reaction with a mortality rate of about 25%. Symptoms include widespread lesions of the skin and mucous membranes, combined with fever, malaise, and toxemia. The reaction is most likely to occur with long-acting sulfonamides, which are now banned in the United States. Short-acting sulfonamides may also induce the syndrome, but the incidence is low. To minimize the risk for severe reactions, sulfonamides should be discontinued immediately

Patient Education

SULFONAMIDES

- Instruct patients to complete the prescribed course of treatment, even though symptoms may abate before the full course is over.
- Patients taking oral sulfonamides should drink at least 8 to 10 glasses of water or other noncaffeinated fluids per day. (Caffeine may be taken in addition to other fluids.)
- To avoid photosensitivity reactions, advise patients to avoid prolonged exposure to sunlight, wear protective clothing, and apply a sunscreen to exposed skin. Avoid tanning beds.
- Instruct patients to observe for alterations that may indicate hypersensitivity (e.g., rash) and to report these promptly if they occur.

if skin rash of any sort is observed. In addition, sulfonamides should not be given to patients with a history of hypersensitivity to chemically related drugs, including thiazide diuretics, loop diuretics, and sulfonylurea-type oral hypoglycemics—although the risk for cross-reactivity with these agents is probably low (see later section "Drug Interactions").

Hematologic Effects

Sulfonamides can cause *hemolytic anemia* in patients with glucose-6-phosphate dehydrogenase (G6PD) deficiency. This inherited trait is most common among blacks and people of Mediterranean origin. Rarely, hemolysis occurs in the absence of G6PD deficiency. Red cell lysis can produce fever, pallor, and jaundice; patients should be observed for these signs. In addition to hemolytic anemia, sulfonamides can cause agranulocytosis, leukopenia, thrombocytopenia, and, very rarely, aplastic anemia. When sulfonamides are used for a long time, periodic blood tests should be obtained.

Kernicterus

Kernicterus is a disorder in newborns caused by deposition of bilirubin in the brain. Bilirubin is neurotoxic and can cause severe neurologic deficits and even death. Under normal conditions, infants are not vulnerable to kernicterus. Any bilirubin present in their blood is tightly bound to plasma proteins and therefore is not free to enter the central nervous system (CNS). Sulfonamides promote kernicterus by displacing bilirubin from plasma proteins. Because the blood-brain barrier of infants is poorly developed, the newly freed bilirubin has easy access to sites within the brain. *Because of the risk for kernicterus, sulfonamides should not be administered to infants younger than 2 months. In addition, sulfonamides should not be given to pregnant patients after 32 weeks of gestation or to those who are breastfeeding.*

Renal Damage From Crystalluria

Because of their low solubility, older sulfonamides tended to come out of solution in the urine, forming crystalline aggregates in the kidneys, ureters, and bladder. These aggregates cause irritation and obstruction, sometimes resulting in anuria and even death. Renal damage is uncommon with today's sulfonamides, owing to their increased water solubility. To minimize the risk for renal damage, adults should maintain a daily urine output of at least 1200 mL. This can be accomplished by consuming 8 to 10 glasses of water each day. Because the solubility of sulfonamides is highest at elevated pH, alkalinization of the urine (e.g., with sodium bicarbonate) can further decrease the chances of crystalluria.

Drug Interactions

Metabolism-Related Interactions

Sulfonamides can intensify the effects of warfarin, phenytoin, and sulfonylurea-type oral hypoglycemics (e.g., glipizide, glyburide). The principal mechanism is inhibition of hepatic metabolism. When combined with sulfonamides, these drugs may require a reduction in dosage to prevent toxicity.

Cross-Hypersensitivity

There is concern that people who are hypersensitive to sulfonamide antibiotics may be cross-hypersensitive to other drugs that contain a sulfonamide moiety (e.g., thiazide diuretics, loop diuretics, sulfonylurea-type oral hypoglycemics). However, there are no good data to show that such cross-hypersensitivity actually exists. In fact, clinical experience has shown that patients with documented allergy to sulfonamide antibiotics have taken other sulfonamide drugs without incident. Still, until more is known regarding cross-hypersensitivity, it is best to avoid taking chances unless the benefits of giving a drug are greater than the risks.

PATIENT-CENTERED CARE ACROSS THE LIFE SPAN

Sulfonamides and Trimethoprim

Life Stage	Patient Care Concerns
Infants	Use of sulfonamides in infants younger than 2 months can cause kernicterus, a potentially fatal condition.
Pregnant women	Systemic sulfonamides are classified in U.S. Food and Drug Administration Pregnancy Risk Category D. They may cause birth defects, especially if taken during the first semester. If taken near term, the infant may develop kernicterus.
Breastfeeding women	Sulfonamides are secreted in breast milk. Breastfeeding women should be warned that breastfeeding an infant younger than 2 months can cause kernicterus.
Older adults	Older patients are more likely to experience adverse effects, and, when experienced, the effects are more likely to be severe. Life-threatening effects, including neutropenia, Stevens-Johnsons syndrome, and toxic epidermal necrolysis, occur more frequently in older adults.

Sulfonamide Preparations

The sulfonamides fall into two major categories: (1) systemic sulfonamides and (2) topical sulfonamides. The systemic agents are used more often.

Systemic Sulfonamides

There are two groups of systemic sulfonamides—short acting and intermediate acting. These differ primarily with regard to dosing interval, which is much shorter for the short-acting drugs.

Sulfamethoxazole

Sulfamethoxazole is the only *intermediate-acting* sulfonamide available. The risk for renal damage from crystalluria can be reduced by maintaining adequate hydration. Sulfamethoxazole is not available for use by itself but *is* available in combination with trimethoprim.

Sulfadiazine

Sulfadiazine is a short-acting sulfonamide. Accordingly, if renal damage is to be avoided, high urine flow must be maintained. Sulfadiazine crosses the blood-brain barrier with ease, so it is the best sulfonamide for prophylaxis of meningitis (although nonsulfonamide antibiotics—ciprofloxacin, ceftriaxone, rifampin—are preferred). When combined with pyrimethamine, sulfadiazine is useful against toxoplasmosis.

Topical Sulfonamides

Topical sulfonamides have been associated with a high incidence of hypersensitivity and are not used routinely. The preparations discussed here have proven utility and a relatively low incidence of hypersensitivity.

Sulfacetamide

Sulfacetamide [Bleph-10] is widely used for superficial infections of the eyes (e.g., conjunctivitis, corneal ulcer). The drug may cause blurred vision, sensitivity to bright light, headache, brow ache, and local irritation. Hypersensitivity is rare, but severe reactions have occurred. Accordingly, sulfacetamide should not be used by patients with a history of severe hypersensitivity to sulfonamides, sulfonylureas, or thiazide or loop diuretics. Sulfacetamide is available in a 10% solution for application to the eyes.

In addition to its ophthalmologic use, topical sulfacetamide is used for dermatologic disorders. The drug is available as a 10% solution in lotions, gels, washes, and shampoos for treating seborrheic dermatitis, acne vulgaris, and bacterial infections of the skin.

Silver Sulfadiazine and Mafenide

These sulfonamides are employed to suppress bacterial colonization in patients with second- and third-degree burns. Mafenide [Sulfamylon] acts by the same mechanism as other sulfonamides. In contrast, antibacterial effects of silver sulfadiazine are due primarily to release of free silver—not to the sulfonamide portion of the molecule. Local application of mafenide is frequently painful, but application of silver sulfadiazine is usually pain free. After application, both agents can be absorbed in amounts sufficient to produce systemic effects. Mafenide, but not silver sulfadiazine, is metabolized to a compound that can suppress renal excretion of acid, causing acidosis. Accordingly, patients receiving mafenide should be monitored for acid-base status. If acidosis becomes severe, mafenide should be discontinued for 1 to 2 days. Silver sulfadiazine [Silvadene, Thermazene, SSD Cream, Flamazine ♣] can cause a blue-green or gray skin discoloration, so facial application should be avoided. A Cochrane review questioned the ability of silver sulfadiazine to promote healing but noted that quality research studies were lacking.

TRIMETHOPRIM

Like the sulfonamides, trimethoprim [Primsol] suppresses synthesis of tetrahydrofolic acid. Trimethoprim is active against a broad spectrum of microbes.

Mechanism of Action

Trimethoprim *inhibits dihydrofolate reductase,* the enzyme that converts dihydrofolic acid to its active form: tetrahydrofolic acid (see Fig. 73.2). Thus, like the sulfonamides, trimethoprim suppresses bacterial synthesis of DNA, RNA, and proteins. Depending on conditions at the site of infection, trimethoprim may be bactericidal or bacteriostatic.

Although mammalian cells also contain dihydrofolate reductase, trimethoprim is selectively toxic to bacteria because bacterial dihydrofolate reductase differs in structure from mammalian dihydrofolate reductase. As a result, trimethoprim inhibits the bacterial enzyme at concentrations about 40,000 times lower than those required to inhibit the mammalian enzyme. This allows suppression of bacterial growth with doses that have essentially no effect on the host.

Microbial Resistance

Bacteria acquire resistance to trimethoprim in three ways: (1) synthesizing increased amounts of dihydrofolate reductase, (2) producing an altered dihydrofolate reductase that has a low affinity for trimethoprim, and (3) reducing cellular permeability to trimethoprim. Resistance has resulted from spontaneous mutation and from transfer of R factors. In the United States bacterial resistance is uncommon.

Antimicrobial Spectrum

Trimethoprim is active against most enteric gram-negative bacilli of clinical importance, including *E. coli, Klebsiella pneumoniae, Proteus mirabilis, Serratia marcescens,* and *Salmonella* and *Shigella* species. The drug is also active against some gram-positive bacilli (e.g., *Corynebacterium diphtheriae, L. monocytogenes*), as well as some pathogenic protozoa (e.g., *Toxoplasma gondii)* and one fungus (*P. jiroveci*).

Therapeutic Uses

Trimethoprim is approved only for initial therapy of acute, uncomplicated UTIs due to susceptible organisms (e.g., *E. coli, P. mirabilis, K. pneumoniae, Enterobacter* species, and coagulase-negative *Staphylococcus* species, including *S. saprophyticus*). When combined with sulfamethoxazole, trimethoprim has considerably more applications, as discussed later.

Patient Education

TRIMETHOPRIM

- Inform patients about early signs of blood dyscrasias (e.g., sore throat, fever, pallor) and instruct them to report these promptly if they occur.

Pharmacokinetics

Trimethoprim is absorbed rapidly and completely from the gastrointestinal (GI) tract. The drug is lipid soluble, and therefore undergoes wide distribution to body fluids and tissues. Trimethoprim readily crosses the placenta. Most of an administered dose is excreted unchanged in the urine. Hence, in the presence of renal impairment, the drug's half-life is prolonged. The concentration of trimethoprim achieved in urine is considerably higher than the concentration in blood.

Adverse Effects and Interactions

Trimethoprim is generally well tolerated. The most frequent adverse effects are itching and rash. GI reactions (e.g., epigastric distress, nausea, vomiting, glossitis, stomatitis) occur occasionally.

Hematologic Effects

Because mammalian dihydrofolate reductase is relatively insensitive to trimethoprim, toxicities related to impaired tetrahydrofolate production are rare. These rare effects—*megaloblastic anemia, thrombocytopenia,* and *neutropenia*—occur only in individuals with preexisting folic acid deficiency. Accordingly, caution is needed when administering trimethoprim to patients in whom folate deficiency might be likely (e.g., alcoholics, pregnant women, debilitated patients). If early signs of bone marrow suppression occur (e.g., sore throat, fever, pallor), complete blood counts should be performed. If a significant reduction in blood cell counts is observed, trimethoprim should be discontinued. Administering leucovorin will restore normal hematopoiesis.

Hyperkalemia

Trimethoprim suppresses renal excretion of potassium and can thereby promote hyperkalemia. Patients at greatest risk are those taking high doses, those with renal impairment, and those taking other drugs that can elevate potassium, including angiotensin-converting enzyme (ACE) inhibitors, angiotensin receptor blockers (ARBs), potassium-sparing diuretics, aldosterone antagonists, and potassium supplements. Patients older than 65 years who are taking an ACE inhibitor or ARB are at especially high risk. Risk can be reduced by checking serum potassium, preferably 4 days after starting treatment (hyperkalemia typically develops within 5 days of starting treatment).

Effects in Pregnancy and Lactation

Large doses of trimethoprim have caused fetal malformations in animals. To date, developmental abnormalities have not been observed in humans. Nonetheless, because trimethoprim readily crosses the placenta, prudence dictates avoiding routine use during pregnancy. The risk for exacerbating pregnancy-related folate deficiency is an additional reason to avoid the drug.

Trimethoprim is excreted in breast milk and may interfere with folic acid utilization by the nursing infant. Administer with caution to women who are breastfeeding.

TRIMETHOPRIM/SULFAMETHOXAZOLE

Trimethoprim (TMP) and sulfamethoxazole (SMZ) are marketed together in a fixed-dose combination product. This combination (TMP/SMZ or one of the variations: TMP/SMX, SMZ/TMP, SMX/TMP) is a powerful antimicrobial preparation whose components act in concert to inhibit sequential steps in tetrahydrofolic acid synthesis. Trade names for TMP/SMZ are *Bactrim* and *Septra.* In many countries, the combination is known generically as *co-trimoxazole.*

Mechanism of Action

The antimicrobial effects of TMP/SMZ result from inhibiting consecutive steps in the synthesis of tetrahydrofolic acid: SMZ acts first to inhibit incorporation of PABA into folic acid; TMP then inhibits dihydrofolate reductase, the enzyme that converts dihydrofolic acid into tetrahydrofolate (see Fig. 73.2). As a result, the ability of the target organism to make nucleic acids and proteins is greatly suppressed. By inhibiting two reactions required for synthesis of tetrahydrofolate, TMP and SMZ potentiate each other's effects. That is, the antimicrobial effect of the combination is more powerful than the sum of the effects of TMP alone plus SMZ alone. TMP/SMZ is selectively toxic to microbes because (1) mammalian cells use preformed folic acid and therefore are not affected by SMZ and (2) dihydrofolate reductases of mammalian cells are relatively insensitive to inhibition by TMP.

Microbial Resistance

Resistance to TMP/SMZ is less than to either drug alone. This is logical in that the chances of an organism acquiring resistance to both drugs are less than its chances of developing resistance to just one or the other.

Antimicrobial Spectrum

TMP/SMZ is active against a wide range of gram-positive and gram-negative bacteria. This should be no surprise in that TMP and SMZ by themselves are broad-spectrum antimicrobial drugs. About 80% of urinary tract pathogens are susceptible. Specific bacteria against which TMP/SMZ is consistently effective include *E. coli, P. mirabilis, L. monocytogenes, S. aureus* (including methicillin-resistant isolates), *C. trachomatis, Salmonella typhi, Shigella* species, *Vibrio cholerae, Haemophilus influenzae,* and *Yersinia pestis*. TMP/SMZ is also active against *Nocardia* species, certain protozoa (e.g., *T. gondii*), and two fungi (*P. jiroveci* and *P. brasiliensis*).

Therapeutic Uses

TMP/SMZ is a preferred or alternative medication for a variety of infectious diseases. The combination is especially valuable for UTIs, otitis media, bronchitis, shigellosis, and pneumonia caused by *P. jiroveci.*

Urinary Tract Infections

TMP/SMZ is indicated for treatment of uncomplicated UTIs caused by susceptible strains of *E. coli, Klebsiella* and *Enterobacter* species, *P. mirabilis, Proteus vulgaris,* and *Morganella morganii.* The combination is particularly useful for chronic and recurrent infections.

Pneumocystis Pneumonia (PCP)

TMP/SMZ is the treatment of choice for PCP, an infection caused by *P. jiroveci,* formerly thought to be *Pneumocystis carinii. P. jiroveci* is an opportunistic fungus that thrives in immunocompromised hosts (e.g., cancer patients, organ transplant recipients, individuals with AIDS). When given to AIDS patients, TMP/SMZ produces a high incidence of adverse effects.

Gastrointestinal Infections

TMP/SMZ is a drug of choice for infections caused by several gram-negative bacilli, including *Yersinia enterocolitica* and *Aeromonas* species. In addition, the combination is a preferred treatment for shigellosis caused by susceptible strains of *Shigella flexneri* and *S. sonnei.*

Other Infections

TMP/SMZ can be used for otitis media and acute exacerbations of chronic bronchitis when these infections are due to susceptible strains of *H. influenzae* or *Streptococcus pneumoniae*. The preparation is also useful against urethritis and pharyngeal infection caused by penicillinase-producing Neisseria gonorrhoeae. Other infections that can be treated with TMP/SMZ include whooping cough, nocardiosis, brucellosis, melioidosis, listeriosis, and chancroid.

Pharmacokinetics

Absorption and Distribution

TMP/SMZ may be administered orally or by IV infusion. Both components of TMP/SMZ are well distributed throughout the body. Therapeutic concentrations are achieved in tissues and body fluids (e.g., vaginal secretions, cerebrospinal fluid, pleural effusions, bile, aqueous humor). Both TMP and SMZ readily cross the placenta, and both enter breast milk.

Plasma Drug Levels

Optimal antibacterial effects are produced when the ratio of TMP to SMZ is 1:20. To achieve this ratio in plasma, TMP and SMZ must be administered in a ratio of 1:5. Hence standard tablets contain 80 mg of TMP and 400 mg of SMZ. Because the plasma half-lives of TMP and SMZ are similar (10 hours for TMP and 11 hours for SMZ), levels of both drugs decline in parallel, and the 1 : 20 ratio is maintained as the drugs are eliminated.

Elimination

Both TMP and SMZ are excreted primarily by the kidneys. About 70% of urinary SMZ is present as inactive metabolites. In contrast, TMP undergoes little metabolism before excretion. Both agents are concentrated in the urine; therefore levels of active drug are higher in the urine than in plasma, despite some conversion to inactive products.

Adverse Effects

TMP/SMZ is generally well tolerated; toxicity from routine use is rare. The most common adverse effects are nausea, vomiting, and rash. However, although infrequent, all of the serious toxicities associated with sulfonamides alone and trimethoprim alone can occur with TMP/SMZ. Like sulfonamides, the combination can cause the following:

- Hypersensitivity reactions (including Stevens-Johnson syndrome)
- Blood dyscrasias (hemolytic anemia, agranulocytosis, leukopenia, thrombocytopenia, aplastic anemia)
- Kernicterus in neonates
- Renal damage

And like trimethoprim, the combination can cause the following:

- Megaloblastic anemia (but only in patients who are folate deficient)
- Hyperkalemia (especially in patients on high doses, in those with renal impairment, and in those taking other drugs that can raise potassium levels)
- Birth defects (especially during the first trimester)

TMP/SMZ may also cause adverse CNS effects (headache, depression, hallucinations). Patients suffering from AIDS are unusually susceptible to TMP/SMZ toxicity. In this group, the incidence of adverse effects (rash, recurrent fever, leukopenia) is about 55%.

Several measures can reduce the incidence and severity of adverse effects. Crystalluria can be avoided by maintaining adequate hydration. Periodic blood tests permit early detection of hematologic disorders. To avoid kernicterus, TMP/SMZ should be withheld from pregnant patients near term, nursing mothers, and infants younger than 2 months. To avoid possible birth defects, TMP/SMZ should be withheld during the first trimester. The risk for megaloblastic anemia can be reduced by withholding sulfonamides from individuals likely to be folate deficient (e.g., debilitated patients, pregnant patients, alcoholics). Hypersensitivity reactions can be minimized by avoiding TMP/SMZ in patients with a history of hypersensitivity to sulfonamides or to chemically related drugs, including thiazide diuretics, loop diuretics, and sulfonylurea-type oral hypoglycemics. Injury from hyperkalemia can be reduced by checking serum potassium and by exercising caution in patients taking other drugs that can elevate potassium.

Drug Interactions

Interactions of TMP/SMZ with other drugs are due primarily to the presence of SMZ. Consequently, like sulfonamides used alone, SMZ in the combination can intensify the effects of warfarin, phenytoin, and sulfonylurea-type oral hypoglycemics (e.g., glipizide). Accordingly, when these drugs are combined with TMP/SMZ, a reduction in their dosage may be needed. TMP/SMZ may also intensify bone marrow suppression in patients receiving methotrexate. As noted, drugs that raise potassium levels can increase the risk for hyperkalemia from TMP.

PRESCRIBING AND MONITORING CONSIDERATIONS FOR SULFONAMIDES

Sulfonamides (Systemic)

The nursing implications summarized here apply only to systemic sulfonamides. Implications specific to topical sulfonamides are not summarized. Dosage and administration are provided in Table 73.1.

Assessment

Therapeutic Goal

Sulfonamides are used primarily for UTIs caused by *E. coli* and other susceptible organisms. Additional indications for TMP/SMZ include shigellosis and PCP.

Identifying High-Risk Patients

Sulfonamides are *contraindicated* for nursing mothers, pregnant women in the first trimester and near term, and infants younger than 2 months. In addition, sulfonamides are contraindicated for patients with a history of severe hypersensitivity to sulfonamides and chemically related drugs, including thiazide diuretics, loop diuretics, and sulfonylurea-type oral hypoglycemics.

Exercise *caution* in patients with renal impairment. They may cause significant hemolysis if prescribed to patients with G6PD deficiency.

In patients with renal impairment (creatinine clearance of 15–30 mL/min), decrease dosage by 50%. If creatinine clearance falls below 15 mL/min, discontinue drug use.

Trimethoprim is *contraindicated* in patients with folate deficiency. If giving TMP/SMZ, it may be important to assess for megaloblastic anemia. This type of anemia is characterized by erythrocytes that have a larger than normal size (elevated mean corpuscular volume).

Metabolism-Related Interactions

Sulfonamides can intensify the effects of *warfarin, phenytoin,* and *sulfonylurea-type oral hypoglycemics* (e.g., glipizide). When combined with sulfonamides, these drugs may require a reduction in dosage

Ongoing Monitoring and Interventions

Hypersensitivity Reactions

Sulfonamides can induce severe hypersensitivity reactions (e.g., Stevens-Johnson syndrome). Assess for early signs of hypersensitivity reaction.

TABLE 73.1 ■ Dosages and Administration

Generic Name	Trade Name	Dosage	Administration
ORAL SULFONAMIDES			
Sulfadiazine	Generic only	Adults: 2–4 g initially, followed by 2–4 g every 24 hours, given as three to six divided doses Children >2 months: *Initial:* 75 mg/kg/day divided into 4–6 doses *Maintenance:* 150 mg/kg (or 4 g/m^2) per day (6 g max.), given as 4–6 divided doses	May be given with or without food. Giving with vitamin C or acidifying drinks such as cranberry juice may increase the risk for crystalluria.
Sulfamethoxazole (+ trimethoprim)	Bactrim, Bactrim DS, Septra, Sulfatrim, Trisulfa ♣	Adults: 800 mg SMZ/160 mg TMP tablets every 12–24 hours × 10–14 days* Children >2 months (based on trimethoprim [TMP]): 4 mg TMP/kg every 12 hours. May be increased to 20 mg TMP/kg/day	Should be taken with a full glass of water May be taken with or without food
TOPICAL SULFONAMIDES			
Silver sulfadiazine	Silvadene, Thermazene, Flamazine ♣	Apply a thin layer to affected skin 1–2 times/day	Do not use on the face; may cause a blue-green or gray discoloration
Mafenide	Sulfamylon	Apply a thin layer to affected skin 1–2 times/day	Cream should cover the burned area at all times. If dressings are used, only a thin, nonocclusive dressing should be used.
Sulfacetamide ophthalmic	Bleph-10, Diosulf ♣, Sodium Sulamyd ♣	Solution: 1–2 drops every 2–3 hours Ointment: ½ inch every 3–4 hours	When tapering off, increase time interval between doses.
TRIMETHOPRIM			
Trimethoprim	Primsol	Adults: 100 mg every 12 hours or 200 mg every 24 hours × 10 days Children >2 months: 4–12 mg/kg/day divided into two 12-hour doses.	Administer with food or milk.

*Dosing is for most infections. Dosing for specific conditions (e.g., shigellosis) and for PCP prophylaxis in patients with AIDS varies.
SMZ, sulfamethoxazole; TMP, trimethoprim

Photosensitivity

Photosensitivity reactions may occur. Observe for evidence of sunburn and reinforce teaching, as necessary.

Hematologic Effects

Sulfonamides can cause hemolytic anemia and other blood dyscrasias (agranulocytosis, leukopenia, thrombocytopenia, aplastic anemia). Observe patients for signs of hemolysis (fever, pallor, jaundice). When sulfonamide therapy is prolonged, periodic blood cell counts should be made.

Renal Damage

Deposition of sulfonamide crystals can injure the kidneys. To minimize crystalluria, it is necessary to maintain hydration sufficient to produce a daily urine flow of 1200 mL in adults. Therefore it is important to ensure that the patient is both able and willing to consume adequate fluid if this drug will be prescribed for other than topical use.

Metabolism-Related Interactions

Sulfonamides can intensify the effects of *warfarin, phenytoin,* and *sulfonylurea-type oral hypoglycemics* (e.g., glipizide). It is important to monitor for increased effects of these drugs and make dosage adjustments accordingly.

Cross-Hypersensitivity

People who are hypersensitive to sulfonamide antibiotics may also be hypersensitive to chemically related drugs—*thiazide diuretics, loop diuretics,* and *sulfonylurea-type oral hypoglycemics*—as well as to *penicillins* and other drugs that induce allergic reactions. Monitor for early evidence of a reaction and select a different drug for management, if needed.

PRESCRIBING AND MONITORING CONSIDERATIONS FOR TRIMETHOPRIM

Assessment

Therapeutic Goal

Initial treatment of uncomplicated UTIs caused by *E. coli* and other susceptible organisms.

Identifying High-Risk Patients

Trimethoprim is *contraindicated* in patients with folate deficiency (manifested as megaloblastic anemia). When possible, the drug should be avoided during pregnancy and lactation.

Patients with renal dysfunction require a reduced dosage.

Ongoing Monitoring and Interventions

Hematologic Effects

Trimethoprim can cause blood dyscrasias (megaloblastic anemia, thrombocytopenia, neutropenia) by exacerbating preexisting folic acid deficiency. Avoid trimethoprim when folate deficiency is likely (e.g., in alcoholics, pregnant women, debilitated patients). Complete blood counts should be performed. If a significant reduction in counts is observed, discontinue trimethoprim. Normal hematopoiesis can be restored with leucovorin.

Hyperkalemia

Trimethoprim can cause hyperkalemia, especially in patients taking high doses, patients with renal impairment, and patients taking ACE inhibitors, ARBs, potassium-sparing diuretics, aldosterone antagonists, and potassium supplements. Risk can be reduced by checking serum potassium 4 days after starting treatment and by exercising caution in patients taking other drugs that can elevate potassium.

CHAPTER

74

Drug Therapy of Urinary Tract Infections

Laura D. Rosenthal, DNP, ACNP, FAANP

Urinary tract infections (UTIs) are one of the most common infections encountered today. In the United States UTIs account for more than 7 million visits to health care providers each year. Among sexually active younger women, 25% to 35% develop at least one UTI a year. Among older women in nursing homes, between 30% and 50% have bacteriuria at any given time. UTIs occur much less frequently in males but are more likely to be associated with complications (e.g., septicemia, pyelonephritis).

Infections may be limited to bacterial colonization of the urine, or bacteria may invade tissues of the urinary tract. When bacteria invade tissues, characteristic inflammatory syndromes result: *urethritis*, *cystitis*, *pyelonephritis*, and *prostatitis*.

UTIs may be classified according to their location, in either the lower urinary tract (bladder and urethra) or upper urinary tract (kidney). Within this classification scheme, *cystitis* and *urethritis* are considered *lower tract infections,* whereas *pyelonephritis* is considered an *upper tract infection.*

UTIs are referred to as *complicated* or *uncomplicated. Complicated* UTIs occur in both males and females and are associated with some predisposing factor, such as calculi, prostatic hypertrophy, an indwelling catheter, or an impediment to the flow of urine (e.g., physical obstruction). *Uncomplicated* UTIs occur primarily in women of childbearing age and are not associated with any particular predisposing factor.

Several classes of antibiotics are used to treat UTIs. Among these are sulfonamides, trimethoprim, penicillins, aminoglycosides, cephalosporins, fluoroquinolones, and two urinary tract antiseptics: nitrofurantoin and methenamine. With the exception of the urinary tract antiseptics, these drugs are discussed in other chapters. The basic pharmacology of the urinary tract antiseptics is introduced here.

ORGANISMS THAT CAUSE URINARY TRACT INFECTIONS

The bacteria that cause UTIs differ between community-associated infections and hospital-associated infections. Most (more than 80%) uncomplicated, community-associated UTIs are caused by *Escherichia coli.* Rarely, other gram-negative bacilli—*Klebsiella pneumoniae* and *Enterobacter, Proteus, Providencia,* and *Pseudomonas* species—are the cause. Gram-positive cocci, especially *Staphylococcus saprophyticus,* account for 10% to 15% of community-associated infections. Hospital-associated UTIs are frequently caused by *Klebsiella, Proteus, Enterobacter* and *Pseudomonas* species, staphylococci, and enterococci; *E. coli* is responsible for less than 50% of these infections. Although most UTIs involve only one organism, infection with multiple organisms may occur, especially in patients with an indwelling catheter, renal stones, or chronic renal abscesses.

SPECIFIC URINARY TRACT INFECTIONS AND THEIR TREATMENT

In this section, we consider the characteristics and treatment of the major UTIs: acute cystitis, acute urethral syndrome, acute pyelonephritis, acute bacterial prostatitis, and recurrent UTIs. Most of these can be treated with oral therapy at home. The principal exception is severe pyelonephritis, which requires intravenous (IV) therapy in a hospital. Drugs and dosages for outpatient therapy in nonpregnant women are shown in Table 74.1.

Acute Cystitis

Acute cystitis is a lower UTI that occurs most often in women of childbearing age. Clinical manifestations are dysuria, urinary urgency, urinary frequency, suprapubic discomfort, pyuria, and bacteriuria (more than 100,000 bacteria per milliliter of urine). It is important to note that many women (30% or more) with symptoms of acute cystitis also have asymptomatic upper UTI (subclinical pyelonephritis). In uncomplicated, community-associated cystitis, the principal causative organisms are *E. coli* (80%), *S. saprophyticus* (11%), and *Enterococcus faecalis.*

For community-associated infections, three types of oral therapy can be employed: (1) single-dose therapy; (2) short-course therapy (3 days); and (3) conventional therapy (7 days). *Single-dose* therapy and *short-course* therapy are recommended only for uncomplicated, community-associated infections in women who are not pregnant and whose symptoms began less than 7 days before starting treatment. As a rule, short-course therapy is more effective than single-dose therapy and hence is generally preferred. Advantages of short-course therapy over conventional therapy are lower cost, greater adherence, fewer side effects, and less potential for promoting emergence of bacterial resistance. *Conventional* therapy is indicated for all patients who do not meet the criteria for short-course therapy. Among these are males, children, pregnant women, and women with suspected upper tract involvement.

Several drugs can be used for treatment (see Table 74.1). For uncomplicated cystitis, trimethoprim/sulfamethoxazole and nitrofurantoin are drugs of first choice. In communities

TABLE 74.1 ■ Regimens for Oral Therapy of Urinary Tract Infections in Nonpregnant Women

Drug	Dose	Duration
ACUTE CYSTITIS		
First-Line Drugs		
Trimethoprim/ sulfamethoxazole	160/800 mg 2 times/day	3 days
Nitrofurantoin (monohydrate/ macrocrystals)	100 mg 2 times/day	5 days
Fosfomycin	3 g once	1 day
Second-Line Drugs		
Ciprofloxacin	250 mg 2 times/day	3 days
Levofloxacin	250 mg once daily	3 days
ACUTE UNCOMPLICATED PYELONEPHRITIS		
First-Line Drugs		
Trimethoprim/ sulfamethoxazole	160/800 mg 2 times/day	14 days
Ciprofloxacin	250–500 mg 2 times/day	7–14 days
Levofloxacin	250 mg once daily*	5–10 days
Second-Line Drugs		
Amoxicillin (with clavulanic acid)	500 mg 3 times/day	10–14 days
Cephalexin	500 mg 4 times/day	10–14 days
Cefotaxime	1 g 3 times/day	10–14 days
Ceftriaxone	1–2 g once daily	10–14 days
COMPLICATED URINARY TRACT INFECTIONS		
Trimethoprim/ sulfamethoxazole	160/800 mg 2 times/day	7–14 days
Ciprofloxacin	500 mg 2 times/day	5–14 days
Levofloxacin	750 mg once daily	5–14 days
Amoxicillin (with clavulanic acid)	500 mg 3 times/day	7–14 days
Cephalexin	500 mg 3 times/day	7–14 days
PROPHYLAXIS OF RECURRENT INFECTIONS		
Trimethoprim/ sulfamethoxazole	40/200 mg† at bedtime 3 times/wk	6 months
Trimethoprim	100 mg at bedtime	6 months
Nitrofurantoin	50–100 mg at bedtime	6 months

*For infection due to *Escherichia coli* without concurrent bacteremia.
†Half of a single-strength tablet.

where resistance to these drugs exceeds 20%, the fluoroquinolones (e.g., ciprofloxacin, norfloxacin) are good alternatives. When adherence is a concern, fosfomycin, which requires just one dose, is a good choice. Beta-lactam antibiotics (e.g., amoxicillin; cephalexin and other cephalosporins) should be avoided because they are less effective than the alternatives, and less well tolerated.

Acute Uncomplicated Pyelonephritis

Acute uncomplicated pyelonephritis is an infection of the kidneys. The disorder is common in young children, older adults, and women of childbearing age. Clinical manifestations include fever, chills, severe flank pain, dysuria, urinary frequency, urinary urgency, pyuria, and, usually, bacteriuria (more than 100,000 bacteria per milliliter of urine). *E. coli* is the causative organism in 90% of initial community-associated infections.

Mild to moderate infection can be treated at home with oral antibiotics. Preferred options are trimethoprim/ sulfamethoxazole, trimethoprim alone, ciprofloxacin, and levofloxacin. Treatment should last 14 days.

Severe pyelonephritis requires hospitalization and IV antibiotics. Options include ciprofloxacin, ceftriaxone, ceftazidime, ampicillin plus gentamicin, and ampicillin/sulbactam. After the infection has been controlled with IV antibiotics, a switch to oral antibiotics should be made, usually within 24 to 48 hours.

Complicated Urinary Tract Infections

Complicated UTIs occur in males and females who have a structural or functional abnormality of the urinary tract that predisposes them to developing infection. Such predisposing factors include prostatic hypertrophy, renal calculi, nephrocalcinosis, renal or bladder tumors, ureteric stricture, or an indwelling urethral catheter. Symptoms of complicated UTIs can range from mild to severe. Some patients even develop systemic illness, manifesting as fever, bacteremia, and septic shock.

The microbiology of complicated UTIs is less predictable than that of uncomplicated UTIs. Although *E. coli* is a common pathogen, it is by no means the only one. Other possibilities include *Klebsiella, Proteus, Pseudomonas, Enterobacter*, *Serratia*, and even *Candida* species, as well as *Staphylococcus aureus*. Accordingly, if treatment is to succeed, we must determine the identity and drug sensitivity of the causative organism. To do so, urine for microbiologic testing should be obtained *before* giving any antibiotics. If symptoms are relatively mild, treatment should wait until test results are available. However, if symptoms are severe, immediate treatment with a broad-spectrum antibiotic can be instituted. After test results are known, a drug specific to the pathogen can be substituted. Duration of treatment ranges from 7 days (for cystitis) to 14 days (for pyelonephritis or when there is systemic involvement).

Recurrent Urinary Tract Infection

Recurrent UTIs result from *relapse* or from *reinfection. Relapse* is caused by recolonization with the same organism responsible for the initial infection. In contrast, *reinfection* is caused by colonization with a new organism.

Reinfection

More than 80% of recurrent UTIs in females are due to reinfection. These usually involve the lower urinary tract and may be related to sexual intercourse or use of a contraceptive diaphragm. If reinfections are *infrequent* (only one or two a year), each episode should be treated as a separate infection. Single-dose or short-course therapy can be used.

When reinfections are *frequent* (three or more a year), long-term prophylaxis may be indicated. Prophylaxis can be achieved with low daily doses of several agents, including trimethoprim (100 mg), nitrofurantoin (50 or 100 mg), or trimethoprim/sulfamethoxazole (40 mg/200 mg). Prophylaxis should continue for at least 6 months. During this time, periodic urine cultures should be obtained. If a symptomatic episode occurs, standard therapy for acute cystitis should be given. If reinfection is associated with sexual intercourse, the risk can be decreased by voiding after intercourse and by single-dose prophylaxis (e.g., trimethoprim/sulfamethoxazole [80 mg/400 mg] taken after intercourse).

Relapse

Recolonization with the original infecting organism accounts for 20% of recurrent UTIs. Symptoms that reappear shortly after completion of a course of therapy suggest either a structural abnormality of the urinary tract, involvement of the kidneys, or chronic bacterial prostatitis, the most common cause of recurrent UTI in males. If obstruction of the urinary tract is present, it should be corrected surgically. If renal calculi are the cause, they should be removed.

Drug therapy is progressive. When relapse occurs in women after short-course therapy, a 2-week course of therapy should be tried. If this fails, an additional 4 to 6 weeks of therapy should be tried. If this, too, is unsuccessful, long-term therapy (6 months) may be indicated. Drugs employed for long-term therapy of relapse include trimethoprim/sulfamethoxazole, norfloxacin, and cephalexin.

Acute Bacterial Prostatitis

Acute bacterial prostatitis is defined as inflammation of the prostate caused by local bacterial infection. Clinical manifestations include high fever, chills, malaise, myalgia, localized pain, and various urinary tract symptoms (dysuria, nocturia, urinary urgency, urinary frequency, urinary retention). In most cases (80%), *E. coli* is the causative organism. Infection is frequently associated with an indwelling urethral catheter, urethral instrumentation, or transurethral prostatic resection. However, in many patients, the infection has no obvious cause.

Bacterial prostatitis responds well to antimicrobial therapy. Because of local inflammation, antibiotics can readily penetrate to the site of infection. (In the absence of inflammation, penetration of the prostate is difficult.) Drug selection and route depend on the causative organism and infection severity. For severe infection with *E. coli,* treatment starts with an IV agent (a fluoroquinolone [e.g., ciprofloxacin]), followed by 2 to 4 weeks with an oral agent (either doxycycline or a fluoroquinolone). For severe infection with vancomycin-sensitive *E. faecalis,* treatment starts with IV ampicillin/sulbactam, followed by 2 to 4 weeks with oral (PO) amoxicillin, levofloxacin, or doxycycline.

URINARY TRACT ANTISEPTICS

Two urinary tract antiseptics are available: nitrofurantoin and methenamine. Both are used only for UTIs. These drugs become concentrated in the urine and are active against the common urinary tract pathogens. Neither drug achieves effective antibacterial concentrations in blood or tissues. Nitrofurantoin is a first-choice drug for uncomplicated cystitis.

Nitrofurantoin

Mechanism of Action

Nitrofurantoin [Furadantin, Macrodantin, Macrobid] is a broad-spectrum antibacterial drug, producing bacteriostatic effects at low concentrations and bactericidal effects at high concentrations. Therapeutic levels are achieved only in urine. Nitrofurantoin can cause serious adverse effects.

Nitrofurantoin injures bacteria by damaging DNA. However, to damage DNA, the drug must first undergo enzymatic conversion to a reactive form. Nitrofurantoin is selectively toxic to bacteria because, unlike mammalian cells, bacteria possess relatively high levels of the enzyme needed for drug activation.

Antimicrobial Spectrum

Nitrofurantoin is active against a large number of gram-positive and gram-negative bacteria. Susceptible organisms include staphylococci, streptococci, *Neisseria* and *Bacteroides* species, and most strains of *E. coli.* These sensitive bacteria rarely acquire resistance. Organisms that are frequently resistant include *Proteus, Pseudomonas, Enterobacter,* and *Klebsiella* species.

Therapeutic Use

Nitrofurantoin is indicated for acute infections of the lower urinary tract caused by susceptible organisms. In addition, the drug can be used for prophylaxis of recurrent lower UTI. Nitrofurantoin is not recommended for infections of the upper urinary tract.

Pharmacokinetics

Absorption and Distribution

Nitrofurantoin is available in three crystalline forms: microcrystals, macrocrystals, and monohydrate/macrocrystals (Table 74.2). The two macrocrystalline forms are absorbed relatively slowly and produce less gastrointestinal (GI) distress than the microcrystalline form. All formulations produce equivalent therapeutic effects. Nitrofurantoin is distributed to tissues, but only in small amounts. Therapeutic concentrations are achieved only in urine.

TABLE 74.2 ▪ Antibiotics Specific for Treatment of Urinary Tract Infection

Drug	Name	Availability	Usual Dose	Use
Nitrofurantoin microcrystals	Furadantin	5 mg/mL oral suspension	50–100 mg four times daily 50–100 mg nightly	Treatment of UTI UTI prophylaxis
Nitrofurantoin macrocrystals	Macrodantin	25-, 50-, 100-mg capsules	50–100 mg four times daily 50–100 mg nightly	Treatment of UTI UTI prophylaxis
Nitrofurantoin monohydrate/ macrocrystals	Macrobid	100-mg extended-release capsules	100 mg twice daily	Treatment of UTI
Methenamine hippurate	Hiprex, Urex	1-g tablets	1 g twice daily	UTI prophylaxis/suppression
Methenamine mandelate	Generic only	0.5-, 1-g tablets	1 g four times daily	UTI prophylaxis/suppression

Metabolism and Excretion

About two thirds of each dose undergoes metabolic degradation, primarily in the liver; the remaining one third is excreted intact in the urine. Nitrofurantoin achieves a urinary concentration of about 200 mcg/mL (compared with less than 2 mcg/mL in plasma). The drug imparts a harmless brown color to the urine; patients should be informed of this effect.

For two reasons, nitrofurantoin should not be administered to individuals with renal impairment (creatinine clearance less than 40 mL/min). First, in the absence of good renal function, levels of nitrofurantoin in the urine are too low to be effective. Second, renal impairment reduces nitrofurantoin excretion, causing plasma levels of the drug to rise, thereby posing a risk for systemic toxicity.

Adverse Effects

Gastrointestinal Effects

The most frequent adverse reactions are GI disturbances (e.g., anorexia, nausea, vomiting, diarrhea). These can be minimized by administering nitrofurantoin with milk or with meals, by reducing the dosage, and by using the macrocrystalline formulations.

Pulmonary Reactions

Nitrofurantoin can induce two kinds of pulmonary reactions: acute and subacute. Acute reactions, which are most common, manifest as dyspnea, chest pain, chills, fever, cough, and alveolar infiltrates. These symptoms resolve 2 to 4 days after discontinuing the drug. Acute pulmonary responses are thought to be hypersensitivity reactions. Patients with a history of these responses should not receive nitrofurantoin again. Subacute reactions are rare and occur during prolonged treatment. Symptoms (e.g., dyspnea, cough, malaise) usually regress over weeks to months after nitrofurantoin withdrawal. However, in some patients, permanent lung damage may occur.

Hematologic Effects

Nitrofurantoin can cause a variety of hematologic reactions, including agranulocytosis, leukopenia, thrombocytopenia, and megaloblastic anemia. In addition, hemolytic anemia may occur in infants and in patients whose red blood cells have an inherited deficiency in glucose-6-phosphate dehydrogenase. Because of the potential for hemolytic anemia in newborns, nitrofurantoin is contraindicated for pregnant women near term and for infants younger than 1 month.

Peripheral Neuropathy

Damage to sensory and motor nerves is a serious concern. Demyelinization and nerve degeneration can occur and may be irreversible. Early symptoms include muscle weakness, tingling sensations, and numbness. Patients should be informed about these symptoms and instructed to report them immediately. Neuropathy is most likely in patients with renal impairment and in those taking nitrofurantoin chronically.

Hepatotoxicity

Rarely, nitrofurantoin has caused severe liver injury, manifesting as hepatitis, cholestatic jaundice, and hepatic necrosis. Deaths have occurred. To reduce risk, patients should undergo periodic tests of liver function. Those who develop liver injury should discontinue nitrofurantoin immediately and never use it again.

Birth Defects

Data are conflicted about the use of nitrofurantoin in pregnancy. Results of the *National Birth Defects Prevention Study,* published in 2009, showed an association between nitrofurantoin and four types of birth defects: anophthalmia (the absence of one or both eyes), hypoplastic left heart syndrome (marked hypoplasia of the left ventricle and ascending aorta), atrial septal defects, and cleft lip with cleft palate. However, owing to limitations of the study, a causal relationship has not been established. Because of the possibility of hemolytic anemia, the drug is contraindicated in pregnant patients at term (38–42 weeks' gestation). Until more is known, it seems prudent to use alternate antibiotics when needed during any gestational age in pregnancy.

Central Nervous System Effects

Nitrofurantoin can cause multiple central nervous system effects (e.g., headache, vertigo, drowsiness, nystagmus). All are readily reversible.

Methenamine

Mechanism of Action

Methenamine [Hiprex, Urex] is a prodrug that, under acidic conditions, breaks down into ammonia and formaldehyde. The formaldehyde denatures bacterial proteins, causing cell death. For formaldehyde to be released, the

PATIENT-CENTERED CARE ACROSS THE LIFE SPAN

Drugs for Urinary Tract Infection

Life Stage	Patient Care Concerns
Infants	Ampicillin and gentamycin are recommended to treat infants with UTI. Often the UTI coincides with other infections or urinary tract abnormalities. The source should be sought immediately.
Children/adolescents	Assess for urinary tract abnormalities in young children with UTI. In sexually active females, assess for birth control methods and complete patient education.
Pregnant women	UTIs in pregnancy must be treated as complicated infections. Nitrofurantoin is contraindicated in the third trimester of pregnancy. Fluoroquinolones should also be avoided in pregnancy.
Breastfeeding women	Administration of nitrofurantoin to infants younger than 1 month is contraindicated. Trimethoprim/sulfamethoxazole should also be avoided in the early stages of infancy. Fluoroquinolones have been detected in breast milk at low doses. Short-term use during breastfeeding is acceptable. For greatest safety, avoid breastfeeding between 4 and 6 hours after a dose.
Older adults	Nitrofurantoin should be avoided in older adults with decreased renal function.

urine must be acidic (pH 5.5 or less). Because formaldehyde is not formed at physiologic systemic pH, methenamine is devoid of systemic toxicity.

Antimicrobial Spectrum

Virtually all bacteria are susceptible to formaldehyde; there is no resistance. Certain bacteria (e.g., Proteus species) can elevate urinary pH (by splitting urea to form ammonia). Because formaldehyde is not released under alkaline conditions, infections with urea-splitting organisms are often unresponsive.

Therapeutic Uses

Methenamine is used for chronic infection of the lower urinary tract. However, trimethoprim/sulfamethoxazole is preferred. Methenamine is not active against upper tract infections because there is insufficient time for formaldehyde to form as the drug passes through. Methenamine does not prevent UTIs associated with catheters.

Pharmacokinetics

Absorption and Distribution

Methenamine is rapidly absorbed after oral administration. However, approximately 30% of each dose may be converted to ammonia and formaldehyde in the acidic environment of the stomach. This can be minimized by using an enteric-coated formulation. The drug is distributed throughout total body water.

Excretion

Methenamine is eliminated by the kidneys. Within the urinary tract, about 20% of the drug decomposes to form formaldehyde. Levels of formaldehyde are highest in the bladder. Because formaldehyde generation takes place slowly, and because transit time through the kidney is brief, formaldehyde levels in the kidney remain subtherapeutic. Ingestion of large volumes of fluid reduces antibacterial effects by diluting methenamine and raising urinary pH. Poorly metabolized acids (e.g., hippuric acid, mandelic acid, ascorbic acid) have been administered with methenamine in attempts to acidify the urine, and thereby increase formaldehyde formation. However, there is no evidence that these acids enhance therapeutic effects.

Adverse Effects and Precautions

Methenamine is relatively safe and generally well tolerated. Gastric distress occurs occasionally, probably from formaldehyde in the stomach. Use of enteric-coated preparations may reduce this effect. Chronic high-dose therapy can cause bladder irritation, manifested as dysuria, frequent voiding, urinary urgency, proteinuria, and hematuria. Because decomposition of methenamine generates ammonia (in addition to formaldehyde), the drug is contraindicated for patients with liver dysfunction. Methenamine salts (methenamine mandelate, methenamine hippurate) should not be used by patients with renal impairment because crystalluria may be caused by precipitating the mandelate or hippurate moiety.

Drug Interactions

Urinary Alkalinizers

Drugs that elevate urinary pH (e.g., acetazolamide, sodium bicarbonate) inhibit formaldehyde production and can thereby reduce the antibacterial effects. Patients taking methenamine should not receive alkalinizing agents.

Sulfonamides

Methenamine should not be combined with sulfonamides because formaldehyde forms an insoluble complex with sulfonamides, thereby posing a risk for urinary tract injury from crystalluria.

CHAPTER

75 Antimycobacterial Agents

Jacqueline Rosenjack Burchum, DNSc, FNP-BC, CNE

Our topic for this chapter is infections caused by two species of mycobacteria: *Mycobacterium tuberculosis* and *Mycobacterium avium.* The mycobacteria are slow-growing microbes, and the infections they cause require prolonged treatment. Because therapy is prolonged, drug toxicity and poor patient adherence are significant obstacles to success. In addition, prolonged treatment promotes the emergence of drug-resistant mycobacteria. Because mycobacteria resist decolorizing by the dilute acid used in some staining protocols, these microorganisms are often referred to as *acid-fast bacteria.*

DRUGS FOR TUBERCULOSIS

Tuberculosis (TB) is a global epidemic. Only AIDs is responsible for more infectious disease–related deaths. According to the World Health Organization, in 2015 there were 10.4 million new TB cases worldwide. Also in 2015, 1.8 million people died from TB worldwide. Most of these (95%) occurred in developing countries.

In the United States we are more fortunate. TB trends have declined over recent decades (down from 20,673 in 1992 to 9421 in 2014). Many of these (66%) occur in people who were born outside of the United States.

There are two reasons for the resurgence in TB. First is the spread of HIV/AIDS and the associated decrease in immunity. The other is the emergence of multidrug-resistant mycobacteria.

Clinical Considerations

Pathogenesis

Tuberculosis is caused by *Mycobacterium tuberculosis,* an organism also known as the tubercle bacillus. Infections may be limited to the lungs or may become disseminated. In most cases the bacteria are quiescent, and the infected individual has no symptoms. However, when the disease is active, morbidity can be significant. In the United States approximately 10 million people harbor tubercle bacilli. However, only a small fraction have symptomatic disease.

Primary Infection

Infection with *M. tuberculosis* is transmitted from person to person by inhaling infected sputum that has been aerosolized, usually by coughing or sneezing. As a result, initial infection is in the lungs. When in the lungs, tubercle bacilli are taken up by phagocytic cells (macrophages and neutrophils). At first, the bacilli are resistant to the destructive activity of phagocytes and multiply freely within them. Infection can spread from the lungs to other organs through the lymphatic and circulatory systems.

In most cases, immunity to *M. tuberculosis* develops within a few weeks, and the infection is brought under complete control. The immune system facilitates control by increasing the ability of phagocytes to suppress multiplication of tubercle bacilli. Because of this rapid response by the immune system, most individuals (90%) with primary infection never develop clinical or radiologic evidence of disease. However, even though symptoms are absent and the progression of infection is halted, the infected individual is likely to harbor tubercle bacilli lifelong, unless drugs are given to eliminate quiescent bacilli. Hence, in the absence of treatment, there is always some risk that latent infection may become active.

If the immune system fails to control the primary infection, clinical disease (tuberculosis) develops. The result is necrosis and cavitation of lung tissue. Lung tissue may also become caseous (cheese-like in appearance). In the absence of treatment, tissue destruction progresses, and death may result.

Reactivation

The term *reactivation* refers to renewed multiplication of tubercle bacilli that had been dormant after control of a primary infection. Until recently, it was assumed that most new cases of symptomatic TB resulted from reactivation of an old (latent) infection. However, we now know that, among some groups, reactivation may be responsible for only 60% of new infections—the remaining 40% result from recent person-to-person transmission.

Diagnosis and Treatment of Active Tuberculosis

Modern antimycobacterial agents have dramatically altered the treatment of TB. In the past, most patients required lengthy hospitalization. Today, hospitalization is generally unnecessary. Prolonged bed rest is neither required nor recommended. To reduce emergence of resistance, treatment is *always* done with two or more drugs. In addition, direct observation of dosing is now considered standard care.

The goals of treatment are to eliminate infection and prevent relapse while preventing the development of drug resistant organisms. To accomplish this, treatment must kill tubercle bacilli that are actively dividing as well as those that are "resting." Success is indicated by an absence of observable mycobacteria in sputum and by the failure of sputum cultures to yield colonies of *M. tuberculosis.*

Diagnosis

Diagnostic testing is indicated for (1) individuals with clinical manifestations that suggest TB and (2) individuals with a positive skin test or blood test (see later section "Diagnosis and Treatment of Latent Tuberculosis"), who are at high risk for developing active disease. A definitive diagnosis is made with a chest radiograph (chest x-ray) and microbiologic evaluation of sputum. A chest radiograph should be ordered for all persons suspected of active infection.

In traditional tests, the presence of *M. tuberculosis* in sputum is evaluated in two ways: (1) microscopic examination of sputum smears and (2) culturing of sputum samples followed by laboratory evaluation. Microscopic examination cannot provide a definitive diagnosis. Why? Because direct observation cannot distinguish between *M. tuberculosis* and other mycobacteria. Furthermore, microscopic examination is much less sensitive than evaluation of cultured samples. Accordingly, sputum cultures are performed to permit a definitive diagnosis. Unfortunately, culturing *M. tuberculosis* is a slow process, taking 2 to 6 weeks to yield results.

With newer technology, known as *nucleic acid amplification (NAA) tests,* we can identify *M. tuberculosis* in sputum rapidly, typically within 24 to 48 hours. Note that this is 1 to 5 *weeks* sooner than when samples are cultured.

Drug Resistance

Drug resistance is a major impediment to successful therapy. Some infecting bacilli are inherently resistant; others develop resistance over the course of treatment. Some bacilli are resistant to just one drug; others are resistant to multiple drugs. Infection with a resistant organism may be acquired in two ways: (1) through contact with someone who harbors resistant bacteria and (2) through repeated ineffectual courses of therapy (see later).

The emergence of *multidrug-resistant TB* (MDR-TB) and *extensively drug-resistant TB* (XDR-TB) is a recent and ominous development. MDR-TB is defined as TB that is resistant to both isoniazid and rifampin, our two most effective antituberculosis (anti-TB) drugs. XDR-TB, a severe form of MDR-TB, is defined as TB that is resistant not only to isoniazid and rifampin but also to all fluoroquinolones (e.g., moxifloxacin) and at least one of the injectable second-line anti-TB drugs (amikacin, kanamycin, or capreomycin). Infection with multidrug-resistant organisms greatly increases the risk for death, especially among patients with AIDS. In addition, multidrug resistance is expensive: the cost of treating one case of resistant TB is about $150,000, compared with $17,000 per case of nonresistant TB. Fortunately, multidrug resistance is rare in the United States: in 2014 there were 91 reported cases of MDR-TB (down from 127 in 2011). In 2011 there were 6 cases of XDR-TB; in 2014 the number was down to 2 cases.

The principal cause underlying the emergence of resistance is inadequate drug therapy. Treatment may be too short; dosage may be too low; patient adherence may be erratic; and, perhaps most important, the regimen may contain too few drugs.

The Prime Directive: Always Treat Tuberculosis With Two or More Drugs

Antituberculosis regimens must always contain two or more drugs to which the infecting organism is sensitive. To understand why this is so, we need to begin with five facts:

- Resistance in *M. tuberculosis* occurs because of spontaneous mutations.
- Each mutational event confers resistance to only one drug.
- Mutations conferring resistance to a single drug occur in about 1 of every 100 million (10^8) bacteria.
- The bacterial burden in active TB is well above 10^8 organisms but far below 10^{16}.
- *M. tuberculosis* grows slowly, and hence treatment is prolonged.

Now, let's assume we initiate therapy with a single drug and that all bacteria present are sensitive when we start. What will happen? Over time, at least one of the more than 10^8 bacteria in our patient will mutate to a resistant form. Hence, as we proceed with treatment, we will kill all sensitive bacteria, but the descendants of the newly resistant bacterium will continue to flourish, thereby causing treatment failure. In contrast, if we initiate therapy with *two* drugs, treatment will succeed. Why? Because failure would require that at least one bacterium undergo *two* resistance-conferring mutations, one for each drug. Because two such mutations occur in only 1 of every 10^{16} bacteria (10^{16} is the product of the probabilities for each mutation), and because the total bacterial load is much less than 10^{16}, the chances of the two events occurring in one of the bacteria in our patient are nil.

Not only do drug combinations decrease the risk for resistance, they also can reduce the incidence of relapse. Because some drugs are especially effective against actively dividing bacilli, whereas other drugs are most active against intracellular (quiescent) bacilli, by using proper combinations of anti-TB agents, we can increase the chances of killing all tubercle bacilli present, whether they are actively multiplying or dormant. Hence, the risk for relapse is lowered.

In Chapter 68, we noted that treatment with multiple antibiotics broadens the spectrum of antimicrobial coverage, thereby increasing the risk for superinfection. This is not the case with multidrug therapy of TB. The major drugs used against *M. tuberculosis* are *selective* for this organism. As a result, these drugs, even when used in combination, do not kill off beneficial microorganisms and therefore do not create the conditions that lead to superinfection.

Because treatment is prolonged, there is a high risk that drug-resistant bacilli will emerge if only one anti-TB agent is employed. Because the chances of a bacterium developing resistance to two drugs are very low, treatment with two or more drugs minimizes the risk for drug resistance. Therefore, when treating TB, we must always use two or more drugs to which the organism is sensitive.

Determining Drug Sensitivity

Because resistance to one or more anti-TB drugs is common, and because many patterns of resistance are possible, it is essential that we determine drug sensitivity in isolates from each patient at treatment onset. How do we test drug sensitivity? The traditional method is to culture sputum samples in the presence of antimycobacterial drugs. Unfortunately, the process is slow, usually taking 6 to 16 weeks to complete. Until test results are available, drug selection must be empiric, based on (1) patterns of drug resistance in the community and (2) the immunocompetence of the patient. However, when test results are available, the regimen should be adjusted accordingly. In the event of treatment failure, sensitivity tests should be repeated.

A new, automated tuberculosis assay, known as *Xpert MTB/RIF,* can identify sensitivity to one key drug—rifampin—in less than 2 hours, while simultaneously confirming the presence of *M. tuberculosis*. This assay uses the NAA technology noted previously. Although the U.S. Food and Drug Administration (FDA) allowed marketing in 2013, use of the Xpert MTB/RIF device is limited owing to its expense.

Treatment Regimens

In August, 2016, joint guidelines from the American Thoracic Society, Centers for Disease Control and Prevention, and the Infectious Diseases Society of America published new clinical practice guidelines (ATS/CDC/IDSA Guidelines) for drug-susceptible tuberculosis treatment. (See http://cid.oxfordjournals.org/content/63/7/e147.full.pdf.) These updates, along with current CDC guidelines for other types of TB, inform TB treatment information in this chapter.

Several regimens may be employed for active TB. Drug selection is based largely on the susceptibility of the infecting organism and the immunocompetence of the host. Life span considerations are also a factor. (See Patient-Centered Care Across the Life Span.) Four drugs — isoniazid, rifampin, pyrazinamide, and ethambutol — are first-line drugs for TB treatment and are used in most treatment regimens. The rifamycin antibiotics rifapentine and rifabutin are also considered first-line drugs. For LTBI, rifapentine replaces rifampin. For patients taking multiple drugs, rifabutin may be used to replace rifampin to reduce drug interactions, but rifampin or rifapentine should be used over rifabutin when possible.

The ATS/CDC/ISDA Guidelines identify the following as second-line drugs for TB treatment: cycloserine; ethionamide; capreomycin; *para*-aminosalicylic acid (PAS); the aminoglycosides streptomycin and amikacin/kanamycin; and the quinolones levofloxacin and moxifloxacin. Additional antibiotics are sometimes employed when necessary due to severe adverse effects or other complications in therapy.

Therapy is usually initiated with a *four-drug* regimen; isoniazid and rifampin are almost always included. In the event of suspected or proved resistance, more drugs are added; the total may be as high as seven. A sample drug regimen is shown in Table 75.1 and discussed later.

Treatment is divided into two phases. The goal of the initial phase (induction phase) is to eliminate actively dividing extracellular tubercle bacilli and thereby render the sputum noninfectious. The goal of the second phase (continuation phase) is to eliminate persistent intracellular organisms.

Drug-Sensitive Tuberculosis. If the infecting organisms are not resistant to isoniazid or rifampin, treatment is relatively simple. The induction phase, which lasts 8 weeks, consists of four drugs: *isoniazid, rifampin, pyrazinamide,* and *ethambutol.* Dosing may be done daily, twice weekly, or thrice weekly. The continuation phase, which lasts 18 weeks, consists of two drugs—*isoniazid* and *rifampin*—administered daily, twice weekly, or thrice weekly. Note that the entire course of treatment is prolonged, making adherence a significant problem.

Isoniazid- or Rifampin-Resistant Tuberculosis. Infections that are resistant to a single drug—isoniazid or rifampin—usually respond well. Isoniazid-resistant TB can be treated for 6 months with three drugs: rifampin, ethambutol, and pyrazinamide. Rifampin-resistant TB can also be treated with three drugs—isoniazid, ethambutol, and pyrazinamide—but the duration is longer: 18 to 24 months, rather than 6 months.

Multidrug-Resistant TB and Extensively Drug-Resistant TB. MDR-TB and XDR-TB are much harder to manage than

TABLE 75.1 ▪ Recommended* Antituberculosis Regimen

Phase of Treatment	Drug Combination	Treatment Intervals	Minimal Length of Treatment
Intensive	Isoniazid Rifampin Pyrazinamide Ethambutol	7 days/wk for 56 doses or 5 days/wk for 40 doses	8 weeks 8 weeks
Continuation	Isoniazid Rifapentine	7 days/wk for 126 doses or 5 days/wk for 90 doses	18 weeks 18 weeks

*Recommendation of the 2016 ATS/CDC/IDSA Clinical Practice Guidelines for Drug-Susceptible TB. Additional regimens are available online at http://www.cdc.gov/tb/publications/guidelines/pdf/clin-infect-dis.-2016-nahid-cid_ciw376.pdf

PATIENT-CENTERED CARE ACROSS THE LIFE SPAN

First-Line Drugs for Tuberculosis

Life Stage	Considerations or Concerns
Children	These drugs are approved for children.
Pregnant women	Rifabutin is FDA Pregnancy Risk Category B. The remaining first-line drugs are Pregnancy Risk Category C; however, there are some differences. The CDC reports that the benefit justifies the risk for isoniazid, rifampin, and pyrazinamide. The CDC does not recommend rifapentine due to insufficient data in pregnant women. Because the animal harm is of a teratogenic nature and there have been reports of eye abnormalities in children, ethambutol should only be taken if benefits are judged to be greater than the risks.
Breastfeeding women	According to the CDC, mothers taking isoniazid and rifampin should be encouraged to breastfeed. For others, it is important to weigh the benefits of breastfeeding against any possible risks to the infant. The amount of drugs excreted in milk are not sufficient for neonatal treatment against TB.
Older adults	No contraindications are identified for these patients. Dosing may need to be adjusted for patients with decreased renal function.

drug-sensitive TB. Treatment is prolonged (at least 24 months) and must use second- and third-line drugs, which are less effective than the first-line drugs (e.g., isoniazid and rifampin) and are generally more toxic. Initial therapy may consist of five, six, or even seven drugs. Hence an initial regimen might include (1) isoniazid; (2) rifampin; (3) pyrazinamide; (4) ethambutol; (5) kanamycin, amikacin, or capreomycin; (6) levofloxacin; and (7) cycloserine, ethionamide, or *para*-aminosalicylic acid (PAS). As a last resort, infected tissue may be removed by surgery. Even with all of these measures, the prognosis is often poor: Among patients with XDR-TB, between 40% and 60% die. Factors that determine outcome include the extent of drug resistance, infection severity, and the immunocompetence of the host.

Patients With TB plus HIV Infection. Between 2% and 20% of patients with HIV infection develop active TB. Because of their reduced ability to fight infection, these patients require therapy that is more aggressive than in immunocompetent patients and that should last several months longer.

Drug interactions are a big problem, especially for patients taking *rifampin.* Why? Because rifampin, a cornerstone of TB therapy, can accelerate the metabolism of antiretroviral drugs that are prescribed to treat HIV and can thereby decrease their effects. Specifically, rifampin can decrease the effects of most protease inhibitors and most nonnucleoside reverse transcriptase inhibitors (NNRTIs). Accordingly, it is best to avoid combining rifampin with these agents. Unfortunately, this means that patients will be denied optimal treatment for one of their infections. That is, if they take rifampin to treat TB, they will be unable to take most protease inhibitors or NNRTIs for HIV. Conversely, if they take protease inhibitors and NNRTIs to treat HIV, they will be unable to take rifampin for TB. This dilemma does not have an easy solution.

Like rifampin, *rifabutin* can accelerate metabolism of antiretroviral drugs. However, the degree of acceleration is much less. As a result, many of the antiretroviral drugs that must be avoided in patients taking rifampin can still be used in patients taking rifabutin.

Duration of Treatment

The ideal duration of treatment has not been established. For patients with drug-sensitive TB, the minimal duration is 6 months. For patients with multidrug-resistant infection and for patients with HIV/AIDS, treatment may last as long as 24 months after sputum cultures have become negative.

Promoting Adherence: Directly Observed Therapy Combined With Intermittent Dosing

Patient nonadherence is the most common cause of treatment failure, relapse, and increased drug resistance. Recall that patients with TB must take multiple drugs for 6 months or more, making adherence a very real problem. Directly observed therapy (DOT), combined with intermittent dosing, helps ensure adherence and thereby increases the chances of success.

In DOT, administration of each dose is done in the presence of an observer, usually a representative of the health department. DOT is now considered the standard of care for TB. In addition to promoting bacterial kill, DOT permits ongoing evaluation of the clinical response and adverse drug effects.

Intermittent dosing is defined as dosing 2 or 3 times a week, rather than every day. Of course, each dose is larger than with daily dosing. Studies have shown that intermittent dosing is just as effective as daily dosing, and no more toxic. The great advantage of intermittent dosing is that it makes DOT more convenient which improves adherence.

Evaluating Treatment

Three modes are employed to evaluate therapy: bacteriologic evaluation of sputum, clinical evaluation, and chest radiographs.

In patients with positive pretreatment sputum tests, sputum should be evaluated every 2 to 4 weeks initially, and then monthly after sputum cultures become negative. With proper drug selection and good adherence, sputum cultures become negative in more than 90% of patients after 3 months of treatment.

Treatment failures should be evaluated for drug resistance and patient adherence. In the absence of demonstrated drug resistance, treatment with the same regimen should continue, using DOT to ensure that medication is being taken as prescribed. In patients with drug-resistant TB, *two* effective drugs should be added to the regimen.

In patients with negative pretreatment sputum tests, treatment is monitored by chest radiographs and clinical evaluation. In most patients, clinical manifestations (e.g., fever, malaise, anorexia, cough) should decrease markedly within 2 weeks. The radiograph should show improvement within 3 months.

After completing therapy, patients should be examined every 3 to 6 months for signs and symptoms of relapse.

Diagnosis and Treatment of Latent Tuberculosis

In the United States an estimated 9 to 14 million people have latent TB infection (LTBI). In the absence of treatment, 5% to 10% of these people will develop active TB. Because LTBI can become active, the condition poses a threat to the infected individual and to the community as well. Accordingly, testing and treatment are clearly desirable—but not for everyone: because treatment of LTBI is often prolonged and carries a risk for drug toxicity, testing and treatment should be limited to people who really need it.

Who Should Be Tested for Latent Tuberculosis?

Testing should be limited to people who are at high risk for either (1) having acquired the infection recently or (2) progressing from LTBI to active TB. Included in this group are people with HIV infection, people receiving immunosuppressive drugs, recent contacts of patients with TB, and people with high-risk medical conditions, such as diabetes, silicosis, or chronic renal failure. Candidates for testing are listed in Table 75.2. Routine testing of low-risk individuals is not recommended.

How Do We Test for Latent Tuberculosis?

There are two types of tests for LTBI: (1) the *tuberculin skin test* (TST), which has been used for more than 100 years; and (2) *interferon gamma release assays* (IGRAs), first approved for American use in 2001.

TABLE 75.2 ▪ Candidates for Targeted Tuberculosis Testing

Individuals at high risk for recent tuberculosis infection	Contacts of tuberculosis (TB) patients Residents and staff of high-risk congregate settings • Prisons and jails • Nursing homes • Hospitals and other health care facilities • Homeless shelters • Residential facilities for patients with AIDS Persons who, in the past 5 years, immigrated from a country where TB is prevalent (The CDC identifies countries in Africa, Asia, the Caribbean, Eastern Europe, Latin America, and Russia as most prevalent.) Staff of mycobacteriology laboratories Infants, children, and adolescents exposed to high-risk adults
Individuals at high risk for progression from latent to active tuberculosis	Infants and children younger than 4 years People with HIV infection People who use illegal IV drugs Patients taking immunosuppressive drugs for 1 month or more Patients with a chest radiograph indicating fibrotic changes consistent with prior TB Patients with high-risk medical conditions, including • Diabetes mellitus • Chronic renal failure • Silicosis • Leukemia or lymphoma • Clinical conditions associated with substantial weight loss, including postgastrectomy state, intestinal bypass surgery, chronic peptic ulcer disease, chronic malabsorption syndromes, and carcinomas of the oropharynx and upper gastrointestinal tract that inhibit adequate nutritional intake

TABLE 75.3 ▪ Tuberculin Skin Test Results That Are Considered Positive (Justifying Treatment) in Patients at Low, Moderate, and High Risk for Latent Tuberculosis

Risk Category	Who Is in the Risk Category?	Test Result Considered Positive
High	People who are HIV-positive People who have had recent contact with someone with tuberculosis (TB) infection People with fibrotic changes on their chest radiograph consistent with prior TB People taking immunosuppressive drugs for more than 1 month People who have had organ transplants	5 mm of induration
Moderate	Recent immigrants from countries with a high prevalence of TB People who use illegal IV drugs Residents and staff of high-risk congregate settings (e.g., prisons, nursing homes, hospitals, homeless shelters) Mycobacteriology laboratory personnel People with high-risk medical conditions (e.g., diabetes mellitus, chronic renal failure, silicosis, leukemia, lymphoma) Children and adolescents exposed to high-risk adults Children younger than 4 years	10 mm of induration
Low	Persons with no risk factors for TB	15 mm of induration

Tuberculin Skin Test. The TST is performed by giving an intradermal injection of a preparation known as *purified protein derivative* (PPD), an antigen derived from *M. tuberculosis.* If the individual has an intact immune system and has been exposed to *M. tuberculosis* in the past, the PPD will elicit a local immune response. The test is read 48 to 72 hours after the injection. A positive reaction is indicated by a region of induration (hardness) around the injection site.

The decision to treat LTBI is based on two factors: (1) the risk category of the individual and (2) the size of the region of induration produced by the TST (Table 75.3). For individuals at high risk, treatment is recommended if the region of induration is relatively small (5 mm). For individuals at moderate risk, treatment is indicated when the region of induration is larger (10 mm). And for individuals at low risk (who should not be routinely tested), the region must be larger still (15 mm) to justify treatment.

Interferon Gamma Release Assays. The IGRAs are *blood* tests for TB, rather than skin tests. These tests are based on the observation that immune white blood cells (WBCs), after exposure to *M. tuberculosis,* will release interferon gamma when exposed to *M. tuberculosis* again. In the IGRAs, a patient's blood (or WBCs isolated from that blood) is exposed to antigens that represent *M. tuberculosis.* If the antigens trigger sufficient release of interferon gamma, the test is considered positive for TB.

In the United States two IGRAs are now in use:

- QuantiFERON-TB Gold In-Tube
- T-SPOT.TB

These IGRAs are as sensitive as the TST and are more specific. Moreover, results with the IGRAs are available faster than with the TST (24 hours vs. 48–72 hours), and only one office visit is required. Current CDC guidelines permit using IGRAs for all situations in which the TST has been used; however, the TST is recommended for children younger than 5 years because there have been limited studies in this population.

How Do We Treat Latent Tuberculosis?

In the United States there are two preferred treatments for LTBI: (1) *isoniazid alone* taken daily for 9 months and (2) *isoniazid plus rifapentine* taken weekly for 3 months. Both treatments are equally effective. Isoniazid alone has been used for decades; isoniazid plus rifapentine is a new option. Because dosing with isoniazid plus rifapentine is so simple—just 12 doses instead of 270—completing the full course is more likely than with isoniazid alone.

Before starting treatment for LTBI, active TB must be ruled out. Why? Because LTBI is treated with just one or two drugs, and hence, if active TB were present, treatment would promote emergence of resistant bacilli. To exclude active disease, the patient should receive a physical examination and chest radiograph; if indicated, bacteriologic studies may also be ordered.

Isoniazid. For more than 30 years, isoniazid has been the standard treatment for LTBI. The drug is effective, relatively safe, and inexpensive. However, isoniazid does have two drawbacks. First, to be effective, isoniazid must be taken for a long time—at least 6 months and preferably 9 months. Second, isoniazid poses a risk for liver damage.

Dosing may be done once daily or twice a week. When twice-weekly dosing is used, each dose should be administered by DOT to ensure adherence. Dosing of this and other drugs used to treat TB are provided in Table 75.4.

Isoniazid Plus Rifapentine. The combination of isoniazid plus rifapentine—taken just *once a week* for *only 3 months*—is just as effective as isoniazid alone taken once a

TABLE 75.4 ▪ Preparation, Dosage, and Administration*

Drug	Preparation	Daily	Three Times a Week	Twice a Week	Weekly	Administration
Isoniazid [generic]	Tablets: 50, 100, 300 mg Oral syrup: 10 mg/mL Solution for injection: 100 mg/mL	Adults: 5 mg/kg/day (usual dose 300 mg) Children: 10–15 mg/kg/day	Adults: 15 mg/kg (usual dose 900 mg) Children: no recommendation	Adults: 15 mg/kg (usual dose 900 mg) Children: 20-30 mg/kg	Adults: 15 mg/kg (usual dose 900 mg) Children: no recommendation	Take with or without food.
Rifampin [Rifadin]	Capsules: 150 mg, 300 mg IV: 600 mg for reconstitution	Adults: 10 mg/kg (usual dose 600 mg) Children: 10–20 mg/kg	Adults: 10 mg/kg (usual dose 600 mg) Children: no recommendation	Adults: 10 mg/kg (usual dose 600 mg) Children: 10–20 mg/kg	Adults: no recommendation Children: no recommendation	Take 1 hour before meals or 2 hours after meals.
Rifapentine [Priftin]	Tablets: 150 mg	Adults: only given weekly in continuation phase Children: not approved for children < 12 years	Adults: only given weekly Children: not approved	Adults: only given weekly Children: not approved	Adults: 20 mg/kg Children: not approved	Take with meals. Tablets may be crushed and added to food.
Rifabutin [Mycobutin]	Capsules: 150 mg	Adults: 5 mg/kg (usual dose 300 mg) Children: 5 mg/kg (suggested)[‡]	Adults: no recommendation Children: no recommendation	Adults: no recommendation Children: no recommendation	Adults: no recommendation Children: no recommendation	May take with food to decrease GI upset.
Pyrazinamide [generic]	Tablet: 500 mg	Adults: Weight 40-55 kg = 1000/mg/kg; Weight 56-75 kg = 1500 mg/kg; Weight 76-90 kg = 2000 mg/kg Children: 30-40 mg/kg	Adults: Weight 40-55 kg = 1500/mg/kg; Weight 56-75 kg = 2500 mg/kg; Weight 76-90 kg = 3000 mg/kg Children: no recommendation	Adults: Weight 40-55 kg = 2000/mg/kg; Weight 56-75 kg = 3000 mg/kg; Weight 76-90 kg = 4000 mg/kg Children: 50 mg/kg	Adults: no recommendation Children: no recommendation	Take on an empty stomach.
Ethambutol [Myambutol]	Tablets: 100 mg, 400 mg	Adults: Weight 40-55 kg = 800 mg/kg; Weight 56-75 kg = 1200 mg/kg; Weight 76-90 kg = 1600 mg/kg Children: 15-25 mg/kg	Adults: Weight 40-55 kg = 1200/mg/kg; Weight 56-75 kg = 2000 mg/kg; Weight 76-90 kg = 2400 mg/kg Children: no recommendation	Adults: Weight 40-55 kg = 2000 mg/kg; Weight 56-75 kg = 2800 mg/kg; Weight 76-90 kg = 4000 mg/kg Children: 50 mg/kg	Adults: no recommendation Children: no recommendation	May take with food if GI upset occurs.

TABLE 75.4 ▪ Preparation, Dosage, and Administration—cont'd

Drug	Preparation	Daily	Three Times a Week	Twice a Week	Weekly	Administration
Para-aminosalicylate [Paser Granules]	Packets: 4-g delayed-release granules	Adults: 4000 mg 2-3 times/day (usual dose 8-12 g/day) Children: 100 mg/kg given 2-3 times/day (usual total dose 200-300 mg/kg/day)	Adults: no recommendation Children: no recommendation	Adults: no recommendation Children: no recommendation	Adults: no recommendation Children: no recommendation	If stomach upset occurs, PAS may be administered with food.
Ethionamide [Trecator]	Tablets: 250 mg	Adults: 15-20 mg/kg/day (usual dose 250-500 mg 1-2 times daily) Children: 15-20 mg/kg/day total in 1-2 doses	Adults: no recommendation Children: no recommendation	Adults: no recommendation Children: no recommendation	Adults: no recommendation Children: no recommendation	Take with or without food. Taking at bedtime may decrease GI effects.
Cycloserine [generic]	Capsules: 250 mg	Adults: 10-15 mg/kg/day (usual dose 250-500 mg 1-2 times daily) Children: 15-20 mg/kg/day in 1-2 doses	Adults: no recommendation Children: no recommendation	Adults: no recommendation Children: no recommendation	Adults: no recommendation Children: no recommendation	Take with or without food.
Capreomycin [Capastat]	Solution for injection: 1 g vial	Adults: 15 mg/kg Children: 15-20 mg/kg	Adults: 25 mg/kg Children: no recommendation	Adults: no recommendation Children: 25-30 mg/kg	Adults: no recommendation Children: no recommendation	IM or IV administration
Streptomycin (generic)	Solution for injection: 1 g vial	Adults: 15 mg/kg Children: 15-20 mg/kg	Adults: 25 mg/kg Children: no recommendation	Adults: no recommendation Children: 25-30 mg/kg	Adults: no recommendation Children: no recommendation	IM or IV administration
Amikacin/kanamycin	Solution for injection: 500 mg, 1 g vial	Adults: 15 mg/kg Children: 15-20 mg/kg	Adults: 25 mg/kg Children: no recommendation	Adults: no recommendation Children: 25-30 mg/kg	Adults: no recommendation Children: no recommendation	IM or IV administration
Levofloxacin [Levaquin]	Tablets: 250, 500, 750 mg Solution for injection: 500 mg vial	Adults: 500-1000 mg Children: ±15-20 mg/kg (suggested)[±]	Adults: no recommendation Children: no recommendation	Adults: no recommendation Children: no recommendation	Adults: no recommendation Children: no recommendation	Take with or without food
Moxifloxacin [Avelox, Avelox ABC Pack]	Tablets: 400 mg Solution for injection: 400 mg/250 mL	Adults: 400 mg Children: ±10 mg/kg (suggested)[±]	Adults: no recommendation Children: no recommendation	Adults: no recommendation Children: no recommendation	Adults: no recommendation Children: no recommendation	Take with or without food

IM, intramuscular; IV, intravenous; PAS, *para*-aminosalicylic acid; TB, tuberculosis.
*Alternate dosing is often used as treatment regimens are commonly individualized.
[±]Optimal dosing unknown; dosing is suggested by experts in the field.

day for 9 months, as shown in the PREVENT TB trial. Accordingly, the CDC has recommended isoniazid plus rifapentine as an equal alternative to 9 months of daily isoniazid. Because dosing is done just once a week, isoniazid plus rifapentine *must be administered by DOT.* In contrast, daily isoniazid is self-administered, without oversight by a health-care provider.

Who can use the new regimen? Isoniazid plus rifapentine is recommended for people 12 years and older, including those with HIV infection who are *not* taking antiretroviral drugs. As a rule, children aged 2 to 11 years should use 9 months of daily isoniazid, and not isoniazid plus rifapentine. Because of its simplicity, the new regimen may be especially useful in correctional institutions, clinics for recent immigrants, and homeless shelters.

Who should *not* use the new regimen? The regimen should not be used by (1) children younger than 2 years because the safety and kinetics of rifapentine are unknown in this group, (2) HIV-infected patients taking antiretroviral drugs because drug interactions have not been studied, (3) women who are pregnant or expecting to become pregnant during treatment because safety in pregnancy is unknown, and (4) patients with LTBI with presumed resistance to isoniazid or rifapentine.

Vaccination Against Tuberculosis

Protection against TB can be conferred by inoculation with bacillus Calmette-Guérin (BCG) vaccine, a freeze-dried preparation of attenuated Mycobacterium bovis. In countries where TB is endemic, the World Health Organization recommends BCG vaccination in infancy, to protect children against severe, life-threatening TB infection (i.e., miliary TB and tuberculous meningitis). In the United States routine vaccination is not done because there is a low risk for infection with M. tuberculosis and protection against pulmonary TB in adulthood is variable. Furthermore, vaccination with BCG can produce a false-positive result in the TST, which can't distinguish between antigens from M. bovis and antigens from M. tuberculosis. (Because the IGRAs are highly specific for antigens from M. tuberculosis, vaccination with BCG does not affect the results of these tests.)

Pharmacology of Individual Antituberculosis Drugs

As mentioned earlier, the anti-TB drugs are divided into two groups: first-line drugs and second-line drugs. The first-line drugs are *isoniazid, rifampin, pyrazinamide,* and *ethambutol (with rifapentine or rifabutin sometimes substituting for rifampin).* Of these, isoniazid and rifampin are the most important. The second-line drugs are generally less effective, more toxic, and more expensive than the primary drugs. Second-line agents are used in combination with the primary drugs to treat disseminated TB and TB caused by organisms resistant to first-line drugs. Adverse effects and routes of administration of the anti-TB drugs are shown in Table 75.5.

Prototype Drugs

DRUGS FOR TUBERCULOSIS

Isoniazid
Rifampin
Pyrazinamide
Ethambutol

TABLE 75.5 ■ Antituberculosis Drugs: Routes and Major Adverse Effects

Drug	Route	Major Adverse Effects
FIRST-LINE DRUGS		
Isoniazid	PO, IM	Hepatotoxicity, peripheral neuritis
Rifampin	PO, IV	Hepatotoxicity
Rifapentine	PO	Hepatotoxicity
Rifabutin	PO	Hepatotoxicity
Pyrazinamide	PO	Hepatotoxicity, polyarthritis
Ethambutol	PO	Optic neuritis
SECOND-LINE DRUGS		
Fluoroquinolones		
Levofloxacin	PO, IV	GI intolerance
Moxifloxacin	PO, IV	GI intolerance
Injectable Drugs		
Capreomycin	IM	Eighth nerve damage, nephrotoxicity
Kanamycin	IM, IV	Eighth nerve damage, nephrotoxicity
Amikacin	IM, IV	Eighth nerve damage, nephrotoxicity
Streptomycin	IM	Eighth nerve damage, nephrotoxicity
Others		
Para-aminosalicylic acid	PO	GI intolerance
Ethionamide	PO	GI intolerance, hepatotoxicity
Cycloserine	PO	Psychoses, seizure, rash

GI, gastrointestinal; IM, intramuscular; IV, intravenous; PO, oral.

Isoniazid

Isoniazid [generic in United States, Isotamine ♣] is the primary agent for treatment and prophylaxis of TB. This drug has early bactericidal activity and is superior to alternative drugs with regard to efficacy, toxicity, ease of use, patient acceptance, and affordability. With the exception of patients who cannot tolerate the drug, isoniazid should be taken by all individuals infected with isoniazid-sensitive strains of *M. tuberculosis.*

Antimicrobial Spectrum and Mechanism of Action

Isoniazid is highly selective for *M. tuberculosis.* The drug can kill tubercle bacilli at concentrations 10,000 times lower than those needed to affect gram-positive and gram-negative bacteria. Isoniazid is bactericidal to mycobacteria that are actively dividing but is only bacteriostatic to "resting" organisms.

Although the mechanism by which isoniazid acts is not known with certainty, available data suggest the drug suppresses bacterial growth by inhibiting synthesis of mycolic acid, a component of the mycobacterial cell wall. Because mycolic acid is not produced by other bacteria or by cells of the host, this mechanism would explain why isoniazid is so selective for tubercle bacilli.

Resistance

Tubercle bacilli can develop resistance to isoniazid during treatment. Acquired resistance results from spontaneous mutation. The precise mechanism underlying resistance has not been established. Emergence of resistance can be decreased through multidrug therapy. Organisms resistant to isoniazid are cross-resistant to ethionamide, but not to other drugs used for TB.

Pharmacokinetics

Absorption and Distribution. Isoniazid is administered orally and intramuscularly. Absorption is good with both routes. Following absorption, isoniazid is widely distributed to tissues and body fluids, including cerebrospinal fluid (CSF).

Metabolism. Isoniazid is inactivated in the liver, primarily by acetylation. The ability to acetylate isoniazid is genetically determined: about 50% of people in the United States are rapid acetylators, and the other 50% are slow acetylators. The drug's half-life is about 1 hour in rapid acetylators and 3 hours in slow acetylators. It is important to note that differences in rates of acetylation generally have little effect on the efficacy of isoniazid, provided patients are taking the drug daily. However, nonhepatic toxicities may be more likely in slow acetylators because drug accumulation is greater in these patients.

Excretion. Isoniazid is excreted in the urine, primarily as inactive metabolites. In patients who are slow acetylators and who also have renal insufficiency, the drug may accumulate to toxic levels.

Therapeutic Use

Isoniazid is indicated only for treating active and LTBI. When used for LTBI, the drug is administered alone or combined with rifapentine. When used for active TB, it must be taken in combination with at least one other agent (e.g., rifampin). For patient convenience, isoniazid is available in two fixed-dose combinations: (1) capsules, sold as Rifamate, containing 150 mg of isoniazid and 300 mg of rifampin; and (2) tablets, sold as Rifater, containing 50 mg of isoniazid, 120 mg of rifampin, and 300 mg of pyrazinamide.

Adverse Effects

Hepatotoxicity. Isoniazid can cause hepatocellular injury and multilobular necrosis. Consequently, the FDA has issued a Black Box Warning. Deaths have occurred. Liver injury is thought to result from production of a toxic isoniazid metabolite. The greatest risk factor for liver damage is advancing age: the incidence is extremely low in patients younger than 20 years, 1.2% in those aged 35 to 49 years, 2.3% in those aged 50 to 64 years, and 8% in those older than 65 years. Patients should be informed about signs and symptoms of hepatitis and instructed to notify the provider immediately if these develop. Patients should also undergo monthly evaluation for these signs. Some clinicians perform monthly determinations of serum aspartate aminotransferase (AST) activity because elevation of AST activity is indicative of liver injury. However, because AST levels may rise and then return to normal, despite continued isoniazid use, increases in AST may not be predictive of clinical hepatitis. It is recommended that isoniazid be withdrawn if signs of hepatitis develop or if AST activity exceeds 3 to 5 times the pretreatment baseline. Caution should be exercised when giving isoniazid to alcoholics and individuals with preexisting disorders of the liver.

BLACK BOX WARNING: ISONIAZID [GENERIC]

Isoniazid therapy may cause severe hepatitis. Fatalities have been reported.

Peripheral Neuropathy. Dose-related peripheral neuropathy is the most common adverse event. Principal symptoms are symmetric paresthesias (tingling, numbness, burning, pain) of the hands and feet. Clumsiness, unsteadiness, and muscle ache may develop. Peripheral neuropathy results from isoniazid-induced deficiency in pyridoxine (vitamin B_6). Prophylactic use of pyridoxine at 25-50 mg/day can decrease the risk of acquiring peripheral neuropathy. Preventive supplementation is especially important for at-risk people with diabetes or with high alcohol intake. If peripheral neuropathy develops, it can be reversed by administering pyridoxine, however, higher doses are required (typically 100 mg daily).

Other Adverse Effects. Because isoniazid crosses the blood-brain barrier, a variety of central nervous system (CNS) effects can occur, including optic neuritis, seizures, dizziness, ataxia, and psychological disturbances (depression, agitation, impairment of memory, hallucinations, toxic psychosis). Gastrointestinal (GI) distress, dry mouth, and urinary retention occur on occasion. Allergy to isoniazid can produce fever and rashes. Antinuclear antibodies develop in 20% of patients taking this drug.

Drug Interactions

Interactions From Inhibiting Drug Metabolism. Isoniazid is a strong inhibitor of three cytochrome P450 isoenzymes, namely CYP2C9, CYP2C19, and CYP2E1. By inhibiting these isoenzymes, isoniazid can raise levels of drugs that are metabolized by these isoenzymes, including phenytoin, carbamazepine, diazepam, and triazolam. Phenytoin is of particular concern. Plasma levels of phenytoin should be monitored, and phenytoin dosage should be reduced as appropriate. Dosage of isoniazid should not be changed.

Alcohol, Rifampin, Rifapentine, Rifabutin, and Pyrazinamide. Daily ingestion of alcohol or concurrent therapy with rifampin, rifapentine, rifabutin, or pyrazinamide increases the risk for hepatotoxicity. Patients should be encouraged to reduce or eliminate alcohol intake.

Rifampin

Rifampin [Rifadin] equals isoniazid in importance as an anti-TB drug. Before the appearance of resistant tubercle bacilli, the combination of rifampin plus isoniazid was the most frequently prescribed regimen for uncomplicated pulmonary TB.

Antimicrobial Spectrum

Rifampin is a broad-spectrum antibiotic. The drug is active against most gram-positive bacteria as well as many gram-negative bacteria. The drug is bactericidal to *M. tuberculosis* and *Mycobacterium leprae.* Other bacteria that are highly sensitive include *Neisseria meningitidis, Haemophilus influenzae, Staphylococcus aureus,* and *Legionella* species.

Mechanism of Action and Bacterial Resistance

Rifampin inhibits bacterial DNA-dependent RNA polymerase and thereby suppresses RNA synthesis and, consequently, protein synthesis. The results are bactericidal. The drug is lipid soluble and hence has ready access to intracellular bacteria. Because mammalian RNA polymerases are not affected, rifampin is selectively toxic to microbes. Bacterial resistance to rifampin results from production of an altered form of RNA polymerase.

Pharmacokinetics

Absorption and Distribution. Rifampin is well absorbed if taken on an empty stomach. However, if dosing is done with or shortly after a meal, both the rate and extent of absorption can be significantly lowered. Rifampin is distributed widely to tissues and body fluids; however, CSF distribution is only 10-20% of that in the systemic circulation.

Elimination. Rifampin is eliminated primarily by hepatic metabolism. Only about 20% of the drug leaves in the urine. Rifampin induces hepatic drug-metabolizing enzymes, including those responsible for its own inactivation. As a result, the rate at which rifampin is metabolized increases over the first weeks of therapy, causing the half-life of the drug to decrease—from an initial value of about 4 hours down to 2 hours at the end of 2 weeks.

Therapeutic Use

Tuberculosis. Rifampin is one of our most effective anti-TB drugs. This agent is bactericidal to tubercle bacilli at extracellular and intracellular sites. Rifampin is a drug of choice for treating pulmonary TB and disseminated disease. Because resistance can develop rapidly when rifampin is employed alone, the drug is always given in combination with at least one other anti-TB agent. Despite the capacity of rifampin to produce a variety of adverse effects, toxicity rarely requires discontinuing treatment.

Leprosy. Rifampin is bactericidal to *M. leprae* and has become an important agent for treating leprosy. (In 2015, the CDC reported 100 people in the United States had leprosy.)

Meningococcus Carriers. Rifampin is highly active against *N. meningitidis* and is indicated for short-term therapy to eliminate this bacterium from the nasopharynx of asymptomatic carriers. Because resistant organisms emerge rapidly, rifampin should not be used against active meningococcal disease.

Adverse Effects

Rifampin is generally well tolerated. When employed at recommended dosages, the drug rarely causes significant toxicity.

Hepatotoxicity. Rifampin can cause hepatotoxicity, posing a risk for jaundice and even hepatitis. Asymptomatic elevation of liver enzymes occurs in about 14% of patients; however, the incidence of overt hepatitis is less than 1%. Hepatotoxicity is most likely in people who abuse alcohol and patients with preexisting liver disease. These individuals should be monitored closely for signs of liver dysfunction. Tests of liver function (serum aminotransferase levels) should be made before treatment and every 2 to 4 weeks thereafter. Patients should be informed about signs of hepatitis (jaundice, anorexia, malaise, fatigue, nausea) and instructed to notify the prescriber if they develop.

Discoloration of Body Fluids. Rifampin frequently imparts a red-orange color to urine, sweat, saliva, and tears. Patients should be informed of this harmless effect. Permanent staining of soft contact lenses has occurred on occasion, and hence the patient should consult an ophthalmologist regarding contact lens use.

Other Adverse Effects. Gastrointestinal disturbances (anorexia, nausea, abdominal discomfort) and cutaneous reactions (flushing, itching, rash) occur occasionally. Rarely, intermittent high-dose therapy has produced a flu-like syndrome, characterized by fever, chills, muscle aches, headache, and dizziness. This reaction appears to have an immunologic basis. In some patients, high-dose therapy has been associated with shortness of breath, hemolytic anemia, shock, and acute renal failure.

Drug Interactions

Accelerated Metabolism of Other Drugs. Rifampin is a powerful inducer of CYP1A2, CYP2A6, CYP2B6, CYP2C19, CYP2C8, CYP2C9, and CYP3A4 cytochrome P450 isoenzymes. It can hasten the metabolism of many drugs, thereby reducing their effects. This interaction is of special concern with *oral contraceptives, warfarin* (an anticoagulant), and certain *protease inhibitors* and *NNRTIs* used for HIV infection. Women taking oral contraceptives should consider a nonhormonal form of birth control. The dosage of warfarin may need to be increased.

Isoniazid and Pyrazinamide. Rifampin, isoniazid, and pyrazinamide are all hepatotoxic. Hence, when these drugs are used in combination, as they often are, the risk for liver injury is greater than when they are used alone.

Rifapentine

Rifapentine [Priftin] is a long-acting analog of rifampin. Both drugs have the same mechanism of action, adverse effects, and drug interactions. When rifapentine was approved in 1998, it was the first new drug for TB in more than 25 years.

Actions and Uses

Rifapentine is indicated only for pulmonary TB. At therapeutic doses, the drug is lethal to *M. tuberculosis*. The mechanism underlying cell kill is inhibition of DNA-dependent RNA polymerase. To minimize emergence of resistance, rifapentine must always be combined with at least one other anti-TB drug.

Pharmacokinetics

Rifapentine is well absorbed from the GI tract, especially in the presence of food. Plasma levels peak 5 to 6 hours after dosing. In the liver, rifapentine undergoes conversion to 25-desacetyl rifapentine, an active metabolite. Excretion is primarily (70%) fecal. Rifapentine and its metabolite have the same half-life—about 13 hours.

Adverse Effects

Rifapentine is well tolerated at recommended doses. Like rifampin, the drug imparts a red-orange color to urine, sweat, saliva, and tears. Permanent staining of contact lenses can occur.

Hepatotoxicity is the principal concern. In clinical trials, serum transaminase levels increased in 5% of patients. However, overt hepatitis occurred in only one patient. Because of the risk for hepatotoxicity, liver function tests (bilirubin, serum transaminases) should be performed at baseline and monthly thereafter. Patients should be informed about signs of hepatitis (jaundice, anorexia, malaise, fatigue, nausea) and instructed to notify the prescriber if these develop.

Drug Interactions

Like rifampin, rifapentine is a powerful inducer of cytochrome P450 drug-metabolizing enzymes. As a result, it can decrease the levels of other drugs. Important among these are protease inhibitors and NNRTIs (used for HIV infection), oral contraceptives, and warfarin.

Rifabutin

Actions and Uses

Rifabutin [Mycobutin] is a close chemical relative of rifampin. Like rifampin, rifabutin inhibits mycobacterial DNA-dependent RNA polymerase and thereby suppresses protein synthesis. The drug is approved for prevention of disseminated *M. avium* complex (MAC) disease in patients with advanced HIV infection (CD4 lymphocyte counts below 200 cells/mm^3). In addition to this approved application, rifabutin is used off-label as an alternative to rifampin to treat TB in patients with HIV infection. Rifabutin is preferred to rifampin in HIV patients because it has less effect on the metabolism of protease inhibitors and NNRTIs.

Pharmacokinetics

Rifabutin is administered orally. Absorption is unaffected by food. Plasma levels peak in 2 to 3 hours. The drug is widely distributed and achieves high concentrations in the lungs. Rifabutin is metabolized in the liver and excreted in the urine, bile, and feces. Its half-life is 45 hours.

Adverse Effects

Rifabutin is generally well tolerated. The most common side effects (affecting less than 5% of patients) are rash, GI disturbances, and neutropenia. Like rifampin, rifabutin can impart a harmless red-orange color to urine, sweat, saliva, and tears; soft contact lenses may be permanently stained. Rifabutin poses a risk for uveitis and hence should be discontinued if ocular pain or blurred vision develops. Other adverse effects include myositis, hepatitis, arthralgia, chest pain with dyspnea, and a flu-like syndrome.

Drug Interactions

Like rifampin, rifabutin induces cytochrome P450 isoenzymes, although less strongly than rifampin does. By increasing enzyme activity, rifabutin can decrease blood levels of other drugs, especially oral contraceptives and delavirdine, an NNRTI (see Chapter 79). Women using oral contraceptives should be advised to use a nonhormonal method of birth control.

Pyrazinamide

Antimicrobial Activity and Therapeutic Use

Pyrazinamide is bactericidal to *M. tuberculosis.* How it kills bacteria is unknown. Currently, the combination of pyrazinamide with rifampin, isoniazid, and ethambutol is a preferred regimen for initial therapy of active disease caused by drug-sensitive *M. tuberculosis.* In addition, pyrazinamide, in combination with rifampin, may be used for short-course therapy of LTBI, although other regimens are preferred.

Pharmacokinetics

Pyrazinamide is well absorbed after oral administration and undergoes wide distribution to tissues and body fluids. In the liver, the drug is converted to pyrazinoic acid, an active metabolite, and then to 5-hydroxypyrazinoic acid, which is inactive. Excretion is renal, primarily as inactive metabolites.

Adverse Effects and Interactions

Hepatotoxicity. Pyrazinamide is the most hepatotoxic of all the first-line drugs. High-dose therapy has caused hepatitis and, rarely, fatal hepatic necrosis. The earliest manifestations of liver damage are elevations in serum levels of transaminases (AST and alanine aminotransferase [ALT]). Levels of these enzymes should be measured before treatment and every 2 weeks thereafter. Patients should be informed about signs of hepatitis (e.g., malaise, anorexia, nausea, vomiting, jaundice) and instructed to notify the prescriber if they develop. Pyrazinamide should be discontinued if significant injury to the liver occurs. The drug should not be used by patients with preexisting liver disease.

The risk for liver injury is increased by concurrent therapy with isoniazid or rifampin, both of which are hepatotoxic. Pyrazinamide plus rifampin is contraindicated for patients with active liver disease or a history of isoniazid-induced liver injury and should be used with caution in patients who are taking hepatotoxic drugs or who drink alcohol in excess.

Nongouty Polyarthralgias. Polyarthralgias develop in 40% of patients, but only occasionally during the initial phase of treatment. Pain can usually be managed with a nonsteroidal antiinflammatory drug (NSAID), such as aspirin or ibuprofen. A few patients may need to reduce the dosage of pyrazinamide or discontinue treatment.

Other Adverse Effects. Pyrazinamide and its metabolites can inhibit renal excretion of uric acid, causing hyperuricemia. Although usually asymptomatic, pyrazinamide-induced hyperuricemia has (rarely) resulted in gouty arthritis. Additional adverse effects include GI disturbances (nausea, vomiting, diarrhea), rash, and photosensitivity with associated dermatitis.

Ethambutol

Antimicrobial Action

Ethambutol [Myambutol, Etibi ♣] is active only against mycobacteria; nearly all strains of *M. tuberculosis* are sensitive. The drug is bacteriostatic, not bactericidal. In most cases, ethambutol is active against tubercle bacilli that are resistant to isoniazid and rifampin. Although we know that ethambutol can suppress incorporation of mycolic acid in the cell wall, the precise mechanism by which it suppresses bacterial growth has not been established.

Therapeutic Use

Ethambutol is an important anti-TB drug. This agent is employed for initial treatment of TB and for treating patients who have received therapy previously. Like other drugs for TB, ethambutol is always employed as part of a multidrug regimen.

Pharmacokinetics

Ethambutol is readily absorbed after oral administration. The drug is widely distributed to most tissues and body fluids. Levels in CSF, however, remain low. Ethambutol undergoes little hepatic metabolism and is excreted primarily in the urine. The half-life is 3 to 4 hours in patients with healthy kidneys and increases to 8 hours in those with significant renal impairment.

Adverse Effects

Ethambutol is generally well tolerated. The most significant adverse effect is optic neuritis.

Optic Neuritis. Ethambutol can produce dose-related optic neuritis, resulting in blurred vision, constriction of the visual field, and disturbance of color discrimination. The mechanism underlying these effects is unknown. Symptoms usually resolve on discontinuation of treatment. Fortunately, this adverse effect is uncommon; however, for some patients, visual disturbance may persist. Color discrimination and visual acuity should be assessed before treatment and monthly thereafter. Patients should be advised to report any alteration in vision. If ocular toxicity develops, ethambutol should be withdrawn immediately. Because visual changes can be difficult to monitor in pediatric patients, ethambutol is not usually recommended for children younger than 8 years.

Other Adverse Effects. Ethambutol can produce allergic reactions (dermatitis, pruritus), GI upset, and confusion. The drug inhibits renal excretion of uric acid, causing asymptomatic hyperuricemia in about 50% of patients; occasionally, elevation of uric acid levels results in acute gouty arthritis. Rare adverse effects include peripheral neuropathy, renal damage, and thrombocytopenia.

Second-Line Antituberculosis Drugs

The group of second-line anti-TB drugs consists of two fluoroquinolones (levofloxacin and moxifloxacin), four injectable drugs (kanamycin, capreomycin, amikacin, streptomycin), and three other drugs (PAS, ethionamide, and cycloserine). In general, these drugs are less effective, more toxic, and more expensive than the first-line drugs. As a result, their principal indication is TB caused by organisms that have proved resistant to first-line agents. In addition, second-line drugs are used to treat severe pulmonary TB as well as disseminated (extrapulmonary) infection. The second-line drugs are always employed in conjunction with a major anti-TB drug.

Fluoroquinolones

Levofloxacin [Levaquin] and moxifloxacin [Avelox] are fluoroquinolone antibiotics indicated for a wide variety of bacterial infections (see Chapter 76). Both drugs have good activity against *M. tuberculosis.* As therapy for

TB, these drugs are reserved for infection caused by multidrug-resistant organisms. Both drugs are generally well tolerated, although GI disturbances are relatively common. Tendon rupture occurs rarely but may result in permanent damage, especially in patients more than 60 years old. The FDA has issued a Black Box Warning to address this concern. These drugs are not recommended for children.

BLACK BOX WARNING: FLUOROQUINOLONES

Systemic fluoroquinolones (e.g. levofloxacin and moxifloxacin) may cause tendinitis, tendon rupture, and permanent and disabling adverse effects of the tendons, muscles, joints, nerves, and CNS.

Fluoroquinolones may worsen myasthenia gravis-associated muscle weakness.

Injectable Drugs

Capreomycin. Capreomycin [Capastat Sulfate] is an antibiotic derived from a species of *Streptomyces*. Antibacterial effects probably result from inhibiting protein synthesis. The drug is bacteriostatic to *M. tuberculosis*. Capreomycin is used only for TB resistant to primary agents. The principal toxicity is renal damage, and hence the drug should not be taken by patients with kidney disease. Capreomycin may also cause eighth cranial nerve damage, resulting in hearing loss, tinnitus, and disturbed balance (see Black Box Warning). Administration is by deep intramuscular (IM) injection (the drug is not absorbed from the GI tract and therefore cannot be administered orally).

BLACK BOX WARNING: CAPREOMYCIN

Capreomycin is nephrotoxic and ototoxic and can cause renal impairment and cranial nerve VIII impairment. It should not be given to patients with renal insufficiency or auditory impairment. It also should not be given with aminoglycosides or other drugs having similar nephrotoxic and ototoxic effects.

Amikacin, Kanamycin, and Streptomycin. Amikacin [Amikin], kanamycin (generic only), and streptomycin (generic only) are aminoglycoside antibiotics with good activity against *M. tuberculosis*. Like other aminoglycosides, these drugs are nephrotoxic and may also damage the eighth cranial nerve. The FDA issued a Black Box Warning regarding this concern. These drugs are not absorbed from the GI tract, and hence administration is parenteral (IM or intravenous [IV]). The pharmacology of these and other aminoglycosides is discussed in Chapter 72.

BLACK BOX WARNING: AMINOGLYCOSIDES

Aminoglycosides (e.g. streptomycin, amikacin, and kanamycin) are ototoxic and can cause permanent hearing loss. Vertigo may occur as a result of vestibular injury. Aminoglycosides are nephrotoxic and may cause renal impairment.

Other Second-Line Drugs

Para-Aminosalicylic Acid

Actions and Uses. PAS [Paser Granules] is similar in structure and actions to the sulfonamides. Like the sulfonamides, PAS exerts its antibacterial effects by inhibiting synthesis of folic acid. However, in contrast to the sulfonamides, which are broad-spectrum antibiotics, PAS is active only against mycobacteria. In the United States PAS has been employed primarily as a substitute for ethambutol in pediatric patients. The drug is always used in combination with other anti-TB agents.

Pharmacokinetics. PAS is administered orally, and absorption is good. The drug is distributed widely to most tissues and body fluids, although levels in CSF remain low. PAS undergoes extensive hepatic metabolism. Metabolites and parent drug are excreted in the urine.

Adverse Effects. PAS is poorly tolerated by adults; children accept the drug somewhat better. The most frequent adverse effects are GI disturbances (nausea, vomiting, diarrhea). Because PAS is administered in large doses as a sodium salt, substantial sodium loading may occur. Additional adverse effects are allergic reactions, hepatotoxicity, and goiter.

Storage. PAS [Paser Granules] loses its effectiveness if exposed to heat. Packets should be stored in a cool location (below 59°F).

Ethionamide

Actions and Uses. Ethionamide [Trecator], a relative of isoniazid, is active against mycobacteria, but less so than isoniazid itself. Ethionamide is administered with other anti-TB drugs to treat TB that is resistant to first-line agents. Gastrointestinal disturbances limit patient acceptance. Ethionamide is the least well tolerated of all anti-TB agents and hence should be used only when there is no alternative.

Pharmacokinetics. Ethionamide is readily absorbed after oral administration. The drug is widely distributed to tissues and body fluids, including the CSF. Ethionamide undergoes extensive metabolism and is excreted in the urine, primarily as metabolites.

Adverse Effects. Gastrointestinal effects (anorexia, nausea, vomiting, diarrhea, metallic taste) occur often; intolerance of these effects frequently leads to discontinuation. Ethionamide is toxic to the liver. Hepatotoxicity is assessed by measuring serum transaminases (AST, ALT) before treatment and periodically thereafter. Additional adverse effects include peripheral neuropathy, CNS effects (convulsions, mental disturbance), and allergic reactions.

Cycloserine

Actions and Uses. Cycloserine [generic] is an antibiotic produced by a species of *Streptomyces*. The drug is bacteriostatic and acts by inhibiting cell wall synthesis. Cycloserine is used against TB resistant to first-line drugs.

Pharmacokinetics. Cycloserine is rapidly absorbed after oral administration. The drug is widely distributed to tissues and body fluids, including the CSF. Elimination is by hepatic metabolism and renal excretion; about 50% of the drug leaves unchanged in the urine. Cycloserine may accumulate to toxic levels in patients with renal impairment.

Adverse Effects. CNS effects occur frequently and can be severe. Possible reactions include anxiety, depression, confusion, hallucinations, paranoia, hyperreflexia, and seizures. Psychotic episodes occur in approximately 10% of patients; symptoms usually subside within 2 weeks after drug withdrawal. Pyridoxine may prevent neurotoxic effects. Other adverse effects include peripheral neuropathy, hepatotoxicity, and folate deficiency. To minimize the risk for adverse effects, serum concentrations of cycloserine should be measured periodically; peak concentrations, measured 2 hours after dosing, should be 25 to 35 mcg/mL.

Bedaquiline

When the FDA granted accelerated approval of bedaquiline [Sirturo] in December 2012, it was heralded as the first unique drug in the anti-TB arsenal to emerge in more than 40 years. The drug appears to work faster and better than all other anti-TB drugs. In addition, bedaquiline does not accelerate the metabolism of other drugs and hence can be used in patients taking drugs for HIV. That being said, it is not among those drugs recommended as first or second-line drugs in the ATS/CDC/IDSA Guidelines pending results of additional clinical trials. It also has some serious adverse effects and costs approximately $36,000 for 100 tablets.

BLACK BOX WARNING: BEDAQUILINE [SIRTURO]

Subjects in a bedaquiline clinical trial had an increased mortality rate: 11.4% died compared with 2.5% in the group taking a placebo.

Bedaquiline can cause QT prolongation. Discontinue the drug if QT prolongation exceeds 500 msec.

Bedaquiline is highly effective. In a mouse model of TB, a three-drug regimen consisting of bedaquiline plus rifampin and pyrazinamide was compared with a conventional three-drug regimen consisting of isoniazid plus rifampin and pyrazinamide. The result? After 1 month with the bedaquiline regimen, bacterial load was as low as seen after 2 months with the conventional regimen, indicating accelerated bacterial kill. And after 2 months with the bedaquiline regimen, mycobacteria were cleared entirely from the lungs, an unprecedented outcome. In laboratory tests, bedaquiline was bactericidal to all isolates of *M. tuberculosis* resistant to conventional therapy, including multidrug-resistant strains.

Actions and Uses

This drug has a unique mechanism of action: bacterial kill results from inhibiting adenosine triphosphate (ATP) synthase, an enzyme required by

M. tuberculosis to make ATP. No other drug shares this mechanism, which explains why there's no cross-resistance between bedaquiline and conventional drugs. Because humans make ATP by a different pathway, bedaquiline does not interfere with ATP synthesis in humans.

Bedaquiline is approved for multidrug-resistant pulmonary TB in patients at least 18 years of age. It is not approved for treatment of latent, nonpulmonary, or drug-sensitive tuberculosis (i.e., TB that is effectively treated by other drugs). It also should not be used for mycobacterial infections other than TB.

Pharmacokinetics

Bedaquiline has desirable kinetics. The drug undergoes rapid absorption after oral dosing and distributes to all tissues. Of particular importance, it concentrates in cells of the lungs, reaching levels 10 times those in blood. Furthermore, it remains in the body for days, permitting continued bactericidal effects with just once-a-week dosing.

Interaction with rifampin may be a concern. Why? Because rifampin induces the activity of CYP3A4, the isoenzyme of cytochrome P450 that metabolizes bedaquiline. In a clinical trial, rifampin significantly reduced blood levels of bedaquiline.

Although resistance to bedaquiline is uncommon, it does occur: about 1 in 200 million tubercle bacilli make a form of ATP synthase that is not inhibited by the drug. Accordingly, to prevent overgrowth with these resistant microbes, the regimen should always contain other anti-TB drugs.

Adverse Effects

Bedaquiline labeling includes a black box warning related to the risk for prolonged QT interval and risk for hepatotoxicity. In clinical trials, there was an increased risk for death in patients taking bedaquiline compared with those taking a placebo. Subsequently, labeling recommends bedaquiline only if there is no other effective treatment. Beyond the adverse effects listed in the black box warning, bedaquiline has few adverse effects. Approximately 10% to 40% of patients may experience nausea, arthralgia, headache, chest pain, and hemoptysis. Fewer than 10% experience rash and anorexia. It has an FDA Pregnancy Risk Category B designation.

DRUGS FOR *MYCOBACTERIUM AVIUM* COMPLEX INFECTION

MAC consists of two nearly indistinguishable organisms: *M. avium* and *M. intracellulare*. Colonization with MAC begins in the lungs or GI tract, but then may spread to the blood, bone marrow, liver, spleen, lymph nodes, brain, kidneys, and skin. Disseminated infection is common in patients infected with HIV; the incidence at autopsy is 50%. Among immunocompetent patients, symptomatic MAC infection is usually limited to the lungs. Signs and symptoms of disseminated MAC infection include fever, night sweats, weight loss, lethargy, anemia, and abnormal liver function tests.

Drugs are used for prophylaxis and to treat active infection. Preferred agents for prophylaxis of disseminated infection are azithromycin and clarithromycin. Regimens for treating active infection in immunocompetent hosts should include (1) azithromycin or clarithromycin plus (2) ethambutol plus (3) rifampin or rifabutin. Additional drugs may be added as needed; options include streptomycin and amikacin. Treatment of active infection in immunocompetent patients should continue for 12 months after cultures become negative. Representative regimens for immunocompetent patients are shown in Table 75.6. Regimens for patients with HIV infection are discussed in Chapter 79.

PRESCRIBING AND MONITORING CONSIDERATIONS

The following discussion is limited to the drug therapy of TB. Patient education for these drugs is provided in the Patient Education box.

Implications That Apply to All Antituberculosis Drugs

Promoting Adherence for All Drugs

Treatment of active TB is prolonged and demands concurrent use of two or more drugs; as a result, adherence can be a

Patient Education

DRUGS FOR TUBERCULOSIS

To promote adherence, educate the patient about the rationale for multidrug therapy and the need for long-term treatment. Encourage patients to take their medication exactly as prescribed and to continue treatment until the infection has resolved.

All first-line drugs except ethambutol carry a risk of hepatotoxicity; therefore, the combination of drugs for TB increases the risk for liver damage. Inform patients about signs of hepatitis (jaundice, anorexia, malaise, fatigue, nausea) and instruct them to report any of these signs and symptoms if these develop. Urge patients who drink alcohol to minimize or eliminate alcohol consumption. Instruct patients to avoid acetaminophen and other drugs that can cause liver damage.

Inform patients taking isoniazid about symptoms of peripheral neuropathy (tingling, numbness, burning, or pain in the hands or feet) and instruct them to report symptoms if these occur.

Inform patients taking rifampin that it may impart a harmless red-orange color to urine, sweat, saliva, and tears. Warn patients that soft contact lenses may undergo permanent staining. Advise them to consult their eye care specialist (optometrist or ophthalmologist) about continued use of the lenses.

When prescribing rifampin, advise women taking oral contraceptives to use a nonhormonal form of birth control.

Advise patients taking pyrazinamide who develop polyarthralgias to take an NSAID (e.g., aspirin, ibuprofen) to relieve pain.

Instruct patients taking ethambutol to report any alteration in vision (e.g., blurring of vision, reduced color discrimination).

TABLE 75.6 ■ Regimens for *Mycobacterium avium* Complex Infection in Immunocompetent Adults

PULMONARY MAC	
Daily regimen	Clarithromycin (500 mg twice daily) *or* azithromycin (250 mg) *plus* Ethambutol (25 mg/kg for 2 months, then 15 mg/kg thereafter) *plus* Rifampin (600 mg) *or* rifabutin (300 mg) *may also add* Streptomycin (15 mg/kg 3 times a week for 2–6 months)
Duration	Treat until cultures remain negative for 12 months
DISSEMINATED MAC	
Daily regimen	Clarithromycin (500 mg twice daily) *or* azithromycin (250–500 mg) *plus* Ethambutol (15 mg/kg) *plus* Rifampin (600 mg) *or* rifabutin (300 mg) *may also add* Streptomycin (15 mg/kg 3 times a week for 2–6 months)
Duration	Treat until cultures remain negative for 12 months

MAC, Mycobacterium avium complex.

significant problem. Adherence can be greatly increased by using DOT combined with intermittent dosing (rather than daily dosing).

Evaluating Treatment

Success is indicated by (1) reductions in fever, malaise, anorexia, cough, and other clinical manifestations of TB (usually within weeks); (2) radiographic evidence of improvement (usually in 3 months); and (3) an absence of *M. tuberculosis* in sputum (usually after 3–6 months).

Treatment evaluation must also consider adverse events. The most concerning adverse effects shared by two or more drugs are presented next.

Hepatotoxicity. All first-line drugs except ethambutol can cause hepatocellular damage. Diligence is assessment for hepatic injury is paramount. Daily ingestion of alcohol increases the risk for liver injury; therefore, efforts taken to help patients to decrease alcohol intake will decrease this risk.

Rash. All drugs for TB can cause rashes. While this effect may be insignificant for a single drug, when combined this can be especially concerning for patients. Use of sunscreen may be beneficial. Care will need to be individualized depending on the presentation.

The ATS/CDC/IDSA Guidelines recommend additional periodic screening to monitor patients receiving treatment. See Table 75.7.

In the following section, we review the most pertinent information, not previously mentioned, about selected drugs for TB.

TABLE 75.7 ▪ Monitoring Recommendations

Providers should assess the following prior to beginning treatment with first-line drugs for TB. Follow-up recommendations should be obtained periodically as indicated.

Assessment	Timing
Sputum smears and culture	Baseline then monthly until two consecutive specimens are negative
Drug susceptibility	Baseline then repeat at 3 months if sputum cultures remain positive
Chest radiograph	Baseline then repeat 2 months following negative sputum cultures
Weight	Baseline then monthly
Symptom assessment	Baseline them monthly
Adherence to treatment	Baseline then monthly
Visual acuity and color discrimination	Baseline then monthly if taking ethambutol
AST, ALT, bilirubin, alkaline phosphate	Baseline then monthly if baseline abnormal, if signs or symptoms of liver injury develop, or for patients at high risk of liver injury (e.g. high alcohol intake, HIV infection, taking drugs associated with liver injury)
Creatinine	Baseline than as indicated
Platelet count	Baseline then monthly if abnormal
HIV	Baseline then, if HIV positive, obtain CD4 lymphocyte count and HIV RNA load
Hepatitis B and C screen	Baseline for patients with risk factors
Diabetes screen	Baseline for patients with risk factors

ALT, alanine aminotransferase; AST, aspartate aminotransferase.

Isoniazid

Identifying High-Risk Patients

Isoniazid is *contraindicated* for patients with acute liver disease or a history of isoniazid-induced hepatotoxicity.

Use with *caution* in alcohol abusers, diabetic patients, patients with vitamin B_6 deficiency, patients older than 50 years, and patients who are taking phenytoin, rifampin, rifabutin, rifapentine, or pyrazinamide.

Ongoing Monitoring and Interventions

Minimizing Adverse Effects

Peripheral Neuropathy. Peripheral neuritis can be reversed by prescribing daily doses of pyridoxine (vitamin B_6). This is especially important for patients at high risk for neuropathy (e.g., patients with diabetes or patients with high alcohol intake).

Minimizing Adverse Interactions

Phenytoin. Isoniazid can suppress the metabolism of phenytoin, thereby causing phenytoin levels to rise. Plasma phenytoin should be monitored. If necessary, phenytoin dosage should be reduced.

Rifampin

Identifying High-Risk Patients

Rifampin is *contraindicated* for patients taking delavirdine (an NNRTI) and most protease inhibitors.

Use with *caution* in alcohol abusers, patients with liver disease, and patients taking warfarin.

Ongoing Monitoring and Interventions

Minimizing Adverse Effects

Discoloration of Body Fluids. Rifampin may impart a harmless red-orange color to urine, sweat, saliva, and tears. If your patient wears soft contact lenses, be certain that they are aware that permanent staining may occur.

Minimizing Adverse Interactions

Accelerated Metabolism of Other Drugs. Rifampin can accelerate the metabolism of many drugs, thereby reducing their effects. This action is of particular concern with *oral contraceptives, warfarin, most protease inhibitors,* and *delavirdine* (an NNRTI). Monitor warfarin effects and increase dosage as needed. Do not combine protease inhibitors or NNRTIs with rifampin. Recommend alternative birth control for women of childbearing age.

Pyrazinamide and Isoniazid. These hepatotoxic anti-TB drugs can increase the risk for liver injury when used with rifampin.

Pyrazinamide

Identifying High-Risk Patients

Pyrazinamide is *contraindicated* for patients with severe liver dysfunction or acute gout.

Use with *caution* in alcohol abusers.

Ongoing Monitoring and Interventions

Minimizing Adverse Effects

Nongouty Polyarthralgias. Polyarthralgias develop in 40% of patients. Some patients may need to stop pyrazinamide, or at least reduce the dosage.

Ethambutol

Identifying High-Risk Patients

Ethambutol is *contraindicated* for patients with optic neuritis.

Ongoing Monitoring and Interventions

Minimizing Adverse Effects

Optic Neuritis. Ethambutol can cause dose-related optic neuritis. Symptoms include blurred vision, altered color discrimination, and constriction of visual fields. Baseline vision tests are required. If ocular toxicity develops, ethambutol should be withdrawn at once.

CHAPTER

76 Miscellaneous Antibacterial Drugs

Laura D. Rosenthal, DNP, ACNP, FAANP

FLUOROQUINOLONES

The fluoroquinolones are fluorinated analogs of nalidixic acid, a narrow-spectrum quinolone antibiotic used only for urinary tract infections (UTIs). However, unlike nalidixic acid, the fluoroquinolones are broad-spectrum agents that have multiple applications. Benefits derive from disrupting DNA replication and cell division. Fluoroquinolones do not disrupt synthesis of proteins or the cell wall. All of the systemic fluoroquinolones can be administered orally. As a result, these drugs are attractive alternatives for people who might otherwise require intravenous antibacterial therapy. Although side effects are generally mild, all fluoroquinolones can cause tendinitis and tendon rupture, usually of the Achilles tendon. Fortunately, the risk is low. Bacterial resistance develops slowly but has become common in *Neisseria gonorrhoeae,* and hence these drugs are no longer recommended for this infection. Five fluoroquinolones are currently available for systemic therapy. Fluoroquinolones used solely for topical treatment of the eyes are discussed in Chapter 84.

Ciprofloxacin

Ciprofloxacin [Cipro] was among the first fluoroquinolones available and will serve as our prototype for the group. The drug is active against a broad spectrum of bacterial pathogens and may be administered by the oral (PO) or intravenous (IV) route. Oral ciprofloxacin has been used as an alternative to parenteral antibiotics for treatment of several serious infections. Because it can be administered by mouth, patients receiving ciprofloxacin can be treated at home, rather than going to the hospital for IV antibacterial therapy.

Mechanism of Action

Ciprofloxacin inhibits two bacterial enzymes: *DNA gyrase* and *topoisomerase IV.* Both are needed for DNA replication and cell division. DNA gyrase converts closed circular DNA into a supercoiled configuration. In the absence of supercoiling, DNA replication cannot take place. Topoisomerase IV helps separate daughter DNA strands during cell division. Because the mammalian equivalents of DNA gyrase and topoisomerase IV are largely insensitive to fluoroquinolones, cells of the host are spared. Ciprofloxacin is rapidly bactericidal.

Antimicrobial Spectrum

Ciprofloxacin is active against a broad spectrum of bacteria, including most aerobic gram-negative bacteria and some gram-positive bacteria. Most urinary tract pathogens, including *Escherichia coli* and *Klebsiella* species, are sensitive. The drug is also highly active against most bacteria that cause enteritis (e.g., *Salmonella* and *Shigella* species, *Campylobacter jejuni, E. coli*). Other sensitive organisms include *Bacillus anthracis, Pseudomonas aeruginosa, Haemophilus influenzae*, meningococci, and many streptococci. Activity against anaerobes is fair to poor. *Clostridium difficile* is resistant.

Bacterial Resistance

Resistance to fluoroquinolones has developed during treatment of infections caused by *Staphylococcus aureus, Serratia marcescens, C. jejuni, P. aeruginosa,* and *N. gonorrhoeae*. Two mechanisms appear responsible: (1) alterations in DNA gyrase and topoisomerase IV and (2) increased drug export. Bacteria do not directly inactivate fluoroquinolones, and there have been no reports of resistance through transfer of R factors.

Pharmacokinetics

Ciprofloxacin may be given by PO or IV route. After oral dosing, the drug is absorbed rapidly but incompletely. High concentrations are achieved in urine, stool, bile, saliva, bone, and prostate tissue. Drug levels in cerebrospinal fluid remain low. Ciprofloxacin has a plasma half-life of about 4 hours. Elimination is by hepatic metabolism and renal excretion.

Therapeutic Uses

Ciprofloxacin is approved for a wide variety of infections. Among these are infections of the respiratory tract, urinary tract, gastrointestinal (GI) tract, bones, joints, skin, and soft tissues. Also, ciprofloxacin is a preferred drug for preventing anthrax in people who have inhaled anthrax spores. Because ciprofloxacin is active against a variety of pathogens and can be given orally, the drug represents an alternative to parenteral treatment for many serious infections. Owing to high rates of resistance, ciprofloxacin is a poor choice for staphylococcal infections. The drug is not useful against infections caused by anaerobes.

Because of concerns about tendon injury (see later), *systemic* ciprofloxacin is generally avoided in children younger than 18 years. Nonetheless, the drug does have two approved pediatric uses: (1) treatment of complicated urinary tract and kidney infections caused by *E. coli* and (2) postexposure treatment of inhalational anthrax.

Adverse Effects

Ciprofloxacin can induce a variety of mild adverse effects, including GI reactions (nausea, vomiting, diarrhea, abdominal pain) and central nervous system (CNS) effects (dizziness, headache, restlessness, confusion). *Candida* infections of the pharynx and vagina may develop during treatment. Very rarely, seizures have occurred. In older adults, ciprofloxacin poses a significant risk for confusion, somnolence, psychosis, and visual disturbances.

Fluoroquinolones damage tendons by disrupting the extracellular matrix of cartilage in immature animals. A similar mechanism may underlie tendon rupture in humans. Because tendon injury is reversible if diagnosed early, fluoroquinolones should be discontinued at the first sign of tendon pain, swelling, or inflammation. In addition, patients should refrain from exercise until tendinitis has been ruled out. Although there are no controlled studies on the use of ciprofloxacin during pregnancy or lactation, limited data indicate that such use poses little or no risk for tendon damage to either the fetus or nursing infant. Because of the relative lack of data, alternative drugs should be given if possible.

Ciprofloxacin and other fluoroquinolones pose a risk for *phototoxicity* (severe sunburn), characterized by burning, erythema, exudation, vesicles, blistering, and edema. These can occur after exposure to direct sunlight, indirect sunlight, and sunlamps—even if a sunscreen has been applied. Patients should be warned about phototoxicity and advised to avoid sunlight and sunlamps. People who must go outdoors should wear protective clothing and apply a sunscreen. Ciprofloxacin should be withdrawn at the first sign of a phototoxic reaction (e.g., burning sensation, redness, rash).

Ciprofloxacin and other fluoroquinolones increase the risk for developing *C. difficile* infection (CDI), a potentially severe infection of the bowel. CDI results from killing off intestinal bacteria that normally keep *C. difficile* in check.

Prototype Drugs

MISCELLANEOUS ANTIBACTERIAL DRUGS

Fluoroquinolone

Ciprofloxacin

Cyclic Lipopeptide

Daptomycin

BLACK BOX WARNING: FLUROQUINALONES AND TENDON RUPTURE

Rarely, ciprofloxacin and other fluoroquinolones have caused tendon rupture, usually of the Achilles tendon. The incidence is 1 in 10,000 or less. People at highest risk are those 60 years and older, those taking glucocorticoids, and those who have undergone heart, lung, or kidney transplantation.

BLACK BOX WARNING: CIPROFLOXACIN AND MYASTHENIA GRAVIS

Ciprofloxacin and other fluoroquinolones can exacerbate muscle weakness in patients with myasthenia gravis. Accordingly, patients with a history of myasthenia gravis should not receive these drugs.

Drug and Food Interactions

Cationic Compounds

Absorption of ciprofloxacin can be reduced by compounds that contain cations. Among these are (1) aluminum- or magnesium-containing antacids, (2) iron salts, (3) zinc salts, (4) sucralfate, (5) calcium supplements, and (6) milk and other dairy products, all of which contain calcium ions. These cationic agents should be administered at least 6 hours before ciprofloxacin or 2 hours after.

Elevation of Drug Levels

Ciprofloxacin can increase plasma levels of several drugs, including *theophylline* (used for asthma), *warfarin* (an anticoagulant), and *tinidazole* (an antifungal drug). Toxicity could result. For patients taking theophylline, drug levels should be monitored and the dosage adjusted accordingly. For patients taking warfarin, prothrombin time should be monitored and the dosage of warfarin reduced as appropriate.

Preparations, Dosage, and Administration

Preparations

Ciprofloxacin is available for PO and IV administration. For PO therapy, ciprofloxacin is supplied in immediate-release tablets (100, 250, 500, and 750 mg) sold as Cipro, a 500 mg/5 mL suspension, and extended-release tablets (500 and 1000 mg) sold as Cipro XR. For IV therapy, ciprofloxacin is supplied in solution (400 mg/200 mL) sold as Cipro I.V.

Dosage and Administration

Oral. Dosing may be done with or without food. The dosage for complicated UTIs is 250 or 500 mg 2 times a day, usually for 7 to 14 days. For other infections, dosages range from 500 to 750 mg 2 times a day. Dosage should be reduced for patients with renal impairment. Dosages for anthrax prevention are presented later.

Intravenous. Intravenous dosages range from 200 to 400 mg every 12 hours. Dosages for anthrax prevention are presented later.

Inhalational Anthrax. Ciprofloxacin is used to reduce the incidence of anthrax or prevent anthrax progression in people who have inhaled *B. anthracis* spores. The dosage for adults is 500 mg PO (or 400 mg IV) every 12 hours for 60 days. The dosage for children is 15 mg/kg PO (or 10 mg/kg IV) every 12 hours for 60 days (with the provision that individual oral doses not exceed 500 mg, and individual IV doses not exceed 400 mg).

PATIENT-CENTERED CARE ACROSS THE LIFE SPAN

Antibacterial Drugs

Life Stage	Patient Care Concerns
Infants	See later entry "Breastfeeding women."
Children/adolescents	Ciprofloxacin and levofloxacin are the only fluoroquinolones approved for use in children. Because of concerns regarding tendon injury, fluoroquinolones are generally avoided in this population.
Pregnant women	Although data reveal little potential for fluoroquinolone toxicity in the fetus, these data are limited. Risks and benefits must be considered for administration during pregnancy.
Breast-feeding women	Effects of fluoroquinolones on the nursing infant are largely unknown. Consider other medications if possible.
Older adults	Fluoroquinolones are generally well tolerated in older adults. Calculate creatinine clearance for safe dosing.

Other Systemic Fluoroquinolones

Ofloxacin

Basic Pharmacology

Ofloxacin is similar to ciprofloxacin in mechanism of action, antimicrobial spectrum, therapeutic applications, and adverse effects. Like ciprofloxacin, the drug is administered orally. Bioavailability is high (90%) in the absence of food and is greatly reduced in the presence of food. Ofloxacin is widely distributed to tissues and excreted in the urine. Like ciprofloxacin, ofloxacin can cause a variety of mild adverse effects, including nausea, vomiting, headache, and dizziness. In addition, ofloxacin may intensify sensitivity to sunlight, thereby increasing the risk for severe sunburn. Like other fluoroquinolones, ofloxacin can (1) exacerbate muscle weakness in patients with myasthenia gravis; (2) increase the risk for CDI; and (3) cause tendinitis and tendon rupture, especially among those older than 60 years, those taking glucocorticoids, and those who have undergone a heart, lung, or kidney transplantation. Ofloxacin elevates plasma levels of warfarin, but, in contrast to ciprofloxacin, has little effect on levels of theophylline. Absorption of oral ofloxacin is reduced by cationic substances: milk, milk products, sucralfate, iron and zinc salts, and magnesium- and aluminum-containing antacids.

Preparations, Dosage, and Administration

Ofloxacin is available in tablets (200, 300, and 400 mg) for dosing with or without food. The usual daily dosage is 200 to 400 mg every 12 hours. Treatment duration ranges from 1 day to 6 weeks. Dosage should be reduced in patients with renal impairment.

Moxifloxacin

Basic Pharmacology

Moxifloxacin [Avelox] is a broad-spectrum fluoroquinolone indicated for respiratory tract infections (community-associated pneumonia [CAP], acute sinusitis, acute exacerbations of chronic bronchitis), intraabdominal infections, and infections of the skin and skin structures. Administration is PO or IV. The drug is well absorbed from the GI tract, undergoes wide distribution, and is eliminated by hepatic metabolism and renal excretion. Side effects are generally mild, the most common being nausea, vomiting, diarrhea, stomach pain, dizziness, and altered sense of taste. Like other fluoroquinolones, moxifloxacin can promote development of CDI, exacerbate muscle weakness in patients with myasthenia gravis, and cause tendinitis and tendon rupture. The drug may also pose a risk for phototoxicity. Moxifloxacin does not increase levels of warfarin or digoxin, but does prolong the QT interval, and hence may pose a risk for serious dysrhythmias. Accordingly, the drug should be used with great caution, if at all, in patients taking prodysrhythmic drugs or in those with hypokalemia or preexisting QT prolongation.

Preparations, Dosage, and Administration

For systemic therapy, moxifloxacin [Avelox, Avelox I.V.] is available in 400-mg tablets and in solution (400 mg/250 mL) for slow IV infusion. PO and IV dosages are the same and should be reduced in patients with renal impairment. The usual dosage for sinusitis and pneumonia is 400 mg once a day for 10 days; the usual dosage for bronchitis is 400 mg once a day for 5 days. Oral dosing may be done with or without food. However, because absorption can be reduced by cationic substances (e.g., milk, sucralfate, iron and zinc salts, magnesium- or aluminum-containing antacids), moxifloxacin should be administered at least 4 hours before these agents or 8 hours after.

Levofloxacin

Levofloxacin [Levaquin] is active against *Streptococcus pneumoniae* (also known as pneumococcus), *H. influenzae, S. aureus, Enterococcus faecalis, Streptococcus pyogenes*, and *Proteus mirabilis*. Approved indications include UTIs, chronic bacterial prostatitis, inhalational anthrax, complicated skin and skin structure infections, and certain respiratory tract infections: acute maxillary sinusitis, acute bacterial exacerbations of chronic bronchitis, and CAP, including CAP caused by penicillin-resistant pneumococci. Possible adverse effects include peripheral neuropathy, rhabdomyolysis, tendinitis, tendon rupture, phototoxicity, and CDI, as well as muscle weakness in patients with myasthenia gravis. To treat systemic infections, levofloxacin may be administered PO or IV. Absorption from the GI tract is reduced by cationic substances (e.g., magnesium- and aluminum-containing antacids, zinc and iron salts, sucralfate, milk and milk products), but not by most foods. Levofloxacin is available in tablets (250, 500, and 750 mg), an oral solution (25 mg/mL), and a solution for slow IV infusion (5 and 25 mg/mL). The usual dosage is 500 mg once a day for 7 to 14 days. In patients with renal impairment, the dosage is 500 mg every 48 hours. Oral doses may be taken with or without food.

Gemifloxacin

Therapeutic Use

Gemifloxacin [Factive] is an oral fluoroquinolone approved for two respiratory tract infections in adults: (1) mild to moderate CAP and (2) acute bacterial exacerbations of chronic bronchitis (ABECB). The drug is active against *H. influenzae, Moraxella catarrhalis, Chlamydia pneumoniae, Mycoplasma pneumoniae, Legionella pneumophila,* and *S. pneumoniae*, including strains that are multidrug resistant. Gemifloxacin causes a high incidence of rash and, compared with older fluoroquinolones used for respiratory infections, has no significant advantages and costs more. Accordingly, the older agents—levofloxacin and moxifloxacin—are preferred.

Adverse Effects

Gemifloxacin is generally well tolerated. The most common reactions are diarrhea, rash, nausea, headache, abdominal pain, vomiting, dizziness, and altered sense of taste. In addition, the drug may cause tendinitis, tendon injury, phototoxicity, hypersensitivity reactions, liver damage, and CDI, as well as muscle weakness in patients with myasthenia gravis. Like some other fluoroquinolones, gemifloxacin can prolong the QT interval, thereby posing a risk for dysrhythmias. Accordingly, the drug should not be used by patients taking prodysrhythmic drugs or those with hypokalemia or preexisting QT prolongation.

The incidence of rash with gemifloxacin is much higher than with other fluoroquinolones. Women younger than 40 years are at greatest risk. Symptoms are severe in about 10% of patients who develop a rash; in the rest, symptoms are mild to moderate. As a rule, gemifloxacin-induced rash resolves spontaneously in 1 to 2 weeks, although some patients require treatment with systemic glucocorticoids. If rash develops, gemifloxacin should be discontinued.

Drug Interactions

As with ciprofloxacin, absorption of gemifloxacin can be reduced by compounds that contain cations. Among these are iron salts, zinc salts, sucralfate, aluminum- or magnesium-containing antacids, and milk and other dairy products, which contain calcium ions. To ensure adequate absorption, these cationic agents should be administered at least 6 hours before gemifloxacin or 2 hours after.

Preparations, Dosage, and Administration

Gemifloxacin [Factive] is available in 320-mg tablets for oral dosing, with or without food. The dosage for CAP is 320 mg once a day for 7 days, and the dosage ABECB is 320 mg once a day for 5 days. For patients with severe renal impairment, the dosage should be reduced. To prevent high concentrations in the urine, all patients should consume liberal amounts of fluid.

ADDITIONAL ANTIBACTERIAL DRUGS

Metronidazole

Metronidazole [Flagyl] is used for protozoal infections and infections caused by obligate anaerobic bacteria. The basic pharmacology of metronidazole is discussed in Chapter 81, as is the drug's use against protozoal infections. Consideration here is limited to antibacterial applications.

Mechanism of Antibacterial Action

Metronidazole is lethal to anaerobic organisms only. To exert bactericidal effects, metronidazole must first be taken up by cells and then converted into its active form; only anaerobes can perform the conversion. The active form interacts with DNA to cause strand breakage and loss of helical structure, effects that result in inhibition of nucleic acid synthesis and, ultimately, cell death. Because aerobic bacteria are unable to activate metronidazole, they are insensitive to the drug.

Antibacterial Spectrum

Metronidazole is active against obligate anaerobes only. Sensitive bacterial pathogens include *Bacteroides fragilis* (and other *Bacteroides* species), *C. difficile* (and other *Clostridium* species), *Fusobacterium* species, *Gardnerella vaginalis, Peptococcus* species, and *Peptostreptococcus* species.

Therapeutic Uses

Metronidazole is active against a variety of anaerobic bacterial infections, including infections of the CNS, abdominal organs, bones and joints, skin and soft tissues, and genitourinary tract. Frequently, these infections also involve aerobic bacteria, and hence therapy must include a drug active against them. Metronidazole is a drug of choice for CDI, as discussed in Chapter 70. In addition, the drug is employed for prophylaxis in surgical procedures associated with a high risk for infection by anaerobes (e.g., colorectal surgery, abdominal surgery, gynecologic surgery). Metronidazole is also used in combination with a tetracycline and bismuth subsalicylate to eradicate *Helicobacter pylori* in people with peptic ulcer disease. Development of resistance to metronidazole is rare.

Preparations, Dosage, and Administration

For initial treatment of serious bacterial infections, metronidazole is administered by IV infusion. Under appropriate conditions, the patient may switch to oral therapy.

Intravenous Formulations
Metronidazole is available in solution for IV use. The solution (generic only) contains 5 mg of metronidazole per milliliter and is ready for IV use.

Intravenous Dosage and Administration
Therapy of anaerobic infections in adults is initiated with a loading dose of 15 mg/kg. After this, maintenance doses of 7.5 mg/kg are given every 6 to 8 hours. Treatment duration is usually 1 to 2 weeks.

Oral Preparations and Dosage
Metronidazole [Flagyl, Flagyl ER] is supplied in capsules (375 mg), immediate-release tablets (250 and 500 mg), and extended-release tablets (750 mg). The adult dosage for anaerobic infections is 7.5 mg/kg every 6 hours. For bacterial vaginosis in adults, a dosage of 750 mg (extended-release formulation) once daily for 7 days is effective. The dosage for CDI is 500 mg 3 times a day for 10 to 14 days.

BLACK BOX WARNING: METRONIDAZOLE

Metronidazole has been associated with increased carcinogenic risk in mice and rats. Avoid unnecessary use.

Daptomycin

Daptomycin [Cubicin] is the first representative of a new class of antibiotics, the *cyclic lipopeptides*. The drug has a unique mechanism and can rapidly kill virtually all clinically relevant gram-positive bacteria, including methicillin-resistant *S. aureus*. Daptomycin is devoid of significant drug interactions, and the only notable side effect is possible muscle injury. The drug is given once daily by IV infusion, and there is no need to monitor its plasma level.

Mechanism of Action

Daptomycin has a novel mechanism of action. The drug inserts itself into the bacterial cell membrane and thereby forms channels that permit efflux of intracellular potassium (and possibly other cytoplasmic ions). Loss of intracellular ions has two effects. First, it depolarizes the cell membrane. And second, it inhibits synthesis of DNA, RNA, and proteins and thereby causes cell death.

Antibacterial Spectrum

Daptomycin is active only against gram-positive bacteria. The drug cannot penetrate the outer membrane of gram-negative bacteria and hence cannot harm them. Daptomycin is rapidly bactericidal to staphylococci (including methicillin- and vancomycin-resistant *S. aureus* and methicillin-resistant *Staphylococcus epidermidis*), enterococci (including vancomycin-resistant *Enterococcus faecium and E. faecalis*), streptococci (including penicillin-resistant *S. pneumoniae*), and most other aerobic and anaerobic gram-positive bacteria. As a rule, daptomycin is more rapidly bactericidal than either vancomycin, linezolid, or quinupristin/dalfopristin.

Therapeutic Use

Daptomycin has two approved indications: (1) bloodstream infection with *S. aureus* and (2) complicated skin and skin structure infections caused by susceptible strains of the following gram-positive bacteria: *S. aureus* (including methicillin-resistant strains), *S. pyogenes, Streptococcus agalactiae, Streptococcus dysgalactiae* subspecies *equisimilis*, and *E. faecalis* (vancomycin-susceptible strains only). The drug is being tested for other possible uses, including endocarditis and infections caused by vancomycin-resistant enterococci. Daptomycin should not be used for CAP. Clinical trials have shown that, in CAP patients receiving daptomycin, the rate of death and serious cardiorespiratory events is higher than in patients receiving equally effective alternatives.

Resistance

Out of more than 1000 patients receiving daptomycin in clinical trials, only 2 had infections resistant to the drug. The mechanism of resistance has not been identified. There is no known mechanism by which resistance can be transferred from one bacterium to another. Also, there is no cross-resistance between daptomycin and any other class of antibiotics.

Pharmacokinetics

Daptomycin is administered by IV infusion, and a significant fraction (92%) becomes bound to plasma proteins. The drug undergoes minimal metabolism. Most of each dose is excreted unchanged in the urine. In patients with normal renal function, the half-life is 9 hours. However, in those with severe renal impairment (creatinine clearance less than 30 mL/min) and in those on hemodialysis or continuous ambulatory peritoneal dialysis (CAPD), the half-life increases threefold. As a result, if the dosage is not reduced, plasma drug levels can rise dangerously high.

Adverse Effects

Daptomycin is generally well tolerated. The most common adverse effects are constipation, nausea, diarrhea, injection-site reactions, headache, insomnia, and rash.

Daptomycin may pose a small risk for myopathy (muscle injury). In clinical trials with doses that were larger and more frequent than those used now, patients often experienced muscle pain and weakness in association with increased levels of creatine phosphokinase (CPK), a marker for muscle injury. However, with currently approved doses, elevation of CPK is rare.

Patient Education

Patients should be warned about possible muscle injury, and told to report any muscle pain or weakness.

In addition, CPK levels should be measured weekly. If the level rises markedly (to more than 10 times the upper limit of normal), daptomycin should be discontinued. Daptomycin should also be discontinued in patients who report muscle pain or weakness in conjunction with a more moderate rise in CPK.

Daptomycin may cause eosinophilic pneumonia, a rare but serious condition in which eosinophils (white blood cells) accumulate in the lungs and thereby impair lung function. Symptoms include fever, cough, and shortness of breath. Left untreated, the condition can rapidly progress to respiratory failure and death.

Drug Interactions

Daptomycin appears devoid of significant drug interactions. It does not induce or inhibit cytochrome P450 and should not affect drugs that are metabolized by this enzyme system. In clinical studies, daptomycin did not affect the kinetics of warfarin, simvastatin, or aztreonam. Concurrent use of daptomycin plus tobramycin caused a moderate increase in daptomycin levels and a moderate decrease in tobramycin levels. Accordingly, caution is needed when these drugs are combined.

Like daptomycin, the HMG-CoA reductase inhibitors (e.g., simvastatin [Zocor]) can cause myopathy. However, in clinical trials, no patient receiving simvastatin plus daptomycin developed signs of muscle injury. Nonetheless, given our limited experience with daptomycin, it may be prudent to suspend HMG-CoA reductase inhibitors while daptomycin is used.

Preparations, Dosage, and Administration

Daptomycin [Cubicin] is available as a powder in 500-mg single-use vials. For patients with normal renal function, the dosage is 4 or 6 mg/kg once every 24 hours. For patients with severe renal impairment and for those on hemodialysis or CAPD, the dosage is 4 to 6 mg/kg once every 48 to 72 hours.

Rifampin

Rifampin [Rifadin] is a broad-spectrum antibacterial agent employed primarily for tuberculosis (see Chapter 75). However, the drug is also used against several nontuberculous infections. Rifampin is useful for treating asymptomatic carriers of *Neisseria meningitidis*, but is not given to treat active meningococcal infection. Unlabeled uses include treatment of leprosy, gram-negative bacteremia in infancy, and infections caused by *S. epidermidis* and *S. aureus* (e.g., endocarditis, osteomyelitis, prostatitis). Rifampin has also been employed for prophylaxis of meningitis due to *H. influenzae*. Because resistance can develop rapidly, established bacterial infections should not be treated with rifampin alone. The basic pharmacology of rifampin and its use in tuberculosis are presented in Chapter 75.

Rifaximin

Rifaximin [Xifaxan] is an oral, nonabsorbable analog of rifampin used to kill bacteria in the gut. Like rifampin, rifaximin inhibits bacterial DNA-dependent RNA polymerase and thereby inhibits RNA synthesis, resulting in inhibition of protein synthesis and subsequent bacterial death.

Rifaximin has three approved uses. The drug was approved initially for traveler's diarrhea caused by *E. coli* in patients at least 12 years old. Rifaximin is not effective against severe diarrhea associated with fever or bloody stools and should not be used if these are present. Rifaximin is also indicated for prevention of hepatic encephalopathy in patients with chronic liver disease. Rifaximin helps prevent encephalopathy by killing the intestinal bacteria that produce ammonia. More recently, rifaximin was approved for the treatment of irritable bowel syndrome with diarrhea (IBS-D) and is marketed under the name Xifaxan. Off-label uses for rifaximin include recurrent *C. difficile* infection.

Rifaximin is administered by mouth, and very little (less than 0.4%) is absorbed. As a result, the drug achieves high concentrations in the intestinal tract and then is excreted unchanged in the stool.

Rifaximin is well tolerated. Gastrointestinal effects—nausea, flatulence, defecation urgency—occur in some patients. Because so little drug is absorbed, systemic effects are minimum. However, studies in rats and rabbits indicate that rifaximin is teratogenic and hence should not be used by pregnant or breastfeeding women. There have been postmarketing reports of hypersensitivity reactions (rash, allergic dermatitis, urticaria, pruritus, angioneurotic edema), but rifaximin has not been clearly identified as the cause.

Rifaximin is available in 200- and 550-mg tablets for oral dosing, with or without food. For traveler's diarrhea, the dosage is 200 mg 3 times a day for 3 days. To prevent hepatic encephalopathy, the dosage is 550 mg 2 times a day for as long as needed. In the treatment of IBS-D, the dose is 550 mg 3 times a day for 2 weeks. This course may be repeated twice for recurrent disease.

Fidaxomicin

Fidaxomicin [Dificid] is a narrow-spectrum, bactericidal, macrocyclic antibiotic indicated only for diarrhea associated with CDI. In one trial, fidaxomicin was compared with vancomycin, a standard treatment for CDI. The cure rate with fidaxomicin was higher than with vancomycin, and the recurrence rate was lower. Like rifaximin, fidaxomicin inhibits DNA-dependent RNA polymerase and thereby inhibits RNA synthesis, causing inhibition of protein synthesis and subsequent bacterial death. Fidaxomicin is administered by mouth, and systemic absorption is low. As a result, the drug achieves high concentrations in the intestine, where it acts to kill *C. difficile*. The most common adverse effects are nausea, vomiting, abdominal pain, GI hemorrhage, anemia, and neutropenia. Fidaxomicin is supplied in 200-mg tablets for dosing with or without food. The dosage for CDI is 200 mg twice daily for 10 days. A course of treatment with fidaxomicin is more expensive than with vancomycin: $5900 vs. $2050.

Bacitracin

Bacitracin is a polypeptide antibiotic produced by a strain of *Bacillus subtilis*. Administration is topical. Because systemic administration can cause serious toxicity, and because superior systemic agents are available, bacitracin is no longer available for systemic infections.

Mechanism of Action and Antimicrobial Spectrum

Bacitracin inhibits synthesis of the bacterial cell wall, thereby promoting cell lysis and death. The drug is active against most gram-positive bacteria, including staphylococci, streptococci, and *C. difficile*. *Neisseria* species and *H. influenzae* are also susceptible, but most other gram-negative bacteria are resistant. Acquisition of resistance by sensitive organisms is uncommon.

Therapeutic Uses

Bacitracin is used for topical treatment of bacterial infections. The drug is very active against staphylococci and group A streptococci, the pathogens that cause most acute infections of the skin. Because of this activity, bacitracin has been marketed in a variety of topical preparations for treatment of skin infections. Many of these preparations contain additional antibiotics, usually polymyxin B, neomycin, or both.

Polymyxin B

Polymyxin B is a bactericidal drug employed primarily for local effects. Because of serious systemic toxicity, parenteral administration is rare.

Antibacterial Spectrum and Mechanism of Action

Polymyxin B is bactericidal to a broad spectrum of aerobic, gram-negative bacilli. Gram-positive bacteria and most anaerobes are resistant.

Bactericidal effects result from binding of polymyxin B to the bacterial cell membrane, an action that disrupts membrane structure and thereby increases membrane permeability. The increase in permeability leads to inhibition of cellular respiration and cell death. The resistance displayed by gram-positive bacteria has been attributed to the thick gram-positive cell wall, a structure that may block access of polymyxin B to the cell membrane.

Therapeutic Uses

Polymyxin B is used primarily for topical treatment of the eyes, ears, and skin. Preparations designed for application to the skin frequently contain other antibiotics, such as bacitracin and neomycin. In addition to its topical uses, polymyxin B (together with neomycin) has been employed as a bladder irrigant to prevent infection in patients with indwelling catheters.

Parenteral use is extremely limited; polymyxin B is not a drug of choice for any systemic infection. The primary indication for parenteral polymyxin B is serious infection caused by *P. aeruginosa*. Polymyxin B may be given when preferred drugs have been ineffective or intolerable.

BLACK BOX WARNING: NEUROTOXICITY AND NEPHROTOXICITY WITH POLYMYXIN B

The major adverse effects associated with parenteral therapy are neurotoxicity and nephrotoxicity. Both occur frequently and limit systemic use of the drug.

CHAPTER

77 Antifungal Agents

Laura D. Rosenthal, DNP, ACNP, FAANP

The antifungal agents fall into two major groups: drugs for *systemic mycoses* (i.e., systemic fungal infections) and drugs for *superficial mycoses.* A few drugs are used for both. Systemic infections occur much less frequently than superficial infections but are much more serious. Accordingly, therapy of systemic mycoses is our main focus.

DRUGS FOR SYSTEMIC MYCOSES

Systemic mycoses can be subdivided into two categories: opportunistic infections and nonopportunistic infections. The opportunistic mycoses—*candidiasis, aspergillosis, cryptococcosis,* and *mucormycosis*—are seen primarily in debilitated or immunocompromised hosts. In contrast, nonopportunistic infections can occur in any host. These latter mycoses, which are relatively uncommon, include *sporotrichosis, blastomycosis, histoplasmosis,* and *coccidioidomycosis.* Treating systemic mycoses can be difficult: these infections often resist treatment and hence may require prolonged therapy with drugs that frequently prove toxic. Drugs of choice for systemic mycoses are shown in Table 77.1.

The systemic antifungal drugs fall into four classes: polyene antibiotics, azoles, echinocandins, and pyrimidine analogs. Class members and mechanisms of action are shown in Table 77.2.

Amphotericin B, a Polyene Antibiotic

Amphotericin B [Abelcet, Amphotec, AmBisome, Fungizone ♣] belongs to a drug class known as *polyene antibiotics,* so named because their structures contain a series of conjugated double bonds. Nystatin, another antifungal drug, is in the same family.

Amphotericin B is active against a broad spectrum of pathogenic fungi and is a drug of choice for most systemic mycoses. Unfortunately, amphotericin B is highly toxic: infusion reactions and renal damage occur in many patients. Because of its potential for harm, amphotericin B should be employed only against infections that are progressive and potentially fatal.

Amphotericin B is available in four formulations: a conventional formulation (amphotericin B deoxycholate) and three lipid-based formulations. The lipid-based formulations are as effective as the conventional formulation and cause less toxicity—but are much more expensive. For treatment of systemic mycoses, all formulations are administered by intravenous (IV) infusion. Infusions are given daily or every other day for several months.

Mechanism of Action

Amphotericin B binds to components of the fungal cell membrane, increasing permeability. The resultant leakage of intracellular cations (especially potassium) reduces viability. Depending on the concentration of amphotericin B and the susceptibility of the fungus, the drug may be fungistatic or fungicidal.

The component of the fungal membrane to which amphotericin B binds is *ergosterol,* a member of the *sterol* family of compounds. Hence, for a cell to be susceptible, its cytoplasmic membrane must contain sterols. Because bacterial membranes lack sterols, bacteria are not affected.

Much of the toxicity of amphotericin is attributable to the presence of sterols (principally cholesterol) in mammalian cell membranes. When amphotericin binds with cholesterol in mammalian membranes, the effect is similar to that seen in fungi. However, there *is* some degree of selectivity: amphotericin binds more strongly to ergosterol than it does to cholesterol, so fungi are affected more than we are.

Microbial Susceptibility and Resistance

Amphotericin B is active against a broad spectrum of fungi. Some protozoa (e.g., *Leishmania braziliensis*) are also susceptible. As noted, bacteria are resistant.

Emergence of resistant fungi is extremely rare and occurs only with long-term amphotericin use. In all cases of resistance, the fungal membranes had reduced amounts of ergosterol or none at all.

Therapeutic Uses

Amphotericin B is a drug of choice for most systemic mycoses. Before this drug became available, systemic fungal infections usually proved fatal. Treatment is prolonged; 6 to 8 weeks is common. In some cases, treatment may last for 3 or 4 months. In addition to its antifungal applications, amphotericin B is a drug of choice for leishmaniasis.

Pharmacokinetics

Absorption and Distribution

Amphotericin is poorly absorbed from the gastrointestinal (GI) tract, and hence oral therapy cannot be used for systemic infection. Rather, amphotericin must be administered intravenously. When the drug leaves the vascular system, it undergoes extensive binding to sterol-containing membranes of tissues. Levels about half those in plasma are achieved in aqueous humor and in peritoneal, pleural, and joint fluids. Amphotericin B does not readily penetrate to the cerebrospinal fluid (CSF).

TABLE 77.1 ▪ Drugs of Choice for Systemic Mycoses

Infection	Causative Organism	Drugs of Choice	Alternative Drugs
Aspergillosis	*Aspergillus* spp.	Voriconazole	Amphotericin B, isavuconazonium, itraconazole, posaconazole, caspofungin, micafungin
Blastomycosis	*Blastomyces dermatitidis*	Amphotericin B *or* itraconazole	No alternative recommended
Candidiasis	*Candida* spp.	Amphotericin B *or* fluconazole, either one ± flucytosine	Itraconazole, voriconazole, caspofungin
Coccidioidomycosis	*Coccidioides immitis*	Amphotericin B *or* fluconazole	Itraconazole, ketoconazole
Cryptococcosis	*Cryptococcus neoformans*	Amphotericin B ± flucytosine	Itraconazole
Chronic suppression		Fluconazole	Amphotericin B
Histoplasmosis	*Histoplasma capsulatum*	Amphotericin B *or* itraconazole	Fluconazole, ketoconazole
Chronic suppression		Itraconazole	Amphotericin B
Mucormycosis	*Mucor*	Amphotericin B	Isavuconazonium
Paracoccidioidomycosis	*Paracoccidioides brasiliensis*	Amphotericin B *or* itraconazole	Ketoconazole
Sporotrichosis	*Sporothrix schenckii*	Amphotericin B *or* itraconazole	Fluconazole

TABLE 77.2 ▪ Classes of Systemic Antifungal Drugs

Drug Class	Mechanism of Action	Class Members
Polyene antibiotics	Bind to ergosterol and disrupt the fungal cell membrane	Amphotericin B
Azoles	Inhibit synthesis of ergosterol and disrupt the fungal cell membrane	Fluconazole Isavuconazonium Itraconazole Ketoconazole Posaconazole Voriconazole
Echinocandins	Inhibit synthesis of beta-1,3-d-glucan and disrupt the fungal cell wall	Anidulafungin Caspofungin Micafungin
Pyrimidine analogs	Disrupt synthesis of RNA and DNA	Flucytosine

Metabolism and Excretion

Little is known about the elimination of amphotericin B. We do not know if the drug is metabolized or if it is ultimately removed from the body. Renal excretion of unchanged amphotericin is minimal. However, dose or frequency reduction may be considered in patients with preexisting renal impairment. Complete elimination of amphotericin takes a long time; the drug has been detected in tissues more than a year after cessation of treatment.

Adverse Effects

Amphotericin can cause a variety of serious adverse effects. Patients should be under close supervision, preferably in a hospital.

BLACK BOX WARNING: AMPHOTERICIN TOXICITY

Because of its toxicity, amphotericin should be used only in the setting of a potentially life-threatening infection.

Infusion Reactions

Intravenous amphotericin frequently produces fever, chills, rigors, nausea, and headache. These reactions are caused by release of proinflammatory cytokines (tumor necrosis factor, interleukin-1, interleukin-6) from monocytes and macrophages. Symptoms begin 1 to 3 hours after starting the infusion and persist about an hour. Mild reactions can be reduced by pretreatment with diphenhydramine plus acetaminophen. Aspirin can also help, but it may increase kidney damage (see later). Intravenous meperidine or dantrolene can be given if rigors occur. If other measures fail, hydrocortisone can be used to decrease fever and chills. However, because glucocorticoids can reduce the patient's ability to fight infection, routine use of hydrocortisone should be avoided. Infusion reactions are less intense with lipid-based amphotericin formulations than with the conventional formulation.

Amphotericin infusion produces a high incidence of phlebitis. This can be minimized by changing peripheral venous sites often, administering amphotericin through a large central vein, and pretreatment with heparin.

Nephrotoxicity

Amphotericin is toxic to cells of the kidneys. Renal impairment occurs in practically all patients. The extent of kidney damage is related to the total dose administered over the full course of treatment. In most cases, renal function normalizes after amphotericin use stops. However, if the total dose exceeds 4 g, residual impairment is likely. Kidney damage can be minimized by infusing 1 L of saline on the days amphotericin is given. Other nephrotoxic drugs (e.g., aminoglycosides, cyclosporine, nonsteroidal antiinflammatory drugs [NSAIDs]) should be avoided. To evaluate renal injury, tests of kidney function should be performed every 3 to 4 days, and intake and output should be monitored. If plasma creatinine content rises above 3.5 mg/dL, amphotericin dosage should be reduced. As noted, the degree of renal damage is less with lipid-based amphotericin than with the conventional formulation.

Hypokalemia

Damage to the kidneys often causes hypokalemia. Potassium supplements may be needed to correct the problem. Potassium levels and serum creatinine should be monitored often.

Hematologic Effects

Amphotericin can cause bone marrow suppression, resulting in normocytic, normochromic anemia. Hematocrit determinations should be conducted to monitor red blood cell status.

Effects Associated With Intrathecal Injection

Intrathecal administration may cause nausea, vomiting, headache, and pain in the back, legs, and abdomen. Rare reactions include visual disturbances, impairment of hearing, and paresthesias (tingling, numbness, or pain in the hands and feet).

Drug Interactions

Nephrotoxic Drugs

Use of amphotericin with other nephrotoxic drugs (e.g., aminoglycosides, cyclosporine, NSAIDs) increases the risk for kidney damage. Accordingly, these combinations should be avoided if possible.

Flucytosine

Amphotericin potentiates the antifungal actions of flucytosine, apparently by enhancing flucytosine entry into fungi. Thanks to this interaction, combining flucytosine with low-dose amphotericin can produce antifungal effects equivalent to those of high-dose amphotericin alone. By allowing a reduction in amphotericin dosage, the combination can reduce the risk for amphotericin-induced toxicity.

Preparations, Dosage, and Administration

Preparations

Amphotericin B is available in a conventional formulation—amphotericin B deoxycholate [Fungizone ♣]—and three lipid-based formulations: liposomal amphotericin B [AmBisome], amphotericin B cholesteryl sulfate complex [Amphotec], and amphotericin B lipid complex [Abelcet]. The lipid-based formulations cause less nephrotoxicity and fewer infusion reactions than the conventional formulation.

Routes

For treatment of systemic mycoses, amphotericin B is almost always administered intravenously. Infusions should be performed slowly (over 2–4 hours) to minimize phlebitis and cardiovascular reactions. Alternate-day dosing can reduce adverse effects. For most patients, several months of therapy are required. Because amphotericin B does not readily enter the CSF, intrathecal injection is used for fungal meningitis.

Intravenous Dosage and Administration

Fungal Infections. Dosage is individualized and based on disease severity and the patient's ability to tolerate treatment. Optimal dosage has not been established. A small test dose is often infused to assess patient reaction. After this, therapy is initiated with a dosage of 0.25 mg/kg/day. Maintenance dosages range from 1.5 to 6 mg/kg/day, depending on the severity of the infection and the form of amphotericin used. Dosage should be reduced in patients with renal impairment.

Leishmaniasis. Leishmaniasis can be treated with amphotericin B deoxycholate or liposomal amphotericin B [AmBisome]. For conventional amphotericin B deoxycholate, the dosage is 0.25 to 1 mg/kg daily for up to 8 weeks. For AmBisome, the dose in immunocompetent individuals is 3 mg/kg on days 1, 2, 3, 4, 5, 14, and 21. However, a single infusion of 10 mg/kg may be just as effective.

Azoles

Like amphotericin B, the azoles are broad-spectrum antifungal drugs. As a result, azoles represent an alternative to amphotericin B for most systemic fungal infections. In contrast to amphotericin, which is highly toxic and must be given intravenously, the azoles have lower toxicity and can be given by mouth. However, azoles do have one disadvantage: they inhibit hepatic cytochrome P450 drug-metabolizing enzymes and can increase the levels of many other drugs. Of the azoles in current use, only six—itraconazole, ketoconazole, fluconazole, voriconazole, posaconazole, and isavuconazonium—are indicated for systemic mycoses. Azoles used for superficial mycoses are discussed separately later.

Itraconazole

Itraconazole [Sporanox] is an alternative to amphotericin B for several systemic mycoses and will serve as our prototype for the azole family. The drug is safer than amphotericin B and has the added advantage of oral dosing. Principal adverse effects are cardiosuppression and liver injury. Like other azoles, itraconazole can inhibit drug-metabolizing enzymes and raise levels of other drugs.

Prototype Drugs

ANTIFUNGAL AGENTS

Polyene Macrolide
Amphotericin B

Azole
Itraconazole

Echinocandin
Caspofungin

Mechanism of Action

Itraconazole inhibits the synthesis of *ergosterol,* an essential component of the fungal cytoplasmic membrane. The result is increased membrane permeability and leakage of cellular components. Accumulation of ergosterol precursors may also contribute to antifungal actions. Itraconazole suppresses ergosterol synthesis by inhibiting fungal cytochrome P450–dependent enzymes.

Therapeutic Use

Itraconazole is active against a broad spectrum of fungal pathogens. At this time, it is a drug of choice for *blastomycosis, histoplasmosis, paracoccidioidomycosis,* and *sporotrichosis* and is an alternative to amphotericin B for *aspergillosis, candidiasis,* and *coccidioidomycosis.* Itraconazole may also be used for superficial mycoses.

Pharmacokinetics

Itraconazole is administered orally, in capsules or suspension. Food increases absorption of capsules but decreases absorption of suspension. Interestingly, administration with cola enhances absorption. When absorbed, the drug is widely distributed to lipophilic tissues. Concentrations in aqueous fluids (e.g., saliva, CSF) are negligible. The drug undergoes extensive hepatic metabolism. About 40% of each dose is excreted in the urine as inactive metabolites.

Adverse Effects

Itraconazole is well tolerated in usual doses. Gastrointestinal reactions (nausea, vomiting, diarrhea) are most common. Other reactions include rash, headache, abdominal pain, and edema. Itraconazole may also cause two potentially serious effects: cardiac suppression and liver injury.

BLACK BOX WARNING: NEGATIVE INOTROPIC ACTIONS WITH ITRACONAZOLE

Because of its negative inotropic actions, itraconazole should not be used for superficial fungal infections (dermatomycoses, onychomycosis) in patients with heart failure, a history of heart failure, or other indications of ventricular dysfunction.

Cardiac Suppression. Itraconazole has negative inotropic actions that can cause a transient decrease in ventricular ejection fraction. Cardiac function returns to normal by 12 hours after dosing. The drug may still be used to treat serious fungal infections in patients with heart failure, but only with careful monitoring and only if the benefits clearly outweigh the risks. If signs and symptoms of heart failure worsen, itraconazole should be stopped.

Liver Injury. Itraconazole has been associated with rare cases of liver failure, some of which were fatal. Although a causal link has not been established, caution is nonetheless advised. Patients should be informed about signs of liver impairment (persistent nausea, anorexia, fatigue, vomiting, right upper abdominal pain, jaundice, dark urine, pale stools) and, if they appear, should seek medical attention immediately.

Drug Interactions

Inhibition of Hepatic Drug Metabolizing Enzymes. Itraconazole inhibits CYP3A4 (the 3A4 isoenzyme of cytochrome P450) and thus can increase levels of many other drugs (Table 77.3). The most important are cisapride, pimozide, dofetilide, and quinidine. When present at high levels, these drugs can cause potentially fatal ventricular dysrhythmias. Accordingly, concurrent use with itraconazole is contraindicated. Other drugs of concern include cyclosporine, digoxin, warfarin, and sulfonylurea-type oral hypoglycemics. In patients taking cyclosporine or digoxin, levels of these drugs should be monitored; in patients taking warfarin, prothrombin time should be monitored; and in patients taking sulfonylureas, blood glucose levels should be monitored.

Drugs that Raise Gastric pH. Drugs that decrease gastric acidity—antacids, histamine-2 (H_2) antagonists, and proton pump inhibitors—can greatly reduce absorption of oral itraconazole. Accordingly, these agents should be administered at least 1 hour before itraconazole or 2 hours after. (Because proton pump inhibitors have a prolonged duration of action, patients using these drugs may have insufficient stomach acid for itraconazole absorption, regardless of when the proton pump inhibitor is given.)

TABLE 77.3 ■ Some Drugs Whose Levels Can Be Increased by Azole Antifungal Drugs

Target Drug	Class	Consequence of Excessive Level
Pimozide [Orap]	Antipsychotic	Fatal dysrhythmias
Dofetilide [Tikosyn]	Antidysrhythmic	Fatal dysrhythmias
Quinidine	Antidysrhythmic	Fatal dysrhythmias
Cisapride [Propulsid]*	Prokinetic agent	Fatal dysrhythmias
Warfarin [Coumadin]	Anticoagulant	Bleeding
Sulfonylureas	Oral hypoglycemic	Hypoglycemia
Phenytoin [Dilantin]	Antiseizure drug	Central nervous system toxicity
Cyclosporine [Sandimmune]	Immunosuppressant	Increased nephrotoxicity
Tacrolimus [Prograf]	Immunosuppressant	Increased nephrotoxicity
Lovastatin [Mevacor]	Antihyperlipidemic	Rhabdomyolysis
Simvastatin [Zocor]	Antihyperlipidemic	Rhabdomyolysis
Eletriptan [Relpax]	Antimigraine	Coronary vasospasm
Fentanyl [Duragesic, others]	Opioid analgesic	Fatal respiratory depression
Calcium channel blockers	Antihypertensive, antianginal	Cardiosuppression

*In 2000, cisapride was voluntarily withdrawn from the U.S. market. It is now available only through an investigational limited-access program.

Preparations, Dosage, and Administration

Itraconazole [Sporanox] is available in suspension (10 mg/mL) and capsules (100 mg) for oral use. The capsules should be taken with food or a cola beverage to increase absorption. The recommended dosage is 200 mg once a day. If needed, the dosage may be increased to 200 mg twice a day.

Fluconazole

Actions and Uses

Fluconazole [Diflucan], a member of the azole family, is an important antifungal drug. It has the same mechanism as itraconazole: inhibition of cytochrome P450–dependent synthesis of ergosterol, with resultant damage to the cytoplasmic membrane and accumulation of ergosterol precursors. The drug is primarily fungistatic. Fluconazole is used for blastomycosis; histoplasmosis; meningitis caused by *Cryptococcus neoformans* and *Coccidioides immitis;* and vaginal, oropharyngeal, esophageal, and disseminated *Candida* infections. In addition, fluconazole is used investigationally for leishmaniasis.

Pharmacokinetics

Fluconazole is well absorbed (90%) after oral dosing and undergoes wide distribution to tissues and body fluids, including the CSF. Most of each dose is eliminated unchanged in the urine. Fluconazole has a half-life of 30 hours, making once-a-day dosing sufficient.

Adverse Effects

Fluconazole is generally well tolerated. The most common reactions are nausea, headache, rash, vomiting, abdominal pain, and diarrhea. Rarely, treatment has been associated with hepatic necrosis, Stevens-Johnson syndrome, and anaphylaxis.

Use in Pregnancy

When taken in high doses (400–800 mg/day) throughout all or most of the first trimester, fluconazole can cause serious birth defects, including cleft palate, femoral bowing, congenital heart disease, and facial abnormalities. By contrast, treatment of vaginal candidiasis with a single low dose (150 mg) appears to be safe. High-dose therapy is now classified in U.S. Food and Drug Administration (FDA) Pregnancy Risk Category D, whereas low-dose therapy remains in Category C.

Drug Interactions

Like other azole antifungal drugs, fluconazole can inhibit CYP3A4 and increase levels of other drugs, including warfarin, phenytoin, cyclosporine, zidovudine, rifabutin, and sulfonylurea oral hypoglycemics.

Preparations, Dosage, and Administration

Fluconazole [Diflucan] is available in solution (2 mg/mL) for IV infusion and in tablets (50, 100, 150, and 200 mg) and suspension (10 and 40 mg/mL) for oral use. Because oral absorption is rapid and nearly complete, oral and IV dosages are the same. For treatment of oropharyngeal and esophageal candidiasis, the usual dosage is 200 mg on the first day, followed by 100 mg once daily thereafter. For treatment of systemic candidiasis and cryptococcal meningitis, the usual dosage is 400 mg on the first day, followed by 200 mg once daily thereafter. Duration of treatment ranges from 3 weeks to more than 3 months, depending on the infection.

Voriconazole

Actions and Uses

Voriconazole [Vfend], a member of the azole family, is an important drug for treating life-threatening fungal infections. Like other azoles, voriconazole inhibits cytochrome P450–dependent enzymes, suppressing synthesis of ergosterol, a critical component of the fungal cytoplasmic membrane. As a result, voriconazole is active against a broad spectrum of fungal pathogens, including *Aspergillus* species, *Candida* species, *Scedosporium* species, *Fusarium* species, *Histoplasma capsulatum, Blastomyces dermatitidis,* and *C. neoformans.* At this time, voriconazole has four approved indications: (1) candidemia, (2) invasive aspergillosis, (3) esophageal candidiasis, and (4) serious infections caused by *Scedosporium apiospermum* or *Fusarium* species in patients unresponsive to or intolerant of other drugs.

According to guidelines from the Infectious Disease Society of America, voriconazole has replaced amphotericin B as the drug of choice for invasive aspergillosis. Voriconazole is just as effective as amphotericin B and poses a much lower risk for kidney damage. However, voriconazole does have its own set of adverse effects, including hepatotoxicity, visual disturbances, hypersensitivity reactions, hallucinations, and fetal injury. In addition, like other azoles, voriconazole can interact with many drugs.

Pharmacokinetics

Voriconazole may be administered intravenously or orally. With oral dosing, bioavailability is high (96%) but can be reduced by food. Plasma levels peak 2 hours after ingestion. The drug's half-life is dose dependent and can range from 6 hours up to 24 hours. Voriconazole undergoes extensive metabolism by hepatic cytochrome P450 isoenzymes.

Adverse Effects

The most common adverse effects are visual disturbances, fever, rash, nausea, vomiting, diarrhea, headache, sepsis, peripheral edema, abdominal pain, and respiratory disorders. During clinical trials, the effects that most often led to discontinuing treatment were liver damage, visual disturbances, and rash.

Hepatotoxicity. Voriconazole can cause hepatitis, cholestasis, and fulminant hepatic failure. Fortunately, these events are both uncommon and generally reversible. To monitor for injury, liver function tests should be obtained before treatment and periodically thereafter.

Visual Disturbances. Reversible, dose-related visual disturbances develop in 30% of patients. Symptoms include reduced visual acuity, increased brightness, altered color perception, and photophobia. As a rule, these begin within 30 minutes of dosing and then greatly diminish over the next 30 minutes. Owing to the risk for visual impairment, patients should be warned against driving, especially at night.

Hypersensitivity Reactions. Voriconazole may cause dermatologic reactions, ranging from rash to life-threatening Stevens-Johnson syndrome. During infusion, anaphylactoid reactions have occurred, manifesting with tachycardia, chest tightness, dyspnea, faintness, flushing, fever, and sweating. If these symptoms develop, the infusion should stop.

Teratogenicity. Voriconazole is teratogenic in rats and can cause fetal harm in humans. The drug is classified in FDA Pregnancy Risk Category D and hence should not be used during pregnancy unless the potential benefits are deemed to outweigh the risk to the fetus. Women taking the drug should use effective contraception.

Drug Interactions

Voriconazole can interact with many other drugs. Several mechanisms are involved. Voriconazole is both a substrate for and inhibitor of hepatic cytochrome P450 isoenzymes. As a result, drugs that inhibit P450 can raise voriconazole levels, and drugs that induce P450 can lower voriconazole levels. On the other hand, because voriconazole itself can inhibit P450, voriconazole can raise levels of other drugs. Therefore the following precautions should be taken when administering voriconazole:

- To ensure that voriconazole levels are adequate, voriconazole should not be combined with powerful P450 inducers, including rifampin, rifabutin, carbamazepine, and phenobarbital.
- To avoid excessive voriconazole levels, voriconazole should not be combined with powerful P450 inhibitors.
- To avoid toxicity from accumulation of other drugs, voriconazole should not be combined with some agents that are P450 substrates, including cisapride, pimozide, and sirolimus.

Preparations, Dosage, and Administration

Voriconazole [Vfend] is available in 200-mg, single-use vials for IV infusion and in two oral formulations: tablets (50 and 200 mg) and a powder for oral suspension (40 mg/mL after reconstitution). Treatment is initiated with IV voriconazole and later can be switched to oral voriconazole as appropriate.

IV therapy consists of two loading doses (6 mg/kg each given 12 hours apart) followed by maintenance doses of 4 mg/kg every 12 hours. All IV doses should be infused slowly, over 1 to 2 hours (maximal rate, 3 mg/kg/hr). If the response is inadequate, maintenance doses can be increased by 50%. Patients with mild to moderate hepatic cirrhosis should receive the standard two loading doses, but maintenance doses should be halved. (There are no data on dosing in patients with severe cirrhosis.) Patients with significant renal impairment (creatinine clearance less than 50 mL/min) should use oral voriconazole, not IV voriconazole, because in the absence of adequate kidney function, the solubilizing agent in the IV formulation can accumulate to dangerous levels.

After receiving IV loading doses, patients who can tolerate oral therapy may be switched to voriconazole tablets. The usual dosage is 200 mg every 12 hours for patients who weigh more than 40 kg and 100 mg every 12 hours for patients who weight less than 40 kg. If the response is inadequate, doses can be increased by 50%. Oral dosing should be done 1 hour before meals or 1 hour after.

Ketoconazole

Actions and Antifungal Spectrum

Ketoconazole belongs to the azole family of antifungal agents. Benefits derive from inhibiting synthesis of ergosterol, an essential component of the fungal cytoplasmic membrane. Ketoconazole is active against most fungi that cause systemic mycoses, as well as fungi that cause superficial infections (dermatophytes and *Candida* species).

Therapeutic Use

Ketoconazole is an alternative to amphotericin B for systemic mycoses. The drug is much less toxic than amphotericin and only somewhat less effective. Responses to ketoconazole are slow. Accordingly, the drug is less useful for severe, acute infections than for long-term suppression of chronic infections. Topical ketoconazole is also a valuable drug for superficial mycoses.

Pharmacokinetics

Absorption. Ketoconazole is a weak base and hence requires an acidic environment for dissolution and absorption. Oral ketoconazole is well absorbed from the GI tract, provided that gastric acid levels are normal. In patients with achlorhydria (absence of gastric acid), absorption is low. Drugs that reduce gastric acidity (e.g., antacids, H_2 blocking agents, proton pump inhibitors) decrease absorption.

PATIENT-CENTERED CARE ACROSS THE LIFE SPAN

Antifungal Agents

Life Stage	Patient Care Concerns
Infants	Nystatin is used to treat oral candidiasis in premature and full-term infants. Fluconazole is also used safely to treat systemic candidiasis in newborn infants.
Children/adolescents	Many antifungal agents are used safely in children, in lower doses. Side-effect profiles are similar to those of adults.
Pregnant women	Many of the azole antifungals are classified in FDA Pregnancy Risk Category C or D. Risks and benefits must be considered for administration during pregnancy.
Breastfeeding women	Data are lacking regarding most antifungals and breastfeeding. Most antifungals are considered safe in lower doses. The exception to this is ketoconazole. Because it has high potential for hepatotoxicity, it should be avoided in breastfeeding women.
Older adults	Older adults have a higher risk for achlorhydria than do younger individuals and may not predictably absorb some antifungal agents. In addition, common drugs prescribed to older adults, including warfarin, phenytoin, and oral hypoglycemic agents, are increased by azoles.

Distribution. Most ketoconazole in the blood is bound to plasma proteins. The drug crosses the blood-brain barrier poorly, and concentrations in the CSF remain low. In contrast, high levels of ketoconazole are achieved in the skin, making oral ketoconazole useful against superficial mycoses.

Elimination. Ketoconazole is eliminated by hepatic metabolism. Its half-life is approximately 3 hours. In patients with liver impairment, the half-life can be substantially prolonged. Because elimination is hepatic, renal impairment does not influence the intensity or duration of effects. Hence no dosage adjustment is needed in patients with kidney disease.

Adverse Effects

Ketoconazole is generally well tolerated. The most common adverse reactions—nausea and vomiting—can be reduced by giving the drug with food. The most serious effects involve the liver.

BLACK BOX WARNING: KETOCONAZOLE HEPATIC TOXICITY

Effects of ketoconazole on the liver are rare but potentially severe. Fatal hepatic necrosis has occurred. Because of the risk for serious harm, oral ketoconazole should be used only for systemic infections, not superficial fungal infections.

Hepatotoxicity. Liver function should be evaluated at baseline and at least monthly thereafter. Ketoconazole should be discontinued at the first sign of liver injury. The drug should be employed with caution in patients with a history of hepatic disease. Patients should be advised to notify the prescriber if they experience symptoms suggesting liver injury (e.g., unusual fatigue, anorexia, nausea, vomiting, jaundice, dark urine, pale stools).

Effects on Sex Hormones. Just as ketoconazole inhibits steroid synthesis in fungi, the drug can inhibit steroid synthesis in humans. In males, inhibition of testosterone synthesis has caused gynecomastia, decreased libido, and reduced potency; reversible sterility has occurred with high doses. In females, reduction of estradiol synthesis has caused menstrual irregularities.

Other Adverse Effects. Ketoconazole can produce a variety of relatively mild adverse effects, including rash, itching, dizziness, fever, chills, constipation, diarrhea, photophobia, and headache. Rarely, ketoconazole has caused anaphylaxis, severe epigastric pain, and altered adrenal function.

Drug Interactions

Drugs that decrease gastric acidity—antacids, H_2 antagonists, proton pump inhibitors—can greatly reduce ketoconazole absorption. Accordingly, these agents should be administered no sooner than 2 hours after ingestion of ketoconazole.

Like other azoles, ketoconazole inhibits CYP3A4 and can increase levels of other drugs.

Rifampin reduces plasma levels of ketoconazole, apparently by enhancing hepatic metabolism. If these drugs are used concurrently, ketoconazole dosage should be increased—and even then it may be impossible to achieve therapeutic levels.

BLACK BOX WARNING: KETOCONAZOLE FATAL CARDIAC DYSRHYTHMIAS

Use of ketoconazole with drugs that prolong the QT (quinidine, methadone, dronedarone, ranolazine) is contraindicated because these combinations can lead to fatal cardiac dysrhythmias.

Preparations, Dosage, and Administration

Ketoconazole is supplied in 200-mg oral tablets. The recommended adult dosage is 200 to 400 mg once a day. To treat severe infection, daily doses of 400 to 800 mg may be required. The dosage for children older than 2 years is 3.3 to 6.6 mg/kg/day in a single dose. Duration of treatment is 6 months or longer. Because an acidic environment is needed for ketoconazole absorption, patients with achlorhydria should dissolve the tablets in acidic liquid and then sip the solution through a plastic or glass straw to avoid damaging the teeth.

Posaconazole

Actions and Uses

Like other azoles, posaconazole [Noxafil, Posanol ♣] binds with ergosterol in the fungal cell membrane, compromising membrane integrity. In vitro, posaconazole has strong activity against *Aspergillus* and *Candida* species, and good activity against several other fungi. Currently, the drug has only two indications: (1) treatment of oropharyngeal candidiasis, including infections resistant to itraconazole or fluconazole; and (2) prophylaxis of invasive *Aspergillus* and *Candida* infection in immunocompromised patients.

Pharmacokinetics

Posaconazole is administered by mouth, and food greatly enhances absorption. For example, when dosing is done with a low-fat meal or liquid nutritional supplement, peak plasma levels are 3 times higher than when dosing is done on an empty stomach. In the blood, posaconazole is highly (over 98%) protein bound. In the liver, posaconazole undergoes a process known as UDP glucuronidation, rather than metabolism by cytochrome P450 isoenzymes (although it can inhibit CYP3A4). Elimination is mainly fecal (71%) and partly urinary (13%). The mean elimination half-life is 35 hours.

Adverse Effects

Posaconazole can cause a variety of adverse effects, which are usually mild. In clinical trials, adverse effects were similar to those seen with itraconazole and fluconazole. The most common reactions were nausea, vomiting, and headache. Like other azoles, posaconazole can cause liver injury. In addition, there have been reports of QT prolongation and dysrhythmias.

Drug Interactions

Like other azoles, posaconazole inhibits CYP3A4 and can increase levels of many other drugs. Two immunosuppressants—cyclosporine and tacrolimus—are of particular concern. If posaconazole is combined with cyclosporine or tacrolimus, their dosages should be reduced by 25% and 66%, respectively. Combined use of posaconazole with pimozide or quinidine is contraindicated (because raising levels of these drugs can lead to QT prolongation and dysrhythmias), as is combined use with ergot alkaloids (because raising their levels can lead to ergotism).

Two drugs—rifabutin and phenytoin—can induce UDP glucuronidase (the hepatic enzyme that metabolizes posaconazole) and reduce posaconazole levels by nearly 50%. Accordingly, an increase in posaconazole dosage may be needed.

Esomeprazole (a proton pump inhibitor) and cimetidine (an H_2 receptor antagonist), both given to lower gastric acidity, can reduce levels of posaconazole by nearly 50%. Therapeutic failure could result. Whether other proton pump inhibitors and H_2 receptor antagonists also reduce posaconazole levels has not been determined.

Preparations, Dosage, and Administration

Posaconazole is supplied as a 40-mg/mL oral suspension and a delayed-release tablet (100 mg). To promote absorption, each dose should be taken with a full meal or a liquid nutritional supplement. Dosages are as follows:

- *Prophylaxis of invasive fungal infections*—Suspension: 200 mg 3 times a day for as long as neutropenia or immunosuppression persists. Tablet: 300 mg twice daily on day 1, followed by 300 mg daily for as long as neutropenia or immunosuppression persists
- *Oropharyngeal candidiasis*—100 mg of oral suspension twice daily on day 1, followed by 100 mg once daily for 13 days
- *Oropharyngeal candidiasis refractory to itraconazole and/or fluconazole*—400 mg of oral suspension twice daily for as long as indicated

Isavuconazonium

Actions and Uses

Isavuconazonium [Cresemba] is the prodrug of isavuconazole and is the newest member of the azole family. Isavuconazonium inhibits the synthesis of ergosterol, a key component of the fungal cell membrane. Isavuconazonium has only two indications: treatment of invasive aspergillosis and invasive mucormycosis.

Pharmacokinetics

Isavuconazonium is administered by mouth and intravenously. After oral administration, the drug is highly bioavailable (98%), and the drug can be taken with or without food. The drug is highly protein bound to albumin (99%). Elimination is evenly split between the fecal (46%) and urinary (46%) routes. The mean elimination half-life is 130 hours.

Drug Interactions

Like other azoles, use of isavuconazonium with other CYP3A4 inhibitors or inducers can alter the plasma levels of isavuconazonium other drugs.

Preparations, Dosage, and Administration

Isavuconazonium is supplied as 186-mg capsules for oral administration and in a single dose vial containing 372 mg for intravenous reconstitution.

- Loading doses—372 mg every 8 hours for 6 doses
- Maintenance doses—372 mg once daily starting 12 to 24 hours after the last loading dose

Echinocandins

The echinocandins are the newest class of antifungal drugs. In contrast to amphotericin B and the azoles, which disrupt the fungal cell membrane, the echinocandins disrupt the fungal cell wall. Echinocandins cannot be dosed orally, and their antifungal spectrum is narrow, being limited mainly to *Aspergillus* and *Candida* species. Three echinocandins are available: caspofungin, micafungin, and anidulafungin. When dosage is appropriate, all three appear therapeutically equivalent.

Caspofungin

Actions and Uses

Caspofungin [Cancidas] was the first echinocandin available. Antifungal effects result from inhibiting the biosynthesis of beta-1,3-d-glucan, an essential component of the cell wall of some fungi, including *Candida* and *Aspergillus.* Caspofungin is approved for IV therapy of (1) invasive aspergillosis in patients unresponsive to or intolerant of traditional agents (e.g., amphotericin B, itraconazole) and (2) systemic *Candida* infections, including candidemia and *Candida*-related peritonitis, pleural space infections, and intraabdominal abscesses. The drug is better tolerated than amphotericin B and appears just as effective.

Pharmacokinetics

Caspofungin is not absorbed from the GI tract and hence must be given parenterally (by IV infusion). In the blood, 97% of the drug is protein bound. Caspofungin is cleared from the blood with a half-life of 9 to 11 hours. The principal mechanism of plasma clearance is redistribution to tissues, not metabolism or excretion. Over time, the drug undergoes gradual metabolism followed by excretion in the urine and feces.

Adverse Effects

Caspofungin is generally well tolerated. The most common adverse effects are fever and phlebitis at the injection site. Less common reactions include headache, rash, nausea, and vomiting. In addition, caspofungin can cause effects that appear to be mediated by histamine release. Among these are rash, facial flushing, pruritus, and a sense of warmth. One case of anaphylaxis has been reported.

Use in Pregnancy

Caspofungin is embryotoxic in rats and rabbits. To date, there are no adequate data on effects in pregnant women. Currently, the drug is classified in FDA Pregnancy Risk Category C and hence should be avoided during pregnancy unless the potential benefits outweigh the potential risks to the fetus.

Drug Interactions

Drugs that induce cytochrome P450 may decrease levels of caspofungin. Powerful inducers include efavirenz, nelfinavir, rifampin, carbamazepine, dexamethasone, and phenytoin. Patients taking these drugs may need to increase caspofungin dosage.

Caspofungin can decrease levels of tacrolimus [Prograf], an immunosuppressant. If these drugs are taken concurrently, levels of tacrolimus should be monitored and dosage increased as needed.

Combining caspofungin with cyclosporine [Sandimmune, others] increases the risk for liver injury, as evidenced by a transient elevation in plasma levels of liver enzyme. Accordingly, the combination should generally be avoided.

Preparations, Dosage, and Administration

Caspofungin [Cancidas] is supplied as a powder (50 and 70 mg) to be reconstituted in sterile saline for IV infusion. Treatment for adults consists of a 70-mg loading dose followed by daily maintenance doses of 50 mg each. All doses should be infused slowly (over 1 hour). Treatment duration depends on infection severity and the clinical response. For patients with moderate liver impairment, maintenance doses should be reduced to 35 mg. There are no data on dosage for patients with severe liver impairment.

Micafungin

Actions and Uses

Micafungin [Mycamine] was the second echinocandin antifungal agent available for general use. Like caspofungin, micafungin inhibits synthesis of beta-1,3-d-glucan, an essential component of the cell wall of *Candida.* Micafungin, administered intravenously, is indicated for (1) prevention of *Candida* infection in patients undergoing a bone marrow transplantation; (2) treatment of esophageal candidiasis; (3) treatment of candidemia, the fourth most common bloodstream infection among hospitalized patients in the United States; and (4) treatment of disseminated infection, peritonitis, or abscesses caused by *Candida.* For all four indications, fluconazole and itraconazole are preferred.

Pharmacokinetics

Like caspofungin, micafungin is not absorbed from the GI tract and hence is given intravenously. Protein binding in blood exceeds 99%. Micafungin undergoes hepatic metabolism—mainly by pathways that do not involve cytochrome P450—followed by excretion in the feces. The elimination half-life is 11 to 17 hours.

Adverse Effects

Micafungin is generally well tolerated. The most common side effects are headache, nausea, vomiting, diarrhea, fever, and phlebitis at the infusion site. Elevation of liver enzymes has occurred, suggesting injury to the liver. Patients may also experience histamine-mediated reactions, including rash, itching, facial swelling, and vasodilation. There have been isolated reports of severe allergic reactions, including life-threatening anaphylaxis.

Drug Interactions

Micafungin appears largely devoid of significant drug interactions. Micafungin can intensify the effects of sirolimus (an immunosuppressant) and nifedipine (a calcium channel blocker). Accordingly, patients treated with sirolimus or nifedipine should be monitored closely for signs of toxicity. Because micafungin does not interact very much with the cytochrome P450 system, it is unlikely to alter the effects of drugs that do.

Preparations, Dosage, and Administration

Micafungin is supplied as a lyophilized powder (50 and 100 mg) in single-use, light-protected vials and must be reconstituted before infusion. The recommended dosage is 50 mg once a day to prevent *Candida* infection, 100 mg once a day to treat candidemia, and 150 mg once a day to treat esophageal candidiasis. All doses are given by a 1-hour IV infusion. Faster infusion rates increase the risk for a histamine reaction.

Anidulafungin

Actions and Uses

Anidulafungin [Eraxis] has good activity against *Candida* species and poor activity against most other fungi. Indications are limited to IV therapy of esophageal candidiasis, candidemia, and other serious *Candida* infections. Like caspofungin and micafungin, anidulafungin inhibits synthesis of beta-1,3-d-glucan, disrupting the *Candida* cell wall.

Pharmacokinetics

Like other echinocandins, anidulafungin is not absorbed from the GI tract and hence must be given intravenously. In the blood, 84% of the drug is protein bound. Clearance is the result of slow, spontaneous chemical degradation, followed by excretion in the feces. The plasma half-life is 40 to 50 hours.

Adverse Effects

Anidulafungin is generally well tolerated. The most common side effects are diarrhea, hypokalemia, and headache. Possible histamine-mediated reactions (rash, urticaria, pruritus, flushing, dyspnea, hypotension) have been reported, especially at higher infusion rates. Accordingly, the infusion rate should not exceed 1.1 mg/min. A few patients have developed signs of liver damage (hepatitis, elevation of circulating liver enzymes, worsening of hepatic failure).

Drug Interactions

No clinically relevant drug interactions have been reported. Anidulafungin is neither a substrate for, inducer of, nor inhibitor of hepatic cytochrome P450 drug-metabolizing enzymes and so will not interact with other drugs affected by this system.

Preparations, Dosage, and Administration

Anidulafungin [Eraxis] is available as a powder (50 and 100 mg) to be reconstituted in the supplied diluent and then further diluted before IV infusion. To minimize histamine-related reactions, the infusion rate should not exceed 1.1 mg/min. Dosages are as follows:

- *Esophageal candidiasis*—Infuse a single 100-mg loading dose on day 1, followed by 50 mg once a day thereafter, continuing for at least 14 days and at least 7 days after the last positive culture.
- *Candidemia and other serious* Candida *infections*—Infuse a single 200-mg loading dose on day 1, followed by 100 mg once a day thereafter, continuing for at least 14 days after the last positive culture.

Flucytosine, a Pyrimidine Analog

Flucytosine [Ancobon], a pyrimidine analog, is employed for serious infections caused by susceptible strains of *Candida* and *C. neoformans.* Because development of resistance is common, flucytosine is almost always used in combination with amphotericin B. Extreme caution is needed in patients with renal impairment and hematologic disorders.

Mechanism of Action

Flucytosine is taken up by fungal cells, which then convert it to 5-fluorouracil (5-FU), a powerful antimetabolite. The ultimate effect is disruption of fungal DNA and RNA synthesis. Flucytosine is relatively harmless to us because mammalian cells lack cytosine deaminase, the enzyme that converts flucytosine to 5-FU.

Fungal Resistance

Development of resistance during therapy is common and constitutes a serious clinical problem. Several mechanisms have been described, including (1) a reduction in cytosine permease (needed for fungal uptake of flucytosine) and (2) loss of cytosine deaminase (needed to convert flucytosine to its active form).

Antifungal Spectrum and Therapeutic Uses

Flucytosine has a narrow antifungal spectrum. Fungicidal activity is highest against *Candida* species and *C. neoformans.* Most other fungi are resistant. Because of this narrow spectrum, flucytosine is indicated only for candidiasis and cryptococcosis. For treatment of serious infections (e.g., cryptococcal meningitis, systemic candidiasis), flucytosine should be combined with amphotericin B. This combination offers two advantages over flucytosine alone: (1) antifungal activity is enhanced and (2) emergence of resistant fungi is reduced.

Pharmacokinetics

Flucytosine is readily absorbed from the GI tract and is well distributed throughout the body. The drug has good access to the central nervous system; levels in the CSF are about 80% of those in plasma. Flucytosine is eliminated by the kidneys, principally as unchanged drug. The half-life is about 4 hours in patients with normal renal function. However, in patients with renal insufficiency, the half-life is greatly prolonged, and hence dosage must be reduced.

Adverse Effects

Hematologic Effects

Bone marrow suppression is the most serious complication of treatment. Marrow suppression usually manifests as reversible neutropenia or thrombocytopenia. Rarely, fatal agranulocytosis develops. Platelet and leukocyte counts should be determined weekly. Adverse hematologic effects are most likely when plasma levels of flucytosine exceed 100 mcg/mL. Accordingly, the dosage should be adjusted to keep drug levels below this value. Flucytosine should be used with caution in patients with preexisting bone marrow suppression.

Hepatotoxicity

Mild and reversible liver dysfunction occurs frequently, but severe hepatic injury is rare. Liver function should be monitored (by making weekly determinations of serum transaminase and alkaline phosphatase levels).

BLACK BOX WARNING: FLUCYTOSINE AND RENAL IMPAIRMENT

Flucytosine should be used with extreme caution in patients with renal impairment.

Drug Interactions

Flucytosine is often combined with amphotericin B. As noted, this combination offers several advantages. However, the combination can also be detrimental. Because amphotericin B is nephrotoxic, and because flucytosine is eliminated by the kidneys, amphotericin B–induced kidney damage may suppress flucytosine excretion, promoting flucytosine toxicity. Therefore it is important to monitor renal function and flucytosine levels when amphotericin B and flucytosine are combined.

Like itraconazole, flucytosine inhibits hepatic drug-metabolizing enzymes and can raise levels of several other drugs. With at least four drugs—cisapride, pimozide, dofetilide, and quinidine—elevated levels can lead to potentially fatal dysrhythmias. Accordingly, flucytosine must not be combined with these drugs.

Preparations, Dosage, and Administration

Flucytosine [Ancobon] is available in 250- and 500-mg oral capsules. The usual dosage for patients with normal kidney function is 50 to 150 mg/kg/day administered in four divided doses at 6-hour intervals. At this dosage, some patients must ingest 10 or more capsules 4 times a day. Dosages must be reduced for patients with renal insufficiency. Nausea and vomiting associated with drug administration can be decreased by swallowing the capsules over a 15-minute interval.

DRUGS FOR SUPERFICIAL MYCOSES

The superficial mycoses are caused by two groups of organisms: (1) *Candida* species and (2) dermatophytes (species of *Epidermophyton, Trichophyton,* and *Microsporum*). *Candida* infections usually occur in mucous membranes and moist skin; chronic infections may involve the scalp, skin, and nails. Dermatophytoses are generally confined to the skin, hair, and nails. Superficial infections with dermatophytes are more common than superficial infections with *Candida.*

Overview of Drug Therapy

Superficial mycoses can be treated with a variety of topical and oral drugs. For mild to moderate infections, topical agents are generally preferred. Specific indications for the drugs used against superficial mycoses are shown in Table 77.4 Some of these drugs are also used for systemic mycoses.

Dermatophytic Infections (Ringworm)

Dermatophytic infections are commonly referred to as *ringworm.* There are four principal dermatophytic infections, defined by their location: *tinea pedis* (ringworm of the foot,

TABLE 77.4 ■ Drugs for Superficial Fungal Infections

Drug	Route	Ringworm*	*Candida* Infection			Onychomycosis†
			Skin	Mouth	Vulvovaginal	
AZOLES						
Clotrimazole	Topical	✔	✔	✔		
Econazole	Topical	✔	✔			
Efinaconazole	Topical					✔
Fluconazole	Oral	✔		✔	✔	✔
Itraconazole	Oral	✔				✔
Ketoconazole	Oral	✔	✔	✔		✔
	Topical	✔				
Miconazole	Topical	✔	✔		✔	
Oxiconazole	Topical	✔				
Sertaconazole	Topical	✔				
Sulconazole	Topical	✔				
ALLYLAMINES						
Butenafine	Topical	✔				
Naftifine	Topical	✔				
Terbinafine	Oral	✔				✔
	Topical	✔				
OTHERS						
Amphotericin B	Topical		✔			
Ciclopirox	Topical	✔	✔			✔
Griseofulvin	Oral	✔				✔
Nystatin	Topical		✔	✔		
Tavaborole	Topical					✔
Tolnaftate	Topical	✔				
Undecylenate	Topical	✔				

**Ringworm* is a popular term for dermatophytic infections, including tinea pedis, tinea cruris, tinea corporis, and tinea capitis.
†*Onychomycosis* is a clinical term for fungal infection of the toenails and fingernails.

or "athlete's foot"), *tinea corporis* (ringworm of the body), *tinea cruris* (ringworm of the groin), and *tinea capitis* (ringworm of the scalp).

Tinea Pedis

Tinea pedis, the most common fungal infection, generally responds well to topical therapy. Patients should be advised to wear absorbent cotton socks, change their shoes often, and dry their feet after bathing.

Tinea Corporis

Tinea corporis usually responds to a topical azole or allylamine. Treatment should continue for at least 1 week after symptoms have cleared. Severe infection may require a systemic antifungal agent (e.g., griseofulvin).

Tinea Cruris

Tinea cruris responds well to topical therapy. Treatment should continue for at least 1 week after symptoms have cleared. If the infection is severely inflamed, a systemic antifungal drug (e.g., clotrimazole) may be needed; topical or systemic glucocorticoids may be needed as well.

Tinea Capitis

Tinea capitis is difficult to treat. Topical drugs are not likely to work. Oral griseofulvin, taken for 6 to 8 weeks, is considered standard therapy. However, oral terbinafine, taken for only 2 to 4 weeks, may be more effective.

Candidiasis

Vulvovaginal Candidiasis

Vulvovaginal candidiasis is very common, occurring in 75% of women at least once in their life. Most cases are caused by *Candida albicans,* and many of the rest are caused by *Candida glabrata,* especially in patients with HIV/AIDS. Factors that predispose to *Candida* infection include pregnancy, obesity, diabetes, debilitation, HIV infection, and use of certain drugs, including oral contraceptives, systemic glucocorticoids, anticancer agents, immunosuppressants, and systemic antibiotics. With current drugs, just 1 or 3 days of *topical* therapy can be curative. In addition, *oral* therapy may be used: a single 150-mg dose of fluconazole can be curative—but it causes more side effects (headache, rash, GI disturbance) than topical agents. For women with recurrent vulvovaginal candidiasis, weekly prophylaxis with oral fluconazole is highly effective—but relapse is common when treatment is stopped. Major drugs for uncomplicated vulvovaginal candidiasis are shown in Table 77.4. All appear equally effective, so drug selection is based largely on patient preference. Longer regimens have no demonstrated advantage over shorter ones.

Oral Candidiasis

Oral candidiasis, also known as *thrush,* is seen often. Topical agents—*nystatin, clotrimazole,* and *miconazole*—are generally effective. In the immunocompromised host, oral therapy with *fluconazole* or *ketoconazole* is usually required.

Onychomycosis (Fungal Infection of the Nails)

Fungal infection of the nails, known as onychomycosis, is difficult to eradicate and requires prolonged treatment. Infections may be caused by dermatophytes or *Candida* species. Because onychomycosis is largely a cosmetic concern, treatment is usually optional.

Onychomycosis may be treated with oral antifungal drugs or with topical ciclopirox. Success rates with oral therapy are quite low, and rates with topical therapy are even lower.

Oral Therapy

The drugs used most often are *terbinafine* [Lamisil] and *itraconazole* [Sporanox]. Both are active against *Candida* species and dermatophytes. When in the body, these drugs become incorporated into keratin as the nails grow. Drug may also diffuse into the nails from the tissue below. Side effects include headache, GI disturbances (e.g., nausea, vomiting, abdominal pain), and skin reactions (e.g., itching, rash). Treatment generally lasts 3 to 6 months. Unfortunately, even with this prolonged therapy, the cure rate is relatively low (about 50%).

Topical Therapy

Ciclopirox. *Ciclopirox* [Penlac Nail Lacquer] is one of three topical agents for onychomycosis available in the United States. In contrast to oral terbinafine or itraconazole, which are active against *Candida* species and several dermatophytes, topical ciclopirox is active against only one dermatophyte—*Trichophyton rubrum*—and has no activity against *Candida.* Ciclopirox is applied once a day to the nails and immediately adjacent skin. New coats are applied over old ones. Once a week, all coats are removed with alcohol. Side effects are minimal and localized. Unfortunately, despite prolonged use (up to 48 weeks), ciclopirox confers only modest benefits: complete cure occurs in less than 12% of patients, and, even when complete cure *does* occur, the recurrence rate is high—about 40%. Compared with oral therapy, topical ciclopirox is safer and cheaper but is much less effective.

Use of ciclopirox for superficial fungal infections of the *skin* is discussed later.

Tavaborole. Tavaborole [Kerydin] is an oxaborole antifungal medication that treats onychomycosis from the dermatophytes *T. rubrum* and *Trichophyton mentagrophytes.* An oxaborole antifungal contains Boron, which is thought to decrease fungal protein synthesis. Tavaborole is available in a 5% solution for topical application. Patients should apply tavaborole to the entire nail surface and under the tip of affected toenails once daily for 48 weeks.

Efinaconazole. Efinaconazole [Jublia] was approved for the topical treatment of onychomycosis in 2014. Efinaconazole belongs to the azole family of antifungal medications. Efinaconazole is available as a 10% gel. Patients cover the entire nail, including the folds, bed, and undersurface of the toenail plate, with the brush applicator supplied with the medication. Like tavaborole, the dosing is one application to affected nails daily for 48 weeks.

Azoles

Twelve members of the azole family are used for superficial mycoses. The usual route is topical. Three of the 12—itraconazole, fluconazole, and ketoconazole—are also used for systemic mycoses (see earlier).

The azoles are active against a broad spectrum of pathogenic fungi, including dermatophytes and *Candida* species. Antifungal effects result from inhibiting the biosynthesis of ergosterol, an essential component of the fungal cytoplasmic membrane.

Clotrimazole

Therapeutic Uses

Topical clotrimazole is a drug of choice for dermatophytic infections and candidiasis of the skin, mouth, and vagina.

Adverse Effects

When applied to the skin, clotrimazole can cause stinging, erythema, edema, urticaria, pruritus, and peeling. However, the incidence is low. Intravaginal administration occasionally causes a burning sensation and lower abdominal cramps. Oral clotrimazole can cause GI distress.

Preparations, Dosage, and Administration

Clotrimazole is available as an oral troche, as a cream or suppository for intravaginal use, and in three formulations for application to the skin: cream, lotion, and solution. For fungal infections of the skin, the drug is applied twice daily for 2 to 4 weeks. For vulvovaginal candidiasis, several dosing schedules have been employed, including (1) insertion of one 100-mg vaginal tablet for 7 days, (2) insertion of one 200-mg vaginal tablet for 3 days, and (3) application of a 2% vaginal cream for 3 days. Trade names for dermatologic products are Desenex, Micatin, Lotrimin, and Canesten ♣, and the trade name for vaginal products is Gyne-Lotrimin.

Ketoconazole

Ketoconazole [Extina, Nizoral, Xolegel, Ketoderm ♣] is approved for oral and topical therapy of superficial mycoses. Oral ketoconazole provides effective treatment of dermatophytic infections as well as candidiasis of the skin, mouth, and vagina. However, because of the toxicity associated with oral use, this route should be reserved for infections that have failed to respond to topical agents. Ketoconazole for topical use is available in five formulations: 2% foam [Extina] and 2% gel [Xolegel] for seborrheic dermatitis, 1% shampoo [Nizoral-AD] for dandruff, 2% shampoo [Nizoral] for tinea versicolor, and 2% cream [Ketoderm ♣] for dermatophytic infections and candidiasis of the skin. The basic pharmacology of ketoconazole was discussed earlier in the section "Drugs for Systemic Mycoses."

Miconazole

Therapeutic Uses

Miconazole [Micatin, Monistat 3, Monistat 7, Oravig, others] is an azole antifungal drug available for topical and systemic administration. Topical miconazole is a drug of choice for dermatophytic infections and for cutaneous and vulvovaginal candidiasis. A new buccal tablet is used for oropharyngeal candidiasis.

Adverse Effects

Adverse effects of topical miconazole are generally mild. Intravaginal administration causes burning, itching, and irritation in about 7% of users. When applied to the skin, miconazole occasionally causes irritation, burning, and maceration. Topical application is not associated with systemic toxicity.

Drug Interactions

Intravaginal miconazole can intensify the anticoagulant effects of warfarin. We have long known that systemic miconazole can inhibit metabolism of warfarin, causing warfarin levels to rise. Apparently, intravaginal miconazole can be absorbed in amounts sufficient to do the same. Because of this interaction, those taking warfarin should not use intravaginal miconazole. If the drugs must be used concurrently, anticoagulation should be monitored closely and warfarin dosage reduced as indicated.

Preparations, Dosage, and Administration

Miconazole is available in cream, liquid spray, and powder formulations for application to the skin; in cream and suppository formulations for intravaginal application; and as a 50-mg buccal tablet [Oravig] for oropharyngeal candidiasis. Cutaneous mycoses are treated with twice-daily applications for 2 to 4 weeks. Oropharyngeal candidiasis is treated by placing a buccal tablet to the upper gum once daily for 14 days.

Itraconazole

Itraconazole [Sporanox] can be used for oral therapy of onychomycosis of the toenails or fingernails. For infection of the toenails, the dosage is 200 mg once daily for 12 weeks. For infection of the fingernails, dosing is done in repeating cycles consisting of 1 week of treatment (200 mg twice daily) followed by 3 weeks off. The basic pharmacology of itraconazole was discussed earlier in the section "Drugs for Systemic Mycoses."

Fluconazole

Fluconazole [Diflucan] can be used for oral therapy of vulvovaginal candidiasis, oropharyngeal candidiasis, and onychomycosis. For vulvovaginal candidiasis, the dosage for treating ongoing infection is 150 mg once; the dosage for preventing recurrent infection is 150 mg once a week for 6 months. The dosage for oropharyngeal candidiasis is 200 mg on day 1 followed by 100 mg daily for 2 weeks. The dosage for onychomycosis is 100 mg daily for 3 to 12 weeks. The basic pharmacology of fluconazole was discussed earlier in the section "Drugs for Systemic Mycoses."

Newer Azole Drugs

Econazole

Econazole [Ecoza] is available for topical application only. The drug is indicated for ringworm infections and superficial candidiasis. Local adverse effects (burning, erythema, stinging, itching) occur in about 3% of patients. Less than 1% of topical econazole is absorbed, and systemic toxicity has not been reported. Econazole is supplied in a 1% foam [Ecoza] or cream. The foam is applied once daily for 4 weeks. The cream is applied once or twice daily for 2 to 4 weeks depending on the indication for treatment.

Oxiconazole and Sulconazole

Oxiconazole [Oxistat] and sulconazole [Exelderm] are broad-spectrum antifungal drugs. Both are approved for topical treatment of tinea infections. Local adverse effects (itching, burning, irritation, erythema) occur in less than 3% of patients. Neither drug is absorbed to a significant degree. Systemic toxicity has not been reported. Oxiconazole is supplied as a cream and lotion applied once daily for 2 to 4 weeks. Sulconazole is supplied as a cream and solution applied once or twice daily for 2 to 4 weeks.

Butoconazole, Terconazole, and Tioconazole

These azole drugs are approved only for topical treatment of vulvovaginal candidiasis. All three are fungicidal. Local adverse effects (burning, itching) occur in 2% to 6% of users. Absorption after intravaginal administration is low, and systemic reactions are rare (except for headache with terconazole). Owing to a small risk for fetal injury, these drugs are not recommended for use during the first trimester of pregnancy.

Sertaconazole

Sertaconazole [Ertaczo], available by prescription, is indicated for topical therapy of tinea pedis. The 2% cream is applied twice daily for 4 weeks. Mild local reactions (itching, burning, irritation, erythema) occur in 2% of patients. Blood levels are undetectable after repeated applications, and systemic effects have not been reported. Cure rates are like those seen with generic clotrimazole and miconazole—older azoles that are much cheaper and can be purchased without a prescription.

Griseofulvin

Griseofulvin [Grifulvin V, Gris-PEG] is administered orally to treat superficial mycoses. The drug is inactive against organisms that cause systemic mycoses.

Mechanism of Action

After absorption, griseofulvin is deposited in the keratin precursor cells of skin, hair, and nails. Because griseofulvin is present, newly formed keratin is resistant to fungal invasion. Hence, as infected keratin is shed, it is replaced by fungus-free tissue.

Griseofulvin kills fungi by inhibiting fungal mitosis by binding to components of microtubules, the structures that form the mitotic spindle. Because griseofulvin acts by disrupting mitosis, the drug only affects fungi that are actively growing.

Pharmacokinetics

Administration is oral, and absorption can be enhanced by dosing with a fatty meal. As noted, griseofulvin is deposited in the keratin precursor cells of skin, hair, and nails. Elimination is by hepatic metabolism and renal excretion.

Therapeutic Uses

Griseofulvin is employed orally to treat dermatophytic infections of the skin, hair, and nails. The drug is not active against *Candida* species, nor is it useful against systemic mycoses. Dermatophytic infections of the skin respond relatively quickly (in 3–8 weeks). However, infections of the palms may require 2 to 3 months of treatment, and a year or more may be needed to eliminate infections of the toenails.

Adverse Effects

Most untoward effects are not serious. Transient headache is common. Other mild reactions include rash, insomnia, tiredness, and GI effects (nausea, vomiting, diarrhea). Griseofulvin may cause hepatotoxicity and photosensitivity in patients with porphyria. The drug is contraindicated for individuals with a history of porphyria or hepatocellular disease.

Drug Interactions

Griseofulvin induces hepatic drug-metabolizing enzymes and can decrease the effects of warfarin. When this combination is used, the dosage of warfarin may need to be increased.

Preparations, Dosage, and Administration.

Griseofulvin is formulated in a solution (125 mg/5 mL) and in two particle sizes: microsized and ultramicrosized. The microcrystalline form [Grifulvin V] is supplied in 500 mg tablets. The ultramicrocrystalline form [Gris-PEG] is supplied in tablets (125 and 250 mg).

Dosage depends to some degree on the formulation (microsized or ultramicrosized). With microsized formulations, the usual adult dosage is 500 mg to 1 g/day, and the usual pediatric dosage is 11 mg/kg/day. The ultramicrosized particles are better absorbed than the microsized particles, and hence doses of ultramicrocrystalline griseofulvin are about 30% lower than doses of microcrystalline griseofulvin.

Polyene Antibiotics

Nystatin

Actions, Uses, and Adverse Effects

Nystatin [Mycostatin, Nyaderm ♣] is a polyene antibiotic used only for candidiasis. Nystatin is the drug of choice for intestinal candidiasis and is also employed to treat candidal infections of the skin, mouth, esophagus, and vagina. Nystatin can be administered orally and topically. There is no significant absorption from either route. Oral nystatin occasionally causes GI disturbance (nausea, vomiting, diarrhea). Topical application may produce local irritation.

Preparations, Dosage, and Administration

For oral administration, nystatin is supplied as a suspension and in tablets and lozenges; dosages range from 400,000 to 1 million units 3 to 4 times a day. Vaginal tablets are employed for vaginal candidiasis; the usual dosage is 100,000 units once a day for 2 weeks. Nystatin is supplied as a cream, ointment, and powder to treat candidiasis of the skin. The cream and ointment formulations are applied twice daily; the powder is applied 3 times daily.

Allylamines

Naftifine

Naftifine [Naftin] was the first allylamine available. Although approved only for topical treatment of dermatophytic infections, naftifine is active against a broad spectrum of pathogenic fungi. The drug works by inhibiting squalene epoxidase, thus inhibiting synthesis of ergosterol, a key component of the fungal cell membrane. The most common adverse effects are burning and stinging. Absorption after topical administration is relatively low (about 6%). Systemic effects have not been reported. Naftifine is supplied in two formulations: 1% and 2% cream and 1% gel. The cream is applied once daily, the gel twice daily. Treatment usually lasts 2 to 4 weeks.

Terbinafine

Actions and Uses

Terbinafine [Lamisil] belongs to the same chemical family as naftifine and has the same mechanism of action: inhibition of squalene epoxidase with resultant inhibition of ergosterol synthesis. The drug is highly active against dermatophytes and less active against *Candida* species. Terbinafine is available in topical and oral formulations. Topical therapy is used for ringworm infections (e.g., tinea corporis, tinea cruris, tinea pedis). Oral therapy is used for ringworm and onychomycosis (fungal infection of the nails).

Adverse Effects

Adverse effects with topical terbinafine are minimal. The discussion that follows applies to oral therapy. The most common side effects are headache, diarrhea, dyspepsia, and abdominal pain. Oral terbinafine may also cause skin reactions and disturbance of taste. Of much greater concern, terbinafine may pose a risk for liver failure. Some terbinafine users have died of liver failure, and others have required a liver transplantation. However, a causal link has not been established. Nonetheless, caution is advised. Baseline tests for serum alanine and aspartate aminotransferases are recommended. In addition, patients should be informed about signs of liver dysfunction (persistent nausea, anorexia, fatigue, vomiting, jaundice, right upper abdominal pain, dark urine, pale stools) and, if they appear, should discontinue terbinafine immediately and undergo evaluation of liver function. Terbinafine is not recommended for patients with preexisting liver disease.

Preparations, Dosage, and Administration

Terbinafine for oral therapy is available in tablets (250 mg). The oral dosage for nail infections is 250 mg/day for 6 to 12 weeks, and the dosage for ringworm is 250 mg/day for 2 to 6 weeks. Terbinafine for topical therapy is available as a gel, spray, powder, and cream, all with strength of 1%. Application is done once or twice daily for 1 to 4 weeks.

Butenafine

Butenafine [Lotrimin Ultra Cream, Mentax] is chemically similar to naftifine and terbinafine, although butenafine is not a true allylamine. However, it does have the same mechanism of action: inhibition of squalene epoxidase with resultant inhibition of ergosterol synthesis. Butenafine is indicated for topical therapy of tinea pedis, tinea corporis, tinea cruris, and tinea versicolor. Absorption is minimum, and systemic side effects have not been reported. Local reactions include burning, stinging, erythema, irritation, and itching. Butenafine 1% cream is applied once daily for 2 to 4 weeks.

Other Drugs for Superficial Mycoses

Tolnaftate

Tolnaftate [Tinactin, others] is employed topically to treat a variety of superficial mycoses. The drug is active against dermatophytes, but not against *Candida* species. The mechanism of antifungal action is unknown. Adverse effects (sensitization, irritation) are extremely rare. Tolnaftate is available in several formulations. Creams, powders, and solutions are most effective; powders are used adjunctively. The drug is applied twice daily for 2 to 4 weeks.

Undecylenic Acid

Undecylenic acid [Fungi-Nail, others] is a topical agent used to treat superficial mycoses. The drug is active against dermatophytes but not *Candida* species. Its major indication is tinea pedis (athlete's foot). However, other drugs (tolnaftate, the azoles) are more effective.

Ciclopirox

Ciclopirox [Loprox, Penlac Nail Lacquer] is a broad-spectrum, topical antifungal drug. Benefits derive from chelating iron and aluminum present in metal-dependent enzymes that protect fungi from peroxides. Ciclopirox is used for infections of the skin (discussed here) and for infections of the fingernails and toenails (discussed earlier in the section "Onychomycosis"). The formulations used for skin infections are marketed as Loprox. The formulation used for nail infections is marketed as Penlac Nail Lacquer.

When applied to the skin, ciclopirox is active against dermatophytes and *Candida* species. The drug is effective against superficial candidiasis and tinea pedis, tinea cruris, and tinea corporis. Ciclopirox penetrates the epidermis to the dermis, but systemic absorption is minimum, and hence no significant systemic accumulation occurs. There is no toxicity from local application. For treatment of skin infections, ciclopirox is available as a 1% shampoo and as a 0.77% cream, gel, and suspension. The shampoo is used twice weekly for 4 weeks. The cream, gel, and suspension are applied twice daily for 2 to 4 weeks.

CHAPTER

78

Antiviral Agents I: Drugs for Non-HIV Viral Infections

Jacqueline Rosenjack Burchum, DNSc, FNP-BC, CNE

Antiviral drugs are discussed in this chapter and Chapter 79. Here, we consider drugs used to treat infections caused by viruses other than human immunodeficiency virus (HIV). In Chapter 79, we consider drugs used against HIV infection. Drugs for non-HIV infections are shown in Table 78.1.

Although antiviral therapy has made significant advances, our ability to treat viral infections remains limited. Compared with the dramatic advances made in antibacterial therapy over the past half-century, efforts to develop safe and effective antiviral drugs have been less successful. A major reason for this lack of success resides in the process of viral replication: viruses are obligate intracellular parasites that use the biochemical machinery of host cells to reproduce. Because the viral growth cycle employs host-cell enzymes and substrates, it is difficult to suppress viral replication without doing significant harm to the host. The antiviral drugs used clinically act by suppressing biochemical processes unique to viral reproduction. As our knowledge of viral molecular biology expands, additional virus-specific processes will be discovered, giving us new targets for drugs.

DRUGS FOR INFECTION WITH HERPES SIMPLEX VIRUSES AND VARICELLA-ZOSTER VIRUS

Herpes simplex virus (HSV) and *varicella-zoster virus* (VZV) are members of the herpesvirus group. HSV causes infection of the genitalia, mouth, face, and other sites. VZV is the cause of *varicella* (chickenpox) and *herpes zoster* (shingles), a painful condition resulting from reactivation of VZV that had been dormant within sensory nerve roots. Both conditions are discussed in Chapter 53, along with the vaccine used to prevent chickenpox. Drugs for infection with HSV and VZV are shown in Table 78.2, genital herpes is discussed in Chapter 80, and lifespan considerations are provided in Box 78.1.

Acyclovir

Acyclovir [Zovirax] is the agent of first choice for most infections caused by HSV and VZV. The drug can be administered topically, orally, and intravenously. Serious side effects are uncommon.

Antiviral Spectrum

Acyclovir is active only against members of the herpesvirus family, a group that includes *herpes simplex viruses, varicella-zoster virus,* and *cytomegalovirus* (CMV). Of these, HSVs are most sensitive, VZV is moderately sensitive, and most strains of CMV are resistant.

Mechanism of Action

Acyclovir inhibits viral replication by suppressing synthesis of viral DNA. To exert antiviral effects, acyclovir must first undergo activation. The critical step in activation is conversion of acyclovir to acyclo–guanosine monophosphate (GMP) by *thymidine kinase.* When formed, acyclo-GMP is converted to acyclo–guanosine triphosphate (GTP), the compound directly responsible for inhibiting DNA synthesis. Acyclo-GTP suppresses DNA synthesis by (1) inhibiting viral DNA polymerase and (2) becoming incorporated into the growing strand of viral DNA, which blocks further strand growth.

The selectivity of acyclovir is based in large part on the ability of certain viruses to activate the drug. HSVs are especially sensitive to acyclovir because the drug is a much better substrate for thymidine kinase produced by HSVs than it is for mammalian thymidine kinase. Hence formation of acyclo-GMP, the limiting step in the activation of acyclovir, occurs almost exclusively in cells infected with HSV. CMV is inherently resistant to the drug because acyclovir is a poor substrate for the form of thymidine kinase produced by this virus.

Resistance

Herpesviruses develop resistance to acyclovir by three mechanisms: (1) decreased production of thymidine kinase, (2) alteration of thymidine kinase such that it no longer converts acyclovir to acyclo-GMP, and (3) alteration of viral DNA polymerase such that it is less sensitive to inhibition. Of these mechanisms, thymidine kinase deficiency is the most common. Resistance is rare in immunocompetent patients, but many cases have been reported in transplant recipients and patients with AIDS. Lesions caused by resistant HSVs can be extensive and severe, progressing despite continued acyclovir therapy. Acyclovir-resistant HSVs and VZV usually respond to intravenous (IV) foscarnet or cidofovir, which are primarily used for treatment of CMV infection (see later discussion).

Therapeutic Uses

Mucocutaneous Herpes Simplex Infections

Herpes infections of the face and oropharynx are usually caused by HSV type 2 (HSV-2). For immunocompetent patients, *oral* acyclovir can be used to treat primary infections of the gums and mouth. Oral acyclovir can also be taken *prophylactically* to prevent episodes of *recurrent* herpes labialis (cold sores). However, there is no truly effective treatment

TABLE 78.1 ▪ Major Drugs for Non-HIV Viral Infections

Drug	Antiviral Spectrum
DRUGS FOR HSV AND VZV INFECTIONS	
Systemic Drugs	
Acyclovir	HSV, VZV
Famciclovir	HSV, VZV
Foscarnet	HSV, VZV
Valacyclovir	HSV, VZV
Topical Drugs	
Vidarabine	HSV, VZV
Penciclovir	HSV
Trifluridine	HSV keratitis
Docosanol	HSV keratitis
Ganciclovir	HSV keratitis
DRUGS FOR HEPATITIS	
Alfa Interferons	
Interferon alfa-2b	HCV, HBV
Interferon alfacon-1	HCV
Peginterferon alfa-2a	HCV, HBV
Peginterferon alfa-2b	HCV
Protease Inhibitors (PIs)	
Boceprevir	HCV
Grazoprevir	HCV
Paritaprevir	HCV
Simeprevir	HCV
NS5A Inhibitors	
Daclatasvir	HCV
Elbasvir	HCV
Ledipasvir	HCV
Ombitasvir	HCV
NS5B Nucleoside Polymerase Inhibitors	
Sofosbuvir	HCV
NS5B Nonnucleoside Polymerase Inhibitors	
Dasabuvir	HCV
Nucleoside Analogs	
Ribavirin (oral)	HCV
Adefovir	HBV*
Entecavir	HBV*
Lamivudine	HBV*
Telbivudine	HBV
Tenofovir	HBV*
DRUGS FOR CYTOMEGALOVIRUS INFECTION	
Ganciclovir	CMV
Valganciclovir	CMV
Cidofovir	CMV
Foscarnet	CMV
DRUGS FOR INFLUENZA	
Oseltamivir	Influenza A and B
Zanamivir	Influenza A and B

CMV, cytomegalovirus; HBV, hepatitis B virus; HCV, hepatitis C virus; HSV, herpes simplex virus; VZV, varicella-zoster virus.
*Also active against HIV.

for active herpes labialis. Mucocutaneous herpes infections can be especially severe in immunocompromised patients. For these people, *intravenous* acyclovir is the treatment of choice.

Varicella-Zoster Infections

High doses of *oral* acyclovir are effective for herpes zoster (shingles) in older adults. Oral therapy is also effective for varicella (chickenpox) in children, adolescents, and adults, provided that dosing is begun early (within 24 hours of rash onset). *Intravenous* acyclovir is the treatment of choice for VZV infection in the immunocompromised host.

Herpes Simplex Genitalis

The characteristics and treatment of genital HSV infection are discussed in Chapter 80.

Pharmacokinetics

Acyclovir may be administered topically, orally, and intravenously. Oral bioavailability is low, ranging from 15% to 30%. No significant absorption occurs with topical use. When in the blood, acyclovir is distributed widely to body fluids and tissues. Levels achieved in cerebrospinal fluid are 50% of those in plasma. Elimination is renal, primarily as the unchanged drug. In patients with normal kidney function, acyclovir has a half-life of 2.5 hours. The half-life is prolonged by renal impairment, reaching 20 hours in anuric patients. Accordingly, dosages should be reduced in patients with kidney disease.

Adverse Effects

Intravenous Therapy

Intravenous acyclovir is generally well tolerated. The most common reactions are *phlebitis* and *inflammation* at the infusion site. Reversible *nephrotoxicity,* indicated by elevations in serum creatinine and blood urea nitrogen, occurs in some patients. The cause is deposition of acyclovir in renal tubules. The risk for renal injury is increased by dehydration and by use of other nephrotoxic drugs. Kidney damage can be minimized by infusing acyclovir slowly (over 1 hour) and by ensuring adequate hydration during the infusion and for 2 hours after.

Neurologic toxicity—agitation, tremors, delirium, hallucinations, and myoclonus—occurs rarely, primarily in patients with renal impairment. In patients on dialysis, very low doses can cause severe neurotoxicity, characterized by delirium and coma.

Oral and Topical Therapy

Oral acyclovir is devoid of serious adverse effects. Renal impairment has not been reported. The most common reactions are nausea, vomiting, diarrhea, headache, and vertigo. Topical acyclovir frequently causes transient local burning or stinging; systemic reactions do not occur. Oral acyclovir is safe during pregnancy, so it can be used to suppress recurrent genital herpes near term.

Preparations, Dosage, and Administration

Topical Ointment. Acyclovir [Zovirax] is supplied as a 5% ointment for topical therapy of herpes genitalis and mild mucocutaneous HSV infection in the immunocompromised host. Application is done 6 times a day at 3-hour intervals for 7 days. Patients should use a finger cot or rubber glove to avoid viral transfer to other parts of the body or to other people.

TABLE 78.2 ▪ Treatment of Herpes Simplex Virus and Varicella-Zoster Virus Infections

Infection	Drug	Route	Dosage	Duration
HERPES SIMPLEX VIRUS INFECTIONS				
Encephalitis	Acyclovir	IV	10–15 mg/kg every 8 hr	14–21 days
Mucocutaneous in ICH	Acyclovir	IV	5 mg/kg every 8 hr	7–10 days
	Acyclovir	PO	400 mg 5 times/day	7–14 days
	Valacyclovir	PO	*Initial episode:* 1 g twice daily for 10 days *Recurrent episode:* 500 mg twice daily for 3 days *Reduction of transmission:* 500 mg once daily *Suppressive therapy:* Immunocompetent patients: 1 g once daily (500 mg once daily in patients with <9 recurrences per year) HIV-infected patients (CD4 ≥100 cells/mm^3): 500 mg twice daily	7–10 days
	Famciclovir	PO	500 mg 2 times/day	7–10 days
	Foscarnet*	IV	400 mg 2–3 times/day	7–21 days
Neonatal	Acyclovir	IV	5–10 mg/kg every 8 hr	7 days
Orolabial	Acyclovir	Topical	5% cream 5 times/day	4 days
	Penciclovir	Topical	1% cream every 2 hr	4 days
	Docosanol	Topical	10% cream 5 times/day	4 days or until lesions have healed
Keratoconjunctivitis	Ganciclovir	Topical	See text	
	Trifluridine	Topical	See text	
	Vidarabine	Topical	See text	
Genital infections	See Chapter 80			
VARICELLA-ZOSTER VIRUS INFECTIONS				
Varicella	Acyclovir	PO	800 mg 4 times/day	5 days
Varicella in ICH*	Acyclovir	IV	10 mg/kg every 8 hr	7 days
Herpes zoster	Acyclovir	PO	800 mg 5 times/day	7–10 days
	Valacyclovir	PO	1 g 3 times/day	7 days
	Famciclovir	PO	500 mg 3 times/day	7 days
Herpes zoster in ICH*	Acyclovir	IV	10 mg/kg every 8 hr	7 days
Acyclovir-resistant zoster	Foscarnet	IV	40 mg/kg every 8–12 hr	10 days

*Reserve foscarnet for acyclovir-resistant infection.
ICH, immunocompromised host; IU, international units; IV, intravenous; PO, oral.

PATIENT-CENTERED CARE ACROSS THE LIFE SPAN

Antiviral Drugs Prescribed for Herpes Virus and Cytomegalovirus Infections

Life Stage	Considerations or Concerns
Children	Ganciclovir and valganciclovir are approved for use in children for selected conditions. Valacyclovir is also approved for children according to diagnosis: it may be given to neonates for HSV suppressive therapy, to children 2 years or older with chicken pox, and to children 12 years or older for cold sores. Adequate studies have not been conducted in children for most of these drugs. Careful weighing of benefits versus risks is advised.
Pregnant women	Acyclovir, famciclovir, valacyclovir, are in FDA Pregnancy Risk Category B. Foscarnet is in FDA Pregnancy Risk Category C. Cidofovir, ganciclovir, and valganciclovir (a prodrug of ganciclovir) are categorized in FDA Pregnancy Risk Category C; however, in these both caused structural abnormalities in animal studies and are not recommended for pregnant women.
Breastfeeding women	Breastfeeding is not contraindicated; however, because inadequate studies are available and serious adverse events could occur, caution is recommended.
Older adults	There are no contraindications for this age group; however, those with renal impairment should be started on lower doses, with dosage adjustments made cautiously.

Patient Education

ACYCLOVIR

Advise patients to apply the drug with a finger cot or rubber glove to avoid viral transfer to other body sites or other people.

Inform patients with herpes simplex genitalis that acyclovir only decreases symptoms; it does not eliminate the virus and does not produce cure. Advise patients to cleanse the affected area with soap and water 3 to 4 times a day, drying thoroughly after each wash. Advise patients to avoid all sexual contact while lesions are present and to use a condom even when lesions are absent.

Topical Cream. Acyclovir [Zovirax] is supplied as a 5% cream for topical therapy of recurrent herpes labialis (cold sores) in patients at least 12 years old. Application is done 5 times a day for 4 days.

Oral. Oral acyclovir [Zovirax] is available in capsules (200 mg), tablets (400 and 800 mg), and a suspension (200 mg/5 mL). Dosages for patients with normal kidney function are given here. Dosages must be reduced for patients with renal impairment.

- For *initial episodes of herpes genitalis,* the usual dosage is 400 mg 3 times a day for 7 to 10 days.
- For *episodic recurrences of herpes genitalis,* the usual dosage is 400 mg 3 times a day for 5 days.
- For *long-term suppressive therapy of recurrent genital infections,* the usual dosage is 400 mg twice daily for up to 12 months.
- For *acute therapy of herpes zoster,* the dosage is 800 mg 5 times a day (at 4-hour intervals) for 7 to 10 days.
- For *VZV* (chickenpox), the dosage is 20 mg/kg (but no more than 800 mg) 4 times a day for 5 days. Treatment should begin at the earliest sign of rash.

Prototype Drugs

DRUGS FOR NON-HIV VIRAL INFECTIONS

Drugs for Herpes Simplex Virus Infection

Acyclovir
Ganciclovir

Drug for Cytomegalovirus Infection

Ganciclovir

Drugs for Hepatitis

Peginterferon alfa-2b
Lamivudine (nucleoside analog)
Peginterferon alfa-2a
Ribavirin (oral nucleoside analog)
Simeprevir (protease inhibitor)
Daclatasvir (NS5A inhibitor)
Sofosbuvir (NS5B inhibitor)

Drugs for Influenza

Influenza vaccine
Oseltamivir

Drugs for Respiratory Syncytial Virus Infection

Ribavirin (inhaled)
Palivizumab

Intravenous. For IV dosing, acyclovir is available in solution (50 mg/mL). Administration is by slow infusion (over 1 hour or more). Parenteral acyclovir must not be given by IV bolus or by intramuscular (IM) or subcutaneous (subQ) injection. To minimize the risk for renal damage, hydrate the patient during the infusion and for 2 hours after. Dosages for patients with normal kidney function are given here. Dosages should be reduced for patients with renal impairment.

- For *mucocutaneous HSV infection in the immunocompromised host,* the adult dosage is 5 mg/kg infused every 8 hours for 7 days. The dosage for children under 12 years is 10 mg/kg infused every 8 hours for 7 days.
- For *VZV infection in the immunocompromised host,* the adult dosage is 10 mg/kg infused every 8 hours for 7 days. The dosage for children under 12 years is 20 mg/kg infused every 8 hours for 7 days.
- For *severe episodes of herpes genitalis in the immunocompetent host,* the adult dosage is 5 to 10 mg/kg infused every 8 hours for 5 to 7 days (or until symptoms resolve). The dosage for children younger than 12 years is 15 to 20 mg/kg/day divided into three doses to be infused every 8 hours for 5 days.

Valacyclovir

Actions and Uses

Valacyclovir [Valtrex], a prodrug form of acyclovir, is approved for management of four conditions: (1) herpes zoster (shingles), (2) herpes simplex genitalis (genital herpes), (3) herpes labialis (cold sores), and (4) varicella (chickenpox). With the exception of herpes labialis, there are limits on use for each condition. For herpes zoster, valacyclovir is indicated only for immunocompetent patients. For varicella, the patients must be immunocompetent children. For herpes simplex genitalis, valacyclovir is indicated for treatment of initial and recurrent episodes for immunocompetent patients; however, for suppressive therapy, this drug is approved for management in immunocompetent and HIV-infected adults with a CD4+ cell count of at least 100 cells/mm3.

Valacyclovir is sometimes used off-label for prophylaxis of HSV, VZV, and CMV infections in patients with cancer. It is also sometimes used for treatment of cancer-related HSV and VZV.

Pharmacokinetics

Oral valacyclovir undergoes rapid absorption followed by rapid and essentially complete conversion to acyclovir. When acyclovir itself is given orally, bioavailability is only 15% to 30%. In contrast, when valacyclovir is given orally, the effective bioavailability of acyclovir is greatly increased—to about 55%. Therefore valacyclovir represents a more efficient way of getting acyclovir into the body. After conversion of valacyclovir to acyclovir, the kinetics are the same as if acyclovir itself had been given.

Adverse Effects

No doubt you noticed the emphasis on using valacyclovir primarily for immunocompetent patients. Why? In some immunocompromised patients, valacyclovir has produced a syndrome known as thrombotic thrombocytopenic purpura/hemolytic uremic syndrome (TTP/HUS). This syndrome, which can be fatal, has not occurred in immunocompetent patients. Aside from causing TTP/HUS, valacyclovir is generally well tolerated, producing the same side effects seen with oral acyclovir (e.g., nausea, vomiting, diarrhea, headache, vertigo).

Preparations, Dosage, and Administration

Valacyclovir [Valtrex] is available in 500- and 1000-mg oral capsules. Dosing may be done without regard to meals. In patients with renal impairment, dosages should be reduced.

For patients with herpes zoster, the recommended dosage is 1000 mg 3 times a day for 7 days. Therapy should begin as soon as possible after symptom onset.

For patients with herpes simplex genitalis, the dosage is 1 g twice daily for 10 days (for the initial episode), or 500 mg twice daily for 3 days (for episodic recurrences). For suppressive therapy, the recommended dosage for immunocompetent patients is 500 to 1000 mg once daily and, for patients with HIV infection, 500 mg twice a day.

For patients with herpes labialis, 2 g/dose should be taken 12 hours apart for 1 day. Dosing should begin as soon as possible after onset of symptoms.

For immunocompetent children aged 2 to 18 years with chickenpox, dosage is 20 mg/kg (up to a maximum of 1 g) 3 times a day.

Famciclovir

Famciclovir [Famvir] is a prodrug used to treat acute herpes zoster and genital herpes infection. Benefits are equivalent to those of acyclovir. Adverse effects are minimal.

Pharmacokinetics

Famciclovir undergoes rapid absorption from the gastrointestinal (GI) tract followed by enzymatic conversion to penciclovir, its active form. Food decreases the rate of famciclovir absorption but not the extent. As a result, the amount of penciclovir produced is the same whether famciclovir is taken with or without food. Penciclovir is excreted in the urine, largely unchanged. The plasma half-life of penciclovir is about 2.5 hours. However, the half-life of penciclovir within cells is much longer. In patients with renal impairment, the plasma half-life of penciclovir is prolonged.

Mechanism of Action and Antiviral Spectrum

Penciclovir undergoes intracellular conversion to penciclovir triphosphate, a compound that inhibits viral DNA polymerase, and thereby prevents replication of viral DNA. Under clinical conditions, formation of penciclovir triphosphate requires viral thymidine kinase. As a result, inhibition of DNA synthesis is limited to cells that are infected, leaving most host cells unharmed. In vitro, penciclovir is active against HSV type 1 (HSV-1), HSV-2, and VZV.

Therapeutic Use

Famciclovir is approved for treatment of acute herpes zoster (shingles) and herpes simplex genitalis. In patients with herpes zoster, the drug can decrease the time to full crusting from 7 days down to 5 days. Famciclovir does not decrease the incidence of postherpetic neuralgia but can decrease the duration (from 112 days down to 61 days).

In patients with genital herpes simplex infection, famciclovir is active against the first episode and recurrent episodes. In addition, it can be used for long-term suppression.

Adverse Effects

Famciclovir is very well tolerated. In clinical trials, the only headache and nausea were reported by more than 10% of the subjects. If given in higher than recommended doses, acute renal failure can occur.

Preparations, Dosage, and Administration

Preparations

Famciclovir [Famvir] is supplied in tablets (125, 250, and 500 mg) for oral dosing, with or without food.

Acute Herpes Zoster

The recommended dosage is 500 mg every 8 hours for 7 days. Treatment should start no later than 72 hours after symptom onset. In patients with renal impairment, the dose should be reduced and the interval between doses should be increased to 12 hours or 24 hours, depending on the degree of impairment.

Herpes Simplex Genitalis

For initial episodes, the dosage is 250 mg 3 times a day for 7 to 10 days. For episodic recurrence, there are three dosage regimens available: (1) 125 mg twice a day for 5 days; (2) 500 mg as a single dose on day 1 followed by 250 mg twice a day on day 2, or (3) two 1000-mg doses 12 hours apart. For long-term suppression, the dosage is 250 mg twice daily for a year.

Herpes Labialis

For cold sores that are recurrent, the dosage is a single 1500-mg dose at the first signs of symptoms.

Topical Drugs for Herpes Labialis

We have three topical drugs for recurrent herpes labialis (cold sores). Two of these drugs—penciclovir and docosanol—are discussed next. The third drug—acyclovir—was discussed earlier.

Penciclovir Cream

Penciclovir [Denavir] is a topical drug indicated for recurrent herpes labialis, an infection caused by HSV-1 and HSV-2. The drug suppresses viral replication by inhibiting DNA polymerase, the enzyme that makes DNA. Penciclovir is supplied as a 1% cream to be applied every 2 hours (except when sleeping) for 4 days. In clinical trials, benefits were modest: the average time to healing and duration of pain were decreased by just half a day, from 5 days down to 4.5 days. The only common adverse effect is mild local erythema.

Docosanol Cream

Docosanol [Abreva] is a topical preparation indicated for recurrent herpes labialis. The drug is available over the counter as a 10% cream. Application is done 5 times a day, beginning at the first sign of recurrence. Benefits are modest. In one trial, treatment reduced the time to healing from 4.8 days down to 4.1 days—about the same response seen with penciclovir. Docosanol cream appears devoid of adverse effects.

Docosanol has a broad antiviral spectrum and a unique mechanism of action. Unlike penciclovir, which inhibits viral DNA synthesis (and thereby suppresses replication), docosanol blocks viral entry into host cells. The drug does not kill viruses and does not prevent them from binding to cells. As a result, viable virions can remain attached to the cell surface for a long time. Because docosanol does not affect processes of replication, it is unlikely to promote resistance.

Topical Drugs for Ocular Herpes Infections

Trifluridine Ophthalmic Solution

Trifluridine [Viroptic] is indicated only for topical treatment of ocular infections caused by HSV-1 and HSV-2. The drug is given to treat acute keratoconjunctivitis and recurrent epithelial keratitis. Antiviral actions result from inhibiting DNA synthesis. The most common side effects are localized burning and stinging. Edema of the eyelid occurs in about 3% of patients. Systemic absorption is minimal after topical administration, so the drug is devoid of systemic toxicity. Trifluridine is supplied as a 1% ophthalmic solution. Treatment consists of placing 1 drop on the cornea every 2 hours while the patient is awake, for a maximum of 9 drops/day. After reepithelialization of the cornea has occurred, the dosage is reduced to 1 drop every 4 hours and continues for an additional 7 days.

Ganciclovir Gel

Ganciclovir 0.15% ophthalmic gel [Zirgan] is indicated for acute herpetic keratitis (inflammation and ulceration of the cornea caused by infection with a herpes simplex virus). As discussed later (see "Ganciclovir"), benefits derive from suppressing viral replication. Principal adverse effects are blurred vision, eye irritation, and red eyes. Systemic effects are absent. The recommended dosage is 1 drop in the affected eye 5 times a day until symptoms abate, followed by 1 drop 3 times a day for 7 days. Instruct patients to apply drops directly to the affected eye and to avoid contact lenses until lesions heal.

DRUGS FOR CYTOMEGALOVIRUS INFECTION

Cytomegalovirus is a member of the herpesvirus group, which includes HSV-1 and HSV-2, VZV (the cause of chickenpox), and Epstein-Barr virus (the cause of infectious mononucleosis). Transmission of CMV occurs person to person—through direct contact with saliva, urine, blood, tears, breast milk, semen, and other body fluids. Infection can also be acquired by way of blood transfusion or organ transplantation. Infection with CMV is very common: between 50% and 85% of Americans 40 years and older harbor the virus. After the initial infection, which has minimal symptoms in healthy people, the virus remains dormant within cells for life, without causing detectable injury or clinical illness. Hence, for most healthy people, CMV infection is of little concern. By contrast, people who are immunocompromised—owing to HIV infection, cancer chemotherapy, or use of immunosuppressive drugs—are at high risk for serious morbidity and even death, both from initial CMV infection and from reactivation of dormant CMV. Common sites for infection are the lungs, eyes, and GI tract. Among people with AIDS, CMV retinitis is the principal reason for loss of vision (see Chapter 79). The four drugs used against CMV are discussed next.

Ganciclovir

Ganciclovir [Cytovene, Vitrasert, Zirgan] is a synthetic antiviral agent with activity against herpesviruses, including CMV. Because the drug can cause serious adverse effects, especially granulocytopenia and thrombocytopenia, it should be used only for prevention and treatment of CMV infection in the immunocompromised host.

Mechanism of Action

Ganciclovir is converted to its active form, ganciclovir triphosphate, inside infected cells. As ganciclovir triphosphate, it suppresses replication of viral DNA by (1) inhibiting viral DNA polymerase and (2) undergoing incorporation into the growing DNA chain, which causes premature chain termination.

Pharmacokinetics

Bioavailability of oral ganciclovir is low: only 5% under fasting conditions and 9% when taken with food. When in the blood, the drug is widely distributed to body fluids and tissues. Ganciclovir is excreted unchanged in the urine. In patients with normal renal function, the half-life is about 3 hours. In patients with renal impairment, the half-life is prolonged. Accordingly, dosages should be reduced in patients with kidney disease.

Therapeutic Use

Ganciclovir is approved only to prevent and treat CMV infection in immunocompromised patients, including transplant recipients, those with HIV infection, and those receiving immunosuppressive drugs.

In patients with AIDS, CMV retinitis has an incidence of 15% to 40%. Although most AIDS patients respond initially, the relapse rate is high. Accordingly, for most patients, maintenance therapy should continue indefinitely. The risk for relapse is higher with oral ganciclovir than with IV ganciclovir. Because viral resistance can develop during treatment, this possibility should be considered if the patient responds poorly.

Patient Education

GANCICLOVIR

Advise patients against becoming pregnant. Inform male patients about possible sterility.

Teach patients to report symptoms of bone marrow suppression (anemia, leukocytopenia, and thrombocytopenia) such as pallor, weakness, fever, chills, increased bruising, or petechiae.

When topical ophthalmic gel drops are prescribed, teach proper methods of administration and instruct patients to avoid use of contact lenses.

Adverse Effects

Granulocytopenia and Thrombocytopenia

The adverse effect of greatest concern is bone marrow suppression, which can result in granulocytopenia and thrombocytopenia. These effects, which are usually reversible, are more likely with IV therapy than with oral therapy. These hematologic responses can be exacerbated by concurrent therapy with zidovudine. Conversely, granulocytopenia can be reduced with granulocyte colony-stimulating factors. Because of the risk for adverse hematologic effects, blood cell counts must be monitored. Treatment should be interrupted if the absolute neutrophil count falls below 500/mm^3 or if the platelet count falls below 25,000/mm^3. Cell counts usually begin to recover within 3 to 5 days. Ganciclovir should be used with caution in patients with preexisting cytopenias, in those with a history of cytopenic reactions to other drugs, and in those taking other bone marrow suppressants (e.g., zidovudine).

BLACK BOX WARNING: GANCICLOVIR AND ITS PRODRUG VALGANCICLOVIR

Ganciclovir may cause anemia, granulocytopenia, and thrombocytopenia. In animal studies, ganciclovir was associated with teratogenic effects, carcinogenic effects, and inhibited sperm formation.

Reproductive Toxicity

Ganciclovir is teratogenic and embryotoxic in laboratory animals and probably in humans. Women should be advised to avoid pregnancy during therapy and for 90 days after ending treatment. At doses equivalent to those used therapeutically, ganciclovir inhibits spermatogenesis in mice; sterility is reversible with low doses and irreversible with high doses. Female infertility may also occur. Patients should be forewarned of these effects.

Other Adverse Effects

Incidental effects include nausea, fever, rash, anemia, liver dysfunction, and confusion and other central nervous system (CNS) symptoms.

Preparations, Dosage, and Administration

Intravenous

Ganciclovir [Cytovene] is available as a powder (500 mg) to be reconstituted for IV infusion. Solutions are alkaline and must be infused into a freely flowing vein to avoid local injury. For treatment of CMV retinitis, the initial dosage for adults with normal renal function is 5 mg/kg (infused over 1 hour) every 12 hours for 14 to 21 days. Two maintenance dosages can be used: (1) 5 mg/kg infused over 1 hour once every day of the week or (2) 6 mg/kg infused over 1 hour once a day, 5 days a week. Dosages must be reduced for patients with renal impairment. Because many patients with AIDS must continue maintenance therapy for life, they need a permanent IV access and equipment for home infusion. Adequate hydration must be maintained in all patients to ensure renal excretion of ganciclovir.

Oral

Ganciclovir is supplied in 250- and 500-mg tablets for maintenance therapy in patients with CMV retinitis. The usual dosage is 1000 mg 3 times daily with food.

Ocular Implant

The ganciclovir ocular implant [Vitrasert] is indicated for CMV retinitis in patients with AIDS. Surgical implantation, which takes about 1 hour, is performed under local anesthesia on an outpatient basis. Vision is usually blurred for 2 to 4 weeks after the procedure. The implant must be replaced every 5 to 8 months. Clinical trials indicate that CMV retinitis progresses more slowly in patients who receive intraocular ganciclovir compared with those on IV ganciclovir.

Ocular Gel

As discussed earlier (under "Topical Drugs for Ocular Herpes Infections"), ganciclovir is available in a 0.15% gel, marketed as Zirgan, for treating herpetic keratitis.

Valganciclovir

Basic and Clinical Pharmacology

Valganciclovir [Valcyte] is a prodrug version of ganciclovir [Cytovene] with greater oral bioavailability (60% vs. 9%). After absorption from the GI tract, valganciclovir is rapidly metabolized to ganciclovir, its active form—and eventually undergoes excretion as unchanged ganciclovir in the urine. Indications are CMV retinitis and prevention of CMV disease in high-risk organ transplant recipients. In patients with active CMV retinitis, oral valganciclovir is just as effective as intravenous ganciclovir—and much more convenient.

Adverse effects are the same as with ganciclovir. The principal concern is blood dyscrasias—granulocytopenia, anemia, and thrombocytopenia—secondary to bone marrow suppression. In addition, any of the following adverse effects typically occur in 20% to 40% of patients: diarrhea, nausea, vomiting, fever, and headache. Valganciclovir is presumed to pose the same risks for mutagenesis, aspermatogenesis, and carcinogenesis as ganciclovir.

Preparations, Dosage, and Administration

Valganciclovir [Valcyte] is available in (1) 450-mg tablets and (2) a powder that makes a 50-mg/mL oral solution when reconstituted with 91 mL of purified water. All doses should be taken with food to enhance bioavailability.

For treatment of CMV retinitis, the adult dosage is 900 mg twice daily for 21 days, followed by 900 mg once daily for maintenance. Dosage must be reduced for patients with renal impairment.

For prevention of CMV disease in transplant recipients, the adult dosage is 900 mg once daily, starting within 10 days of transplantation and continuing until 100 days posttransplantation (or 200 days after transplantation in kidney recipients).

Because valganciclovir has the potential for mutagenesis and carcinogenesis, the powder and tablets should be handled carefully. Tablets should be ingested intact, without crushing or chewing. Direct contact with the powder or broken tablets should be avoided. If contact does occur, the area should be washed with soap and water. When handling or disposing of the drug, healthcare workers should follow the same guidelines established for cytotoxic anticancer drugs.

Cidofovir

Cidofovir [Vistide] is an IV drug with just one indication: CMV retinitis in patients with AIDS who have failed on ganciclovir or foscarnet. Alternative drugs for this infection are foscarnet, which is given intravenously, and ganciclovir, which may be administered intravenously, orally, or by ocular insert. Compared with IV foscarnet or IV ganciclovir, cidofovir has the distinct advantage of needing fewer infusions: Whereas foscarnet and ganciclovir must be infused daily, cidofovir is infused just once a week or every other week. The major adverse effect of the drug is kidney damage.

BLACK BOX WARNING: CIDOFOVIR [VISTIDE]

Cidofovir has been associated with severe renal impairment. Dialysis has been required after only one or two doses.

Cidofovir neutropenia. In animal studies, cidofovir was associated with teratogenic effects, carcinogenic effects, and inhibited sperm formation.

Mechanism of Action

When inside cells, cidofovir is converted to cidofovir diphosphate, its active form. As the diphosphate, cidofovir causes selective inhibition of viral DNA polymerase and thereby inhibits viral DNA synthesis. Intracellular concentrations of cidofovir diphosphate are too low to inhibit human DNA polymerases; thus host cells are spared.

Antiviral Spectrum and Therapeutic Use

Cidofovir is active against herpesviruses, including CMV, HSV-1, HSV-2, and VZV. However, the drug is approved only for CMV retinitis in patients with AIDS. Whether cidofovir is active against CMV infections in other patients or at other sites (e.g., GI tract, lungs) is unknown. In clinical trials in patients with AIDS and established CMV retinitis, cidofovir significantly delayed progression of retinitis.

Pharmacokinetics

Cidofovir is administered by IV infusion and undergoes excretion by the kidneys. Probenecid competes with cidofovir for renal tubular secretion and thereby delays elimination. Cidofovir has a prolonged intracellular half-life (17–65 hours), and hence a long interval (2 weeks) can separate doses. In contrast, IV foscarnet and ganciclovir must be infused daily.

Adverse Effects

Nephrotoxicity

The principal adverse effect is dose-dependent nephrotoxicity, manifesting as decreased renal function and symptoms of a Fanconi-like syndrome (proteinuria, glucosuria, bicarbonate wasting). To reduce the risk for renal injury, all patients must receive probenecid and IV hydration therapy with each infusion. Also, serum creatinine and urine protein should be checked within 48 hours before each dose, and, if these values indicate kidney damage, cidofovir should be withheld or the dosage reduced. Cidofovir is contraindicated for patients taking other drugs that can injure the kidney and for patients with proteinuria (2+ or greater) or baseline serum creatinine greater than 1.5 mg/dL.

Other Adverse Effects

Neutropenia develops in about 20% of patients, so neutrophil counts should be monitored. Ocular disorders—iritis, uveitis, or ocular hypotony (low intraocular pressure)—can also occur. In animal studies, cidofovir was carcinogenic and teratogenic and caused hypospermia. Adverse effects are more likely in patients taking antiretroviral drugs (i.e., drugs for HIV).

Preparations, Dosage, and Administration

Cidofovir [Vistide] is supplied in solution (75 mg/mL) in 5-mL ampules. To reduce the risk for renal injury, cidofovir infusions must be accompanied by IV hydration therapy and oral (PO) probenecid.

Each cidofovir dose—for induction or maintenance—consists of 5 mg/kg by IV infusion over 1 hour. For induction, two doses are given 1 week apart. For maintenance, one dose is given every 2 weeks. The size of each dose must be reduced for patients with renal impairment. If impairment is severe, cidofovir should be withheld.

Oral probenecid must accompany each infusion. The dosage is 2 g given 3 hours before the infusion, 1 g given 1 hour after the infusion, and another 1 g given 8 hours after that. Ingesting food before each dose can decrease probenecid-induced nausea and vomiting. An antiemetic may also be used.

Hydration is accomplished by infusing 1 L of 0.9% saline solution over 1 to 2 hours immediately before infusing cidofovir. For patients who can tolerate it, 1 L more can be infused over 1 to 3 hours, beginning when the cidofovir infusion begins or as soon as it is over.

Foscarnet

Foscarnet is an IV drug active against all known herpesviruses, including CMV, HSV-1, HSV-2, and VZV. Compared with ganciclovir, foscarnet is more difficult to administer, less well tolerated, and much more expensive. The major adverse effect is renal injury.

Mechanism of Action

Foscarnet, an analog of pyrophosphate, inhibits viral DNA polymerases and reverse transcriptases and thereby inhibits synthesis of viral nucleic acids. At the concentrations achieved clinically, the drug does not inhibit host DNA replication. Unlike many other antiviral drugs, which must undergo conversion to an active form, foscarnet is active as administered.

Therapeutic Use

Foscarnet has two approved indications: (1) CMV retinitis in patients with AIDS and (2) acyclovir-resistant mucocutaneous HSV and VZV infection in the immunocompromised host. CMV retinitis resistant to ganciclovir may respond to foscarnet.

Pharmacokinetics

Foscarnet has low oral bioavailability and must be administered intravenously. The drug is poorly soluble in water and does not penetrate cells easily. As a result, it must be given in large doses with large volumes of fluid. Between 10% and 28% of each dose is deposited in bone; the remainder is excreted unchanged in the urine. Because foscarnet is eliminated by the kidneys, dosages must be reduced in patients with renal impairment. The plasma half-life is 3 to 5 hours.

Adverse Effects and Interactions

In general, foscarnet is less well tolerated than ganciclovir. However, unlike ganciclovir, foscarnet does not cause granulocytopenia or thrombocytopenia.

Nephrotoxicity

Renal injury, as evidenced by a rise in serum creatinine, is the most common dose-limiting toxicity. Most patients develop some degree of renal impairment. Renal injury occurs most often during the second week of therapy. The risk for nephrotoxicity is increased by concurrent use of other nephrotoxic drugs, including amphotericin B, aminoglycosides (e.g., gentamicin), and pentamidine. Prehydration with IV saline may reduce the risk for renal injury. Renal function (creatinine clearance) should be monitored closely, and the dosage should be reduced if renal impairment develops.

BLACK BOX WARNING: FOSCARNET [FOSCAVIR]

Renal impairment has occurred. Seizures have occurred in relation to alterations in electrolytes and mineral composition in plasma.

Electrolyte and Mineral Imbalances

Foscarnet frequently causes hypocalcemia, hypokalemia, hypomagnesemia, and hypophosphatemia or hyperphosphatemia. Ionized serum calcium may be reduced despite normal levels of total serum calcium. Patients should be informed about symptoms of low ionized calcium (e.g., paresthesias, numbness in the extremities, perioral tingling) and instructed to report these. Severe hypocalcemia can result in dysrhythmias, tetany, and seizures. Serum levels of calcium, magnesium, potassium, and phosphorus should be measured frequently. Special caution is required in patients with preexisting electrolyte, cardiac, or neurologic abnormalities. The risk for hypocalcemia is increased by concurrent use of pentamidine.

Other Adverse Effects

Common reactions (occurring in 25%–50% of patients) include fever, nausea, anemia, diarrhea, vomiting, and headache. In addition, foscarnet can cause fatigue, tremor, irritability, genital ulceration, abnormal liver function tests, neutropenia, and seizures.

Preparations, Dosage, and Administration

Foscarnet is supplied in solution (24 mg/mL) for IV infusion. An infusion pump is essential to reduce the risk for dosing errors. Infusions may be administered through a central venous line or a peripheral vein. When a central line is used, a concentrated (24 mg/mL) solution may be given. When a peripheral vein is used, the solution should be diluted to 12 mg/mL. For patients with normal kidney function, the initial dosage is 60 mg/kg (for CMV infection) or 40 mg/kg (for HSV infection) infused over 1 hour (or longer) every 8 hours for 2 to 3 weeks. The maintenance dosage (for CMV or HSV infection) is 90 to 120 mg/kg infused over 2 hours once daily. All dosages must be reduced for patients with renal impairment.

DRUGS FOR HEPATITIS

Viral hepatitis is the most common liver disorder, affecting millions of Americans. The disease can be caused by six different hepatitis viruses, labeled A, B, C, D, E, and G. All six can cause *acute* hepatitis, but only B, C, and D also cause *chronic* hepatitis. Acute hepatitis lasts for 6 months or less and is characterized by liver inflammation, jaundice, and elevation of serum alanine aminotransferase (ALT) activity. In most cases, acute hepatitis resolves spontaneously, so intervention is generally unnecessary. In contrast, chronic hepatitis can lead to cirrhosis, hepatocellular carcinoma, and life-threatening liver failure, and hence treatment should be considered.

Most cases (90%) of chronic hepatitis are caused by either hepatitis B virus (HBV) or hepatitis C virus (HCV). Accordingly, our discussion focuses on hepatitis B and hepatitis C. About 1.5% of Americans are infected with HBV or HCV, which is 5 times more than the number infected with HIV. Vaccines for hepatitis A and B are discussed in Chapter 53. Drugs for hepatitis B and C are discussed here.

Hepatitis C

The Centers for Disease Control and Prevention (CDC) estimate that about 3.9 million Americans have chronic hepatitis C. Transmission occurs primarily through exchange of blood, with injection drug use being the most common means. Transmission may also occur as the result of sex with an HCV-infected partner, although this occurs far less frequently. Pregnant women who are infected can transfer the virus to their offspring. Among people who acquire HCV, 75% to 85% develop active infection. However, most people with chronic hepatitis C have no symptoms, although they can transmit HCV to others. Chronic HCV infection undergoes slow progression and, in some people, eventually causes liver failure, cancer, and death. Chronic hepatitis C is the leading reason for liver transplantations and kills about 15,000 Americans each year—more than are killed by HIV.

It is important to note that not all hepatitis C viruses are the same. There are 6 genotypes of HCV, and more than 50 subtypes. In the United States 75% of HCV infections are caused by HCV genotype 1, which, unfortunately, is less responsive to treatment than other HCV genotypes.

The options for hepatitis C management increased dramatically between 2011 and 2016 as new categories of antiviral drugs were developed and added to the arsenal of agents targeting HCV infection. New guidelines were developed and then updated and then updated yet again. In 2015 the European Association for the Study of Liver (EASL) released their groundbreaking recommendations for treatment of HCV infection (available online at http://www.easl.eu/medias/cpg/HEPC-2015/Full-report.pdf). The first sentence following the introduction was astounding: "The primary goal of HCV therapy is to cure the infection." For the patients, their families, and the health care providers who had accepted the long-held belief that there is no cure, hope had truly arrived.

At the time of this writing, joint guidelines by the American Association for the Study of Liver Diseases (AASLD) and the Infectious Diseases Society of America (IDSA) have just been released (see http://www.hcvguidelines.org). These guidelines complement those of the EASL. Like the EASL guidelines, they focus on genotype-specific treatment that considers liver status (i.e., presence of cirrhosis) and treatment history (i.e., treatment-naïve and previous treatment failure) to optimize therapy. (See Fig. 78.1.)

It is quite likely that, by the time you read this, there will be new updates in treatment of HCV infection. The most current recommendations are maintained at the AASLD/IDSA website at http://www.hcvguidelines.org.

The ultimate goal of HCV therapy is cure of HCV infection. This is manifested by a sustained virologic response (SVR), which represents elimination of HCV RNA. The SVR occurs if there is no detectable HCV RNA at 12 weeks (SVR12) or 24 weeks (SVR24) after therapy.

Treatment of HCV infection is typically managed in specialty practices. Rather than give detailed information about drugs that nonspecialist providers may never prescribe or encounter, our goal will be to provide a summary of information that will benefit health care providers who see these patients for other conditions.

For years, dual therapy with *pegylated interferon alfa (peginterferon alfa) plus ribavirin* was the standard of care. The expanse in knowledge and understanding of the HCV

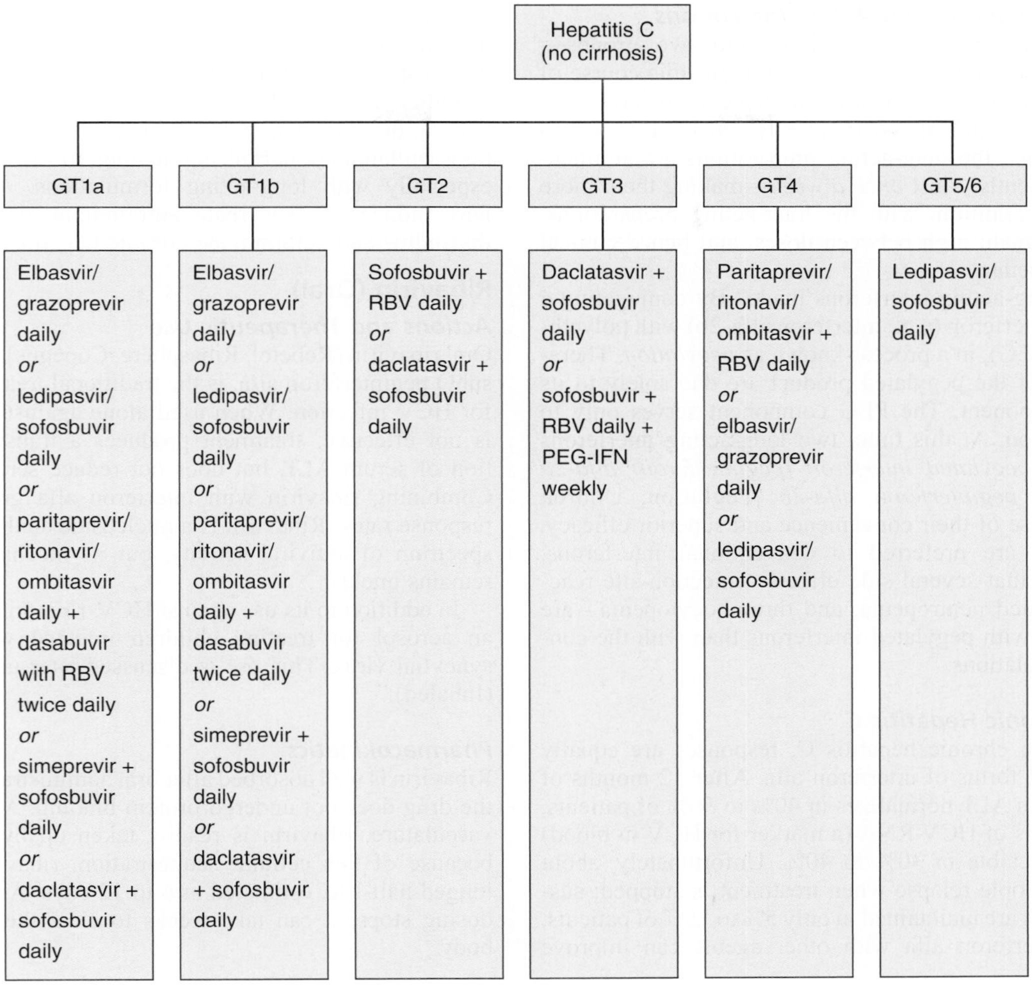

Figure 78.1 ▪ Drug selection for initial treatment of hepatitis C virus (HCV) infection by genotype in the patient without cirrhosis.
* Prescribed to be taken for 12 weeks. (Based on joint recommendations of the American Association for the Study of Liver Diseases [AASLD] and Infectious Diseases Society of America [IDSA]. Summary of recommendations for patients who are initiating therapy for HCV infection by HCV genotype. 2016. http://www.hcvguidelines.org/full-report/initial-treatment-box-summary-recommendations-patients-who-are-initiating-therapy-hcv.)

genome led to the development of direct-acting antiviral (DAA) drugs. These highly effective drugs have largely replaced the older regimen. Moreover, through the carefully orchestrated HCV treatment that these drugs allow, outcomes have greatly improved.

DAAs are drugs that target specific steps in the process of HCV replication. Because the mechanisms of action are directed toward the virus, the drugs avoid the sometimes dangerous adverse effects associated with interferon therapy. To decrease the development of viral resistance and to increase the likelihood of successful outcomes, all of these drugs are used in combination therapy. There are currently four categories of DAAs: NS3/4A protease inhibitors (PIs), NS5A inhibitors, NS5B nucleoside polymerase inhibitors (NPIs), and NS5B nonnucleoside polymerase inhibitors (NNPIs).

For our discussion, we will first examine interferon alfa and ribavirin. Thereafter, we will discuss the DAA drugs.

Interferon Alfa

Human interferons are naturally occurring compounds with complex antiviral, immunomodulatory, and antineoplastic actions. The interferon family has three major classes, designated alpha, beta, and gamma. All of the interferons used for hepatitis belong to the alpha class. In the following discussion, these compounds are referred to collectively as *interferon alfa.* None of these agents can be used orally, and hence administration is parenteral—almost always subQ. Commercial production is by recombinant DNA technology.

Mechanism of Action

Interferon alfa has multiple effects on the viral replication cycle. After binding to receptors on host cell membranes, the drug blocks viral entry into cells, synthesis of viral messenger RNA and viral proteins, and viral assembly and release.

Conventional Versus Long-Acting Interferons

The alfa interferons can be divided into two groups—conventional and long acting—based on their time course of action. The conventional preparations have short half-lives, so they must be administered frequently—at least *3 times a week.* In contrast, the long-acting preparations are administered less frequently—just *once a week*—making them more convenient. In addition, with the long-acting preparations, blood levels remain high between doses, and hence clinical responses are better.

How are long-acting interferons made? By conjugating a conventional interferon (e.g., interferon alfa-2b) with polyethylene glycol (PEG), in a process known as *pegylation.* Therapeutic effects of the pegylated product are due solely to its interferon component. The PEG component serves only to delay elimination. At this time, two long-acting interferons are available: *pegylated interferon (peginterferon) alfa-2a* [Pegasys] and *peginterferon alfa-2b* [PegIntron, Unitron PEG ♣]. Because of their convenience and superior efficacy, these products are preferred to conventional interferons. However, note that several side effects—injection-site reactions, dose-related neutropenia, and thrombocytopenia—are more common with pegylated interferons than with the conventional formulations.

Effects in Chronic Hepatitis C

In patients with chronic hepatitis C, responses are equally modest with all forms of interferon alfa. After 12 months of treatment, serum ALT normalizes in 40% to 50% of patients, and serum levels of HCV-RNA (a marker for HCV in blood) become undetectable in 30% to 40%. Unfortunately, about half of these people relapse when treatment is stopped; sustained responses are maintained in only 5% to 15% of patients. Combining interferon alfa with other agents can improve response rates.

Adverse Effects

All formulations of interferon alfa produce the same spectrum of adverse effects, some of which can be life threatening. The incidence is higher with the long-acting preparations.

BLACK BOX WARNING: INTERFERON ALFA [INTRON A, PEGASYS, OTHERS]

Alpha interferons may cause or worsen life-threatening disorders, including autoimmune, infectious, and ischemic conditions. Serious neuropsychiatric conditions have also occurred.

The most common side effect is a *flu-like syndrome* characterized by fever, fatigue, myalgia, headache, and chills. The incidence is about 50%. Fortunately, symptoms tend to diminish with continued therapy. Some symptoms (fever, headache, myalgia) can be reduced with acetaminophen.

Interferon alfa frequently causes *neuropsychiatric effects*—especially *depression.* Suicidal ideation and suicide have occurred. The risk for depression is increased by large doses and prolonged treatment. The mechanism underlying depression is unknown. In many patients, depression responds to antidepressant drugs (e.g., paroxetine). If depression persists, a reduction in dosage or cessation of treatment is indicated.

Prolonged or high-dose therapy can cause fatigue, thyroid dysfunction, heart damage, and bone marrow suppression, manifesting as neutropenia and thrombocytopenia.

Other adverse effects include alopecia and GI effects: nausea, diarrhea, anorexia, and vomiting. Injection-site reactions (inflammation, bruising, itching, irritation) are common, especially with long-acting formulations. Also, interferon may induce or exacerbate autoimmune diseases, such as thyroiditis and autoimmune chronic hepatitis.

Ribavirin (Oral)

Actions and Therapeutic Use

Oral ribavirin [Rebetol, Ribasphere, Copegus], combined with subQ peginterferon alfa, is the traditional treatment of choice for HCV infection. When used alone against HCV, ribavirin is not effective: treatment produces a transient normalization of serum ALT, but does not reduce serum HCV-RNA. Combining ribavirin with interferon alfa greatly improves response rates. Ribavirin is a nucleoside analog with a broad spectrum of antiviral activity, but its mechanism of action remains unclear.

In addition to its use against HCV, ribavirin is available as an aerosol for treating children infected with respiratory syncytial virus. This use is discussed later under "Ribavirin (Inhaled)."

Pharmacokinetics

Ribavirin is well absorbed after oral administration. In plasma, the drug does not undergo protein binding. After leaving the vasculature, ribavirin is readily taken up by cells. Perhaps because of this cellular sequestration, ribavirin has a prolonged half-life, estimated at 6 to 12 days. As a result, when dosing stops, it can take weeks to clear the drug from the body.

Adverse Effects

Although ribavirin and interferon alfa are generally well tolerated, both drugs can cause significant adverse effects. As noted earlier, interferon alfa frequently causes *flu-like symptoms* and occasionally causes *severe depression.* The principal concerns with ribavirin are *hemolytic anemia* and *fetal injury.*

BLACK BOX WARNING: RIBAVIRIN

Ribavirin may cause hemolytic anemia and cardiac decompensation secondary to hemolytic anemia.

Hemolytic Anemia. Hemolytic anemia, characterized by a hemoglobin (Hb) level below 10 g/dL, develops in 10% to 13% of patients receiving dual therapy with ribavirin/interferon alfa. Onset is typically 1 to 2 weeks after starting treatment. Hemolytic anemia can worsen heart disease and may lead to nonfatal or fatal myocardial infarction. Owing to the risk for anemia, ribavirin should be avoided in patients with significant heart disease and in those with hemoglobinopathies, including sickle cell anemia and thalassemia major. Because anemia can develop rapidly, Hb determinations should be made before treatment, 2 weeks and 4 weeks into treatment, and periodically thereafter.

Fetal Injury. Ribavirin is both embryolethal and teratogenic. In laboratory animals, the drug has caused fetal death as well as malformations of the skull, palate, eyes, jaw, limbs, GI tract, and skeleton—all at doses as low as one-twentieth of those used to treat humans. Accordingly, *ribavirin is classified in U.S. Food and Drug Administration (FDA) Pregnancy Risk Category X and therefore is contraindicated for use during pregnancy.* Pregnancy must be ruled out before starting ribavirin. Also, pregnancy testing must be done every month during treatment and for 6 months after treatment stops. To avoid pregnancy, couples should use *two* reliable forms of birth control during treatment and for 6 months after stopping. Furthermore, if ribavirin is used in conjunction with a *protease inhibitor,* hormonal contraceptives may not work, and hence two *barrier* contraceptives should be used, as discussed later under "Protease Inhibitors."

Among men being treated, ribavirin can be present in sperm. We don't know whether ribavirin-containing sperm will be teratogenic upon fertilizing an ovum. Until more is known, prudence dictates that couples avoid pregnancy if the male partner is receiving ribavirin.

Other Adverse Effects. In addition to flu-like symptoms, depression, anemia, and birth defects, ribavirin/interferon alfa can cause many other adverse effects. Among these are autoimmune disorders, infections, pancreatitis, neutropenia, and injury to the eyes and lungs.

Protease Inhibitors

In 2011, the FDA approved two PIs—boceprevir and telaprevir—for treatment of chronic hepatitis C, making them the first new drugs for hepatitis C in 20 years. These were the first of the direct-acting antivirals that would revolutionize hepatitis C treatment. (Telaprevir was subsequently withdrawn from the market in 2014 by the manufacturer who cited dwindling sales of this first-generation DAA among increased competition from new products, including DAAs with fewer interactions and fewer adverse effects.)

PIs inhibit viral protease, an enzyme required for HCV replication. There are currently three "second wave" PIs approved in the United States: grazoprevir, paritaprevir, and simeprevir. Of these, only simeprevir is available as a single agent (with indications to only use it in combination with other drugs). Grazoprevir and paritaprevir are available in combination with other drugs. There are at least four other protease inhibitors in clinical trials.

For our discussion, we will examine the first generation PI boceprevir and the second wave PI simeprevir. Properties of the combination drugs will be presented in Table 78.3.

Boceprevir

Therapeutic Use. Boceprevir [Victrelis] is first-generation protease inhibitor indicated for chronic hepatitis C caused by genotype 1 HCV in adults with compensated (stable) liver disease. Its approval included a caveat that it is only to be used in conjunction with peginterferon alfa and ribavirin. It must never be used alone.

Triple therapy with boceprevir/peginterferon alfa/ribavirin is much more effective than traditional dual therapy with

TABLE 78.3 ▪ Properties of Anti-HCV Direct-Acting Antiviral Drug Combinations

Drug Combinations	Elbasvir/Grazoprevir [Zepatier]	Ledipasvir/Sofosbuvir [Harvoni]	Ombitasvir/ Paritaprevir/Ritonavir* [Technivie]	Ombitasvir/Paritaprevir/ Ritonavir* With Dasabuvir [Viekira Pak]
Classification	NS5A inhibitor + PI	NS5A inhibitor + NPI	NS5A inhibitor + PI + CYP3A inhibitor	NS5A inhibitor + PI + CYP3A inhibitor + NNPI
HCV genotype treated	1a, 1b, & 4	1a, 1b, 4, 5, 6	4	1a, 1b
Adverse effects	Significant ALT elevations have occurred. The most common adverse reactions are headache, nausea, and fatigue. About 5% develop anemia	Common adverse effects are headache, fatigue, and weakness	ALT elevations up to 5 times normal have occurred. Patients with cirrhosis may develop hepatic failure. Common adverse reactions are nausea, fatigue, insomnia, weakness	Significant ALT elevations have occurred. Hepatic failure has occurred, primary in patients with advanced cirrhosis. Common adverse reactions include nausea, fatigue, insomnia, weakness, pruritus, and skin reactions
Contraindications	Moderate to severe hepatic impairment	Administration with amiodarone can cause dangerous symptomatic bradycardia	Moderate to severe hepatic impairment	Moderate to severe hepatic impairment
Monitoring	Check liver enzymes before initiating therapy, after 2 months, and if s/s of liver complications develop. Check baseline CBC and recheck if s/s anemia develop	Cardiac monitoring recommended if administration with amiodarone is necessary	Check liver enzymes before initiating therapy, within 4 weeks of therapy, and if s/s of liver complications develop	Check liver enzymes before initiating therapy, within 4 weeks of therapy, and if s/s of liver complications develop
Administration	Administer with or without food	Administer with or without food	Administer with meals (increases absorption)	Administer with meals (increases absorption)

*Ritonavir is an HIV protease inhibitor with no inherent anti-HCV activity. It boosts the HCV antiviral drugs through its CYP3A inhibitor activity. ALT, alanine aminotransferase; CBC, complete blood count; HCV, hepatitis C virus; NNPI, nonnucleoside polymerase inhibitor; NPI, nucleoside polymerase inhibitor; PI, protease inhibitor; s/s, signs or symptoms.

interferon alfa/ribavirin. In a trial known as SPRINT-2, in patients of African ancestry who received triple therapy, 47% obtained an SVR compared to only 23% of those receiving dual therapy. Results were even more dramatic among the other patients: an SVR was obtained in 68% of those receiving triple therapy compared with only 40% of those receiving dual therapy. The benefits of boceprevir triple therapy are especially dramatic in previously treated patients who failed to respond to dual therapy. For example, in the RESPOND-2 trial, which enrolled 403 patients who had failed with dual therapy, an SVR was obtained in 59% to 66% of those given boceprevir triple therapy compared with only 21% of those retreated with dual therapy.

Mechanism of Action. Boceprevir inhibits a protease specific to HCV (NS3/4A serine protease) and thereby arrests HCV replication. As discussed in Chapter 79, viral proteases act during the replication cycle to cleave large polypeptides into their smaller, functional forms. Hence, by inhibiting protease activity, boceprevir prevents replicating HCV from progressing to its mature, infectious state.

Pharmacokinetics. Boceprevir is administered orally, and plasma levels peak about 2 hours after dosing. Any food, be it low fat or high fat, increases absorption by about 65%. Boceprevir undergoes metabolism in the liver—partly by CYP3A4 (the 3A4 isoenzyme of cytochrome P450) and partly by other pathways—followed by excretion in the feces. The half-life is 3.4 hours.

Adverse Effects. Among patients receiving triple therapy with boceprevir/interferon alfa/ribavirin, the most common adverse effects, occurring in approximately 20% to 60% of patients, are fatigue, nausea, altered taste, chills, insomnia, vomiting, anemia, and neutropenia. Anemia and neutropenia are significantly more common than when peginterferon and ribavirin are used without boceprevir. To monitor for hematologic effects, complete blood counts should be obtained at baseline and then at weeks 4, 8, and 12 of treatment.

Effect in Pregnancy. Boceprevir *alone* is safe during pregnancy (FDA Pregnancy Risk Category B). However, the drug is not used alone. Rather, it is always combined with ribavirin (a teratogenic, embryolethal drug) plus peginterferon. The triple combination—ribavirin, peginterferon, and boceprevir—is very dangerous to the fetus and is classified in FDA Pregnancy Risk Category X. Accordingly, before women use the combination, pregnancy must be ruled out and two effective forms of contraception must be implemented. Furthermore, because the triple combination can render hormonal contraceptives ineffective, two nonhormonal contraceptives should be employed. Options include a copper-T intrauterine device, a diaphragm with spermicidal jelly, a cervical cap with spermicidal jelly, a male condom with spermicidal jelly, and a female condom with spermicidal jelly (but not a male condom combined with a female condom).

Not only is the drug combination dangerous for women should they become pregnant while using it, it is also dangerous for a pregnant woman whose male partner is using it. Accordingly, the combination is contraindicated for any man whose female partner is pregnant.

Drug Interactions. Boceprevir is subject to *many* drug interactions. Why? First, boceprevir is a substrate for CYP3A4. Therefore drugs that induce CYP3A4 isoenzyme activity will lower boceprevir levels, and drugs that inhibit CYP3A4 isoenzymes will increase boceprevir levels. Further, boceprevir is also an inhibitor of CYP3A4 isoenzymes; therefore boceprevir can increase levels of other drugs that are CYP3A4 substrates. Second, boceprevir inhibits P-glycoprotein, the transporter that pumps drugs out of cells in the intestine, liver, kidney, and other sites (see Chapter 4). By doing so, boceprevir can alter levels of drugs that are P-glycoprotein substrates. To list all the possible interactions would not be feasible, and it would be impossible to expect you to remember those. It is wise to always use a drug interaction checker (software application or online) before administering unfamiliar drugs, especially those, like this one, that have so many possible interactions.

Simeprevir

Action and Use. Simeprevir [Olysio, Galexos ♣] is a second-wave protease inhibitor and DAA against HVC. Simeprevir is approved for treatment of chronic hepatitis C for HCV genotype 1 or 4. It must always be used in combination with other anti-HCV drugs.

Adverse Effects. FDA labeling warns of the potential for hepatic injury, significant photosensitivity, and severe rashes. The most common adverse effects experienced are headache, nausea, and fatigue.

Pharmacokinetics. Taking simeprevir with food will enhance its absorption to 62% bioavailability. Metabolism is primarily by CYP3A4 isoenzymes. Half-life is 10 to 13 hours in healthy individuals, but in HCV-infected patients, the half-life may be as long as 41 hours. Excretion is primarily in the feces (91%), with less than 1% eliminated in the urine.

Contraindications. There are no absolute contraindications for simeprevir. Although not contraindicated, simeprevir is not recommended for patients with severe liver impairment and should not be administered with peginterferon and ribavirin if the patient has decompensated cirrhosis. Also, simeprevir contains a component of sulfonamide, so caution is advised for patients who have had previous reactions to sulfonamides.

Drug Interactions. Simeprevir exerts mild inhibition of CYP1A2 isoenzyme activity, but it is unlikely to have a significant effect. On the other hand, it is a substrate of CYP3A4 isoenzymes; therefore drugs that are CYP3A4 inducers may lower simeprevir levels, whereas CYP3A4 inhibitors may raise levels. Significant adverse effects may occur when given with amiodarone (serious symptomatic bradycardia). It may elevate levels of HMG CoA reductase inhibitors, so lower doses of statin drugs may be necessary. It may also raise levels of sedative anxiolytics such as midazolam and triazolam, which both have a narrow therapeutic index. Labeling warns against coadministration of a number of drugs. As with any drug, it is important to consult drug interaction software before prescribing a new drug to patients taking anti-HCV therapy.

Monitoring. Serum HCV-RNA should be obtained before initiating treatment; at 4, 12, and 24 weeks; and during follow-up after the end of treatment. Because simeprevir can cause liver injury, liver enzymes, bilirubin, and uric acid should be checked before initiating therapy and repeated as indicated. Simeprevir is in FDA Pregnancy Risk Category C; monthly pregnancy tests are indicated if pregnancy status is a concern for ongoing therapy.

NS5A Inhibitors

NS5A inhibitors target a nonstructural protein, NS5A, that is necessary for HCV RNA replication and assembly. In so doing, these drugs prevent replication and construction of HCV. Unfortunately, resistance can build easily to these agents. Hence, as with other HCV regimens, they should never be given alone.

There are currently four NS5A inhibitors approved for use in the United States. Daclatasvir is approved as a single agent to be added to other anti-HCV regimens. Elbasvir, ledipasvir, and ombitasvir are combined in fixed dosages with other antiviral drugs. As with our previous classification, those in combined combinations will be summarized in tables.

Daclatasvir

Action and Use. Daclatasvir [Daklinza] is an NS5A inhibitor antiviral drug approved for treatment of chronic hepatitis C infection with HCV genotype 1 or 3. It should be used with sofosbuvir, with or without the addition of ribavirin.

Adverse Effects. The most common adverse reactions are headache and fatigue (in combination with sofosbuvir). With the addition of ribavirin, nausea and anemia also occurred in at least 10% of those taking the triple therapy.

Pharmacokinetics. Absorption is essentially unaffected by food intake. Metabolism occurs through CYP3A isoenzymes with CYP3A4 predominating. About 88% of the drug is eliminated in the feces and 7% in the urine.

Contraindications. There are no absolute contraindications. However, product labeling includes drug interactions with strong CYP3A inducers and amiodarone here (see "Drug Interactions" next).

Drug Interactions. Because daclatasvir is a CYP3A substrate, strong CYP3A inducers can significantly lower daclatasvir levels. Examples of strong inducers include the antiepileptic drugs carbamazepine and phenytoin and the herbal supplement St. John's wort. Similarly, CYP3A inhibitors can raise daclatasvir levels. Both situations may require dosage adjustments of daclatasvir. Although not a contraindication per se, there is a strong warning and recommendation against adding the daclatasvir/sofosbuvir combination to amiodarone because dangerous symptomatic bradycardia may occur. In addition to the interactions mentioned as contraindications, a large number of others can occur. Most notably, substances that induce or inhibit CYP3A isoenzymes may affect daclatasvir levels. Others, when given together, include elevations of HMG CoA reductase inhibitors (statins) and elevations of digoxin. Use of drug interaction software is needed to screen potential interactions when prescribing new drugs to patients taking daclatasvir.

Monitoring. Monitoring of HCV RNA should be undertaken to assess outcomes. Cardiac monitoring should be undertaken if it becomes necessary to administer amiodarone while the patient is taking daclatasvir. If digoxin is administered, because it has a narrow therapeutic index, it is important to monitor patient status and serum digoxin levels.

NS5B Inhibitors

NS5B is a nonstructural HCV protein that, like NS5A, is vital for HCV RNA replication. There are two classes of drugs that target this protein: NS5B NPIs and NS5B NNPIs. Beyond structural composition, they differ primarily in respect to properties of resistance and genotype. NPIs have a low likelihood of development of viral resistance, whereas the likelihood of viral resistance is high for NNPIs. In contrast, NPIs have high efficacy for all genotypes, whereas the NNPIs have lower efficacy and are effective for fewer genotypes.

The only NPI currently approved is sofosbuvir [Sovaldi]. The only NNPI is dasabuvir, which is only available in a fixed-dose combination with ombitasvir, paritaprevir, and ritonavir. As before, we will examine sofosbuvir as an individual drug, whereas dasabuvir will be examined in the combined form. It is important to note that ritonavir has an associated black box warning.

BLACK BOX WARNING: RITONAVIR [NORVIR]

Life-threatening adverse effects can occur when ritonavir is administered with sedative hypnotics, antidysrhythmics, and ergot preparations.

Sofosbuvir

Action and Use. Sofosbuvir [Sovaldi] is an NS5B NPI. It is activated by metabolism, after which it incorporates into the HCV RNA through NS5B polymerase. It is approved as a component of antiviral treatment for chronic hepatitis C of HCV genotype 1, 2, 3, or 4.

Adverse Effects. Headaches and fatigue affect about 20% of patients when given in combination with ribavirin. When interferon alfa is added to the combination, nausea, anemia, and insomnia may also occur.

Pharmacokinetics. Food does not significantly alter absorption. Sofosbuvir is a prodrug that is metabolized to its active form through intracellular processes. Elimination is primarily through urine (80%), followed by feces and the respiratory system.

Contraindications. There are no contraindications for sofosbuvir. Those mentioned in product labeling apply only to drugs with which sofosbuvir may be combined.

Drug Interactions. If sofosbuvir is administered with amiodarone, dangerous symptomatic bradycardia may occur. Sofosbuvir is a substrate of P-glycoprotein (P-gp), a drug transporter with a role in determining the amount of drug that is absorbed and distributed. If administered with P-gp inducers such as St. John's wort, the level of sofosbuvir may decrease.

Monitoring. HCV RNA should be monitored to determine outcomes. Cardiac monitoring is needed if amiodarone must be administered to the patient taking sofosbuvir.

Hepatitis B

In the United States about 1.4 million people have chronic hepatitis B. Transmission is primarily through exchange of blood or semen. Between 45% and 60% of exposed adults develop acute hepatitis. Of these, about 11,000 require hospitalization for deep fatigue, muscle pain, and jaundice. In adults, acute infection usually leads to viral clearance by the immune system. As a result, only 3% to 5% of infected adults develop chronic infection. However, when chronic infection does develop, it can lead to cirrhosis, hepatic failure, hepatocellular carcinoma, and death. The best strategy against HBV is prevention: all children should receive HBV vaccine before entering school (see Chapter 53).

Seven drugs are used for chronic HBV. Two are alfa interferons—*interferon alfa-2b* [Intron A] and *peginterferon alfa-2a* [Pegasys]—and five are nucleoside analogs: *lamivudine* [Epivir HBV, Heptovir ♣], *adefovir* [Hepsera], *entecavir* [Baraclude], *telbivudine* [Tyzeka, Sebivo ♣], and *tenofovir* [Viread]. The alfa interferons are administered subcutaneously; the nucleoside analogs are administered orally. The interferons are more effective than the nucleoside analogs but are also more expensive and less well tolerated. Development of resistance is common with lamivudine and telbivudine and relatively rare with the other five drugs. Four agents—lamivudine, adefovir, entecavir, and tenofovir—are also active against HIV and hence may promote emergence of resistant HIV in people coinfected with that virus.

With all seven drugs—and especially the nucleoside analogs—the rate of relapse after cessation of treatment is high. As a result, treatment is usually prolonged, thereby amplifying concerns about adverse effects and drug cost. To decrease unnecessary drug exposure and expense, current guidelines recommend treatment only for patients at highest risk, indicated by elevated aminotransferase levels, or with histologic evidence of moderate or severe hepatic inflammation or advanced fibrosis. We do not yet know whether treatment should continue lifelong or whether clinical benefit is sustained if treatment is stopped after several years. Given that relapse is common, patients should be followed closely if these drugs *are* withdrawn. Comparisons between the seven drugs are shown in Table 78.4.

Interferon Alfa

Only two forms of interferon alfa—interferon alfa-2b [Intron A] and peginterferon alfa-2a [Pegasys]—are approved for chronic hepatitis B. Both preparations are administered subcutaneously. In clinical trials, treatment for 4 months reduced serum ALT and improved liver histology in about 40% of recipients. Remissions have been prolonged in some patients, and resistance has not been reported. Unfortunately, although alfa interferons are effective, they are also expensive, and adverse effects—flu-like syndrome, depression, fatigue, and leukopenia—are common. The basic pharmacology of interferon alfa and its use in hepatitis C were discussed previously.

Nucleoside Analogs

Lamivudine

Lamivudine [Epivir HBV, Heptovir ♣] is a nucleoside analog approved for infections caused by HBV or HIV. The drug was originally developed for HIV infection and was later approved for HBV. Formulations and dosages for treating HIV and HBV infections differ, so they must not be considered interchangeable. Discussion here is limited to treatment of HBV.

Lamivudine suppresses HBV replication by inhibiting viral DNA synthesis. The process begins with intracellular conversion of lamivudine to lamivudine triphosphate, the drug's active form. As the triphosphate, lamivudine undergoes incorporation into the growing DNA chain and thereby causes premature chain termination.

Lamivudine offers at least some benefit to most patients. In one trial, 52 weeks of daily lamivudine normalized serum ALT in 72% of patients and reduced liver inflammation and fibrosis in 56%. Unfortunately, the rate of relapse is high when treatment stops. Also, emergence of resistance is a concern: resistant isolates appear in 24% of patients after 1 year of continuous treatment, 42% after 2 years, 53% after 3 years, and 70% after 4 years.

At the dosage employed to treat hepatitis B, side effects are minimal. In clinical trials, the incidence of most side effects was no greater than with placebo. *Lactic acidosis, pancreatitis,* and *severe hepatomegaly* are rare but dangerous complications. If one of these conditions develops, lamivudine should be discontinued.

For treatment of HBV, lamivudine [Epivir HBV, Heptovir ♣] is formulated in 100-mg tablets and a 5-mg/mL oral solution. The adult dosage is 100 mg once daily (compared with 150 mg twice daily for HIV). The pediatric dosage is 3 mg/kg once daily (compared with 4 mg/kg twice daily for HIV). Because lamivudine is eliminated primarily by renal excretion, dosage must be reduced in patients with renal impairment.

TABLE 78.4 ▪ Drugs for Chronic Hepatitis B

Drug	Route	Relapse Rate*	Adverse Effects	Resistance Rate	Active Against HIV
INTERFERON ALFA PREPARATIONS					
Interferon alfa-2b [Intron A]	SubQ	Moderate	Flu-like symptoms, fatigue, neutropenia, depression	Zero	No
Peginterferon alfa-2a [Pegasys]	SubQ	Moderate	Same as interferon alfa-2b	Zero	No
NUCLEOSIDE ANALOGS					
Lamivudine [Epivir HBV, Heptovir ♣]	PO	High	Well tolerated; lactic acidosis and hepatomegaly are possible	15%–30% in yr 1; 70% by yr 5	Yes
Adefovir [Hepsera]	PO	High	Nephrotoxic at high doses; lactic acidosis and hepatomegaly are possible	Zero in yr 1; 29% by yr 5	Yes
Entecavir [Baraclude]	PO	High	Well tolerated; lactic acidosis and hepatomegaly are possible	Zero in yr 1; 1% or less by yr 3	Yes
Tenofovir [Viread]	PO	High	Weakness, headache, gastrointestinal reactions; lactic acidosis and hepatomegaly are possible	—	Yes
Telbivudine [Tyzeka, Sebivo ♣]	PO	Moderate	Myopathy, lactic acidosis, hepatomegaly are possible	6%–12% in yr 1; 9%–22% by yr 2	No

*After discontinuation of treatment.

Adefovir

Therapeutic Use. Adefovir [Hepsera] is indicated for oral therapy of chronic hepatitis B. The drug was originally developed to fight HIV infection but was not approved owing to a high incidence of nephrotoxicity at the doses required. The doses used for hepatitis B are much lower, and thus the risk for renal injury is lower too.

Mechanism of Action. Adefovir is a nucleoside analog with a mechanism similar to that of acyclovir. Both drugs inhibit viral DNA synthesis, and both must be converted to their active form within the body. Activation of adefovir is mediated by cellular kinases—enzymes that convert the drug into adefovir diphosphate, a compound with two actions: (1) it directly inhibits viral DNA polymerase (by competing with deoxyadenosine triphosphate, a natural substrate for the enzyme) and (2) it undergoes incorporation into the growing strand of viral DNA, and thereby causes premature strand termination. Host cells are spared because adefovir diphosphate is a poor inhibitor of human DNA polymerase.

Pharmacokinetics. Bioavailability is about 60% after oral administration, both in the presence and absence of food. Plasma levels peak about 2 hours after dosing. Elimination is renal, by a combination of glomerular filtration and active tubular secretion. In patients with normal kidney function, the half-life is 7.5 hours. In patients with renal impairment, the half-life is significantly increased.

Adverse Effects. Nephrotoxicity is the principal concern. Increased serum creatinine, a sign of kidney damage, was seen in 4% of patients who received 48 weeks of therapy and in 9% of patients who received 96 weeks of therapy. To reduce risk, kidney function should be assessed at baseline and periodically thereafter, paying special attention to patients at high risk (i.e., patients with preexisting renal impairment and those taking nephrotoxic drugs [e.g., cyclosporine, tacrolimus, aminoglycosides, vancomycin, aspirin, and other nonsteroidal antiinflammatory drugs]).

When adefovir is discontinued, patients may experience acute exacerbation of hepatitis B. In clinical trials, serum ALT levels rose dramatically in 25% of patients when treatment was stopped. Liver function should be assessed periodically after adefovir withdrawal.

Drug Interactions. Drugs that are eliminated by active tubular secretion can compete with adefovir for renal excretion. As a result, if one of these agents were combined with adefovir, excretion of adefovir, the other drug, or both could be decreased, causing their plasma levels to rise.

Precautions. Because adefovir is related to the nucleoside analogs used against HIV, there is a concern that, if the patient were infected with HIV, giving adefovir in the low doses employed against HBV could allow emergence of HIV viruses resistant to nucleoside analogs. Accordingly, HIV infection should be ruled out before adefovir is used.

The nucleoside analogs used to treat HIV infection can cause lactic acidosis and severe hepatomegaly. There is concern that adefovir can cause these effects, too. If the patient develops clinical or laboratory findings that suggest lactic acidosis or pronounced hepatotoxicity, adefovir should be withdrawn.

Preparations, Dosage, and Administration. Adefovir [Hepsera] is supplied in 10-mg tablets. For patients with good kidney function, the dosage is 10 mg once a day, taken with or without food. For patients with impaired kidney function, as indicated by reduced creatinine clearance (CrCl), the dosing interval should be increased.

Entecavir

Therapeutic Use. Entecavir [Baraclude] is indicated for oral therapy of chronic hepatitis B. Candidates for treatment should have evidence of active viral replication along with persistently elevated serum aminotransferases or histologic evidence of active disease. In clinical trials, entecavir was more effective than lamivudine. In patients with lamivudine-resistant HBV, responses to entecavir were somewhat reduced, but were still better than responses to lamivudine. Recent evidence indicates that, with long-term use (3 years), entecavir can reverse fibrosis and cirrhosis.

Mechanism of Action. Entecavir is a nucleoside analog that undergoes conversion to entecavir triphosphate (its active form) within the body. As entecavir triphosphate, the drug inhibits HBV DNA polymerase and thereby prevents viral replication. Entecavir triphosphate is a weak inhibitor of human DNA polymerases, both nuclear and mitochondrial, and hence host cells are spared. Like lamivudine and adefovir, entecavir may impede HIV replication, so it may promote emergence of resistant HIV.

Pharmacokinetics. Entecavir is available in tablets and solution for oral dosing. Bioavailability with both formulations is the same. Plasma levels peak 0.5 to 1.5 hours after dosing. Entecavir undergoes extensive distribution to body tissues, with little binding to plasma proteins. Metabolism is minimal. Entecavir is neither a substrate for, inhibitor of, nor inducer of cytochrome P450 enzymes. Excretion is through the urine, primarily as unchanged drug. The half-life is about 5.5 days.

Adverse Effects and Precautions. Entecavir is very well tolerated. The most common adverse effects are dizziness, headache, fatigue, and nausea—and even these occur in less than 5% of patients.

Patients treated with other nucleoside analogs have developed lactic acidosis and severe hepatomegaly, and hence there is concern that entecavir may cause these effects, too. If the patient develops clinical or laboratory findings that suggest lactic acidosis or pronounced hepatotoxicity, entecavir should be withdrawn.

Acute severe exacerbations of hepatitis B have developed after discontinuation of entecavir and other drugs for hepatitis B. Accordingly, if entecavir is discontinued, liver function should be monitored closely for several months.

Preparations, Dosage, and Administration. Entecavir [Baraclude] is available in tablets (0.5 and 1 mg) and an oral solution (0.05 mg/mL). Dosing is done once a day, either 2 hours before eating or 2 hours after. Dosage depends on renal function (as indicated by CrCl) and on the infection's sensitivity to lamivudine. Typical doses are 0.5 mg once daily for patients who are nucleoside treatment naïve; 1 mg once daily for patients with viremia that is lamivudine refractory or lamivudine resistant; and 1 mg once daily for those with decompensated liver disease.

Telbivudine

Therapeutic Use. Telbivudine [Tyzeka, Sebivo 🍁] is a nucleoside analog indicated for chronic HBV infection in adults and adolescents age 16 years or older. Patients must have evidence of active HBV replication, plus either persistent elevations in serum ALT or aspartate aminotransferase (AST) or histologic evidence of active liver disease. In nucleoside-naïve patients, telbivudine is at least as effective as lamivudine (as indicated by suppression of HBV DNA and either normalization of ALT or loss of serum HBeAg, a hepatitis B antigen). As with lamivudine, resistance can be significant: after 2 years of treatment with telbivudine, resistance develops in 9% to 22% of patients. Patients resistant to telbivudine show cross-resistance to lamivudine. In contrast to lamivudine, entecavir, and adefovir, telbivudine is not active against HIV.

Mechanism of Action. Telbivudine is a thymidine nucleoside analog that undergoes intracellular conversion to its active form: telbivudine triphosphate. As the triphosphate, it inhibits HBV replication in two ways. First, it directly inhibits HBV DNA polymerase (by competing with the natural substrate, thymidine triphosphate). Second, it undergoes incorporation into the growing viral DNA chain and thereby causes chain termination.

Adverse Effects. The most common adverse effects are fever, fatigue/malaise, arthralgia, myalgia, cough, headache, and GI symptoms (e.g., abdominal pain, nausea, vomiting, diarrhea, dyspepsia). Some patients have developed symptomatic myopathy, characterized by persistent muscle pain, tenderness, or weakness. Lactic acidosis and severe hepatomegaly have occurred with other nucleoside analogs but have not been reported with telbivudine. As with other drugs for hepatitis B, severe exacerbations can occur when treatment is discontinued.

Drug Interactions. No significant interactions have been reported. However, because telbivudine is eliminated primarily by renal excretion, drugs that impair renal function may raise its level. Also, other drugs that cause muscle injury may increase risk in patients taking telbivudine. Telbivudine is neither a substrate for nor inhibitor of CYP isoenzymes and hence will not be affected by drugs that inhibit or induce CYP isoenzymes, nor will it affect drugs that are metabolized by these isoenzymes.

Preparations, Dosage, and Administration. Telbivudine [Tyzeka, Sebivo 🍁] is supplied in 600-mg tablets. The usual dosage for adults and children is 600 mg once a day, taken with or without food. For patients with renal impairment, as indicated by reduced CrCl, the dosing interval should be increased. For patients with hepatic impairment, no dosage adjustment is required.

Tenofovir

Like lamivudine and adefovir, tenofovir [Viread] was originally approved for HIV infection, and then later approved for HBV in adults. When compared directly with adefovir in patients with HBV, tenofovir was considerably more effective. However, as with other nucleoside analogs, discontinuation of treatment is followed by exacerbation of hepatitis. Adverse effects include weakness, headache, lactic acidosis with hepatomegaly, and GI reactions: diarrhea, vomiting, and flatulence. Like some other nucleoside analogs, tenofovir can impede HIV replication and hence may promote emergence of resistant HIV. Tenofovir is supplied in 150-, 200-, 250-, and 300-mg tablets and in a 40-mg/g powder for oral dosing. The recommended dosage for HBV is 300 mg once daily, the same dosage we use for HIV. Dosage should be reduced for patients with renal impairment.

DRUGS FOR INFLUENZA

Influenza is a serious respiratory tract infection that constitutes a major cause of morbidity and mortality worldwide. During the 1918 to 1919 global pandemic, more than 500,000 people died in the United States and up to 50 million people died worldwide. Complications of influenza (e.g., bronchitis, pneumonia) cause up to 300,000 American hospitalizations a year. Annual deaths vary widely, depending on the strain of flu in circulation. For example, between 1976 and 2007, annual deaths ranged from a low of 3300 to a high of 49,000. The cost of influenza is huge: direct and indirect expenses total between $3 billion and $5 billion annually.

Influenza is caused by influenza viruses, of which there are two major types: *influenza A* and *influenza B.* Type A influenza viruses cause far more infections than type B influenza viruses (about 96% vs. 4%). The influenza A viruses are further subclassified on the basis of two types of surface antigens: hemagglutinin (H) and neuraminidase (N). The predominant subgroups of seasonal influenza A viruses in circulation today are known as H1N1 and H3N2, because of the specific types of hemagglutinin and neuraminidase that they carry. Keep in mind, however, that viral strains undergo constant evolution. As a result, the strains of H1N1 and H3N2 in circulation this year are likely to differ from the strains of H1N1 and H3N2 in circulation next year.

Influenza is a highly contagious infection spread by aerosolized droplets produced by coughing or sneezing. The virus enters the body through mucous membranes of the nose, mouth, or eyes. Viral replication takes place in the respiratory tract. Symptoms begin 2 to 4 days after exposure and last 5 to 6 days. Influenza is characterized by fever, cough, chills, sore throat, headache, and myalgia (muscle pain). For typical patients, infection results in 5 to 6 days of restricted activity, 3 to 4 days of bed disability, and 3 days of absence from work or school. In the United States the influenza "season" begins in November and extends through March or April.

Influenza is managed by vaccination and with drugs. Vaccination is the primary management strategy; drug therapy is secondary. For very current information on influenza vaccines and drugs, see www.cdc.gov/flu, a comprehensive website maintained by the CDC.

Influenza Vaccines

Annual vaccination is the best protection against influenza. Because influenza viruses are constantly evolving, influenza vaccines must continuously change too. Each year, manufacturers produce a new vaccine directed against the three (trivalent) or four (quadrivalent) strains of influenza virus deemed most likely to cause disease during the upcoming flu season. Identification of the strains is done jointly by the CDC, FDA, and World Health Organization.

Types of Influenza Vaccines

Two basic kinds of flu vaccine are available: (1) *inactivated influenza vaccine* and (2) *live, attenuated influenza vaccine,* also known as LAIV. The inactivated vaccine is administered by *IM or intradermal injection.* The live, attenuated vaccine is administered by *intranasal spray.* Both kinds of vaccine are directed against the same three influenza strains, and both are reformulated annually.

At this time, there are nine influenza vaccines on the market (Table 78.5). The vaccines differ regarding the age groups for which they are approved. This is discussed later.

TABLE 78.5 ■ Influenza Vaccines

Vaccine	Route	Formulation	Mercury Content* (Mcg/0.5-mL Dose)	Ovalbumin Content (Mcg/0.5-mL Dose)	Approved Age Group
INACTIVATED INFLUENZA VACCINES					
Afluria	IM	0.5-mL single-dose syringe	None	1 or less	6 mo and older†
		5-mL multidose vial	25	1 or less	6 mo and older†
Flucelvax	IM	0.5-mL single-dose syringe	None	—‡	18 yr and older
Fluarix	IM	0.5-mL single-dose syringe	None	0.05 or less	3 yr and older
FluLaval	IM	5-mL multidose vial	25	1 or less	18 yr and older
Fluvirin	IM	0.5-mL single-dose syringe	1 or less	1 or less	4 yr and older
		5-mL multidose vial	25	1 or less	4 yr and older
Fluzone	IM	0.25-mL single-dose syringe	None	—‡	6–35 months
		0.5-mL single-dose syringe	None	—‡	3 yr and older
		0.5-mL single-dose vial	None	—‡	3 yr and older
		5-mL multidose vial	24	—‡	3 yr and older
Fluzone High-Dose	IM	0.5-mL single-dose syringe	None	—‡	65 yr and older
Fluzone Intradermal	ID	0.1-mL single-dose syringe	None	—‡	18–64 yr
LIVE, ATTENUATED INFLUENZA VACCINE					
FluMist	Nasal	0.2-mL single-dose sprayer	None	—§	2–49 yr

ID, intradermal; IM, intramuscular.

*Mercury, in the form of thimerosal, is used as a preservative in some vaccines.

†Although Afluria is approved for children as young as 6 months, ACIP recommends avoiding Afluria in children younger than 9 years, owing to a possible risk for fever and febrile seizures in younger children.

‡Information not included in the package insert.

§Insufficient data available to use FluMist in egg-allergic persons.

Efficacy

Protection begins 1 to 2 weeks after vaccination and generally lasts 6 months or longer. However, among older vaccine recipients, protection may be lost in 4 months or even less. Efficacy of vaccination depends not only on the age and health status of the vaccinee but also on how well the vaccine matches the strains of influenza virus in circulation that year. Efficacy of the inactivated vaccine and the LAIV had been considered about equal until retrospective studies determined that the effectiveness of the LAIV vaccine, which is administered by nasal spray, was lower during the 2013–2014 and 2014–2015 flu seasons. For this reason, the CDC recommended that LAIV vaccine not be administered for the 2016–2017 influenza season. Whether it will continue to be recommended in the future remains to be seen.

Because the influenza virus evolves rapidly, influenza vaccines are reformulated annually. Accordingly, to maintain protection, revaccination is required each year. Furthermore, because antibody titers can decline fairly quickly, annual revaccination is recommended even if the formulation does *not* change, as sometimes occurs.

Adverse Effects

Adverse effects differ for the inactivated vaccine versus the LAIV. However, with both vaccines, significant adverse effects are rare.

Inactivated Influenza Vaccine

Adverse effects are uncommon, except for possible soreness at the site of IM or intradermal injection. People who have not been vaccinated previously may experience fever, myalgia, and malaise lasting 1 or 2 days.

Influenza vaccination may carry a very small risk for *Guillain-Barré syndrome* (GBS), a severe, paralytic illness. In 1976 swine flu vaccine was associated with GBS. However, there has been no clear link between GBS and influenza vaccines used since then. If there *is* a risk, it is very small, estimated at 1 to 2 cases per million vaccine recipients—much smaller than the risk posed by severe influenza.

Live, Attenuated Influenza Vaccine

LAIV has been given to millions of people since it was first approved in 2003, and reports of serious adverse events have been relatively rare. The most common side effects for all ages are nasal congestion with rhinorrhea, lethargy, headache, sore throat, and decreased appetite. There have been reports of rare neurological events (most commonly seizures and GBS) and respiratory events (most commonly pneumonia and reactive airway disease).

Precautions and Contraindications

People with acute febrile illness should defer vaccination until symptoms abate. Minor illnesses (e.g., common cold), with or without fever, do not preclude vaccination.

Special considerations are indicated for persons with hypersensitivity to eggs. Why? Because the vaccines are produced from viruses grown in eggs and hence may contain trace amounts of egg proteins. According to 2014 recommendations from the CDC, patients who have egg allergies manifested by hives may take the influenza vaccine; however, those who have had more serious reactions (e.g., angioedema, respiratory distress) or those who have required emergency medical intervention should be referred to an allergist for risk assessment before receiving vaccination. In any case, emergency equipment should be available whenever vaccinations are given.

Who Should Be Vaccinated?

The Advisory Committee on Immunization Practices (ACIP) now recommends annual vaccination for *all people 6 months and older.* Although an annual flu shot is recommended for everyone, an annual shot is especially important for persons at high risk for flu complications and for those who live with or care for persons at high risk. Persons at high risk include the following:

- Children younger than 5 years, and especially children younger than 2 years
- Children age 18 years or younger receiving long-term aspirin therapy
- Pregnant women
- People 65 years and older
- People who are morbidly obese
- People who live in nursing homes and other long-term care facilities
- American Indians/Alaskan Natives
- People who are immunosuppressed (e.g., owing to HIV infection or use of immunosuppressant drugs)
- People with certain chronic medical conditions, including spinal cord injury; asthma; anemia; diabetes; heart, kidney, or lung disease; and neurologic disorders, such as epilepsy or cerebral palsy, that can lead to breathing or swallowing problems

Important note: These people at high risk should only receive the *inactivated* influenza vaccine. They should not receive the live influenza vaccine. Why? Because safety of the live vaccine has not been evaluated in this population.

Who Should NOT Be Vaccinated?

As noted earlier, people at high risk for flu complications, including pregnant women, should not receive the *live* influenza vaccine. Instead, they should receive the *inactivated* vaccine. In addition, some people should not receive *either* vaccine without a specialist's approval. In this group are the following:

- People who have a *severe* allergic reaction (e.g., angioedema, respiratory distress) to chicken eggs
- People who have had a severe reaction to influenza vaccination in the past
- People who have experienced GBS

When Should Vaccination Be Administered?

In the United States flu season usually peaks in January or February but can also peak as early as October or as late as May. To ensure full protection, the best time to vaccinate is October or November. However, for people who missed the best time, vaccinating as late as April may be of benefit. Influenza vaccine may be given at the same time as other vaccines, including pneumococcal vaccine.

Dosage and Administration

Inactivated Influenza Vaccine: Intramuscular

Inactivated influenza vaccines for IM dosing are available under seven trade names: Afluria, Fluarix, Flucelvax, FluLaval, Fluvirin, Fluzone, and Fluzone High-Dose. Fluzone High-Dose is approved only for patients 65 years and older. Only Afluria and Fluzone are approved for patients as young as

6 months. However, although Afluria is approved for younger children, ACIP recommends using it only for children 9 years and older. Why? Because Afluria may increase the risk for fever and febrile seizures in younger children.

Dosage is a function of age and vaccination history. Dosages and routes of these and other forms of influenza vaccine are available in Table 78.5.

Inactivated Influenza Vaccine: Intradermal

Fluzone Intradermal is the first influenza vaccine formulated for intradermal injection. Compared with the IM flu vaccines, the intradermal vaccine contains less antigen/dose (9 mcg vs. 15 mcg) and is injected in a smaller volume (0.1 mL vs. 0.5 mL). The preferred injection site is over the deltoid muscle.

Live, Attenuated Influenza Vaccine

LAIV [FluMist] is supplied in a single-dose, 0.2-mL sprayer for intranasal administration to persons aged 2 through 49 years. This live virus drug should not be administered to people who are immunocompromised, pregnant, or otherwise at high risk for influenza complications. Most vaccine recipients get just one dose a year. However, children aged 2 through 8 years who have not been vaccinated before require two doses, administered at least 1 month apart. FluMist is unstable at room temperature and hence must be stored frozen.

Avian Influenza

The FDA has approved an inactivated vaccine against avian H5N1 influenza. It is not available commercially in the United States but is being included in the CDC Strategic National Stockpile in case H5N1 avian influenza strains become able to spread efficiently between humans. The vaccine is given as 2 IM injections, 1 month apart.

Neuraminidase Inhibitors

The neuraminidase inhibitors are active against influenza A and influenza B. At this time, three neuraminidase inhibitors are available: oseltamivir, peramivir, and zanamivir. Peramivir [Rapivab] is only available for IV delivery. For this reason, most providers do not routinely offer this in nonacute settings. Our focus will be on examining oseltamivir and zanamivir.

Both oseltamivir and zanamivir are approved for influenza prophylaxis and treatment. Although approved for prophylaxis, these drugs are not as adequate as vaccination and should not be considered as a substitute for annual vaccination against influenza. However, because it takes about 2 weeks after vaccination for antibodies to develop against the influenza virus, oseltamivir can provide some protection for unvaccinated people during a community outbreak.

When used for treatment, dosing must begin early—no later than 2 days after symptom onset, and preferably much sooner. Why? Because benefits decline greatly when treatment is delayed: when treatment is started within 12 hours of symptom onset, symptom duration is reduced by more than 3 days; when started within 24 hours, symptom duration is reduced by less than 2 days; and when started within 36 hours, symptom duration is reduced by only 29 hours. In addition to reducing symptom duration, oseltamivir can reduce symptom severity and the incidence of complications (sinusitis, bronchitis). Unfortunately, in the real world, patients may be unable to obtain and fill a prescription soon enough for the drug to be of significant benefit.

Oseltamivir

Actions and Uses

Oseltamivir [Tamiflu] is an oral drug approved for prevention and treatment of influenza in patients 1 year and older. Antiviral effects derive from inhibiting *neuraminidase,* a viral enzyme required for replication. As a result of neuraminidase inhibition, newly formed viral particles are unable to bud off from the cytoplasmic membrane of infected host cells. Hence, viral spread is stopped. Oseltamivir is active against most strains of influenza A and influenza B responsible for seasonal influenza, as well as most isolates of influenza A type H5N1 (the cause of *avian flu*). In addition, the drug is active against the so-called *swine flu,* the variant of influenza A type H1N1 that caused the influenza pandemic in 2009. Emergence of resistance over the course of treatment is rare.

Pharmacokinetics

Oseltamivir is well absorbed after oral administration. In the liver, the drug undergoes conversion to oseltamivir carboxylate, its active form. Bioavailability of the carboxylate is 80%. Plasma levels of active drug peak 2.5 to 6 hours after dosing. The plasma half-life is 6 to 10 hours. The drug is eliminated in the urine, primarily as the carboxylate form.

Adverse Effects

Oseltamivir is generally well tolerated. The most common side effects are nausea and vomiting. Nausea can be reduced by giving oseltamivir with food.

Rarely, oseltamivir has caused *severe hypersensitivity reactions,* including anaphylaxis and serious skin reactions (e.g., toxic epidermal necrolysis, erythema multiforme, Stevens-Johnson syndrome). If an allergic reaction develops, oseltamivir should be discontinued.

Rarely, oseltamivir has been associated with *neuropsychiatric effects,* mainly in younger patients. Reported reactions include delirium and abnormal behavior, which has led to injury and even death. However, because influenza itself can cause these reactions, they cannot be ascribed with certainty to oseltamivir.

Interaction With Live Influenza Vaccine

In theory, oseltamivir can blunt responses to LAIV. Accordingly, oseltamivir should be discontinued at least 2 days before giving LAIV. After dosing with LAIV, at least 2 weeks should elapse before starting oseltamivir.

Preparations, Dosage, and Administration

Oseltamivir [Tamiflu] is available in capsules (30, 45, and 75 mg) and as a powder (360 mg) to be reconstituted to a 6-mg/mL oral suspension. Dosing can be done with or without food, although dosing with food can reduce nausea.

Treatment of Influenza. For treatment, the dosage for patients 13 years and older is 75 mg twice daily for 5 days, beginning no later than 2 days after the onset of symptoms. Dosage should be reduced to 75 mg once daily in patients with significant renal impairment. The dosage for children 1 year old through 12 years old is based on body weight as follows: 15 kg or less, 30 mg twice daily; 15.1 to 23 kg, 45 mg twice daily; 23.1 to 40 kg, 60 mg twice daily; and more than 40 kg, 75 mg twice daily.

Prevention of Influenza. For prevention, the dosage is one half the dosage used for treatment. This is accomplished by switching from twice-daily dosing to once-daily dosing. For patients 13 years and older, the dosage is 75 mg once a day. The dosage for children 1 year old through 12 years old is based on body weight as follows: 15 kg or less, 30 mg once daily; 15 to 23 kg, 45 mg once daily; 23.1 to 40 kg, 60 mg once daily; and more than 40 kg, 75 mg once daily.

Candidates for prophylactic therapy include family members of someone with flu and residents of nursing homes. To protect family members, dosing should begin within 48 hours of exposure and should continue for 10 days. To protect residents of nursing homes or high-risk members of the community at large, dosing can be done continuously for up to 42 days.

Zanamivir

Actions and Uses

Zanamivir [Relenza], administered by oral inhalation, is approved for treatment of acute uncomplicated influenza in patients at least 7 years old, and for prophylaxis of influenza in people at least 5 years old. As with oseltamivir, benefits derive from inhibiting viral neuraminidase, an enzyme required for viral replication. Like oseltamivir, zanamivir is well tolerated, except in patients with underlying airway disease.

Pharmacokinetics

Zanamivir is formulated as a dry powder for oral inhalation. The drug is poorly absorbed from the GI tract, so it cannot be administered by mouth. Most (70%–90%) of an inhaled dose is deposited in the oropharynx and throat. About 10% to 20% reaches the tracheobronchial tree and lungs. Between 4% and 17% of each dose undergoes absorption into the systemic circulation. Zanamivir has a plasma half-life of 2.5 to 5 hours and is eliminated unchanged in the urine. No metabolites have been detected.

Adverse Effects and Interactions

In patients with healthy lung function, serious adverse effects are uncommon. Because zanamivir is administered as an inhaled powder, patients may experience cough or throat irritation. Also, as with oseltamivir, there have been rare reports of severe allergic reactions and neuropsychiatric effects.

In patients with preexisting lung disorders (e.g., asthma, chronic obstructive pulmonary disease), zanamivir may cause severe bronchospasm and respiratory decline. Some patients have required immediate treatment or hospitalization. Deaths have occurred. However, given the effect of flu itself on lung function, it's not clear that zanamivir was the cause. Nonetheless, owing to the potential risk, zanamivir is not recommended for patients with underlying airway disease.

Zanamivir appears devoid of drug interactions. However, like oseltamivir, zanamivir may blunt responses to LAIV, and hence should be stopped 2 days before giving LAIV, and should not be started for 2 weeks after giving LAIV.

Preparations, Dosage, and Administration

Zanamivir [Relenza] is supplied in blister packs that contain 5 mg of powdered drug. Administration is by oral inhalation using the Diskhaler provided by the manufacturer.

Influenza Treatment. The dosage for adults and children is 10 mg (two 5-mg inhalations) twice daily for 5 days. Each 10-mg dose should be separated by 12 hours. However, on the first day of treatment, less separation (as little as 2 hours) is permitted if the first dose cannot be taken early enough in the day to allow 12 hours between doses. Patients who are using an inhaled bronchodilator (e.g., albuterol) should administer the bronchodilator before inhaling zanamivir.

Influenza Prevention. The dosage for adults and children is 10 mg (two 5-mg inhalations) once daily. Note that this is one half the dosage used for treatment.

Adamantanes

The adamantanes—amantadine [Symmetrel] and rimantadine [Flumadine]—were the first influenza drugs available. Although they remain on the market and were approved for influenza infection, because most current strains of influenza A are resistant, and because all strains of influenza B are resistant, the CDC recommends against using these drugs for any influenza patients, whether infected with influenza A or influenza B.

PRESCRIBING AND MONITORING CONSIDERATIONS

Acyclovir

Therapeutic Goal

Treatment of infections caused by HSV and VZV.

Identifying High-Risk Patients

Use with *caution* in patients with dehydration or renal impairment and in those taking other nephrotoxic drugs.

Administration Considerations

Routes

Topical, oral, IV.

Dosage

Oral and IV dosages must be reduced in patients with renal impairment.

Administration

Topical. During administration care must be taken to avoid viral transfer to other body sites or to other people.

Oral. Dosages vary widely for different indications (see Table 78.2).

Intravenous. Give by slow IV infusion (over 1 hour or more). Never give by IV bolus.

Ongoing Monitoring and Interventions

Evaluating Therapeutic Effects

Observe for decreased clinical manifestations of HSV and VZV infections. Virologic testing may also be performed.

Minimizing Adverse Effects

Nephrotoxicity. Intravenous acyclovir can precipitate in renal tubules, causing reversible kidney damage. To minimize risk, infuse acyclovir slowly and ensure adequate hydration during the infusion and for 2 hours after. Exercise caution in patients with preexisting renal impairment and in those who are dehydrated or taking other nephrotoxic drugs.

Ganciclovir

Therapeutic Goal

Treatment and prevention of CMV infection in immunocompromised patients, including those with AIDS and those taking immunosuppressive drugs after an organ transplantation.

Topical treatment of acute keratitis caused by HSV.

Baseline Data

Obtain a complete blood count and platelet count.

Identifying High-Risk Patients

Ganciclovir is *contraindicated* during pregnancy and for patients with neutrophil counts below $500/mm^3$ or platelet counts below $25,000/mm^3$.

Use with *caution* in patients taking zidovudine or nephrotoxic drugs (e.g., amphotericin B, cyclosporine) and in patients with a history of cytopenic reactions to other drugs.

Administration Considerations

Routes

Oral, IV, intraocular, topical to the eye.

Dosage

Oral and IV dosages must be reduced in patients with renal impairment. AIDS patients with CMV retinitis must take ganciclovir for life.

Administration

Intravenous. Give by slow IV infusion (over 1 hour or more). Ensure adequate hydration to promote renal excretion.

Intraocular Implants. Surgical implants are replaced every 5 to 8 months.

Topical to the Eye. Advise patients to apply ganciclovir gel drops directly to the affected eye and to avoid contact lenses until lesions heal.

Ongoing Evaluation and Interventions

Minimizing Adverse Effects

Granulocytopenia and Thrombocytopenia. Ganciclovir suppresses bone marrow function when given intravenously or orally. Obtain complete blood counts and platelet counts frequently. Discontinue ganciclovir if the neutrophil count falls below 500/mm^3 or the platelet count falls below 25,000/mm^3. The risk for granulocytopenia can be reduced by giving granulocyte colony-stimulating factors. The risk for granulocytopenia is increased by concurrent therapy with zidovudine (a drug for AIDS).

Reproductive Toxicity. In animals, ganciclovir is teratogenic and embryotoxic and suppresses spermatogenesis. These risks should be shared with patients and the need for birth control strongly advised.

CHAPTER

79

Antiviral Agents II: Drugs for HIV Infection and Related Opportunistic Infections

Jacqueline Rosenjack Burchum, DNSc, FNP-BC, CNE

In this chapter we discuss drug therapy of infection with the *human immunodeficiency virus* (HIV), the microbe that causes *acquired immunodeficiency syndrome* (AIDS). Pharmacologic management of HIV/AIDS is typically carried out by HIV specialists. Still, because a vast number of people have HIV/AIDS, it is important that all providers be familiar with these drugs and their effects on patients even if it is unlikely that they will be prescribing them. Our focus will be on providing generalized information.

HIV promotes immunodeficiency by killing CD4 T lymphocytes (CD4 T cells), which are key components of the immune system (see Chapter 52). As a result of HIV-induced immunodeficiency, patients are at risk for opportunistic infections and certain neoplasms.

It is important to appreciate that HIV infection is not synonymous with AIDS, which develops years after HIV infection is acquired. The definition of AIDS, established by the Centers for Disease Control and Prevention (CDC), is a syndrome in which the individual is HIV positive and has either (1) CD4 T-cell counts below 200 cells/mL or (2) an AIDS-defining illness. Included in the CDC's long list of AIDS-defining illnesses are *Pneumocystis* pneumonia, cytomegalovirus retinitis, disseminated histoplasmosis, tuberculosis, and Kaposi's sarcoma.

Since being identified as a new disease in 1981, AIDS has become a global epidemic. According to the 2014 HIV Surveillance Report, in the United States, approximately 1.2 million people are now infected and about 50,000 more become infected each year. More than 658,000 have died since the epidemic began. The World Health Organization (WHO) reports that, worldwide, an estimated 36.9 million people are now infected, and approximately 34 million have died. However, there is good news: according to a United Nations report released in 2014, the number of new HIV infections has declined by 35%, and AIDs-related deaths declined by 42% in the previous decade, owing in large part to more widespread use of HIV drugs.

Therapy of HIV infection has made dramatic advances. Today, standard *antiretroviral therapy* (ART) consists of three or four drugs. These combinations, often referred to as *HAART* (for *highly active antiretroviral therapy*), can decrease plasma HIV to levels that are undetectable with current technology and can thus delay or reverse loss of immune function, decrease certain AIDS-related complications, preserve health, prolong life, and decrease HIV transmission. However, these benefits have not come without a price: ART is expensive, poses a risk for long-term side effects and serious drug interactions, and must continue lifelong. Accordingly, if treatment is to succeed, patients must be highly motivated and well informed about all aspects of the treatment program. A strong support network is extremely valuable, too.

ART cannot cure HIV infection. Although treatment *can* greatly reduce HIV levels—often rendering the virus undetectable—discontinuation has consistently been followed by a rebound in HIV replication. Because ART does not eliminate HIV, patients continue to be infectious and must be warned to avoid behaviors that can transmit the virus to others.

Understanding this chapter requires a basic understanding of the immune system. Accordingly, you may find it helpful to read Chapter 52 before proceeding.

PATHOPHYSIOLOGY

Characteristics of HIV

HIV is a *retrovirus.* Like all other viruses, retroviruses lack the machinery needed for self-replication and thus are obligate intracellular parasites. However, in contrast to other viruses, retroviruses have positive-sense, single-stranded RNA as their genetic material. Accordingly, in order to replicate, retroviruses must first transcribe their RNA into DNA. The enzyme employed for this process is viral *RNA-dependent DNA polymerase,* commonly known as *reverse transcriptase.* (The enzyme is called reverse transcriptase to distinguish it from DNA-dependent RNA polymerase, the host enzyme that transcribes DNA into RNA, which is the usual ["forward"] transcription process.) The name *retrovirus* is derived from the first two letters of *reverse* and *transcriptase.*

There are two types of HIV, referred to as HIV-1 and HIV-2. HIV-1 is found worldwide, whereas HIV-2 is found mainly in West Africa. Although HIV-1 and HIV-2 differ with respect to genetic makeup and antigenicity, they both cause similar disease syndromes. Not all drugs that are effective against HIV-1 are also effective against HIV-2.

Target Cells

The principal cells attacked by HIV are *CD4 T cells* (helper T lymphocytes). As discussed in Chapter 52, these cells are essential components of the immune system. They are required for production of antibodies by B lymphocytes and for activation of cytolytic T lymphocytes. Accordingly, as HIV kills CD4 T cells, the immune system undergoes progressive decline. As a result, infected individuals become increasingly vulnerable to opportunistic infections, a major cause of death among people with AIDS. HIV targets CD4 T cells because the CD4 proteins on the surface of these cells provide points of attachment for HIV (see later). Without such a receptor, HIV would be unable to connect with and penetrate these cells. After HIV has infected a CD4 T cell, the cell dies in about 1.25 days. It is important to appreciate that only a few percent of CD4 T cells circulate in the blood; most reside in lymph nodes and other lymphoid tissues.

In addition to infecting CD4 T cells, HIV infects *macrophages* and *microglial cells* (the central nervous system [CNS] counterparts of macrophages), both of which carry CD4 proteins. Because macrophages and microglial cells are resistant to destruction by HIV, they can survive despite being infected. As a result, they serve as a reservoir of HIV during chronic infection.

Structure of HIV

The structure of HIV is very simple. As shown in Fig. 79.1, the HIV *virion* (i.e., the entire virus particle) consists of *nucleic acid* (RNA) surrounded by *core proteins,* which in turn are surrounded by a *capsid* (protein shell), which in turn is surrounded by a *lipid bilayer envelope* (derived from the membrane of the host cell).

The central core contains two separate but identical single strands of RNA, each with its own molecule of *reverse transcriptase* attached. The RNA serves as the template for DNA synthesis.

The outer envelope of HIV contains *glycoproteins* that are needed for attachment to host cells. Each glycoprotein (gp) consists of two subunits, known as *gp41* and *gp120.* The smaller protein (gp41) is embedded in the lipid bilayer of the viral envelope; the larger protein (gp120) is connected firmly to gp41. (The numbers 41 and 120 simply indicate the mass of these glycoproteins in thousands of daltons.)

Replication Cycle of HIV

The replication cycle of HIV is shown in Fig. 79.2. The numbered steps listed here correspond to the numbers in the figure.

- *Step 1*—The cycle begins with attachment of HIV to the host cell. The primary connection takes place between *gp120* on the HIV envelope and a *CD4* protein on the host cell membrane. Other host proteins, known as coreceptors, act in concert with CD4 to tighten the bond with HIV. Two of these coreceptors—known as CCR5 and CXCR4—are of particular importance. (One drug—maraviroc—blocks HIV entry by binding CCR5.)
- *Step 2*—The lipid bilayer envelope of HIV fuses with the lipid bilayer of the host cell membrane. Fusion is followed by release of HIV RNA into the host cell. (One drug—enfuvirtide—works by blocking the fusion process.)

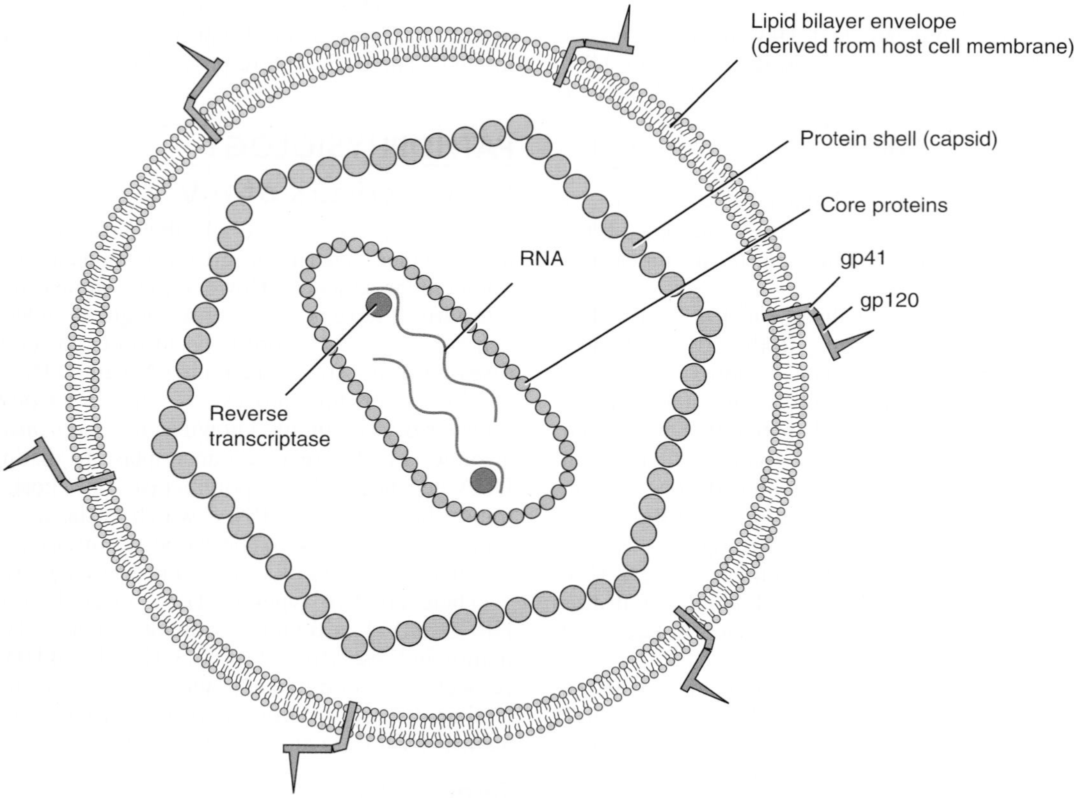

Figure 79.1 ▪ Structure of the human immunodeficiency virus.
Note that HIV has two single strands of RNA and that each strand is associated with a molecule of reverse transcriptase. gp41, glycoprotein 41; gp120, glycoprotein 120.

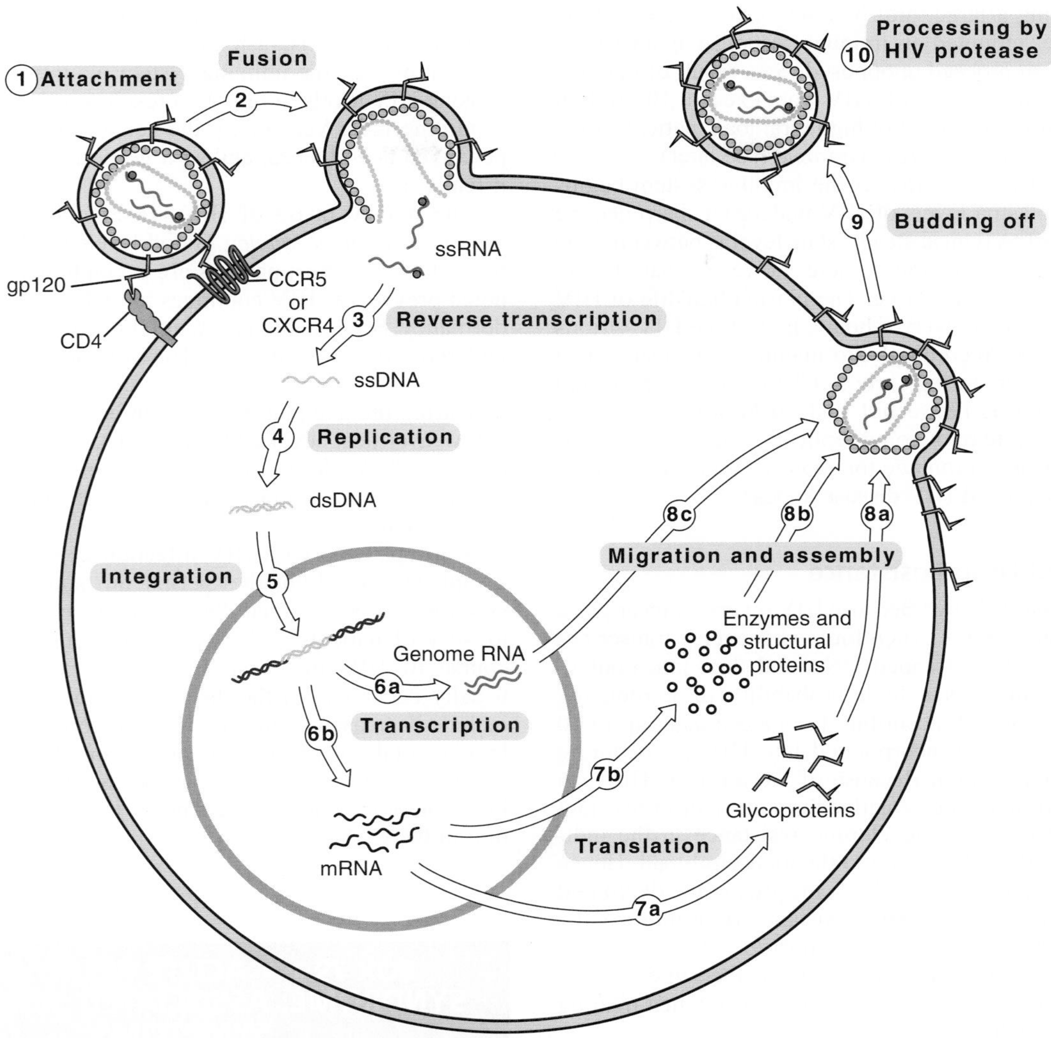

Figure 79.2 ▪ Replication cycle of the human immunodeficiency virus. See text for description of events. CCR5, CCR5 coreceptor; CD4, CD4 receptor; CXCR4, CXCR4 coreceptor; dsDNA, double-stranded DNA; gp120, glycoprotein 120; mRNA, messenger RNA; ssDNA, single-stranded DNA; ssRNA, single-stranded RNA.

- *Step 3*—HIV RNA is transcribed into single-stranded DNA by HIV *reverse transcriptase.*
- *Step 4*—Reverse transcriptase converts the single strand of HIV DNA into double-stranded HIV DNA.
- *Step 5*—Double-stranded HIV DNA becomes integrated into the host's DNA, under the direction of a viral enzyme known (aptly) as *integrase.* (One drug—raltegravir—inhibits this enzyme.)
- *Step 6*—HIV DNA undergoes transcription into RNA. Some of the resulting RNA becomes the genome for daughter HIV virions (step 6a). The rest of the RNA is messenger RNA that codes for HIV proteins (step 6b).
- *Step 7*—Messenger RNA is translated into HIV glycoproteins (step 7a) and HIV enzymes and structural proteins (step 7b).
- *Step 8*—The components of HIV migrate to the cell surface and assemble into a new virus. Before assembly, HIV glycoproteins become incorporated into the host cell membrane (step 8a). In steps 8b and 8c, the other components of the virion migrate to the cell surface, where they undergo assembly into the new virus.
- *Step 9*—The newly formed virus buds off from the host cell. As indicated, the outer envelope of the virion is derived from the cell membrane of the host.
- *Step 10*—In this step, which occurs either during or immediately after budding off, HIV undergoes final maturation under the influence of *protease,* an enzyme that cleaves certain large polyproteins into their smaller, functional forms. If protease fails to cleave these proteins, HIV will remain immature and noninfectious. HIV protease is the target of several important drugs.

Replication Rate

HIV replicates rapidly during *all* stages of the infection. During the initial phase of infection, replication is massive. Why? Because (1) the population of CD4 cells is still large, thereby providing a large viral breeding ground; and (2) the host has not yet mounted an immune response against HIV, so replication can proceed unopposed. As a result of massive replication, plasma levels of HIV can exceed 10 million virions/mL. During this stage of high viral load, patients often experience an *acute retroviral syndrome* (see later).

Over the next few months, as the immune system begins to attack HIV, plasma levels of HIV undergo a sharp decline and then level off. A typical steady-state level is between 1000 and 100,000 virions/mL. Please note, however, that steady-state numbers can be deceptive. The plasma half-life of HIV is only 6 hours; that is, every 6 hours, half of the HIV virions in plasma are lost. Accordingly, to maintain the steady-state levels typically seen during chronic HIV infection, the actual rate of *replication* is between 1 and 10 *billion* virions/day. Despite this high rate of ongoing replication, infected persons typically remain asymptomatic for about 10 years, after which symptoms of advanced HIV disease appear.

Mutation and Drug Resistance

HIV mutates rapidly. Why? Because HIV reverse transcriptase is an error-prone enzyme. Therefore, whenever it transcribes HIV RNA into single-stranded DNA and then into double-stranded DNA, there is a high probability of introducing base-pair errors. In fact, according to one estimate, up to 10 incorrect bases may be incorporated into HIV DNA during each round of replication. Because of these errors, HIV can rapidly mutate from a drug-sensitive form into a drug-resistant form. The probability of developing resistance in the individual patient is directly related to the total viral load. Hence the more virions the patient harbors, the greater the likelihood that at least one will become resistant. To minimize the emergence of resistance, patients must be treated with a combination of antiretroviral drugs. This is the same strategy we employ to prevent emergence of resistance when treating tuberculosis (see Chapter 75).

Transmission of HIV

HIV is transmitted sexually and by other means. The virus is present in all body fluids of infected individuals. Transmission can be by intimate contact with semen, vaginal secretions, and blood. The disease can be transmitted by sexual contact, transfusion, sharing intravenous (IV) needles, and accidental needle sticks. In addition, it can be transmitted to the fetus by an infected mother, usually during the perinatal period. Initially, HIV infection was limited largely to homosexual males, injection-drug users, and hemophiliacs. However, the disease can now be found routinely in the population at large. The risk for acquiring HIV sexually can be reduced by male circumcision, limiting sexual partners, and use of condoms—as well as by complete sexual abstinence. In addition, infection can be prevented with drugs, as discussed later under "Preventing HIV Infection with Drugs."

Clinical Course of HIV Infection

HIV infection follows a triphasic clinical course. During the initial phase, HIV undergoes massive replication, causing blood levels of HIV to rise very high. As a result, between 50% and 90% of patients experience a flu-like *acute retroviral syndrome.* Signs and symptoms include fever, lymphadenopathy, pharyngitis, rash, myalgia, and headache (Box 79.1). Soon, however, the immune system mounts a counterattack, causing HIV levels to fall. As a result, symptoms of the acute syndrome fade. Very often, the acute retroviral syndrome is perceived as influenza, and so it goes unrecognized for what it really is.

The middle phase of HIV infection is characterized by prolonged *clinical latency.* Blood levels of HIV remain relatively low, and most patients are asymptomatic. However, as noted previously, HIV continues to replicate despite apparent dormancy. Because of persistent HIV replication, CD4 T cells undergo progressive decline. The average duration of clinical latency is 10 years.

During the late phase of HIV infection, CD4 T cells drop below a critical level (200 cells/mL), rendering the patient highly vulnerable to opportunistic infections and certain neoplasms (e.g., Kaposi sarcoma). The late phase is when AIDS occurs.

Many patients with HIV infection experience neurologic complications. Both the peripheral and central nervous systems may be involved. *Peripheral neuropathies* affect 20% to 40% of patients and may develop at any time over the course of HIV infection. In contrast, *CNS complications* usually occur late in the disease. Symptoms of CNS injury include decreased cognition, reduced concentration, memory loss, mental slowness, and motor complaints (e.g., ataxia, tremors). Neuronal injury may be the direct result of HIV infection or may develop secondary to an opportunistic infection in the CNS.

BOX 79.1 ■ ACUTE RETROVIRAL SYNDROME: ASSOCIATED SIGNS AND SYMPTOMS

- Fever (96%)
- Lymphadenopathy (74%)
- Pharyngitis (70%)
- Rash and mucocutaneous ulceration (70%)
- Erythematous maculopapular rash with lesions on face and trunk and sometimes extremities, including palms and soles
- Mucocutaneous ulceration involving mouth, esophagus, or genitals
- Myalgia or arthralgia (54%)
- Diarrhea (32%)
- Headache (32%)
- Nausea and vomiting (27%)
- Hepatosplenomegaly (14%)
- Weight loss (13%)
- Thrush (12%)
- Neurologic symptoms (12%)
- Meningoencephalitis or aseptic meningitis
- Peripheral neuropathy or radiculopathy
- Facial palsy
- Guillain-Barré neuritis
- Brachial neuritis
- Cognitive impairment or psychosis

DRUG INTERACTIONS

Before we begin our discussion of the different classes of antiretroviral drugs, it will be wise to explore a topic of great concern. Drug interactions are common and significant with these drugs. Many are inducers or inhibitors of one or more (and sometimes many) CYP450 isoenzymes. Many are also substrates of one or more of these. As a result, interactions are common. Some drugs have the same adverse effect, and giving them together can intensify an effect so that it becomes dangerous. Moreover, when we consider all the various combinations of these drugs plus drugs taken for other conditions and illnesses the patient may have, the possibility of dangerous drug interactions increases dramatically. Simple lists of common drug interactions are inadequate to address this issue.

Every provider needs access to reliable drug interaction software that is capable of simultaneously checking for interactions among multiple drugs. These are widely available online and as downloads for mobile devices.

CLASSIFICATION OF ANTIRETROVIRAL DRUGS

At this time, we have five types of antiretroviral drugs. Three types—*reverse transcriptase inhibitors, integrase strand transfer inhibitors* (INSTIs), and *protease inhibitors* (PIs)—inhibit enzymes required for HIV replication. The other two types—*fusion inhibitors* and *chemokine receptor 5 (CCR5) antagonists*—block viral entry into cells. As discussed later, the reverse transcriptase inhibitors are subdivided into two groups: *nucleoside/nucleotide reverse transcriptase inhibitors* (NRTIs), which are structural analogs of nucleosides or nucleotides; and (2) *nonnucleoside reverse transcriptase inhibitors* (NNRTIs). Drugs that belong to these groups are shown in Table 79.1.

Nucleoside/Nucleotide Reverse Transcriptase Inhibitors

The NRTIs were the first drugs used against HIV infection and remain mainstays of therapy today. In fact, these drugs constitute the backbone of all treatment regimens. As their name suggests, the NRTIs are chemical relatives of naturally occurring nucleosides or nucleotides, the building blocks of DNA. Antiretroviral effects derive from suppressing synthesis of viral DNA by reverse transcriptase. All are prodrugs; to be effective, all of the NRTIs must first undergo intracellular conversion to their active (triphosphate) forms. At this time, seven NRTIs are available: abacavir, didanosine, emtricitabine, lamivudine, stavudine, tenofovir, and zidovudine. The availability of combination antiretroviral products has simplified treatment. The fixed-dose combinations are shown in Table 79.1. Pharmacokinetic properties of NRTIs are shown in Table 79.2. Significant adverse effects are provided in Table 79.3. Important properties of these drugs, as well as drugs of other categories, are provided in the "Prescribing and Monitoring Considerations" at the end of this chapter.

TABLE 79.1 ▪ Classification of Antiretroviral Drugs

Generic Name	Trade Name	Abbreviation
DRUGS THAT INHIBIT HIV ENZYMES		
Nucleoside/Nucleotide Reverse Transcriptase Inhibitors (NRTIs)		
Single-Drug Products		
Abacavir	Ziagen	ABC
Didanosine	Videx	ddI
Emtricitabine	Emtriva	FTC
Lamivudine	Epivir	3TC
Stavudine	Zerit	d4T
Tenofovir	Viread	TDF
Zidovudine	Retrovir	ZDV
Fixed-Dose Combinations		
Abacavir 600 mg Lamivudine 300 mg	Epzicom	ABC/3TC
Abacavir 300 mg Lamivudine 150 mg Zidovudine 300 mg	Trizivir	ABC/3TC/ZDV
Zidovudine 300 mg Lamivudine 150 mg	Combivir	ZDV/3TC
Emtricitabine 200 mg Tenofovir 300 mg	Truvada	FTC/TDF
Emtricitabine 200 mg Tenofovir 300 mg Efavirenz* 600 mg	Atripla	FTC/TDF/EFV
Emtricitabine 200 mg Tenofovir 300 mg Rilpivirine† 25 mg	Complera	FTC/TDF/RPV
Efavirenz* 600 mg Tenofovir 300 mg Emtricitabine 200 mg	Atripla	EFV/TDF/FTC
Elvitegravir‡ 150 mg Cobicistat§ 150 mg Emtricitabine 200 mg Tenofovir 300 mg	Stribild	N/A
Nonnucleoside Reverse Transcriptase Inhibitors (NNRTIs)		
Delavirdine	Rescriptor	DLV
Efavirenz	Sustiva	EFV
Etravirine	Intelence	ETR
Nevirapine	Viramune	NVP
Rilpivirine	Edurant	RPV
Protease Inhibitors		
Atazanavir	Reyataz	ATV
Darunavir	Prezista	DRV
Fosamprenavir	Lexiva, Telzir ♣	FPV
Indinavir	Crixivan	IDV
Nelfinavir	Viracept	NFV
Ritonavir	Norvir	RTV
Saquinavir	Invirase	SQV
Tipranavir	Aptivus	TPV
Lopinavir/ritonavir	Kaletra	LPV/r
Integrase Strand Transfer Inhibitor		
Raltegravir	Isentress	RAL
Elvitegravir	Vitekta	EVG
DRUGS THAT BLOCK HIV ENTRY INTO CELLS		
Fusion Inhibitor		
Enfuvirtide	Fuzeon	T-20
CCR5 Antagonist		
Maraviroc	Selzentry, Celsentri ♣	MVC

*Efavirenz is an NNRTI, not an NRTI.
†Rilpivirine is an NNRTI, not an NRTI.
‡Elvitegravir is an INSTI, not an NRTI.
§Cobicistat is a CYP3A inhibitor.

PATIENT-CENTERED CARE ACROSS THE LIFE SPAN

Nucleoside Reverse Transcriptase Inhibitors

Life Stage	Considerations or Concerns
Children	Pediatric dosing is available for all NRTIs.
Pregnant women	Didanosine, emtricitabine, and tenofovir are in FDA Pregnancy Risk Category B. Lamivudine, stavudine, and zidovudine are in FDA Pregnancy Risk Category C. Current labeling for abacavir does not include a risk category. The choice of antiretroviral drug for the pregnant woman must consider not only the risk for harm to the fetus from the drug but also the risk for harm to the fetus from the adverse effects tied to the drug. Although it is categorized in FDA Pregnancy Risk Category C, zidovudine is the drug of choice for preventing mother-to-infant HIV transmission during labor and delivery.
Breastfeeding women	Breastfeeding should be avoided by women with HIV because there is a danger of transmitting the virus.
Older adults	Older patients taking didanosine have a higher risk for developing pancreatitis than younger patients. Peripheral neuropathy may be increased for older patients taking stavudine.

TABLE 79.2 ▪ Pharmacokinetic Properties of Nucleoside/Nucleotide Reverse Transcriptase Inhibitors

	Abacavir (ABC)	Didanosine (ddI)	Emtricitabine (FTC)	Lamivudine (3TC)	Stavudine (d4T)	Tenofovir (TDF)	Zidovudine (ZDV)
Trade name	Ziagen	Videx, Videx EC	Emtriva	Epivir	Zerit	Viread	Retrovir
Bioavailability	83%	30%–40%	93%	86%	86%	39% (with food)	60%
Serum half-life	1.5 hr	1.5 hr	10 hr	5–7 hr	1 hr	17 hr	1.1 hr
Intracellular half-life	12–26 hr	More than 20 hr	More than 20 hr	18–22 hr	7.5 hr	More than 60 hr	7 hr
Elimination	Metabolized by alcohol dehydrogenase, then excreted in the urine	Partial metabolism followed by renal excretion	Renal excretion	Renal excretion (unchanged)	Partial metabolism followed by renal excretion	Renal excretion	Hepatic metabolism followed by renal excretion

EC, enteric coated.

TABLE 79.3 ▪ Significant Adverse Effects of Antiretroviral Drugs

NUCLEOSIDE/NUCLEOTIDE REVERSE TRANSCRIPTASE INHIBITORS	
Abacavir [ABC]	Lactic acidosis,* severe hepatomegaly with steatosis,* severe hypersensitivity reactions,* headache, nausea, vomiting, fatigue, malaise, sleep disorders
Didanosine [ddI]	Lactic acidosis,* severe hepatomegaly with steatosis,* severe pancreatitis,* hepatotoxicity,† noncirrhotic portal hypertension,† immune reconstitution syndrome,† redistribution of adipose tissue,† peripheral neuropathy,† retinal disorders and/or optic neuritis,† headache, nausea, vomiting, rash
Emtricitabine [FTC]	Lactic acidosis,* severe hepatomegaly with steatosis,* hepatitis B exacerbations,* immune reconstitution syndrome,† redistribution of adipose tissue,† headache, nausea, fatigue, malaise, weakness, sleep disorders, depression, rash, dermal hyperpigmentation, rhinitis, cough, abdominal discomfort, diarrhea
Lamivudine [3TC]	Lactic acidosis,* severe hepatomegaly with steatosis,* hepatitis B exacerbations,* risk for HIV-1 resistance if used in a patient with untreated HIV-1 infection,* ENT infections, sore throat, diarrhea
Stavudine [d4T]	Lactic acidosis,* severe hepatomegaly with steatosis,* severe pancreatitis,* hepatotoxicity,† immune reconstitution syndrome,† redistribution of adipose tissue,† neurologic symptoms (e.g., motor weakness, peripheral neuropathy),† headache, nausea, vomiting, rash, diarrhea
Tenofovir [TDF]	Lactic acidosis,* severe hepatomegaly with steatosis,* hepatitis B exacerbations,* immune reconstitution syndrome,† redistribution of adipose tissue,† renal impairment,† decreased BMD,† headache, nausea, weakness, depression, rash, diarrhea
Zidovudine [ZDV]	Lactic acidosis,* severe hepatomegaly with steatosis,* severe anemia and neutropenia,* serious myopathy and myositis,* immune reconstitution syndrome,† redistribution of adipose tissue,† headache, nausea, vomiting, anorexia, malaise, fever, cough
NONNUCLEOSIDE REVERSE TRANSCRIPTASE INHIBITORS	
Delavirdine [Rescriptor]	Rash ranging from erythema and pruritus (16.7%) to desquamation and ulceration (4.4%), headache, nausea, vomiting, fatigue, weakness, diarrhea
Efavirenz [Sustiva]	Rash,† hepatotoxicity,† severe depression with/without suicidal ideation,† nervous system symptoms,† convulsions,† immune reconstitution syndrome,† redistribution of adipose tissue,† hyperlipidemia,† headache, nausea, vomiting, fatigue, dizziness, impaired concentration, sleep disorders

TABLE 79.3 ▪ Significant Adverse Effects of Antiretroviral Drugs—cont'd

Etravirine [Intelence]	Severe rashes, including SJS and TEN,† peripheral neuropathy
Nevirapine [Viramune]	Life-threatening skin reactions,* hepatotoxicity,* immune reconstitution syndrome,† redistribution of adipose tissue†
Rilpivirine [Edurant]	Rash,† hypersensitivity reactions,† hepatotoxicity,† immune reconstitution syndrome,† redistribution of adipose tissue,† depression,† headache, sleep disorders
PROTEASE INHIBITORS	
Atazanavir [Reyataz]	Dangerous drug interactions,† severe skin reactions,† PR interval prolongation,† hepatotoxicity,† hyperbilirubinemia,† kidney stones and gallstones,† diabetes (new onset or exacerbation),† immune reconstitution syndrome,† redistribution of adipose tissue,† renewed bleeding in patients with hemophilia,† headache, dizziness, nausea, vomiting, abdominal discomfort, fever, rash, peripheral neurologic symptoms, depression, sleep disorders
Darunavir [Prezista]	Dangerous drug interactions,† severe skin reactions, including SJS and TEN, hepatitis, diabetes (new onset or exacerbation),† immune reconstitution syndrome,† redistribution of adipose tissue,† renewed bleeding in patients with hemophilia,† headache, nausea, vomiting, abdominal discomfort, diarrhea, rash
Fosamprenavir [Lexiva]	Dangerous drug interactions,† severe skin reactions, including SJS and TEN, transaminase elevations (especially in patients with hepatitis B or C),† diabetes (new onset or exacerbation),† immune reconstitution syndrome,† redistribution of adipose tissue,† hyperlipidemia,† hemolytic anemia,† renewed bleeding in patients with hemophilia,† kidney stones,† headache, nausea, vomiting, diarrhea, rash
Indinavir [Crixivan]	Dangerous drug interactions,† hepatitis, including reports of liver failure,† hyperglycemia or diabetes (new onset or exacerbation),† hemolytic anemia,† renewed bleeding in patients with hemophilia,† kidney stones,† hyperbilirubinemia, headache, nausea, vomiting, abdominal pain, back pain
Lopinavir (with ritonavir) [Kaletra]	Dangerous drug interactions,† hepatotoxicity,† pancreatitis,† PR interval prolongation,† QT interval prolongation,† hyperglycemia or diabetes (new onset or exacerbation),† immune reconstitution syndrome,† redistribution of adipose tissue,† hyperlipidemia,† renewed bleeding in patients with hemophilia,† headache, nausea, vomiting, abdominal discomfort, indigestion, weakness
Nelfinavir [Viracept]	Dangerous drug interactions,† diabetes (new onset or exacerbation),† diarrhea
Ritonavir [Norvir]	Dangerous drug interactions,* hepatotoxicity,† pancreatitis,† severe hypersensitivity reactions,† PR interval prolongation,† hyperlipidemia,† diabetes (new onset or exacerbation),† immune reconstitution syndrome,† redistribution of adipose tissue,† renewed bleeding in patients with hemophilia,† nausea, vomiting, abdominal discomfort, diarrhea, fatigue, weakness, paresthesias, rash
Saquinavir [Invirase]	Dangerous drug interactions (including danger with ritonavir),† PR interval prolongation,† QT interval prolongation,† diabetes (new onset or exacerbation),† immune reconstitution syndrome,† redistribution of adipose tissue,† renewed bleeding in patients with hemophilia,† exacerbation of comorbid hepatic disease,† hyperlipidemia,† nausea, vomiting, abdominal pain, diarrhea, fatigue
Tipranavir [Aptivus]	Hepatotoxicity,* intracranial hemorrhage,* dangerous drug interactions,† renewed bleeding in patients with hemophilia,† serious rash,† hyperglycemia and diabetes (new onset or exacerbation),† immune reconstitution syndrome,† redistribution of adipose tissue,† renewed bleeding in patients with hemophilia,† increased bleeding risk in the absence of hemophilia,† hyperlipidemia,† headache, nausea, vomiting, indigestion, diarrhea
INTEGRASE STRAND TRANSFER INHIBITORS	
Raltegravir [Isentress]	Immune reconstitution syndrome,† headache, nausea, insomnia, fatigue, weakness, CK elevations
Elvitegravir [Viteka]	Immune reconstitution syndrome,† diarrhea
HIV FUSION INHIBITORS	
Enfuvirtide [Fuzeon]	Injection site reactions (98%),† hypersensitivity,† postinjection bleeding,† immune reconstitution syndrome,† pneumonia, nausea, diarrhea, fatigue
CCR5 ANTAGONISTS	
Maraviroc [Selzentry, Celsentri ♣]	Hepatotoxicity,* myocardial ischemia or infarction,† orthostatic hypotension (in patients with impaired renal function),† immune reconstitution syndrome,† increased risk for infection,† potential risk for malignancy,† fever, upper respiratory infections, cough, rash, dizziness

Note: Immune reconstitution syndrome describes the paradoxical inflammatory response to and exacerbation of preexisting infections after initiation of antiretroviral therapy. *Redistribution of adipose tissue* results in increased fat deposits in the trunk, abdomen, and dorsocervical region ("buffalo hump") and decreased body fat in the extremities and face.

*Black box warnings issued.

†Warnings issued.

BMD, bone mineral density; CK, creatine kinase; ENT, ear nose throat; SJS, Stevens-Johnson syndrome; TEN, toxic epidermal necrolysis.

Nonnucleoside Reverse Transcriptase Inhibitors

The NNRTIs differ from the NRTIs in structure and mechanism of action. As their name suggests, the NNRTIs have no structural relationship with naturally occurring nucleosides. Also, in contrast to the NRTIs, which inhibit synthesis of HIV DNA primarily by causing premature termination of the growing DNA strand, the NNRTIs bind to the active center of reverse transcriptase and thereby cause direct inhibition. Furthermore, whereas all NRTIs must undergo intracellular conversion to their active forms, the NNRTIs are active as administered. At this time, five NNRTIs are available: efavirenz [Sustiva], nevirapine [Viramune], delavirdine [Rescriptor], etravirine [Intelence], and rilpivirine [Edurant]. Pharmacokinetic properties of the NNRTIs are shown in Table 79.4. Significant adverse effects are provided in Table 79.3.

Protease Inhibitors

The PIs are among the most effective antiretroviral drugs available. When used in combination with NRTIs, they can reduce viral load to a level that is undetectable with current assays.

All of the PIs are substrates of (i.e., metabolized by) cytochrome P450 enzymes. Additionally, they all act as both inhibitors of some isoenzymes and inducers of others. Sometimes they may even act both as inhibitors and inducers of the same isoenzymes. For example, ritonavir is a PI commonly given with other PIs because it is a very strong inhibitor of CYP3A4, and all PIs are substrates of CYP3A4. But that isn't all! Ritonavir itself is primarily metabolized by CYP3A4 isoenzymes, plus it is a substrate of CYP1A2, CYP2B6, and CYP2D6 isoenzymes. In addition to its strong inhibition of CYP3A4, ritonavir also strongly inhibits CYP2C8 and CYP2D6 isoenzymes. To a lesser extent, it inhibits CYP2C19, CYP2C9, and CYP2E1 isoenzymes. Finally, ritonavir is a weak to moderate inducer of CYP1A2, CYP2C9, and CYP3A4 isoenzymes. But wait! Add to this that ritonavir is commonly given with other PIs that have their own functions as substrates, inducers, and inhibitors. Certainly it is easy to understand why PIs are subject to a bewildering array of drug interactions.

As with other antiretroviral drugs, HIV resistance can be a significant problem. Mutant strains of HIV that are resistant to one PI are likely to be cross-resistant to other PIs. In contrast, because PIs do not share the same mechanism as the reverse transcriptase inhibitors, fusion inhibitors, INSTIs, or CCR5 antagonists, cross-resistance between PIs and these other antiretroviral drugs does not occur. To reduce the risk for resistance, PIs should never be used alone; rather, they should always be combined with at least one reverse transcriptase inhibitor, and preferably two.

Nine PIs are available: atazanavir, darunavir, fosamprenavir, indinavir, lopinavir (with ritonavir), nelfinavir, ritonavir, saquinavir, and tipranavir. Pharmacokinetic properties of PIs are shown in Table 79.5. Significant adverse effects are provided in Table 79.3.

Integrase Strand Transfer Inhibitors

Actions and Use

HIV integrase strand transfer inhibitors, or simply *integrase inhibitors,* target HIV by terminating the integration of HIV into DNA. Integrase is one of three viral enzymes needed for HIV replication. As its name implies, integrase inserts HIV genetic material into the DNA of CD4 cells. By inhibiting integrase, these drugs prevent insertion of HIV DNA and thereby stop HIV replication. We currently have two approved INSTIs: raltegravir and elvitegravir. Both are indicated for combined use with other antiretroviral agents to treat adults infected with HIV-1. *Elvitegravir* is incapable of achieving therapeutic levels when given alone, owing to extensive metabolism by the P450 enzyme system, especially CYP3A

TABLE 79.4 ▪ Pharmacokinetic Properties of Nonnucleoside Reverse Transcriptase Inhibitors

	Delavirdine (DLV)	Efavirenz (EFV)	Etravirine (ETR)	Nevirapine (NVP)	Rilpivirine (RPV)
Trade name	Rescriptor	Sustiva	Intelence	Viramune, Viramune XR	Edurant
Bioavailability	85%	Data not available	Data not available	More than 90%	Data not available
Serum half-life	5.8 hr	40–55 hr	41 hr	25–30 hr	50 hr
Metabolism	Metabolized by CYP3A and possibly CYP2D6	Metabolized by CYP3A4 and CYP2B6	Metabolized by CYP3A4, CYP2C9, and CYP2C19	Metabolized by P450	Metabolized by CYP3A4
Elimination	Urine (51%) and feces (44%)	Urine (14%–34%) and feces (16%–61%)	Urine (1.2%) and feces (93.7%)	Urine (80%) and feces (10%)	Urine (6.1%) and feces (85%)

IR, immediate release; XR, extended release.

TABLE 79.5 ▪ Pharmacokinetic Properties of Protease Inhibitors

	Atazanavir (ATV)	Darunavir (DRV)	Fosamprenavir (FPV)	Indinavir (IDV)
Trade name	Reyataz	Prezista	Lexiva, Telzir ♣	Crixivan
Bioavailability	Not determined	82% (with ritonavir)	Not determined	65%
Serum half-life	7 hr	15 hr (with ritonavir)	7.7 hr	1.5–2 hr
Metabolism	Hepatic, primarily by CYP3A	Hepatic CYP3A	Metabolized to amprenavir in the gastrointestinal system; hepatic metabolism primarily by CYP3A4	Hepatic by CYP3A4
Elimination	Primarily in feces (20% unmetabolized) then urine (7% unmetabolized)	Primarily in feces (41% unmetabolized) then urine (8% unmetabolized)	Primarily in feces then urine (1% unmetabolized)	Primarily in feces (19% unmetabolized) then urine (9% unmetabolized)

PATIENT-CENTERED CARE ACROSS THE LIFE SPAN

Nonnucleoside Reverse Transcriptase Inhibitors

Life Stage	Considerations or Concerns
Children	The safety of rilpivirine has not been adequately evaluated in children younger than 12 years. Delavirdine is approved for children 16 years and older. Children taking efavirenz have had a greater incidence of rash than did adults. It is not recommended for children younger than 3 months or weighing less than 3.5 kg.
Pregnant women	Etravirine, nevirapine, and rilpivirine are in FDA Pregnancy Risk Category B. Delavirdine is in FDA Pregnancy Risk Category C. Neural tube defects have been associated with efavirenz; contraception is recommended during treatment and for 3 months after treatment is discontinued.
Breastfeeding women	Breastfeeding should be avoided by women with HIV because there is a danger of transmitting the virus.
Older adults	Each drug in this category identified insufficient numbers of older adults in clinical trials. Individual patient status regarding cardiac, hepatic, and renal status or comorbidities.

PATIENT-CENTERED CARE ACROSS THE LIFE SPAN

Protease Inhibitors

Life Stage	Considerations or Concerns
Children	Pediatric dosing is available for all drugs in this category. Unlike most, darunavir is indicated only for children 6 years and older; although it is sometimes prescribed for younger children, it should not be used for children younger than 3 years because of increased risks for toxicity. Children taking indinavir are at increased risk for nephrolithiasis.
Pregnant women	Nelfinavir, ritonavir, and saquinavir are in FDA Pregnancy Risk Category B. Darunavir, fosamprenavir, indinavir, lopinavir/ritonavir, and tipranavir are in FDA Pregnancy Risk Category C. Updated labeling for atazanavir does not include a risk category (see new FDA guidelines in Chapter 7) but reports that there is no evidence that atazanavir causes major birth defects. Labeling emphasizes that atazanavir should be accompanied by ritonavir when prescribed for pregnant women.
Breastfeeding women	Breastfeeding should be avoided by women with HIV because there is a danger of transmitting the virus.
Older adults	Clinical trials did not enroll sufficient numbers of patients 65 years and older to adequately determine comparative responses to younger subjects. Consider hepatic, renal, or cardiac function and comorbidity in monitoring.

PATIENT-CENTERED CARE ACROSS THE LIFE SPAN

Integrase Strand Inhibitors, HIV Fusion Inhibitors, and CCR5 Antagonists

Life Stage	Considerations or Concerns
Children	Safety of elvitegravir has not been adequately evaluated for patients younger than 12 years. Maraviroc is not indicated for children younger than 16 years.
Pregnant women	Elvitegravir, enfuvirtide, and maraviroc are in FDA Pregnancy Risk Category B. Raltegravir is in FDA Pregnancy Risk Category C.
Breastfeeding women	Breastfeeding should be avoided by women with HIV because there is a danger of transmitting the virus.
Older adults	Clinical trials did not enroll sufficient numbers of patients 65 years and older to adequately determine comparative responses to younger subjects. Consider hepatic, renal, or cardiac function and comorbidity in considering therapy.

Lopinavir/Ritonavir (LPV/r)	Nelfinavir (NFV)	Ritonavir (RTV)	Saquinavir (SQV)	Tipranavir (TPV)
Kaletra	Viracept	Norvir	Invirase	Aptivus
Not determined	20%–80%	Adequate	Low (4%) and erratic	Not determined
5–6 hr	3.5–5 hr	3–5 hr	1–2 hr	6 hr
Hepatic by CYP3A4	Hepatic by CYP2C19 and CYP3A4	Hepatic by CYP3A4 and CYP2D6	Hepatic by CYP3A4	Hepatic by CYP3A4
Primarily in feces (20% unmetabolized) then urine (3% unmetabolized)	Feces (22% unmetabolized) with only 1%–2% excretion in urine	Primarily in feces (34% unmetabolized) then urine (4% unmetabolized)	Primarily in feces then urine (extensively metabolized before excretion)	Primarily in feces then urine (most unmetabolized when administered with ritonavir)

TABLE 79.6 ▪ Pharmacokinetic Properties of Integrase Strand Inhibitors, HIV Fusion Inhibitors, and CCR5 Antagonists

	Raltegravir	Elvitegravir	Enfuvirtide	Maraviroc
Trade name	Isentress	Viteka	Fuzeon	Selzentry, Celsentri ♣
Bioavailability	Not established	Unknown	SubQ: 84.3% (±) 15.5%	23%–33%
Serum half-life	9 hr	9 hr	4 hr	14–18 hr
Metabolism	Hepatic glucuronidation	CYP3A isoenzymes and hepatic glucuronidation	Peptidase and proteinases in liver and kidneys	CYP3A isoenzymes
Elimination	Feces (unchanged) followed by urine (9% unchanged)	Predominantly feces (5%–7% urine)	Unknown*	Predominantly feces (25% unchanged) followed by urine (8% unchanged

*The most recent product labeling states, "Mass balance studies to determine elimination pathway(s) of enfuvirtide have not been performed in humans."
SubQ, subcutaneous.

isoenzymes. It must be combined with a drug that boosts the activity of elvitegravir by inhibiting CYP3A isoenzymes. Most often it is available in combination with cobicistat, a CYP3A inhibitor that has no intrinsic activity against HIV. It is also available as a single agent, Vitekta. Product labeling for Vitekta specifies that it must be given with an HIV protease inhibitor and an HIV antiretroviral drug such as ritonavir; however, it should not be administered with cobicistat. Pharmacokinetic properties for these drugs, as well as for the representative drugs in the two categories that follow, are provided in Table 79.6. Significant adverse reactions are detailed in Table 79.3.

HIV Fusion Inhibitors

HIV fusion inhibitors are reserved for treating HIV-1 infection that has become resistant to other antiretroviral agents. Specifically, the drug is indicated for HIV-1 infection in patients 6 years and older who are treatment experienced and have evidence of HIV replication despite ongoing antiretroviral therapy.

Enfuvirtide [Fuzeon], widely known as T-20, is the first and only HIV fusion inhibitor. Unlike most other drugs for HIV, which inhibit essential viral enzymes—either reverse transcriptase, integrase, or protease—enfuvirtide blocks entry of HIV into CD4 T cells.

Enfuvirtide prevents the HIV envelope from fusing with the cell membrane of CD4 cells (see Fig. 79.2, step 2) and thereby blocks viral entry and replication. Fusion inhibition results from binding of enfuvirtide to gp41, a subunit of the glycoproteins embedded in the HIV envelope (see Fig. 79.1). As a result of enfuvirtide binding, the glycoprotein becomes rigid and hence cannot undergo the configurational change needed to permit fusion of HIV with the cell membrane.

Chemokine Receptor 5 (CCR5) Antagonists

Actions

Maraviroc [Selzentry, Celsentri ♣] is the first representative of a new class of antiretroviral drugs: the *chemokine receptor 5* (CCR5) *antagonists.* As discussed previously, CCR5 is a coreceptor that some strains of HIV must bind with to enter CD4 cells. Maraviroc binds with CCR5 and thereby blocks viral entry. HIV strains that require CCR5 for entry are referred to as being *CCR5 tropic.* Between 50% and 60% of patients are infected with this type of HIV. Maraviroc and enfuvirtide (a fusion inhibitor) are the only antiretroviral drugs that block HIV entry. All other agents inhibit HIV enzymes, either reverse transcriptase, integrase, or protease.

MANAGEMENT OF HIV INFECTION

Thanks to the drugs we have today, HIV infection has been transformed from a near-certain death sentence to a manageable chronic disease. Most patients take several antiretroviral drugs—typically two NRTIs combined with either a PI or NNRTI. These highly effective regimens can reduce plasma HIV to undetectable levels, causing CD4 T-cell counts to return toward normal and thereby restoring some immune function. However, despite these advances, treatment cannot cure HIV. In all cases, discontinuation of antiretroviral drugs has led to a rebound in plasma HIV.

Therapy of HIV disease is often complex. Patients take a combination of drugs for HIV itself—and may take additional drugs to manage treatment side effects (e.g., hyperlipidemia, lipodystrophy, depression) along with drugs to prevent or treat opportunistic infections. As a result, the potential for adverse effects and drug interactions is large. Also, among the drugs used for HIV, emergence of resistance is common. Furthermore, adverse effects and pill burden make adherence difficult. Because of these complexities, management is best done by a specialist with extensive experience in treating HIV.

Because HIV infection is usually managed by specialists, we will not delve into management in this chapter. For those who would like to know more, treatment guidelines developed by the Panel on Clinical Practices for Treatment of HIV Infection, convened by the U.S. Department of Health and Human Services (DHHS), are available online. Two primary documents—*Guidelines for the Use of Antiretroviral Agents in HIV-1–Infected Adults and Adolescents* (updated January 28, 2016) and *Guidelines for the Use of Antiretroviral Agents in Pediatric HIV Infection* (updated March 1, 2016)—are available online at https://aidsinfo.nih.gov/guidelines, along with companion guidelines for treating pediatric and pregnant patients, and for prophylaxis after HIV exposure.

PREVENTING HIV INFECTION WITH DRUGS

Although nonspecialists are less likely to manage HIV infection, they may be commonly involved in treating patients prophylactically. The following section focuses on prevention of HIV infection.

Treatment as Prevention

Treatment of HIV-positive people with ART greatly reduces the risk for transmitting HIV to their sexual partners. There are indications for both preexposure and postexposure prophylaxis.

Preexposure Prophylaxis

The term *preexposure prophylaxis* (PrEP) refers to the use of antiretroviral drugs to *prevent* HIV infection, rather than treat it. In this section, we consider the ability of antiretroviral drugs to reduce HIV *acquisition* when given to an HIV-*negative* person.

Oral Preexposure Prophylaxis

In 2010, results of the *Pre-Exposure Prophylaxis Initiative* study, a study of HIV-negative men also known as iPrEx, demonstrated that tenofovir/emtricitabine [Truvada] could reduce infection risk by 44% to 73%. These results led the CDC to recommend use of tenofovir/emtricitabine for PrEP. Current indications are only for those considered at high risk for HIV acquisition. Those identified at high risk are people who (1) have sexual partners with known HIV-1 infection *or* are sexually active with people who belong to social networks with high HIV-1 prevalence *and* (2) have one or more of the following risk factors:

- Do not regularly use condoms
- Have sexually transmitted infections
- Engage in sex for money, drugs, or other supplies
- Use recreational drugs or are dependent on alcohol
- Are imprisoned

Preexposure guidelines were updated in 2014. The guidelines–*Clinical Practice Guideline: Pre-Exposure Prophylaxis for the Prevention of HIV Infection in the United States*—are available at https://aidsinfo.nih.gov/guidelines.

Postexposure Prophylaxis

One-time exposure to HIV carries a small, but nonetheless real, risk for infection. Sources of exposure include unprotected vaginal or anal intercourse, receptive oral intercourse, sharing a contaminated needle, accidental needle sticks, and being splashed with blood and other body fluids. Risk is especially high after exposure to a large quantity of infected blood or blood with a high virus titer, and after deep percutaneous penetration with a needle recently removed from the vein of an infected person.

The risk for developing HIV disease after a single exposure can be reduced—but not eliminated—with prophylactic antiretroviral drugs. Presumably, protection results from preventing initial cellular infection and local propagation of HIV, thereby allowing host immune defenses to eliminate the virus before it can become established. To be effective, postexposure prophylaxis (PEP) should be initiated as soon as possible after HIV exposure—preferably within 1 or 2 hours, and no later than 72 hours—and should continue for 28 days. All patients should undergo testing for antibodies against HIV, preferably at the time of exposure, and then 6 weeks, 12 weeks, and 6 months after exposure.

Recommendations for PEP are based on whether the exposure was nonoccupational or occupational, defined as exposure of health care personnel while on the job.

Nonoccupational Postexposure Prophylaxis

For nonoccupational PEP, current guidelines recommend ART regimens much like those employed for initial therapy of established HIV infection. Two three-drug regimens are preferred:

- *NNRTI-based:* efavirenz + (lamivudine or emtricitabine) + (zidovudine or tenofovir)
- *PI-based:* lopinavir/ritonavir + (lamivudine or emtricitabine) + zidovudine

Detailed information on nonoccupational PEP is available in a document titled *Antiretroviral Postexposure Prophylaxis After Sexual, Injection-Drug Use, or Other Nonoccupational Exposure to HIV in the United States* (revised January 21, 2005), which can be found online at https://aidsinfo.nih.gov/guidelines.

Occupational Postexposure Prophylaxis

Recommendations for occupational PEP are based on the risk for acquiring HIV, which is determined by multiple factors, including (1) the nature of the exposure (skin penetration vs. body fluid splashed onto nonintact skin or mucous membrane); (2) the severity of the exposure (e.g., shallow skin penetration with a solid probe, deep skin penetration with a large-bore hollow needle, surface exposure to small volume of sputum, surface exposure to a large volume of blood); and (3) the HIV status of the exposure source (e.g., asymptomatic with a low viral load, symptomatic with a high viral load). Preferred regimens, based on risk for transmission, may involve one of the following options:

- No PEP
- 2 NRTIs (e.g., emtricitabine plus tenofovir)
- PI-based regimen (e.g., lopinavir/ritonavir plus emtricitabine plus tenofovir)

Please note that our discussion of this important topic is greatly simplified. For detailed information, you can refer to a document titled *Updated U.S. Public Health Service Guidelines for the Management of Occupational Exposures to HIV and Recommendations for Postexposure Prophylaxis* (revised November 2013), which is available at https://aidsinfo.nih.gov/guidelines. Another valuable resource for recommendations on managing PEP (occupational, nonoccupational, or perinatal) is a 24-hour National HIV/AIDS Clinicians' Consultative Center through the University of California, San Francisco. Information is available by calling the PEP hotline at 1-888-448-4911.

HIV VACCINES

Development of an HIV vaccine is critical to controlling the AIDS epidemic worldwide. Although HIV infection can now be managed with ART, treatment is expensive and potentially dangerous and must continue lifelong. Furthermore, ART is largely unavailable in developing countries, where most AIDS cases occur. Accordingly, vaccine development has been assigned high priority.

Obstacles to Vaccine Development

Making a safe and effective vaccine against HIV has proved exceedingly and unexpectedly difficult. Obstacles include the wide global variation in HIV strains, lack of information on natural immunity to HIV, multiple modes of HIV transmission, and lack of an ideal animal model for studying vaccine efficacy. Also, scientists are concerned that the vaccine may need to (1) *prevent* HIV infection, rather than minimize it, and may need to (2) stimulate cell-mediated immunity in addition to humoral immunity. These two concerns are discussed next.

Vaccines do not prevent infection—they only attenuate it. By priming the immune system, vaccines reduce microbial replication and accelerate microbial kill. As a result, infection does not spread as far as it would in an unvaccinated person and does not injure as many cells. Unfortunately, HIV is different from all other pathogens: HIV kills the very cells that are meant to attack it and that vaccination is meant to stimulate. Given the nature of HIV, we must ask, "Will a vaccine that permits HIV to infect even a small number of immune cells be able to contain the infection—or will HIV eventually break through?" The answer is unknown.

Vaccines elicit two kinds of immune responses: *humoral immunity* (production of antibodies) and *cell-mediated immunity* (activation of cytotoxic T lymphocytes, also known as killer T cells). Most authorities agree that, to be effective, an HIV vaccine should elicit both types of responses. Why? The answer is simple: We already know that HIV-positive people produce billions of antibodies against HIV, and yet the infection progresses relentlessly; hence, a vaccine that only stimulates humoral immunity would seem likely to fail. Unfortunately, although it's relatively easy to make a safe vaccine that stimulates humoral immunity, it's much harder to make a safe vaccine that stimulates cellular immunity. Why? Because the best way to stimulate cellular immunity is with a *live virus* vaccine—in this case, a vaccine made from HIV that has been attenuated by removing some of its genes, but has not been killed. The problem is that live virus vaccines pose a risk for infection—a risk that is unacceptable with HIV. The potential danger of this approach was underscored when monkeys were given a simian version of such a vaccine and subsequently developed simian AIDS, presumably from the vaccine itself.

Current Status of Vaccine Development

To date, only one vaccine—AIDSVAX—has undergone a phase 3 trial. AIDSVAX is a bivalent vaccine composed of gp120 proteins, which are found in the outer envelope of HIV. The vaccine activates the antibody-producing arm of the immune system, but does not activate killer T cells. The phase 3 trial enrolled 5095 HIV-negative men and 308 HIV-negative women, all considered at high risk for acquiring HIV. One third of participants received placebo, and two thirds were injected with vaccine. The result? HIV infection developed in 5.8% of placebo recipients and 5.7% of those given the vaccine. Clearly, AIDSVAX didn't work. These results were especially disappointing in that, in an earlier trial, the vaccine elicited production of neutralizing antibodies in 99% of study subjects. Apparently, although antibodies were made, they were unable to prevent infection.

The current best hope for protection is to combine a vaccine similar to AIDSVAX (i.e., a purified HIV envelope protein) with a "vectored" vaccine, consisting of a harmless virus, such as canarypox, that has been genetically engineered to produce HIV proteins. In phase 1 and 2 clinical trials, this approach appeared safe and elicited both antibody production and activation of killer T cells.

KEEPING CURRENT

Drug therapy of HIV infection is continuously evolving. New drugs are being developed, knowledge of existing drugs is expanding, and new drug combinations are being studied. The following websites are good sources of current information:

- **AIDSinfo (aidsinfo.nih.gov).** This site, maintained by the DHHS, has information on treatment guidelines, drugs, vaccines, and clinical trials. Links to other HIV/AIDS-related sites are there, too. Content is presented in English and Spanish. You can sign up for e-mail notification of updates.
- **HIV and AIDS Activities (http://www.fda.gov/forhealthprofessionals/liaisonactivities/ucm404963.htm).** This page on the U.S. Food and Drug Administration (FDA) website offers the latest information on approved drugs, drug development, and drugs in clinical trials.

PRESCRIBING AND MONITORING CONSIDERATIONS

When patients are taking antiretroviral drugs, always use a drug interaction checker (software application or online) to verify safety before prescribing any new drug.

Instruct the patient not to take any over-the-counter drugs or supplements without first checking with the provider to verify safety.

Nucleoside/Nucleotide Reverse Transcriptase Inhibitors

Therapeutic Goals

Treatment has six goals: maximal and durable suppression of viral load, restoration and/or preservation of immune function, improvement of quality of life, reduction of HIV-related morbidity and mortality, reduction of HIV sexual transmission, and prevention of vertical HIV transmission.

Baseline Data

All NRTIs

Assess the patient's clinical status and obtain a plasma HIV RNA level and CD4 T-cell count.

Zidovudine. Obtain a hemoglobin value and granulocyte count.

Abacavir. Screen for HLA-B*5701, which indicates abacavir hypersensitivity.

Identifying High-Risk Patients

Didanosine

The risk for pancreatitis is increased by a history of alcoholism or pancreatitis and by use of IV pentamidine.

Zidovudine

The risk for hematologic toxicity is increased by a low granulocyte count; low levels of hemoglobin, vitamin B_{12}, or folic acid; and concurrent use of drugs that are myelosuppressive, nephrotoxic, or toxic to circulating blood cells.

Ongoing Monitoring and Interventions

Evaluating Therapeutic Effects

Plasma HIV RNA. Success is indicated by a reduction in plasma HIV RNA. With ART, plasma HIV RNA should decline to 10% of baseline within 2 to 8 weeks. After 16 to 20 weeks of treatment, plasma HIV RNA should reach its minimum. Ideally, the minimum will be undetectable with sensitive assays.

CD4 T-Cell Counts. As viral load decreases, CD4 T-cell counts may rise, indicating some restoration of immune function.

Minimizing Adverse Effects

All NRTIs. Giving a combination of NRTIs to a pregnant patient may increase the risk for lactic acidosis and hepatic steatosis. Accordingly, it would seem prudent to avoid these combinations during pregnancy.

Anemia and Neutropenia. *Zidovudine* can cause severe anemia and neutropenia. Determine hematologic status before treatment and at least every 4 weeks thereafter. In the event of severe anemia (hemoglobin below 7.5 g/dL or down 25% from the pretreatment baseline) or severe neutropenia (granulocyte count below 750 cells/mL or down 50% from the pretreatment baseline), interrupt treatment until there is evidence of bone marrow recovery. If neutropenia and anemia are less severe, a reduction in dosage may be sufficient. Some patients may require multiple transfusions. Granulocyte colony-stimulating factors can be used to reverse neutropenia. Epoetin alfa (recombinant erythropoietin) can be given to reduce transfusion requirements in patients with anemia, provided endogenous erythropoietin levels are not already elevated.

Lactic Acidosis With Hepatic Steatosis. Potentially fatal lactic acidosis and hepatic steatosis can occur with *all NRTIs.* Diagnosis is done by measuring lactate in arterial blood. If lactic acidosis is present, the NRTI should be discontinued.

Pancreatitis. *Didanosine* can cause potentially fatal pancreatitis. Monitor patients for signs of developing pancreatitis (elevated serum amylase in association with elevated serum triglycerides, decreased serum calcium, and nausea, vomiting, or abdominal pain). If evolving pancreatitis is diagnosed, didanosine should be withdrawn.

Peripheral Neuropathy. *Didanosine* and *stavudine* can cause painful peripheral neuropathy. Opioid analgesics may be required to treat pain of *severe* neuropathy. Neuropathy may reverse if didanosine and stavudine are withdrawn early.

Patient Education

NUCLEOSIDE/NUCLEOTIDE REVERSE TRANSCRIPTASE INHIBITORS

Instruct patients to adhere closely to the prescribed dosing schedule. Emphasize the need to avoid taking any over-the-counter drugs or supplements without first checking with the provider to verify safety.

All NRTIs, except didanosine, may be taken without regard to meals.

Patients taking NRTIs are at risk of lactic acidosis and hepatic steatosis. Inform patients about symptoms—nausea, vomiting, abdominal pain, malaise, fatigue, anorexia, and hyperventilation—and instruct them to report these immediately.

Inform patients that, even when HIV RNA is undetectable, they are still infectious and hence should avoid behaviors that can transmit HIV.

Abacavir. Inform patients of hypersensitivity reactions that are possible with this abacavir. Teach them common symptoms—fever, rash, myalgia, arthralgia, nausea, vomiting, diarrhea, abdominal pain, pharyngitis, dyspnea, and cough—and instruct them to report these immediately.

Didanosine. Instruct patients to take didanosine 30 minutes before meals or 2 hours after. Instruct patients taking powdered didanosine to pour the contents of one packet into 4 ounces of water (not fruit juice or any other acid-containing beverage), stir the mixture until the drug dissolves (about 2–3 minutes), and then drink the solution immediately. Also, inform patients about early signs of neuropathy (numbness, tingling, or pain in hands and feet) and instruct them to report these immediately.

Zidovudine. Instruct patients to report new or worsening symptoms of anemia (e.g. pallor, weakness) or neutropenia (evidence of infection). To prevent exposure to illness, patients should be cautioned to avoid contact with people who are ill and to avoid areas where people may congregate in large numbers.

Hypersensitivity Reactions. *Abacavir* can cause potentially fatal hypersensitivity reactions. Before using abacavir, screen for HLA-B*5701 (a genetic variant associated with abacavir hypersensitivity), and don't use the drug if the variant is detected.

If a hypersensitivity reaction is diagnosed—or even strongly suspected—abacavir should be discontinued and never used again.

Exacerbation of Hepatitis. In patients coinfected with HBV, withdrawal of *emtricitabine, lamivudine,* or *tenofovir* may result in severe exacerbation of hepatitis. Inform patients of this possibility.

HIV Transmission. Reduction of plasma HIV RNA may create a false sense of safety. Accordingly, inform patients that, even when HIV RNA is undetectable, they are still infectious and hence should avoid behaviors that can transmit HIV.

Minimizing Adverse Interactions

Zidovudine. Drugs that are myelosuppressive, nephrotoxic, or directly toxic to circulating blood cells can increase the risk for hematologic toxicity. Drugs of concern include ganciclovir, dapsone, pentamidine, pyrimethamine, trimethoprim/

sulfamethoxazole, amphotericin B, flucytosine, vincristine, vinblastine, and doxorubicin.

Ribavirin and Allopurinol. Ribavirin and allopurinol can increase levels of the active form of *didanosine,* thereby posing a risk for toxicity. Avoid these combinations.

Nonnucleoside Reverse Transcriptase Inhibitors

Therapeutic Goals

Treatment has six goals: maximal and durable suppression of viral load, restoration and/or preservation of immune function, improvement of quality of life, reduction of HIV-related morbidity and mortality, reduction of HIV sexual transmission, and prevention of vertical HIV transmission.

Baseline Data

Assess the patient's clinical status and obtain a plasma HIV RNA level, CD4 T-cell count, and liver function tests. Perform a pregnancy test before giving efavirenz.

Ongoing Monitoring and Interventions

Evaluating Therapeutic Effects

See information for NRTIs.

Minimizing Adverse Effects

Rash and Other Hypersensitivity Reactions. Rash is common and may range from mild to severe. Rarely, rash evolves into a life-threatening reaction: Stevens-Johnson syndrome, toxic epidermal necrolysis, or erythema multiforme. Mild rash can be treated with an antihistamine or topical glucocorticoid. If a severe reaction develops, the NNRTI should be withdrawn immediately. To minimize risk, use a low dosage for the first 14 days of treatment, and then increase the dosage if rash has not occurred.

Hepatotoxicity. NNRTIs can cause hepatotoxicity, which may be severe. Risk is greatest with nevirapine. Perform liver function tests at baseline and periodically thereafter. Interrupt treatment if tests indicate significant liver injury.

CNS Symptoms. Efavirenz frequently causes CNS symptoms (e.g., dizziness, insomnia, impaired consciousness, drowsiness, vivid dreams, nightmares). If severe symptoms occur (e.g., delusions, hallucinations, severe acute depression), efavirenz should be withdrawn.

Depression. Rilpivirine can cause depression. Assess for evidence of depression at each clinical encounter.

Birth Defects. Efavirenz is teratogenic. Perform a pregnancy test before treatment and ensure that the female patient had adequate contraception.

HIV Transmission. Reduction of plasma HIV RNA may create a false sense of safety. Accordingly, inform patients that, even when HIV RNA is undetectable, they are still infectious and hence must avoid behaviors that can transmit HIV.

Minimizing Adverse Interactions

Nevirapine. Nevirapine *induces* cytochrome P450 and can thereby decrease levels of other drugs. Effects on PIs, hormonal contraceptives, and methadone are of particular concern.

Combining nevirapine with *St. John's wort* or *rifampin,* which also induce P450, can decrease nevirapine levels, and hence these combinations should be avoided.

Delavirdine. Delavirdine *inhibits* P450 and can thereby increase levels of other drugs. To avoid toxicity from excessive drug levels, patients must not take cisapride, alprazolam, midazolam, triazolam, lovastatin, or simvastatin—or astemizole or terfenadine, which are no longer available in the United States. In addition, the following drugs should be used with caution: indinavir, saquinavir, clarithromycin, dapsone, warfarin, quinidine, ergot alkaloids, phosphodiesterase type 5 inhibitors (e.g., sildenafil [Viagra]), and the dihydropyridine-type calcium channel blockers.

Antacids, histamine-2 receptor blockers, proton pump inhibitors, and *buffered formulations of didanosine* can decrease absorption of delavirdine.

Efavirenz. Efavirenz *competes with other drugs for metabolism by P450* and can thereby increase their levels. To avoid toxicity from excessive drug levels, the patient must not take astemizole, terfenadine, cisapride, midazolam, triazolam, dihydroergotamine, or ergotamine.

Efavirenz *induces P450* and can thereby accelerate metabolism of other drugs, including two PIs: *saquinavir* and *indinavir.* Avoid combined use with saquinavir. Increase indinavir dosage.

By inducing P450, efavirenz can decrease the efficacy of *hormonal contraceptives.* Contraceptive failure can result.

St. John's wort induces P450 and can reduce levels of efavirenz. The combination should not be used.

Etravirine. Etravirine competes with other drugs for metabolism by P450 and can thereby increase their levels.

Patient Education

NONNUCLEOSIDE REVERSE TRANSCRIPTASE INHIBITORS

Explain the need to adhere closely to the prescribed dosing schedule.

Inform patients about signs and symptoms of an evolving hypersensitivity reaction—severe rash, or rash accompanied by fever, malaise, fatigue, blisters, oral lesions, conjunctivitis, facial edema, hepatitis, muscle aches, or joint aches—and instruct them to report these immediately.

Explain to patients that, even when HIV RNA is undetectable, they are still infectious and hence should avoid behaviors that can transmit HIV.

Delavirdine. Inform patients that delavirdine may be taken with or without food. Inform patients who cannot swallow delavirdine tablets whole that they can mix the 100-mg tablets (but not the 200-mg tablets) with 3 or more ounces of water. Advise patients with achlorhydria to take delavirdine with an acidic beverage, such as orange or cranberry juice.

Efavirenz. Inform patients that CNS symptoms typically resolve in 2 to 4 weeks, despite ongoing efavirenz use, and that taking efavirenz at bedtime can minimize CNS effects. Also, inform women about the potential for fetal harm, and instruct them to use effective contraception, preferably a barrier method of birth control (e.g., condom) in conjunction with a hormonal method (e.g., oral contraceptive) unless contraindicated.

Rilpivirine. Instruct patients to contact their provider immediately if they start feeling sad, hopeless, or suicidal.

The plasma concentration of etravirine is lowered by use of St. John's wort, anticonvulsants, darunavir/ritonavir, systemic dexamethasone, rifampin, rifapentine, ritonavir, saquinavir/ritonavir, and tipranavir/ritonavir.

Rilpivirine. All of the following drugs significantly *reduce* rilpivirine levels and hence are *contraindicated:* (1) antiseizure drugs (carbamazepine, oxcarbazepine, phenobarbital, phenytoin); (2) rifamycins (rifabutin, rifampin, rifapentine); (3) proton pump inhibitors (esomeprazole, lansoprazole, omeprazole, pantoprazole, rabeprazole); (4) glucocorticoids (when given in repeated doses); and (5) St. John's wort.

Antacids (e.g., aluminum hydroxide, magnesium hydroxide, calcium carbonate) can reduce rilpivirine levels. If taken by patients, write prescription so that antacids are taken at least 2 hours before rilpivirine or 4 hours after.

Histamine-2 receptor blockers (e.g., cimetidine, famotidine, ranitidine) can reduce rilpivirine levels. If these drugs are needed, write prescription to take histamine-2 blockers at least 12 hours before rilpivirine or 4 hours after.

Azole antifungal drugs (e.g., ketoconazole, itraconazole, fluconazole) and macrolide antibiotics (e.g., erythromycin, clarithromycin, troleandomycin) can increase rilpivirine levels. Use with caution.

Patient Education

PROTEASE INHIBITORS

All PIs can cause hyperglycemia and diabetes. Instruct patients to report any new symptoms (e.g., polydipsia, polyphagia, polyuria).

Forewarn patients that all PIs may cause accumulation of fat on the waist, stomach, breasts, and back of the neck, and loss of fat from the face, arms, buttocks, and legs.

To reduce risk of bone loss, encourage patients to ensure adequate intake of calcium and vitamin D.

St. John's wort induces P450 and can reduce levels of PIs. Warn patients not to use St. John's wort.

Inform patients that, even when HIV RNA is undetectable, they are still infectious and hence should avoid behaviors that can transmit HIV.

Indinavir and fosamprenavir: Inform patients that these drugs may cause kidney stones. Instruct patients to report symptoms: pain in the abdomen, groin, testicles, or side of the back. To decrease the risk for nephrolithiasis, instruct patients to consume at least 48 ounces (1.5 L) of water daily.

Protease Inhibitors

Therapeutic Goals

Treatment has six goals: maximal and durable suppression of viral load, restoration and/or preservation of immune function, improvement of quality of life, reduction of HIV-related morbidity and mortality, reduction of HIV sexual transmission, and prevention of vertical HIV transmission.

Baseline Data

Assess the patient's clinical status and obtain a plasma HIV RNA level and CD4 T-cell count. Measure serum transaminases and blood glucose.

Identifying High-Risk Patients

Lopinavir/ritonavir oral solution is contraindicated for full-term infants (until 14 days after birth) and preterm infants (until 14 days after their predicted due date).

Use *atazanavir, saquinavir,* and *lopinavir/ritonavir* with caution in patients with structural heart disease, cardiac conduction disturbances, and ischemic heart disease, and in those taking other drugs that prolong the PR interval.

Avoid *lopinavir/ritonavir* and *saquinavir* in patients with congenital long QT syndrome and in those taking drugs that prolong the QT interval.

Ongoing Monitoring and Interventions

Evaluating Therapeutic Effects

See information for NRTIs.

Minimizing Adverse Effects

Hyperglycemia/Diabetes. All PIs can cause hyperglycemia and diabetes. In patients with existing diabetes, monitor blood glucose closely. To detect new-onset diabetes, measure blood glucose at baseline, every 3 to 4 months during the first year of treatment, and less frequently thereafter. Diabetes can be treated with insulin and oral antidiabetic agents (e.g., metformin).

Fat Redistribution. PIs may cause accumulation of fat on the waist, stomach, breasts, and back of the neck, and loss of fat from the face, arms, buttocks, and legs. Drug withdrawal may cause symptoms to resolve, but is not recommended. Injections of Sculptra can be used to compensate for loss of facial fat. Injection of tesamorelin [Egrifta] can reduce excess visceral abdominal fat.

Hyperlipidemia. All PIs can elevate cholesterol and triglycerides, thereby posing a risk for cardiovascular events and pancreatitis. Monitoring plasma cholesterol and triglycerides every 3 to 4 months may be wise. If drugs are given to lower lipid levels, two agents—lovastatin and simvastatin—should be avoided.

Increased Bleeding in Patients With Hemophilia. PIs may increase the risk for bleeding in patients with hemophilia. Higher doses of coagulation factors may be needed.

Increased Transaminase Levels. PIs can increase serum levels of transaminases. Exercise caution in patients with chronic liver disease (e.g., hepatitis B or C, cirrhosis). Measure serum transaminases before treatment and periodically thereafter.

Nephrolithiasis. Indinavir and *fosamprenavir* can cause nephrolithiasis. Management consists of hydration and interruption or discontinuation of the PI.

Bone Loss. PIs may promote bone loss. A diet that provides adequate calcium and vitamin D may decrease risk. Osteoporosis can be treated with bisphosphonates, raloxifene, calcitonin, teriparatide, or denosumab.

Diarrhea. Nelfinavir causes diarrhea in 20% to 32% of patients. Diarrhea can usually be managed with loperamide or some other over-the-counter antidiarrheal drug.

Cardiac Effects. Atazanavir, saquinavir, and *lopinavir/ritonavir* prolong the PR interval and can thereby promote atrioventricular block. Use with caution in patients with structural heart disease, cardiac conduction disturbances, and ischemic heart disease and in those taking other drugs that prolong the PR interval.

Lopinavir/ritonavir and *saquinavir* prolong the QT interval, and thereby pose a risk for torsades de pointes. Avoid these drugs in patients with congenital long QT syndrome and in those taking other drugs that prolong the QT interval.

Toxicity in Newborns. *Lopinavir/ritonavir oral solution* can be lethal to newborns, owing to its propylene glycol content. Accordingly, the oral solution should be avoided in full-term infants (for the first 14 days after birth) and in preterm infants (until 14 days after their predicted due date).

Indirect Hyperbilirubinemia. *Atazanavir* and *indinavir* can raise plasma levels of unconjugated bilirubin (indirect bilirubin). Be alert for jaundice (yellowing of the skin) and icterus (yellowing of the eyes), which reverse on drug withdrawal.

HIV Transmission. Reduction of plasma HIV RNA may create a false sense of safety. Accordingly, inform patients that, even when HIV RNA is undetectable, they may still be infectious and so should avoid behaviors that can transmit HIV.

Minimizing Adverse Interactions

Interactions Resulting From Inhibition of P450. All PIs inhibit cytochrome P450 and can thereby increase levels of other drugs. To avoid serious toxicity from excessive drug levels, patients must not take *cisapride, alprazolam, triazolam, midazolam, ergot alkaloids, lovastatin,* or *simvastatin*—or *astemizole* or *terfenadine,* which are no longer available in the United States.

RITONAVIR BOOSTING. Because ritonavir is a powerful inhibitor of P450, the drug is often combined with other PIs to raise their blood levels, and thereby boost antiviral effects.

DIDANOSINE. Buffered formulations of didanosine decrease absorption of *indinavir* and *ritonavir.* Accordingly, buffered didanosine should be administered 1 or 2 hours apart from these drugs.

RIFAMPIN. Rifampin induces P450 and can thereby reduce levels of the PIs. Concurrent use with all PIs should be avoided.

ORAL CONTRACEPTIVES. *Fosamprenavir, lopinavir/ritonavir, nelfinavir, ritonavir,* and *tipranavir/ritonavir* can reduce levels of ethinyl estradiol, a component of many oral contraceptives. An alternative form of birth control must be prescribed.

ST. JOHN'S WORT. St. John's wort induces P450 and can reduce levels of PIs. Warn patients not to use St. John's wort.

SULFONAMIDES. Darunavir and fosamprenavir, and tipranavir contain a sulfonamide component and hence should be used with caution in patients with sulfonamide allergy.

Enfuvirtide, an HIV Fusion Inhibitor

Therapeutic Goals

Enfuvirtide is indicated for HIV infection that is resistant to traditional antiretroviral drugs.

Treatment has six goals: maximal and durable suppression of viral load, restoration and/or preservation of immune function, improvement of quality of life, reduction of HIV-related morbidity and mortality, reduction of HIV sexual transmission, and prevention of vertical HIV transmission.

Baseline Data

Assess the patient's clinical status and obtain a plasma HIV RNA level and CD4 T-cell count.

Identifying High-Risk Patients

Use enfuvirtide with *caution* in patients who have pneumonia risk factors: low initial CD4 cell counts, high initial viral load, IV drug use, smoking, and a history of lung disease.

Ongoing Monitoring and Interventions

Evaluating Therapeutic Effects

See information for NRTIs.

Patient Education

ENFUVIRTIDE

Inform patients about manifestations of ISRs—pain, tenderness, erythema, induration, nodules, cysts, pruritus, and ecchymosis—and forewarn them that these occur in nearly everyone. Inform patients that they can reduce the risk for a severe ISR by rotating the injection site, avoiding sites with an active ISR and avoiding unnecessarily deep injections. Instruct patients to seek immediate medical attention if a severe ISR occurs or if local infection develops.

Explain that the risk for bacterial pneumonia is increased. Inform patients about signs of pneumonia—cough, fever, and breathing difficulties—and instruct them to report these immediately.

Inform patients about signs of hypersensitivity and advise them to report them immediately.

Minimizing Adverse Effects

Injection-Site Reactions. ISRs occur in nearly all patients using this enfuvirtide. Instruct patients to seek immediate medical attention if a severe ISR occurs or if local infection develops.

Pneumonia. Enfuvirtide may increase the risk for bacterial pneumonia. Use enfuvirtide with caution in patients who have pneumonia risk factors.

Hypersensitivity Reactions. Enfuvirtide may cause hypersensitivity reactions, manifesting as rash, fever, nausea, vomiting, chills, rigors, hypotension, or elevated serum transaminases, or possibly as respiratory distress, glomerulonephritis, Guillain-Barré syndrome, or primary immune complex reaction. If a systemic hypersensitivity reaction occurs, enfuvirtide should be discontinued and never used again.

HIV Transmission. Reduction of plasma HIV RNA may create a false sense of safety. Accordingly, inform patients that, even when HIV RNA is undetectable, they are still infectious and hence must avoid behaviors that can transmit HIV.

Maraviroc, a CCR5 Antagonist

Therapeutic Goals

Maraviroc, in combination with other antiretroviral drugs, is indicated for treating patients 16 years and older who are infected with CCR5-tropic HIV-1 strains.

Treatment has six goals: maximal and durable suppression of viral load, restoration and/or preservation of immune function, improvement of quality of life, reduction of HIV-related morbidity and mortality, prevention of HIV sexual transmission, and prevention of vertical HIV transmission.

Baseline Data

Assess the patient's clinical status and obtain the following laboratory data: HIV RNA level, CD4 T-cell count, serum transaminases, and proof that the infecting HIV strain is CCR5 tropic.

Identifying High-Risk Patients

Patients with elevated liver function and cardiovascular disease must be monitored carefully.

Ongoing Monitoring and Interventions

Evaluating Therapeutic Effects

See information for NRTIs.

> **Patient Education**
>
> **MARAVIROC**
>
> Advise patients that, if they forget to take a dose, they should take the missed dose as soon as possible and take the next scheduled dose at its regular time. If the time to the next dose is less than 6 hours, the patient should skip the missed dose and take the next dose as scheduled.
>
> Inform patients about signs of an evolving reaction (itchy rash, yellow skin, dark urine, and vomiting and/or abdominal pain) and instruct them to stop maraviroc and seek medical attention.

Minimizing Adverse Effects

Hepatotoxicity. Liver injury has been seen in some patients and may be preceded by evidence of an allergic reaction. To identify early, question patient about signs and symptoms at each encounter.

Cardiovascular Events. During clinical trials, a few patients experienced cardiovascular events, including myocardial ischemia and myocardial infarction. Exercise caution in patients with cardiovascular risk factors.

HIV Transmission. Reduction of plasma HIV RNA may create a false sense of safety. Accordingly, inform patients that, even when HIV RNA is undetectable, they are still infectious and must avoid behaviors that can transmit HIV.

Raltegravir, an Integrase Strand Transfer Inhibitor

Therapeutic Goals

Raltegravir is indicated for combined use with other antiretroviral drugs to treat adults infected with HIV-1.

Treatment has six goals: maximal and durable suppression of viral load, restoration and/or preservation of immune function, improvement of quality of life, reduction of HIV-related morbidity and mortality, reduction of HIV sexual transmission, and prevention of vertical HIV transmission.

Baseline Data

Assess the patient's clinical status and obtain a plasma HIV RNA level and CD4 T-cell count.

Ongoing Evaluation and Interventions

Evaluating Therapeutic Effects

See information for NRTIs.

> **Patient Education**
>
> **RALTEGRAVIR**
>
> Inform patients about signs of a hypersensitivity reaction (e.g., severe rash, or rash associated with blisters, fever, malaise, fatigue, oral lesions, facial edema, hepatitis, angioedema, or muscle or joint aches) and instruct them to discontinue raltegravir immediately.

Minimizing Adverse Effects

Severe Hypersensitivity Reactions. Raltegravir can cause potentially fatal hypersensitivity reactions, including Stevens-Johnson syndrome and toxic epidermal necrolysis. The drug should be discontinued if signs and symptoms develop.

HIV Transmission. Reduction of plasma HIV RNA may create a false sense of safety. Accordingly, inform patients that, even when HIV RNA is undetectable, they are still infectious and hence must avoid behaviors that can transmit HIV.

CHAPTER

80 Drug Therapy of Sexually Transmitted Diseases

Jacqueline Rosenjack Burchum, DNSc, FNP-BC, CNE

Sexually transmitted diseases (STDs), also known as *sexually transmitted infections,* are infectious diseases transmitted primarily through sexual contact. STDs are very common in the United States and constitute a major public health problem. In 2014 the Centers for Disease Control and Prevention (CDC) reported sharp increases in the number of reported STDs for the first time since 2006. For three STDs in particular, the increase from 2013 to 2014 alone was dramatic: syphilis rates increased 15.1%; congenital syphilis rates increased 27.5%; gonorrhea rates increased 5.1%, and chlamydia rates increased 2.8%. Bear in mind that those are known reported STDs. Because most STDs go unreported, the actual incidence is much higher, estimated at 20 million new infections a year, more than 50% of which occur in people younger than 25 years. According to the CDC, Americans now have a 25% lifetime risk for contracting an STD.

Our objective in this chapter is to describe the principal STDs and provide an overview of their treatment (Table 80.1). The basic pharmacology of these drugs is discussed in other chapters. HIV infection is covered separately in Chapter 79.

In 2015, the CDC updated its *Sexually Transmitted Diseases Treatment Guidelines*. The treatment recommendations presented in this chapter reflect those guidelines, which are available at http://www.cdc.gov/std/tg2015.

CHLAMYDIA TRACHOMATIS INFECTIONS

Characteristics

Chlamydia trachomatis is the most frequently reported bacterial STD (Fig. 80.1). The various strains of *Chlamydia* can cause genital tract infections, proctitis, conjunctivitis, and lymphogranuloma venereum (LGV), as well as ophthalmia and pneumonia in infants. Infection is frequently asymptomatic in women and may also be asymptomatic in men. In women, untreated infection can cause pelvic inflammatory disease (PID), ectopic pregnancy, and infertility. The CDC estimates that chlamydial infections cause sterility in up to 50,000 women each year, primarily from fallopian tube scarring. Because infection is often asymptomatic in women, and because sequelae can be serious, the CDC now recommends annual screening for all sexually active women 25 years or younger. Screening is also recommended for women older than 25 years who have a new sex partner, multiple partners, or a partner with a history of an STD.

Treatment

Adults and Adolescents

For uncomplicated urethral, cervical, or rectal infections in adults or adolescents, treatment with either *azithromycin* [Zithromax] or *doxycycline* [Vibramycin, others] is recommended. Patients who are unable to take these medications may take erythromycin, levofloxacin [Levaquin], or ofloxacin [generic]. Table 80.1 provides a detailed summary of specific dosages of drugs used to treat chlamydia and other STDs.

Infection in Pregnancy

Azithromycin is the preferred treatment for *C. trachomatis* infection. Although doxycycline and other tetracyclines are active against *C. trachomatis,* these drugs are contraindicated because they can damage fetal teeth and bones. If the patient cannot take azithromycin, the approved alternatives are amoxicillin, erythromycin base, or erythromycin ethylsuccinate.

Infants

About half the infants born to women with cervical *C. trachomatis* acquire the infection during delivery, putting them at risk for *pneumonia* and *conjunctivitis* (ophthalmia neonatorum). Pneumonia is generally not severe and lasts about 6 weeks. Conjunctivitis does not result in blindness and spontaneously resolves in 6 months. The preferred treatment for both infections is oral *erythromycin base* or *erythromycin ethylsuccinate.* Azithromycin suspension may be given as an alternative. Although topical erythromycin, tetracycline, or silver nitrate may be given to prevent conjunctivitis, these drugs are not completely effective—and they have no effect on pneumonia.

Preadolescent Children

Although infection in preadolescent children can result from perinatal transmission, sexual abuse is the more likely cause, especially in children older than 2 years. Because of the legal implications, diagnosis must be definitive. Treatment depends on the age and weight of the child. For children who weigh less than 45 kg, the preferred treatment is oral *erythromycin base* or *erythromycin ethylsuccinate.* For children who weigh 45 kg or more, but are younger than 8 years, the preferred treatment is *azithromycin.* For children at least 8 years old, the preferred treatments are *azithromycin* or *doxycycline.*

TABLE 80.1 ▪ Drug Therapy Recommendations for Sexually Transmitted Diseases*

Disease or Syndrome	Recommended Treatment	Causative Organism(s)
Chlamydia trachomatis **infections**		*Chlamydia trachomatis*
Adults and adolescents	Azithromycin, 1 g PO once *or* Doxycycline, 100 mg PO 2 times/day × 7 days	
Children		
<45 kg	Erythromycin base/ethylsuccinate, 12.5 mg/kg PO 4 times/day × 14 days	
≥45 kg but <8 yr old	Azithromycin, 1 g PO once	
≥8 yr old	Azithromycin, 1 g PO once *or* Doxycycline, 100 mg PO 2 times/day × 7 days	
Pregnant women	Azithromycin, 1 g PO once	
Newborns: ophthalmia or pneumonia	Erythromycin base/ethylsuccinate, 12.5 mg/kg PO 4 times/day × 14 days	
Lymphogranuloma venereum	Doxycycline, 100 mg PO 2 times/day × 21 days	
Gonococcal infections (gonorrhea)		*Neisseria gonorrhoeae*
Urethritis, cervicitis, proctitis	Ceftriaxone, 250 mg IM once, *plus* azithromycin, 1 g PO once	
Pharyngitis	Ceftriaxone, 250 mg IM once, *plus* azithromycin, 1 g PO once	
Disseminated gonococcal infection (DGI) in adults	Ceftriaxone, 1 g IM or IV every 24 hr, *plus* azithromycin, 1 g PO once	
DGI with meningitis	Ceftriaxone, 1–2 g IV every 12 hr × 10–14 days, *plus* azithromycin, 1 g PO once	
DGI with endocarditis	Ceftriaxone, 1–2 g IV every 12 hr × 28 days or more, *plus* azithromycin, 1 g PO once	
Conjunctivitis	Ceftriaxone, 1 g IM once, *plus* azithromycin 1 g PO once	
Newborns		
Ophthalmia neonatorum prophylaxis	Erythromycin 0.5% ophthalmic ointment in each eye at birth	
Ophthalmia neonatorum	Ceftriaxone 25–50 mg/kg (not to exceed 125 mg) IM or IV once	
Disseminated infection or scalp abscess	Ceftriaxone, 25–50 mg/kg IM or IV once daily × 7 days *or* Cefotaxime, 25 mg/kg IM or IV every 12 hr × 7 days (Dosing of both drugs is increased to 10–14 days if meningitis is present.)	
Children		
Arthritis, bacteremia	If 45 kg or less, ceftriaxone, 50 mg/kg IM or IV once daily × 7 days, not to exceed 1 g If more than 45 kg, ceftriaxone 1 g IM or IV once daily × 7 days	
Vulvovaginitis, cervicitis, proctitis, pharyngitis, urethritis	If 45 kg or less, ceftriaxone 25–50 mg/kg (not to exceed 125 mg) IM or IV once If more than 45 kg, same as adult	
Nongonococcal urethritis		*Chlamydia trachomatis, Ureaplasma urealyticum, Trichomonas vaginalis, Mycoplasma genitalium*
Acute infection	Azithromycin, 1 g PO once *or* Doxycycline, 100 mg PO 2 times/day × 7 days	
Recurrent/persistent	Azithromycin, 1 g PO once if original treatment was with doxycycline Moxifloxacin 400 mg PO daily × 7 days if original treatment was azithromycin Metronidazole (2 g PO once) or tinidazole (2 g PO once) in areas where *Trichomonas* outbreaks are common	
Pelvic inflammatory disease		*Neisseria gonorrhoeae, Chlamydia trachomatis,* others
Inpatients	Doxycycline (100 mg IV or PO every 12 hr), *plus* either cefoxitin (2 g IV every 6 hr) or cefotetan (2 g IV every 12 hr); or clindamycin (900 mg IV every 8 hr), *plus* gentamicin (3–5 mg/kg IM or IV once or 2 mg/kg IM or IV once then 1.5 mg/kg every 8 hr)	
Outpatients	Doxycycline (100 mg PO 2 times/day × 14 days), *plus* either cefoxitin (2 g IM once, boosted with probenecid 1 g PO once) or ceftriaxone (250 mg IM once), *with or without* metronidazole (500 mg PO 2 times/day × 14 days)	
Sexually acquired epididymitis		*Chlamydia trachomatis, Neisseria gonorrhoeae,* enteric organisms
Sexually acquired epididymitis without history of insertive anal sex	Ceftriaxone (250 mg IM once) *plus* doxycycline (100 mg PO 2 times/day × 10 days)	
Sexually acquired epididymitis with history of insertive anal sex	Ceftriaxone (250 mg IM once) *plus either* levofloxacin (500 mg PO daily × 10 days) or ofloxacin (300 mg PO 2 times/day × 10 days)	

TABLE 80.1 ▪ Drug Therapy Recommendations for Sexually Transmitted Diseases*—cont'd		
Disease or Syndrome	**Recommended Treatment**	**Causative Organism(s)**
Syphilis		*Treponema pallidum*
Primary syphilis, secondary syphilis, and early latent syphilis	*Adults:* Benzathine penicillin G, 2.4 million units IM once *Children:* Benzathine penicillin G, 50,000 units/kg IM once (up to a max. of 2.4 million units)	
Late latent syphilis or latent syphilis of unknown duration	*Adults:* Benzathine penicillin G, 2.4 million units IM once/week for 3 weeks *Children:* Benzathine penicillin G, 50,000 units/kg IM once/week for 3 weeks (up to a max. of 7.2 million units over the course of treatment)	
Tertiary syphilis	Benzathine penicillin G, 2.4 million units IM once/week for 3 weeks (must rule out CNS involvement)	
Neurosyphilis	Aqueous crystalline penicillin G, 18–24 million units IV daily for 10–14 days, administered by continuous infusion or in separate doses of 3–4 million units each every 4 hr	
Congenital syphilis	Aqueous crystalline penicillin G, 50,000 units/kg IV every 12 hr for the first 7 days of life, followed by 50,000 units/kg every 8 hr for the next 3 days *or* Procaine penicillin G, 50,000 units/kg IM once daily for 10 days	
Acquired immunodeficiency syndrome (AIDS)	*See* Chapter 79	Human immunodeficiency virus (HIV)
Bacterial vaginosis	Metronidazole, 500 mg PO 2 times/day × 7 days *or* Metronidazole gel (0.75%), 1 full applicator (5 g) intravaginally once/day × 5 days *or* Clindamycin cream (2%), 1 full applicator (5 g) intravaginally at bedtime × 7 days	*Gardnerella vaginalis, Mycoplasma hominis,* various anaerobes
Trichomoniasis	Metronidazole, 2 g PO once *or* Tinidazole, 2 g PO once	*Trichomonas vaginalis*
Chancroid	Azithromycin, 1 g PO once *or* Ceftriaxone, 250 mg IM once *or* Ciprofloxacin, 500 mg PO 2 times/day × 3 days *or* Erythromycin base, 500 mg PO 3 times/day × 7 days	*Haemophilus ducreyi*
Genital herpes simplex virus infections		Herpes simplex virus
First episode, genital herpes	Acyclovir, 400 mg PO 3 times/day × 7–10 days (or longer) *or* Acyclovir, 200 mg PO 5 times/day × 7–10 days (or longer) *or* Famciclovir, 250 mg PO 3 times/day × 7–10 days (or longer) *or* Valacyclovir, 1 g PO 2 times/day × 7–10 days (or longer)	
Severe infection	Acyclovir, 5–10 mg/kg IV every 8 hr for 2–7 days or until clinical improvement, then PO acyclovir to complete at least 10 days	
Recurrent episodes	Acyclovir, 800 mg PO 2 times/day × 5 days *or* Acyclovir, 800 mg PO 3 times/day × 2 days *or* Acyclovir, 400 mg PO 3 times/day × 5 days *or* Famciclovir, 125 mg PO 2 times/day × 5 days *or* Famciclovir, 1 g 2 times/day × 1 day *or* Famciclovir, 500 mg once, followed by 200 mg 2 times/day for 2 days *or* Valacyclovir, 500 mg PO 2 times/day × 3 days *or* Valacyclovir, 1 g PO once/day × 5 days	
Daily suppressive therapy	Acyclovir, 400 mg PO 2 times/day *or* Famciclovir, 250 mg PO 2 times/day *or* Valacyclovir, 500 mg PO once/day *or* Valacyclovir, 1 g PO once/day	
Neonatal herpes	Acyclovir, 20 mg/kg IV every 8 hr × 14 days (for skin or mucous membrane infection) or × 21 days (for disseminated or CNS infection)	
Proctitis	Ceftriaxone (250 mg IM once) *plus* doxycycline (100 mg PO 2 times/day × 7 days)	*Chlamydia trachomatis, Neisseria gonorrhoeae, Treponema pallidum,* herpes simplex virus
Venereal warts	*See* Chapter 85	Human papillomavirus

*Recommendations from Centers for Disease Control and Prevention: Sexually transmitted diseases treatment guidelines, 2015. MMWR Morb Mortal Wkly Rep 2016;64:1-137. Dosing for alternative regimens is available at http://www.cdc.gov/std/tg2015/tg-2015-print.pdf.
CNS, central nervous system.

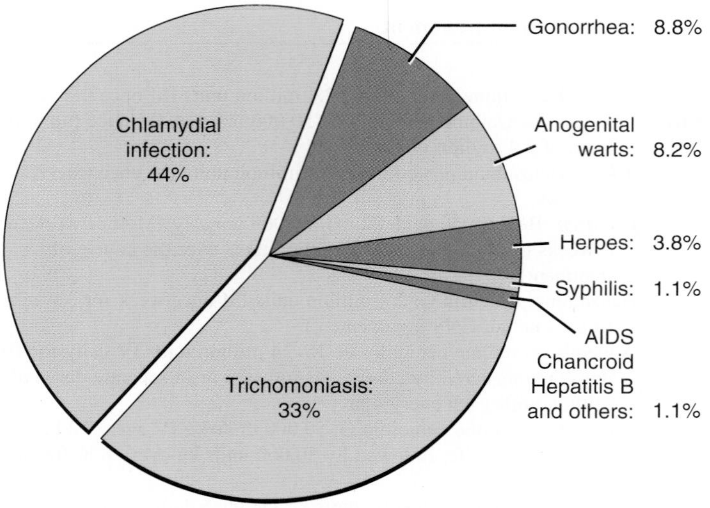

Figure 80.1 ■ Incidence of sexually transmitted diseases.

Lymphogranuloma Venereum

LGV is caused by a unique strain of *C. trachomatis*. Transmission is strictly by sexual contact. LGV is most common in tropical countries but does occur in the United States, especially in the South. Infection begins as a small erosion or papule in the genital region. From this site, the organism migrates to regional lymph nodes, causing swelling, tenderness, and blockage of lymphatic flow. Tremendous enlargement of the genitalia may result. The enlarged nodes, called buboes, may break open and drain. The treatment of choice for genital, inguinal, and anorectal LGV is *doxycycline*. Erythromycin base serves as an alternative for those who cannot take tetracycline antibiotics.

GONOCOCCAL INFECTIONS

Characteristics

Gonorrhea is caused by *Neisseria gonorrhoeae,* a gram-negative diplococcus, often referred to as the gonococcus. Gonorrhea is second only to chlamydia as our most common STD. Gonorrhea is transmitted almost exclusively by sexual contact.

The intensity of symptoms differs between men and women. In men, the main symptoms are a burning sensation during urination and a pus-like discharge from the penis. In contrast, gonorrhea in women is often asymptomatic or may present as mild cervicitis. However, serious infection of female reproductive structures (vagina, urethra, cervix, ovaries, fallopian tubes) can occur, ultimately resulting in sterility. Among people who engage in oral sex, the mouth and throat can become infected, causing sore throat and tonsillitis. Among people who engage in receptive anal sex, the rectum can become infected, causing a purulent discharge and constant urge to move the bowels (tenesmus). Bacteremia can develop in males and females, causing cutaneous lesions, arthritis, and, rarely, meningitis and endocarditis.

Treatment

Owing to antibiotic resistance, treatment of gonorrhea has changed over the years—and undoubtedly will continue to evolve. In the 1930s, virtually all strains of the gonococcus were sensitive to sulfonamides. However, within a decade, sulfonamide resistance had become common. Fortunately, by that time penicillin had become available, and the drug was active against all gonococcal strains. However, in 1976, organisms resistant to penicillin began to emerge. More recently, resistance to fluoroquinolones has become common. As a result, in 2007 *the CDC recommended against using fluoroquinolones for gonorrhea,* leaving cephalosporins as the preferred treatments. This recommendation was changed yet again in 2012, also triggered by antimicrobial resistance—this time to oral cephalosporins.

Urethral, Cervical, and Rectal Infection

Because of increasing resistance to cephalosporins, preferred treatment now consists of a combination of two drugs: *ceftriaxone* [Rocephin] intramuscular (IM) plus *azithromycin*. If a patient refuses IM therapy, oral (PO) cefixime can be substituted for IM ceftriaxone; however, the CDC recommends not routinely substituting this drug because resistance to cefixime has been documented and is anticipated to increase. If a patient is allergic to azithromycin, a 7-day course of doxycycline may be substituted. For patients with cephalosporin allergies, the options are not as clear. Although prescribing double the azithromycin dose as monotherapy will cure gonorrhea in most cases, the CDC does not recommend this because of treatment failures and rapid development of resistance. Although acknowledging a lack of data for recommendation, the CDC suggests substituting gemifloxacin for the cephalosporin component, despite having recommended against using quinolones to treat gonorrhea. Spectinomycin, an aminoglycoside, has also been suggested; however, it is not currently available in the United States. For additional information on this dilemma, see http://www.cdc.gov/std/tg2015/gonorrhea.htm.

Pharyngeal Infection

Gonococcal infection of the pharynx is more difficult to treat than infection of the urethra, cervix, or rectum; therefore, parenteral therapy is recommended for all patients. The preferred treatment is *ceftriaxone* combined with *azithromycin.* Azithromycin is preferred over doxycycline because patients are more likely to adhere to a single-dose regimen of azithromycin than the full-week regimen of doxycycline taken twice a day.

Conjunctivitis

Gonococcal conjunctivitis can be reliably eradicated with *ceftriaxone* plus azithromycin. Treatment also includes washing the infected eye with saline solution once.

Disseminated Gonococcal Infection

Disseminated gonococcal infection (DGI) occurs secondary to gonococcal bacteremia. Symptoms include petechial or pustular skin lesions, arthritis, arthralgia, and tenosynovitis. Endocarditis and meningitis occur rarely. Strains of *N. gonorrhoeae* that cause DGI are uncommon in the United States. In the absence of endocarditis or meningitis, treatment consists of IM or intravenous (IV) *ceftriaxone* plus azithromycin. For patients with endocarditis or meningitis, the preferred treatment is IV *ceftriaxone* plus azithromycin.

Neonatal Infection

Neonatal gonococcal infection is acquired through contact with infected cervical exudates during delivery. Infection can be limited to the eyes or it may be disseminated.

Gonococcal *neonatal ophthalmia* is a serious infection. The initial symptom is conjunctivitis. Over time, other structures of the eye become involved. Blindness can result. The recommended therapy is a single dose of *ceftriaxone* given by either IM or IV injection.

To protect against neonatal ophthalmia, a topical antibiotic should be instilled into both eyes immediately postpartum—as required by law in most states. According to the 2015 CDC guidelines, the only approved topical agent is *0.5% erythromycin* ophthalmic ointment. If this antimicrobial is not available, parenteral therapy with ceftriaxone is to be used.

In neonates, *DGI* is rare. Possible manifestations include sepsis, arthritis, meningitis, and scalp abscesses. There are two recommended treatments: *ceftriaxone and cefotaxime.* If meningitis is present, dosing is prolonged from 7 days to 10 to 14 days.

Preadolescent Children

Among preadolescent children, the most common cause of gonococcal infection is sexual abuse. Vaginal, anorectal, and pharyngeal infections are most common. Because of legal implications, diagnosis must be definitive. Growing a specimen in culture is the preferred technique.

Treatment depends on the type of infection and the weight of the child. For children who have localized infection (vulvovaginitis, cervicitis, urethritis, pharyngitis, proctitis) and who weigh 45 kg or less, the preferred treatment is a single dose of IM or IV *ceftriaxone.* For children with localized infection who weigh more than 45 kg, treatment is the same as for adults. For children of any weight who have systemic infection (bacteremia, arthritis), the preferred treatment is IM or IV *ceftriaxone,* once daily for 7 days. Specific dosing is provided in Table 80.1.

NONGONOCOCCAL URETHRITIS

Nongonococcal urethritis (NGU) is defined as urethritis caused by any organism other than *N. gonorrhoeae,* the gonococcus. The most common infectious agent is *C. trachomatis* (15%–55%). Other likely agents are *Ureaplasma urealyticum, Trichomonas vaginalis,* and *Mycoplasma genitalium.* NGU is diagnosed by the presence of polymorphonuclear leukocytes and a negative culture for *N. gonorrhoeae.* The infection is especially prevalent among sexually active adolescent girls. The recommended treatment is either *azithromycin* [Zithromax] or *doxycycline* [Vibramycin]. Alternative regimens are erythromycin base, erythromycin ethylsuccinate, levofloxacin, or ofloxacin. For persistent or recurrent NGU, one of two drugs, *metronidazole* [Flagyl] or *tinidazole* [Tindamax], is recommended if *T. vaginalis* transmission is a suspected cause. *Azithromycin* should be added to the regimen if it had not been used during initial therapy. If the infection still fails to respond, the cause may be *M. genitalium.* Unfortunately, we have no easy tests for this bacterium, and hence definitive diagnosis may not be possible. Nonetheless, when *M. genitalium* is suspected, a trial with *moxifloxacin* [Avelox] may be warranted.

PELVIC INFLAMMATORY DISEASE

Acute PID is a syndrome that includes endometritis, pelvic peritonitis, tuboovarian abscess, and inflammation of the fallopian tubes. Infertility can result. Prominent symptoms are abdominal pain, vaginal discharge, and fever. Most frequently, PID is caused by *N. gonorrhoeae, C. trachomatis,* or both. However, *Mycoplasma hominis,* as well as assorted anaerobic and facultative bacteria, may also be present. In recent years, the United States has experienced an almost 40% decrease in PID despite the increase in diseases that cause this condition. This may be attributable to intensified patient education efforts, increased and improved screening practices, or improved adherence to single-dose treatment.

Because multiple organisms are likely to be involved, drug therapy must provide broad coverage. Because no single drug can do this, combination therapy is required. For the *hospitalized patient,* treatment can be initiated with either *cefoxitin* or *cefotetan,* combined with *doxycycline.* After symptoms resolve, IV therapy can be discontinued—but must be followed by oral *doxycycline* to complete a 14-day course of treatment. An alternative recommended regimen consists of IV *clindamycin* plus IV or IM *gentamicin.*

Outpatients can be treated with either *ceftriaxone* or *cefoxitin.* Treatment should also include *doxycycline,* with or without *metronidazole*). Because PID can be difficult to treat, and because the consequences of failure can be severe (e.g., sterility), many experts recommend that *all* patients receive IV antibiotics in a hospital.

ACUTE EPIDIDYMITIS

Epididymitis may be acquired by sexual contact or nonsexually. Sexually acquired epididymitis is usually caused by *N. gonorrhoeae, C. trachomatis,* or both. The syndrome occurs primarily in young adults (under 35 years old) and may be associated with urethritis. Primary symptoms are fever accompanied by pain in the back of the testicles that develops over the course of several hours. For patients with gonococcal or chlamydial infection, the recommended treatment is *ceftriaxone* [Rocephin] plus *doxycycline* [Vibramycin, others]. For patients who engage in insertive anal sex, the addition of levofloxacin or ofloxacin is recommended to target enteric bacteria. Testicular pain can be managed with analgesics, bed rest, and ice packs.

Non–sexually transmitted epididymitis generally occurs in older men and in men who have had urinary tract instrumentation. Causative organisms are gram-negative enteric bacilli and *Pseudomonas* species. Ofloxacin can be used for treatment.

SYPHILIS

Syphilis is caused by the spirochete *Treponema pallidum.* In the United States the incidence of syphilis has risen steadily since 2000. In 2012 reported cases of primary and secondary syphilis totaled 15,667. In 2014 reported cases increased to 19,999. Approximately two thirds of cases occur in men who have sex with men. Fortunately, *T. pallidum* has remained highly responsive to penicillin, the treatment of choice.

Characteristics

Syphilis develops in three stages, termed *primary, secondary,* and *tertiary. T. pallidum* enters the body by penetrating the mucous membranes of the mouth, vagina, or urethra of the penis. After an incubation period of 1 to 4 weeks, a primary lesion, called a chancre, develops at the site of entry. The chancre is a hard, red, protruding, painless sore. Nearby lymph nodes may become swollen. Within a few weeks the chancre heals spontaneously, although *T. pallidum* is still present. In clinical practice, chancres are rarely seen, especially in females.

Two to 6 weeks after the chancre heals, secondary syphilis develops. Symptoms result from spread of *T. pallidum* through the bloodstream. Skin lesions and flu-like symptoms (fever, headache, reduced appetite, general malaise) are typical. Enlarged lymph nodes and joint pain may also be present. The symptoms of secondary syphilis resolve in 4 to 8 weeks—but may recur episodically over the next 3 to 4 years.

Tertiary syphilis develops 5 to 40 years after the initial infection. Almost any organ can be involved. Infection of the brain—neurosyphilis—is common and can cause senility, paralysis, and severe psychiatric symptoms. The heart valves and aorta can be damaged. Lesions can also occur in the skin, bones, joints, and eyes. The risk for neurosyphilis is increased in individuals with HIV infection.

Infants exposed to *T. pallidum* in utero can be born with syphilis. Early signs of congenital syphilis include sores, rhinitis, and severe tenderness over bones.

Treatment

Penicillin G is the drug of choice for all stages of syphilis. The form and dosage of penicillin G depend on the disease stage. *Early syphilis* (primary, secondary, or latent syphilis of less than 1 year's duration) is treated with a single IM dose of benzathine penicillin G. *Late latent syphilis* (more than 1 year's duration) and tertiary syphilis are also treated with IM benzathine penicillin G. However, instead of receiving a single dose, adults and children receive three doses 1 week apart. *Neurosyphilis* requires more aggressive therapy. The recommended treatment is IV penicillin G daily for 10 to 14 days, administered either by continuous infusion or in separate doses every 4 hours. For *congenital syphilis,* treatment options are either IV penicillin G or IM procaine penicillin. *Syphilis in pregnancy* should be treated with penicillin G, using a dosage appropriate to the stage of the disease.

How should patients with *penicillin allergy* be treated? For *nonpregnant* patients with early or late syphilis, either *doxycycline* or *tetracycline* may be used. For patients with *neurosyphilis,* ceftriaxone can be effective, but possible cross-reactivity with penicillin is a concern. If the patient is a child or a pregnant woman, the CDC recommends a penicillin-allergy desensitization protocol to permit penicillin use, rather than substituting another drug for penicillin.

BACTERIAL VAGINOSIS

Bacterial vaginosis is a common vaginal infection in women of childbearing age. The condition results from an alteration in vaginal microflora. Organisms responsible for the syndrome include *Gardnerella vaginalis* (also known as *Haemophilus vaginalis*), *Mycoplasma hominis,* and various anaerobes. The syndrome occurs most commonly in sexually active women, although it may be transmitted in other ways. Bacterial vaginosis is characterized by a malodorous vaginal discharge, elevation of vaginal pH (above 4.5), and generation of a fishy odor when vaginal secretions are mixed with 10% potassium hydroxide. Clue cells (epithelial cells whose borders are obscured by bacteria) are typically found on microscopic examination of vaginal secretions.

The recommended therapy for bacterial vaginosis is either oral or vaginal *metronidazole* [Flagyl] or vaginal clindamycin cream. Clindamycin cream is available as a *short-acting 2% clindamycin cream* [Cleocin] and a *long-acting 2% clindamycin cream* [Clindesse]. Clindesse cream is formulated to adhere to the vaginal mucosa for several days and hence can clear bacterial vaginosis with just one application. Approved alternative regimens are tinidazole [Tindamax], oral clindamycin, or clindamycin ovules (intravaginal suppositories). Unlike the other drugs approved for bacterial vaginosis, tinidazole should not be prescribed for pregnant women.

TRICHOMONIASIS

Trichomoniasis, caused by *T. vaginalis,* is the most common nonviral STD in the United States. In men, infection is usually asymptomatic. In women, infection may be asymptomatic or may cause a diffuse, malodorous, yellow-green vaginal discharge, along with burning and itching. The rapid movement of *T. vaginalis* protozoa are notable on microscopic examination of vaginal secretions.

Most infections can be eliminated with a single, 2-g oral dose of either *metronidazole* [Flagyl, others] or *tinidazole* [Tindamax]. Dosing can be repeated in the event of treatment failure. Male partners of infected women should always be treated, even if free of symptoms. Although some clinicians remain concerned about giving metronidazole during pregnancy, there is no evidence that the drug causes birth defects in humans. Tinidazole, on the other hand, should not be prescribed for pregnant women.

CHANCROID

Chancroid, also known as soft chancre, is one of the few STDs for which prevalence has declined both in the United States and worldwide. It is caused by *Haemophilus ducreyi.* Transmission is primarily by sexual contact. The infection is characterized by a painful, ragged ulcer at the site of inoculation, usually the external genitalia. Regional lymph nodes may be swollen. Multiple secondary lesions may develop. There are four antibiotics recommended for treatment: (1) *azithromycin* [Zithromax], (2) *ceftriaxone* [Rocephin], (3) *ciprofloxacin* [Cipro], and (4) *erythromycin base.*

HERPES SIMPLEX VIRUS INFECTIONS

Characteristics

Most genital herpes infections are caused by herpes simplex virus type 2 (HSV-2). However, an increasing number of anogenital infections are caused by HSV-1, the herpesvirus that causes cold sores. In the United States the infection has reached epidemic proportions: more than 50 million people are affected.

Symptoms of primary infection develop 6 to 8 days after contact. Some people with HSV infection are asymptomatic or have relatively mild symptoms; however, for others there is a common presentation. In females, blisters or vesicles can appear on the perianal skin, labia, vagina, cervix, and foreskin of the clitoris. In males, vesicles develop on the penis and occasionally on the testicles. Painful urination and a watery discharge can occur in both sexes. Also, the patient may experience systemic symptoms: fever, headache, myalgia, and tender, swollen lymph nodes in the affected region. Within days, the original blisters can evolve into large, painful, ulcer-like sores. Over the next 2 to 3 weeks, all symptoms resolve spontaneously. However, this does not indicate cure: the virus remains present in a latent state and can cause recurrence. Because available drugs can't eliminate the virus, there is no cure. Symptoms may recur for life; however, for some patients, subsequent episodes become progressively shorter and less severe, and in rare cases they may cease entirely.

Neonatal Infection

Genital herpes in pregnant women can be transmitted to the infant. Transmission can occur in utero, which is very rare, or during delivery. Infection acquired in utero can result in spontaneous abortion or fetal malformation. Infection acquired during delivery can cause blindness, severe neurologic damage, and even death. To protect the infant during delivery, birth should be accomplished by cesarean delivery if the mother has an active infection. Infants who acquire the infection should be treated with acyclovir.

Treatment

Genital herpes can be treated with three drugs: *acyclovir* [Zovirax], *famciclovir* [Famvir], and *valacyclovir* [Valtrex] at dosage regimens recommended in Table 80.1. These agents cannot eliminate the virus, but they can reduce symptoms and shorten the duration of pain and viral shedding. Patients with recurrent infections may take these drugs every day (suppressive therapy) or just when symptoms appear (episodic therapy). Continuous daily administration reduces the frequency and intensity of episodes, whereas episodic treatment reduces symptom intensity after an episode has begun.

Reduction of Transmission

Transmission of HSV can occur when symptoms are absent as well as when symptoms are present. *Valacyclovir* (500 mg once daily) can decrease transmission of genital herpes by 50%. No other drug has been shown to reduce transmission of this STD, or any other STD, for that matter. Valacyclovir only *reduces* transmission, it doesn't stop it entirely. Accordingly, patients must continue to use condoms. Because viral shedding is increased when the infection is active, it is advisable to abstain from sex during breakouts.

PROCTITIS

Sexually acquired proctitis (inflammation of the rectum) results primarily from receptive anal intercourse. Symptoms include anorectal pain, tenesmus (a sensation of the need to have a bowel movement when the bowel and rectum are empty), and rectal discharge. Usual causative organisms are *N. gonorrhoeae, C. trachomatis, T. pallidum,* and HSV. Empiric treatment is *ceftriaxone* plus *doxycycline.* If perianal ulcers are present, treatment for HSV should also be included.

VENEREAL WARTS

Genital and perianal warts are caused by human papillomaviruses (HPVs). Characteristics of these warts and their treatment are presented in Chapter 85. As discussed in Chapter 53, an HPV vaccine, sold as *Gardasil,* can protect against both venereal warts and cervical cancer. Another HPV vaccine, sold as *Cervarix,* protects against cervical cancer, but not against venereal warts.

CHAPTER

81 Anthelmintics

Jacqueline Rosenjack Burchum, DNSc, FNP-BC, CNE

Helminths are parasitic worms, and *anthelmintics* are the drugs used against them. Helminthiasis (worm infestation) is the most common affliction of humans, affecting more than 2 billion people worldwide. The intestine is a frequent site of infestation. Other sites include the liver, lymphatic system, and blood vessels. Infestation is frequently asymptomatic. However, infestation with some parasites can cause severe complications. Helminthiasis is most prevalent where sanitation is poor. Cleanliness greatly reduces infestation risk.

Treatment of helminthiasis is not always indicated. Most parasitic worms do not reproduce in the human body. Therefore, in the absence of reinfestation, many infections simply subside as adult worms die. Accordingly, treatment may be optional. In countries where providers and medication are readily available, drug therapy is definitely indicated. However, in less fortunate locales, several factors—cost of medication, limited medical facilities, and high probability of reinfestation—may render individual treatment impractical. In these places, preventative measures, such as improved hygiene and elimination of carriers, may be the most valuable interventions.

In approaching the anthelmintic drugs, we begin by reviewing classification of the parasitic worms. Next we briefly discuss the characteristics of the more common helminthic infestations. After this, we discuss preferred drugs for treatment.

CLASSIFICATION OF PARASITIC WORMS

The most common parasitic worms belong to three classes: Nematoda (roundworms), Cestoda (tapeworms), and Trematoda (flukes). Nematodes belong to the phylum Nemathelminthes. Cestodes and trematodes belong to the phylum Platyhelminthes (flat worms).

Nematodes (Roundworms)

Parasitic nematodes can be subdivided into two groups: (1) those that infest the intestinal lumen and (2) those that inhabit tissues. There are five major species of intestinal nematodes. Their common names are giant roundworm, pinworm, hookworm, whipworm, and threadworm. Official names (e.g., Ascaris lumbricoides) are shown in Table 81.1. Two types of nematodes invade tissues: (1) pork roundworms (responsible for trichinosis) and (2) filariae. The three species of filariae encountered most commonly are also found in Table 81.1.

Cestodes (Tapeworms)

Three species of cestodes infest humans. Common names for these parasites are beef tapeworm, pork tapeworm, and fish tapeworm. Their official names appear in Table 81.1.

Trematodes (Flukes)

Five species of trematodes infest humans. These organisms fall into four groups having the following common names: blood fluke, liver fluke, intestinal fluke, and lung fluke. Official names of the five species belonging to these groups are given in Table 81.1.

HELMINTHIC INFESTATIONS

This section describes the major characteristics of infestation by specific helminths. These infestations can differ with respect to anatomic site and danger to the host. Infestations also differ with respect to the drugs employed for treatment.

The name applied to an infestation is based on the official name of the invading organism. For example, infestation with the giant roundworm, whose official name is *Ascaris lumbricoides*, is referred to as ascariasis.

In the following discussion, the helminthic infestations are grouped in four categories: (1) nematode infestations of the intestine, (2) nematode infestations of extraintestinal sites, (3) cestode infestations, and (4) trematode infestations.

Nematode Infestations (Intestinal)

Ascariasis (Giant Roundworm Infestation)

Ascariasis is the most prevalent helminthic infestation. Worldwide, one of every three people is affected. Adult worms inhabit the small intestine. Ascariasis is usually asymptomatic. However, serious complications can result if worms migrate into the pancreatic duct, bile duct, gallbladder, or liver. In addition, if infestation is extremely heavy, intestinal blockage may occur. Because of these potential hazards, ascariasis should always be treated. Drugs of choice are albendazole, mebendazole, and ivermectin.

Enterobiasis (Pinworm Infestation)

Enterobiasis is the most common helminthic infestation in the United States. Adult pinworms inhabit the ileum and large intestine. Their life span is approximately 2 months. Although usually asymptomatic, some patients experience intense perianal itching. Serious complications are rare. Drugs of choice are albendazole, mebendazole, and pyrantel pamoate. Because enterobiasis is readily transmitted, all family members of an infected individual should be treated simultaneously.

Ancylostomiasis and Necatoriasis (Hookworm Infestation)

Hookworm infestation is most common in rural areas where hygiene is poor and people go barefoot. Adult hookworms attach to the wall of the small intestine and suck blood. As a result, infestation is associated with chronic blood loss and progressive anemia. Symptomatic anemia is most likely in menstruating women and undernourished individuals. Nausea, vomiting, and abdominal pain may accompany the infestation. Albendazole, mebendazole, and pyrantel pamoate are treatments of choice.

Trichuriasis (Whipworm Infestation)

Trichuriasis is extremely common, affecting about 1 billion people worldwide. Larvae and adult worms inhabit the large intestine. Mature worms may live for 10 years or more. The disease is usually devoid of symptoms. However, when the worm burden is very large, rectal prolapse may occur. Patients with severe infestation require therapy. Albendazole is the treatment of choice.

TABLE 81.1 ■ Drugs of Choice for Parasitic Worms

Worm Class	Parasitic Organism: Common Name	Parasitic Organism: Official Name	Drugs of Choice
Nematodes (roundworms): intestinal	Giant roundworm	*Ascaris lumbricoides*	Albendazole *or* mebendazole *or* ivermectin
	Pinworm	*Enterobius vermicularis*	Albendazole *or* mebendazole *or* pyrantel pamoate
	Hookworm	*Ancylostoma duodenale, Necator americanus*	
	Whipworm	*Trichuris trichiura*	Albendazole
	Threadworm	*Strongyloides stercoralis*	Ivermectin
Nematodes (roundworms): extraintestinal	Pork roundworm	*Trichinella spiralis*	Albendazole*
	Filariae	*Brugia malayi, Loa loa, Wuchereria bancrofti*	Diethylcarbamazine†
		Onchocerca volvulus	Ivermectin
Cestodes (tapeworms)	Beef tapeworm	*Taenia saginata*	Praziquantel*
	Pork tapeworm	*Taenia solum*	
	Fish tapeworm	*Diphyllobothrium latum*	
Trematodes (flukes)	Blood fluke	*Schistosoma* species	Praziquantel
	Intestinal fluke	*Fasciolopsis buski*	
	Lung fluke	*Paragonimus westermani*	
	Liver flukes	*Fasciola hepatica* (sheep liver fluke)	Triclabendazole‡
		Clonorchis sinensis (Chinese liver fluke)	Praziquantel *or* albendazole*

*Not approved by the U.S. Food and Drug Administration for this indication.
†Available from the Centers for Disease Control and Prevention.
‡Not available in the United States.

Strongyloidiasis (Threadworm Infestation)

Strongyloidiasis is common in the southern United States. Larval and adult threadworms inhabit the small intestine. The disease can be very dangerous, although symptoms are usually absent. Mild infestation may cause abdominal pain and occasional diarrhea. Severe infestation can cause vomiting, massive diarrhea, dehydration, electrolyte imbalance, and secondary bacteremia. Death has occurred. Affected individuals should always be treated. Ivermectin is the treatment of choice.

Nematode Infestations (Extraintestinal)

Trichinosis (Pork Roundworm Infestation)

Trichinosis, also called trichinellosis, is acquired by eating undercooked pork that contains encysted larvae of *Trichinella spiralis*. Adult worms reside in the intestine, whereas larvae migrate to skeletal muscle and become encysted. Some encysted larvae live for years; others die and calcify within months. Symptoms of trichinosis include gastrointestinal (GI) upset, fever, muscle pain, and sore throat. Potentially lethal complications (heart failure, meningitis, neuritis) arise in some patients. Albendazole is the drug of choice for killing adult worms and migrating larvae. However, this agent may not be active against larvae that have become encysted. Prednisone (a glucocorticoid) is given to reduce inflammation during larval migration.

Wuchereriasis and Brugiasis (Lymphatic Filarial Infestation)

Wuchereria bancrofti and *Brugia malayi* are filarial nematodes that invade the lymphatic system. Infestation with either organism can cause severe complications. When infestation is heavy, lymphatic obstruction occurs, resulting in elephantiasis (usually of the scrotum or legs). In addition, "filarial fever" may develop. Symptoms include chills, fever, headache, nausea, vomiting, constipation, and lymphadenitis. The drug of choice for killing both filarial species is diethylcarbamazine.

Onchocerciasis (River Blindness)

Onchocerca volvulus is a filarial nematode found in streams and rivers of Mexico, Guatemala, northern South America, and equatorial Africa. The parasite is transmitted to humans by the bite of certain flies. Heavy infestation with *O. volvulus* causes dermatologic and ophthalmic symptoms. Dermatologic manifestations include subcutaneous nodules (filled with adult worms) and persistent pruritic dermatitis. Ocular lesions, caused by the infiltration and death of microfilariae, result in optic neuritis, optic atrophy, and then blindness. The drug of choice for treating onchocerciasis is ivermectin.

Cestode Infestations

Taeniasis (Beef and Pork Tapeworm Infestation)

Taeniasis is acquired by eating undercooked beef or pork that contains tapeworm larvae. Adult tapeworms live attached to the wall of the small intestine. Infestation is usually asymptomatic. Taeniasis is treated with praziquantel.

Diphyllobothriasis (Fish Tapeworm Infestation)

Diphyllobothriasis is acquired by ingestion of undercooked fish that is infested with tapeworm larvae. Adult worms inhabit the ileum. Infestation is usually devoid of symptoms. Worms can be killed with praziquantel.

Trematode Infestations

Schistosomiasis (Blood Fluke Infestations)

The term schistosomiasis refers to infestation with blood flukes of any species (e.g., *Schistosoma mansoni, S. japonicum*). Specific snails serve as intermediate hosts for these flukes. Schistosomiasis cannot be acquired in the continental United States because the appropriate snails are not indigenous.

Schistosomiasis has an acute and a chronic phase. The acute phase subsides in 3 to 4 months. Symptoms during this phase include lymphadenopathy, fever, anorexia, malaise, muscle pain, and rash. During the chronic phase, schistosomes take up residence in the vascular system, primarily in veins of the intestines and liver. This late infestation can produce intestinal polyposis, hepatosplenomegaly, and portal hypertension. For either the acute or the chronic stage, praziquantel is the treatment of choice.

Fascioliasis (Liver Fluke Infestation)

Fascioliasis is caused by two liver flukes: *Fasciola hepatica* (sheep liver fluke) and *Clonorchis sinensis* (Chinese liver fluke). Both parasites inhabit the biliary tract. Symptoms (anorexia, mild fever, fatigue, aching in the region of the liver) are delayed for 1 to 3 months.

Liver flukes differ in drug sensitivity. The preferred drug for use against *F. hepatica* is triclabendazole (a veterinary anthelmintic). It is not U.S. Food and Drug Administration (FDA) approved, but it is available through the Centers for Disease Control and Prevention (CDC) under an investigational drug protocol. The preferred drugs for use against *C. sinensis* are praziquantel and albendazole.

Fasciolopsiasis (Intestinal Fluke Infestation)

Fasciolopsiasis is most common in Southeast Asia. Adult worms inhabit the small intestine. The disease is usually asymptomatic. However, some people experience ulcer-like pain; some develop constipation or diarrhea; and, in the presence of massive infestation, bowel obstruction may occur, requiring surgery for clearance. Praziquantel is the treatment of choice.

DRUGS OF CHOICE FOR HELMINTHIASIS

The major anthelmintic drugs are considered next. These agents differ in antiparasitic spectra: some are active against several worms; others are more selective. Because of these differences, it is important to identify the invading organism so that the most appropriate drug can be chosen. Table 81.2 lists the major anthelmintic drugs and indicates the parasites against which each is most effective. Although the discussion that follows is limited to drugs of choice, be aware that additional anthelmintics are available.

Mebendazole

Target Organisms

Mebendazole [Vermox] is a drug of choice for most intestinal roundworms. This agent clears infestation with pinworms, hookworms, and giant roundworms. Because of its relatively broad spectrum of action, mebendazole is especially useful for treatment of mixed infestations.

Mechanism of Action

Mebendazole prevents uptake of glucose by susceptible intestinal worms. Glucose deprivation results in immobilization followed by slow death. Because the worms die slowly, up to 3 days may elapse between treatment onset and complete clearance of parasites. Mebendazole does not influence glucose uptake or utilization by humans.

Pharmacokinetics

Only a small fraction (5%–10%) of orally administered mebendazole is absorbed, and this fraction undergoes rapid metabolism. Consequently, plasma levels of mebendazole remain low.

Adverse Effects

Systemic effects are rare at usual doses, perhaps because the drug is so poorly absorbed. In patients with massive parasitic infestations, transient abdominal pain and diarrhea may occur.

Relatively low doses are embryotoxic and teratogenic in rats. However, these effects have not been observed in dogs, sheep, or horses. Limited experience with mebendazole in pregnant patients has shown no increase in

TABLE 81.2 ▪ First-Choice Anthelmintic Drugs: Target Organisms and Dosages

Generic Name [Trade Name]	Target Organism	Adult and Pediatric Dosages	Administration
Mebendazole [Vermox]	Roundworm	100 mg 2 times/day for 3 days *or* 500 mg once	May be taken with or without food. May be swallowed whole or crushed and mixed with food.
	Hookworm	500 mg once	
	Pinworm	100 mg; repeat in 2 weeks	
Albendazole [Albenza]	Giant roundworm	400 mg once	Take with high-fat food. May be swallowed whole or crushed and mixed with food.
	Hookworm		
	Whipworm	400 mg/day for 3 days	
	Pork roundworm	400 mg 2 times/day for 8–14 days	
	Pinworm	400 mg; repeat in 2 weeks	
	Chinese liver fluke	10 mg/kg/day for 7 days	
Triclabendazole*	Sheep liver fluke	10 mg/kg once or twice	Take with food
Pyrantel pamoate [Pin-X, others]	Hookworm	11 mg/kg (max. 1 g) for 3 days	May be taken with or without food. Chewable tablets must be chewed thoroughly. Suspensions should be shaken well.
	Pinworm	11 mg/kg (max. 1 g); repeat in 2 weeks	
Praziquantel [Biltricide]	Beef tapeworm†	5–10 mg/kg once	Take with food. Do not chew or crush. Swallow quickly to prevent nausea or vomiting due to taste.
	Pork tapeworm†		
	Fish tapeworm†		
	Blood flukes (*Schistosoma*)	20 mg/kg 3 doses 4–6 hours apart	
	S. japonicum, S. mekongi	20 mg/kg 3 times/day for 1 day	
	S. mansoni, S. haematobium	20 mg/kg 2 times/day for 1 day	
	Intestinal fluke	25 mg/kg 3 times/day for 1 day	
	Chinese liver fluke	25 mg/kg 3 times/day for 2 days	
	Lung fluke		
Diethylcarbamazine‡	*Wuchereria bancrofti*	Day 1: 50 mg	Take immediately after meals
	Brugia malayi	Day 2: 50 mg 3 times/day Day 3: 100 mg 3 times/day Days 4–21: 6 mg/kg/day in 3 divided doses	
	Loa loa	Day 1: 50 mg Day 2: 50 mg 3 times/day Day 3: 100 mg 3 times/day Days 4–21: 9 mg/kg/day in 3 divided doses	
Ivermectin [Stromectol]	Threadworm	200 mcg/kg/day for 2 days	Take on an empty stomach with water.
	Giant roundworm	150–200 mcg/kg once	
	Onchocerca volvulus	150 mcg/kg every 6–12 months until asymptomatic	

*Not available in the United States.
†Treatment of adult (intestinal) stage.
‡Available from the Centers for Disease Control and Prevention.

spontaneous abortion or fetal malformation. Nonetheless, pregnant patients should avoid this drug, especially during the first trimester.

Albendazole

Target Organisms

Albendazole [Albenza] is active against many cestode and nematode parasites, including larval forms of *Taenia solium* and *Echinococcus granulosus*. In the United States the drug is approved only for (1) parenchymal neurocysticercosis caused by larval forms of the pork tapeworm, *T. solium*; and (2) cystic hydatid disease of the liver, lung, and peritoneum caused by larval forms of the dog tapeworm, *E. granulosus*. However, despite lack of FDA approval, albendazole is considered a drug of choice for infestation with hookworms, pinworms, whipworms, Chinese liver flukes, giant roundworms, and pork roundworms, the cause of trichinosis.

Mechanism of Action

Albendazole inhibits polymerization of tubulin and thereby prevents formation of cytoplasmic microtubules. As a result, microtubule-dependent uptake of glucose is prevented.

Pharmacokinetics

Albendazole is poorly absorbed from the GI tract, owing largely to low solubility in water. Absorption is enhanced by administration with a fatty meal. After absorption, albendazole is rapidly converted to albendazole sulfoxide, its active form. Albendazole sulfoxide is distributed widely to body fluids and tissues and undergoes excretion in the bile. The half-life is 8 to 12 hours.

Adverse Effects

Albendazole is generally well tolerated. Mild to moderate liver impairment has occurred in 16% of patients, as indicated by elevation of liver transaminases in plasma. Liver function should be assessed before each cycle of treatment and 14 days later.

Albendazole suppresses bone marrow function and can thereby cause granulocytopenia, agranulocytosis, and even pancytopenia. Liver impairment may increase risk. Blood cell counts should be obtained before each cycle of treatment and 14 days later.

Albendazole is teratogenic in animals and hence should not be used during pregnancy. If pregnancy occurs, the drug should be discontinued immediately.

For neurocysticercosis or cystic hydatid disease, each dose is 400 mg (for patients greater than 60 kg) or 7.5 mg/kg (for patients less than 60 kg). The dosing schedule for neurocysticercosis is two doses twice daily with meals for 8 to 30 days. Dosing for cystic hydatid disease is done in three consecutive cycles, each consisting of two doses twice daily with meals for 28 days, followed by 14 days with no drug.

Pyrantel Pamoate

Target Organisms

Pyrantel pamoate [Pamix, Pin-X, Reese's Pinworm, Combantrin ♣] is active against intestinal nematodes. The drug is an alternative to mebendazole or albendazole for infestations with hookworms or pinworms.

Mechanism of Action

Pyrantel is a depolarizing neuromuscular blocking agent that causes spastic paralysis of intestinal parasites. The paralyzed worms are cleared in the feces.

Pharmacokinetics

Pyrantel is poorly absorbed, and plasma levels remain low. Most of an administered dose is excreted unchanged in the feces.

Adverse Effects

Serious reactions are rare. The most common effects are GI reactions (nausea, vomiting, diarrhea, stomach pain, cramps). Possible central nervous system effects include dizziness, drowsiness, headache, and insomnia.

Praziquantel

Target Organisms

Praziquantel [Biltricide] is very active against flukes and cestodes (tapeworms), and is the drug of choice for tapeworms, schistosomiasis, and other fluke infestations.

Mechanism of Action

Praziquantel is readily absorbed by helminths. At low therapeutic concentrations, the drug produces spastic paralysis, causing detachment of worms from body tissues. At high therapeutic concentrations, praziquantel disrupts the integument of the worms, rendering the parasites vulnerable to lethal attack by host defenses.

Pharmacokinetics

Praziquantel is rapidly absorbed from the GI tract. The drug undergoes extensive hepatic metabolism, followed by excretion in the urine. The half-life is short (about 1.5 hours).

Adverse Effects

Praziquantel is relatively free of toxicity. Transient headache and abdominal discomfort are the most frequent reactions. Drowsiness may occur, and hence patients should avoid driving and other hazardous activities.

Diethylcarbamazine

Target Organisms

Diethylcarbamazine [Hetrazan] is the drug of choice for filarial infestations. The drug destroys microfilariae of *W. bancrofti, B. malayi,* and *Loa loa*. In addition, it kills adult females of these species.

Mechanism of Action

Diethylcarbamazine has two antifilarial actions. First, it reduces muscular activity, causing parasites to be dislodged from their site of attachment. Second, by altering the surface properties of the parasites, it renders the organisms more vulnerable to attack by host defenses.

Pharmacokinetics

Diethylcarbamazine is readily absorbed and undergoes rapid and extensive metabolism. Metabolites are excreted in the urine.

Adverse Effects

Adverse effects caused directly by diethylcarbamazine are minor (headache, weakness, dizziness, nausea, vomiting). Indirect effects, occurring secondary to death of the parasites, can be more serious. These include rashes, intense itching, encephalitis, fever, tachycardia, lymphadenitis, leukocytosis, and proteinuria. Fortunately, these reactions are transient, lasting just a few days—and can be minimized by pretreatment with glucocorticoids.

Ivermectin

Target Organisms

Ivermectin [Stromectol] is active against many nematodes. Currently, the drug has two approved indications: onchocerciasis (a major cause of blindness worldwide) and intestinal strongyloidiasis. Ivermectin is active against the tissue microfilariae of *O. volvulus* (the cause of onchocerciasis), but not against the adult form. Ivermectin can also be used to kill mites and lice, although these parasites are not approved targets. In addition to its use in humans, ivermectin is used widely in veterinary medicine.

Mechanism of Action

Ivermectin disrupts nerve traffic and muscle function in target parasites. How? By opening chloride channels on the cell surface, which allows chloride ions to rush into nerve and muscle cells. The resultant hyperpolarization of these cells causes paralysis followed by death. Host cells are not affected because ivermectin is selective for chloride channels in parasites.

Pharmacokinetics

Ivermectin is administered orally and achieves peak plasma levels in 4 hours. Distribution to the central nervous system is poor. The drug is metabolized in the liver and excreted in the feces. Less than 1% of each dose appears in urine. The half-life is 16 hours.

Adverse Effect: Mazotti Reaction

The Mazotti reaction occurs in patients treated for onchocerciasis. Principal symptoms are pruritus, rash, fever, lymph node tenderness, and bone and joint pain. The apparent cause is an allergic and inflammatory response to the death of microfilariae. Mazotti-type reactions do not occur in patients treated for strongyloidiasis. Abdominal pain and headache are seen in less than 5% of patients. Hypotension develops rarely.

Use in Pregnancy

Ivermectin is teratogenic in mice, rats, and rabbits. Cleft palate is the most common effect. There are no adequate data on teratogenesis in humans. Until more is known, ivermectin should be avoided during pregnancy.

UNIT XIX

Drug Therapy for Patients with Cancer

CHAPTER 82

Anti-Cancer Drugs for the Nonspecialist

Jacqueline Rosenjack Burchum, DNSc, FNP-BC, CNE

BASIC PRINCIPALS OF CANCER CHEMOTHERAPY

THE ROLE OF THE NONSPECIALIST

Oncologists and affiliated specialists oversee cancer treatment. Although the nonspecialist provider does not typically have an active role in deciding how to treat cancer, as part of the interdisciplinary team caring for the patient, it remains essential to provide preventive care and to promote optimal well-being for those patients who receive treatment. Hence it is important to have a basic understanding of cancer, drugs used to treat cancer, and the effects that anticancer drugs have on patients.

WHAT IS CANCER?

In the discussion that follows, we consider properties shared by neoplastic cells as a group. However, although the discussion addresses cancers in general, be aware that the term *cancer* refers to a large group of disorders and not to a single disease: there are more than 100 different types of cancer, most of which have multiple subtypes. These various forms of cancer differ in clinical presentation, aggressiveness, drug sensitivity, and prognosis. Because of this diversity, treatment is individualized, based on the specific biology of the cells involved.

Characteristics of Neoplastic Cells

Persistent Proliferation

Unlike normal cells, whose proliferation is carefully controlled, cancer cells undergo unrestrained growth and division. This capacity for persistent proliferation is the most distinguishing property of malignant cells. In the absence of intervention, cancerous tissues will continue to grow until they cause death.

It was once believed that cancer cells divided more rapidly than normal cells and that this excessive rate of division was responsible for the abnormal growth patterns of cancerous tissues. We now know that this concept is not correct. The correct explanation for the relentless growth of tumors is that *malignant cells are unresponsive to the feedback mechanisms that regulate cellular proliferation in healthy tissue.* As a result, cancer cells are able to continue multiplying under conditions that would suppress further growth and division of normal cells. In other words, instead of dividing more rapidly, they divide more frequently than normal cells.

Invasive Growth

In the absence of malignancy, the various types of cells that compose a tissue remain segregated from one another; cells of one type do not invade territory that belongs to cells of a different type. In contrast, malignant cells are free of the constraints that inhibit invasive growth. As a result, cells of a solid tumor can penetrate adjacent tissues, thereby allowing the cancer to spread.

Formation of Metastases

Metastases are secondary tumors that appear at sites distant from the primary tumor. Metastases result from the unique ability of malignant cells to break away from their site of origin, migrate to other parts of the body (through the lymphatic and circulatory systems), and then reimplant to form a new tumor.

Immortality

Unlike normal cells, which are programmed to differentiate and eventually die, cancer cells can undergo endless divisions. The underlying cause for this difference is *telomerase,* an enzyme that is active in most cancers, and expressed only rarely in normal cells. Telomerase permits repeated division by preserving *telomeres*—the DNA-protein "caps" found on the end of each chromosome. As normal cells divide and differentiate, their telomeres become progressively shorter. When telomeres have lost a critical portion of their length, the cell is unable to keep on dividing. In cancer cells, telomerase continually adds back lost pieces of the telomere, and thereby preserves or extends telomere length. As a result, cancer cells can divide indefinitely.

Etiology of Cancer

The abnormal behavior of cancer cells results from alterations in their DNA. Specifically, malignant transformation results from a combination of activating *oncogenes* (cancer-causing genes) and inactivating *tumor suppressor genes* (genes that prevent replication of cells that have become cancerous). These genetic alterations are caused by chemical carcinogens, viruses, and radiation (x-rays, ultraviolet light, radioisotopes). Malignant transformation occurs in three major stages, called initiation, promotion, and progression. These stages suggest that DNA in cancer cells undergoes a series of small modifications, rather than a single large change. This accumulated genetic damage leads to dysregulation of cell division and protection against cell death.

It is important to appreciate that the changes in cellular function caused by malignant transformation are primarily *quantitative* rather than *qualitative.* That is, malignant transformation simply results in the overexpression or underexpression of the same gene products made by normal cells. As a result, cancer cells employ the same metabolic machinery as normal cells, use the same signaling pathways as normal cells, and express the same surface antigens as normal cells. Nonetheless, even though these changes in cellular function are only quantitative, they are still sufficient to allow unrestrained growth and avoidance of cell death.

Epidemiology

The American Cancer Society estimated that 589,430 Americans died from cancer in the year 2015. Cancer is a leading cause of death among all age groups, including children aged 1 to 18 years, in whom it is the leading nonaccidental cause of death. Among women, the most common cancers are breast, lung, and colorectal cancer. Among men, the most common cancers are prostate, lung, and colorectal cancer (Table 82.1).

For patients with some forms of cancer (see Table 82.1), drugs can often be curative. Cancers with a high cure rate include Hodgkin disease, testicular cancer, and acute lymphocytic leukemia. For many patients whose cancer is not yet curable, chemotherapy can still be of value, offering realistic hopes of palliation and prolonged life. However, although progress in chemotherapy has been encouraging, the ability to cure most cancers with drugs alone remains elusive.

TABLE 82.1 ▪ Estimated New Cancer Cases and Deaths, United States, 2015

	Females		Males	
Type of Cancer	New Cases	Deaths	New Cases	Deaths
All types	810,170	277,280	848,200	312,150
Breast	231,840	40,290	2350	440
Prostate			220,800	27,540
Lung and bronchus	105,590	71,660	115,610	86,380
Colon and rectum	63,610	23,600	69,090	26,100
Leukemia	23,370	10,240	30,900	14,210
Lymphoma	35,950	8,800	44,950	12,140
Endometrium	54,870	10,170		
Cervix	12,900	4100		
Ovary	21,290	14,180		
Melanoma of skin	31,200	3300	42,670	6640
Pancreas	24,120	19,850	24,840	20,710
Urinary bladder	17,680	4490	56,320	11,510
Kidney	23,290	5010	38,270	9070
Oral cavity and pharynx	13,110	2640	32,670	6010
Stomach	9050	4220	15,540	6500
Esophagus	3410	2990	13,570	12,600
Liver	10,150	7520	25,510	17,030
Brain and other central nervous system	9950	6380	12,900	8940
Multiple myeloma	12,760	5000	14,090	6240
Thyroid	47,230	1080	15,220	870

Data from American Cancer Society: Cancer Facts & Figs. 2015. Atlanta: American Cancer Society, 2015. http://www.cancer.org/acs/groups/content/@editorial/documents/document/acspc-044552.pdf (p. 4).

TREATMENT OF CANCER

We have three major modalities for treating cancer: *surgery, radiation therapy,* and *drug therapy.* Surgery is the most common treatment for *solid* cancers. In contrast, drug therapy is the treatment of choice for *disseminated* cancers (leukemias, disseminated lymphomas, and metastases) along with several localized cancers (e.g., choriocarcinoma, testicular carcinoma). Drug therapy also plays an important role as an adjunct to surgery and irradiation: by suppressing or killing malignant cells that surgery and irradiation leave behind, adjuvant drug therapy can reduce recurrence and improve survival.

Anticancer drugs fall into four major classes: *cytotoxic agents* (i.e., drugs that kill cells directly), *hormones and hormone antagonists, biologic response modifiers* (e.g., immunomodulating agents), and *targeted drugs* (i.e., drugs that bind with specific molecules [targets] that promote cancer growth). Of the four classes, the cytotoxic agents are used most often. You should note that the term *cancer chemotherapy* applies *only to the cytotoxic drugs*—it does not apply to the use of hormones, biologic response modifiers, or targeted drugs.

Introduction to the Cytotoxic Anticancer Drugs

The cytotoxic agents constitute the largest class of anticancer drugs. As their name implies, these agents act directly on cancer cells to cause their death. The cytotoxic drugs can be subdivided into eight major groups: (1) alkylating agents, (2) platinum compounds, (3) antimetabolites, (4) hypomethylating agents, (5) antitumor antibiotics, (6) mitotic inhibitors, (7) topoisomerase inhibitors, and (8) miscellaneous cytotoxic drugs. Individual cytotoxic agents are shown in Table 82.2.

Mechanisms of Cytotoxic Action

Table 82.2 shows the principal mechanisms by which the cytotoxic anticancer drugs act. As the table shows, most cytotoxic agents disrupt processes related to synthesis of DNA

TABLE 82.2 ■ Cytotoxic Anticancer Drugs

Generic Name	Trade Name	Cell-Cycle Phase Specificity	Route	Dose-Limiting Toxicity
ALKYLATING AGENTS				
Nitrogen Mustards				
Bendamustine	Treanda	Phase nonspecific	IV	Bone marrow suppression, infusion reactions
Chlorambucil	Leukeran	Phase nonspecific	PO	Bone marrow suppression
Cyclophosphamide	Generic only	Phase nonspecific	PO, IV	Bone marrow suppression
Ifosfamide	Ifex	Phase nonspecific	IV	Bone marrow suppression, hemorrhagic cystitis
Mechlorethamine	Mustargen	Phase nonspecific	IV, IC, IP	Bone marrow suppression
Melphalan	Alkeran	Phase nonspecific	PO, IV	Bone marrow suppression
Nitrosoureas				
Carmustine	BiCNU, Gliadel	Phase nonspecific	IV, CNS implant	Bone marrow suppression
Lomustine	CeeNU	Phase nonspecific	PO	Bone marrow suppression
Streptozocin	Zanosar	Phase nonspecific	IV	Nephrotoxicity
Others				
Busulfan	Myleran, Busulfex	Phase nonspecific	PO, IV	Bone marrow suppression, pulmonary fibrosis
Temozolomide	Temodar, Temodal ♣	Phase nonspecific	PO	Bone marrow suppression
Platinum Compounds				
Carboplatin	Generic only	Phase nonspecific	IV	Bone marrow suppression
Cisplatin	Generic only	Phase nonspecific	IV	Nephrotoxicity
Oxaliplatin	Eloxatin	Phase nonspecific	IV	Peripheral neuropathy
ANTIMETABOLITES				
Folic Acid Analogs				
Methotrexate	Rheumatrex, Trexall	S-phase specific	IV, IM, PO, IT	Bone marrow suppression, mucositis
Pemetrexed	Alimta	S-phase specific	IV	Bone marrow suppression
Pralatrexate	Folotyn	S-phase specific	IV	Bone marrow suppression, mucositis
Pyrimidine Analogs				
Capecitabine	Xeloda	Kills dividing cells only, mainly in S phase	PO	Bone marrow suppression, diarrhea, hand-and-foot syndrome
Cytarabine	DepoCyt, Tarabine PFS ♣	S-phase specific	IV, subQ, IT	Bone marrow suppression
Floxuridine	FUDR	Kills dividing cells only, mainly in S phase	IA	Bone marrow suppression, oral and GI ulceration
Fluorouracil	Adrucil	Kills dividing cells only, mainly in S phase	IV	Bone marrow suppression, oral and GI ulceration
Gemcitabine	Gemzar	S-phase specific	IV	Bone marrow suppression
Purine Analogs				
Cladribine	Generic only	Kills dividing cells only, mainly in S phase	IV	Bone marrow suppression
Clofarabine	Clolar	S-phase specific	IV	Bone marrow suppression
Fludarabine	Fludara	S-phase specific	IV	Bone marrow suppression
Mercaptopurine	Purinethol	S-phase specific	PO	Bone marrow suppression
Nelarabine	Arranon, Atriance ♣	S-phase specific	IV	Neurotoxicity
Pentostatin	Nipent	S-phase specific	IV	Bone marrow suppression
Thioguanine	Tabloid, Lanvis ♣	S-phase specific	PO, IV	Bone marrow suppression
Hypomethylating Agents				
Azacitidine	Vidaza	S-phase specific	SubQ	Bone marrow suppression
Decitabine	Dacogen	S-phase specific	IV	Bone marrow suppression
ANTITUMOR ANTIBIOTICS				
Anthracyclines				
Daunorubicin (conventional)	Cerubidine	Phase nonspecific	IV	Bone marrow suppression, cardiotoxicity
Daunorubicin (liposomal)	DaunoXome	Phase nonspecific	IV	Bone marrow suppression, cardiotoxicity
Doxorubicin (conventional)	Adriamycin	Phase nonspecific	IV	Bone marrow suppression, cardiotoxicity

Continued

TABLE 82.2 ▪ Cytotoxic Anticancer Drugs—cont'd

Generic Name	Trade Name	Cell-Cycle Phase Specificity	Route	Dose-Limiting Toxicity
Doxorubicin (liposomal)	Doxil, Caelyx ♣	Phase nonspecific	IV	Bone marrow suppression, heart failure
Epirubicin	Ellence	Phase nonspecific, but S and G_2 most sensitive	IV	Bone marrow suppression, cardiotoxicity
Idarubicin	Idamycin	Phase nonspecific, but S most sensitive	IV	Bone marrow suppression, cardiotoxicity
Valrubicin	Valstar	G_2-phase specific	Intravesical	Dysuria inadequately controlled by phenazopyridine, hematuria lasting more than 2 days
Mitoxantrone*	Novantrone	Phase nonspecific	IV	Bone marrow suppression, cardiotoxicity
Nonanthracyclines				
Bleomycin	Generic only	G_2-phase specific	IV, IM, subQ, IP	Pneumonitis and pulmonary fibrosis
Dactinomycin	Cosmegen	Phase nonspecific	IV	Bone marrow suppression, mucositis
Mitomycin	Generic only in United States, Mutamycin ♣	Phase nonspecific, but G_1 and S most sensitive	IV	Bone marrow suppression
MITOTIC INHIBITORS				
Vinca Alkaloids				
Vinblastine	Velban	M-phase specific	IV	Bone marrow suppression
Vincristine (conventional)	Oncovin, Vincasar PFS	M-phase specific	IV	Peripheral neuropathy
Vincristine (liposomal)	Marqibo	M-phase specific	IV	Peripheral neuropathy
Vinorelbine	Navelbine	M-phase specific	IV	Bone marrow suppression
Taxanes				
Cabazitaxel	Jevtana	G_2/M-phase specific	IV	Bone marrow suppression, diarrhea
Docetaxel	Docefrez, Taxotere	G_2/M-phase specific	IV	Bone marrow suppression
Paclitaxel	Abraxane, Onxol, Taxol ♣	G_2/M-phase specific	IV	Bone marrow suppression
Others				
Eribulin	Halaven	G_2/M-phase specific	IV	Bone marrow suppression, peripheral neuropathy
Estramustine	Emcyt	M-phase specific	PO	Nausea and vomiting
Ixabepilone	Ixempra	G_2/M-phase specific	IV	Bone marrow suppression, neurotoxicity
Topoisomerase Inhibitors				
Etoposide	Toposar	S and G_2 most sensitive	IV, PO	Bone marrow suppression
Irinotecan	Camptosar	S-phase specific	IV	Bone marrow suppression and late diarrhea
Teniposide	Vumon	S and G_2 most sensitive	IV	Bone marrow suppression
Topotecan	Hycamtin	S-phase specific	IV	Bone marrow suppression
Miscellaneous				
Altretamine	Hexalen	Specificity unknown	PO	Bone marrow suppression
Asparaginase	Elspar, Erwinase ♣, Kidrolase ♣	G_1-phase specific	IV, IM	None
Dacarbazine	DTIC-Dome	Phase nonspecific	IV	Bone marrow suppression
Hydroxyurea	Hydrea	S-phase specific	PO	Bone marrow suppression
Mitotane	Lysodren	Phase nonspecific	PO	CNS depression
Pegaspargase	Oncaspar	G_1-phase specific	IV, IM	None
Procarbazine	Matulane	Phase nonspecific	PO	Bone marrow suppression

*Mitoxantrone is classified chemically as an anthracenedione, which is very similar to an anthracycline.
CNS, central nervous system; GI, gastrointestinal; IA, intraarterial; IC, intracavitary; IM, intramuscular; IP, intrapleural; IT, intrathecal; IV, intravenous; PO, oral; subQ, subcutaneous.

or its precursors. In addition, some agents (e.g., vinblastine, vincristine) act specifically to block mitosis, and one drug—asparaginase—disrupts synthesis of proteins. Note that, with the exception of asparaginase, all of the cytotoxic drugs disrupt processes carried out exclusively by cells that are undergoing replication. As a result, these drugs are most toxic to tissues that have a high growth fraction (i.e., a high proportion of proliferating cells).

Cell-Cycle Phase Specificity

Some anticancer agents, known as *cell-cycle phase–specific drugs,* are effective only during a specific phase of the cell cycle. (See Box 82.1.) Other anticancer agents, known as cell-cycle phase–nonspecific drugs, can affect cells during any phase of the cell cycle. About half of the cytotoxic anticancer drugs are phase specific, and the other half are phase nonspecific. The phase specificity of individual cytotoxic agents is shown in Table 82.2.

Cell-Cycle Phase–Specific Drugs

Phase-specific agents are toxic only to cells that are passing through a particular phase of the cell cycle (see Fig. 82.1). Vincristine, for example, acts by causing mitotic arrest and hence is effective only during M phase. Other agents act by disrupting DNA synthesis and hence are effective only during S phase. Because of their phase specificity, these drugs are toxic only to cells that are active participants in the cell cycle; cells that are "resting" in G_0 will not be harmed. Obviously, if these drugs are to be effective, they must be present as neoplastic cells cycle through the specific phase in which they act. Accordingly, these drugs must be present for an extended time. To accomplish this, phase-specific drugs are often administered by prolonged infusion. Alternatively, they can be given in multiple doses at short intervals over an extended time. Because the dosing schedule is so critical to therapeutic response, phase-specific drugs are also known as *schedule-dependent drugs.*

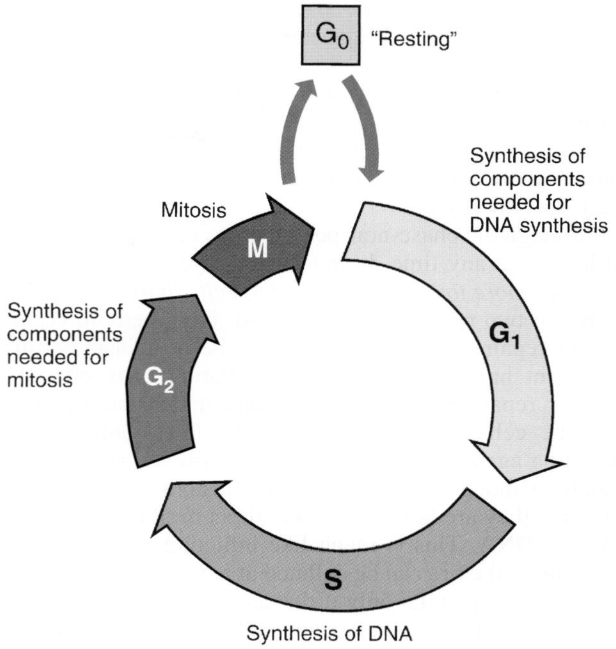

Figure 82.1 ▪ The cell cycle.

BOX 82.1 ▪ THE GROWTH FRACTION AND ITS RELATIONSHIP TO CHEMOTHERAPY

The growth fraction of a tissue is a major determinant of its responsiveness to chemotherapy. Consequently, before we discuss the anticancer drugs, we must first understand the growth fraction. To define the growth fraction, we must review the cell cycle.

The Cell Cycle

The cell cycle is the sequence of events that a cell goes through from one mitotic division to the next. As shown in Fig. 82.1, the cell cycle consists of four major phases, named G_1, S, G_2, and M. (The length of the *arrows* in the figure is proportional to the time spent in each phase.) For our purpose, we can imagine the cycle as beginning with G_1, the phase in which the cell prepares to make DNA. After G_1, the cell enters S phase, the phase in which DNA synthesis actually takes place. After synthesis of DNA is complete, the cell enters G_2 and prepares for mitosis (cell division). Mitosis occurs next during M phase. On completing mitosis, the resulting daughter cells have two options: they can enter G_1 and repeat the cycle, or they can enter the phase known as G_0. Cells that enter G_0 become mitotically dormant; they do not replicate and are not active participants in the cycle. Cells may remain in G_0 for days, weeks, or even years. Under appropriate conditions, resting cells may leave G_0 and resume active participation in the cycle.

The Growth Fraction

In any tissue, some cells are going through the cell cycle, whereas others are "resting" in G_0. The ratio of proliferating cells to G_0 cells is called the *growth fraction.* A tissue with a large percentage of proliferating cells and few cells in G_0 has a *high* growth fraction. Conversely, a tissue composed mostly of G_0 cells has a *low* growth fraction.

Impact of Tissue Growth Fraction on Responsiveness to Chemotherapy

As a rule, *chemotherapeutic drugs are much more toxic to tissues that have a high growth fraction than to tissues that have a low growth fraction.* Why? Because most cytotoxic agents are more active against proliferating cells than against cells in G_0. Proliferating cells are especially sensitive to chemotherapy because cytotoxic drugs usually act by disrupting either DNA synthesis or mitosis—activities that only proliferating cells carry out. Unfortunately, toxicity of anticancer drugs is not restricted to cancers: These drugs are also toxic to normal tissues that have a high growth fraction (e.g., bone marrow, GI epithelium, hair follicles, sperm-forming cells).

Having established the relationship between growth fraction and drug sensitivity, we can apply this knowledge to predict how specific cancers will respond to chemotherapy. As a rule, *the most common cancers*—solid tumors of the breast, lung, prostate, colon, and rectum—have a *low* growth fraction, so they *respond poorly to cytotoxic drugs.* In contrast, only some rarer cancers—such as acute lymphocytic leukemia, Hodgkin disease, and certain testicular cancers—have a *high* growth fraction, so they tend to respond *well to cytotoxic drugs.* In practical terms, this means that the most common cancers, which don't respond well to drugs, must be managed primarily with surgery. Only a few cancers can be managed primarily with drugs.

Cell-Cycle Phase–Nonspecific Drugs

The phase-nonspecific drugs can act during any phase of the cell cycle, including G_0. Among the phase-nonspecific drugs are the alkylating agents and most antitumor antibiotics. Because phase-nonspecific drugs can injure cells throughout the cell cycle, whereas phase-specific drugs cannot, phase-nonspecific drugs can increase cell kill when combined with phase-specific drugs.

Although the phase-nonspecific drugs can cause biochemical lesions at any time during the cell cycle, *as a rule these drugs are more toxic to proliferating cells than to cells in* G_0. There are two reasons why this is so. First, cells in G_0 have time to repair drug-induced damage before it can result in significant harm. In contrast, proliferating cells often lack time for repair. Second, toxicity may not become manifest until the cells attempt to proliferate. For example, many alkylating agents act by producing cross-links between DNA strands. Although these biochemical lesions can be made at any time, they are largely without effect until cells attempt to replicate DNA. This is much like inflicting a flat tire on an automobile: the tire can be deflated at any time; however, loss of air is consequential only if the car is moving. Carrying the analogy further, if the flat occurs while the car is stopped, and is repaired before travel is attempted, the flat will have no functional effect at all.

It should be noted that some dividing cells are more vulnerable than others. Specifically, cells that divide frequently are harmed more readily than cells that divide infrequently because the cytotoxic drugs have more opportunities to act.

Toxicity to Normal Cells

Toxicity to normal cells is a major barrier to successful chemotherapy. Injury to normal cells occurs primarily in tissues where the growth fraction is high: bone marrow, gastrointestinal (GI) epithelium, hair follicles, and germinal epithelium of the testes. Drug-induced injury to each of these tissues is discussed in detail later. For now, let's consider injury to normal cells as a group.

Toxicity to normal cells is dose limiting. That is, dosage cannot exceed an amount that produces the maximally tolerated injury to normal cells. Although very large doses of cytotoxic drugs might be able to produce cure, these doses cannot be given because they are likely to kill the patient.

Why are cytotoxic anticancer drugs so harmful to normal tissues? Because these drugs lack *selective toxicity.* That is, *they cannot kill target cells without also killing other cells with which the target cells are in intimate contact.* We encountered this concept in Chapter 68. As noted there, successful antimicrobial therapy is possible because antimicrobial drugs are highly selective in their toxicity. Penicillin, for example, can readily kill invading bacteria while being virtually harmless to cells of the host. This high degree of selective toxicity stands in sharp contrast to the lack of selectivity displayed by cytotoxic anticancer drugs.

Why have we been unable to develop drugs that selectively kill neoplastic cells? Because neoplastic cells and normal cells are very similar: differences between them are quantitative rather than qualitative. To make a cytotoxic drug that is truly selective, the target cell must have a biochemical feature that normal cells lack. Unfortunately, we have yet to identify unique biochemical features that would render cancer cells vulnerable to selective attack. Nevertheless, there is reason for hope: our expanding knowledge of cancer biology is revealing potential new targets for anticancer drugs. Exploiting these targets may lead to anticancer drugs that are more selective than the drugs we have now.

Major Toxicities of Chemotherapeutic Drugs

The agents used for cancer chemotherapy constitute our most toxic group of medicines. In the discussion that follows, we consider the more common toxicities of the *cytotoxic* anticancer drugs along with steps that can be taken to minimize harm and discomfort.

Bone Marrow Suppression

Chemotherapeutic drugs are highly toxic to the bone marrow, a tissue with a high proportion of proliferating cells. Myelosuppression reduces the number of circulating neutrophils, platelets, and erythrocytes. Loss of these cells has three major consequences: (1) infection (from loss of neutrophils); (2) bleeding (from loss of platelets); and (3) anemia (from loss of erythrocytes).

Neutropenia

Neutrophils (neutrophilic granulocytes) are white blood cells that play a critical role in fighting infection. In patients with neutropenia (a reduction in circulating neutrophils), both the incidence and severity of infection are increased. Infections that are normally benign (e.g., candidiasis) can become life-threatening. Infection secondary to neutropenia is one of the most serious complications of chemotherapy.

With most anticancer drugs, onset of neutropenia is rapid and recovery develops relatively quickly. Neutropenia begins to develop a few days after dosing, and the lowest neutrophil count, called the *nadir,* occurs between days 10 and 14. Neutrophil counts then recover a week or so later. Patients are at highest risk during the nadir. Accordingly, special care should be taken to prevent infection.

With some anticancer drugs, neutropenia is *delayed.* Neutrophil counts begin to fall in 1 to 2 weeks and reach their nadir between weeks 3 and 4. Full recovery may not occur until after week 7.

Neutrophil counts must be monitored. Normal counts range from 2500 to 7000 cells/mm^3. If neutropenia is substantial (absolute neutrophil count below 500/mm^3), chemotherapy should be withheld until neutrophil counts return toward normal. Fortunately, normal cells such as neutrophils repopulate faster than malignant cells (see Fig. 82.2).

Lack of neutrophils confounds the diagnosis of infection. Why? Because the usual signs of infection (e.g., pus, abscesses, infiltrates on the chest radiograph) depend on neutrophils being present. In the absence of neutrophils, *fever* is the principal early sign of infection.

Patients must be their own first line of defense against infection. They should be made aware of their elevated risk for infection and taught how to minimize contagion. They should be informed that fever may be the only indication of infection and instructed to report immediately if fever develops. Because infection is commonly acquired through contact with other people, hospitalized patients should be instructed to refuse direct contact with anyone who has not washed his or her hands in the patient's presence. This rule applies not

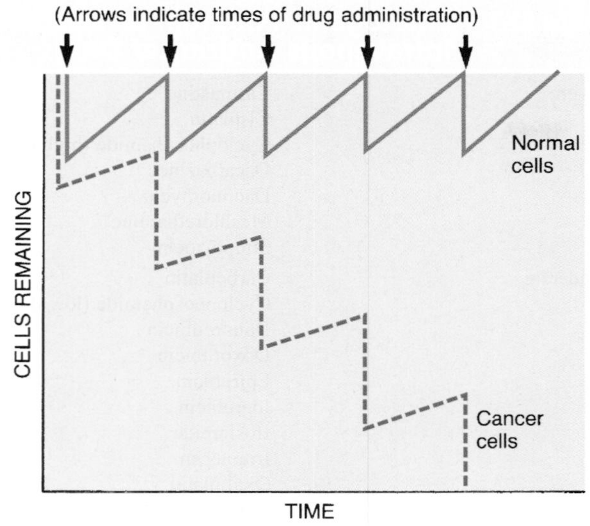

Figure 82.2 ■ Recovery of critical normal cells. Cancer cells and normal cells (e.g., cells of the bone marrow) are killed each time cytotoxic drugs are given. In the interval between doses, both types of cells proliferate. Because normal cells repopulate faster than the cancer cells, normal cells are able to recover in higher numbers between doses, whereas regrowth of the cancer cells is slower.

only to visiting friends and relatives but also to nurses, physicians, and all other hospital staff. The normal flora of the body is a major source of infection; the risk for acquiring an infection with these microbes can be reduced by daily examination and cleansing of the skin and oral cavity.

Hospitalization of the infection-free neutropenic patient is controversial. Some providers feel that hospitalization *increases* the risk for acquiring a serious infection. Why? Because hospitals harbor drug-resistant microbes, which can make hospital-acquired (nosocomial) infections especially difficult to treat. Accordingly, these providers recommend that neutropenic patients stay at home as long as they remain infection free.

If neutropenic patients *are* hospitalized, every precaution must be taken to prevent nosocomial infection. Patients should be given an isolation room and monitored frequently for fever. Certain foods (e.g., lettuce) abound in pathogenic bacteria and must be avoided.

When a neutropenic patient develops an infection, immediate and vigorous intervention is required. Specimens for culture should be taken to determine the identity and drug sensitivity of the infecting organism. While awaiting reports on the cultures, empiric therapy with intravenous (IV) antibiotics should be instituted. Initial therapy is usually done with a single drug active against *Pseudomonas* species and other gram-negative bacteria. Options include ceftazidime, imipenem, and doripenem. If the patient develops sepsis, an aminoglycoside (e.g., tobramycin, amikacin) is added. If the patient remains febrile, vancomycin is added (for gram-positive coverage).

Colony-stimulating factors can minimize neutropenia. Three preparations are available: *granulocyte colony-stimulating factor* (filgrastim), long-acting granulocyte colony-stimulating factor (pegfilgrastim), and *granulocyte-macrophage colony-stimulating factor* (GM-CSF) (sargramostim). All three drugs act on the bone marrow to enhance granulocyte (neutrophil) production. Colony-stimulating factors can decrease the incidence, magnitude, and duration of neutropenia. As a result, they can decrease the incidence and severity of infection as well as the need for IV antibiotics and hospitalization.

Thrombocytopenia

Bone marrow suppression can cause thrombocytopenia (a reduction in circulating platelets), thereby increasing the risk for serious bleeding. Bleeding from the nose and gums is relatively common. Bleeding from the gums can be reduced by avoiding vigorous tooth brushing. Drugs that promote bleeding (e.g., aspirin, anticoagulants) should not be used. When a mild analgesic is required, acetaminophen, which does not promote bleeding, is preferred to aspirin. For patients with severe thrombocytopenia, platelet infusions are the mainstay of treatment. Platelet production can be stimulated with *oprelvekin* [Neumega]. However, owing to limited efficacy and flu-like reactions, oprelvekin is not often used.

Caution should be exercised when performing procedures that might promote bleeding. IV needles should be inserted with special care, and intramuscular (IM) injections should be avoided. Blood pressure cuffs should be applied cautiously because overinflation may cause bruising or bleeding.

Anemia

Anemia is defined as a reduction in the number of circulating erythrocytes (red blood cells). Although anticancer drugs can suppress erythrocyte production, anemia is much less common than neutropenia or thrombocytopenia. Why? Because circulating erythrocytes have a long life span (120 days), which usually allows erythrocyte production to recover before levels of existing erythrocytes fall too low.

If anemia does develop, it can be treated with a transfusion or with erythropoietin (*epoetin alfa* or *darbepoetin alfa*), a hormone that stimulates production of red blood cells. Because transfusions require hospitalization, whereas epoetin can be administered at home, epoetin therapy can spare the patient inconvenience. However, erythropoietin has two huge drawbacks. First, it cannot be used in patients with leukemias and other myeloid malignancies (because it can stimulate proliferation of these cancers). Second, it *shortens* survival in all cancer patients and hence is indicated only when the treatment goal is *palliation.* Clearly, erythropoietin should not be used when the goal is cure or prolongation of life. The basic pharmacology of erythropoietin is discussed in Chapter 45.

Digestive Tract Injury

The epithelial lining of the GI tract has a very high growth fraction, so it is exquisitely sensitive to cytotoxic drugs. Stomatitis and diarrhea are common. Severe GI injury can be life-threatening.

Stomatitis

Stomatitis (inflammation of the oral mucosa) often develops a few days after the onset of chemotherapy and may persist for 2 or more weeks after treatment has ceased. Inflammation can progress to denudation and ulceration and is often complicated by infection. Pain can be severe, inhibiting eating, speaking, and swallowing. Management includes good oral hygiene and a bland diet. Topical antifungal drugs may be needed to control infection with *Candida albicans.* For patients with mild stomatitis, pain can be managed with a mouthwash containing a topical anesthetic (e.g., lidocaine) plus an antihistamine (e.g., diphenhydramine). For patients with severe stomatitis, a systemic opioid is needed for pain. In some cases, stomatitis is so severe that chemotherapy has to be interrupted. For patients being treated for hematologic malignancies, *palifermin* [Kepivance], a chemoprotective agent and keratinocyte growth factor, can decrease the severity of stomatitis.

Diarrhea

By injuring the epithelial lining of the intestine, anticancer drugs can impair absorption of fluids and other nutrients, thereby causing diarrhea. Diarrhea can be reduced with oral loperamide, a nonabsorbable opioid that slows gut motility by activating local opioid receptors.

Nausea and Vomiting

Nausea and vomiting are common sequelae of cancer chemotherapy. These responses, which result in part from direct stimulation of the chemoreceptor trigger zone, can be both immediate and dramatic and may persist for hours or even days. In some cases, discomfort is so great as to prompt refusal of further treatment.

You should appreciate that nausea and vomiting associated with chemotherapy are much more severe than with other medications. Whereas these reactions are generally unremarkable with most drugs, they must be considered major and characteristic toxicities of cytotoxic drugs. The emetogenic potential of several intravenous agents is shown in Table 82.3.

Nausea and vomiting can be reduced by premedication with antiemetics. These drugs offer three benefits: (1) reduction of anticipatory nausea and vomiting, (2) prevention of dehydration and malnutrition secondary to frequent nausea and vomiting, and (3) promotion of compliance with chemotherapy by reducing discomfort. Combinations of antiemetics are more effective than single-drug therapy. The regimen of choice for patients taking highly emetogenic drugs consists of *aprepitant* [Emend], *dexamethasone,* and a *serotonin antagonist,* such as *ondansetron* [Zofran]. The use of antiemetics for chemotherapy-induced nausea and vomiting is discussed in Chapter 64.

TABLE 82.3 ▪ Emetogenic Potential of Selected Intravenous Anticancer Drugs

Severe	Carmustine Cisplatin Cyclophosphamide (high dose) Dacarbazine Dactinomycin Mechlorethamine Streptozocin
Moderate	Carboplatin Cyclophosphamide (low dose) Daunorubicin Doxorubicin Epirubicin Idarubicin Ifosfamide Irinotecan Oxaliplatin
Low	Cytarabine Docetaxel Etoposide Fluorouracil Gemcitabine Methotrexate (high dose) Mitomycin Mitoxantrone Paclitaxel Pemetrexed Topotecan Trastuzumab
Minimal	Bevacizumab Bleomycin Busulfan Cetuximab Fludarabine Pralatrexate Rituximab Vinblastine Vincristine Vinorelbine

Other Important Toxicities

Alopecia

Reversible alopecia (hair loss) results from injury to hair follicles. Alopecia can occur with most cytotoxic anticancer drugs. Hair loss begins 7 to 10 days after the onset of treatment and reaches maximal loss in 1 to 2 months. Regeneration begins 1 to 2 months after the last course of treatment.

Although alopecia is not dangerous, it is nonetheless very upsetting. In fact, for many cancer patients, alopecia is second only to vomiting as their greatest treatment-related fear. If drugs are expected to cause hair loss, the patient should be forewarned. For patients who choose to wear a hairpiece or wig, one should be selected before hair loss occurs. Hairpieces are tax deductible as medical expenses and are covered by some insurance plans.

To some degree, hair loss can be prevented by cooling the scalp while chemotherapy is being administered. Cooling causes vasoconstriction and thereby reduces drug delivery to hair follicles. Unfortunately, scalp cooling is uncomfortable, causes headache, and creates a small risk for cancer recurrence in the scalp (because drug delivery is reduced).

Reproductive Toxicity

The developing fetus and the germinal epithelium of the testes have high growth fractions. As a result, both are highly susceptible to injury by cytotoxic drugs, especially the alkylating agents. These drugs can interfere with embryogenesis, causing death of the early embryo. They may also cause fetal malformation. Risk is highest during the first trimester, and hence chemotherapy should generally be avoided during this time. However, after 18 weeks of gestation, risk appears to be very low: according to a 2012 report in *Lancet,* exposure during this time does not cause neurologic, cardiac, or any other fetal abnormalities. Drug effects on the ovaries may result in amenorrhea, menopausal symptoms, and atrophy of the vaginal epithelium.

Cytotoxic drugs can cause irreversible sterility in males. Men should be forewarned and counseled about sperm banking.

Hyperuricemia

Hyperuricemia is defined as an excessive level of uric acid in the blood. Uric acid, a compound with low solubility, is formed by the breakdown of DNA after cell death. Hyperuricemia is especially common after treatment for leukemias and lymphomas (because therapy results in massive cell kill). The major concern with hyperuricemia is injury to the kidneys secondary to deposition of uric acid crystals in renal tubules. The risk for crystal formation can be reduced by increasing fluid intake. In patients with leukemias and lymphomas, in whom hyperuricemia is likely, prophylaxis with *allopurinol* is the standard of care. (As discussed in Chapter 58, allopurinol prevents hyperuricemia by inhibiting xanthine oxidase, an enzyme involved in converting nucleic acids to uric acid.) If hyperuricemia develops despite use of allopurinol, it can be managed with *rasburicase,* an enzyme that catalyzes uric acid degradation).

Local Injury From Extravasation of Vesicants

Certain anticancer drugs, known as *vesicants,* are highly chemically reactive. These drugs can cause severe local injury if they make direct contact with tissues. Vesicants are administered intravenously, usually into a central line (because rapid dilution in venous blood minimizes the risk for injury). When a peripheral line is used, administration is by IV push into a freely flowing IV line. Sites of previous irradiation should be avoided. Extreme care must be exercised to prevent extravasation because leakage can produce high local concentrations, resulting in prolonged pain, infection, and loss of mobility. Severe injury can lead to necrosis and sloughing, requiring surgical débridement and skin grafting. If extravasation occurs, the infusion should be stopped immediately. Because of the potential for severe tissue damage, vesicants should be administered only by clinicians specially trained to handle them safely.

Unique Toxicities

In addition to the toxicities discussed previously, which generally apply to the cytotoxic drugs as a group, some agents produce unique toxicities. For example, a number of drugs can cause peripheral sensory neuropathy, manifesting as numbness or tingling in the fingers and toes and around the mouth and throat. Neuropathy may impede activities of daily living, such as buttoning clothing, writing, or just holding things. Anthracyclines such as daunorubicin and doxorubicin can cause serious injury to the heart. Ifosfamide, a nitrogen mustard, can cause severe hemorrhagic cystitis.

Carcinogenesis

Along with their other adverse actions, anticancer drugs have one final and ironic toxicity: these drugs, which are used to treat cancer, have caused cancer in some patients. Cancer results from drug-induced damage to DNA and is most likely to occur with alkylating agents. Cancers caused by anticancer drugs may take many years to appear and are hard to treat.

MAKING THE DECISION TO TREAT

From the preceding discussion of toxicities, it is clear that cytotoxic anticancer drugs can cause great harm. Given the known dangers of these drugs, we must ask why such toxic substances are given to sick people at all. The answer lies with the primary rule of therapeutics, which states that the benefits of treatment must outweigh the risks. For most patients undergoing chemotherapy, the conditions of this rule are met. That is, although the toxicities of the anticancer drugs can be significant, the potential benefits (cure, prolonged life, palliation) justify the risks. However, the desirability of treating cancer with drugs is not always obvious. There are patients whose chances of being helped by chemotherapy are remote, whereas the risk for serious toxicity is high. Because the potential benefits for some patients are small and the risks are large, the decision to institute chemotherapy must be made with care.

Before a decision to treat can be made, the patient must be given some idea of the benefits the proposed therapy might offer. Three basic benefits are possible: cure, prolongation of life, and palliation. For treatment to be justified, there should be reason to believe that at least one of these benefits will be forthcoming. If a patient cannot be offered some reasonable hope of cure, prolonged life, or palliation, it would be difficult to justify treatment.

The most important factors for predicting the outcome of chemotherapy are (1) the general health of the patient and (2) the responsiveness of the type of cancer the patient has. General health status is assessed by measuring performance status, frequently using the Karnofsky Performance Scale (Table 82.4). A Karnofsky score of less than 40 indicates the patient is debilitated and not likely to tolerate the additional stress of chemotherapy. Accordingly, patients with a low

TABLE 82.4 ▪ Karnofsky Performance Scale

Definition	Percentage	Criteria
Able to carry on normal activity and work; no special care needed	100	Normal; no complaints; no evidence of disease
	90	Able to carry on normal activity; minor signs or symptoms of disease
	80	Normal activity with effort; some signs or symptoms of disease
Unable to work; able to live at home and care for most personal needs; a varying amount of assistance needed	70	Cares for self; unable to carry on normal activity or do active work
	60	Requires occasional assistance; able to care for most needs
	50	Requires considerable assistance and frequent medical care
Unable to care for self; requires equivalent of institutional or hospital care; disease may be progressing rapidly	40	Disabled; requires special care and assistance
	30	Severely disabled; hospitalization is indicated although death not imminent
	20	Very sick, hospitalization necessary; active supportive treatment necessary
	10	Moribund; fatal processes progressing rapidly
	0	Dead

Karnofsky rating should not receive anticancer drugs—unless their cancer is known to be especially responsive.

The responsiveness of specific cancers is not highly predictable: some patients with a specific type of cancer may respond well, but others may not. Nonetheless, we should still try to assess whether treatment is likely to produce cure, palliation, or prolonged life. If a positive outcome is deemed likely, the patient should almost always be treated, even if his or her Karnofsky score is low. In contrast, if a positive outcome is deemed highly unlikely, the patient should be treated only after careful consideration, so as to avoid the discomforts of a course of treatment that has little to offer.

An important requirement for deciding in favor of chemotherapy is that the effect of treatment be measurable. That is, there must be some objective means of determining the cancer's response to drugs. For solid tumors, we should be able to measure a decrease in tumor size (or at least inhibition of further growth). For hematologic cancers, we should be able to measure a decrease in neoplastic cells in blood and bone marrow. If we have no way to measure the response of a cancer, then we have no way of knowing if treatment has done any good. If we cannot determine that drugs are doing something beneficial, there is little justification for giving them.

Clearly, not all patients are candidates for chemotherapy. The decision to institute treatment must be individualized. Patients should be informed as accurately as possible about the potential risks and benefits of the proposed therapy. When the decision to treat is made, it should be the result of collaboration between the patient, family, and physician and should reflect a conviction on the part of the patient that, within his or her set of values, the potential benefits outweigh the inherent risks.

CYTOTOXIC AGENTS

ALKYLATING AGENTS

The family of alkylating agents consists of nitrogen mustards, nitrosoureas, and other compounds. The alkylating agents are shown in Table 82.2.

Shared Properties

Mechanism of Action

The alkylating agents are highly reactive compounds that can transfer an alkyl group to various cell constituents. Cell kill results primarily from alkylation of DNA. As a rule, alkylating agents interact with DNA by forming a covalent bond with a specific nitrogen atom in guanine.

Some alkylating agents have two reactive sites, whereas others have only one. Alkylating agents with two reactive sites (*bifunctional* agents) are able to bind DNA in two places to form *cross-links.* These bridges may be formed within a single DNA strand or between parallel DNA strands. Fig. 82.3 shows the production of interstrand cross-links by nitrogen mustard. Alkylating agents with only one reactive site (*monofunctional* agents) lack the ability to form cross-links but can still bind to a single guanine in DNA.

The consequences of guanine alkylation are miscoding, scission of DNA strands, and, if cross-links have been formed, inhibition of DNA replication. Because cross-linking of DNA is especially injurious, cell death is more likely with bifunctional agents than with monofunctional agents.

Because alkylation reactions can take place at any time during the cell cycle, alkylating agents are considered *cell-cycle phase nonspecific.* However, *most of these drugs are more toxic to dividing cells—especially cells that divide rapidly—than they are to cells in G_0.* Why? Because (1) alkylation of DNA produces its most detrimental effects when cells attempt to replicate DNA and (2) quiescent cells are often able to repair damage to DNA before it can affect cell function.

Toxicities

Alkylating agents are toxic to tissues that have a high growth fraction. Accordingly, these drugs may injure cells of the bone marrow, hair follicles, GI mucosa, and germinal epithelium. Blood dyscrasias—neutropenia, thrombocytopenia, and anemia—caused by bone marrow suppression are of greatest concern. Nausea and vomiting occur with all alkylating agents. Also, several of these drugs are vesicants and hence must be administered through a free-flowing IV line. The major dose-limiting toxicities of individual drugs are provided in Table 82.2.

Nitrosoureas

The nitrosoureas are bifunctional alkylating agents and are active against a broad spectrum of neoplastic diseases. Cell kill results from cross-linking DNA. Unlike many anticancer drugs, the nitrosoureas are highly lipophilic and hence can readily penetrate the blood-brain barrier. As a result, these drugs are especially useful against *cancers of the CNS.* The major dose-limiting toxicity is *delayed bone marrow suppression.*

PLATINUM COMPOUNDS

The platinum-containing anticancer drugs—cisplatin, carboplatin, and oxaliplatin—are similar to the alkylating agents and are often classified as such. Like the bifunctional alkylating agents, the platinum compounds produce cross-links in DNA and hence are cell-cycle phase nonspecific.

ANTIMETABOLITES

Antimetabolites are structural analogs of important natural metabolites. Because they resemble natural metabolites, these drugs are able to disrupt critical metabolic processes. Some antimetabolites inhibit enzymes that synthesize essential cellular constituents. Others undergo incorporation into DNA and thereby disrupt DNA replication and function.

Antimetabolites are effective only against cells that are active participants in the cell cycle. Most antimetabolites are S-phase specific, although some can act during any phase of the cycle, except G_0. To be effective, agents that are S-phase specific must be present for an extended time.

There are three classes of antimetabolites: (1) folic acid analogs, (2) pyrimidine analogs, and (3) purine analogs. Members of each class, along with their dose-limiting toxicities, are shown in Table 82.2.

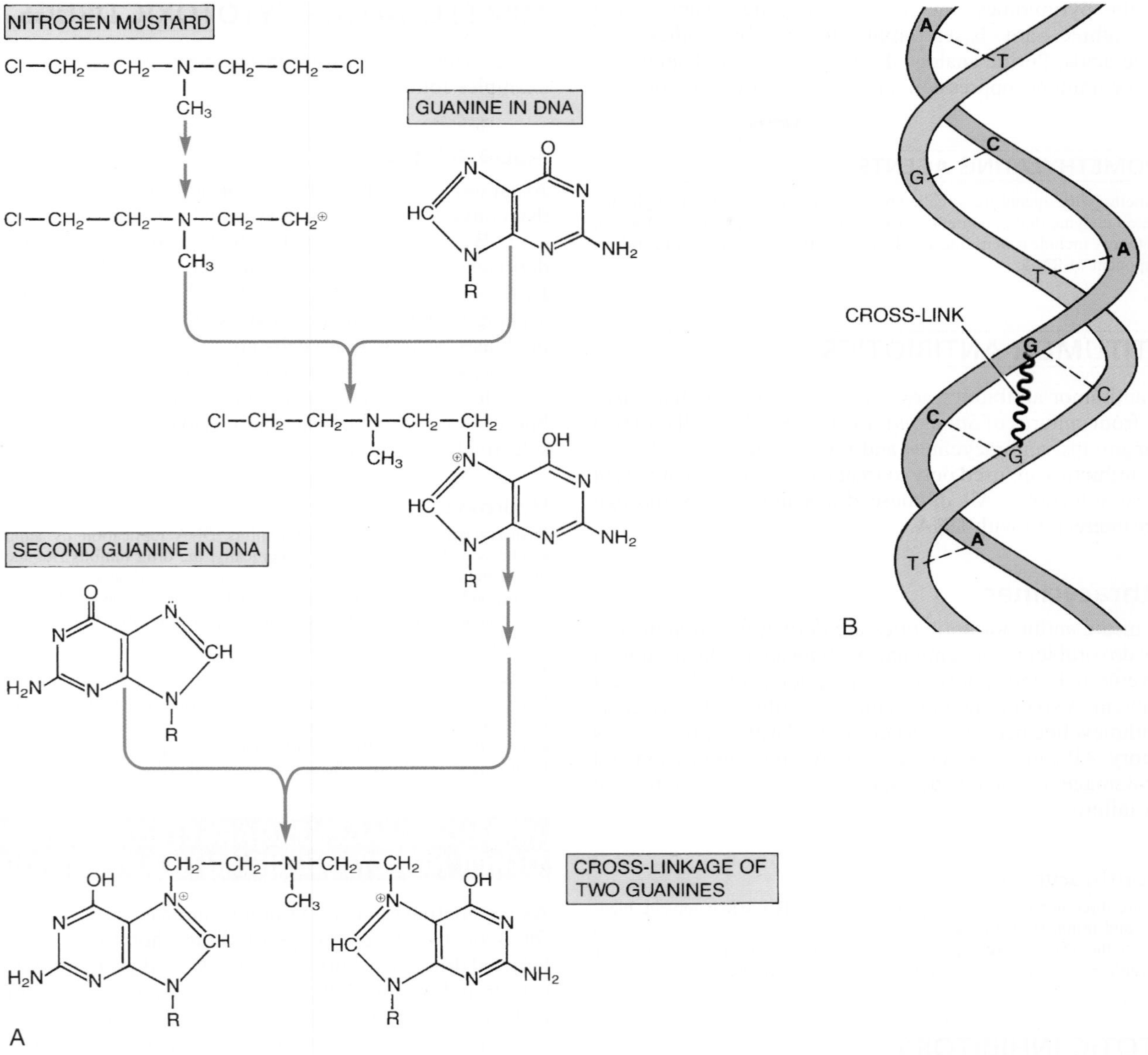

Figure 82.3 ■ Cross-linking of DNA by an alkylating agent.
A, Reactions leading to cross-linkage between guanine moieties in DNA. **B,** Schematic representation of interstrand cross-linking within the DNA double helix. A, adenine; C, cytosine; G, guanine; T, thymine.

Folic Acid Analogs

Folic acid, in its active form, is needed for several essential biochemical reactions. The folic acid analogs block the conversion of folic acid to its active form. At this time, three analogs of folic acid are used against cancer: methotrexate, pemetrexed, and pralatrexate. Other folate analogs are used to treat bacterial infections (trimethoprim), malaria (pyrimethamine), and *Pneumocystis jiroveci* pneumonia (trimetrexate).

Pyrimidine Analogs

The pyrimidine analogs are cytarabine, fluorouracil, *capecitabine,* floxuridine, and gemcitabine.

Pyrimidines—cytosine, thymine, and uracil—are bases employed in the biosynthesis of DNA and RNA. The pyrimidine analogs, because of their structural similarity to naturally occurring pyrimidines, can act in several ways: (1) they can inhibit biosynthesis of pyrimidines, (2) they can inhibit biosynthesis of DNA and RNA, and (3) they can undergo incorporation into DNA and RNA and thereby disrupt nucleic acid function. All of the pyrimidine analogs are prodrugs that must be converted to their active forms in the body.

Purine Analogs

The purine analogs are cladribine, clofarabine, fludarabine, mercaptopurine, nelarabine, pentostatin, and thioguanine.

Like the pyrimidines, the purines—adenine, guanine, and hypoxanthine—are bases employed for biosynthesis of nucleic acids. Purine analogs discussed in other chapters are used for immunosuppression, antiviral therapy, and gout.

HYPOMETHYLATING AGENTS

Hypomethylating agents are so-called because they inhibit DNA methyltransferase, an enzyme that puts methyl groups onto DNA components. Drugs in this category include azacitidine and decitabine. Both are analogs of cytidine, a component of RNA.

ANTITUMOR ANTIBIOTICS

The antitumor antibiotics are cytotoxic drugs originally isolated from cultures of *Streptomyces* species. They fall into two major groups: anthracyclines and nonanthracyclines. Antitumor antibiotics are used only to treat cancer; they are not used to treat infections. All of these drugs injure cells through direct interaction with DNA.

Anthracyclines

Five of the antitumor antibiotics are derivatives of anthracycline: doxorubicin (conventional and liposomal), daunorubicin (conventional and liposomal), epirubicin, idarubicin, and valrubicin. A sixth drug, mitoxantrone, is often categorized as an anthracycline because of its close similarity to drugs in this category. All can cause severe bone marrow suppression and heart damage. In some patients, cardiotoxicity has led to fatal heart failure.

Nonanthracyclines

There are three nonanthracycline antitumor antibiotics: dactinomycin, bleomycin, and mitomycin. In contrast to anthracyclines, nonanthracyclines do not injure the heart. However, these drugs do have serious toxicities of their own. Table 82.2 details dose-limiting toxicities of each drug.

MITOTIC INHIBITORS

Mitotic inhibitors are drugs that act during M phase to prevent cell division. There are two major groups of these drugs—vinca alkaloids and taxanes—as well as three other drugs that belong to neither group. Of these, vincristine is unique in that it spares the bone marrow and thus causes very little damage with regard to hematopoiesis.

TOPOISOMERASE INHIBITORS

Topoisomerases are nuclear enzymes that alter the shape (topology) of supercoiled DNA. Without the actions of topoisomerases, the double helix would be too tangled to permit DNA replication, RNA synthesis, or DNA repair. How do topoisomerases alter DNA configuration? They make a cut in the DNA strand—which permits the strand to relax in the vicinity of the cut—and then later they reseal the cut. There are two types of topoisomerase, known as topoisomerase I and topoisomerase II. Topoisomerase I makes single-strand cuts, and topoisomerase II makes double-strand cuts. Of the four topoisomerase inhibitors in current use, two—topotecan and irinotecan—inhibit topoisomerase I, and the other two—etoposide and teniposide—inhibit topoisomerase II. The actions of these drugs are partly like those of the antitumor antibiotics discussed previously, which inhibit topoisomerase II and intercalate DNA.

MISCELLANEOUS CYTOTOXIC DRUGS

Some cytotoxic drugs are in categories of their own. A few examples follow.

Asparaginase

Asparaginase [Elspar, Erwinase ♣, Kidrolase ♣] is an enzyme that converts asparagine, an essential amino acid, into aspartic acid. By converting asparagine to aspartic acid, the drug deprives cells of asparagine needed to synthesize proteins. However, not all cells are affected. In fact, toxicity from asparaginase is limited almost exclusively to leukemic lymphoblasts because these cells are unable to manufacture their own asparagine like normal cells can. Therefore normal cells are able to replace the asparagine that asparaginase took away, but leukemic lymphoblasts can't. Asparaginase appears to act selectively during G_1.

Hydroxyurea

Hydroxyurea [Hydrea, Droxia] inhibits DNA replication by suppressing synthesis of DNA precursors. Specifically, the drug inhibits ribonucleoside diphosphate reductase, the enzyme that converts ribonucleotides into their corresponding deoxyribonucleotides. In the absence of deoxyribonucleotides, DNA cannot be made. Hydroxyurea is S-phase specific.

Mitotane

Mitotane [Lysodren] is a structural analog of two insecticides: DDD and DDT. For reasons that are not understood, the drug is selectively toxic to cells of the adrenal cortex, both normal and neoplastic. The only indication for mitotane is palliative therapy of inoperable adrenocortical carcinoma.

HORMONAL AGENTS, TARGETED DRUGS, AND OTHER NONCYTOTOXIC ANTICANCER DRUGS

As we continue our discussion of anticancer agents, we will focus on two large groups of drugs: hormonal agents and targeted drugs. The hormonal agents, used primarily for breast cancer and prostate cancer, mimic or suppress the actions of endogenous hormones. The so-called targeted drugs bind with specific molecular targets on cancer cells and thereby suppress tumor growth and promote cell death. Unlike the cytotoxic agents discussed previously, many of which are cell-cycle phase specific, the drugs addressed here lack phase specificity. In addition, many of these drugs lack the serious toxicities associated with cytotoxic agents, including bone marrow suppression, stomatitis, alopecia, and severe nausea and vomiting. Nonetheless, most of these have severe toxicities of their own.

DRUGS FOR BREAST CANCER

Principal treatment modalities for breast cancer treatment are *surgery, radiation, cytotoxic drugs (chemotherapy),* and *hormonal drugs.* Surgery and radiation are considered primary therapy; chemotherapy and hormonal therapy are used as adjuvants. For a woman with early breast cancer, treatment typically consists of surgery (using total mastectomy or partial mastectomy [lumpectomy]) followed by local radiation. After that, chemotherapy is used to kill cells left behind after surgery and radiation and to kill cells that may have metastasized to other sites. Finally, hormonal agents are taken for several years to reduce recurrence. Increasingly, chemotherapy is used *before* surgery—so-called neoadjuvant therapy—to shrink large tumors, and thereby permit lumpectomy in women who would otherwise require mastectomy. Drugs for adjuvant therapy are shown in Table 82.5.

Hormonal agents for breast cancer fall into two major groups: *antiestrogens* (e.g., tamoxifen [Nolvadex]) and *aromatase inhibitors* (e.g., anastrozole [Arimidex]). Antiestrogens block receptors for estrogen, whereas aromatase inhibitors block estrogen biosynthesis. In both cases, tumor cells are deprived of the estrogen they need for growth. However, there is a caveat: for these drugs to work, tumor cells must have estrogen receptors (ERs). Fortunately, most breast cancers are ER positive.

In addition to chemotherapy and hormonal therapy, four other drugs—*trastuzumab* [Herceptin], *ado-trastuzumab emtansine* [Kadcyla], *pertuzumab* [Perjeta], and *lapatinib* [Tykerb]—can be used for adjuvant treatment. Trastuzumab, pertuzumab, and ado-trastuzumab emtansine block receptors known as human epidermal growth factor receptor type 2 (HER2). In addition, when ado-trastuzumab emtansine binds with HER2 receptors, it releases cytotoxic catabolites that cause cell apoptosis. Lapatinib inhibits two enzymes, known as HER2 tyrosine kinase and epidermal growth factor receptor (EGFR) tyrosine kinase. These drugs are indicated only for cancers that are HER2 positive. Lastly, patients may take *denosumab* [Xgeva] or *zoledronate* [Zometa] to minimize hypercalcemia (caused by bone metastases) and fractures (caused by bone metastases as well as hormonal therapy).

What about breast cancer *prevention*? Currently, two drugs are approved for preventing breast cancer in women at high risk. Both drugs are *selective estrogen receptor modulators,* or SERMS. One of the drugs—*raloxifene* [Evista]—is approved only for postmenopausal women. The other drug—*tamoxifen* [Nolvadex]—is approved for premenopausal *and* postmenopausal women. Raloxifene is discussed in Chapter 59. Tamoxifen is discussed later in this chapter. Another drug—*exemestane* [Aromasin] (discussed later)—can also prevent breast cancer, but currently it is only approved for breast cancer treatment.

Antiestrogens

Antiestrogens are drugs that block ERs and hence only work against cells that are ER positive. Benefits derive from depriving tumor cells of the growth-promoting influence of estrogen. Three antiestrogens—tamoxifen, toremifene, and fulvestrant—are approved for adjuvant treatment. Of these, tamoxifen is by far the most widely used.

Tamoxifen

Tamoxifen [Nolvadex] is considered the gold standard for endocrine treatment of breast cancer. The drug is approved for treating established disease and for primary prevention in women at high risk. As discussed later, tamoxifen is a prodrug that must be converted to active metabolites.

Overview of Actions

Tamoxifen blocks ERs in some tissues and activates them in others. Receptor *blockade* underlies benefits in breast cancer and also underlies some adverse effects (especially hot flashes). Receptor *activation* leads to other beneficial effects (increased bone mineral density, reduction of low-density lipoprotein cholesterol, elevation of high-density lipoprotein cholesterol) as well as certain adverse effects (endometrial cancer and blood clots). Because tamoxifen can cause receptor activation as well as blockade, the drug is often classified as a SERM.

Mechanism of Action in Breast Cancer

Tamoxifen is a prodrug that undergoes hepatic conversion to active metabolites. These metabolites then block ERs on breast cancer cells and thereby prevent receptor activation by estradiol, the principal endogenous estrogen. Estrogen acts on tumor cells to stimulate growth and proliferation. Hence, in the absence of the influence of estradiol, the rate of tumor cell proliferation declines. Tumors regress in size as the rate of cell death outpaces new cell production. Obviously, if treatment is to be effective, target cells must be ER positive.

Use for Treatment of Breast Cancer

Tamoxifen has two treatment applications: (1) as adjuvant therapy to suppress growth of residual cancer cells after surgery and (2) as treatment of metastatic disease. Tamoxifen can be used in both premenopausal and postmenopausal women.

Use for Prevention of Breast Cancer

Tamoxifen is approved for reducing the development of breast cancer in healthy women at high risk. Unfortunately, tamoxifen *increases* the incidence of endometrial cancer, pulmonary embolism, and deep vein thrombosis. Hence women considering tamoxifen for chemoprevention must carefully weigh the benefits of treatment (reduced risk for breast cancer) against the risks (increased risk for endometrial cancer and thromboembolic events). According to guidelines issued in 2013 by the U.S. Preventive Services Task Force (USPSTF), tamoxifen chemoprevention is appropriate only for women at *high* risk, and not for women at low to moderate risk.

To help determine who is at high risk for breast cancer, the National Cancer Institute has created an Internet-based Breast Cancer Risk Assessment Tool. You can access the tool at www.cancer.gov/bcrisktool.

Pharmacokinetics

Tamoxifen is readily absorbed after oral administration. In the liver, CYP2D6 (the 2D6 isoenzyme of cytochrome P450) converts tamoxifen to two active metabolites: 4-hydroxy-*N*-desmethyltamoxifen (endoxifen) and 4-hydroxytamoxifen. The half-lives of tamoxifen and its metabolites range from 1 to 2 weeks. Because clearance is slow, once-daily dosing is adequate. When treatment is stopped, tamoxifen and its metabolites can be detected in serum for weeks.

Not surprisingly, benefits of tamoxifen are greatly reduced in women with an inherited deficiency in the gene that codes for CYP2D6. Cancer recurrence rate in poor metabolizers may be higher than in good metabolizers. Between 8% and 10% of white women have gene variants that prevent them from converting tamoxifen to its active metabolites. However, at this time, the U.S. Food and Drug Administration (FDA) neither requires nor recommends testing for variants in the *CYP2D6* gene, although a test kit *is* available.

TABLE 82.5 ▪ Drugs for Adjuvant Therapy of Breast Cancer

Generic Name	Trade Name	Route	Mechanism	Indications	Major Adverse Effects
HORMONAL THERAPIES					
Antiestrogens					
Tamoxifen	Nolvadex	PO	Blockade of estrogen receptors	ER-positive breast cancer in premenopausal and postmenopausal women	Increased risk for endometrial cancer and thrombosis Hot flashes, fluid retention, vaginal discharge, nausea, vomiting, and menstrual irregularities
Toremifene	Fareston	PO	Blockade of estrogen receptors	ER-positive breast cancer in postmenopausal women only	
Fulvestrant	Faslodex	IM	Blockade of estrogen receptors	ER-positive breast cancer in postmenopausal women only	
Aromatase Inhibitors					
Anastrozole Letrozole Exemestane	Arimidex Femara Aromasin	PO PO PO	Inhibition of estrogen synthesis	ER-positive breast cancer in postmenopausal women only	Musculoskeletal pain, osteoporosis and related fractures
OTHER DRUGS FOR BREAST CANCER					
Anti-HER2 Antibodies					
Trastuzumab	Herceptin	IV	Blockade of HER2 receptors	HER2-positive breast cancer in premenopausal and postmenopausal women	Cardiotoxicity and hypersensitivity reactions
Ado-trastuzumab	Kadcyla	IV	Blockade of HER2 receptors	HER2-positive breast cancer	Hepatotoxicity, cardiotoxicity, neurotoxicity
Pertuzumab	Perjeta	IV	Blockade of HER2 receptors	HER2-positive breast cancer	Cardiotoxicity, hypersensitivity reactions
Kinase Inhibitor					
Lapatinib	Tykerb	PO	Inhibits HER2 tyrosine kinase and EGFR tyrosine kinase	HER2-positive breast cancer in premenopausal and postmenopausal women	Diarrhea, hepatotoxicity, cardiotoxicity, interstitial lung disease
Cytotoxic Drugs (Representative Agents)					
Doxorubicin *plus* cyclophosphamide	Adriamycin; Cytoxan, Neosar	IV	Direct cell kill by DNA intercalation, topoisomerase II inhibition, and DNA alkylation	Breast cancer in all women, regardless of ER, HER2, or menopausal status	Together, these drugs can cause cardiotoxicity, bone marrow suppression, alopecia, oral and GI ulceration, and hemorrhagic cystitis
Paclitaxel	Taxol 🍁, Onxol, Abraxane	IV	Direct cell kill by mitotic arrest	Breast cancer in all women, regardless of ER, HER2, or menopausal status	Bone marrow suppression, peripheral neuropathy, alopecia, cardiotoxicity, muscle and joint pain Severe hypersensitivity reactions with Taxol 🍁 and Onxol, but not Abraxane
Eribulin	Halaven	IV	Direct cell kill by mitotic arrest	Breast cancer in all women, regardless of ER, HER2, or menopausal status	Bone marrow suppression, peripheral neuropathy
Drugs to Delay Skeletal Events					
Zoledronate	Zometa*	IV	Inhibits osteoclast function	Hypercalcemia of malignancy, prevention of malignancy-related skeletal events	Kidney damage, osteonecrosis of the jaw, rare atrial fibrillation
Denosumab	Xgeva†	SubQ	Inhibits osteoclast function and production	Hypercalcemia of malignancy, prevention of malignancy-related skeletal events	Hypocalcemia, serious infections, skin reactions, osteonecrosis of the jaw

*Zoledronate is also available as *Reclast* for treating osteoporosis and Paget disease.
†Denosumab is also available as *Prolia* for treating postmenopausal osteoporosis.
EGFR, epidermal growth factor receptor; ER, estrogen receptor; GI, gastrointestinal; HER2, human epidermal growth factor receptor 2; IM, intramuscular; IV, intravenous; PO, oral; subQ, subcutaneous.

Adverse Effects

The most common adverse effects are hot flashes, fluid retention, vaginal discharge, nausea, vomiting, and menstrual irregularities. In women with bone metastases, tamoxifen may cause transient hypercalcemia and a flare in bone pain. Because of its estrogen agonist actions, tamoxifen poses a small risk for *thromboembolic events,* including deep vein thrombosis, pulmonary embolism, and stroke.

Perhaps the biggest concern is *endometrial cancer.* Tamoxifen acts as an estrogen agonist at receptors in the uterus, causing proliferation of endometrial tissue. Proliferation initially results in endometrial hyperplasia and may eventually lead to endometrial cancer. In women taking tamoxifen to *treat* breast cancer, the benefits clearly outweigh this risk. However, in women taking the drug to *prevent* breast cancer, the risk/benefit balance is less obvious. In postmenopausal women, endometrial cancer is usually caught early, owing to abnormal menstrual bleeding.

Tamoxifen can harm the developing fetus and hence is classified in FDA Pregnancy Risk Category D. Accordingly, women using the drug should avoid getting pregnant.

Interaction With CYP2D6 Inhibitors

Inhibitors of CYP2D6 can prevent activation of tamoxifen and can thereby negate the benefits of treatment. Put another way, when tamoxifen is combined with a CYP2D6 inhibitor, the risk for breast cancer recurrence is greater than when tamoxifen is used alone. Accordingly, women using tamoxifen should avoid strong CYP2D6 inhibitors. Important among these are *fluoxetine* [Prozac], *paroxetine* [Paxil, Pexeva], and *sertraline* [Zoloft]—selective serotonin reuptake inhibitors (SSRIs) taken by many women to suppress tamoxifen-induced hot flashes. Fortunately, alternatives with less effect on CYP2D6 are available. Among these are *escitalopram* [Lexapro, Cipralex] (an SSRI) and *venlafaxine* [Effexor] (a serotonin/norepinephrine reuptake inhibitor).

Toremifene

Actions and Use

Toremifene [Fareston] is an antiestrogen indicated for metastatic breast cancer in postmenopausal women with ER-positive tumors or tumors for which ER status is unknown. The drug is a structural analog of tamoxifen and shares most of that drug's properties. Like tamoxifen, toremifene is a SERM with antiestrogenic actions in some tissues and estrogenic actions in others. In women with breast cancer, toremifene blocks ERs on tumor cells, thereby depriving them of estrogen's growth-promoting effects.

Pharmacokinetics

Toremifene is well absorbed after oral administration. Plasma levels peak in 3 hours. The drug undergoes extensive hepatic metabolism, primarily by CYP3A4 (the 3A4 isoenzyme of cytochrome P450). Metabolites are excreted in the feces. The half-life is prolonged (about 5 days), owing to enterohepatic recirculation. As with tamoxifen, drugs that induce CYP3A4 will reduce toremifene levels, and drugs that inhibit the enzyme will raise toremifene levels.

Adverse Effects

Adverse effects are like those of tamoxifen. Hot flashes are most common. Other common reactions are sweating, nausea, and vaginal discharge. Patients may also experience dizziness, vomiting, and vaginal bleeding. Hypercalcemia may occur in women with bone metastases. There is a small risk for thromboembolic events. Cataracts and elevation of liver enzymes have been reported.

Toremifene prolongs the QT interval and thereby poses a risk for potentially fatal dysrhythmias. To reduce risk, toremifene should be avoided in patients with hypokalemia, hypomagnesemia, or preexisting QT prolongation and in those taking other QT drugs.

Like tamoxifen, toremifene activates ERs in the uterus. As a result, the drug can promote uterine hyperplasia and uterine cancer.

Fulvestrant

Actions and Use

Fulvestrant [Faslodex] is an antiestrogen indicated for metastatic ER-positive breast cancer in postmenopausal women. Unlike tamoxifen and toremifene, which block some ERs and activate others, fulvestrant is a pure estrogen receptor antagonist—the first one available. As with other antiestrogens, benefits derive from depriving breast cancer cells of required hormonal stimulation.

Pharmacokinetics

Plasma levels peak about 7 days after IM injection and remain therapeutic for at least 1 month. Steady-state levels are reached after three to six monthly doses. The drug undergoes hepatic metabolism followed by renal excretion. The apparent half-life is 40 days.

Adverse Effects and Drug Interactions

Fulvestrant is generally well tolerated. The most common adverse effects are GI disturbances, hot flashes, headache, pharyngitis, and bone and back pain. Thromboembolism can occur but is uncommon. In contrast to tamoxifen, fulvestrant poses no risk for endometrial cancer. Fulvestrant has no known drug interactions.

Aromatase Inhibitors

The aromatase inhibitors are used to treat ER-positive breast cancer in *postmenopausal* women. These drugs block the production of estrogen from androgenic precursors and thereby deprive breast cancer cells of the estrogen they need for growth. Aromatase inhibitors do not block production of estrogen by the ovaries and hence are of little benefit in premenopausal women. In fact, aromatase inhibitors may cause a compensatory rise in estradiol in premenopausal patients. Aromatase inhibitors are more effective than tamoxifen and have a different toxicity profile. Unlike tamoxifen, aromatase inhibitors pose no risk for endometrial cancer and only rarely cause thromboembolism. However, they *can* increase the risk for fractures and have been associated with moderate to severe myalgias.

Anastrozole

Actions and Use

Anastrozole [Arimidex] is approved for first-line oral therapy of *postmenopausal* women with early or advanced *ER-positive breast cancer.* The drug works by depriving breast cancer cells of estrogen. In postmenopausal women, the major source of estrogen is adrenal androgens, which are converted into estrogen by the enzyme *aromatase* in peripheral tissues. Anastrozole inhibits aromatase and thereby reduces estrogen production. With regular use, the drug lowers estrogen to undetectable levels. In women with estrogen-dependent cancer, estrogen deprivation can arrest tumor growth and may cause outright cell death. Anastrozole may be used as initial therapy or as a follow-up to therapy with tamoxifen.

Adverse Effects

Anastrozole is generally well tolerated. At a daily dose of 1 mg, the most common adverse effects are musculoskeletal pain, asthenia, headache, and menopausal symptoms, including hot flashes, vaginal dryness, and GI disturbances. Other reactions include anorexia, vomiting, diarrhea, constipation, dyspnea, peripheral edema, vaginal hemorrhage, and hypertension.

Up to 50% of women experience *musculoskeletal pain,* often described with the statement, "Every bone in my body hurts." The cause may be estrogen deprivation. Persistent or severe pain drives about 5% of users to discontinue treatment. For women who choose to continue anastrozole, pain can often be managed with a mild analgesic (e.g., acetaminophen, ibuprofen). High-dose vitamin D may help, too.

Estrogen depletion increases the risk for *osteoporosis and related fractures*. To reduce bone loss, women should ensure adequate intake of calcium and vitamin D. Women at high risk should take a bisphosphonate (e.g., zoledronate [Zometa]) or denosumab [Prolia].

Comparison With Tamoxifen

Anastrozole is more effective than tamoxifen. Anastrozole is less likely to cause hot flashes, weight gain, or vaginal bleeding—although it may cause more nausea and irritability. In contrast to tamoxifen, anastrozole is devoid of all estrogenic activity and hence does not promote endometrial cancer or thromboembolic events—although it does increase the risk for fractures. Because of their superior efficacy and tolerability, aromatase inhibitors have replaced tamoxifen as the drug of first choice for treating ER-positive breast cancer in postmenopausal women.

Letrozole

Letrozole [Femara], a selective aromatase inhibitor, is indicated for (1) first-line therapy of early and advanced ER-positive breast cancer in postmenopausal women and (2) extended adjuvant therapy of early breast cancer after 5 years of adjuvant therapy with tamoxifen. Like anastrozole, letrozole blocks conversion of androgens into estrogens and thereby deprives breast cancer cells of estrogen's growth-promoting influence. Letrozole's most common adverse effects are musculoskeletal pain and nausea. Other reactions include headache, arthralgia, fatigue, constipation, dyspnea, cough, vomiting, diarrhea, and hot flashes. Extremely low doses are embryotoxic and fetotoxic in animals. Like anastrozole, and unlike tamoxifen, letrozole poses no risk for endometrial cancer. However, it can cause osteoporosis and fractures and, rarely, thromboembolism. Osteoporosis can be managed with denosumab [Prolia] or a bisphosphonate (e.g., zoledronate [Zometa]). No significant drug interactions have been reported.

Exemestane

Exemestane [Aromasin] is indicated for oral therapy of (1) advanced ER-positive breast cancer in postmenopausal women whose disease has progressed despite treatment with tamoxifen and (2) early ER-positive breast cancer in postmenopausal women who have received 2 to 3 years of tamoxifen therapy and then are switched to adjuvant exemestane to complete a 5-year course of treatment. Like anastrozole, exemestane inhibits aromatase and thereby reduces estrogen levels. A dosage of 25 mg once daily (administered after a meal) can reduce circulating estrogen by 85% to 95%. In the absence of sufficient estrogen, estrogen-dependent tumors cannot thrive. In addition to treating breast cancer, exemestane can be effective for breast cancer prevention; however, it does not yet have approval for this indication.

Exemestane is rapidly absorbed after oral dosing and is widely distributed to tissues. In the liver, the drug undergoes extensive metabolism, mainly by CYP3A4. Excretion is through the urine and feces. Its half-life is about 24 hours.

Exemestane is generally well tolerated. The most common adverse effects are fatigue, nausea, hot flashes, depression, and weight gain. Like anastrozole and letrozole, exemestane often causes musculoskeletal pain. Increased risk for osteoporosis and fractures is a concern. Women at high risk for osteoporosis can be treated with denosumab [Prolia] or a bisphosphonate (e.g., zoledronate [Zometa]).

Drugs that induce CYP3A4 (e.g., phenytoin, phenobarbital, rifampin, St. John's wort) can cause a significant drop in exemestane levels. Accordingly, if these drugs are combined, exemestane dosage may need to increase.

Trastuzumab

Actions and Use

Trastuzumab [Herceptin] is a monoclonal antibody originally approved for *HER2-positive metastatic breast cancer* and for *adjuvant therapy of HER2-positive breast cancer*. Trastuzumab is also approved for treatment of *HER2-positive metastatic gastric cancer*. Discussion here is limited to breast cancer.

Trastuzumab is only effective against tumors that overexpress *HER2*, a transmembrane receptor that helps regulate cell growth. Trastuzumab binds with HER2 and thereby (1) inhibits cell proliferation and (2) promotes antibody-dependent cell death. Between 25% and 30% of metastatic breast cancers produce excessive HER2. High numbers of HER2 receptors are associated with unusually aggressive tumor growth. For treatment of breast cancer, trastuzumab may be used (1) alone in women who failed to respond to prior chemotherapy, (2) in combination with paclitaxel as first-line therapy, and (3) for adjuvant treatment as part of a regimen containing doxorubicin, cyclophosphamide, and paclitaxel.

Adverse Effects

The principal concern with trastuzumab is *cardiotoxicity*, manifesting as ventricular dysfunction and congestive heart failure. Because of cardiotoxicity, trastuzumab should be used with caution in women with preexisting heart disease. Concurrent use with other drugs that can cause cardiotoxicity such as doxorubicin and other anthracyclines should generally be avoided. In contrast to the cytotoxic anticancer drugs, trastuzumab does not cause bone marrow suppression or alopecia.

Many patients experience a *flu-like syndrome*, which also occurs with other monoclonal antibodies. Symptoms include chills, fever, pain, weakness, nausea, vomiting, and headache. The syndrome develops in 40% of patients receiving their first infusion and then diminishes with subsequent infusions.

Ado-Trastuzumab Emtansine

Actions and Use

Ado-trastuzumab emtansine [Kadcyla] is a monoclonal antibody approved for *HER2-positive metastatic breast cancer* in patients previously treated with trastuzumab and/or a taxane.

Like trastuzumab, ado-trastuzumab emtansine is only effective against tumors that overexpress *HER2*. Ado-trastuzumab emtansine binds with HER2 and releases cytotoxic catabolites, thereby (1) inhibiting the cell cycle and (2) promoting cell death. In addition, ado-trastuzumab emtansine inhibits HER2 receptor signaling and shedding of HER2 in breast cancer cells.

Adverse Effects

Ado-trastuzumab emtansine can cause hepatotoxicity, cardiotoxicity, and neurotoxicity. Serious hepatotoxicity, including liver failure and death, have been reported. Liver function tests should be obtained before each dose. Left ventricular dysfunction was seen in 1.8% of patients. Ejection fraction should be monitored at regular intervals. The incidence of neurotoxicity, expressed as peripheral neuropathy, was 2.2%.

Ado-trastuzumab emtansine can also cause embryo and fetal toxicity. Because exposure can result in birth defects or death of the fetus, ado-trastuzumab emtansine is classified in FDA Pregnancy Risk Category D and should be avoided by pregnant women and nursing mothers.

The most common reactions include nausea, fatigue, musculoskeletal pain, headache, and constipation. Other common, but more serious, reactions include thrombocytopenia, increases in liver function test results, anemia, and hypokalemia.

Like trastuzumab, ado-trastuzumab emtansine can cause potentially fatal *hypersensitivity reactions, infusion reactions,* and *pulmonary events.* If a patient experienced trastuzumab-related infusion reactions, ado-trastuzumab emtansine should be avoided.

Pertuzumab

Pertuzumab [Perjeta] is used in combination with trastuzumab and docetaxel for the treatment of women with *HER2-positive metastatic breast cancer* who have not received prior therapy for metastatic disease. Like trastuzumab, pertuzumab is an antibody that blocks HER2 receptors, resulting in cell growth arrest and cell death.

Adverse effects include infusion-related reactions. Patients should be closely monitored for 60 minutes after the first infusion and for 30 minutes after subsequent infusions. Other adverse effects include cardiotoxicity, diarrhea, leukopenia, and neuropathy. Oligohydramnios has been reported in pregnancy, so pregnant women should avoid use of pertuzumab.

Lapatinib

Actions and Use

Lapatinib [Tykerb] is an oral inhibitor of two enzymes—HER2 tyrosine kinase and EGFR tyrosine kinase—that are involved in cell signal transduction. Enzyme inhibition results in apoptosis and suppression of tumor cell growth. Lapatinib is approved for treating advanced HER2-positive breast cancer, but only in combination with either (1) capecitabine (in patients who have received prior therapy with multiple drugs, including an anthracycline, a taxane, and trastuzumab) or (2) letrozole (in postmenopausal women for whom estrogen deprivation therapy is indicated). EGFR tyrosine kinase is discussed further in the later section "EGFR Tyrosine Kinase Inhibitors."

Adverse Effects

The most common adverse effects of lapatinib plus capecitabine are GI disturbances (diarrhea, nausea, vomiting), fatigue, rash, and palmar-plantar erythrodysesthesia (swelling and numbness of the hands and feet). The most common adverse effects of lapatinib plus letrozole are diarrhea, rash, nausea, and fatigue. Diarrhea occurs in 65% of patients and is the most common reason for stopping treatment. Like other HER2 inhibitors, lapatinib may pose a risk for cardiotoxicity. Accordingly, the drug should be used with caution in patients with existing cardiac impairment. Rarely, letrozole has been associated with severe liver injury. Liver function tests should be performed at baseline and periodically throughout treatment. When used alone and together with other drugs, letrozole has been associated with interstitial lung disease and pneumonitis. In laboratory animals, giving letrozole during pregnancy resulted in death of the pups a few days after birth. Women using the drug should avoid getting pregnant.

Drug Interactions

Lapatinib is metabolized by CYP3A4, and hence CYP3A4 inducers (e.g., phenytoin, carbamazepine, rifampin, rifabutin, phenobarbital, St. John's wort) can lower lapatinib levels, and CYP3A4 inhibitors (e.g., ketoconazole, itraconazole, erythromycin, indinavir, nelfinavir) can raise lapatinib levels. If possible, CYP3A4 inducers and inhibitors should be avoided.

Cytotoxic Drugs (Chemotherapy)

Cytotoxic drugs may be used before breast surgery or after. When used before surgery, chemotherapy can shrink large tumors, thereby permitting lumpectomy in women who would otherwise require a mastectomy. When used after surgery, chemotherapy can kill cancer cells that remain in the breast as well as cells that may have metastasized to distant sites. A common regimen for breast cancer consists of doxorubicin (an anthracycline-type anticancer antibiotic) plus cyclophosphamide (an alkylating agent) followed by paclitaxel (a mitotic inhibitor).

Denosumab and Bisphosphonates for Skeletal-Related Events

Women with breast cancer are at risk for skeletal-related events (SREs), especially hypercalcemia and fractures. There are two causes: the cancer itself and the drugs used for treatment. In breast cancer, most metastases occur in bone. These metastases promote hypercalcemia by increasing the activity of osteoclasts, the cells that promote bone resorption. Not only does resorption promote hypercalcemia, it also weakens bone and thereby increases the risk for fractures. Fracture risk is further increased by use of antiestrogens and aromatase inhibitors. As we discussed in Chapter 48, estrogens promote bone health by inhibiting bone resorption and promoting bone deposition. Hence, by removing the influence of estrogen, the antiestrogens and aromatase inhibitors accelerate bone resorption and reduce bone deposition. Both actions weaken bone and thereby increase the risk for fractures. To reduce the risk for SREs, we can treat patients with denosumab or a bisphosphonate (usually zoledronate).

Zoledronate and Other Bisphosphonates

In women with breast cancer, bisphosphonates can help preserve bone integrity and can thereby decrease the risk for hypercalcemia and fractures. Benefits derive from inhibiting the activity of osteoclasts. At this time, two bisphosphonates—*zoledronate* [Zometa] and *pamidronate* [Aredia]—are approved for hypercalcemia of malignancy, and one of them—pamidronate—is also approved for managing osteolytic bone metastases. However, although zoledronate is not *approved* for osteolytic bone metastases, it is just as effective as pamidronate. Furthermore, compared with pamidronate, zoledronate has three advantages: onset is faster, duration is longer, and infusion time is shorter (15 minutes vs. 2–4 hours). Accordingly, zoledronate is generally preferred to pamidronate. Principal adverse effects of the bisphosphonates are kidney damage and osteonecrosis of the jaw.

In addition to reducing fractures and hypercalcemia, bisphosphonates may actually prevent metastases and prolong life. How do bisphosphonates suppress metastases? When cancer cells spread to bone, they stimulate the activity of osteoclasts, the cells responsible for bone resorption. In turn, osteoclasts release growth factors that stimulate the cancer cells, thereby setting up a self-reinforcing cycle. Bisphosphonates interrupt the cycle by inhibiting osteoclast function and blocking tumor adhesion to bone. The basic pharmacology of the bisphosphonates is discussed in Chapter 59.

Denosumab

Denosumab, marketed as *Xgeva,* is indicated for preventing (delaying) SREs in patients with breast cancer and other solid tumors that have metastasized to bone. Benefits derive from inhibiting the formation and function of osteoclasts. Principal adverse effects of denosumab are hypocalcemia, serious infections, skin reactions, and osteonecrosis of the jaw. The pharmacology of denosumab is presented in Chapter 59.

DRUGS FOR PROSTATE CANCER

Cancer of the prostate is the most common cancer among men in the United States. In 2013 an estimated 238,590 new cases were diagnosed, and 29,720 were fatal. For men with *localized* prostate cancer, the preferred treatments are surgery and radiation, with or without adjunctive use of drugs. For men with *metastatic* prostate cancer, drug therapy and castration are the only options. Among the drugs employed, agents for *androgen deprivation therapy* (ADT) comprise the largest and most widely used group. The only other choices are cytotoxic drugs and a new immunotherapy known as sipuleucel-T [Provenge]. As with breast cancer, most metastases (65%–75%) go to bone. To minimize hypercalcemia and fractures caused by bone metastases, men may take *zoledronate* [Zometa] or *denosumab* [Xgeva] (see previous discussion of breast cancer). The drugs used to treat prostate cancer are shown in Table 82.6.

Androgen Deprivation Therapy

The term *androgen deprivation therapy* refers to the use of castration, drugs, or both to deprive prostate cancers of the androgens they need for growth. By implementing ADT, we can slow disease progression and increase comfort. Initially, ADT was reserved for patients with metastatic disease. However, ADT is now used as an adjuvant in earlier stage disease. Unfortunately, the benefits of ADT are time limited: after 18 to 24 months of treatment, disease progression often resumes. Side effects of ADT include hot flashes, reduced libido, erectile dysfunction, gynecomastia, decreased muscle mass, and decreased bone mass with associated increased risk for fractures.

Where do androgens come from, and how can we reduce their influence? About 90% of circulating androgens are produced by the testes. The remaining 10% are produced by the adrenal glands and by the prostate cancer itself. Accordingly, we can reduce the influence of androgens in three ways. Specifically, we can block testosterone receptors with drugs; we can lower testosterone production with drugs; and we can lower testosterone production by castration. Drug therapy is more effective than castration because castration only eliminates testicular androgens, leaving androgen synthesis by the adrenal glands and cancer cells intact. In contrast, by using drugs to block testosterone receptors and testosterone synthesis, we can reduce the influence of testosterone from all sources (testes, adrenal glands, prostate cancer).

Gonadotropin-Releasing Hormone Agonists

The gonadotropin-releasing hormone (GnRH) agonists suppress production of androgens by the testes—but not by the adrenal glands and prostate cancer cells. Currently, four

TABLE 82.6 ▪ Drugs for Prostate Cancer

Generic Name	Trade Name	Route	Major Adverse Effects
DRUGS FOR ANDROGEN DEPRIVATION THERAPY			
GnRH Agonists*			
Leuprolide	Lupron ♣, Lupron Depot Eligard Viadur	IM SubQ SubQ implant	Hot flashes, erectile dysfunction, decreased libido, decreased muscle mass, gynecomastia, osteoporosis
Triptorelin	Trelstar	IM	
Goserelin	Zoladex	SubQ	
Histrelin	Vantas	SubQ implant	
GnRH Antagonist			
Degarelix	Firmagon	SubQ	Same as the GnRH agonists *plus* hepatotoxicity
Androgen Receptor Blockers			
Flutamide	Generic only	PO	Same as the GnRH agonists *plus* hepatotoxicity
Bicalutamide	Casodex	PO	Same as the GnRH agonists *plus* hepatotoxicity
Nilutamide	Nilandron, Anandron ♣	PO	Same as the GnRH agonists *plus* hepatotoxicity and interstitial pneumonitis
CYP17 Inhibitor			
Abiraterone	Zytiga	PO	Same as the GnRH agonists *plus* hepatotoxicity, edema, hypertension, hypokalemia, glucocorticoid insufficiency
OTHER DRUGS FOR PROSTATE CANCER			
Immunotherapy			
Sipuleucel-T	Provenge	IV	Infusion reactions, fatigue, fever
Cytotoxic Drugs			
Cabazitaxel	Jevtana	IV	Neutropenia, hypersensitivity reactions, diarrhea
Docetaxel	Taxotere	IV	Neutropenia, anemia, hypersensitivity reactions, fluid retention
Estramustine	Emcyt	PO	Gynecomastia, thrombosis
Drugs to Delay Skeletal Events			
Zoledronate	Zometa†	IV	Kidney damage, osteonecrosis of the jaw, rare atrial fibrillation
Denosumab	Xgeva‡	SubQ	Hypocalcemia, serious infections, skin reactions, osteonecrosis of the jaw

*Gonadotropin-releasing hormone agonists, also known as luteinizing hormone–releasing hormone (LHRH) agonists.
†Zoledronate is also available as *Reclast* for treating osteoporosis and Paget disease.
‡Denosumab is also available as *Prolia* for treating postmenopausal osteoporosis.
IM, intramuscular; IV, intravenous; PO, oral; subQ, subcutaneous.

GnRH agonists are available: leuprolide, triptorelin, goserelin, and histrelin. All four are indicated for cancer of the prostate. In addition, leuprolide is used for endometriosis.

Leuprolide

Therapeutic Use. Leuprolide [Eligard, Lupro ♣, Lupron Depot, Viadur] is a synthetic analog of GnRH, also known as *luteinizing hormone–releasing hormone* (LHRH). Leuprolide is indicated for *advanced carcinoma of the prostate.* Palliation is the primary benefit. For patients with prostate cancer, leuprolide represents an alternative to orchiectomy (surgical castration). Leuprolide may be administered daily (subQ); monthly (IM); every 3, 4, or 6 months (IM); or once a year (subQ implant).

Mechanism of Action. Cells of the prostate, both normal and neoplastic, are androgen dependent. Leuprolide provides palliation by suppressing androgen production in the *testes.* During the initial phase of treatment, leuprolide *mimics* GnRH. That is, the drug acts on the pituitary to *stimulate* release of interstitial cell–stimulating hormone (ICSH), which acts on the testes to *increase* production of testosterone. As a result, there may be a transient "flare" in prostate cancer symptoms. However, with continuous exposure to leuprolide, GnRH receptors in the pituitary become desensitized. As a result, release of ICSH declines, causing testosterone production to decline, too. After several weeks of treatment, testosterone levels are equivalent to those seen after surgical castration. Because leuprolide therapy mimics the effects of orchiectomy, treatment is often referred to as *chemical castration.*

It is important to note that leuprolide does *not* decrease production of androgens made by the adrenal glands or by the prostate cancer itself. As noted, these nontesticular sources account for about 10% of the androgens in circulation. Hence, even though production of testicular androgens is essentially eliminated, adrenal and prostatic androgens can still provide some support for prostate cancer cells.

Cotreatment With an Androgen Receptor Blocker. In patients receiving leuprolide, an androgen receptor blocker can help in two ways. Specifically, (1) it can prevent cancer cells from undergoing increased stimulation during the initial phase of GnRH therapy, when androgen production is increased; and (2) it can block the effects of adrenal and prostatic androgens, whose production is not reduced by GnRH agonists. The current trend is to use an androgen receptor blocker during the first weeks of leuprolide therapy (to prevent leuprolide-induced tumor flare), after which the drug is discontinued unless there is tumor progression despite continued leuprolide treatment.

Adverse Effects. Leuprolide is generally well tolerated. Hot flashes are the most common adverse effect, but these usually decline as treatment continues. Reduced testosterone may also lead to erectile dysfunction, loss of libido, gynecomastia, reduced muscle mass, new-onset diabetes, myocardial infarction, and stroke. During the initial weeks of treatment, elevation of testosterone levels may aggravate bone pain and urinary obstruction caused by prostate cancer. As a result, patients with vertebral metastases or preexisting obstruction of the urinary tract may find treatment intolerable. As noted, concurrent treatment with an androgen receptor blocker can minimize these problems.

By suppressing testosterone production, leuprolide may increase the risk for osteoporosis and related fractures. Bone loss can be minimized by consuming adequate calcium and vitamin D and by performing regular weight-bearing exercise. In addition, a bisphosphonate (e.g., zoledronate [Zometa]) or denosumab [Xgeva] can be used to preserve bone and reduce fracture risk (see earlier discussion of breast cancer).

Triptorelin, Goserelin, Histrelin

Triptorelin, goserelin, and histrelin are GnRH analogs indicated for palliative treatment of advanced prostate cancer. All three have the same mechanism and adverse effects of leuprolide, our prototype GnRH agonist.

Gonadotropin-Releasing Hormone Antagonists

Like the GnRH agonists, the GnRH *antagonists* suppress production of androgens by the testes. However, in contrast to the GnRH agonists, the GnRH antagonists do not produce an initial tumor flare. Currently, only one GnRH antagonist—degarelix—is available.

Degarelix

Degarelix [Firmagon] is a synthetic decapeptide GnRH antagonist indicated for palliative therapy of *advanced prostate cancer* in men who are not candidates for a GnRH agonist and who do not want surgical castration. Benefits derive from suppressing testosterone production by the testes. The underlying mechanism is blockade of GnRH receptors in the anterior pituitary, which decreases release of luteinizing hormone and follicle-stimulating hormone, which in turn deprives the testes of the stimulus they need for testosterone production. Because degarelix works through direct blockade of GnRH receptors, the drug does not cause the initial surge in testosterone production seen with GnRH agonists, and hence there is no early tumor flare.

Degarelix is administered subcutaneously, and absorption is slow. Plasma levels peak in 2 days. Elimination is primarily by peptide bond hydrolysis, a process that occurs in the liver but does not involve cytochrome P450 enzymes. The drug's half-life is long: 53 days.

As with other drugs for ADT, major side effects are hot flashes, reduced libido, erectile dysfunction, gynecomastia, decreased muscle mass, and decreased bone mass with associated increased risk for fractures. In addition, degarelix often causes injection-site reactions (pain, erythema, swelling), weight gain, and elevation of liver transaminases. After a year of treatment, about 10% of patients develop antibodies against degarelix. However, the antibodies do not reduce the effectiveness of treatment.

Androgen Receptor Blockers

Androgen receptor blockers, or simply *antiandrogens,* are indicated only for advanced androgen-sensitive prostate cancer—and only in combination with surgical castration or chemical castration using a GnRH agonist. Currently, three androgen receptor blockers are available: flutamide, bicalutamide, and nilutamide.

Flutamide

Flutamide is indicated for *prostate cancer* only. Benefits derive from blocking androgen receptors in tumor cells, thereby depriving them of needed androgenic support. In patients taking a GnRH agonist, flutamide can serve two purposes: (1) it can prevent tumor flare when GnRH therapy is started, and (2) it can block the effects of adrenal and prostatic androgens. As a rule, the combination of an androgen antagonist plus a GnRH agonist—so-called complete androgen blockade—is reserved for suppressing the initial flare and for suppressing the tumor after it has stopped responding to a GnRH agonist alone. The combination is not used continuously because it does not increase survival, but it does increase toxicity.

Flutamide is administered orally and undergoes rapid and complete absorption. Most of each dose is converted to an active metabolite on the first pass through the liver. Parent drug and metabolites are excreted in the urine.

As with other drugs for ADT, prominent side effects are hot flashes, reduced libido, erectile dysfunction, gynecomastia, decreased muscle mass, and decreased bone mass with associated increased risk for fractures. Nausea, vomiting, and diarrhea are also common. Rarely, potentially fatal liver toxicity has occurred. To reduce the risk for serious harm, liver function should be assessed at baseline, monthly during the first 4 months of treatment, and periodically thereafter.

Flutamide may cause fetal harm and hence is classified in FDA Pregnancy Risk Category D. Accordingly, the drug should not be used during pregnancy. Of course, because flutamide is approved only for prostate cancer, it should not be used during pregnancy anyway.

Bicalutamide

Like flutamide, bicalutamide [Casodex] is an androgen receptor blocker used for advanced androgen-sensitive prostate cancer in men undergoing therapy with a GnRH agonist (e.g., leuprolide). The rationale for the combination is explained in the discussion of flutamide. When bicalutamide is used alone, the most common side effects are breast pain and gynecomastia. When the drug is combined with leuprolide, the most common side effect is hot flashes. Like all other drugs used for ADT, bicalutamide can also cause reduced libido, erectile dysfunction, decreased muscle mass, and decreased bone mass with associated increased risk for fractures. Also, like flutamide, bicalutamide poses a small risk for liver injury, and hence liver function should be monitored. Bicalutamide poses a significant risk for fetal harm and hence is classified in FDA Pregnancy Risk Category X. Bicalutamide is just as effective as flutamide, and dosing is more convenient. As a result, bicalutamide is preferred.

Nilutamide

Like flutamide and bicalutamide, nilutamide [Nilandron, Anandron ♣] blocks receptors for androgens. The drug is approved for metastatic prostate cancer in men who have undergone surgical castration. Benefits derive from blocking the actions of adrenal androgens, which are not reduced by castration.

Although nilutamide is structurally similar to flutamide, the drug is not as well tolerated. The most common adverse effects are hot flashes, delayed adaptation to darkness, nausea, constipation, insomnia, and gynecomastia. In addition, nilutamide can cause reduced libido, erectile dysfunction, decreased muscle mass, and decreased bone mass with associated increased risk for fractures. Other reactions occur less frequently but are more dangerous. About 2% of patients experience dyspnea secondary to interstitial pneumonitis. If this develops, nilutamide should be withdrawn. About 1% of patients develop hepatitis. To ensure early diagnosis, liver function should be monitored.

Abiraterone, a CYP17 Inhibitor

Actions and Use

Abiraterone [Zytiga] is indicated for combined use with prednisone to treat *metastatic castration-resistant prostate cancer* in men previously treated with docetaxel. Benefits derive from inhibiting production of androgens by the adrenal gland and by the prostate cancer itself. (If castration has not been done, abiraterone can also inhibit androgen production by the testes.) In all cases, the underlying mechanism is inhibition of the cytochrome P450 enzyme 17 (CYP17), an enzyme needed by the adrenals, testes, and prostate tumors for androgen synthesis. When tested in men with metastatic castration-resistant prostate cancer, the combination of abiraterone plus prednisone increased overall survival by nearly 4 months and progression-free survival by 2 months.

Adverse Effects

The most common adverse effects are hypokalemia, edema, joint swelling and discomfort, muscle discomfort, hot flashes, diarrhea, urinary tract infection, cough, and hypertension. Like all other drugs for ADT, abiraterone can also decrease libido, muscle mass, and bone mass and can cause erectile dysfunction and gynecomastia.

Inhibition of CYP17 in the adrenals can lead to overproduction of mineralocorticoids and underproduction of glucocorticoids. High levels of mineralocorticoids can cause retention of sodium and loss of potassium, leading to fluid retention, edema, hypertension, and hypokalemia. Low levels of glucocorticoids can increase the risk for death from traumatic events. Cotreatment with prednisone (a glucocorticoid) helps compensate for reduced production of glucocorticoids by the adrenal glands, and, by suppressing release of adrenocorticotropic hormone from the pituitary, prednisone can reduce excessive production of mineralocorticoids.

Hepatotoxicity, manifesting as a marked elevation of liver transaminases—alanine aminotransferase (ALT) and aspartate aminotransferase (AST)—develops in about 30% of patients. To monitor liver status, ALT and AST should be measured at baseline, every 2 weeks for the first 3 months of treatment, and once a month thereafter. If these tests indicate significant liver injury, abiraterone should be discontinued or the dosage reduced.

Abiraterone can harm the developing fetus and hence is classified in FDA Pregnancy Risk Category X. Accordingly, the drug should be avoided by women who are pregnant. Of course, because abiraterone is approved only for prostate cancer, use during pregnancy should not be an issue.

Drug Interactions

Abiraterone is a substrate for CYP3A4, and hence its levels can be raised by CYP3A4 inhibitors (e.g., ketoconazole, clarithromycin, ritonavir) and lowered by CYP3A4 inducers (e.g., phenytoin, carbamazepine, rifampin). Abiraterone inhibits hepatic CYP2D6 and hence can raise levels of CYP2D6 substrates (e.g., dextromethorphan, thioridazine).

Ketoconazole

Ketoconazole [Nizoral], used primarily for fungal infections (see Chapter 77), can be used off-label for prostate cancer. As with abiraterone, benefits derive from inhibiting testicular, adrenal, and prostatic production of androgens. Ketoconazole is employed as secondary therapy in men who have rising prostate-specific antigen levels despite treatment with a GnRH agonist plus an antiandrogen. Dosages are higher than those used for antifungal therapy, and hence side effects are common. Among these are nausea, vomiting, fatigue, skin changes, liver damage, and gynecomastia. Because high-dose ketoconazole can suppress adrenal production of glucocorticoids, the drug is usually combined with hydrocortisone (to avoid adrenal insufficiency).

Other Drugs for Prostate Cancer

Sipuleucel-T

Sipuleucel-T [Provenge] is the name for a patient-specific form of immunotherapy designed to stimulate an immune attack against prostate cancer cells. Each dose is custom made from the patient's own immune cells and hence cannot be used by any other patient. Unfortunately, sipuleucel-T is very expensive—and only moderately effective. Nonetheless, sipuleucel-T is of great interest in that it represents an entirely new approach to cancer treatment.

Therapeutic Use

Sipuleucel-T is indicated for treatment of asymptomatic or minimally symptomatic metastatic castration-resistant (hormone-refractory) prostate cancer. Treatment consists of three infusions given 2 weeks apart. Of note, although sipuleucel-T improves survival, it does not cause measurable tumor regression, nor does it delay the time to tumor progression—suggesting that the mechanism underlying prolonged survival may be something other than immune-mediated injury to cancer cells.

Production

Sipuleucel-T is produced in two steps: collection of circulating immune cells (macrophages) from the patient, followed by modification of those cells in the laboratory. This process—cell collection plus modification—takes about 2 days and must be done for *each dose.*

Macrophage collection is done by *leukapheresis,* a process in which venous blood is circulated from the patient, through a machine, and then back into the patient. The machine separates out macrophages (along with some platelets and other blood cells) and then returns the remaining cells and serum to the patient. The whole procedure takes 3 to 4 hours.

In the laboratory, the macrophages—also known as *antigen-presenting cells,* or *APCs*—are modified by incubation with a recombinant human protein consisting of prostatic acid phosphatase (PAP) linked with GM-CSF. PAP is a protein that is highly expressed by more than 95% of prostate cancer cells. GM-CSF is a blood growth factor that stimulates the production and function of macrophages and some other blood cells. During incubation, the APCs engulf the PAP–GM-CSF, break it into small peptides, and then express those peptides on the APC surface. The modified APCs can now activate cytolytic T cells (killer T cells), causing them to attack prostate cancer cells by recognizing the PAP molecules on their surface.

Adverse Effects

Sipuleucel-T can cause multiple adverse effects. The most common are chills, fatigue, fever, back pain, nausea, joint ache, and headache. Other common reactions include paresthesias, vomiting, anemia, constipation, dizziness, weakness, and extremity pain.

Acute infusion reactions develop in more than 70% of patients. Symptoms include fever, chills, nausea, vomiting, fatigue, hypertension, tachycardia, and respiratory reactions (dyspnea, hypoxia, and bronchospasm). Severe reactions may require hospitalization. Infusion reactions can be reduced by premedication with acetaminophen plus an antihistamine, such as diphenhydramine [Benadryl].

Cytotoxic Drugs

Docetaxel and Cabazitaxel

Docetaxel [Taxotere] and cabazitaxel [Jevtana] are cytotoxic anticancer drugs indicated for hormone-refractory prostate cancer (i.e., prostate cancer that no longer responds to ADT). Either drug (in combination with prednisone) can prolong overall survival as well as progression-free survival. At this time, docetaxel is considered a first-line drug for hormone-refractory prostate cancer. Cabazitaxel is reserved for patients who have already been treated with docetaxel. The major adverse effects of docetaxel are neutropenia, hypersensitivity reactions, and fluid retention. The major adverse effects of cabazitaxel are neutropenia, hypersensitivity reactions, anemia, and diarrhea. With both drugs, benefits derive from causing mitotic arrest.

Estramustine

Estramustine [Emcyt] is a hybrid molecule composed of estradiol (an estrogen) coupled to nitrogen mustard (an alkylating agent). The only indication for the drug is palliative therapy of advanced prostate cancer. Estramustine is administered orally and becomes concentrated in prostate cells, apparently through the actions of a unique "estramustine-binding protein." Injury to prostate cells appears to result from three mechanisms. First, estramustine acts as a weak alkylating agent. Second, hydrolysis of estramustine releases free estradiol, which suppresses ICSH release by the pituitary, thereby depriving prostate cells of hormonal support. Third, and most important, the drug binds to microtubules of mitotic spindles and thereby disrupts mitosis. As a result, estramustine has M-phase specificity.

Adverse effects are caused primarily by free estradiol. Gynecomastia is common. The most serious effect is thrombosis, with resultant myocardial infarction and stroke. Other adverse effects include fluid retention, nausea, vomiting, diarrhea, and hypercalcemia.

TARGETED ANTICANCER DRUGS

Targeted anticancer drugs are designed to bind with specific molecules (targets) with the goal of suppressing tumor growth. The hope is that these drugs will be more selective than hormones and cytotoxic anticancer drugs and hence will be able to destroy cancer cells while leaving normal cells untouched. A few targeted drugs, such as imatinib [Gleevec], have been remarkably successful, producing complete responses with relatively mild adverse effects. Unfortunately, with many other targeted drugs, responses have been less impressive, whereas adverse effects have been more severe. Nonetheless, the concept of targeted therapy has great appeal, and intensive research is underway to make it more of a reality.

How do targeted drugs work? Many of these drugs are *antibodies* that bind with specific antigens on tumor cells; others are *small molecules* that inhibit intracellular enzymes. Some antibodies mark cancer cells for immune attack, some block cell-surface receptors, some deliver toxic drugs or radioactivity, and some inhibit angiogenesis and thereby deprive tumor cells of their blood supply. Most of the small molecules inhibit specific tyrosine kinases and thereby disrupt intracellular signaling pathways. Properties of the targeted drugs are shown in Table 82.7.

Kinase Inhibitors

A kinase is an enzyme that catalyzes the transfer of a phosphate group from a nucleoside triphosphate donor (e.g., adenosine triphosphate [ATP]) to an acceptor molecule, often a protein involved in regulation of cell behavior. This process, known as phosphorylation, alters the structure of the acceptor protein and thereby increases or decreases its activity. Put another way, the result of phosphorylation is like flipping a switch, turning it on or turning it off. Of interest to us are the protein "switches" that help promote cancer growth. For example, certain regulatory proteins, when phosphorylated, activate signaling pathways that increase cell proliferation and cell survival. Accordingly, if we prevent phosphorylation with a kinase inhibitor, we can shut down the signaling pathway and thereby inhibit proliferation and promote apoptosis (programmed cell death).

TABLE 82.7 ▪ Targeted Anticancer Drugs

Drug	Molecular Target	Drug Structure	Indications	Major Toxicities
KINASE INHIBITORS				
EGFR Tyrosine Kinase Inhibitors				
Cetuximab [Erbitux]	Inhibits EGFR	Antibody	EGFR-positive colorectal cancer and head and neck cancer	Rash, infusion reactions, interstitial lung disease
Panitumumab [Vectibix]	Inhibits EGFR	Antibody	EGFR-positive colorectal cancer	Rare infusion reactions, rash, rare interstitial pneumonitis
Gefitinib [Iressa]	Inhibits EGFR tyrosine kinase	Small molecule	Non–small cell lung cancer	Rash, diarrhea, interstitial lung disease
Erlotinib [Tarceva]	Inhibits EGFR tyrosine kinase	Small molecule	Non–small cell lung cancer	Blistering, GI perforation, interstitial lung disease, corneal ulceration/perforation
Afatinib [Gilotrif]	Inhibits EGFR tyrosine kinase, HER2 and HER4 tyrosine kinase	Small molecule	Metastatic non–small cell lung cancer	Diarrhea, cutaneous reactions, keratitis
Lapatinib [Tykerb]	Inhibits EGFR tyrosine kinase and HER2 tyrosine kinase	Small molecule	HER2-positive breast cancer	Diarrhea, hepatotoxicity, cardiotoxicity, interstitial lung disease
BCR-ABL Tyrosine Kinase Inhibitors				
Imatinib [Gleevec]	Inhibits BCR-ABL tyrosine kinase	Small molecule	Chronic myeloid leukemia, GI stromal tumors	Nausea, diarrhea, myalgia, edema, liver injury
Dasatinib [Sprycel]	Inhibits BCR-ABL tyrosine kinase	Small molecule	Chronic myeloid leukemia	Myelosuppression, QT prolongation, fluid retention, pulmonary arterial hypertension
Nilotinib [Tasigna]	Inhibits BCR-ABL tyrosine kinase	Small molecule	Chronic myeloid leukemia	Myelosuppression, QT prolongation
Bosutinib [Bosulif]	Inhibits BCR-ABL tyrosine kinase	Small molecule	Philadelphia chromosome–positive chronic myelogenous leukemia	Myelosuppression, hepatotoxicity, anaphylactic shock
Ponatinib [Iclusig]	Inhibits BCR-ABL tyrosine kinase	Small molecule	Chronic myeloid leukemia or Philadelphia chromosome–positive lymphoblastic leukemia	Venous thromboembolism, cardiotoxicity, pancreatitis, cardiac dysrhythmias
Multi–Tyrosine Kinase Inhibitors				
Sorafenib [Nexavar]	Inhibits multiple cell-surface and intracellular tyrosine kinases	Small molecule	Renal cell carcinoma, hepatocellular carcinoma	Rash, diarrhea, hand-and-foot syndrome, bleeding, QT prolongation, hypertension
Sunitinib [Sutent]	Inhibits multiple tyrosine kinases	Small molecule	Renal cell carcinoma, GI stromal tumors, pancreatic neuroendocrine tumors	Hepatotoxicity, heart failure, QT prolongation, hypertension, hemorrhage
Pazopanib [Votrient]	Inhibits multiple tyrosine kinases	Small molecule	Renal cell carcinoma	Bone marrow suppression, hepatotoxicity
Vandetanib [Caprelsa]	Inhibits multiple tyrosine kinases	Small molecule	Medullary thyroid cancer	QT prolongation, rash, diarrhea/colitis
Axitinib [Inlyta]	Inhibits multiple tyrosine kinases	Small molecule	Advanced renal cell carcinoma	Hypertensive crisis, venous thromboembolism, hypothyroidism
Cabozantinib [Cometriq]	Inhibits multiple tyrosine kinases	Small molecule	Metastatic medullary thyroid cancer	Thromboembolism, GI perforation, posterior leukoencephalopathy
Regorafenib [Stivarga]	Inhibits multiple tyrosine kinases	Small molecule	Metastatic colon cancer, metastatic GI stromal cancer	Hepatotoxicity, toxic cutaneous reactions, cardiotoxicity
mTOR Kinase Inhibitors				
Temsirolimus [Torisel]	Inhibits mTOR kinase	Small molecule	Renal cell carcinoma	Mucositis, bone marrow suppression, metabolic abnormalities
Everolimus [Afinitor]	Inhibits mTOR kinase	Small molecule	Renal cell carcinoma	Oral ulceration, bone marrow suppression, metabolic abnormalities

TABLE 82.7 ▪ Targeted Anticancer Drugs—cont'd

Drug	Molecular Target	Drug Structure	Indications	Major Toxicities
BRAF V600E Kinase Inhibitors				
Vemurafenib [Zelboraf]	Inhibits BRAF V600E kinase	Small molecule	BRAF V600E-positive melanoma	Cutaneous squamous cell carcinoma, arthralgia, QT prolongation, severe skin reactions, photosensitivity
Dabrafenib [Tafinlar]	Inhibits BRAF V600E kinase	Small molecule	BRAF V600E–positive melanoma	Retinal vein occlusion, cutaneous malignancies
Trametinib [Mekinist]	Inhibits BRAF V600E pathway through inhibition of MEK1 and MEK2	Small molecule	BRAF V600E–positive melanoma	Cutaneous malignancies, hemorrhage, thromboembolism, retinal vein occlusion
Anaplastic Lymphoma Kinase (ALK) Inhibitor				
Crizotinib [Xalkori]	Inhibits ALK	Small molecule	ALK-positive non–small cell lung cancer	Pneumonitis, hepatotoxicity, QT prolongation
OTHER TARGETED DRUGS				
CD20-Directed Antibodies				
Rituximab [Rituxan]	Binds CD20 antigen, causing apoptosis and immune attack	Antibody	B-cell chronic lymphocytic leukemia, B-cell non-Hodgkin lymphoma	Severe infusion reactions, severe mucocutaneous reactions, tumor lysis syndrome, PML
Ofatumumab [Arzerra]	Binds CD20 antigen, causing apoptosis and immune attack	Antibody	B-cell chronic lymphocytic leukemia	Severe infusion reactions, cytopenias, PML
Ibritumomab tiuxetan/ yttrium-90 [Zevalin]	Binds CD20 antigen, causing radiation injury	Antibody/ yttrium-90 hybrid	B-cell non-Hodgkin lymphoma	Bone marrow suppression and infusion reactions
Tositumomab/^{131}I-tositumomab [Bexxar]	Binds CD20 antigen, causing immune attack and radiation injury	Antibody/iodine-131 hybrid	B-cell non-Hodgkin lymphoma	Bone marrow suppression, infusion reactions, hypersensitivity reactions
Antibody-Drug Conjugate				
Brentuximab vedotin [Adcetris]	Binds CD30 antigen, to deliver a toxin that causes mitotic arrest	Antibody/drug hybrid	Hodgkin lymphoma, anaplastic large cell lymphoma	Peripheral neuropathy, neutropenia
Angiogenesis Inhibitor				
Bevacizumab [Avastin]	Binds VEGF and thereby inhibits angiogenesis	Antibody	Colorectal cancer, non–small cell lung cancer, glioblastoma, renal cell carcinoma	Hypertension, GI perforation, impaired wound healing, hemorrhage, thromboembolism, nephrotic syndrome
Proteasome Inhibitors				
Bortezomib [Velcade]	Inhibits proteasome activity	Small molecule	Multiple myeloma	Bone marrow suppression, GI disturbances, peripheral neuropathy, weakness
Carfilzomib [Kyprolis]	Inhibits proteasome activity	Small molecule	Multiple myeloma	Cardiac arrest, cardiotoxicity, infusion reactions
Histone Deacetylase (HDAC) Inhibitors				
Vorinostat [Zolinza]	Inhibits HDAC	Small molecule	Cutaneous T-cell lymphoma	Pulmonary embolism, bone marrow suppression, fatigue, nausea, diarrhea
Romidepsin [Istodax]	Inhibits HDAC	Small molecule	Cutaneous T-cell lymphoma	Bone marrow suppression, infection, QT prolongation
Additional Targeted Anticancer Drugs				
Ipilimumab [Yervoy]	Binds CTLA-4 to unleash an immune attack	Antibody	Melanoma	Severe immune-mediated enterocolitis, hepatitis, dermatitis, neuropathies, endocrinopathies
Alemtuzumab [Campath]	Binds CD52 antigen	Antibody	B-cell chronic lymphocytic leukemia	Bone marrow suppression, infusion reactions, infection

CTLA-4, cytotoxic T lymphocyte–associated antigen-4; EGFR, epidermal growth factor receptor, which is coupled with tyrosine kinase; GI, gastrointestinal; HER2, human epidermal growth factor receptor 2; MEK, MAP (mitogen-activated protein)/ERK (extracellular signal–regulated) kinase; mTOR, mammalian target of rapamycin; PML, progressive multifocal leukoencephalopathy; VEGF, vascular endothelial growth factor.

Most of the drugs discussed next inhibit *tyrosine kinases* of one type or another. What's a tyrosine kinase? It's simply a kinase that transfers a phosphate group specifically to tyrosine, one of the amino acid components of the protein undergoing phosphorylation. Other kinases phosphorylate different amino acids, often serine or threonine.

EGFR Tyrosine Kinase Inhibitors

The *epidermal growth factor receptor* is a transmembrane regulatory molecule that works through activation of intracellular tyrosine kinase. The receptor portion of EGFR, which is found on the outer surface of the cell membrane, is coupled with tyrosine kinase on the inner surface of the cell membrane. Binding of an agonist to EGFR activates tyrosine kinase, which in turn activates signaling pathways that regulate cell proliferation and survival. EGFRs are expressed constitutively in many normal epithelial tissues (e.g., skin, hair follicles) and are overexpressed in several cancers, including cancers of the lung, breast, prostate, bladder, ovary, colon, and rectum. Overexpression is associated with unregulated cell growth and poor prognosis. Drugs that inhibit EGFR suppress cell proliferation and promote apoptosis. At this time, we have six EGFR tyrosine kinase inhibitors. Two of these drugs—cetuximab and panitumumab—are monoclonal antibodies that bind with the receptor portion of EGFR tyrosine kinase and thereby prevent its activation by agonists. The other four drugs—erlotinib, gefitinib, afatinib, and lapatinib—are small molecules that work inside the cell to inhibit tyrosine kinase directly. It should be noted that EGFRs belong to the same receptor family as HER2, the target that trastuzumab [Herceptin] works through.

Cetuximab

Cetuximab [Erbitux] is a monoclonal antibody that blocks EGFRs. The drug is approved for refractory colorectal cancer and for carcinoma of the head and neck. Infusion reactions, acneiform rash, low magnesium, and GI symptoms are common.

Mechanism of Action. Cetuximab acts as a competitive antagonist at EGFRs. As noted, these receptors, which help regulate cell growth, are overexpressed in certain cancers, including those of the colon and rectum. EGFR blockade inhibits cell growth and promotes apoptosis. In animal studies, cetuximab decreased growth and survival of cancer cells that overexpress EGFR, but had no effect on cancer cells that lack EGFR.

Therapeutic Uses

COLORECTAL CANCER. Cetuximab is approved for metastatic, EGFR-positive colorectal cancer. The drug may be added to an irinotecan-based regimen (if the cancer has progressed despite irinotecan treatment), or it may be used alone (in patients who cannot tolerate irinotecan). Treatment improves quality of life and can improve survival rate at 3 years.

HEAD AND NECK CANCER. Cetuximab, in combination with radiation, is approved for initial treatment of locally or regionally advanced squamous cell carcinoma of the head and neck. In addition, the drug can be used for recurrent or metastatic cancers that have progressed despite treatment with a platinum-based regimen.

Adverse Effects. Cetuximab causes adverse effects in most patients. The effects of greatest concern are severe infusion reactions, severe rash, and interstitial lung disease (ILD).

Cetuximab causes severe *infusion reactions* in 2% to 5% of patients. Manifestations include rapid-onset airway obstruction, hypotension, shock, loss of consciousness, myocardial infarction, and cardiopulmonary arrest. Severe reactions can happen with any infusion, but most (90%) occur with the first infusion. If a severe reaction develops, cetuximab should be discontinued immediately and never used again. Agents for medical management—epinephrine, glucocorticoids, IV antihistamines, bronchodilators, and oxygen—should always be on hand. To reduce the risk for a severe reaction, premedication with an IV antihistamine (e.g., 50 mg diphenhydramine) is recommended.

Acne-like rash, mainly on the face and upper torso, develops in 88% of patients and is severe in 12%. Severe rash has led to *Staphylococcus aureus* sepsis and abscesses that require incision and drainage. Sunlight can exacerbate dermatologic reactions, and hence patients should limit sun exposure, use a sunblock, and wear protective clothing.

Very rarely, cetuximab has been associated with *interstitial lung disease,* characterized by inflammation, scarring, and hardening of the lungs. One case of fatal interstitial pneumonitis with pulmonary edema has been reported. Whether cetuximab is truly the cause of these lung disorders has not been established.

The combination of cetuximab and irinotecan often causes *GI toxicity,* manifesting as diarrhea, nausea, abdominal pain, vomiting, anorexia, and constipation.

Hypomagnesemia is common. Magnesium supplements are often required.

Cetuximab can cross the placenta, but whether it causes fetal harm has not been studied in humans. Animal studies do show adverse fetal effects. Until more is known, prudence dictates avoiding cetuximab during pregnancy. Cetuximab is classified in FDA Pregnancy Risk Category C.

Panitumumab

Panitumumab [Vectibix] is a monoclonal antibody similar to cetuximab with respect to mechanism, indications, and adverse effects. The principal difference between the drugs is that panitumumab is a fully human antibody, whereas cetuximab is not. Like cetuximab, panitumumab blocks EGFRs, causing inhibition of tyrosine kinase and, ultimately, apoptosis. At this time, the drug has only one indication: treatment of EGFR-expressing metastatic colorectal cancer in patients who have already received chemotherapy. The most common adverse effect is acne-like rash. Other adverse effects include fatigue, nausea, diarrhea, and hypomagnesemia. Because panitumumab is a fully human antibody, severe infusion reactions are less frequent than with cetuximab (1% vs. 3%).

Gefitinib

Therapeutic Use. Gefitinib [Iressa] is approved for oral therapy of advanced non–small cell lung cancer (NSCLC) that has been refractory to first-line treatment (platinum- or docetaxel-based therapy). Unfortunately, postmarketing studies failed to show any survival benefit. As a result, gefitinib is restricted to patients enrolled in a medical trial in the United States. NSCLC is the most common form of lung cancer, and cells of this cancer often overexpress EGFRs.

Mechanism of Action. Like cetuximab, gefitinib disrupts cellular processes regulated by EGFRs. However, unlike cetuximab, which acts on the cell surface to block EGFRs, gefitinib acts within the cell to inhibit tyrosine kinase that is linked with EGFR. Under normal conditions, activation of EGFR leads to activation of tyrosine kinase, which in turn activates signaling pathways that regulate cell proliferation and survival. By inhibiting EGFR-linked tyrosine kinase, gefitinib has the same effect as EGFR blockade: suppression of cell proliferation and promotion of apoptosis.

Responding Populations. A mutation in the EGFR tyrosine kinase gene predicts who will respond to gefitinib. This mutation is more likely in women, Asians, and patients with the adenocarcinoma subtype of NSCLC. People in these populations are more likely to respond.

Pharmacokinetics. Gefitinib is slowly absorbed from the GI tract. Plasma levels peak 3 to 7 hours after dosing. The drug undergoes extensive hepatic metabolism, primarily by CYP3A4, followed by excretion in the feces. The elimination half-life is 48 hours.

Adverse Effects. Gefitinib is generally well tolerated. As with cetuximab, the most frequent reactions are diarrhea and acne-like rash. Other fairly common reactions are dry skin, nausea, and vomiting. Ocular effects—amblyopia, conjunctivitis, eye pain, and corneal erosion or ulceration—occur infrequently. Asymptomatic elevation of liver transaminases has been reported.

Interstitial lung disease is the most serious adverse effect. This condition begins with acute-onset dyspnea, sometimes with cough or fever. Rapid deterioration may ensue. The overall incidence is about 1%, with one third of cases being fatal. If respiratory symptoms develop, gefitinib should be interrupted and the patient evaluated. If ILD is diagnosed, gefitinib should not be used again. The risk for ILD is highest among patients with prior radiation or chemotherapy.

Drug and Herb Interactions. Drugs that inhibit CYP3A4 (e.g., itraconazole, ketoconazole) can decrease gefitinib metabolism and may thereby increase its plasma level. Conversely, agents that induce CYP3A4 (e.g., rifampin, phenytoin, carbamazepine, St. John's wort) can accelerate gefitinib metabolism and may thereby reduce its level. (For patients taking a potent inducer of CYP3A4, dosage may be increased.) Furthermore, drugs that lower gastric pH (e.g., histamine-2 antagonists, proton pump inhibitors, antacids) can decrease gefitinib absorption and may thereby lower its level.

Use in Pregnancy and Lactation. Gefitinib can harm the developing fetus and hence should not be used by pregnant women. In laboratory animals, the drug decreased the number of live births, increased neonatal mortality, and reduced fetal weight. We don't know if gefitinib is safe during breastfeeding.

Erlotinib

Actions and Use. Erlotinib [Tarceva] has three indications: (1) advanced NSCLC after previous chemotherapy has failed; (2) maintenance therapy of advanced NSCLC when the disease has remained stable after four cycles of platinum-based first-line therapy, and (3) first-line treatment of inoperable pancreatic cancer in combination with gemcitabine.

Like gefitinib, erlotinib inhibits tyrosine kinase coupled with EGFR and thereby suppresses cell proliferation and promotes apoptosis. However, in contrast to gefitinib, erlotinib has been shown to prolong survival. Survival was longest among patients who had never smoked and those with high levels of EGFR.

Responding Populations. As with gefitinib, a mutation in the EGFR tyrosine kinase gene predicts who will respond to erlotinib. As noted, this mutation is more likely in women, Asians, and patients with the adenocarcinoma subtype of NSCLC, and hence people in these populations are more likely to respond.

Pharmacokinetics. Oral bioavailability is 60% in the absence of food and nearly 100% in the presence of food. Plasma levels peak about 4 hours after dosing. In the blood, erlotinib is 93% bound to proteins. The drug undergoes extensive metabolism by hepatic CYP3A4, followed by excretion in the bile.

Adverse Effects. Although erlotinib is generally well tolerated, adverse effects occur often. The most common are rash, diarrhea, nausea, and vomiting. Diarrhea can usually be managed with loperamide. Rarely, patients develop ILD, a potentially fatal condition that begins with dry cough and sudden onset of dyspnea (or sudden worsening of existing dyspnea). Hepatotoxicity, manifesting as asymptomatic elevation of liver transaminases, occurs in some patients. Rarely, erlotinib causes GI perforation or severe skin reactions, both of which can be fatal. The drug can also cause ocular disorders, including corneal perforation, corneal ulceration, and abnormal eyelash growth. In animal studies, erlotinib caused fetal death and abortion and hence should not be used during pregnancy.

Drug Interactions. Strong inhibitors of CYP3A4 (e.g., itraconazole, clarithromycin, ritonavir) can decrease metabolism of erlotinib, causing its level to rise. Conversely, inducers of CYP3A4 (e.g., rifampin, carbamazepine) can accelerate metabolism of erlotinib, causing its level to fall, sometimes dramatically. Erlotinib may increase the risk for bleeding in patients taking warfarin; close monitoring of prothrombin time or the international normalized ratio (INR) is recommended.

Afatinib

Actions and Use. Afatinib [Gilotrif] is approved for treatment of metastatic NSCLC in patients whose tumors have EGFR deletions or other mutations as detected by an FDA-approved test.

Like gefitinib and erlotinib, afatinib inhibits tyrosine kinase coupled with EGFR and thereby suppresses cell proliferation and promotes apoptosis. In addition, afatinib also inhibits tyrosine kinase coupled with HER2 and HER4.

Pharmacokinetics. The half-life of afatinib is 37 hours. Despite this long half-life, plasma levels peak about 4 hours after dosing. In the blood, afatinib is 95% bound to proteins. The drug undergoes minimal metabolism and is highly excreted in the feces.

Adverse Effects. Afatinib has caused severe diarrhea leading to dehydration and death. Diarrhea can usually be managed with loperamide. Skin and eye reactions have also occurred. These are characterized by blistering or exfoliating lesions as well as keratitis of the eye. Afatinib should be withheld in these cases. Liver test abnormalities have been seen. Periodic liver testing should be completed to monitor for this adverse effect. Afatinib may cause fetal harm and should be avoided in pregnancy.

Drug Interactions. As with erlotinib, strong inhibitors of CYP3A4 (e.g., itraconazole, clarithromycin, ritonavir) can decrease metabolism of afatinib, causing its level to rise. Conversely, inducers of CYP3A4 (e.g., rifampin, carbamazepine) can accelerate metabolism of afatinib, causing its level to fall, sometimes dramatically.

Lapatinib

Lapatinib [Tykerb] is a small-molecule inhibitor of EGFR tyrosine kinase and HER2 tyrosine kinase. Lapatinib and its use in breast cancer were discussed earlier.

BCR-ABL Tyrosine Kinase Inhibitors

The BCR-ABL tyrosine kinase inhibitors are the preferred agents for treating *chronic myeloid leukemia* (CML). Five of these drugs are available: imatinib, dasatinib, bosutinib, ponatinib, and nilotinib. Imatinib is the "gold standard" for CML therapy. Unfortunately, relapse can occur, owing to evolution of subclones that have imatinib-resistant BCR-ABL mutations. The other drugs—dasatinib, bosutinib, ponatinib, and nilotinib—are active against all but one of these resistant subclones and hence can be effective even in patients who no longer respond to imatinib.

Imatinib

Indications. Imatinib [Gleevec] was approved for oral therapy of CML, but only after treatment with interferon alfa had failed. Because of clear superiority, imatinib had displaced interferon alfa as the initial treatment of choice. Imatinib may be continued as long as there is no evidence of disease progression and as long as side effects remain tolerable.

Imatinib is also approved for *myelodysplastic/myeloproliferative diseases, aggressive systemic mastocytosis, acute lymphoblastic leukemia, dermatofibrosarcoma protuberans, hypereosinophilic syndrome, chronic eosinophilic leukemia,* and unresectable or metastatic malignant *gastrointestinal stromal tumor,* a rare form of stomach and intestinal cancer. These applications are not discussed further.

CML and Its Treatment. CML is a cancer in which myeloid cells undergo massive clonal expansion. The disease begins with a chronic phase, progresses through an accelerated phase, and ends with the blast crisis phase. The underlying cause is a genetic abnormality known as the *Philadelphia chromosome,* which is produced by translocation of genetic material between chromosomes 9 and 22. Because of this genetic change, CML cells make an abnormal, continuously active enzyme, called *BCR-ABL tyrosine kinase.* This enzyme phosphorylates, and thereby activates, as-yet unidentified regulatory proteins, which in turn inhibit apoptosis and stimulate cell proliferation. Major treatment options are the BCR-ABL tyrosine kinase inhibitors, interferon-based regimens, and stem cell transplantation (the only potentially curative treatment).

Mechanism of Action and Clinical Effects. Imatinib is a highly specific competitive inhibitor of BCR-ABL tyrosine kinase. By inhibiting this enzyme, imatinib prevents the phosphorylation and resultant activation of regulatory proteins and thereby suppresses proliferation of CML cells and promotes apoptosis. Imatinib is selective for cells that express BCR-ABL tyrosine kinase; normal cells are not affected. When tested during the chronic phase of CML, imatinib was superior to the combination of interferon alfa plus cytarabine. After 18 months, disease progression was stopped in 92% of imatinib users, compared with 74% of those getting interferon. Furthermore, imatinib was better tolerated. Long-term follow-up is needed to determine how long responses to imatinib will last and whether imatinib prolongs survival.

Over time, resistance to imatinib may develop because the genes that code for BCR-ABL can mutate, causing production of imatinib-resistant forms of the enzyme.

Pharmacokinetics. Imatinib is well absorbed after oral administration. Bioavailability is 98%. In the blood, the drug is highly protein bound. Imatinib undergoes extensive metabolism, primarily by hepatic CYP3A4, followed by excretion in the feces. The elimination half-lives of imatinib and its major active metabolite are 18 hours and 40 hours, respectively.

Adverse Effects. Imatinib causes adverse effects in most patients. The incidence and severity of adverse effects is lowest during the chronic phase of CML, higher during the accelerated phase, and highest during blast crisis. Common reactions include nausea, vomiting, diarrhea, rash, headache, fatigue, fever, and musculoskeletal complaints, including muscle cramps, muscle pain, and arthralgia. Fluid retention occurs in 52% to 68% of patients and may lead to pleural effusion, pericardial effusion, pulmonary edema, or ascites. Neutropenia and thrombocytopenia develop often, posing a risk for infection and bleeding. Accordingly, complete blood counts should be obtained weekly during the first month of treatment, biweekly during the second month, and periodically thereafter. Hepatotoxicity, indicated by severe elevations of transaminases or bilirubin, develops in 1.1% to 3.5% of patients. Other reported effects include severe congestive heart failure, serious skin reactions (e.g., erythema multiforme, Stevens-Johnson syndrome), and hypothyroidism in thyroidectomy patients receiving thyroid hormone replacement therapy.

Effects in Pregnancy and Breastfeeding. In animal studies, doses equivalent to those used clinically have caused major fetal malformations. Accordingly, imatinib is classified in FDA Pregnancy Risk Category D and should be avoided during pregnancy. Women of childbearing age should use adequate contraception.

Imatinib achieves high concentrations in breast milk and poses a risk to the breastfed infant. The manufacturer recommends against breastfeeding while taking the drug.

Drug Interactions. Imatinib is a substrate for and competitive inhibitor of CYP3A4, CYP2C9, and CYP2D6. By inhibiting these CYP isoenzymes, imatinib can raise levels of warfarin and other drugs that are metabolized by them. Drugs that inhibit CYP3A4 (e.g., ketoconazole, erythromycin) can raise levels of imatinib. Conversely, drugs that induce CYP3A4 (e.g., carbamazepine, rifampin, St. John's wort) can reduce levels of imatinib.

Dasatinib

Dasatinib [Sprycel] is indicated for all three phases of CML: chronic, accelerated, and blast crisis. Initially, the drug was approved only for patients who were unresponsive to or intolerant of imatinib. Soon after, the FDA approved dasatinib as first-line therapy.

Dasatinib inhibits BCR-ABL tyrosine kinase more effectively than imatinib. First, dasatinib binds to both the active and inactive conformations of BCR-ABL tyrosine kinase, whereas imatinib only binds to the inactive conformation. Second, dasatinib binds the enzyme with greater affinity than imatinib. Third, dasatinib binds a wider variety of protein kinases. As a result of these differences, dasatinib is active against nearly all imatinib-resistant mutant clones. In fact, the only exception is the T315I mutation, which is resistant to all available drugs.

Adverse effects of dasatinib are much like those of imatinib, with one important exception: dasatinib produces more myelosuppression and thereby poses a risk for severe neutropenia, thrombocytopenia, and anemia. Fluid retention is seen in about 35% of patients. Severe cases can cause pulmonary edema. Rarely, dasatinib has been associated with pulmonary arterial hypertension, although a causal relationship has not been established. Dasatinib has the potential to prolong the QT interval, but the clinical significance is unclear.

Levels of dasatinib can be affected by other drugs. Dasatinib is a substrate for CYP3A4; therefore drugs that induce CYP3A4 can lower dasatinib levels, and drugs that inhibit CYP3A4 can raise dasatinib levels. Solubility of dasatinib is pH dependent, so drugs that raise gastric pH (antacids, proton pump inhibitors, histamine-2 receptor blockers) can reduce dasatinib absorption.

Nilotinib

Nilotinib [Tasigna] is indicated for (1) accelerated-phase CML in patients resistant to or intolerant of imatinib and (2) chronic-phase CML in treatment-naïve patients as well as patients previously treated with imatinib. Like imatinib, nilotinib binds to the inactive form of BCR-ABL. However, the binding affinity is much greater. Like dasatinib, nilotinib is active against all imatinib-resistant clones, except those with the T315I mutation.

In general, patients tolerate nilotinib better than imatinib. The most common adverse effects are thrombocytopenia, neutropenia, rash, pruritus, nausea, fatigue, headache, and constipation. Of much greater concern, nilotinib prolongs the QT interval, posing a risk for severe dysrhythmias and sudden cardiac death. Accordingly, the drug should not be used in patients with hypokalemia, hypomagnesemia, or long QT syndrome. Also, it should not be combined with other QT drugs or with strong inhibitors of CYP3A4 (e.g., ketoconazole, clarithromycin, ritonavir).

Like dasatinib, nilotinib is a substrate for CYP3A4; therefore drugs that induce CYP3A4 can lower nilotinib levels, and drugs that inhibit CYP3A4 can raise nilotinib levels.

Bosutinib

Bosutinib [Bosulif] has one indication: treatment of adults with Philadelphia chromosome–positive CML resistant to prior therapy. Bosutinib inhibits the tyrosine kinase that promotes CML.

Myelosuppression has occurred in patients taking bosutinib. A complete blood count should be performed weekly during the first month and then monthly thereafter. Because of the potential for hepatotoxicity, liver function tests should be obtained monthly for the first 3 months. Bosutinib can result in fetal harm and should be avoided in pregnancy.

As bosutinib is metabolized by the CYP3A system, drugs that affect this system may alter the metabolism of bosutinib. Taking CYP3A inhibitors (clarithromycin, grapefruit juice, ketoconazole, ritonavir) and CYP3A inducers (carbamazepine, phenytoin, rifampin) in conjunction with bosutinib may increase adverse reactions.

Ponatinib

Ponatinib [Iclusig] is indicated for (1) treatment of adults with CML that is resistant to or intolerant of prior therapy and (2) treatment of Philadelphia chromosome–positive lymphoblastic leukemia resistant to prior therapy with tyrosine kinase inhibitors.

Ponatinib, like dasatinib, inhibits multiple tyrosine kinases and is therefore used as an alternative treatment after use of other tyrosine kinase inhibitors such as imatinib.

Venous thromboembolic events have been reported in patients taking ponatinib. Reduction or cessation of the drug should be considered in patients who develop serious thromboembolism. Other adverse effects include pancreatitis, hypertension, cardiotoxicity, heart dysrhythmias, GI perforation, and myelosuppression. Blood pressure, complete blood counts, and ejection fraction should be closely followed during treatment with ponatinib.

Like bosutinib, ponatinib is metabolized by the CYP3A system. Drugs that affect this system may alter the metabolism of ponatinib.

Ponatinib is available in 15- and 45-mg tablets. Dosing is 45 mg daily. Treatment should be continued until the disease progresses or unacceptable toxicity is experienced.

Multi–Tyrosine Kinase Inhibitors

In contrast to the EGFR tyrosine kinase inhibitors and the BCR-ABL tyrosine kinase inhibitors, which inhibit just one type of tyrosine kinase, the drugs in this section inhibit several types of tyrosine kinase. However, despite their diverse actions, the multi–tyrosine kinase inhibitors have limited indications: four of the available agents—sorafenib, sunitinib, axitinib, and pazopanib—are approved for advanced renal cell carcinoma. In addition, sorafenib is approved for hepatocellular carcinoma, and sunitinib is approved for GI stromal tumor and PNET. Two additional drugs—vandetanib and cabozantinib—are approved for medullary thyroid cancer. A seventh drug—regorafenib—is approved for metastatic colon cancer and metastatic GI stromal tumor.

Sorafenib

Sorafenib [Nexavar] is an oral multi–tyrosine kinase inhibitor approved for advanced renal cell carcinoma, recurrent thyroid carcinoma refractory to iodine treatment, and unresectable hepatocellular carcinoma. The drug inhibits multiple cell-surface and intracellular kinases that are associated with angiogenesis, apoptosis, and cell proliferation.

The most common adverse effects are diarrhea, rash, fatigue, and hand-and-foot syndrome. Between 15% and 20% of patients develop hypertension. Nausea and vomiting are usually mild. Sorafenib prolongs the QT interval and thereby poses a risk for serious dysrhythmias. In addition, the drug doubles the risk for bleeding (by inhibiting vascular endothelial growth factor [VEGF] tyrosine kinase). Myocardial ischemia and GI perforation occur rarely. Sorafenib (in low doses) is teratogenic and embryolethal in animals and hence should be avoided during pregnancy (FDA Pregnancy Risk Category D).

Sunitinib

Sunitinib [Sutent] is an oral multi–tyrosine kinase inhibitor with three indications: advanced renal cell carcinoma, pancreatic neuroendocrine tumor (PNET), and GI stromal tumor in patients unresponsive to or intolerant of imatinib. The drug inhibits multiple tyrosine kinases and thereby disrupts angiogenesis, cellular growth, and tumor metastasis.

Adverse effects are very common. Twenty percent or more of patients experience fatigue, weakness, anorexia, altered taste, fever, dyspnea, cough, GI disturbances (nausea, vomiting, diarrhea, dyspepsia, abdominal pain, mucosis), pain (headache, back pain, arthralgia, extremity pain), and skin reactions (rash, dryness, hand-and-foot syndrome, discolored skin and hair). Of much greater concern, sunitinib can cause heart damage, liver damage, and hemorrhage. About 15% of patients develop irreversible heart failure, and hence cardiac function should be monitored closely. Like sorafenib, sunitinib prolongs the QT interval and hence can cause severe dysrhythmias. Sunitinib can cause potentially fatal liver injury. Accordingly, liver function tests should be conducted at baseline and periodically throughout the treatment period. By suppressing platelet production, sunitinib can cause hemorrhage. To reduce risk, serial blood counts should be conducted. About 25% of patients develop mild to moderate hypertension, which responds to standard antihypertensive drugs. Other serious effects include impairment of wound healing, adrenal function, and thyroid function. In animal studies, sunitinib has been teratogenic and fetotoxic and hence is classified in FDA Pregnancy Risk Category D.

Sunitinib is a substrate for CYP3A4, so medications that inhibit CYP3A4 (e.g., ketoconazole, erythromycin) can raise levels of sunitinib and increase toxicity. Conversely, drugs that induce CYP3A4 (e.g., carbamazepine, rifampin, St. John's wort) can reduce levels and thereby decrease efficacy.

Pazopanib

Pazopanib [Votrient] is an oral multi–tyrosine kinase inhibitor indicated only for advanced renal cell carcinoma. Like sunitinib and sorafenib, pazopanib disrupts tumor growth and angiogenesis by inhibiting multiple forms of tyrosine kinase.

Adverse effects are common and sometimes severe. Effects seen often include hepatotoxicity, diarrhea, hypertension, hyperglycemia, change in hair color, leukopenia, and thrombocytopenia, sometimes associated with hemorrhage. Rarely, pazopanib has caused fatal GI perforation, fatal thrombotic events, and potentially fatal torsades de pointes secondary to prolonging the QT interval. In pregnant animals, pazopanib has been teratogenic, embryolethal, and abortifacient. Accordingly, the drug is classified in FDA Pregnancy Risk Category D.

Like sunitinib, pazopanib is metabolized by CYP3A4, and hence medications that inhibit CYP3A4 can raise levels of pazopanib (and thus increase toxicity), and medications that induce CYP3A4 can reduce levels of pazopanib (and thus decrease efficacy).

Vandetanib

Vandetanib [Caprelsa] is indicated for advanced medullary thyroid cancer, a rare disease that accounts for just 3% to 5% of all thyroid cancers. In the United States this translates to about 1300 to 2200 cases a year. Benefits of vandetanib appear to result from inhibiting multiple tyrosine kinases, including EGFR tyrosine kinase.

The most common adverse effects are diarrhea/colitis, rash, acne, nausea, hypertension, headache, fatigue, decreased appetite, and abdominal pain. More important, vandetanib poses a significant risk for QT prolongation, which can lead to potentially fatal dysrhythmias. Furthermore, because vandetanib has a long half-life (19 days), this risk can persist long after dosing is stopped. To monitor QT effects, an electrocardiogram should be obtained at baseline, between weeks 2 and 4, between weeks 8 and 12, and every 3 months thereafter. Other drugs that prolong the QT interval should be avoided. In laboratory animals, low-dose vandetanib is fetotoxic and teratogenic. Accordingly, the drug is classified in FDA Pregnancy Risk Category D and hence should be avoided by women who are pregnant.

Axitinib

Axitinib [Inlyta] is approved for treatment of advanced renal cell carcinoma after failure of one prior systemic therapy. Axitinib inhibits VEGF receptors, resulting in inhibition of cell proliferation, survival, and tumor growth.

Hypertension and hypertensive crises have been reported with use of axitinib. Blood pressure should be monitored closely, and dosage should be reduced if persistent hypertension occurs. As there is potential for hepatotoxicity, liver function should also be monitored periodically.

Cabozantinib

Cabozantinib [Cometriq], like pazopanib, is an oral multi–tyrosine kinase inhibitor. Cabozantinib is indicated for the treatment of metastatic medullary thyroid cancer.

Common adverse effects include diarrhea, stomatitis, nausea, and fatigue. More concerning adverse effects include posterior leukoencephalopathy syndrome. Patients present with seizures, headache, confusion, or visual disturbances. Osteonecrosis of the jaw has also been reported with cabozantinib use. If these adverse effects are present, treatment should cease. Fetal harm has been reported with cabozantinib, so it is classified in FDA Pregnancy Risk Category D and should be avoided in pregnant women. As with other kinase inhibitors, cabozantinib interacts with strong inducers and inhibitors of CYP3A4.

Regorafenib

Regorafenib [Stivarga] is a multi–tyrosine kinase inhibitor approved for the treatment of metastatic colorectal cancer previously treated with chemotherapy. Regorafenib is also indicated for the treatment of unresectable GI stromal tumor previously treated with imatinib and sunitinib.

Severe and sometimes fatal hepatotoxicity has occurred with regorafenib. Liver function tests should be monitored every 2 weeks for the first 2 months of therapy, then monthly thereafter. Severe skin reactions, including Stevens-Johnson syndrome, have been reported. As with the other kinase inhibitors, regorafenib should be avoided in combination with CYP3A4 inhibitors or inducers. Patients on warfarin should also have frequent international normalized ratio (INR) monitoring.

mTOR Kinase Inhibitors

Temsirolimus

Temsirolimus [Torisel] is indicated for IV therapy of advanced renal cell carcinoma. After conversion to its active form—sirolimus—the drug inhibits mTOR (mammalian target of rapamycin), a protein kinase that helps regulate cell growth, proliferation, and survival. Inhibition of mTOR leads to G_1 arrest and apoptosis. Adverse effects, which are common, include weakness, rash, mucositis, nausea, edema, anorexia, dyspnea, pain, and fever. Common laboratory abnormalities include anemia, neutropenia, hyperglycemia, and increases in cholesterol, triglycerides, and alkaline phosphatase. Sirolimus (the active metabolite of temsirolimus) is metabolized by CYP3A4, and hence levels of sirolimus can be altered by drugs that induce or inhibit CYP3A4.

Everolimus

Everolimus [Afinitor] has four anticancer indications: (1) advanced renal cell carcinoma after failure with sorafenib or sunitinib; (2) subependymal giant cell astrocytoma (SEGA) in patients who are not candidates for curative surgical resection; (3) advanced hormone receptor–positive, HER2-negative breast cancer in postmenopausal women; and (4) PNETs that are unresectable, locally advanced, or metastatic. As with temsirolimus, benefits derive from inhibiting mTOR kinase. In addition to its use in cancer, everolimus, sold as Zortress, is used to prevent organ rejection in transplant recipients.

Everolimus causes multiple adverse effects, including weakness, fatigue, diarrhea, nausea, cough, dyspnea, rash, and peripheral edema. Hematologic effects include reduced hemoglobin levels, reduced lymphocyte counts, and reduced platelet counts. Neutropenia predisposes to infections. Metabolic abnormalities include elevations of cholesterol, triglycerides, and glucose. About 44% of patients develop oral mucositis, stomatitis, or mouth and tongue ulcers. Everolimus is toxic to the developing fetus and so is classified in FDA Pregnancy Risk Category D.

BRAF V600E Kinase Inhibitors

Vemurafenib

Actions and Use. Vemurafenib [Zelboraf] is a kinase inhibitor indicated for patients with unresectable or metastatic *melanoma* that expresses *BRAF V600E kinase,* a variant form of BRAF kinase that is found in 30% to 60% of melanoma cells. In healthy cells, BRAF kinase (a cell-membrane protein) stimulates cell proliferation, but only when activated by specific growth factors. BRAF V600E differs from normal BRAF kinase in that BRAF V600E is highly active in the *absence* of stimulation by growth factors. As a result, cells with the BRAF V600E mutation undergo excessive proliferation and metastasis. Vemurafenib is a small molecule that inhibits BRAF V600E kinase activity and thereby suppresses tumor growth. Before vemurafenib is used, the BRAF V600E mutation must be confirmed using an FDA-approved assay, such as the *cobas 4800 BRAF V600 Mutation Test.*

Adverse Effects. Vemurafenib can cause serious adverse effects. *Cutaneous squamous cell carcinoma,* seen in 24% of patients, is of greatest concern. Other serious effects include hepatotoxicity, severe hypersensitivity reactions (e.g., anaphylaxis), severe skin reactions (e.g., Stevens-Johnson syndrome, toxic epidermal necrolysis), serious ophthalmic reactions (e.g., uveitis, iritis, retinal vein occlusion), and QT prolongation, which poses a risk for severe dysrhythmias. Less serious effects include arthralgia, hair loss, fatigue, rash, photosensitivity reactions, itching, nausea, and diarrhea. Because of its mechanism, vemurafenib is likely to cause fetal harm and hence is classified in FDA Pregnancy Risk Category D. Accordingly, women using the drug should avoid getting pregnant.

Drug Interactions. Vemurafenib is subject to multiple drug interactions, which could be hard to predict. Vemurafenib is a substrate for CYP3A4 and P-glycoprotein (a transporter that pumps drugs out of cells), and hence levels of vemurafenib can be altered by drugs that induce or inhibit these pathways. Also, vemurafenib itself is an inhibitor of P-glycoproteins as well as several CYP isoenzymes, and hence vemurafenib can increase levels of drugs that employ these pathways. Lastly, vemurafenib can induce CYP3A4 and hence can reduce levels of CYP3A4 substrates.

Dabrafenib

Dabrafenib [Tafinlar] is used as a single agent or in combination with trametinib for the treatment of unresectable metastatic *melanoma* with BRAF V600E mutation. Dabrafenib acts as a kinase inhibitor that inhibits melanoma cell growth.

In addition to fatigue, rash, diarrhea, and nausea, dabrafenib is associated with retinal vein occlusion and venous thromboembolism. Providers should assess for changes in vision. Also of concern is the potential development of new cutaneous malignancies. Dermatologic evaluations should be performed at the beginning and throughout therapy. Cardiomyopathy may also occur with dabrafenib use. Ejection fraction should be assessed before initiation as well as periodically during treatment. Dabrafenib is classified in FDA Pregnancy Risk Category D and should be avoided during pregnancy and breastfeeding. Like vemurafenib, dabrafenib metabolism is altered when combined with drugs that inhibit the cytochrome systems.

Trametinib

Trametinib [Mekinist] is an inhibitor of the MAP (mitogen-activated protein)/ERK (extracellular signal–regulated) kinases 1 and 2 (MEK1 and MEK2). Because MEK1 and MEK2 are part of the BRAF pathway, trametinib is an indirect inhibitor of the BRAF V600E kinase. Trametinib is used to treat unresectable or metastatic *melanoma* with BRAF V600E or V600K mutations.

Adverse effects are similar to those of dabrafenib, including thromboembolism, new cutaneous malignancies, and retinal vein occlusion. Increased toxicity has been reported when trametinib is used in conjunction with other kinase inhibitors and cytotoxic agents. Trametinib should not be used in pregnancy.

Crizotinib, an Anaplastic Lymphoma Kinase Inhibitor

Crizotinib [Xalkori] is indicated for advanced non–small cell lung cancer that is anaplastic lymphoma kinase (ALK) positive. Benefits derive from inhibiting ALK, a tyrosine kinase found in normal and cancerous cells. However, the form of ALK found in normal cells differs from the form found in cancer cells. Because of this difference, ALK activity in normal cells is low, whereas ALK activity in certain cancer cells is high—so high, in fact, that it drives proliferation and prolongs survival. Hence, by inhibiting ALK, crizotinib can suppress tumor growth. Because crizotinib is approved only for NSCLC that is ALK positive, the cancer must be tested for ALK before treatment. Among patients with NSCLC, about 2% to 10% have the ALK-positive type.

Crizotinib is generally well tolerated. The most common adverse effects are nausea, diarrhea, vomiting, constipation, edema, fatigue, dizziness, and neuropathies. Elevation of liver enzymes is seen in 4% to 7% of patients. Crizotinib prolongs the QT interval and hence poses a risk for serious dysrhythmias. The most serious adverse effect—potentially fatal pneumonitis—develops in 1.6% of patients. If pneumonitis is diagnosed, crizotinib should be stopped and never used again. In laboratory animals, crizotinib was fetotoxic at doses close to those used clinically. Accordingly, women using the drug should avoid pregnancy.

Crizotinib is a substrate for and inhibitor of CYP3A4. Accordingly, crizotinib levels can be increased by CYP3A4 inhibitors (e.g., ketoconazole, clarithromycin, ritonavir) and can be decreased by CYP3A4 inducers (e.g., carbamazepine, phenytoin, St. John's wort). By inhibiting CYP3A4, crizotinib can raise levels of CYP3A4 substrates, including cyclosporine, fentanyl, and alfentanil.

Other Targeted Drugs

CD20-Directed Antibodies

Antibodies directed against CD20 are used to treat B-cell non-Hodgkin lymphoma and B-cell chronic lymphocytic leukemia. CD20 is a molecule found on the cell membrane surface of B lymphocytes (B cells). When antibodies bind with CD20, they trigger an immune attack against the B cell itself. Because most other cells do not have CD20, injury is limited to normal and malignant B lymphocytes.

At this time, four products containing anti-CD20 antibodies are available. Two of these products—ibritumomab [Zevalin] and tositumomab [Bexxar]—consist of a monoclonal antibody that has been linked with a radioactive isotope. With these drugs, cell kill results largely from radiation damage, rather than from immune attack. The other two drugs—rituximab [Rituxan] and ofatumumab [Arzerra]—have no radioactivity and thus cell kill results from immune attack promoted by the antibody.

Rituximab

Actions and Use. Rituximab [Rituxan] is a monoclonal antibody indicated for IV therapy of *B-cell non-Hodgkin lymphoma* and *B-cell chronic lymphocytic leukemia.* The antibody is directed against the CD20 antigen, found on the surface of most normal and malignant B cells. Binding of rituximab recruits components of the immune system, which then cause cell lysis.

In addition to its use in cancer, rituximab is used for rheumatoid arthritis (see Chapter 57) and for two inflammatory disorders of blood vessels: microscopic polyangiitis and Wegener granulomatosis.

Adverse Effects

INFUSION REACTIONS. Rituximab can cause severe infusion-related hypersensitivity reactions. Prominent symptoms are hypotension, bronchospasm, and angioedema. Deaths have occurred. Management includes slowing or discontinuing the infusion and injecting epinephrine.

TUMOR LYSIS SYNDROME (TLS). Rapid and massive death of tumor cells can lead to TLS, characterized by acute renal failure, hyperkalemia, hypocalcemia, hyperuricemia, or hyperphosphatemia. Rarely, the syndrome proves fatal. TLS begins within 12 to 24 hours of the first rituximab infusion. The risk for TLS is increased by a high tumor burden. Management includes dialysis and correction of fluid and electrolyte abnormalities.

MUCOCUTANEOUS REACTIONS. Rituximab has been associated with severe mucocutaneous reactions, including Stevens-Johnson syndrome, lichenoid dermatitis, vesiculobullous dermatitis, and toxic epidermal necrolysis. Deaths have occurred. Reaction onset is typically 1 to 3 weeks after rituximab exposure. Patients who experience these reactions should seek immediate medical attention and should not receive rituximab again.

HEPATITIS B REACTIVATION. There have been reports of hepatitis B virus (HBV) reactivation, leading to fulminant hepatitis, hepatic failure, and death. Patients at high risk for HBV should be screened before getting rituximab. Asymptomatic carriers should be closely monitored for clinical and laboratory signs of active HBV infection while taking rituximab and for several months after stopping.

PROGRESSIVE MULTIFOCAL LEUKOENCEPHALOPATHY (PML). Rituximab has been associated with rare cases of PML, a severe infection of the central nervous system (CNS) caused by reactivation of the JC virus, an opportunistic pathogen resistant to all available drugs.

OTHER ADVERSE EFFECTS. Like other monoclonal antibodies, rituximab can cause a flu-like syndrome, especially during the initial infusion. Symptoms include fever, chills, nausea, vomiting, and myalgia. Rituximab causes transient neutropenia, but this does not appear to increase the risk for infection.

Ofatumumab

Actions and Use. Ofatumumab [Arzerra] is a monoclonal antibody directed against the CD20 antigen on B lymphocytes. The drug was approved as second-line therapy for B-cell chronic lymphocytic leukemia in patients refractory to fludarabine [Fludara] and alemtuzumab [Campath]. Like rituximab, ofatumumab binds with CD20 antigens on B cells and thereby promotes immune-mediated cell lysis. In patients refractory to fludarabine and alemtuzumab, the overall response rate to ofatumumab is 42%, with a median response duration of 6.5 months.

Adverse Effects. Ofatumumab can cause severe adverse effects. Like rituximab, the drug can cause infusion reactions, PML, and reactivation of HBV. In addition, ofatumumab can cause severe neutropenia and thrombocytopenia, increasing the risk for infections and bleeding. Intestinal obstruction may also occur. Common, but less serious effects include fever, cough, dyspnea, diarrhea, fatigue, rash, and nausea.

Zevalin (Ibritumomab Tiuxetan Linked With Yttrium-90)

Description, Actions, and Use. Ibritumomab tiuxetan (IT), marketed as Zevalin, is a compound molecule composed of ibritumomab (a monoclonal antibody) that has been covalently bound with tiuxetan. Like rituximab, IT binds selectively with the CD20 antigen present on most normal and malignant B cells. However, unlike rituximab, which is used by itself to treat cancer, IT is first linked with yttrium-90 (Y90), a beta particle–emitting radioisotope. When the IT-Y90 complex binds with cellular CD20 antigens, cell kill results from radiation-induced injury, rather than from injury caused by ibritumomab itself. Because beta particles have a relatively short path length (about 5 mm), injury is restricted to CD20-containing cells and to neighboring cells within a 5-mm radius. The radioactive drug poses no danger to persons in proximity. IT-Y90 was the first anticancer treatment to employ an antibody complexed with a radioactive compound. IT-Y90 was originally approved for low-grade, B-cell non-Hodgkin lymphoma and then later was approved for follicular non-Hodgkin lymphoma.

Before patients receive IT-Y90, they are given two small doses of rituximab, 7 to 9 days apart. The contribution of rituximab is twofold. First, it binds with circulating B cells and thereby greatly reduces their numbers. Second, it occupies nonspecific binding sites that could otherwise attract IT-Y90 and hence would reduce the amount of IT-Y90 available to bind with target cells. For the purpose of diagnostic imaging, the first dose of rituximab is accompanied by a small dose of IT that has been linked to radioactive indium-111.

Adverse Effects. Adverse effects of treatment are due to IT-Y90 itself and to the rituximab given before it. As noted above, rituximab can cause severe infusion reactions. With IT-Y90, hematologic toxicity is the major concern: severe, prolonged cytopenias develop in more than 50% of patients. Counts of neutrophils and platelets reach their nadir 7 to 9 weeks after treatment and take 3 to 7 weeks to recover. Infection risk is high. Deaths have occurred. Because of its hematologic toxicity, IT-Y90 is contraindicated for patients with (1) lymphoma bone marrow involvement of 25% or more or (2) limited bone marrow reserve (e.g., platelet count below 100,000/mm^3 or neutrophil count below 1500/mm^3; history of prior myeloablative therapy).

Bexxar (Tositumomab Linked With ^{131}I-Tositumomab)

Description, Actions, and Use. Bexxar is the trade name for a regimen that consists of (1) tositumomab, a monoclonal antibody, and (2) ^{131}I-tositumomab, tositumomab covalently linked with radioactive iodine-131. This regimen, which was the second to employ a radiolabeled antibody, is very similar in mechanism and uses to the Zevalin regimen (ibritumomab tiuxetan/yttrium-90), the first to employ a radiolabeled antibody.

Bexxar kills cancer cells through a combination of immune activation and radiation damage. Like ibritumomab and rituximab, tositumomab binds selectively with the CD20 antigen found on the surface of most normal and malignant B cells. This binding stimulates an immune attack on the cell, with three possible results: complement-dependent cytotoxicity, antibody-dependent cytotoxicity, and induction of apoptosis (programmed cell death). Cell death also results when ^{131}I-tositumomab binds with the CD20 antigen, thereby exposing target cells to a high dose of ionizing radiation.

Treatment is performed in two steps, called the dosimetric step and the therapeutic step. The dosimetric step is conducted to determine, for each patient, the specific dose of radiation to be given in the therapeutic step.

Bexxar is approved for CD20-positive follicular B-cell non-Hodgkin lymphoma, a form of low-grade B-cell non-Hodgkin lymphoma. However, the drug should be used only if the cancer (1) is refractory to rituximab and (2) has relapsed after chemotherapy.

Adverse Effects. Like Zevalin, Bexxar can cause severe, prolonged cytopenias. Neutropenia and thrombocytopenia are most common, often leading to infections and hemorrhage. Management may require infusion of blood products (platelets and red blood cells [RBCs]) as well as treatment with a hematologic growth factor (epoetin alfa, granulocyte colony-stimulating factor). To monitor hematologic status, complete blood counts should be obtained at baseline and then weekly for 10 to 12 weeks. Like Zevalin, Bexxar is contraindicated for patients with lymphoma bone marrow involvement of 25% or more and for those with limited bone marrow reserve.

Hypersensitivity reactions, including anaphylaxis, occur in 6% of patients. Medication for treating severe reactions (epinephrine, antihistamines, glucocorticoids) should be immediately available.

Many patients experience infusional toxicity, either during the infusion or within 48 hours after. Symptoms include fever, rigors, chills, sweating, hypotension, dyspnea, nausea, and bronchospasm. Pretreatment with acetaminophen or diphenhydramine may help.

The radioactive iodine in ^{131}I-tositumomab can damage the thyroid gland, causing hypothyroidism. To protect the thyroid, patients should take oral potassium iodide (tablets or solution), starting at least 24 hours before the dosimetric dose and continuing for 2 weeks after the therapeutic dose.

Gastrointestinal toxicity is seen in 38% of patients. Symptoms include nausea, vomiting, abdominal pain, and diarrhea.

Secondary malignancies—myelodysplastic syndrome (MDS) and/or acute leukemia—occur in 2% to 3% of patients, usually within 3 years of treatment.

Use in Pregnancy and Lactation. Radioactive iodine can harm the developing thyroid gland. Irreversible hypothyroidism may result. Accordingly, Bexxar is classified in FDA Pregnancy Risk Category D and hence should not be used during pregnancy. Radioiodine and (probably) tositumomab are excreted in breast milk, posing a risk to the breastfed infant. Mothers should be warned not to breastfeed while receiving Bexxar.

Elimination of Iodine-131. Elimination of iodine-131 occurs by radioactive decay and excretion in the urine. About 67% is cleared by 5 days after the infusion. Of the amount not eliminated through radioactive decay, 98% is eliminated in the urine.

For several days after treatment, persons in close proximity to the patient receiving Bexxar could be harmed by radiation from iodine-131. Therefore, before discharge, the patient should be given oral and written instruction on how to minimize exposure of family, friends, and the general public. Specific measures include staying at least 9 feet away from others, sleeping alone, maintaining sole bathroom use (owing to urinary radiation excretion), avoiding contact with children and pregnant women, refraining from travel by plane or mass transit, and avoiding prolonged car travel with other people.

Brentuximab Vedotin, an Antibody-Drug Conjugate

Brentuximab vedotin [Adcetris] is an antibody-drug conjugate (ADC), composed of brentuximab coupled with monomethyl auristatin E (MMAE). Brentuximab is a monoclonal antibody that selectively binds with CD30, an antigen expressed on the surface of certain cancer cells. MMAE is a toxic compound that binds with intracellular tubulin. Cell kill results as follows: after binding with CD30 on the cell surface, the entire ADC is rapidly internalized and then cleaved to release free MMAE, which then binds with tubulin to cause mitotic arrest.

Brentuximab vedotin has two indications: *Hodgkin lymphoma* after failure of autologous stem cell transplantation or after failure of at least two multidrug chemotherapy regimens and (2) systemic *anaplastic large cell lymphoma* after failure of at least one multidrug chemotherapy regimen. In clinical trials, the drug demonstrated response rates that were higher than those produced with any available chemotherapy regimen.

Adverse effects are generally "manageable." The most common are peripheral sensory neuropathy, neutropenia, anemia, fatigue, nausea, diarrhea, and fever. Of these, neuropathy and neutropenia are the greatest concerns. If neuropathy or neutropenia develops, dosage should be reduced or the dosing interval increased.

In laboratory animals, low-dose brentuximab vedotin was teratogenic and fetotoxic. Accordingly, the drug should be avoided in women who are pregnant (FDA Pregnancy Risk Category D).

Angiogenesis Inhibitors

Angiogenesis inhibitors suppress formation of new blood vessels and thereby deprive solid tumors of the expanding blood supply they need for continued growth. It is important to note, however, that although tumor growth is suppressed, angiogenesis inhibitors, by themselves, cannot kill tumor cells that already exist. At this time, only one angiogenesis inhibitor—bevacizumab—is approved for treating cancer.

Bevacizumab

Bevacizumab [Avastin] became the first angiogenesis inhibitor approved for clinical use. In patients with metastatic colorectal cancer or nonsquamous NSCLC, the drug can delay tumor progression and prolong life. Unfortunately, bevacizumab can also cause life-threatening side effects, including GI perforation, hemorrhage, and thromboembolism.

Mechanism of Action. Bevacizumab is a monoclonal antibody that binds with VEGF, an endogenous compound that stimulates blood vessel growth. Binding with bevacizumab prevents VEGF from binding with its receptors on vascular endothelial cells, preventing VEGF from promoting new vessel formation. As a result, further tumor growth is suppressed.

Therapeutic Use. Bevacizumab has four approved uses:

- Metastatic *cancer of the colon or rectum,* in combination with a regimen based on IV 5-fluorouracil (5-FU)
- *Nonsquamous non–small cell lung cancer,* in combination with carboplatin and paclitaxel
- Metastatic *renal cell carcinoma,* in combination with interferon alfa
- *Glioblastoma,* as a single agent after prior therapy

In addition to its use in cancer, bevacizumab is used off-label to treat the neovascular form of *age-related macular degeneration* (see Chapter 84).

Pharmacokinetics. The pharmacokinetics of bevacizumab are poorly understood. We do know that the drug has an average half-life of 20 days and that clearance occurs faster in males and in patients with a high tumor burden. However, there is no evidence that faster clearance reduces the clinical response. How clearance occurs is unknown.

Adverse Effects. The most serious adverse effects are GI perforation, hemorrhage, thromboembolism, nephrotic syndrome, disruption of wound healing, and hypertensive crisis. Less serious effects include diarrhea, rhinitis, proteinuria, taste alteration, dry skin, headache, and back pain.

Some cases of GI perforation have been fatal. Primary symptoms are abdominal pain in association with constipation and vomiting. If GI perforation occurs, bevacizumab should be stopped and never used again.

Bevacizumab greatly increases the risk for *severe or fatal hemorrhage.* Patients have experienced GI bleeding, intracranial bleeding, vaginal bleeding, and nosebleeds. In addition, patients with NSCLC have experienced life-threatening *pulmonary hemorrhage.* The risk for a life-threatening or fatal lung bleed is very high (31%) in patients with squamous cell histology and much lower (4%) in those with non–squamous cell histology. Onset of pulmonary bleeding is sudden and presents as major or massive hemoptysis (expectoration of blood). Bevacizumab should be avoided in patients with recent hemoptysis or serious hemorrhage.

When added to a regimen based on 5-FU, bevacizumab doubles the risk for *arterial thromboembolic events,* including ischemic stroke, myocardial infarction, and transient ischemic attacks. Deaths have occurred. Patients who experience a thromboembolic event should stop bevacizumab and never use it again.

Bevacizumab *impairs wound healing* and can induce wound dehiscence (splitting open). Because of these effects, if bevacizumab is initiated too soon after surgery, or if it is not discontinued soon enough before surgery, impaired wound healing can result. To minimize healing complications, guidelines suggest waiting at least 28 days after surgery before using the drug and stopping the drug at least 28 days before elective surgery.

Bevacizumab can cause *severe hypertension* that may persist for months after the drug is withdrawn. Some patients have experienced hypertensive encephalopathy and subarachnoid hemorrhage. Blood pressure should be monitored in all patients. If severe hypertension develops, bevacizumab should be permanently discontinued.

Nephrotic syndrome may develop. Patients should be monitored for development or worsening of proteinuria, a sign of kidney injury. If moderate to severe proteinuria occurs, bevacizumab should be withdrawn.

Effect in Pregnancy. Angiogenesis is critical to fetal development, and hence angiogenesis inhibition is likely to cause fetal harm. Although human data are lacking, animal studies indicate that bevacizumab decreases fetal weight, increases fetal resorption, and can promote gross malformations. Currently, bevacizumab is classified in FDA Pregnancy Risk Category C and should be used only if the benefits to the mother are judged to outweigh the risks to the fetus.

Proteasome Inhibitors

Proteasomes are intracellular multienzyme complexes that degrade proteins. Their physiologic role is to rid cells of proteins that are not needed, including proteins that regulate transcription, cell adhesion, apoptosis, and progression through the cell cycle. Proteasome inhibitors can cause these proteins to accumulate and can thereby disrupt various aspects of cell physiology. In cancer cells, these drugs appear to promote accumulation of proteins that promote apoptosis (programmed cell death). Why this effect is limited largely to cancer cells is not clear but may be related to inhibition of NF-kappa B, a transcription factor critical to the growth of several types of cancer, including multiple myeloma.

Bortezomib

Actions. Bortezomib [Velcade] is the first proteasome inhibitor available for general use. The drug inhibits a specific proteasome, known as the 26S proteasome, and thereby alters the concentration of proteins that regulate cell growth and division. The result is reduced cell viability, increased apoptosis, and increased sensitivity to the lethal effects of radiation and cytotoxic anticancer drugs. Does bortezomib hurt normal cells too? Yes. However, in vitro studies suggest that normal cells are less vulnerable than cancer cells.

Therapeutic Use. Bortezomib is approved for (1) multiple myeloma, both as first-line therapy and for patients who have not responded adequately to other therapies (e.g., thalidomide, autologous stem cell transplantation); and (2) mantle cell lymphoma in patients with at least 1 prior year of therapy.

Adverse Effects. Adverse effects are common and often serious. The most frequent reactions are weakness, nausea, and diarrhea. Also common are hematologic effects—thrombocytopenia, anemia, and neutropenia—as well as constipation, anorexia, peripheral neuropathy, fever, and postural hypotension. Bortezomib is fetotoxic in rabbits and has been classified in FDA Pregnancy Risk Category D. Accordingly, pregnancy should be avoided.

Drug Interactions. St. John's wort may decrease levels of bortezomib, so this combination should be avoided. Both hypoglycemia and hyperglycemia were reported in patients taking oral antidiabetic agents in conjunction with bortezomib. Blood glucose levels should be monitored closely. Bortezomib is metabolized in the liver by CYP isoenzymes. Accordingly, inhibitors or inducers of these isoenzymes might be expected to alter bortezomib levels.

Carfilzomib

Carfilzomib [Kyprolis] works similarly to bortezomib by binding to the active sites of the core particle within the 26S proteasome. It is approved for treatment of patients with multiple myeloma who have received at least two prior therapies.

A serious adverse effect of carfilzomib is cardiac arrest. This can occur within 1 day of administration. Cardiac function should be monitored closely during treatment with carfilzomib. Other infusion reactions have also occurred, including shortness of breath, chest tightness, fever, and chills. Dexamethasone can be administered before treatment in an attempt to reduce infusion-associated incidences. Like bortezomib, carfilzomib should be avoided in pregnancy. There are no reported drug interactions known at this time.

Carfilzomib is initially administered intravenously at a dose of 20 mg/m^2 over 2 to 10 minutes on 2 consecutive days. If this dose is tolerated, subsequent doses may be increased to 27 mg/m^2. These doses are administered weekly for 3 weeks on days 1, 2, 8, 9, 15, and 16. These doses are followed by a 12-day rest period (days 17–28). Each 28-day period is considered one cycle of treatment.

Histone Deacetylase Inhibitors

The histone deacetylase (HDAC) inhibitors are a relatively new class of targeted anticancer drugs. Vorinostat and romidepsin were the first approved drugs in this class. Both drugs are indicated only for cutaneous T-cell lymphoma (CTCL), a rare form of cancer with only 1500 new cases a year in the United States. As their name implies, these drugs inhibit HDAC and thereby increase the acetylation of histones, regulatory proteins in the cell nucleus that help control DNA transcription. When histones are in their acetylated state, they turn on gene transcription. In tumor cells, increased transcription leads to cell-cycle arrest and apoptosis.

Vorinostat

Vorinostat [Zolinza], the first HDAC inhibitor available, is indicated for oral therapy of CTCL that has progressed or returned after treatment with two systemic therapies. Unfortunately, benefits of vorinostat are modest. The most common adverse effects are fatigue, diarrhea, nausea, altered taste, anorexia, weight loss, thrombocytopenia, and anemia. Pulmonary embolism is the most common serious effect. When used with warfarin, prolonged levels of prothrombin time and INR have been noted. These levels should be monitored closely. Severe thrombocytopenia has also occurred when vorinostat is combined with valproic acid. Platelet levels should be checked every 2 weeks for the first 2 months.

Romidepsin

Romidepsin [Istodax] is indicated for intravenous therapy of CTCL and peripheral T-cell lymphoma that has progressed or returned despite treatment with at least one systemic agent. As with vorinostat, benefits are modest.

Romidepsin can cause multiple adverse effects. The most common are nausea, vomiting, fatigue, anorexia, taste disturbance, and hematologic deficits: anemia, leukopenia, and thrombocytopenia. Because of leukopenia, patients are at increased risk for serious infections. Primary cardiac effects are electrocardiographic T-wave changes and QT prolongation. Romidepsin can harm the developing fetus and hence should not be used during pregnancy. In contrast to vorinostat, romidepsin has not been associated with pulmonary embolism.

Romidepsin undergoes extensive metabolism by CYP3A4, and hence strong inhibitors (e.g., clarithromycin) and inducers (e.g., carbamazepine) should be avoided. Romidepsin binds with receptors for estrogen and can thereby reduce the effects of estrogen-containing contraceptives.

Ipilimumab

Ipilimumab [Yervoy] is indicated for unresectable or metastatic melanoma. Benefits derive from unleashing an immune attack on cancer cells. Here's how it works. Ipilimumab is a monoclonal antibody directed against cytotoxic T-lymphocyte–associated antigen 4 (CTLA-4), a regulatory molecule that puts a brake on T-cell function. When ipilimumab binds with CTLA-4, it releases the brake, thereby allowing T cells to attack and kill cancer cells.

By promoting T-cell activation and proliferation, ipilimumab can cause severe or fatal immune-mediated effects. Among these are enterocolitis, hepatitis, dermatitis (including toxic epidermal necrolysis), neuropathies (both motor and sensory), and endocrinopathies (e.g., hypopituitarism, hypothyroidism, adrenal insufficiency). Patients should be closely monitored for signs and symptoms. If a severe immune-mediated reaction is diagnosed, ipilimumab should be immediately and permanently discontinued, and patients should be treated with high-dose systemic glucocorticoids.

IMMUNOSTIMULANTS

As their name implies, the immunostimulants enhance the body's immune attack on cancer cells. In the following discussion, we focus on three agents: interferon alfa-2b, aldesleukin, and BCG vaccine. Indications and routes are shown in Table 82.8.

Interferon Alfa-2b

Interferons are naturally occurring proteins with complex antiviral, anticancer, and immunomodulatory actions. Release of endogenous interferons is triggered by viral infections and other stimuli. Interferons are active against a variety of solid tumors and hematologic malignancies.

Discussion here is limited to two interferons: interferon alfa-2b [Intron A] and peginterferon alfa-2b [Sylatron]. (Peginterferon alfa-2b is simply a long-acting form of interferon alfa-2b produced by a process known as pegylation, in which a polymer of polyethylene glycol [PEG] is attached to native interferon alfa-2b.) Although the active component of interferon alfa-2b and peginterferon alfa-2b is the same, these preparations have different indications. Specifically, interferon alfa-2b is approved for melanoma, hairy cell leukemia, chronic myelogenous leukemia, follicular lymphoma, and AIDS-related Kaposi sarcoma, whereas peginterferon alfa-2b is approved only for melanoma.

Anticancer effects of interferon alfa-2b are thought to result from two basic processes: (1) enhancement of host immune responses and (2) direct antiproliferative effects on cancer cells. Both processes are mediated by binding of interferon alfa-2b to cell-surface receptors, with resultant increased expression of certain genes and reduced expression of others. Interferon alfa-2b can cause G_0 cells to remain dormant, preventing proliferation. In addition, it can cause proliferating cells to differentiate into nonproliferative mature forms.

Interferon alfa can cause multiple adverse effects. The most common is a flu-like syndrome characterized by fever, fatigue, myalgia, headache, and chills. Symptoms tend to diminish with continued therapy. Some symptoms (fever, headache, myalgia) can be reduced with acetaminophen. Other common effects include anorexia, weight loss, diarrhea, abdominal pain, dizziness, and cough. Prolonged or high-dose therapy can cause fatigue, cardiotoxicity, thyroid dysfunction, and bone marrow suppression, manifesting as neutropenia and thrombocytopenia. Neuropsychiatric effects—especially depression—are a serious concern, owing to a risk for death by suicide.

The pharmacology of interferon alfa-2b and peginterferon alfa-2b is discussed in Chapter 78.

Aldesleukin (Interleukin-2)

Aldesleukin [Proleukin], also known as interleukin-2 (IL-2), is an immunostimulant indicated for advanced renal carcinoma and melanoma. Because severe adverse effects occur often, the drug must be administered in a hospital that has an intensive care facility; a specialist in cardiopulmonary or intensive care medicine must be available.

Description and Actions

Aldesleukin is a large glycoprotein nearly identical in structure and actions to human IL-2. The drug is produced by recombinant DNA technology. Like IL-2, aldesleukin stimulates immune function. Specific responses include enhanced production and cytotoxicity of lymphocytes; increased production of IL-1, interferon gamma, and tumor necrosis factor; and induction of lymphokine-activated killer cell activity. These powerful immunostimulant actions are believed to underlie antitumor effects.

Therapeutic Use

Aldesleukin has two approved uses: metastatic renal cell carcinoma and metastatic melanoma. Among patients with renal cell cancer, 4% respond completely and 11% respond partially. The median response duration is 2 years.

Pharmacokinetics

Aldesleukin is administered by IV infusion and distributes throughout the extracellular space. About 70% of each dose undergoes preferential uptake by the liver, kidneys, and lungs. Renal enzymes convert the drug into inactive metabolites, which are excreted in the urine. The drug's half-life is short—just 85 minutes.

Adverse Effects

Practically all patients experience significant toxicity. The fatality rate is high (4%). Effects seen most frequently are fever and chills, nausea and vomiting, hypotension, anemia, diarrhea, altered mental status, sinus tachycardia, impaired renal function, impaired liver function, pulmonary congestion, dyspnea, and pruritus. Depression may also occur.

Capillary leak syndrome (CLS) is of particular concern. This potentially fatal reaction is characterized by hypotension and reduced organ perfusion (secondary to loss of vascular tone and extravasation of plasma proteins and fluid). Symptoms begin to develop immediately after treatment. CLS may be associated with angina pectoris, cardiac dysrhythmias, myocardial infarction, pronounced respiratory insufficiency, renal insufficiency, GI bleeding, and altered mental status. Because of the risk for CLS, aldesleukin must not be given to patients with cardiac, pulmonary, renal, hepatic, or CNS impairment. Careful monitoring is essential.

BCG Vaccine

Description and Therapeutic Use

BCG vaccine [TheraCys, TICE BCG] is a freeze-dried preparation of live, attenuated *Mycobacterium bovis* (bacillus of Calmette and Guérin [BCG]). The vaccine is approved for primary and relapsed carcinoma in situ of the bladder, in both the presence and absence of associated papillary tumors. To treat bladder cancers, BCG vaccine is administered intravesically (i.e., directly into the bladder through a urethral catheter). In addition to its use in cancer therapy, BCG vaccine is used to protect against tuberculosis (see Chapter 75).

Mechanism of Action

BCG vaccine is a nonspecific immunostimulant. Instillation in the bladder produces a local inflammatory response that, by an unknown mechanism, promotes regression of tumors in the urothelial lining.

Adverse Effects

The most common adverse effects, which result from bladder irritation, are dysuria, urinary frequency, urinary urgency, and hematuria. Urinary status

TABLE 82.8 ▪ Immunostimulants

Generic Name	Trade Name	Route	Indications
Interferon alfa-2b	Intron A	SubQ, IM, IV	Melanoma, hairy cell leukemia, chronic myelogenous leukemia, follicular lymphoma, AIDS-related Kaposi's sarcoma
Peginterferon alfa-2b	Sylatron*	SubQ	Melanoma
Aldesleukin (interleukin-2)	Proleukin	IV	Metastatic renal cell cancer, metastatic melanoma
BCG vaccine	TheraCys, TICE BCG	Intravesical	*In situ* bladder cancer

*Peginterferon alfa-2b is also marketed as *PegIntron* for treatment of hepatitis.
BCG, bacillus of Calmette and Guérin; IM, intramuscular; IV, intravenous; subQ, subcutaneous.

should be monitored closely. The most common systemic reactions are malaise, fatigue, fever, and chills.

Because BCG vaccine consists of live *M. bovis*, therapy carries a risk for systemic infection, including fatal septic shock. Accordingly, the vaccine is contraindicated for (1) immunocompromised patients (e.g., those taking immunosuppressant drugs, those with symptomatic or asymptomatic HIV infection); (2) patients with fever of unknown origin (because it may signify infection); and (3) patients with urinary tract infections (because there is an increased risk for systemic absorption of BCG vaccine).

Because BCG vaccine is infectious, it must be handled using aseptic technique. All materials employed during administration should be disposed of in plastic bags labeled "Infectious Waste." Urine voided within 6 hours of BCG instillation should be disinfected with an equal volume of 5% hypochlorite before flushing.

OTHER NONCYTOTOXIC ANTICANCER DRUGS

Glucocorticoids

The basic pharmacology of the glucocorticoids is discussed in Chapter 56. Discussion here is limited to their use in cancer. To benefit patients with cancer, dosages must be high, and hence, with long-term use, adverse effects are a concern.

Glucocorticoids (e.g., prednisone, dexamethasone) are used in combination with other agents to treat cancers arising from lymphoid tissue. Specific indications are *acute and chronic lymphocytic leukemias, Hodgkin disease, non-Hodgkin lymphomas,* and *multiple myeloma.* Glucocorticoids are beneficial in these cancers because they are directly toxic to lymphoid tissues: high-dose therapy causes suppression of mitosis, dissolution of lymphocytes, regression of lymphatic tissue, and cell death. When glucocorticoids are used acutely, toxicity is limited and manageable. However, with prolonged treatment, multiple serious toxicities can occur, including osteoporosis, adrenal insufficiency, increased susceptibility to infection, GI ulcers, fluid and electrolyte disturbances, myopathy, growth delay in children, cutaneous atrophy, and diabetes. Unlike the short-term toxicities, these long-term toxicities are hard to manage.

In addition to their use against lymphoid-derived cancers, glucocorticoids are used to manage complications of cancer and cancer therapy. Specific benefits include suppression of chemotherapy-induced nausea and vomiting, reduction of cerebral edema (caused by brain metastasis and irradiation to the brain), reduction of pain (caused by nerve compression or edema), and suppression of hypercalcemia in patients with steroid-responsive tumors. In addition, glucocorticoids can improve appetite and promote weight gain.

Retinoids

Retinoids are derivatives of retinol (vitamin A) that bind to and activate retinoid receptors. In their active state, retinoid receptors regulate the proliferation and differentiation of cells, both normal and neoplastic. In patients with cancer, retinoids inhibit cancer cell growth.

Alitretinoin

Alitretinoin [Panretin], an analog of retinol, is indicated for topical therapy of cutaneous lesions in patients with AIDS-related Kaposi sarcoma. When alitretinoin is added to Kaposi sarcoma cells in culture, it inhibits their growth.

The drug should be applied only to cutaneous Kaposi sarcoma lesions, not to normal skin. After application, the area should be allowed to dry for 3 to 5 minutes before putting clothing over it. Occlusive dressings should be avoided.

Adverse effects are limited to the site of application. Local reactions—erythema, scaling, irritation, rash, and dermatitis—occur in 25% to 77% of patients. The incidence of severe reactions is 10%. Other retinoids are known to cause photosensitivity reactions. Although photosensitivity has not been reported with alitretinoin, exposing the treated area to sunlight or sunlamps should nonetheless be minimized. Retinoids are highly teratogenic. Accordingly, women using alitretinoin should avoid getting pregnant (even though systemic absorption of alitretinoin appears to be minimal).

Bexarotene

Mechanism and Use

Bexarotene [Targretin] is indicated for oral therapy of cutaneous T-cell lymphoma in patients who have been refractory to prior systemic therapy. Like alitretinoin, bexarotene is an analog of vitamin A (retinol) and can activate retinoid receptors. The result is altered regulation of cellular proliferation and differentiation. In vitro, bexarotene can inhibit growth of some tumor cell lines.

Pharmacokinetics

Plasma levels peak 2 hours after oral administration. Taking the drug with a high-fat meal increases absorption. Bexarotene undergoes metabolism by CYP3A4 followed by excretion in the bile.

Adverse Effects and Interactions

Major lipid abnormalities are common. Plasma triglycerides rise to a level 2.5 times above the upper limit of the normal range in 70% of patients. Sixty percent of patients have significant elevations in total cholesterol and low-density lipoprotein cholesterol. Levels of high-density lipoprotein cholesterol (good cholesterol) are reduced.

Bexarotene frequently causes headache, asthenia, leukopenia, anemia, infection, rash, and photosensitivity. The incidence of clinically significant hypothyroidism is 30%. Fatal pancreatitis and fatal cholestasis have been reported.

Bexarotene and other retinoids are powerful teratogens. Accordingly, bexarotene is absolutely contraindicated for use during pregnancy. Women taking the drug must ensure that pregnancy does not occur.

In theory, drugs that inhibit CYP3A4 can increase bexarotene levels, and drugs that induce CYP3A4 can reduce its levels. Combining vitamin A with bexarotene could result in increased toxicity.

Tretinoin

Tretinoin [Vesanoid], also known as all-trans retinoic acid (ATRA), is approved for induction of remission in patients with acute promyelocytic leukemia (APL). Rates of complete remission are high. Unfortunately, although tretinoin can be very effective, it can also cause severe toxicity, and hence the benefits of treatment must be carefully weighed against the risks. The mechanism underlying beneficial effects is not well established.

The most common adverse effects are rash, dry skin, and CNS toxicity, manifesting as headache, depression, confusion, and anxiety. The most serious effect, seen in 25% of patients, is retinoic acid–APL syndrome, characterized by fever, pleural and pericardial effusions, and hypoxia. In its most severe form, the syndrome can lead to respiratory failure and death. Milder reactions generally respond to high-dose IV glucocorticoids, without interruption of tretinoin. In severe cases, tretinoin should be withdrawn.

Tretinoin is a substrate for hepatic CYP enzymes, and hence CYP inducers (e.g., rifampin, phenytoin, St. John's wort) and inhibitors (e.g., erythromycin, azole antifungals, diltiazem) should be avoided.

The use of tretinoin for dermatologic disorders is discussed in Chapter 85.

Arsenic Trioxide

Arsenic trioxide [Trisenox] is approved for APL, a rare subtype of acute myelogenous leukemia in which myeloid cells are blocked from undergoing normal differentiation and apoptosis. In patients who have relapsed after standard therapy for APL, arsenic trioxide has produced a high rate of complete remission. The drug appears to work by reversing the blockade on myeloid differentiation and apoptosis and by inhibiting angiogenesis.

Toxicity occurs in most patients. Common side effects include nausea, vomiting, diarrhea, fatigue, edema, hyperglycemia, dyspnea, cough, rash, headache, and dizziness. Leukocytosis (elevation of white blood cell counts) occurs in 50% of patients. Of greater concern, about 23% experience a potentially fatal condition known as APL differentiation syndrome, characterized by fever, weight gain, pulmonary infiltrates, dyspnea, musculoskeletal pain, and pleural and pericardial effusions. Symptoms can be reduced by immediate therapy with high-dose glucocorticoids. Prolongation of the QT interval is common and can lead to life-threatening dysrhythmias. An electrocardiogram should be obtained before treatment and at least weekly thereafter. If possible, drugs known to cause QT prolongation should be withdrawn. Among these are class I and class III antidysrhythmics, clarithromycin, daunorubicin, mesoridazine, and thioridazine. Arsenic trioxide has the potential to cause fetal harm and hence is classified in FDA Pregnancy Risk Category D. In contrast to cytotoxic anticancer drugs, arsenic trioxide does not cause alopecia or mucositis.

Denileukin Diftitox

Therapeutic Use

Denileukin diftitox [Ontak] is an IV drug approved for cutaneous T-cell lymphoma. Unfortunately, adverse events are very common and sometimes severe. Denileukin can cause life-threatening hypersensitivity reactions and hence must be administered in a facility equipped for cardiopulmonary resuscitation.

Description and Mechanism of Action

Denileukin is a hybrid molecule consisting of IL-2 coupled to diphtheria toxin. The IL-2 portion of the molecule enables it to bind with CTCL cells that have IL-2 receptors. After the drug is bound, the diphtheria toxin moiety inhibits protein synthesis, causing cell death within hours. Denileukin is produced by recombinant DNA technology.

Adverse Effects

Acute hypersensitivity reactions occur in 69% of patients. Prominent symptoms are hypotension, back pain, dyspnea, vasodilation, rash, chest pain, and tachycardia. Management consists of stopping the infusion and, if necessary, administering IV epinephrine, antihistamines, and glucocorticoids.

Denileukin can cause potentially fatal capillary leak syndrome, characterized by hypoalbuminemia, edema, and hypotension. Onset usually occurs during the first or second week of treatment. Because of vascular leak, hypoalbuminemia occurs in 83% of patients. Serum albumin should be monitored, and, if it falls below 3 g/dL, the next round of treatment should be postponed.

A flu-like syndrome occurs in 91% of patients. Symptoms include fever or chills, asthenia, nausea and vomiting, myalgia, and arthralgia. Diarrhea occurs in 29% of patients and leads to dehydration in 9%.

Denileukin can cause eye damage, manifesting as a decrease in color vision and vision acuity. For a few patients, these effects are irreversible. However, most report persistent impairment.

Thalidomide

Thalidomide [Thalomid] is a drug with complex pharmacologic actions, including the ability to cause severe birth defects. In the United States thalidomide has two approved indications: (1) erythema nodosum leprosum, a complication of leprosy; and (2) multiple myeloma, a cancer of the bone marrow. Promising results have also been seen with other cancers, including plasma cell leukemia and various solid tumors, including renal cell carcinoma, AIDS-related Kaposi sarcoma, and cancers of the brain, breast, ovary, prostate, and colon. Anticancer effects are thought to derive from (1) effects on the immune system and (2) inhibition of angiogenesis. Compared with cytotoxic anticancer drugs, thalidomide is relatively well tolerated but can cause clinically important neuropathy, sedation, and constipation. Neuropathy can be a chronic dose-limiting toxicity. Because thalidomide is a powerful teratogen, patients must comply with a strict set of FDA-mandated safeguards, known as the System for Thalidomide Education and Prescribing Safety, or S.T.E.P.S.

Lenalidomide

Lenalidomide [Revlimid], an analog of thalidomide, is indicated for (1) multiple myeloma, (2) relapsed mantle cell lymphoma after two prior therapies, and (3) raising red blood cell (RBC) counts in patients with transfusion-dependent anemia due to myelodysplastic syndrome—but only if their MDS is associated with a specific cytogenetic abnormality known as a 5q deletion, which is seen in up to 30% of MDS patients. In these patients, lenalidomide increases RBC production and greatly reduces the need for RBC transfusions. The mechanism underlying benefits in multiple myeloma and MDS is unclear.

Lenalidomide has serious toxicities, including thrombocytopenia and neutropenia. In patients with multiple myeloma, the drug has caused deep vein thrombosis and pulmonary embolism. Like thalidomide, lenalidomide is teratogenic in primates and thus must not be used during pregnancy. To reduce risk, the drug is available only through a restricted distribution program, known as RevAssist, similar to the S.T.E.P.S. program used for thalidomide.

Progestins

Two progestins can be employed to treat cancer: medroxyprogesterone acetate [Depo-Provera] and megestrol acetate [Megace]. Medroxyprogesterone is indicated for advanced endometrial and renal cancer. Megestrol is indicated for advanced endometrial and breast cancer. In women with metastatic endometrial cancer, progestins promote palliation and tumor regression. About 30% of patients have an objective response. Among those who respond, survival time is increased to about 2 years. This compares with survival times of 6 months among nonresponders. Benefits appear to derive from depriving these cancers of estrogen by inducing enzymes that metabolize estradiol, the primary endogenous estrogen. The principal adverse effects of progestins are fluid retention and nonfluid weight gain. Hypercalcemia may occur if bone metastases are present. Progestins may be teratogens and hence should be avoided during pregnancy. The basic pharmacology of the progestins is discussed in Chapter 48.

CHAPTER

83 Pain Management in Patients With Cancer

Laura D. Rosenthal, DNP, ACNP, FAANP

Our topic—management of cancer pain—is of note both for its good news and its bad news. The good news is that cancer pain can be relieved with simple interventions in 90% of patients. The bad news is that, despite the availability of effective treatments, pain goes unrelieved far too often. Multiple factors contribute to undertreatment (Box 83.1). Important among these are inadequate prescriber training in pain management; unfounded fears of addiction (shared by prescribers, patients, and families); and a health care system that focuses more on treating disease than relieving suffering.

Pain has a profound effect on both the patient and family. Pain undermines quality of life for the patient and puts a heavy burden on the family. Unrelieved pain compromises the patient's ability to work, enjoy leisure activities, and fulfill his or her role in the family and in society at large. Furthermore, pain can impede recovery, hasten death from cancer, and possibly even create a risk for suicide.

Every patient has the right to expect that pain management will be an integral part of treatment throughout the course of his or her disease. The goal is to minimize pain and thereby maintain a reasonable quality of life, including the ability to function at work and at play and within the family and society. In addition, if the cancer is incurable, treatment should permit the patient a relatively painless death when that time comes.

PATHOPHYSIOLOGY OF PAIN

What Is Pain?

The International Association for the Study of Pain defines pain as "an unpleasant sensory and emotional experience associated with actual or potential tissue damage, or described in terms of such damage." Note that, by this definition, pain is not simply a sensory experience resulting from activation of pain receptors. Rather, it also includes the patient's emotional and cognitive responses to both the sensation of pain and the underlying cause (e.g., tissue damage caused by cancer). Most important, we must appreciate that pain is inherently *personal and subjective.* Hence, when assessing pain, the most reliable method is to have the patient describe his or her experience.

Neurophysiologic Basis of Painful Sensations

The following discussion is a simplified version of how we perceive pain. Nonetheless, it should be adequate as a basis for understanding the interventions used for pain relief.

Sensation of pain is the net result of activity in two opposing neuronal pathways. The first pathway carries pain impulses from their site of origin to the brain and thereby generates pain sensation. The second pathway, which originates in the brain, suppresses impulse conduction along the first pathway and thereby diminishes pain sensation.

Pain impulses are initiated by activation of pain receptors, which are simply free nerve endings. These receptors can be activated by three types of stimuli: mechanical (e.g., pressure), thermal, and chemical (e.g., bradykinin, serotonin, histamine). In addition, *prostaglandins* and *substance P* can enhance the sensitivity of pain receptors to activation, although these compounds do not activate pain receptors directly.

Conduction of pain impulses from the periphery to the brain occurs by way of a multineuron pathway. The first neuron carries impulses from the periphery to a synapse in the spinal cord, where it releases either *glutamate* or *substance P* as a transmitter. The next neuron carries the impulse up the cord to a synapse in the thalamus. And the next neuron carries impulses from the thalamus to the cerebral cortex.

The brain is able to suppress pain conduction using endogenous opioid compounds, especially *enkephalins* and *beta-endorphin.* These compounds are released at synapses in the brain and spinal cord. Release within the spinal cord is controlled by a descending neuronal pathway that originates in the brain. The opioids that we give as drugs (e.g., morphine) produce analgesia by activating the same receptors that are activated by this endogenous pain-suppressing system.

Nociceptive Pain Versus Neuropathic Pain

In patients with cancer, pain has two major forms, referred to as *nociceptive* and *neuropathic.* Nociceptive pain results from injury to *tissues,* whereas neuropathic pain results from injury to *peripheral nerves.* These two forms of pain respond differently to analgesic drugs. Accordingly, it is important to differentiate between them. Among cancer patients, nociceptive pain is more common than neuropathic pain.

Nociceptive pain has two forms, known as *somatic* and *visceral.* Somatic pain results from injury to somatic tissues (e.g., bones, joints, muscles), whereas visceral pain results from injury to visceral organs (e.g., small intestine). Patients generally describe somatic pain as localized and sharp. In contrast, they describe visceral pain as vaguely localized with a diffuse, aching quality. Both forms of nociceptive pain respond well to *opioid analgesics* (e.g., morphine). In addition, they may respond to *nonopioids* (e.g., ibuprofen).

BOX 83.1 ▪ BARRIERS TO CANCER PAIN MANAGEMENT

Barriers Related to Health Care Professionals

Inadequate knowledge of pain management
- Poor assessment of pain
- Concerns stemming from regulations on controlled substances
- Fear of patient addiction
- Concern about side effects of analgesics
- Concern about tolerance to analgesics

Barriers Related to Patients

Reluctance to report pain
- Fear of distracting physicians from treating the cancer
- Fear that pain means the cancer is worse
- Concern about not being a "good" patient
- Reluctance to take pain medication
- Fear of addiction or being thought of as an addict
- Worries about unmanageable side effects
- Concern about becoming tolerant to pain medications
- Inability to pay for treatment

Barriers Related to the Health Care System

Low priority given to cancer pain management
- Inadequate reimbursement: the most appropriate treatment may not be reimbursed
- Restrictive regulation of controlled substances
- Treatment is unavailable or access is limited

Adapted from Jacox A, Carr DB, Payne R, et al. Management of Cancer Pain (Clinical Practice Guideline No. 9; AHCPR Publication No. 94-0592). Rockville, MD: Agency for Health Care Policy and Research, 1994.

Neuropathic pain produces different sensations than does nociceptive pain and responds to a different group of drugs. Patients describe neuropathic pain with such words as "burning," "shooting," "jabbing," "tearing," "numb," "dead," and "cold." Unlike nociceptive pain, neuropathic pain responds poorly to opioid analgesics. However, it does respond to drugs known collectively as *adjuvant analgesics.* Among these are certain antidepressants (e.g., imipramine), anticonvulsants (e.g., carbamazepine, gabapentin), and local anesthetics/antidysrhythmics (e.g., lidocaine).

Pain in Cancer Patients

Among patients with cancer, pain can be caused by the cancer itself and by therapeutic interventions. Cancer can cause pain through direct invasion of surrounding tissues (e.g., nerves, muscles, visceral organs) and through metastatic invasion at distant sites. Metastases to bone are very common, causing pain in up to 50% of patients. Cancer can cause neuropathic pain through infiltration of nerves, and visceral pain through infiltration, obstruction, and compression of visceral structures.

The incidence and intensity of cancer-induced pain is a function of cancer type and the stage of disease progression. Among patients with advanced disease, about 75% experience significant pain. Of these, 40% to 50% report moderate to severe pain, and 25% to 30% report very severe pain.

Therapeutic interventions—especially chemotherapy, radiation, and surgery—cause significant pain in at least 25% of patients, and probably more. Chemotherapy can cause painful mucositis, diffuse neuropathies, and aseptic necrosis of joints. Radiation can cause osteonecrosis, chronic visceral pain, and peripheral neuropathy (secondary to causing fibrosis of nerves). Surgery can cause a variety of pain syndromes, including phantom limb syndrome and postmastectomy syndrome.

MANAGEMENT STRATEGY

Management of cancer pain is an ongoing process that involves repeating cycles of assessment, intervention, and reassessment. The goal is to create and implement a flexible treatment plan that can meet the changing needs of the individual patient. Fig. 83.1 shows the steps involved. Management begins with a comprehensive assessment. After the nature of the pain has been determined, a treatment modality is selected. Analgesic drugs are preferred and hence are usually tried first. If drugs are ineffective, other modalities can be implemented. Among these are radiation, surgery, and nerve blocks. After each intervention, pain is reassessed. When relief has been achieved, the effective intervention is continued, accompanied by frequent reassessments. If severe pain returns or new pain develops, a new comprehensive assessment should be performed—followed by appropriate interventions and reassessment. Throughout this process, the health care team should make every effort to ensure active involvement of the patient and his or her family. Without their involvement, maximal benefits cannot be achieved. The importance of patient and family involvement is reflected in the clinical approach to pain management recommended by the Agency for Healthcare Research and Quality:

A **Ask** about pain regularly. **Assess** pain systematically.
B **Believe** the patient and family in their reports of pain and what relieves it.
C **Choose** pain control options appropriate for the patient, family, and setting.
D **Deliver** interventions in a timely, logical, and coordinated fashion.
E **Empower** patients and their families. **Enable** patients to control their treatment to the greatest extent possible.

ASSESSMENT AND ONGOING EVALUATION

Assessment is the foundation of treatment. In the absence of thorough assessment, effective pain management is impossible. Assessment begins with a comprehensive evaluation and then continues with regular follow-up evaluations. The initial assessment provides the basis for designing the treatment program. Follow-ups let us know how well treatment is working.

Comprehensive Initial Assessment

The initial assessment employs an extensive array of tests. The primary objective is to characterize the pain and identify its cause. This information provides the basis for designing a pain management plan. In addition, by documenting the

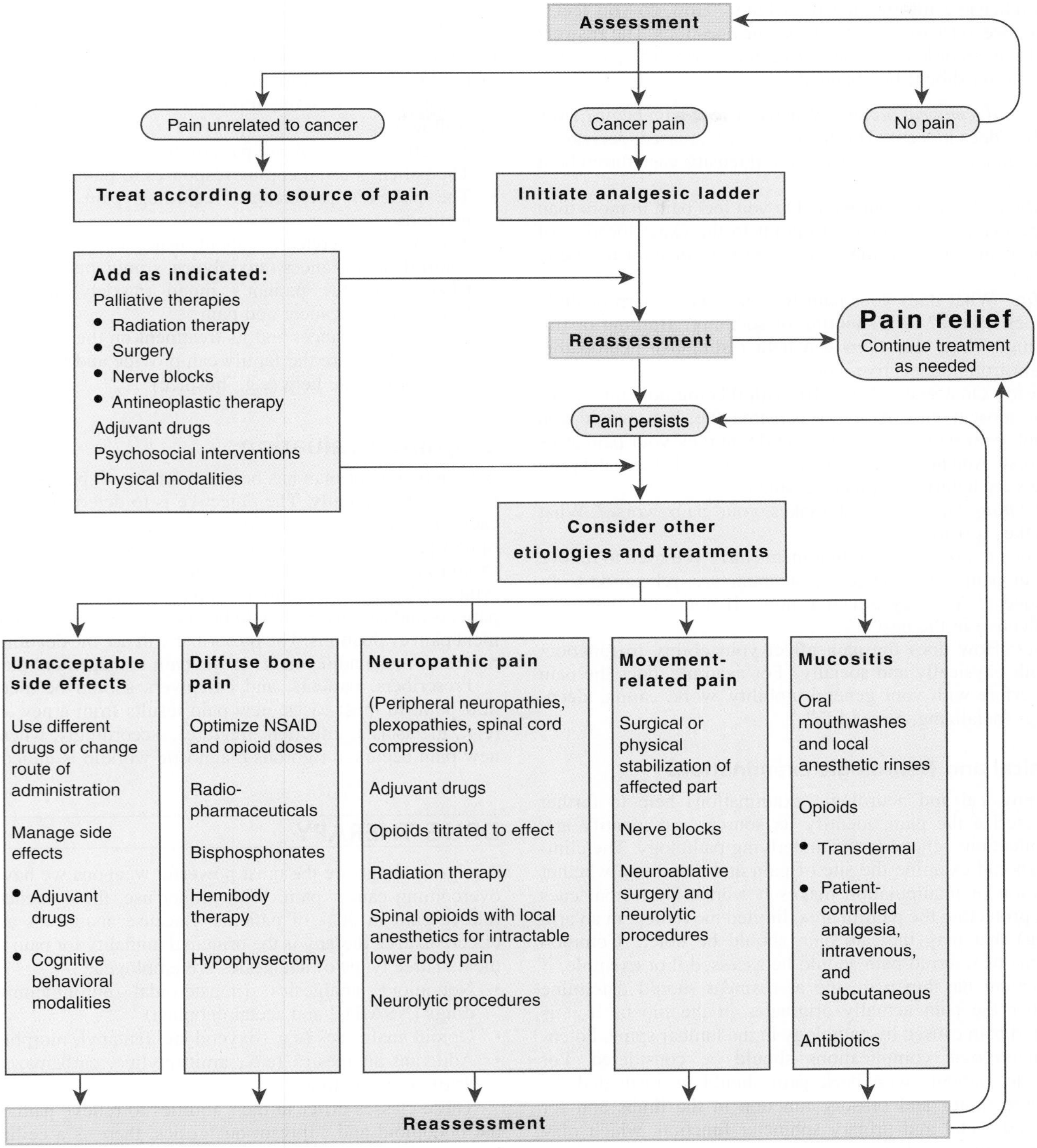

Figure 83.1 ▪ Flow chart for pain management in patients with cancer.
NSAID, nonsteroidal antiinflammatory drug. (Adapted from Jacox A, Carr DB, Payne R, et al. Management of Cancer Pain [Clinical Practice Guideline No. 9; AHCPR Publication No. 94-0592]. Rockville, MD: Agency for Health Care Policy and Research, 1994.)

patient's baseline pain status, the initial assessment provides a basis for evaluating the efficacy of treatment.

Assessment of Pain Intensity and Character: The Patient Self-Report

The patient's description of his or her pain is the cornerstone of pain assessment. No other component of assessment is more important! Remember, pain is a personal experience. Accordingly, if we want to assess pain, we must rely on the patient to tell us about it. Furthermore, we must act on what the patient says—even if we personally believe the patient may not be telling the truth.

The best way to ensure an accurate report is to ask the right questions and listen carefully to the answers. We cannot elicit comprehensive information by asking, "How do you feel?" Rather, we must ask a series of specific questions. The answers should be recorded on a pain inventory form. The following information should be obtained:

Onset and temporal pattern: When did your pain begin? How often does it occur? Has the intensity increased, decreased, or remained constant? Does the intensity vary throughout the day?

Location: Where is your pain? Do you feel pain in more than one place? Ask patients to point to the exact location of the pain, either on themselves, on you, or on a full-body drawing.

Quality: What does your pain feel like? Is it sharp or dull? Does it ache? Is it shooting or stabbing? Burning or tingling? These questions can help distinguish neuropathic pain from nociceptive pain.

Intensity: On a scale of 0 to 10, with 0 being no pain and 10 the most intense pain you can imagine, how would you rank your pain now? How would you rank your pain at its worst? And at its best? A pain intensity scale (see later) can be very helpful for this assessment.

Modulating factors: What makes your pain worse? What makes it better?

Previous treatment: What treatments have you tried to relieve your pain (e.g., analgesics, acupuncture, relaxation techniques)? Are they effective now? If not, were they ever effective in the past?

Impact: How does the pain affect your ability to function, both physically and socially? For example, does the pain interfere with your general mobility, work, eating, sleeping, socializing, or sex life?

Physical and Neurologic Examinations

The physical and neurologic examinations help to further characterize the pain, identify its source, and identify any complications related to the underlying pathology. The clinician should examine the site of pain and determine whether palpation or manipulation makes it worse. Nonverbal cues (e.g., protecting the painful area, limited movement in an arm or leg) that may indicate pain should be noted. Common patterns of referred pain should be assessed. For example, if the patient has hip pain, the assessment should determine whether the pain actually originates in the hip or if it is referred pain caused by pathology in the lumbar spine. Potential neurologic complications should be considered. For example, patients with back pain should be evaluated for impaired motor and sensory function in the limbs and for impaired rectal and urinary sphincter function, which may indicate spinal cord involvement.

Diagnostic Tests

Diagnostic tests are performed to identify the underlying cause of pain (e.g., progression of cancer, tissue injury caused by cancer treatments). The battery of diagnostic tests includes imaging studies (e.g., computed tomography scan, magnetic resonance imaging), neurophysiologic tests, and tests for tumor markers in blood. To ensure that abnormalities identified in the diagnostic tests really do explain the patient's pain, these findings should be correlated with findings from the physical and neurologic examinations.

Psychosocial Assessment

Psychosocial assessment is directed at both the patient and his or her family. The information is used in making pain management decisions. Some important issues to address include the following:

- The effect of significant pain on the patient in the past
- The patient's usual coping responses to pain and stress
- The patient's preferences regarding pain management methods
- The patient's concerns about using opioids and other controlled substances (anxiolytics, stimulants)
- Changes in the patient's mood (anxiety, depression) brought on by cancer and pain
- The effect of cancer and its treatment on the family
- The level of care the family can provide and the potential need for outside help (e.g., hospice)

Ongoing Evaluation

After a treatment plan has been implemented, pain should be reassessed frequently. The objective is to determine the efficacy of treatment and to allow early diagnosis and treatment of new pain. Each time an analgesic drug is administered, pain should be evaluated after sufficient time has elapsed for the drug to take effect. Because most patients are treated at home, patients and caregivers should be taught to conduct and document pain evaluations. The prescriber will use the documented record to make adjustments to the pain management plan.

Prescribers, patients, and caregivers should be alert for new pain. In most cases, new pain results from a new cause (e.g., metastasis, infection, fracture). Accordingly, whenever new pain occurs, a rigorous diagnostic workup is indicated.

DRUG THERAPY

Analgesic drugs are the most powerful weapons we have for overcoming cancer pain. With proper use, these agents can relieve pain in 90% of patients. Because analgesics are so effective, drug therapy is the principal modality for pain treatment. Three types of analgesics are employed:

- Nonopioid analgesics (nonsteroidal antiinflammatory drugs [NSAIDs] and acetaminophen)
- Opioid analgesics (e.g., oxycodone, fentanyl, morphine)
- Adjuvant analgesics (e.g., amitriptyline, carbamazepine, dextroamphetamine)

These classes differ in their abilities to relieve pain. With the nonopioid and adjuvant analgesics, there is a ceiling to how much relief we can achieve. In contrast, there is no ceiling to relief with the opioids.

Selection among the analgesics is based on pain intensity and pain type. To help guide drug selection, the World Health Organization (WHO) devised a drug selection ladder (Fig. 83.2). The first step of the ladder—for mild to moderate pain—consists of nonopioid analgesics: NSAIDs and acetaminophen. The second step—for more severe pain—*adds* opioid analgesics of moderate strength (e.g., oxycodone, hydrocodone). The top step—for severe pain—substitutes powerful opioids (e.g., morphine, fentanyl) for the weaker ones. Adjuvant analgesics, which are especially effective against neuropathic pain, can be used on any step of the ladder. Specific drugs to *avoid* are listed in Table 83.1.

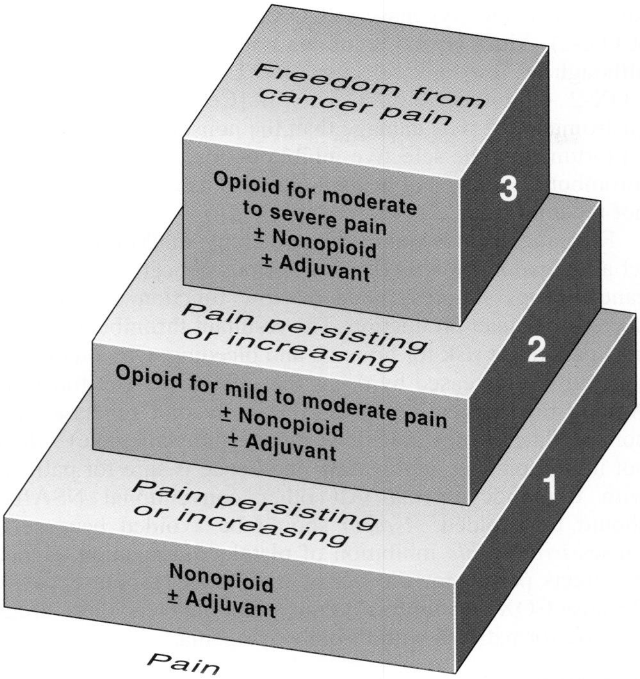

Figure 83.2 ■ The World Health Organization analgesic ladder for cancer pain management.
Note that steps represent pain intensity. Accordingly, if a patient has intense pain at the outset, then treatment can be initiated with an opioid (step 2), rather than trying a nonopioid first (step 1). (Adapted from Cancer Pain Relief, 2nd ed. Geneva: World Health Organization, 1996.)

Traditionally, patients have been given opioid analgesics only after a trial with nonopioids has failed. Guidelines from the National Comprehensive Cancer Network (NCCN) recommend a different approach, in which initial drug selection is based on pain intensity. Specifically, if the patient reports pain in the 4 to 10 range, then treatment should start directly with an opioid; an initial trial with a nonopioid is considered unnecessary. If the patient reports pain in the 1 to 3 range, then treatment usually begins with a nonopioid, although starting with an opioid remains an alternative.

It is common practice to combine an opioid with a nonopioid because the combination can be more effective than either drug alone. When pain is only moderate, opioids and nonopioids can be given in a fixed-dose combination formulation, thereby simplifying dosing. However, when pain is severe, these drugs must be given separately because, with a fixed-dose combination, side effects of the nonopioid would become intolerable as the dosage grew large and hence would limit how much opioid could be given.

Drug therapy of cancer pain should adhere to the following principles:

- Perform a comprehensive pretreatment assessment to identify pain intensity and the underlying cause.
- Individualize the treatment plan.
- Use the WHO analgesic ladder and NCCN guidelines to guide drug selection.
- Use oral therapy whenever possible.
- Avoid intramuscular (IM) injections whenever possible.

TABLE 83.1 ■ Drugs That Are Not Recommended for Treating Cancer Pain

Drug Class	Drug	Why the Drug Is Not Recommended
OPIOIDS		
Pure agonists	Meperidine	A toxic metabolite accumulates with prolonged use
	Codeine	Maximal pain relief is limited owing to dose-limiting side effects
Agonist-antagonists	Buprenorphine Butorphanol Nalbuphine Pentazocine	Ceiling to analgesic effects; can precipitate withdrawal in opioid-dependent patients; cause psychotomimetic reactions
OPIOID ANTAGONISTS	Naloxone Naltrexone	Can precipitate withdrawal in opioid-dependent patients; limit use to reversing life-threatening respiratory depression caused by opioid overdose
BENZODIAZEPINES	Diazepam Lorazepam others	Sedation from benzodiazepines limits opioid dosage; no demonstrated analgesic action
BARBITURATES	Amobarbital Secobarbital Others	Sedation from barbiturates limits opioid dosage; no demonstrated analgesic action
MISCELLANEOUS	Marijuana	Side effects (dysphoria, drowsiness, hypotension, bradycardia) preclude routine use as an analgesic

- For persistent pain, administer analgesics on a fixed schedule around-the-clock (ATC), and provide additional rescue doses of a short-acting agent if breakthrough pain occurs.
- Evaluate the patient frequently for pain relief and drug side effects.

Nonopioid Analgesics

The nonopioid analgesics—NSAIDs and acetaminophen—constitute the first rung of the WHO analgesic ladder. These agents are the initial drugs of choice for patients with mild pain. There is a ceiling to how much pain relief nonopioid drugs can provide, so there is no benefit to exceeding recommended dosages (Table 83.2). Acetaminophen is about equal to the NSAIDs in *analgesic* efficacy but lacks *antiinflammatory* actions. Because of this difference and others, acetaminophen is considered separately later. The NSAIDs and acetaminophen are discussed in Chapter 55.

Nonsteroidal Antiinflammatory Drugs

NSAIDs (e.g., aspirin, ibuprofen) can produce a variety of effects. Primary beneficial effects are pain relief, suppression

TABLE 83.2 ▪ Dosages for Nonopioid Analgesics: Acetaminophen and Selected NSAIDs

	Usual Adult Dosage*	
Drug	**Body Weight 50 kg or More**	**Body Weight Less Than 50 kg**
Acetaminophen	650 mg every 4 hr *or* 975 mg every 6 hr	10–15 mg/kg every 4 hr *or* 15–20 mg/kg every 4 hr (rectal)
NSAIDS: SALICYLATES		
Aspirin	650 mg every 4 hr *or* 975 mg every 6 hr	10–15 mg/kg every 4 hr *or* 15–20 mg/kg ever 4 hr (rectal)
Magnesium salicylate [Magan]†	650 mg every 4 hr	—
NSAIDS: PROPIONIC ACID DERIVATIVES		
Fenoprofen	300–600 mg every 6 hr	—
Ibuprofen [Motrin, Advil, others]	400–800 mg every 6 hr	10 mg/kg every 6–8 hr
Ketoprofen	25–60 mg every 6–8 hr	—
Naproxen [Naprosyn]	250–275 mg every 6–8 hr	5 mg/kg every 8 hr
Naproxen sodium [Anaprox, Aleve, Naprelan, others]	275 mg every 6–8 hr	—
NSAIDS: SELECTIVE COX-2 INHIBITORS		
Celecoxib [Celebrex]	200 mg every 12 hr	—
NSAIDS: MISCELLANEOUS		
Diflunisal	500 mg every 12 hr	—
Etodolac	200–400 mg every 6–8 hr	—
Meclofenamate sodium	50–100 mg every 6 hr	—
Mefenamic acid [Ponstel, Ponstan ♣]	250 mg every 6 hr	—

*All dosages are oral except where indicated.
†Magnesium salicylate is nonacetylated and hence, unlike aspirin, is safe for patients with thrombocytopenia.
NSAID, nonsteroidal anti-inflammatory drug.

of inflammation, and reduction of fever. Primary adverse effects are gastric ulceration, acute renal failure, and bleeding. In addition, all NSAIDs *except aspirin* increase the risk for thrombotic events (e.g., myocardial infarction, stroke). In contrast to opioids, NSAIDs do not cause tolerance, physical dependence, or psychological dependence.

NSAIDs are effective analgesics that can relieve mild to moderate pain. All of the NSAIDs have essentially equal analgesic efficacy, although individual patients may respond better to one NSAID than to another. NSAIDs relieve pain by a mechanism different from that of the opioids. As a result, combined use of an NSAID with an opioid can produce greater pain relief than either agent alone.

NSAIDs produce their effects—both good and bad—by inhibiting cyclooxygenase (COX), an enzyme that has two forms, known as cyclooxygenase-1 (COX-1) and cyclooxygenase-2 (COX-2). Most NSAIDs inhibit both COX-1 and COX-2, although a few are selective for COX-2. The selective COX-2 inhibitors (e.g., celecoxib [Celebrex]) cause less gastrointestinal (GI) damage than the nonselective inhibitors. Unfortunately, the selective inhibitors pose a greater risk for thrombotic events, and hence long-term use of these drugs is not recommended.

For patients undergoing chemotherapy, inhibition of platelet aggregation by NSAIDs is a serious concern. Many anticancer drugs suppress bone marrow function and thereby decrease platelet production. The resultant thrombocytopenia puts patients at risk for bruising and bleeding. Obviously, this risk will be increased by drugs that inhibit platelet function. Among the conventional NSAIDs, only one subclass—the nonacetylated salicylates (e.g., magnesium salicylate)—does not inhibit platelet aggregation and hence is safe for patients with thrombocytopenia. All other conventional NSAIDs should be avoided. *Aspirin* should be avoided because it causes *irreversible* inhibition of platelet aggregation. Hence its effects persist for the life of the platelet (about 8 days). Because COX-2 inhibitors do not affect platelets, these drugs are safe for patients with thrombocytopenia.

Acetaminophen

Acetaminophen [Tylenol, others] is similar to the NSAIDs in some respects and different in others. Like the NSAIDs, acetaminophen is an effective analgesic and hence can relieve mild to moderate pain. Benefits derive from inhibiting COX in the central nervous system (CNS), but not in the periphery. Combining acetaminophen with an opioid can produce greater analgesia than either drug alone (because acetaminophen and opioids relieve pain by different mechanisms).

Acetaminophen differs from the NSAIDs in several important ways. Because it does not inhibit COX in the periphery, acetaminophen lacks antiinflammatory actions, does not inhibit platelet aggregation, and does not promote gastric ulceration, renal failure, or thrombotic events. Because acetaminophen does not affect platelets, the drug is safe for patients with thrombocytopenia.

Acetaminophen has important interactions with two other drugs: alcohol and warfarin (an anticoagulant). Combining acetaminophen with alcohol, even in moderate amounts, can result in potentially fatal liver damage. Accordingly, patients taking acetaminophen should minimize alcohol consumption. Acetaminophen also can increase the risk for bleeding in patients taking warfarin. The mechanism appears to be inhibition of warfarin metabolism, which causes warfarin to accumulate to toxic levels.

Opioid Analgesics

Opioids are the most effective analgesics available and hence are the primary drugs for treating moderate to severe cancer pain. With proper dosing, opioids can safely relieve pain in about 90% of cancer patients. Unfortunately, many patients are denied adequate doses, owing largely to unfounded fears of addiction.

Opioids produce a variety of pharmacologic effects. In addition to analgesia, they can cause sedation, euphoria, constipation, respiratory depression, urinary retention, and miosis. With continuous use, tolerance develops to most of these effects, with the notable exceptions of constipation and miosis. Continuous use also results in physical dependence, which must not be equated with addiction.

The opioids are discussed in Chapter 22. Discussion here focuses on their use in patients with cancer.

Mechanism of Action and Classification

Opioid analgesics relieve pain by mimicking the actions of endogenous opioid peptides (enkephalins, dynorphins, endorphins), primarily at mu receptors and partly at kappa receptors.

Based on their actions at mu and kappa receptors, the opioids fall into two major groups: (1) *pure (full) agonists* (e.g., morphine) and (2) *agonist-antagonists* (e.g., butorphanol). The pure agonists can be subdivided into (1) agents for mild to moderate pain and (2) agents for moderate to severe pain. The pure agonists act as agonists at mu receptors *and* at kappa receptors. In contrast, the agonist-antagonists act as agonists only at kappa receptors; at mu receptors, these drugs act as *antagonists*. Because their agonist actions are limited to kappa receptors, the agonist-antagonists have a ceiling to their analgesic effects. Furthermore, because of their antagonist actions, the agonist-antagonists can block access of the pure agonists to mu receptors, and can thereby prevent the pure agonists from relieving pain. Accordingly, agonist-antagonists are not recommended for managing cancer pain.

Tolerance and Physical Dependence

Over time, opioids cause tolerance and physical dependence. These phenomena, which are generally inseparable, reflect neuronal adaptations to prolonged opioid exposure. Some degree of tolerance and physical dependence develops after 1 to 2 weeks of opioid use.

Tolerance

Tolerance can be defined as a state in which a specific dose (e.g., 10 mg of morphine) produces a smaller effect than it could when treatment began. Put another way, tolerance is a state in which dosage must be increased to maintain the desired response. In patients with cancer, however, a need for larger doses isn't always a sign of tolerance. In fact, it's usually a sign that pain is getting worse (owing to disease progression).

Tolerance develops to some opioid effects but not to others. Tolerance develops to analgesia, euphoria, respiratory depression, and sedation. In contrast, little or no tolerance develops to constipation or miosis.

There is cross-tolerance among opioids. Accordingly, significant tolerance to one opioid confers a similar degree of tolerance to all others.

Physical Dependence

Physical dependence is a state in which an abstinence syndrome will occur if a drug is abruptly withdrawn. With opioids, the abstinence syndrome can be very unpleasant—but not dangerous. The intensity and duration of the abstinence syndrome are determined in part by the duration of drug use and in part by the half-life of the drug taken. Because drugs with a short half-life leave the body rapidly, the abstinence syndrome is brief but intense. Conversely, for drugs with long half-lives, the syndrome is prolonged but relatively mild. The abstinence syndrome can be minimized by withdrawing opioids slowly (i.e., by giving progressively smaller doses over several days). Please note that *physical dependence is not the same as addiction!*

Addiction

Opioid addiction is an important issue in pain management—not because addiction occurs (it rarely does), but because *inappropriate fears of addiction* are a major cause for undertreatment.

The American Society of Addiction Medicine defines addiction as *a disease process characterized by continued use of a psychoactive substance despite physical, psychological, or social harm.* According to this definition, addiction is primarily a *behavior pattern*—and is *not* equated with physical dependence. Although it is true that physical dependence can contribute to addictive behavior, other factors—especially *psychological dependence*—are the primary underlying cause. All cancer patients who take opioids chronically develop substantial physical dependence, but only a few (<1%) develop addictive behavior. Most patients, if their cancer were cured, would simply go through gradual withdrawal and never think about or use opioids again. Clearly, these patients cannot be considered addicted, despite their physical dependence.

Because of misconceptions about opioid addiction, prescribers often order lower doses than patients need, nurses administer lower doses than were ordered, patients report less pain than they actually have, and family members discourage opioid use. The end result? Most cancer patients receive lower doses of opioids than they need. We can improve this unacceptable situation by educating providers, nurses, patients, and family members. Specifically, we must teach them about the nature of addiction and inform them that development of addiction in the therapeutic setting is very rare. Hopefully, this information will dispel unfounded fears of addiction and will thereby help ensure delivery of opioids in doses that are sufficient to relieve suffering.

Drug Selection

Preferred Opioids

For all cancer patients, *pure opioid agonists* are preferred to the agonist-antagonists. If pain is not too intense, a moderately strong opioid (e.g., oxycodone) is appropriate. If pain is moderate to severe, a strong opioid (e.g., morphine) should be used. Because morphine is inexpensive, available in multiple dosage forms, and clinically well understood, this opioid is used more than any other. Preferred opioids are listed in Table 83.3.

Opioid Rotation

Opioid rotation—switching from one opioid to another—is now an accepted practice. Because opioids have different side-effect profiles, rotation can help minimize adverse effects while maintaining good analgesia. To make the switch, the current opioid is stopped abruptly and immediately replaced with an equianalgesic dose of an alternative opioid.

Opioids to Use With Special Caution

Methadone [Dolophine, Methadose] and *levorphanol* must be used with caution. Both drugs have prolonged half-lives, which makes dosage titration difficult. If dosing is not done skillfully, these drugs can accumulate to dangerous levels, causing excessive sedation and respiratory depression.

TABLE 83.3 ■ Equianalgesic Doses of Pure Opioid Agonists and Tramadol

Drug	Equianalgesic Dose[a] Parenteral	Oral	Duration (Hours)[b]
AGENTS FOR MILD TO MODERATE PAIN			
Codeine[c,d]	130 mg	200 mg	3–4
Hydrocodone[e]	NA	30–45 mg	3–4
Oxycodone[f]	NA	20 mg	3–4
Tramadol[f,g]	NA	50–100 mg	3–7
AGENTS FOR MODERATE TO SEVERE PAIN			
Morphine[c,h]	10 mg	30 mg	3–4
Fentanyl[i,j]	100 mcg	NA	1–3
Hydromorphone[c]	1.5 mg	7.5 mg	2–3
Levorphanol[k]	2 mg	4 mg	3–6
Methadone[k,l]	Variable	Variable	Variable
Oxymorphone[f]	1 mg	10 mg	3–6

NA, not available.
[a]Equianalgesic dose = dose that will produce the same degree of analgesia as 10 mg of parenteral morphine.
[b]Shorter time generally applies to parenteral opioids. Longer time generally applies to immediate-release oral opioids. Sustained-release oral opioids have a prolonged duration.
[c]Codeine, morphine, and hydromorphone should be used with caution in patients with impaired renal function owing to potential accumulation of renally cleared metabolites. Monitor for neurologic adverse effects.
[d]Codeine is not generally recommended for chronic therapy because the doses required to produce significant analgesia also produce significant side effects.
[e]Equivalence data not substantiated. Usually combined with aspirin or acetaminophen.
[f]Available in a sustained-release formulation administered every 12 hours.
[g]Tramadol is a weak opioid agonist with some antidepressant activity. Reserve for mild to moderate pain. The recommended dosage is 100 mg 4 times a day. At the maximal dosage of 400 mg/day, tramadol is less effective than morphine and other strong pure opioid agonists.
[h]Available in sustained-release formulations administered every 12 or 24 hours.
[i]The equianalgesic dose listed applies to IV fentanyl compared with other IV opioids.
[j]Available in a long-acting transdermal system (applied every 48–72 hours) for around-the-clock pain relief and in short-acting transmucosal and intranasal formulations for breakthrough pain.
[k]Has a long half-life, so observe for adverse effects after 2 to 5 days. May need to be dosed every 4 hours initially and then every 6 to 8 hours after steady state is achieved (in 1–2 weeks).
[l]For patients converting from morphine to methadone, choosing the proper methadone dosage is complex and should be done with the advice of a pain specialist familiar with methadone prescribing.
Modified from NCCN Clinical Practice Guidelines in Oncology: Adult Cancer Pain, Version1.2011. Atlanta: National Comprehensive Cancer Network, Inc., 2011.

Codeine deserves special comment. Although codeine is capable of producing significant analgesia, side effects limit the dose that can be given. As a result, the degree of pain relief that can be achieved safely is quite low.

Opioids to Avoid

Meperidine [Demerol], a pure opioid agonist, may be used for a few days, but no longer. When the drug is taken chronically, a toxic metabolite—normeperidine—can accumulate, thereby posing a risk for adverse CNS effects (dysphoria, agitation, seizures).

The *agonist-antagonists*—buprenorphine, butorphanol, nalbuphine, and pentazocine—should be avoided for several reasons. First, they are less effective than pure opioid agonists, and hence, there is little reason to choose them. Second, if given to a patient who is physically dependent on a pure opioid agonist, these drugs can prevent the pure agonist from working and can thereby block analgesia and precipitate withdrawal. Third, the agonist-antagonists can cause adverse psychological reactions (nightmares, hallucinations, dysphoria).

Dosage

Dosage must be individualized. The objective is to find a dosage that can relieve pain without causing intolerable side effects. For patients with moderate pain and low opioid tolerance, very low doses (e.g., 2 mg of parenteral morphine every 4 hours) can be sufficient. In contrast, when pain is severe or tolerance is high, much larger doses (e.g., 600 mg of parenteral morphine every few hours) may be required. The upper limit to dosage is determined only by the intensity of side effects. Accordingly, as pain or tolerance increases, dosage should be increased until pain is relieved—unless intolerable side effects (e.g., excessive respiratory depression) occur first.

The dosing schedule is determined by the temporal pattern of the pain. If pain is intermittent and infrequent, PRN dosing can suffice. However, because most patients have persistent pain, PRN dosing is inappropriate. Instead, dosing should be done *on a fixed schedule* ATC. A fixed schedule can prevent opioid levels from becoming subtherapeutic and can thereby prevent pain recurrence. As a result, the patient is spared needless suffering, both from the pain itself and from anxiety about its return.

What dose should be used when switching from one opioid to another, or from one route of administration to another? To help make this decision, an equianalgesia table such as Table 83.3 should be consulted. Equianalgesia tables indicate equivalent analgesic doses for different opioids and for the same opioid administered by different routes. Let's assume, for example, that our patient has been getting 10 mg of IV morphine every 4 hours, and we want to switch to oral hydromorphone. Table 83.3 shows that 7.5 mg of oral hydromorphone is about equivalent to 10 mg of parenteral morphine, with both drugs being given every 4 hours. Hence we might begin oral hydromorphone at 7.5 mg. However, there is a caveat: because cross-tolerance among opioids is incomplete, the listed equianalgesic dose may actually produce a *stronger* effect than advertised. Accordingly, when switching drugs, it is safer to use a dose that is somewhat *lower* than the equianalgesic dose, and then titrate up.

Routes of Administration

Because most patients with cancer pain must take analgesics continuously, the route should be as convenient, affordable, and noninvasive as possible. Oral administration meets these criteria best and hence is preferred for most patients. If oral medication cannot be used, the preferred alternative routes are rectal and transdermal: both are relatively convenient, affordable, and noninvasive. If these routes are ineffective or inappropriate, then parenteral administration (intravenous [IV] or subcutaneous [subQ]) is indicated (IM injections should be avoided). For patients who cannot be managed with IV or subQ therapy, more invasive routes—intraspinal or intraventricular—can be tried.

Oral

Oral administration is the preferred route for chronic therapy because oral dosing is cheap, convenient, and noninvasive. Accordingly, in the absence of contraindications (e.g., vomiting, inability to swallow), oral therapy should be considered for all patients. Opioids are available in several formulations (e.g., tablets, capsules, solution) for oral use. To reduce the number of daily doses, a long-acting formulation (e.g., controlled-release morphine) can be used. Because oral opioids undergo substantial first-pass metabolism, oral doses must be larger than parenteral doses to achieve equivalent analgesic effects.

Rectal

Rectal administration is a preferred alternative for patients who cannot take drugs by mouth. Two opioids—morphine and hydromorphone—are available in rectal formulations (suppositories). When switching from oral to rectal administration, dosing is begun with the same dose that was used orally and then adjusted as needed. Rectal administration is inappropriate for patients with diarrhea or lesions of the rectum or anus. Also, children frequently object to this route.

Transdermal

Transdermal administration is a preferred alternative to oral therapy. Only one pure opioid agonist—fentanyl [Duragesic]—is available for chronic transdermal use. Fentanyl patches provide steady analgesia for 72 hours and hence are appropriate for patients with pain that is continuous and does not fluctuate much in intensity. Absorption from the patch is very slow. As a result, when the first patch is applied, effective analgesia may take 12 to 24 hours to develop. During this time, PRN therapy with a short-acting opioid may be required. Fentanyl patches are available in five strengths, allowing dosage to be matched with pain intensity. As with other long-acting opioids, rescue doses with a short-acting opioid are needed when breakthrough pain occurs.

Intravenous and Subcutaneous

IV and subQ administrations are acceptable alternatives when less invasive routes (oral, transdermal, rectal) cannot be used. The IV and subQ routes have two advantages: (1) onset of analgesia is quick and (2) these routes permit rapid escalation of dosage. Obvious disadvantages are inconvenience and increased cost. In addition, frequent subQ dosing is uncomfortable. Conditions that might justify IV or subQ administration include the following:

- Persistent nausea and vomiting (which preclude oral dosing)
- Inability to swallow (which precludes oral dosing)
- Delirium or stupor (which precludes oral dosing)
- Pain that requires a large number of pills (which makes oral dosing inconvenient)
- Unstable pain that requires rapid dosage escalation (which precludes oral, rectal, and transdermal administration)

Dosages for IV and subQ administration are the same.

Intramuscular

IM administration should be avoided. IM injections are painful and hence unacceptable for repeated dosing. In addition, absorption from IM sites is inconsistent, so pain relief is unpredictable.

Intraspinal

Intraspinal administration is reserved for patients with intractable pain that cannot be controlled with less invasive routes (e.g., IV, subQ). In this technique, opioids are delivered to the epidural or subarachnoid space through a percutaneous catheter connected to an infusion pump or injection port. By using this route, we can achieve high opioid concentrations at receptors on pain pathways in the spinal cord. It is important to note, however, that effects will not be limited to the spinal cord: intraspinal opioids undergo absorption into the blood in amounts sufficient to cause systemic effects. In fact, blood levels may be equivalent to those achieved with conventional routes (e.g., subQ). Intraspinal administration is especially useful for patients with severe pain in the lower body: pain is relieved in up to 90% of appropriate candidates. Patients who are tolerant to opioids delivered by other routes will also be tolerant to opioids given intraspinally, and hence dosage should be adjusted accordingly. Patients should have access to rescue medication in case breakthrough pain occurs, owing either to delivery system malfunction or inadequate dosing. Side effects with intraspinal administration are the same as with other routes. In addition, there is a risk for *delayed* respiratory depression as well as infection associated with the catheter.

Intraventricular

Like intraspinal administration, intraventricular administration is reserved for patients whose pain cannot be controlled with less invasive routes. In this procedure, morphine is delivered to the cerebral ventricles through a catheter connected to an external infusion pump (for continuous administration) or a subcutaneous reservoir (for intermittent administration). Because morphine is delivered directly to the brain, bypassing the blood-brain barrier, analgesia can be achieved with extremely low doses (e.g., 5 mg daily). Pain is relieved in 90% of patients. Intraventricular administration is especially helpful for patients with intractable pain caused by head and neck malignancies or tumors that affect the brachial plexus.

Managing Breakthrough Pain

Many patients whose pain is well controlled most of the day experience transient episodes of moderate to severe pain, known as breakthrough pain. Breakthrough pain develops quickly, reaches peak intensity in minutes, and may persist from minutes to hours (the median duration is 30 minutes). At least 50% of cancer patients experience these episodes, typically 1 to 4 times a day. Breakthrough pain may occur spontaneously, or it may be precipitated by coughing or other movements. In contrast to end-of-dose pain, which occurs because analgesic levels are lowest at that time, breakthrough pain can occur at any time during the dosing interval.

All patients receiving ATC opioids for persistent pain should have access to a rescue medication to manage breakthrough pain. Because breakthrough pain is both severe and self-limited, the best medication is a strong opioid with a rapid onset and short duration. The rapid onset permits speedy relief, and the short duration facilitates dosage titration. For ease of administration, oral, transmucosal, and intranasal formulations are preferred; examples include immediate-release oral morphine, transmucosal fentanyl [Abstral, Actiq, Fentora, Subsys], and fentanyl nasal spray [Lazanda]. The dosage, as recommended by the American Pain Society and the WHO, should be equivalent to one sixth (17%) of the total daily opioid dose, repeated in 2 hours if needed.

Managing Side Effects

Side effects of the opioids include respiratory depression, constipation, sedation, orthostatic hypotension, miosis, nausea, and vomiting. All can be effectively managed. In many patients, side effects can be reduced simply by decreasing the dosage (typically by 25%). If dosage reduction causes pain to return, adding a nonopioid analgesic may take care of the problem. Over time, tolerance develops to sedation, respiratory depression, nausea, and vomiting—but not to constipation or miosis.

Respiratory Depression

Respiratory depression is the most serious side effect of the opioids; death can result. Fortunately, when dosage and monitoring are appropriate, significant respiratory depression is rare. Pain counteracts the depressant actions of opioids. Hence, as pain decreases, respiratory depression may deepen.

Respiratory depression is greatest at the outset of treatment and then decreases as tolerance develops. As a result, small initial doses of opioids (e.g., 5 mg of IV morphine every hour) can pose a greater risk than much larger doses (e.g., 1000 mg of IV morphine every hour) later on.

Significant respiratory depression is most likely when dosage is being titrated up. The best way to assess the risk for impending respiratory depression is to monitor opioid-induced sedation. An increase in sedation generally precedes an increase in respiratory depression, so if excessive sedation is observed, further dosing should be delayed.

Respiratory depression is increased by other drugs with CNS-depressant actions (e.g., alcohol, barbiturates, benzodiazepines). Accordingly, these agents should be avoided.

Severe respiratory depression can be reversed with *naloxone* [Narcan], a pure opioid antagonist. However, caution is required: excessive dosing will reverse analgesia, thereby putting the patient in great pain. Accordingly, naloxone dosage must be titrated carefully.

When death is near, should opioids be withheld out of fear that respiratory depression may bring death sooner? For several reasons, the answer is no. First, significant respiratory depression is rare in the tolerant patient. Hence concerns about hastening death are largely unfounded. Second, unrelieved pain can itself hasten death. Third, when death is imminent, it is more important to provide comfort than prolong life. Accordingly, adequate opioids should be provided, even if doing so means life ends a bit sooner.

Constipation

Constipation occurs in most patients. Opioids promote constipation by decreasing propulsive intestinal contractions, increasing nonpropulsive contractions, increasing the tone of the anal sphincter, and reducing fluid secretion into the intestinal lumen. No tolerance to these effects develops. To reduce constipation, all patients should increase dietary fiber and fluid. However, most patients also need pharmacologic help. Options include stool softeners (e.g., docusate), stimulant laxatives (e.g., senna), osmotic laxatives (e.g., sodium phosphate), and methylnaltrexone [Relistor], which blocks opioid receptors in the intestine. For prophylaxis of constipation, current guidelines recommend daily therapy with a combination product, such as Senokot-S, which contains both senna and docusate. Strong osmotic laxatives are reserved for severe constipation. Methylnaltrexone [Relistor] is indicated only for constipation in patients with end-stage disease. Drugs with anticholinergic properties (e.g., tricyclic antidepressants, antihistamines) can exacerbate opioid-induced constipation (by further depressing bowel function) and hence should be avoided.

Sedation

Sedation is common early in therapy, but tolerance develops quickly. If sedation persists, it can be reduced by giving smaller doses of the opioid more frequently, while keeping the total daily dose the same. This dosing schedule decreases peak opioid levels and reduces excessive CNS depression. If necessary, sedation can be opposed with a CNS stimulant (e.g., caffeine, methylphenidate, dextroamphetamine, modafinil).

Nausea and Vomiting

Initial doses of opioids may cause nausea and vomiting. Fortunately, tolerance develops rapidly. Nausea and vomiting can be minimized by pretreatment with an antiemetic (e.g., prochlorperazine, metoclopramide). A serotonin antagonist (e.g., granisetron, ondansetron) may also be tried, but these drugs may increase constipation.

Other Side Effects

Opioids promote histamine release and can thereby cause *itching,* which can be relieved with an antihistamine (e.g., diphenhydramine).

Opioids increase the tone in the urinary bladder sphincter and can thereby cause *urinary retention.* Benign prostatic hypertrophy and use of anticholinergic drugs will exacerbate the problem. Patients should be monitored for urinary retention and encouraged to void every 4 hours.

Opioids can cause *orthostatic hypotension.* Patients should be informed about symptoms of hypotension (lightheadedness, dizziness) and instructed to sit or lie down if they occur. Orthostatic hypotension can be minimized by moving slowly when changing from a supine or seated position to an upright posture.

Opioid-induced *neurotoxicity* is a recently recognized syndrome. Symptoms include delirium, agitation, myoclonus, and hyperalgesia. Primary risk factors are renal impairment, preexisting cognitive impairment, and prolonged, high-dose opioid use. Management consists of hydration, dose reduction, and opioid rotation.

Adjuvant Analgesics

Adjuvant analgesics are used to *complement* the effects of opioids. Accordingly, these drugs are employed in *combination* with opioids—not as substitutes. Adjuvant analgesics can (1) enhance analgesia from opioids, (2) help manage concurrent symptoms that exacerbate pain, and (3) treat side effects caused by opioids. Several of the adjuvants are especially useful for *neuropathic pain.* The adjuvant analgesics differ from opioids in that pain relief is limited and less predictable and often develops slowly.

Adjuvant agents may be employed at any step on the analgesic ladder. The adjuvants are interesting in that, although they can relieve pain, all of them were developed to treat other conditions (e.g., depression, seizures, dysrhythmias). Accordingly, it is important to reassure patients that the adjuvant is being used to alleviate pain, and not for its original purpose. Dosages for the adjuvant analgesics are shown in Table 83.4.

Antidepressants

Tricyclic Antidepressants

Amitriptyline [Elavil] and other tricyclic antidepressants (TCAs) can reduce pain of *neuropathic* origin. TCAs have analgesic effects of their own, and they enhance the effects of opioids and may thereby allow a reduction in opioid dosage. As a side benefit, TCAs can elevate mood. Important adverse effects are orthostatic hypotension, sedation, anticholinergic effects (dry mouth, urinary retention, constipation), and weight gain (secondary to improved appetite). Dosing at bedtime takes advantage of sedative effects and minimizes hypotension during the day. Effects begin in 1 to 2 weeks and reach their maximum in 4 to 6 weeks. The TCAs are discussed in Chapter 25.

Other Antidepressants

In addition to the tricyclic agents, certain other antidepressants (e.g., bupropion, duloxetine, venlafaxine) can help with neuropathic pain.

Antiseizure Drugs

Certain antiseizure drugs can help relieve *neuropathic pain.* Acute pain (sharp, darting pain) is especially responsive, although other forms of neuropathic pain (cramping pain, aching pain, burning pain) also respond. Analgesia is thought to result from suppressing spontaneous neuronal firing. Of the available antiseizure drugs, *carbamazepine* [Tegretol] has been used most widely. Because carbamazepine is myelosuppressive, it must be used with caution in patients receiving anticancer drugs that suppress bone marrow function. As discussed in Chapter 19, caution is also needed in patients of Asian descent, owing to an increased risk for severe dermatologic reactions. Another drug—*gabapentin* [Neurontin]—is also very effective and causes fewer side effects than carbamazepine. Dosage should be low initially (100 mg once a day) and then gradually increased; dosages as high as 1200 mg 3 times a day have been employed. Antiseizure drugs are discussed in Chapter 19.

Local Anesthetics/Antidysrhythmics

Lidocaine (a local anesthetic and antidysrhythmic) and *mexiletine* (an antidysrhythmic related to lidocaine) are considered second-line agents for *neuropathic pain.* IV infusion of lidocaine produces analgesia in 10 to 15 minutes. The drug may be most appropriate for rapidly escalating neuropathic pain. Both lidocaine and mexiletine are discussed in Chapter 41. Lidocaine is also discussed in Chapter 21.

Central Nervous System Stimulants

The CNS stimulants, such as *dextroamphetamine* [Dexedrine] and *methylphenidate* [Ritalin], have two beneficial effects:

TABLE 83.4 ■ Adjuvant Drugs for Cancer Pain

Drug	Usual Adult Dosage	Beneficial Actions
TRICYCLIC ANTIDEPRESSANTS		
Amitriptyline [Elavil]	25–150 mg/day PO	Reduce neuropathic pain
Desipramine [Norpramin]*	10–150 mg/day PO	
Doxepin [Sinequan]*	25–150 mg/day PO	
Imipramine [Tofranil]	20–100 mg/day PO	
Nortriptyline [Aventyl, Pamelor]*	10–150 mg/day PO	
OTHER ANTIDEPRESSANTS		
Duloxetine [Cymbalta]	30–60 mg/day PO	Reduce neuropathic pain
Venlafaxine [Effexor]*	37.5–225 mg/day PO	
ANTISEIZURE DRUGS		
Carbamazepine [Tegretol]	200–1600 mg/day PO	Reduce neuropathic pain
Gabapentin [Neurontin]	300–3600 mg/day PO	
Lamotrigine [Lamictal]*	25–400 mg/day PO	
Phenytoin [Dilantin]*	300–500 mg/day PO	
Pregabalin [Lyrica]	100–600 mg/day PO	
LOCAL ANESTHETICS/ANTIDYSRHYTHMICS		
Lidocaine	5 mg/kg/day IV or subQ Apply topical patch for up to 12 hours daily	Reduce neuropathic pain
Mexiletine [Mexitil]	450–600 mg/day PO	
CNS STIMULANTS		
Dextroamphetamine [Dexedrine]	5–10 mg/day PO	Enhance analgesia and reduce sedation from opioids
Methylphenidate [Ritalin]	10–15 mg/day PO	
ANTIHISTAMINE		
Hydroxyzine [Vistaril]	300–450 mg/day IM	Reduces anxiety, insomnia, and nausea
GLUCOCORTICOIDS		
Dexamethasone [Decadron, others]	16–96 mg/day PO or IV	Reduce pain associated with brain metastases and epidural spinal cord compression
Prednisone	40–100 mg/day PO	
BISPHOSPHONATES		
Etidronate [Didronel]	7.5 mg/kg IV for 3 days	Reduce hypercalcemia and possibly bone pain
Pamidronate	60–90 mg IV once	

*Off-label use.

IM, intramuscular; IV, intravenous; PO, oral; subQ, subcutaneous.

they can enhance opioid-induced analgesia, and they can counteract opioid-induced sedation. In addition, they can be used for rapid elevation of mood. Principal adverse effects are weight loss (from appetite suppression) and insomnia (from CNS stimulation). To minimize interference with sleep, dosing late in the day should be avoided. The CNS stimulants are discussed in Chapter 29.

Antihistamines

Hydroxyzine [Vistaril], an antihistamine, promotes drowsiness and reduces anxiety. Hydroxyzine can be useful for nausea and vomiting as well as insomnia. Although widely believed to enhance analgesia, proof is lacking. Drawbacks include worsening of constipation, urinary retention, and cognitive impairment. The antihistamines are discussed in Chapter 54.

Glucocorticoids

Although glucocorticoids lack direct analgesic actions, they can help manage painful cancer-related conditions. Because glucocorticoids can reduce cerebral and spinal edema, they are essential for the emergency management of elevated intracranial pressure and epidural spinal cord compression. Similarly, glucocorticoids are part of the standard therapy for tumor-induced spinal cord compression. In addition to these benefits, glucocorticoids can improve appetite and impart a general sense of well-being; both actions help in managing anorexia and cachexia-associated with terminal illness.

Glucocorticoids are very safe when used short term (even in high doses) and very dangerous when used long term (even in low doses). In particular, long-term therapy can cause adrenal insufficiency, osteoporosis, glucose intolerance (hyperglycemia), increased vulnerability to infection, thinning of the skin, and, possibly, peptic ulcer disease. The risk for osteoporosis can be reduced by giving calcium supplements and vitamin D along with calcitonin or a bisphosphonate (e.g., etidronate). The glucocorticoids are discussed in Chapter 56.

Bisphosphonates

Bisphosphonates, such as *etidronate* [Didronel] and *pamidronate*, can reduce cancer-related *bone pain* in some patients. Bone pain is common when cancers metastasize to bone. The cause of pain may be tumor-induced bone resorption, which can also cause hypercalcemia, osteoporosis, and related fractures. Bisphosphonates inhibit bone resorption and are approved for treating hypercalcemia of malignancy and bone metastases in breast cancer—but not bone pain itself. However, when these drugs are given to treat hypercalcemia, many patients report a reduction in bone pain, although others do not. Hence, although these drugs appear promising, their use for management of bone pain is still considered investigational. The bisphosphonates are discussed in Chapter 59.

NONDRUG THERAPY

Neurolytic Nerve Block

The goal of this procedure is to destroy neurons that transmit pain from a limited area, thereby providing permanent pain relief. Nerve destruction is accomplished through local injection of a neurolytic (neurotoxic) substance, typically alcohol or phenol. To ensure that the correct nerves are destroyed, reversible nerve block is done first, using a local anesthetic. If the local anesthetic relieves the pain, a neurolytic agent is then applied to the same site. Neurolytic nerve block can eliminate pain in up to 80% of patients. However, even if pain relief is only partial, the procedure can still permit some reduction in opioid dosage and can thereby decrease side effects, such as sedation and constipation. When nerve block is successful and opioids are discontinued, opioid dosage should be tapered gradually to avoid withdrawal. Nerve block is not without risk. Potential complications include hypotension, paresis (slight paralysis), paralysis, and disruption of bowel and bladder function (e.g., diarrhea, incontinence). The incidence of complications ranges from 0.5% to 2%.

Radiation Therapy

Radiation therapy relieves pain by causing tumor regression. Palliative treatment can be directed at primary tumors and at metastases anywhere in the body.

Radiation can be delivered in four forms: *brachytherapy* (implanted radioactive pellets), *teletherapy* (external beam radiation therapy), *radiofrequency ablation,* and *IV radiopharmaceuticals.* With brachytherapy, cell kill is limited to the immediate area of the implanted pellets; hence the technique is suited only for localized tumors. With teletherapy, cell kill can be localized or widespread, depending on the size of the beam employed; hence the technique can be used for both localized tumors and metastases. Radiofrequency ablation uses a thin, needle-like probe inserted into a tumor through an incision in the skin. The probe extends electrodes that emit high-frequency electrical current, producing heat to destroy cancer cells; hence the technique is best suited for localized tumors. IV radiopharmaceuticals travel throughout the body and hence are best suited for widespread metastases.

With radiation therapy, as with chemotherapy, damage to normal tissue is dose limiting. Therefore the challenge is to deliver a dose of radiation that is large enough to kill cancer cells, but not so large that it causes intolerable damage to healthy tissue.

Some side effects of radiation occur early, and some are late. Early effects develop during or immediately after radiation exposure. Late reactions develop months or years later. The most common early effects are skin inflammation and lesions of the GI mucosa. Fortunately, in the regimens employed for palliation, these acute effects are generally mild. The most common late reaction is fibrosis, which occurs mainly in tissues that have a limited ability to regenerate (e.g., brain, peripheral neurons, lung). Late reactions are of limited concern, however, because most patients die of their cancer before late reactions can develop.

PAIN MANAGEMENT IN SPECIAL POPULATIONS

Older Adults

In older-adult patients, two issues are of special concern: (1) undertreatment of pain and (2) increased risk for adverse effects. Paradoxically, a third issue—heightened drug sensitivity—contributes to both problems.

Heightened Drug Sensitivity

Older adults are more sensitive to drugs than are younger adults, owing largely to a decline in organ function. In particular, rates of hepatic metabolism and renal excretion decline with age. As a result, drugs tend to accumulate in the body, causing responses to be more intense and prolonged.

Undertreatment of Pain

Undertreatment is common in older adults. In addition to the usual reasons (fears about tolerance, addiction, adverse effects, and regulatory actions), older adults are denied adequate medication for two more reasons: difficulties with assessment and erroneous ideas about "old age."

Assessment is made difficult by cognitive impairment (e.g., delirium, dementia) and by impairment of vision and hearing. As a result, self-reporting of pain may be inaccurate or even impossible. Because of these obstacles, special effort must be made to help ensure that assessment is accurate. However, because accuracy cannot be guaranteed, frequent reassessment is recommended.

Misconceptions about older adults contribute to undertreatment. Specifically, providers may believe (incorrectly) that dosage should be low because (1) older adults are relatively insensitive to pain; (2) if pain occurs, older adults can tolerate it well; and (3) older adults are highly sensitive to opioid side effects. The first two concepts have no basis in fact, and therefore must not be allowed to influence treatment. Although there is some truth to the third concept, concern about side effects is no excuse for inadequate dosing.

Increased Risk for Side Effects and Adverse Interactions

For several reasons, older-adult patients may experience more side effects than younger adults. As noted, drug elimination in older adults is impaired, posing a risk that drug levels may rise dangerously high. However, with careful dosing, drug levels can be kept within a range that is both safe and effective. Drugs with prolonged half-lives (e.g., methadone) pose an increased risk for excessive accumulation and should be avoided.

The risk for gastric ulceration and renal toxicity from NSAIDs is increased in older patients. Gastric erosion can be reduced by concurrent therapy with misoprostol or a proton pump inhibitor (e.g., esomeprazole). There is no specific way to prevent renal toxicity. The best we can do is monitor closely for evolving kidney damage.

Older-adult patients are at increased risk for adverse drug-drug interactions. In addition to the disorder that's causing pain, older adults are likely to have other disorders and require more drugs than younger adults. The risk for serious injury from drug interactions can be reduced by careful drug selection and by monitoring for potential reactions.

Young Children

Management of cancer pain in children is much like management in adults. The principal difference is that assessment in children is more difficult. In addition, children frequently experience more pain from chemotherapy and other interventions than from the cancer itself.

Assessment

Assessment must be tailored to the child's developmental level and personality. Selecting an appropriate assessment method is especially important for children with developmental delays, learning disabilities, and emotional disturbances. Assessment can be greatly facilitated by open communication about pain between the child, family, and health care team.

Assessment methods include self-reporting, behavioral observation, and measurement of physiologic parameters (e.g., heart rate, blood pressure, respiratory rate, sweating). As stressed earlier, self-reporting is preferred and should be employed whenever appropriate. Behavioral observation is a distant second choice. Because many factors other than pain can alter physiologic parameters, measuring these is the least reliable way to assess pain.

Verbal Children

For children who can verbalize and are older than 4 years, self-reporting is the most reliable way to assess pain. Because children rarely claim to have pain that isn't there, there is little risk for error from overreporting. However, there *is* a significant risk for error from underreporting. Children may report less pain than they have for several reasons. These include (1) fear that revealing their pain will lead to additional injections and other painful procedures, (2) lack of awareness that we can help their pain go away, (3) a desire to protect their parents from the knowledge that their cancer is getting worse, and (4) a desire to please. Because the self-report may conceal pain, it can be helpful to supplement the self-report with behavioral observation (see later).

Preverbal and Nonverbal Children

Because preverbal and nonverbal children cannot self-report pain, a less reliable method must be used for assessment. The principal alternative is *behavioral observation.* Behavioral cues suggesting pain include vocalization (crying, whining, groaning), facial expression (grimacing, frowning, reduced affect), muscle tension, inability to be consoled, protection of body areas, and reduced activity. The biggest drawback to behavioral observation is the risk for a false-negative conclusion. That is, a child may be in pain although his or her behavior may lead the observer to conclude otherwise. For example, sleeping, watching TV, or laughing may suggest that a child is comfortable. However, these behaviors can actually represent an attempt to control pain. Similarly, although sitting quietly might indicate comfort, it could also mean that moving and talking are painful. When behavioral observation leaves doubt about whether the child is in pain, a trial with an analgesic can help confirm the assessment.

Treatment

Therapy of cancer pain in children is essentially the same as in adults. As in adults, drugs are the cornerstone of treatment; nondrug therapies are used only as supplements. Drug selection is guided by the WHO analgesic ladder. Because of the risk for Reye syndrome, children with influenza or chickenpox should not receive NSAIDs, including aspirin. Acetaminophen is a safe alternative. As in adults, oral dosing is preferred. More invasive routes should be reserved for patients who cannot take drugs by mouth. Children generally object to rectal administration and may refuse treatment by this route. Administration with a patient-controlled analgesia (PCA) device is an option for children older than 7 years.

Neonates and infants are highly sensitive to drugs and hence must be treated with special caution. Drug sensitivity occurs for two reasons: (1) the blood-brain barrier is incompletely formed, giving drugs ready access to the CNS; and (2) the kidneys and liver are poorly developed, causing drug elimination to be slow. Because of heightened drug sensitivity, neonates and infants are at increased risk for respiratory depression from opioids. Accordingly, when opioids are given to nonventilated infants, the initial dosage should be very low (about one third the dosage employed for older children). Furthermore, use of opioids should be accompanied by intensive monitoring of respiration.

Opioid Abusers

When treating cancer pain in opioid abusers, we have two primary obligations: we must try to (1) relieve the pain and (2) avoid giving opioids simply because the patient wants to get high. Both obligations are difficult to meet. Because of the challenge, treatment should be directed by a clinician trained in substance abuse as well as pain management.

Concerns about abuse can result in undertreatment of pain. This must be avoided. Remember, abusers feel pain like everyone else and therefore need opioids like everyone else. Clinicians must take special care not to withhold opioids because they have confused relief-seeking behavior with drug-seeking behavior. In the end, we have little choice but to base treatment on the patient's self-report of pain. Hence, if the patient tells us that pain is persisting, adequate doses of opioids should be provided.

Because of opioid tolerance, initial doses in abusers must be higher than in nonabusers. To estimate how high the initial dosage should be, we must try to estimate the existing degree of tolerance by interviewing the patient about the extent of opioid use.

As with other adults, drug selection can be guided by the WHO analgesic ladder and the NCCN guidelines. If pain is sufficient to justify opioids, then opioids should be used; nonopioids (NSAIDs and acetaminophen) should not be substituted for opioids out of concern for addiction. If the patient is on methadone maintenance, methadone can be used for the pain. However, because regulations limit the dosage of methadone that drug-abuse clinics can dispense, the increased dosage required to manage pain will have to come from another source. One group of opioids—the agonist-antagonists—will precipitate withdrawal in opioid abusers and hence must never be prescribed for these patients.

PATIENT EDUCATION

Patient education is an integral part of cancer pain management. When education is successful, it can help reduce anxiety, dispel hopelessness, facilitate assessment, enhance compliance, decrease complications, provide a sense of control, and enable patients to take an active role in their care. All of these will promote pain relief.

General Issues

Common sense tells us that patient education should be accurate, comprehensive, and understandable. To reinforce communication, information should be presented at least twice and in more than one way. Major topics to discuss are (1) the nature and causes of pain, (2) assessment and the importance of honest self-reporting, and (3) plans for drug and nondrug therapy. Patients should be encouraged to express their fears and concerns about cancer, cancer pain, and pain treatment—and they should be reassured that pain can be effectively controlled in most cases. All patients should receive a written pain management plan. To facilitate ongoing education, patients should be invited to contact care providers whenever they feel the need—be it to discuss specific concerns with treatment or simply to acquire new information. Finally, patients should know when and how to contact the prescriber to report treatment failure, serious side effects, or new pain.

Drug Therapy

The goal in teaching patients about analgesic drugs is to maximize pain relief and minimize harm. To help achieve this goal, patients should know the following about each drug they take:

- Drug name and therapeutic category
- Dosage size and dosing schedule
- Route and technique of administration
- Expected therapeutic response and when it should develop
- Duration of treatment
- Method of drug storage and disposal
- Symptoms of major adverse effects and measures to minimize discomfort and harm
- Major adverse drug-drug and drug-food interactions
- Whom to contact in the event of therapeutic failure, severe adverse effects, or severe adverse interactions

The dosing schedule should be discussed. Patients should understand that PRN dosing is appropriate only if pain is intermittent. When pain is persistent, as it is for most patients, the objective is to *prevent* pain from returning. Hence dosing should be done on a fixed schedule ATC, not PRN. However, even with ATC dosing, breakthrough pain can occur. Hence patients should be taught what drug and dosage to use for rescue treatment.

Fears based on misconceptions about opioids can impair compliance and can thereby impair pain control. The misconceptions that influence compliance the most relate to tolerance, physical dependence, addiction, and side effects. To correct these misconceptions, and thereby dispel fears and improve compliance, the following topics should be discussed:

- *Tolerance*—Some patients fear that, because of tolerance, taking opioids now will decrease their effectiveness later. Hence, to help ensure pain relief in the future, they limit opioid use now and thus suffer needless pain. These patients should be reassured that, if tolerance does develop, efficacy can be restored by increasing the dosage; tolerance does not mean that efficacy is lost.
- *Physical dependence and addiction*—Many patients fear opioid addiction and hence are reluctant to take these drugs. This fear is based largely on the misconception

that physical dependence (which eventually develops in all patients) equals addiction. Patients should be taught that physical dependence is not the same as addiction and that physical dependence itself is nothing to fear. In addition, they should be taught that the behavior pattern that constitutes addiction rarely develops in people who take opioids in a therapeutic setting.

- *Fear of severe side effects*—Some patients fear that opioids cannot relieve pain without causing severe side effects. These patients should be reassured that, when used correctly, opioids are both safe and effective. The most dangerous side effect—respiratory depression—is uncommon.

The rationale for using an adjuvant analgesic should be discussed. With all of the adjuvants, the objective is to *complement* the effects of opioid and nonopioid analgesics. Adjuvants are not intended to substitute for these drugs. Furthermore, because the drugs we use as adjuvants were originally developed to treat disorders other than pain, the rationale for prescribing specific adjuvants should be explained. For example, when imipramine is prescribed, the patient should understand that the objective is to relieve neuropathic pain and not depression, the disorder for which this drug was originally developed.

Basic issues related to patient education in drug therapy are discussed in Chapter 3

THE JOINT COMMISSION PAIN MANAGEMENT STANDARDS

The Joint Commission (TJC) established a set of standards designed to make assessment and management of pain a priority in the nation's health care system. Under the standards, *accountability for pain management is shifted from individual practitioners to the institution as a whole.* Compliance is mandatory: health care organizations that fail to meet the standards will lose accreditation. Loss of accreditation would mean loss of insurance reimbursement and would disqualify teaching hospitals from offering training programs. Hence, thanks to the enforcement power wielded by TJC, health care institutions in the United States now have a very real incentive to correct the persistent problem of pain undertreatment. It should be noted that the standards are *not* a guideline on how to treat specific kinds of pain. Rather, they focus on (1) the rights of patients to receive appropriate assessment and management of pain and (2) ways for institutions to establish a formalized, systematic approach to pain management that involves interdisciplinary teams whose members have clearly identified responsibilities. Specific provisions include the following:

- Institutions must recognize assessment and management of pain as a right of all patients.
- Institutions must assess all patients for pain and, if pain is present, identify its nature and intensity.
- Pain must be regarded as a "fifth vital sign," and pain intensity must be quantified and recorded along with blood pressure, heart rate, respiration, and temperature.
- Institutions must educate patients and their families about pain management and must provide ready access to educational materials.
- Institutions must educate clinical staff about assessment and management of pain and must document the education provided.
- Institutions must establish a system to monitor pain management, including a system of checks and balances in which individuals who assess and manage pain are monitored for compliance with standards set by the institution.
- Institutions must monitor patient satisfaction with pain management.
- Discharge planning must provide for continuing reassessment and management of pain.

TJC has inserted content related to pain management throughout existing manuals, as well as on their website. Current TJC resources regarding pain can be found at http://www.jointcommission.org/pain_management/.

UNIT XX

Drugs for Eyes, Ears, and Skin

CHAPTER 84

Drugs for the Eye

Jacqueline Rosenjack Burchum, DNSc, FNP-BC, CNE

The drugs addressed in this chapter are used to diagnose and treat disorders of the eye. Our primary focus is on glaucoma. Many of the drugs considered here are discussed in other chapters, so discussion in this chapter is limited to ophthalmologic applications.

DRUGS FOR GLAUCOMA

Glaucoma refers to a group of diseases characterized by a decrease in peripheral vision secondary to optic nerve damage. The most common forms of glaucoma are primary open-angle glaucoma and acute angle-closure glaucoma. These forms differ with respect to underlying pathology and treatment.

In the United States glaucoma is the leading cause of preventable blindness. Of the 120,000 Americans blinded each year by glaucoma, 90% could have saved their sight with timely treatment. Unfortunately, many afflicted persons are unaware of their condition: of the 4 million Americans with glaucoma, only 50% are diagnosed.

Before discussing glaucoma, we need to review the role of aqueous humor in maintaining intraocular pressure (IOP). As shown in Fig. 84.1, aqueous humor is produced by the ciliary body and secreted into the posterior chamber of the eye. From there it circulates around the iris into the anterior chamber and then exits the anterior chamber through the trabecular meshwork and canal of Schlemm. If outflow from the anterior chamber is impeded, back-pressure will develop, and IOP will rise. Conversely, if production of aqueous humor falls, IOP will decline.

Pathophysiology and Treatment Overview

Primary Open-Angle Glaucoma

Characteristics

Primary open-angle glaucoma (POAG) is the most common form of glaucoma in the United States. About 90% of people with glaucoma have this type. POAG is a leading cause of blindness in the United States.

POAG is characterized by progressive optic nerve damage with eventual impairment of vision. Visual loss develops first in the peripheral visual field. As the disease advances, loss occurs in the central visual field. The pathologic process that leads to optic nerve damage is not understood. IOP is often elevated, but it may also be normal. POAG is a painless, insidious disease in which injury develops over years. Symptoms are absent until extensive optic nerve damage has been produced.

Risk Factors

The major risk factors for POAG are the following:

- Elevated IOP
- African or South American ancestry
- Family history of POAG
- Advancing age

Of these, elevated IOP is most important. Please note, however, that glaucomatous optic nerve damage can develop even when IOP is normal (i.e., below 20 mm Hg). Furthermore, some individuals can have very high IOP (e.g., 30 mm Hg) with no associated injury to the optic nerve. These individuals are said to have *ocular hypertension*—not glaucoma.

Screening

Because POAG has no symptoms (until significant and irreversible optic nerve injury has occurred), regular testing for early POAG is important among individuals at high risk. With early detection and treatment, blindness can usually be prevented.

Management

Treatment of POAG is directed at reducing elevated IOP, the only risk factor we can modify. Although POAG has no cure, reduction of IOP can slow or even stop disease progression. Management is usually initiated by specialists; however, primary care providers often play a role in ongoing monitoring and follow-up of patients taking these medications.

The principal method for reducing IOP is chronic therapy with drugs. Drugs lower IOP by either (1) facilitating aqueous humor outflow or (2) reducing aqueous humor production. As indicated in Table 84.1, the first-line drugs for glaucoma belong to three classes: *beta-adrenergic blocking agents* (beta blockers), *alpha$_2$-adrenergic agonists,* and *prostaglandin analogs.* Other options—*cholinergic drugs* and *carbonic anhydrase inhibitors*—are considered second-line choices. All of the

Patient Education

GLAUCOMA

- It is important to take the prescribed medications according to schedule. If days are skipped or if prescriptions are not refilled, loss of vision may occur.
- Notify the provider immediately if experiencing vision loss, severe eye pain, headache, or nausea and vomiting. These could indicate angle-closure glaucoma.
- If photophobia is a problem when outdoors, sunglasses, wide-brimmed hats, visors, or baseball caps may be helpful.
- Check labels of ophthalmic drugs to see if they contain benzalkonium as a preservative. These drugs may be absorbed by soft contact lenses. Allow at least 15 minutes to elapse between administration and insertion of the lenses.

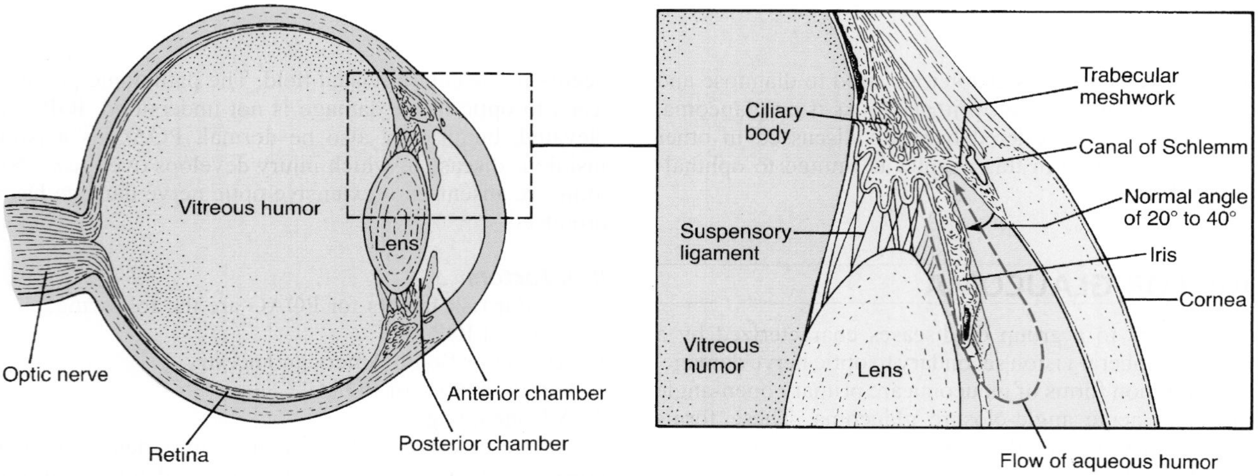

Figure 84.1 ■ Anatomy of the normal eye.

TABLE 84.1 ■ Topical Drugs for Open-Angle Glaucoma

Class	Drugs	Mechanism	Adverse Effects
FIRST-LINE AGENTS			
Beta blockers		Decreased aqueous humor formation	
Nonselective	Timolol Carteolol Levobunolol Metipranolol		Heart block, bradycardia, bronchospasm
$Beta_1$ selective	Betaxolol		Heart block, bradycardia, hypotension
Prostaglandin analogs	Latanoprost Travoprost Bimatoprost	Increased aqueous humor outflow	Heightened brown pigmentation of the iris and eyelid
$Alpha_2$-adrenergic agonists	Apraclonidine* Brimonidine	Decreased aqueous humor formation	Headache, dry mouth, dry nose, altered taste, conjunctivitis, lid reactions, pruritus
SECOND-LINE AGENTS			
Cholinergic drugs		Increased aqueous humor outflow	
Muscarinic agonists	Pilocarpine		Miosis, blurred vision
Cholinesterase inhibitors	Echothiophate		Miosis, blurred vision
Carbonic anhydrase inhibitors	Dorzolamide Brinzolamide	Decreased aqueous humor formation	Ocular stinging, bitter taste, conjunctivitis, lid reactions

*Apraclonidine is indicated for short-term use only and therefore is *not* a first-line drug for glaucoma.

antiglaucoma drugs are available for topical administration, which is the preferred route. For more than 25 years, the beta blockers (e.g., timolol) have been considered drugs of first choice. However, the $alpha_2$ agonists (e.g., brimonidine) and prostaglandin analogs (e.g., latanoprost) are just as effective as the beta blockers and have a more desirable side-effect profile. Accordingly, these drugs have joined the beta blockers as first-choice agents. Because drugs in different classes lower IOP by different mechanisms, combined therapy can be more effective than monotherapy. Because all of these drugs are applied topically, systemic effects are relatively uncommon. Nonetheless, serious systemic reactions *can* occur if sufficient absorption takes place.

If drugs are unable to reduce IOP to an acceptable level, surgical intervention to promote outflow of aqueous humor is indicated. Options include trabeculectomy and laser trabeculoplasty.

Angle-Closure Glaucoma

Angle-closure glaucoma is precipitated by displacement of the iris such that it covers the trabecular meshwork, thereby preventing exit of aqueous humor from the anterior chamber. As a result, IOP increases rapidly and to dangerous levels. This disorder is referred to as *angle-closure* or *narrow-angle* glaucoma because the angle between the cornea and the iris is greatly reduced (Fig. 84.2). Angle-closure glaucoma develops suddenly and is extremely painful. In the absence of treatment, irreversible loss of vision occurs in 1 to 2 days. This disorder is much less common than open-angle glaucoma.

Treatment consists of *drug therapy* (to control the acute attack) followed by *corrective surgery.* A combination of drugs (osmotic agents, short-acting miotics, carbonic anhydrase inhibitors, topical beta-adrenergic blocking agents) is employed to suppress symptoms. After IOP has been reduced with drugs, definitive treatment can be rendered with surgery. Options include *iridectomy* and *laser iridotomy.* Both procedures alter the iris to permit unimpeded outflow of aqueous humor.

Drugs Used to Treat Glaucoma

Beta-Adrenergic Blocking Agents

Actions and Use in Glaucoma

Five beta blockers—*betaxolol, carteolol, levobunolol, metipranolol,* and *timolol*—are approved for use in glaucoma. Dosing is topical. These agents cause minimal disturbance of vision and are considered first-line drugs for glaucoma, although prostaglandin analogs are becoming favored. Formulations and dosages of the beta blockers are shown in Table 84.2.

The beta-adrenergic blockers lower IOP by decreasing production of aqueous humor. Reductions in IOP occur with

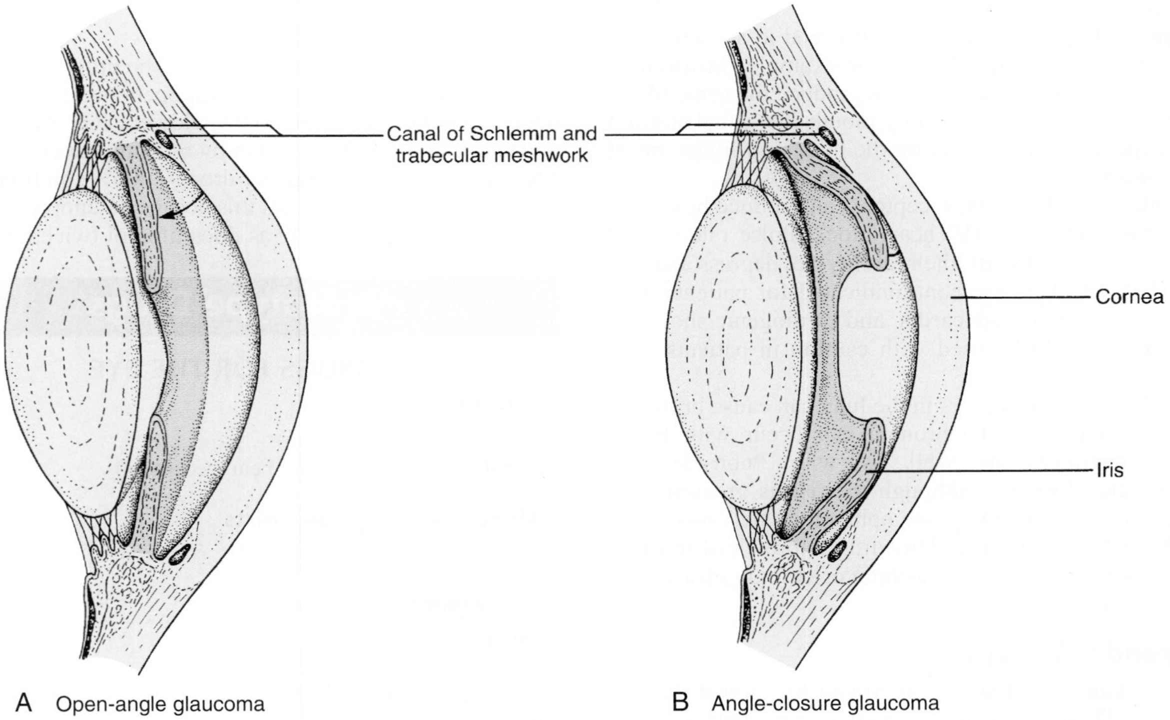

Figure 84.2 ■ Comparative anatomy of the eye in open-angle and angle-closure glaucoma.
A, Note that the angle between the iris and cornea is open in open-angle glaucoma, permitting unimpeded outflow of aqueous humor through the canal of Schlemm and trabecular meshwork. **B,** Note that the angle between the iris and cornea is constricted in angle-closure glaucoma, thereby blocking outflow of aqueous humor through the canal of Schlemm and trabecular meshwork.

TABLE 84.2 ▪ Beta Blockers Used in Glaucoma

Drug	Receptor Specificity	Formulation	Usual Dosage
Betaxolol [Betoptic S]	$Beta_1$	0.25% suspension	1 drop twice a day
Carteolol	$Beta_1$, $beta_2$	1% solution	1 drop twice a day
Levobunolol [Betagan Liquifilm, AKBeta]	$Beta_1$, $beta_2$	0.25% solution	1 drop twice a day
		0.5% solution	1 drop once or twice a day
Metipranolol [OptiPranolol]	$Beta_1$, $beta_2$	0.3% solution	1 drop twice a day
Timolol [Timoptic, Betimol, Istalol]	$Beta_1$, $beta_2$	0.25% solution	1 drop once or twice a day
		0.5% solution	1 drop once or twice a day
		0.25% gel	1 drop once a day
		0.5% gel	1 drop once a day

"nonselective" beta blockers (drugs that block $beta_1$ *and* $beta_2$ receptors) as well as with "cardioselective" beta blockers (drugs that block $beta_1$ receptors only).

Beta blockers are used primarily for open-angle glaucoma. They are suitable for initial therapy as well as maintenance therapy. Beta blockers, in combination with other drugs, are also employed for emergency management of acute angle-closure glaucoma.

The basic pharmacology of the beta blockers is discussed in Chapter 14.

Adverse Effects

Local. Local effects are generally minimal, although patients commonly complain of transient ocular stinging. Beta blockers occasionally cause conjunctivitis, blurred vision, photophobia, and dry eyes.

Systemic. Beta blockers can be absorbed in amounts sufficient to cause systemic effects. For example, instilling 1 drop of 0.5% timolol in each eye can produce the same blood level as taking 10 mg of timolol by mouth (the usual starting dose for hypertension). Effects on the heart and lungs are of greatest concern.

Blockade of cardiac $beta_1$ receptors can produce bradycardia and atrioventricular (AV) heart block. Pulse rate should be monitored. Because of their ability to depress cardiac function, beta blockers are contraindicated for patients with AV heart block, sinus bradycardia, and cardiogenic shock. In addition, they should be used with caution in patients with heart failure.

Blockade of $beta_2$ receptors in the lung can cause bronchospasm. Constriction of the bronchi can occur with $beta_1$-selective antagonists as well as with "nonselective" beta-adrenergic blockers—although the risk is greatest with the nonselective agents. Only one ophthalmic beta blocker—betaxolol—is $beta_1$ selective. This drug is preferred to other beta blockers for patients with asthma or chronic obstructive pulmonary disease.

Prostaglandin Analogs

Four prostaglandin analogs are approved for topical therapy of glaucoma. These drugs are as effective as the beta blockers and cause fewer side effects. Accordingly, they are considered first-line medications for glaucoma. Formulations and dosages are shown in Table 84.3.

Latanoprost

Latanoprost [Xalatan], an analog of prostaglandin F_2 alpha, was the first prostaglandin approved for glaucoma and will serve as our prototype for the group. The drug is applied topically to lower IOP in patients with open-angle glaucoma and ocular hypertension. Latanoprost lowers IOP by facilitating aqueous humor outflow, in part by relaxing the ciliary muscle. The recommended dosage is 1 drop (0.005% solution) applied once daily in the evening. At this dosage, latanoprost produces the same reduction in IOP as does timolol twice daily.

TABLE 84.3 ▪ Prostaglandin Analogs Used in Glaucoma

Generic Name	Trade Name	Formulation	Usual Dosage
Latanoprost	Xalatan	0.005% solution	1 drop once daily in the evening
Travoprost	Travatan	0.004% solution	1 drop once daily in the evening
Bimatoprost	Lumigan	0.01% solution	1 drop once daily in the evening
		0.03% solution	1 drop once daily in the evening
Tafluprost	Zioptan	0.0015% solution	1 drop once daily in the evening

Prototype Drugs

DRUGS FOR THE EYE

Beta Blockers

Betaxolol ($beta_1$ selective)
Timolol (blocks $beta_1$ and $beta_2$ receptors)

Alpha-Adrenergic Agonists

Brimonidine

Prostaglandin Analogs

Latanoprost

Angiogenesis Inhibitors

Ranibizumab

Latanoprost is generally well tolerated, and systemic reactions are rare. The most significant side effect is a harmless heightened brown pigmentation of the iris, which is most noticeable in patients whose irides are green-brown, yellow-brown, or blue/gray-brown. The effect is rare in patients whose irides are blue, green, or blue-green. Heightened pigmentation stops progressing when latanoprost is discontinued but does not usually regress. Topical latanoprost may also increase pigmentation of the eyelid and may increase the length, thickness, and pigmentation of the eyelashes. Other side effects include blurred vision, burning, stinging, conjunctival hyperemia, and punctate keratopathy. Rarely, latanoprost may cause migraine.

Other Prostaglandin Analogs

In addition to latanoprost, three other topical prostaglandins are approved for topical therapy of glaucoma. Like latanoprost, these drugs—travoprost [Travatan], bimatoprost [Lumigan], and tafluprost [Zioptan]—reduce IOP by increasing aqueous humor outflow. In clinical trials, these agents were at least as effective as timolol, a representative beta blocker. Interestingly, one drug—travoprost—was more effective in blacks than in nonblacks. Like latanoprost, these prostaglandins can cause a gradual increase in brown pigmentation of the iris, which may be irreversible. In addition, these drugs can increase pigmentation of the eyelid and growth of the eyelashes. In fact, bimatoprost, marketed as Latisse, is used for the specific purpose of increasing eyelash length, darkness, and thickness. With prostaglandins used to treat glaucoma, the most common adverse effect is ocular hyperemia (engorgement of ocular blood vessels). Less commonly, these drugs cause blurred vision, eye discomfort, ocular pruritus, conjunctivitis, dry eye, light intolerance, and tearing.

Alpha$_2$-Adrenergic Agonists

Two alpha$_2$ agonists are approved for glaucoma. One agent—apraclonidine—is used only for short-term therapy. The other agent—brimonidine—has emerged as a first-line drug for long-term therapy.

Brimonidine

Brimonidine [Alphagan P, Alphagan ♣] is the first and only topical alpha$_2$-adrenergic agonist approved for *long-term* reduction of elevated IOP in patients with open-angle glaucoma or ocular hypertension. Effects on IOP are similar to those achieved with timolol. The drug lowers IOP by reducing aqueous humor production and perhaps by increasing outflow. In addition to lowering IOP, brimonidine may delay optic nerve degeneration and may protect retinal neurons from death. This possibility arises from the ability of alpha$_2$ agonists to protect neurons from injury caused by ischemia. The most common adverse effects are dry mouth, ocular hyperemia, local burning and stinging, headache, blurred vision, foreign body sensation, and ocular itching. In contrast to apraclonidine (see later), brimonidine can cross the blood-brain barrier and hence can cause drowsiness, fatigue, and hypotension. (Recall from Chapter 13 that activation of alpha$_2$ receptors in the brain decreases sympathetic outflow to blood vessels, and thereby lowers blood pressure.) Brimonidine can be absorbed onto soft contact lenses. Accordingly, at least 15 minutes should elapse between drug administration and lens installation.

Apraclonidine

Apraclonidine [Iopidine], a topical alpha$_2$-adrenergic agonist, lowers IOP by reducing aqueous humor production and possibly by increasing outflow. The drug is indicated only for (1) short-term therapy of open-angle glaucoma in patients who have not responded adequately to maximal doses of other IOP-lowering drugs and (2) preoperative medication before laser trabeculoplasty or iridotomy. Side effects include headache, dry mouth, dry nose, altered taste, conjunctivitis, lid reactions, pruritus, tearing, and blurred vision. Apraclonidine does not cross the blood-brain barrier and thus does not promote hypotension.

Alpha$_2$ Agonist/Beta Blocker Combination

A fixed-dose combination of brimonidine (an alpha$_2$ agonist) and timolol (a nonselective beta blocker) is available for lowering IOP in patients with glaucoma or ocular hypertension. Benefits and adverse effects are about equal to those seen when the two drugs are applied separately. Formulations and dosages for the alpha$_1$ agonist and the alpha$_2$ agonist/beta blocker combination are shown in Table 84.4.

Pilocarpine, a Direct-Acting Muscarinic Agonist

Pilocarpine is a direct-acting muscarinic agonist (parasympathomimetic agent). Administration is topical. The basic pharmacology of the muscarinic agonists is discussed in Chapter 12. Consideration here is limited to the use of pilocarpine in glaucoma.

Effects on the Eye

By stimulating cholinergic receptors in the eye, pilocarpine produces two direct effects: (1) miosis (constriction of the pupil secondary to contraction of the iris sphincter) and (2) contraction of the ciliary muscle (an action that focuses the lens for near vision). IOP is lowered indirectly. In patients with open-angle glaucoma, IOP is reduced because the tension generated by contracting the ciliary muscle promotes widening of the spaces within the trabecular meshwork, thereby facilitating outflow of aqueous humor. In angle-closure glaucoma, contraction of the iris sphincter pulls the iris away from the pores of the trabecular meshwork, thereby removing the impediment to aqueous humor outflow.

Therapeutic Uses

Although used widely in the past, pilocarpine is now considered a second-line drug for open-angle glaucoma. Pilocarpine can also be used for emergency treatment of acute angle-closure glaucoma.

Adverse Effects

The major side effects of pilocarpine concern the eye. Contraction of the ciliary muscle focuses the lens for near vision; corrective lenses can provide partial compensation for this problem. Occasionally, sustained contraction of the ciliary muscle causes retinal detachment. Constriction of the pupil, caused by contraction of the iris sphincter, may decrease visual acuity. Pilocarpine may also produce local irritation, eye pain, and brow ache.

Rarely, pilocarpine is absorbed in amounts sufficient to cause systemic effects. Stimulation of muscarinic receptors throughout the body can produce a variety of responses, including bradycardia, bronchospasm, hypotension, urinary urgency, diarrhea, hypersalivation, and sweating. Caution should be exercised in patients with asthma or bradycardia. Systemic toxicity can be reversed with a muscarinic antagonist (e.g., atropine).

Pilocarpine is available in solution and a gel for topical use. Pilocarpine solutions have a relatively short duration of action and must be administered more frequently than the gel. Formulations and dosages are shown in Table 84.5.

TABLE 84.4 ▪ Alpha$_2$ Agonists Used in Glaucoma

Generic Name	Trade Name	Formulation	Usual Dosage
Brimonidine	Alphagan P	0.1% and 0.15% solutions (0.2% solution available in Canada)	1 drop approximately every 8 hr
Apraclonidine	Iopidine	0.5% solution	1–2 drops approximately every 8 hr
Brimonidine + timolol (a beta blocker)	Combigan	0.2% brimonidine + 0.5% timolol	1 drop approximately every 12 hr

Echothiophate, a Cholinesterase Inhibitor

Only one cholinesterase inhibitor—echothiophate [Phospholine Iodide]—is available for glaucoma. The drug has a long duration of action. The basic pharmacology of echothiophate and other cholinesterase inhibitors is discussed in Chapter 12. Consideration here is limited to its use in glaucoma.

Effects on the Eye

Cholinesterase inhibitors inhibit breakdown of acetylcholine by cholinesterase and thereby promote accumulation of acetylcholine at muscarinic receptors. As a result, they can produce the same ocular effects as pilocarpine (i.e., miosis, focusing of the lens for near vision, reduction of IOP).

Use in Glaucoma

Echothiophate is indicated for POAG. However, because of concerns about adverse effects, the drug is not a first-choice agent. Rather, it is reserved for patients who have responded poorly to preferred medications (e.g., beta blockers, $alpha_2$ agonists, prostaglandins).

Adverse Effects

Like pilocarpine, echothiophate can cause myopia (secondary to contraction of the ciliary muscle) and excessive pupillary constriction. However, of much greater concern is the association between long-acting cholinesterase inhibitors and development of cataracts. Absorption of echothiophate into the systemic circulation can produce typical parasympathomimetic responses, including bradycardia, bronchospasm, sweating, salivation, urinary urgency, and diarrhea.

Preparations, Dosage, and Administration

Echothiophate iodide [Phospholine Iodide] is supplied as a powder for reconstitution to solution. Formulations and dosages are shown in Table 84.5.

Carbonic Anhydrase Inhibitors: Topical

Dorzolamide

Dorzolamide [Trusopt] was the first carbonic anhydrase inhibitor available for topical administration. The drug is used to reduce IOP in patients with open-angle glaucoma and ocular hypertension. Dorzolamide lowers IOP by decreasing production of aqueous humor. Responses are similar to those produced with beta blockers.

Dorzolamide is generally well tolerated. The most common side effects are ocular stinging and bitter taste immediately after dosing. Between 10% and 15% of patients experience allergic reactions, primarily conjunctivitis and lid reactions. If these occur, the patient should stop dorzolamide and contact the prescriber. Other reactions include blurred vision, tearing, eye dryness, and photophobia. In contrast to systemic carbonic anhydrase inhibitors, dorzolamide does not produce acidosis or electrolyte imbalance.

Dorzolamide is also available in a fixed-dose combination with timolol, marketed as Cosopt. The combination produces a greater reduction in IOP than either component used alone. Formulations and dosages for these products as well as other carbonic anhydrase inhibitors shown in Table 84.6.

Brinzolamide

Brinzolamide [Azopt] is approved for topical treatment of elevated IOP in patients with open-angle glaucoma or ocular hypertension. The drug is as effective as dorzolamide and better tolerated. Like other carbonic anhydrase inhibitors, brinzolamide reduces IOP by slowing production of aqueous humor. The most common adverse effects are bitter aftertaste and transient blurred vision. Brinzolamide causes less ocular stinging and burning than dorzolamide. Both brinzolamide and dorzolamide contain the preservative benzalkonium chloride. This is absorbed by soft contact lenses. Patients wearing these should wait 15 minutes after administration before inserting contact lenses.

Carbonic Anhydrase Inhibitors: Systemic

Two carbonic anhydrase inhibitors—acetazolamide and methazolamide—are available for systemic therapy of glaucoma. Acetazolamide is used more often.

Actions and Uses in Glaucoma

Carbonic anhydrase inhibitors lower IOP by decreasing production of aqueous humor. Maximally effective doses reduce aqueous flow by 50%. Administration is oral.

Carbonic anhydrase inhibitors are employed primarily for long-term treatment of open-angle glaucoma. They are not drugs of first choice. Rather, they should be reserved for patients who have been refractory to preferred medications (e.g., beta blockers, $alpha_2$ agonists, prostaglandin analogs). Carbonic anhydrase inhibitors may also be given (in combination with other antiglaucoma drugs) to produce rapid lowering of IOP in patients with angle-closure glaucoma.

Adverse Effects

Systemic carbonic anhydrase inhibitors can produce a variety of adverse effects. Effects on the central nervous system (CNS), which are relatively common, include malaise, anorexia, fatigue, and paresthesias. The sense of malaise causes many patients to discontinue treatment. Reduced appetite,

TABLE 84.5 ▪ Direct and Indirect Parasympathomimetic Preparations Used in Glaucoma

Generic Name	Trade Name	Formulation	Usual Dosage
Pilocarpine solution	Isopto Carpine, Akarpine ♣, Diocarpine ♣	0.5%–8% solution	Open-angle maintenance: 1 drop of solution (0.5%–4%) 4 times daily Acute angle-closure: 1 drop every 5–10 minutes for three to six doses, then 1 drop every 1–3 hr
Pilocarpine Ophthalmic Gel	Pilopine HS	4% pilocarpine hydrochloride in an aqueous gel base	½-inch ribbon at bedtime
Echothiophate	Phospholine Iodide	0.03%–0.25% reconstituted solution	1 drop twice daily Maintenance may be once daily, twice daily, or every other day

TABLE 84.6 ▪ Carbonic Anhydrase Inhibitors Used in Glaucoma

Generic Name	Trade Name	Formulation	Usual Dosage
Dorzolamide	Trusopt	2% solution	1 drop three times daily
Dorzolamide + timolol (a beta blocker)	Cosopt	2% dorzolamide + 0.5% timolol	1 drop twice daily
Brinzolamide	Azopt	1% solution	3 times daily
Acetazolamide	Diamox, Diamox Sequels, Acetazolam ♣	125- and 250-mg tablets 500-mg sustained-release capsules	250 mg to 1 g daily
Methazolamide	Neptazane	25- and 50-mg tablets	50–100 mg 2–3 times daily

coupled with GI disturbances (nausea, vomiting, diarrhea), may result in weight loss. Carbonic anhydrase inhibitors are teratogenic in animals and should be avoided during pregnancy, especially the first trimester. Additional concerns are acid-base disturbances, electrolyte imbalance, and nephrolithiasis.

PRESCRIBING AND MONITORING CONSIDERATIONS FOR GLAUCOMA

Therapeutic Goal

The goal of glaucoma treatment is to prevent progressive visual field loss and acute symptoms (if present) through the reduction of IOP. Because POAG is often asymptomatic, primary care providers have important roles in identifying patients with risk factors. These patients are then screened for glaucoma through visual field testing, funduscopic examination for optic nerve cupping, and tonometry to determine IOP, if available.

Definitive diagnosis and treatment decisions are typically carried out by ophthalmologists. Primary care providers need to be prepared to monitor for outcomes or adverse effects that may indicate a need for a change in management.

Ongoing Monitoring and Interventions

Pharmacologic therapy for POAG is lifelong. Meanwhile, nonadherence to medication regimens is high. Various reasons for high rates of nonadherence have been proposed. These include the asymptomatic nature of the condition, frequent dosing intervals, and age-related issues. Age-related issues may include forgetfulness associated with dementia or failure of providers to continue medications when admitted to tertiary facilities. For these reasons, monitoring is especially important. Outcomes monitoring by the primary care provider may include funduscopic examination and visual field testing. Monitoring of pharmacologic effects depends on the drug prescribed.

Patients taking ophthalmic beta-blockers will need to be assessed for systemic effects. These include hypotension, bradycardia, AV block, and wheezing due to bronchoconstriction.

Prostaglandins have few adverse effects. They are expensive, however, and this may create an adherence issue for patients with limited income.

Patients taking the $alpha_2$ agonist brimonidine should be assessed for CNS effects (e.g., excessive drowsiness) and hypotension. Verify that patients who wear soft contact lenses allow at least 15 minutes to elapse between administration and lens insertion.

Assessment of visual acuity can be important for patients taking the parasympathomimetics pilocarpine and echothiophate. If changes are noted, referral to an optometrist for new glasses may be in order. These patients should also be assessed for cholinergic effects (e.g., wheezing, slowed heart rate, decreased blood pressure, urinary urgency, diarrhea, excessive salivation, and excessive perspiration).

Finally, it is important to remember that a large number of patients will have an allergic response to the topical carbonic anhydrase inhibitor dorzolamide. This will necessitate changing medications. Systemic drugs in this class may need to be discontinued if they cause significant CNS effects such as malaise.

DRUGS FOR ALLERGIC CONJUNCTIVITIS

Pathophysiology

Allergic conjunctivitis (AC) is defined as inflammation of the conjunctiva in response to an allergen. AC may be seasonal or perennial (chronic). Primary symptoms are itching, burning, and a thin, watery discharge. In addition, the conjunctivae are usually red and congested.

Symptoms of AC result from a biphasic immune response. Initially, symptoms are caused by release of inflammatory mediators—histamine, prostaglandins, leukotrienes, and kinins—from mast cells. These mediators stimulate mucus production (and thereby cause discharge), activate nerve endings (and thereby cause itching and burning sensations), and promote vasodilation and increase capillary permeability (and thereby cause redness and congestion). These symptoms peak about 20 minutes after allergen exposure and abate 20 minutes later. After this early response, symptoms typically reappear 6 or more hours later. The late phase is due to recruitment of immune cells—eosinophils, neutrophils, and macrophages—that amplify the inflammatory response.

Drugs Used to Manage Allergic Conjunctivitis

AC can be managed with a variety of topical drugs (Table 84.7). *Mast cell stabilizers* (e.g., cromolyn, lodoxamide) prevent release of inflammatory mediators. Patients should be

Patient Education

ALLERGIC CONJUNCTIVITIS

- Allergen avoidance can reduce the severity of symptoms; for example, avoid being outside on windy days during pollen season if allergic to pollen.
- Mast cell stabilizers, if prescribed, should not be abandoned prematurely. They require several days to develop symptom relief and several weeks to achieve maximal benefit.
- If oral antihistamines are taken for allergy symptoms, they will probably cause eye dryness. Artificial tears or other eye lubricants may provide relief from dryness and the associated discomfort.
- Artificial tears will help flush out allergens that are causing symptoms. These are available over the counter. Application of cold compresses for 5 to 10 minutes at a time may help if discomfort is severe.
- Rubbing eyes and wearing contact lenses may result in worsening of symptoms.
- Notify the provider if symptoms worsen or if there is no relief after 2 weeks of therapy. (This could indicate an underlying problem other than allergic conjunctivitis.)
- Benzalkonium is a common preservative in over-the-counter and prescription eye drops. These drugs may be absorbed by soft contact lenses. Allow at least 15 minutes to elapse between administration and insertion of the lenses.

TABLE 84.7 ▪ Topical Drugs for Allergic Conjunctivitis

Class and Generic Name	Trade Name	Concentration	Usual Daily Dosage
MAST CELL STABILIZERS			
Cromolyn sodium	Crolom, Opticrom	4%	1–2 drops every 4–6 hr
Lodoxamide tromethamine	Alomide	0.1%	1–2 drops 4 times daily
Nedocromil sodium	Alocril	2%	1–2 drops twice daily
H_1-RECEPTOR BLOCKER			
Emedastine difumarate	Emadine	0.05%	1 drop 4 times daily
MAST CELL STABILIZERS/H_1 BLOCKERS			
Alcaftadine	Lastacaft	0.25%	1 drop once daily
Azelastine hydrochloride	Optivar	0.05%	1 drop twice daily
Epinastine	Elestat	0.05%	1 drop twice daily
Ketotifen fumarate	Zaditor, Alaway	0.025%	1 drop every 8–12 hr
Olopatadine hydrochloride	Patanol	0.1%	1 drop twice daily
	Pataday	0.2%	1 drop once daily
Bepotastine besylate	Bepreve	1.5%	1 drop twice daily
NSAIDS			
Ketorolac tromethamine	Acular LS	0.4%	1 drop 4 times daily
	Acuvail	0.45%	1 drop twice daily
	Acular, Acular PF	0.5%	1 drop 4 times daily
GLUCOCORTICOIDS			
Loteprednol etabonate	Alrex	0.2%	1 drop 4 times daily
	Lotemax	0.5%	1–2 drops 4 times daily
Dexamethasone sodium phosphate	Various	0.1%	1 drop every 6–8 hr
Fluorometholone	FML (ointment)	0.1%	½ inch ribbon 1–3 times daily
	Flarex (suspension)	0.1%	1 drop every 4 hr × 24–48 hr, then 1–2 drops 4 times daily
Prednisolone acetate	Various	1%	2 drops every 6–12 hr
Prednisolone sodium phosphate	Various	1%	1 drop every 6–8 hr
Rimexolone*	Vexol	1%	1–2 drops every 1–4 hr
DECONGESTANTS (VASOCONSTRICTORS)			
Naphazoline	Clear Eyes	0.012%	1–2 drops up to 4 times daily
Oxymetazoline	Visine L.R., OcuClear	0.025%	1–2 drops 4 times daily
Phenylephrine	Neo-Synephrine	0.12%	1–2 drops 4 times daily
Tetrahydrozoline	Visine Moisturizing	0.05%	1–2 drops 4 times daily
DECONGESTANT/H_1 BLOCKER			
Naphazoline/pheniramine	Naphcon-A	0.025%/0.3%	1–2 drops 1–4 times daily
Naphazoline/pheniramine	Opcon-A	0.27%/0.325%	1–2 drops 1–4 times daily

*Off-label use.
NSAIDs, nonsteroidal antiinflammatory drugs.

informed that benefits take several days to develop and several weeks to become maximal. In contrast to mast cell stabilizers, *histamine-1* (H_1)*-receptor antagonists* (antihistamines) can provide immediate symptomatic relief. Some drugs (e.g., azelastine, olopatadine) have two actions: they prevent mediator release from mast cells, and they block H_1 receptors. Ketorolac, a *nonsteroidal antiinflammatory drug* (NSAID), reduces symptoms by inhibiting cyclooxygenase, an enzyme required for synthesis of prostaglandins.

Like the NSAIDs, *glucocorticoids* (e.g., loteprednol) inhibit production of prostaglandins. In addition, glucocorticoids inhibit production of leukotrienes and thromboxane. As a result, these drugs are highly effective. Because they have been associated with serious adverse effects, prescribing should be done by a specialist with the equipment to verify that symptoms are not caused by an underlying infection such as herpes. Unfortunately, with prolonged use, they can cause serious adverse effects, including cataracts, eye infection, and elevation of IOP. Accordingly, glucocorticoids are generally reserved for short-term therapy in patients who have not responded adequately to safer drugs.

The *ocular decongestants* (e.g., naphazoline, phenylephrine) decrease redness and edema by activating alpha$_1$-adrenergic receptors on blood vessels, thereby causing vasoconstriction. Benefits are only symptomatic; these drugs do not interrupt any phase of the immune response. Furthermore, with regular use, rebound congestion is likely. For this reason, short-term use of no longer than 2 weeks is recommended. Fortunately, that gives time for drugs such as mast cell stabilizers to become effective.

PRESCRIBING AND MONITORING CONSIDERATIONS

Assessment

Therapeutic Goal

The goal of treatment is to decrease inflammation and discomfort associated with the allergic conjunctivitis. Early intervention may also decrease associated complications that occur secondary to dry eyes or vigorous eye rubbing.

Before making a decision for therapy, it is important to determine the severity of symptoms. This can be used to guide treatment decisions (Fig. 84.3).

- Mild symptoms: mild pruritus that is intermittent or short lived
- Moderate symptoms: mild to severe pruritus lasting a few days to 2 weeks without eye redness
- Severe symptoms: moderate to severe pruritus that is chronic with eye redness

Identifying High-Risk Patients

The ocular decongestants are contraindicated for the patient with a history of angle-closure glaucoma.

Ongoing Monitoring and Interventions

Monitoring is needed to identify the success of interventions and the need to take therapy to a higher or lower level. Ideally, the least amount of drugs necessary to control symptoms should be used for the shortest time necessary.

If ocular decongestants (e.g., naphazoline, phenylephrine) have been prescribed, these need to be discontinued after a couple of weeks. Failure to do so may result in rebound congestion.

Most medications used to manage AC do not have significant adverse-effect profiles. The exception is glucocorticoids. Prescribing should be restricted to specialists in eye care such as ophthalmologists. Because it decreases immune responses, it is important to consider whether new symptoms may indicate an infection. If prescribed long-term, monitoring should include assessment for cataract development and elevation of IOP.

ADDITIONAL OPHTHALMIC DRUGS

Drugs for Dry Eyes

Ophthalmic demulcents (artificial tears) are isotonic solutions employed as substitutes for natural tears. Most preparations contain polyvinyl alcohol, cellulose esters, or both. Artificial tears are indicated for relieving dry-eye syndromes and discomfort and dryness caused by irritants, wind, and sun. In addition, demulcents may be used to lubricate artificial eyes. Artificial tears are devoid of adverse effects and hence may be administered as often and as long as desired.

Topical cyclosporine ophthalmic emulsion [Restasis] is prescribed for dry eyes due to inflammation. It suppresses the immune response, thereby promoting resumption of tear production.

Ocular Decongestants

Ocular decongestants are weak solutions of adrenergic agonists applied topically to constrict dilated conjunctival blood vessels. These preparations are used to reduce redness of the eye caused by minor irritation. The adrenergic

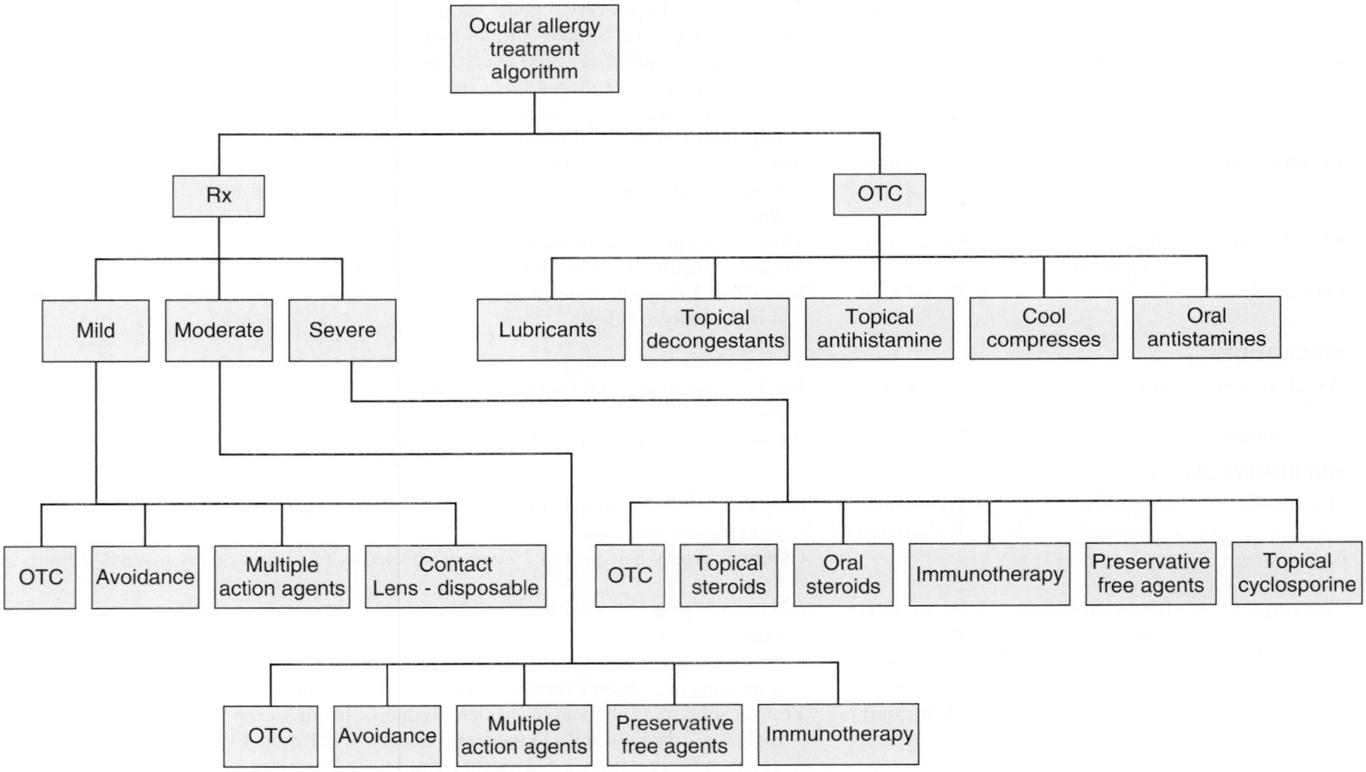

Figure 84.3 ■ Management of allergic conjunctivitis.
(From Bielory L, Meltzer EO, Nichols KK, et al. An algorithm for the management of allergic conjunctivitis. Allergy Asthma Proc 2013;34:408–420. Copyright © 2013, OceanSide Publications, Inc., U.S.A.)

agents employed as decongestants are phenylephrine, naphazoline, oxymetazoline, and tetrahydrozoline. When applied to the eye in the low concentrations found in decongestant products, adrenergic agonists rarely cause adverse effects. Local reactions (stinging, burning, reactive hyperemia) may occur with overuse. The adrenergic agonists are discussed in Chapter 13.

Glucocorticoids

Glucocorticoids are used for inflammatory disorders of the eye (e.g., uveitis, iritis, conjunctivitis). Short-term therapy, in the absence of infection, is generally devoid of adverse effects. In contrast, prolonged therapy may cause cataracts, reduced visual acuity, and glaucoma. In addition, there is an increased risk for infection secondary to glucocorticoid-induced suppression of host defenses. The glucocorticoids are discussed in Chapter 56.

Dyes

Fluorescein is a water-soluble dye that produces an intense green color. This agent is applied to the surface of the eye to detect lesions of the corneal epithelium; intact areas of the cornea remain uncolored, whereas abrasions and other defects turn bright green. Intravenous (IV) fluorescein is used to facilitate visualization of retinal blood vessels; IV fluorescein has been employed to help evaluate diabetic retinopathy and other abnormalities of the retinal vasculature. Fluorescein can also be used topically and intravenously to assess flow of aqueous humor. Adverse effects from systemic administration include nausea, vomiting, paresthesias, and pruritus. Severe reactions (anaphylaxis, pulmonary edema, cardiac arrest) are rare.

Rose bengal is applied topically to visualize abrasions of the corneal and conjunctival epithelium. Injured tissue appears rose colored when viewed with a slit lamp. The dye is also employed for diagnosis of dryness of conjunctival tissue.

Lissamine green, another topical dye, turns bright green in the presence of conjunctival defects and dryness. Because it is less likely to cause stinging, it is beginning to replace rose bengal as a diagnostic tool.

Topical Drugs for Ocular Infections

Topical drugs are available for treating viral and bacterial infections of the eye. Four antiviral drugs—trifluridine, vidarabine, ganciclovir, and idoxuridine—are employed. The pharmacology of antiviral drugs is discussed in Chapter 78. Important antibacterial drugs are shown in Table 84.8. These drugs are used to treat serious ophthalmic infections and to prevent infection after ocular surgery. As a rule, antiinfective drugs are not needed for simple conjunctivitis. Patients should be made aware that bacterial and viral infections are contagious. Bacterial infections will remain contagious until treated for 24 to 48 hours. Viral infections may remain contagious until they are completely gone. Patients should not use contact lenses while they have an eye infection and while they are treating the infection with a topical drug.

TABLE 84.8 ▪ Some Topical Ophthalmic Antibacterial Agents

Class and Generic Name	Trade Name	Formulation	Typical Dosage*
FLUOROQUINOLONES			
Besifloxacin	Besivance	0.6% suspension	Instill 1 drop in affected eye 3 times daily administered 4–12 hours apart x 7 days
Ciprofloxacin	Ciloxan	0.3% solution, 0.3% ointment	Solution: Instill 1 or 2 drops in affected eye every 2 hours while awake x 2 days, then 1 or 2 drops every 4 hours while awake x 5 days Ointment: Apply 1/2" ribbon 3 times daily x 2 days, then 2 times daily x 5 days
Gatifloxacin	Zymar ♣	0.3% solution	Instill 1 drop in affected eye(s) every 2 hours while awake x 2 days (maximum 8 times daily), then 1 drop 4 times daily while awake x 5 days
	Zymaxid	0.5% solution	Instill 1 drop in affected eye every 2 hours while awake (maximum 8 times) the first day, then 1 drop 2–4 times daily while awake for 6 days.
Levofloxacin	Quixin	0.5% solution	Instill 1 to 2 drops in affected eye every 2 hours while awake x 2 days (maximum 8 times daily), then 1 to 2 drops every 4 hours while awake for 5 days (maximum 4 times daily)
Moxifloxacin	Moxeza, Vigamox	0.5% solution	Moxeza: Instill 1 drop in affected eye 2 times daily x 7 days Vigamox: Instill 1 drop in affected eye 3 times daily x 7 days
Ofloxacin	Ocuflox	0.3% solution	Instill 1 to 2 drops in affected eye every 2 to 4 hours x 2 days, then instill 1–2 drops 4 times daily x 5 days
MACROLIDES			
Azithromycin	Azasite	1% solution	Instill 1 drop in affected eye(s) twice daily x 2 days, then 1 drop in affected eye once daily x 5 days.
Erythromycin	Ilotycin	0.5% ointment	Apply 1 cm in affected eye up to 6 times daily x 7 days
AMINOGLYCOSIDES			
Gentamicin	Diogent ♣, Gentak	0.3% solution, 0.3% ointment	Solution: Instill 1–2 drops in affected eye every 4 hours or 2 drops every hour for more severe infection Ointment: Apply half-inch (1.25 cm) in affected eye 2–3 times daily given 3–4 hours apart
Tobramycin	Tobrex, Tobrexan ♣	0.3% solution, 0.3% ointment 0.3% viscous solution (Tobrexan)	Ointment: Apply half-inch in affected eye 2 or 3 times daily or every 3 to 4 hours if infection is severe. Solution: Instill 1 to 2 drops in affected eye every 4 hours for mild to moderate infections or 2 drops every hour for severe infections. Viscous solution (Tobrexan [Canadian product]): Instill 1 drop in affected eye twice daily for 7 days for mild to moderate infections or1 drop 4 times daily on the first day then twice daily for 5 days for more severe infections.
SULFONAMIDES			
Sulfacetamide	Bleph-10, Sodium Sulamyd ♣	10% solution, 10% ointment	Solution: Instill 1 to 2 drops every 2 or 3 hours Ointment: Apply $^1/_2$-inch every 3 to 4 hours and at bedtime

TABLE 84.8 ▪ Some Topical Ophthalmic Antibacterial Agents—cont'd

Class and Generic Name	Trade Name	Formulation	Typical Dosage*
POLYMYXIN B–CONTAINING MIXTURES			
Polymyxin B/ bacitracin	AK-Poly-Bac	Ointment	Apply the ointment every 3 or 4 hours x 7–10 days, depending on the severity of the infection.
Polymyxin B/ bacitracin/ neomycin	Neo-Polycin	Ointment	Apply 0.5 inch to affected eye every 3–4 hours for acute infections, or 2 to 3 times daily for mild to moderate infections x 7–10 days
Polymyxin B/ gramicidin/ neomycin	Neosporin, Optimyxin ♣	Solution	Instill 1–2 drops to affected eye every 4 hours or 2 drops per hour x 7–10 days
Polymyxin B/ trimethoprim	Polytrim	Solution	Instill 2 drops in the affected eye every 3 hours (maximum of 6 doses/day) x 7–10 days.

*Dosage is typical for infections such as bacterial conjunctivitis and does not include treatment of corneal ulcers or prophylaxis of neonatal conjunctivitis secondary to sexually transmitted infections.

CHAPTER

85 Drugs for the Skin

Jacqueline Rosenjack Burchum, DNSc, FNP-BC, CNE

When one considers the vast number of skin conditions and the even greater number of pharmacologic agents used in their management, it is easy to see that the topic of dermatologic conditions alone could comprise a separate textbook. Our objective is to discuss dermatologic drugs used to manage a select group of conditions commonly managed by nonspecialists. Most are dosed topically; some are given systemically. Before discussing the dermatologic drugs, we review the anatomy of the skin.

ANATOMY OF THE SKIN

The skin is composed of three distinct layers: the epidermis, the dermis, and a layer of subcutaneous fat. These layers and other features of the skin are shown in Fig. 85.1.

Epidermis

The epidermis is the outermost layer of the skin and is composed almost entirely of closely packed cells. As indicated in Fig. 85.1B, the epidermis itself consists of several layers. The deepest, known as the *basal layer* or *stratum germinativum,* contains the only epidermal cells that are mitotically active. All cells of the epidermis arise from this layer. Production of new cells within the basal layer pushes older cells outward. During their migration, these cells become smaller and flatter. As epidermal cells near the surface of the skin, they die and their cytoplasm is converted to *keratin,* a hard, proteinaceous material. Because of its high content of keratin, the outer layer of the epidermis has a rough, horny texture. Because of its texture, this layer is referred to as the *cornified layer* or *stratum corneum.* The surface of the stratum corneum undergoes continuous exfoliation (shedding). This shedding completes the epidermal growth cycle.

In addition to germinal cells, the basal layer of the epidermis contains *melanocytes.* These cells, which are few in number, produce *melanin,* the pigment that determines skin color. After its synthesis within melanocytes, melanin is transferred to other cells of the epidermis. Melanin protects the skin against ultraviolet (UV) radiation, which is the principal stimulus for melanin production.

Dermis

The dermis underlies the epidermis and is composed largely of connective tissue, primarily collagen. A major function of the dermis is to provide support and nourishment for the epidermis. Structures found in the dermis include blood vessels, nerves, and muscle. The dermis also contains sweat glands, sebaceous glands, and hair follicles. Sebaceous glands secrete an oily composite known as sebum. Almost all sebaceous glands are associated with hair follicles (see Fig. 85.1A).

Subcutaneous Tissue

Subcutaneous tissue consists largely of fat. This fatty layer provides protection and insulation. In addition, the stored fat constitutes a reserve source of calories.

TOPICAL DRUG FORMULATIONS

Topical drugs are provided through a number of vehicles. The most popular are ointments, creams, lotions, gels, foams, powders, and pastes.

Ointments are thick, greasy preparations with an oil or petroleum jelly base and little, if any, water. They provide the highest medication absorption of all formulations. The enhanced penetration makes it especially useful in management of conditions with thickened skin (e.g., with lichenification secondary to prolonged scratching) or inflamed skin. Because it provides an occlusive film that retains moisture, it is not a good choice for weeping or oozing skin conditions or in areas prone to heavy perspiration. It is often an excellent choice, however, for dry skin conditions.

Creams are an oil and water emulsion. Some contain more oil than water, whereas others contain more water than oil. This affects the thickness of their consistency and how oily or sticky they feel on the skin. They are not as thick as ointments, but they are thicker than lotions. Creams tend to be good for inflamed skin and dry sensitive skin. It may or may not be useful for oozing lesions depending on the ratio of water to oil. Creams tend to be more appropriate than ointments for intertriginous areas.

Lotions are water based. Some may contain alcohol or acids, which can cause a burning sensation. They have little, if any, oil; as a result, they have a lighter feel than creams. Lotions are nongreasy, which tends to promote more patient satisfaction. Another advantage of lotions is that they are easy to spread, which makes them a good choice for large areas or for hairy areas. They are suitable for intertriginous areas. Unlike ointments and creams, they are suitable for oily skin and may even decrease oiliness depending on the ingredients.

Gels are transparent preparations that usually contain cellulose with a water or alcohol base. They liquefy on skin contact and often have a cooling effect as they dry. Because they are nongreasy and tend to have drying effects, gels are good choices for oily skin. They spread easily, so they are good for covering large or hairy areas. Because they dry clear and invisible, they may be more acceptable for facial regions.

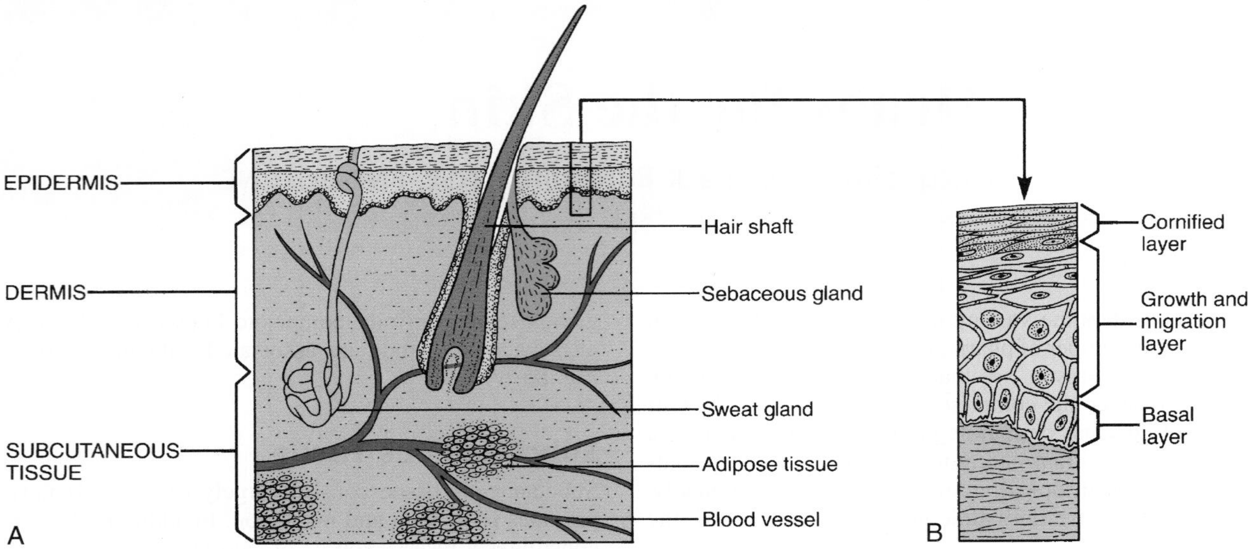

Figure 85.1 ■ Anatomy of the skin.
A, Major structures of the skin. **B,** Growth layers of the epidermis.

These may cause burning, but when this occurs, it is often the fault of the inactive ingredients rather than the medication.

Foams are aerated solutions. They spread easily, dry quickly, and leave negligible residue. They tend to be good choices for oily skin and large or hairy areas.

Most powders have a talc or cornstarch base. They are dry with a silky feel that reduces friction between surfaces. This can make them useful between skin folds. The dryness of the vehicle can be helpful when applied to regions that tend to perspire, such as the feet or axillae.

Pastes are mixtures of an ointment and a powder. The addition of a powder increases adherence to the skin. Because the powder disrupts the occlusive nature of an ointment, allowing for air to reach the covered skin, most pastes can be used safely in areas that are occluded, such as use of Desitin diaper rash paste beneath a diaper.

Topical Glucocorticoids

The basic pharmacology of the glucocorticoids is discussed in Chapter 56. Consideration here is limited to their use for skin disorders.

Actions and Uses

Topical glucocorticoids are employed to relieve inflammation and itching associated with a variety of dermatologic conditions (e.g., insect bites, dermatitis, psoriasis, eczema, pemphigus).

The vehicle in which a glucocorticoid is dispersed (e.g., cream, ointment, gel) can enhance the therapeutic response by helping the glucocorticoid penetrate to its site of action. The vehicle may provide additional benefits by acting as a drying agent or an emollient.

Relative Potency

Glucocorticoid preparations vary widely in potency. As indicated in Table 85.1, these drugs can be assigned to groups that range in potency from low to super high. Preparations within each group are equipotent.

It is important to note that the intensity of the response to topical glucocorticoids depends not only on the concentration and inherent activity of the glucocorticoid but also on the vehicle employed and the method of application. Occlusive dressings can enhance percutaneous absorption by as much as 10-fold, thereby greatly increasing pharmacologic effects.

Absorption

Topical glucocorticoids can be absorbed into the systemic circulation. The extent of absorption is proportional to the duration of use and the surface area covered. Absorption is higher from regions where the skin is especially permeable (axilla, face, eyelids, neck, perineum, genitalia) and lower from regions where penetrability is poor (palms, soles). Absorption through intact skin is lower than through inflamed skin. As noted, absorption is influenced by the vehicle and can be greatly increased by an occlusive dressing.

Adverse Effects

Adverse effects may be local or systemic. Factors that increase the risk for adverse effects include use of a high-potency glucocorticoid, use of an occlusive dressing, prolonged therapy, and application over a large area.

Local Reactions

Glucocorticoids increase the risk for local infection and may also produce irritation. With prolonged use, glucocorticoids can cause atrophy of the dermis and epidermis, resulting in thinning of the skin, striae, purpura, and telangiectasis. Long-term therapy may induce acne and hypertrichosis (excessive growth of hair, especially on the face).

Systemic Toxicity

Topical glucocorticoids can be absorbed in amounts sufficient to produce systemic toxicity. Principal concerns are growth

TABLE 85.1 ■ Relative Potency of Topical Glucocorticoids

Potency Class and Drug	Formulation	Concentration
SUPER-HIGH POTENCY		
Betamethasone dipropionate [Diprolene]	Ointment, lotion, gel	0.05%
Clobetasol propionate [Clobex, Cormax, Temovate]	Cream, ointment, gel, spray, foam, lotion, shampoo	0.05%
Diflorasone diacetate ointment [Psorcon]	Ointment	0.05%
Fluocinonide [Vanos]	Cream	0.1%
Flurandrenolide [Cordran tape]	Tape	4 mcg/m^2
Halobetasol propionate [Ultravate]	Cream, ointment	0.05%
HIGH POTENCY		
Amcinonide [Cyclocort]	Cream, ointment, lotion	0.1%
Betamethasone dipropionate [Diprolene, Diprolene AF]	Cream, ointment, lotion	0.05%
Desoximetasone [Topicort]	Cream, ointment, gel, spray	0.5%, 0.25%
Diflorasone diacetate cream [ApexiCon, Florone, Maxiflor, Psorcon]	Cream	0.05%
Fluocinonide [Fluonex, Lidex, Vanos]	Cream, ointment, gel, solution	0.05%
Halcinonide [Halog]	Cream, ointment	0.1%
Triamcinolone acetonide	Ointment	0.5%
MEDIUM TO HIGH POTENCY		
Amcinonide cream [Cyclocort]	Cream	0.1%
Betamethasone dipropionate cream [Diprosone]	Cream	0.05%
Diflorasone diacetate [ApexiCon, Psorcon]	Cream, ointment	0.05%
Fluocinonide emollient cream [Lidex E]	Cream	0.05%
Fluticasone propionate ointment [Cutivate]	Ointment	0.005%
Triamcinolone acetonide ointment [Aristocort A]	Ointment	0.01%
Triamcinolone high-potency cream [Aristocort-HP]	Cream	0.05%
MEDIUM POTENCY		
Betamethasone dipropionate	Lotion	0.05%
Betamethasone valerate [Beta-Val, Luxiq, Valisone]	Cream, ointment, lotion, foam	0.1%, 0.12%
Clocortolone pivalate [Cloderm]	Cream	0.1%
Desoximetasone [Topicort LP]	Cream, ointment, gel, spray	0.05%
Fluocinolone acetonide [Synalar]	Cream, ointment	0.025%, 0.2%
Flurandrenolide [Cordran, Cordran SP]	Cream, lotion	0.05%
Fluticasone propionate [Cutivate]	Cream	0.05%
Hydrocortisone butyrate [Locoid, Locoid Lipocream]	Cream, ointment, lotion, solution	0.1%
Hydrocortisone valerate [Westcort]	Cream, ointment	0.2%
Mometasone furoate [Elocon]	Cream, ointment, lotion, solution	0.1%
Prednicarbate [Dermatop]	Cream, ointment	0.1%
Triamcinolone acetonide [Kenalog]	Cream, lotion	0.1%
	Ointment	0.025%
	Aerosol	0.2%
LOW POTENCY		
Alclometasone dipropionate [Aclovate]	Cream, ointment	0.05%
Desonide [DesOwen, LoKara, Verdeso]	Cream, ointment, gel, lotion, foam	0.05%
Fluocinolone acetonide [Capex, Synalar]	Cream, oil, shampoo, solution	0.01%
Hydrocortisone acetate [Lanacort 10, U-Cort]	Cream, ointment	1%
Hydrocortisone butyrate [Locoid]	Cream, ointment, lotion, solution	0.1%
Triamcinolone acetonide [Kenalog]	Cream, ointment, lotion	0.025%
LEAST POTENCY		
Hydrocortisone [Ala-Cort, Anusol-HC, Cortaid, Cortizone-10, Hytone]	Cream, ointment, lotion	1%, 2.5%

delay (in children) and adrenal suppression (in all age groups). Systemic toxicity is more likely under extreme conditions of use (prolonged therapy in which a large area is treated with big doses of a high-potency agent covered with an occlusive dressing). When these conditions are present, adrenal suppression can occur.

Administration

Topical glucocorticoids should be applied in a thin film and gently rubbed into the skin. Patients should be advised not to use occlusive dressings (bandages, plastic wraps) unless the prescriber tells them to. Tight-fitting diapers and plastic pants can act as occlusive dressings and should not be worn when glucocorticoids are applied to the diaper region of infants. The same would be true of adults who wear diapers owing to urinary or bowel incontinence.

Keratolytic Agents

Keratolytic agents are drugs that promote shedding of the horny layer of the skin. They are used to treat conditions where there is an overgrowth or abnormal thickening of the skin. Effects range from peeling to extensive desquamation of the stratum corneum. Two keratolytic compounds—*salicylic acid* and *sulfur*—are considered next. A third agent—*benzoyl peroxide*—is discussed later under "Topical Drugs for Acne."

Salicylic Acid

Salicylic acid promotes desquamation by dissolving the intracellular cement that binds scales to the stratum corneum. Keratolytic effects are achieved with concentrations between 3% and 6%. At concentrations above 6%, tissue injury is likely. Low (3%–6%) concentrations are used to treat dandruff, seborrheic dermatitis, acne, and psoriasis. Higher concentrations (up to 40%) are used to remove warts and corns.

Salicylic acid is readily absorbed through the skin. Though rare, systemic salicylate toxicity (salicylism) can result when large amounts are used for a prolonged period. Symptoms of salicylism include tinnitus, hyperpnea, and psychological disturbances. Systemic effects can be minimized by avoiding prolonged use of high concentrations over large areas.

Sulfur

Sulfur promotes peeling and drying. Compounds containing sulfur have been used to treat acne, dandruff, psoriasis, and seborrheic dermatitis. Sulfur is available in lotions, gels, and shampoos. It is commonly combined with salicylic acid for the additive effects (e.g., Sebex shampoo). Concentrations range from 2% to 10%.

ACNE

Acne is the most common dermatologic disease. About 85% of teenagers develop acne, which often persists into adulthood. Acne accounts for more visits to dermatologists than any other disorder. In the United States the direct costs of acne exceed $1 billion a year, including about $100 million spent on acne products sold over the counter.

Prototype Drugs

DRUGS FOR ACNE

Topical Drug for Acne

Benzoyl peroxide
Tretinoin

Oral Drugs for Acne

Isotretinoin
Doxycycline

Pathophysiology

Acne is a chronic skin disorder that usually begins during puberty. The disease is more common and more severe in males. Lesions typically develop on the face, neck, chest, shoulders, and back. In mild acne, *open comedones* (blackheads) are the most common lesion. A comedo forms when sebum combines with keratin to create a plug within a pore (oxidation of the sebum causes the exposed surface of the plug to turn black). *Closed comedones* (whiteheads) develop when pores become blocked with sebum and scales below the skin surface. In its most severe form, acne is characterized by abscesses and inflammatory cysts. As a rule, acne begins to improve after puberty and, for some, clears entirely during the early 20s. However, with some people, the disease continues for decades.

Onset of acne is initiated by increased production of androgens during adolescence. Under the influence of androgens, sebum production and turnover of follicular epithelial cells are increased, leading to plugging of pores. Symptoms are intensified by the activity of *Propionibacterium acnes,* a microbe that converts sebum into irritant fatty acids. This bacterium also releases chemotactic factors that promote inflammation. Oily skin and a genetic predisposition also contribute.

Overview of Treatment

Because acne is a chronic disease, treatment is prolonged. Fortunately, almost all patients respond well. Effective treatment will prevent scarring and limit the duration of symptomatic disease and will thereby minimize the psychological effect of acne.

Nonpharmacologic Therapy

Nonpharmacologic measures can help minimize acne lesions, especially in patients with milder acne. Surface oiliness should be reduced by cleansing with a gentle nonirritant soap a couple of times a day. Care should be taken to avoid irritation from vigorous scrubbing or use of abrasives. Oil-based make-up or moisturizing products should not be used. Additional measures (e.g., comedo extraction, dermabrasion) may be indicated for some individuals. Research has demonstrated that dietary changes provide no benefit.

Drug Therapy

Drugs for acne fall into two major groups: topical drugs and oral drugs (Table 85.2). The topical drugs have two principal subgroups: antibiotics and retinoids. Likewise, the oral drugs have two principal subgroups: antibiotics and retinoids. Occasionally, other agents, such as keratolytic agents (e.g., salicylic or azelaic acid) or hormonal agents (e.g., oral contraceptives [OCs]) may be used.

Drug selection is based on symptom severity. For patients with relatively mild symptoms, topical therapy can suffice. When symptoms are more severe, oral therapy is required. *Mild* acne can be managed with *topical* antibiotics and topical retinoids. *Moderate* acne can be treated with *oral* antibiotics (e.g., doxycycline, minocycline) and comedolytics (retinoids and azelaic acid). In addition, hormonal agents—combination OCs and spironolactone—can be used in young women whose

TABLE 85.2 ▪ Drugs for Acne

TOPICAL DRUGS	
Antibiotics	Benzoyl peroxide (generic only) Clindamycin [Cleocin, others] Erythromycin [Eryderm, others] Dapsone [Aczone] Benzoyl peroxide/clindamycin [BenzaClin, Clindoxyl ♣] Benzoyl peroxide/erythromycin [Benzamycin]
Retinoids	Tretinoin [Atralin, Avita, Retin-A, Retin-A Micro] Adapalene [Differin] Tazarotene [Avage, Tazorac]
Retinoid/antibiotic combinations	Tretinoin/clindamycin [Veltin Gel, Ziana] Adapalene/benzoyl peroxide [Epiduo]
Others	Azelaic acid [Azelex, Finacea ♣]
ORAL DRUGS	
Antibiotics	Doxycycline [Vibramycin, others] Minocycline [Minocin, others] Tetracycline (generic only) Erythromycin [Ery-Tab, others]
Retinoids	Isotretinoin [Amnesteem, Claravis]
Hormonal agents	Combination oral contraceptives Spironolactone [Aldactone]

acne is unresponsive to other drugs. The principal agent for *severe* acne is isotretinoin.

Topical Drugs for Acne

Antibiotics

Benzoyl Peroxide

Benzoyl peroxide, a first-line drug for mild to moderate acne, is both an antibiotic and keratolytic. Improvement can be seen within days of starting treatment. Benefits derive primarily from suppressing growth of *P. acnes.* The presumed mechanism is release of active oxygen. In addition to suppressing *P. acnes,* benzoyl peroxide can reduce inflammation and promote keratolysis (peeling of the horny layer of the epidermis).

Unlike other topical antimicrobials, benzoyl peroxide does not promote emergence of resistant *P. acnes.* In fact, the drug is often combined with clindamycin or erythromycin to protect against resistance to those drugs, which can occur when those antibiotics are used alone.

Benzoyl peroxide may produce drying and peeling of the skin. If signs of severe local irritation occur (e.g., burning, blistering, scaling, swelling), the frequency of application should be reduced. Benzoyl peroxide has been associated with potentially serious hypersensitivity reactions, especially in patients with asthma. In Canada, 131 instances of severe allergies experienced by patients using benzoyl peroxide and/or salicylic acid prompted a safety review. In December, 2015, Health Canada issued a public warning. A revised drug monographs will include information on sensitivity testing. (See http://healthycanadians.gc.ca/recall-alert-rappel-avis/hc-sc/2015/56268a-eng.php.)

Benzoyl peroxide is available in a variety of formulations (e.g., lotion, cream, gel, foam). Concentrations range from 2.5% to 10%. For initial therapy, once-daily application is recommended. Over time, the frequency of administration can be increased (to a maximum of 3 times a day) as tolerance permits. Patients should be advised to keep the drug away from the eyes, mouth, and mucous membranes as well as inflamed or denuded skin.

Clindamycin and Erythromycin

Like benzoyl peroxide, topical clindamycin [Cleocin, others] and erythromycin [Eryderm, others] suppress growth of *P. acnes.* In addition, these drugs can decrease inflammation. Monotherapy with either drug quickly leads to resistance. To protect against emergence of resistance, these drugs can be combined with benzoyl peroxide. Two fixed-dose combinations are available: clindamycin/benzoyl peroxide, sold as *BenzaClin* and *Clindoxyl* ♣; and erythromycin/benzoyl peroxide, sold as *Benzamycin.*

Dapsone

Dapsone [Aczone] has been used for oral therapy of leprosy for decades. In patients with acne, the drug yields a modest decrease in inflammation and number of lesions. The mechanism of action underlying antiacne benefits has not been established. Dapsone is available as a 5% gel in 30-, 60-, and 90-g tubes for twice-daily application. The site should be washed and dried before applying the drug, and the hands should be washed afterward. The most common side effects of dapsone gel are oiliness, peeling, dryness, and erythema. These effects are caused primarily by the gel vehicle, and not by dapsone. Oral dapsone, but not topical dapsone, poses a risk for hemolytic anemia and peripheral neuropathy. Combining dapsone with benzoyl peroxide can turn the skin yellow or orange. Until more is known, dapsone should be reserved for patients who can't tolerate traditional topical treatments.

Retinoids

The topical retinoids—derivatives of vitamin A (retinol)—are a cornerstone of acne therapy. These drugs can unplug existing comedones and prevent development of new ones. In addition, they can reduce inflammation and improve penetration of other topical agents. Topical retinoids currently approved for acne use are tretinoin, adapalene, and tazarotene. They may be used alone or in combination with other drugs, including topical and oral antimicrobials.

Tretinoin

Tretinoin, a topical derivative of vitamin A, is used for acne and to remove fine wrinkles. Formulations for acne are marketed as Atralin, Avita, Retin-A, and Retin-A Micro. The formulation for wrinkles, which is nearly identical to one of the formulations for acne, is marketed as Renova. Tretinoin should not be confused with isotretinoin, a powerful *oral* antiacne medicine (see later discussion).

Use for Acne. Tretinoin is approved for topical treatment of mild to moderate acne. Benefits derive from normalizing hyperproliferation of epithelial cells within hair follicles. Tretinoin also causes thinning of the stratum corneum and can thereby facilitate penetration of other drugs. Therapeutic effects can be enhanced by combining tretinoin with benzoyl peroxide, topical antibiotics, and oral antibiotics.

Use for Fine Wrinkles. Tretinoin is approved for reducing fine wrinkles, tactile roughness, and mottled hyperpigmentation ("liver spots," age spots) in facial skin. Benefits may derive from suppressing genes that code for specific proteases that break down collagen and elastin. In clinical trials, responses to tretinoin were modest. In fact, many patients achieved equivalent effects with a program of comprehensive skin care and sun protection. It is important to appreciate that tretinoin does *not* repair deep, coarse wrinkles and other damage caused by chronic sun exposure. Furthermore, the drug does not reverse photoaging or restore the microscopic structure of skin to a more youthful pattern. Benefits in patients older than 50 years have not been established.

Adverse Effects. Tretinoin can cause *localized* reactions, but absorption is insufficient to cause systemic toxicity. In patients with sensitive skin, tretinoin may induce blistering, peeling, crusting, burning, and edema. These effects can be intensified by concurrent use of abrasive soaps and keratolytic agents (e.g., sulfur, resorcinol, benzoyl peroxide, salicylic acid). Accordingly, these preparations should be discontinued before beginning tretinoin therapy. Skin reactions with two formulations—Avita and Retin-A Micro—may be less intense than those caused by Retin-A, an older formulation.

Tretinoin increases susceptibility to sunburn. Patients should be warned to apply a sunscreen with a sun protection factor (SPF) of 15 or greater and wear protective clothing. Patients with existing sunburn should not apply the drug.

Preparations, Dosage, and Administration. For treatment of acne, tretinoin is available under four trade names: Retin-A, Retin-A Micro, Atralin, and Avita. Products marketed as Retin-A are available in two formulations: cream (0.025%, 0.05%, and 0.1%) and gel (0.01% and 0.025%). Retin-A Micro is supplied as a gel (0.04% and 0.1%), Atralin as a 0.05% gel, and Avita as a 0.025% cream or gel. All products are administered topically, usually once a day at bedtime. Before application, the skin should be washed, toweled dry, and allowed to dry fully for 20 to 30 minutes. Tretinoin should not be applied to open wounds or to areas of sunburn or windburn. Contact with the eyes, nose, ears, and mouth should be avoided.

For fine wrinkles of the face, tretinoin is available in a 0.02% cream, sold as Renova. Application is done once daily at bedtime. Cosmetics should be washed off before use. Up to 6 months of treatment may be needed to see a response, and treatment must continue to maintain the response.

Adapalene

Adapalene [Differin] is a topical antiacne drug similar to tretinoin. Through actions in the cell nucleus, adapalene modulates inflammation, epithelial keratinization, and differentiation of follicular cells. As a result, the drug reduces formation of comedones and inflammatory lesions. Benefits take 8 to 12 weeks to develop. During the early weeks, adapalene may appear to exacerbate acne by affecting previously invisible lesions. In clinical trials, 0.1% adapalene gel was as effective as 0.025% tretinoin gel in reducing the total number of comedones, and it was more effective than tretinoin in reducing the total number of acne lesions and inflammatory lesions.

Adverse effects are limited to sites of application. The drug is not absorbed in quantifiable amounts, so systemic effects are absent. Common side effects include burning, pruritus or burning immediately after application, erythema, dryness, and scaling. These are most likely during the first 2 to 4 weeks of treatment and tend to subside as treatment continues.

Adapalene increases the risk for developing sunburn and can intensify existing sunburn. Accordingly, all patients should apply a sunscreen and wear protective clothing. In addition, adapalene should not be used until existing sunburn has resolved.

Adapalene, by itself, is available in three 0.1% and 0.3% formulations—gel, cream, and lotion—for once-daily application in the evening. In addition, adapalene is available in a fixed-dose combination with benzoyl peroxide. Contact with the eyes, lips, angles of the nose, and mucous membranes should be avoided. It is also important to avoid contact with abraded, sunburned, or eczematous skin.

Tazarotene

Tazarotene [Avage, Tazorac] is indicated for topical therapy of acne, wrinkles, and psoriasis. Like tretinoin and adapalene, tazarotene is a derivative of vitamin A. For treatment of acne, tazarotene is available in a gel (0.05%, 0.1%) and cream (0.05%, 0.1%). The gel or cream is applied to affected areas of the face each evening. The face should be cleaned and dried before application. The most common side effects—itching, burning, and dry skin—occur more often with tazarotene than with tretinoin or adapalene. Like other retinoids, tazarotene sensitizes the skin to UV light, and hence patients should be advised to use a sunscreen and wear protective clothing.

Azelaic Acid

Azelaic acid [Azelex, Finacea ♣] is a topical keratolytic drug for mild to moderate acne. It appears to work by suppressing growth of *P. acnes* and by decreasing proliferation of keratinocytes, thereby decreasing the thickness of the stratum corneum. In clinical trials, topical azelaic acid (20% cream) was as effective as 5% benzoyl peroxide, 0.05% tretinoin, or 2% erythromycin. For severe acne, azelaic acid was much less effective than oral isotretinoin. Adverse effects—which are uncommon and less intense than with tretinoin or benzoyl peroxide—include pruritus, burning, stinging, tingling, and erythema. Azelaic acid may reduce pigmentation in patients with dark complexions, so people using this product should be monitored for hypopigmentation. Azelaic acid 20% cream is applied twice daily by gently massaging a thin film into the affected area. Contact with the eyes, nose, and mouth should be avoided. Before application, the skin should be washed and patted dry.

Salicylic Acid

Salicylic acid is another topical keratolytic drug for mild to moderate acne. For acne, 0.5% to 2% strengths are used. It is available in multiple formulations: cleanser, cream, gel, liquid, lotion, and impregnated pads. As with azelaic acid, it is important to avoid contact with the eyes, nose, and mouth. Adverse effects such as local irritation and peeling are usually mild, but recall that Health Canada has issued safety alerts regarding the association between salicylic acid and severe allergic reactions. Salicylate toxicity is not a problem when applied only to the face; however, if acne is extensive and the drug is applied to the trunk, back, and other locations, this could possibly occur. Monitoring for signs and symptoms of salicylism (e.g., hyperpnea, tinnitus, nausea and vomiting, and mental status changes) is indicated.

Oral Drugs for Acne

Antibiotics

Oral antibiotics are used for moderate to severe acne. These drugs suppress growth of *P. acnes* and directly suppress inflammation. Oral antibiotics can be combined with a topical retinoid.

Doxycycline [Vibramycin, others] and minocycline [Minocin, others] are considered agents of choice. Tetracycline [generic] and erythromycin [Ery-Tab, others] are alternatives, but resistance to these drugs is common. With all antibiotics, benefits develop slowly, taking 3 to 6 months to become maximal. After symptoms have been controlled with an oral antibiotic, patients should switch to a topical antibiotic for long-term maintenance.

Isotretinoin

Actions and Use. Isotretinoin [Amnesteem, Claravis], a derivative of vitamin A, is used to treat *severe nodulocystic acne vulgaris,* a condition for which this drug is highly effective. For most patients, a single course of therapy can produce complete and prolonged remission. Because isotretinoin can cause serious side effects, use is restricted to patients with severe, disfiguring acne that has not responded to more conventional agents, including oral antibiotics. Isotretinoin is highly teratogenic and hence must not be used during pregnancy.

Isotretinoin has several actions that may contribute to antiacne effects. The drug decreases sebum production, sebaceous gland size, inflammation, and keratinization. In addition, by decreasing availability of sebum, a nutrient for *P. acnes,* isotretinoin lowers the skin population of this microbe.

Pharmacokinetics. Absorption from the gastrointestinal (GI) tract is rapid but incomplete. Food greatly increases absorption. In the blood, isotretinoin is nearly 100% bound to albumin. The drug undergoes metabolism in the liver and possibly in cells of the intestinal wall. Excretion is by renal and biliary processes. The drug's half-life is 10 to 20 hours.

Adverse Effects

COMMON EFFECTS. The most common reactions are nosebleeds (80%), inflammation of the lips (90%), inflammation of the eyes (40%), and dryness or itching of the skin, nose, and mouth (80%). About 15% of patients experience pain, tenderness, or stiffness in muscles, bones, and joints. Among pediatric patients, nearly 30% experience back pain. Less common reactions include skin rash, headache, hair loss, and peeling of skin from the palms and soles. Reduction in night vision has occurred, sometimes with sudden onset. The skin may become sensitized to UV light; patients should be advised to wear protective clothing or a sunscreen if responses to sunlight become exaggerated. Rarely, isotretinoin causes cataracts, optic neuritis, papilledema (edema of the optic disk), and pseudotumor cerebri (benign elevation of intracranial pressure).

Triglyceride levels may become elevated. Blood triglyceride content should be measured before treatment and periodically thereafter until effects on triglycerides have been evaluated. Alcohol can potentiate hypertriglyceridemia and should be avoided.

Although these adverse effects occur frequently, they usually reverse on stopping treatment.

DEPRESSION. Isotretinoin may pose a risk for depression and suicide, although proof of a causal relationship is lacking. Nonetheless, because the potential consequences of depression are severe, steps should be taken to minimize risk. Accordingly, providers should ask patients to report signs of depression (e.g., depressed mood, loss of interest or pleasure) or thoughts of suicide. If these occur, isotretinoin should be withdrawn, and psychiatric evaluation should be considered.

Drug Interactions. Adverse effects of isotretinoin can be increased by *tetracyclines* and *vitamin A*. Tetracyclines increase the risk for pseudotumor cerebri and papilledema. Vitamin A, a close relative of isotretinoin, can produce generalized intensification of isotretinoin toxicity. Because of the potential for increased toxicity, tetracyclines and vitamin A supplements should be discontinued before isotretinoin therapy.

Contraindication: Pregnancy. Isotretinoin is teratogenic and must not be used during pregnancy. The drug is classified in U.S. Food and Drug Administration (FDA) Pregnancy Risk Category X: the risks for use during pregnancy clearly outweigh any possible benefits. Major fetal abnormalities that have occurred include hydrocephalus, microcephaly, facial malformation, cleft palate, cardiovascular defects, and abnormal formation of the outer ear.

iPLEDGE Program. iPLEDGE is a very strict risk management program designed to ensure that no woman starting isotretinoin *is* pregnant and that no woman taking isotretinoin *becomes* pregnant. The iPLEDGE program, which went into effect December 31, 2005, replaced all other programs designed to guard against use of isotretinoin during pregnancy. Under iPLEDGE, all transactions involving isotretinoin must be processed through a *central automated system,* which tracks and verifies critical elements that control access to the drug. The program has rules that apply to the prescriber, patient, pharmacist, and wholesaler. Details regarding iPLEDGE are available online at www.ipledgeprogram.com.

Requirements for Female Patients. Each patient must receive oral and written warnings about the high risk for fetal harm if isotretinoin is taken during pregnancy.

Pregnancy must be ruled out before the initial prescription and again before each monthly refill. Before the initial prescription, the patient must undergo *two* pregnancy tests, both of which must be negative. For the monthly refills, only one negative test result is required.

Each patient must use *two* effective forms of birth control, even if one of them is tubal ligation or vasectomy of the male partner. In addition, the patient must review educational material, provided through iPLEDGE, on contraceptive methods, possible reasons for contraceptive failure, and the importance of using effective contraception while taking a teratogenic drug. Birth control measures must be implemented at least 1 month before starting isotretinoin and must continue at least 1 month after stopping. Birth control is not required after hysterectomy or for women who commit to total abstinence from sexual intercourse.

Each patient must sign a Patient Information/Informed Consent document, designed to reinforce the benefits and risks of isotretinoin use.

Each patient must be registered with iPLEDGE by her prescriber and must contact iPLEDGE (through the Internet or by phone) before starting treatment, once a month during treatment, and, finally, 1 month after stopping treatment. At each contact, the patient must answer questions on program requirements and must indicate her two chosen methods of birth control.

Requirements for Prescribers. Prescribers must register with iPLEDGE and must agree to follow key points of the iPLEDGE program, as described in the *iPLEDGE Program Guide to Best Practices for Isotretinoin.* Also, the prescriber must register each patient with iPLEDGE, enter the results of each monthly pregnancy test, and indicate what methods of contraception the patient is using. The initial prescription for isotretinoin and each monthly refill must be entered into the iPLEDGE system.

Requirements for Pharmacists. To dispense isotretinoin, pharmacists must be registered with iPLEDGE and must obtain the drug through an iPLEDGE-registered wholesaler. Every time a prescription for isotretinoin is filled, the pharmacist must do the following:

- Contact iPLEDGE for authorization
- Confirm with iPLEDGE that the prescription is no more than 7 days old
- Dispense no more than a 30-day supply
- Write the risk management authorization (RMA) number on the prescription

Preparations, Dosage, and Administration. Isotretinoin is available in standard capsules (10, 20, 30, and 40 mg) sold as Amnesteem and Claravis. The usual course of treatment is 0.5 to 1 mg/kg/day (taken in two divided doses with food) for 15 to 20 weeks. If needed, a second course may be given, but no sooner than 2 months after completing the first course.

Hormonal Agents

Hormonal therapies can be used for acne in young women. Combination oral contraceptives and spironolactone are the main agents employed. In both cases, benefits derive from decreasing androgen activity, leading to decreased production of sebum.

Oral Contraceptives

Four combination OCs—Estrostep, Ortho Tri-Cyclen, Beyaz, and YAZ—are approved for managing acne in women.

Treatment is limited to females at least 15 years old who want contraception, have reached menarche, and have not responded to topical drugs. Acne may take 6 or more months to improve. Benefits are due primarily to the *estrogen* in combination OCs, not the progestin. Two mechanisms are involved: (1) suppression of ovarian androgen production and (2) increased production of *sex hormone–binding globulin,* a protein that binds androgens and thereby renders them inactive. By decreasing androgen availability, estrogens decrease production of sebum. Although only four OCs are approved for acne, all estrogen-containing OCs should work. Accordingly, selection among them should be based primarily on tolerability.

Spironolactone

Spironolactone [Aldactone] blocks a variety of steroid receptors, including those for aldosterone and sex hormones. Blockade of aldosterone receptors underlies the drug's use as a diuretic (see Chapter 35) as well as its use in heart failure (see Chapter 40). Blockade of androgen receptors underlies benefits in females with acne. As a rule, spironolactone is added to the regimen after an OC has proved inadequate. This sequence makes sense because spironolactone is teratogenic, and hence contraception should be implemented before taking the drug. Adverse effects include menstrual irregularities, breast tenderness, and hyperkalemia.

In 2016, the American Academy of Dermatology published *Guidelines of Care for the Management of Acne Vulgaris.* Their algorithm for acne management is included in this chapter. (See Fig. 85.2.) The complete guidelines are available online at https://www.aad.org/File%20Library/Main%20navigation/Practice%20tools/Quality%20care%20and%20guidelines/Acne-guideline.pdf.

SUNSCREENS

Sunlight has multiple effects on the skin. In addition to promoting tanning, solar radiation can cause burns, premature aging of the skin, skin cancer, and immunosuppression. Sun exposure can also induce photosensitivity reactions to drugs. All of these effects are caused by UV radiation, and all can be greatly reduced by using a sunscreen.

Types of Ultraviolet Radiation: UVB and UVA

Solar UV radiation that reaches the earth's surface is classified by wavelength into two basic types: ultraviolet B (UVB: 290–320 nm) and ultraviolet A (UVA: 320–400 nm). UVA can be further subdivided into UVA2 (320–340 nm) and UVA1 (340–400 nm). Most (95%) of terrestrial UV radiation is UVA; only 5% is UVB. The intensity of UVA is fairly constant from morning to evening and from one day to the next throughout the year. In contrast, UVB is significant only between late spring and early fall and, on any given day, is moderate in the morning and evening, and most intense around noon. UVA can penetrate glass; UVB can't.

Diagnosis of acne

	Mild	Moderate	Severe
1st Line treatment	Benzoyl peroxide (BP) or topical retinoid -or- Topical combination therapy** BP + antibiotic or retinoid + BP or retinoid + BP + antibiotic	Topical combination therapy** BP + antibiotic or retinoid + BP or retinoid + BP + antibiotic -or- Oral antibiotic + topical retinoid + BP -or- Oral antibiotic + topical retinoid + BP + topical antibiotic	Oral antibiotic + Topical combination therapy** BP + antibiotic or retinoid + BP or retinoid + BP + antibiotic -or- Oral isotretinoin
Alternative treatment	Add topical retinoid or BP (if not on already) -or- Consider alternate retinoid -or- Consider topical dapsone	Consider alternate combination therapy -or- Consider change in oral antibiotic -or- Add combined oral contraceptive or oral spironolactone (females) -or- Consider oral isotretinoin	Consider change in oral antibiotic -or- Add combined oral contraceptive or oral spironolactone (females) -or- Consider oral isotretinoin

Figure 85.2 ■ Treatment of acne vulgaris.
(From https://www.aad.org/File%20Library/Main%20navigation/Practice%20tools/Quality%20care%20and%20guidelines/Acne-guideline.pdf, page 4.)

The dermatologic effects of UVA and UVB differ. UVA penetrates the epidermis and deep into the dermis. In contrast, UVB penetrates into the epidermis but goes no deeper. Tanning and sunburn are caused primarily by UVB. Because UVA penetrates much deeper than UVB, UVA is the primary cause of immunosuppression, photosensitive drug reactions, and photoaging of the skin (wrinkling, thickening, yellowing, breakdown of elastic fibers). Both UVA and UVB promote damage to DNA, and hence both can cause premalignant actinic keratoses, basal cell carcinoma, squamous cell carcinoma, and malignant and nonmalignant melanoma. Properties of UVA and UVB are shown in Table 85.3.

Benefits of Sunscreens

Sunscreens impede penetration of UV radiation to viable cells of the skin. As a result, sunscreens can protect against sunburn, photoaging of the skin, and photosensitivity reactions to certain drugs (e.g., tricyclic antidepressants, phenothiazines, sulfonamides, sulfonylureas). Sunscreens can also decrease the risk for actinic keratoses, squamous cell carcinoma, and melanoma. Whether sunscreens protect against basal cell carcinoma is unclear.

Compounds Employed as Sunscreens

There are two categories of sunscreens: *organic* screens (also known as *chemical* screens) and *inorganic* screens (also known as *physical* screens). Organic screens *absorb* UV radiation and then dissipate it as heat. Inorganic screens *scatter* UV radiation. At this time, 17 compounds are FDA approved for use as sunscreens (Fig. 85.3).

Organic (Chemical) Screens

Most (15) of the approved sunscreens are organic. Almost all of them absorb UVB, but only six absorb UVA. Of these six, five absorb UVA2, and only one—*avobenzone*—absorbs UVA1. Therefore, to provide protection against the full range of UV radiation, products must contain a mixture of compounds, one of which must be avobenzone.

Inorganic (Physical) Screens

Physical screens act primarily as barriers to the sun's rays. Hence, rather than absorbing solar radiation, they *reflect and scatter* sunlight, thereby preventing penetration to the skin. Only two agents are employed as physical screens: *titanium dioxide* and *zinc oxide.* Preparations containing these compounds are especially useful for protecting limited areas (e.g., nose, lips, tips of ears). In the formulations used today, titanium dioxide and zinc oxide are "micronized." As a result, they are clear when applied to the skin, unlike older formulations, which were white.

TABLE 85.3 ■ Properties of UVB and UVA Radiation

Property	Type of UV Radiation: UVB	UVA
Wavelength (nm)	290–320	320–400
Can penetrate glass	No	Yes
Skin penetration	Epidermis only	Epidermis/dermis
Effects on the skin:		
Burning	Major cause	Minor cause
Tanning	Major cause	Minor cause
Cancer	Major cause	Major cause
Photoaging		Sole cause
Photosensitive drug reactions		Sole cause

UV, ultraviolet.

Sun Protection Factor

All sunscreen products are labeled with an SPF. The SPF is an index of protection against UVB. The SPF says nothing about protection against UVA.

The SPF is determined by shining UV light on adjacent regions of protected and unprotected skin and recording the time required for erythema (redness) to develop in both areas. The SPF is calculated by dividing the time required for erythema to develop in the protected region by the time required for erythema to develop in the unprotected region. For example, if the unprotected region developed erythema in 15 minutes, and the protected region developed erythema in 150 minutes, the sunscreen would have an SPF of 10 (150 divided by 15). Be aware that the methods for determining the SPF are not very precise. Hence, all products labeled with the same SPF may not provide an equal degree of protection.

The relationship between SPF and protection against sunburn is not linear. That is, an SPF of 30 does not indicate twice as much protection as an SPF of 15. In fact, as the SPF increases, the increment in protection gets progressively smaller. For example, SPF 15 indicates 93% block of UVB, SPF 30 indicates 96.7% block, and SPF 40 indicates 97.5% block. Because SPF values above 30 provide only a small additional benefit, the FDA no longer allows companies to

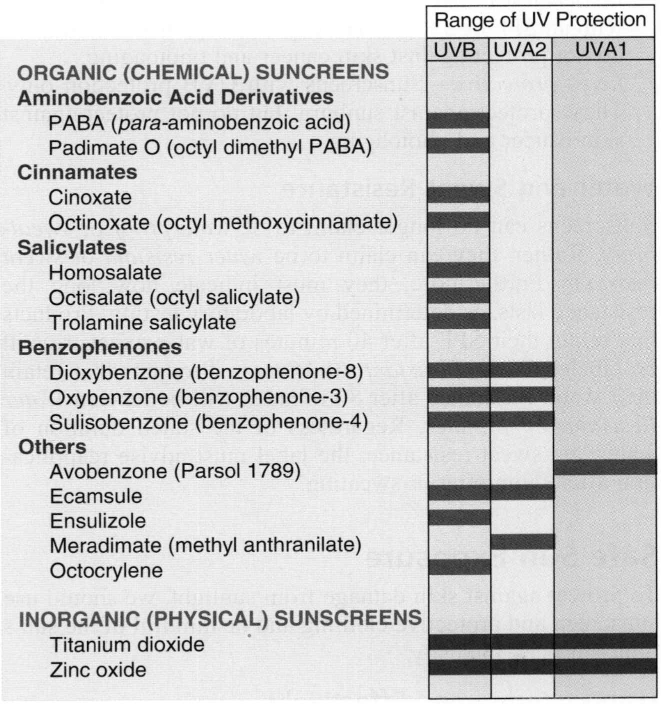

Figure 85.3 ■ Range of ultraviolet B and ultraviolet A protection conferred by U.S. Food and Drug Administration–approved sunscreens.

advertise high SPF values (e.g., SPF 80). Instead, products with an SPF greater than 50 can only be labeled as SPF 50+.

Adverse Effects of Sunscreens

Contact dermatitis and photosensitivity reactions can occur, especially with products that contain *para*-aminobenzoic acid (PABA) derivatives. PABA-containing products should be avoided by people with allergies to benzocaine, sulfonamides, or thiazides, all of which can cross-react with PABA.

Rules for Sunscreen Labeling

In 2011, the FDA released new rules for labeling sunscreens. Under these rules, the label must indicate (1) the range of UV radiation protection and (2) the degree of water/sweat resistance. As in the past, labels will continue to indicate the SPF.

Range of UV Protection and SPF

All sunscreens protect against UVB radiation, but only some protect against UVA, too. Products that protect against UVA *and* UVB are labeled BROAD SPECTRUM. The label also shows the SPF, indicating the degree of UVB protection. Broad-spectrum sunscreens that have an SPF of 15 or higher can claim to protect against skin cancer and photoaging. Broad-spectrum agents with an SPF below 15 cannot make this claim. In fact, these products must carry a warning that they do *not* protect against skin cancer or photoaging. Products that only protect against UVB must carry the same warning. In summary, the new labels will allow consumers to distinguish between three basic groups of sunscreens:

- *Highly protective*—BROAD SPECTRUM sunscreens with an SPF of 15 or higher. These protect against sunburn, skin cancer, and photoaging.
- *Moderately protective*—BROAD SPECTRUM sunscreens with an SPF of 2 to 14. These protect against sunburn, but do not protect against skin cancer and photoaging.
- *Least protective*—Sunscreens with UVB protection only. These protect against sunburn, but do not protect against skin cancer and photoaging.

Water and Sweat Resistance

Sunscreens can no longer claim to be *waterproof* or *sweatproof.* Rather, they can claim to be *water resistant* or *sweat resistant.* Furthermore, they must indicate how long the resistance lasts, as determined by laboratory testing. Products that retain their SPF after 40 minutes of water exposure will be labeled *Water Resistant 40 Minutes.* Products that retain their water resistance after 80 minutes will be labeled *Water Resistant 80 Minutes.* Regardless of the stated duration of water and sweat resistance, the label must advise reapplication after swimming or sweating.

Safe Sun Exposure

To protect against skin damage from sunlight, we should use sunscreen and protective clothing and be mindful of the sun's hours of peak intensity.

Using a Sunscreen Effectively

Sunscreens must be used properly to achieve maximal benefit. The American Academy of Dermatology recommends using a sunscreen with coverage against both UVB and UVA. The SPF should be at least 15. Individuals who burn easily should use a higher SPF product. Protection is greatest when a sunscreen has been allowed to penetrate the skin in advance of exposure to the sun. Accordingly, sunscreens should be applied at least 30 minutes before going outdoors; sunscreens containing PABA or padimate O should be applied up to 2 hours in advance. The amount applied is an important determinant of protection; 1 ounce applied liberally to the body is considered adequate. Sunscreens should be reapplied after swimming and profuse sweating; failure to do so reduces the duration of protection. However, it is important to note that reapplication will not extend the period of protection beyond that indicated by the SPF. That is, if treated skin can be expected to burn when sun exposure exceeds 2 hours, no amount of reapplication can prevent burning if the duration of exposure exceeds the limit.

Environmental factors play a part in sunscreen use. The intensity of UVB radiation is greatest between the hours of 10:00 AM and 4:00 PM. Accordingly, the need for a sunscreen is correspondingly high during this time. UV radiation can be reflected by painted surfaces, white sand, and snow, thereby augmenting total UV exposure. Accordingly, the contribution of reflected radiation should be considered when choosing a sunscreen. Clouds can filter out UV radiation. Nonetheless, the amount of UV light reaching the ground on a bright day with thin cloud cover can be as much as 80% of that reaching the ground on days that are sunny and clear. UV radiation can penetrate at least several centimeters of clear water; swimmers should be made aware of this fact.

Other Protection Measures

Sunscreens alone cannot completely protect against sun damage. Accordingly, to further reduce risk, you should wear sunglasses, protective clothing, and a wide-brimmed hat. In addition, you should avoid sun exposure in the middle of the day, especially between 10:00 AM and 4:00 PM. If you must be outside at these times, try to stay in the shade as much as possible.

DRUGS FOR ATOPIC DERMATITIS (ECZEMA)

Atopic dermatitis, also known as eczema, is a chronic inflammatory skin disease. The condition is characterized by dry, scaly skin and intense pruritus that often leads to scratching and rubbing, which in turn can lead to erythema, abrasions, rash, erosions with an exudate, and increased susceptibility to skin infection. Continued scratching will typically result in lichenification of the affected skin. The underlying cause is abnormal activity of T lymphocytes. First-line therapy consists of moisturizers (e.g., Cetaphil Moisturizing Cream, Eucerin Original Cream) and topical glucocorticoids. Unfortunately, the glucocorticoids can cause skin atrophy, hypopigmentation, telangiectasis (permanent focal red lesions), and, in high doses, possible systemic effects, including adrenal suppression. If topical glucocorticoids are insufficient, patients may be treated with a topical immunosuppressant (see later). A sedating antihistamine can help control itching and can facilitate sleeping at night.

Topical Immunosuppressants

Two topical immunosuppressants—tacrolimus and pimecrolimus—are approved for atopic dermatitis. Both drugs are calcineurin inhibitors. Although effective against atopic dermatitis, both drugs may pose a risk for skin cancer and lymphoma. Because of this potential for serious harm, tacrolimus and pimecrolimus are considered second-line drugs for atopic dermatitis and should be reserved for patients who have not responded to glucocorticoids.

Tacrolimus Ointment

Tacrolimus [Protopic] is available as an ointment for moderate to severe atopic dermatitis. The drug relieves symptoms by attenuating local immune responses. Specifically, the drug inhibits calcineurin and thereby suppresses the activity of T cells and decreases the release of inflammatory mediators from cutaneous mast cells and basophils. The result is reduced inflammation.

Systemic absorption of topical tacrolimus is low, and it gets even lower as the skin heals. Absolute bioavailability is less than 0.05%. Blood levels of tacrolimus are usually low.

Tacrolimus ointment is generally well tolerated. The most common side effects are erythema, pruritus, and burning sensations at the application site. As the skin heals, these local reactions abate. In children, tacrolimus may increase the risk for varicella-zoster virus infection. Adverse effects associated with systemic tacrolimus (nephrotoxicity, neurotoxicity, hypertension, diarrhea, nausea) have not occurred with topical therapy. Unlike topical glucocorticoids, tacrolimus does not cause thinning of the skin.

There is concern that tacrolimus may pose a risk for cancer. The drug increases the incidence of skin cancer in laboratory animals exposed to UV light. In mice, tacrolimus increases the incidence of lymphoma. There have been reports of skin cancer and lymphoma in humans, although a causal relationship has not been established. To reduce any risk for skin cancer, patients should protect treated areas from direct sunlight and should avoid sunlamps and tanning beds.

Tacrolimus ointment [Protopic] is available in two concentrations: 0.03% and 0.1%. Adults may use either formulation; children ages 2 to 16 years should use the 0.03% formulation; and children younger than 2 years should not use the drug. All patients should apply a thin layer twice daily. Occlusive dressings should be avoided. Treatment should be intermittent or short term.

Pimecrolimus Cream

Pimecrolimus 1% cream [Elidel] is a topical immunosuppressant approved for mild to moderate atopic dermatitis. The drug is very similar to tacrolimus with regard to mechanism, therapeutic effects, and adverse effects. In clinical trials, twice-daily application for 3 weeks reduced signs and symptoms of eczema by 72%. Initial improvement could be seen in 2 days. Pimecrolimus may be less effective than topical glucocorticoids. Although studies comparing pimecrolimus directly with tacrolimus have not been done, clinical efficacy of the drugs appears similar.

Pimecrolimus is generally well tolerated. The most common adverse effects are erythema, pruritus, and burning sensations at the application site, especially during the first few days of treatment. As with tacrolimus, there have been reports of skin cancer and lymphoma, but a causal relationship has not been established. Like tacrolimus, pimecrolimus sensitizes the skin to UV light, and hence patients should use a sunscreen and should limit exposure to natural and artificial sunlight. Systemic absorption of pimecrolimus is minimal; in clinical trials, blood levels were at or below the limit of detection. As with tacrolimus, prolonged treatment should be avoided.

AGENTS USED TO REMOVE WARTS

Warts are small, benign tumors that form in the skin and mucous membranes. They are caused by infection of squamous epithelial cells with human papillomavirus (HPV), of which there are roughly 100 types. Most warts resolve spontaneously within a few months, but some can last for years. Discussion below focuses primarily on management of venereal warts.

Venereal Warts

Venereal warts form around the cervix, vulva, urethra, glans penis, and anus and anal canal. Most are caused by two types of HPV, known as HPV-6 and HPV-11. Two other types—HPV-16 and HPV-18—are responsible for most cervical cancers. As discussed in Chapter 53, an HPV vaccine, sold as Gardasil, can protect against all four HPV types and hence can help prevent venereal warts as well as cancer of the cervix. Another HPV vaccine, sold as Cervarix, only protects against HPV-16 and HPV-18, so it can help prevent cervical cancer but not venereal warts.

Infection with HPV can be transmitted by sexual contact. Individuals with anogenital warts should be warned that they can transmit the infection to sexual partners. Partners of infected individuals should be examined for warts. Using a condom can reduce the risk for transmission.

Genital warts can be removed in two basic ways: with topical drugs or with physical measures such as cryotherapy (freezing), electrodesiccation (destruction with an electric current), laser surgery, and conventional surgery. Physical measures are much faster than drugs but also more painful. Neither drugs nor physical measures can eradicate the virus because, even after successful wart removal, the virus remains. Treatments for genital warts are shown in Table 85.4.

The drugs used to remove venereal warts can be divided into two groups: agents that must be administered by a health care provider and agents that can be applied at home. With both groups, application is done repeatedly until the warts disappear. Provider-applied drugs are podophyllin, trichloroacetic acid, and bichloroacetic acid. Drugs for home application are podofilox, imiquimod, and kunecatechins. All of these drugs act slowly, and they all cause local irritation. The pharmacology of six topical drugs is discussed later.

TABLE 85.4 ▪ Treatment and Prevention of Venereal Warts

TREATMENT	
External genital	*Patient administered:* Podofilox 0.5% solution or gel (topical) *or* Imiquimod 3.75% or 5% cream (topical) *or* Kunecatechins (sinecatechins) 15% ointment (topical) *Provider administered:* Cryotherapy with liquid nitrogen or cryoprobe *or* Podophyllin 10%–25% (topical) *or* TCA or BCA 80%–90% (topical) *or* Surgical excision
Anal	Cryotherapy with liquid nitrogen *or* TCA or BCA (80%–90%) applied to warts *or* Surgical excision
Vaginal	Cryotherapy with liquid nitrogen *or* TCA or BCA (80%–90%) applied to warts
Urethral meatus	Cryotherapy with liquid nitrogen *or* Podophyllin resin 10%–25% (topical)
PREVENTION	
All sites	*Gardasil* vaccine: protects against HPV-6 and HPV-11, which cause 90% of venereal warts, as well as HPV-16 and HPV-18, which cause 70% of cervical cancers

BCA, bichloroacetic acid; TCA, trichloroacetic acid.

Provider-Applied Drugs

Podophyllin

Podophyllin (podophyllum resin) [Podocon-25, Podofilm ♣] is used primarily for perianal and venereal warts. The drug is not very effective against common warts. Podophyllin is a mixture of resins from the May apple or mandrake (*Podophyllum peltatum* Linne). The active ingredient in the resin is podophyllotoxin, a compound that inhibits DNA synthesis and mitosis. These actions eventually lead to cell death and erosion of warty tissue. Formulations employed to remove warts contain 25% podophyllum resin. These preparations are highly caustic and should be applied only by a trained clinician. To minimize the risk for toxicity from systemic absorption, the resin should be washed off with alcohol or soap and water a few hours after application. Each treatment should be limited to a small surface area and to a small number of warts.

Podophyllin can be absorbed in amounts sufficient to cause systemic toxicity. Potential reactions include central and peripheral neuropathy, kidney damage, and blood dyscrasias. These effects are most likely when the drug is applied to large areas in excessive amounts. Podophyllin is teratogenic and must not be used during pregnancy.

Podophyllin is supplied in a 25% solution for topical use. Application should be limited to small areas. The drug should not be applied to moles or birthmarks, nor should it be applied to warts that are bleeding or friable (easily crumbled) or that have undergone recent biopsy. When used to remove venereal warts, podophyllin should be washed off 1 to 4 hours after application. Treatment may be repeated at weekly intervals for up to 4 weeks.

Bichloroacetic Acid (BCA) and Trichloroacetic Acid (TCA)

When applied in high concentration (80%–90%), BCA and TCA can destroy warts by chemical coagulation. Application is repeated weekly if needed.

Solutions of these acids are very watery and hence can easily spread to and thereby injure surrounding tissue. To minimize spread, the solution should be allowed to dry before the patient sits or stands. If pain develops, BCA and TCA can be neutralized with liquid soap or sodium bicarbonate (baking soda). If too much solution is applied, it should be neutralized with soap or sodium bicarbonate, or removed by applying talc.

Patient-Applied Drugs

Patient-applied drugs are used for topical therapy of external genital and perianal warts. Like podophyllin, these drugs require a prescription. Because they are applied at home, these drugs are more convenient than the provider-applied drugs.

Imiquimod

Imiquimod cream [Aldara, Zyclara] stimulates production of interferon alpha, TNF, and several interleukins and thereby intensifies immune responses to HPV, the virus that causes venereal warts. Imiquimod has no direct antiviral effects of its own. Principal adverse effects are erythema, erosion, and flaking at the site of administration. Local itching, burning, and pain may occur, too. Imiquimod undergoes minimal absorption, and hence systemic effects are usually absent.

Imiquimod cream is available in two formulations: a 3.75% cream sold as Zyclara, and a 5% cream sold as Aldara. Zyclara is applied once a day for up to 8 weeks; Aldara is applied 3 times a week for up to 16 weeks. Both formulations are applied at bedtime and washed off in the morning. Imiquimod use for actinic keratoses was discussed earlier.

Podofilox

Like podophyllin, podofilox [Condylox] inhibits mitosis. Whether this action underlies beneficial effects (erosion of warty tissue) is unknown. Podofilox is supplied as a 0.5% gel or 0.5% solution to be applied twice daily for 3 consecutive days followed by 4 days off. This pattern is repeated 4 times or until the warts are gone—whichever comes first. Patients should wash their hands before and after applying the drug. However, unlike imiquimod, podofilox needn't be washed from the site of application. Treatment frequently causes local inflammation, burning, erosion, pain, itching, and bleeding. These can be minimized by limiting the application area to 10 cm^2, applying no more than 0.5 g/day, and avoiding application to normal skin. Podofilox causes more discomfort than imiquimod but works faster and costs less.

Kunecatechins (Sinecatechins) Ointment

Kunecatechins [Veregen] is made by extraction from the leaves of Camellia sinensis (green tea). The primary active component in this extract is epigallocatechin, a compound in the catechin family. The extract also contains small amounts of gallic acid and three methylxanthines: caffeine, theophylline, and theobromine. Although the mechanism of action has not been determined, possibilities include antioxidative effects, induction of apoptosis (programmed cell death), and inhibition of telomerase (an enzyme cells use to extend the telomere cap on DNA). Kunecatechins is supplied as a 15% ointment to be applied 3 times daily until all warts clear, or for 16 weeks, whichever comes first. In one trial, treatment for 16 weeks produced complete wart removal in 53.6% of patients, compared with 35.3% in those treated with placebo. Adverse effects, which are common, include erythema (70%), pruritus (69%), burning (67%), pain (56%), erosion or ulceration (49%), edema (45%), induration (35%), and rash (2%). Moderate reactions develop in 37% of patients, and severe reactions develop in 30%. Kunecatechins is only indicated for external genital and perianal warts. It should not be inserted into the vagina or rectum and should not be applied to open wounds. Patients should avoid sexual contact while the ointment is present. Kunecatechins is not recommended for HIV-infected patients, immunocompromised patients, or patients with genital herpes infection. Why? Because safety and efficacy in these patients has not been established.

Common Warts

Common warts—also known as verruca vulgaris—manifest as hard, rough, horny papules. These benign lesions may appear anywhere on the body but are most common on the hands and feet. Most common warts are caused by just three types of HPV, known as HPV-1, HPV-2, and HPV-3.

Like venereal warts, common warts may be removed by physical procedures and with topical drugs. The physical methods are cryotherapy, electrodesiccation, curettage (surgical removal with a loop-shaped cutting tool), and laser therapy. Pharmacologic agents include salicylic acid, podophyllin, podofilox, imiquimod, trichloroacetic acid, and topical fluorouracil.

DRUGS FOR NONSURGICAL COSMETIC PROCEDURES

OnabotulinumtoxinA [Botox] is an acetylcholine release inhibitor and neuromuscular blocking agent. Botulinum toxin type A is a protein produced by the gram-negative bacterium *Clostridium botulinum*. This is the same powerful toxin that causes botulism, a potentially fatal condition brought on by eating foods contaminated with *C. botulinum*; however, the doses approved for cosmetic use are much too small to produce toxic effects.

In the United States two licensed Botox products are available: Botox and Botox Cosmetic. Botox Cosmetic is approved only for treating frown lines, whereas plain Botox is approved for treating cervical dystonia, detrusor overactivity, upper limb spasticity, strabismus, blepharospasm, and hyperhidrosis, and for migraine headache prophylaxis. However, except for the packaging, both Botox products are identical. The drug is available as a powder in 100-unit vials under the name Botox. Immediately before use, the powder is reconstituted with 2.5 mL of preservative-free normal saline to form a clear, colorless solution. According to the package label, reconstituted botulinum toxin is unstable and hence should be stored cold and used within 4 hours. However, data indicate that, if the drug is diluted in normal saline that contains the preservative benzyl alcohol, it retains its potency for 5 weeks and causes less pain when injected.

How does Botox work? OnabotulinumtoxinA is a neurotoxin that acts on cholinergic neurons to block release of acetylcholine. After injection, the drug is taken up by cholinergic nerve terminals, where it inactivates SNAP-25, a protein critical to the function of acetylcholine-containing vesicles. In the absence of SNAP-25, the vesicles are unable to fuse with the terminal membrane and hence cannot release their acetylcholine. Restoration of neuronal function requires sprouting of new terminals, a process that can take several months. Botulinum toxin blocks transmission at neuromuscular junctions and at cholinergic synapses of the autonomic nervous system, including synapses in autonomic ganglia.

The FDA has approved Botox for reducing frown lines, known formally as "glabellar" lines (because they appear on the glabella—the smooth area located between the eyebrows, directly above the nose). Botox is also used to soften lines on the forehead and neck and to diminish "crow's feet" (lines that form near the outer corners of our eyes when we squint).

Botox is administered by injection. (Pretreatment with a topical anesthetic cream is commonly done to reduce discomfort.) To reduce frown lines, for example, Botox is injected directly into the small muscles that produce a frown when they contract. Five injections are made, each consisting of 4 units of botulinum toxin in 0.1 mL of fluid. Two injections go into each corrugator muscle and one into the procerus muscle. The whole procedure takes just a few minutes.

Results are neither instantaneous nor permanent. Rather, muscle paralysis develops slowly—over 3 to 10 days—and fades within 3 to 6 months. Botox injections may be repeated to maintain cosmetic benefits. However, at least 3 months should separate treatments. There are no data on long-term effects.

The FDA has issued a black box warning related to spread of the toxin from the site of injection to other areas, leading to life-threatening injuries; however, this has not occurred with the small doses used for cosmetic treatment. For cosmetic treatment, the most common side effects are headache, facial pain, swelling, and bruising. Swelling and bruising can be reduced by applying ice to the site and by avoiding alcohol, vitamin E, and aspirin (and related NSAIDs) for the week before treatment.

Injection into the wrong site, or diffusion from the right site into surrounding tissues, can weaken muscles that were not intended as targets, causing multiple undesired effects. Ptosis (droopy eyelids) occurs in about 5% of patients and can persist for 3 to 6 months. Injections in the lower face can result in drooling, an asymmetric smile, drooping mouth, and biting of the inside of the cheek. Injections in the neck can make swallowing difficult and can change vocal pitch.

Who should not use Botox? The drug should be avoided by women who are pregnant or breastfeeding and by patients who may be allergic to human albumin, a protein in Botox preparations. In addition, Botox should be avoided by people using aminoglycoside antibiotics or any other agent that has neuromuscular blocking properties. The drug should be used with caution in patients with myasthenia gravis and other neuromuscular disorders that can intensify muscle paralysis. Lastly, Botox should be avoided by people older than 65 years. Why? Because it's unlikely to help: in older people, the major cause of lines and wrinkles is loss of elasticity in the skin—a phenomenon that can't be reversed by neuromuscular blockade.

Over time, some patients develop antibodies against botulinum toxin type A. The only consequence is a reduction in Botox benefits. The risk for antibody production may be increased by using high doses and short dosing intervals. If antibodies do develop, patients may still respond to a product known as Myobloc, which consists of botulinum toxin type B (instead of botulinum toxin type A).

ANTIPERSPIRANTS AND DEODORANTS

Perspiration is produced by two types of sweat glands: eccrine glands and apocrine glands. The eccrine glands secrete profuse, watery perspiration. The apocrine glands secrete a small volume of fluid rich in organic compounds. The unpleasant odor associated with sweating results from chemical and bacterial degradation of the compounds in apocrine sweat. Eccrine glands contribute to odor by creating a moist environment that favors bacterial growth. Perspiration odor can be reduced with antiperspirants (agents that decrease flow of eccrine sweat) and deodorants (antiseptics that suppress growth of skin-dwelling bacteria).

Antiperspirants

The principal compounds employed as antiperspirants are aluminum chlorohydrate, aluminum chloride, and buffered aluminum sulfate. These agents can decrease flow of eccrine sweat by 20% to 50%. Reduced flow appears to result from inhibition of sweat production and from partial occlusion of sweat glands. Topical antiperspirants can cause stinging, burning, itching, and irritation. Dermatitis and ulceration occur rarely.

Severe sweating can be reduced with botulinum toxin type A [Botox], the same drug used to smooth facial wrinkles. Botulinum toxin inhibits release of acetylcholine from sympathetic neurons that innervate sweat glands and thereby reduces sweat volume. To treat axillary hyperhidrosis (severe underarm sweating), 10 to 15 intradermal injections (0.1–0.2 mL apiece) are made into each armpit. The needle employed is very fine (30 gauge) to minimize discomfort. One set of injections can markedly decrease sweating for 6 or more months.

Deodorants

Deodorants inhibit growth of the surface bacteria that degrade components of apocrine sweat into malodorous products; deodorants do not suppress sweat formation. Agents employed as deodorants include carbanilide, triclocarban, and triclosan. These antiseptics are the active ingredients in deodorant soaps, such as Dial, Lever, Tom's of Maine, and Irish Spring.

DRUGS FOR SEBORRHEIC DERMATITIS AND DANDRUFF

Seborrheic dermatitis is a chronic, relapsing condition characterized by inflammation and scaling of the scalp and face. Skin of the underarms, chest, and anogenital region may also be affected. Symptoms result from an inflammatory reaction to infection with *Malassezia* (formerly *Pityrosporum*), a microbe in the yeast family.

Symptoms respond rapidly to topical treatment with ketoconazole, an antifungal drug with activity against yeast (see Chapter 77). For treatment of seborrhea, ketoconazole is available in a 2% cream [Ketoderm ♣], 2% foam [Extina], 2% gel [Xolegel], and 1% and 2% shampoos [Nizoral]. The cream and foam formulations are applied twice daily for 4 weeks. The gel is more convenient, being applied just daily and for only 2 weeks. Concurrent use of topical glucocorticoids can accelerate initial responses. After the yeast infection has been controlled, remission can be maintained by periodic use of a shampoo that contains a yeast-suppressing drug, such as ketoconazole (in Nizoral), pyrithione zinc (in Head & Shoulders), or selenium sulfide (in Selsun Blue and Head & Shoulders Intensive Treatment).

DRUGS FOR HAIR LOSS

Two drugs are available to promote hair growth: minoxidil and finasteride. Minoxidil is applied topically; finasteride is taken orally. Neither drug was originally developed for baldness: minoxidil was developed for hypertension and finasteride for benign prostatic hyperplasia (BPH).

Topical Minoxidil

Minoxidil is a direct-acting vasodilator used primarily to treat severe hypertension. The drug's basic pharmacology is discussed in Chapter 38. Consideration here is limited to its use against patterned hair loss in men and women.

Minoxidil for baldness is available in three formulations, a 2% solution (generic only), a 5% solution [Rogaine Extra Strength for Men], and a 5% foam [Rogaine Men's Extra Strength]. All formulations are approved for men, but only the 2% solution is approved for women. Nonetheless, all formulations are routinely prescribed for women. All formulations are applied to the scalp twice a day.

The mechanism by which minoxidil promotes hair growth is unknown. One possibility is that it causes resting hair follicles to enter a state of active growth. Improved cutaneous blood flow secondary to vasodilation does not seem to be involved.

Minoxidil can delay loss of hair and stimulate hair growth. Benefits take several months to develop. Unfortunately, response rates are somewhat disappointing: only about one-third of patients experience significant restoration of hair to regions of baldness. Hair regrowth is most likely when baldness has developed recently and has been limited to a small area. Responses with the 5% solution are only 50% greater than with the 2% solution. When minoxidil is discontinued, newly gained hair is lost in 3 to 4 months, and the natural progression of hair loss resumes. In some cases, beneficial effects may decline even with uninterrupted treatment.

Topical minoxidil is generally devoid of adverse effects. A few patients have reported pruritus and local allergic responses (e.g., rash, swelling, burning sensation). Absorption is low, and hence systemic reactions (e.g., hypotension, headache, flushing) are rare.

Finasteride

Finasteride is an oral drug with two indications: androgenic alopecia (male-pattern baldness) and BPH. For treatment of androgenic alopecia, finasteride is sold in 1-mg tablets under the trade name Propecia. For treatment of BPH, the drug is sold in 5-mg tablets under the trade name Proscar (see Chapter 51).

Male-pattern baldness is caused by dihydrotestosterone (DHT), a powerful androgenic hormone formed from testosterone. In balding men, the scalp has high levels of DHT, which acts on hair follicles to induce shrinkage. Finasteride promotes hair growth by inhibiting the enzyme that converts testosterone into DHT. A 1-mg dose reduces serum levels of DHT by 65% after 24 hours. In the prostate gland, levels of testosterone increase by sixfold (because conversion of testosterone into DHT has been suppressed).

Regrowth of hair with finasteride is very modest. The drug has been evaluated in men 18 to 41 years old. Only 50% grew any hair. Furthermore, even when hair growth did occur, the amount was small: 1 year of treatment with 1 mg/day increased hair count by only 12% (in a 5.1-cm^2 circle on the scalp, the average hair count rose by 107 hairs, up from a baseline of 867 hairs). In older men taking 5 mg/day to treat BPH, no hair growth has been reported.

At the dosage employed to treat baldness (1 mg/day), adverse effects are few. About 4% of men experience reduced libido, erectile dysfunction, impaired ejaculation, and reduced ejaculate volume. Orthostatic hypotension and dizziness may occur. Finasteride is a teratogen that can cause genitourinary abnormalities in males exposed to the drug in utero. Accordingly, women who are or may become pregnant should not take finasteride, nor should they handle tablets that are crushed or broken.

EFLORNITHINE FOR UNWANTED FACIAL HAIR

Eflornithine [Vaniqa] is an old drug with a new indication and new formulation. It has been available since 1990 for systemic therapy of African trypanosomiasis (sleeping sickness). Now, the drug is also available in a 13.9% cream, for use by women to remove facial hair. Topical eflornithine acts on cells in hair follicles to inhibit ornithine decarboxylase, an enzyme required for synthesis of polyamines, which in turn are required for cell division and subsequent hair growth.

In clinical trials, eflornithine cream was moderately effective in some women and had no effect in others. All subjects had beards or mustaches that required removal (e.g., by shaving, waxing, tweezing,) at least twice a week. Participants were randomized to receive either (1) eflornithine cream twice a week or (2) the vehicle alone (i.e., the cream without eflornithine). What happened? Substantial hair reduction occurred in 40% of treated women in one study and 20% of treated women in another, compared with a 10% response in women receiving the vehicle alone. Among the women who did respond, benefits developed slowly—over 4 to 8 weeks or more—and then faded entirely within 8 weeks of stopping treatment. It should be noted that eflornithine does not remove facial hair entirely. Rather, it slows hair growth, causes hair to be finer and lighter, and decreases (but does not eliminate) the need for shaving and other hair-removal procedures. Because effects are not permanent, continuous treatment is required.

Very little of topical eflornithine gets absorbed: about 1% of each dose reaches the systemic circulation. Absorbed drug is eliminated intact in the urine. No metabolism occurs.

Eflornithine cream is generally well tolerated—although there is some concern about possible fetal harm. The most common reactions are transient stinging, burning, tingling, or rash at the application site. Although eflornithine absorption is minimal, it may still be sufficient to cause fetal injury. In animal studies, there was no evidence that topical eflornithine is teratogenic or fetotoxic. However, of the 19 pregnancies that occurred during clinical trials, there were 4 spontaneous abortions and 1 birth defect (Down syndrome). Until more is known, avoiding pregnancy would seem prudent.

Eflornithine is supplied in 45-g tubes (a 2-month supply). Applications are made twice daily, 8 hours apart. Women should rub the cream in thoroughly and should not wash the treated area for at least 4 hours. Cosmetics and sunscreens can be applied as soon as the cream dries.

DRUGS FOR IMPETIGO

Impetigo is the most common bacterial infection of the skin. The usual pathogen is Staphylococcus aureus. Most cases are seen in children 2 to 5 years old, although all age groups are susceptible. Impetigo is highly contagious and usually spread by person-to-person contact. Fortunately, the infection is superficial and usually is self-limited.

Impetigo has two forms: bullous and nonbullous. Bullous impetigo is caused by a toxin from *S. aureus* and manifests as rapidly spreading papules that may evolve into large, thin-walled vesicles. The usual location is a warm, moist area of the skin. Nonbullous impetigo, also known as crusted impetigo, is caused by *S. aureus* and/or *Streptococcus pyogenes*. This infection typically manifests as a single small macule or papule that evolves into a vesicle that oozes a yellow-brown exudate, which then dries into a honey-colored crust. The usual location is skin of the hands, feet, and legs. Most (70%) impetigo cases are nonbullous.

Impetigo is treated with antibiotics. Mild to moderate infection can be treated with topical agents. More serious infection is treated with oral agents. Dosages for representative antibiotics are shown in Table 85.5.

LOCAL ANESTHETICS

Local anesthetics (e.g., benzocaine, lidocaine, pramoxine) can be applied topically to relieve pain and itching associated with various skin disorders, including sunburn, plant poisoning, fungal infection, diaper rash, and eczema. Selection of a topical anesthetic is based on duration of action, desired vehicle (cream, ointment, solution, gel), and prior history of hypersensitivity reactions. The pharmacology of the local anesthetics is discussed in Chapter 21.

Table 85.6 shows patient concerns across the life span for many of the drugs discussed in this chapter.

TABLE 85.5 ▪ Some Antibiotics for Impetigo

			Dosage	
Generic Name	**Trade Name**	**Formulation**	**Pediatric**	**Adult**
TOPICAL				
Mupirocin	Bactroban	Ointment, cream	Apply 3 times a day for 3–5 days	Apply 3 times a day for 3–5 days
Retapamulin	Altabax	Ointment	Apply 2 times a day for 5 days	Apply 2 times a day for 5 days
ORAL				
Cephalexin	Keflex	Capsules, suspension	6.25 mg/kg 4 times a day	500 mg every 6–12 hr
Dicloxacillin	Generic only	Capsules	6.25 mg/kg 4 times a day	250 mg 4 times a day
Clindamycin	Cleocin	Capsules, suspension	10–20 mg/kg/day in three doses	300–450 mg 3 times a day
Amoxicillin/clavulanate	Augmentin	Tablets, suspension	*3 months and older and under 40 kg:* 20–40 mg/kg/day (amoxicillin component) divided every 8 hr *or* 25–45 mg/kg/day (amoxicillin component) divided every 12 hr *40 kg and greater:* 500 mg every 12 hr *or* 250 mg every 8 hr *Severe infections, 40 kg and greater:* 875 mg every 12 hr *or* 500 mg every 8 hr	875 mg amoxicillin/125 mg clavulanate twice daily

TABLE 85.6 ▪ Life Span Considerations of Selected Drugs for the Skin

Drug/Drug Category	Children	FDA Pregnancy Risk Category	Breastfeeding Women	Adults 65 Years or Older
Glucocorticoids, topical	Children <12 years old should use lower potency formulations	C	It is unknown whether topical glucocorticoids are excreted in breast milk; no adverse effects have been noted	Skin atrophy may be pronounced
Dapsone [Aczone]	Approved for children ≥12 years old	C	Not recommended	No age-specific precautions
Tretinoin [Retin-A, Renova]	Approved for children >12 years old	C	Enters breast milk; not recommended	Safety and efficacy not established
Adapalene [Differin]	Approved for children >12 years old	C	Excretion in breast milk unknown; manufacturer recommends caution	Not indicated for this age group
Tazarotene [Tazorac]	Approved for children ≥12 years old	X	Excretion in breast milk unknown; caution recommended	No age-specific precautions
Azelaic acid [Azelex]	Approved for children ≥12 years old	B	Enters breast milk; caution recommended	Not indicated for this age group
Isotretinoin [Claravis]	Approved for patients 12–17 years old	X	Excretion in breast milk unknown; not recommended	Not indicated for this age group
Oral contraceptives		X	May decrease milk production and protein content†	Not indicated for this age group
Fluorouracil, topical	Not approved for children	X	Excretion in breast milk unknown; not recommended	No age-specific precautions
Imiquimod [Aldara]	Approved for children ≥12 years old	C	Excretion in breast milk unknown; caution recommended	No age-specific precautions
Tacrolimus topical [Protopic]	Approved for children >2 years old	C	Can enter breast milk; not recommended	No age-specific precautions
Pimecrolimus cream [Elidel]	Approved for children ≥2 years old	C	Excretion in breast milk unknown; not recommended	No age-specific precautions
HPV Vaccine [Gardasil, Cervarix]	Approved for children ≥9 years old	B	Excretion in breast milk unknown; caution recommended	Not indicated for this age group
Podophyllin [Podocon-25]	Approved for use in children	X	Excretion in breast milk unknown; breastfeeding contraindicated	No age-specific precautions
Podofilox [Condylox]	Not approved for use in children	C	Excretion in breast milk unknown; breastfeeding contraindicated	No age-specific recommendations
Kunecatechins [Veregen]	Safety not established for patients <18 years old	C	Excretion in breast milk unknown; caution recommended	No age-specific recommendations
OnabotulinumtoxinA [Botox]	Not approved for purposes in this chapter‡	C	Excretion in breast milk unknown; caution recommended	No age-specific recommendations
Ketoconazole topical	Approved for children >12 years old	C	Excretion in breast milk unknown; caution recommended	No age-specific recommendations
Minoxidil [Rogaine]	Not approved for hair regrowth in children	C	Excretion in breast milk unknown; caution recommended	May have additive effects with antihypertensives
Finasteride [Propecia]	Not approved for use in children	X*	Excretion in breast milk unknown; breastfeeding contraindicated	No age-specific recommendations
Eflornithine [Vaniqa]	Approved for children >12 years old	C	Excretion in breast milk unknown; caution recommended	No age-specific precautions

*Women who are or plan to become pregnant should avoid handling broken finasteride tablets.
†According to the American Academy of Pediatrics, use of combination oral contraceptives is compatible with breastfeeding.
‡OnabotulinumtoxinA is approved for children for strabismus and for spasticity associated with cerebral palsy.

CHAPTER

86 Drugs for the Ear

Jacqueline Rosenjack Burchum, DNSc, FNP-BC, CNE

In this chapter, we discuss drugs for disorders of the middle ear and external ear. Information on the drugs discussed in this chapter is provided in Unit XVIII: Therapy of Infectious and Parasitic Diseases.

ANATOMY OF THE EAR

The ear has three major divisions: the external ear, middle ear, and inner ear (Fig. 86.1). Their primary features are as follows:

- The *external ear* consists of (1) the auricle or pinna (the cartilaginous flap visible on the side of the head that serves to collect sound waves) and (2) the external auditory canal (EAC), a skin-lined tube that directs sound waves from the auricle to the tympanic membrane (eardrum). The surface of the EAC is coated with cerumen (earwax), a hydrophobic substance that blocks penetration of water and helps protect against bacterial and fungal infection.
- The *middle ear* is the chamber that houses the malleus, incus, and stapes—three tiny bones that transmit sound vibrations from the eardrum to the inner ear. The middle ear is bounded laterally by the tympanic membrane, which walls off the middle ear from the external ear. The eustachian tube (auditory tube) connects the middle ear with the nasopharynx and thereby allows air pressure within the middle ear to equalize with air pressure in the environment. The mucociliary epithelium that lines the eustachian tube sweeps bacteria out of the middle ear into the nasopharynx.
- The *inner ear* consists of the semicircular canals and the cochlea. The canals provide our sense of balance. The cochlea houses the apparatus of hearing.

OTITIS MEDIA AND ITS MANAGEMENT

Otitis media (OM), defined as an inflammation of the middle ear, is the most prevalent disorder of childhood. The condition affects more than 75% of children by age 3 years and about 95% by age 12 years. In the United States OM is responsible for more than 16 million clinic visits a year.

OM may result from bacterial or viral infection or from noninfectious causes. Only bacterial OM responds to antibiotics. Furthermore, most cases resolve spontaneously, making antibiotics largely unnecessary—even when bacteria *are* the cause. Nonetheless, antibiotics have been used routinely. In fact, OM is the most common reason antibiotics are prescribed for children—at an estimated cost of $5 billion a year.

Acute Otitis Media

Characteristics, Pathogenesis, and Microbiology

Acute OM (AOM) is defined by *infection, inflammation,* and *fluid in the middle ear.* Otalgia (ear pain) is characteristic, often causing the young child to tug at or hold the affected ear. Other signs and symptoms accompanying AOM may include fever, vomiting, anorexia, irritability, sleeplessness, and diarrhea.

AOM results from a bacterial or viral infection of the middle ear. It occurs most commonly among children. The middle ear is filled with purulent fluid, which can cause the tympanic membrane to bulge outward. If the membrane is perforated, purulent otorrhea results.

AOM commonly develops after a viral upper respiratory infection, which can cause inflammation, swelling, and subsequent blockage of the eustachian tube. This results in negative pressure in the middle ear that, in turn, leads to fluid accumulation in the middle ear. When the eustachian tube opens, causing pressure equalization, bacteria and viruses can be sucked in. If the mucociliary system is sufficiently impaired, it will be unable to transport these pathogens back to the nasopharynx. OM results when bacteria colonize the fluid of the middle ear or when viruses colonize cells of the middle-ear mucosa. Common pathogens are provided in Table 86.1.

Diagnosis

To diagnose AOM, three elements must be present: (1) acute onset of signs and symptoms; (2) middle-ear effusion (MEE) or, if the tympanic membrane is ruptured, purulent otorrhea; and (3) middle-ear inflammation. The presence of MEE is indicated by limited mobility of the tympanic membrane on pneumatic otoscopy or tympanometry. (The best predictor of AOM is a bulging tympanic membrane.) Middle-ear inflammation is indicated by either (1) distinct erythema of the tympanic membrane or (2) distinct otalgia.

It is important to distinguish between AOM and otitis media with effusion (OME). As discussed later, children with OME have fluid in the middle ear but no signs of local or systemic illness. Prolonged OME is common after resolution of AOM.

Standard Treatment

All children with AOM should receive pain medication, and *some* should receive antibiotics. Prescribing antibiotics for *all* children should be discouraged because most (over 80%) of AOM episodes resolve spontaneously within a week. If

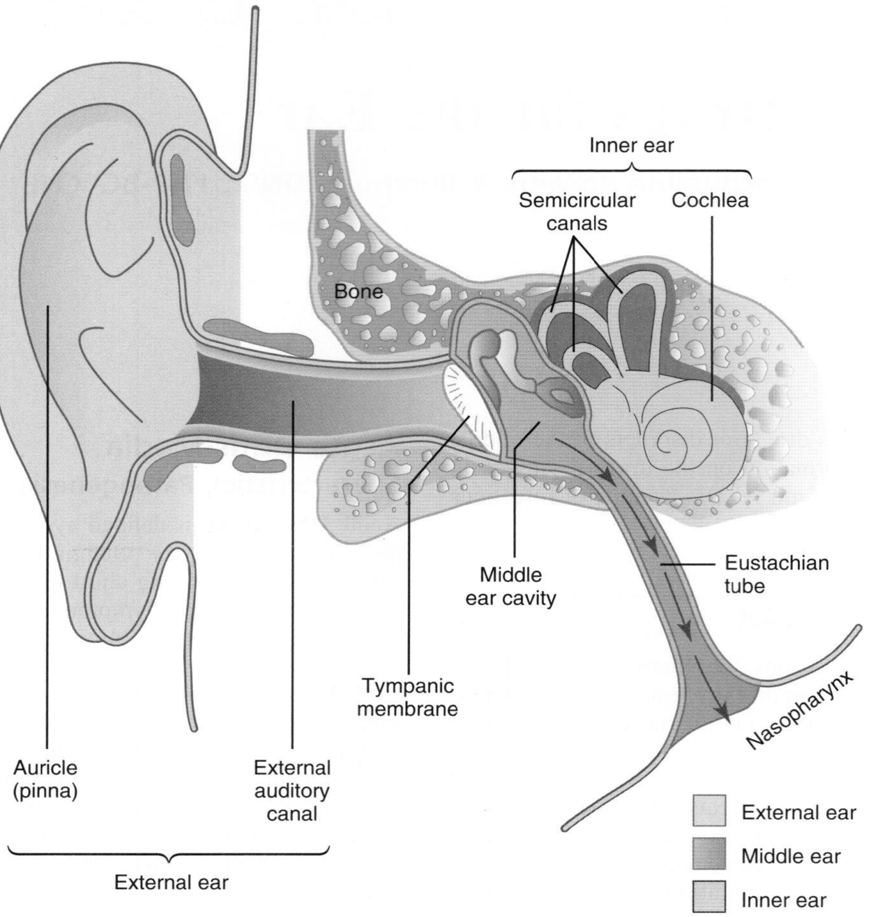

Figure 86.1 ■ Anatomy of the ear.
The *purple arrows* indicate flow of the mucociliary system, which can transport bacteria out of the middle ear.

TABLE 86.1 ■ Primary Pathogens Found in Fluid From the Middle Ear of Children With Acute Otitis Media

Pathogen	Children With the Pathogen (%)
Streptococcus pneumoniae	12
Haemophilus influenzae	56
Moraxella catarrhalis	22
Others (e.g., *Streptococcus pyogenes, Staphylococcus aureus*, gram-negative bacilli)	Uncommon
No bacteria found	10–30
Both bacteria and viruses	66
Viruses alone*	4

*It is uncommon for viruses to be present in the absence of bacteria.

antibiotics are prescribed routinely, most recipients will be taking drugs they don't really need. Not only does this generate unnecessary expense, worse yet, it puts children at needless risk for adverse drug effects, increases their risk for recurrent AOM, and accelerates the emergence of antibiotic-resistant bacteria.

In 2013, the American Academy of Pediatrics (AAP) released guidelines for treating AOM in children. (See Fig. 86.2.) These build on earlier guidelines developed jointly by the AAP and the American Academy of Family Physicians. For many patients, the guidelines include an important option—*observation*—rather than immediate treatment with antibiotics. Observation is defined as management by symptomatic relief alone for 48 to 72 hours, thereby allowing time for AOM to resolve on its own. If symptoms persist or worsen, antibacterial therapy is then started. As part of this strategy, parents are informed about (1) the high probability of spontaneous AOM resolution and (2) the drawbacks of giving antibiotics when they are not needed. Observation is considered appropriate only when follow-up can be ensured. The recommendation for observation is based on studies showing the following:

- Most episodes of AOM resolve spontaneously.
- Immediate antibacterial therapy is only marginally superior to observation at causing AOM resolution and is no better at relieving pain or distress.
- Parents find the observation approach acceptable.
- Delaying antibacterial therapy does not significantly increase the risk for mastoiditis, which can occur when bacteria invade the mastoid bone.

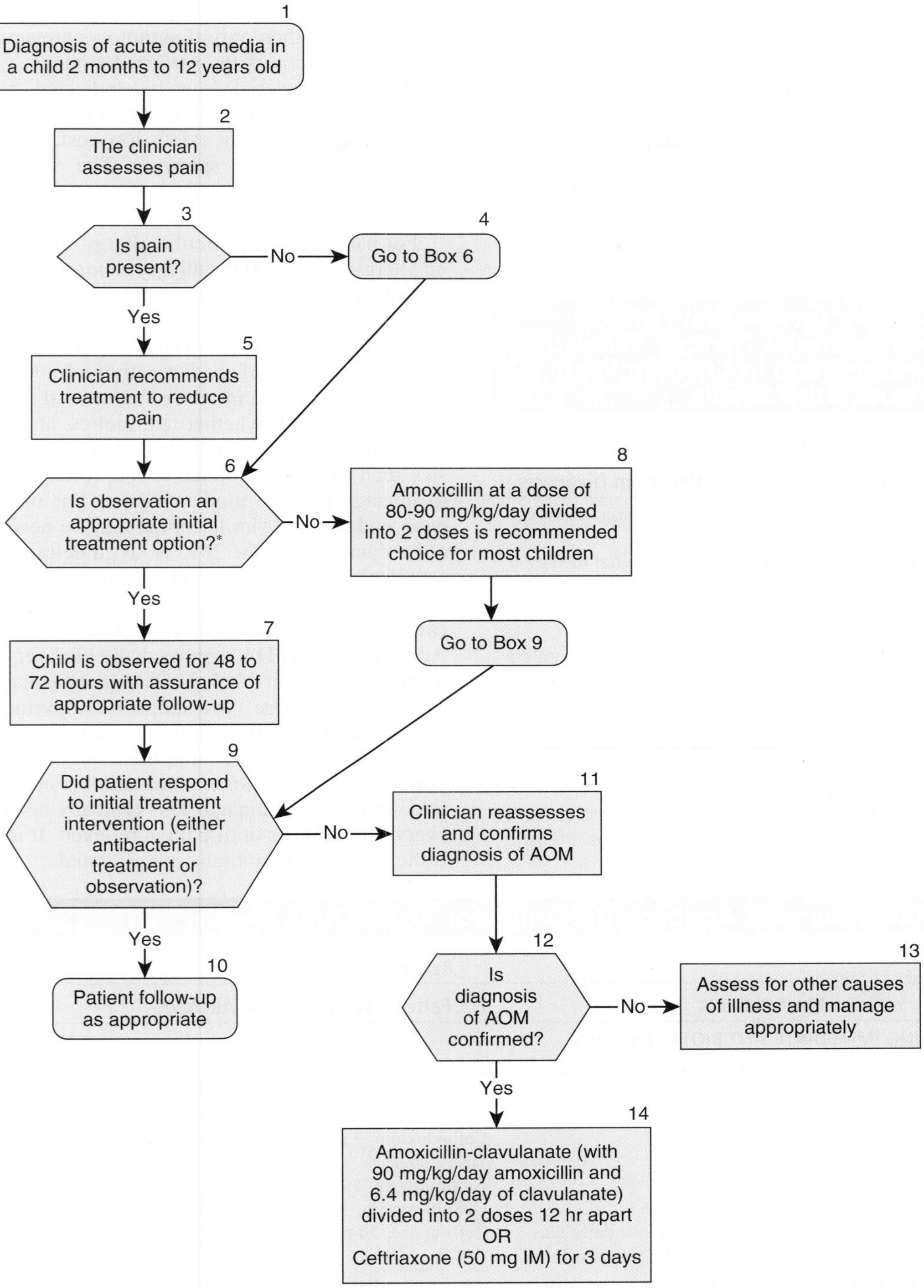
1
Diagnosis of acute otitis media in a child 2 months to 12 years old
2
The clinician assesses pain
3
Is pain present?
No
4
Go to Box 6
Yes
5
Clinician recommends treatment to reduce pain
6
Is observation an appropriate initial treatment option?*
No
8
Amoxicillin at a dose of 80-90 mg/kg/day divided into 2 doses is recommended choice for most children
Go to Box 9
Yes
7
Child is observed for 48 to 72 hours with assurance of appropriate follow-up
9
Did patient respond to initial treatment intervention (either antibacterial treatment or observation)?
No
11
Clinician reassesses and confirms diagnosis of AOM
Yes
10
Patient follow-up as appropriate
12
Is diagnosis of AOM confirmed?
No
13
Assess for other causes of illness and manage appropriately
Yes
14
Amoxicillin-clavulanate (with 90 mg/kg/day amoxicillin and 6.4 mg/kg/day of clavulanate) divided into 2 doses 12 hr apart
OR
Ceftriaxone (50 mg IM) for 3 days

* Criteria for antibacterial treatment or observation in children with uncomplicated AOM**

1) <6 mo: antibacterial treatment
2) 6 mo - 2 yr: antibacterial treatment if AOM diagnosis is certain unless AOM is unilateral without otorrhea
3) 2 yr and older: antibacterial treatment if severe pain >48 hours, fever ≥39°C (102.2°F) during the preceding 48 hours, or if there is a possibility that the caregiver may not reliably arrange for follow-up, if needed. For mild earache of <48 hours or if temperature is <39°C, observation is appropriate

**Caregiver is informed and agrees to the option of observation.
Caregiver is able to monitor child and return should condition worsen.
Systems are in place for ready communication with the clinician, evaluation, and obtaining medication if necessary.

*Appropriate medication alternatives should be used for the child with penicillin allergy.

Figure 86.2 ■ Management of acute otitis media.
(Data from http://pediatrics.aappublications.org/content/113/5/1451.figures-only; http://pediatrics.aappublications.org/content/pediatrics/early/2013/02/20/peds.2012-3488.full.pdf.)

Criteria for choosing between observation and initial antibacterial therapy are shown in Table 86.2. As indicated, all children younger than 6 months should receive antibiotics, regardless of diagnostic certainty or symptom severity. Among children 6 months to 2 years old, antibiotics are indicated whenever the diagnosis is certain. For children 2 years and older, antibacterial therapy is indicated only if the diagnosis is certain, and then only if symptoms are severe. In all other cases, observation is the preferred strategy.

When antibacterial drugs *are* indicated, *high-dose amoxicillin* is the treatment of choice (Table 86.3). Benefits of amoxicillin are efficacy, safety, low cost, acceptable taste, and narrow microbiologic spectrum. The duration of treatment ranges from 5 to 10 days, depending on patient age and illness severity.

For patients with penicillin allergy, drug selection depends on allergy severity. If the allergy is *not* severe (type II allergy), a cephalosporin may be used (e.g., cefdinir, cefuroxime). However, if the allergy is *severe* (type I allergy, causing urticaria or anaphylaxis), cephalosporins should be avoided, owing to concerns of cross-reactivity. In this case azithromycin and clarithromycin are recommended.

Regardless of whether antibiotics are prescribed, pain management must be included when treating AOM. Analgesics such as acetaminophen or ibuprofen are commonly used to manage mild to moderate pain. For moderate to severe pain, codeine and similar drugs may be needed. For children older than 5 years, the 2013 AAP guidelines also recommend a topical anesthetic such as procaine or lidocaine drops for pain relief. (The 2013 guidelines also recommended benzocaine; however, because it lacked U.S. Food and Drug Administration (FDA) approval, the FDA required its removal from the market in 2015. In Canada, benzocaine is still available for this purpose. An example is antipyrine and benzocaine [Auralgan ♣]. Both antipyrine and benzocaine are local anesthetics.) To relieve pain, the EAC is filled with the solution and then a solution-soaked cotton pledget is placed in the EAC to prevent drainage. This typically needs to be repeated every 1 to 2 hours until pain is relieved. It is contraindicated if the tympanic membrane is perforated.

TABLE 86.2 ▪ Criteria for Choosing Initial Antibacterial Therapy Versus Observation in Children With Acute Otitis Media

	Management Recommendation	
Age	**Certain Diagnosis**	**Uncertain Diagnosis**
Less than 6 months	Antibacterial therapy	Antibacterial therapy
6 months to 2 years	Antibacterial therapy*	Antibacterial therapy if illness is severe; observation if illness is not severe†
2 years and older	Antibacterial therapy if illness is severe; observation if illness is not severe†	Observation, regardless of symptom severity

*If AOM is unilateral without otorrhea and with mild symptoms, observation may be appropriate.
†Severe illness = moderate to severe otalgia or fever of 39°C (102.2°F) or higher; nonsevere illness = mild otalgia and fever below 39°C in the past 24 hours.

TABLE 86.3 ▪ Recommended Antibacterial Drugs for Acute Otitis Media

	Recommended Drugs	
Patient Group and Illness Severity	**For Most Patients**	**For Patients With Penicillin Allergy***
PATIENTS RECEIVING IMMEDIATE ANTIBIOTIC THERAPY		
Nonsevere illness	Amoxicillin, 40–45 mg/kg twice daily	*Non–type I allergy:* Cefdinir, 14 mg/kg/day in 1 or 2 divided doses *or* Cefuroxime, 15 mg/kg twice daily *or* Cefpodoxime, 5 mg/kg twice daily *Type I allergy:* Azithromycin, 10 mg/kg on day 1, then 5 mg/kg on days 2, 3, 4, and 5 *or* Clarithromycin, 7.5 mg/kg twice daily
Severe illness	Amoxicillin, 45 mg/kg twice daily *plus* clavulanate, 3.2 mg/kg twice daily†	Ceftriaxone, 50 mg/kg IM for 1 or 3 days
PATIENTS WITH PERSISTENT SYMPTOMS AFTER 48–72 HOURS OF OBSERVATION (WITH NO ANTIBIOTIC THERAPY)		
	Same as for patients receiving immediate antibiotic therapy	
PATIENTS WITH PERSISTENT SYMPTOMS AFTER 48–72 HOURS OF ANTIBIOTIC THERAPY (INDICATING DRUG RESISTANCE)		
Nonsevere illness	Amoxicillin, 45 mg/kg twice daily *plus* clavulanate, 3.2 mg/kg twice daily†	*Non–type I allergy:* Ceftriaxone, 50 mg/kg IM or IV for 3 days *Type I allergy:* Clindamycin, 30–40 mg/kg/day in 3 divided doses
Severe illness	Ceftriaxone, 50 mg/kg IM for 3 days	Clindamycin (plus a third-generation cephalosporin if non–type I penicillin allergy), tympanocentesis

*Type I allergy is severe (urticaria or anaphylaxis); type II is less severe.
†This ratio of amoxicillin to clavulanate can be achieved with Augmentin ES-600, a fixed-dose combination containing amoxicillin and clavulanic acid.
IM, intramuscular; IV, intravenous.

Treatment of Antibiotic-Resistant AOM

Antibiotic resistance is indicated by persistence of symptoms (fever, earache, otorrhea, a red and bulging tympanic membrane) for 2 to 3 days despite antibiotic therapy. Major risk factors for developing resistant AOM are the following:

- Day care attendance
- Age younger than 2 years
- Exposure to antibiotics in the prior 1 to 3 months
- Winter and spring seasons

In the United States the incidence of resistant AOM is on the rise because overuse of antibiotics has favored emergence of resistant pathogens. Resistance among strains of *Haemophilus influenzae* and *Moraxella catarrhalis* is limited to beta-lactam antibiotics. The mechanism is production of beta-lactamase, an enzyme that inactivates amoxicillin and certain other beta-lactam antibiotics. In contrast, strains of *Streptococcus pneumoniae* are resistant to multiple antibiotics, including erythromycin and trimethoprim/sulfamethoxazole, as well as amoxicillin and other beta-lactam antibiotics. Interestingly, *S. pneumoniae* resistance to amoxicillin does not result from beta-lactamase production. Rather, it results from synthesis of altered penicillin-binding proteins (PBPs), whose affinity for amoxicillin is much lower than that of normal PBPs.

How should resistant AOM be treated? Using a high dose of amoxicillin increases activity against resistant *S. pneumoniae.* For *H. influenzae* and *M. catarrhalis,* the preferred approach is oral therapy with *high-dose amoxicillin/clavulanate.* The clavulanate (clavulanic acid) in the combination inhibits beta-lactamase and thereby increases activity against resistant *H. influenzae* and *M. catarrhalis.* Because the clavulanate in the combination can cause diarrhea, the dosage of clavulanate should be low. It is important to be aware that the ratio of amoxicillin to clavulanate is not constant. For example, Augmentin (amoxicillin with clavulanate) is available as tablets containing 250 mg amoxicillin with 125 mg clavulanate and as tablets containing 500 mg amoxicillin with 125 mg clavulanate. If two tablets containing 250 mg amoxicillin are administered to give a patient a 500-mg dose of the amoxicillin component, the excess of clavulanate can result in worsening diarrhea. Alternatives to amoxicillin/clavulanate include *intramuscular (IM) ceftriaxone* and *oral clindamycin.* All three regimens are recommended for (1) children with acute AOM that has not responded to standard antibiotic therapy and (2) initial therapy of AOM in children with risk factors for resistant infection.

Prevention

The risk for acquiring AOM can be decreased in several ways. Breastfeeding for at least 6 months seems to reduce early episodes of AOM. During infancy and early childhood, AOM can be significantly reduced by avoiding childcare centers, if possible, when respiratory infections are prevalent. Measures believed to help prevent AOM include eliminating exposure to tobacco smoke, reducing pacifier use in the second 6 months of life, and avoiding supine bottle feeding. Two additional measures are prevention and treatment of influenza and vaccination against pneumococcal infection.

Prevention and Treatment of Influenza

As noted, influenza and other viral infections of the respiratory tract predispose children to developing bacterial and viral OM. Accordingly, measures that reduce influenza can reduce OM risk. Two methods are available: (1) vaccination against influenza and (2) treatment of active influenza infection. Although both immunization against and treatment of influenza can help during the flu season, they do nothing to alter AOM risk the rest of the year.

Vaccination Against Streptococcus Pneumoniae

Vaccination with *pneumococcal conjugate vaccine* (PCV) [Prevnar] can reduce the risk for AOM. Of note, *S. pneumoniae* was once responsible for 40% to 50% of bacterial AOM. This has decreased significantly since the first PCV was introduced in 2000. Unfortunately, there has now been an increase in strains that are not included in PCV.

Recurrent Otitis Media

Recurrent AOM can be defined as AOM that occurs 3 or more times within 6 months, or 4 or more times within 12 months. Four management strategies are available: (1) short-term antibacterial therapy, (2) prophylactic antibacterial therapy, (3) prevention and treatment of influenza, and (4) placement of a tympanostomy tube.

Short-Term Antibacterial Therapy

There is disagreement among experts regarding antibacterial therapy. Some authorities recommend antibiotics for each recurrent episode, regardless of presentation. Others recommend reserving antibiotics for episodes in which symptoms are severe. In both cases, high-dose amoxicillin is the treatment of choice. If resistance is suspected, amoxicillin/clavulanate can be used.

Prophylactic Antibacterial Therapy

Antibacterial prophylaxis is *not* generally recommended. An analysis of several studies indicates that, for each year of prophylaxis (with *trimethoprim/sulfamethoxazole,* or *amoxicillin*), only 1.3 episodes of AOM are prevented. This small benefit is largely outweighed by the risk for promoting antibiotic resistance. If prophylaxis *is* elected, it should be conducted only during the upper respiratory infection season. The preferred drug for prophylaxis is amoxicillin because, compared with sulfonamides, amoxicillin is more active against multidrug-resistant strains of *S. pneumoniae.*

Prevention and Treatment of Influenza

As discussed previously, AOM occurrence can be reduced by vaccinating against the influenza virus and by treating active influenza infection. However, benefits are seen only during the flu season.

Tympanostomy Tubes

A tympanostomy tube permits drainage and aeration of the middle ear. Tube insertion is performed under general anesthesia. In children with recurrent AOM, the procedure can significantly reduce AOM episodes. Complications of the procedure include obstruction of the tube, secondary infection with otorrhea, and premature tube extrusion.

Otitis Media With Effusion

OME (previously called secretory or serous otitis media) is more common than AOM. It often occurs with upper respiratory tract infections and may precede or follow an episode of AOM. The condition is characterized by fluid in the middle ear but without evidence of local or systemic illness. OME may cause mild hearing loss, but not pain. The condition can persist for weeks to months after AOM has resolved. Because it is not caused by a bacterial infection, antibiotics have no effect on OME and should not be used.

OTITIS EXTERNA AND ITS MANAGEMENT

Otitis externa (OE) is an inflammation of the EAC. The usual cause is bacterial infection, which may be limited to the EAC or may spread to adjacent tissues. Most cases of OE respond to topical drugs.

Acute Otitis Externa

Characteristics, Pathogenesis, and Microbiology

Acute otitis externa (AOE), also known as "swimmer's ear," is a bacterial infection of the EAC. The most common pathogens are *Pseudomonas aeruginosa* and *Staphylococcus aureus*. Other pathogens include *Staphylococcus epidermidis* and *Microbacterium otitidis*. Patients who have AOE present with one or more of the following: rapid-onset ear pain associated with pruritus, a sensation of ear fullness, tenderness on manipulation of the external ear, or edema or erythema of the EAC. Impaired hearing and purulent discharge may occur.

Susceptibility to AOE is precipitated primarily by two factors: abrasion and excessive moisture. Both facilitate bacterial colonization. Abrasion of the epithelium creates a site for bacterial entry. Most often, abrasion results from cleaning or scratching the EAC with a cotton-tipped swab or some other foreign object (e.g., finger, pencil, toothpick). Abrasion can also be caused by hearing aids and earplugs. Moisture can wash away the protective layer of cerumen. As a result, keratin debris in the EAC is able to absorb water, thereby creating a nourishing medium for bacterial growth. Moisture in the EAC may come from swimming, perspiration, and even high humidity.

Treatment

AOE is a painful condition, often severely so, so analgesics are indicated. The same analgesics used for AOM are appropriate for AOE pain management.

AOE usually responds well to simple treatment. The goal is to eradicate the pathogen and reduce pain. For most patients, cleaning and use of topical antimicrobials will suffice. If the infection is extensive, oral antibiotics may be needed. To facilitate healing, the ear should be kept as dry as possible. Most infections begin to improve in 3 days and resolve completely by 10 days.

Topical Medications

The most recent (2014) AOE clinical practice guidelines published by the American Academy of Otolaryngology recommend topical antimicrobials over systemic drugs for uncomplicated AOE. (See Fig. 86.3.) There are two reasons for this recommendation. First, topical agents achieve very high local concentrations (often 100–1000 times the concentration achieved with systemic drugs), antibacterial effects are superior, disease persistence is lower, and recurrence is less likely. Second, with topical therapy, systemic side effects are absent. Exceptions are made for patients with diabetes, immune deficiencies, or those who would have difficulty with proper administration of topical drugs. These patients should have systemic therapy. Systemic therapy should also be prescribed if the infection has spread beyond the EAC. In severe cases, both systemic and topical antibiotics are needed.

A variety of topical medications can be used. A *2% solution of acetic acid* is safe, effective, and inexpensive. A solution of *alcohol plus acetic acid* offers the additional benefit of promoting tissue drying. For many patients, acidification and drying are all that is needed.

If the infection is more extensive or cannot be cleared with acetic acid and alcohol, a topical antibiotic should be employed. In the past, a three-drug combination—*hydrocortisone, neomycin,* and *polymyxin B*—was considered standard therapy. The hydrocortisone reduces inflammation and edema; neomycin and polymyxin kill bacterial pathogens. Unfortunately, although this combination is effective and inexpensive, it has drawbacks. Specifically, the neomycin component is ototoxic and causes local swelling and erythema in about 15% of patients. Today, *quinolones* (e.g., ciprofloxacin) are preferred because these drugs are highly effective, do not cause local reactions, and are not ototoxic. Unlike many otic preparations, quinolones and quinolone/glucocorticoid combinations are safe for patients who have perforated tympanic membranes. The glucocorticoid has the added benefit of decreasing pain by reducing swelling caused by inflammation. Options include Cipro HC (*ciprofloxacin plus hydrocortisone*), Ciprodex (*ciprofloxacin plus dexamethasone*), and Floxin Otic (*ofloxacin* alone). Principal drawbacks of these preparations are expense and the potential to promote resistance to quinolone antibiotics.

Applying ear drops correctly can improve outcomes and reduce drug-related discomfort. Instillation of cold solutions can cause dizziness; therefore, ear drops should be warmed before administration. Wiggling the earlobe, if tolerated, can facilitate transit of solutions down the EAC. If edema results in EAC closure that is sufficient to impede drug penetration, insertion of a wick can help. A wick is like a very tiny elongated tampon. After it is carefully inserted into the edematous EAC, ear drops are applied to the exposed tip. (It will be important to apply enough medication to keep the wick moist.) Drug solutions are absorbed into the wick, which then delivers them to the epithelium of the entire canal. The wick should be replaced at least every 48 hours to allow cleaning and to determine whether further wicking is still needed.

Oral Medications

Oral antibacterials are indicated if the infection extends beyond the EAC to involve the pinna. For adults, *ciprofloxacin* [Cipro] is a good choice; however, because oral quinolones can cause tendon rupture in younger patients, it should not be given to patients younger than 18 years. For children, *cephalexin* [Keflex] is preferred.

Necrotizing Otitis Externa

Necrotizing OE is a rare but potentially fatal complication of AOE that develops when bacteria in the EAC invade the mastoid or temporal bone. Spread of infection to the skull base can affect cranial nerves, and spread to the dura mater

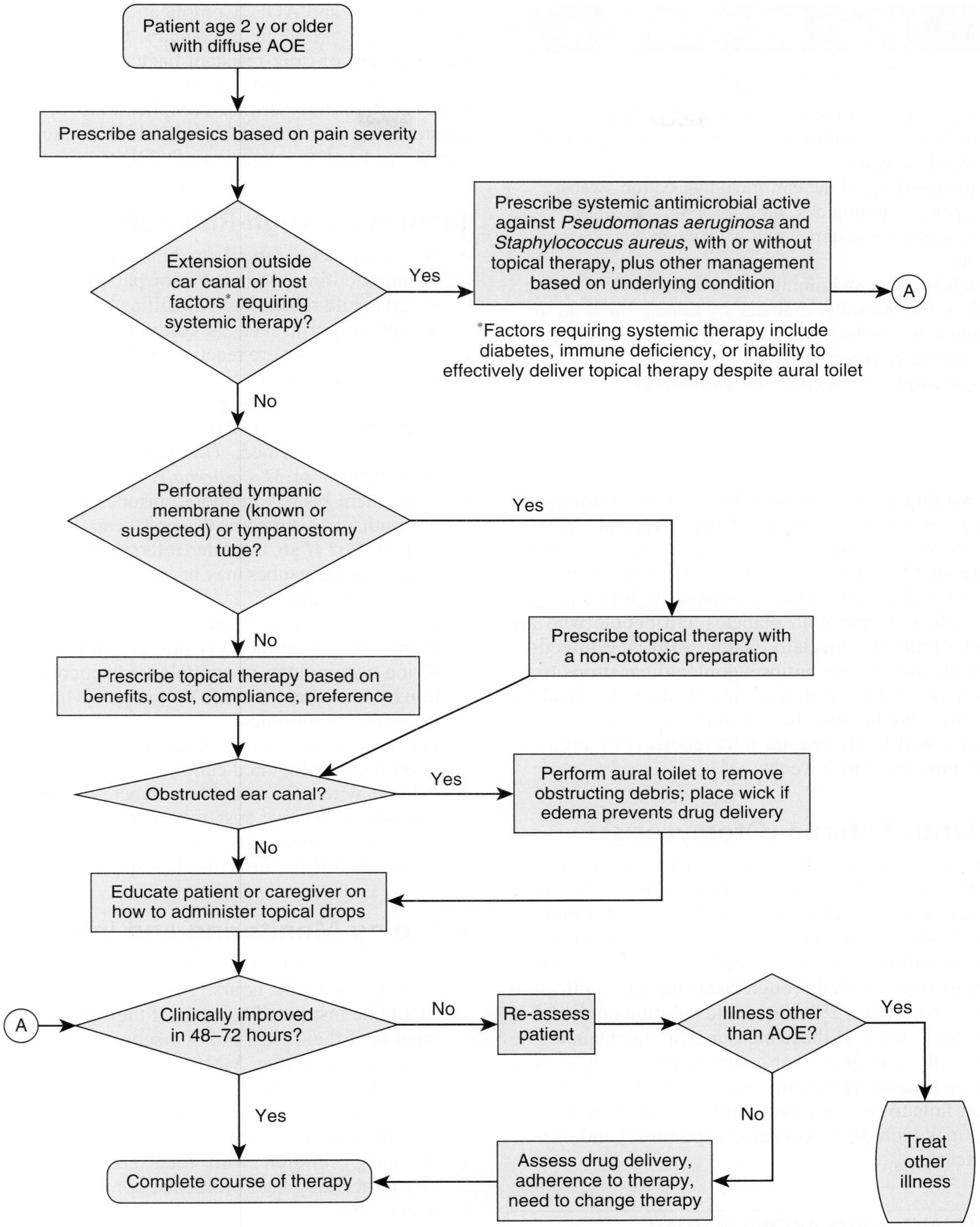

Figure 86.3 ■ Management of acute otitis externa.
(From Rosenfeld RM, Schwartz SR, Cannon CR, et al. Clinical practice guideline: acute otitis externa. Otolaryngol Head Neck Surg 2014;150(1 Suppl):S1–S24. © American Academy Otolaryngology—Head and Neck Surgery Foundation 2014. Reprints and permission: sagepub.com/journalsPermissions.nav.)

Patient Education

PREVENTION

The best way to prevent bacterial AOE is to keep the natural defenses of the EAC healthy. Ear hygiene can be promoted by following these rules:

- Don't put *anything* in the ear, including cotton swabs, fingers, pencils, toothpicks, liquids, or sprays, all of which can remove cerumen and/or damage the epithelium.
- Dry the EAC after swimming and showering by toweling off and promoting water drainage by tipping the head to each side while pulling the auricle in different directions.
- Don't remove cerumen (earwax).
- Don't use earplugs (except when swimming).

can cause meningitis and possibly lateral sinus thrombosis. The usual pathogen is *P. aeruginosa.* Patients typically present with progressive severe otic pain, purulent discharge from the ear, and granulation of tissue in the EAC. Necrotizing OE occurs almost exclusively in two groups of high-risk people, specifically, older people with diabetes and people who are immunocompromised, especially people with HIV infection. All patients should receive antipseudomonal ear drops (e.g., ofloxacin solution) along with oral ciprofloxacin. Referral for specialist care should also be considered. Progression to severe disease will likely require intravenous (IV) antipseudomonal therapy for 4 to 6 weeks.

Fungal Otitis Externa (Otomycosis)

In about 10% of patients, OE is caused by fungi and not bacteria. The two most common pathogens are *Aspergillus,* which causes 80% to 90% of otomycoses, and *Candida.* Fungal OE typically manifests as intense pruritus and erythema, with or without pain or hearing loss. As a rule, otomycosis can be managed with thorough cleansing and application of acidifying drops (e.g., 2% acetic acid solution applied 3–4 times a day for 7 days). If these measures are inadequate, the patient can apply a solution that contains an antifungal drug (e.g., *1% clotrimazole* [Lotrimin] twice daily for 7 days). If the infection fails to respond, *oral* antifungal therapy may be needed. Options include *itraconazole* [Sporanox] and *fluconazole* [Diflucan].

PRESCRIBING AND MONITORING CONSIDERATIONS

Therapeutic Goal

The goals of management of ear infections are to reduce inflammation, eliminate infection, and prevent complications due to AOM and AOE. Complications include development of language problems secondary to hearing deficits and development of drug-resistant bacteria (primarily as a result of not taking medication as directed or stopping them prematurely). Rare but serious complications of AOM include mastoiditis and meningitis. As noted, necrotizing otitis externa can occur from an extension of AOE.

Identifying High-Risk Patients

- Assess for penicillin allergy before prescribing amoxicillin or amoxicillin/clavulanate. For patients who have experienced a mild reaction to penicillins, guidelines recommend a cephalosporin such as cefdinir, cefuroxime, or cefpodoxime. For a severe reaction such as anaphylaxis, azithromycin or clarithromycin is recommended.
- Determine whether the patient with AOM has taken amoxicillin in the past 30 days. If so, amoxicillin/clavulanate should be prescribed. This should also be prescribed if *H. influenzae* or *M. catarrhalis* is suspected.
- Have there been 3 or more episodes of AOM in the past 6 months or 4 times in the past year (indicative of recurrent AOM)? If so, consider referral to an otolaryngologist. Tympanostomy tubes may be indicated, especially if hearing loss is a concern.
- Is the tympanic membrane intact? If not, avoid ototoxic drops such as aminoglycoside preparations. Instead, prescribe a quinolone or quinolone/glucocorticoid combination because these are safe for patients who have perforated tympanic membranes.
- For AOE, if the canal is significantly swollen, insert a wick to ensure that the medication reaches all affected tissues.
- Patients with AOE who have diabetes or immune deficiencies should receive systemic therapy or a combination of systemic and topical therapy. Systemic therapy or referral is indicated if the infection has spread beyond the EAC.

Ongoing Monitoring and Interventions

- Patients with both AOM and AOE should have improvement in 48 to 72 hours. Before leaving the clinic, they should be instructed to return if they do not have improvement or if their condition worsens.
- Keep in mind that MME will continue long after the AOM has resolved. For this reason, tympanometry and pneumatic otoscopy will not reflect a normal response to pressure changes for several weeks or even months.
- If young children with recurrent or prolonged AOM experience language problems, consider early referral for intervention.

UNIT XXI

Drug Therapy in Acute Care

CHAPTER 87

Agents Affecting the Volume and Ion Content of Body Fluids

Laura D. Rosenthal, DNP, ACNP, FAANP

The drugs discussed in this chapter are used to correct disturbances in the volume and ionic composition of body fluids. Standard guidelines do not exist for electrolyte and fluid replacement. Most facilities will have their own protocols regarding recommended replacement. Many of these protocols allow for the replacement of electrolytes by the registered nurse. Three groups of agents are considered for replacement: (1) drugs used to correct disorders of fluid volume and osmolality, (2) drugs used to correct disturbances of hydrogen ion concentration (acid-base status), and (3) drugs used to correct electrolyte imbalances.

DISORDERS OF FLUID VOLUME AND OSMOLALITY

Good health requires that both the volume and osmolality of extracellular and intracellular fluids remain within a normal range. If a substantial alteration in either the volume or osmolality of these fluids develops, significant harm can result.

Maintenance of fluid volume and osmolality is primarily the job of the kidneys, and, even under adverse conditions, renal mechanisms usually succeed in keeping the volume and composition of body fluids within acceptable limits. However, circumstances can arise in which the regulatory capacity of the kidneys is exceeded. When this occurs, disruption of fluid volume, osmolality, or both can result.

Abnormal states of hydration can be divided into two major categories: volume contraction and volume expansion. *Volume contraction* is defined as a *decrease* in total body water; conversely, *volume expansion* is defined as an *increase* in total body water. States of volume contraction and volume expansion have three subclassifications based on alterations in extracellular osmolality. For volume contraction, the subcategories are *isotonic contraction, hypertonic contraction,* and *hypotonic contraction.* Volume expansion may also be subclassified as *isotonic, hypertonic,* or *hypotonic.* Descriptions and causes of these abnormal states are discussed later.

In the clinical setting, changes in osmolality are described in terms of the sodium content of plasma. Sodium is used as the reference for classification because this ion is the principal extracellular solute. In most cases, the total osmolality of plasma is about 2 times the osmolality of sodium. That is, total plasma osmolality usually ranges from 280 to 300 mOsm/kg water.

Volume Contraction

Isotonic Contraction

Definition and Causes

Isotonic contraction is defined as volume contraction in which *sodium and water are lost in isotonic proportions.* Hence, although there is a decrease in the total volume of extracellular fluid, there is no change in osmolality. Causes of isotonic contraction include vomiting, diarrhea, kidney disease, and misuse of diuretics.

Treatment

Lost volume should be replaced with fluids that are isotonic to plasma. This can be accomplished by infusing isotonic (0.9%) sodium chloride in sterile water, a solution in which both sodium and chloride are present at a concentration of 145 mEq/L.

Hypertonic Contraction

Definition and Causes

Hypertonic contraction is defined as volume contraction in which *loss of water exceeds loss of sodium.* Hence there is a reduction in extracellular fluid volume coupled with an increase in osmolality. Because of extracellular hypertonicity, water is drawn out of cells, thereby producing intracellular dehydration and partial compensation for lost extracellular volume.

Causes of hypertonic contraction include excessive sweating, osmotic diuresis, and feeding excessively concentrated foods to infants. Hypertonic contraction may also develop secondary to extensive burns or disorders of the central nervous system (CNS) that render the patient unable to experience or report thirst.

Treatment

Volume replacement in hypertonic contraction should be accomplished with hypotonic fluids (e.g., 0.45% sodium chloride) or with fluids that contain no solutes at all. Initial therapy may consist simply of drinking water. Alternatively, 5% dextrose can be infused intravenously. (Because dextrose is rapidly metabolized to carbon dioxide and water, dextrose solutions can be viewed as the osmotic equivalent of water alone.) Volume replenishment should be done in stages. About 50% of the estimated loss should be replaced during the first 24 hours of treatment. The remainder should be replenished over the next 1 to 2 days.

Hypotonic Contraction

Definition and Causes

Hypotonic contraction is defined as volume contraction in which *loss of sodium exceeds loss of water.* Hence both the volume and osmolality of extracellular fluid are reduced. Because intracellular osmolality now exceeds extracellular osmolality, extracellular volume becomes diminished further by movement of water into cells.

The principal cause of hypotonic contraction is excessive loss of sodium through the kidneys. This may occur because of diuretic therapy, chronic renal insufficiency, or lack of aldosterone (the adrenocortical hormone that promotes renal retention of sodium).

Treatment

If hyponatremia is mild, and if renal function is adequate, hypotonic contraction can be corrected by infusing *isotonic* sodium chloride solution for injection. When this is done, plasma tonicity will be adjusted by the kidneys. However, if the sodium loss is severe, a *hypertonic* (e.g., 3%) solution of sodium chloride should be infused. Administration should continue until plasma sodium concentration has been raised to about 130 mEq/L. Patients should be monitored for signs of fluid overload (distention of neck veins, peripheral or pulmonary edema). When hypotonic contraction is due to aldosterone insufficiency, patients should receive hormone replacement therapy along with intravenous (IV) infusion of isotonic sodium chloride.

Volume Expansion

Volume expansion is defined as an *increase in the total volume of body fluid.* As with volume contraction, volume expansion may be *isotonic, hypertonic,* or *hypotonic.* Volume expansion may result from an overdose with therapeutic fluids (e.g., sodium chloride infusion) or may be associated with disease states, such as heart failure, nephrotic syndrome, or cirrhosis of the liver with ascites. The principal drugs employed to correct volume expansion are *diuretics* and the *agents used for heart failure.* These drugs are discussed in Chapters 35 and 40, respectively.

ACID-BASE DISTURBANCES

Maintenance of acid-base balance is a complex process, the full discussion of which is beyond the scope of this text. Hence, discussion here is condensed.

Acid-base status is regulated by multiple systems. The most important are (1) the bicarbonate–carbonic acid buffer system, (2) the respiratory system, and (3) the kidneys. The respiratory system influences pH through control of CO_2 exhalation. Because CO_2 represents volatile carbonic acid, exhalation of CO_2 tends to elevate pH (reduce acidity), whereas retention of CO_2 (secondary to respiratory slowing) tends to lower pH. The kidneys influence pH by regulating bicarbonate excretion. By *retaining* bicarbonate, the kidneys can raise pH. Conversely, by increasing bicarbonate *excretion,* the kidneys can lower pH, and thereby compensate for alkalosis.

There are four principal types of acid-base imbalance: (1) respiratory alkalosis, (2) respiratory acidosis, (3) metabolic alkalosis, and (4) metabolic acidosis. Causes and treatments are discussed next.

Respiratory Alkalosis

Causes

Respiratory alkalosis is produced by hyperventilation. Deep and rapid breathing increases CO_2 loss, which in turn lowers the P_{CO_2} (partial pressure of carbon dioxide) of blood and increases pH. Mild hyperventilation may result from a number of causes, including hypoxia, pulmonary disease, and drugs (especially aspirin and other salicylates). Severe hyperventilation can be caused by CNS injury and hysteria.

Treatment

Management of respiratory alkalosis is dictated by the severity of pH elevation. When alkalosis is mild, no specific treatment is indicated. Severe respiratory alkalosis resulting from hysteria can be controlled by having the patient rebreathe his or her CO_2-laden expired breath. This can be accomplished by holding a paper bag over the nose and mouth. Although this technique has been used for many years, there remains a lack of evidence regarding its efficacy in respiratory alkalosis. A sedative (e.g., diazepam [Valium]) can help suppress the hysteria.

Respiratory Acidosis

Causes

Respiratory acidosis results from retention of CO_2 secondary to hypoventilation. Reduced CO_2 exhalation raises plasma P_{CO_2}, which in turn causes plasma pH to fall. Primary causes of impaired ventilation are (1) depression of the medullary respiratory center and (2) pathologic changes in the lungs (e.g., status asthmaticus, airway obstruction). Over time, the kidneys compensate for respiratory acidosis by excreting less bicarbonate.

Treatment

Primary treatment of respiratory acidosis is directed at correcting respiratory impairment. The patient may also need oxygen and ventilatory assistance. Infusion of sodium bicarbonate may be indicated if acidosis is severe (pH $\leq$6.9).

Metabolic Alkalosis

Causes

Metabolic alkalosis is characterized by increases in both the pH and bicarbonate content of plasma. Causes include excessive loss of gastric acid (through vomiting or suctioning) and administration of alkalinizing salts (e.g., sodium bicarbonate). The body compensates for metabolic alkalosis by (1) hypoventilation (which causes retention of CO_2), (2) increased renal excretion of bicarbonate, and (3) accumulation of organic acids.

Treatment

In most cases, metabolic alkalosis can be corrected by targeting the specific cause of the acidosis (e.g., medicating for vomiting or decreasing gastric suction). One may also consider infusing a solution of *sodium chloride plus potassium chloride*. This facilitates renal excretion of bicarbonate and thereby promotes normalization of plasma pH.

Metabolic Acidosis

Causes

Principal causes of metabolic acidosis are chronic renal failure, loss of bicarbonate during severe diarrhea, and metabolic disorders that result in overproduction of lactic acid (lactic acidosis) or ketoacids (ketoacidosis). Metabolic acidosis may also result from poisoning by methanol and certain medications (e.g., aspirin and other salicylates).

Treatment

Treatment consists of correcting the underlying cause of acidosis, and, if the acidosis is severe, administering an alkalinizing salt (e.g., sodium bicarbonate, sodium carbonate).

When an alkalinizing salt is indicated, *sodium bicarbonate* is generally preferred. Administration may be oral or IV. If acidosis is mild, oral administration is preferred. IV infusion is usually reserved for severe reductions of pH. When sodium bicarbonate is given intravenously to treat acute, severe acidosis, caution must be exercised to avoid excessive elevation of plasma pH because rapid conversion from acidosis to alkalosis can be hazardous. Also, because of the sodium content of sodium bicarbonate, care should be taken to avoid hypernatremia.

POTASSIUM IMBALANCES

Potassium is the most abundant *intracellular* cation, having a concentration within cells of about 150 mEq/L. In contrast, *extracellular* concentrations are low (4–5 mEq/L). Potassium plays a major role in conducting nerve impulses and maintaining the electrical excitability of muscle. Potassium also helps regulate acid-base balance.

Regulation of Potassium Levels

Serum levels of potassium are regulated primarily by the kidneys. Under steady-state conditions, urinary output of potassium equals intake. Renal excretion of potassium is increased by aldosterone, an adrenal steroid that promotes conservation of sodium while increasing potassium loss. Potassium excretion is also increased by most diuretics. Potassium-sparing diuretics (e.g., spironolactone) are the exception.

Potassium levels are influenced by extracellular pH. In the presence of extracellular *alkalosis,* potassium uptake by cells is *enhanced,* causing a *reduction* in extracellular potassium levels. Conversely, extracellular *acidosis* promotes the exit of potassium from cells, thereby causing extracellular *hyperkalemia.*

Insulin has a profound effect on potassium: in high doses, insulin stimulates potassium uptake by cells. This ability has been used to treat hyperkalemia.

Hypokalemia

Causes and Consequences

Hypokalemia exists when serum potassium levels fall below 3.5 mEq/L. The most common cause is treatment with a thiazide or loop diuretic (see Chapter 35). Other causes include insufficient potassium intake; alkalosis and excessive insulin (both of which decrease extracellular potassium levels by driving potassium into cells); increased renal excretion of potassium (e.g., as caused by aldosterone); and potassium loss associated with vomiting, diarrhea, and abuse of laxatives. Hypokalemia may also occur because of excessive potassium loss in sweat. As a rule, potassium depletion is accompanied by loss of chloride. Insufficiency of both ions produces *hypokalemic alkalosis.*

Prevention and Treatment

Potassium depletion can be treated with four potassium salts: potassium chloride, potassium phosphate, potassium gluconate, and potassium bicarbonate. These may also be used for prophylaxis against potassium insufficiency. For either treatment or prophylaxis, the preferred salt is *potassium chloride* because chloride deficiency frequently coexists with potassium deficiency.

Potassium chloride may be administered orally or intravenously. Oral therapy is preferred for prophylaxis and for treating mild deficiency. IV therapy is reserved for severe deficiency and for patients who cannot take potassium by mouth.

Oral Potassium Chloride

Uses, Dosage, and Preparations. Oral potassium chloride may be used for both prevention and treatment of potassium deficiency. Dosages for prevention range from 16 to 24 mEq/day. Dosages for deficiency range from 40 to 100 mEq/day (Table 87.1). In a perfect world, giving 10 mEq of potassium should raise the serum potassium level by about 0.1 mEq/L.

Adverse Effects. Potassium chloride irritates the gastrointestinal (GI) tract, frequently causing abdominal discomfort, nausea, vomiting, and diarrhea. With the exception of the sustained-release tablets, solid formulations can produce high local concentrations of potassium, resulting in severe intestinal injury (ulcerative lesions, bleeding, perforation); death has occurred. To minimize GI effects, oral potassium chloride should be taken with meals or a full glass of water. If symptoms of irritation occur, dosing should be discontinued. Rarely, oral potassium chloride produces hyperkalemia. This dangerous development is much more likely with IV therapy.

The principal complication is *hyper*kalemia, which can prove fatal. To reduce the risk for hyperkalemia, serum potassium levels should be measured before the infusion and periodically throughout the treatment interval. Also, renal function should be assessed before and during treatment to ensure adequate output of urine. If renal failure develops, the infusion should be stopped immediately. Changes in the electrocardiogram (ECG) can be an early indication that potassium toxicity is developing.

TABLE 87.1 ■ Potassium Chloride Uses, Dosage, and Preparations

Drug	Forms	Uses	Usual Adult Doses
K-Dur	Tablets	Prevention of hypokalemia	20–40 mEq/day PO in 1–2 divided doses
Micro-K	Powder	Treatment of mild hypokalemia	40–100 mEq/day PO in 2–5 divided doses
Klor-Con	Intravenous solution	Treatment of mild to moderate hypokalemia	120–240 mEq/day PO in 3–4 divided doses
Potassium chloride		Treatment of moderate to severe hypokalemia	10 mEq/hr IV Maximum 24-hr dose: 200 mEq

Contraindications to Potassium Use. Potassium should be avoided under conditions that predispose to hyperkalemia (e.g., severe renal impairment, use of potassium-sparing diuretics, hypoaldosteronism). Potassium must also be avoided when hyperkalemia already exists.

Hyperkalemia

Causes

Hyperkalemia (excessive elevation of serum potassium) can result from a number of causes. These include severe tissue trauma, untreated Addison disease, acute acidosis (which draws potassium out of cells), acute renal failure, misuse of potassium-sparing diuretics, and overdose with IV potassium.

Consequences

The most serious consequence of hyperkalemia is disruption of the electrical activity of the heart. Because hyperkalemia alters the generation and conduction of cardiac impulses, alterations in the ECG and cardiac rhythm are usually the earliest signs that potassium levels are growing dangerously high. With mild elevation of serum potassium (5–7 mEq/L), the T wave heightens and the PR interval becomes prolonged. When serum potassium reaches 8 to 9 mEq/L, cardiac arrest can occur, possibly preceded by ventricular tachycardia or fibrillation.

Effects of hyperkalemia are not limited to the heart. Noncardiac effects include confusion, anxiety, dyspnea, weakness or heaviness of the legs, and numbness or tingling of the hands, feet, and lips.

Treatment

Treatment is begun by withholding any foods that contain potassium and any medicines that promote potassium accumulation (e.g., potassium-sparing diuretics, potassium supplements). After this, management consists of measures that (1) counteract potassium-induced cardiotoxicity and (2) lower extracellular levels of potassium. Specific steps include infusion of a *calcium salt* (e.g., calcium gluconate) to offset effects of hyperkalemia on the heart and infusion of *glucose* and *insulin* to promote uptake of potassium by cells and thereby decrease extracellular potassium levels. If these measures prove inadequate, steps can be taken to remove potassium. These include (1) oral or rectal administration of *sodium polystyrene sulfonate* [Kayexalate, Kionex], an exchange resin that absorbs potassium; and (2) peritoneal or extracorporeal dialysis.

In 2015, the U.S. Food and Drug Administration approved the first new drug to treat hyperkalemia in many years. Patiromer [Veltassa] is a powder that works by decreasing absorption of potassium by binding potassium within the GI tract. Patiromer is useful in reducing potassium levels in patients with chronic kidney disease or patients treated with a drug that affects the renin-angiotensin-aldosterone system. Because of its slower onset, patiromer is not approved for the treatment of acute hyperkalemia.

MAGNESIUM IMBALANCES

Magnesium is required for the activity of many enzymes and for binding of messenger RNA to ribosomes. In addition, magnesium helps regulate neurochemical transmission and the excitability of muscle. The concentration of magnesium within cells is about 40 mEq/L, much higher than its concentration outside cells (about 2 mEq/L).

Hypomagnesemia

Causes and Consequences

Low levels of magnesium may result from a variety of causes, including diarrhea, hemodialysis, kidney disease, and prolonged IV feeding with magnesium-free solutions. Hypomagnesemia may also be seen in people with chronic alcoholism, diabetes, or pancreatitis. Frequently, patients with magnesium deficiency also present with hypocalcemia and hypokalemia.

Prominent symptoms of hypomagnesemia involve cardiac and skeletal muscle. In the presence of low levels of magnesium, release of acetylcholine at the neuromuscular junction is enhanced. This can increase muscle excitability to the point of tetany. Hypomagnesemia also increases excitability of neurons in the CNS, causing disorientation, psychoses, and seizures.

Prevention and Treatment

Frank hypomagnesemia is treated with parenteral magnesium sulfate. For prophylaxis against magnesium deficiency, an oral preparation (magnesium oxide) may be used (Table 87.2).

Adverse Effects

Excessive levels of magnesium cause *neuromuscular blockade.* Paralysis of the respiratory muscles is of particular concern. By suppressing neuromuscular transmission, magnesium excess can intensify the effects of neuromuscular blocking agents (e.g., succinylcholine, atracurium). Hence caution must be exercised in patients receiving these drugs. The neuromuscular blocking actions of magnesium can be counteracted with calcium. Accordingly, when parenteral magnesium

TABLE 87.2 ■ Magnesium Uses, Dosage, and Preparations

Drug	Forms	Uses	Usual Adult Doses
Magnesium oxide	Tablets	Prevention of hypomagnesemia	400–800 mg/day PO in 1–2 divided doses
Magnesium sulfate	Intravenous solution	Treatment of mild hypomagnesemia	1–2 g IV as indicated by serum magnesium concentrations
		Treatment of moderate hypomagnesemia	2–4 g IV as indicated by serum magnesium concentrations
		Treatment of severe hypomagnesemia	4–8 g IV as indicated by serum magnesium concentrations

is being employed, an injectable form of calcium (e.g., calcium gluconate) should be immediately available.

In the heart, excessive magnesium can suppress impulse conduction through the atrioventricular (AV) node. Accordingly, magnesium sulfate is contraindicated for patients with AV heart block.

To minimize the risk for toxicity, serum magnesium levels should be monitored. Respiratory paralysis occurs at 12 to 15 mEq/L. When magnesium levels exceed 25 mEq/L, cardiac arrest may set in.

Hypermagnesemia

Toxic elevation of magnesium levels is most common in patients with renal insufficiency, especially when magnesium-containing antacids or cathartics are being used. Symptoms of mild intoxication include muscle weakness (resulting from inhibition of acetylcholine release), hypotension, sedation, and ECG changes. As noted, respiratory paralysis is likely when plasma levels reach 12 to 15 mEq/L. At higher magnesium concentrations, there is a risk for cardiac arrest. Muscle weakness and paralysis can be counteracted with IV calcium.

CHAPTER 88

Management of ST-Segment Elevation Myocardial Infarction

Laura D. Rosenthal, DNP, ACNP, FAANP

Myocardial infarction (MI), also known as heart attack, is defined as necrosis of the myocardium (heart muscle) resulting from local ischemia (deficient blood flow). The underlying cause is partial or complete blockage of a coronary artery. When blockage is complete, the area of infarction is much larger than when the blockage is partial. In this chapter, discussion is limited to acute MI caused by *complete* interruption of regional myocardial blood flow. This class of MI is called *ST-segment elevation myocardial infarction* (STEMI) because it causes elevation of the ST segment on the electrocardiogram (ECG). Management of STEMI differs from management of non–ST-elevation MI, which occurs when blockage of blood flow is only partial.

In the United States STEMI strikes about 250,000 people each year and is the most common cause of death. Between 20% and 30% of STEMI victims die before reaching the hospital, another 5% to 6% die in the hospital, and 7% to 18% die within a year of hospital discharge. Risk factors for STEMI include advanced age, a family history of MI, sedentary lifestyle, high serum cholesterol, hypertension, smoking, and diabetes. The objectives of this chapter are to describe the pathophysiology of STEMI and to discuss interventions that can help reduce morbidity and mortality.

PATHOPHYSIOLOGY OF STEMI

Acute MI occurs when blood flow to a region of the myocardium is stopped owing to platelet plugging and thrombus formation in a coronary artery—almost always at the site of a fissured or ruptured atherosclerotic plaque. Myocardial injury is ultimately the result of an imbalance between oxygen demand and oxygen supply.

In response to local ischemia, a dramatic redistribution of ions takes place. Hydrogen ions accumulate in the myocardium, and calcium ions become sequestered in mitochondria. The resultant acidosis and functional calcium deficiency alter the distensibility of cardiac muscle. Sodium ions accumulate in myocardial cells and promote edema. Potassium ions are lost from myocardial cells, setting the stage for dysrhythmias.

Local metabolic changes begin rapidly after coronary arterial occlusion. Within seconds, metabolism shifts from aerobic to anaerobic. High-energy stores of adenosine triphosphate (ATP) and creatine phosphate become depleted. As a result, contraction ceases in the affected region.

If blood flow is not restored, cell death begins within 20 minutes. Clear indices of cell death—myocyte disruption, coagulative necrosis, elevation of cardiac proteins in serum—are present by 24 hours. By 4 days, monocyte infiltration and removal of dead myocytes weaken the infarcted area, making it vulnerable to expansion and rupture. Structural integrity is partially restored with deposition of collagen, which begins in 10 to 12 days and ends with dense scar formation by 4 to 6 weeks.

Myocardial injury also triggers ventricular remodeling, a process in which ventricular mass increases and the chambers change in volume and shape. Remodeling is driven in part by local production of angiotensin II. Ventricular remodeling increases the risk for heart failure and death.

The degree of residual cardiac impairment depends on how much of the myocardium was damaged. With infarction of 10% of left ventricular (LV) mass, the ejection fraction is reduced. With 25% LV infarction, cardiac dilation and heart failure occur. With 40% LV infarction, cardiogenic shock and death are likely.

MANAGEMENT OF STEMI

The acute phase of management refers to the interval between the onset of symptoms and discharge from the hospital (usually 6–10 days). The goal is to bring cardiac oxygen supply back in balance with oxygen demand. This can be accomplished by reperfusion therapy, which restores blood flow to the myocardium, and by reducing myocardial oxygen demand. The first few hours of treatment are most critical. The major threats to life during acute STEMI are ventricular dysrhythmias, cardiogenic shock, and heart failure.

To aid clinicians in the management of STEMI, the American College of Cardiology Foundation (ACCF), the American Heart Association (AHA), and the Society for Cardiovascular Angiography and Interventions (SCAI) have updated a series of evidence-based guidelines, including the following:

- *2013 ACCF/AHA Guideline for the Management of ST-Elevation Myocardial Infarction: A Report of the American College of Cardiology Foundation/American Heart Association Task Force on Practice Guidelines*
- *2015 ACC/AHA/SCAI Focused Update on Primary Percutaneous Coronary Intervention for Patients with ST-Elevation Myocardial Infarction: An Update of the 2011 ACCF/AHA/SCAI Guideline for Percutaneous Coronary Intervention and the 2013 ACCF/AHA Guideline for the Management of ST-Elevation Myocardial Infarction*

These guidelines are available at circ.ahajournals.org. The following discussion reflects recommendations in these documents.

Routine Drug Therapy

When a patient presents with suspected STEMI, several interventions should begin immediately. The objective is to minimize possible myocardial necrosis while waiting for a clear diagnosis. After STEMI has been diagnosed, more definitive therapy—reperfusion—can be implemented (see later).

Oxygen

Supplemental oxygen, administered by nasal cannula, can increase arterial oxygen saturation and can thereby increase oxygen delivery to the ischemic myocardium. Accordingly, current guidelines recommend giving oxygen to all patients with reduced arterial oxygen saturation (below 90%). However, although oxygen is recommended, and using it seems to make sense, the practice is not evidence based. That is, we have no hard evidence to show that oxygen is beneficial. In fact there is some evidence that oxygen may actually be harmful, causing mortality to increase rather than decline.

Aspirin

Aspirin suppresses platelet aggregation, producing an immediate antithrombotic effect. In the Second International Study of Infarct Survival (ISIS-2), aspirin caused a substantial reduction in mortality. Moreover, benefits were synergistic with fibrinolytic drugs: mortality was 13.2% with fibrinolytics alone, and dropped to 8% with the addition of aspirin. Because of these benefits, virtually all patients with evolving STEMI should get aspirin. Therapy should begin immediately after onset of symptoms and should continue indefinitely. The first dose (162–325 mg) should be chewed to allow rapid absorption across the buccal mucosa. Prolonged therapy (with 81–162 mg/day) reduces the risk for reinfarction, stroke, and death.

Nonaspirin Nonsteroidal Antiinflammatory Drugs

According to the 2013 guideline updates, routine use of nonsteroidal antiinflammatory drugs (NSAIDs) other than aspirin should be *discontinued.* Unlike aspirin, these agents increase the risk for mortality, reinfarction, hypertension, heart failure, and myocardial rupture.

Morphine

Intravenous morphine is the treatment of choice for STEMI-associated pain. In addition to relieving pain, morphine can improve hemodynamics. By promoting venodilation, the drug reduces cardiac preload. By promoting modest arterial dilation, morphine may cause some reduction in afterload. The combined reductions in preload and afterload lower cardiac oxygen demand, helping preserve the ischemic myocardium.

Beta Blockers

When given to patients undergoing acute STEMI, beta blockers (e.g., atenolol, metoprolol) reduce cardiac pain, infarct size, and short-term mortality. Recurrent ischemia and reinfarction are also decreased. Reduction in myocardial wall tension may decrease the risk for myocardial rupture. Continued use of an oral beta blocker increases long-term survival. Unfortunately, although nearly all patients can benefit from beta blockers, many don't get them. Furthermore, among patients who *do* get a beta blocker, the dosage is often too low.

Benefits result from several mechanisms. As STEMI evolves, traffic along sympathetic nerves to the heart increases greatly, as does the number of beta receptors in the heart. As a result, heart rate and force of contraction rise substantially, increasing cardiac oxygen demand. By preventing beta receptor activation, beta blockers reduce heart rate and contractility and thereby reduce oxygen demand. They reduce oxygen demand even more by lowering blood pressure. By prolonging diastolic filling time, beta blockers increase coronary blood flow and myocardial oxygen supply. Additional benefits derive from antidysrhythmic actions.

Beta blockers should be used routinely in the absence of specific contraindications (e.g., bradycardia, significant LV dysfunction). The initial dose may be oral or IV; oral dosing is used thereafter. Treatment with an oral beta blocker should begin within 24 hours. Beta blockers are especially good for patients with reflex tachycardia, systolic hypertension, atrial fibrillation, and atrioventricular conduction abnormalities. Contraindications include overt severe heart failure, pronounced bradycardia, persistent hypotension, advanced heart block, and cardiogenic shock. The basic pharmacology of the beta blockers is presented in Chapter 14.

Nitroglycerin

In patients with STEMI, nitroglycerin has several beneficial effects: it can (1) reduce preload and thereby reduce oxygen demand; (2) increase collateral blood flow in the ischemic region of the heart; (3) control hypertension caused by STEMI-associated anxiety; and (4) limit infarct size and improve LV function. However, despite these useful effects, nitroglycerin does not reduce mortality. Nonetheless, because the drug is easily administered, offers hemodynamic benefits, and helps relieve ischemic chest pain, it continues to be used. According to the current guidelines, patients with ongoing ischemic discomfort should be given sublingual nitroglycerin (0.4 mg) every 5 minutes for a total of three doses, and then be assessed to determine whether IV nitroglycerin should be given. Indications for IV therapy include persisting ischemic discomfort, hypertension, and pulmonary congestion. Nitroglycerin should be avoided in patients with hypotension (systolic pressure below 90 mm Hg), severe bradycardia (heart rate below 50 beats/min), marked tachycardia (heart rate above 100 beats/min), or suspected right ventricular infarction. In addition, nitroglycerin should be avoided in patients who have taken sildenafil, avanafil, or vardenafil for erectile dysfunction or pulmonary hypertension within the last 24 hours, or tadalafil within the last 48 hours.

Reperfusion Therapy

The goal of reperfusion therapy is to restore blood flow through the blocked coronary artery. Reperfusion is the most effective way to preserve myocardial function and limit infarct size. How do we accomplish reperfusion? Either with fibrinolytic drugs (also known as thrombolytic drugs) or with percutaneous coronary intervention (PCI), usually balloon angioplasty coupled with placement of a stent. Both options are very effective. However, PCI is generally preferred. The relative advantages of fibrinolytic therapy and primary PCI are shown in Table 88.1. With either intervention, rapid implementation is essential.

TABLE 88.1 ▪ Comparison of Fibrinolytic Therapy With Primary PCI

Advantages of fibrinolytic therapy	• More universal access • Shorter time to treatment • Results less dependent on physician experience • Lower system cost
Advantages of primary PCI	• Higher initial reperfusion rates • Less residual stenosis • Lower recurrence rates of ischemia/infarction • Does not promote intracranial bleeding • Defines coronary anatomy and LV function • Can be used when fibrinolytic therapy is contraindicated

LV, left ventricular; PCI, percutaneous coronary intervention.

Primary Percutaneous Coronary Intervention

The term *primary PCI* refers to the use of angioplasty, rather than fibrinolytic therapy, to recanalize an occluded coronary artery. In almost all cases, PCI consists of balloon angioplasty coupled with placement of a drug-eluting stent. Under current guidelines, the institutional goal is to implement PCI within 90 minutes of initial patient contact. As discussed later, all patients undergoing PCI should receive an anticoagulant (IV heparin, bivalirudin) combined with antiplatelet drugs: aspirin plus either clopidogrel, ticagrelor, or prasugrel, and perhaps a glycoprotein (GP) IIb/IIIa inhibitor.

The success rate with primary PCI is somewhat higher than with fibrinolytic therapy. Moreover, studies indicate that the benefits of PCI last longer. After 30 days, the rate of death, reinfarction, or disabling stroke after PCI is 8%, versus 13.7% after fibrinolytic therapy using tissue plasminogen activator (tPA). After 7.8 years, the rate of all-cause mortality after PCI is 34.88%, versus 41.3% with streptokinase—the difference being due entirely to lower cardiovascular mortality in PCI-treated patients. Benefits of primary PCI over fibrinolytic therapy are greatest in high-risk patients.

Fibrinolytic Therapy

Fibrinolytic drugs dissolve clots by converting plasminogen into plasmin, a proteolytic enzyme that digests the fibrin meshwork that holds clots together. In the United States three fibrinolytic drugs are available: *alteplase (tPA), reteplase,* and *tenecteplase.* The basic pharmacology of these drugs is discussed in Chapter 89. Discussion here is limited to their use in STEMI.

Fibrinolytic therapy is most effective when presentation is early. When thrombolytics are given soon enough, the occluded artery can be opened in 80% of patients. Current guidelines suggest a target of 30 minutes or less for the time between entering the emergency department and starting fibrinolysis. Clinical trials have shown that timely therapy improves ventricular function, limits infarct size, and reduces mortality. Restoration of blood flow reduces or eliminates chest pain and often reduces ST elevation. Current guidelines restrict fibrinolytic therapy to patients with ischemic pain that has been present no more than 12 to 24 hours. Patients for whom fibrinolytic therapy is contraindicated are listed in Table 88.2.

Under *typical* conditions, all fibrinolytics are equally beneficial. However, under *ideal* conditions (i.e., treatment within 4–6 hours of pain onset), alteplase is most effective, especially in patients younger than 75 years as shown in a trial known as GUSTO-I. Unfortunately, alteplase is very expensive.

The major complication of fibrinolytic therapy is bleeding, which occurs in 1% to 5% of patients. Intracranial hemorrhage (ICH) is the greatest concern. ICH has an incidence of 0.5% to 1%, and is most likely in older adults. Nonetheless, the benefits of fibrinolysis generally outweigh the risks.

As discussed later, all patients undergoing fibrinolytic therapy should receive an anticoagulant (IV heparin, bivalirudin, enoxaparin, fondaparinux) plus antiplatelet drugs (aspirin plus clopidogrel—but not a GP IIb/IIIa inhibitor, such as abciximab).

TABLE 88.2 ▪ Contraindications and Cautions Regarding Fibrinolytic Use for Myocardial Infarction

Absolute contraindications	• Any prior intracranial hemorrhage • Known structural cerebrovascular lesion • Ischemic stroke within last 3 months *except* ischemic stroke within 4.5 hours • Known intracranial neoplasm • Active internal bleeding (other than menses) • Severe uncontrolled hypertension (unresponsive to emergency therapy) • Suspected aortic dissection • For streptokinase, prior treatment within the previous 6 months • Intracranial or intraspinal surgery within 2 months • Significant closed head or facial trauma within 3 months
Relative contraindications and cautions	• Severe, uncontrolled hypertension on presentation (blood pressure above 180/110 mm Hg) • History of chronic, severe, poorly controlled hypertension • History of prior ischemic stroke (>3 months ago), dementia, or known intracerebral pathology not covered in contraindications • Current use of anticoagulants in therapeutic doses (INR 2–3 or greater); known bleeding diathesis • Traumatic or prolonged (>10 minutes) CPR or major surgery (<3 weeks ago) • Recent internal bleeding (within 2–4 weeks) • Noncompressible vascular punctures • Pregnancy • Active peptic ulcer • Oral anticoagulant therapy

CPR, cardiopulmonary resuscitation; INR, international normalized ratio.
Adapted from O'Gara PT, Kushner FG, Ascheim DD, et al. 2013 ACCF/AHA Guideline for the Management of ST-Elevation Myocardial Infarction: a report of the American College of Cardiology Foundation/American Heart Association Task Force on Practice Guidelines. J Am Coll Cardiol 2013;61:e78–e140.

Adjuncts to Reperfusion Therapy

Anticoagulants

Heparin

Heparin is a parenteral anticoagulant that was used widely to treat MI before fibrinolytics and primary PCI became available. The drug was shown to decrease mortality, reinfarction, stroke, pulmonary embolism, and deep vein thrombosis. Today, heparin is used in conjunction with fibrinolytics and PCI to reduce the risk for thrombosis. The main complication of heparin is bleeding.

Heparin is recommended for all STEMI patients undergoing fibrinolytic therapy or PCI. For those receiving fibrinolytic drugs, treatment should begin before giving the fibrinolytic and should continue for at least 48 to 72 hours after. For patients undergoing PCI, heparin is given once, immediately before the procedure.

Heparin is available as the intact (unfractionated) drug and in low-molecular-weight (LMW) forms. When heparin is used as an adjunct to fibrinolytic therapy, selection of a heparin product depends on duration of use. For treatment lasting less than 48 hours, *unfractionated* heparin can be employed. However, for treatment lasting more than 48 hours, enoxaparin [Lovenox], an *LMW* heparin, should be chosen because prolonged use of unfractionated heparin poses a risk for heparin-induced thrombocytopenia (Table 88.3).

Antiplatelet Drugs

Thienopyridines: Clopidogrel, Ticagrelor, and Prasugrel

Clopidogrel [Plavix], ticagrelor [Brilinta], and prasugrel [Effient] suppress platelet aggregation by blocking receptors for adenosine diphosphate. These drugs are recommended for all MI patients undergoing PCI. In all cases, clopidogrel, ticagrelor, or prasugrel should be *combined* with aspirin. In patients undergoing PCI with stenting, duration of treatment should be at least 12 months, unless the risk for bleeding outweighs the benefits of continued drug use. In patients undergoing fibrinolytic therapy, clopidogrel is the only recommended antiplatelet drug. Dosing should continue for at least 14 days up to a period of 1 year. These drugs are discussed in detail in Chapter 44.

Glycoprotein IIb/IIIa Inhibitors

The GP IIb/IIIa inhibitors (e.g., abciximab [ReoPro]) are powerful, intravenous antiplatelet drugs that inhibit the final step in platelet aggregation. These drugs are recommended for patients undergoing PCI, but not for those undergoing fibrinolytic therapy. Of the three GP IIb/IIIa inhibitors available, abciximab is preferred. Treatment should begin as soon as possible before PCI and should continue for 12 hours after. For further information, refer to Chapter 89.

Aspirin

As discussed earlier, *low-dose* aspirin (81–162 mg/day) should be taken indefinitely by all people who have had an MI. This should be combined with antiplatelet drugs (clopidogrel, ticagrelor, prasugrel) for a period of 1 year. The duration of therapy does not change with placement of a drug-eluting stent or bare metal stent.

Increased Risk for Bleeding

All of the anticoagulant and antiplatelet drugs mentioned increase the risk for bleeding. The nurse must be diligent in assessing for and reporting any signs and symptoms of bleeding, including decreased level of consciousness, painful or swollen joints, oozing gums, hematuria, or decrease in platelet or hemoglobin values.

Angiotensin-Converting Enzyme Inhibitors and Angiotensin II Receptor Blockers

When used after acute STEMI, angiotensin-converting enzyme (ACE) inhibitors (e.g., captopril, lisinopril) decrease short-term mortality in all patients and long-term mortality in patients with reduced LV function. Benefits derive from reducing preload and afterload, promoting water loss, and favorably altering ventricular remodeling. Because of their benefits, ACE inhibitors are recommended for all STEMI patients in the absence of specific contraindications. Treatment should start within 24 hours of symptom onset. The possibility that long-term therapy may also benefit patients who do not have LV dysfunction is being evaluated in large-scale trials. The major adverse effects of ACE inhibitors are hypotension and cough. Contraindications to ACE inhibitors are hypotension, bilateral renal artery stenosis, renal failure,

TABLE 88.3 ▪ Adjuncts to Reperfusion Therapy

Drug	Class	Usual Adult Dose	Preferred Use	Contraindications
Enoxaparin [Lovenox]	Low-molecular-weight heparin	30-mg IV bolus followed by 1 mg/Kg every 12 hours subcutaneously Continue until revascularization or a period of 8 days	Treatment lasting >48 hours	Patients >75 years should not receive IV bolus Adjust dose for CrCl <30 mL/min
Fondaparinux [Arixtra]	Factor Xa inhibitor	2.5 mg IV followed by 2.5 mg daily subcutaneously Continue until revascularization or a period of 8 days	Alternative to therapy with heparin in patients undergoing reperfusion with thrombolytics	Not recommended as sole anticoagulant in PCI Do not use in patients with CrCl <30 mL/min
Bivalirudin [Angiomax]	Direct thrombin inhibitor	0.75-mg/Kg bolus IV followed by continued infusion at 1/75 mg/kg/hr	Preferred agent with GP IIb/IIIa inhibitors in patients undergoing PCI Alternative to heparin in patients with heparin-induced thrombocytopenia	Reduce doses for patients with CrCl <30 mL/min

CrCl, creatinine clearance; PCI, percutaneous coronary intervention.

and a history of ACE inhibitor–induced cough or angioedema. The basic pharmacology of the ACE inhibitors is described in Chapter 36

Therapy with angiotensin II receptor blockers (ARBs) in STEMI patients has not been studied as extensively as has therapy with ACE inhibitors. However, one major trial—Valsartan in Acute Myocardial Infarction Trial (VALIANT)—demonstrated that, in patients with post-MI heart failure or LV dysfunction, valsartan (an ARB) was as effective as captopril (an ACE inhibitor) at reducing short-term and long-term mortality. In the current guidelines, ARBs are recommended for STEMI patients who are intolerant of ACE inhibitors and have heart failure or reduced LV function.

Calcium Channel Blockers

Because of their antianginal, vasodilatory, and antihypertensive actions, calcium channel blockers (CCBs) were presumed beneficial for patients with acute STEMI and were once used widely. However, in large-scale controlled trials, CCBs failed to decrease mortality during or after acute STEMI. Accordingly, CCBs are not recommended for routine use. However, because the effects of CCBs on the heart are nearly identical to those of beta blockers, current guidelines state that it is reasonable to use two CCBs—verapamil or diltiazem—when beta blockers are either ineffective or contraindicated to relieve ongoing ischemia or control a rapid ventricular rate caused by atrial fibrillation or atrial flutter. CCBs should not be used if the patient has heart failure, LV dysfunction, or atrioventricular block.

COMPLICATIONS OF STEMI

MI predisposes the heart and vascular system to serious complications. Among the most severe are ventricular dysrhythmias, cardiogenic shock, and heart failure.

Ventricular Dysrhythmias

These dysrhythmias develop frequently and are the major cause of death after MI. Sudden death from dysrhythmias occurs in 15% of patients during the first hour. Ultimately, ventricular dysrhythmias cause 60% of infarction-related deaths. Acute management of ventricular fibrillation consists of defibrillation followed by IV amiodarone for 24 to 48 hours. Programmed ventricular stimulation with guided antidysrhythmic therapy may be lifesaving for some patients.

Attempts to prevent dysrhythmias by giving antidysrhythmic drugs *prophylactically* have failed to reduce mortality. Worse yet, attempted prophylaxis of ventricular dysrhythmias with two drugs—encainide and flecainide—actually *increased* mortality. Similarly, when quinidine was employed to prevent supraventricular dysrhythmias, it too increased mortality. Therefore, because prophylaxis with antidysrhythmic drugs does not reduce mortality—and may in fact increase mortality—antidysrhythmic drugs should be withheld until a dysrhythmia actually occurs.

Cardiogenic Shock

Shock results from greatly reduced tissue perfusion secondary to impaired cardiac function. Shock develops in 7% to 10% of patients in the first few days after MI and has a mortality rate of up to 50% in hospitalized patients. Patients at highest risk are those with large infarcts, a previous infarct, a low ejection fraction (less than 35%), diabetes, and advanced age. Drug therapy includes inotropic agents (e.g., dopamine, dobutamine) to increase cardiac output and vasodilators (nitroglycerin, nitroprusside) to improve tissue perfusion and reduce cardiac work and oxygen demand. Unfortunately, although these drugs can improve hemodynamic status, they do not seem to reduce mortality. Restoration of cardiac perfusion with PCI or coronary artery bypass grafting may be of value.

Heart Failure

Heart failure secondary to acute MI can be treated with a combination of drugs. A diuretic (e.g., furosemide) is given to decrease preload and pulmonary congestion. Inotropic agents (e.g., digoxin) increase cardiac output by enhancing contractility. Vasodilators (e.g., nitroglycerin, nitroprusside) improve hemodynamic status by reducing preload, afterload, or both. ACE inhibitors (or ARBs), which reduce both preload and afterload, can be especially helpful. Beta blockers may also improve outcome. Drug therapy of heart failure is discussed in Chapter 40

Cardiac Rupture

Weakening of the myocardium predisposes the heart wall to rupture. After rupture, shock and circulatory collapse develop rapidly. Death is often immediate. Fortunately, cardiac rupture is relatively rare (less than 2% incidence). Patients at highest risk are those with a large anterior infarction. Cardiac rupture is most likely within the first days after MI. Early treatment with vasodilators and beta blockers may reduce the risk for wall rupture.

SECONDARY PREVENTION OF STEMI

As a rule, patients who survive the acute phase of STEMI can be discharged from the hospital as early as 72 hours after admission, if they remain free from complications. However, they are still at risk for reinfarction (5%–15% incidence within the first year) and other complications (e.g., dysrhythmias, heart failure). Outcome can be improved with risk factor reduction, exercise, and long-term therapy with drugs.

Reduction of risk factors for MI can increase long-term survival. Patients who smoke must be encouraged to quit; the goal is total cessation. Patients with high serum cholesterol should be given an appropriate dietary plan and treated with a high-dose statin. Hypertension and diabetes increase the risk for mortality and must be controlled. For patients with hypertension, blood pressure should be decreased to below 140/90 mm Hg. For patients with diabetes, the goal is a level of hemoglobin A_{1c} below 7%.

Exercise training can be valuable for two reasons: it reduces complications associated with prolonged bed rest, and it accelerates return to an optimal level of functioning. The goal is 30 minutes of exercise at least 3 to 4 days a week. Although exercise is safe for most patients, there is concern about cardiac risk and impairment of infarct healing in patients whose infarct is large.

All post-MI patients should take four drugs: (1) a beta blocker; (2) an ACE inhibitor or an ARB; either (3a) an antiplatelet drug (aspirin or clopidogrel, ticagrelor, or prasugrel) or (3b) an anticoagulant (warfarin); and (4) a statin. All four should be taken indefinitely.

Estrogen therapy for postmenopausal women is not effective as secondary prevention and should not be initiated.

CHAPTER

89 Drugs for Acute Care

Laura D. Rosenthal, DNP, ACNP, FAANP

Most of the medications discussed throughout this book are available in oral form or are used in primary care settings. There are a few medications that are reserved for the hospital setting. These medications are given to treat acute illness.

DRUGS FOR ANEMIA

Parenteral Iron Preparations

Iron is available in four forms for parenteral therapy. However, only one of these forms—iron dextran—is approved for iron deficiency of all causes. Approval of the other three forms—iron sucrose, sodium–ferric gluconate complex, and ferumoxytol—is limited to treating iron deficiency anemia in patients with chronic kidney disease.

Iron Dextran

Iron dextran [INFeD, Dexferrum, Infufer, Dexiron] is the most frequently used parenteral iron preparation. The drug is a complex consisting of ferric hydroxide and dextrans (polymers of glucose). The rate of response to parenteral iron is equal to that of oral iron.

Indications

Iron dextran is reserved for patients with a clear diagnosis of iron deficiency and for whom oral iron is either ineffective or intolerable. Primary candidates for parenteral iron are patients who, because of intestinal disease, are unable to absorb iron taken orally. Iron dextran is also indicated when blood loss is so great (500–1000 mL/wk) that oral iron cannot be absorbed fast enough to meet hematopoietic needs. Parenteral iron may also be employed when there is concern that oral iron might exacerbate preexisting disease of the stomach or bowel. Lastly, parenteral iron can be given to the rare patient for whom the gastrointestinal (GI) effects of oral iron are intolerable.

Adverse Effects

Anaphylactic Reactions. Potentially fatal anaphylaxis is the most serious adverse effect. Anaphylactic reactions are triggered by dextran in the product, not by the iron. Although these reactions are rare, their possibility demands that iron dextran be used only when clearly required. Furthermore, whenever iron dextran is administered, injectable epinephrine and facilities for resuscitation should be at hand. To reduce risk, each full dose must be preceded by a small test dose. However, be aware that even the test dose can trigger anaphylactic and other hypersensitivity reactions. In addition, even when the test dose is uneventful, patients can still experience anaphylaxis.

Other Adverse Effects. Hypotension is common in patients receiving parenteral iron. In addition, iron dextran can cause headache, fever, urticaria, and arthralgia. More serious reactions—circulatory failure and cardiac arrest—may also occur. When administered intramuscularly, iron dextran can cause persistent pain and prolonged, localized discoloration. Very rarely, tumors develop at sites of intramuscular (IM) injection. Intravenous (IV) administration may result in lymphadenopathy and phlebitis.

Preparations, Dosage, and Administration

Preparations. Iron dextran [INFeD, Dexferrum, Infufer, Dexiron] is available in single-dose vials (1 and 2 mL) that contain 50 mg/mL of elemental iron.

Dosage. Dosage determination is complex. Dosage depends on the degree of anemia, the weight of the patient, and the presence of persistent bleeding. A suggested calculation is [0.0442 × (desired Hgb – observed Hgb) × LBW] = (0.26 × LBW), where Hgb is hemoglobin and LBW is lean body weight in kilograms. The maximal safe dose is 100 mg.

Administration. Iron dextran may be administered by IM or IV route. IV administration is preferred. This route is just as effective as IM administration but causes fewer anaphylactic reactions and other adverse effects.

Intravenous. To minimize anaphylactic reactions, IV iron dextran should be administered by the following protocol: (1) administer a small test dose (25 mg over 5 minutes) and observe the patient for at least 15 minutes; (2) if the test dose appears safe, slowly administer a larger dose (over a 10- to 15-minute interval); and (3) additional doses may be given as needed on a daily basis.

Intramuscular. IM iron dextran has significant drawbacks and should be avoided. Disadvantages include persistent pain and discoloration at the injection site, possible development of tumors, and a greater risk for anaphylaxis. As with IV iron dextran, a small test dose should precede the full therapeutic dose.

Sodium–Ferric Gluconate Complex, Iron Sucrose, and Ferumoxytol

Sodium–ferric gluconate complex (SFGC), iron sucrose, and ferumoxytol represent alternatives to iron dextran for parenteral iron therapy. With all three drugs, the risk for anaphylaxis is very low, so there is little or no need for giving test doses. As a result, these drugs are more convenient than iron dextran. Unfortunately, indications for these drugs are limited to treatment of iron deficiency anemia in patients with chronic kidney disease (CKD). They are not approved for iron deficiency from other causes.

Sodium–Ferric Gluconate Complex

SFGC, sold under the trade name Ferrlecit, is a parenteral iron product indicated for iron deficiency anemia in patients with CKD who are undergoing chronic hemodialysis. The drug is always used in conjunction with erythropoietin, an agent that stimulates RBC production.

BLACK BOX WARNING: IRON DEXTRAN

This preparation should be used for treatment of iron deficiency only in patients in whom oral administration is infeasible or ineffective due to increased risk for anaphylaxis. A test dose is required before administration.

SFGC can cause transient flushing and hypotension, associated with lightheadedness, malaise, fatigue, weakness, and severe pain in the chest, back, flanks, or groin. This reaction can be minimized by infusing the drug slowly. In contrast to iron dextran, SFGC poses little risk for anaphylaxis. SFGC is supplied in 5-mL ampules that contain 62.5 mg of elemental iron. For most patients, a single dose consists of 125 mg. The typical patient requires a cumulative dose of 1 g (eight 125-mg infusions on separate days). Every time the drug is administered, facilities for cardiopulmonary resuscitation should be immediately available.

Iron Sucrose

Like SFGC, iron sucrose [Venofer] is a parenteral form of iron indicated for iron deficiency anemia in patients with CKD. However, in contrast to SFGC, whose indications are limited to CKD patients undergoing hemodialysis in conjunction with erythropoietin therapy, iron sucrose is indicated for a broader range of CKD patients, specifically the following:

- Non–dialysis-dependent (NDD) patients receiving erythropoietin
- NDD patients *not* receiving erythropoietin
- Hemodialysis-dependent (HDD) patients receiving erythropoietin
- Peritoneal dialysis–dependent (PDD) patients receiving erythropoietin

The most common adverse effects of iron sucrose are hypotension and cramps. The drug has also been associated with heart failure (HF), sepsis, and taste perversion. Life-threatening hypersensitivity reactions are very rare: no cases were observed during clinical trials, and only 27 cases (out of 450,000 patients) were reported during postmarketing surveillance. Nonetheless, facilities for cardiopulmonary resuscitation should be available during administration. However, in contrast to iron dextran, no test dose is needed.

Iron sucrose is supplied in 2.5-, 5-, and 10-mL single-dose vials. Administration is IV, either by (1) slow injection (1 mL/min) or (2) infusion. Iron sucrose should not be mixed with other drugs or with parenteral nutrition solutions. All patients should receive a total dose of 1000 mg, but the dosing schedule and administration technique depend on the patient as follows:

- HDD patients—Give ten 100-mg doses during each of 10 consecutive dialysis sessions. Administer by slow IV injection or IV infusion.
- NDD patients—Give five 200-mg doses on separate occasions over a 14-day span. Administer by slow IV injection.
- PDD patients—Give two 300-mg doses 14 days apart, then one 400-mg dose 14 days later. Administer by slow IV infusion.

Ferumoxytol

Ferumoxytol [Feraheme] is a parenteral form of iron indicated for iron deficiency anemia in all patients with CKD, whether or not they are on dialysis or using erythropoietin. Compared with SFGC and iron sucrose, ferumoxytol is much more convenient because it requires only 2 doses (given over 3–8 days), whereas SFGC and iron sucrose require 3 to 10 doses (given over several weeks).

Ferumoxytol is generally well tolerated. The most common adverse effects are nausea, dizziness, hypotension, headache, vomiting, and edema. In clinical trials, about 0.2% of patients experienced serious hypersensitivity reactions. Accordingly, facilities for cardiopulmonary resuscitation should be immediately available. However, in contrast to iron dextran, no test dose is needed.

Because of its unique composition (ferumoxytol is a superparamagnetic form of iron oxide), the drug can interfere with magnetic resonance imaging studies. This interference is most profound 1 to 2 days after dosing but can persist for up to 3 months. Fortunately, ferumoxytol does not interfere with other forms of diagnostic imaging, including x-rays, computed tomography, positron emission tomography, ultrasound, or nuclear medicine imaging.

Ferumoxytol [Feraheme] is supplied in 17-mL single-dose vials (30 mg elemental iron/mL). Administration is by slow IV injection. The usual dosage is 510 mg on day 1, followed by another 510 mg 3 to 8 days later. Additional doses may be given as needed. After each injection, patients should be monitored for at least 30 minutes for hypotension and hypersensitivity reactions. For patients on dialysis, dosing should be done at least 1 hour after starting dialysis, and only after blood pressure (BP) has stabilized.

INPATIENT ANESTHESIA

Intravenous Regional Anesthesia

IV regional anesthesia is employed to anesthetize the extremities—hands, feet, arms, and lower legs, but not the entire leg (because too much anesthetic would be needed). Anesthesia is produced by injection into a distal vein of an arm or leg. Before giving the anesthetic, blood is removed from the limb (by gravity or by application of an Esmarch bandage), and a tourniquet is applied to the limb (proximal to the site of anesthetic injection) to prevent anesthetic from entering the systemic circulation. To ensure complete blockade of arterial flow throughout the procedure, a double tourniquet is used. After injection, the anesthetic diffuses out of the vasculature and becomes evenly distributed to all areas of the occluded limb. When the tourniquet is loosened at the end of surgery, about 15% to 30% of administered anesthetic is released into the systemic circulation. Lidocaine—without epinephrine—is the preferred agent for this type of anesthesia.

Alfentanil and Sufentanil

Alfentanil [Alfenta] and sufentanil are IV opioids related to fentanyl. Both drugs are used for induction of anesthesia, for maintenance of anesthesia (in combination with other agents), and as sole anesthetic agents. Pharmacologic effects are like those of morphine. Sufentanil has an especially high milligram potency (about 1000 times that of morphine). Alfentanil is about 10 times more potent than morphine. Both drugs have a rapid onset, and both are Schedule II agents.

Remifentanil

Remifentanil [Ultiva] is an IV opioid with a rapid onset and brief duration. The brief duration results from rapid metabolism by plasma and tissue esterases, and not from hepatic metabolism or renal excretion. Like fentanyl, remifentanil is about 100 times more potent than morphine. Remifentanil is approved for analgesia during surgery and during the immediate postoperative period. Administration is by continuous IV infusion. Effects begin in minutes and terminate 5 to 10 minutes after the infusion is stopped. For surgical analgesia, the infusion rate is 0.05 to 2 mcg/kg/min. For postoperative analgesia, the infusion rate is 0.025 to 0.2 mcg/kg/min. Adverse effects during the infusion include respiratory depression, hypotension, bradycardia, and muscle rigidity sufficient to compromise breathing. Postinfusion effects include nausea, vomiting, and headache. Remifentanil is regulated as a Schedule II substance.

Dexmedetomidine

Actions and Therapeutic Use

Dexmedetomidine [Precedex], like clonidine, is a selective $alpha_2$-adrenergic agonist. The drug acts in the central nervous system (CNS) to cause sedation and analgesia. The drug has two approved indications: (1) short-term sedation in critically ill patients who are initially intubated and undergoing mechanical ventilation and (2) sedation for nonintubated patients before and/or during surgical and other procedures. However, in addition to these approved uses, dexmedetomidine has a variety of off-label uses, including sedation during awake craniotomy, prevention and treatment of postanesthetic shivering, and enhancement of sedation and analgesia in patients undergoing general anesthesia. In contrast to clonidine, which is administered by epidural infusion, dexmedetomidine is administered by IV infusion.

Pharmacokinetics

With IV infusion, dexmedetomidine undergoes wide distribution to tissues. In the blood, the drug is 94% protein bound. Dexmedetomidine undergoes rapid and complete hepatic metabolism, followed by excretion in the urine. The elimination half-life is 2 hours.

Adverse Effects

The most common adverse effects are hypotension and bradycardia. The mechanism is activation of alpha$_2$-adrenergic receptors in the CNS and periphery, which results in decreased release of norepinephrine from sympathetic neurons innervating the heart and blood vessels. If these cardiovascular effects are too intense, they can be managed in several ways, including (1) decreasing or stopping the infusion, (2) infusing fluid, and (3) elevating the lower extremities. Giving a muscarinic antagonist (e.g., atropine) can increase heart rate.

Additional adverse effects include nausea, dry mouth, and transient hypertension. Importantly, dexmedetomidine does not cause respiratory depression.

Drug Interactions

Dexmedetomidine can enhance the actions of anesthetics, sedatives, hypnotics, and opioids. Excessive CNS depression can be managed by reducing the dosage of dexmedetomidine or the other agents.

Preparations, Dosage, and Administration

Dexmedetomidine [Precedex] is supplied in solution (100 mcg/mL), which must be diluted to 4 mcg/mL before use. Administration is by IV infusion. For intensive care sedation, treatment consists of a loading dose (1 mcg/kg infused over 10 minutes) followed by a maintenance infusion of 0.2 to 0.7 mcg/kg/hr for no more than 24 hours. For procedural sedation, treatment typically consists of a loading dose (1 mcg/kg infused over 10 minutes) followed by a maintenance infusion of 0.2 to 1 mcg/kg/hr.

Epidural Anesthesia

Epidural anesthesia is achieved by injecting a local anesthetic into the epidural space (i.e., within the spinal column but outside the dura mater). A catheter placed in the epidural space allows administration by bolus or by continuous infusion. After administration, diffusion of anesthetic across the dura into the subarachnoid space blocks conduction in nerve roots and in the spinal cord. Diffusion through intervertebral foramina blocks nerves located in the paravertebral region. With epidural administration, anesthetic can reach the systemic circulation in significant amounts. As a result, when the technique is used during delivery, neonatal depression may result. Lidocaine and bupivacaine are popular drugs for epidural anesthesia. Because of the risk for death from cardiac arrest, the concentrated (0.75%) solution of bupivacaine must not be used in obstetric patients.

Spinal (Subarachnoid) Anesthesia

Technique

Spinal anesthesia is produced by injecting local anesthetic into the subarachnoid space. Injection is made in the lumbar region below the termination of the cord. Spread of anesthetic within the subarachnoid space determines the level of anesthesia achieved. Movement of anesthetic within the subarachnoid space is determined by two factors: (1) the density of the anesthetic solution and (2) the position of the patient. Anesthetics employed most commonly are bupivacaine, lidocaine, and tetracaine. All must be free of preservatives.

Adverse Effects

The most significant adverse effect of spinal anesthesia is hypotension. Blood pressure is reduced by venous dilation secondary to blockade of sympathetic nerves. (Loss of venous tone decreases the return of blood to the heart, causing a reduction in cardiac output and a corresponding fall in BP.) Loss of venous tone can be compensated for by placing the patient in a 10- to 15-degree head-down position, which promotes venous return to the heart. If BP cannot be restored through head-down positioning, drugs may be indicated; ephedrine and phenylephrine have been employed to promote vasoconstriction and enhance cardiac performance.

Autonomic blockade may disrupt function of the intestinal and urinary tracts, causing fecal incontinence and either urinary incontinence or urinary retention. The prescriber should be notified if the patient fails to void within 8 hours of the end of surgery.

Spinal anesthesia frequently causes headache. These "spinal" headaches are posture dependent and can be relieved by having the patient assume a supine position.

ANTICOAGULANTS AND THROMBOLYTICS

Continuous Unfractionated Heparin Intravenous Infusion

IV infusion provides steady levels of heparin and therefore is preferred to intermittent injections. Indications for the use of heparin infusion include treatment of deep vein thrombosis (DVT) or pulmonary embolism (PE), or in patients with myocardial ischemia or infarction. Dosing may consist of an initial weight-based bolus followed by a weight-based infusion titrated to laboratory results. Whether or not a bolus is indicated depends on the indication for treatment and the facility policy. During the initial phase of treatment, the activated partial thromboplastin time (aPTT) should be measured once every 4 to 6 hours and the infusion rate adjusted accordingly. For additional information on unfractionated heparin, see Chapter 44.

Low-Dose Unfractionated Heparin Therapy

Heparin in low doses is given for prophylaxis against thromboembolism in hospitalized patients. Doses of 5000 units are given subcutaneously every 8 to 12 hours depending on patient weight. During low-dose therapy, monitoring of the aPTT is not usually required.

Protamine Sulfate for Heparin Overdose

Protamine sulfate is an antidote to severe heparin overdose. Protamine is a small protein that has multiple positively charged groups. These groups bond ionically with the negative groups on heparin, thereby forming a heparin-protamine complex that is devoid of anticoagulant activity. Neutralization of heparin occurs immediately and lasts for 2 hours, after which additional protamine may be needed. Protamine is administered by slow IV injection. Dosage is based on the fact that 1 mg of protamine will inactivate 100 units of heparin. Hence, for each 100 units of heparin in the body, 1 mg of protamine should be injected.

Direct Thrombin Inhibitors

Bivalirudin

Bivalirudin [Angiomax], an IV direct thrombin inhibitor, has actions like those of dabigatran (see Chapter 44). The drug is a synthetic drug chemically related to hirudin, an anticoagulant isolated from the saliva of leeches.

Bivalirudin is given in combination with aspirin, clopidogrel, or prasugrel to prevent clot formation in patients undergoing coronary angioplasty. At this time, the standard therapy for these patients is aspirin combined with a platelet glycoprotein (GP) IIb/IIIa inhibitor combined with low-dose, unfractionated heparin. Bivalirudin, an alternative to heparin in this regimen, has been studied in combination with aspirin as well as GP IIb/IIIa inhibitors. In one trial—the Hirulog Angioplasty Study—bivalirudin plus aspirin was compared with heparin plus aspirin. Bivalirudin was at least as effective as heparin at preventing ischemic complications (myocardial infarction [MI], abrupt vessel closure, death) and caused fewer bleeding complications. In a subgroup of patients—those with postinfarction angina—bivalirudin was significantly more effective than heparin.

Adverse Effects

The most common side effects are back pain, nausea, hypotension, and headache. Other relatively common effects (incidence greater than 5%) include vomiting, abdominal pain, pelvic pain, anxiety, nervousness, insomnia, bradycardia, and fever.

Bleeding is the effect of greatest concern. However, compared with heparin, bivalirudin causes fewer incidents of major bleeding (3.7% vs. 9.3%), and fewer patients require transfusions (2% vs. 5.7%). Coadministration of bivalirudin with heparin, warfarin, or thrombolytic drugs increases the risk for bleeding.

Pharmacokinetics

With IV dosing, anticoagulation begins immediately. Drug levels are maintained by continuous infusion. Bivalirudin is eliminated primarily by renal excretion and partly by proteolytic cleavage. The half-life is short (25 minutes) in patients with normal renal function but may be longer in patients with renal impairment. Coagulation returns to baseline about 1 hour after stopping the infusion. Anticoagulation can be monitored by measuring activated clotting time.

Comparison With Heparin

Bivalirudin is just as effective as heparin and has several advantages: it works independently of antithrombin (AT), inhibits clot-bound thrombin as well as free thrombin, and causes less bleeding and fewer ischemic events. However, the drug has one disadvantage: bivalirudin is more expensive than heparin. One single-use vial, good for a full course of treatment, costs about $1000, compared with $10 for an equivalent course of heparin. However, the manufacturer estimates that reductions in bleeding and ischemic complications would save, on average, $1000 per patient, which would offset the greater cost of bivalirudin. The bottom line? Bivalirudin works as well as heparin, is safer, and may be equally cost effective—and hence is considered an attractive alternative to heparin for use during angioplasty.

Preparations, Dosage, and Administration

Bivalirudin [Angiomax] dosing consists of an initial IV bolus (0.75 mg/kg) followed by continuous infusion (1.75 mg/kg/hr) for the duration of the procedure and up to 4 hours after. If necessary, bivalirudin may be infused for up to 20 additional hours at a rate of 0.2 mg/kg/hr. Treatment should begin just before angioplasty. Dosage should be reduced in patients with severe renal impairment. All patients should take aspirin (300–325 mg).

Argatroban

Like bivalirudin, argatroban is an IV anticoagulant that works by direct inhibition of thrombin. The drug is indicated for prophylaxis and treatment of thrombosis in patients with heparin- induced thrombocytopenia (HIT). In clinical trials, argatroban reduced development of new thrombosis and permitted restoration of platelet counts. Like other anticoagulants, argatroban poses a risk for hemorrhage. About 12% of patients experience hematuria. Allergic reactions (dyspnea, cough, rash), which develop in 10% of patients, occur almost exclusively in those receiving either thrombolytic drugs (e.g., alteplase) or contrast media for coronary angioplasty. Argatroban has a short half-life (about 45 minutes), owing to rapid metabolism by the liver. Treatment is monitored by measuring the aPTT. When infusion of argatroban is discontinued, the aPTT returns to baseline in 2 to 4 hours.

Argatroban dosage depends on the setting as follows:

- *For prophylaxis and treatment of thrombosis in patients with HIT and normal liver function* (but who are *not* undergoing percutaneous coronary intervention [PCI])—The initial infusion rate is 2 mcg/kg/min. In patients with liver dysfunction, the initial rate is only 0.5 mcg/kg/min. Dosage is adjusted to maintain the aPTT at 1.5 to 3 times the baseline value.
- *For prevention of thrombosis in patients with or at risk for HIT who are undergoing PCI*—Give an IV bolus (350 mcg/kg) followed by continuous IV infusion (25 mcg/kg/min). Adjust the infusion rate (and perhaps give a second IV bolus) to achieve the desired activated clotting time.

Antithrombin

AT is an endogenous compound that suppresses coagulation, primarily by inhibiting thrombin and factor Xa. Clinically, AT is used to prevent thrombosis in patients with inherited AT deficiency. Currently, we have two AT preparations, marketed as ATryn and Thrombate III. Atryn is made by recombinant DNA technology; Thrombate III is made by extraction from human plasma. Nonetheless, the actions of both products are the same: suppression of coagulation mediated by thrombin and factor Xa.

Recombinant Human Antithrombin

Production. Recombinant human AT (rhAT), sold as ATryn, is produced in goats that have been given the DNA sequence for human AT, along with genetic instructions that cause the AT to be expressed into their milk. The rhAT produced in goats is nearly identical to endogenous AT.

Therapeutic Use. rhAT is approved for prevention of perioperative or peripartum thromboembolic events in patients with inherited AT deficiency, a disorder that puts these people at high risk for VTE. In fact, to protect against thromboembolism, these people typically require lifelong therapy with an anticoagulant, usually warfarin. During surgery or childbirth, the risk for thrombosis increases. However, there is also an obvious increase in the risk for serious bleeding. Accordingly, when patients with hereditary AT deficiency are facing childbirth or surgery, anticoagulant therapy is usually discontinued—reducing the risk for bleeding but increasing the risk for thrombosis. To reduce the risk for thrombosis, rhAT is given until anticoagulant therapy can be safely resumed. In clinical trials, rhAT prevented thromboembolism associated with childbirth or surgery in 30 of 31 patients with inherited AT deficiency.

Adverse Effects. The principal concern is hemorrhage. To minimize risk, AT activity should be monitored and, if it rises too high, the rhAT dosage should be reduced. In addition to causing outright hemorrhage, rhAT may cause hematoma, hematuria, and hemarthrosis. Infusion-site reactions are common.

Because rhAT is derived from goats' milk, there is a risk for hypersensitivity reactions. Accordingly, patients should be closely observed during the infusion period. If signs of a hypersensitivity reaction develop (e.g., hives, generalized urticaria, wheezing, hypotension), rhAT should be discontinued immediately.

Interaction With Heparin. As discussed in Chapter 44, heparin produces its anticoagulant effects by enhancing the actions of AT. Accordingly, if rhAT is given to a patient taking heparin, anticoagulation will be greatly increased, thereby posing a risk for bleeding. Accordingly, if heparin is used with rhAT, tests for anticoagulation should be performed often, especially during the first hours after the initiation or termination of rhAT use.

Preparations, Dosage, and Administration. Treatment consists of a 15-minute loading infusion followed immediately by a continuous maintenance infusion. The loading infusion should begin before delivery or 24 hours before surgery and should continue until normal maintenance coagulation can be reestablished. Dosage size is based on the patient's AT activity and body weight. The goal is to maintain AT activity between 80% and 120% of normal. During the maintenance infusion, AT activity should be monitored periodically and the dosage adjusted accordingly. Treatment with rhAT is hugely expensive: the drug costs $2.34/unit, and a full course of treatment may require 40,000 units to more than 250,000 units. Financial assistance is available from the manufacturer.

Plasma-Derived Antithrombin. Plasma-derived AT [Thrombate III] is made by extraction from the plasma of human volunteers. Thrombate III is like rhAT in most regards: Both drugs share the same indication (prevention of thromboembolic events associated with surgery or childbirth in patients with inherited AT deficiency), both pose a risk for hemorrhage, both increase the anticoagulant effects of heparin, and both are given by IV infusion. The drugs differ primarily in that plasma-derived AT carries a risk for hepatitis C and other infections, whereas rhAT does not. As with rhAT, dosage is based on AT activity and body weight.

Glycoprotein IIb/IIIa Receptor Antagonists

Group Properties

The GP IIb/IIIa receptor antagonists, sometimes called "super aspirins," are the most effective antiplatelet drugs on the market. Three agents are available: abciximab, tirofiban, and eptifibatide. All three are administered intravenously, usually in combination with aspirin and low-dose heparin. Dosages are shown in Table 89.1.

Actions

The GP IIb/IIIa antagonists cause *reversible* blockade of platelet GP IIb/IIIa receptors and thereby inhibit the final step in aggregation. As a result, these drugs can prevent aggregation stimulated by all factors, including collagen, thromboxane A_2 adenosine diphosphate, thrombin, and platelet activation factor.

Therapeutic Use

The GP IIb/IIIa antagonists are used short term to prevent ischemic events in patients with acute coronary syndrome (ACS) and those undergoing PCI.

Acute Coronary Syndromes

ACSs have two major manifestations: unstable angina and non–ST-segment elevation myocardial infarction (non-STEMI). In both cases, symptoms result from thrombosis triggered by disruption of atherosclerotic plaque. When added to traditional drugs for ACS (heparin and aspirin), GP IIb/IIIa antagonists reduce the risk for ischemic complications.

Percutaneous Coronary Intervention

GP IIb/IIIa antagonists reduce the risk for rapid reocclusion after coronary artery revascularization with PCI (balloon or laser angioplasty, or atherectomy using an intraarterial rotating blade). Reocclusion is common because PCI damages the arterial wall, encouraging platelet aggregation.

Properties of Individual Glycoprotein IIb/IIIa Antagonists

Abciximab

Description and Use. Abciximab [ReoPro] is a purified Fab fragment of a monoclonal antibody. The drug binds to platelets in the vicinity of GP IIb/IIIa receptors and thereby prevents the receptors from binding fibrinogen. Abciximab, in conjunction with aspirin and heparin, is approved for IV therapy of ACS and for patients undergoing PCI. In addition, studies indicate it can accelerate revascularization in patients undergoing thrombolytic therapy for acute MI. Antiplatelet effects persist for 24 to 48 hours after stopping the infusion.

Adverse Effects and Interactions. Abciximab doubles the risk for major bleeding, especially at the PCI access site in the femoral artery. The drug may also cause GI, urogenital, and retroperitoneal bleeds. However, it does not increase the risk for fatal hemorrhage or hemorrhagic stroke. In the event of severe bleeding, infusion of abciximab and heparin should be discontinued. Other drugs that impede hemostasis will increase bleeding risk.

Eptifibatide

Eptifibatide [Integrilin] is a small peptide that causes reversible and highly selective inhibition of GP IIb/IIIa receptors. The drug is approved for patients with ACS and those undergoing PCI. Antiplatelet effects reverse within 4 hours of stopping the infusion. The most important adverse effect is bleeding, which occurs most often at the site of PCI catheter insertion, and in the GI and urinary tracts. As with other GP IIb/IIIa inhibitors, the risk for bleeding is increased by concurrent use of other drugs that impede hemostasis.

TABLE 89.1 ▪ Dosages for Glycoprotein IIb/IIIa Receptor Antagonists

Application	Tirofiban [Aggrastat]	Eptifibatide [Integrilin]	Abciximab [ReoPro]
Acute coronary syndrome (ACS)	0.4 mcg/kg/min for 30 min, then 0.1 mcg/kg/min for 48–108 hr	180-mcg/kg bolus, then 2 mcg/kg/min for up to 72 hr	0.25-mg/kg bolus, then 10 mcg/kg/min for 18–24 hr
Percutaneous coronary intervention* (PCI) after treatment for ACS	Continue 0.1 mcg/kg/min for the procedure and 12–24 hr after	Consider decreasing the infusion rate to 0.5 mcg/kg/min for the procedure and 20–24 hr after	Continue 10 mcg/kg/min for the procedure and 1 hr after
PCI without prior treatment for ACS	Not FDA approved for this application	135-mcg/kg bolus before procedure, then 0.5 mcg/kg/min for 20–24 hr	0.25-mg/kg bolus 10–60 min before procedure, then 0.125 mcg/kg/min (max.,10 mcg/min) for 12 hr

*Balloon or laser angioplasty, or atherectomy.
FDA, U.S. Food and Drug Administration.

Tirofiban

Tirofiban [Aggrastat] causes selective and reversible inhibition of GP IIb/IIIa receptors. The drug—neither an antibody nor a peptide—was modeled after a platelet inhibitor isolated from the venom of the saw-scaled viper, a snake indigenous to Africa. Like other GP IIb/IIIa inhibitors, tirofiban is used to reduce ischemic events associated with ACS and PCI. Platelet function returns to baseline within 4 hours of stopping the infusion. Bleeding is the primary adverse effect. The risk for bleeding can be increased by other drugs that suppress hemostasis.

Thrombolytic (Fibrinolytic) Drugs

As their name implies, thrombolytic drugs are given to remove thrombi that have already formed. This contrasts with the anticoagulants, which are given to prevent thrombus formation. In the United States three thrombolytic drugs are available: alteplase, reteplase, and tenecteplase. These drugs are employed acutely and only for severe thrombotic disease: acute MI, PE, and ischemic stroke. Principal differences among the drugs concern specific uses, duration of action, and ease of dosing. All thrombolytics pose a risk for serious bleeding and hence should be administered only by clinicians skilled in their use. Because of their mechanism, thrombolytic drugs are also known as *fibrinolytics* (and informally as *clot busters*). Properties of individual agents are shown in Table 89.2.

Alteplase (Tissue Plasminogen Activator)

Alteplase [Activase, Cathflo Activase]—also known as *tissue plasminogen activator (tPA)*—is identical to naturally occurring human tPA. The drug is manufactured using recombinant DNA technology.

The drug first binds with *plasminogen* to form an active complex. The alteplase-plasminogen complex then catalyzes the conversion of other plasminogen molecules into *plasmin,* an enzyme that digests the fibrin meshwork of clots. In addition to digesting fibrin, plasmin degrades fibrinogen and other clotting factors. These actions don't contribute to lysis of thrombi, but they do increase the risk for hemorrhage.

Therapeutic Uses

Alteplase has three major indications: (1) acute MI, (2) acute ischemic stroke, and (3) acute massive PE. In all three settings, timely intervention is essential: the sooner alteplase is administered, the better the outcome.

The importance of early intervention was first demonstrated in GUSTO-I (Global Utilization of Streptokinase and tPA for Occluded Coronary Arteries), a huge trial that evaluated the benefits of two thrombolytic drugs—alteplase (tPA) and streptokinase—in patients with acute MI. Results for alteplase were as follows: among patients treated within 2 hours of symptom onset, the death rate was only 5.4%; among those treated 2 to 4 hours after symptom onset, the rate increased to 6.6%; and among those treated 4 to 6 hours after symptom onset, the rate jumped to 9.4%. Clearly, outcomes are best when thrombolytic therapy is started quickly, preferably within 2 to 4 hours of symptom onset, and even earlier if possible. Thrombolytic therapy of acute MI is discussed further in Chapter 88.

In addition to its use for acute thrombotic disease, alteplase can be used to restore patency in a clogged central venous catheter.

Pharmacokinetics

Alteplase is a large molecule that must be administered parenterally, almost always by IV infusion. The drug has a very short half-life (5 minutes), owing to rapid hepatic

TABLE 89.2 ▪ Properties of Thrombolytic (Fibrinolytic) Drugs

	Alteplase (tPA)	Tenecteplase	Reteplase
Trade name	Activase, Cathflo Activase	TNKase	Retavase
Description	A compound identical to human tPA	Modified form of tPA with a prolonged half-life	A compound that contains the active sequence of amino acids present in tPA
Source	All three drugs are made using recombinant DNA technology		
Mechanism	All three drugs promote conversion of plasminogen to plasmin, an enzyme that degrades the fibrin matrix of thrombi		
INDICATIONS:			
Acute MI	Yes	Yes	Yes
Acute ischemic stroke	Yes	No	No
Acute pulmonary embolism	Yes	No	No
Clearing a blocked central venous catheter	Yes	No	No
Adverse effect: bleeding	With all three drugs, bleeding is the primary adverse effect		
Half-life (min)	5	20–24	13–16
Dosage and administration for acute MI	*Intravenous:* 15-mg bolus, then 50 mg infused over 30 min, then 35 mg infused over 60 min*	*Intravenous:* Single bolus based on body weight (see text)	*Intravenous:* 10-unit bolus 2 times, separated by 30 min

MI, myocardial infarction; tPA, tissue plasminogen activator.
*Dosage for patients who weigh more than 67 kg.

inactivation. Within 5 minutes of stopping an infusion, 50% of the drug is cleared from the blood. About 80% is cleared within 10 minutes.

Adverse Effect

Bleeding. Bleeding is the major complication of treatment. Intracranial hemorrhage (ICH) is by far the most serious concern. Bleeding occurs for two reasons: (1) plasmin can destroy preexisting clots and can thereby promote recurrence of bleeding at sites of recently healed injury; and (2) by degrading clotting factors, plasmin can disrupt coagulation and can thereby interfere with new clot formation in response to vascular injury. Likely sites of bleeding include recent wounds, sites of needle puncture, and sites at which an invasive procedure has been performed. Anticoagulants and antiplatelet drugs further increase hemorrhage risk. Accordingly, high-dose therapy with these drugs must be avoided until thrombolytic effects of alteplase have abated.

Management of bleeding depends on severity. Oozing at sites of cutaneous puncture can be controlled with a pressure dressing. If severe bleeding occurs, alteplase should be discontinued. Patients who require blood replacement can be given whole blood or blood products (packed red blood cells, fresh-frozen plasma). As a rule, blood replacement restores hemostasis. However, if this approach fails, excessive fibrinolysis can be reversed with IV *aminocaproic acid* [Amicar], a compound that prevents activation of plasminogen and directly inhibits plasmin.

The risk for bleeding can be lowered by the following:

- Minimizing physical manipulation of the patient
- Avoiding subcutaneous (subQ) and IM injections
- Minimizing invasive procedures
- Minimizing concurrent use of anticoagulants (e.g., heparin, warfarin, dabigatran)
- Minimizing concurrent use of antiplatelet drugs (e.g., aspirin, clopidogrel)

Owing to the risk for hemorrhage, alteplase and other thrombolytic drugs must be avoided in patients at high risk for bleeding complications and must be used with great caution in patients at lower risk for bleeding. Absolute and relative contraindications to thrombolytic therapy are shown in Table 89.3.

Preparations

Alteplase is available under two trade names: Activase and Cathflo Activase. Activase is used to treat thrombotic disorders. Cathflo Activase is used to clear clogged central venous catheters.

Dosage and Administration

Acute Myocardial Infarction (Activase Only). Alteplase is usually given by an "accelerated" or "front-loaded" schedule, in which the infusion time is only 90 minutes, compared with 3 hours as routinely done in the past. Dosage is based on patient weight but should not exceed 100 mg because doses in excess of 100 mg are associated with an increased risk for intracranial bleeding.

For patients who weigh more than 67 kg, the total dose is 100 mg, administered in three phases: a 15-mg IV bolus, followed by 50 mg infused over 30 minutes, followed in turn by 35 mg infused over 60 minutes.

For patients who weigh less than 67 kg, the maximal dose is 100 mg, administered in three phases: a 15-mg IV bolus, followed by 0.75 mg/kg (maximum, 50 mg) infused over 30 minutes, followed in turn by 0.5 mg/kg (maximum, 35 mg) infused over 60 minutes.

Acute Ischemic Stroke (Activase Only). The recommended dosage is 0.9 mg/kg (maximum, 90 mg) infused IV over 60 minutes, with 10% of the dose given as an initial IV bolus over 1 minute.

TABLE 89.3 ▪ Contraindications and Cautions Regarding Thrombolytic Use for Myocardial Infarction

Absolute contraindications	• Any prior intracranial hemorrhage • Known structural cerebral vascular lesion • Ischemic stroke within last 3 months *except* ischemic stroke within 4.5 hr • Known intracranial neoplasm • Active internal bleeding (other than menses) • Suspected aortic dissection
Relative contraindications/ cautions	• Severe, uncontrolled hypertension on presentation (blood pressure above 180/110 mm Hg) • History of chronic, severe, poorly controlled hypertension • History of prior ischemic stroke, dementia, or known intracerebral pathology not covered in absolute contraindications • Current use of anticoagulants in therapeutic doses (INR 2–3 or greater); known bleeding diathesis • Traumatic or prolonged (more than 10 min) CPR or major surgery (less than 3 wk ago) • Recent internal bleeding (within 2–4 wk) • Noncompressible vascular punctures • Pregnancy • Active peptic ulcer

CPR, cardiopulmonary resuscitation; INR, international normalized ratio.

Pulmonary Embolism (Activase Only). The recommended dosage is 100 mg infused IV over 2 hours.

Tenecteplase

Tenecteplase [TNKase], a variant of human tPA (alteplase), is approved only for acute MI. Except for the substitution of three amino acids, the drug is structurally identical to tPA. However, because of this small structural change, the pharmacokinetics of tenecteplase are much different. Specifically, tenecteplase is 80 times more resistant than tPA to circulating inhibitors and has a much longer half-life (20–24 minutes vs. 5 minutes for tPA). Like tPA, tenecteplase acts by converting plasminogen into plasmin, an enzyme that digests fibrin clots. Tenecteplase is just as safe and effective as tPA, but much easier to use: whereas tPA must be infused over 90 minutes, tenecteplase is given as a single IV bolus. As a result, thrombolysis develops faster, and emergency personnel are spared the trouble of monitoring a prolonged infusion. Because tenecteplase is so easy to administer, it has the potential to allow dosing before the patient reaches a hospital.

Tenecteplase was compared with tPA in the second Assessment of the Safety and Efficacy of a New Thrombolytic (ASSENT-2) study, which enrolled 16,949 patients. Tenecteplase was given as a 5-second IV bolus; tPA was infused over 90 minutes. The median time between symptom onset and starting treatment was 2.7 hours for tenecteplase and 2.8 hours for tPA. Thirty days after treatment, outcomes were equivalent with respect to mortality (6.2% with each drug), ICH (0.93% with tenecteplase vs. 0.94% with tPA), and total stroke (1.78% vs. 1.66% with tPA). Of significance, the incidence of major hemorrhage (other than intracranial) was lower with tenecteplase (4.7% vs. 5.9%).

Tenecteplase dosage is based on body weight as follows:

- Less than 60 kg: dose 30 mg
- 60 to 69.9 kg: dose 35 mg
- 70 to 79.9 kg: dose 40 mg
- 80 to 89.9 kg: dose 45 mg
- More than 90 kg: dose 50 mg

Reteplase

Reteplase [Retavase] is a derivative of tPA produced by recombinant DNA technology. Like tPA, reteplase converts plasminogen to plasmin, which in turn digests the fibrin matrix of the thrombus. Reteplase has a short half-life (13–16 minutes), owing to rapid clearance by the liver and kidneys. As with other thrombolytic drugs, bleeding is the major adverse effect. The risk for bleeding is increased by concurrent use of heparin, aspirin, and other drugs that impair hemostasis.

Reteplase is approved only for acute MI. Treatment consists of two 10-unit doses separated by 30 minutes. Each dose is given by IV bolus injected over a 2-minute interval.

ANTIDYSRHYTHMICS

Lidocaine

Lidocaine [Xylocaine], an IV agent, is used only for ventricular dysrhythmias. In addition to its antidysrhythmic applications, lidocaine is employed as a local anesthetic (see Chapter 21).

Effects on the Heart and Electrocardiogram

Lidocaine has three significant effects on the heart: (1) like other class I drugs, lidocaine blocks cardiac sodium channels and thereby *slows conduction* in the atria, ventricles, and His-Purkinje system; (2) the drug *reduces automaticity* in the ventricles and His-Purkinje system by a mechanism that is poorly understood; and (3) lidocaine *accelerates repolarization* (shortens the action potential duration and event-related potential). In contrast to quinidine and procainamide, lidocaine is devoid of anticholinergic properties. Also, lidocaine has no significant effect on the electrocardiogram (ECG): a small reduction in the QT interval may occur, but there is no QRS widening.

Pharmacokinetics

Lidocaine undergoes rapid hepatic metabolism. If the drug were administered orally, most of each dose would be inactivated on its first pass through the liver. For this reason, administration is parenteral, almost always by IV infusion.

Because lidocaine is rapidly degraded, plasma drug levels can be easily controlled: if levels climb too high, the infusion can be slowed and the liver will quickly remove excess drug from the circulation. The therapeutic range for lidocaine is 1.5 to 5 mcg/mL.

Antidysrhythmic Use

Antidysrhythmic use of lidocaine is limited to short-term therapy of *ventricular dysrhythmias* (Table 89.4). Lidocaine is not active against supraventricular dysrhythmias.

Adverse Effects

Lidocaine is generally well tolerated. However, adverse CNS effects can occur. High therapeutic doses can cause *drowsiness, confusion,* and *paresthesias.* Toxic doses may produce *seizures* and *respiratory arrest.* Consequently, whenever lidocaine is used, equipment for resuscitation must be available. Seizures can be managed with diazepam.

Preparations, Dosage, and Administration.

Administration is parenteral only. The usual route is IV. IM injection can be used in emergencies. Blood pressure and the ECG should be monitored for signs of toxicity.

TABLE 89.4 ▪ Properties of Antidysrhythmic Drugs

Drug	Acute Care Route	Effects on the ECG	Major Antidysrhythmic Applications
CLASS IA			
Procainamide	IV	Widens QRS, prolongs QT	Broad spectrum: similar to quinidine, but toxicity makes it less desirable for long-term use
CLASS IB			
Lidocaine	IV	No significant change	Ventricular dysrhythmias
CLASS II			
Esmolol	IV	Prolongs PR, bradycardia	Control of ventricular rate in patients with supraventricular tachydysrhythmias
CLASS III			
Amiodarone	IV	Prolongs QT and PR, widens QRS	Life-threatening ventricular dysrhythmias, atrial fibrillation*
Ibutilide	IV	Prolongs QT	Atrial flutter, atrial fibrillation
CLASS IV			
Diltiazem	IV	Prolongs PR, bradycardia	Control of ventricular rate in patients with supraventricular tachydysrhythmias
OTHERS			
Adenosine	IV	Prolongs PR	Termination of paroxysmal supraventricular tachycardia

*Amiodarone is widely used for atrial fibrillation, but it is not approved for this use.
IV, intravenous.

Intravenous

Lidocaine [Xylocaine] preparations intended for IV administration are clearly labeled as such. They contain no preservatives or catecholamines. (Lidocaine used for local anesthesia frequently contains epinephrine.) Preparations that contain epinephrine or another catecholamine must never be administered intravenously because doing so can cause severe hypertension and life-threatening dysrhythmias.

IV therapy is initiated with a loading dose followed by continuous infusion for maintenance. The usual loading dose is 50 to 100 mg (1 mg/kg) administered at a rate of 25 to 50 mg/min. An infusion rate of 1 to 4 mg/min is used for maintenance; the rate is adjusted on the basis of cardiac response. IV lidocaine should be discontinued as soon as possible, usually within 24 hours.

To avoid toxicity, dosage should be reduced in patients with impaired hepatic function or impaired hepatic blood flow (e.g., older-adult patients; patients with cirrhosis, shock, or HF).

Intramuscular

Lidocaine is available in an automatic injection device [LidoPen Auto-Injector] for IM administration. A dose of 300 mg is injected into the deltoid muscle. This dose can be repeated in 60 to 90 minutes if necessary. The patient should be switched to IV lidocaine as soon as possible.

Procainamide

Procainamide blocks cardiac sodium channels, thereby decreasing conduction velocity in the atria, ventricles, and His-Purkinje system. Also, the drug delays repolarization. In contrast to quinidine, procainamide is only weakly anticholinergic and hence is not likely to increase ventricular rate.

Procainamide is effective against a broad spectrum of atrial and ventricular dysrhythmias. Like quinidine, the drug can be used for long-term suppression (Table 89.4). However, because prolonged therapy is often associated with serious adverse effects, procainamide is less desirable than quinidine for long-term use. In contrast to quinidine, procainamide can be used to terminate ventricular tachycardia and ventricular fibrillation.

Procainamide is available in solution for IM and IV administration. IM injection is made deep into the gluteal muscle; dosage is 0.5 to 1 g repeated every 4 to 8 hours.

IV infusion may be performed at an initial rate of 20 to 50 mg/min (maximal loading dose is 1500 mg). After the loading period, an infusion rate of 2 to 6 mg/min should be employed. When the dysrhythmia has been controlled, the patient should be switched to oral procainamide. Three hours should elapse between terminating the infusion and the first oral dose.

Esmolol

Esmolol [Brevibloc] is a cardioselective beta blocker with a very short half-life (9 minutes). Administration is by IV infusion. The drug is employed for immediate control of ventricular rate in patients with supraventricular tachycardia (SVT), atrial flutter, and atrial fibrillation. Use is short term only (e.g., in patients with dysrhythmias associated with surgery). The most common adverse reaction is hypotension. However, like other beta blockers, esmolol can also cause bradycardia, heart block, HF, and bronchospasm (at higher doses). In addition, pain can occur at the infusion site. Treatment begins with a loading dose (500 mcg/kg) infused over 1 minute. The usual maintenance infusion rate is 100 mcg/kg/min.

Amiodarone

IV amiodarone is approved only for initial treatment and prophylaxis of recurrent ventricular fibrillation and hemodynamically unstable ventricular tachycardia in patients refractory to safer drugs. For these indications, amiodarone may be lifesaving.

In addition to its approved uses, IV amiodarone has been used with success against other dysrhythmias, including atrial fibrillation, atrioventricular (AV) nodal reentrant tachycardia, and shock-resistant ventricular fibrillation.

Effects on the Heart and Electrocardiogram

In contrast to oral amiodarone (discussed in Chapter 41, which affects multiple aspects of cardiac function, IV amiodarone affects primarily the AV node. Specifically, the drug slows AV conduction and prolongs AV refractoriness. Both effects probably result from antiadrenergic actions. The mechanism underlying antidysrhythmic effects is unknown.

Adverse Effects

The most common adverse effects are hypotension and bradydysrhythmias. Hypotension develops in 15% to 20% of patients and may require discontinuation of treatment. Bradycardia or AV block occurs in 5% of patients; discontinuation of treatment or insertion of a pacemaker may be needed. Infusions containing more than 2 mg/mL (in 5% dextrose in water) produce a high incidence of phlebitis and therefore should be administered through a central venous line. Torsades de pointes in association with QT prolongation occurs rarely.

Dosage

Dosing is complex. During the first 24 hours, a total dose of 1050 mg is infused. After that, a maintenance infusion (0.5 mg/min) is given around-the-clock. The usual duration of treatment is 2 to 4 days. However, maintenance infusions may be continued for up to 3 weeks before switching to oral amiodarone.

Ibutilide

Ibutilide [Corvert] is an IV agent used to terminate atrial flutter and atrial fibrillation of recent onset (i.e., that has been present no longer than 90 days). Conversion to sinus rhythm occurs during the infusion or within 90 minutes of its termination. Ibutilide is more effective against atrial flutter (49%–70% success) than atrial fibrillation (22%–43% success). Like other class III agents, ibutilide blocks potassium channels and thereby prolongs the action potential duration and QT interval. Up to 8% of patients develop torsades de pointes, frequently in association with QT prolongation. Oral doses are teratogenic and embryocidal in rats. For patients who weigh more than 60 kg, the dosage is 1 mg infused over 10 minutes. If the dysrhythmia does not convert within 10 minutes of terminating the infusion, a second 1-mg infusion may be tried.

Verapamil

The pharmacology of verapamil, a calcium channel blocker, is discussed in Chapter 37. Dosing of verapamil may be IV or oral. IV therapy is preferred for initial treatment. Oral therapy is used for maintenance. The initial IV dose is 5 to 10 mg injected slowly. If the dysrhythmia persists, an additional 10 mg may be administered in 30 minutes. An IV infusion (0.375 mg/min) can be used for maintenance. IV verapamil can cause serious cardiovascular effects. Accordingly, BP and the ECG should be monitored, and equipment for resuscitation should be immediately available.

Diltiazem

Like verapamil, diltiazem is also a calcium channel blocker. Diltiazem may be given by IV or oral route and is discussed in Chapter 37. IV therapy is preferred for initial treatment, and oral therapy is used for maintenance. IV therapy is initiated with an IV bolus (0.25 mg/kg). If the response is inadequate, a second bolus (0.35 mg/kg) may be administered in 15 minutes. If appropriate, initial therapy may be followed with a continuous IV infusion (up to 24 hours' duration) at a rate of 5 to 15 mg/hr.

Adenosine

Adenosine [Adenocard], a naturally occurring nucleotide, is a drug of choice for terminating paroxysmal SVT. Adenosine has an extremely short half-life and thus must be administered intravenously. Adverse effects are minimum because adenosine is rapidly cleared from the blood.

Effects on the Heart and Electrocardiogram

Adenosine decreases automaticity in the sinoatrial (SA) node and greatly slows conduction through the AV node. The most prominent ECG change is prolongation of the PR interval, brought on by delayed AV conduction. Adenosine works in part by inhibiting cyclic adenosine monophosphate (cAMP)-induced calcium influx, thereby suppressing calcium-dependent action potentials in the SA and AV nodes.

Therapeutic Use

Adenosine is approved only for termination of paroxysmal SVT, including Wolff-Parkinson-White syndrome. The drug is not active against atrial fibrillation, atrial flutter, or ventricular dysrhythmias.

Pharmacokinetics

Adenosine has an extremely short half-life (estimated at 1.5–10 seconds), owing primarily to rapid uptake by cells and partly to deactivation by circulating adenosine deaminase. Because of its rapid clearance, adenosine must be administered by IV bolus, as close to the heart as possible.

Adverse Effects

Adverse effects are short lived, lasting less than 1 minute. The most common are sinus bradycardia, dyspnea (from bronchoconstriction), hypotension and facial flushing (from vasodilation), and chest discomfort (perhaps from stimulation of pain receptors in the heart).

Drug Interactions

Methylxanthines (aminophylline, theophylline, caffeine) block receptors for adenosine. Hence asthma patients taking aminophylline or theophylline need larger doses of adenosine, and even then adenosine may not work.

Dipyridamole, an antiplatelet drug, blocks cellular uptake of adenosine and can thereby intensify its effects.

Preparations, Dosage, and Administration

Adenosine [Adenocard] is supplied in solution (3 mg/mL) for bolus IV administration. The injection should be made as close to the heart as possible, and should be followed by a saline flush. The initial dose is 6 mg. If there is no response in 1 or 2 minutes, 12 mg may be tried and repeated once. If a response is going to occur, it should happen as soon as the drug reaches the AV node.

DRUGS FOR HYPERTENSIVE EMERGENCIES

A hypertensive emergency exists when systolic BP exceeds 180 mm Hg, diastolic BP exceeds 100 mm Hg, and there is evidence of end organ damage. When excessive BP is associated with papilledema (edema of the retina), ICH, MI, or acute congestive heart failure (CHF), a severe emergency exists—and BP must be lowered rapidly (within 1 hour). If severe hypertension is present but does not yet pose an immediate threat of organ damage, reducing BP more slowly (over 24–48 hours) is preferable. This situation is often referred to as hypertensive urgency. Because rapid reductions can cause cerebral ischemia, MI, and renal failure, pressure should be reduced gradually whenever possible.

The major drugs used for hypertensive emergencies are discussed next. All reduce BP by causing vasodilation, and all are given intravenously.

Sodium Nitroprusside

When acute, severe hypertension demands a rapid but controlled reduction in BP, IV nitroprusside [Nitropress] is usually the drug of first choice. Effects begin in seconds and then fade rapidly when administration ceases.

Cardiovascular Effects

Nitroprusside is a direct-acting vasodilator that relaxes smooth muscle of arterioles and veins. Curiously, although nitroprusside is an effective arteriolar dilator, reflex tachycardia is minimal. Nitroprusside can trigger retention of sodium and water; furosemide can help counteract this effect.

Mechanism of Action

When in the body, nitroprusside breaks down to release nitric oxide, which then activates guanylate cyclase, an enzyme present in vascular smooth muscle (VSM). Guanylate cyclase catalyzes the production of cyclic GMP, which, through a series of reactions, causes vasodilation. This mechanism is similar to that of nitroglycerin.

Metabolism

Nitroprusside contains five *cyanide groups,* which are split free in the first step of nitroprusside metabolism. *Nitric oxide,* the active component, is released next. Both reactions take place in smooth muscle. When freed, the cyanide groups are converted to *thiocyanate* by the liver, using *thiosulfate* as a cofactor. Thiocyanate is eliminated by the kidneys over several days.

Adverse Effects

Excessive Hypotension

If administered too rapidly, nitroprusside can cause a precipitous drop in blood pressure, resulting in headache, palpitations, nausea, vomiting, and sweating. Blood pressure should be monitored continuously.

Cyanide Poisoning

Rarely, lethal amounts of cyanide have accumulated. Cyanide buildup is most likely in patients with liver disease and in those with low stores of thiosulfate, the cofactor needed for cyanide detoxification. The chances of cyanide poisoning can be minimized by avoiding rapid infusion (faster than 5 mcg/kg/min) and by coadministering thiosulfate. If cyanide toxicity occurs, nitroprusside should be withdrawn.

Thiocyanate Toxicity

When nitroprusside is given for several days, thiocyanate may accumulate. Although much less hazardous than cyanide, thiocyanate can also cause adverse effects. These effects, which involve the CNS, include disorientation, psychotic behavior, and delirium. To minimize toxicity, patients receiving nitroprusside for more than 3 days should undergo monitoring of plasma thiocyanate, which must be kept below 0.1 mg/mL.

Preparations, Dosage, and Administration

Sodium nitroprusside [Nitropress] initial infusion rate is 0.3 mcg/kg/min. The maximal rate is 10 mcg/kg/min. If infusion at the maximal rate for 10 minutes fails to produce an adequate drop in blood pressure, administration should stop. During the infusion, blood pressure should be monitored continuously, with either an arterial line or an electronic monitoring device. No other drugs should be mixed with the nitroprusside solution

Fenoldopam

Fenoldopam [Corlopam] is an IV drug indicated for short-term management of hypertensive emergencies. Benefits equal those of nitroprusside. Fenoldopam lowers BP by activating dopamine-1 receptors on arterioles to cause vasodilation. In animal models, the drug dilates renal, coronary, mesenteric, and peripheral vessels.

Fenoldopam differs from other antihypertensives in that it helps maintain (or even improve) renal function. Two mechanisms are involved. First, the drug dilates renal blood vessels, increasing renal blood flow (despite reducing arterial pressure). Second, fenoldopam promotes sodium and water excretion through direct effects on renal tubules.

Fenoldopam has a rapid onset and short duration. Effects begin in less than 5 minutes. The drug undergoes rapid hepatic metabolism followed by renal excretion. Its plasma half-life is only 5 minutes.

Fenoldopam is generally well tolerated. The most common side effects are hypotension, headache, flushing, dizziness, and reflex tachycardia—all of which occur secondary to vasodilation. Tachycardia may cause ischemia in patients with angina. Combined use with a beta blocker can minimize tachycardia, but may also result in excessive lowering of BP. Fenoldopam can elevate intraocular pressure and hence should be used with caution in patients with glaucoma.

Fenoldopam is administered by continuous IV infusion. To minimize tachycardia, the initial dosage should be low. The typical infusion rate is 0.25 to 0.5 mcg/kg/min. With continuous 24-hour infusion, no tolerance develops to antihypertensive effects, and there is no rebound increase in BP when the infusion is stopped. With a 48-hour infusion, some tolerance may develop. Oral antihypertensive therapy can be added as soon as BP has stabilized.

Labetalol

Labetalol blocks alpha- and beta-adrenergic receptors. Blood pressure is reduced by arteriolar dilation secondary to alpha blockade. Beta blockade prevents reflex tachycardia in response to reduced arterial pressure, and hence the drug is probably safe for patients with angina or MI. Beta blockade can aggravate bronchial asthma, HF, AV block, cardiogenic shock, and bradycardia. Accordingly, labetalol should not be given to patients with these disorders. Administration is by slow IV injection.

Clevidipine

Clevidipine [Cleviprex] is a dihydropyridine calcium channel blocker with an ultrashort half-life (about 1 minute). Administration is by IV infusion. As with nitroprusside, effects begin rapidly and then fade rapidly when the infusion is slowed or stopped. As a result, BP can be easily titrated. For patients with severe hypertension, the infusion rate is 1 to 2 mg/hr initially and can be doubled every 3 minutes up to a maximum of 32 mg/hr. In clinical trials, the average time to reach the target BP was 10.9 minutes. The most common side effects are headache, nausea, and vomiting. The basic pharmacology of clevidipine is discussed in Chapter 37.

BENZODIAZEPINE REVERSAL

Flumazenil

Flumazenil [Romazicon] is a competitive benzodiazepine receptor antagonist. The drug can reverse the sedative effects of benzodiazepines, but may not reverse respiratory depression. Flumazenil is approved for benzodiazepine overdose and for reversing the effects of benzodiazepines after general anesthesia. The principal adverse effect is precipitation of seizures. This is most likely in patients taking benzodiazepines to treat epilepsy and in patients who are physically dependent on benzodiazepines. Flumazenil is administered intravenously. Doses are injected over 15 seconds and may be repeated every minute as needed up to a dose of 3 mg. The first dose is 0.2 mg, the second is 0.3 mg, and all subsequent doses are 0.5 mg. Effects of flumazenil fade in about 1 hour, hence repeated doses may be required.

DIABETES

Intravenous Insulin

Infusion

IV insulin infusion is reserved for emergencies that require a rapid reduction in blood glucose and for people being managed in the inpatient setting during hospitalization. Not long ago, regular insulin (U-100 strength) was the only formulation considered safe for IV use. Today, three other short-acting insulins—insulin aspart [Novolog], insulin lispro [Humalog], and insulin glulisine [Apidra]—may also be used. Regular insulin is most commonly used because it is less expensive. An initial infusion rate of 0.1 unit/kg/hr is often recommended, but infusion rates and insulin doses must be individualized based on individual needs.

IV insulin is used to treat *diabetic ketoacidosis*. Because of its ability to promote cellular uptake of potassium and thereby lower plasma potassium levels, insulin infusion is employed to treat *hyperkalemia*. The properties of insulin are discussed fully in Chapter 46.

Acute Complications of Poor Glycemic Control

Uncontrolled diabetes will lead to hyperglycemia, which in turn can lead to *diabetic ketoacidosis* (DKA) or *hyperosmolar hyperglycemic state* (HHS). The cardinal feature of both conditions is hyperglycemic crisis and associated loss of fluid and electrolytes. Both conditions can be life-threatening, and hence immediate treatment should be implemented. As indicated in Table 89.5, these disorders have two principal differences. First, hyperglycemia is more severe in HHS. Second, whereas ketoacidosis is characteristic of DKA, it is absent in HHS. Treatment of both disorders is similar.

Diabetic Ketoacidosis

DKA is a severe manifestation of insulin deficiency. This syndrome is characterized by hyperglycemia, production of ketoacids, hemoconcentration, acidosis, and coma. These symptoms typically evolve quickly, over a period of several hours to a couple of days. Before insulin became available, practically all patients with type 1 diabetes died from ketoacidosis. Today, DKA remains a common complication in pediatric patients and is the leading cause of diabetes-related death in this group. DKA occurs much more often in patients with type 1 diabetes than in those with type 2 diabetes.

TABLE 89.5 ■ Contrasts Between Diabetic Ketoacidosis and Hyperosmolar Hyperglycemic State

Characteristic	Diabetic Ketoacidosis	Hyperosmolar Hyperglycemic State
Patient population	Mainly in type 1 diabetes	More likely in type 2 diabetes
Onset	Rapid	Gradual
Blood glucose (mg/dL)	≥250	≥600
Plasma osmolality (mOsm/L)*	<320	>320
pH of arterial blood	≤7.3	≥7.3
Blood ketones	Large increase	Little or no change
Urine ketones	Large increase	Normal or small increase
Urine and breath odor	Urine smells like rotten apples; breath smells sweet or like acetone (nail polish)	Normal

Pathogenesis

DKA is brought on by derangements of glucose and fat metabolism. Altered glucose metabolism causes hyperglycemia, water loss, and hemoconcentration. Altered fat metabolism causes production of ketoacids. Note that, in its final stages, the syndrome consists of hemoconcentration and shock in addition to ketoacidosis. The alterations in fat and glucose metabolism that lead to ketoacidosis are described in detail later.

Treatment

DKA is a life-threatening emergency. Treatment is directed at correcting hyperglycemia and acidosis, replacing lost water and sodium, and normalizing potassium balance. We begin with IV fluids and electrolytes, followed as soon as possible by IV insulin. Although it might seem reasonable to drive glucose levels down quickly with lots of insulin, doing so is unsafe and should be avoided. Instead, glucose levels should be reduced slowly, by about 50 mg/dL/hr.

Insulin Replacement

Insulin levels are restored with an initial IV bolus of regular insulin (0.1–0.15 unit/kg body weight) followed by continuous infusion at a rate of 0.1 unit/kg/hr. When plasma glucose has fallen to 200 mg/dL, the infusion rate should be reduced to 0.02 to 0.05 unit/kg/hr. Thereafter the insulin dosage should be adjusted as needed to maintain plasma glucose levels between 150 and 200 mg/dL until acidosis has resolved. Switching to subQ insulin is common and acceptable after the patient recovers from the acute episode.

IV insulin is preferred to subQ insulin for initial management. In patients with DKA, absorption of subQ insulin is apt to be both slow and erratic, making accurate dosing difficult. Also, when insulin is administered subQ, insulin levels cannot be lowered quickly in response to inadvertent excessive dosing, and hence avoiding hypoglycemia may be difficult. IV dosing avoids these problems: blood levels of insulin are established immediately; there is no uncertainty about the amount "absorbed"; and, if the blood level of insulin is too high, it can be quickly lowered by stopping the infusion, thereby permitting good control of blood glucose content.

Bicarbonate for Acidosis

Treating acidosis with bicarbonate is controversial. Studies have failed to demonstrate any benefit of giving bicarbonate to patients with severe acidosis (blood pH 6.9–7.1). Nonetheless, some authorities recommend empiric therapy with bicarbonate if blood pH is below 6.9. Because bicarbonate promotes hypokalemia, potassium should be infused along with the bicarbonate, as noted earlier, unless hyperkalemia (serum potassium above 5.5 mEq/L) is present.

Water and Sodium Replacement

Dehydration and sodium loss are both corrected with IV saline. Depending on the specific needs of the patient, either 0.9% or 0.45% saline is employed. Adults usually require between 8 and 10 L of fluid during the first 12 hours of treatment. In older-adult patients and patients with heart disease, central venous pressure should be monitored.

Potassium Replacement

Hypokalemia of DKA is a serious problem and must be corrected. As a rule, potassium is replenished by IV administration. Because hypokalemia predisposes the patient to dysrhythmias, electrocardiographic monitoring is essential.

Treatment of potassium loss is tricky because plasma potassium levels may be normal even though intracellular potassium is very low. When insulin is administered, causing cellular uptake of potassium to increase, severe hypokalemia can develop as plasma potassium rushes into potassium-depleted cells. Because of this relationship between insulin administration and plasma potassium levels, the following guidelines apply: (1) if plasma potassium is normal, no potassium should be administered until plasma potassium declines in response to insulin; (2) if plasma potassium is low, potassium should be given immediately (and then readministered if potassium levels fall after insulin administration).

Normalization of Glucose Levels

Treatment of ketoacidosis with insulin may convert hyperglycemia into hypoglycemia. Because cellular uptake of glucose is impaired by insulin deficiency, ketoacidosis is likely to be associated with a reduction in intracellular glucose—despite elevations in plasma glucose content. Under these conditions, giving insulin will cause plasma glucose to rush into the glucose-depleted cells, thereby causing plasma levels of glucose to drop precipitously. If insulin therapy induces hypoglycemia, plasma glucose can be restored by giving glucagon or glucose.

Hyperosmolar Hyperglycemic State

HHS, also known as hyperglycemic hyperosmolar nonketotic syndrome (HHNS), is similar to DKA in some respects and different in others. As noted, the central characteristic in both disorders is severe hyperglycemia brought on by insulin deficiency. In HHS, as in DKA, a large amount of glucose is excreted in the urine, carrying a large volume of water with it. The result is dehydration and loss of blood volume, which greatly increases the blood concentrations of electrolytes and nonelectrolytes (particularly glucose)—hence the term hyperosmolar. Loss of blood volume also increases the hematocrit. As a result, the blood "thickens" and blood flow becomes sluggish. How does HHS differ from DKA? As its name indicates, HHS is nonketotic: there is little or no change in ketoacid levels in blood and hence little or no change in blood pH. In contrast, blood levels of ketoacids rise dramatically in DKA, causing blood pH to fall. Because ketone levels remain close to normal in HHNS, the sweet or acetone-like smell imparted to the urine and breath of the DKA patient is absent. Finally, whereas DKA occurs mainly in patients with type 1 diabetes and develops quickly (usually in association with infection, acute illness, or some other stress), HHS occurs more often in patients with type 2 diabetes and evolves slowly: metabolic changes typically begin a month or two before signs and symptoms become apparent. If HHS goes untreated, severe dehydration will eventually lead to coma, seizures, and death. As with DKA, management of HHS is directed at correcting hyperglycemia and dehydration by use of IV insulin, fluids, and electrolytes.

DIURETICS

Furosemide

Furosemide is usually given intravenously for the treatment of pulmonary edema or acute decompensated HF in the hospital setting. Furosemide (discussed further in Chapter 35) is available in solution for IV and IM administration. The usual dosage for adults is 20 to 40 mg, repeated in 1 or 2 hours if needed. For high-dose therapy, furosemide can be administered by continuous infusion at a rate of 4 mg/min or slower.

Mannitol, an Osmotic Diuretic

Osmotic diuretics differ from other diuretics with regard to mechanism and uses. At this time, mannitol is the only osmotic diuretic available in the United States. Mannitol [Osmitrol] is a simple six-carbon sugar that embodies the following four properties of an ideal osmotic diuretic:

- Is freely filtered at the glomerulus
- Undergoes minimal tubular reabsorption
- Undergoes minimal metabolism
- Is pharmacologically inert (i.e., it has no direct effects on the biochemistry or physiology of cells)

After IV administration, mannitol is filtered by the glomerulus. However, unlike other solutes, the drug undergoes minimal reabsorption. As a result, most of the filtered drug remains in the nephron, creating an osmotic force that inhibits passive reabsorption of water. Hence urine flow increases. The degree of diuresis produced is directly related to the concentration of mannitol in the filtrate: the more mannitol present, the greater the diuresis. Mannitol has no significant effect on the excretion of potassium and other electrolytes.

Pharmacokinetics

Mannitol does not diffuse across the GI epithelium and cannot be transported by the uptake systems that absorb dietary sugars. Accordingly, to reach the circulation, the drug must be given parenterally. After IV injection, mannitol distributes freely to extracellular water. Diuresis begins in 30 to 60 minutes and persists 6 to 8 hours. Most of the drug is excreted intact in the urine.

Therapeutic Uses

Prophylaxis of Renal Failure

Under certain conditions (e.g., dehydration, severe hypotension, hypovolemic shock), blood flow to the kidney is decreased, causing a great reduction in filtrate volume. When the volume of filtrate is this low, transport mechanisms of the nephron are able to reabsorb virtually all of the sodium and chloride present, causing complete reabsorption of water as well. As a result, urine production ceases, and kidney failure ensues. The risk for renal failure can be reduced with mannitol. Here's how. Because filtered mannitol is not reabsorbed—even when filtrate volume is small—filtered mannitol will remain in the nephron, drawing water with it. Hence mannitol can preserve urine flow and may thereby prevent renal failure. Thiazides and loop diuretics are not as effective for this application because, under conditions of low filtrate production, there is such an excess of reabsorptive capacity (relative to the amount of filtrate) that these drugs are unable to produce sufficient blockade of reabsorption to promote diuresis.

Reduction of Intracranial Pressure

Intracranial pressure (ICP) that has been elevated by cerebral edema can be reduced with mannitol. The drug lowers ICP because its presence in the blood vessels of the brain creates an osmotic force that draws edematous fluid from the brain into the blood. There is no risk for increasing cerebral edema because mannitol cannot exit the capillary beds of the brain.

Reduction of Intraocular Pressure

Mannitol and other osmotic agents can lower intraocular pressure (IOP) by rendering the plasma hyperosmotic with respect to intraocular fluids. The hyperosmotic plasma creates an osmotic force that draws ocular fluid into the blood. Use of mannitol to lower IOP is reserved for patients who have not responded to more conventional treatment.

Adverse Effects

Edema

Mannitol can leave the vascular system at all capillary beds except those of the brain. When the drug exits capillaries, it draws water along, causing edema. Mannitol must be used with extreme caution in patients with heart disease because it may precipitate CHF and pulmonary edema. If signs of pulmonary congestion or CHF develop, use of the drug must cease immediately. Mannitol must also be discontinued in patients with HF or pulmonary edema who develop renal failure because the resultant accumulation of mannitol would increase the risk for cardiac or pulmonary injury.

Other Adverse Effects

Common responses include headache, nausea, and vomiting. Fluid and electrolyte imbalance may also occur.

Preparations, Dosage, and Administration

Mannitol [Osmitrol] is administered by IV infusion. Solutions for IV use range in concentration from 5% to 25%. Dosing is complex and varies with the objective of therapy (prevention of renal failure, lowering of ICP, lowering of IOP). The usual adult dosage for preventing renal failure is 50 to 100 g over 24 hours. The infusion rate should be set to elicit a urine flow of at least 30 to 50 mL/hr. If urine flow declines to a very low rate or ceases entirely, the infusion should be stopped.

ACUTE DECOMPENSATED HEART FAILURE

Inotropic Agents

In addition to digoxin, we have two other types of inotropic drugs: sympathomimetics and phosphodiesterase (PDE) inhibitors. Unlike digoxin, which can be taken orally, these other inotropics must be given by IV infusion. Accordingly, their use is restricted to acute care of hospitalized patients. Because digoxin can be given orally, it is the only inotropic agent suited for long-term therapy.

Sympathomimetic Drugs: Dopamine and Dobutamine

The basic pharmacology of dopamine and dobutamine is presented in Chapter 13. Discussion here is limited to their use in HF. Both drugs are administered by IV infusion.

Dopamine

Dopamine is a catecholamine that can activate (1) beta_1-adrenergic receptors in the heart, (2) dopamine receptors in the kidney, and (3) at high doses, alpha_1-adrenergic receptors in blood vessels. Activation of beta_1 receptors increases myocardial contractility, thereby improving cardiac performance. Beta_1 activation also increases heart rate, creating a risk for tachycardia. Activation of dopamine receptors dilates renal blood vessels, thereby increasing renal blood flow and urine output. Activation of alpha_1 receptors increases vascular resistance (afterload) and can thereby reduce cardiac output. Dopamine is administered by continuous infusion. Constant monitoring of blood pressure, the ECG, and urine output is required. Dopamine is employed as a short-term rescue measure for patients with severe, acute cardiac failure.

Dobutamine

Dobutamine is a synthetic catecholamine that causes selective activation of beta_1-adrenergic receptors. By doing so, the drug can increase myocardial contractility and can thereby improve cardiac performance. Like dopamine, dobutamine can cause tachycardia and induce myocardial ischemia. In contrast to dopamine, dobutamine does not activate alpha_1 receptors and therefore does not increase vascular resistance. As a result, the drug is generally preferred to dopamine for short-term treatment of acute HF. Administration is by continuous infusion.

Phosphodiesterase Inhibitors

Milrinone

Milrinone has been called an inodilator because it increases myocardial contractility and promotes vasodilation. Increased contractility results from accumulation of cAMP secondary to inhibition of PDE-3, an enzyme that degrades cAMP. Milrinone is administered by IV infusion and is indicated only for short-term therapy of severe HF. The initial dose is 25 to 75 mcg/kg over 10 to 20 minutes. The maintenance infusion is 0.375 to 0.75 mcg/kg/min. Use should be reserved for patients with severe reduction in cardiac output resulting in decreased organ perfusion because ionotropes can induce dysrhythmias and cause myocardial ischemia from increased metabolic demand.

Intravenous Vasodilators

Nitroglycerin

IV nitroglycerin is a powerful venodilator that produces a dramatic reduction in venous pressure. Effects have been described as being equivalent to "pharmacologic phlebotomy." In HF, nitroglycerin is used to relieve acute severe pulmonary edema. Principal adverse effects are hypotension and resultant reflex tachycardia. The basic pharmacology of nitroglycerin is discussed in Chapter 43.

Nesiritide

Nesiritide [Natrecor] is a synthetic form of human brain natriuretic peptide (BNP) indicated only for short-term, IV therapy of hospitalized patients with acutely decompensated HF, characterized by increased pulmonary capillary wedge pressure (PCWP) and dyspnea at rest. Nesiritide is produced by recombinant DNA technology and has the same amino acid sequence as naturally occurring BNP. The drug was approved after a relatively small trial showed a modest decrease in dyspnea and PCWP. However, after 10 years of use, a much larger trial—Acute Study of Clinical Effectiveness of Nesiritide in Decompensated Heart Failure (ASCEND-HF)—failed to show any benefit: The incidence of dyspnea, rehospitalization, and 30-day mortality was the same for patients receiving nesiritide as it was for patients receiving placebo. Worse yet, although nesiritide offered no benefit, it nearly doubled the incidence of hypotension. These results led the authors to conclude that "Nesiritide cannot be recommended for routine use in the broad population of patients with heart failure."

Mechanism of Action

Nesiritide affects hemodynamics by three mechanisms: suppression of the renin-angiotensin-aldosterone system suppression of sympathetic outflow from the central nervous system (CNS), and direct dilation of arterioles and veins. In patients with HF, benefits derive primarily from direct vasodilation. To promote vasodilation, nesiritide binds with receptors on VSM and thereby stimulates production of cyclic guanosine monophosphate (cGMP), a second messenger that causes VSM to relax. This mechanism is similar to that of nitroglycerin, which also stimulates cGMP production. However, whereas nitroglycerin acts primarily on veins, nesiritide dilates arterioles as well. By dilating arterioles and veins, nesiritide reduces both preload and afterload. The net result is a decrease in PCWP and increased cardiac output. Also, by dilating afferent renal arterioles, nesiritide increases glomerular filtration rate, and thereby increases excretion of sodium and water. The result is a reduction in blood volume, which further reduces cardiac preload.

Pharmacokinetics

With continuous infusion, nesiritide achieves steady-state levels that are 3 to 6 times greater than the level of endogenous BNP present at baseline. Nesiritide is eliminated by three mechanisms: (1) proteolytic cleavage by endopeptidases present on the luminal surface of blood vessels; (2) binding to clearance receptors on the surface of cells, followed by cellular uptake and proteolytic cleavage; and (3) renal filtration. The drug's half-life is short, about 18 minutes.

Adverse Effects

The principal adverse effect is symptomatic hypotension. In the ASCEND-HF trial, hypotension developed in 26.6% of patients receiving nesiritide, compared with 15.3% of those receiving placebo. The risk for hypotension is increased by high doses of nesiritide and by concurrent use of angiotensin-converting enzyme inhibitors and other vasodilators. In addition to causing hypotension, nesiritide can cause ventricular tachycardia, headache, back pain, dizziness, and nausea. An analysis of several clinical trials suggested that nesiritide might cause renal damage. However, ASCEND-HF revealed no evidence of renal harm.

Preparations, Dosage, and Administration

Nesiritide [Natrecor] dosing consists of an initial IV bolus (2 mcg/kg) followed by continuous infusion (0.01 mcg/kg/min), typically lasting 48 hours or less. If symptomatic hypotension develops, the infusion should be slowed or stopped.

ACUTE MANAGEMENT OF PAIN

Acetaminophen

IV acetaminophen [Ofirmev] is indicated for fever and mild to moderate pain (when used alone) and for moderate to severe pain (when combined with an opioid). Dosages are as follows:

- Adults and children 13 years and older who weigh more than 50 kg—1000 mg every 6 hours or 650 mg every 4 hours as needed. Daily maximum is 4000 mg.
- Children 2 to 12 years old, and children 13 years and older who weigh less than 50 kg—15 mg/kg every 6 hours or 12.5 mg/kg every 4 hours as needed. Daily maximum is 75 mg/kg.

Acetaminophen Overdose—Acetylcysteine

For IV therapy, acetylcysteine is supplied in solution (200 mg/mL), sold as Acetadote, and should be diluted in 5% dextrose. Three doses are given in sequence. The first dose—150 mg/kg (in 200 mL of 5% dextrose)—is infused over 15 minutes to 1 hour. The second dose—50 mg/kg (in 500 mL of 5% dextrose)—is infused over 4 hours. And the third dose—100 mg/kg (in 1000 mL of 5% dextrose)—is infused over 16 hours. Rarely, IV acetylcysteine causes allergic reactions (rash, itching, angioedema, bronchospasm, hypotension), most often in response to the first dose. Fortunately, these reactions tend to be mild and self-limited and can be minimized by infusing the initial dose slowly (over a 1-hour interval).

Opioids

Morphine

Intravenous

IV morphine should be injected slowly (over 4–5 minutes). Rapid IV injection can cause severe adverse effects (profound hypotension, cardiac arrest, respiratory arrest) and should be avoided. When IV injections are made, an opioid antagonist (e.g., naloxone) and facilities for respiratory support should be available. The usual dose for adults is 4 to 10 mg (diluted in 4–5 mL of sterile water for injection). The usual pediatric dose is 0.05 to 0.1 mg/kg.

Epidural and Intrathecal

When morphine is employed for spinal analgesia, epidural injection is preferred to intrathecal. With either route, onset of analgesia is rapid and the duration prolonged (up to 24 hours). The most troubling side effects are delayed respiratory depression and delayed cardiac depression. Be alert for possible late reactions. The usual adult epidural dose is 5 mg. Intrathecal doses are much smaller—about $\frac{1}{10}$ the epidural dose.

The extended-release liposomal formulation [DepoDur], used only for postsurgical pain, is intended for epidural use only. Inadvertent intrathecal and subarachnoid administration has been associated with profound and prolonged respiratory depression, which can be managed with a naloxone infusion. Dosing is highly individualized and must account for age, body mass, physical status, history of opioid use, risk factors for respiratory depression, and medications to be coadministered before and during surgery.

Fentanyl

Parenteral fentanyl [generic], administered IM or IV, is employed primarily for induction and maintenance of surgical anesthesia. The drug is well suited for these applications, owing to its rapid onset and short duration. Most effects are like those of morphine. In addition, fentanyl can cause muscle rigidity, which can interfere with induction of anesthesia.

Nalbuphine

Nalbuphine is an agonist at kappa receptors and an antagonist at mu receptors. At low doses, nalbuphine has analgesic actions equal to those of morphine. However, as dosage increases, a ceiling to analgesia is reached. As a result, the maximal pain relief that can be produced with nalbuphine is much lower than with morphine. As with pain relief, there is also a ceiling to respiratory depression. Like pentazocine, nalbuphine can cause psychotomimetic reactions. With prolonged treatment, physical dependence can develop. Symptoms of abstinence are less intense than with morphine but more intense than with pentazocine. When used during labor and delivery, nalbuphine has caused serious adverse effects, including bradycardia in the fetus and apnea, cyanosis, and hypotonia in the neonate. Accordingly, use during labor and delivery should be avoided. Nalbuphine has a low abuse potential and is not regulated under the Controlled Substances Act. As with the pure opioid agonists, toxicity can be reversed with naloxone. Like pentazocine, nalbuphine will precipitate a withdrawal reaction if administered to an individual physically dependent on a pure opioid agonist. Nalbuphine is supplied in solution for IV, IM, and subQ injection. The usual adult dosage is 10 mg repeated every 3 to 6 hours as needed.

Patient-Controlled Analgesia

Patient-controlled analgesia (PCA) is a method of drug delivery that permits the patient to self-administer parenteral (transdermal, IV, subQ, epidural) opioids on an "as-needed" basis. PCA has been employed primarily for relief of pain in postoperative patients. Other candidates include patients experiencing pain caused by cancer, trauma, MI, vasoocclusive sickle cell crisis, and labor. As discussed later, PCA offers several advantages over opioids administered by the nurse.

Patient-Controlled Analgesia Devices

PCA was made possible by the development of reliable PCA devices. At this time, only one kind of PCA device is available: an electronically controlled infusion pump that can be activated by the patient to deliver a preset bolus dose of an opioid, which is delivered through an indwelling catheter. In addition to providing bolus doses on demand, some PCA pumps can deliver a basal infusion of opioid.

An essential feature of all PCA pumps is a timing control. This control limits the total dose that can be administered each hour, thereby minimizing the risk for overdose. In addition, the timing control regulates the minimum interval (e.g., 10 minutes) between doses. This interval, referred to as the "lock-out" or "delay" interval, prevents the patient from administering a second dose before the first has had time to produce its full effect.

Drug Selection and Dosage Regulation

The opioid used most extensively for PCA is morphine. Other pure opioid agonists (e.g., methadone, hydromorphone, fentanyl) have also been employed, as have agonist-antagonist opioids (e.g., nalbuphine, buprenorphine).

Before starting PCA, the postoperative patient should be given an opioid loading dose (e.g., 2–10 mg of morphine). After effective opioid levels have been established with the loading dose, PCA can be initiated, provided the patient has recovered sufficiently from anesthesia. For PCA with morphine, initial bolus doses of 1 mg are typical. The size of the bolus should be increased if analgesia is inadequate and decreased if excessive sedation occurs. The size of the bolus dose is usually increased during sleeping hours, thereby promoting rest by prolonging the interval between doses.

Comparison of Patient-Controlled Analgesia and Traditional Intramuscular Therapy

The objective of therapy with analgesics is to provide comfort while minimizing sedation and other side effects, especially respiratory depression. This objective is best achieved by maintaining plasma levels of opioids that have minimal fluctuations. In this manner, side effects from excessively high levels can be avoided, as can the return of severe pain when levels dip too low.

In the traditional management of postoperative pain, patients are given an IM injection of an opioid every 3 to 4 hours. With this dosing schedule, plasma drug levels can vary widely. Shortly after the injection, plasma levels may rise very high, causing excessive sedation and possibly respiratory depression. Late in the dosing interval, pain may return as plasma levels drop to their lowest point. In addition, multiple IM injections can be painful to the patient and cause negative side effects, including bruising and hematoma formation.

In contrast to traditional therapy, PCA is ideally suited to maintain steady levels of opioids because it relies on small doses given frequently (e.g., 1 mg of morphine every 10 minutes) rather than on large doses given infrequently (e.g., 20 mg of morphine every 3 hours). Maintenance of steady drug levels can be facilitated further if the PCA device is capable of delivering a basal infusion. Because plasma drug levels remain relatively steady, PCA can provide continuous pain control while avoiding the adverse effects associated with excessive drug levels.

An additional advantage of PCA is rapid relief. Because the patient can self-administer a parenteral dose of opioid as soon as pain begins to return, there is minimal delay between detection of pain and restoration of an adequate drug level. With traditional therapy, the patient must wait for the nurse to respond to a request for more drug; this delay allows pain to grow more intense.

Studies indicate that PCA is associated with accelerated recovery. Compared with patients receiving traditional IM analgesia, postoperative patients receiving PCA show improved early mobilization, greater cooperation during physical therapy, and a shorter hospital stay.

Patient and Family Education

Patient education is important for successful PCA. Surgical patients should be educated preoperatively. Education should include an explanation of what PCA is, along with instruction on how to activate the PCA device.

Patients should be told not to fear overdose; the PCA device will not permit self-administration of excessive doses. Families should be informed that activating the device for the patient while he or she is sleeping can lead to drug overdose.

Patients should be informed that there is a time lag (about 10 minutes) between activation of the device and production of maximal analgesia. To reduce discomfort associated with physical therapy, changing of dressings, ambulation, and other potentially painful activities, patients should be taught to activate the pump prophylactically (e.g., 10 minutes before the anticipated activity). Patients should be informed that, at night, the PCA device will be adjusted to deliver larger doses than during waking hours. This will prolong the interval between doses and thereby facilitate sleep.

Using Opioids for Specific Kinds of Pain

Postoperative Pain

Opioid analgesics offer several benefits to the postoperative patient. The most obvious is increased comfort through reduction of pain. In addition, by reducing painful sensation, opioids can facilitate early movement and intentional cough. In patients who have undergone thoracic surgery, opioids permit chest movement that would otherwise be too uncomfortable for adequate ventilation. By promoting ventilation, opioids can reduce the risk for hypoxia and pneumonitis.

Opioids are not without drawbacks for the postoperative patient. These agents can cause constipation and urinary retention. Suppression of reflex cough can result in respiratory tract complications. In addition, analgesia may delay diagnosis of postoperative complications—because pain will not be present to signal them.

Obstetric Analgesia

When administered to relieve pain during delivery, opioids such as morphine or meperidine may depress fetal respiration and uterine contractions when administered parenterally. Although these drugs are still used for relief of labor pain, regional and epidural modes of analgesia are often favored for pain relief in childbirth. For patients who are hesitant to use these more invasive methods, providers are employing newer opioid medications. Fentanyl, sufentanil, alfentanil, and remifentanil have a short duration of action and should not produce significant neonatal depression. The mixed opioid agonist-antagonists—nalbuphine, butorphanol, pentazocine, and buprenorphine—offer increased pain relief without causing further respiratory depression in higher doses. Even if these newer medications are used, however, respiration in the neonate should be monitored closely after delivery. Naloxone can reverse respiratory depression and should be on hand.

Reversal of Opioid Effects

Naloxone

Naloxone may be employed to reverse excessive respiratory and CNS depression caused by opioids. Dosage should be titrated with care; the objective is to achieve adequate ventilation and alertness without reversing opioid actions to the point of unmasking pain. The initial dose is 0.4 mg for adults and 10 mcg/kg for children. The preferred route is IV.

If IV administration is not possible, then IM or subQ injection may be employed. Dosing is repeated at 2- to 3-minute intervals until a satisfactory response has been achieved. Additional doses may be needed at 1- to 2-hour intervals for up to 72 hours, depending on the duration of the offending opioid.

Alvimopan

Alvimopan [Entereg] is a selective, peripherally acting mu opioid antagonist developed to counteract the adverse effects of opioids on bowel function. At therapeutic doses, alvimopan does not reduce opioid-mediated analgesia, in part because of limited ability to cross the blood-brain barrier. In contrast to methylnaltrexone, which is approved for long-term therapy of constipation in patients taking opioids for chronic pain, alvimopan is approved only for short-term therapy of opioid-induced ileus after partial small or large bowel resection with primary anastomosis. The goal is to accelerate time to recovery of upper and lower bowel function, which can be impaired by opioids used for analgesia during and after surgery.

When used short term in postoperative patients, alvimopan is very well tolerated. However, when used long term in patients taking opioids for chronic pain, the drug has been associated with an increased incidence of MI, although a causal relationship has not been established. Because MI may be a risk with prolonged dosing, the drug is approved only for short-term (7-day) use, and only for hospitalized patients. Furthermore, hospitals that dispense the drug must enroll in the Entereg Access Support and Education program, designed to minimize risk for MI.

Alvimopan is available in 12-mg capsules for oral dosing. The regimen consists of 12 mg given 0.5 to 5 hours before surgery, followed by 12 mg twice daily (beginning the day after surgery) for a total of 15 doses or less.

Nonsteroidal Antiinflammatory Drugs

Ibuprofen

An IV formulation of ibuprofen is sold as Caldolor. Caldolor is indicated for fever and pain in adults. The drug may be used alone for mild to moderate pain or combined with an opioid for moderate to severe pain. Caldolor is supplied as a concentrated solution (100 mg/mL) that must be diluted (to 4 mg/mL or less) before use. Infusions are done slowly (over 30 minutes or longer). For patients with pain, the usual dosage is 400 to 800 mg every 6 hours as needed. For patients with fever, treatment consists of an initial 400-mg dose, followed by either (1) 400 mg every 4 to 6 hours or (2) 100 to 200 mg every 4 hours as needed.

Ketorolac

Parenteral therapy with ketorolac can be accomplished with one injection or with several. When a single injection is used, the IM dose is 30 or 60 mg, and the IV dose is 15 or 30 mg. When multiple injections are given, the dosage (IM or IV) is 15 or 30 mg every 6 hours as needed. In all cases, the smaller dosage option is employed for patients older than 65 years, patients with impaired kidney function, and patients who weigh less than 50 kg (110 pounds). IV doses should be administered over 15 seconds or longer. IM injections should be done slowly and deep in the muscle. Treatment should not exceed 5 days.

PEPTIC ULCER DISEASE

Antagonists

Cimetidine

Parenteral cimetidine (discussed in Chapter 62) is reserved for patients with hypersecretory conditions (e.g., Zollinger-Ellison syndrome) and ulcers that have failed to respond to oral therapy. The usual dosage (IM or IV) is 300 mg every 6 to 8 hours. IM injections are made with a concentrated solution (300 mg/2 mL). For IV administration, two concentrations may be employed: (1) 300 mg may be diluted in 20 mL of 0.9% sodium chloride and injected slowly (over 2 minutes) or (2) 300 mg may be diluted in 100 mL of 0.9% sodium chloride and infused over 15 minutes.

Proton Pump Inhibitors

Esomeprazole

For IV therapy, esomeprazole (discussed further in Chapter 62) is indicated only for gastroesophageal reflux disease with a history of erosive gastritis. For adults, dosing is done by either injection or infusion. For children, dosing is done by infusion only. For all patients, dosing is done once a day for up to 10 days. For adults, the daily dose is 20 or 40 mg. For children aged 1 month to less than 1 year, the daily dose is 0.5 mg/kg. For children aged 1 year to 17 years, the daily dose is either 10 mg (for those who weigh less than 55 kg) or 20 mg (for those who weigh 55 kg or more).

STATUS EPILEPTICUS

Status epilepticus (SE) is defined as a continuous series of tonic-clonic seizures that lasts for at least 30 minutes. Consciousness is lost during the entire attack. Tachycardia, elevation of blood pressure, and hyperthermia are typical. Between 50,000 and 150,000 Americans experience SE each year. About 30% of adults and 3% of children die as a result.

Generalized convulsive SE is a medical emergency that requires immediate treatment. Ideally, treatment should commence within 5 minutes of seizure onset. Speed is important because, as time passes, SE becomes more and more resistant to therapy.

Our management is based on the latest 2016 clinical guidelines released by the American Epilepsy Society. These guidelines are available online at www.epilepsycurrents.org/doi/pdf/10.5698/1535-7597-16.1.48.

The goals of treatment are to maintain ventilation, correct hypoglycemia and precipitating factors, and terminate the seizure as quickly as possible. After 30 minutes, continued seizure activity can cause permanent neurologic injury (cognitive impairment, memory loss, worsening of the underlying seizure disorder) and even death.

Clinical guidelines propose a stabilization phase followed by three therapy phases. In the stabilization phase, an IV line is established to draw blood for analysis of glucose levels, electrolyte levels, and drug levels. The line is also used to administer glucose and antiepileptic drugs (AEDs).

The initial therapy phase centers on choice and administration of an AED. One of three benzodiazepine options is recommended for first choice: IV lorazepam (0.1 mg/kg), IV diazepam (0.15–0.2 mg/kg), or IM midazolam (5 mg if 13–40 kg or 10 mg if >40 kg). All of these drugs can terminate seizures quickly: however, lorazepam is generally preferred for its longer duration of action. Each IV drug may be repeated once before moving to the second therapy phase. (See algorithm provided in Chapter 19.) Detailed information for AEDs is presented in Chapter 19.

UNSTABLE ANGINA

Unstable angina is a medical emergency. Symptoms result from severe CAD complicated by vasospasm, platelet aggregation, and transient coronary thrombi or emboli. The patient may present with either symptoms of angina at rest, new-onset exertional angina, or intensification of existing angina. Unstable angina poses a much greater risk for death than stable angina, but a smaller risk for death than MI. The risk for dying is greatest initially and then declines to baseline in about 2 months.

In March of 2012, the American College of Cardiology (ACC) and the American Heart Association (AHA) issued updated guidelines for the diagnosis and management of unstable angina. The document—*2012 ACCF/AHA Focused Update Incorporated Into the ACC/AHA 2007 Guidelines for the Management of Patients with Unstable Angina and Non–ST-Segment Elevation Myocardial Infarction*—is available free at www.acc.org and www.americanheart.org. According to the guideline, the treatment strategy is to maintain oxygen supply and decrease oxygen demand. The goal is to reduce pain and prevent progression to MI or death. All patients should be hospitalized. Acute management consists of antiischemic therapy combined with antiplatelet and anticoagulation therapy.

Antiischemic therapy consists of the following:

- Nitroglycerin—give three doses sublingually every 5 minutes (tablet or spray) and follow with IV therapy in the event of persistent ischemia or hypertension.
- A beta blocker—give the first dose IV if chest pain is ongoing. If beta blockers are contraindicated, substitute a nondihydropyridine calcium channel blocker (verapamil or diltiazem).
- Supplemental oxygen—for patients with cyanosis or respiratory distress
- IV morphine sulfate—if pain is not relieved immediately by nitroglycerin, or if pulmonary congestion or severe agitation is present
- An angiotensin-converting enzyme inhibitor—for patients with left ventricular dysfunction or CHF. Angiotensin receptor blockers are a reasonable alternative in patients who have intolerance to angiotensin-converting enzyme inhibitors.

Antiplatelet therapy, which should be started promptly, consists of the following:

- Aspirin—continue indefinitely
- Clopidogrel [Plavix], prasugrel [Effient], or ticagrelor [Brilinta]—continue for up to 2 months
- Abciximab [ReoPro], a GP IIb/IIIa inhibitor—but only if angioplasty is planned
- Eptifibatide [Integrilin] or tirofiban [Aggrastat] (both are GP IIb/IIIa inhibitors)—but only in high-risk patients with continuing ischemia, and only if angioplasty is *not* planned

Anticoagulant therapy consists of subcutaneous low-molecular-weight heparin (e.g., enoxaparin [Lovenox]), direct thrombin inhibitors (bivalirudin [Angiomax]), factor Xa inhibitors (fondaparinux [Arixtra]), or IV unfractionated heparin.

Intravenous Nitroglycerin

Intravenous Therapy

IV nitroglycerin is indicated for perioperative control of blood pressure, production of controlled hypotension during surgery, and treatment of HF associated with acute MI. In addition, IV nitroglycerin is used to treat unstable angina and chronic angina when symptoms cannot be controlled with preferred medications.

IV nitroglycerin is employed only rarely to treat angina pectoris. When used for angina, IV nitroglycerin is limited to patients who have failed to respond to other medications. Additional uses of IV nitroglycerin include treatment of HF associated with acute MI, treatment of perioperative hypertension, and production of controlled hypotension for surgery.

IV nitroglycerin has a very short duration, so continuous infusion is required. The infusion rate is 5 mcg/min initially and then is increased gradually until an adequate response has been achieved. Heart rate and blood pressure must be monitored continuously.

Appendix A

Canadian Drug Information

Courtney Quiring, BSP, BCGP

CANADIAN DRUG LEGISLATION

Two acts form the basis of the drug laws in Canada: the Food and Drugs Act and the Controlled Drugs and Substance Act. The Health Products and Food Branch within Health Canada is responsible for ensuring that health products and foods approved for sale to Canadians are safe and of high quality. The Therapeutic Products Directorate (TPD) is responsible for pharmaceutical drugs and medical devices. The Biologics & Genetic Therapies Directorate regulates biologic drugs (drugs derived from living sources) and radiopharmaceuticals. Examples of biologic products are insulin analogues, blood products, and vaccines. The Natural and Non-prescription Health Products Directorate is the regulating authority for natural health products for sale in Canada. Natural Health Products (NHPs) are a class of health products which include vitamin and mineral supplements, herbal preparations, traditional and homeopathic medicines, probiotics, and enzymes.

The Food and Drug Act (1927), accompanied by the Food and Drug Regulations (1953, 1954, 1979), reviews the safety and efficacy of drugs before they are marketed, and the legislation determines whether the medicine is classified as prescription or nonprescription status. The Act controls the requirements for good manufacturing practices, labeling, distribution, and sale, including advertising of the drug. They also prescribe the standards of composition, strength, potency, purity, and quality of drugs in Canada.

Prescription Drugs (Schedule F)

All drugs that require a prescription, except for narcotics and controlled substances, are listed in Schedule F of the Food and Drug Regulations. Prescriptions for Schedule F medications may be written, including facsimiles and electronic prescriptions (depending on the province), or transmitted verbally (i.e. telephone order directly to the pharmacist) by a duly qualified medical practitioner, dentist, veterinarian, or other healthcare professional authorized to issue prescriptions. The symbol [Pr] must appear on all manufacturing labels. Individual provinces can legislate more restrictive control and require a prescription for a medication classified by the TPD as a nonprescription drug (e.g. digoxin). Provinces cannot legislate less restrictive control on any drug.

The Controlled Drugs and Substances Act (1997) establishes the requirements for the control and sale of narcotics, controlled drugs, and substances of abuse in Canada. The Controlled Drugs and Substances Act lists eight schedules of controlled substances. Assignment to a schedule is based on potential for abuse and the ease with which illicit substances can be manufactured in illegal laboratories. The degree of control, the conditions of record keeping, and other regulations depend on the specific schedule. For example, Schedule I, which includes the narcotic agents, requires written orders only, and no repeat prescriptions are allowed. Some provinces require prescriptions for certain narcotics, such as morphine, to be written on a triplicate prescription form with one copy to be sent to the practitioner's regulatory body. The symbol Ⓒ must appear on the labels of controlled products, while the letter N is printed on the label of all the narcotic agents. Schedules I through VIII are defined below. Benzodiazepines are classified as Targeted Substances, and the symbol [T/C] must appear on all the labels.

- Schedule I: Opium poppy and its derivatives (eg, morphine, heroin); methadone; coca and its derivatives (eg, cocaine)
- Schedule II: Cannabis and its derivatives (eg, marijuana, hashish)
- Schedule III: Amphetamines, methylphenidate, lysergic acid diethylamide (LSD), methaqualone, psilocybin, mescaline
- Schedule IV: Sedative-hypnotic agents (eg, barbiturates, benzodiazepines); anabolic steroids
- Schedule V: Propylhexedrine and any salt thereof
- Schedule VI: Compounds that can serve as precursors for manufacturing controlled substances
  - *Part 1: Class A Precursors.* Acetic anhydride, N-acetylanthranilic acid, anthranilic acid, ephedrine, ergometrine, ergotamine, isosafrole, lysergic acid, 3,4-methylenedioxyphenyl-2-propanone, norephedrine, 1-phenyl-2-propanone, phenylacetic acid, piperidine, piperonal, potassium permanganate, pseudoephedrine, safrole, gamma-butyrolactone, 1,4-butanediol, red and white phosphorus, hypophosphorous acid, hydriodic acid
  - *Part 2: Class B Precursors.* Acetone, ethyl ether, hydrochloric acid, methyl ethyl ketone, sulphuric acid, toluene
  - *Part 3:* Any preparation or mixture that contains a precursor set out in Part 1 or in Part 2
- Schedule VII: Cannabis resin 3 kg; Cannabis (marijuana) 3 kg
- Schedule VIII: Cannabis resin 1 g; Cannabis (marijuana) 30 g

The Controlled Drugs and Substance Act also provides for the nonprescription sale of certain codeine preparations. The content must not exceed the equivalent of 8 mg codeine phosphate per solid dosage unit or 20 mg/30 mL of a liquid, and the preparation must also contain two additional non-narcotic medicinal ingredients (usually acetylsalicylic acid or acetaminophen and caffeine). These preparations may not be advertised or displayed and may be sold only by pharmacists. Some provinces choose to restrict the amount that can be sold at any given time. The Royal Canadian Mounted Police

(RCMP) is responsible for enforcing the Controlled Drugs and Substances Act and related sections of the *Criminal Code*.

Nonprescription Medications—National Drug Schedules

As previously mentioned, individual provinces have enacted their own legislation controlling the sale of both prescription and nonprescription products. As a result, the National Association of Pharmacy Regulatory Authorities (NAPRA) endorsed a proposal for a national drug scheduling model. This model attempts to align the provincial drug schedules so that the conditions for the sale of drugs will be consistent across the country. The harmonized model includes all classes of medications. Narcotics, controlled substances, and prescription medications are listed in Schedule I, while nonprescription medications are assigned to one of the three categories described below. There is general support among the provincial regulatory bodies for the National Drug Schedules, although there are some differences from province to province of the actual list of drugs in each schedule. For a complete drug list proposed by NAPRA, visit their web site at *www.napra.ca:*

- **Schedule I** drugs require a prescription for sale and are provided to the public by the pharmacist following the diagnosis and professional intervention of a practitioner. The sale is controlled in a regulated environment as defined by provincial pharmacy regulation.
- **Schedule II** drugs, while less strictly regulated, do require professional intervention from the pharmacist at the point of sale and possibly referral to a practitioner. While a prescription is not required, the drugs are available only from the pharmacist and must be retained within an area of the pharmacy where there is no public access and no opportunity for patient self-selection.
- **Schedule III** drugs may present risks to certain populations in self-selection. Although available without a prescription, these drugs are to be sold from the self-selection area of the pharmacy which is operated under the direct supervision of the pharmacist, subject to any local professional discretionary requirements which may increase the degree of control. Such an environment is accessible to the patient and clearly identified as the "professional services area" of the pharmacy. The pharmacist is available, accessible, and approachable to assist the patient in making an appropriate self-medication selection.
- **Unscheduled** drugs can be sold without professional supervision. Adequate information is available for the patient to make a safe and effective choice and labeling is deemed sufficient to ensure the appropriate use of the drug. These drugs are not included in Schedules I, II, or III and may be sold from any retail outlet.

New-Drug Development in Canada

The process for approving a new drug in Canada is very similar, if not identical, to the process in the United States. The same drug data that are required for approval by the Food and Drug Administration in the United States are required by the TPD in Canada. The principal difference between Canada and the United States is one of nomenclature: Once preclinical testing is completed, the manufacturer in Canada applies for a Preclinical New Drug Submission, versus an Investigational New Drug in the United States. At the end of clinical testing, the manufacturer in Canada seeks a New Drug Submission (NDS), versus a New Drug Application in the United States.

After all the information on a new drug has been submitted—including results of preclinical and clinical testing, method of manufacturing, packaging, labeling, and results of stability testing—the pharmaceutical company receives a Notice of Compliance (NOC) from the TPD, and the drug enters the market.

Although data collection for a new drug is thorough, there is no guarantee that all adverse reactions are known, especially when the drug is used concurrently with other drugs. Also, long-term effects are not fully appreciated. For these reasons, post-market surveillance plays a major role in monitoring new drugs. The Canada Vigilance Program is Health Canada's post-market surveillance program that collects and assesses reports of suspected adverse reactions to health products marketed in Canada. Post-market surveillance enables Health Canada to monitor the safety profile of health products once they are marketed to ensure that the benefits of the products continue to outweigh the risks. The manufacturer and all healthcare practitioners must immediately report any new clinical findings, unexpected adverse effects, or therapeutic failures to the TPD. The Canada Vigilance Program also collects information for non-prescription drugs, natural health products, biologics, radiopharmaceuticals, and disinfectants and sanitizers with disinfectant claims.

Patent Laws

In 1969, the Patent Act was changed to include compulsory licensing. This new provision allowed generic drug companies to manufacture and distribute patented drugs in Canada, provided that a minimal 4% royalty fee was paid to the patent holder. This system was introduced to help control drug prices. Unfortunately, the system caused a decline in revenue to "innovative" pharmaceutical companies, with a resultant decline in research on new drug development. After much debate, and retroactive to June 1987, the Patent Act was amended to give patent holders market exclusivity either (1) for 7 to 10 years or (2) until the 17-year patent (from date of filing) expires, whichever comes first. The Patent Act was then further amended to "make Canada's intellectual property legislation more in line with that of the major industrialized countries."

In response to provisions of the North American Free Trade Agreement (NAFTA) and the General Agreement on Tariffs and Trade (GATT), Bill C-91 was introduced in 1993. This bill (1) eliminated compulsory licensing and (2) extended patent protection on brand-name drugs to 20 years, thereby making Canadian patent laws similar to those of the United States and other industrialized nations. Section 14 of Bill C-91 called for a parliamentary review of legislation in 1997. A special committee reviewed the impact of Bill C-91 on such factors as drug prices, drug research and development, and job creation. No changes to the legislation were made.

In order to respond to concerns arising from changes in the Patent Act, a Patented Medicine Prices Review Board was created. Its mandate is to (1) ensure that prices of patented medicines are not excessive and (2) report on the ratios of research and development expenditures relative to sales for individual patentees and for the pharmaceutical industry as a whole. There is, however, some pressure by the pharmaceutical industry to adopt worldwide patent laws for pharmaceutical products.

DRUG ADVERTISING

Direct-to-consumer advertising is restricted in Canada to giving names of prescription drugs only, which is different from the United States. Advertisements to health professionals are permitted to contain claims for product effectiveness and prescribing information. The Pharmaceutical Advertising Advisory Board (PAAB) and Advertising Standards Canada (ASC) review and clear advertisements according to standards set by the Food and Drugs Act.

INTERNATIONAL SYSTEM OF UNITS

In an attempt to standardize the large number of different units used worldwide and thus improve communication, the Système International d'Unités (International System of Units; SI) was recommended in 1954. In 1971, the mole (mol) was adopted as the standard for designating the amount of substance present, and the liter (L) was adopted as the standard for designating volume. The World Health Organization recommended the adoption of SI units in 1977. However, Canada had already implemented an equivalent system in 1971.

In the area of therapeutics, the major change caused by adopting the SI was to express drug concentrations present in body fluids in molar units (eg, mmol/L) rather than in mass units (eg, mg/L). This allows a better comparison between the pharmacologic and pharmacodynamic effects of different drugs, since these properties are relative to the number of molecules (eg, mmol) of drug present rather than to the number of mass units (eg, mg).

DRUG SERUM CONCENTRATIONS

Many drugs have known therapeutic or toxic levels that are monitored in patients to ensure safety and efficacy. In Canada, clinical laboratories report these levels in SI units. Levels traditionally reported as milligrams per milliliter (mg/mL) can be converted to millimoles per liter (mmol/L) using the conversion factor (CF) for that specific drug:

$$CF = 1000/\text{molecular weight of the drug}$$

To convert from micrograms per milliliter to SI units, the following equation is used:

$$\text{mcg/mL} \times CF = \text{micromoles/L}$$

To convert from SI units to micrograms per milliliter, the following equation is used:

$$(\text{micromoles/L})/CF = \text{mcg/mL}$$

Table A.1 shows some important drugs for which therapeutic or toxic levels have been established. For most of these drugs, the levels presented are trough (minimum) values,

TABLE A.1 ▪ Therapeutic Serum Drug Concentrations

Drugs	SI Reference Interval	SI Unit	Conversion Factor	Traditional Reference Interval	Traditional Reference Unit
Acetaminophen	13–40	micromol/L	66.15	0.2–0.6	mg/dL
Acetylsalicylic acid	7.2–21.7	micromol/L	0.0724	100–300	mg/dL
Amikacin*	—	—	—	15–25†; <8‡	mcg/mL
Amitriptyline	430–9000§	mmol/L	3.605	120–250§	ng/mL
Carbamazepine	17–42	micromol/L	4.233	4–10	mcg/mL
Desipramine	430–750	nmol/L	3.754	115–200	ng/mL
Digoxin	0.6–2.8	nmol/L	1.282	0.5–2.2	ng/mL
Disopyramide	6–18	micromol/L	2.946	2–6	mcg/mL
Gentamicin*	—	—	—	6–10†; <2‡	mcg/mL
Imipramine	640–1070§	nmol/L	3.566	180–300§	ng/mL
Lidocaine	4.5–21.5	micromol/L	4.267	1–5	mcg/mL
Lithium	0.4–1.2	mmol/L	1	0.4–1.2	mEq/L
Netilmicin*	—	—	—	6–10†; <2‡	mcg/mL
Nortriptyline	190–570	nmol/L	3.797	50–150	ng/mL
Phenobarbital	65–170	micromol/L	4.306	15–40	mcg/mL
Phenytoin	40–80	micromol/L	3.964	10–20	mcg/mL
Primidone	25–46	micromol/L	4.582	6–10	mcg/mL
Procainamide	17–34§	micromol/L	4.249	4–8§	mcg/mL
Quinidine	4.6–9.2	micromol/L	3.082	1.5–3	mcg/mL
Theophylline	55–110	micromol/L	5.55	10–20	mcg/mL
Tobramycin*	—	—	—	6–10†; <2‡	mcg/mL
Valproic acid	300–700	micromol/L	6.934	50–100	mcg/mL
Vancomycin*	—	—	—	25–40†; <10‡	mcg/mL

*Aminoglycosides (amikacin, gentamicin, netilmicin, tobramycin) and vancomycin are not reported in SI units because of the variability of their molecular weights.
†Peak drug level.
‡Trough drug level.
§Drug level reported as the total of the parent drug and its active metabolite.

which are measured in blood samples drawn just prior to the next dose. For the aminoglycosides and vancomycin, two levels are listed: a trough level and a peak (maximum) level. Levels must remain between the peak and trough to ensure efficacy of these drugs and at the same time to minimize toxicity.

REFERENCES

Bachynsky J: Nonprescription drugs in health care. *In* Nonprescription Drug Reference for Health Professionals. Ottawa: Canadian Pharmaceutical Association, 1996.

Canada Vigilance Program web site: http://www.hc-sc.gc.ca/dhp-mps/medeff/vigilance-eng.php

Controlled Drugs and Substances Act, S.C. 1996, c. 19.

Evans WE, Schentag JJ, Jusko WJ (eds): Applied Pharmacokinetics: Principles of Therapeutic Drug Monitoring. Spokane, WA: Applied Therapeutics, Inc., 1992.

Food and Drugs Act, R.S.C., 1985, c. F-27.

Health Protection and Drug Laws. Ottawa: Health and Welfare Canada, Canadian Publishing Center, 1988.

Health Protection Branch: Information Newsletter No. 798, 1991.

Johnson GE, Hannah KJ, Zerr SR: Pharmacology and the Nursing Process, 3rd ed. Philadelphia: WB Saunders, 1992.

Mailhot R: The Canadian drug regulatory process. J Clin Pharmacol 26:232, 1986.

McLeod DC: SI units in drug therapeutics. Drug Intell Clin Pharm 22:990, 1988.

National Association of Pharmacy Regulatory Authorities web site: www.napra.ca.

Subcommittee of Metric Commission Canada, Sector 9.10: SI Manual in Health Care, 2nd ed. Ottawa: Health and Welfare Canada, 1982.

Sullivan P: CMA to support increased patent protection for drugs but will attach strong qualifications. CMAJ 147:1669, 1992.

Index

Page numbers followed by "*f*" indicate figures, "*t*" indicate tables, and "*b*" indicate boxes.

T